Mastery of Surgery

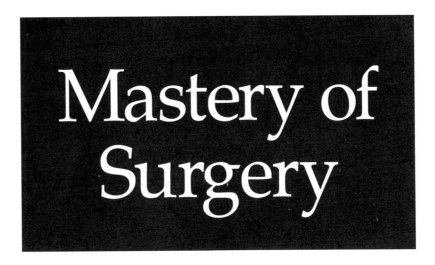

Mastery of Surgery

Third Edition
Volume I

Edited by

Lloyd M. Nyhus, M.D.

Warren H. Cole Professor of Surgery, Emeritus, University of Illinois College of Medicine;
Surgeon-in-Chief Emeritus, University of Illinois Hospital, Chicago

Robert J. Baker, M.D.

Professor and Vice Chairman of Surgery, University of Chicago, Pritzker School of Medicine;
Attending Surgeon, University of Chicago Hospitals, Chicago

Josef E. Fischer, M.D.

Christian R. Holmes Professor and Chairman of Surgery, University of Cincinnati College of Medicine;
Surgeon-in-Chief, Department of Surgery, University Hospital, Cincinnati

In conjunction with

Anne Greene, M.A., C.M.I.
Art Editor and Medical Illustrator

Steve Wiesner
Editorial Coordinator
Department of Surgery
University of Cincinnati College of Medicine
Cincinnati

Little, Brown and Company
Boston   New York   Toronto   London

Library of Congress Cataloging-in-Publication Data

Mastery of surgery / edited by Lloyd M. Nyhus, Robert J. Baker, Josef
   E. Fischer ; in conjunction
  with Anne Greene, art editor and medical illustrator. —3rd ed.
     p. cm.
   Includes bibliographical references and index.
   ISBN 0-316-617466-2 (set)
   1. Surgery.   I. Nyhus, Lloyd M. (Lloyd Milton), 1923–
  II. Baker, Robert J., 1927– . III. Fischer, Josef E., 1937–
   [DNLM: 1. Surgery.   WO 100 M423 1996]
  RD11.M29 1996
  617—dc20
  DNLM/DLC
  for Library of Congress   96-9115
                                      CIP

Vol. I ISBN 0-316-617512-2
Vol. II ISBN 0-316-617571-2

Printed in the United States of America
EB-M

Editorial: Nancy E. Chorpenning, Richard L. Wilcox
Copyeditors: Libby Dabrowski, June Goldstein, Anne Miller, and David March
Indexer: Herr's Indexing Service
Production Supervisor/Designer: Mike Burggren

Contents

THREE. HEAD AND NECK

II. The Stomach and Duodenum

[†]Deceased

Volume II

[†]Deceased

EIGHT. NONGASTROINTESTINAL TRANSABDOMINAL SURGERY

I. Surgery of the Urinary Tract and Bladder

Preface
to the
Third Edition

It has been a source of continuous pleasure and, frankly, some pride that the first two editions of *Mastery of Surgery* have now become well established as a significant reference in the well-rounded surgical library, both institutional and personal. This is reflected by the many positive comments that we have heard over the past 13 years. This has occurred despite an increasing number of surgeons limiting their practice to a particular subspecialty. Nevertheless, it is our conviction that the focusing of interest on the part of a given surgeon does not negate the need for a comprehensive text encompassing a broad cross-section of that which the general surgeon is apt to encounter. Rather, it affirms the desirability of having a wide range of procedures detailed in such a way that both the practitioner of surgery and the surgeon in training can understand the technical nuances. *Mastery of Surgery* particularly appeals to the surgeon who does not practice in a major urban setting and, therefore, cannot readily refer patients to subspecialists, as well as to residents rotating through specialty services.

With the third edition, the time has come to introduce a new spectrum of operations and procedures performed with newer techniques, most prominently videoscopic surgery, which represents one of the most sweeping changes in general surgery in the past several decades. In keeping with this philosophy of modernization and updating, our first approach was to invite a third editor to join us. Dr. Josef E. Fischer, one of the most active and experienced surgical educators, investigators, and authors in American surgery today. Dr. Fischer accepted our proposal with enthusiasm and promptly threw himself into the rigorous requirement of selecting and inviting authors, editing manuscripts, and doing the myriad other tasks required to

produce a worthwhile and valuable text. Many of the chapters are new, with a significant number of new authors, not because our previous contributors were anything other than stellar, but simply to expand the scope and develop new points of view about certain operations. In some cases, the chapters have proven to be so classic that it was desirable to invite a few returning authors to update their earlier work.

Our contributing authors continue to be acknowledged national and international authorities where they provide the benefit of their vast personal experience and technical expertise. We have selected "Masters" of proven talent and skill, who are renowned not only as leaders in their field, but also for their unique abilities to convey information and to teach their craft. We are extremely grateful for the time and effort that has gone into the production of each of these chapters, and know that the reader will find these contributions to be of great help in placing into proper perspective both the approach to the clinical problem and the technique of solving that problem.

The editor's comments section at the end of each chapter are in no way to be interpreted as being critical of the author's technique or principles. The editors have simply added their own observations, or have abstracted those from the literature, in order to either contribute or emphasize some of the salient points of practice to provide a slightly different approach or counterpoint, in an attempt to underscore another way to solve a problem.

We miss our late colleague, Dr. Harry Monsen, whose contributions to anatomic accuracy and completeness will be sorely missed, as is he. Our new editorial colleague, Steven Wiesner, of the University of Cincinnati, has exercised great patience and intestinal fortitude in working with us to develop this compendium, and to keep manuscripts flowing to the publisher.

Part of our enthusiasm for this project has been generated by our fine colleagues at Little, Brown and Company, including Nancy Chorpenning, Richard Wilcox, Anne Greene, and numerous others who have exercised great restraint and allowed us significant latitude in producing this work, but most important have provided the editing and publishing expertise without which this entire project would not have been possible.

It is often said that much research educates the researcher more thoroughly than anyone else; by the same token, having had the opportunity to edit manuscripts such as the ones that appear in this text has been of enormous value to all three of us; and we have learned a great deal. We hope that it is likewise of substantial benefit to you, the reader.

L.M.N.

R.J.B.

J.E.F.

Preface
to the
First Edition

This work is a product, or natural result, of a total of more than 50 years spent by the two editors teaching residents and other students the intricacies of surgical technique. As all who teach and learn and perform operations know, teaching surgical technique must be a labor of love because the intellectual and emotional effort put into such endeavors is incalculable. Literally thousands of surgeons have been taught technique by a like number of preceptors, since teaching technique in the operating room is almost invariably a one-on-one experience.

Because of the time and effort involved in teaching surgical skills, it was decided to take the format of this work beyond that of an atlas that would simply show the steps in an operation. Instead, the format is directed toward showing the reader how to improve performance of the procedures described by emphasizing the refinements of technique developed by the respective authors and which they, through personal experience, have found to work well. In some instances, the entire procedure has been described in detail; in others the focus is on prevention of common mistakes or a guide to nuances of the procedure that will save time or trauma to both patient and surgeon. Knowledge of important anatomic concepts is a critical ingredient in surgical technique, and important areas have been highlighted in chapters at the beginning of most sections describing the pertinent anatomic landmarks and interrelationships useful to know in performing certain procedures.

Editor's comments are provided to emphasize important points or, frequently, to add a contrapuntal view. In no instance are these comments intended to criticize or refute the author's approach, but rather to add a second view of possible strategies for a successful approach to a surgical problem. In several instances, two chapters on the same topic are provided by different authors to describe essentially the same frequently performed operation but with somewhat disparate points of emphasis so as to highlight several effective ways to accomplish the surgical objectives.

The contributing authors are acknowledged authorities in the areas in which they have written, but, more important, they are skilled, experienced teachers of surgery. We are deeply indebted to each of them for producing a worthy contribution and for their patience in tolerating the countless delays and myriad requests from our editorial office for more, different, or revised information.

Our deep appreciation must be expressed to our colleague, Dr. Harry Monsen, who reviewed every manuscript in order to provide anatomic accuracy and continuity. Similarly, our other colleague, Ms. Catherine Judge, has kept us grammatically and conceptually honest. Zelda Oser Zelinsky, our consulting artist, has been most gracious with her time and talent in standardizing portions of the art-work. The "family" at Little, Brown and Co., Lin Paterson, Fred Belliveau, George McKinnon, and Anne Najarian-Merian, has contributed greatly, not only in editing and publishing expertise, but also in encouragement, patience, and general good humor. Finally, we sincerely hope our readers derive as much pleasure and benefit from reading this book as we have from compiling and editing it.

L.M.N.

R.J.B.

Contributing Authors

Hiroshi Akiyama, M.D.

Professor of Surgery, Tokyo Medical College; Chairman, Department of Surgery, Toranomon Hospital, Tokyo, Japan

Mario Albertucci, M.D.

Assistant Professor of Surgery, Division of Cardiac Surgery, University of Chicago, Pritzker School of Medicine, Chicago

Robert J. Albo, M.D.

Clinical Professor of Surgery, University of California, San Francisco School of Medicine, San Francisco; Chief of Surgery, Student Health Department, University of California, Berkeley, Berkeley, California

J. Wesley Alexander, M.D.

Professor of Surgery, University of Cincinnati College of Medicine; Director, Transplantation Division, University Hospital, Cincinnati

Brent T. Allen, M.D.

Associate Professor of Surgery, Washington University School of Medicine; Attending Surgeon, Barnes-Jewish Hospital, St. Louis

R. Peter Altman, M.D.

Professor of Surgery, Columbia University College of Physicians and Surgeons; Surgeon-in-Chief and Director, Pediatric Surgery, Babies and Children's Hospital of New York, New York

Jose C. Alves, M.D.

Research Associate, Vascular Surgery, University of Utah Health Sciences Center, Salt Lake City, Utah

Teruaki Aoki, M.D.

Professor of Surgery, Jikei University School of Medicine; Director, Department of General and Digestive Surgery, Tokyo, Japan

Richard B. Arenas, M.D.

Assistant Professor of Surgery, University of Chicago, Pritzker School of Medicine; Attending Physician, Department of Surgery, University of Chicago Hospitals and Clinics, Chicago

Robert M. Arensman, M.D.

Professor of Surgery, Northwestern University Medical School; Surgeon-in-Chief, Department of Pediatric Surgery, Children's Memorial Hospital, Chicago

Joseph N. Attie, M.D.

Clinical Professor of Surgery, Albert Einstein College of Medicine of Yeshiva University, Bronx; Director, Head and Neck Surgery, Long Island Jewish Medical Center, New Hyde Park, New York

Hervy E. Averette, M.D.

Professor of Clinical Oncology, Department of Obstetrics and Gynecology, Jackson Memorial Hospital; Professor of Clinical Oncology, Division of Gynecologic Oncology, Sylvester Comprehensive Cancer Center, Miami

Timothy J. Babineau, M.D.

Assistant Professor of Surgery, Harvard Medical School, and New England Deaconess, Boston

Ronald J. Baird, M.D.

Professor Emeritus, Department of Surgery, University of Toronto Faculty of Medicine; Senior Surgeon, Department of Cardiovascular Surgery, Toronto General Hospital, Toronto, Ontario, Canada

Robert J. Baker, M.D. Professor and Vice Chairman of Surgery, University of Chicago, Pritzker School of Medicine; Attending Surgeon, University of Chicago Hospitals, Chicago

William H. Baker, M.D. Professor and Chief, Division of Peripheral Vascular Surgery, Loyola University of Chicago Stritch School of Medicine; Attending Staff, Division of Peripheral Vascular Surgery, Foster G. McGaw Hospital of Loyola University, Maywood, Illinois

Joseph P. Bannon, M.D. Staff Surgeon, Mercy Hospital, Scranton, Pennsylvania

Philip S. Barie, M.D. Associate Professor of Surgery, Cornell University Medical College; Associate Attending Surgeon and Director, Anne and Max M. Cohen Surgical Intensive Care Unit, New York Hospital-Cornell Medical Center, New York

Robert H. Bartlett, M.D. Professor of Surgery, University of Michigan Medical School; Chief, Division of Critical Care, University of Michigan Medical Center, Ann Arbor, Michigan

Francesco Battocchio, M.D. Professor of General Surgery, Facolta Medicina e Chirurgia Universita; Aiuto Corresponsabile, Department of Geriatric Surgery, Azienda Ospedaliera, Padova, Italy

Robert W. Beart, M.D. Director of Colorectal Surgery, University of Southern California School of Medicine; Surgeon, USC University Hospital, Norris Cancer Center, Los Angeles

Dennis G. Begos Chief Resident of Surgery, Yale University School of Medicine, New Haven, Connecticut

Michael Belkin, M.D. Assistant Professor of Surgery, Harvard Medical School; Staff Surgeon, Brigham and Women's Hospital, Boston

Richard H. Bell, Jr., M.D. Professor and Vice Chairman of Surgery, University of Washington School of Medicine; Chief, Surgical Service, VA Puget Sound Health Care System, Seattle

Robert Bendavid, M.D. Attending Surgeon, Shouldice Hospital, Thornhill, Toronto, Ontario, Canada

Marshall E. Benjamin, M.D. Vascular Fellow, Department of Surgery, Bowman Gray School of Medicine of Wake Forest University; Vascular Fellow, Department of Surgery, North Carolina Baptist Hospitals, Inc., Winston-Salem, North Carolina

Jeffrey Berger, M.D. Assistant Professor of Surgery, Eastern Virginia Medical School, Norfolk; Attending Surgeon, Department of Surgery, Virginia Beach General Hospital, Virginia Beach, Virginia

Ramon Berguer, M.D., Ph.D. Professor of Surgery, Wayne State University School of Medicine; Chief of Vascular Surgery, Harper Hospital, Detroit

Yacov Berlatzky, M.D. Associate Professor of Surgery, Department of Vascular Surgery and Transplantation, Hebrew University-Hadassah Medical School; Chief of Vascular Surgery and Transplantation, Hadassah University Medical Center, Jerusalem, Israel

Thomas V. Berne, M.D. Professor of Surgery, University of Southern California School of Medicine; Associate Director of Surgery, LAC-USC Medical Center, Los Angeles

Victor M. Bernhard, M.D. Vice President for Medical Affairs, EndoVascular Technologies, Inc., Menlo Park, California

Mitchell A. Bernstein, M.D. Staff Surgeon, Columbia University College of Physicians and Surgeons; Attending Surgeon, Division of Colon and Rectal Surgery, St. Luke's Roosevelt Hospital Center, New York

Pr Henri Bismuth — Professor, Hepatobiliary Center, University of Paris-Sud, Kremlin-Bicetre; Head, Hepatobiliary Center, Paul Brousse Hospital, Villejuif, France

Kirby I. Bland, M.D. — J. Murray Beardsley Professor and Chairman of Surgery, Brown University School of Medicine; Executive Surgeon-in-Chief, Brown University Affiliated Hospitals, Providence, Rhode Island

Leslie H. Blumgart, M.D. — Professor of Surgery, Cornell University Medical College; Chief of Hepatobiliary Service, Department of Surgery, Memorial Sloan Kettering Cancer Center, New York

John W. Braasch, M.D., Ph.D. — Associate Professor of Surgery, Harvard Medical School, Boston; Senior Staff Consultant, Department of General Surgery, Lahey Hitchcock Medical Center, Burlington, Massachusetts

R. Bruce Bracken, M.D. — Professor and Director of Surgery, Division of Urology, University of Cincinnati College of Medicine; Director, Division of Urology, University of Cincinnati Medical Center, Cincinnati

Edward L. Bradley III, M.D. — Professor and Vice Chairman of Surgery, State University of New York at Buffalo; Chief of Surgery, Buffalo General Hospital, Buffalo, New York

Frank James Branicki, M.B.B.S., D.M. — Reader in Surgery, University of Hong Kong; Honorary Consultant, Department of Surgery, Queen Mary Hospital, Pokfulam, Hong Kong

Bruce J. Brener, M.D. — Clinical Professor of Surgery, UMDNJ-New Jersey Medical School; Chief, Vascular Surgery, Newark Beth Israel Medical Center, Newark, New Jersey

Murray F. Brennan, M.D. — Professor of Surgery, Cornell University Medical College; Chairman, Department of Surgery, Memorial Sloan Kettering Cancer Center, New York

David C. Brewster, M.D. — Clinical Professor of Surgery, Harvard Medical School; Senior Attending Surgeon, Division of Vascular Surgery, Massachusetts General Hospital, Boston

Donald K. Brief, M.D. — Clinical Professor of Surgery, UMDNJ-New Jersey Medical School; Chairman of Surgery, Newark Beth Israel Hospital, Newark, New Jersey

L. D. Britt, M.D., M.P.H. — Brickhouse Professor and Chairman of Surgery, Eastern Virginia Medical School; Chief, Division of Trauma and Critical Care, Department of Surgery/Burn Trauma Unit, Sentara Norfolk General Hospital, Norfolk, Virginia

Henry Buchwald, M.D., Ph.D. — Professor of Surgery and Biomedical Engineering, University of Minnesota Medical School—Minneapolis; Surgeon, University of Minnesota Hospital and Clinic of the University of Minnesota Health Sciences Center, Minneapolis

Larry C. Carey, M.D. — Chairman and Professor of Surgery, University of South Florida College of Medicine; Chief of Surgery, Tampa General Hospital, Tampa, Florida

Denis Castaing, M.D.

Frank B. Cerra, M.D. — Dean of the Medical School, University of Minnesota Medical School—Minneapolis; Professor of Surgery, University of Minnesota Hospital and Clinic of the University of Minnesota Health Sciences Center, Minneapolis

Benjamin B. Chang, M.D. — Provost, Academic Health Center, University of Minnesota Medical School—Minneapolis; Professor of Surgery, University of Minnesota Hospital and Clinic of the University of Minnesota Health Sciences Center, Minneapolis

Alfred M. Cohen, M.D.	Professor of Surgery, Cornell University Medical Center; Chief, Colorectal Service, Department of Surgery, Memorial Sloan Kettering Cancer Center, New York
Mimis Cohen, M.D.	Professor of Surgery, University of Illinois College of Medicine; Chief, Divisions of Plastic Surgery, University of Illinois Hospital and Cook County Hospital, Chicago
Gene L. Colborn, Ph.D.	Director, Center for Clinical Anatomy and Professor of Anatomy and Surgery, The Medical College of Georgia, Augusta, Georgia
Michael D. Colburn, M.D.	Clinical Instructor in Surgery, University of California Los Angeles, UCLA School of Medicine, Los Angeles
Anthony J. Comerota, M.D.	Professor of Surgery, Temple University School of Medicine; Chief, Section of Vascular Surgery, Temple University Hospital, Philadelphia
Robert E. Condon, M.D.	Professor of Surgery, Medical College of Wisconsin; Staff Surgeon, Department of General Surgery, Froedtert Memorial Lutheran Hospital, Milwaukee
Edward E. Cornwell III, M.D.	Assistant Professor of Surgery, University of Southern California School of Medicine; Associate Chief, Trauma Service "B", Department of Surgery, LAC-USC Medical Center, Los Angeles
John M. Daly, M.D.	Lewis Atterbury Stimson Professor of Surgery, Cornell University Medical College; Surgeon-in-Chief, New York Hospital-Cornell Medical Center, New York
R. Clement Darling III, M.D.	Associate Professor of Surgery, Albany Medical College; Attending, Department of Vascular Surgery, Albany Medical Center Hospital, Albany, New York
Nina S. Davis, M.D.	Assistant Professor of Surgery and Urology, University of Cincinnati Medical College, Cincinnati
Richard H. Dean, M.D.	Director of Surgical Sciences, Department of Surgery, Bowman Gray School of Medicine of Wake Forest University; Chief of Surgery, North Carolina Baptist Hospitals, Inc., Winston-Salem, North Carolina
Malcolm M. DeCamp, Jr., M.D.	Assistant Professor of Surgery, Harvard Medical School; Associate Surgeon, Division of Thoracic Surgery, Brigham and Women's Hospital, Boston
Eric J. DeMaria, M.D.	Assistant Professor of Surgery, Medical College of Virginia; Director, Center for Minimally Invasive Surgery, Medical College of Virginia Hospitals, Richmond, Virginia
Tom R. DeMeester, M.D.	Professor and Chairman of Surgery, University of Southern California School of Medicine, Los Angeles
Lawrence W. DeSanto, M.D.	Associate Professor, Department of Otorhinolaryngology, Mayo Clinic; Staff Surgeon Department of Surgery, Scottsdale Memorial Hospital, Scottsdale, Arizona
Daniel J. Deziel, M.D.	Associate Professor of General Surgery, Rush Medical College of Rush University; Associate Attending Surgeon, Department of General Surgery, Rush-Presbyterian-St. Luke's Medical Center, Chicago
Christopher S. Dickson, M.D.	Vascular Fellow, Department of Vascular Surgery, Eastern Virginia Medical School of the Medical College of Hampton Roads, Norfolk, Virginia
Yves-Marie Dion, M.D.	Assistant Professor of Surgery, Université Laval, Quebec, Canada; Staff Surgeon, Hôpital St. François d'Assise, Quebec, Canada

Rudolph F. Dolezal, M.D.
Associate Professor of Surgery, University of Illinois College of Medicine; Attending Surgeon, Division of Plastic Surgery, University of Illinois Hospital and Lutheran General Hospital, Chicago

Philip E. Donahue, M.D.
Professor of Surgery, University of Illinois College of Medicine; Chairman, Division of General Surgery, Cook County Hospital, Chicago

Daniel M. Donato, M.D.
Associate Professor of Gynecologic Oncology, University of Virginia School of Medicine; Director, Gynecologic Oncology, Department of Obstetrics and Gynecology, Community Hospital, Roanoke, Virignia

Richard Drake, Ph.D.
Professor and Associate Director, Department of Cell Biology, Neurobiology and Anatomy, University of Cincinnati College of Medicine, Cincinnati

Stephen P. Dretler, M.D.
Professor of Surgery and Urology, Harvard Medical School; Director, MGH Kidney Stone Center, Department of Urology, Massachusetts General Hospital, Boston

Stanley J. Dudrick, M.D.
Clinical Professor of Surgery, Yale University School of Medicine, New Haven, Connecticut; Program Director and Associate Chairman, Department of Surgery, St. Mary's Hospital, Waterbury, Connecticut

Joseph R. Durham, M.D.
Visiting Professor of Surgery, University Illinois College of Medicine, Chicago; Attending Vascular Surgeon, Ingalls Memorial Hospital, Harvey, Illinois

E. Christopher Ellison, M.D.
Zollinger Professor of Surgery, Ohio State University College of Medicine and Ohio State University Medical Center, Columbia, Ohio

Donald A. Elmajian, M.D.
Fellow of Urologic Oncology, University of Southern California School of Medicine, Los Angeles

Scott A. Engum, M.D.
Assistant Professor of Surgery, Indiana University School of Medicine; Active Staff, Pediatric Surgery, James Whitcomb Riley Hospital for Children, Indianapolis

Douglas B. Evans, M.D.
Associate Professor of Surgery, University of Texas Medical School at Houston; Associate Professor of Surgery, Department of Surgical Oncology, M. D. Anderson Cancer Center, Houston

Cheryl A. Ewing, M.D.
Assistant Professor of Surgery, University of Chicago, Pritzker School of Medicine; Attending Surgeon, Department of Surgery, University of Chicago Hospitals and Clinics, Chicago

Augustine R. Eze, M.D.
Clinical Instructor of Surgery, Temple University School of Medicine; General Vascular Surgery Fellow, Temple University Hospital, Philadelphia

Samir M. Fakhry, M.D.
Associate Professor of Surgery and Chief, Surgical Critical Care, University of North Carolina at Chapel Hill, School of Medicine; Medical Director, Surgical Intensive Care Unit, UNC Hospitals, Chapel Hill, North Carolina

Diana Farmer, M.D.
Assistant Professor of Surgery, Wayne State University School of Medicine; Associate Attending Surgeon, Children's Hospital of Michigan, Detroit

Victor W. Fazio, M.D.
Professor of Surgery, Cleveland Clinic Health Sciences; Rupert B. Turnbull, Jr. Chairman, Department of Colon and Rectal Surgery, Cleveland Clinic Foundation, Cleveland

Gregory M. Fedele, M.D.
Senior Resident, Department of Surgery, Case Western Reserve University School of Medicine, and University Hospitals of Cleveland, Cleveland

Francis D. Ferdinand, M.D. Chief Resident of Thoracic Surgery, Sections of Cardiac and Thoracic Surgery, University of Chicago, Pritzker School of Medicine, Chicago

Mark K. Ferguson, M.D. Associate Professor of Surgery, University of Chicago, Pritzker School of Medicine; Chief, Section of Thoracic Surgery, University of Chicago Hospitals, Chicago

Abe Fingerhut, M.D. Professor of Surgery, Louisiana State University School of Medicine in New Orleans, New Orleans, Louisiana; Chief of Surgery, Department of Digestive Surgery, Centre Hospitalier Intercommunal, Poissy, France

Josef E. Fischer, M.D. Christian R. Holmes Professor and Chairman of Surgery, University of Cincinnati College of Medicine; Surgeon-in-Chief, Department of Surgery, University Hospital, Cincinnati

Robert J. Fitzgibbons, Jr., M.D. Professor of Surgery, Creighton University School of Medicine, Omaha, Nebraska; Clinical Professor of Vascular Surgery, University of California, Irvine

D. Preston Flanigan, M.D. Clinical Professor of Surgery, University of California, Irvine, College of Medicine, Irvine; Codirector, Vascular Laboratory, St. Joseph Hospital, Orange, California

Linda Flesch, M.S.N., R.N., C.S. Clinical Nurse Specialist, Department of Nursing Consultation, University Hospital, Cincinnati

Thomas J. Fogarty, M.D. Professor of Surgery, Division of Vascular Surgery, Stanford University Medical Center, Stanford, California

Manson Fok, F.R.C.S.E. Honorary Clinical Lecturer, Department of Surgery, The University of Hong Kong, Hong Kong

Yuman Fong, M.D. Assistant Professor of Surgery, Cornell University Medical College; Assistant Attending Surgeon, Memorial Sloan Kettering Cancer Center, New York

James H. Foster, M.D. Emeritus Professor of Surgery, University of Connecticut School of Medicine, Farmington, Connecticut

Herbert R. Freund, M.D. Professor of Surgery, Hebrew-University Hadassah Medical School, Jerusalem; Chief of Surgery, University Hospital, Mt. Scopus, Israel

Thomas R. Gadacz, M.D. Professor and Chairman of Surgery, Medical College of Georgia School of Medicine, Augusta, Georgia

Michel Gagner, M.D. Staff Surgeon, Department of General Surgery, The Cleveland Clinic Foundation, Cleveland

Irwin M. Gelernt,[†] M.D. Dean of Hospital and Medical Affairs, and Clinical Professor of Surgery, Mount Sinai School of Medicine of the City University of New York; Attending Surgeon, Mount Sinai Medical Center, New York

Bruce L. Gewertz, M.D. Dallas B. Phemister Professor and Chairman of Surgery, University of Chicago, Pritzker School of Medicine; Surgeon-in-Chief, University of Chicago Hospitals and Medical Center, Chicago

Clare R. Giegerich, M.D. Clinical Assistant Professor of Orthopedic Surgery, Northwestern University Medical School; Attending Surgeon, Department of Orthopedic Surgery, Northwestern Memorial Hospital, Chicago

[†]Deceased

Jean Warren Gillon, M.D.

Assistant Professor of Surgery, University of California, San Francisco, School of Medicine; Assistant Professor of Surgery, Division of Vascular Surgery, San Francisco General Hospital Medical Center, San Francisco

Lyon L. Gleich, M.D.

Assistant Professor of Otolaryngology and Head and Neck Surgery, University of Cincinnati College of Medicine, Cincinnati

Jack L. Gluckman, M.D.

Professor of Otolaryngology, University of Cincinnati College of Medicine; Chairman, Department of Otolaryngology, University Hospital, Cincinnati

Ricardo N. Goes, M.D.

Assistant Professor of Surgery, State University of Campinas School of Medicine; Surgeon, Colorectal Division, Clinical Hospital of the State University of Campinas School of Medicine, Campinas, São Paulo, Brazil

Stanley Morton Goldberg, M.D.

Clinical Professor of Surgery, Division of Colon and Rectal Surgery, University of Minnesota Medical School—Minneapolis, Minneapolis

Philip H. Gordon, M.D.

Professor of Surgery and Oncology, McGill University Faculty of Medicine; Director, Colon and Rectal Surgery, Sir Mortimer B. Davis-Jewish General Hospital, Montreal, Quebec, Canada

Stephen R. Gorfine, M.D.

Assistant Clinical Professor of Surgery, Mount Sinai School of Medicine of the City University of New York; Attending Surgeon, Mount Sinai Medical Center, New York

Robert C. Gorman, M.D.

Instructor of Surgery, University of Pennsylvania School of Medicine; Surgical Resident, Hospital of the University of Pennsylvania, Philadelphia

Clive S. Grant, M.D.

Professor of Surgery, Mayo Medical School; Vice Chairman, Department of Surgery, Mayo Clinic, Rochester, Minnesota

Richard M. Green, M.D.

Associate Professor of Surgery, University of Rochester School of Medicine and Dentistry; Attending Surgeon, The Strong Memorial Hospital, Rochester, New York

A. Gerson Greenburg, M.D., Ph.D.

Professor of Surgery, Brown University School of Medicine; Surgeon-in-Chief, Miriam Hospital, Providence, Rhode Island

Charles A. Griffith[†], M.D.

Late Clinical Professor of Surgery, University of Washington School of Medicine, St. Louis

Hermes Grillo, M.D.

Professor of Surgery, Harvard Medical School; Emeritus, Chief of General Thoracic Surgery, Thoracic Surgical Unit, Massachusetts General Hospital, Boston

Jay L. Grosfeld, M.D.

Chairman, Department of Surgery, Indiana University School of Medicine; Surgeon-in-Chief and Director, Section of Pediatric Surgery, James Whitcomb Riley Hospital for Children, Indianapolis

Jeffrey A. Hagen, M.D.

Assistant Professor of Surgery, Division of Cardiothoracic Surgery, University of Southern California School of Medicine; Chief of Foregut/Pulmonary Service, LA County General Hospital, Los Angeles

Thomas E. Hamilton, M.D.

Assistant Clinical Instructor in Surgery, University of Pennsylvania School of Medicine, Philadelphia

Douglas W. Hanto, M.D., Ph.D.

Associate Professor of Surgery, University of Cincinnati College of Medicine; Director, Liver Transplant Services, University Hospital, Cincinnati

Per-Olof Hasselgren, M.D., Ph.D.

Professor of Surgery, University of Cincinnati College of Medicine, Cincinnati

[†]Deceased

Daniel H. Hechtman, M.D.

Assistant Professor of Surgery, Division of Pediatric Surgery, Medical College of Pennsylvania, Philadelphia; Attending Pediatric Surgeon, Division of Pediatric Surgery, Allegheny General Hospital, Pittsburgh

Thomas G. Heffron, M.D.

Associate Professor of Surgery, University of Nebraska College of Medicine; Director of Pediatric and Living Related Transplantation, Department of Surgery, University of Nebraska Medical Center, Omaha, Nebraska

W. Hardy Hendren, M.D.

Professor of Surgery, Harvard Medical School; Chief, Department of Surgery, Children's Hospital, Boston

William N. P. Herbert, M.D.

Professor of Obstetrics and Gynecology, Duke University School of Medicine; Director, Division of Maternal-Fetal Medicine, Duke University Medical Center, Durham, North Carolina

Steven M. Hertz, M.D.

Associate Director, Division of Vascular Surgery, Newark Beth Israel Medical Center, Newark, New Jersey

Graham L. Hill, M.D.

Professor of Surgery, School of Medicine, Aukland, New Zealand; Colorectal Surgeon, Department of Surgery, Aukland Hospital, Aukland, New Zealand

Frank Hinman, Jr., M.D.

Clinical Professor of Urology, University of California, San Francisco School of Medicine, San Francisco

Arnulf H. Hölscher, M.D.

Professor of Surgery, University of Cologne; Director, Department of Visceral and Vascular Surgery, Klinikum Lindenthal der Universität Köln, Cologne, Germany

Tracy L. Hull, M.D.

Staff Surgeon, Department of Colorectal Surgery, The Cleveland Clinic Foundation, Cleveland

Kelly K. Hunt, M.D.

Assistant Professor of Surgery, Department of Surgical Oncology, University of Texas Medical School at Houston; M. D. Anderson Cancer Center, Houston

John G. Hunter, M.D.

Associate Professor of Surgery, Emory University School of Medicine; Vice Chairman of Surgery and Chief of Gastrointestinal Surgery, Emory University Hospital, Atlanta

Roger D. Hurst, M.D.

Assistant Professor of Surgery, University of Chicago, Pritzker School of Medicine; Assistant Professor of Surgery, University of Chicago Hospitals, Chicago

David A. Iannitti, M.D.

Assistant Instructor in Surgery, Brown University School of Medicine; Chief Resident in Surgery, Rhode Island Hospital and Affiliated Institutions, Providence, Rhode Island

Timothy D. Jacob, M.D.

Assistant Professor of Surgery, University of Pittsburgh School of Medicine; Staff Surgeon, Department of Surgery, University of Pittsburgh Medical Center, Pittsburgh

Juan Carlos Díaz Jeraldo, M.D.

Instructor in Surgery, Clinical Hospital University of Chile, Santiago, Chile

Jerry M. Jesseph, M.D.

Associate Clinical Professor of Surgery and Anatomy, Indiana University School of Medicine; Staff Surgeon, Bloomington Hospital, Bloomington, Indiana

Daniel B. Jones, M.D.

Chief Resident, Department of Surgery, Washington University School of Medicine; Senior Resident, Department of Surgery, Barnes-Jewish Hospital, St. Louis, Missouri

Glyn Jones, M.D.

Assistant Professor of Plastic Surgery, Emory University School of Medicine; Attending Plastic Surgeon, Emory Affiliated Hospitals, Atlanta

R. Scott Jones, M.D.	Professor and Chairman, Department of Surgery, University of Virginia School of Medicine, Charlottesville, Virginia
Attila Csendes Juhasz, M.D.	Professor of Surgery, University of Chile; Chairman, Department of Surgery, Hospital J.J. Aguirre, Santiago, Chile
Maurice J. Jurkiewicz, M.D.	Emeritus Professor of Surgery, Emory University School of Medicine; Attending Surgeon, Emory Affiliated Hospitals, Atlanta
Robert J. Keenan, M.D.	Assistant Professor of Surgery, University of Pittsburgh School of Medicine; Head, Section of Thoracic Surgery, Presbyterian-University Hospital, Pittsburgh
M. R. B. Keighley, M.S.	Barling Professor of Surgery, University of Birmingham; Head of the University Department of Surgery, Queen Elizabeth Hospital, Birmingham, England
Keith A. Kelly, M.D.	Professor of Surgery, Mayo Medical School, Rochester, Minnesota; Chair, Department of Surgery, Mayo Clinic Scottsdale, Scottsdale, Arizona
W. John Kitzmiller, M.D.	Assistant Professor, Division of Plastic Surgery, University of Cincinnati College of Medicine; Active Staff, Division of Plastic Surgery, University Hospital, Cincinnati
Jake E. J. Krige, M.B.Ch.B.	Associate Professor of Surgery, University of Cape Town; Senior Surgeon and Associate Professor of Surgery, Groote Schuur Hospital, Cape Town, South Africa
Rodney J. Landreneau, M.D.	Associate Professor of Surgery, University of Pittsburgh; Director, Allegheny Center for Lung and Thoracic Disease, Pittsburgh
Gregory J. Landry, M.D.	Resident, Department of Surgery, Division of Vascular Surgery, Oregon Health Sciences University School of Medicine, Portland, Oregon
Ian C. Lavery, M.B.B.S.	Staff Surgeon, Colorectal Surgery, Clinic Foundation, Cleveland
Peter F. Lawrence, M.D.	Professor of Surgery, University of Utah School of Medicine; Chief, Division of Vascular Surgery, University of Utah Hospital, Salt Lake City
Gary P. Lawton, M.D.	Resident, Department of Surgery, Yale University School of Medicine, New Haven, Connecticut
Robert P. Leather, M.D.	Professor of Surgery, Albany Medical College; Chief, Department of Vascular Surgery, Albany Medical Center Hospital, Albany, New York
Jeffrey E. Lee, M.D.	Assistant Professor of Surgical Oncology, University of Texas Medical School at Houston; Assistant Surgeon, Department of Surgical Oncology, University of Texas M. D. Anderson Cancer Center, Houston
Raymond A. Lee, M.D.	Professor of Obstetrics and Gynecology, Mayo Medical School, Rochester; Consultant, Departments of Obstetrics and Gynecology and Surgery, Mayo Clinic and Mayo Foundation, Rochester, Minnesota
Eric G. LeVeen, M.D.	Attending Physician, Bon Secour St. Francis Xavier Hospital, Charleston, South Carolina
Harry H. LeVeen, M.D.	Professor of Surgery, Emeritus, Medical University of South Carolina College of Medicine, Charleston, South Carolina

Keith D. Lillemoe, M.D.	Professor of Surgery, Johns Hopkins University School of Medicine; Full-Time Staff, Department of Surgery, Johns Hopkins Hospital, Baltimore
Bruce W. Lindgren, M.D.	Chief Resident of Urology, Loyola University of Chicago Stritch School of Medicine, Maywood, Illinois
Michael J. Liptay, M.D.	Fellow in Thoracic Surgery, Harvard Medical School; Fellow in Thoracic Surgery, Brigham and Women's Hospital, Boston
Alex G. Little, M.D.	Professor and Chairman of Surgery, University of Nevada School of Medicine; Chief of Surgery, University Medical Center of Southern Nevada, Las Vegas
Fred N. Littooy, M.D.	Professor of Surgery, Loyola University of Chicago Stritch School of Medicine; Chief, Division of Peripheral Vascular Surgery, Hines VA Medical Center, Hines, Illinois
Elizabeth G. Livingston, M.D.	Assistant Professor of Obstetrics and Gynecology, Duke University School of Medicine; Assistant Professor, Duke University Medical Center, Durham, North Carolina
Susan M. Love, M.D.	Associate Professor of Clinical Surgery, University of California, Los Angeles, UCLA School of Medicine; Director, Revlon/ UCLA Breast Center, University of California, Los Angeles, Los Angeles
David W. Low, M.D.	Assistant Professor of Surgery, University of Pennsylvania School of Medicine, Philadelphia
Dana C. Lynge, M.D.	Instructor, Department of Surgery, University of Washington School of Medicine; Staff Surgeon, Surgical Service, Veterans Affairs Medical Centers, Seattle
Junji Machi, M.D., Ph.D.	Associate Professor of Surgery, University of Hawaii at Manca, Manca; Attending Surgeon, Queen's Medical Center, and Kuakini Medical Center, Honolulu
Gerald J. Marks, M.D.	Edgar J. Deissler Professor of Surgery, Medical College of Pennsylvania and Hahnemann University School of Medicine; Director, Comprehensive Rectal Cancer Center, and Director of Gastrointestinal Surgical Endoscopy, Hahnemann University Hospital, Philadelphia
John H. Marks, M.D.	Instructor, Department of Surgery, Medical College of Pennsylvania and Hahnemann University School of Medicine; Staff, Department of Surgery, Hahnemann University Hospital, Philadelphia
Lester W. Martin, M.D.	Professor of Surgery and Pediatrics, Emeritus, University of Cincinnati College of Medicine; Emeritus Director of Pediatric Surgery, Children's Hospital Medical Center, Cincinnati
Philippe A. Masser, M.D.	Attending Surgeon, Salem Hospital, Salem, Oregon
Douglas J. Mathisen, M.D.	Associate Professor of Surgery, Harvard Medical School; Chief of Thoracic Surgery and Visiting Surgeon, Division of Thoracic Surgery, Massachusetts General Hospital, Boston
Kenneth L. Mattox, M.D.	Professor and Vice Chairman of Surgery, Baylor College of Medicine; Chief of Staff and Surgery, Ben Taub General Hospital, Houston
Jaime Lopez Mayoral, M.D.	Medical Fellow of Surgery, Division of Colon and Rectal Surgery, University of Minnesota Medical School—Minneapolis, Minneapolis
James F. McKinsey, M.D.	Assistant Professor of Surgery, University of Chicago, Pritzker School of Medicine; Attending Surgeon, University of Chicago Medical Center, Chicago

Donald G. McQuarrie, M.D., Ph.D. — Professor and Vice Chairman, Department of Surgery, University of Minnesota Medical School—Minneapolis; Chief of Surgical Services, Department of Surgery, Veterans Affairs Center, Minneapolis

Jonathan L. Meakins, M.D., D.Sc. — Archibald Professor of Surgery, McGill University Faculty of Medicine; Chief of Surgery, Royal Victoria Hospital Montreal, Quebec, Canada

Dorothea Liebermann-Meffert, M.D. — Professor of Surgery, Technical University, München, Germany; Professor of Surgery, Kantonsspital, University Hospital, Basel, Switzerland

W. Scott Melvin, M.D. — Assistant Professor of Surgery, Ohio State University College of Medicine, Columbus, Ohio

W. J. Messick, M.D. — Assistant Clinical Professor of Surgery, University of North Carolina School of Medicine; Director, Surgical Critical Care, Carolinas Medical Center, Charlotte, North Carolina

Fabrizio Michelassi, M.D. — Professor of Surgery, University of Chicago, Pritzker School of Medicine; Professor of Surgery, University of Chicago, Chicago

Carmelo A. Milano, M.D. — Chief Resident in Surgery, Duke University School of Medicine; Chief Resident in Surgery, Duke University Medical Center, Durham, North Carolina

Bertrand Millat, M.D. — Professor of Digestive Surgery, Université de Montpellier; Chief of Surgery, Department of Digestive Surgery, Hôpital St. Eloi, Montpellier, France

Italo Braghetto Miranda, M.D. — Professor of Surgery, University of Chile, Santiago, Chile

Irvin M. Modlin, M.D. — Professor of Surgery, Yale University School of Medicine; Director, Gastric Hepatobiliary Research Group, Yale University School of Medicine, New Haven, Connecticut

Robert M. Moldwin, M.D. — Assistant Professor of Urology, Long Island Jewish Medical Center, New Hyde Park, New York

Gregory L. Moneta, M.D. — Associate Professor of Surgery, Division of Vascular Surgery, Oregon Health Sciences University School of Medicine, Portland, Oregon

Stephen G. Moon, M.S. — Instructor of Allied Medicine, Ohio State University College of Medicine, Columbus, Ohio

Wesley S. Moore, M.D. — Professor of Surgery, University of California School of Medicine, Los Angeles, UCLA School of Medicine; Chief, Section of Vascular Surgery, University of California Medical Center, Los Angeles

Monica Morrow, M.D. — Associate Professor of Surgery, Northwestern University Medical School; Director, Lynn Sage Comprehensive Breast Program, Northwestern Memorial Hospital, Chicago

Joseph L. Mulherin, Jr., M.D. — Associate Clinical Professor of Surgery, Vanderbilt University School of Medicine; Attending Physician, Edwards-Eve Clinic, Nashville, Tennessee

Kenric M. Murayama, M.D. — Assistant Professor of Surgery, University of Nebraska College of Medicine, Omaha, Nebraska

Leslie Karl Nathanson, M.D. — Associate Professor of Surgery, University of Queensland; Reader, Department of Clinical Sciences, Royal Brisbane Hospital, Herston, Queensland, Australia

Henry W. Neale, M.D. — Professor and Chairman, Division of Plastic Surgery, University of Cincinnati College of Medicine; Director, Division of Plastic Surgery, University Hospital, Cincinnati

David H. Nichols, M.D. — Visiting Professor of Obstetrics, Gynecology and Reproductive Biology, Harvard Medical School; Visiting Professor of Obstetrics, Gynecology and Reproductive Biology, and Reproductive Biology, Massachusetts General Hospital, Boston

Santhat Nivatvongs, M.D.	Professor of Surgery, Mayo Medical School; Consultant in Colon and Rectal Surgery, Mayo Clinic, Rochester, Minnesota
Jeffrey A. Norton, M.D.	Professor of Surgery and Chief of Endocrine and Oncologic Surgery, University of Washington School of Medicine; Attending Surgeon, Barnes Hospital, St. Louis
Michael S. Nussbaum, M.D.	Assistant Professor of Surgery, University of Cincinnati College of Medicine; Director, Department of Surgical Endoscopy, University of Cincinnati Medical Center, Cincinnati
Lloyd M. Nyhus, M.D.	Warren H. Cole Professor of Surgery, Emeritus, University of Illinois College of Medicine; Surgeon-in-Chief Emeritus, University of Illinois Hospital, Chicago
Theodore K. Oates, M.D.	Clinical Assistant Professor of Surgery, University of Rochester School of Medicine and Dentistry; Attending Surgeon, Rochester General Hospital, Rochester, New York
Jae-Wook Oh, M.D., Ph.D.	Assistant Professor of Plastic Surgery, Inje University Medical School, Pusan, Korea; Clinical Fellow in Plastic Surgery, University of Alabama Hospital, Birmingham, Alabama
Jemi Olak, M.D.	Assistant Professor of Surgery, University of Chicago, Pritzker School of Medicine, Chicago
Keith T. Oldham, M.D.	Professor of Surgery, Duke University School of Medicine; Chief, Division of Pediatric Surgery, Duke University Medical Center, Durham, North Carolina
Michael P. O'Leary, M.D., M.P.H.	Assistant Professor of Surgery, Harvard Medical School; Urologist, Brigham and Women's Hospital, Boston
Kerry D. Olsen, M.D.	Professor of Otorhinolaryngology, Head and Neck Surgery, Mayo Medical School; Consultant, Otorhinolaryngology, Head and Neck Surgery, Mayo Clinic, Rochester, Minnesota
Eduardo Orihuela, M.D.	Associate Professor of Urology, University of Texas Medical School at Galveston, Galveston, Texas
Adrian Ortega, M.D.	Assistant Professor of Surgery, University of Southern California School of Medicine, Los Angeles
David M. Ota, M.D.	Professor and Chief of Surgical Oncology, University of Missouri—Columbia School of Medicine; Medical Director, Department of Surgery, University of MO-Ellis Fischel Cancer Center, Columbia, Missouri
Kenneth Ouriel, M.D.	Associate Professor of Surgery, University of Rochester School of Medicine and Dentistry; Attending Surgeon, The Strong Memorial Hospital, Rochester, New York
Edward Passaro, Jr., M.D.	Professor of Surgery, University of California, Los Angeles, UCLA School of Medicine; Chief, Surgical Services, Veteran's Affairs Medical Center West Los Angeles, Los Angeles
William H. Pearce, M.D.	Professor of Surgery, Northwestern University Medical School; Interim Director, Blood Flow Laboratory, Northwestern Memorial Hospital, Chicago
Manuel A. Penalver, M.D.	Assistant Professor of Surgery, University of Miami School of Medicine, Miami
Israel Penn, M.D.	Professor of Surgery, University of Cincinnati School of Medicine; Professor of Surgery, University Hospital, Cincinnati
Arvin I. Philippart, M.D.	Professor of Surgery, Wayne State University School of Medicine; Surgeon-in-Chief, Children's Hospital of Michigan, Detroit

Giancarlo Piano, M.D.	Assistant Professor of Surgery, University of Chicago, Pritzker School of Medicine; Attending Surgeon, University of Chicago Medical Center, Chicago
Jack R. Pickleman, M.D.	Dr. and Mrs. John Igini Professor of Surgery, Loyola University of Chicago Stritch School of Medicine; Chief, Division of General Surgery, Loyola University Medical Center, Maywood, Illinois
Patricio Burdiles Pinto, M.D.	Assistant Professor of Surgery, University of Chile, Santiago, Chile
Peter W. T. Pisters, M.D.	Assistant Professor of Surgical Oncology, University of Texas Medical School at Houston, Houston
M. Steven Piver, M.D.	Professor of Clinical Gynecology, Department of Obstetrics and Gynecology, State University of New York at Buffalo; Chief, Department of Gynecologic Oncology, Roswell Park Cancer Institute, Buffalo, New York
Raymond Pollak, M.B.	Professor of Surgery, University of Illinois College of Medicine; Director, Transplant Service, University of Illinois Hospital, Chicago
Stephen F. Ponchak, M.D.	Assistant Clinical Professor of Obstetrics and Gynecology, Tufts University School of Medicine, Boston
Jeffrey L. Ponsky, M.D.	Professor and Vice Chairman of Surgery, Case Western Reserve University School of Medicine; Director of Surgery, Mount Sinai Medical Center, Cleveland
John M. Porter, M.D.	Professor and Head, Division of Vascular Surgery, Oregon Health Sciences University School of Medicine, Portland, Oregon
Richard A. Prinz, M.D.	Helen Shedd Keith Professor and Chairman, Department of General Surgery, Rush Medical College of Rush University; Chairman of General Surgery, Rush-Presbyterian-St. Luke's Medical Center, Chicago
David A. Provost, M.D.	Assistant Professor of General Surgery-Burns/Trauma Critical Care, University of Texas Southwestern Medical Center at Dallas Southwestern Medical School, Dallas
Joseph S. Raccuia, M.D.	
Jayant Radhakrishnan, M.D.	Professor of Surgery and Urology, University of Illinois College of Medicine; Chief of Pediatric Surgery, University of Illinois Hospital, Chicago
Seshadri Raju, M.D.	Professor of Surgery, Emeritus, and Attending Surgeon, University of Mississippi School of Medicine, Jackson, Mississippi
Sai S. Ramasastry, M.D.	Associate Professor of Plastic Surgery, University of Illinois College of Medicine; Attending Plastic Surgeon, Cook County Hospital and University of Illinois Hospital, Chicago
Raymond C. Read, M.D.	Professor of Surgery, University of Arkansas for Medical Sciences College of Medicine; Chief, General Thoracic Surgery, Veteran's Administration Medical Center, Little Rock, Arkansas
Howard A. Reber, M.D.	Professor of Surgery, Division of General Surgery, University of California, Los Angeles, UCLA School of Medicine; Chief of Surgery, Sepulveda Veteran's Administration Medical Center, Los Angeles
Jeffrey M. Reilly, M.D.	Assistant Professor of Surgery, Washington University School of Medicine; Attending Surgeon, Barnes-Jewish Hospital, St. Louis
Joseph M. Reising, M.D.	Assistant Professor of Surgery, University of Cincinnati College of Medicine; Director of Thoracic Surgery, University of Cincinnati Medical Center, Cincinnati

Petachia Reissman, M.D. — Senior Lecturer in Surgery, Hadassah Hebrew University; Staff Surgeon, Hadassah Hebrew University Hospital, Jerusalem, Israel

Harry M. Richter III, M.D. — Assistant Professor of Surgery, University of Illinois College of Medicine; Attending Surgeon and Chief of Surgical Research, Cook County Hospital, Chicago

Layton F. Rikkers, M.D. — Professor and Chairman of Surgery, University of Wisconsin School of Medicine Madison, Wisconsin

Michael Rodriguez, M.D. — Assistant Professor of Obstetrics and Gynecology, Case Western Reserve School of Medicine, and University Hospital of Cleveland, Cleveland

John L. Rombeau, M.D. — Professor of Surgery, University of Pennsylvania School of Medicine, Philadelphia

Glorianne V. Ropchan, M.D. — Assistant Professor of Surgery, Queen's University Faculty of Medicine; Staff Surgeon, Department of Cardiovascular Surgery, Kingston General and Hotel Dieu Hospital, Kingston, Ontario, Canada

Ernest F. Rosato, M.D. — Professor of Surgery, University of Pennsylvania School of Medicine; Chief, Division of Gastrointestinal Surgery, Hospital of the University of Pennsylvania, Philadelphia

Alexander S. Rosemurgy II, M.D. — Professor of Surgery, University of South Florida College of Medicine; Chief of General Surgery, Tampa General Hospital, Tampa, Florida

Michael Rosenbloom, M.D. — Assistant Professor of Surgery, Washington University School of Medicine, St. Louis

Mario E. Rossetti, M.D. — Professor Emeritus, University of Basel, Basel; Chairman Emeritus, Department of Surgery, Kantonsspital, Liestal, Switzerland

Aaron Ruhalter, M.D. — Professor of Surgery and Anatomy, Volunteer Faculty, University of Cincinnati College of Medicine; Director of Medical Education, Ethicon Endo-Surgery, Cincinnati

Benjamin F. Rush, Jr., M.D. — Distinguished Professor of Surgery and Attending Surgeon, UMDNJ-New Jersey Medical School, Newark, New Jersey

Robb H. Rutledge, M.D. — Clinical Professor of Surgery, University of Texas Southwestern Medical Center at Dallas Southwestern Medical School, Dallas; Attending Surgeon, John Peter Smith Hospital, Fort Worth, Texas

Frederick C. Ryckman, M.D. — Associate Professor of Surgery, University of Cincinnati College of Medicine; Pediatric Surgeon, Children's Hospital Medical Center, Cincinnati

David C. Sabiston, Jr., M.D., Sc.D. — James Buchanan Duke Professor of Surgery, Duke University School of Medicine; Director, International Programs, Department of Surgery, Duke University Medical Center, Durham, North Carolina

Farrokh Saidi, M.D. — Professor of General and Thoracic Surgery, Beheshti University School of Medicine; Chief, Department of General and Thoracic Surgery, Modarress Hospital, Tehran, Iran

Atef A. Salam, M.D. — Professor of Surgery, Emory University School of Medicine; Professor of Surgery and General Vascular Surgeon, Emory University Hospital, Atlanta

Kaoru Sano, M.D. — Second Department of Surgery, Kyoto University; Second Department of Surgery, Kyoto University Hospital, Kyoto, Japan

John L. Sawyers, M.D. — Professor of Surgery, Emeritus, Vanderbilt University School of Medicine, Nashville, Tennessee

William P. Schecter, M.D.	Professor of Clinical Surgery, University of California, San Francisco, School of Medicine; Chief of Surgery, San Francisco General Hospital, San Francisco
Richard T. Schlinkert, M.D.	Associate Professor of Surgery, Mayo Medical School, Rochester, Minnesota; Consultant, Department of General Surgery, Mayo Clinic Scottsdale, Scottsdale, Arizona
Theodore R. Schrock, M.D.	Professor and Interim Chair, Department of Surgery, University of California, San Francisco, School of Medicine; Attending Surgeon, Moffitt/Long Hospital, San Francisco
Seymour I. Schwartz, M.D.	Distinguished Alumni Professor and Chair, Department of Surgery, University of Rochester School of Medicine and Dentistry; Surgeon-in-Chief, The Strong Memorial Hospital, Rochester, New York
James Sciubba, DMD, Ph.D.	Professor of Oral Biology and Pathology, State University of New York at Stony Brook; Chairman, Department of Dental Medicine, Long Island Jewish Medical Center, New Hyde Park, New York
Andrew Seely, M.D.	Resident, Department of Surgery, McGill University Faculty of Medicine, Montreal, Quebec, Canada
Bernd-Uwe Sevin, M.D., Ph.D.	Professor of Gynecology and Oncology, University of Miami School of Medicine, Miami
Dhiraj M. Shah, M.D.	Professor of Surgery, Albany Medical College; Head, Department of General Surgery, Albany Medical Center Hospital, Albany, New York
Charles J. Shanley, M.D.	Assistant Professor of Surgery, University of Michigan Medical School; Associate Director, Surgical Intensive Care Unit and Critical Care Residency Program, University of Michigan Medical Center, Ann Arbor, Michigan
Byers W. Shaw, Jr., M.D.	Professor of Surgery and Chief of Transplantation, University of Nebraska Medical Center, Omaha, Nebraska
George F. Sheldon, M.D.	Professor and Chairman of Surgery, University of North Carolina at Chapel Hill School of Medicine; Professor and Chairman of Surgery, UNC Hospitals, Chapel Hill, North Carolina
Jerry M. Shuck, M.D., D.Sc.	Oliver H. Payne Professor and Chairman, Department of Surgery, Case Western Reserve University School of Medicine; Director of Surgery, University Hospitals of Cleveland, Cleveland
Gregorio A. Sicard, M.D.	Professor of Surgery, Washington University School of Medicine; Director, Vascular Service, Department of Surgery, Barnes-Jewish Hospital, St. Louis
J. Rüdiger Siewert, M.D.	Full Professor of Surgery, Technische Universität München; Director, Department of Surgery, Klinikum rechts der Isar of the Technische Universität München, München, Germany
Bernard Sigel, M.D.	Professor of Surgery, Medical College of Pennsylvania, Philadelphia
Donald Silver, M.D.	Professor and Chairman, Department of Surgery, University of Missouri—Columbia School of Medicine; Chief of Surgery, University of Missouri—Columbia Hospitals and Clinics, Columbia, Missouri
Richard L. Simmons, M.D.	Professor and Chairman of Surgery, University of Pittsburgh School of Medicine; Chairman of Surgery, University of Pittsburgh Medical Center, Pittsburgh
Rakesh Sindhi, M.D.	Assistant Professor of Surgery, University of California, Davis, School of Medicine, Davis, California

Adolf Singer, M.D.	Emeritus Associate Clinical Professor of Surgery, Albert Einstein College of Medicine of Yeshiva University, Bronx, New York
John E. Skandalakis, M.D.	Chris Carlos Distinguished Professor, Emeritus, of Surgical Anatomy and Technique and Director of Centers for Surgical Anatomy and Technique, Emory University School of Medicine; Senior Attending Surgeon, Piedmont Hospital, Atlanta
Lee J. Skandalakis, M.D.	Clinical Assistant Professor of Surgical Anatomy and Technique, Emory University School of Medicine; Attending Surgeon, Piedmont Hospital, Atlanta
Donald G. Skinner, M.D.	Professor and Chairman, Department of Urology, University of Southern California School of Medicine; Medical Director, Kenneth Norris Jr. Cancer Hospital and Research Institute, Los Angeles
Milton M. Slocum, M.D.	Chief Vascular Resident, Department of Surgery, University of Missouri—Columbia School of Medicine; Chief Vascular Resident, University of Missouri Hospitals and Clinics, Columbia, Missouri
H. Wayne Slone, M.D.	Clinical Instructor of Radiology, The Ohio State University Medical Center, Columbus, Ohio
Arthur D. Smith, M.D.	Professor of Surgery, Albert Einstein College of Medicine of Yeshiva University, Bronx; Professor and Chairman, Department of Urology, Long Island Jewish Medical Center, New Hyde Park, New York
Stephen L. Smith, M.D.	Instructor in Surgery, Mayo Medical School, Rochester, Minnesota; Staff Surgeon, St. Luke's Hospital, Jacksonville, Florida
Nathaniel J. Soper, M.D.	Professor of Surgery, Washington University School of Medicine; Director, Washington University Institute for Minimally Invasive Surgery, St. Louis
Dimitrios G. Spigos, M.D.	Professor and Chairman of Radiology, The Ohio State University Medical Center, Columbus, Ohio
Ronald H. Spiro, M.D.	Clinical Professor of Surgery, Cornell University Medical College; Attending Surgeon, Head and Neck Service, Memorial Sloan Kettering Cancer Center, New York
James C. Stanley, M.D.	Professor of Surgery, University of Michigan Medical School; Head, Section of Vascular Surgery, University Hospital, Ann Arbor, Michigan
Mindy B. Statter, M.D.	Assistant Professor of Surgery and Pediatrics, University of Chicago, Pritzker School of Medicine; Attending Surgeon, Department of Pediatric Surgery, Wyler Children's Hospital, Chicago
Glenn D. Steele, Jr., M.D., Ph.D.	Dean and Richard T. Crane Professor of Surgery, University of Chicago, Pritzker School of Medicine; Vice President for Medical Affairs, University of Chicago Hospitals, Chicago
Felicien M. Steichen, M.D.	Professor of Surgery, New York Medical College, Valhalla, New York; Director, Institute for Minimally Invasive Surgery, St. Agnes Hospital, White Plains, New York
Ronald J. Stoney, M.D.	Professor of Surgery, Emeritus, Division of Vascular Surgery, University of California, San Francisco, School of Medicine; Attending Vascular Surgeon, Long/Moffitt Hospitals, San Francisco
René E. Stoppa, M.D.	Professor Emeritus, Clinique Chirurgicale, Faculté de Médecine; Director (Honorary), Department of Digestive Surgery, Centre Hospitalier Universitaire, Amiens, France
David J. Sugarbaker, M.D.	Associate Professor of Surgery, Division of Thoracic Surgery, Harvard Medical School; Chief, Division of Thoracic Surgery, Brigham and Women's Hospital, Boston

Harvey J. Sugarman, M.D. David M. Hume Professor of Surgery, Virginia Commonwealth University Medical College of Virginia School of Medicine, Richmond, Virginia

David S. Sumner, M.D. Distinguished Professor of Surgery, Southern Illinois University School of Medicine, Springfield, Illinois

Richard E. Symmonds, M.D. Emeritus Professor of Obstetrics and Gynecology, Mayo Medical School; Emeritus Consultant, Department of Obstetrics and Gynecology, Mayo Clinic and Foundation, Rochester, Minnesota

Sumio Takayama, M.D. Lecturer, Department of Surgery, Jikei University School of Medicine; Chief Surgeon, Department of General and Digestive Surgery, Jikei University Hospital, Tokyo, Japan

Lloyd M. Taylor, Jr., M.D. Professor of Surgery, Division of Vascular Surgery, Oregon Health Sciences University School of Medicine, Portland, Oregon

John Terblanche, Ch.M. Professor and Chairman, Department of Surgery, University of Cape Town; Professor and Surgeon-in-Chief, Groote Schuur Hospital Teaching Hospital Group, Cape Town, South Africa

Oreste Terranova, M.D. Professor of General Surgery, Universitá di Padova, Padova, Italy

Erwin R. Thal, M.D. Professor of Surgery, University of Texas Southwestern Medical Center and Parkland Memorial Hospital, Dallas

Robert G. Thompson, M.D. Clinical Professor, Emeritus, Department of Orthopedic Surgery, Northwestern University Medical School; Emeritus Attending Surgeon, Department of Orthopedic Surgery, Northwestern Memorial Hospital, Chicago

Greg Tiao, M.D. Resident, Department of Surgery, University of Cincinnati College of Medicine, Cincinnati

Joe J. Tjandra, M.D. Senior Lecturer, Department of Surgery, University of Melbourne; Staff Colorectal Surgeon, Royal Melbourne Hospital, Parkville, Victoria, Australia

Sidney Trodgon, M.D. Assistant Professor of Surgery, Eastern Virginia Medical School of the Medical College of Hampton Roads, Norfolk, Virginia

Donald D. Trunkey, M.D. Professor and Chairman, Department of Surgery, Oregon Health Sciences University School of Medicine, Portland, Oregon

Ted Trus, M.D. Instructor in Surgery, Emory University School of Medicine, Atlanta

BaoLien Nguyen Tu, M.D. Research Fellow, Department of Surgery, Mayo Clinic Scottsdale, Scottsdale, Arizona

Kenan M. Ulualp, M.D. Associate Professor of Surgery, Istanbul University Cerrahpasa Faculty, Istanbul, Turkey

Joseph P. Vacanti, M.D. Associate Professor of Surgery, Harvard Medical School; Director of Organ Transplantation and Senior Associate in Surgery, Children's Hospital, Boston

John F. Valente, M.D. Assistant Professor of Surgery, University of Cincinnati College of Medicine; Transplant Surgeon, University Hospital, Cincinnati

Jon A. van Heerden, M.B., Ch.B. Professor of Surgery, Mayo Medical School; Consultant, Department of General Surgery, Mayo Clinic and Mayo Foundation, Rochester, Minnesota

Luis O. Vasconez, M.D. Professor and Chief, Division of Plastic Surgery, University of Alabama School of Medicine, Birmingham, Alabama

Michael P. Vezeridis, M.D.

Professor of Surgery, Brown University School of Medicine; Associate Director, Division of Surgical Oncology, Roger Williams Medical Center, Providence, Rhode Island

Stephen B. Vogel

Professor of Surgery, University of Florida College of Medicine, Gainesville, Florida

Daniel von Allmen, M.D.

Assistant Professor in General and Pediatric Surgery, University of North Carolina at Chapel Hill School of Medicine, Chapel Hill, North Carolina; Fellow in Pediatric Surgery, Children's Hospital Medical Center, Cincinnati

Matthew J. Wall, Jr., M.D.

Associate Professor of Surgery, Baylor College of Medicine; Chief of General Surgery, Ben Taub General Hospital, Houston

Brad W. Warner, M.D.

Assistant Professor of Surgery, University of Cincinnati College of Medicine; Attending Surgeon, Department of Pediatric Surgery, Children's Hospital Medical Center, Cincinnati

W. Bedford Waters, M.D.

Professor of Urology, Loyola University Stritch School of Medicine, Maywood; Associate Chief of Urology, Department of Surgical Service, Hines Veteran's Administration Medical Center, Hines, Illinois

John A. Weigelt, M.D.

Professor and Vice Chairman, Department of Surgery, University of Minnesota Medical School—Minneapolis, Minneapolis; Chairman, Department of Surgery, Saint Paul-Ramsey Medical Center, St. Paul, Minnesota

Samuel A. Wells, Jr., M.D.

Bixby Professor and Chairman, Department of Surgery, Washington University School of Medicine; Surgeon-in-Chief, Barnes-Jewish Hospital, St. Louis

Steven D. Wexner, M.D.

Chairman and Residency Program Director, Department of Colorectal Surgery, Cleveland Clinic Florida, Fort Lauderdale, Florida

Jock R. Wheeler, M.D.

Dean and Provost, Eastern Virginia Medical School of the Medical College of Hampton Roads, Norfolk, Virginia

Anthony D. Whittemore, M.D.

Professor of Surgery, Harvard Medical School; Chief, Vascular Surgery, Brigham and Women's Hospital, Boston

Catherine M. Wittgen, M.D.

Assistant Professor of Surgery, University of Minnesota Medical School—Minneapolis, Minneapolis; SICU Medical Director, Department of Surgery, Saint Paul-Ramsey Medical Center, St. Paul, Minnesota

Dietmar H. Wittmann, M.D., Ph.D.

Professor of Surgery, Medical College of Wisconsin; Director, Surgical Critical Care Program, Froedtert Memorial Lutheran Hospital, Milwaukee, Wisconsin

John Wong, M.D., Ph.D.

Professor and Head, Department of Surgery, The University of Hong Kong Medical Center; Chief of Service, Department of Surgery, Queen Mary Hospital, Hong Kong

Thomas F. Wood, M.D.

Resident in General Surgery, University of California Los Angeles Medical Center, Los Angeles

James S. T. Yao, M.D., Ph.D.

Magerstadt Professor of Surgery, Northwestern University Medical School; Chief, Division of Vascular Surgery, Northwestern Memorial Hospital, Chicago

Christopher K. Zarins, M.D.

Chidester Professor and Acting Chairman, Department of Surgery, Division of Vascular Surgery, Stanford University School of Medicine; Chief of Vascular Surgery, Stanford University Medical Center, Stanford, California

Moritz M. Ziegler, M.D.

Professor of Surgery, University of Cincinnati College of Medicine; Director and Surgeon-in-Chief, Division of Pediatric Surgery, Children's Hospital Medical Center, Cincinnati

ONE

PERIOPERATIVE CARE OF THE SURGICAL PATIENT

1

Metabolic Response to Trauma and Infection

Per-Olof Hasselgren   *Greg Tiao*

Trauma and infection initiate changes in metabolism that can affect virtually all organs and tissues by altering carbohydrate, lipid, and protein metabolism. The metabolic response to injury and sepsis is usually divided into an ebb and a flow phase followed by a convalescence phase (Fig. 1-1). This metabolic pattern is better defined following injury than during sepsis since a well-characterized series of events occur beginning at the time of injury. The metabolic course during sepsis is more convoluted because the septic insult is usually more insidious in its onset and can vary in its duration and intensity. This variability of the metabolic response was illustrated in a recent report of patients with severe sepsis (Voerman et al, 1993). Individuals with severe sepsis or septic shock display many of the characteristics of the ebb phase while patients with a more chronic, less severe sepsis display the hypermetabolism and catabolism of the flow phase ("hypermetabolic sepsis").

The ebb phase is dominated by glycogenolysis and lipolysis, which provide the organism with energy substrates for "fight or flight." This is followed by the flow phase, a state of catabolism manifested by elevated metabolic rate and increases in body temperature, pulse rate, urinary nitrogen excretion, and muscle catabolism. The subsequent anabolic "recovery" phase can last from weeks to months.

It is the purpose of this chapter to describe the characteristic changes in carbohydrate, lipid, and protein metabolism that occur in trauma and sepsis with an emphasis placed on metabolic mediators including hormones, cytokines, and nitric oxide (NO). In addition, intracellular mechanisms, including molecular regulation, of

metabolic consequences of injury and severe infection are discussed.

Understanding the metabolic response to injury and sepsis is important from a clinical perspective for several reasons. Some of the metabolic alterations that occur following injury and severe infection are essential for survival. For example, several studies, including that of Dominioni and associates (1987), have found a correlation between survival and maintenance of the acute-phase response in the liver. In contrast, the excessive muscle catabolism that occurs during sepsis may be detrimental to patients, delaying recovery, slowing ambulation, and increasing the risk of pulmonary complications if the respiratory muscles are involved. Identifying methods to limit excessive catabolism may therefore be essential. By understanding the mediators and mechanisms of the metabolic response to trauma and infection, novel therapeutic strategies targeting specific metabolic alterations may be developed, possibly resulting in improved survival, as discussed in more detail in the last section of this chapter.

Release of Metabolic Mediators

Many of the metabolic alterations that occur in response to trauma and infection are regulated by hormones, cytokines, and NO. Frequently, these substances interact with each other to induce a complete metabolic response. Before the role of these mediators in the regulation of metabolism is discussed, the influence of injury and sepsis on their release is reviewed. It should be noted that although a number

of other biologically active substances, such as oxygen radicals, prostaglandins, leukotrienes, and complement components, are released following injury and sepsis, this chapter focuses on hormones, cytokines, and NO since they have been studied most extensively as metabolic regulators.

Hormones

Frayn (1986) found that injury and sepsis are associated with a pronounced neuroendocrine response with an initial sympathoadrenal discharge, stimulating the release of the counterregulatory hormones glucagon, epinephrine, norepinephrine, growth hormone (GH), and cortisol. According to Gann and associates (1987), the stimuli that activate the neuroendocrine response during trauma and infection include hemodynamic changes (caused by hemorrhage, dehydration, third space losses, and so forth), changes in pH, PO_2, PCO_2, ambient or body temperature, substrate availability (e.g., plasma glucose and amino acids), pain, and anxiety. The regulation of the neuroendocrine system is illustrated in Fig. 1-2.

The counterregulatory hormones respond to hypoglycemia and play a role in glucose "counterregulation." Several of the counterregulatory hormones have a catabolic effect and are called "catabolic hormones." The counterregulatory hormones are usually elevated during the ebb phase following injury, but can remain increased into the flow phase during sustained injury, such as burn injury, and during sepsis.

There are numerous reports in the literature of increased levels of cortisol, glucagon, catecholamines, and GH following

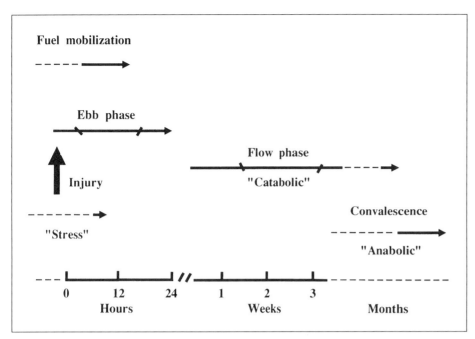

Fig. 1-1. The metabolic response to injury can be divided into an early ebb phase, followed by a flow phase and a convalescence (anabolic) phase. The duration of each phase is variable and only approximate figures are given. The response to infection and sepsis is seldom as well defined as outlined in the figure. (Redrawn with permission from KN Frayn, Hormonal control of metabolism and sepsis. Clin Endocrinol 24:577, 1986.)

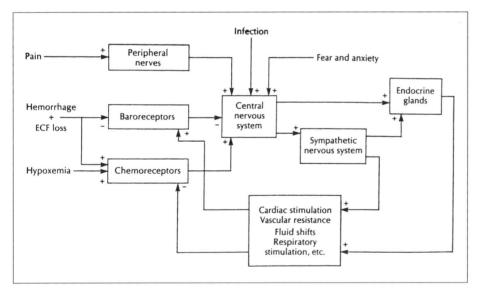

Fig. 1-2. Neuroendocrine reflexes induced by shock and trauma. Pain, reduction of circulating volume (caused by hemorrhage or other extracellular fluid loss), hypoxemia, infection, fear, and anxiety are stimuli to the neuroendocrine response. ECF = extracellular fluid. (From DS Gann, JF Amaral, MD Caldwell. Neuroendocrine response to stress, injury, and sepsis. In JH Davis (ed), Clinical Surgery. St. Louis: Mosby, 1987. Reproduced with permission.)

trauma, burn injury, infection and and sepsis. From a metabolic standpoint, cortisol is probably the most important among the counterregulatory hormones, with widespread effects on glucose, amino acid, and fatty acid metabolism. The release of glucocorticoids in trauma and sepsis is centrally regulated. Thus, stress results in hypothalamic release of corticotropin releasing factor, which in turn stimulates pituitary release of adrenocorticotropic hormone (ACTH). ACTH regulates cortisol synthesis and release from the adrenal cortex. The importance of the role of the central nervous system during trauma and infection is illustrated by the fact that the glucocorticoid response can be abolished by blocking afferent nervous stimuli.

Recent evidence from Molina and Abumrad (1994) suggests a role for endogenous opiates and opioids as contributing mediators in the neuroendocrine response. It is likely that central nervous system hypoglycemia during the early part of the ebb phase causes increased release of central nervous system morphine. The elevated morphine levels may play a role in mediating metabolic alterations, including intestinal proteolysis.

In addition to the catabolic hormones, trauma and infection influence other hormones as well, most notably insulin, insulin-like growth factor (IGF-I), and thyroid hormone. Frayn found that plasma insulin levels decrease during the ebb phase and rise during the catabolic flow phase. Despite high levels of plasma insulin during the flow phase, plasma glucose levels remain elevated, supporting the concept of "insulin resistance" in peripheral tissues, in particular in skeletal muscle, during sepsis and following trauma. There is evidence that the insulin resistance in these conditions is at the postreceptor level and may be mediated by beta-adrenergic receptor activity and tumor necrosis factor (TNF) (Lang et al, 1992; Hasselgren and Fischer, 1992).

Ross and colleagues found that circulating IGF-I levels decrease in septic and critically ill patients. IGF-I and insulin are anabolic hormones that promote protein and glycogen synthesis and block protein breakdown. Diminished influence of the anabolic hormones, in addition to increased levels of the catabolic hormones, may represent an important mechanism by which metabolic alterations occur during trauma and infection. Both IGF-I and insulin have been used as therapeutic agents in an effort to reduce postinjury catabolism (Ziegler et al, 1994).

Serum levels of triiodothyronine (T3) are frequently reduced in injured and septic patients without clinical signs of hypothyroidism. The predominant mechanism of this "low T3 syndrome" is probably a defect in the peripheral conversion of thyroxine to T3. Alternatively, increased cellular uptake of T3 may be responsible, at least in part, for decreased circulating levels of the hormone and could explain the increased tissue concentrations of T3 that have been reported in sepsis by Hasselgren and associates (1987). Interestingly, catecholamines stimulate cellular uptake of thyroid hormone following trauma. Many of the catabolic changes that occur during sepsis are similar to those seen during hyperthyroidism, suggesting that increased tissue T3 concentrations may be one of the mechanisms (albeit not a major mechanism) of the catabolic response to injury and sepsis.

Cytokines

Cytokines are biologically extremely potent proteins of low molecular weight (the majority less than 20 kD) that can be released from a variety of cells. Following trauma and sepsis, macrophages are probably the predominant source. Cytokines were first described as mediators of the immune system but have been increasingly recognized as key regulators of a variety of metabolic processes. Although cytokines are thought to act primarily in an autocrine or paracrine fashion, several studies, including those of Pinsky and associates (1993), and of Drost and colleagues (1993), have found a correlation between high levels of plasma cytokines and high mortality following injury and sepsis, suggesting that the cytokines may have a systemic effect as well. Circulating cytokines may also represent an overflow phenomenon, reflecting leakage of the substances into the bloodstream from tissues with extremely high local production.

Among the proinflammatory cytokines, TNF, interleukin-1, and interleukin-6 (IL-1 and IL-6) have been most widely studied with respect to metabolic regulation following injury, inflammation, and infection. Other cytokines that may be involved in the metabolic response to injury and infection include IL-4, IL-7, IL-8, and interferon (IFN)γ. This list will probably grow longer as new cytokines and their functions continue to be identified. Increased circulating levels of TNF, IL-1, and IL-6 following trauma and infection have been reported in a number of previous studies, including those by Pinsky (1993) and associates, and by Drost and colleagues (1993). Evidence for local production of cytokines in response to endotoxemia has been found in liver, intestinal mucosa, and brain (Keogh et al, 1990; Mester et al, 1993;

Gatti and Bartkin, 1993). Recent studies in our laboratory (Meyer et al, 1994, 1995) suggest that endotoxin has a direct effect on intestinal epithelial cells, stimulating the release of IL-6. In the same studies, NO downregulated and prostaglandin E_2 upregulated the endotoxin-induced release of IL-6 from the enterocytes, consistent with a complex interaction among different mediators released during sepsis and endotoxemia. The mucosa of small intestine as a source of cytokines in trauma, sepsis, and shock has attracted increasing interest in recent years.

The pattern of cytokine release during sepsis and endotoxemia and following severe injury is that of an early release of TNF followed by subsequent production of IL-1 and IL-6. This cascade-like cytokine response in part reflects the fact that TNF stimulates the release of IL-1 and that both TNF and IL-1 stimulate the relase of IL-6.

Several recent studies, including those of Pinsky and associates (1993), and of Drost and colleagues (1993), have found a correlation between plasma levels of cytokines, in particular TNF and IL-6, and mortality in sepsis. Such results may be consistent with the concept that cytokines are responsible for the high mortality in these conditions. It is possible that the persistence of TNF and IL-6 in serum, rather than the peak levels of the cytokines, is important in predicting a poor outcome in patients with septic shock. Because of the correlation between high mortality and increased cytokine levels, cytokine antibodies or receptor antagonists have been tested in the treatment of sepsis and endotoxemia. Both anti-TNF and anti-IL-6 antibodies improve survival in experimental endotoxemia and sepsis. Results from animal experiments and initial human studies suggested that IL-1 receptor antagonist (IL-1ra) may improve survival in sepsis and endotoxemia. A subsequent controlled, multicenter clinical study by Fisher et al (1994), however, failed to demonstrate a significant overall improvement of survival in patients with sepsis. The use of cytokine antibodies or receptor antagonists in the treatment of septic patients remains controversial and it is possible that this type of treatment is of value only in specific subgroups of septic patients.

The potentially deleterious effects of high concentrations of cytokines are blunted by

endogenous inhibitors released concomitantly with the cytokines. For example, cytokine receptors are shed from cell surfaces during sepsis and endotoxemia. Receptor shedding reduces cytokine action by removing binding sites from the target cells and by providing soluble inhibitors that bind to circulating cytokines. Soluble forms of receptors for TNF, IL-1, IL-6, and IFNγ have been identified. Two structurally distinct soluble TNF receptors have been found and both these binding proteins protect cells from TNF-mediated toxicity. The cDNAs for the two soluble TNF receptors have been cloned and expressed as recombinant soluble TNF binding proteins by Gray and associates (1990). Release of IL-1ra offers an additional example of a naturally occurring inhibitor. Interleukin-1 and IL-1ra are released from the same cells during sepsis and endotoxemia. The balance between the cytokines and their natural inhibitors is probably important both for the regulation of metabolism and for the outcome following severe injury and sepsis. The role of cytokines and cytokine inhibitors in the regulation of postinjury and sepsis-related metabolic changes is discussed in subsequent sections of this chapter.

Nitric Oxide

Nitric oxide was initially identified as an important mediator of smooth-muscle relaxation (Moncada, 1992). Since then, its role in a variety of physiologic and pathophysiologic processes, including some of the metabolic changes that occur following trauma and sepsis, has become increasingly recognized. Nitric oxide can probably be regarded as the "molecule of the decade" as far as the regulation of the inflammatory process is concerned.

Nitric oxide is derived from L-arginine in a reaction catalyzed by the rate-limiting enzyme nitric oxide synthase (NOS). Nitric oxide is extremely labile, with a half-life measured in minutes. Degradation of NO results in the stable end products nitrite and nitrate (NO_2/NO_3), which are often quantitated as an indirect measure of NO production. Nitric oxide is generated by a number of different cell types including endothelial cells, Kupffer cells, macrophages, and cerebellar neurons and neutrophils. Nitric oxide synthase has two isoforms, a calcium-independent inducible (iNOS) and a calcium-dependent constitutive (cNOS) form. The inducible NOS is probably the most important of the enzymes in mediating metabolic alterations during trauma and infection. Recently, the human form of this enzyme was cloned by Geller and associates (1993). Both forms of NOS can be inhibited by using competitive analogs, such as N-monomethyl-L-arginine (NMA) and N-nitro-L-arginine (NNA). NMA has been used extensively in characterizing the role of NO and has been tested as a therapeutic agent during sepsis.

Nitric oxide mediates most of its cellular effects by activation of soluble guanylate cyclase, which in turn increases levels of cyclic guanine monophosphate (cGMP). The physiologic effects of NO include relaxation of smooth muscle, inhibition of platelet aggregation and adherence and inactivation of complex I and II of the electron transport chain (Moncada, 1992).

It has been shown both in experimental animals and in patients that sepsis and injury are associated with increased production of NO as evidenced by elevated levels of circulating NO_2/NO_3. In two patients with septic shock, administration of NMA improved hemodynamic parameters, suggesting that NO may mediate some of the hemodynamic consequences of sepsis (Nava et al, 1991). The exact role of blockade of NO production during injury and sepsis is not clear, however, and several studies, including that of Tiao and associates (1994), suggest that inhibition of NOS during sepsis and endotoxemia may be detrimental. It is possible that worsened outcome following treatment with arginine analogs reflects the fact that most of these drugs are nonspecific NOS inhibitors, blocking both iNOS and cNOS. Specific iNOS inhibitors may prove more efficient in preventing mortality from severe injury and sepsis.

Interaction Between Mediators

Although, in the previous section of this chapter, the release of hormones, cytokines, and NO during trauma and infection was treated as if each were independent systems, in reality, there is close interaction among the different types of mediators. For example, TNF, IL-1, and IL-6 stimulate the hypothalamus-pituitary-adrenal axis, resulting in the release of ACTH and glucocorticoids (Del Rey and Besedovsky, 1992). All three cytokines stimulate the pituitary-adrenal axis, but

IL-1 is most potent. In addition to stimulating the hypothalamus-pituitary-adrenal axis, there is evidence that at least IL-1 has a direct effect on the adrenals. In normal human subjects, TNF administration induces a stress hormone response with elevated plasma levels of ACTH, cortisol, catecholamines, growth hormone, and glucagon.

The interaction between the two systems is further illustrated by downregulated cytokine release from macrophages following treatment with glucocorticoids, consistent with a negative feedback mechanism. This regulation occurs at the transcriptional level as evidenced by reduced cytokine mRNA concentrations in different tissues following treatment with glucocorticoids. In studies such as that of Ray and associates (1990), using cultured HeLa cells, evidence was found that glucocorticoid repression of IL-6 gene expression involves direct binding of the glucocorticoid receptor to functional DNA elements in the IL-6 promoter. The negative feedback between glucocorticoids and cytokines may protect the body from dangerously high levels of cytokines during trauma and sepsis.

Reduced T3 levels after treatment with TNF or IL-1 demonstrate another link between hormones and cytokines. Hormones can also influence each other as catecholamines increase cellular uptake of T3. The "low T3 syndrome" in sepsis and following trauma may be due to a combination of cytokine and catecholamine effects.

There is also evidence for an interaction between hormones, cytokines, and NO. With the cloning of iNOS, studies have begun to identify the regulators of its expression. For example, NO production and the mRNA for iNOS are induced by a mixture of TNFα, IL-1β, and IFNγ in hepatocytes (Geller et al, 1993). Glucocorticoids may downregulate iNOS expression as suggested by in vivo experiments in which administration of glucocorticoids decreased endotoxin-induced NO production.

Nitric oxide, in turn, may regulate cytokine production. In studies from our laboratory (Meyer et al, 1995), endotoxin-induced production of IL-6 in intestinal epithelial cells was downregulated by NO. Similar findings have been reported in Kupffer cells by Stadler and associates (1993). In other experiments, TNF and IL-

6 levels were substantially increased in endotoxemic rats following treatment with NNA, supporting the concept that NO downregulates cytokine release (Tiao et al, 1994).

The complex interaction between the different types of mediators may at least in part explain why treatment directed against individual mediators following trauma or sepsis has not always been successful and has sometimes even resulted in increased mortality. It is possible that a broader therapeutic approach will be required, taking the interaction between the different mediators into account, before improved clinical outcome can be achieved.

Mechanisms of Hormonal and Cytokine Action

Hormones and cytokines can act on cells remote from the production site (endocrine effect), on adjacent cells (paracrine effect), or on the secretory cell itself (autocrine effect). In general, hormones and cytokines induce intracellular changes in the target cells by binding to specific receptors located on the cell membrane or in the cytoplasm. Receptor binding results in the activation of second messenger systems, such as the diacylglycerol–protein kinase C pathway, the cyclic adenosine monophosphate (cAMP)–protein kinase A pathway, and the receptor tyrosine kinase pathway. The second messenger systems alter intracellular function by affecting gene expression or by modifying preexisting proteins, resulting in changes in their activity or function, or both.

An example of a hormone that induces modification of preexisting proteins is insulin. Insulin influences amino acid and glucose transport by activating transporters that are already present in the cell. Catecholamines can modulate ion transport through their G protein–coupled alpha and beta receptors.

Cytokines frequently exert their biologic activity by altering gene expression and may do so by interacting with hormones. The molecular regulation of acute-phase protein synthesis by IL-6 in the hepatocyte has been studied extensively in recent years and is briefly summarized here as an example of how cytokines can cause gene activation. Following binding of IL-6 to its receptor on the hepatocyte, a cascade of

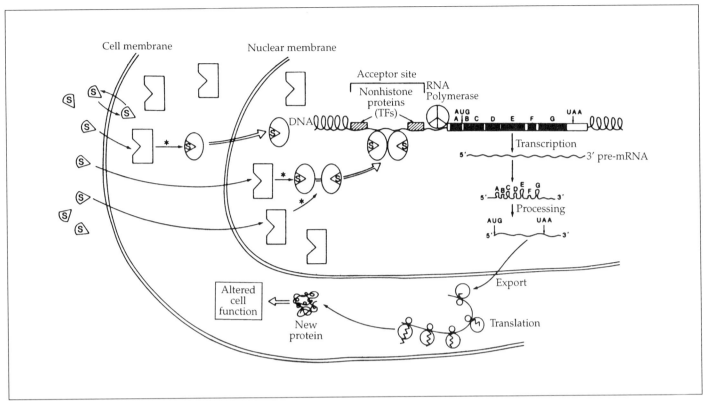

Fig 1-3. Scheme of the molecular pathway of steroid hormone action. Steroids bind to receptors in the cytoplasm or in the nucleus. The receptor undergoes conformational changes after binding to the hormone. The activated hormone-receptor complex stimulates gene transcription after binding to a response element (receptor site) in the promoter. (From JH Clark, WT Schrader, BW O'Malley. Mechanisms of action of steroid hormones. In JD Wilson, DW Foster (eds), Williams Textbook for Endocrinology. Philadelphia: Saunders, 1992. Reproduced with permission.)

intracellular protein phosphorylations occurs, resulting in activation of nuclear transcription factors. Recent work characterized two of these cascades, the mitogen-activated protein kinase (MAPK) pathway, described by Egan and Weinberg (1993), and the Jak (Janus kinase)–STAT (signal transducer and activator of transcription) pathway, discussed by Darnell and associates (1994). These pathways transfer activity at the cell surface to the nucleus. Interleukin-6 is believed to mainly activate the Jak-STAT pathway.

The activated transcription factor binds to a so-called response element in the promoter of the target gene. For example, the IL-6 response element (IL-6RE) is present in the promoter of several of the acute-phase genes, including human and rat haptoglobin, human hemopexin, human C-reactive protein (CRP), and rat α_2-macroglobulin. Binding of the transcription factor to the response element activates gene transcription. The result is

newly synthesized mRNA, which in turn is translated to a protein that can influence cellular metabolism and function.

Other hormones bind to intracellular receptors, which are found both in the cytoplasm and the nucleus. Steroid hormones enter most cells by diffusion, whereas thyroid hormones are actively transported across both the cellular and nuclear membrane before binding to the receptor. Binding of the hormone to the receptor results in conformational changes of the receptor. The activated hormone-receptor complex acts as a transcription factor and stimulates gene expression by binding to a specific hormone receptor binding site (Clark et al, 1992) (Fig. 1-3). The hormone response elements are enhancer elements with profound effect on transcriptional activity when stimulated by the hormone-receptor complex. Hormone response elements have been described for each of the known ligand-activated cytoplasmic and nuclear receptors

and have been identified as glucocorticoid response element (GRE), thyroid hormone reponse element (TRE), and so forth.

The Metabolic Response to Injury and Infection

Trauma and sepsis induce substantial changes in carbohydrate, lipid, and protein metabolism in most organs and tissues. In addition, important changes in fluid balance, electrolytes, acid base balance, and tissue oxygenation occur, but these are not covered in this chapter.

Carbohydrate Metabolism

Early in the course of sepsis and endotoxemia, serum glucose levels rise, mainly reflecting increased hepatic glucose production caused by stimulated glycogenolysis and gluconeogenesis. Concomitant with the increased hepatic glucose production

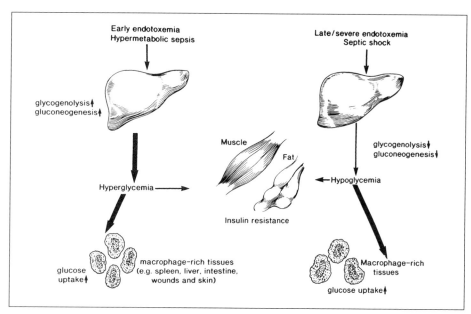

Fig. 1-4. Summary of carbohydrate metabolism during early endotoxemia-hypermetabolic sepsis (left panel) and left endotoxemia–septic shock (right panel). Increased hepatic glucose production results in hyperglycemia during early endotoxemia–hypermetabolic sepsis despite stimulated uptake of glucose in macrophage-rich tissues. During late/severe endotoxemia, hypoglycemia develops secondary to reduced hepatic glucose production and continued high glucose uptake by macrophage-rich tissues.

is increased glucose utilization in multiple tissues, including liver, spleen, small intestine, skin, and some (but not all) muscles. A common feature of several of these tissues is a high content of macrophages. Studies have shown that in the liver the high glucose uptake reflects increased utilization of glucose by Kupffer cells. In addition, endotoxemia is associated with a substantial inflow of neutrophils into the liver and these cells as well contribute to the increase in glucose uptake. Interestingly, the hepatocyte uptake of glucose does not change, suggesting a dichotomy in glucose kinetics between the hepatocyte and the Kupffer cell during sepsis and endotoxemia. Because the rate of glucose production exceeds the rate of glucose disposal during this phase of sepsis and endotoxemia, serum glucose levels are elevated. Another contributing factor to increased serum glucose is the insulin resistance in muscle and fat, resulting in a relative inhibition of glucose uptake by these tissues.

If sepsis is prolonged, hypoglycemia usually develops as hepatic glucose production fails. Hepatic glycogen is depleted during protracted sepsis and the liver has to rely on gluconeogenesis for glucose production. There is evidence that gluconeogenesis can also be inhibited during sepsis

secondary to decreased gluconeogenic substrates and altered enzyme function. Some studies suggest that decreased phosphoenolpyruvate carboxykinase activity is a mechanism of reduced hepatic gluconeogenesis whereas other reports have implied stimulated phosphofructokinase-1 activity.

Lang and Dobrescu (1991) found that, despite decreased glucose production, uptake remains high in macrophage-rich tissues, further exacerbating hypoglycemia. This in turn may contribute to mortality during septic shock. The changes in glucose metabolism during early and late sepsis-endotoxemia are summarized in Fig. 1-4.

Lipid Metabolism

Circulating levels of free fatty acids, triglycerides, and cholesterol are increased during injury and sepsis. The mechanism of these changes is multifactorial with stimulated synthesis in the liver of apolipoproteins and triglycerides being the major mechanism of hypertriglyceridemia. Contributing factors include reduced activity of the enzyme lipoprotein lipase in muscle and adipose tissue, decreasing the clearance of triglyceride-rich lipoproteins, and increased lipolysis in adipose tissue.

Although it is fairly well accepted that hepatic synthesis of triglycerides increases during sepsis, the influence of sepsis and endotoxemia on the secretion of triglycerides is more controversial, with studies showing both unchanged and reduced secretion.

Although plasma levels of free fatty acids and triglycerides are usually elevated during sepsis and endotoxemia, this is not always the case. One reason for this may be decreased perfusion of adipose tissue during severe sepsis or endotoxic shock, resulting in reduced lipolysis and decreased plasma levels of free fatty acids. Fatty acids are also used as an alternative energy source by peripheral tissues following injury and sepsis, and if the rate of fatty acid clearance (peripheral oxidation) is higher than the rate of appearance (lipolysis) or production (hepatic lipogenesis), plasma fatty acid concentrations do not increase.

Alterations in lipid metabolism as manifested by increased lipolysis and stimulated hepatic production of triglycerides and fatty acids are beneficial to the injured and septic organism for several reasons. By providing lipid substrates as an alternative energy source for peripheral tissues, including muscle and the immune system, glucose is spared for the nervous system. In addition, lipoproteins can bind endotoxin and a number of different viruses. Increased plasma lipoproteins may therefore help protect the organism from the toxic and lethal effects of endotoxin and infectious agents (Read et al, 1995).

Protein Metabolism

Among the metabolic alterations that occur following injury and infection, those that affect protein metabolism have probably been studied most extensively. This section of the chapter focuses on changes in protein metabolism in skeletal muscle, liver, and intestine, and argues for the concept that these changes are part of an integrated metabolic response to injury and sepsis.

Muscle

Interest in protein metabolism following trauma began more than 60 years ago, when studies by Sir David Cuthbertson (1932) demonstrated increased urinary excretion of nitrogen, phosphate, and sulfate in injured patients. A number of subsequent studies have provided evidence that skeletal muscle is the major source of increased urinary nitrogen secretion following injury and sepsis. Negative nitrogen balance and muscle catabolism are now well-recognized metabolic responses to these conditions. The catabolic condition in muscle that develops during critical illness is multifactorial and is caused by a combination of reduced protein synthesis, increased protein breakdown, and inhibited amino acid uptake (Fig. 1-5). From a quantitative standpoint, the increase in protein breakdown, in particular the breakdown of the myofibrillar proteins actin and myosin, is the most prominent component of muscle catabolism following injury and sepsis. Increased myofibrillar protein breakdown results in increased urinary excretion of 3-methylhistidine (3-MH) in injured and septic patients and increased release of 3-MH by incubated muscles from septic animals. The breakdown of myofibrillar proteins may in part explain the muscle weakness typically seen in patients with severe trauma and sepsis and may severely impair recovery in these patients. The net result of decreased protein synthesis and increased protein breakdown is the release of amino acids from muscle, in particular glutamine. Inhibited cellular uptake of amino acids contributes to the peripheral release of amino acids in injury and sepsis. Skel-

etal muscle can be viewed as an endogenous source of amino acids for the rest of the body during infection and injury, which is of particular importance for protein synthesis and function in liver, intestine, and cells of the immune system.

Glutamine is the most important amino acid released from skeletal muscle both from a quantitative and qualitative standpoint. Intestinal epithelial cells and cells in the immune system rely on glutamine for optimal function and energy production. Increased efflux of glutamine from muscle may in part explain the reduced intracellular glutamine levels reported in the muscle following trauma and infection. Reduced glutamine levels may be one of the mechanisms of increased muscle proteolysis and inhibited protein synthesis in these conditions although the role of glutamine in the regulation of muscle protein turnover in sepsis is controversial (Fang et al, 1995).

Recent studies have clarified some of the intracellular mechanisms of muscle proteolysis during sepsis and following injury (Tiao et al, 1994). Intracellular protein breakdown is regulated by lysosomal and nonlysosomal mechanisms (Table 1-1). Among the nonlysosomal pathways, the energy-ubiquitin-dependent protein degradation is particularly important in various catabolic conditions, including sepsis, burn injury, cancer, starvation, and metabolic acidosis. Before proteins are degraded by this mechanism, they are first conjugated to ubiquitin, which is a small, 76–amino acid protein. The ubiquitin-protein conjugate is recognized by the large proteolytic complex, the 26 S proteasome, which catalyzes the breakdown of the ubiquitin-conjugated protein (Hershko and Ciechanover, 1992). In recent studies we found evidence that ubiquitin mRNA levels are increased in skeletal muscle during sepsis (Tiao et al, 1994) and following burn injury (Fang et al, 1995), suggesting that muscle proteolysis in these conditions is, at least in part, regulated by increased transcription of the ubiquitin gene.

Liver
The bulk of amino acids released from muscle during sepsis and injury are taken up by the liver (Rosenblatt et al, 1983). These amino acids support hepatic gluconeogenesis and, perhaps more importantly, the synthesis of acute-phase proteins. Increased hepatic protein synthesis

Table 1-1. Different Intracellular Proteolytic Pathways in Skeletal Muscle

Pathway	Enzymes
LYSOSOMAL	Cathepsin
NONLYSOSOMAL	
Energy dependent	
Ubiquitin dependent	26 S protease
Ubiquitin independent	600-kDa protease
Energy independent	
Calcium dependent	Calpain I, II

has been reported following trauma and during sepsis in a number of previous studies, both in patients and in experimental animals. As mentioned earlier, maintenance of a sustained acute-phase response in the liver is critical to survival in sepsis and severe injury (Dominioni et al, 1987).

An acute-phase protein is usually defined as a plasma protein, the concentration of which is increased by 25 percent or more following stimulus. The acute-phase proteins are essential in the restoration of homeostasis following injury and sepsis; their biologic functions were reviewed previously by Kushner (1988). The plasma concentrations of other proteins produced in the liver, most notably albumin, are decreased in injury and sepsis. These proteins are referred to as "negative" acute-phase proteins and are consistent with reprioritization of liver protein synthesis in critical illness.

The genes for several acute-phase proteins have been cloned, making it possible to study the molecular regulation of the acute-phase response. In humans, CRP is a major acute-phase reactant. C-reactive protein mRNA is detectable in liver tissue of individuals during inflammation but not in liver samples of normal subjects, suggesting that the CRP gene is activated during inflammation. Increased acute-phase protein mRNA during trauma and infection can be caused by upregulated transcription of the corresponding gene or increased stability of the mRNA molecule. Interestingly, there is evidence that both mechanisms may be involved. For example, in experiments by Northemann and associates (1985) in rats, plasma levels of α_2-macroglobulin were elevated nearly 100-fold during the acute-phase response. This increase was preceded by an approximately 70-fold increase in hepatocyte

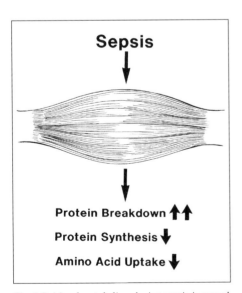

Fig. 1-5. Muscle catabolism during sepsis is caused by a combination of increased protein breakdown, reduced protein synthesis, and inhibited amino acid uptake. From a quantitative standpoint, the increase in protein breakdown is probably most important, in particular the breakdown of myofibrillar proteins.

mRNA concentration. Nuclear run-on experiments showed that the α_2-macroglobulin gene transcription rate was increased only to 4- to 5-fold, suggesting that in addition to stimulated transcription rate, α_2-macroglobulin mRNA stability was also enhanced, thus accounting for the 70-fold increase in mRNA levels.

The intracellular regulation of protein secretion is a complex, tightly regulated process. Acute-phase proteins are secretory proteins and the regulation of their secretion may be as important as the regulation of the synthesis itself. The intracellular mechanisms involved in the secretion of proteins were reviewed recently by Halban and Irminger (1994). After synthesis in the rough endoplasmic reticulum, secretory proteins are transported into the Golgi network. The Golgi network is comprised of three areas, the cis-Golgi network, the Golgi stacks, and the trans-Golgi network (Fig. 1-6). Proteins can be secreted either by a constitutive or a regulated pathway. Alternatively, proteins may be retained in the Golgi network or transported to lysosomes. In the trans-Golgi network, proteins are sorted as to which pathway they will follow. In the constitutive pathway, secretory rates are constant and the amount of protein released is limited only by the availability of the protein. In contrast, proteins secreted by the regulated pathways can be stored, and large amounts of protein can be released with the appropriate stimulus. The influence of injury and infection on the secretory processes is currently unknown, but regulation of these mechanisms may have a significant impact on the acute-phase response during injury and infection and is an important area for future research.

In recent work, such as that of Clemens and associates (1994), the importance of the microanatomy of the liver in the response to injury and infection has been recognized. The liver contains several different cell types (hepatocytes, Kupffer cells, endothelial cells, Ito cells, pit cells, and neutrophils) arranged in well-organized repeating units (Fig. 1-7). The morphologic arrangement of these cells plays a critical role in the response to trauma and infection, as these cells communicate with each other via mediators, modulating the metabolic response in the liver. In particular, the interaction between hepatocytes and Kupffer cells has been extensively studied as an important component of the inflammatory response in the liver.

At least during the initial phase of sepsis and inflammation, hepatocytes function in a heterogeneous fashion, in part reflecting gradients of oxygen, nutrients, and inflammatory mediators. For example, the periportal hepatocytes are recruited first for the acute-phase response following stimulus. Each individual hepatocyte that is involved is capable of exhibiting a full acute-phase response, that is, simultaneously increasing the synthesis of multiple acute-phase proteins and reducing the production of albumin. [*Editor's note:* "Downregulation" of albumin synthesis seems almost an article of faith nowadays. However, reduction in plasma level may reflect not only decreased synthesis but redistribution of albumin. Albumin synthesis probably returns to normal 2–3 days after the insult.]

Located within the sinusoids, Kupffer cells represent the largest class of fixed macrophages in the body. They release cytokines, prostaglandins, oxygen radicals, and NO when stimulated with endotoxin. The interaction between hepatocytes and Kupffer cells plays a key role in the regulation of the acute-phase response. These two cell types communicate in a paracrine fashion, with bidirectional signaling via different mediators.

Intestine

Despite the fact that the intestinal mucosa has one of the highest protein turnover rates in the body and is the production site of a number of biologically important proteins, it is only recently that the influence of injury and sepsis on protein metabolism in the intestine has been investigated. Studies suggest that hypermetabolic sepsis stimulates protein synthesis in the mucosa of the small intestine and colon (von Allmen et al, 1992; Higashiguchi et al, 1994). The mechanism(s) by which this occurs is not yet clear, but increased cellular turnover secondary to cell loss may be a partial explanation. Other studies suggest that the

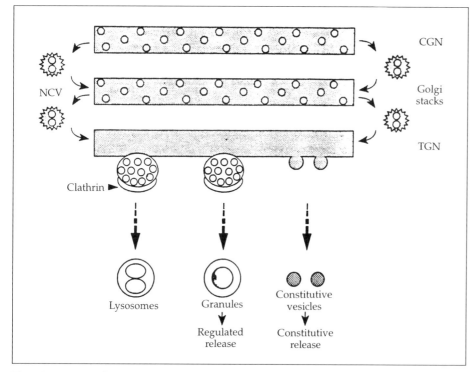

Fig. 1-6. Processing of secretory proteins in the Golgi complex. Proteins received from the rough endoplasmic reticulum are transferred from the cis-Golgi network (CGN) to the trans-Golgi network (TGN) via the Golgi stacks in non–clathrin-coated vesicles (NCV). In the TGN, lysosomal proteins and regulated secretory proteins are actively sorted to corresponding clathrin-coated vesicles. Delivery to the constitutive release takes place by default. (From PA Halban, JC Irminger. Sorting and processing of secretory proteins. Biochem J 299:1, 1994. Reproduced with permission.)

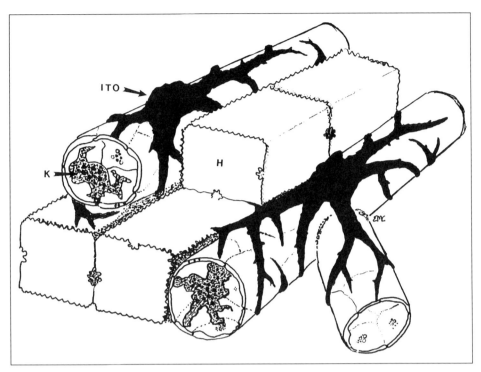

Fig. 1-7. Three-dimensional view of the microanatomy of the liver. The hepatocytes (H) are arranged in cords surrounded by sinusoids. The sinusoids are lined by a discontinuous endothelium, allowing for communication between the vascular and perisinusoidal (Disse's space) spaces. The Kupffer cells (K) are present in the sinusoidal lumen. The Ito cells are located in Disse's space, where they wrap around the sinusoid. Interaction and signaling between the different cell types, in particular between the Kupffer cells and hepatocytes, are important for the metabolic response to inflammation, shock, and sepsis. (From MG Clemens, M Bauer, C Gingalewski, et al. Hepatic intracellular communication in shock and inflammation. Shock 2:1, 1994. Reproduced with permission.)

Alterations in protein metabolism in various organs and tissues during trauma and infection can be looked on as an integrated response supporting the body's defense against invading bacteria and tissue injury. This concept of an integrated response is discussed in more detail elsewhere (Hasselgren 1993) and is summarized in Fig. 1-8. The fact that the same control mechanisms (discussed below) regulate different aspects of the alterations in protein metabolism in different tissues gives further credence to this concept. During protracted and more severe sepsis and other critical illness, multiple organ failure may occur and the metabolic regulation may "get out of control." For example, in the liver, acute-phase reactants may be synthesized at the expense, as it were, of structural hepatic proteins. Loss of the structural proteins may contribute to the hepatic failure of severe sepsis.

Regulation of Metabolism During Trauma and Infection

In this section, the role of hormones, cytokines, and NO in the regulation of metabolism following trauma and infection is described. Interaction between the different mediators in the metabolic control is also elucidated. Among the mediators, hormones and cytokines regulate changes in carbohydrate, lipid, and protein metabolism, whereas NO has been studied most extensively in the control of protein metabolism.

Carbohydrate Metabolism

The hormones involved in the regulation of carbohydrate metabolism during trauma and infection include the counterregulatory hormones and insulin. In this respect, catecholamines and glucagon are the major counterregulatory hormones in humans. Evidence in support of the role of the counterregulatory hormones was found in early experiments by Bessey and associates (1984) in which intravenous infusion of a combination of glucagon, epinephrine, and cortisol ("triple hormone infusion") resulted in alterations in whole-body carbohydrate metabolism similar to those seen in sepsis and other critical illness.

production of specific proteins may be increased. These proteins include the gut hormones vasoactive intestinal peptide and peptide YY, in part explaining why circulating levels of these and other gut peptides are increased during sepsis and endotoxemia. These observations suggest that the intestine may have an endocrine function during injury and infection and support the concept that the gut is an active participant in the metabolic response to critical illness rather than a passive bystander.

In addition to the enterocytes, the intestinal mucosa contains a number of other cell types, including lymphocytes, macrophages, and endothelial cells. Measurement of protein turnover rates in isolated jejunal enterocytes demonstrated that both sepsis (induced by cecal ligation and puncture in rats) and endotoxemia stimulate protein synthesis in enterocytes from all levels of the villi, although the increase in protein synthesis was most pronounced in

cells from the lower parts of the villi and the crypts (unpublished observations). Protein turnover in cell types other than the enterocyte during sepsis and injury has not yet been reported.

Recent work by Molina and Abumrad (1994) suggests that intestinal proteolysis, measured as splanchnic efflux of amino acids, increases during the ebb phase of injury. Increased intestinal proteolysis was also noted in a model of insulin-induced hypoglycemia and the mediator of this increased proteolysis appeared to be central nervous system glucopenia. Associated with the central nervous system glucopenia was an increase in the production of endogenous opioids and opiates, including morphine. It was speculated that the elevated levels of morphine mediate intestinal proteolysis following injury. Further studies will be needed to define in which cell type of the intestinal tract the stimulated protein breakdown takes place following injury.

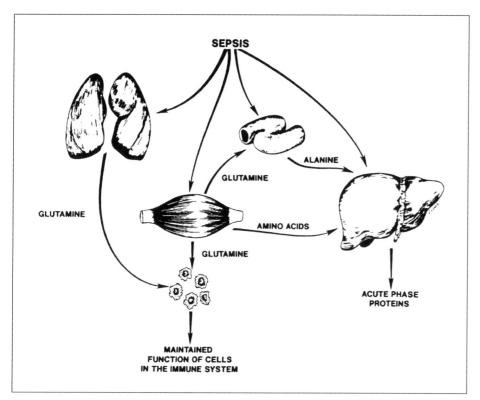

Fig. 1-8. Integrated concept of sepsis-induced changes in protein metabolism. The catabolic response in muscle and lungs results in release of glutamine and other amino acids, which are used by cells in the immune system, intestinal mucosa, and liver. (From PO Hasselgren. Protein Metabolism in Sepsis. *Austin, TX: RG Landes, 1993. (Reproduced with permission.)*

Catecholamine regulation of carbohydrate metabolism is well recognized. Epinephrine influences carbohydrate metabolism by increasing hepatic glycogenolysis, followed by stimulated gluconeogenesis and by inhibiting the metabolic clearance rate of glucose, further increasing serum glucose levels. In addition, epinephrine modulates other glucose-regulating hormones, stimulating release of glucagon while inhibiting release of insulin. In burned patients, treatment with phentolamine and propranolol reduced whole-body metabolic rate, further illustrating the role of catecholamines in the regulation of metabolism following injury.

Glucagon plays a more important role in the control of carbohydrate metabolism during sepsis, at least in the regulation of hepatic glucose production. The important role of hyperglucagonemia seen during sepsis was demonstrated in experiments by Lang and associates (1989) in which the hormone was blocked by infusion of somatostatin in septic rats and the elevated rate of glucose production was reduced to control values. In contrast, treatment with

somatostatin did not decrease sepsis-induced increase in glucose disposal, suggesting that the two aspects of carbohydrate metabolism (hepatic glucose production and glucose clearance) are controlled by different mechanisms during sepsis. Glucagon probably does not act alone during sepsis but instead acts synergistically with other mediators, such as glucocorticoids and catecholamines.

Insulin also plays a key role in the regulation of carbohydrate metabolism in injury and sepsis. Insulin levels vary depending on the phase of injury. During the ebb phase, insulin levels are reduced despite hyperglycemia (Frayn, 1986; Gann et al, 1987). The combined effects of catecholamines, somatostatin, glucocorticoids, and reduced pancreatic blood flow may reduce pancreatic beta-cell sensitivity to glucose. During the flow phase, beta-cells regain their sensitivity and insulin concentrations rise. Despite increased insulin concentrations, however, hyperglycemia may persist, consistent with insulin resistance. Clinically, the presence of insulin resistance is evident from reduced hormone

response when exogenous insulin is administered to septic or injured patients. As previously mentioned, this insulin resistance is secondary to a postreceptor alteration resulting in decreased cellular responsiveness to insulin, possibly mediated by TNF and catecholamines.

The most extensively studied cytokine in terms of regulation of carbohydrate metabolism is TNF. van der Poll and Sauerwein (1993) reported that changes in glucose metabolism during endotoxemia and sepsis are mirrored by the in vivo administration of TNF with increased hepatic production of glucose, hyperglycemia, and stimulated glucose utilization by macrophage-rich tissues and diaphragm. The effect of TNF on glucose kinetics is dose dependent, with relatively modest doses causing hyperglycemia and larger doses inducing hypoglycemia. The hypoglycemia seen after high doses of TNF can at least in part be explained by increased peripheral glucose utilization, although impaired hepatic gluconeogenesis may contribute.

The data from in vivo studies do not define whether TNF has a direct or indirect effect on hepatic glucose metabolism. It is important to recognize that administration of TNF induces a stress response and it is possible that the effects of TNF are secondary to release of counterregulatory hormones. Indeed, infusion of phentolamine and propranolol prevented the increase in glucose appearance noted in rats treated with TNF, suggesting that the TNF-induced increase in hepatic glucose production is at least in part mediated by catecholamines (Bagby et al, 1992). In a recent study by Bagby and associates (1993), pretreatment of septic or endotoxemic rats with anti-TNF antibodies did not modify the changes in whole-body carbohydrate metabolism assessed from measurements of plasma glucose and lactate levels and rates of glucose appearance and clearance. The results were interpreted as indicating that endogenous production of TNF is not a requirement for the increase in hepatic glucose production and whole-body glucose disposal seen in endotoxemia and hypermetabolic sepsis. An integrated picture of the role of TNF and its interaction with counterregulatory hormones in hepatic gluconeogenesis was provided recently by van der Poll and Sauerwein (1993) (Fig. 1-9).

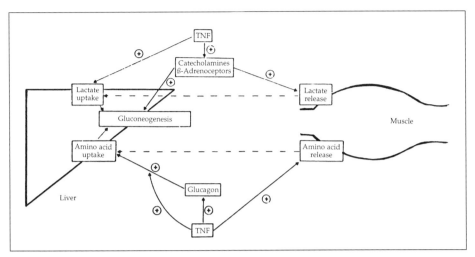

Fig. 1-9. Interaction between TNF, catecholamines, and glucagon in the regulation of hepatic gluconeogenesis. The supply of the gluconeogenic precursors alanine and lactate is increased by the stimulation of their release from muscle by TNF (possibly mediated by glucocorticoids). Tumor necrosis factor increases hepatic uptake of amino acids and lactate by increasing glucagon levels and potentiating the effect of glucagon on the liver. (From T van der Poll, HP Sauerwein. Tumour necrosis factor-α: its role in the metabolic response to sepsis. Clin Sci *84:247, 1993. Reproduced with permission.)*

In contrast to the liver, TNF may have a direct effect on cellular glucose kinetics in muscle and adipose tissue. In recent experiments, Cornelius and associates (1990) demonstrated how this regulation occurs. In their studies, exposure of cultured murine 3T3-L1 preadipocytes to TNF resulted in a dose- and time-dependent increase in glucose transport, measured as uptake of 2-deoxyglucose. The molecular regulation of the TNF-induced glucose transport was multifaceted; TNF caused an initial translocation of the glucose transporter to the cell surface, followed by an increased transcription rate of the glucose transporter gene, stabilization of glucose transporter mRNA, and increased production of the glucose transporter protein.

In addition to TNF, IL-1 can also influence carbohydrate metabolism. Del Rey and Besedovsky (1992) found that plasma glucose levels decreased significantly following administration of IL-1 in rats and this effect of IL-1 was even more pronounced than that of TNF. Results in the same study suggest that IL-1 may mediate its effects through the central nervous system. When equal doses of IL-1 were injected intracerebroventricularly versus intraperitoneally, only the intracerebroventricularly injected group demonstrated hypoglycemia. Decreased hepatic glucose production and increased peripheral glucose transport and utilization may be the mechanisms by which IL-1 induces hypoglycemia.

Lipid Metabolism

Hormones regulate lipid metabolism both in adipose and other tissues. The role of hormonal control of lipid metabolism in injury and infection, however, is probably less prominent than that of other mediators, such as cytokines. An exception to this may be the catecholamines. For example, the sepsis-induced increase in palmitate appearance can be inhibited by combined alpha- and beta-adrenergic blockade. This is consistent with other reports that catecholamines stimulate lipolysis in adipose tissue.

There is evidence that cytokines may participate in the regulation of lipid metabolism following injury and infection. Tumor necrosis factor has received most attention in this respect, in part because of work done in the characterization of the cause of cancer cachexia. A factor, cachectin, was identified from the serum of patients with cancer and shown to be an inducer of both the cachexia and hyperlipidemia that accompany some tumors. Subsequent studies have shown that cachectin and TNF are the same substance.

TNF infusion in vivo causes several changes in lipid metabolism that are similar to those that occur during sepsis and injury. One mechanism by which TNF may alter lipid metabolism is reduction of lipoprotein lipase activity, thus decreasing degradation of lipoproteins. This regulation probably occurs at the molecular level by downregulated lipoprotein lipase gene expression in adipose tissue. Downregulation of lipoprotein lipase activity, however, may not be the only mechanism by which TNF induces hypertriglyceridemia because in some studies, serum levels of triglycerides were increased before a decreased lipoprotein lipase activity could be detected in adipose tissue following administration of TNF.

The liver is probably the major site at which TNF influences lipid metabolism. There is evidence that TNF stimulates both synthesis and secretion of triglycerides in the liver. Fatty acids are the rate-limiting substrates in triglyceride synthesis. Tumor necrosis factor treatment does not change activities of the enzymes involved in the esterification of fatty acids to glycerol, suggesting that the stimulated triglyceride production in the liver is due primarily to availability of fatty acids. In addition to stimulated liver synthesis of fatty acids, increased lipolysis in adipose tissue can also increase fatty acid availability. There is evidence that TNF stimulates both these processes. Interestingly, the effect of TNF on fatty acid synthesis is site specific. Thus, whereas TNF increases fatty acid synthesis in the liver, it does not influence this process in muscle, fat tissue, or small intestine. The mechanism for this differential effect is not clear but may reflect differences between tissues in the activity of enzymes responsible for fatty acid synthesis.

Other factors may contribute to the ability of TNF to alter lipid metabolism. For example, there is evidence that the catecholamines and TNF act synergistically to increase lipolysis. Nutritional status may also be important in TNF-induced hypertriglyceridemia. Feingold and associates (1990) found that in chow-fed rats, lipolysis in adipose tissue was stimulated following TNF administration, increasing the availability of fatty acids. In contrast, in sucrose-fed rats, TNF markedly stimulated hepatic de novo synthesis of fatty acids. Both conditions resulted in increased triglyceride production by the liver. The observation that TNF can stimulate hepatic triglyceride synthesis and increase plasma triglyceride levels through multiple mechanisms supports the concept that changes in lipid metabolism play an important role in the overall response to infection and inflammation.

Although TNF has been most extensively studied in the regulation of lipid metabolism, there is evidence that other cytokines as well may influence lipid metabolism, including IL-1, IFN-α, IFN-β, and IFN-γ. Interestingly, the mechanism by which different cytokines alter fatty acid synthesis varies. Grunfeld and associates (1990) found that citrate levels increase following TNF, IL-1, and IL-6 treatment of adipocytes in culture. Citrate is an activator of acetyl–coenzyme A (CoA) carboxylase, the rate-limiting enzyme in fatty acid synthesis. Interferon α treatment does not increase citrate levels, suggesting an alternative mechanism. These different mechanisms may explain the results of simultaneous cytokine treatment. Thus, IFN-α and either TNF or IL-1 resulted in an additive effect on fatty acid synthesis. In contrast, maximal doses of TNF and IL-1 given together (presumably working through the same mechanism) did not further increase fatty acid synthesis.

Not all cytokines stimulate fatty acid synthesis. Recent studies, by Grunfeld and associates (1991), suggest that IL-4 inhibits TNF-, IL-1–, or IL-6–induced hepatic fatty acid synthesis. Interleukin-4 alone had no effect and did not influence the IFNα-stimulated hepatic fatty acid synthesis. These results are further support of the concept that different cytokines induce hepatic lipogenesis through distinct mechanisms.

Protein Metabolism

Both hormones, cytokines and NO, regulate protein metabolism following injury and during sepsis. The hormonal regulation may reflect a balance between catabolic hormones, such as glucocorticoids and anabolic hormones, such as insulin and IGF-I. During trauma and infection, both types of hormones probably play a role in protein regulation. The role of the various mediators in protein metabolism following injury and infection has been most extensively studied in skeletal muscle and liver, although there is emerging evidence that the same substances regulate protein metabolism in other organs and tissues as well.

Muscle

Among the "counterregulatory" hormones, glucocorticoids probably play the most important role in the regulation of

muscle protein and amino acid metabolism during trauma and infection. Treatment with glucocorticoids results in increased muscle protein breakdown, especially myofibrillar protein breakdown, similar to the effects of sepsis and injury. In a previous study by Hall-Angerås and associates (1991), the glucocorticoid receptor antagonist RU 38486 reduced the sepsis-induced increase in total and myofibrillar proteolysis, supporting the role of glucocorticoids in mediating muscle proteolysis. In more recent studies in our laboratory (unpublished) we found evidence that the glucocorticoids may regulate muscle proteolysis during sepsis at the molecular level. Thus, treatment of rats with RU 38486 abolished the sepsis-induced increase in muscle ubiquitin mRNA levels (Fig. 1-10). When normal rats were treated with dexamethasone, a dose-dependent increase in ubiquitin mRNA levels was noticed, suggesting that glucocorticoids stimulate muscle proteolysis by upregulating the expression of the ubiquitin gene.

In addition to regulating muscle protein breakdown, glucocorticoids may also influence the metabolism of amino acids, in particular, glutamine. Skeletal muscle glu-

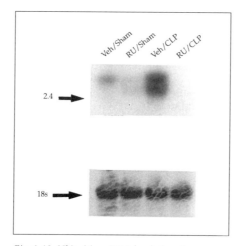

Fig. 1-10. Ubiquitin mRNA levels in extensor digitorum muscles from sham-operated and septic (induced by cecal ligation and puncture, CLP) rats determined by Northern blot. Groups of rats were treated with 10 mg/kg of the glucocorticoid receptor antagonist RU 38486 or solvent by gavage 2 hours before sham operation or CLP. The sepsis-induced increase in ubiquitin mRNA was almost abolished by RU 38486, suggesting that increased transcription of the ubiquitin gene in skeletal muscle during sepsis is regulated by glucocorticoids.

tamine concentrations decrease following dexamethasone treatment, similar to the effect of sepsis and severe injury. Although somewhat controversial (Fang et al, 1995), there is evidence that reduced intracellular glutamine levels may be a mechanism of stimulated muscle proteolysis. Reduced glutamine levels may be due to a combination of decreased uptake (as evidenced by inhibited activity of the muscle glutamine transporter) and increased release of glutamine from skeletal muscle. Both phenomena increase the release of glutamine from muscle into the central circulation. Thus, glucocorticoids may stimulate muscle proteolysis both by a direct effect on the proteolytic process, perhaps at the molecular level by stimulating transcription of the ubiquitin gene, and by reducing muscle glutamine levels.

The catabolic state in skeletal muscle induced by injury and infection may also reflect a decreased influence of anabolic hormones. Growth hormone promotes protein synthesis but does not block protein degradation in skeletal muscle. In a variety of catabolic conditions, such as surgical injury, burn, critical illness, in patients receiving parenteral nutrition, and in healthy volunteers treated with glucocorticoids, improved nitrogen balance has been documented following the administration of GH (Jiang et al, 1989; Harber and Haymond, 1990).

Insulin-like growth factor-I probably mediates most of the anabolic effects of GH. The majority of IGF-I is produced in the liver in response to GH but IGF-I is produced in other tissues as well, including skeletal muscle. Recently, Ross and associates (1991) showed that IGF-I levels are reduced in critically ill patients, suggesting a possible mechanism of muscle catabolism in trauma and infection. Interestingly, in the same study, GH levels were high, indicating that the biosynthesis of IGF-I in the liver becomes resistant to GH during catabolic conditions. In other studies, administration of IGF-I prevented weight loss after burn injury, inhibited protein breakdown during starvation, and blocked protein loss induced by TNF (Strock et al, 1990; Douglas et al, 1991). IGF-I probably has a direct effect on skeletal muscle since abundant IGF-I receptors are found in muscle tissue and IGF-I increases protein synthesis and decreases protein breakdown in incubated rat muscles and cultured myoblasts.

Insulin has been recognized as a regulator of muscle protein turnover for many years. Protein synthesis is stimulated by insulin mainly at the translational level by enhanced peptide chain initiation, although increased capacity for protein synthesis, secondary to increased amounts of ribosomes, may also play a role. The inhibitory effect of insulin on muscle protein breakdown reflects inhibition of lysosomal proteolysis as well as reduced formation of autophagosomes. These mechanisms may be impaired during infection and injury, resulting in insulin resistance.

Although the phenomenon of insulin resistance has been most extensively studied with respect to glucose metabolism, there is evidence that other metabolic events also become resistant to insulin in injury and sepsis. We found evidence of insulin resistance in muscle from septic rats with respect to the regulation of protein degradation (Hasselgren et al, 1987). Dose response curves for insulin concentration in incubation medium and the inhibition of protein degradation in incubated muscles suggested that the insulin resistance of protein breakdown in septic muscle reflected a reduced responsiveness; that is, it was caused by a postreceptor defect. We further supported this with the finding that the stimulatory effects of the hormone on protein synthesis and amino acid uptake were not impaired in septic muscle.

In addition to hormones, cytokines play an important role in the regulation of muscle protein metabolism in trauma and sepsis. A role for cytokines, in particular IL-1, in mediating muscle proteolysis during sepsis and injury was first proposed by Clowes and associates (1983) and by Baracos and colleagues (1983) in the early 1980s. Since then, the evidence for a role of cytokines in the regulation of protein and amino acid metabolism has continued to expand.

There are mainly three lines of evidence to support the role of cytokines in the regulation of muscle protein turnover in injury and sepsis. First, increased cytokine levels have been reported in a number of studies, including those of Pinsky and associates and of Drost and colleagues, following injury and sepsis. Second, sepsis-like metabolic changes can be induced by the administration of cytokines (Zamir, Hasselgren, Kunkel, et al, 1992; Zamir, Hasselgren, Higashiguchi, et al, 1992). Fi-nally, sepsis-induced muscle catabolism can be blocked by cytokine antibodies or receptor antagonists (Zamir, Hasselgren, Kunkel, et al, 1992; Zamir, Hasselgren, O'Brien, et al, 1992).

In experiments in our laboratory (Zamir, Hasselgren, Kunkel, et al, 1992; Zamir, Hasselgren, Higashiguchi, et al, 1992), treatment of rats with rTNFα resulted in increased muscle protein breakdown, in particular myofibrillar protein breakdown, a response identical to that seen during sepsis. Pretreatment of septic rats with anti-TNF antibodies blunted the sepsis-induced increase in muscle protein breakdown, providing further evidence that TNF participates in the regulation of muscle proteolysis in sepsis (Zamir, Hasselgren, Kunkel, et al, 1992). When endotoxemic or septic rats were treated with a recombinant form of IL-1ra, muscle proteolysis was inhibited (Zamir, Hasselgren, O'Brien, et al, 1992), suggesting that IL-1 as well may regulate muscle protein breakdown during sepsis.

In contrast to protein degradation, the sepsis-induced decrease in muscle protein synthesis does not appear to be regulated by cytokines. Infusion of TNF or IL-1 in normal rats does not influence muscle protein synthesis rates. Pretreatment with anti-TNF antibodies did not influence the reduced muscle protein synthesis noted in septic rats (Zamir, Hasselgren, Kunkel, et al, 1992). These data suggest that muscle protein synthesis and breakdown are subject to different control mechanisms during sepsis.

It is important to recognize that cytokines are released in a cascade-like fashion. Although there is evidence in support of TNF and IL-1 in mediating protein breakdown during sepsis and endotoxemia, it should be noted that TNF induces release of IL-1. It is possible, therefore, that the effects caused by injection of TNF in normal rats or by administration of anti-TNF antibodies in septic rats reflected a regulatory role of IL-1. It is also possible that both TNF and IL-1 exert their effects through another downstream mediator or mediators, for example, cytokines such as IL-6, or hormones induced by the cytokines.

Indeed, treatment of rats with RU 38486 prevented the TNF-induced increase in muscle proteolysis, suggesting that the catabolic response to TNF is mediated by glucocorticoids (Zamir, Hasselgren, Higa-shiguchi, et al, 1992). In addition, there is evidence that glucocorticoids potentiate the effect of TNF in a synergistic fashion at the cellular level, further illustrating the important interaction between hormones and cytokines in the metabolic response to sepsis and injury. In contrast, IL-1 probably mediates its effect on muscle proteolysis independently of glucocorticoids since RU 38486 did not block muscle protein breakdown induced by IL-1 (Zamir, Hasselgren, Higashiguchi, et al, 1992). The interaction between TNF, IL-1, and glucocorticoids in the regulation of muscle proteolysis is summarized in Fig. 1-11.

Although IL-1 stimulates muscle proteolysis independently of glucocorticoids, it is not likely that IL-1 (or any other known proinflammatory cytokine) exerts its catabolic effect via a direct effect on muscle. A number of studies have failed to demonstrate increased protein breakdown in isolated muscles incubated in the presence of various cytokines, individually or in combinations and at high concentrations.

Impaired response to anabolic hormones may be an alternative mechanism by which cytokines exert their catabolic effect on protein metabolism. As described previously, IGF-I inhibits muscle protein breakdown and stimulates protein synthesis. Lazarus and colleagues (1993) found that cytokines, especially TNF, inhibited the anabolic effects of IGF-I in rat chondrocytes. Further studies will be important to define the interaction between IGF-I and cytokines in the regulation of muscle proteolysis.

Liver

A large body of evidence suggests that hormones, cytokines, and NO regulate protein metabolism in the liver, and frequently, these mediators interact to induce an hepatic acute-phase response. Although the interaction between the different mediators is probably essential for acute-phase protein synthesis during sepsis, some of the mediators can induce at least a partial acute-phase response. Both catecholamines, glucagon and glucocorticoids, regulate acute-phase protein synthesis and amino acid transport in the liver.

Glucocorticoids mainly act as an important, and probably essential, cofactor in the acute-phase response, since by themselves they do not stimulate acute-phase protein

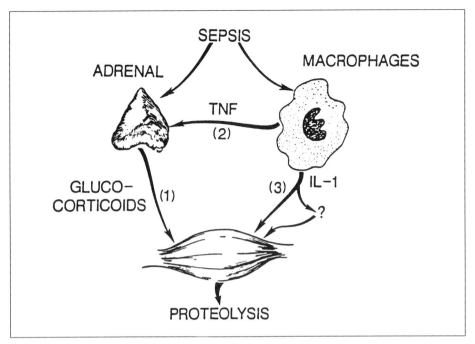

Fig. 1-11. Interaction between (1) glucocorticoids, (2) TNF, and (3) IL-1 in the regulation of sepsis-induced muscle proteolysis. The effect of TNF on muscle proteolysis is primarily mediated by glucocorticoids, whereas IL-1 regulates muscle proteolysis by glucocorticoid-independent pathway(s). (From O Zamir et al. Tumor necrosis factor [TNF] and interleukin-1 [IL-1] induce muscle proteolysis through different mechanisms. *Mediat Inflam 1:247, 1992. Reproduced with permission.)*

synthesis. Many of the acute-phase proteins have glucocorticoid response elements in their gene promoters, strongly suggesting a role for glucocorticoids in gene regulation. Glucocorticoids may also regulate amino acid transport. In vitro experiments in isolated rat hepatocytes suggest that system A amino acid transport is stimulated by dexamethasone and that this hormonal effect is caused by synthesis of new transporter proteins, perhaps regulated at the transcriptional level. In addition to system A amino acid transport, there is evidence that system N is also stimulated by steroids.

Growth hormone does not appear to have a direct effect on acute-phase protein synthesis but affects amino acid transport by systems A and N in liver. The effect of GH is biphasic with an acute (within hours) increase in hepatic amino acid transport and a delayed (following treatment for days) inhibition of amino acid transport.

Even more important than hormones are cytokines, in particular, IL-6, for regulation of the acute-phase response in the liver. The role in the acute-phase response of IL-6, previously also called hepatocyte-stimulating factor (HSF) or interferon β_2,

was reviewed more extensively elsewhere by Heinrich and associates (1990).

Acute-phase proteins can be induced by IL-6 infusion in vivo. Hepatic mRNA levels for the acute-phase proteins, α_2-macroglobulin, beta fibrinogen, cysteine protease inhibitor, and α_1-acid glycoprotein are increased and albumin mRNA is decreased following administration of IL-6, indicating that an almost complete acute-phase response can be induced by this cytokine. This appears to be a direct effect of the cytokine because IL-6, added in vitro to cultured human hepatocytes, stimulates acute-phase protein synthesis. This direct effect is probably receptor mediated, as hepatocytes possess IL-6 receptors on their cell surface. Clinical studies have further documented the important role of IL-6 in the acute-phase response. High circulating levels of IL-6 were observed in patients with severe sepsis, and Damas and associates (1992) found a correlation between cytokine levels and CRP concentrations.

Kupffer cells are the most important source of IL-6 during sepsis and inflammation, although other cell types, including the hepatocyte itself, have been found

to secrete IL-6. Recent studies in our laboratory, by Meyer and associates (1994, 1995), suggest that the enterocyte is another potential source of IL-6. This may be of biological significance since IL-6 produced in the intestine reaches the liver directly through the portal vein and there is abundant evidence of the importance of gut flow on hepatic function, particularly biosynthetic activity.

In addition to IL-6, other cytokines may contribute to the acute-phase response. In studies using recombinant forms of IL-1α, a partial acute-phase response was generated, supporting a role of this cytokine in the control of acute-phase protein synthesis. Serum amyloid A mRNA levels increased in liver following treatment of mice with rIL-1α. When rIL-1α was administered to rats over a 3-day course, the synthesis of total secreted proteins, complement component C3, and α_1-acid glycoprotein was increased in perfused liver whereas the synthesis of albumin was unchanged and not reduced as expected. These results suggest that IL-1 regulates part of, but not the complete, acute-phase response.

Tumor necrosis factor may also regulate acute-phase protein synthesis. In unpublished experiments in our laboratory, pretreatment of endotoxemic rats with anti-TNF antibodies almost completely abolished the increase of hepatic protein synthesis. This result is consistent with TNF being a "proximal" mediator in the cytokine cascade. Rat hepatoma cells treated with TNF increase synthesis of α_1-acid glycoprotein and reduce production of albumin. These changes may be regulated at the transcriptional level since mRNA levels for α_1-acid glycoprotein and albumin were increased and reduced, respectively. Because TNF has no effect on fibrinogen mRNA hepatoma cells, the acute-phase response induced by TNF is probably only partial.

Based on studies like those already described and analysis of acute-phase protein gene promoters, two major classes of acute-phase protein genes have been identified. Those induced by IL-1, combinations of IL-1 and IL-6, and combinations of these two cytokines with glucocorticoids are grouped in class 1; this class includes the rat haptoglobin, C3, α_1-acid glycoprotein, and the human C-reactive protein.

Genes induced primarily by IL-6, its related factors such as leukemia inhibitory factor, and combinations of these cytokines and glucocorticoids are grouped as class 2; this class includes fibrinogen, α_1-antitrypsin, α_1-antichymotrypsin, and α_2-macroglobulin.

In addition to IL-6, IL-1, and TNF, other cytokines as well may be involved in the regulation of acute-phase protein synthesis. Those cytokines include IFNγ, transforming growth factor-β, leukemia inhibiting factor, IL-11, and oncostatin M. The large number of substances that modulate the acute-phase response illustrates the complexity of this system.

As discussed earlier in this chapter, an interaction between cytokines and glucocorticoids is important for the induction of a complete acute-phase response. Cytokines from endotoxin-stimulated human monocytes increase the production of α_2-macroglobulin and fibrinogen and inhibit albumin synthesis in isolated rat hepatocytes only when dexamethasone is present in the medium. Baumann and associates (1987) found that dexamethasone alone does not affect the production of acute-phase proteins in human hepatoma cells, but potentiates the effect of IL-1 or IL-6 severalfold. The molecular basis for this interaction lies within the promoter regions of the various acute-phase genes. Cytokine and glucocorticoid response elements have been found in many of the promoters, suggesting that an interaction between the transcription factors activated by these mediators is necessary to maximally stimulate transcription of the acute-phase protein genes. This interaction is supported by in vivo work where administration of IL-6 or IL-1 to rats stimulated the acute-phase protein expression in liver, but glucocorticoids were necessary to achieve maximal response.

The fact that some acute-phase proteins are induced by single mediators while others require combinations of mediators further illustrates the complexity involved in the metabolic control of the acute-phase response. For example, while fibrinogen mRNA levels increased severalfold in a rat hepatoma cell line after the addition of IL-6, other cytokines (IL-1 and TNF) had no effect on fibrinogen gene transcription, but instead led to a substantial increase in α_1-acid glycoprotein mRNA. All three

cytokines reduced albumin mRNA concentrations. In the same experiments, dexamethasone potentiated the induction of fibrinogen mRNA and was required for the increase in α_1-acid glycoprotein mRNA.

In addition to hormones and cytokines, several recent studies suggest that NO plays an important role in the regulation of hepatic protein synthesis. The role of NO in the regulation of hepatic protein synthesis, however, is complicated by the fact that the substance does not only have a direct effect on hepatocyte protein synthesis but may also have indirect effects, secondary to hemodynamic changes. This probably explains why the influence of NO on hepatic protein synthesis in vitro is apparently different from the influence of NO in vivo.

Curran and associates (1991) found evidence that NO decreases protein synthesis in vitro in cultured hepatocytes. Initially it was thought that Kupffer cells were the only source of NO production. However, subsequent experiments have provided evidence that the hepatocyte as well can produce NO under certain circumstances. Supernatant from Kupffer cells, stimulated by endotoxin and IFNγ, induces release of NO from cultured hepatocytes and, at the same time, inhibits protein synthesis. These results suggest that hepatocyte protein synthesis may be regulated by NO in an autocrine fashion in addition to the paracrine effect of NO released from Kupffer cells. Also, following in vivo stimulation, evidence has been found that both Kupffer cells and hepatocytes can produce NO.

In contrast to the in vitro effect of NO, the substance may have a protective effect on hepatic protein synthesis in vivo. For example, we found evidence that NO may participate in the upregulation of hepatic protein synthesis during sepsis and endotoxemia (Frederick et al). In those experiments, circulating levels of NO_2/NO_3 and hepatic protein synthesis rates were increased following injection of endotoxin in rats. When NO production was blocked with NNA, plasma levels of NO_2/NO_3 in endotoxemic rats were almost normalized and hepatic protein synthesis decreased rather than increased as would have been expected if NO inhibits protein synthesis. The mechanism of the stimulatory effect of NO on hepatic protein synthesis in vivo is

not known but may reflect improved liver blood flow at the microcirculatory level, secondary to the vasodilatory effect of the substance, or to prevention of platelet aggregation and adhesion. Other studies as well suggest that NO has a protective effect on the liver in vivo by reducing sepsis-induced hepatocyte damage.

Other Tissues

Although less well established than for muscle and liver, there is evidence that hormones and cytokines may regulate amino acid and protein metabolism following injury and sepsis in other organs and tissues as well. Regulation by hormones in the intestine of the transport and metabolism of amino acids, in particular glutamine, has received a significant amount of attention. Glucocorticoids have been most extensively studied in this respect. The in vivo role of glucocorticoids remains unclear, however, as administration of dexamethasone has caused both increased, decreased, and unchanged intestinal glutamine uptake. The direct effects of glucocorticoids in vitro on enterocyte amino acid transport have also been contradictory. Thus, dexamethasone inhibited glutamine transport when added to cultured Caco-2 cells (a human intestinal epithelial cell line), but did not influence glutamine transport when added to perfused small intestine. In other studies, the Na^+-dependent transport of alanine in the small intestine was stimulated by dexamethasone, whereas the Na^+-independent alanine uptake and lysine transport (probably by systems L and y^+) were unaffected. These results suggest that glucocorticoids may regulate the activity of different intestinal amino acid transporters individually.

In addition to regulating amino acid transport, glucocorticoids may regulate enzymes involved in the metabolism of amino acids in the gut. Intestinal glutaminase and glutamine synthetase both appear to be regulated by glucocorticoids and there is evidence that regulation may occur at the level of transcription. For example, Sarantos and associates (1994) found that glutaminase activity and mRNA levels increase following treatment with dexamethasone and the endotoxin-induced increase in mucosal glutamine synthetase activity is inhibited by the glucocorticoid receptor antagonist RU 38486.

In the same study, Caco-2 cells treated with dexamethasone increased both glutamine synthetase mRNA levels and the activity of the enzyme.

The role of glucocorticoids in the stimulated mucosal protein synthesis observed during sepsis and endotoxemia is not fully known but may not be important. Thus, in experiments in our laboratory (unpublished), treatment of rats with RU 38486 did not influence the sepsis-induced increase in mucosal protein synthesis and treatment of normal rats with dexamethasone did not influence protein synthesis in small intestine.

In contrast, there is stronger evidence that cytokines may participate in the regulation of intestinal protein synthesis. van Allmen and associates (1992) found that administration of IL-1 or TNF to rats resulted in increased protein synthesis in the mucosa of the small intestine, similar to the response seen during sepsis and endotoxemia. In other studies, IL-1 (but not TNF) induced a sepsis-like increase in the biosynthesis of intestinal polyamines. The increased intracellular polyamine levels may be a mechanism of stimulated mucosal protein synthesis during sepsis. In vitro treatment of cultured rat intestinal epithelial cells with IL-1 stimulated the expression and activity of ornithine decarboxylase, the rate-limiting enzyme in the polyamine biosynthesis, further supporting a role of cytokines (at least IL-1) in sepsis-induced metabolic changes in the intestinal mucosa.

Intestinal amino acid transport and metabolism may also be regulated by IL-1. There is evidence that IL-1 inhibits intestinal glutaminase activity and glutamine uptake. This effect of the cytokine is probably caused by reduced extraction of glutamine since intestinal blood flow is not affected by IL-1. In contrast, TNF does not influence intestinal glutamine uptake or glutaminase activity, suggesting that amino acid metabolism in the intestinal mucosa may be selectively regulated by IL-1.

Increased pulmonary efflux of amino acids, in particular glutamine and alanine, suggests that the lungs respond to injury and infection with protein catabolism. This response has been observed both in patients with sepsis and in experimental animals with sepsis and endotoxemia. A contributing factor to the increased efflux of glutamine from the lungs may be enhanced de novo synthesis of the amino acid as suggested by stimulated glutamine synthetase activity in lung tissue during sepsis and endotoxemia.

There is evidence that glucocorticoids may regulate the catabolic response in the lungs. Dexamethasone treatment of rats results in increased pulmonary release of glutamine and alanine. This treatment also stimulates glutamine synthetase activity by 20 to 30 percent in the lungs. In subsequent experiments by Sarantos and associates (1993), it was found that the increase in enzyme activity is preceded by increased levels of glutamine synthetase mRNA, suggesting that dexamethasone stimulates enzyme gene transcription.

The role of cytokines in the regulation of amino acid and protein metabolism in the lungs during sepsis and injury is not known. There is evidence, however, that cytokines may influence amino acid transport and metabolism in different cell types present in the lungs.

Therapeutic Implications

As the understanding of the metabolic response to injury and infection has evolved, new strategies have been developed in an effort to modulate this response. Most of these strategies have focused on attenuating protein catabolism following severe injury and sepsis. Although muscle catabolism provides the liver, intestine, and cells in the immune system with amino acids for protein synthesis and other functions (see Fig. 1-8), a sustained catabolic response in muscle may be deleterious to the organism. In general, three types of treatments have been tested in recent years to reduce the catabolic response to injury and infection: 1) nutritional, 2) hormonal, and 3) biologic. In this section, we discuss some of these novel therapeutic strategies, in particular with respect to metabolic changes (Table 1-2).

Nutritional Intervention

Over the past 25 years, the field of nutrition has evolved from nutritional supplementation to nutritional pharmacology. This is especially apparent with regard to

Table 1-2. Therapeutic Strategies Based on the Metabolic Response to Injury and Infection

NUTRITIONAL TREATMENT
Enteral vs parenteral
Supplements
    Glutamine
    Branched chain amino acids
    Arginine
    Omega-3 polyunsaturated fatty acids
    RNA

HORMONAL TREATMENT
GH
IGF-I
Insulin

BIOLOGIC TREATMENT
Antibodies to endotoxin and TNF
IL-1ra
NO inhibitors
"Gene therapy"

the metabolic response to injury and infection, for which specialized nutritional formulations have been developed and tested in an effort to improve survival.

When nutritional intervention is being considered, three important questions need to be addressed: 1) route of administration (enteral vs parenteral), 2) timing (early vs late feeding), and 3) composition of the feeding. Since the pioneering work by Alexander and colleagues (1980) 15 years ago, it has been recognized that enteral nutrition can limit the hypermetabolism of injury and infection. In other studies, using animal models, evidence has been found that enteral nutrition may improve protein balance, especially in the liver and the intestine. Improvement of intestinal mucosal function following enteral feeding may reflect synthesis of specific proteins, such as immunoglobulin A (IgA), which in turn may decrease bacterial translocation following injury and sepsis. Fong and associates (1989) found that enteral nutrition may also decrease the release of counterregulatory hormones and cytokines, especially TNF. Although studies in humans are not as clear, protein balance is usually improved in patients receiving enteral as compared to parenteral nutrition.

It should be noted that the major advantage of enteral versus parenteral nutrition has not been manifested in metabolic effects but in improved clinical outcome with increased survival rates and reduced infectious complications following severe injury, as shown by Moore and associates (1992). It is also important to remember that conflicting results have been reported, with some studies finding no advantage of enteral versus parenteral feeding, perhaps reflecting different patient populations and different nutritional regimens in different studies.

When enteral nutrition is administered in injured patients, it should be started early after trauma. There is experimental evidence that early enteral feeding (started within hours after injury) is superior to delayed enteral feeding (started several days after trauma) in its effect on the catabolic and hypermetabolic response to injury. More recently, specific components have been added to nutritional formulations in an effort to improve outcome. Glutamine, because of its use as an energy source by the immune system and intestinal mucosa, has been tested in a variety of situations both for enteral and parenteral nutrition. In a recent clinical trial by Ziegler and associates (1992), glutamine-supplemented TPN reduced infectious complications, improved nitrogen balance and shortened hospital stay in patients undergoing bone marrow transplantation. Alexander (1993) has provided evidence that oral glutamine supplementation improves bacterial killing and decreases translocation.

Interest in the use of the branched chain amino acids (BCAA) leucine, valine, and isoleucine as a therapeutic supplement dates back to early studies in which leucine inhibited protein breakdown in skeletal muscle. Whereas BCAA-enriched diets were efficacious in some studies, other reports found only marginal effects of BCAA-enriched solutions in septic patients. One reason why BCAA-enriched nutritional formulas have not always been successful in blocking muscle catabolism in critically ill patients may be that muscle becomes resistant to the effect of leucine during sepsis (Hasselgren et al, 1988).

Kirk and Barbul (1990) reported arginine stimulates GH and IGF-I release and is the rate-limiting substrate for NO production. Arginine supplementation of nutritional formulas may therefore be beneficial. Arginine at high doses promotes wound healing and immune function.

Another group of substances that have been used recently to supplement nutritional support are omega-3 polyunsaturated fatty acids. Some of the mechanisms by which they exert their effects include decreased cytokine and prostaglandin production, which may explain why they reduce the hypermetabolism seen following injury and sepsis. In more recent years, supplementation of nutritional formulas with RNA has been tested. The presumed beneficial effects of dietary nucleotides may reflect improved cell-mediated immunity.

A combination of arginine, omega-3 polyunsaturated fatty acids, and nucleotides has been used in "immune enhancing" diets and tested in clinical trials by Daly and colleagues (1992), and by Bower and associates (1993). Reduced infectious complications and shortened hospital stay were reported following enteral administration of the immune enhancing diets. The influence of these diets on metabolic changes induced by injury and sepsis are not known.

Hormonal Treatment

Administration of the anabolic hormones, GH, IGF-I, and insulin promotes positive nitrogen balance. All three hormones have been tested as an adjunct to nutritional support in injured and septic patients.

Supplementation of nutritional support with GH increased whole-body protein synthesis rates and nitrogen balance and decreased muscle amino acid efflux and urea generation in a variety of clinical conditions (Jiang et al, 1989; Harber and Haymond, 1990). In addition to the metabolic effects, Herndon and associates (1990) found evidence that GH supplementation improves wound healing and decreases postoperative wound infection rates and length of hospital stay in patients with burn injury. The benefits of GH administration must be weighed against its physiologic "side effects." Hyperglycemia, insulin resistance, and fluid retention are normal metabolic responses to GH and make it necessary to monitor administration of GH carefully.

There is evidence that IGF-I mediates most of the anabolic effects of GH. Because IGF-I levels are decreased in critically ill patients, it has been proposed that treatment with IGF-I may be of benefit. Recent studies, such as those by Strock and associates (1990) and by Douglas and colleagues (1991), suggest that IGF-I reverses the catabolic effects of hypocaloric diets in normal healthy adults and improves nitrogen balance following burn injury or treatment with TNF. More studies are needed to define the therapeutic role of IGF-I in patients with sepsis.

Insulin, as the major anabolic hormone of the body, has also been tested as a supplement to nutritional support. Both Hinton and associates (1971) and Brooks and colleagues found that insulin infusion in burn and trauma patients improved nitrogen balance during high-dose dextrose parenteral nutrition; however, because of the risk of hypoglycemia, the clinical usefulness of insulin during critical illness is limited.

Biologic Treatment

Biologic treatment of patients with sepsis and other critical illnesses can be directed either at altering circulating levels of endotoxin, or at reducing the levels and effects of mediators released in response to endotoxin. Strategies have included treatment with antibodies to endotoxin, TNF, or IL-6 and treatment with IL-1ra. Although most studies have focused on complications and survival rates, some information is available regarding the effect on metabolic events. For example, as discussed previously, Zamir et al (1992) found that treatment of experimental animals with anti-TNF antibodies or IL-1ra blocks sepsis-induced muscle proteolysis.

One of the problems with this type of treatment is that most patients with sepsis already have elevated levels of cytokines and other mediators when they are initially seen. In fact, in most previous experimental studies in which biologic treatment was successful, animals were pretreated with antibodies or receptor antagonists before the induction of sepsis or endotoxemia. It is possible that patients who are at particularly high risk of developing gram-negative sepsis, for example, those undergoing major surgical procedures, may benefit most from anticytokine treatment since it can be given as "prophylaxis" in these patients.

With the fast-developing field of molecular biology, it has been recognized that there are genetic alterations during injury and infection, as exemplified on several occasions in this chapter. Although speculative at this point, it is possible that "gene therapy" will eventually be applied to critical illness.

Suggested Reading

Alexander JW. Immunoenhancement via enteral nutrition. *Arch Surg* 128:1242, 1993.

Alexander JW, MacMillan BG, Stinnett JD, et al. Beneficial effects of aggressive protein feeding in severely burned children. *Ann Surg* 192:505, 1980.

Bagby GJ, Lang CH, Skrepnik N, et al. Attenuation of glucose metabolic changes resulting from TNF-α administration by adrenergic blockage. *Am J Physiol* 262:R628, 1992.

Bagby GJ, Lang CH, Skrepnik N, et al. Regulation of glucose metabolism after endotoxin and during infection is largely independent of endogenous tumor necrosis factor. *Circ Shock* 39:211, 1993.

Baracos V, Rodemann HP, Dinarello CA, et al. Stimulation of protein degradation and prostaglandin E_2 release by leukocyte pyrogen (interleukin-1). *N Engl J Med* 308:553, 1983.

Baumann H, Richards C, Gauldie J. Interaction among hepatocyte-stimulating factors, interleukin-1, and glucocorticoids for regulation of acute phase plasma proteins in human hepatoma (Hep G2) cells. *J Immunol* 139:4122, 1987.

Bessey PQ, Watters JM, Aoki TT, et al. Combined hormonal infusion stimulates the metabolic response to injury. *Ann Surg* 200:264, 1984.

Bower RH, Lavin PT, Licari JJ, et al. A modified enteral formula reduces hospital length of stay in intensive care units (abstract). *Crit Care Med* 21:S275, 1993.

Brooks DC, Bessey PO, Black PR, et al. Insulin stimulates branched chain amino acid uptake and diminishes nitrogen flux from skeletal muscle of injured patients. *J Surg Res* 40:395, 1986.

Clark JH, Schrader WT, O'Malley BW. Mechanisms of action of steroid hormones. In JD Wilson, DW Foster (eds), *Williams Textbook for Endocrinology*. Philadelphia: Saunders, 1992.

Clemens MG, Bauer M, Gingalewski C, et al. Hepatic intracellular communication in shock and inflammation. *Shock* 2:1, 1994.

Clowes GHA, George BC, Villee CA, et al. Muscle proteolysis induced by a circulating peptide in patients with sepsis or trauma. *N Engl J Med* 308:545, 1983.

Cornelius P, Marolow M, Lee MD, et al. The growth factor–like effects of tumor necrosis factor-α. Stimulation of glucose transport activity and induction of glucose transporter and im-

mediate early gene expression in 3T3-L1 preadipocytes. *J Biol Chem* 265:20506, 1990.

Curran RD, Ferrari FC, Kispert PH, et al. Nitric oxide and nitric oxide generating compounds inhibit hepatocyte protein synthesis. *FASEB J* 5:2085, 1991.

Cuthbertson DP. Observations on the disturbance of metabolism produced by injury to the limbs. *Q J Med* 1:233, 1932.

Daly JM, Lieberman MD, Goldfine J, et al. Enteral nutrition with supplemental arginine, RNA and omega-3 fatty acids in patients after operation: Immunologic, metabolic and clinical outcome. *Surgery* 112:56, 1992.

Damas P, Ledoux D, Nys M, et al. Cytokine serum levels during severe sepsis in human: IL-6 as a marker of severity. *Ann Surg* 215:356, 1992.

Darnell JE, Kerr IM, Stark G. Jak-STAT pathways and transcriptional activation in response to IFNs and other extracellular signaling proteins. *Science* 264:1415, 1994.

Del Ray A, Besedovsky HO. Metabolic and neuroendocrine effects of pro-inflammatory cytokines. *Eur J Clin Invest* 22(Suppl 1):10, 1992.

Dominioni L, Dionigi H, Zanello M, et al. Sepsis score and acute phase protein response as predictors of outcome in septic surgical patients. *Arch Surg* 122:141, 1987.

Douglas RG, Gluckman PD, Breier BH, et al. Effects of recombinant IGF-1 on protein and glucose metabolism in rTNF-infused lambs. *Am J Physiol* 261:E606, 1992.

Drost AC, Burleson DG, Cioffi WG, et al. Plasma cytokines after thermal injury and their relationship to infection. *Ann Surg* 218:74, 1993.

Egan SE, Weinberg RA. The pathway to signal achievement. *Nature* 365:781, 1993.

Fang CH, James CH, Fischer FE, et al. Is muscle protein turnover regulated by intracellular glutamine during sepsis? *J Parent Ent Nutr* 19:279, 1995.

Fang Ch, Tiao G, James H, et al. Burn injury stimulates multiple proteolytic pathways in skeletal muscle, including the ubiquitin-energy-dependent pathway. *J Am Coll Surg* 180:161, 1994.

Feingold KR, Adi S, Staprans I, et al. Diet affects the mechanisms by which TNF stimulates hepatic triglyceride production. *Am J Physiol* 259:E177, 1990.

Fisher CJ, Dhainaut JFA, Opal SM, et al. Recombinant human interleukin-1 receptor antagonist in the treatment of patients with sepsis syndrome. Results from a randomized, double-blind, placebo-controlled trial. *JAMA* 271:1836, 1994.

Fong Y, Marano MA, Barber, et al. Total parenteral nutrition and bowel rest modify the met-

abolic response to endotoxin in humans. *Ann Surg* 210:449, 1989.

Frayn KN. Hormonal control of metabolism in trauma and sepsis. *Clin Endocrinol* 24:577, 1986.

Frederick JA, Hasselgren PO, Davis S, et al. Nitric oxide may upregulate *in vivo* hepatic protein synthesis during endotoxemia. *Arch Surg* 128:152, 1993.

Gann DS, Amaral JF, Caldwell MD. Neuroendocrine response to stress, injury, and sepsis. In JH Davis (ed). *Clinical Surgery*. St. Louis: Mosby, 1987.

Gatti S, Bartkin T. Induction of tumor necrosis factor-α mRNA in the brain after peripheral endotoxin treatment: comparison with interleukin-1 family and interleukin-6. *Brain* 624:291, 1993.

Geller DA, Lowenstein CJ, Shapiro RA, et al. Molecular cloning and expression of inducible nitric oxide synthase from human hepatocytes. *Proc Natl Acad Sci USA* 90:3491, 1993.

Gray PW, Barrett K, Chantry D, et al. Cloning of human tumor necrosis factor (TNF) receptor cDNA and expression of recombinant soluble TNF-binding protein. *Proc Natl Acad Sci USA* 87:7380, 1990.

Grunfeld C, Soued M, Adi S, et al. Evidence for two classes of cytokines that stimulate hepatic lipogenesis: Relationships among tumor necrosis factor, interleukin-1 and interferon-α. *Endocrinology* 127:46, 1990.

Grunfeld C, Soued M, Adi S, et al. Interleukin-4 inhibits stimulation of hepatic lipogenesis by tumor necrosis factor, interleukin-1 and interleukin-6 but not by interferon-α_1. *Cancer Res* 51:2803, 1991.

Halban PA, Irminger JC. Sorting and processing of secretory proteins. *Biochem J* 299:1, 1994.

Hall-Angerås M, Angerås U, Zamir O, et al. Effect of the glucocorticoid receptor antagonist RU 38486 on muscle protein breakdown in sepsis. *Surgery* 109:468, 1991.

Harber FF, Haymond MW. Human growth hormone prevents the protein catabolic side-effects of prednisolone in humans. *J Clin Invest* 86:265, 1990.

Hasselgren PO. *Protein Metabolism in Sepsis*. Austin, TX: RG Landes, 1993.

Hasselgren PO, Fischer JE. Regulation by insulin of muscle protein metabolism during sepsis and other catabolic conditions. *Nutrition* 8:434, 1992.

Hasselgren PO, Chen IW, James JH, et al. Studies on the possible role of thyroid hormone in altered muscle protein turnover during sepsis. *Ann Surg* 206:18, 1987.

Hasselgren PO, James JH, Warner BW, et al. Protein synthesis and degradation in skeletal muscle from septic rats. Response to leucine and α-ketoisoaproic acid. *Arch Surg* 123:640, 1988.

Hasselgren PO, Warner BW, James JH, et al. Effect of insulin on amino acid uptake and protein turnover in skeletal muscle from septic rats. Evidence from insulin resistance of protein breakdown. *Arch Surg* 122:228, 1987.

Heinrich PC, Castell JV, Andus T. Interleukin-6 and the acute phase response. *Biochem J* 265:621, 1990.

Herndon DN, Barrow RE, Kunkel KR, et al. Effects of recombinant human growth hormone on donor-site healing in severely burnt children. *Ann Surg* 212:424, 1990.

Hershko A, Ciechanover A. The ubiquitin system for protein degradation. *Annu Rev Biochem* 61:761, 1992.

Higashiguchi T, Noguchi Y, O'Brien W, et al. Effect of sepsis on mucosal protein synthesis in different parts of the gastrointestinal tract in rats. *Clin Sci* 87:207, 1994.

Hinton P, Allison SP, Littlejohn S, et al. Insulin and glucose to reduce catabolic response to injury in burned patients. *Lancet* 1:767, 1971.

Jiang ZM, He GZ, Zhang SY, et al. Low-dose growth hormone and hypocaloric nutrition attenuate the protein-catabolic response after major operation. *Ann Surg* 210:513, 1989.

Keogh C, Fong Y, Marano MA, et al. Identification of a novel tumor necrosis factor α-cachectin from the livers of burned and infected rats. *Arch Surg* 125:79, 1990.

Kirk SJ, Barbul A. Role of arginine in trauma, sepsis and immunity. *JPEN* 14:226S, 1990.

Kushner I. The acute phase response: An overview. *Methods Enzymol* 163:373, 1988.

Lang CH, Dobrescu C. Sepsis-induced increases in glucose uptake by macrophage-rich tissues persist during hypoglycemia. *Metabolism* 40:585, 1991.

Lang CH, Dobreson C, Bagby GJ. Tumor necrosis factor impairs insulin action on peripheral glucose disposal and hepatic glucose disposal and hepatic glucose output. *Endocrinology* 130:43, 1992.

Lang CH, Bagby GJ, Blakesley HL, et al. Importance of hyperglucagonemia in eliciting the sepsis-induced increase in glucose production. *Circ Shock* 29:181, 1989.

Lazarus DD, Moldawer LL, Lowry SF. Insulin-like growth factor-1 activity is inhibited by interleukin-1α, tumor necrosis factor-α and interleukin-6. *Lymphokine Cytokine Res* 12:219, 1993.

Mester M, Tompkins RG, Gelfand JA, et al. Intestinal production of interleukin-1α during endotoxemia in the mouse. *J Surg Res* 54:584, 1993.

Meyer TA, Noguchi Y, Ogle C, et al. Endotoxin stimulates IL-6 production in intestinal epithelial cells: A synergistic effect with PGE_2. *Arch Surg* 129:1290, 1994.

Meyer TA, Tiao G, James JH, et al. Nitric oxide inhibits LPS-induced IL-6 production in enterocytes. *J Surg Res* 58:570, 1995.

Molina PE, Abumrad N. Gut-derived proteolysis during insulin-induced hypoglycemia: The pain that breaks down the gut. *JPEN* 18:549, 1994.

Moncada S. The L-arginine:nitric oxide pathway. *Acta Physiol Scand* 145:201, 1992.

Moore FA, Feliciano DV, Andrassy RJ, et al. Early enteral feeding compared with parenteral reduces post-operative septic complications. The result of meta-analysis. *Ann Surg* 216:172, 1992.

Nava E, Palmer RM, Moncada S. Inhibition of nitric oxide synthesis in septic shock: how much is beneficial? *Lancet* 338:1555, 1991.

Northemann W, Heisig M, Kunz D, et al. Molecular cloning of cDNA sequences for rat $α_2$-macroglobulin and measurement of its transcription during experimental inflammation. *J Biol Chem* 260:6200, 1985.

Pinsky MR, Vincent JL, Deviere J, et al. Serum cytokine levels in human septic shock: Relation to multiple system organ failure and mortality. *Chest* 103:565, 1993.

Ray A, LaForage KS, Sehgal PB. On the mechanism for efficient repression of the interleukin-6 promoter by glucocorticoids: Enhancer, TATA box, and RNA start site (infr motif) inclusion. *Mol Cell Biol* 10:5736, 1990.

Read TE, Grunfeld C, Kumwenda Z, et al. Triglyceride-rich lipoproteins improve survival when given after endotoxin in rats. *Surgery* 117:62, 1995.

Rosenblatt S, Clowes GHA, George BC, et al. Exchange of amino acids by muscle and liver in sepsis. *Arch Surg* 118:167, 1983.

Ross R, Miell J, Freeman E, et al. Critically ill patients have high basal growth hormone levels with attenuated oscillatory activity associated with low levels of insulin like growth factor-I. *Clin Endocrinol* 35:47, 1991.

Sarantos P, Howard D, Souba WW. Dexamethasone regulates glutamine synthetase expression in rat lung. *Metabolism* 42:795, 1993.

Sarantos P, Abouhamze A, Chakrabarti R, et al. Glucocorticoids regulate intestinal glutamine synthetase gene expression in endotoxemia. *Arch Surg* 129:59, 1994.

Stadler J, Harbrecht BG, DiSilvio M, et al. Endogenous nitric oxide inhibits the synthesis of cyclooxygenase products and interleukin-6 by rat Kupffer cells. *J Leuk Biol* 53:165, 1993.

Strock LL, Sing H, Abdulla A, et al. The effect of insulin-like growth factor I on post-burn hypermetabolism. *Surgery* 108:161, 1990.

Tiao G, Fagan JM, Samuels N, et al. Sepsis stimulates nonlysosomal, energy-dependent proteolysis and increases ubiquitin mRNA levels in rat skeletal muscle. *J Clin Invest* 94:2255, 1994.

Tiao G, Rafferty J, Ogle CK, et al. Detrimental effect of nitric oxide synthase inhibition during endotoxemia may be caused by high levels of TNF and IL-6. *Surgery* 116:332, 1994.

van der Poll T, Sauerwein HP. Tumour necrosis factor-α: its role in the metabolic response to sepsis. *Clin Sci* 84:247, 1993.

Voerman HJ, Groeneveld ABJ, de Boer H, et al. Time course and variability of the endocrine and metabolic response to severe sepsis. *Surgery* 114:951, 1993.

von Allmen D, Hasselgren PO, Higashiguchi T, et al. Increased intestinal protein synthesis during sepsis and following the administration of tumor necrosis factor-α or interleukin-1α. *Biochem J* 286:585, 1992.

Zamir O, Hasselgren PO, Higashiguchi T, et al. Tumor necrosis factor (TNF) and interleukin-1 (IL-1) induce muscle proteolysis through different mechanisms. *Mediat Inflam* 1:247, 1992.

Zamir O, Hasselgren PO, Kunkel SL, et al. Evidence that tumor necrosis factor participates in the regulation of muscle proteolysis during sepsis. *Arch Surg* 127:170, 1992.

Zamir O, Hasselgren PO, O'Brien W, et al. Muscle protein breakdown during endotoxemia in rats and after treatment with interleukin-1 receptor antagonist (IL-1ra). *Ann Surg* 216:381, 1992.

Ziegler TR, Gatzen CG, Wilmore DW. Strategies for attenuating protein-catabolic responses in critically ill. *Ann Rev Med* 45:459, 1994.

Ziegler TR, Young LS, Benfell K, et al. Clinical and metabolic efficacy of glutamine-supplemented parenteral nutrition after bone marrow transplantation: A randomized, double-blind, controlled study. *Ann Intern Med* 116:821, 1992.

2

Preparation of the Patient

John M. Daly   Philip S. Barie   Stanley J. Dudrick

Comprehensive preparation of a patient for a surgical procedure involves both physiologic and psychological support and initiates the development of trust, which is essential to an optimal physician-patient relationship. Appropriate preoperative preparation requires gaining a thorough knowledge of the natural history of the patient's disease, evaluating his or her surgical risk, making decisions relevant to the need and timing of surgical intervention, estimating the potential for physiologic stress imposed by the operation, and quantitatively assessing the patient's physiologic status.

Psychological preparation should proceed concomitantly with physiologic preoperative support. Although problematic to a large degree when preparations are made urgently, the need to provide information regarding the benefits, risks, alternatives, and expected outcome of the proposed surgery cannot be dismissed. Apart from being a legal obligation on the part of the surgeon, the process of informed consent provides an opportunity to address concerns, allay anxiety, and gain the patient's trust. Once accomplished, proper informed consent improves the patient's perception, as well as decreasing the possibility of an adversarial process between patient and surgeon. Informed consent should only be provided by a member of the operating team with sufficient expertise and knowledge of the planned operation to be able to provide accurate information. The responsibility, ultimately, lies with the operating surgeon. Patient recall of specific details is highly variable, and is influenced by age, the interval between the discussion and the operation, cognitive impairment, and the patients' perceptions

regarding the degree to which they control their own health. Providing more, rather than less, detail does not appear to increase patient anxiety. Written summaries of the elements of informed consent are well received by patients and do increase recall. These can be prepared by the surgeon for any of a number of commonly performed operations, and given to patients beforehand.

The aim of all treatment during the preoperative period is to prepare the patient to withstand the stresses or surgery and to minimize the risks of the surgical procedure. The appropriate duration of preoperative preparation depends on the relative urgency of the procedure, whereas the urgency of any surgical procedure depends on the surgical risk and the natural history of the disease without surgical intervention. Factors such as the chronologic and physiologic age of the patient, the degree of physiologic derangements and nutritional deficits, the presence of organ system failure or insufficiency, the presence of obesity, and the stage of the primary disease must be considered in the decision of when, how, and why to perform an operative procedure. Although the urgency of surgical intervention may limit both the length of preoperative preparation and the methods available to the physician for correcting preexisting abnormalities, partial repair of deficiencies should be initiated promptly with the understanding that more complete correction will be undertaken during and after the operation. Months of chronic undernutrition cannot be corrected in a matter of hours, but anemia, dehydration, and electrolyte abnormalities can be ameliorated with early initiation of intensive intrave-

nous support and appropriate laboratory monitoring.

Cost-Effective Patient Preparation in an Era of Economic Constraints

The elaborate preparatory maneuvers to be described in the following sections, however necessary for the best possible outcome for the patient, may not be possible in a leisurely manner for emergencies, or even in an inpatient setting in anticipation of elective surgery. For emergencies, resuscitation must be compressed into hours or even minutes of preoperative preparation, with resuscitation ongoing throughout surgery and into the postoperative period. The decision to proceed with surgery at an intermediate point in the resuscitation is based on a risk-benefit analysis of the individual scenario. In contrast, elective operations can often be preceded by a focused laboratory evaluation. If so, it is dependent on the surgeon to take the history and perform the physical examination with particular care, so as to avoid overlooking comorbidity of potential importance. Asking a new patient to come to the office with ample time allotted for completion of a detailed health questionnaire, with a focused review of affirmative responses during the consultation itself, can be a cost-effective method of screening.

Minor operations (e.g., breast biopsy, inguinal herniorrhaphy) performed under local anesthesia in healthy ambulatory patients require a minimum of laboratory testing. Our own practice is to screen such patients with only a hematocrit determination and a urinalysis. Similar patients, if over the age of 40 years and scheduled to undergo intravenous sedation as part of their surgery, are also screened by resting electrocardiography. Even a general anesthetic for relatively small procedures in young, healthy patients requires no additional preparation. In particular, the yield of chest x-ray in patients without a suggestive history or current symptoms is very low for findings of importance. The screening of coagulation-related tests (e.g., prothrombin time, partial thromboplastin time, platelet count) has a similarly low yield. There may be no correlation between the number and function of circulating platelets, but even in patients in whom iatrogenic platelet dysfunction is present (i.e., ingestion of aspirin or nonsteroidal anti-inflammatory drugs) the template bleeding time usually yields no useful information.

In many patients with mild or well-controlled illness that will not preclude safe surgery, additional screening is important. Hypertensive or diabetic patients require a biochemical profile. Cigarette smokers or asthmatic patients should have a chest x-ray, but formal pulmonary function testing may not be necessary for the asymptomatic or minimally symptomatic patient who is not undergoing a major operation. For cigarette smokers, cessation of smoking for even a few days before general anesthesia is highly desirable, but will yield no meaningful improvement in pulmonary function (other than perhaps for local tracheobronchial mucociliary host defenses) unless it is stopped several weeks beforehand. The patient with asthma or chronic obstructive pulmonary disease (COPD) may benefit from a short course of inhaled bronchodilators if suggested by pulmonary function testing. The patient with COPD and an exacerbation of acute bronchitis can be treated with a short preoperative course of oral antibiotics.

Mild hypertension (diastolic blood pressure ≤115 mm Hg) poses little additional risk, and surgery may proceed safely. It is now standard practice to maintain patients on their antihypertensive medications through the perioperative period, with the possible exception of diuretics (if the patient is volume depleted or hypokalemic, diuretics may need to be held). It is especially important to maintain patients on beta-blocker drugs, as abrupt withdrawal can precipitate a rebound increase in myocardial work and oxygen consumption.

Drugs that interfere with platelet function are ubiquitous in the outpatient setting. Many patients take aspirin daily for its benefit for the coronary circulation. Nonsteroidal anti-inflammatory agents, available over the counter, are self-prescribed for headache, arthritis, sports injuries, dysmenorrhea, and other common problems. A single dose of any one of those drugs irreversibly impairs platelet function. Given the normal 7- to 10-day half-life of a circulating platelet, it is recommended that such drugs be held for at least 3 full days before an elective operation. A longer period may be advisable for patients with low-normal platelet counts.

The management of insulin therapy requires careful attention, especially now that regimens to achieve close control of plasma glucose by frequent insulin injections are standard practice. Even patients undergoing ambulatory surgery take nothing by mouth for several hours surrounding their procedures. If such a patient takes a single injection of insulin in the morning, hypoglycemia may result. Our practice is to recommend that the patient administer one-half of the total daily insulin dose as regular (short-acting) insulin at the usual time of his or her morning injection. Unless the surgery is very minor (i.e., excision of a small skin lesion), an infusion of 5% dextrose in water is advisable during the procedure. An intravenous catheter should also be inserted in the preparation or "holding" area if unforeseen delays are encountered with the operating room schedule. Most patients undergoing ambulatory surgery are able to resume their diabetic management regimen the next day. Inpatients will require tailored coverage, depending upon the type and magnitude of their procedure and the status of their nutritional support requirement.

Cardiac Risk Assessment and Preparation

Three million Americans with coronary artery disease (CAD) undergo anesthesia and surgery each year. As many as 50,000 of those patients sustain a perioperative myocardial infarction (MI), which may be increasing in incidence because of an aging population and patients at increasingly high risk. Overall mortality remains nearly 40 percent despite improvements in preoperative assessment and perioperative critical care. The cardiac risk of noncardiac surgery is caused by exacerbation of occult or symptomatically stable CAD due to the stress of the perioperative period.

Aortic and peripheral vascular surgery, orthopedic surgery, and major intrathoracic and intraperitoneal procedures are more frequently associated with perioperative cardiac mortality than are other types of surgery. The association with peripheral vascular surgery relates in part to the known, high incidence of CAD in those patients, whereas major orthopedic, general, aortic, and thoracic surgical procedures may impose additional stresses from blood loss, fluid shifts, vasoactive drug therapy, or prolonged circulatory support. The incidence of nonlethal MI is reported to be between 4 and 6 percent in most series of elective aortic aneurysm repair. However, the incidence has been reported to be 17 percent or more when evidence of MI was specifically sought by serial electrocardiograms (ECGs) and creatine kinase isoenzyme determinations.

Critical to the task of risk-benefit analysis is identification of the patient at risk for a perioperative cardiac complication. In the setting of proposed vascular surgery, one can make a reasonable presumption of the presence of CAD. Only 8 percent of patients who undergo general vascular surgery have normal coronary arteries. Severe but surgically correctable CAD is present in about 30 percent of patients with an aortic aneurysm, 25 percent of patients with cerebrovascular disease, and 20 percent of patients with peripheral occlusive disease, respectively. In the absence of a history of heart disease, men are at increased risk above 35 years of age, whereas female patients are at increased risk above age 40. Cardiac mortality risk increases markedly in patients over age 70. Cigarette smoking also confers increased risk. The perioperative history and physical examination must also ascertain the presence of valvular heart disease (particularly aortic stenosis in the asymptomatic patient), congestive heart failure, or arrhythmias.

A history of congestive heart failure (CHF) is strongly predictive of perioperative pulmonary edema, as are signs of decompensation in the preoperative period. Retrospective data indicate that 35 percent of patients with a preoperative S_3 gallop will develop perioperative pulmonary edema, and that 6 percent of patients with a history of CHF but no perioperative signs will do so. A prospective study of 254 predominantly hypertensive, diabetic patients undergoing elective general surgery operations revealed a 17 percent incidence of perioperative CHF among patients with cardiac disease (previous MI, valvular disease, or CHF). Patients with diabetes and heart disease were at especially high risk. In contrast, CHF developed in fewer than 1 percent of patients without prior cardiac disease.

Cardiac arrhythmias also pose a substantial risk of perioperative cardiac complications. Perioperative arrhythmias are common even in the absence of heart disease, although the incidence may be decreasing with the use of newer anesthetic agents. The high incidence of minor arrhythmias reflects the alterations in metabolism, autonomic tone, and pharmacologic manipulations characteristic of the perioperative period. In one series, patients with prior heart disease had a 32 percent incidence of perioperative arrhythmias, but only 14 patients (3%) had serious rhythm disturbances. Retrospective data show that 33 percent of patients with a preoperative arrhythmia will have a perioperative cardiac complication, as compared to a 9 percent incidence of complications in patents in normal sinus rhythm.

Supraventricular tachyarrhythmias (SVT) are generally of little consequence, and are unusual in patients free of arrhythmia preoperatively. Goldman found a 4 percent incidence of SVT in 916 patients over age 40; only 2 of the 35 patients required electrical cardioversion and 14 (40%) converted back to sinus rhythm without intervention. Patients with five or more ventricular premature depolarizations (VPDs) are at increased risk for perioperative cardiac morbidity, but their importance appears to be as a marker for myocardial dysfunction rather than as an inherent danger. Patients with complex ventricular arrhythmias without structural heart disease do not appear to be at increased risk. The patient with VPDs and myocardial dysfunction is at increased risk, but the risk is a reflection of the underlying state of the myocardium.

Severe aortic stenosis (AS) must be detected preoperatively, if possible. The risk of perioperative mortality from severe AS has been estimated to be 13 percent. The increased mortality results from limited capacity to increase cardiac output in response to stress, vasodilation, or hypovolemia. Patients with AS tolerate poorly the development of hypovolemia, tachycardia, or new-onset atrial fibrillation. Moreover, left ventricular hypertrophy decreases ventricular compliance and leads to decreased diastolic filling. Elective aortic valve replacement before noncardiac surgery may be indicated in severe AS (generally defined as a pressure gradient of 50 mm Hg or greater by Doppler echocardiography or cardiac catheterization) if the patient has any symptoms of syncope, angina, or CHF. Patients with less critical AS require invasive hemodynamic monitoring in the perioperative period, and caution with the use of afterload-reducing agents.

Aortic and mitral insufficiency subject the left ventricle to high volume loads that may impair contractility, but such patients are not as sensitive to hemodynamic insults as are patients with AS. These patients also require close monitoring as occult ventricular dysfunction may be present in the asymptomatic patient, but patients can be expected to tolerate surgery well if they are not in CHF at the time of the preoperative evaluation. Patients with mitral stenosis (MS) or hypertrophic cardiomyopathy are at increased risk of perioperative pulmonary edema. Pulmonary edema usually develops in MS because of tachycardia and decreased left atrial emptying. Perioperative fluid shifts of little consequence to the healthy patient may wreak havoc with MS, where careful fluid balance must be maintained. Hypovolemia and a resultant low flow state may occur despite relatively high pulmonary vascular pressures, but overzealous volume or blood replacement may cause pulmonary edema rapidly. In contrast, pulmonary vascular congestion in hypertrophic obstructive cardiomyopathy is due to left ventricular stiffness with impaired filling, and sometimes to a provocable subvalvular pressure gradient. Such patients tolerate beta-adrenergic agonists, hypovolemia, vasodilation, and atrial fibrillation poorly.

Chest pain requires very careful consideration if the history suggests an atypical or unstable pattern. Stable chest pain is not a perioperative risk factor, as opposed to a pattern of unstable disease manifested by new-onset or crescendo angina, a recent MI, or recent or current heart failure. As a consequence, the preoperative evaluation of a patient with stable angina should determine whether the patient's ischemic symptoms are truly stable. If deemed so, surgery can generally proceed with the maintenance of an effective antianginal regimen during and after operation. Similarly, asymptomatic or only minimally symptomatic patients who have previously undergone coronary bypass grafting tolerate surgery well. Perioperative mortality overall is 1 percent or less for elective surgery in these patients, but this may argue more for the favorable prognosis of successful bypass operations than for an aggressive policy of preparatory myocardial revascularization.

A recent MI is the single most important risk for perioperative infarction. The risk is greatest within the first 3 months following an infarction. One retrospective review of 587 patients who underwent general anesthesia following an MI indicated a perioperative risk of reinfarction of 27 percent within 3 months, 11 percent between 3 and 6 months, and 5 percent after a 6-month interval. Patients who suffer subendocardial (non-Q wave) infarctions appear to be at identical risk. However, recent data suggest that cardiac risk management strategies may be succeeding. One recent study found a 5.8 percent reinfarction rate with perioperative invasive hemodynamic monitoring within 3 months of the first MI, and only a 2.3 incidence within 3 to 6 months, whereas another recent study reported no perioperative infarctions in 48 patients within 3 months of the previous infarction.

Such data suggest that purely elective surgery should be postponed for 6 months following an acute MI. When major emergency surgery is necessary, full hemodynamic monitoring is essential. When operation is urgent, as for a potentially resectable malignant tumor, it can be undertaken from 4 to 6 weeks after infarction if the patient has had an uncomplicated recent course or a favorable exercise tolerance test or radionuclide study in the interim.

Quantitative Evaluation of Cardiac Risk

Further study of CAD serves primarily to quantify risk in patients with identified risk factors. In patients under age 70 without additional risk factors, the risk of a perioperative cardiac event is small (4–8%) and mortality is very unlikely. For patients at moderate or higher clinical risk who undergo a vascular surgical procedure, the incidence of perioperative cardiac events may be 20 percent or greater. The incidence is probably similar for other major operations, but is only 5 to 10 percent for moderate- to high-risk patients who undergo lesser procedures. Whether patients with no cardiac risk factors should undergo additional preoperative testing is still debated, as is the need for additional testing in patients about to undergo a less hazardous surgical procedure. Clinically inapparent myocardial ischemia must be suspected, particularly in patients with diabetes mellitus. Routine laboratory testing may identify additional risk factors, such as hypercholesterolemia. As a consequence, some believe that testing is particularly important in patients with diabetes or hypertension. If the surgeon has any doubt regarding the presence of CAD, such concern can only be assuaged by further investigation.

The routine clinical evaluation, including a resting ECG and a biochemistry profile, can be a powerful predictor alone, without need to resort to additional testing. The cardiac risk index system (CRIS) was developed after multivariate analysis of preoperative clinical data from 1001 consecutive patients aged 40 years or greater who underwent noncardiac surgery. Risk factors with independent predictive value were weighted according to risk; risk classes (I–IV) are assigned based on accumulated points (Table 2-1). According to CRIS, any elective operation is contraindicated if the patient falls within class IV. A number of independent studies have validated CRIS in general terms, and the risk of major cardiac complications from even minor surgical procedures can be estimated without additional corroborative tests.

The routine resting ECG remains the primary screening modality for virtually all patients over age 40 who are to undergo general anesthesia. In one retrospective study, patients with an abnormal perioperative ECG were more than three times as likely to suffer a fatal perioperative infarction. However, the resting ECG may be normal in as many as one-half of patients with CAD, and is nondiagnostic in additional patients because of conduction abnormalities such as left bundle branch block. However, evidence of a prior MI (a Q wave 0.04 sec or wider, and at least one-third the height of the R wave) is nearly indisputable evidence of CAD. Important information, such as cardiomegaly or parenchymal evidence of pulmonary edema, can sometimes be obtained from chest radiography. However, a normal chest radiograph may coexist with markedly abnormal cardiac function.

A wide array of other tests have been employed for the preoperative assessment of cardiac risk, including ambulatory ECG, exercise ECG, echocardiography, radionuclide imaging, and coronary angiography. Costs would be prohibitive if these modalities were employed in every patient. Noninvasive tests appear sufficiently sensitive to identify most patients at increased risk. The ambulatory ECG has been recommended because of relatively modest cost and widespread availability. Ambulatory monitoring indicates that the incidence of silent ischemia in patients with known, stable CAD may be 75 percent or greater. However, the ambulatory ECG has limited detection capability in patients without CAD and suffers from some of the interpretive limitations of the resting ECG, limiting its appeal.

Exercise ECG (exercise stress testing) is the historic standard to unmask myocardial ischemia, and is recognized to be safe. There is ample clinical evidence that patients with abnormal exercise ECG are at increased risk of perioperative cardiovascular complications. Retrospective exercise ECG data reveal otherwise occult ischemia in as many as 25 percent of asymptomatic patients. Exercise ECG is reasonably accurate, and has clinically practical precision and the advantage of low cost. The sensitivity for detection of CAD ranges up to 81 percent, whereas specificity varies up to 96 percent, depending on the testing protocol. Testing has important prognostic value when ST-

Table 2-1. Cardiac Risk Index System (CRIS)

	Factors	Points
History	Age > 70 yr	5
	Myocardial infarction < 6 mo ago	10
	Aortic stenosis	3
Physical Examination	S_3 gallop, jugular venous distention, or congestive heart failure	11
	Bedridden	3
Laboratory	PO_2 < 60 mm Hg	3
	PCO_2 > 50 mm Hg	3
	Potassium < 3 meq/dl	3
	Blood urine nitrogen > 50 mg/dl	3
	Creatinine > 3 mg/dl	3
Operation	Emergency	4
	Intrathoracic	3
	Intra-abdominal	3
	Aortic	3

APPROXIMATE CARDIAC RISK (PERCENT INCIDENCE OF MAJOR COMPLICATIONS)

		Class*			
	Baseline	I	II	III	IV
Minor surgery	1	0.3	1	3	19
Major noncardiac surgery, age > 40	4	1.2	4	12	48
Abdominal aortic surgery, or age > 40 with other characteristics	10	3	10	30	75

*CRIS class I: 0–5 points; class II: 6–12 points; class III: 13–25 points; class IV: ≥26 points.

segment depression of 1.5 mm or greater occurs early during testing, is sustained into the recovery period, is associated with a submaximal increase in heart rate or blood pressure, or is accompanied by angina or an arrhythmia. However, false-negative studies are problematic. As many as one-third of patients who undergo coronary artery bypass grafting for anatomically demonstrable lesions have negative exercise ECG results. Moreover, the test has limited value as a screening procedure for healthy, asymptomatic individuals. The usefulness and, indeed, the interpretability of exercise ECG in the setting of a preoperative evaluation is a matter of debate. Detractors argue that exercise testing may add little beyond the information obtainable from the routine clinical evaluation, in that a history of typical exercise-induced chest pain may be more specific for CAD. Moreover, inability to exercise is an important predictor of a poor outcome, but patients with lower-extremity ischemia or orthopedic problems may be physically unable to exercise, and submaximal exercise may confound interpretation of the test results. Exercise ECG may be most beneficial in those patients in whom the history is believed to be an unreliable indicator of functional status.

Echocardiography may be a valuable modality in selected circumstances, with advantages of simplicity, ready availability, and low cost. Two-dimensional echocardiography records lateral wall motion and axial motion in multiple planes. Pharmacologic stress testing is also being employed as an adjunct to echocardiography. Wall motion and wall thickening can be quantified, and an estimate of left ventricular ejection fraction (LVEF) can be made from measurements of end-systolic and end-diastolic areas. Echocardiographic estimates of ventricular function correlate well with angiographic and radionuclide data. Such information can be of great value, as reduced LVEF correlates strongly with perioperative myocardial events. Segmental wall motion abnormalities define the presence of ischemia by echocardiography, although wall thickening may be a better indicator because a number of extraneous factors, such as temperature, intracardiac volume, or conduction abnormalities, may interfere with wall motion.

Radionuclide cardiac imaging represents the current standard for preoperative evaluation of cardiac disease. Radionuclide imaging takes many forms, including radionuclide cineangiography and thallium perfusion scanning, both of which can be performed at rest, during exercise, or during a pharmacologically induced exercise equivalent. Radionuclide (technetium-99m) cineangiography (RNCA) can be performed either as first-pass angiography or as gated blood-pool imaging. Each technique has diagnostic advantages. Both techniques provide an accurate assessment of global LVEF and are useful for exercise testing or detection of ventricular dyskinesis, whereas the first-pass technique is capable of assessing right ventricular EF and the presence of intracardiac shunt. The correlation between the two methods is high. Practicality has led to the dominance of gated blood-pool scanning as an evaluation tool. Technetium-99m (^{99m}Tc) is labeled to red blood cells or albumin, which remain intravascular during gated scanning. The gamma camera identifies end systole and end diastole by gating to the R wave of the ECG. Data from up to 500 cardiac cycles are averaged, producing very high resolution. Using this technique, a prospective study of 100 patients who underwent lower-extremity revascularization revealed no perioperative infarctions in 50 patients with an LVEF of greater than 55 percent, whereas the incidence of perioperative infarction was 19 percent in 42 patients with LVEF between 36 and 55 percent, and 75 percent in 8 patients with LVEF between 26 and 35 percent. Decreased LVEF also indicates a high incidence of severe CAD in patients scheduled for aortic surgery. The long-term prognosis of patients with CAD and LV dysfunction is poorer than that for patients with CAD alone.

Myocardial perfusion imaging using intravenous thallium-201 (^{201}Th) analyzes the extent and localization of CAD, the reversibility of the lesions, and the stress response of the coronary circulation. The isotope is taken up by myocytes in a manner analogous to potassium. Rapid uptake allows visualization of ischemic or unperfused myocardium. Normal coronary blood flow is relatively homogeneous, such that perfusion deficits cannot be detected in the resting state unless severe (90% or greater) coronary artery stenosis is present. Heterogeneity can therefore be enhanced by superimposed myocardial stress, which reflects ischemia. Because myocardial clearance of ^{201}Th is rapid, redistribution during reperfusion of ischemic myocardium can also be observed. The test can be performed during maximal exercise or after infusion of a coronary vasodilator, such as dipyridamole, is given to simulate exercise. The accuracy of dipyridamole-thallium scanning (DTS) for detection of CAD is high. Sensitivity averages 85 percent and specificity averages nearly 91 percent in collected series of DTS, and agreement between exercise-induced ^{201}Th scanning and DTS is very high. Distinctions between ischemic areas and scar from a previous infarction in patients with regional wall motion abnormalities can be made with DTS, as can the distinction between ischemic and nonischemic cardiomyopathy. Boucher and co-workers were first to report the utility of DTS for preoperative risk stratification. In a prospective study of 54 patients with stable CAD, no cardiac events were observed in 32 patients with either normal perfusion or persistent defects on DTS. In contrast, 8 of 18 patients with ^{201}Th redistribution, who did not undergo preparatory myocardial revascularization, suffered postoperative infarctions. Subsequently, Eagle and Bonchers found that 50 percent of patients with at least one clinical risk factor for CAD had ischemia by DTS, and that such patients had a 50 percent risk of a perioperative ischemic event. Similarly, patients without ^{201}Th redistribution had a low incidence of postoperative events.

Performance of DTS can be limited by, among other things, lower sensitivity with lesser degrees of coronary stenosis. Single-vessel disease involving the circumflex or right coronary circulations may not be detected, and disease in the left anterior descending artery may go unrecognized if redistribution occurs in other segmental circulations. Although the negative predictive value of DTS is high (90%), the presence of DTS redistribution is identified so often, particularly in vascular surgical patients, that its positive predictive value is low (30%). Certain patients may therefore still require coronary angiography, particularly those with clinical or laboratory evidence of unstable or disabling CAD, such as those with multiple areas of DTS redistribution or decreased LVEF, or those with very high-risk clinical profiles. However, patients over the age of 65 years or those with peripheral vascular disease are at increased risk of morbidity from cardiac catheterization, including such complications as reaction to the contrast material, ventricular fibrillation, vascular thrombosis, MI, hemorrhage, cerebral embolization, or pseudoaneurysm formation.

Preparation of the High-Risk Cardiac Patient for Surgery

Determination of the indications for surgery and quantitation of cardiac risk in the at-risk patient are essential, but there is more to proper preparation for surgery. In order to minimize risk, the patient must be in optimal medical condition. Such optimization is ultimately the responsibility of the operating surgeon, but may often be undertaken by the referring physician or a consultant. Obvious among such preparations are the need for stabilization of medical conditions such as congestive heart failure, or poorly controlled hypertension or diabetes, before an elective procedure is undertaken. A pragmatic approach is essential. Evaluation of certain problems might safely be deferred to the postoperative period. For example, postponing surgery to achieve better control of stable, mild hypertension (diastolic blood pressure 110 mm Hg or less) does not reduce perioperative risk. Most tachyarrhythmias do not require aggressive preoperative control. The patient with ventricular arrhythmias and myocardial dysfunction is at increased risk, but the risk is probably due to poor ventricular function rather than the arrhythmia. Prophylactic antiarrhythmic therapy will not eliminate the underlying ventricular arrhythmia, and may be proarrhythmic. Such therapy is best reserved for patients with hemodynamically important arrhythmias or a history of sudden death.

Placement of a prophylactic temporary pacemaker for conduction abnormalities is indicated rarely. Pacemaker placement should not be entertained unless the patient had an indication for a permanent pacemaker, in which case it is ideally placed beforehand. An exception to this rule can be made for patients with preoperative left bundle branch block who require perioperative placement of a pulmonary artery catheter, because right bundle branch block occurs during approximately 5 percent of catheterizations and complete heart block may ensue. For patients with permanent pacemakers, the intraoperative use of electrocautery is po-

tentially dangerous and should be avoided. Bipolar electrocautery may be safer. Demand pacemakers may be inhibited by electrocautery, but placement of a magnet or programmer on the skin directly over the generator converts many pacemakers to a fixed rate regardless of the electrical activity sensed by the pacemaker. Because pacemaker programming varies widely, reprogramming methods must be reviewed individually before surgery.

Continuation of antihypertensive therapy throughout the preoperative period does not contribute to hemodynamic instability, although the data are conflicting as to whether continuation of antihypertensive therapy actually decreases perioperative morbidity. Discontinuation of antihypertensive therapy does pose potential hazards. Rebound hypertension has been reported in the postoperative period when centrally acting α_2-adrenergic agonists (e.g., clonidine) are withheld. There is a possibility of congestive heart failure in the perioperative period when angiotensin-converting enzyme inhibitors used preoperatively for that indication are withheld, although perioperative hypertension is less of a problem. Diuretic therapy may cause hypovolemia or hypokalemia, but neither problem poses major difficulties if recognized and treated.

There is widespread agreement that beta-adrenergic blockade should be continued throughout the perioperative period. Abrupt discontinuation of most beta blockers, except perhaps those with partial intrinsic agonist activity, is associated with a hyperadrenergic withdrawal syndrome characterized by unstable angina, tachyarrhythmias, MI, or sudden death in both surgical and nonsurgical settings. Calcium slow-channel blocking drugs are now employed for a panoply of clinical disorders, which is a reflection of the variable properties of individual agents within this class of compounds. Continuation of these drugs in the perioperative period has been controversial. Rebound phenomena associated with abrupt drug discontinuance are less common than with beta blockers. On the other hand, patients receiving combined therapy with beta-adrenergic and calcium channel blockers, which may synergistically produce conduction abnormalities or left ventricular dysfunction, may be at further risk from the cardiodepressant effects of inhalational anesthetics. If

patients are doing well on chronic therapy with these drugs, continuation in the perioperative period is reasonable. However, these drugs should probably not be relied upon alone to prevent myocardial ischemia in patients at increased risk.

Digoxin therapy for chronic congestive heart failure, particularly with complicating supraventricular tachyarrhythmias, should be continued through the perioperative period. Optimal perioperative management includes a careful preoperative search for the sometimes subtle signs of digitalis toxicity (arrhythmias, nausea, vomiting, headache, dizziness, and visual disturbances have been described). Serum digoxin levels should be checked, and adjusted if subtherapeutic. However, increased serum levels alone may not indicate toxicity, as toxicity is best defined in terms of drug levels within tissue. For example, control of ventricular rate in chronic atrial fibrillation often requires levels up to 3.0 ng/ml (usual therapeutic range, 0.5–1.5 ng/ml). If the drug is not being used for treatment of arrhythmias, it is probably safe to withhold digoxin on the morning of surgery. Digitalis toxicity may be precipitated by hypo- or hypercalcemia, hypokalemia, or hypomagnesemia. Rapid intravenous administration of calcium may produce serious arrhythmias in a digitalized patient, and should be avoided.

Preoperative Preparation in the Intensive Care Unit

The practice of preoperative admission to the ICU for final preparation for surgery is a relatively recent innovation with distinct advantages, but is not routinely utilized in many centers because of added expense and the chronic shortage of ICU beds and nurses. Thus, there is a paucity of data regarding the benefit of this approach. Only patients in whom active intervention, such as a fluid infusion to increase intravascular volume, is planned, should be considered candidates for preoperative admission to the ICU. Patients likely to benefit from preoperative evaluation in the ICU include those with unstable angina, severe valvular heart disease or decompensated CHF, end-stage renal disease, and perhaps those scheduled for repair of an abdominal aortic aneurysm. Patients at high risk but for whom no short-term interventions can reduce the risk, such as those with chronic obstructive pulmonary disease or chronic renal failure not requiring dialysis, generally are not candidates. The patient should be admitted to the ICU beginning the evening before the scheduled surgery. At least 12 hours of observation are required for proper evaluation of the effects of therapy. It is not known whether it is better to seek to maximize cardiac output, to achieve a particular pulmonary wedge pressure, or to achieve adequate oxygen delivery with minimal stroke work and myocardial oxygen consumption. Administration of fluids before surgery is individualized for each patient. Regardless of the goal, pulmonary wedge pressure may bear little relation to left ventricular end-diastolic volume in the poorly compliant or ischemic ventricle, or the patient with mitral valve disease. Close monitoring of pulmonary wedge pressure may identify a poorly compliant ventricle if a large increase in pressure accompanies infusion of a small volume of fluid.

Preoperative Preparation and Assessment of Pulmonary Function

Many patients who develop acute respiratory failure in the perioperative period do so because of catastrophic illness or injury rather than intrinsic pulmonary disease. For those patients preoperative testing is of no value, or impossible in an emergency situation. However, in patients with a history of lung disease or those in whom a pulmonary resection is contemplated, preoperative assessment of pulmonary function is of great value.

Late postoperative pulmonary complications are leading causes of morbidity and mortality after surgery. Respiratory complications accounted for 24 percent of immediate causes of death in one series of 197 patients who died within 6 days of surgery. A review of 10,000 major operations found that 10 percent of all operative deaths occurred in patients who developed pneumonia, which itself was associated with a 46 percent mortality in the 1.3 percent of patients in whom it developed. Prolonged postoperative decreases in functional residual capacity (FRC) and forced vital capacity (FVC) are associated with atelectasis, decreased pulmonary compliance, increased work of breathing,

and tachypnea at low tidal volumes. Poor cough effort and impaired airway reflexes increase the susceptibility of postoperative patients to retained secretions, bacterial invasion, and pneumonia. Upper abdominal and thoracic incisions, increased operative time (longer than 3 hr), increased severity of underlying pulmonary disease (COPD or chronic bronchitis), cigarette smoking, and poor preoperative nutrition are all independent risk factors for major pulmonary morbidity.

The criteria for anticipation of morbidity after thoracotomy are relatively well established in contrast to those for patients who are to undergo other types of surgery, although the same functional studies are performed in all such patients. Resection of a lung tumor requires removal of functional, albeit abnormal, tissue in patients who have limited pulmonary reserve. Operability is assessed by evaluation of baseline pulmonary function, the contribution of the tissue proposed for resection to overall pulmonary function (by split-function studies), or pulmonary vascular studies, as pulmonary resection can sometimes precipitate cor pulmonale. Preoperative assessment of the candidate for nonthoracic surgery should focus on identification of chronic airway obstruction, possible preoperative therapy to minimize risk, and the choice of surgical incision in the case of celiotomy. However, it should be realized that few data suggest that outcome is improved by optimization of pulmonary function before elective procedures.

Historical information of value includes the frequency and intensity of bronchospasm, and the duration of prior asthma therapy including previous hospitalizations, steroid use, and prior mechanical ventilation. The smoking history should be quantitated as pack-years. Nutritional status, concomitant heart disease, and current therapy (including oxygen use) should be documented, as should changes in cough or sputum production suggestive of an active pulmonary infection.

Notable physical examination findings for severe pulmonary disease are often absent. Use of accessory muscles, a prolonged expiratory phase, a "barrel chest" configuration, and cyanosis are uncommon except in advanced emphysema. A patient with asthma may be normal to chest ausculta-

tion between episodes, or may have wheezing or rhonchi even when clinically asymptomatic. Evidence of right ventricular failure, including peripheral edema, a prominent right ventricular impulse, a loud or widely split P_2 heart sound, or neck vein distention should be sought specifically.

Although the value of the routine, perioperative chest radiograph has been discounted, it is frequently of value with underlying lung disease to evaluate the cause of dyspnea, and to serve as a basis for comparison in the perioperative period should complications occur. Radiographic clues to the presence of airflow obstruction include depression of the right hemidiaphragm at or below the seventh rib anteriorly on a conventional posteroanterior view, a cardiac silhouette with a transverse dimension of less than 11.5 cm, and a retrosternal air space of greater than 4.4 cm on a lateral view. Although specific, these indicators have low sensitivity. Significant airflow obstruction may be associated with a normal x-ray. Hyperlucency and increased bronchial markings are not valuable as indicators of chronic lung disease.

Most laboratory studies are of little benefit for prediction in chronic lung disease. In COPD, an elevated serum bicarbonate suggests chronic respiratory acidosis. Polycythemia may suggest chronic hypoxemia. Arterial blood gas analysis on room air should be performed in patients deemed to be at risk, as an arterial oxygen tension (PaO_2) of less than 60 mm Hg correlates with pulmonary hypertension, and a $PaCO_2$ of greater than 45 mm Hg is associated with increased perioperative morbidity. Electrocardiography should be performed to look for evidence of pulmonary hypertension (right axis deviation, right ventricular hypertrophy, or right atrial enlargement). Supraventricular tachycardias are common during acute exacerbations of chronic disease, and even in patients in stable condition in the postoperative period. However, arrhythmias in patients with COPD are generally associated with a poor overall prognosis.

Spirometry before and after bronchodilators is simple to obtain and very safe for patients. Analysis of forced expiratory volume in one second (FEV_1) and FVC usually provides all of the information that is necessary for clinical decision making.

Dyspnea is assumed to occur when FEV_1 is less than 2 liters, while an FEV_1 less than 50 percent of the predicted value predicts exertional dyspnea. In COPD, the FVC decreases less than the FEV_1, resulting in an FEV_1/FVC ratio of less than 0.8. The degree of spirometric abnormalities correlates with the incidence of postoperative atelectasis and pneumonia, particularly if FEV_1 is less than 1.2 liters or less than 70 percent of predicted, FVC is less than 1.7 liters or less than 70 percent of predicted, or FEV_1/FVC is less than 0.65. If spirometric parameters improve by 15 percent or more after bronchodilator therapy, such therapy should be continued throughout the perioperative period, although many patients will experience subjective improvement that cannot be quantified. If pulmonary resection is contemplated, abnormal spirometry can be followed by split-lung function studies using either bronchospirometry or radionuclide imaging with either xenon-133 (^{133}Xe) or ^{99m}Tc. An FEV_1 from the contralateral lung of more than 800 ml is required to proceed with pneumonectomy, as at an FEV_1 of approximately 800 ml, carbon dioxide retention naturally occurs in patients with COPD. For abdominal surgery, there is no indication for evaluation beyond spirometry and aterial blood gas analysis.

Pulmonary toilet probably accomplishes more by educating the patient about perioperative care and engendering a cooperative attitude about chest physiotherapy than by actually improving gas exchange. Bronchodilator therapy should be continued through the perioperative period if the patient is maintained on therapy chronically. Patients with COPD can be considered for a short course of oral antibiotics before surgery if bronchitis is associated with purulent or tenacious sputum, although expectorants and mucolytic agents are of no value and may actually promote bronchospasm. Cessation of cigarette smoking is very important in all patients who smoke 10 or more cigarettes per day. Even short-term abstinence (48 hr) decreases the carboxyhemoglobin level to that of a nonsmoker, abolishes the effects of nicotine on the cardiovascular system, and improves mucosal ciliary function. Sputum volume decreases after 1 to 2 weeks of abstinence, and spirometry improves after about 6 weeks of abstinence. However, except in the case of abstinence from cigarettes, objective data of good quality that document improved outcome from the provision of preoperative pulmonary toilet are scant.

Correction of Fluid and Electrolyte Disorders
Body Fluid Compartments

To identify and correct preoperative fluid and electrolyte disorders, one must understand thoroughly the size, solute composition, and interchange of the various body fluid compartments. Although normal values vary according to body cell mass, percentage of body fat, weight, age, and sex, these compartments are surprisingly constant in volume and in their relations to each other for individual patients under steady-state conditions.

Total body water constitutes between 55 and 75 percent of body weight in men and between 45 and 60 percent of body weight in women. Males have a greater proportion of muscle mass, which has a high water content. Total body water can be subdivided into the *intracellular* compartment, representing approximatley 40 percent of body weight, and the *extracellular* compartment, representing approximately 20 percent of body weight (Fig. 2-1). The extracellular fluid compartment is composed of the plasma compartment (approximately 5% of body weight) and the interstitial fluid compartment (approximately 15% of body weight). The extracellular fluid compartment is generally in a highly dynamic state compared with the intracellular compartment, but some subdivisions of the extracellular compartment, such as connective tissue water, joint fluid, and cerebrospinal fluid, remain fairly stable for long periods. The major electrolyte components of the intracellular compartment (principal cations are potassium and magnesium and principal anions are phosphates and proteins) are shown in Fig. 2-2. In the extracellular fluid compartment, sodium is the principal cation and chloride and bicarbonate are the principal anions. There is a considerably higher protein content in plasma than in interstitial fluid, which results in a higher total cation concentration (meq/liter) and a lower inorganic ion concentration in plasma compared with interstitial fluid.

Healthy people ingest approximatley 2000 to 2500 ml per day of water. Water from oxidation of carbohydrate, protein, and fat amounts to an additional 250 ml per day. Water intake is usually controlled in conscious patients by the thirst mechanism, activated by the hypertonicity that results when the body's water content decreases without an associated loss of electrolytes.

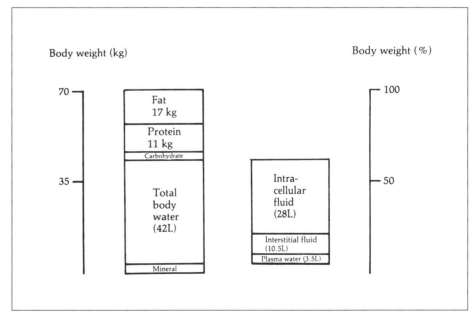

Fig. 2-1. *Sixty percent of body weight is composed of the total body water compartment with its subdivisions as shown.*

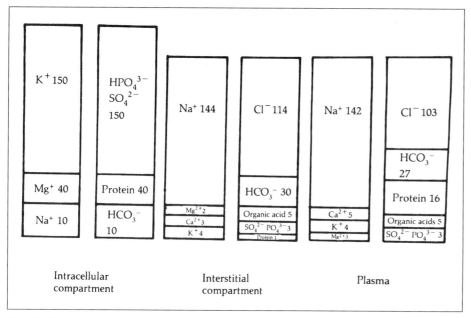

Fig. 2-2. Electrolyte and protein contributions to intracellular and extracellular body compartment solutes.

The change in osmolality stimulates osmoreceptors, which cause an increased release of arginine vasopressin (AVP) and, subsequently, increased renal free-water resorption. Pain, fear, decreased blood or extracellular fluid volumes, and drugs such as morphine, epinephrine, and barbiturates stimulate the release of AVP. Healthy people lose approximately 800 to 1500 ml per day of water as urine, 250 ml as stool, and 600 to 900 ml as insensible loss through the skin (75%) and lungs (25%). A wide range of fluid intake and output occurs under normal conditions; with good renal function, homeostasis generally is assured even during abnormal conditions associated with mild diarrhea, vomiting, or hyperpyrexia, or after mild traumatic injuries.

Healthy people ingest approximately 50 to 90 meq sodium per day. The main function of sodium is the control and distribution of water throughout the body by its effect on osmolality. When the intake of sodium is severely limited or when large extrarenal losses occur, the renal excretion of sodium can decrease to a level of 1 meq per day. The normal daily dietary intake of potassium is approximately 40 to 90 meq. In the body, 98 percent of the potassium is within the intracellular compartment. The total extracellular potassium in a healthy 70-kg adult is approximately 63 meq. Although the amount is small in comparison with the total intracellular potassium, it is

essential to neural, cardiac, and muscular function. Serum concentrations of potassium may not reflect total body content of this ion. For example, potassium is transferred from the intracellular to the extracellular compartment during acidosis or after major trauma and semistarvation, and serum levels do not correlate with intracellular potassium concentrations. In addition, chronic diuretic therapy may result in severe total body potassium depletion in the presence of a normal or slightly low serum potassium concentration.

Preoperative fluid management is normally a hallmark of preparation for urgent or emergency operations, where one needs to replenish existing fluid or electrolyte deficits and to replace ongoing abnormal losses resulting from the patient's disease or therapy. Mechanical bowel preparation can also cause iatrogenic fluid losses. It is less common to need to treat surgical patients for fluid overload, except for cardiac surgery. For patients with heart disease, replacement therapy must sometimes be undertaken with the guidance of invasive hemodynamic monitoring.

Fluid Volume and Concentration Disorders

Shires has classified fluid and electrolyte balance abnormalities into three general categories: disorders of volume, concentration, and composition. These problems may be single or multiple in an individual patient. The most common fluid problem found in the preoperative patient is extracellular fluid volume depletion (Table 2-2). The diagnosis of isotonic volume depletion can be established by a thorough patient history and physical examination. Knowledge of body weight changes, frequency and amount of vomiting and diarrhea, quantity of fistula losses, increases in abdominal girth with ascites, and duration of diuretic therapy can be used to estimate volume deficits. A physical examination may show decreased skin turgor, dry tongue and mucous membranes, and sunken eyes in a patient who is apathetic, oliguric, tachycardic, or hypotensive on standing. Volume depletion may occur not only secondary to external losses due to vomiting, diarrhea, nasogastric suction, or fistula drainage, but also as a result of sequestration of fluid following massive soft-tissue injuries, peritonitis, pancreatitis, or intestinal obstruction or infarction. Such fluid sequestration results in a loss of "functioning" extracellular fluid (third space loss), which ultimately causes a loss of circulating blood volume and adverse cardiovascular symptoms. The major homeostatic response to this disorder is re-

Table 2-2. Causes of Common Volume and Electrolyte Disorders in the Preoperative Patient

Decreased effective volume + normal
  electrolyte concentration (hyperosmolality)
  Major burn, pelvic or long bone fracture
  Duodenal fistula
  Perforated viscus
  Pancreatitis
  Intestinal infarction
  Distal intestinal obstruction
Decreased volume + decreased electrolyte
  concentration (isoosmolality or
  hypoosmolality)
  Proximal intestinal obstruction
  Ileal fistula (moderate output) with water
    ingestion
  Diarrhea secondary to enteritis or colitis
    with water ingestion
  Overzealous administration of diuretics
  Salt-losing nephropathy
Normal or increased water + decreased
  electrolyte concentration (hypoosmolality)
  Inappropriate AVP level
  Chronic renal failure
  Hepatic failure
  Cardiac failure
  Cirrhosis

AVP = arginine vasopressin.

nal, including decreased urine output, increased urine osmolality, and decreased urine sodium concentration. Major elective surgical procedures in a patient suffering moderate to severe isotonic dehydration may result in cardiovascular collapse and shock, further impairing vital functions and resulting in a sequence that leads to multiple organ failure.

Fluid resuscitation of volume-depleted patients should be accompanied by hourly monitoring of urine output through an indwelling bladder catheter. In the presence of normal renal function without glycosuria, a minimal hourly urine output of 0.5 ml/kg signifies restoration of fluid volume toward normal. In elderly patients or those with decreased cardiac reserve, one should also monitor hourly changes in central venous pressure or pulmonary artery wedge pressure; fluid overload is unlikely to occur when the central venous pressure is below 8 to 10 cm H_2O. Determination of arterial blood pH and lactate concentrations and calculations of the base deficit may be helpful in difficult or confusing resuscitations. Even with close monitoring, however, all of the estimated fluid deficit should not be replaced in a matter of a few hours. For example, after a major thermal injury, it is usually advisable to administer one-half the estimated fluid requirement in the first 8 hours and to give the remaining required fluids over the next 16 hours. On the other hand, in an elderly patient with a partial upper small-intestinal obstruction and a 3-day history of vomiting, only one-half the calculated deficit should be given along with maintenance requirements during the first 24 hours, if immediate surgical intervention is not required.

The need for surgical intervention is a major factor that determines the rate of parenteral fluid and electrolyte replacement. Each patient is unique, and good clinical judgment depends on repeated reassessment of urinary output, central venous pressure or pulmonary artery wedge pressure, and the overall clinical response of the patient. The existing volume deficit can be calculated by estimating body weight change, if preillness weight is known; by noting the change in hematocrit value, if preillness values are known; and by physical examination. A deficit of approximately 3 to 5 liters has occurred when a dry tongue and decreased skin turgor are noticed. Parenteral fluid therapy should

begin with lactated Ringer's solution. Correction of all clinical signs of volume deficit (tachycardia, hypotension, oliguria) is the best indication of therapeutic success.

In the preoperative preparation of the surgical patient, emphasis should be placed on correcting existing volume deficits; however, severe electrolyte abnormalities should be corrected as well, particularly if they are symptomatic. Hyponatremia may be caused by an actual loss of sodium from the body (primary hyponatremia) or by an accumulation of water in excess of sodium (secondary hyponatremia). The former could be secondary to vomiting, diarrhea, fistula drainage, diuretics, or adrenal insufficiency. The latter condition may be caused by inappropriate antidiuretic hormone (AVP) syndrome (SIADH). Clinically, the signs and symptoms of primary hypothermia are similar to those of isotonic dehydration (dry tongue and mucous membranes, decreased skin turgor, oliguria, and tachycardia). Secondary hyponatremia (water intoxication) can be associated with nervous system abnormalities such as increased deep tendon reflexes progressing to convulsions; cardiovascular symptoms are less common. The rapidity of the fall in serum sodium concentration, particularly to levels below 120 meq per liter, is correlated directly with the severity of the attendant symptoms.

Primary hyponatremia is treated by salt and volume repletion. An otherwise healthy patient shoulder undergo repletion with isotonic sodium chloride solution to correct both abnormalities at the same time, particularly if a metabolic alkalosis due to volume contraction is present. A patient with neurologic symptoms, an individual without symptoms who has hyponatremia caused by renal salt wasting or inappropriate secretion of AVP, or a patient who has poor cardiac reserve might best have his or her sodium concentration restored initially with isotonic sodium–containing fluids. A modest quantity of 3 or 5% sodium chloride solution, followed by a slower infusion of isotonic sodium chloride, can be used to treat symptoms or restore marked derangements, or for temporary management of SIADH while fluid restriction and oral demeclocycline take effect. The sodium deficit can be calculated by multiplying the decrease in serum sodium concentration below normal (140 meq/liter) by the estimated normal total body water in liters. For example, an 80-

kg man with symptomatic primary hyponatremia and a serum sodium concentration of 115 meq per liter has a sodium deficit calculated as

$$(140 - 115 \text{ meq/L}) \times (80 \text{ kg} \times 0.60)$$
$$= 25 \text{ meq/L} \times 48 \text{ L} = 1200 \text{ meq}$$

Slow infusion of 600 ml of 5% NaCl solution (containing approximately 513 meq Na) should provide relief of symptoms and raise the serum Na^+ concentration to above the usual threshold for seizure activity in the asymptomatic patient. The remaining sodium deficit as well as maintenance sodium requirements can be given as an isotonic sodium chloride infusion over the next 48 hours. When adequate urine volume is ensured, more rapid repletion may itself cause severe neurologic complications, such as central pontine demyelination, as well as volume overload. Replacement of potassium is required because, even though a normal serum potassium level may be present initially, a total body potassium deficit is usually found.

Secondary hyponatremia, which is asymptomatic and is associated with excess total body water, is treated by water restriction. A classic example is the patient with severe hepatic cirrhosis, ascites, peripheral edema, and hyponatremia in the presence of excessive total body sodium and water. Salt and water restriction and close monitoring of urine output permit safe correction of this electrolyte disorder if renal function remains relatively normal. In patients who have a low serum albumin concentration (<2.0 g/dl) in addition to secondary hyponatremia, administration of 25% ("salt-poor") human albumin coupled with water restriction may be appropriate. Such patients should not receive crystalloid fluids containing sodium if at all possible. Administration of sodium to such patients invariably increases ascites, often with no impact on the serum sodium concentration.

Hyponatremia may be factitious in the presence of marked hyperglycemia, and must be taken into account. Such patients must have a correction factor applied (the factitious decrease is 3 meq/100 mg/dl glucose over 100 mg/dl). For example, the diabetic patient admitted with a serious infection and hyperosmolar osmolar nonketotic coma who has a serum glucose of 1100 mg/dl and a serum sodium of 127 meq/dl is actually hypernatremic (about

157 meq/dl), and markedly volume depleted secondary to the osmotic diuresis caused by the hyperglycemia.

Hypernatremia is often iatrogenic, produced by administration of sodium in excess of water. Awake, communicative patients usually complain of thirst and, if able, prevent or correct this disorder themselves. Symptomatic hypernatremia may develop insidiously and accidentally in pediatric patients, semiconscious patients with neurologic disorders, diabetic patients, and patients receiving hypertonic saline solution. Administration of hypertonic tube feedings (usually, 2 kcal/ml) results commonly in this disorder, particularly if added water is not administered. Correction of this abnormality should be initiated by infusion of a 0.45% sodium chloride solution with close monitoring of the serum sodium concentration. If the extracellular osmolality is reduced too rapidly, as it might be when 5% dextrose in water is give intravenously, convulsions and coma may occur secondary to cerebral edema as water rapidly crosses the blood-brain barrier.

Abnormalities of Electrolyte Composition

Isolated potassium, magnesium, and calcium abnormalities are rarely seen in the preoperative patient, and usually occur in association with volume, sodium, chloride, and acid base disorders. Control of potassium levels by the kidney is imprecise, and even in the presence of a deficit in total body potassium concentration, renal excretion of potassium continues. In the presence of metabolic alkalosis, extracellular potassium ions move intracellularly, whereas intracellular hydrogen ions move extracellularly to buffer the extracellular alkalotic state. Often, renal loss of potassium occurs in metabolic alkalosis along with this internal shift, resulting in paradoxical aciduria. Another mechanism for the movement of potassium into the intracellular compartment is by the administration of hypertonic dextrose–amino acid solutions (total parenteral nutrition with inadequate potassium concentration) to malnourished patients. Amino acids, glucose, and potassium move intracellularly to synthesize cellular protein even at the expense of plasma potassium levels.

When hypokalemia is severe enough to cause cardiac abnormalities, potassium chloride can be infused intravenously at the rate of 20 to 40 meq per hour if renal function is adequate and cardiac monitoring is continuous (Table 2-3). Peripheral vein phlebitis can be avoided by administration of 20 meq potassium chloride in 50 ml of 5% dextrose in water or normal saline solution through a central venous catheter. Severe potassium deficiency may be associated with a total body deficit of 400 to 500 meq potassium. When a preoperative patient is found to have hypokalemia, operation should be postponed (unless to correct an immediately life-threatening condition) to allow intensive potassium repletion. Surgery can generally proceed safely when serum potassium is raised to 3.5 meq/dl.

Hyperkalemia can be a life-threatening emergency requiring prompt management. The most common cause is renal failure, but it can also occur secondary to major tissue destruction from trauma, revascularization of a markedly ischemic extremity, massive infusion of stored blood, intravascular hemolysis, sepsis, or iatrogenic infusion of excessive potassium. Management of this problem in the presence of renal failure consists of promoting temporary intracellular transfer of potassium while methods (ion exchange resins, dialysis) are mobilized for increasing potassium loss from the body. Correction of acidosis by administration of sodium bicarbonate promotes intracellular transfer of potassium and lowers plasma levels. Administration of hypertonic dextrose plus insulin (1 unit/10 g dextrose) shifts some potassium intracellularly. Neuromuscular toxicity can be inhibited some-

Table 2-3. Management of
Serum Potassium Disorders

Hypokalemia
  Correct alkalosis (administer 0.9% NaCl or
    0.1 N HCl)
  Administer potassium (up to 20 meq K^+/hr)
    in the presence of good urine output
  Discontinue or change diuretics
Hyperkalemia
  Correct acidosis (administer sodium
    bicarbonate or lactate)
  Inhibit neuromuscular toxicity (administer
    calcium gluconate)
  Encourage intracellular transfer (administer
    50% dextrose in water ± insulin)
  Sodium cation-exchange resins (sodium
    polystyrene sulfonate [Kayexalate])
  Peritoneal dialysis or hemodialysis

what by intravenous administration of calcium gluconate if life-threatening cardiac arrhythmias occur. Sodium cation-exchange resins can be given orally, by nasogastric tube, or rectally to increase excretion of potassium. Hemodialysis or peritoneal dialysis can be used to alleviate life-threatening hyperkalemia if other methods are unavailable or unable to correct the abnormality.

Most of the calcium in the body is present in bone. Plasma calcium is divided into two fractions: One is bound to plasma protein and the other is ionizable and physiologically much more important. Control of calcium metabolism is related to parathormone, calcitonin, and vitamin D. Hypocalcemia is only rarely a problem in the preoperative patient and is most often secondary to hypoparathyroidism, pancreatitis, respiratory alkalosis, or hyperphosphatemia. Treatment of the patient with symptoms of hypoparathyroidism is accomplished by intravenous infusion of 4.4 to 8.8 meq (1–2 g) calcium over 30 minutes or by continuous infusion if ongoing abnormalities are expected, as is sometimes the case in severe pancreatitis. When hypocalcemia is secondary to hypoalbuminemia, it is asymptomatic because ionized calcium levels remain normal and will be corrected by improving nutritional status and albumin levels. Total serum calcium is reduced by 0.8 meq/dl for each 1-g decrease (below 4.0) in serum albumin concentration. Hypercalcemia may be caused by the milk-alkali syndrome, vitamin D intoxication, carcinomatosis, sarcoidosis, hyperparathyroidism, and multiple myeloma (see below).

Preoperative Fluid and Electrolyte Therapy

The length of time available for preoperative preparation is dictated by the underlying disease and the urgency of the indicated surgical procedure. Some situations (e.g., perforated colonic diverticulitis) necessitate almost immediate surgical intervention, but others, such as acute cholecystitis and partial small-intestinal obstruction, often lend themselves to semielective operative therapy. Parenteral fluid and electrolyte therapy can be classified into requirements administered intravenously for maintenance of homeostasis, correction of existing deficits, and replacement of ongoing losses secondary

Table 2-4. Composition and Osmolarity of Gastrointestinal Secretions

Secretion	Volume (ml/24 hr)	Osmolarity (meq/L)	Na (meq/L)	K (meq/L)	Cl (meq/L)	HCO₃ (meq/L)
Salivary	1500 (500–2000)*	—	10 (3–10)	26 (20–30)	10 (8–20)	—
Gastric	1000 (400–4000)	2160	60 (30–116)	10 (0–32)	120 (50–154)	—
Bile	400 (50–800)	300	145 (135–155)	5 (3–10)	75 (83–110)	70 (25–45)
Pancreas	1500 (200–2000)	300	140 (112–185)	5 (3–10)	75 (55–95)	70 (50–85)
Ileum	3000 (100–9000)	240	120 (80–140)	5 (3–7)	105 (60–135)	20 (15–30)
Colon	250 (100–400)	—	60	30	40	—

*Values in parentheses indicate normal ranges.

Table 2-5. Fluid and Electrolyte Requirements for a Patient* with Normal Cardiovascular Status Undergoing an Urgent Operation

	Requirements			
	Water (ml)	Na (meq)	Cl (meq)	K (meq)
Maintenance	2000	80	80	60
Deficit				
Vomiting	1000	60	120	5
Third space sequestration	4000–6000	560–840	400–600	16–20
Electrolyte composition (based on body water)	—	420	420	100+?
Total	7000–9000	1120–1400	1020–1220	181+?

*A 57-year-old man weighing 69 kg (normal wt = 70 kg) with a 72-hr history of no flatus or stool per rectum; a 24-hr history of vomiting; dry mouth; poor skin turgor; distended abdomen; and a tender femoral mass.
Serum electrolyte levels are
Na = 130 meq/L K = 3.2 meq/L Cr = 1.0 mg/dl
Cl = 90 meq/L CO₂ = 33 meq/L BUN = 35 mg/dl

cause of acid base disturbances (alkalosis from loss of gastric juice) or volume changes ("contraction" alkalosis), which may alter compartmental potassium flux and renal potassium secretion. Table 2-4 lists approximate volumes and solute levels of gastrointestinal secretions; precise management can be obtained by direct measurement of the electrolyte composition of the fluid being lost, particularly if management is difficult, large fluid losses are involved, or renal compensatory mechanisms are deranged. Once fluid and electrolyte requirements are calculated, the rate of intravenous administration is determined by the patient's cardiovascular status, the urgency of the operation, renal function, and the severity of preexisting abnormalities.

Fluid abnormalities should be suspected and corrected even in patients scheduled for elective operations. Serum electrolyte concentrations should be measured within 24 hours before the operation, especially in patients who are receiving diuretics or digitalis. Mechanical intestinal preparation with laxatives, for example, often results in mild to moderate dehydration, and at least 1 or 2 liters of isotonic salt solution (Ringer's lactate) should be infused during the 18 hours before the operation to correct body fluid deficits. Preoperative tests such as arteriography and intravenous pyelography may also contribute to mild fluid deficits.

Urgent Operation–Normal Cardiovascular Status

Fluid and electrolyte requirements are determined by adding estimated maintenance needs to calculated deficits (Table 2-5). Because an immediate operation is deemed necessary, ongoing losses (nasogastric suction plus continued sequestered fluid and solute) should be replaced during the operation and the immediate postoperative period. Maintenance requirements have been discussed and listed previously. Deficit requirements are the quantities lost from the body by vomiting and those sequestered within the intestinal lumen or inflamed tissues. Both deficits result in a decrease in effective circulating blood volume. Fluid losses from vomiting probably amount to 1000 ml (1 kg recent loss in body weight); electrolyte losses are estimated from average solute gastric juice content. Greater solute and fluid losses may occur from vomiting, but the patient

to the patient's disease or to the treatment of the disease.

Maintenance fluid requirements for adults can be estimated as 100 ml/kg for the first 10 kg, 50 ml/kg for the second 10 kg, and 10 ml/kg thereafter. Therefore, the typical 70-kg patient may need 2000 ml water per day. Additionally, 60 to 80 meq sodium and 40 to 60 meq potassium per day are required. Maintenance requirements usually are constant but can change under certain conditions, such as hyperthermia and hyperventilation, which may increase fluid requirements by as much as 1000 ml per day. Isotonic hypovolemia, the most common problem in the preoperative patient, is difficult to quantify exactly, but physical assessment of dehydration (poor skin turgor and dry tongue) usually indicates a fluid deficit of at least 3 to 5 liters in adults. Serum electrolyte levels are nor-

mal after isotonic losses, such as those secondary to distal small-intestinal obstruction or pancreatitis, and require balanced salt solutions, such as lactated Ringer's solution.

In addition to providing maintenance requirements and satisfying fluid and solute needs to correct existing abnormalities, ongoing abnormal losses must be replaced with solutions of similar composition. For example, gastrointestinal fluid losses (with the exception of gastric secretions) can usually be replaced with equal volumes of lactated Ringer's solution (Table 2-4). Replacement of gastric juice should be accomplished with 0.45% sodium chloride solutions containing additional potassium (usually 20 meq/liter). Additional potassium chloride (≥209 meq/liter) may be required not only because of potassium loss for gastrointestinal secretions but also be-

probably ingested some water because serum sodium and chloride concentrations were low. The total sodium deficit can be calculated using the formula

$$[\text{NA (normal meq/L)} - \text{Na (current meq/l)}]$$
$$\times [\text{body weight (kg)} \times 0.6 \ (\% \ \text{TBW})]$$
$$= (140 \ \text{meq/L} - 130 \ \text{meq/L}) \times (70 \ \text{kg} \times 0.6)$$
$$= (10 \ \text{meq/L}) \times 42 \ \text{L} = 420 \ \text{meq Na}$$

where TBW = total body weight. The total chloride deficit can be calculated similarly, but the total potassium deficit cannot be determined precisely from the serum potassium concentration. However, the serum potassium decrease of 0.8 meq per liter probably represents a total body deficit of 100 to 200 meq. Sequestered third space losses are difficult to estimate accurately, but a distal small-intestinal obstruction can easily result in the sequestration of 4000 to 6000 ml isotonic fluid with electrolyte concentrations similar to extracellular fluid. Thus, the total *preoperative* fluid and solute requirements are approximately.

Water = 5000–7000 ml
Na = 1040–1320 meq
Cl = 940–1140 meq
K = 120 meq

If surgical intervention is planned within 4 hours of admission, fluid therapy should be initiated promptly with 1000 ml of 0.9% sodium chloride to be infused over the first 30 minutes to 1 hour, with close monitoring of urine output and central venous pressure (CVP). If there is no increase in CVP and urine output is still low (<30 ml/h), 1000 ml Ringer's lactate should be infused during the next hour. At this point, serum electrolyte measurements should be repeated. Depending on the CVP and urine output response, the rate of infusion should either remain at 1000 ml per hour or be decreased to 500 ml per hour. An adult with normal renal function excreting 30 ml urine or more per hour, who is not receiving diuretics and does not have glycosuria, has had volume repletion adequate to withstand a major operation. After an adequate urine output is established, 20 meq of KCl should be added to each liter of the infusate. Close monitoring of central venous and pulmonary capillary wedge pressure prevents the development of pulmonary edema in patients with compromised cardiac function. Thus, during the estimated 4-hour preparatory period, volume replacement

of 3000 to 5000 ml and sodium replacement of 450 to 700 meq can be accomplished. After the operation, fluid and electrolyte requirements not replaced preoperatively are incorporated into the postoperative therapy.

Nonurgent Operation—Normal Cardiovascular Status

Maintenance requirements are calculated as described previously. Deficits can be calculated as fluids lost from the body through diarrhea and fistulous loss plus fluids sequestered in the inflamed intestine (Table 2-6). The electrolyte content of this fluid can be estimated from Table 2-4 (ileal solute content) until accurate laboratory determinations of fistulous electrolyte concentration can be made. Ongoing losses from fistulas must be included in the initial estimate of fluid and solute requirements because that amount is likely to be lost during the ensuing 24 hours.

If no immediate surgical intervention is to be performed, fluid and solute orders should include maintenance requirements and ongoing losses plus one-half the deficit over each of the first 2 days. On each of the first 2 days, therefore, the fluid required can be calculated as

5000 + 2500 ml = 7500 ml;
Na = 440 + 300 meq = 740 meq;
Cl = 395 + 262 meq = 657 meq;
and K = 75 + 12 meq = 87 meq

Thereafter, fluid and solute replacement depends on maintenance requirements, which are usually relatively stable, and measurement of ongoing fistulous losses.

In summary, most preoperative patients have minimal fluid and electrolyte abnormalities, and normal renal function ordinarily compensates for inappropriate parenteral salt and water replacement therapy. In patients with cardiac, renal, or hepatic disease, however, precise determinations of fluid and electrolyte requirements are necessary because compensatory mechanisms are compromised. In these patients meticulous attention to body-weight determinations, intake and output records, CVP measurements, serum electrolyte levels, exogenous fluid and solute losses, and urinary output is imperative.

Hematologic Preparation

Evaluation of the patient's risk of bleeding requires an especially careful history and physical assessment if the evaluation is to be cost-effective, because the yield of positive findings from routine screening tests of hemostasis is very low. Many hematologic tests can be omitted safely from the preparation protocol if there is no clinical suspicion of a coagulopathy, even before many types of major surgery. Notable exceptions are those operations known to affect the coagulation system, including cardiopulmonary bypass procedures, peripheral vascular surgery, and prostatectomy. The major historic topics to be covered include whether the patient or a family member has had a prior episode of bleeding or a thromboembolic event, and whether the patient has a history of prior transfusions, prior surgery, heavy men-

Table 2-6. Fluid and Electrolyte Requirements for a Patient* with Normal Cardiovascular Status Undergoing a Nonurgent Operation

	Requirements			
	Water (ml)	Na (meq)	Cl (meq)	K (meq)
Maintenance	2000	80	80	60
Deficit				
Diarrhea	1000	120	105	5
Fistula	3000	360	105	5
Third space sequestration	1000	360	315	15
Ongoing loss/24 hr (fistula)	3000	360	315	15
Total	10,000	1280	920	100

*A 27-year-old man (70 kg) with inflammatory bowel disease; a 24-hr history of diarrhea associated with sudden development of an enterocutaneous fistula (3000 ml/day); normal serum electrolyte levels; poor skin turgor; tachycardia; and oliguria.

strual bleeding, easy bruising, frequent nosebleeds, bleeding gums after brushing the teeth, coexistent liver or kidney disease, poor dietary habits, recent dieting or excessive ingestion of alcohol, or ingestion of aspirin or other nonsteroidal anti-inflammatory drugs (interference with platelet function), lipid-lowering drugs (possible vitamin K deficiency), or anticoagulants (usually, warfarin) for prophylaxis (e.g., chronic atrial fibrillation). Answers to these 10 sets of questions should uncover most potential problems with hemostasis. If the history is completely negative and the patient has had a previous hemostatic challenge from surgery or trauma, then an important hemostatic defect is extremely unlikely. A mild coagulopathy in the previously unchallenged patient is not excluded; however, the consequences once such a mild defect is unmasked can be managed readily.

The physical examination should focus on the skin and mucous membranes for evidence of ecchymosis or petechiae. The presence of venous stasis changes about the ankles may suggest a prior thrombotic event, and the extremities must also be assessed for the presence of pulses, asymmetric edema or inflammation, or arthropathy suggestive of a previous intra-articular hemorrhage. Stigmata of chronic liver and kidney disease must be sought specifically.

Laboratory testing is overutilized in healthy patients, and almost never yields a finding of importance in patients with a negative history and physical examination. Many screening coagulation tests have major problems with false-positive results that do not translate into increased surgical bleeding. Minor problems, such as oozing from the subcutaneous portion of the incision, can be managed readily by a number of techniques. In the absence of a clinical suggestion of a bleeding disorder, the chance that a patient will have a major clotting disorder during surgery has been estimated to be less than 0.01 percent. When indicated, the usual screening battery of tests includes a prothrombin time (PT), an activated partial thromboplastin time (aPTT), and a platelet count. Even when screening is indicated clinically, important abnormalities are seldom identified. In two retrospective studies in which the prevalence of indicated testing was 61 and 92 percent, abnormalities of importance were identified in only 0.2 percent of

patients. False positives are especially common with the aPTT, where one study found the test to be abnormal 14 percent of the time, but consequential in only 16 percent of positives (2.2% overall). Similarly, elevations of the template bleeding time, as, for example, after aspirin ingestion, do not correlate with increased operative blood loss.

The first step in evaluation of an abnormal PT/aPTT is a mixing experiment, wherein the patient's plasma is mixed in equal volume with normal plasma and the tests are repeated. Complete correction indicates a factor deficiency, because levels of all factors of 50 percent or greater will produce normal tests. The specific deficit is then identified by assay of specific factors. If the PT/aPTT does not correct with mixing, an inhibitor is present, most commonly the lupus-like anticoagulant. Aside from its association with various autoimmune diseases, and various medications (quinidine, procainamide, chlorpromazine), it may also occur as an isolated abnormality without any underlying disease. Its presence does not impair surgical hemostasis, but rather represents a slightly hypercoagulable state. Fibrin degradation products or abnormal fibrinogens produced as a consequence of liver disease may also act as inhibitors. Identification of an abnormality when clinical suspicion is strong but screening tests are negative is complex, and beyond the scope of this chapter. Potential causes include mild hemophilia or von Willebrand's disease, a dysfibrinogenemia, or excessive fibrinolysis. Elective surgery should not proceed until the cause has been elucidated.

Thrombocytopenia may be caused either by decreased production or increased destruction, with a platelet count below $100,000/\mu l$ posing risk and a count below 50,000 making procedure-related bleeding likely. However, the surgeon must also be alert to qualitative disorders of platelet function in which the platelet count may be normal, such as in uremia or after ingestion of nonsteroidal anti-inflammatory agents. In such cases, transfusion of platelets without correction of the underlying problem will result only in inactivation of the transfused cells, a wasted resource, and risk to the patient. Therapeutic strategies for management of various coagulation disorders in preparation for surgery are listed in Table 2-7.

Prophylaxis of Deep Venous Thrombosis and Pulmonary Embolism

The morbidity and mortality of deep venous thrombosis and pulmonary embolism make consideration of prophylaxis mandatory for every major operation. A number of risk factors have been identified, including increasing age, obesity, previous thromboembolic disease or abdominal surgery, varicose veins, cigarette smoking, major surgery (especially pelvic, urologic, orthopedic, and cancer surgery), elevated platelet count, and antithrombin III deficiency (Table 2-8). Among these, age, previous abdominal surgery, varicose veins, antithrombin III concentration, cigarette smoking, and platelet count have been shown to be the most significant risk factors by a discriminant function analysis. The lowest risk patients are those who are undergoing only minor surgery and who have none of the identified risk factors. However, risk is increased somewhat in any patient over the age of 40 who undergoes general anesthesia for more than 30 minutes. Many prophylactic regimens have proved efficacy for patients at moderate risk, and some have negligible morbidity; therefore, standard regimens are employed increasingly for virtually all patients.

Options for prophylaxis of patients at moderate risk that have proved to be of benefit in prospective trials include low-dose heparin or oral anticoagulation (Tables 2-9 and 2-10), but the authors prefer the routine use of intermittent pneumatic compression, which is begun in the operating room immediately on induction of general anesthesia. Compression to a maximum pressure of about 40 cm H_2O over an automatic 45-second cycle is well tolerated by the patient. Mechanical pressure injury to the peroneal nerve has been reported, but is largely of theoretical risk with careful application, as we have observed only a single occurrence in many thousands of applications. Compression is continued until the patient is ambulating. As the primary effect is through stimulation of endothelial cell fibrinolytic activity, one sleeve is probably as effective as two, and they can be placed on an upper extremity if lower-extremity application is contraindicated (e.g., previous major amputation, peripheral vascular insufficiency, lower-extremity fracture). Low-

Table 2-7. Preoperative Management of Selected Coagulation Disorders

Diagnosis	Treatment
FACTOR DEFICIENCIES	
Hemophilia A: (Mild—factor VIII > 10%)	Desmopressin, 0.3 μg/kg IV q12–24 h × 5–7 days for minor surgery
Severe	Factor VIII concentrate (level 50–75% for mild–moderate injury, 75–100% for severe insults) Dose: 1 U will increase F:VIII level by 2% in a 70-kg patient—give one-half IV q12h or ¹⁄₂₄ dose IV q1h by infusion after the initial bolus. Levels should be maintained for 5–7 (moderate injury) or 7–14 days for severe injury, as delayed bleeding is typical. Levels of 25–30% are adequate for a minor operation.
Hemophilia B: Mild	Desmopressin, 0.3 μg/kg IV q12–24h
Severe	Factor IX concentrate (level 50–75% for mild–moderate injury, 75–100% for severe insults) Dose: 1 U will increase F:IX level by 2% in a 70-kg patient—give one-half IV q18–24h after the initial bolus. Levels should be maintained for 5–7 (moderate injury) or 7–14 days for severe injury, as delayed bleeding is typical. Levels of 10–25% are adequate for a minor operation.
von Willebrand's disease: Type 1	Desmopressin, 0.3 μg/kg IV q12–24h × 5–7 days. Tachyphylaxis can be restored by a 24-hr drug holiday to allow repletion of endothelial stores. Keep VIII:vWF 60% for 24–72 hours for minor surgery, 80% for 5–7 days for major surgery.
Type 2	Trial of desmopressin (unpredictable effect) Cryoprecipitate (contains 80–100 units vWF/10 units)
Liver disease (multifactorial)	Based on specific defect Fresh frozen plasma to keep PT/aPTT < 1.3 × control (difficult to correct factor VII deficiency) Vitamin K, 10 mg IM, if vitamin K deficiency suspected Platelet count >100,000 Cryoprecipitate if low fibrinogen, factor VIII
Warfarin (vitamin K deficiency, factor II, VII, IX, X)	Fresh frozen plasma to keep PT < 1.3 × control Vitamin K, 10 mg IM, if the patient does not require immediate correction (<12–48 hr) or short-term anticoagulation
PLATELET ABNORMALITIES	
Thrombocytopenia:	
Idiopathic thrombocytopenic purpura	Intravenous immune globulin, 2 g/kg over 2–4 days Platelet infusion after ligation of the splenic artery if the response to immune globulin is poor
Drug induced	Discontinue all noncritical medications Transfuse platelets only if surgery cannot be delayed to allow spontaneous recovery
Uremia	Aggressive hemodialysis? Transfuse to hematocrit ~30% to allow improved adhesion? Desmopression, 0.3 μg/kg IV q12–24h (rapid effect of short duration) Cryoprecipitate, 10 units (rapid effect of short duration) Conjugated estrogens, 25 mg IV bid for 3 days (slow onset of action but effective for up to 2 weeks)

dose heparin must be administered 2 hours before induction to be effective, making it somewhat inconvenient for use in ambulatory or same-day admission settings. Many surgeons find the increased incidence of wound bleeding (~25%) with low-dose heparin unacceptable, especially in operations with a large amount of dissection (e.g., mastectomy, major flaps). Low-dose heparin is inadvisable in a patient with major fractures (especially pelvic fracture), recent head injury, or gastrointestinal bleeding.

Patients at high risk require aggressive prophylaxis, and may need multimodality therapy (e.g., low-dose oral anticoagulation plus intermittent pneumatic compression). The increased cost and risks of combined-modality prophylaxis are offset by the potential devastation of a pulmonary embolism. The risks must be appreciated for patients being treated nonoperatively or for individuals such as those with major trauma, for whom operation is being delayed for several days for stabilization of the patient. Although the risk is very high in a patient with multiple injuries who may require a period of immobilization, the injuries themselves may preclude use of anticoagulants, even in low dose. In such patients, intermittent pneumatic compression may be insufficient prophylaxis even if it is possible; therefore, some authorities have recommended prophylactic interruption of the inferior vena cava via percutaneous placement of a filter. Percutaneous insertion techniques have made the procedure readily available with minimal morbidity. However, since such ag-

gressive prophylaxis has not yet been shown to be of unequivocal benefit, its use should be reserved for carefully selected patients at very high risk for pulmonary embolism. Appropriate candidates might include those with severe injuries, such as a spinal cord injury or the combination of a head injury with long-bone or pelvic fractures that place them at risk for prolonged bed rest and immobility. Patients undergoing high-risk surgery who have a history of deep venous thrombosis or pulmonary embolism may also be appropriate candidates.

Blood Transfusion Therapy

The issue of blood transfusion is of great concern to patients because of real and perceived risk of infectious disease transmission. Such issues are also of concern to the surgeon, but in preparing the patient for surgery, they must be considered in the context of additional concerns, such as availability of blood, the "optimal" hematocrit for oxygen transport, and alternatives to transfusion itself. Options for

Table 2-8. Individual Risk Factors in Venous Thromboembolism

Age over 40 yr
Prior deep venous thromboembolism
Varicose veins
Extensive trauma
Operations or trauma in lower extremity or pelvis
Prolonged operation
Malignant tumor
Hematologic abnormalities
    Antithrombin III deficiency
    Protein C deficiency
    Protein S deficiency
    Dysfibrinogenemia
    Disorders of plasminogen-plasminogen activation
    Lupus anticoagulant
    Polycythemia vera
Exogenous estrogen therapy
Prolonged immobilization
Acute myocardial infarction
Congestive heart failure
Stroke
Postpartum state
Obesity
Cigarette smoking

Reprinted with permission from HL Bush, Jr. Venous thromboembolic disease. In PS Barie, GT Shires (eds), *Surgical Intensive Care*. Boston: Little, Brown, 1993. Pp 477–518.

blood transfusion therapy currently include no transfusions whatsoever (which may be dictated for religious reasons), a lowering of the transfusion "trigger" such that a lower hematocrit is tolerated in the stable patient, or alternatives for increasing hematocrit such as preparatory therapy with recombinant human erythropoietin. When transfusion is ordered, alternatives to allogeneic (anonymous volunteer donor) transfusion include blood donated from a designated donor (known to the patient, usually a relative or close friend), autologous transfusion of blood donated by the patient and banked in anticipation of surgery, and intraoperative hemodilution with autotransfusion of reserved blood at the end of the case.

The tolerance of the surgeon and the patient for a reduced hematocrit depends on the acuity and activity of ongoing blood loss, if any; the magnitude of the proposed operation and the potential for bleeding during surgery or afterward; and the patient's age and health with particular reference to cardiovascular disease and risk. The clinical issue in transfusion therapy, apart from the arrest of hemorrhage and the proper conduct of resuscitation, is the determination of that critical hemoglobin concentration below which myocardial oxygen delivery (DO_2) is not supported, and myocardial oxygen consumption (VO_2) and cardiac output (Q) decrease. Animal studies suggest that the presence or absence of coronary artery disease is of critical importance in this estimation, as is

the amount of myocardial work required to overcome the insult and the concomitant physiologic stresses. Studies in dogs, whose myocardial glycolytic enzymes and metabolism are similar to those of humans, suggest that myocardial performance is not impaired under isovolemic, resting conditions until hematocrit decreases below 20 percent. Other studies suggest that the healthy canine heart with a stable work requirement can withstand a hematocrit of 10 percent, but that myocardial VO_2 is maintained during simulated coronary insufficiency only when hematocrit is maintained above 17 percent. Whether these resting animal studies are applicable to humans is debatable, but there is a clear inference that hematocrit should be maintained 5 to 10 percentage points higher in patients with known or suspected coronary artery disease than might otherwise be the case.

Continuing blood loss triggers compensatory regional blood flow distribution to counteract the decreased DO_2 that results from decreased Q. This redistribution of blood flow attempts to maintain VO_2 in the face of decreased DO_2 by diverting blood from organs of lesser biologic significance and lower oxygen extraction ratios (that function relatively well under anaerobic conditions), to those organs vital to survival, with high extraction ratios (e.g., heart, brain), that do not tolerate anaerobic conditions. Expressed in terms of the volume of blood loss, these mechanisms fail when acute blood loss exceeds 50 percent

Table 2-9. Prophylactic Methods for Deep Venous Thrombosis

Method	Mechanism	Daily Dose	Route	Complications
Low-dose heparin	Combines with AT III to neutralize factors XIIa, XIa, IXa, and Xa before generation of thrombus	10,000–15,000 units	SC	Minor wound bleeding Heparin sensitivity
Warfarin	Inhibition of synthesis of vitamin K–dependent coagulation factors (II, VII, IX, X)	Adjust prothrombin to 1.5–2× control	PO	Major bleeding Skin necrosis
Dextran 40 (low molecular weight)	Hemodilution Inhibits platelet aggregation, factor VIII aggregation, and fibrin polymerization	10 ml/kg 12 hr preop; IV 7 ml/kg postop	IV	Congestive heart failure Allergic reactions Bleeding Interference with blood cross matching
Antithrombin III	Replaces deficiency to facilitate heparin prophylaxis	1500–3000 units preop; 1000–2000 units postop		Minor wound bleeding
Intermittent pneumatic leg compression	Reduces venous stasis Increased systemic fibrinolysis			Mechanical (pressure) injury to leg
Graded compression stockings	Reduces venous stasis			Lower-extremity ischemia (contraindication)

AT III = antithrombin III.
Reprinted with permission from HL Bush, Jr. Venous thromboembolic disease. In PS Barie, GT Shires (eds), *Surgical Intensive Care*. Boston: Little, Brown, 1993. Pp 477–518.

Table 2-10. Risk Classification and Methods of Prophylaxis for Venous Thromboembolism

| Risk Category* | Risk Without Prophylaxis | | | Prophylaxis Options |
	Calf Vein Thrombosis	Proximal Vein Thrombosis	Pulmonary Embolism	
LOW RISK	<10%	<1%	0.2%	Graded compression stockings
Minor surgery <40 yr of age No additional risk factors				
MODERATE RISK ≥40 yr of age Procedure duration >30 min Uncomplicated myocardial infarction		2–10%	1–8%	Low-dose heparin (q12h) Intermittent pneumatic compression (IPC) Dextran
HIGH RISK >40 yr of age Malignant disease (abdominal, pelvic) Prior history of deep venous thromboembolism Major orthopedic surgery Stroke Major trauma	40–80%	10–20%	5–10%	Warfarin Low-dose heparin *plus* IPC Adjusted-dose heparin (therapeutic anticoagulation) Dextran *plus* IPC

*Risk is defined by advancing age, malignant disease, prolonged immobility, varicose veins, or heart failure.
Reprinted with permission from HL Bush, Jr. Venous thromboembolic disease. In PS Barie, GT Shires (eds), *Surgical Intensive Care*. Boston: Little, Brown, 1993. Pp 477–518.

of blood volume. However, the maintenance of VO_2 at the expense of perfusion of kidney, the splanchnic circulation, or other beds may also be deleterious at smaller volumes of hemorrhage. Thus, both the patient's intravascular volume status and red blood cell mass must be considered when making the decision to transfuse blood.

The flow of blood, particularly through the microcirculation where resistance is greatest, is also an important determinant of DO_2. Microcirculatory vascular resistance is directly proportional to the length of the vessel and the viscosity of the blood, and inversely proportional to the fourth power of the radius of the vessel. Blood viscosity, in turn, is dependent on hematocrit, flow velocity (shear rate), red blood cell deformability, red blood cell aggregation (Rouleaux), the concentration of plasma proteins (principally fibrinogen and α_2-globulins), and temperature. Hematocrit has a disproportionate effect on blood viscosity. As hematocrit increases, viscosity becomes inversely proportional to the flow velocity, but this relationship becomes progressively less important as hematocrit

decreases to 30 percent with hemodilution. Thus, it has been argued that a hematocrit of 30 percent is the "optimal hematocrit" for total body DO_2. Hypothermia increases viscosity by increasing the density of blood. A decrease in temperature from 37 to 25°C increases the viscosity of blood with a hematocrit of 45 percent to such a degree that hematocrit would have to be reduced to 20 percent to negate any effects of hypothermia. For this reason, isovolemic hemodilution is a popular technique in cardiac surgery. Vasoconstriction that accompanies hypothermia or brisk, untreated hemorrhage decreases flow velocity. At low flow velocity, red blood cell aggregation and decreased deformability occur. Frank occlusion of microcirculatory beds may ensue. Resuscitation may restore blood volume but may not completely restore perfusion at the level of the microcirculation (the "no-flow" phenomenon).

Clinical studies have consistently demonstrated increased cardiac performance during acute, progressive isovolemic hemodilution. Hemodynamic improvement is due largely to increased venous return mediated by diminished viscosity. Left

ventricular afterload is also reduced as total peripheral resistance decreases. Normovolemic hemodilution does decrease DO_2, but when hypervolemia is superimposed (as may readily occur, even if only transiently) during acute volume resuscitation, maximal DO_2 is achieved at a hematocrit of 30 percent. Under resting conditions, a 25 percent reduction in hematocrit (to 30%) produces only a 15 percent reduction in DO_2; VO_2 is maintained by the compensatory mechanisms described above. Tissue PO_2 values for skeletal and cardiac muscle, bone, pancreas, small intestine, kidney, and brain remain normal during isovolemic hemodilution down to a hematocrit of 18 to 20 percent.

Acute hemorrhage induces a state of hypovolemia in which hematocrit may vary, depending on the phase of resuscitation and the degree of success with the control of bleeding. Observations of oxygen transport made under isovolemic conditions may be inapplicable. Under these conditions, few clinical observations are available. During hemorrhage (constant mean arterial blood pressure) in dogs, coronary DO_2 is maximal (and essentially unchanged from control values) at a hematocrit of 25 percent, but is reduced to 75 percent of baseline at a hematocrit of 45 percent. Myocardial VO_2 in hemorrhagic hypotension is normal at a hematocrit of 25 percent, and reduced by 20 percent at 45 percent hematocrit. Systemic DO_2, although grossly depressed during hemorrhage, is not further diminished by a hematocrit of 25 percent, although systemic VO_2 remains about 60 percent of normal at hematocrits ranging from 25 to 45 percent. Thus, hemodilution is desirable, if not mandatory, for maintenance of myocardial VO_2 during hemorrhagic hypotension and its immediate aftermath, provided the coronary circulation is normal.

Thus, a hematocrit of approximately 20 percent may be acceptable in a stable young patient with multiple pelvic fractures, and selected patients may tolerate well a hematocrit below 20 percent if normovolemia is maintained. Such a scenario is plausible during some types of elective general surgery. However, such management is probably not prudent in an elderly patient (with presumed coronary disease) who has the same injuries, or is even undergoing the same major elective operation. For the latter patient, a hematocrit of 27 to 30 percent may be desirable. For a patient with a critical disorder of oxygen transport, such as acute respiratory distress syndrome, maintenance of hematocrit near an "optimal" level (i.e., 30%) is highly desirable. However, slavish adherence to a particular level of hematocrit throughout the perioperative period is naive, as clinical circumstances will change with time after the insult and through the period of aftercare.

The Blood Donation Protocol

Although any voluntary donation of blood is a precious gift, allogeneic transfusion for a specific patient (directed donation) is a controversial practice. Current evidence suggests that directed blood transfusions are no safer than transfusions from anonymous volunteer donors. Offers of designated blood donations should be referred to the local blood bank. In contrast, donation of autologous blood is to be strongly encouraged in select circumstances where the likelihood of transfusion is real, as it is safest, adds to overall blood supplies, and reinforces conservative transfusion practices owing to its scarcity as a resource. Acute preoperative hemodilution with reinfusion and perioperative autologous blood salvage ("cell saver") techniques are autologous transfusion practices in essence. However, from the standpoint of patient preparation for elective surgery, preoperative autologous blood donation has become extremely popular. Such a strategy, employed rationally, can decrease the likelihood of allogeneic transfusion by up to 80 percent in elective surgery requiring the transfusion of blood. Successful donation of the requested number of units of blood, based on established maximal surgical blood-ordering schedules maintained by the blood bank, makes allogeneic transfusion significantly less likely, and therefore attention to the mechanics of the donation process is important.

Patients who are not anemic (hematocrit ≥40%) can donate approximately one unit of blood per week, although the final donation can be as little as 3 days before surgery. Anticipated major elective orthopedic or cardiac surgery, for which 4 to 6 units of blood must be provided beforehand in order to indemnify the need for allogeneic blood, therefore requires substantial advance planning. Anemic pa-

tients are less likely to complete the scheduled donations, and more likely to receive allogeneic blood, and therefore may benefit from aggressive and innovative blood procurement strategies. All autotransfusion candidates require a screening hematocrit, and we place all patients accepted by the blood bank on oral iron supplementation (325 mg po tid) before the first scheduled donation. Concomitant ingestion of 500 mg vitamin C with each dose of iron optimizes absorption of iron from the duodenum. A unit of blood can usually be collected twice a week as long as the hematocrit is 33 percent or greater.

Although the overall physiologic benefit of preoperative autologous donation may be partly due to the hemodilution effect, it is primarily a result of the degree to which the patient's bone marrow is stimulated to increase erythropoiesis. Studies in humans indicate that the endogenous erythropoietin response is submaximal in response to the typical stimulus presented by autologous donation. Administration of recombinant human erythropoietin (rHuEPO) has been shown to facilitate collection of blood from patients scheduled to undergo major elective orthopedic surgery. Basal red blood cell production was increased 67 to 100 percent by standard autologous donation schedules, whereas the addition of rHuEPO increased basal red blood cell production rates by approximately 150 percent, or the equivalent of about 2 additional units of blood over a typical donation period. Large-scale clinical trials are under way to define the role of rHuEPO in autologous donation programs for many types of operations. Open questions regarding the efficacy and appropriateness of rHuEPO for this indication include the potential negative impact of iron deficiency on the maximal response to hormone therapy (which may not be prevented even by oral iron supplementation). Optimal dose, route, and timing of administration have yet to be established in the surgical setting. Cost-effectiveness at current prices for rHuEPO will be difficult to justify, as the cost of procurement of one unit of blood is increased approximately 10-fold by the cost of the drug. Serious adverse effects, including a possible relationship with thromboembolic events speculated to be related to increased blood viscosity, also make this approach investigational at the present time.

The desirable avoidance of allogeneic transfusion must be balanced against procurement costs and wastage. A recent survey of autologous blood programs at 612 hospitals, in which blood-ordering practice was based on a maximal blood-ordering schedule designed to meet the needs of 90 percent of patients undergoing elective surgery, found that 9 percent of autologous blood donors subsequently required an allogeneic transfusion. Moreover, 40 to 50 percent of units collected autologously were discarded, because 24 percent of collected units were reserved for procedures in which the transfusion likelihood was less than 10 percent. A program of prioritization in which autologous donations are discouraged in anticipation of surgery with a "low" risk (<5%) of transfusion (Table 2-11), combined with release of autologous units to the volunteer donor pool once potential need has been eliminated, can ensure maximal cost-effectiveness. Enlightened individual and institutional transfusion policies are also important. Published guidelines suggest the same criteria for autologous and allogeneic transfusions, beause the leading causes of acute transfusion reactions, accounting for more than 50 percent of acute transfusion-related mortality, are administrative error and bacterial contamination. Neither is eliminated as a potential problem by an autologous blood transfusion. A unit of autologous blood should not be infused simply because it is available.

Table 2-11. Selected Surgical Procedures and Likelihood of Blood Transfusion

LOW (< %) RISK; NO LIKELY BENEFIT FROM PREOPERATIVE AUTOLOGOUS DONATION
Childbirth
  Cesarean section
  Vaginal
Cholecystectomy
Transurethral prostatectomy
Vaginal hysterectomy

HIGH (>5%) RISK; LIKELY BENEFIT FROM PREOPERATIVE AUTOLOGOUS DONATION
Abdominal hysterectomy
Cardiac surgery
Colorectal surgery
Craniotomy
Mastectomy
Radical prostatectomy
Spinal surgery
Total joint replacement
Vascular graft surgery

Preoperative Management of Therapeutic Anticoagulation

It is often necessary to perform both elective and emergency surgery on a therapeutically anticoagulated patient. In such circumstances it is usually desirable to reverse temporarily the patient's anticoagulation so that hemostasis can be optimized, although vast experience with vascular and cardiac operations shows that good hemostasis can be achieved in patients who undergo surgery while anticoagulated. Procoagulant therapy may sometimes obviate the need for surgery by cessation of bleeding in some patients, such as those with a gastrointestinal hemorrhage. The usual clinical circumstance requiring perioperative anticoagulant management has historically been the need for surgery in a patient with a metal prosthetic heart valve, but the problem will become increasingly commonplace now that the indications for chronic warfarin anticoagulation are expanding to include diseases such as chronic atrial fibrillation. As with many other facets of preoperative preparation, the approach can be individualized based on the urgency and magnitude of the surgery to be performed, and the firmness of the indication for anticoagulant therapy.

Most patients who take warfarin and who are to undergo ambulatory or same-day admission elective surgery can be managed simply by having them hold their warfarin 2 or 3 days before surgery. Most such patients are on a stable dose of warfarin and are sophisticated regarding their medication and diet because of the need for frequent monitoring of their level of anticoagulation. The timing of the medication adjustment depends on the degree of anticoagulation determined by preoperative testing, which in turn depends on the indication for the anticoagulation. For example, a patient with a valve prosthesis can be maintained at an international normalized ratio (INR—a term that is now used widely to compensate for the wide variation of the normal range of PT among clinical laboratories) of 2.0 to 2.5, whereas a patient receiving short-term treatment for thrombophlebitis can be maintained at an INR of 1.5 to 2.0. The goal is to have the PT within 2 seconds of the control value at the time of surgery. A reduction of the PT of 2 seconds per day may reasonably be expected just from holding warfarin. Only the occasional patient will require fresh frozen plasma to prepare for minor surgery, but even then, arrangements for transfusion in the preoperative holding area can usually avoid the need for hospitalization. Avoidance of a plasma transfusion is desirable not only for reasons of infection control and the possibility of a reaction, but because those patients who receive plasma will be more difficult to re-anticoagulate after surgery. However, that difficulty is much less than if anticoagulation is reversed with vitamin K, which should be avoided. Patients who are not reversed actively can be re-anticoagulated over a period of a few days using oral warfarin only, with a 10-mg dose given the evening of surgery followed by resumption of the maintenance dose beginning the next day. The risk of postoperative bleeding is negligible. Heparinization (which requires hospitalization) is an alternative for those cases where warfarin therapy is known to be difficult to manage, when even a brief period of subtherapeutic anticoagulation is deemed hazardous, or when the patient is already hospitalized. The heparin infusion is discontinued approximately 4 hours preoperatively (the half-life of heparin is about 90 minutes), and surgery proceeds with good hemostasis.

In most circumstances, there is probably less urgency for re-anticoagulation than is generally appreciated. Protection of a cardiac valve prosthesis is the most urgent indication, but a metallic valve can be left without anticoagulation for at least 72 hours and perhaps as long as one week, although such a long interval is seldom necessary, if ever. High-risk patients or those who will be unable to take warfarin by mouth for several days can be heparinized with safety as few as 12 hours after almost any operation where operative hemostasis was secure, except neurosurgical procedures and some operations for major trauma.

There are very few indications for active preoperative reversal of heparin with protamine sulfate, as simply stopping the heparin almost always suffices. Moreover, protamine is difficult to dose, causes allergic reactions and vasodilation, and may cause bleeding if given to excess. Protamine sulfate, 1 mg, will reverse 100 units of heparin, but the half-life of the heparin must be taken into account and coagulation must be monitored closely. One-half of the estimated remaining active heparin is generally reversed. Thus, 50 mg protamine sulfate, given no more rapidly than 5 mg per minute, would be appropriate to reverse a 10,000-unit intravenous bolus of heparin given 30 minutes earlier.

Correction of Nutritional Abnormalities

Protein-calorie malnutrition is a common problem in hospitalized medical and surgical patients. Several studies have shown that from 30 to 50 percent of hospitalized patients suffer from moderate to severe malnutrition as a result of their primary disease or of the diagnostic and therapeutic regimens employed in the management of their primary disease. Protein-calorie malnutrition is generally a result of decreased oral intake, increased enteral losses secondary to malabsorption or intestinal fistula, or increased nutritional requirements secondary to hypermetabolism caused by major burns, sepsis, or multiple trauma. All too often a "vicious circle" occurs in which the patient's primary disease leads to malnutrition, which results in impaired wound healing, reduced immunocompetence, anemia, decreased resistance to infection, generalized sepsis, and further malnutrition. The end result may be multiple organ failure and death.

Successful interruption of this circle requires a comprehensive knowledge of body composition and energy requirements, quantitative nutritional assessment techniques, and current methods of enteral and parenteral nutrition support. Although nutritional assessment and therapy represent an essential part of the preparation of select surgical patients (Table 2-12), the reader is invited to look elsewhere in this volume for detailed discussions of assessment techniques and both parenteral and enteral therapy.

Antimicrobial Prophylaxis

Surgery unquestionably induces systemic and local changes in immune function, including suppression of neutrophil function. Some procedures produce greater de-

Table 2-12. Indications for Nutritional Assessment

Patient Unable to Eat	Patient Unwilling to Eat	Patient Unable to Eat Enough	Patient with Specific Nutritional Requirements
Difficulties in swallowing	Anorexia secondary to malignancy, depression, chronic illness	Increased nutritional requirements: severe catabolism secondary to burns, sepsis, multiple trauma	Cardiac failure
Cancer of mouth pharynx, larynx, or esophagus	Anorexia nervosa	Impaired digestion and absorption, short-gut syndrome	Renal failure
Trauma to mouth or throat	Xerostomia		Liver failure
Radiation effects, stomatitis, enteritis	Radiation effects, stomatitis, enteritis, intestinal stricture		
Stupor or coma, stroke, or paralysis	Chemotherapy effects, stomatitis mucositis, enteritis		
Oropharyngeal or esophageal stricture	Acute or chronic inflammatory bowel disease		
Esophageal achalasia	Hyperemesis gravidarum		
Upper gastrointestinal tract fistulas or obstruction			

rangements than others. For example, in cardiac surgery, exposure to hypothermia, bypass, and hypoperfusion can each contribute to increased risk of infection. However, even operations of moderate complexity, such as abdominal hysterectomy, produce measurable immune deficits. After hysterectomy, bacterial killing by neutrophils is reduced by about 25 percent and may take as long as 10 days to recover.

The interaction between bacteria inoculated into the surgical wound and prophylactic antibiotic administration is a critical determinant of the fate of the wound. The efficacy of perioperative antibiotic prophylaxis after many surgical procedures is unquestioned. Marked reductions in wound infection rates have been documented over the past 30 years for a host of surgical procedures, including many procedures considered "clean" (no transection or disease-related disruption of an aerodigestive or genitourinary tract structure). Rational and cost-effective antimicrobial prophylaxis incorporates decisions about whether to treat, the potential pathogens of concern, the timing of the first dose, the duration of the prophylaxis, the type of operation and the potential for bacterial

contamination of the operative field or hemorrhage during surgery, the potential need for an intraoperative dose of antibiotics during long operations, and an effective postoperative wound surveillance program. However, rational antibiotic use is but one important aspect in an effective strategy for the prevention of postoperative infection (Table 2-13).

Most prophylaxis regimens are designed to reduce the risk of surgical wound infection, or infection of prosthetic materials such as vascular grafts, introduced to the patient through the wound. Nonwound nosocomial infections, especially pneumonia and vascular catheter-related infections, are increasingly important in surgical patients, but beside the point in wound prophylaxis. Prophylaxis of endocarditis, with appreciation of the role of enterococci and viridans streptococci, is another special consideration (Table 2-14). Gram-positive infections, most notably due to staphylococci, are the most important consideration in surgery upon the soft tissues, whereas aerobic gram-negative or anaerobic pathogens are of potential importance in surgery of the visceral organs. The cephalosporins are the drugs of choice

for prophylaxis of the vast majority of operative procedures for which antibiotics are of benefit (Table 2-15), based on antibacterial spectrum, safety, and low cost. Because of these features and a relatively long half-life, cefazolin has been the dominant choice for both "clean" and "clean-contaminated" operations, the latter including hysterectomy, high-risk cholecystectomy, and high-risk gastrectomy among many others. Second-generation cephalosporins are appropriate prophylactic agents for colorectal surgery (including appendectomy) and abdominal trauma, among a narrow list of indications. Third-generation agents are expensive, no more effective, and promote the emergence of resistant bacteria. There is no rationale whatsoever for their use as prophylactic agents.

Examples of "clean" operations for which antibiotic prophylaxis is of benefit include open heart operations, operations on the aorta or vessels in the groin (regardless of the type of vascular graft to be used, if any), and open reduction of closed fractures. Although one multicenter study published by Platt and associates provides data to justify antibiotic prophylaxis in clean groin hernia and breast operations, the study has been criticized for a higher than expected incidence of wound and urinary tract infections in the control group and for a small sample size, and the conclusions are not widely accepted as representing a new standard of practice. In-

Table 2-13. Preoperative Maneuvers of Proved or Theoretical Benefit for the Prevention of Surgical Wound Infection

REDUCTION OF WOUND INOCULATION WITH VIRULENT BACTERIA
Minimize preoperative antibiotic therapy
Minimize preoperative hospitalization
Eliminate nasal colonization of *Staphyloccus aureus*
Treat remote sites of infection
Avoid shaving the operative field, or delay until the operating room
Shower or bathe preoperatively with chlorhexidine-containing soap

IMPROVEMENT OF PATIENT'S HOST DEFENSES
Resolve malnutrition or obesity
Discontinue cigarette smoking
Maximize diabetes control
Minimize glucocorticoid dosage
Avoid hypoxemia
Avoid operation through previously (more than several weeks) irradiated tissue

Table 2-14. Indications and Antibiotic Choices for Prophylaxis of Endocarditis

INDICATIONS

Cardiac
   Prosthetic cardiac valves (all types)
   Congenital anomalies
   Surgical pulmonary-systemic shunts
   Valvular stenosis or insufficiency
   Mitral valve prolapse
   Asymmetric septal hypertrophy (idiopathic hypertrophic subaortic stenosis)
   Previous endocarditis

Vascular
   Synthetic vascular grafts

PROCEDURES (IN ADDITION TO THOSE LISTED IN TABLE 2-15)

Dental-oral-pharyngeal
   Any procedure causing bleeding or incision of the mucosa

Thoracic
   Bronchoscopy
   Incision and drainage of infection

Urologic
   Presence of infected urine

Gastrointestinal
   Incision of mucosa
   Endoscopy

ANTIBIOTICS

Drugs of Choice	Penicillin Allergy
Ampicillin, 2 g IV/IM, plus Gentamicin, 1.5 mg/kg IV/IM 30 min preoperatively	Vancomycin, 1 g IV, plus Gentamicin, 1.5 mg/kg IV/IM 1 hr preoperatively
followed by	
Amoxicillin, 1.5 g po 6 hr later, or the above regimen 8 hr later	Repeat of the above regimen 8 hr later

fection from implanted pacemakers or vascular catheters for nutrition or dialysis usually occurs for technical reasons, but can cause major morbidity despite being "clean" procedures. There are no data available to support antibiotic use, but prophylaxis based on local factors and the surgeon's judgment is difficult to criticize.

Animal studies indicate clearly that antibiotic prophylaxis is most effective when the antibiotic is present in tissue before the bacteria are inoculated (i.e., the skin incision is made). Antibiotics are ineffective when administration is delayed for 3 hours, and effectiveness is intermediate when antibiotics are administered within that interval. Administration is ideally complete, or at least under way, when the patient arrives in the operating room. The half-life of cefazolin is sufficiently long that bactericidal tissue levels are still present at incision when the drug is given up to one hour beforehand, affording great flexibility in scheduling. Such flexibility is

necessary now that many operations requiring antibiotic prophylaxis are performed on an ambulatory or same-day admission basis, and an order for administration of antibiotics "on call to the operating room" may afford insufficient time.

Vancomycin is a very popular alternative for surgical prophylaxis against gram-positive bacteria, but its general use must be discouraged. Primary prophylaxis with vancomycin (i.e., for the non–penicillin-allergic patient) may be appropriate for cardiac valve replacement, placement of a nontissue peripheral vascular prosthesis, or total joint replacement in institutions where a high rate of infections with methicillin-resistant *Staphylococcus aureus* or *Staphylococcus epidermidis* is prevalent. A single dose administered immediately before surgery is sufficient unless the operation lasts for more than 6 hours, in which case the dose should be repeated. Prophylaxis should be discontinued after a maxi-

mum of two doses. Too often, vancomycin is prescribed for every patient with a history of a penicillin allergy. In our opinion, such a nonrestrictive policy represents but one of many examples of overuse (Table 2-16). The incidence of clinically important cross reactivity for penicillin allergy with the cephalosporins is less than 10 percent, so that patients who report only a prior maculopapular rash due to penicillin can receive a cephalosporin with safety. Vancomycin is cumbersome to use as a prophylactic agent because a slow infusion rate is necessary to avoid the possibility of marked hypotension or even cardiac arrest. A minimum of one hour is required for the safe infusion of a 1-g dose of vancomycin. Overuse, besides the expense, has led to the emergence of vancomycin-resistant enterococci in many centers. These pathogens are very difficult to treat, and raise concern regarding the possibility that vancomycin-resistant staphylococci may emerge.

Current trends are toward a very limited duration of prophylaxis. Regimens consisting of only a single preoperative dose of antibiotic appear to be as effective as a longer regimen. A second dose may be beneficial after 3 to 4 hours (1–2 half-lives of the drug used) if the operation lasts longer. No data exist to support prophylactic use beyond that point, although many surgeons still prefer to continue the regimen for 24 hours. Regimens that extend beyond 24 hours are unsupportable. In particular, there is no rationale for longer courses of antibiotics because an operation was subjectively more difficult, or because of inadvertent contamination of the operative field.

Bowel Preparation

The patient is protected from a huge reservoir of pathogenic aerobic and anaerobic bacteria present in the colon and distal small intestine by a mucosal membrane. Surgical disruption of the barrier may cause the escape of these pathogens into the peritoneal cavity and the potential for serious infection. Safe elective surgery on these organs was not possible until regimens for reductions of bacterial count and activity were introduced. Results of numerous clinical trials have shown clearly that such reductions must include both mechanical cleansing of the bowel to eliminate bulk feces and reduce bacterial

Table 2-15. Appropriate Cephalosporin Prophylaxis for Selected Operations

Operation	Alternative Prophylaxis in Serious Penicillin Allergy
FIRST GENERATION (I.E., CEFAZOLIN)	
Cardiovascular and thoracic	
Median sternotomy	Vancomycin (for all cases herein)[a]
Pacemaker insertion	
Peripheral vascular reconstruction (except carotid endarterectomy)	
Pulmonary resection	
General	
Cholecystectomy	Gentamicin
(High risk only: age > 60, jaundice, acute, prior biliary procedure)	
Gastrectomy	Gentamicin and metronidazole
(High risk only: not uncomplicated chronic duodenal ulcer)	
Hepatobiliary	Gentamicin and metronidazole
Gynecologic	
Cesarean section (STAT)	Metronidazole (after cord clamping)
Hysterectomy	Doxycycline
Head and neck/oral cavity	
Major procedures	Gentamicin and clindamycin
Neurosurgery	
Craniotomy	Clindamycin, vancomycin
Orthopedics	
Major joint arthroplasty	Vancomycin[a]
Open reduction of closed fracture	Vancomycin
SECOND GENERATION (I.E., CEFOXITIN)	
Lower limb amputation	Gentamicin and metronidazole (for all cases herein)
Appendectomy	Metronidazole with or without gentamicin
Colon surgery[b]	
Surgery for penetrating abdominal trauma	

[a]Primary prophylaxis with vancomycin (i.e., for the non–pencillin-allergic patient) may be appropriate for cardiac valve replacement, placement of a nontissue peripheral vascular prosthesis, or total joint replacement in institutions where a high rate of infections with methicillin-resistant *Staphylococcus aureus* or *Staphylococcus epidermidis* has occurred. A single dose administered immediately before surgery is sufficient unless operation lasts for more than 6 hr, in which case the dose should be repeated. Prophylaxis should be discontinued after a maximum of two doses.
[b]Benefit beyond that provided by bowel preparation with mechanical cleansing and oral neomycin and erythromycin base is debatable.

Table 2-16. Situations in Which the Use of Vancomycin Is Discouraged

Routine surgical prophylaxis in the absence of life-threatening allergy to beta-lactam antibiotics
Empiric therapy of febrile neutropenia in the absence of evidence for a gram-positive infection
Continued empiric use when microbiologic data suggest a reasonable alternative
Systemic or local (i.e., catheter flush) prophylaxis of indwelling vascular catheters
Selective decontamination of the digestive tract
Eradication of colonization of methicillin-resistant staphylococci
Primary treatment of antibiotic-associated colitis due to *Clostridium difficile*
Routine prophylaxis for patients receiving hemodialysis or continuous ambulatory peritoneal dialysis
Use for topical irrigation or application

Table 2-17. Options for Mechanical and Antibiotic Bowel Preparation

MECHANICAL CLEANING
Diet
  Clear liquid diet, or
  Low-residue diet
Cathartics
  Magnesium sulfate, 30 ml, of 50% solution × 3, or
  Magnesium citrate, 240 ml, or
  Whole-gut lavage with electrolyte–polyethylene glycol solution, or
  Fleet Phospho-Soda
Enemas
  None (with whole-gut lavage)
  Fleet Enema
  Tap water or soapsuds enema, for inpatients

ANTIBIOTICS
  Neomycin, 1 g po, at 1 PM, 2 PM, and 11 PM
  Erythromycin base, 1 g po, at 1 PM, 2 PM, and 11 PM
  Metronidazole (can be substituted for erythromycin)
  Second-generation cephalosporin, 1 g IV just before incision (optional)
  Gentamicin and clindamycin or metronidazole, or doxycycline (can be substituted for the cephalosporin)

counts, and administration of antibiotics that act against both aerobic gram-negative bacilli and anaerobic bacteria. The optimal manner to accomplish this universally accepted goal remains a matter of debate, and of preference (Table 2-17).

Mechanical cleaning reduces residual fecal mass, facilitating operative manipulation of the bowel and enhancing the effect of the antibiotics, but alone does not reduce bacterial counts in the residual feces. Mechanical regimens vary, and include more leisurely regimens of dietary restriction, cathartics, and enemas, or more rapid cleaning with whole-gut lavage techniques. The regimens are not necessarily

exclusive, and can be employed in various combinations.

There is even less consensus about the best route and timing of antibiotic administration for bowel preparation. Both oral and parenteral administration have their devotees. Oral administration of neomycin and erythromycin base, introduced in 1972, is the most common regimen in use. The timing of administration appears to be critical for efficacy. It is recommended that 1 g each of neomycin and erythromycin base should be administered orally at 1 PM, 2 PM, and 11 PM of the day before surgery if the operation is scheduled for 8 AM the following day, so that nadir bacterial

counts will coincide with the beginning of surgery. A later operation requires commensurate adjustment in the schedule of administration. More than three doses of antibiotics are unwarranted, and have been shown to produce resistant flora. Recent data suggest that metronidazole can be substituted for erythromycin with equal efficacy. As metronidazole is readily absorbed for the proximal small intestine, it appears that oral antibiotics are effective for reasons other than high intraluminal concentrations at the time of surgery (it remains true that oral neomycin is not appreciably absorbed). Parenteral antibiotics that are effective in bowel preparation for elective colon resection include second-generation cephalosporins, metronidazole, and doxycycline, either alone or in combination with an aminoglycoside. Data are emerging to support mechanical preparation along with a single parenteral dose as effective prophylaxis. Although it is commonplace to combine oral and intravenous antibiotic prophylaxis with the mechanical regimen, few data exist to show enhancement of benefit. If combined routes are chosen, a single dose of parenteral antibiotic is sufficient. The theoretical benefit of the parenteral antibiotic is as a "fail-safe" mechanism when the oral antibiotics are mistimed, or the operation is delayed unexpectedly.

Bowel preparation regimens are changing with the changing times as well. Gone is the era when patients could be admitted to the hospital for complete bowel preparation. Now, some of the mechanical preparation must begin before the patient is admitted, if the patient can be admitted before the day of surgery at all. Even if a hospital bed is available for such purposes, the likelihood is small of admission in the morning or even at a time predictable in advance. Hospital beds sometimes become available with very short notice if hospital census is managed aggressively. The temporal precision necessary for the neomycin-erythromycin regimen may be difficult to achieve. The effectiveness of the oral antibiotic regimen has not been tested with current methods of whole-gut lavage now employed, where the patient rapidly ingests a 4-liter aliquot of a balanced electrolyte–polyethylene glycol solution, and diarrhea until the effluent is clear is the goal. Starting the lavage before admission may produce the unpleasantness of loose stools during the trip to the hospital. Starting coincident with oral antibiotic administration may wash out the antibiotic with a less-than-desired effect. Starting the lavage after an afternoon admission may result in an inadequate clearance of feces if the patient cannot ingest the entire amount or can take it only slowly (e.g., cramps

from lavage in the presence of a partially obstructing lesion, fluid overload in an elderly patient with heart disease) or a patient who must remain in the bathroom for much of the evening. We prefer to perform whole-gut lavage in the hospital, because dehydration is another short-term problem and we usually administer a maintenance infusion of balanced salt solution (Ringer's lactate) during the lavage unless contraindicated by the patient's cardiovascular status. However, lavage can also be performed in the outpatient setting in many healthy patients. Given these many confounding variables, we have adopted a bowel preparation regimen for elective colon surgery that incorporates dietary changes and cathartics or whole-gut lavage on the day before surgery (whether in the hospital or at home, prior to admission) and a perioperative dose of cefoxitin (Table 2-18).

Bowel preparation before emergency surgery is often impossible. The many conditions that may indicate an emergency colectomy, including hemorrhage, obstruction, perforation, ischemia, or trauma, may actually represent contraindications to mechanical preparation. Since oral antibiotics are ineffective without mechanical preparation, parenteral antibiot-

Table 2-18. Author's Regimen for Outpatient* Bowel Preparation for Elective Colon Surgery

DAY MINUS 3
Last full meal at dinnertime

DAY MINUS 2
Clear liquid diet ad libitum, unless the patient is on a medical fluid restriction
Magnesium citrate, 240 ml po, after breakfast

DAY MINUS 1
Clear liquid diet ad libitum, unless the patient is on a medical fluid restriction
Electrolyte-polyethylene glycol solution, 4 L po after breakfast
Neomycin and erythromycin base, 1 g each po, at 1 PM, 2 PM, and 11 PM

DAY 0
Cefoxitin, 1 g IV at 7:30 AM
Skin incision for colectomy at 8 AM
Cefoxitin, 1 g IV 4 hr after completion of the first infusion, if the patient is still undergoing surgery

*If admission is arranged for the day before surgery, whole-gut lavage can be performed either at home or after admission. If lavage is delayed until the afternoon or evening, oral antibiotics can be omitted, as efficacy cannot be assured.

ics become the only option. The choice can be made from among those antibiotics suitable for prophylaxis in elective surgery. Most surgeons would continue parenteral antibiotics for a 24-hour period in this circumstance. Of course, with any prophylactic regimen the indication for antibiotics may change based on the intraoperative identification of infection (e.g., unexpected identification of a perforated viscus), and the distinction between prophylaxis and an appropriate longer course of therapy can be made. Intraoperative lavage of the colon may be appropriate in some emergency circumstances. Many techniques have been described. One convenient technique is the introduction of a Foley urinary catheter into the terminal ileum, or the cecum via the appendiceal stump. When inserted via the ileum, the catheter is positioned so that the ileocecal valve is occluded by the balloon, and the colon is irrigated with 8 to 10 liters of saline for uniform cleaning of the unprepared colon.

Mechanical bowel preparation without oral antibiotics may be elected in preparation for elective noncolonic abdominal surgery. Such preparation facilitates operative manipulation of the colon, may hasten the return of gastrointestinal function after surgery, and may decrease the risk of an inadvertent enterotomy during reoperative abdominal surgery (e.g., repair of an abdominal aortic aneurysm in a patient with a history of an abdominal operation in the past). Preparation in this setting currently usually involves only whole-gut lavage, and not all surgeons embrace the concept.

Endocrine Preparation

Acute derangements of endocrine function pose markedly increased risk in seriously ill patients. Such derangements are usually imposed upon an already unstable patient, and widely variable clinical manifestations may obscure and delay the diagnosis. One endocrinopathy may precipitate a second syndrome, which may be manifested concurrently (e.g., precipitation of thyroid storm by diabetic ketoacidosis [DKA]). Moreover, laboratory tests may be difficult to interpret in critical illness, while emergency therapy may be necessary before test results become available.

Thyroid Storm

Thyroid storm may be precipitated in patients with underlying hyperthyroidism of virtually any cause. Reported precipitants include burns, DKA, hyperglycemic hyperosmolar nonketotic coma (HHNC), hypoglycemia, iodinated radiocontrast agents, pulmonary embolism, sepsis syndrome, major surgery, trauma, and vascular accidents including visceral organ infarction. Clinical manifestations are those of adrenergic hyperactivity. Fever, confusion or agitation, and tachycardia or widened pulse pressure are usually appreciable; seizures, diarrhea, nausea or vomiting, abdominal pain, and congestive heart failure may sometimes develop. Rapid atrial fibrillation is common in elderly patients. The differential diagnosis includes intoxication with anticholinergic or adrenergic agents, malignant hyperthermia syndrome, pheochromocytoma crisis, and sepsis. As the diagnosis of thyroid storm constitutes a true emergency, therapy must begin before the diagnosis is secure. Standard thyroid function tests, elevated in both disorders, do not distinguish storm from uncomplicated thyrotoxicosis.

Treatment of thyroid storm prevents the peripheral tissue effects of thyroid hormone, inhibits tri-iodothyronine (T_3) production from thyroxine (T_4), treats the precipitating or concurrent factors, and provides general supportive care. Beta-adrenergic blockade with propranolol (40–80 mg po q6h or 1–2 mg IV q15min until heart rate is controlled) is central to therapy, and attenuates fever, tachycardia, dysrhythmias, anxiety, and agitation. Patients with congestive heart failure should receive digitalis and either a cardioselective beta blocker such as atenolol or the ultra–short-acting nonselective agent, esmolol, by continuous infusion. Iodine preparations prevent the release of preformed T_3 or T_4 from colloid stores. Propylthiouracil (PTU), 150 mg po/ng q6h, must be begun one hour before iodine administration to prevent organification of the iodine. Ipodate (Orograffin), 500 to 1000 mg po every day, is useful when PTU is contraindicated (severe hepatic disease), as it both decreases secretion of preformed hormone and prevents peripheral conversion of T_4 to T_3 (as does PTU). Dexamethasone, 2 mg IV q6h, also prevents peripheral conversion to T_3 and may be indicated in those patients in whom coexistent adrenal insufficiency is suspected. Salicylates are contraindicated for antipyresis because levels of free thyroid hormone are increased.

Hypercalcemia

Hypercalcemic crisis is an unusual manifestation of hypercalcemia, and constitutes an emergency. Elevated serum levels of calcium combine with marked volume depletion to produce malaise, weakness, prerenal azotemia, and eventual obtundation or coma. Documentation of weakness and obtundation with an elevated serum calcium (>13.0 mg/dl) is sufficient for the diagnosis. Malignant disease is the most common cause of hypercalcemic disease, and may be associated with both lymphoid tumors and metastatic bone disease. Tumors and primary hyperparathyroidism account for 90 percent of all cases of hypercalcemia, but the latter is an unusual cause of hypercalcemia crisis. Hypercalcemia may produce many other signs and symptoms in addition to those associated with crisis. Confusion, headaches, gait disturbance, hypothermia, hyporeflexia, nausea, vomiting, anorexia, constipation, diarrhea, abdominal pain, thirst, polyuria, and musculoskeletal pain are all potential manifestations. Proteinuria, hypokalemia, hypomagnesemia, and hypernatremia may be present, as may a shortened electrocardiographic Q-T interval and various dysrhythmias.

Whenever an obtunded patient presents with a suspected endocrinopathy, a broad panel of blood work (glucose, renal function tests, calcium, thyroid-stimulating hormone [TSH], T_4, cortisol, adrenocorticotropic hormone [ACTH], albumin, total protein, and electrolytes) is obtained. Vigorous hydration with 0.9% NaCl is begun. Confirmation of hypercalcemia indicates continued aggressive fluid repletion with the addition of potassium and magnesium if indicated and if renal function will allow. Calcium should not be present in the intravenous fluids, and therefore lactated Ringer's solution should be avoided. If the patient is making urine after 2 hours of fluid and electrolyte repletion, a vigorous calciuresis is induced with a large (100–200 mg IV) dose of furosemide. Both hemodialysis and peritoneal dialysis offer a rapid means to remove calcium in patients who are intolerant of large volumes of saline solution. Once the elevated serum calcium level has been reduced, chronic therapy is directed toward reduction of calcium reabsorption from bone while the primary problem is also corrected. Pharmacologic agents effective against bone reabsorption include plicamycin, calcitonin, corticosteroids, diphosphonates, and gallium nitrate.

Complications of Diabetes Mellitus

It is advisable to achieve good control of diabetes in all preoperative patients, so as to minimize the potential for postoperative infection from the immunocompromised state. However, many conditions that require urgent or emergency surgery can precipitate a diabetic emergency. The most severe manifestation of insulin deficiency is ketoacidosis (DKA).

Diabetic Ketoacidosis

Insulin deficiency and a synergistic increase in "stress" hormone (epinephrine, cortisol, glucagon) secretion produce a volume-depleted, acidemic, hyperglycemic, and ketonemic state with severe electrolyte abnormalities. Acutely decompensated type 1 diabetes mellitus is the most common underlying problem, and the cause of the destabilization is usually infection. Frequently, DKA is the presenting manifestation of previously undiagnosed diabetes. Other precipitants may include pregnancy, acute myocardial infarction, trauma, acute psychiatric illness, or major surgery. Endocrine precipitants include thyrotoxicosis and pheochromocytoma.

The massive hyperglycemia is due primarily to accelerated gluconeogenesis in the face of reduced peripheral glucose utilization and catabolism of lean tissue and lipid stores. Serum hyperosmolarity precipitates an osmotic diuresis with subsequent volume depletion and paradoxical dilutional hyponatremia. Ketonemia results from the inability to metabolize mobilized long-chain fatty acids via lipogenic pathways.

A high index of suspicion for DKA is indicated in patients with dehydration, vomiting, tachypnea, severe abdominal pain, obtundation, or a combination of those findings. Diagnostic criteria for DKA include a blood glucose greater than 700 mg/dl, serum osmolarity greater than 340 mosm per liter, arterial pH less than 7.30 with an arterial carbon dioxide tension of 40 mm Hg or less, and ketonemia and ketonuria. The differential diagnosis includes lactic acidosis, uremia, various intoxicants (including ethanol), sepsis syndrome, cerebrovascular accident, and intra-abdominal catastrophe. Patients with HHNC by definition do not have ketonemia, although HHNC and DKA may co-exist.

Effective treatment for DKA requires simultaneous metabolic management and a meticulous search for the precipitant. An electrocardiogram must always be obtained to rule out the "silent" myocardial infarction typical of diabetic patients. Patients with DKA may have a volume deficit of up to 10 liters, and therefore vigorous fluid replacement is essential. Hypotonic saline is the treatment of choice. One liter is given in the first 30 minutes, followed by 500 to 1000 ml per hour. Shock or hyponatremia is an indication for isotonic saline. When the blood glucose decreases below 250 mg/dl, resuscitation continues with 5% dextrose in water (D5W) to prevent hypoglycemia and cerebral edema. Central hemodynamic monitoring is used as indicated.

All patients in DKA require prompt insulin treatment. After a bolus dose of 10 to 30 units, a continuous infusion of short-acting (regular) insulin, 5 to 10 units per hour, is effective and safe if monitored closely. Higher doses carry a greater risk of hypokalemia and hypoglycemia. If close monitoring of blood glucose shows that glucose has not decreased by 30 percent or more within 4 hours or by at least 50 percent within 8 hours, the insulin dosage should be doubled. Once blood glucose decreases to 250 mg/dl, the continuous infusion is discontinued and subcutaneous doses of short-acting insulin are substituted. Longer-acting insulin preparations should not be used until the patient's condition has stabilized and he or she can take fluids by mouth. However, persistent ketonemia despite lowered plasma glucose is an indication for continued intravenous insulin.

Bicarbonate therapy in DKA is seldom necessary, because metabolism of acetoacetate and beta-hydroxybutyrate generates HCO_3. Indications for bicarbonate therapy in DKA include arterial pH below 7.1, HCO_3 level below 10 meq/dl, or to re-lieve the discomfort of Kussmaul's respirations. If indicated, 100 meq of $NaHCO_3$ can be added to the first liter of saline. In contrast, potassium supplementation is invariably required. Ketonuria, diuresis, and frequent vomiting can produce marked potassium depletion, which may be masked initially as intracellular stores shift to the extracellular space in response to acidosis. Correction of acidosis will unmask marked hypokalemia. Potassium chloride, 20 to 40 meq, is added to the second liter of resuscitation fluid and supplemented further as appropriate. If the patient is hypokalemic while acidemic at presentation, potassium depletion is profound and replacement (40–60 meq/liter) should begin with the first liter of resuscitation fluid.

Hyperglycemic Hyperosmolar Nonketotic Coma

Patients with HHNC present with very high blood glucose concentrations (sometimes >1000 mg/dl), depressed sensorium, marked dehydration, and prerenal azotemia. By definition, acidosis, ketonemia, and ketonuria are absent. Precipitants include many stresses typical of the surgical patient, including burns, severe infections, pancreatitis, and major surgery. Mortality appears to be higher in cases associated with sepsis or pancreatitis. Therapy with beta blockers, diazoxide, furosemide, glucocorticoids, parenteral nutrition, or thiazides may precipitate HHNC, as may hemodialysis or renal transplantation. Intake of large quantities of dextrose alone, either enterally or parenterally, may be sufficient cause.

Diabetic ketoacidosis and HHNC share two similarities: relative insulin deficiency and marked volume depletion. The diagnosis of HHNC should be suspected in the setting of marked hyperglycemia (>700 mg/dl) and azotemia without ketonemia. The serum sodium concentration may be factitiously normal in the setting of elevated blood glucose (decreased 3 meq/dl per 100 mg glucose elevation). Ketosis is absent because sufficient insulin is present to suppress lipolysis. Hyperglycemia itself suppresses lipolysis, and the stress hormone response in HHNC is modest compared to that in DKA. Changes in mental states can be related directly to the degree of hyperosmolarity. Neurologic abnormalities include lethargy, focal or generalized seizures, or coma.

As with DKA, therapy consists of rehydration, intravenous insulin, electrolyte replacement, and correction of the precipitant. Isotonic saline is the fluid of choice except for the hypernatremic patient. As much as 10 liters may be required in the first 24 hours. Potassium supplementation of up to 20 meq per hour may be necessary as well. Fluid administration is then adjusted based upon the response to resuscitation. Intravenous insulin is given as an infusion of 6 to 10 units per hour until blood glucose decreases to 250 mg/dl, when a change is also made to dextrose-containing fluid to prevent hypoglycemia and cerebral edema.

Adrenal Insufficiency

Adrenal insufficiency in critical illness may precipitate an addisonian crisis, which can be fatal. The diagnosis is difficult, however, and therapy must be instituted before the diagnosis is confirmed. Hypoglycemia can be profound. Hyperpyrexia is a common manifestation even in the absence of infection. Hypotension and hypovolemia may be due either to hypovolemia and decreased vascular tone or to the retroperitoneal (adrenal) hemorrhage that may have precipitated the syndrome. Likewise, abdominal pain may be caused either by hypocortisolism or by the hemorrhage or intra-abdominal infection that precipitated the crisis. The constellation may be difficult to distinguish from that of hypovolemic or septic shock, depending on the predominant manifestation.

The presence of coexisting endocrinopathies must be considered. Diabetes mellitus, hypothyroidism, thyrotoxicosis, and hypoparathyroidism may all be associated with adrenal insufficiency. In diabetic patients with addisonian crisis, DKA may be precipitated. Only a small minority of patients will develop symptomatic mineralocorticoid deficiency. Those that do may manifest severe hyponatremia, hyperkalemia, hypovolemia, and hypotension.

Addisonian crisis should be suspected in a patient with sudden cardiovascular collapse, especially with coexistent signs of chronic adrenal insufficiency (especially hyperpigmentation). Laboratory abnormalities include hyponatremia, hyperkalemia, hypoglycemia, prerenal azotemia, and a low plasma cortisol level. Mild hypercalcemia is unusual. An ECG may thus show low voltage with a peaked T wave and a narrow QRS complex. Measurement of plasma corticotropin is not diagnostic, but administration of cosyntropin (0.25 mg IV, with serum cortisol determinations beforehand and one hour afterward) is the procedure of choice to determine adrenal responsiveness in critically ill patients. The test can be completed in one hour, and glucocorticoid therapy (immediately) thereafter does not interfere with interpretation. Prompt therapy is mandatory. Patients already receiving steroids must have the daily dose increased to 300 mg hydrocortisone or equivalent. Severely ill patients will also require hydration and correction of a multiplicity of 300 mg hydrocortisone or equivalent. Severely ill patients will also require hydration and correction of a multiplicity of electrolyte abnormalities in addition to the search for the precipitant. In these cases, hydrocortisone usually exerts sufficient mineralocorticoid activity, making specific replacement unnecessary. Volume depletion can be profound, but is not of the magnitude seen in the hyperglycemic emergencies unless shock is present. Refractory hypotension suggests an underlying infection, or may be an indication for mineralocorticoid replacement therapy (deoxycorticosterone acetate, 2–3 mg IM, or fluorohydrocortisone, 0.1–0.2 mg po daily).

Perioperative Glucocorticoid Prophylaxis

Recognizing the danger inherent in addisonian crisis and the additional stress posed by surgery, surgeons have been quick to prescribe large doses of glucocorticoids as prophylaxis despite a paucity of supporting evidence and the knowledge that glucocorticoids impair host defenses and wound healing, among other potentially deleterious effects. This is often done not only if the patient is taking steroids currently, but also if he or she received steroids up to 6 months beforehand. Typically, hydrocortisone, 100 mg IV, is given preoperatively and every 8 hours for the first day, with tapering to the equivalent maintenance dose (or zero, as appropriate) within 72 hours thereafter. Unfortunately, such practices are based upon clinical anecdotes that are now more than 40 years old, and result in administration of glucocorticoids far in excess of physiologic rates of production. Salem and associates have argued recently that that practice is obsolete and such dosages are too high.

Perioperative adrenal insufficiency appears to be quite rare, with an incidence of 0.1 percent reported in one series of 4346 cardiac surgical procedures. Another prospective study of 40 renal allograft recipients, maintained on 5 to 10 mg prednisone per day, who were admitted for acute rejection or an operation and who did not receive supplemental steroids, had no evidence of adrenal insufficiency. All but one of the patients had normal or increased urinary cortisol concentrations, suggesting that baseline glucocorticoid therapy is sufficient to prevent adrenal insufficiency even during surgical stress. A cosyntropin stimulation test should be performed in all questioned cases.

Glucocorticoids should be administered if the diagnosis is confirmed or is possible but data are inconclusive or unavailable. Estimates of daily endogenous cortisol production rates range from 50 mg per day for minor surgery (which represents no change from baseline) to 75 to 150 mg per day in response to major surgery. Secretion rates appear to exceed 200 mg per day only rarely. There are no data to support exceeding these endogenous secretion rates with exogenous administration. Salem and associates recommend the supplemental administration of the equivalent of 25 mg hydrocortisone for minor surgical stress, such as an inguinal herniorrhaphy. For moderate surgical stress (open cholecystectomy, lower-extremity revascularization, segmental colectomy), Salem's group recommend 50 to 75 mg per day hydrocortisone equivalent for 1 to 2 days, and for major stress (pancreatic resection, esophagogastrectomy, total proctocolectomy), 100 to 150 mg per day for 2 to 3 days is recommended.

Pheochromocytoma

Aside from catecholamines, other substances reported to be secreted by pheochromocytomas include enkephalins, calcitonin, somatostatin, parathyroid hormone, and atrial natriuretic factor. Patients with pheochromocytoma are also profoundly volume depleted. Some patients may have paroxysmal hypertension or may even be normotensive if vasodilator substances act effectively against vasoconstriction. Thus, there may be marked variation in the clinical presentation. Persistent hypertension is present in 50 percent of patients. Paroxysms of hyperten-

sion, possibly accompanied by headache, dyspnea, chest or abdominal pain, dyspnea, fever, or seizures occur in as many as 75 percent of patients, including those with persistent hypertension. Rarely, newly diagnosed patients may present in a pheochromocytoma crisis characterized by marked hypertension and potentially severe end-organ damage. Even less commonly, a patient with a known pheochromocytoma may become critically ill for other reasons before resection and require management in that setting. Careful preparation is essential for safe resection, as is close intraoperative supervision. Extracellular fluid volume is restored for several days beforehand, and alpha-adrenergic blockade is instituted with phenoxybenzamine (10 mg po q8h) or phentolamine (0.5 to 1.0-mg bolus; then 1.0 mg/min by IV infusion). Postural hypotension is an indication for more fluid, less drug, or both. Propranolol is begun to manage tachyarrhythmias once alpha blockade is achieved, but not beforehand, as it could aggravate hypertension by creating unopposed alpha-adrenergic agonism.

Summary

Preoperative preparation of the patient for surgery depends on the urgency and magnitude of the procedure, the underlying pathophysiologic processes, and the age and medical condition of the patient. Safe, cost-efficient patient management will reduce postoperative derangements and enhance patient outcome.

Suggested Reading

Alford WC Jr, Meador CK, Mihalevich J, et al. Acute adrenal insufficiency following cardiac surgical procedures. *J Thorac Cardiovasc Surg* 78:489, 1979.

Amrein PC, Ellman L, Harrie WH. Aspirin-induced prolongation of bleeding time and perioperative blood loss. *JAMA* 245:1825, 1981.

Barie PS. Emerging problems in gram-positive infections in the postoperative patient. *Surg Gynecol Obstet* 177:S55, 1993.

Barie PS. Acute Respiratory Failure. In PS Barie, GT Shires (eds), *Surgical Intensive Care*. Boston, Little, Brown, 1993. Pp 227–283.

Battathiry MM, Clark OH. Endocrinopathies in the Critically Ill Patient. In PS Barie, GT Shires (eds), *Surgical Intensive Care*. Boston, Little, Brown, 1993. Pp 861–892.

Beller GA. Pharmacologic stress testing. *JAMA* 265:633, 1991.

Bromberg JS, Alfrey EJ, Barker CF, et al. Adrenal suppression and steroid supplementation in renal transplant recipients. *J Transplantation* 51:385, 1991.

Bush HL Jr. Venous Thromboembolic Disease. In PS Barie, GT Shires (eds), *Surgical Intensive Care*. Boston, Little, Brown, 1993. Pp 477–518.

Charlson ME, MacKenzie CR, Gold JP, et al. The preoperative predictors of postoperative myocardial infarction or ischemia in patients undergoing noncardiac surgery. *Ann Surg* 210:637, 1989.

Charlson ME, MacKenzie CR, Gold JP, et al. Risk for postoperative congestive heart failure. *Surg Gynecol Obstet* 172:95, 1991.

Classen DC, Evans RS, Pestotnik SL, et al. The timing of prophylactic administration of antibiotics and the risk of surgical wound infection. *N Engl J Med* 326:281, 1992.

Consensus conference. Prevention of venous thrombosis and pulmonary embolism. *JAMA* 256:744, 1986.

Dawes PJ, Davison P. Informed consent: What do patients want to known? *J R Soc Med* 87:149, 1994.

Dellinger EP, Gross PA, Barrett TL, et al. Quality standard for antimicrobial prophylaxis in surgical procedures. *Clin Infect Dis* 18:422, 1994.

Eagle KA, Bonchers CA. Cardiac risk of noncardiac surgery. *N Engl J Med* 321:1330, 1989.

Gass GD, Olsen GN. Preoperative pulmonary function testing to predict postoperative morbidity and mortality. *Chest* 89:127, 1986.

Goldman L. Cardiac risks and complications of noncardiac surgery. *Ann Intern Med* 98:504, 1983.

Goldman L. Multifactorial index of cardiac risk in noncardiac surgery: Ten-year status report. *J Cardiothor Anesth* 1:237, 1987.

Goldman L, Caldera DL, Nussbaum SR, et al. Multifactorial index of cardiac risk in noncardiac surgical procedures. *N Engl J Med* 297:845, 1977.

Goodnough LT, Bodner MS, Martin JW. Blood conservation and blood salvage. *J Intens Care Med* 9:86, 1994.

Goodnough LT, Saha P, Hirschler N, et al. Autologous blood donation in nonorthopaedic surgery as a blood conservation strategy. *Vox Sang* 63:96, 1992.

Hospital Infection Control Practices Advisory Committee (HICPAC). Recommendations for preventing the spread of vancomycin resistance. *Infect Control Hosp Epidemiol* 16:105, 1995.

Isom OW, Barie PS. Myocardial Ischemia and Infarction. In PS Barie, GT Shires (eds), *Surgical Intensive Care*. Boston: Little, Brown, 1993. Pp 535–575.

Kernodle DS, Kaiser AB. Postoperative Infections and Antimicrobial Prophylaxis. In GL Mandell, JE Bennett, R Dolin (eds), *Mandell, Douglas, and Bennett's Principles and Practice of Infectious Diseases* (4th ed). New York: Churchill Livingstone, 1994. Pp 2742–2756.

Lavelle-Jones C, Byrne DJ, Rice P, Cuschieri A. Factors affecting quality of informed consent. *Br Med J* 306:885, 1993.

Leach TA, Pastena JA, Swan KG, et al. Surgical prophylaxis for pulmonary embolism. *Am Surg* 60:292, 1994.

Lee TH, Goldman L. Cardiac Risk Assessment for Individual Patients. In MJ Breslow, CF Miller, M Rogers (eds), *Perioperative Management*. New York: Mosby, 1990. Pp 22–35.

Mangano DT. Perioperative Assessment of the Patient with Ischemic Heart Disease. In DT Mangano (ed), *Preoperative Cardiac Assessment*. Philadelphia: Lippincott, 1990. Pp 1–55.

Miller CL, Martin JL. Changes in Lung Function Following Anesthesia and Surgery. In MJ Breslow, CF Miller, M Rogers (eds), *Perioperative Management*. New York: Mosby, 1990. Pp 194–210.

Nichols RL. Bowel Preparation. In DW Wilmore, MF Brennan, AH Harken, et al (eds). *Care of the Surgical Patient*. New York: Scientific American, 1990. VI–4:1–10.

Page CP, Bohnen JMA, Fletcher JR, et al. Antimicrobial prophylaxis for surgical wounds. Guidelines for clinical care. *Arch Surg* 128:79, 1992.

Pearce AC, Jones RM. Smoking and anesthesia: Preoperative abstinence and perioperative morbidity. *Anesthesiology* 61:576, 1984.

Platt R, Zucker JR, Zaleznik DF, et al. Perioperative antibiotic prophylaxis for herniorrhaphy and breast surgery. *N Engl J med* 322:153, 1990.

Rapaport SI. Preoperative hemostatic evaluation: Which tests, if any? *Blood* 61:229, 1983.

Rogers FB, Shackford SR, Wilson J, et al. Prophylactic vena cava filter insertion in severely injured trauma patients: Indications and preliminary results. *J Trauma* 35:637, 1993.

Ruggiero JT, Barie PS. Hematologic Disease and Surgical Hemostasis. In PS Barie, GT Shires (eds), *Surgical Intensive Care*. Boston: Little, Brown, 1993. Pp 667–680.

Salem M, Tainish RE Jr, Bromberg J, et al. Perioperative glucocorticoid coverage. A reassessment 42 years after emergence of a problem. *Ann Surg* 219:416, 1994.

Suchman AC, Mashlin AI. How well does the activated partial thromboplastin time predict post-operative hemorrhage? *JAMA* 256:750, 1986.

Sue-Ling MH, Johnson D, MacMahon MJ, et al. Preoperative identification of patients at high risk of deep venous thrombosis after major elective surgery. *Lancet* 1:1173, 1986.

Tinker JH, Tarhan S. Discontinuing anticoagulant therapy in surgical patients with cardiac valve prostheses. *JAMA* 239:738, 1978.

Tisi GM. Preoperative identification and evaluation of the patient with lung disease. *Med Clin North Am* 71:399, 1987.

Van Zee KJ, Barie PS, Lowry SF. Electrolyte Disorders. In JL Cameron (ed), *Current Surgical Therapy* (4th ed). St. Louis: Mosby Year Book, 1992. Pp 1005–1023.

Weitz HH, Goldman L. Noncardiac surgery in the patient with heart disease. *Med Clin North Am* 71:413, 1987.

EDITOR'S COMMENT

Doctors Barie, Dudrick, and Daly have presented an excellent and comprehensive approach to the perioperative preparation of patients. Surgery is details, and the more attention to detail, the better the patient generally does. As with any complicated approach to surgery, everyone develops his or her own system.

As others have emphasized in this volume, the functional status of the patient is most important. This is particularly true of the pulmonary and cardiac situations, and has been emphasized elsewhere by Graham Hill, whose excellent chapter, Nutritional Assessment, is critically important. When functional status is impaired with respect to nutritional status, the patient is likely to experience a complication following surgery.

The advice concerning operative consent is well taken. Today patients demand more and are more questioning than in the past. It is difficult to lie to patients even when they have malignant disease. One is far better off explaining the possibility of malignant disease and indicating what one will do. It also sets the stage for trust, which is important in the future therapy of the patient with malignant disease, and without which therapy is very complicated.

The most dramatic and probably single life-threatening area is preoperative assessment of cardiac risk. Every surgeon should know that risk is diminished after 6 months to approximately 5 percent. Within 3 months it is very high, and, if at all possible, surgery should be put off until after 6 months. Most of us have gone to a preoperative ICU preparation, although as the authors rightly point out, that will be increasingly difficult to justify. In my experience, the occurrence of preoperative CHF is a danger sign that cannot be taken lightly. There should be vigorous investigation of any and all possibilities with respect to cardiac risk following such demonstration. As with other perioperative risk factors, it is entirely possible that preoperative risk has in fact been diminished not only by contemporary monitoring and preparation techniques, but also by changes in some of the anesthesia techniques, which probably reduce the stress of operation, such as release of cytokines and other deleterious factors. Such techniques include the perioperative epidural, the use of local anesthetics, and perhaps the use of morphine sedation, particularly in patients with cardiac disease. It is my impression, as well as that of others, that the traditional nutritional risk factors have diminished over the past decade. Experimental investigation has focused on the epidural and other local catheters, and the same may be true of cardiac stress in cardiac disease.

Preoperative preparation of pulmonary function is well worthwhile. A number of studies have demonstrated that thoracotomy can be performed without mortality even in patients with an FEV_1 of less than 1 liter, including moderate resections. Studies in preparation in this area are very useful. Some of the more expensive and more efficacious forms of physical therapy, such as postural drainage and percussive therapy, have not been emphasized. With cost cuts, incentive spirometry with proper instruction, where possible, appears to be the most cost-effective way of preventing postoperative pneumonia.

While I agree that the judicious correction of primary hyponatremia should be undertaken with a slow infusion of approximately half the calculated deficit of 3% normal saline, the example given for secondary hyponatremia, that of cirrhosis, is not the usual situation encountered clini-

Table 2-19. "Factitious" Values for Common Chemistries and the Appropriate Calculable Corrective Factors

Component	Cause of "Factitious" Value	Correction
Sodium	Hyperglycemia	3 meq/L for each 100 mg glucose/L
Calcium	Hypoalbuminemia	0.8 meq/dl/1 g albumin/dl

cally, which is much more likely to be the inappropriate secretion of antidiuretic hormone (ADH) and hemodilution. Here, water restriction is appropriate. However, when the serum sodium gets to about 115 meq per liter or mental function begins to be a problem, or both, the judicious use of 3% sodium chloride is appropriate. I usually start with about 50 meq of 3% sodium given over 3 hours, and then repeat it in about 6 hours. This may trigger a diuresis and solve the problem, after which food restriction can be utilized. It is important, for reasons mentioned in this chapter, not to proceed with sodium correction too quickly. Judicious use of adjunctive diuretics such as furosemide may be appropriate here as well.

Hypernatremia may complicate tube feeding, particularly when hypercaloric tube feedings are utilized. In my experience, they create so much of a problem that they are hardly worth the effort. Even isotonic tube feedings, however, should be given with free water, and I will rarely use tube feedings at more than three-quarter strength, that is, an osmolality of about 240. This point was first made by Dr. Francis Moore in his landmark book, *The Metabolic Care of the Surgical Patient*, and is good advice that is valid to this day.

Hypokalemia is usually dissociated from the total body deficit and is difficult to calculate. As Dr. Baker suggested in the previous edition of this book, a 1 meq per liter decrease in serum potassium concentration usually reflects a loss of between 200 and 400 meq; a 2-meq sodium potassium deficit suggests 400- to 600-meq losses. A serum potassium of less than 2 may reflect a total deficit of less than 800 meq. I have never been very fond of calculating total body deficits, and I do not believe that they are especially accurate (Table 2-19). They may be used, however, as a guide.

Hyperkalemia constitutes a real surgical emergency. The proposed therapies are all useful, but one should not overlook the use of essential amino acids and hyper-

tonic dextrose, which forces potassium into the cell and keeps it there. Early studies (Abel et al, *Am J Surg* 123:632–638, 1972) indicate that successful use of essential amino acids and hypertonic dextrose may actually require potassium administration even in patients who are close to being anuric.

The use of lactated Ringer's solution has almost become a mythic cult and is probably more balanced than the use of dextrose and saline for initial resuscitation. It is not clear to me why Ringer's lactate rather than acetate has been the favored resuscitative solution, as the acetate would probably be more effective from the standpoint of overall body economy. Nonetheless, in a patient who is severely volume restricted, it is reasonable not to carry out the initial resuscitation with Ringer's lactate until one is certain that a urine output will result. In prolonged vomiting and hypokalemia, Ringer's lactate and the use of potassium may not be adequate. One may reach a point where the paradoxical aciduria may require the administration of hydrogen ion and excessive chloride either in the guise of arginine hydrochloride or 0.1% hydrochloric acid, which must always be administered via central line.

Finally, prophylaxis against pulmonary embolism remains a practice that is relatively underutilized in the United States, as opposed to Europe, where at least for a period of time many of the papers at various meetings concentrated on the prevention of venous thromboembolism. One technique that I like to use in a patient at moderate risk is microheparin at 1 unit/kg/hr, which must be started preoperatively. I differ with the authors on how much one must neutralize warfarin anticoagulation before operation. I am perfectly happy to operate on a patient who is anticoagulated on warfarin (Coumadin) with a prothrombin time of 16 to 18 seconds, which is an INR of 1.5, provided that one relies less on cautery and more on surgical ligature including suture ligature.

J.E.F.

3

Nutritional Assessment and Intravenous Nutritional Support

Graham L. Hill

Protein Energy Malnutrition in Surgical Patients

Because protein energy malnutrition (PEM) may impact adversely on surgical outcome, it is important that the surgeon be able to recognize it when it is present, categorize it accurately, and assess its intensity. It is first necessary, however, to understand the pathogenesis of PEM in surgical patients before a proper assessment can be made.

Pathogenesis of PEM in Surgical Patients

Prolonged starvation of a patient is accompanied by an adaptive response that results in a reduction of loss of protein from body protein stores. However, when major injury or serious sepsis supervenes, this adaptive process is lost and massive losses of body protein occur. The scheme shown in Fig. 3-1 illustrates how two variables, semistarvation and stress (sepsis or injury), determine the degree and type of PEM. A patient with normal fat and protein stores and normal physiologic function who undergoes semistarvation will eventually develop severe PEM with impaired physiologic function (marasmus). Severe stress (that is, from serious sepsis or major trauma) results in expansion of extracellular water, hypoalbuminemia, and rapid consumption of protein stores. A severely stressed patient who is well nourished does not present at first with the physical findings of PEM, for the loss of

fat and protein is masked by an expanded extracellular water (kwashiorkor). Stress of lesser severity (such as major elective surgery, pneumonia, pancreatitis) may produce extracellular water expansion and hypoalbuminemia in a patient with moderate-to-severe marasmus—this is marasmic kwashiorkor. Intermediate states are, of course, common.

Three Basic Types of PEM in Surgical Patients

Marasmus
Marasmus is malnutrition in a patient who has sustained more than 10 percent weight

loss and has clinical signs of reduced stores of fat and protein with accompanying physiologic impairments. There is no evidence of recent injury or sepsis. Metabolic expenditure is normal or low. Plasma albumin is within the normal range.

Other names include

- Moderate to severe PEM without stress
- Moderate to severe protein depletion without raised metabolic expenditure
- Resting semistarvation
- Resting total starvation

Clinical examples include esophageal stricture, carcinoma of the proximal stom-

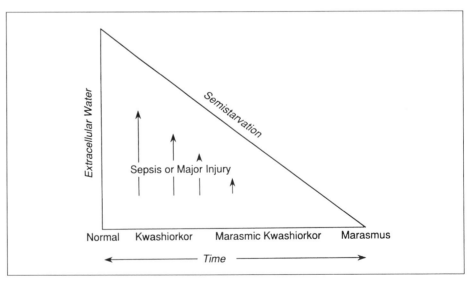

Fig. 3-1. *This scheme shows how semistarvation eventually leads to severe PEM (marasmus). Severe stress from serious sepsis or major injury leads to rapid consumption of host tissues and an expanded extracellular water (kwashiorkor). Intermediate stages, that is, marasmic kwashiorkor, are common. (From GL Hill.* Disorders of Nutrition and Metabolism in Clinical Surgery. *Edinburgh: Churchill Livingstone, 1992. Reproduced with permission.)*

ach, carcinoma of the gastric antrum, pharyngeal pouch, short-gut syndrome, and chronic intestinal obstruction.

Marasmic Kwashiorkor

Marasmic kwashiorkor is malnutrition in a patient who has sustained more than 10 percent weight loss, has clinical evidence of reduced stores of fat and protein, and has accompanying physiologic impairments. A major injury has occurred or the patient is currently septic or has been in the recent past. Metabolic expenditure is usually raised. Plasma levels of albumin are low or are falling.

Other names include

- Moderate-to-severe PEM with stress
- Moderate-to-severe protein depletion with raised metabolic expenditure
- Septic starvation

Clinical examples include a depleted patient with carcinoma of the esophagus or stomach in whom septic complications develop after esophagoscopy or gastrectomy, late stage of pancreatitis with complications, chronic colitis with a prolonged acute exacerbation, and a depleted patient with an acute attack of Crohn's disease.

Kwashiorkor

Kwashiorkor can be said to be present in a hypermetabolic patient early after major injury or serious sepsis when bodily edema and hypoalbuminemia are present. Clinical evidence of depleted protein and fat stores or abnormal physiologic function may not be apparent in the early stage. Metabolic expenditure is raised.

Other names include

- Hypoalbuminemic malnutrition
- Protein depletion with raised metabolic expenditure
- Early posttraumatic catabolic weight loss
- Early septic starvation
- Protein malnutrition—kwashiorkor-like

Clinical examples include acute attacks of severe inflammatory bowel disease in some nondepleted patients, acute severe pancreatitis, major trauma, and serious sepsis.

Definition of Clinically Significant PEM

PEM is important surgically when it is severe enough to impact on physiologic function sufficiently to increase operative risk and/or prolong postoperative recovery and convalescence. This intensity of malnutrition is termed *moderate-to-severe* PEM and is present whenever the tissue loss is associated with clinically obvious physiologic dysfunction. If PEM does not impact on physiologic function, it is termed *mild* PEM and is usually of no surgical importance.

Micronutrient Deficiencies in Surgical Patients

Biochemical evidence of deficiencies of important vitamins, such as vitamin A, vitamins of the B group, folic acid, vitamin C, and vitamin K, or of minerals, such as iron, magnesium, or zinc, is frequently present in surgical patients with moderate-to-severe PEM. All of these deficiencies are accompaniments of the disease causing PEM or of a grossly inadequate diet. They are usually not the cause of PEM. Tables 3-1 and 3-2 show the major vitamins and trace elements, their normal action, the effects of deficiency, and the recommended daily allowances. Recommended intravenous allowances are based on dietary allowances in healthy individuals. The effect of serious illness, sepsis, and trauma on these requirements when the vitamins are given by intravenous and commercial enteral feedings is not fully known.

Static Nutritional Assessment

The Objective of Nutritional Assessment of Surgical Patients

We have found the "concept of circles" developed by Dr. Stephen Heymsfield to de-

Table 3-1. Vitamins: Normal Action, Effects of Deficiency, and Recommended Daily Allowances

Vitamin	Action	Effect of Deficiency	Recommended Daily Allowance	
			Dietary[a]	Intravenous[b]
WATER SOLUBLE				
Thiamine (B₁)	Glucose metabolism	Beriberi	1.4 mg	3 mg/day
Riboflavin (B₂)	Energy transfer	Glossitis, dermatitis	1.6 mg	3.6 mg/day
Nicotinic acid (niacin) (B₃)	Energy transfer	Pellagra	18 mg	40 mg/day
Pyridoxine (B₆)	Decarboxylation and transamination	Muscle weakness, seizures	2.2 mg	4 mg/day
Pantothenic acid	Component of CoA	Fatigue, muscle cramps	7 mg	15 mg/day
Folate	Coenzyme with B₁₂	Anemia	400 μg	400 μg/day
B₁₂	Coenzyme with nucleic acid synthesis	Pernicious anemia	3 μg	5 mg/day
C	Collagen synthesis	Scurvy	60 mg	100 mg/day
FAT SOLUBLE				
A	Glycoprotein synthesis	Night blindness	1000 μg RE[c]	2500 IU/day
D	Calcium and phosphate utilization	Rickets	5 μg	5 μg/day
E	Energy transfer	Neurologic disorder	10 mg[d]	50 mg[d]/day
K	Prothrombin synthesis	Bleeding disorder	NR	10 mg/week

CoA = coenzyme A; NR = no recommendation.
[a]Committee on Dietary Allowances (1980) (men 23–50 years old).
[b]Nutrition Advisory Group (1979).
[c]Retinol equivalents: 1 μg retinol equivalent corresponds to 1 μg retinol or 3.33 IU.
[d]Alpha-tocopherol equivalents: 1 mg alpha-tocopherol equivalent has the same activity as 0.67 mg *d*-alpha-tocopherol.
From GL Hill. *Disorders of Nutrition and Metabolism in Clinical Surgery.* Edinburgh: Churchill Livingstone, 1992. With permission.

Table 3-2. Trace Elements: Effects of Deficiency and Recommended Daily Allowances

Element	Effect of Deficiency	Recommended Daily Allowance	
		Dietary[a]	Intravenous
Iron	Anemia	2 mg	2 mg
Zinc[c]	Impaired wound healing and growth, dermatitis, alopecia	15 mg	4–10 mg[d]
Copper	Anemia, neutropenia, bone demineralization	2–3 mg	0.5 mg[b]
Chromium	Impaired glucose handling	0.05–0.2 mg	10–15 μg[b]
Iodine	Goiter, hypothyroidism	150 μg	150 μg
Fluorine	Dental susceptibility to caries	1.5–4 mg	0.4 mg
Manganese	Vitamin K deficiency	2–3 mg	0.15–0.8 mg[b]
Molybdenum	Neurologic abnormalities	100 μg	100–200 μg
Selenium	Muscle weakness and pain	20–50 μg	40–120 μg

[a]Committee on Dietary Allowances (1980).
[b]Nutrition Advisory Group (1979).
[c]Excessive losses of zinc are not uncommon in surgical patients and clinical zinc deficiency syndromes were first described in such patients. Patients with diarrhea or ileostomies lose about 17 mg zinc per liter of feces, but for patients with a high small-bowel fistula the losses are proportionately less, about 12 mg/L fistula discharge.
[d]If given as zinc sulphate, this needs to be multiplied by 2.5. As only 20% of orally administered zinc is absorbed, a further multiplication by 5 is required if given orally. Zinc levels in the blood reflect zinc ingestion rather than balance, while 4 mg elemental zinc is sufficient for parenteral regimens to maintain most patients in zinc balance. Many surgical patients require more than this and 10 mg as a base requirement is suggested.
From GL Hill. *Disorders of Nutrition and Metabolism in Clinical Surgery.* Edinburgh: Churchill Livingstone, 1992. With permission.

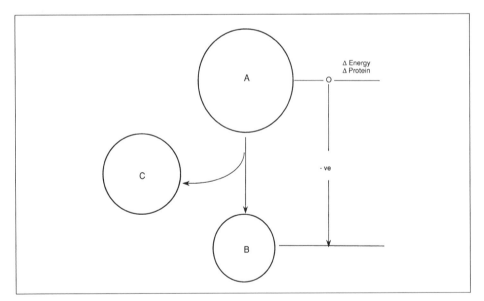

Fig. 3-2. The "concept of circles" is used to describe changes in energy and protein balance, and body composition and function, in protein energy malnutrition. Circle A is the range of body composition and physiologic function of a normal subject. Weight is stable and energy and protein balance is zero. Surgical disease causes negative energy and protein balance with accompanying changes in body composition and physiologic function. Circle B is the minimal range of body composition and function that is compatible with life. The deterioration in the state of a patient passing between A and B may be interrupted by major injury or serious sepsis and the result is depicted by circle C. Assessment of nutritional state aims to determine the location, direction, and rate of change of the patient between circles A, B, and C. (From GL Hill. **Disorders of Nutrition and Metabolism in Clincal Surgery.** *Edinburgh: Churchill Livingstone, 1992. Reproduced with permission.)*

scribe body composition and physiologic function to be a most helpful way of understanding the objective of nutritional assessment. Figure 3-2 describes this concept. Circle A is thought of as encompassing the body composition and physiologic function of a normal healthy subject. Disease causes negative energy and protein balance with accompanying changes in body composition and physiologic function. Circle B is where all reserves of fat and protein have been utilized and physiologic function is barely compatible with life. An alternative outcome is for major injury or serious sepsis to intervene, causing not only consumption of host tissue but also an expansion of extracellular water and profound deficits in physiologic function (circle C). The objective of the nutritional assessment is to determine the location, direction, and rate of change of the patient between circles A, B, and C. For the proper assessment of nutritional status, therefore, four components are necessary: energy and protein balance, body composition, physiologic function, and degree of metabolic stress (injury or sepsis).

Assessment of Energy and Protein Balance

Clinical

In practice the clinician can obtain an overview of energy and protein balance by assessing the frequency and size of the patient's meals and comparing the results obtained with an estimate of rate of loss of body weight. Table 3-3 shows the relationship between meal size and loss of body weight over time (data come from the Min-

Table 3-3. Relationship Between Meal Size and Loss of Body Weight Over Time

Meal Size (% of Normal)	Weight Loss* (%) Over Time		
	3 mo	6 mo	12 mo
20	30	45	—
30	25	35	40
50	15	25	30
70	10	15	20
80	8	12	15

*Weight loss expressed as a percentage of original body weight.
From GL Hill. *Disorders of Nutrition and Metabolism in Clinical Surgery.* Edinburgh: Churchill Livingstone, 1992. With permission.

nesota starvation experiment). It can be seen that if meal size has been only 50 percent of normal over a period of 3 months the patient will have a weight loss of 15 percent. If energy intake is 20 percent of normal over a period of 6 months, the patient will suffer from near lethal loss of body weight (45%).

Over shorter time periods changes in body weight reflect either overhydration or the combined effects of starvation and major metabolic stress. With multiple injury and serious sepsis, negative energy and protein balance are the rule, but simple bedside estimation of body weight loss to assess the magnitude of this imbalance is almost impossible due to the confounding effects on body weight of the overhydration that accompanies resuscitation.

Objective

A more comprehensive assessment of *energy and protein intake* is performed by a dietician. A 24-hour recall with a food frequency cross check is the technique used most frequently, although an analysis of a food record diary or a calorie count is also used. Once the diet information is collected the data are processed by a computer using food composition tables, and the amount and adequacy of the total energy intake and protein intake are assessed by comparison with recommended daily allowances.

For clinical purposes, *energy and protein output* in surgical patients is calculated at the bedside; 40 kcal/kg/body weight and 1.5 g protein/kg/day are reasonable approximations of energy and protein requirements. When the output calculated in this way is related to dietary assessment of intake then an approximation of the energy and protein deficit is obtained.

Research Techniques

For the accurate calculation of energy and protein balance, such as that required for research purposes, a metabolic ward is used. All nutrient intake is precisely and accurately measured and all losses from the body are collected and analyzed. Whole-body calorimetry energy balance techniques using body composition methodology and isotopic methods utilizing double-labeled water allow direct and very accurate measurements of energy balance to be made.

Assessment of Body Composition

Clinical

Body Weight. In the assessment and subsequent evaluation of patients with nutritional and metabolic disorders measurements of body weight should always be made. Body weight can be measured on chair-type ward scales to the nearest 0.1 kg. In some cases scales cannot be used for acutely ill patients and bed-type scales onto which the patient can be moved can be used. Other scales are available that make it possible to weigh the patient without moving the bed, but here it is important to ensure that the same "patient extras," such as sheets and pillows, are included in exactly the same way at each weighing. A clinical protocol for measuring body weight is shown in Table 3-4.

Weight Loss. This can be determined easily if a patient's weight before and after the occurrence of the loss has been measured. Usually, however, patients have already lost weight when they are first seen and the size of the weight loss then needs to be evaluated by comparing the measured weight with some other estimate of well weight. The accuracy of the result depends on the accuracy with which well weight can be measured. There is a lot of research on the measurement of well weight (ideal weight) and it is now clear that it is more reliable to estimate weight loss by using the patient's recalled well weight than by using published tables of ideal weight. Even then, estimating weight loss can be quite misleading in individual subjects, and it is important, therefore, to

Table 3-4. Protocol for Measuring Body Weight

The measurement is made at approximately the same time each day (best first thing in the morning)

The patient should be weighed in the same clothing each day and the bladder should be emptied immediately before weighing

Weighing should always be made on the same properly calibrated scales

If there are any gross or unexpected inconsistencies the measurement should be checked by a second observer

From GL Hill. *Disorders of Nutrition and Metabolism in Clinical Surgery*. Edinburgh: Churchill Livingstone, 1992. With permission.

relate the estimate of weight loss obtained to the physical examination of the patient.

General Appearance. The appearance of the marasmic patient is classic. There are marked decreases in muscle tissue and subcutaneous fat with the patient losing the rounded contours of the body. The face is thin and the cheekbones are prominent; the patient looks haggard and emaciated. The wasting of soft tissues is particularly marked in the region of the buttocks, which are thin and flat. The shoulder girdle is square and prominent. After major injury and serious sepsis, patients may be profoundly protein depleted with severe erosions of muscle mass (kwashiorkor), yet may be without this classic appearance due to an apparent preservation of body fat mass caused by an overlying layer of extracellular water. Patients with marasmic kwashiorkor are wasted but subcutaneous tissues appear to be relatively preserved.

Body Fat Stores—The Finger-Thumb Test. Gross loss of body fat can be observed not only from the patient's appearance but also by palpating a number of skin folds between the finger and thumb. When the dermis can be felt between the finger and thumb on pinching the triceps and biceps skin folds then one can be sure that considerable losses of body fat have occurred. Body composition studies have shown that the body mass of such patients is composed of less than 10 percent fat. It is very difficult to assess fat stores in edematous intensive care patients, however.

Body Protein Stores—The Tendon Bone Test. In a similar manner protein stores can be assessed by inspection and palpation of a number of muscle groups. The temporalis muscles, deltoids, suprascapular and infrascapular muscles, bellies of biceps and triceps, and interossei of the hands should all be looked at and palpated. The long muscles in particular are considered to be profoundly protein depleted when the tendons are prominent to palpation. Similarly when the bony shoulder girdle is sharply outlined beneath the skin there is profound protein depletion. Body composition studies have shown that when the tendons are prominent to palpation and the skeleton is emerging beneath the skin, patients have lost more than 30 percent of their total body protein stores.

Hypoalbuminemia and Excess Body Water.
Plasma albumin levels are of fundamental help in determining the type of protein energy malnutrition. Although albumin is affected by a host of factors unrelated to nutrition, when a patient with protein energy malnutrition has low levels of plasma albumin it usually indicates an expanded extracellular fluid space that may be large enough to be clinically detectable as pitting edema.

Objective

Anthropometry.
Many nutritionists use anthropometry routinely to measure body fat and the fat-free mass. Two types of measurement are usually made: skin fold thicknesses and limb circumferences. Triceps skin fold in particular is used in the clinical setting and the result obtained is compared to reference tables and an estimate of fat depletion is made. A single skin fold thickness is, however, a relatively poor predictor of the absolute amount and rate of change in total body fat in an individual. Combining a limb skin fold thickness with a corresponding circumference allows the calculation of limb fat areas. It is also possible to measure a number of skin folds (usually triceps and biceps and subscapular) and to derive from them an estimate of total body fat. This estimate of total body fat is subtracted from body weight, giving an estimate of the fat-free body mass.

There are limitations in using anthropometry routinely in nutritional assessment because of the large errors both in accuracy and precision that are involved in individual patients. Nevertheless such measurements can be very valuable in patients undergoing long-term nutritional follow-up over months or years or in identifying patients who are profoundly depleted. They can also be used in assessing the incidence of malnutrition in a patient population.

Chemical Methods.
In addition to plasma albumin, which is an indispensable chemical method for identifying the type of malnutrition present, other chemical methods used for nutritional assessment include 24-hour urea-creatinine and creatinine-height index. The levels of plasma transferrin, plasma prealbumin,

and retinol-binding protein are affected by recent changes in energy intake and are also highly correlated with all other commonly used methods of assessing nutritional state. They are valuable as well in following the nutritional status of a patient longitudinally, but only in ward patients (see below).

Research Techniques

Physical Techniques.
A number of research techniques are available for measuring body composition, and some of the more simple ones may soon be applicable to the daily care of the sick. The techniques being used in research laboratories are in vivo neutron activation analysis (IVNAA), multifrequency bioelectrical impedance (BIA), dual-energy x-ray absorptiometry (DEXA), and total body potassium measurements (TBK). BIA measures the resistance and reactance of a current passed through the body between the wrist and the contralateral leg. From the data obtained total body water can be estimated and by using assumptions as to the relationship between body water and the fat-free body mass the latter can be estimated. Some suggest that extracellular water can also be estimated by these techniques. The simplicity and low cost of BIA have made some nutritionists advocate its widespread use, but most restrict its use to estimating the fat-free body mass, while at the same time advising caution in using the technique for following the patient on treatment.

Dual-energy x-ray absorptiometry is a technique that was developed to measure skeletal mineralization, but more recently further development has enabled measurements of body fat, total body soft tissue, and skeletal mass to be obtained. DEXA gives very precise estimates of total body fat.

The technique of combining DEXA with IVNAA to give a comprehensive assessment of body composition is the ultimate in sophistication. Although this is the ideal for a research-based nutritional assessment, the cost and complexity of the combined technique restrict its use clinically. There are also potential developments in in vivo neutron activation analysis (associated particle technique) that may add a new dimension to the precision and accuracy of the measurements of protein and extracellular water. Isotopic dilution meth-

ods using tritium and radioactive sulfate are used to measure body water and its compartments. All these are research techniques and due to their expense and sophistication have not yet found a place in routine patient care.

Growth Hormone—Somatomedin Axis.
Undernutrition reduces the hepatic release of somatomedins even though growth hormone levels may be raised. This is probably due to a metabolic adaptation that allows reduced growth processes from decreased somatomedin activity while direct actions of growth hormone spare muscle protein and mobilize fat. This sensitivity to alterations in nutritional state has led to the use of somatomedin-C (insulin-like growth factor–I, or IGF-I) as a marker of malnutrition where its plasma levels have been shown to be closely correlated with those of transferrin.

Assessment of Physiologic Function

Clinical
Functional impairment secondary to loss of body protein is the msot important part of the assessment of nutritional status. The loss of function to be noted is that which is clinically quite obvious and which has occurred over the same time period as the loss of body weight.

The patient should be questioned about unhealed scratches or sores, easy tiredness, or substantial changes in exercise tolerance. Weight loss without evidence of physiologic abnormality is probably of no consequence. Function is observed while performing the physical examination and by watching the patient's activity around the ward. Grip strength can be assessed by asking the patient to squeeze strongly the surgeon's index and middle fingers for at least 10 seconds. Impairment is judged in the light of the patient's age, sex, and body habitus. Respiratory muscle function is assessed by asking the patient to blow hard, holding a strip of paper 10 cm from the lips; this should normally be blown away with some force, and severe impairment is present when the paper does not move. Shortness of breath is noted at rest. Severe impairment is indicated when normal conversation is not possible. Respiratory excursion is noted by asking the patient to take as deep a breath as possible. When there is virtually no chest expansion, severe impairment exists.

Objective

It is possible to measure the wound healing response directly by a microimplant technique that includes inserting a 1-mm tube of Gore-tex in the subcutaneous tissues and estimating the amount of collagen accumulating in it over a 7-day period. Skeletal muscle function and respiratory function can also be assessed objectively by standard techniques. In clinical practice objective measurement of grip strength by the use of a hand-held vigorimeter has, in some nutritional assessment programs, become a regular and valuable part of nutritional assessment.

Assessment of Metabolic Stress

Clinical

A history and physical examination will reveal evidence of metabolic stress. It is present if the patient has had major trauma or major surgery in the previous week or has evidence of serious sepsis according to the criteria shown in Table 3-5.

Objective

Indirect Calorimetry. Direct measurement of resting metabolic expenditure by indirect calorimetry is the best way of quantifying the intensity of metabolic stress. This is then related to estimated values when well. These are best related to an anthropometric measurement of metabolic body size. Although measurements of total body potassium and, through them, estimates of the body cell mass are the gold standard for metabolic body size, fat-free body mass is more practical in the clinical setting. It is measured by first estimating

total body fat from skin fold measurements, then subtracting the result from body weight. In normal subjects resting metabolic expenditure is related closely to the size of the fat-free body regardless of age and regardless of sex.

From a normal population the following regression equation was obtained:

RME (kcal/24 hr) = 13.6 FFM
+ 550 (males and females)

where RME is resting metabolic expenditure and FFM is fat-free body mass in kilograms. The mean (SD) ratio of the measured RME to predicted RME for normal subjects was 1.00 ± 0.09, and therefore patients with a ratio greater than 1.18 can be considered to have a raised RME and to suffer from metabolic stress.

Catabolic Index. This index separates urinary urea excretion into urea excretion due to dietary protein intake and urea excretion due to increased protein catabolism. Measurements required are 24-hour nitrogen intake and 24-hour urinary urea over the same time period.

The catabolic index (CI) is then calculated as follows:

$$CI = \text{urinary urea N(g)} - \left(\frac{\text{dietary N(g)}}{2} + 3\right)$$

If CI is less than 0, no stress is present; if CI equals 0 to 5, there is moderate stress, and if CI is greater than 5, stress is severe.

Scoring Systems. There are physiologic scoring systems such as the APACHE-II score that give a general measurement of disease severity. [*Editor's Note*: A general indication perhaps, but APACHE-II has been disappointing in rigorously assessing degree of illness in various outcome studies.]

Research. Levels of counterregulatory hormones, acute-phase reactants, and quantification of circulating cytokines are used by some to estimate the degree of metabolic stress or presence of invasive sepsis.

Putting the Components of the Assessment Together

From the clinical estimates of the separate components of the assessment (see Table 3-6 for summary), that is, energy and protein balance, body composition, physiologic function, and metabolic stress, the surgeon will be able to identify the type of malnutrition present, quantify the intensity of the malnutrition, and de-

Table 3-5. Markers of Metabolic Stress

Highest temperature in the last 24 hr > 100°F
Pulse rate > 100/min in the last 24 hr
Respiratory rate > 30 per min in the last 24 hours
White cell count > 12,000 or < 3000 in the last 24 hr
Positive blood culture
Active inflammatory bowel disease
Defined focus of infection

From GL Hill. *Disorders of Nutrition and Metabolism in Clinical Surgery*. Edinburgh: Churchill Livingstone, 1992. With permission.

Table 3-6. Clinical Assessment of Nutritional Status

Component	Method	Suggestive of Moderate-to-Severe PEM
Energy balance	Ask patient about reduction in meal size over time	If meal size 50% or less than usual over the previous 3 mo
Body composition	Weight loss (recalled weight–measured weight)	>15%
	Appearance	Severe marasmus
	Finger-Thumb test	If two layers of dermis can be felt with little or no fat between them
	Tendon bone test	Shoulder girdle prominent
Physiologic function	Exercise tolerance Unhealed scars or wounds Respiratory muscle function Grip strength	Impairments must be clinically obvious and have occurred over same time period as loss of weight
	Plasma albumin level	>2 SDs below normal
Metabolic stress	Fever in last 24 hr	>100°F
	Pulse rate in last 24 hr	>100/min
	Respiratory rate in last 24 hr	>30/min
	White cell count in last 24 hr	>1200 or <3000
	Positive blood culture Trauma Serious sepsis Active inflammatory bowel disease	

cide whether or not metabolic stress is present.

The Type of Protein Malnutrition Present

Marasmus. Patients with marasmus will be found to have an overall deficit in their intake and/or utilization of food. They will also have weight loss of 10 percent or more, marked by clinical evidence of subcutaneous fat loss and wasting of muscle bellies. Plasma albumin remains normal but plasma prealbumin, plasma transferrin, and IGF-I may be low. Indirect calorimetry will demonstrate that resting metabolic expenditure is low normal or low and urinary nitrogen loss will be found to be small.

Marasmic Kwashiorkor. Patients with this type of PEM will be found to have an overall deficit in their intake and/or utilization of food. They will also have weight loss of 10 percent or more, marked by clinical evidence of subcutaneous fat loss and wasting of muscle bellies. Indirect calorimetry may give normal values if the metabolic stress causing the malnutrition has been dealt with. If there is continuing stress, indirect calorimetry will show an increase in the measured compared with the predicted RME. Plasma albumin levels are low, as are levels of plasma transferrin, prealbumin, and IGF-I. There may be evidence of pitting edema.

Kwashiorkor. These patients are easily picked out because currently or in the recent past they have suffered from major trauma or serious sepsis. They are not eating. Massive weight loss may not yet be a feature because of expanded body water, and clinical examination will find near normal stores of muscle and fat, but clear signs of sepsis or major metabolic stress will be present. Plasma levels of albumin will be low, but those for transferrin, prealbumin, and IGF-I will be variable. Edema is frequently present. If this situation persists, muscle wasting follows and extracellular fluid accumulates further, although fat stores appear to be relatively preserved.

Intensity of Malnutrition

Moderate-to-severe protein energy malnutrition has previously been defined as that which is of sufficient intensity to impact on physiologic function. *The definition requires this impact to be clinically obvious.* When PEM of this degree of intensity is present, it has been demonstrated that postoperative complications are more common and hospital stay is prolonged.

Assessment of Metabolic Stress

The importance of identifying metabolic stress is that:

- It gives a clue as to the type of malnutrition that is present or soon will be present
- It indicates that extracellular water is expanded or will be expanding
- The response to nutritional support will be impaired in those in whom metabolic stress is present (Fig. 3-3).

Implications for Patient Management

The Type of Protein Energy Malnutrition

The surgeon needs to identify the type of malnutrition in order to set appropriate nutritional/metabolic goals for treatment. The marasmic patient has less distortion of body compartments but the malnutrition may have developed over a long period of time and hence considerable caution must be taken over the rate of repletion to avoid complications. The patient with marasmic kwashiorkor has an overexpanded extracellular water as well as erosion of body stores and needs careful restriction of sodium and free water to normalize body hydration and avoid the possibility of oversalting and overwatering. The patient with kwashiorkor has a catastrophic illness with massive proteolysis and expansion of extracellular water. The surgeon's eye must be directed toward dealing with the metabolic stress that causes this, as well as management of the developing compositional defect.

The Intensity

There is ample evidence now to suggest that patients without physiologic impairment or in whom physiologic impairment is not expected to occur do not need nutritional repletion.

Metabolic Stress

Patients with metabolic stress have a blunted ability to retain administered protein because of continuing catabolism. Protein synthesis can be increased in patients with trauma and sepsis with adequate nutritional support, but whole-body protein catabolism goes on unabated and is not re-

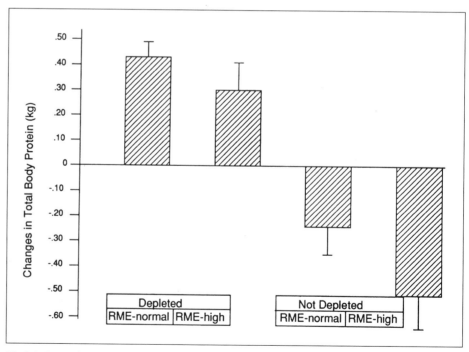

Fig. 3-3. Surgical patients who are depleted of body stores of protein have a marked tendency to gain protein with total parenteral nutrition even when metabolic expenditure is raised. (Data from Hill et al, 1991. From GL Hill. Disorders of Nutrition and Metabolism in Clinical Surgery. Edinburgh: Churchill Livingstone, 1992. Reproduced with permission.)

versed by known nutritional or pharmacologic regimens (Fig. 3-4).

Assessing the Response to Nutritional Support (Dynamic Nutritional Assessment)

Clinical Response

For nutritional therapy to be effective, it is necessary to ensure that the nutrients being provided are adequate and are being utilized effectively. A number of studies show that wound healing, muscle function, and psychological function may be measurably improved with nutritional support, resulting in the clinical observation that the patient looks and feels better and that on examination he or she is physically stronger.

Nitrogen Balance

On the laboratory side nitrogen balance is sometimes used as a marker of dynamic nutritional assessment but in clinical practice the performance of a nitrogen balance is full of difficulties unless very strict attention is paid to measuring *all* losses. In many surgical patients this is quite impractical. If, however, the surgeon can be sure that there has been a complete 24-hour collection of urine, a fair approximation of all nitrogen losses from the body can be made. Generally speaking though, all "clinical nitrogen balances" tend to have cumulative errors that err on the side of being optimistic, and the patient needs to be in a positive nitrogen balance of +5 g N per day to be certain that nitrogen accretion is occurring. The technique of performing a clinical nitrogen balance is as follows:

- The amount of urea passed in the urine in a 24-hour period is calculated by multiplying the 24-hour urine output by the urine urea concentration
- Urea with a molecular weight of 60 is, by weight, about 50 percent nitrogen
- Urea accounts for approximately 80 percent of nitrogen in urine and therefore the urea N must be increased by 20 percent
- In addition 2 g per day of nitrogen is added to account for stool N, and integumentary losses

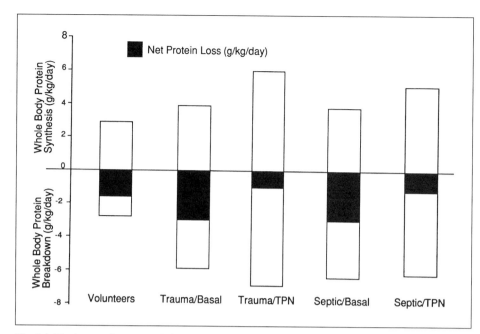

Fig. 3-4. *The increase in net protein loss during trauma and sepsis results from an increase in protein breakdown, not from a decrease in protein synthesis. Here the patients given total parenteral nutrition (TPN) had an increase in synthesis of protein but there was no effect on protein catabolism. Nevertheless, the net result was a halving of the net loss of the protein from the body. A similar effect probably occurs after enteral feeding, and it can be concluded that nutritional support in seriously ill surgical patients reduces protein loss from the body although it cannot be expected to eliminate the loss altogether. (From GL Hill.* Disorders of Nutrition and Metabolism in Clinical Surgery. *Edinburgh: Churchill Livingstone, 1992. Reproduced with permission.)*

Table 3-7. Sensitivity, Specificity, and Predictive Value of Weekly Rise in Plasma Protein Levels in Detecting Positive Nitrogen Balance in Patients Receiving 2 Weeks of TPN

	Albumin	Prealbumin	Transferrin
Sensitivity (%)	61	88	67
Specificity (%)	45	70	55
Positive predictive value (%)	86	93	87
Negative predictive value (%)	17	56	27
Prevalence of rising nitrogen balance	61/72	90/108	90/108

From GL Hill. *Disorders of Nutrition and Metabolism in Clinical Surgery.* Edinburgh: Churchill Livingstone, 1992. With permission.

- Nitrogen balance (g/day) = N intake − N output
- If nitrogen balance is greater than 5 g per day, the patient is in positive N balance

Plasma Proteins and Insulin-Like Growth Factor–I

Ward Patients

As practical alternatives to nitrogen balance, four serum transport proteins have

been suggested as markers of nutritional progress and are now being used in some nutritional assessment programs. These are *albumin, transferrin, prealbumin, and retinol-binding protein.* One study (Table 3-7) showed that in patients who required total parenteral nutrition (TPN) for 2 weeks a positive nitrogen balance was reflected by a rise of prealbumin in 88 percent of cases, whereas a negative nitrogen balance was associated with a falling prealbumin in 70 percent. Predictive values in the group indicate that 93 percent of patients with a rising positive prealbumin had a positive nitrogen balance.

Insulin-like growth factor–I levels have been shown to be low in ward surgical patients with PEM and increase with nutritional repletion, and predict body composition changes better than transferrin levels.

Intensive Care Patients

It has recently been shown that changes in plasma prealbumin, transferrin, and IGF-I levels do not reflect changes in total body protein in intensive care patients, as they do in ward patients.

Assessment of Energy Requirements

Total Energy Requirements

For some time it was thought that energy requirements for sick surgical patients were very high and that large energy intakes (described as hyperalimentation) were necessary in order to gain protein and fat. It is now realized that, apart from being wasteful of resources and money, excessive energy intakes can, by raising the level of catecholamines, be the source of added metabolic stress. Hypercaloric feeding may also increase ventilatory demand, which may be important in patients with borderline respiratory function and imminent respiratory failure and in those with problems in weaning from mechanical ventilation. There is therefore a strong argument for tailoring energy intakes to the patient's requirements.

The total energy requirements of a patient in metabolic balance are the same as his or her total energy expenditure. This includes basal requirements (i.e., the energy necessary for the work of the heart and lungs, work for the synthesis of new chemical bondings, and work to maintain electrochemical gradients in cells), the increased energy requirements brought about by the patient's disease, the energy expended during the process of assimilation of nutrients, and the energy expended on physical work. The only direct way to measure all these components together is by means of a direct calorimeter, which measures all the heat produced by the patient in a 24-hour period. A direct calorimeter is in re-

ality a huge airtight insulated box that completely isolates the patient, and is therefore quite impractical for day-to-day patient management. Total energy requirements can also be measured by the double-labeled water technique, but this is prohibitively expensive. In order to understand how total energy requirements are calculated in clinical practice some definitions are required.

Definitions

Terms currently used by clinical nutritionists for the calculation of total energy expenditure are defined in the following paragraphs.

Basal Metabolic Rate (BMR)

This is the lowest or basal metabolic requirement, which occurs for a period of time when the patient is deeply asleep during the early hours of the morning. These conditions are not often available clinically.

Resting Metabolic Expenditure (RME)

This is a measurement in a fasted patient who has been quietly resting for at least half an hour in a thermoneutral environment. It is 5 to 10 percent higher than BMR and is the measurement used in clinical practice.

Diet-Induced Thermogenesis (DIT)

This is the energy expended in the assimilation of nutrients whether given enterally or parenterally. In a surgical context it is not to be thought of as the energy expended after a bolus of food. Rather, it is the energy expended during the assimilation of a diet that is being administered continuously. It varies with the type of diet being infused and the metabolic state of the patient. In surgery, when nutritional support is usually given continuously in the form of a balanced mixed diet, DIT is calculated by multiplying the RME by 0.1.

Resting Energy Expenditure (REE)

This is the same as RME, except that the patient is being measured during continuous enteral or parenteral infusion. Thus, it includes the additional 10 percent of

RME caused by diet-induced thermogenesis.

Activity Energy Expenditure (AEE)

This depends on the amount of physical work performed and varies in active people from 500 kcal per day in sedentary individuals to 3000 kcal per day for manual laborers. In surgical patients either in the ward or in the intensive care unit, it is calculated by multiplying the REE by 0.3.

Stress Factor

Surgical disease usually raises metabolic rate by a factor of 5 to 10 percent for uncomplicated surgery to more than 100 percent for extensive burns. In practice the stress factors are calculated as follows:

PATIENT STATUS	MULTIPLY REE BY
Skeletal trauma	0.3
Postelective surgery	0.1
Head injury and multiple injury	0.5
Serious sepsis	0.4–0.6
Major burn	Up to 1.0

Clinical Measurement of Total Energy Requirements

In surgical practice there are three ways in which total energy requirements are calculated.

The Surgeon Can Assume that All Surgical Patients Need 35 to 40 kcal/kg/day

A number of studies have shown that for a variety of surgical illnesses total energy expenditure (TEE) is about 35 to 40 kcal/kg/day. This is explained by the fact that those patients whose REE is raised are usually the most ill and, because they are unable to move around the ward, their AEE is low. On the other hand those who are up and about around the ward with a higher AEE are less ill and their REE is not raised. The net effect is that all patients have about the same TEE. This general rule is subject to wide variation, and calculation of TEE in this way frequently leads to overprescription because of the varying proportions of body fat between patients. One study showed that of 50 patients given a prescription of 40 kcal/kg/day one-third received more than 1000 kcal over what they would have been given if their energy requirements had been measured directly.

The Surgeon Can Use Standard Tables and Add Factors for DIT, AEE, and Stress

According to the Harris-Benedict equations the basal metabolic rate can be computed using the following equations:

RME (kcal/day) for males
$$= 66.5 + 13.8 \times W + 5 \times H - 6.8 \times A$$
RME (kcal/day) for females
$$= 655 + 9.6 \times W + 1.9 \times H - 4.7 \times A$$

where W is weight in kilograms, H is height in centimeters, and A is age in years. Having obtained the RME, requirements for DIT, AEE, and stress are added. Thus,

$$TEE = RME + stress\ factor + DIT + AEE$$

Most studies show that energy requirements, for groups of patients in particular, can be fairly accurately calculated in this way. The problem arises because body weight is used in the calculation of RME, and in individual patients, particularly those who are very thin or very fat or who have abnormal degrees of hydration, the results can be quite misleading. Furthermore, the stress factor is not always easy to calculate, leading to a further source of error.

REE and Stress Factor Are Measured Directly Using a Metabolic Cart (Indirect Calorimeter) and AEE Factor Is Added

There are now a number of indirect calorimeters commercially available that have been specially designed for clinical use. These instruments measure oxygen consumption rate (VO_2), carbon dioxide production rate (VCO_2), and respiratory quotient (VCO_2/VO_2). From the VO_2 (assuming the RQ is 0.82) REE is calculated, for the caloric value of 1 liter of oxygen consumed at this RQ is 4.825 kcal. This value for REE in surgical patients includes both diet-induced thermogenesis and the stress factor for the disease and TEE is obtained by adding AEE. In practice REE × 1.3 is very close to the true TEE in all surgical patients.

A number of studies now show the cost-effectiveness of indirect calorimetry in clinical practice. A recent study of the energy requirements of a large number of patients showed that total energy requirements estimated from the Harris-Benedict equations tended to overestimate energy needs in 90 percent of patients, leading to overfeeding of more than 500 kcal per patient per day. It was shown that considerable cost savings could be made by using indirect calorimetry in patients who required intravenous nutrition.

Prescribing Energy Requirements

Having measured the total energy requirements of a patient, the amount of energy prescribed depends on the nutritional/metabolic goal for the individual patient. To preserve total body protein and total body fat at present levels the measured TEE is used. For energy store repletion, that is, gain in body protein and body fat, the TEE is multiplied by 1.2.

For those who have a metabolic cart the process is even simpler. For tissue preservation multiply REE by 1.3; for tissue repletion multiply REE by 1.5.

Assessment of Protein Requirements

Calculating a patient's requirements for protein is a much less precise procedure than that used for the calculation of energy requirements. All current methods are based on body weight and are therefore prone to considerable error.

The recommended daily requirement for protein for healthy adult men is about 50 g per day although the average Western diet may contain more than twice this amount. Patients with moderate to severe protein depletion behave as growing children and may gain body protein at intakes far below that which are required in surgical patients who are not as depleted. Patients with major injury or serious sepsis have increased requirements although in such patients continuing whole-body protein breakdown means that there is a limit above which increased protein intakes are not utilized.

The biologic value of the administered protein (or intravenous amino acid solu-

tion) is important. All diets do not have the same biologic value. This depends on the detailed amino acid composition of the diet in relation to the amino acid composition of the body. The lack of an essential amino acid can considerably decrease the biologic value of an otherwise adequate intake of protein. Egg protein is very effectively utilized by humans and supplementation of its amino acid content does not improve its biologic value. For this reason egg protein is frequently used as a reference protein and comparisons made between its content of amino acids and those in synthetic amino acid mixtures can give a useful guide when selecting a solution for clinical use.

A number of studies have shown that amino acids or protein hydrolysates administered enterally have a similar effect as when these same amino acids or protein hydrolysates are given intravenously. The precise amount of protein intake that an *individual patient* should receive cannot be measured, but three principles apply:

- There is an increasing linear retention of nitrogen with an increasing protein intake over a range of 0.25 to 2.0 g/kg/day.
- 1.5 g protein/kg/day is suggested by some to be the upper limit that surgical patients, even those who are severely septic, are able to utilize.
- Some patients have protein needs over and above those involved in metabolic processes. For instance, patients with inflammatory bowel disease may lose 0.5 to 1.0 g/kg/day in the stool.

With these principles in mind the following recommendations are made:

For maintenance	Prescribe 1.0–1.5 g/kg/day
For repletion	Prescribe 1.5–2.0 g/kg/day
For those with excessive losses	Prescribe 2.0–2.5 g/kg/day

Intravenous Nutrition

Intravenous nutrition (IVN) is primarily used for dysfunction of the gastrointestinal tract. It is particularly applicable to the following situations in surgery:

- *Preoperatively*, to improve surgical outcome
- *Postoperatively*, for patients with ileus or wound infection, or those in whom GI function is not adequate for a prolonged period
- *For inflammatory bowel disease*, pancreatitis, and massive enterectomy
- *For patients with protein energy malnutrtion* who have organ failure, major sepsis, some malignancies, and trauma

Indications for IVN in General Surgical Practice

From the point of view of the general surgeon, it is easier to divide the indications according to the condition of the alimentary tract, as in the following instances.

When the Alimentary Tract Is Obstructed

Patients with esophageal, gastric, or upper GI malignancies who need preoperative nutritional therapy and in whom the enteral route cannot be used are prime examples.

When the Alimentary Tract is Too Short

This includes those patients who have had a massive enterectomy. Generally speaking, when less than 3 meters of small bowel remain, a number of serious metabolic and nutritional abnormalities occur, although these can usually be treated by dietary means. When 2 meters or less of small bowel remain, most patients require a period of IVN but eventually can be weaned from it. On the other hand those patients with less than 1 meter of small bowel remaining need IVN at home on an indefinite basis.

When the Alimentary Tract Is Fistulated

Enterocutaneous fistulas, particularly in the upper small intestine, are particular examples of the value of IVN in modern surgical practice.

When the Alimentary Tract Is Inflamed

The perioperative care of patients with Crohn's disease and ulcerative colitis represent prime examples of the use of IVN in this setting.

When the Alimentary Tract Cannot Cope

Such patients include those with an ileus secondary to major intra-abdominal sepsis or inflammatory processes such as pancreatitis.

The Central Venous Catheter

The development of central venous catheterization has enabled the safe delivery of hypertonic solutions. The glucose, fat, and amino acid admixture is given through a central venous line with its tip in the superior vena cava. The solutions used for central venous nutrient infusion (IVN) usually contain 1 kcal/ml, and water and electrolyte requirements are prescribed to meet the individual patient's needs. The key to successful IVN is in the insertion and care of the central venous cannula.

Insertion of Central Venous Cannula

The Dudrick Technique. A 20-cm-long, 16-gauge, radiopaque silicone catheter passed into the subclavian vein and into the superior vena cava through a 5-cm 14-gauge needle under strict aseptic conditions, a technique described by Stanley

Dudrick, has gained wide acceptance because it is associated with the fewest number of problems. With practice there is almost no occasion on which this route cannot be used.

The initial step is to place the patient on his or her back with the foot of the bed elevated to 15 degrees. A small pad is placed between the shoulder blades to allow the shoulders to drop backward. The skin is prepared with povidone-iodine (Betadine) solution in the same manner as for a surgical operation. The drapes are placed carefully and the operator, who is scrubbed up, wears gown, gloves, and a hat. Local anesthetic is infiltrated into the skin, subcutaneous tissue, and periosteum at the inferior border just lateral to the midpoint of the clavicle. The needle, attached to a small syringe, is advanced toward the tip of the finger, which is placed firmly in the suprasternal notch (Fig. 3-5). The needle should be very close to the inferior surface of the clavicle and penetration of the subclavian vein is signaled by a rush of blood into the syringe. The needle is advanced a few millimeters more to ensure that it is entirely within the vein. The patient is then asked to perform a Valsalva maneuver; the thumb is held over the needle hub as the syringe is removed. The radiopaque catheter is then intro-

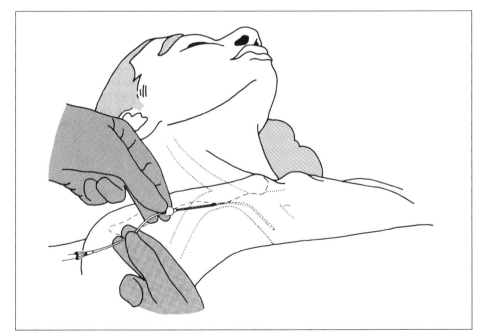

Fig. 3-5. A 16-gauge catheter is advanced into the vein to lie in the superior vena cava. (From GL Hill. Disorders of Nutrition and Metabolism in Clinical Surgery. *Edinburgh: Churchill Livingstone, 1992. Reproduced with permission.)*

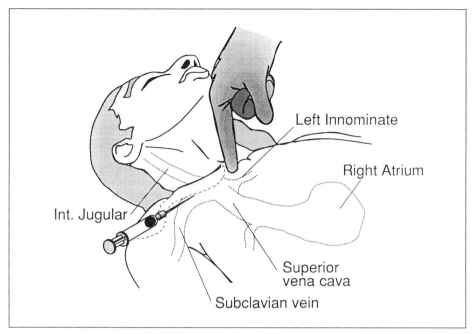

Int. Jugular

Left Innominate

Right Atrium

Superior
vena cava

Subclavian vein

Fig. 3-6. *A 14-gauge needle is inserted just lateral to the midpoint of the clavicle and directed toward the suprasternal notch. Puncture of the subclavian vein is indicated by a flush of blood into the syringe. (From GL Hill.* Disorders of Nutrition and Metabolism in Clinical Surgery. *Edinburgh: Churchill Livingstone, 1992. Reproduced with permission.)*

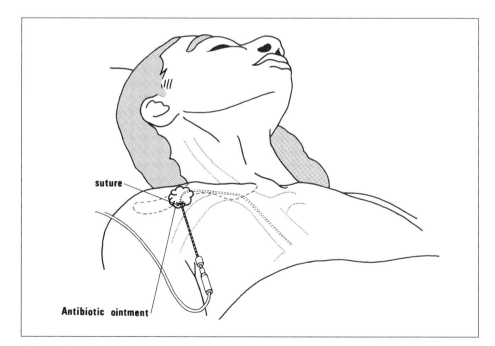

suture

Antibiotic ointment

Fig. 3-7. *The catheter is sutured to the skin and antiseptic ointment is placed around the catheter at the skin entrance site. (From GL Hill.* Disorders of Nutrition and Metabolism in Clinical Surgery. *Edinburgh: Churchill Livingstone, 1992. Reproduced with permission.)*

duced through the needle and threaded into the superior vena cava (Fig. 3-6). The needle is then withdrawn from the patient and a small plastic cuff is fitted over the junction of the catheter and needle tip. The catheter is then connected to an intravenous administration set and a slow infusion of normal saline is begun while the catheter is sewn to the skin (Fig. 3-7). Antiseptic ointment is applied around the entrance of the catheter into the skin, and a dressing is applied over it including the junction of the intravenous tubing and the hub of the catheter (Fig. 3-8). Confirmation that the catheter is in the correct place is obtained first by lowering the saline and seeing blood return up the tubing and secondly by a chest x-ray. If the catheter tip is in the right atrium or ventricle the catheter should be pulled back an appropriate distance so that the tip is positioned in the superior vena cava. If the catheter tip is in the contralateral subclavian vein or directed upward into veins in the neck, attempts are made to reposition it under fluoroscopic control and image intensification.

The Seldinger Technique. Central venous catheterization by the Seldinger technique now has an established place in clinical nutrition. The first step in this approach is to insert a small-diameter needle into the vein (the same way as described above), remove the syringe, and then direct a flexible guidewire through the needle into the vein. The needle is then removed and a dilator is passed over the wire to create a track; finally, the catheter is threaded over the wire into the superior vena cava. The technique is probably safer than the one mentioned above but *all of the time-honored principles of the approach described by Dudrick still apply.*

Other Methods and Types of Catheters to Use

The internal and external jugular veins, the cephalic veins, and the basilic veins are alternate sites for catheter insertion. They provide access for IVN in patients who have undergone head and neck surgery or who have infected tracheostomies. Polyvinyl, Teflon, polyurethane, or silicone rubber catheters can be used; silicone rubber is the most popular and seems to be associated with the lowest incidence of thrombosis.

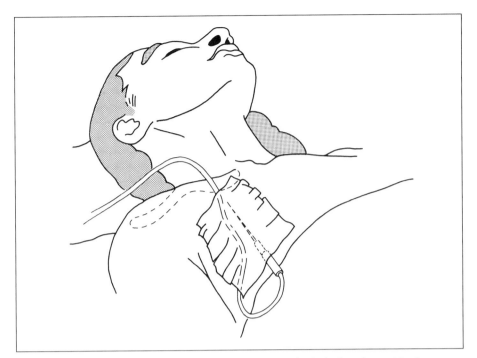

Fig. 3-8. Sterile dressing secures the catheter and tubing in place. The site is cleaned every Monday, Wednesday, and Friday and the infusion tubing is changed. (From GL Hill. Disorders of Nutrition and Metabolism in Clinical Surgery. Edinburgh: Churchill Livingstone, 1992. Reproduced with permission.)

Care of the Central Venous Cannula: Golden Rules

The Catheter Is Used Exclusively for the Nutrient Solution. Once positioned the catheter is used exclusively for the administration of the nutrient solution. Drawing blood, monitoring central venous pressure, administering medications, and the use of this catheter for nutrient administration postoperatively are prohibited. Triple-lumen central venous catheters are now available and if one of the ports is devoted entirely to nutrient administration and the rules above are adhered to reports suggest that the rates of catheter sepsis are the same as when a single-lumen catheter is used.

Strict Rules of Asepsis Must Apply. High standards of maintenance of the catheter are critical for achieving success for IVN. The dressing over the catheter insertion site should be removed each Monday, Wednesday, and Friday. At this time the skin around the catheter exit should be cleaned with ether and acetone and the skin painted again with Betadine solution. Antiseptic ointment should be placed around the catheter exit site and after the tubing is changed a sterile dressing is reapplied.

Catheter-Related Sepsis

The most dangerous part of patient treatment with IVN is catheter-related sepsis.

Definition of Catheter-Related Sepsis. Catheter-related sepsis is present when

- There is clinical evidence of bloodstream infection, that is, fever and a high white cell count.
- There is no clinical evidence of another source of the septicemia.
- There is isolation of the same organism from the catheter tip and from the peripheral blood.

Definition of Catheter Contamination. Catheter contamination is present when there is isolation of an organism from the catheter tip but not from the peripheral blood. The problem clinically is that patients who may have catheter-related sepsis on clinical grounds frequently have only catheter contamination, which is probably of no clinical significance. Catheter removal in these circumstances may be an unnecessary and expensive waste of time. In one study over 90 percent of catheters removed for suspected sepsis were not the cause of catheter-related sepsis.

Protocol When Catheter-Related Sepsis Is Suspected. Failure to recognize catheter-related sepsis and to remove the catheter promptly may prove to be life threatening to the patient. There are two ways of handling the dilemma as to whether the catheter may not be the cause of the sepsis:

1. In the patient suspected of having catheter-related sepsis, the catheter is removed over a guidewire and replaced by a new one. The catheter tip and peripheral blood are cultured and if, when the results are available, both the catheter tip and the peripheral blood are growing the same bacteria the diagnosis of catheter-related sepsis is confirmed and the catheter is removed.
2. The catheter is left in place but blood is taken simultaneously through a peripheral vein and through the suspected central venous catheter and quantitative blood cultures are obtained. Around 16 hours later the results are available and a central venous catheter blood colony count five times (or more) higher than the peripheral vein colony count can be considered as indicating catheter-related sepsis, and the catheter is removed.

Whichever of these two methods is used, the results depend on the local availability of the appropriate microbiologic techniques, but both are now established and safe procedures.

Treatment of Established Catheter-Related Sepsis

Most patients with catheter-related sepsis respond promptly and favorably to removal of the catheter. A favorable response is defined as that which occurs when the temperature and white blood count return to normal and local signs of inflammation at the catheter insertion site resolve within the 24-hour period. No other treatment is necessary and a new catheter can be inserted on the other side when all signs of sepsis have subsided. If the patient continues to show clinical signs of bacteremia after removal, a brief course of antibiotics is indicated and particularly so if the catheter tip culture reveals a large number of colonies of *Staphylococcus aureus*.

The Nutrient Solution

The Role of the Surgeon and the Role of the Pharmacist

Once the intensity and type of malnutrition have been assessed and the nutritional goal has been set, the patient's requirements are calculated. *The daily quantities of energy, protein, water, electrolytes, vitamins, and trace metals are prescribed by the surgeon, and the pharmacist formulates an appropriate nutrient solution.* Some surgeons prefer to prescribe precise types and concentrations of amino acid, dextrose, and fat solutions, but modern pharmacists are better equipped than their surgical counterparts to choose and mix the detailed ingredients to meet the patient's prescribed nutrient needs.

Generally speaking, the pharmacist formulates a solution from commonly available combinations of 70% dextrose, 10% amino acid solutions, and 20% fat emulsions to which electrolytes, vitamins, and trace elements are added. All the nutrients are mixed together in a 3-liter bag and the entire contents of the bag are infused over the 24-hour period. An automated mixing device is available that allows the pharmacist to manufacture a variety of nutrient combinations from these components and at the same time generate a label for the bag that allows its precise contents to be known.

It is important for the surgeon not only to prescribe exactly the quantities of energy, protein, and water to be given but also to state precisely the quantities of cations and anions required to be added to the base formula.

Sodium and potassium are added as the chloride or acetate salts depending on the patient's requirements. Generally there should be equal quantities of chloride and acetate. If there are increased gastric losses, however, the salts should all be in chloride form; it must be remembered that excessive chloride administration can lead to the potentially fatal problem of hyperchloremic metabolic acidosis. Acetate is used whenever extra base is required. Sodium bicarbonate cannot be incorporated into nutrient solutions, and acetate, which is metabolized to bicarbonate, is used instead.

Phosphate, which is essential in patients receiving high glucose intakes, is usually given as the potassium salt. When potassium is contraindicated it is supplied as the sodium salt.

Some amino acid mixtures already contain sodium, potassium, chloride, acetate, and phosphate, so it is only if quantities over and above these are required that additional electrolytes are added. Fat emulsions also contain phosphate.

Commonly available preparations of vitamins and trace elements are also added to the 3-liter bag. Berocca Parenteral Nutrition (Roche) and MVI-12 (Armour) provide fat- and water-soluble vitamins to meet recommended daily requirements. Very depleted patients should receive loading doses of intramuscular vitamin B_{12}, folate, and vitamin K before the commencement of feeding. Patramin-6A (Pentcal) is designed to provide recommended daily requirements of zinc, copper, manganese, iron, chromium, and selenium.

An example of how the nutrient requirements are prescribed and how the nutrient solution is formulated is given in Tables 3-8 and 3-9.

Special Additions and Deletions from the Nutrient Solution

Albumin. Severe hypoalbuminemia, that is, plasma albumin, 30 g per liter or less, is best treated at the commencement and throughout the course of TPN. Salt-poor albumin, 25 to 50 g per day given during the first few days of replenishment, may restore the colloid osmotic pressure and gastrointestinal function in patients in whom sepsis has been eliminated or controlled. It probably is wasteful to give albumin in critically ill patients who suffer from continuing sepsis.

Potassium and Phosphorus. It is important to remember that the need for potassium and phosphorus may be quite high in very debilitated patients. In order to achieve positive nitrogen balance and tissue synthesis, not only must adequate calories and sufficient nitrogen be provided but also potassium and phosphorus must be supplied in sufficient quantities to support cellular growth without causing hypokalemia or hypophosphatemia. The recommended daily doses of potassium and phosphorus may be insufficient in severely depleted patients, and the exact requirement can best be controlled according to daily plasma levels.

Table 3-8. Prescription for the Maintenance of the Nutritional State of a 54-Year-Old 71-kg Man

	24-Hour Nutritional Requirement
Energy	2866 kcal/day (40 kcal/kg/day)
Protein	106 g/day (1.5 g/kg/day)
Water	2500 (35 ml/kg/day)
Na	75 meq
K	75 meq
P	37.5 mmole
Mg	12.5 meq
Calcium	11.8 meq
Chloride	125 meq
Acetate	175 meq
1 ampule of MVI	12
1 ampule of trace element solution	7

Note: Approximately 30% of nonprotein energy should be supplied as fat.
From GL Hill. *Disorders of Nutrition and Metabolism in Clinical Surgery.* Edinburgh: Churchill Livingstone, 1992. With permission.

Table 3-9. Pharmacologic Formulation of the Nutrient Admixture

	Volume (ml)	Content (g)	kcal
Amino acids (10%)	1000	100	400
Dextrose (70%)	700	490	1666
Fat emulsion (20%)	400	800	800
Free water	400		
Total Volume	2500 ml		
Protein	100g		
Energy	2866 kcal		

To this were added electrolytes, vitamins, and trace elements as above

From GL Hill. *Disorders of Nutrition and Metabolism in Clinical Surgery.* Edinburgh: Churchill Livingstone, 1992. With permission.

Sodium. Wasted patients with hypoalbuminemia usually have an expanded extracellular water space and require little or no sodium in the nutrient solution until body hydration is normalized.

Insulin. This is added in sufficient quantities to the nutrient solution to keep the blood sugar within the normal range.

Other Medications. Other medications that are commonly added to the nutrient solution include the H_2 blockers, ranitidine and cimetidine.

Administration of Nutrient Solution

Great care must be taken in delivering the nutrient solution, which is usually given over a 24-hour period. Some authorities use cyclical parenteral feeding but in ordinary surgical practice it is simpler to continue feeding at a constant rate throughout the day and night using a volumetric infusion pump. It is usual to give 1.0 to 1.5 liters in the first 24-hour period, followed by the administration of a further liter every 12 hours for the next 48-hour period or until requirements are met. Supplemental water, sodium, and potassium are given separately as indicated from balance studies and plasma levels. This careful administration of moderate increments avoids hyperosmolarity problems and gives the pancreas time to adapt with increased insulin output in response to the glucose load. Within 2 or 3 days, most patients cope well with their full requirement.

Monitoring

Intravenous nutrition is not the sort of treatment that can be given casually. The patient should be weighed daily and an accurate intake and output record should be kept. Each time the patient passes urine it should be tested for glucosuria. If this is present blood glucose should be monitored until the situation is under control,

either by reducing intake or giving added insulin.

A monitoring schedule that is used widely is shown in Table 3-10.

Complications

Numerous complications may occur during the administration of IVN (Table 3-11) but with experience and proper management most of these can be avoided, or if they happen they can be detected early and treated properly and successfully.

Before patients undergo surgical procedures, IVN should be tapered and during the operation itself the line should be kept

open with a 10% dextrose solution. Before IVN is commenced again when the patient's condition is stable after surgery, it is necessary to change the catheter over a guideline because catheter-related sepsis occurs frequently if that is not done.

Special Conditions

Several conditions are encountered in general surgical practice that sometimes require modification of the nutrient regimen.

Hepatic Failure

In patients with fulminant hepatic failure administration of conventional amino acid solutions may worsen the encephalopathy.

Table 3-10. Monitoring Patients on TPN

Measurement	Frequency Required	
	First Week	Thereafter if Patient's Condition is Stable
Body weight	Daily	Daily
Volume of infusate	Daily	Daily
Oral intake	Daily	Daily
Urine output	Daily	Daily
Plasma electrolytes	Daily	3×/wk
Plasma osmolality	Daily	3×/wk
Blood glucose	Daily	3×/wk
Hemoglobin	3×/wk	Weekly
Calcium	3×/wk	Weekly
Magnesium	3×/wk	Weekly
Triglycerides	3×/wk	Weekly
Urine		
Glucose	4–6×/day	2×/day
Sodium	As indicated	As indicated
Potassium	As indicated	As indicated

From GL Hill. *Disorders of Nutrition and Metabolism in Clinical Surgery.* Edinburgh: Churchill Livingstone, 1992. With permission.

Table 3-11. Common Metabolic Complications of TPN

Complication	Usual Cause	Treatment
Hyperglycemia	Too-rapid infusion, developing sepsis	Slow rate, add insulin, treat sepsis
Hypoglycemia	Rapid cessation of nutrient infusion	When infusion stopped give 10% dextrose solution for ~8 hr
Hypertriglyceridemia	Too much fat being administered	Discontinue fat infusion
Hyperchloremic metabolic acidosis	Too much chloride	Na^+ + K^+ administered as acetate salts
Prerenal azotemia	Excessive amino acid infusion	Reduce intake or increase free water
Hypophosphatemia	Insufficient phosphorus in infusate	Stop infusion and ensure that 20 mmole phosphate is being given for every 1000 kcal
Hypokalemia	Very depleted patient with insufficient K in infusate	Slow administration and add more K^+
Hyperkalemia	Metabolic acidosis, renal failure	Stop all K^+ intake; treat cause

From GL Hill. *Disorders of Nutrition and Metabolism in Clinical Surgery.* Edinburgh: Churchill Livingstone, 1992. With permission.

Hepatic encephalopathy has been related to the high levels of aromatic amino acids (phenylalanine, tyrosine, and tryptophan) in the plasma, acting as precursors of false neurotransmitter amines in the central and peripheral nervous systems. Administration of branched-chain amino acid solutions (enriched with leucine, isoleucine, and valine) will normalize the plasma aminogram and possibly reverse the coma in patients with chronic encephalopathy. Glucose should be used as the energy source in hepatic failure but it needs careful monitoring. Blood levels may fluctuate widely because carbohydrate tolerance is impaired as a result of peripheral insulin resistance. Intravenous lipid infusions are contraindicated as they have a synergistic effect in producing coma particularly with ammonia and they may exacerbate coma by displacing tryptophan from plasma protein binding sites. Patients with chronic hepatic failure should also receive increased amounts of vitamins. In spite of several trials, which together show that such solutions do indeed improve encephalopathy, there continues to be concern over the possibility that they may be associated with an increased mortality.

Renal Failure

Patients with acute renal failure are usually hypercatabolic and have increased requirements for energy and nitrogen. They have a high mortality. Generally, they suffer from serious surgical problems or major trauma, or both, and are often unable to eat. They frequently need IVN. Because of limited fluid volumes and the increased blood urea from protein administration, modified nutritional regimens have been suggested for such patients. However, with the early use of dialysis many of these problems can be overcome and a full nutritional regimen prescribed. It has been suggested that the use of essential amino acids alone may improve survival as well as improve blood urea levels. Others have shown that the administration of adequate amounts of protein and energy with hemodialysis is more important in improving survival than the use of essential or nonessential amino acids. In fact there are some data to suggest that recovery of renal function is enhanced when the amino acid load is reduced. Careful monitoring of potassium, phosphate, hydrogen, magnesium, and calcium ions in patients with renal failure who are receiving TPN is essential. Thus, the composition of nutri-

ent solution used in patients with acute renal failure should take into account the patient's nutritional status and ability to tolerate amino acids, fluids, and electrolytes.

Respiratory Failure

Administration of high doses of glucose to patients with borderline respiratory function may increase their carbon dioxide production to the point of compromising respiratory function. Such patients in intensive care may benefit from the replacement of some glucose energy intake with fat. High rates of infusion of amino acids may increase respiratory drive in some patients; this may be important therapeutically.

Cardiac Failure

The goals of IVN in patients with cardiac failure are to provide adequate nutritional requirements in a concentrated form and with lower sodium intakes than usual.

Major Injury or Sepsis

Branched-chain amino acids (leucine, isoleucine, valine) are essential amino acids that can be used primarily as fuel for skeletal muscle. Leucine in particular stimulates protein synthesis and inhibits protein breakdown in muscle. It has therefore been proposed that amino acid solutions for stressed patients should be fortified with leucine, isoleucine, and valine. Such solutions are now available and are used to enrich standard solutions up to 46%. Some clinical studies have noted improved nitrogen retention with such solutions but no major effect on outcome has been demonstrable.

Short-Chain Peptides in IVN

The very low solubility of cysteine and tyrosine and the instability of cysteine and glutamine in aqueous solutions prevent addition of these amino acids to nutrient solutions. A way has now been found of supplementing commonly available synthetic amino acid solutions with synthetic dipeptides. For instance the synthetic dipeptide L-alanyl-L-glutamine can be used as a safe and efficient source of free glutamine as part of a commercial solution. Glutamine, apart from its use as a "gut fuel," which has potential as a general anabolic mediator, and in the future it will be a standard component of parenteral nutrient solutions.

Growth Factors and Parenteral Nutrition

Growth hormone has anabolic, lipolytic, and diabetogenic properties. Early studies with pituitary extracts showed its anabolic effects in convalescent patients and those with burns, but until the production of growth hormone by recombinant DNA methods began, the small supply of pituitary-derived human growth hormone limited its use to the treatment of children with growth hormone deficiency. The wide availability of synthetic human growth hormone has raised the question as to its role in clinical nutrition. Low-dose growth hormone and hypocaloric nutrition (20 kcal/kg/day, 1 g protein/kg/day) has been found to attenuate the loss of protein after elective gastrointestinal surgery. This effect of growth hormone was achieved through increased protein synthesis and was also associated with increased muscular strength.

As we have seen, patients with sepsis or trauma, or both, continue to lose body protein in spite of IVN. The administration of recombinant human growth hormone increases whole-body protein synthesis and the net loss of protein is decreased.

More comprehensive studies are now under way both with growth hormone and its mediator (insulin-like growth factor–I) to see if the combined effect of hypocaloric feeding can reduce morbidity and length of hospital stay for surgical patients.

Suggested Reading

ASPEN Board of Directors. Guidelines for the use of parenteral and enteral nutrition in adult and paediatric patients. *J Parenteral Enteral Nutr* 17 (Suppl), 1993.

Haydock DA, Hill GL. Improved wound healing response in surgical patients receiving intravenous nutrition. *Br J Surg* 74:320, 1987.

Hill GL. Body composition research: Implications for the practice of clinical nutrition. *J Parenteral Enteral Nutr* 16:197, 1992.

Hill GL. Impact of nutritional support on the clinical outcome of the surgical patient. *Clin Nutr* 13:331, 1994.

Jeejeebhoy KN. Bulk or bounce—the object of nutritional support. *J Parenteral Enteral Nutr* 12:539, 1988.

Jiang Z-M, He GZ, Zhang S-Y, et al. Low dose growth hormone and hypocaloric nutrition attenuate the protein-catabolic response after major operation. *Ann Surg* 210:513, 1989.

Long CL, Schaffel N, Geiger JW, et al. Metabolic response to injury and illness: estimation of energy and protein needs from indirect calorimetry and nitrogen balance. *J Parenteral Enteral Nutr* 3:452, 1979.

Mansfield PF, Hohn DC, Fornage BD, et al. Complications and failures of subclavian catheterization. *N Engl J Med* 331:1735, 1994.

Streat SJ, Hill GL. Nutritional support in the management of critically ill patients in surgical intensive care. *World J Surg* 11:194, 1987.

Windsor JA, Hill GL. Grip strength: a measure of the proportion of protein loss in surgical patients. *Br J Surg* 75:880, 1988.

Windsor JA, Hill GL. Weight loss with physiologic impairment—a basic indicator of surgical risk. *Ann Surg* 207:290, 1988.

EDITOR'S COMMENT

Professor Hill has provided an excellent chapter in which the emphasis, as in his various studies, is on identification of the patient at risk by physiologic impairment. Other studies from two groups in the United States have identified patients at risk on the basis of two very simple parameters: (1) weight loss of 10 to 15 percent and (2) a serum albumin in the normovolemic state of less than 3.0 mg/dl. Two entirely different bodies of investigations have come together to yield this assessment of the patient at risk.

Nutritional assessment, a clinical term, is a method of estimating changes in body nutritional composition in order to predict risk for a given treatment, usually surgical treatment but at times chemotherapy or radiation, or both. Nutritional assessment at present is disappointing but shows some hope of improvement. Although the ability to predict risk in a large population, such as severely malnourished populations in Third World countries, has been well established in the nonsurgical nutritional literature, risk for an individual patient cannot be predicted accurately in a United States hospital setting. In other words, outcome has not been predictable except in a statistical sense.

It is thought that confusion in this area is due to inaccuracies of concept, such as confusion between measuring structure and function. Theoretically, one should

measure lean body mass functionally. For example, how does loss of lean body mass affect muscular, respiratory, cardiac, hepatic, and renal functions? More importantly, how have immunologic and host defense functions, including neutrophil function, been affected?

If one views current practices in the light of the aforementioned goals, the parameters commonly used are disappointing. Structural measurements, including midarm muscle circumference and height-weight ratio, indicate stores but do not reflect function, and triceps skin fold thickness measures fat stores, which has little to do with function. Neutrophil function is at least one order of magnitude removed from cell-mediated immunity, most commonly tested by delayed hypersensitivity to skin recall antigens. Although recent reviews discounted the value of skin recall antigen testing, better-directed studies may identify the individual patient at risk.

Acceptable studies, in my opinion, should be randomized and prospective, include a large number of *consecutive* nonselected patients, and have blinded observers. When these criteria are applied, few studies qualify. Most published studies are retrospective for selected patients, usually specifically those patients judged severely at risk. More recent studies that emphasize hepatic synthesis of short-turnover proteins, immunologically related proteins, and neutrophil function may be more successful in identifying patients at risk for infection. Buzby, Mullen, and coworkers have suggested a "prognostic nutritional index," but their patients were selected nonconsecutively and studied retrospectively (*Ann Surg* 192:604, 1980). Consecutive patients studied prospectively in equally large numbers failed to reveal a group at risk. Other investigators have convincingly shown that accurate observation by experienced observers not particularly skilled in "nutritional assessment" provides the same accuracy as extensive tests.

Recent studies, especially those by Hill and colleagues, and summarized here, have stressed the importance of a careful functional history, which makes sense since it is not the malnutrition per se, but apparently an immunologic defect associated with severe malnutrition that places

patients at risk. Once this subset of patients can be identified, one can then concentrate on repairing the defect. Buzby and coworkers, in the recent Veterans Administration Hospital cooperative study, have identified a group of severely malnourished patients at risk, and decreased operative morbidity with perioperative parenteral nutrition (*N Engl J Med* 325:525, 1991). If all of these studies are collated, the potential for identification of the patient at risk is quite close. Clearly, while many of the large demographic studies using commercially available skin-testing apparatus are nonspecific, carefully done studies may soon identify the individual patient at risk, which is the goal of nutritional assessment.

When all studies are evaluated, the patient at risk can be recognized, in the reviewer's opinion, in the following manner:

1. Recent weight loss of greater than 15 percent body weight and/or body weight of 80 to 85 percent ideal body weight
2. Serum albumin in a stable, hydrated patient of less than 3.0 g/dl.

These two simple parameters will probably define the population at risk. Additional corroborative information includes

3. Anergy to *injected* skin recall antigen by the injection technique
4. True transferrin of less than 200 mg/dl
5. A history of functional impairment
6. Significant deficits in hand dynamometry or muscle response to nerve stimulation

The critical importance of albumin is shown by juxtaposing two logit functions that attempt to identify the patient at risk: (1) From Mullen and coworkers:

$$PNI = 158 - 16.6\ ALB - 0.78\ \text{triceps skinfold} - 0.20\ TFN - 5.8\ DTH$$

where PNI is prognostic nutritional index, TH is delayed-type hypersensitivity, and TNF is transferrin. (2) From Christou's work:

$$P\ |death|$$
$$= 1 + e^{(-3-45+1.75*(ALB)+0.3*(In[DTH\ score]))}$$

What is it about albumin that figures so prominently in both bodies of work that determine nutritional risk? In subsequent studies from the Montreal group, it appears that the same individuals who are anergic also have an exchangeable sodium-potassium ratio of greater than 1.22, making them malnourished. This in itself is not surprising. However, there is another implication for an increased exchangeable sodium-potassium ratio of greater than 1.22, and that is an increase in extravascular volume. If there is a greater extravascular volume, there is likely to be a greater amount of albumin in the extravascular space; since the serum concentration of albumin is directly proportional to its degradation, increasing the amount of albumin in the extravascular space will increase the rate of its degradation, thus decreasing serum concentration.

There has always been controversy over what the lowered serum albumin means in patients who are ostensibly malnourished.

While some have said that serum albumin is low because of decreased synthesis, others have claimed that there is a greater volume of distribution and increased degradation. Yet others have suggested that perhaps there is low-grade sepsis and that the synthesis of albumin is downregulated. The author does not believe this latter point to be tenable because in a long-term sepsis model, von Allmen and associates, working in our laboratory, found that whereas albumin synthesis was downregulated for the first 24 hours, after 3 or 4 days it was actually increased (*J Surg Res* 48:476, 1990).

Thus, decreased albumin synthesis because of downregulation is not tenable in long-term malnutrition. The fact that there is increased albumin in the extravascular space with an increased rate of degradation may very well explain the lowered serum albumin in patients who are at risk. What is of interest is that it took two different bodies of work coming together to come to this conclusion.

However, both of these approaches, and particularly that of Christou and Meakins, identify only a population at risk. Within that population, the immunologic defect associated with malnutrition will result in impaired outcome in approximately 60 percent of the patients. Thus, even when one is injecting antigens and obtaining anergy, only 60 percent of those patients will be at risk. The advantage of the approach that Professor Hill espouses is that it will usually identify the individual patient at risk. Albumin is not foolproof, as Professor Hill indicates, depending on the evolution of the nutritional impairment. Particular attention as to whether the patient can do ordinary tasks or if ordinary tasks have been limited over the past several months, such as the ability to breathe, ambulate, give hand grip, and so forth, will reveal the patient who is in jeopardy from a major surgical procedure.

J.E.F.

4

Enteral Nutritional Support

John L. Rombeau   Thomas E. Hamilton

Enteral nutrition is the provision of liquid formula diets into the gastrointestinal tract. When compared to total parenteral nutrition (TPN), enteral nutrition significantly increases intestinal growth and function and is less expensive. Due to the recognition of these important benefits, enteral nutrition is being prescribed with increasing frequency in surgical patients. It is therefore incumbent on surgeons to be familiar with the rationale, administration, and prevention of complications of enteral nutrition.

Rationale

Effects on Intestinal Growth and Function

The presence of nutrients in the lumen of the gut provides the most important stimulus for gut growth and function. Enteral nutrients mediate their effects on the gut directly and indirectly. The mechanical contact of enteral nutrients with the apex of the intestinal villus directly increases epithelial desquamation, thereby stimulating mucosal cell renewal in the villus crypt. Atrophy of the small and large bowel occurs when luminal stimuli or intestinal nutrients are absent. These atrophic changes occur in absorptive cells, mucus-secreting goblet cells, gut-associated lymphoid tissue, and brush border enzymes, all of which are integral components of the intestinal barrier against bacteria, endotoxins, and other antigenic macromolecules. Maintenance of the intestinal barrier is one of the reasons for administering small volumes of continuous enteral feeding even when parenteral feeding is required to meet total nutrient needs.

Many indirect effects of enteral nutrients are mediated by enterotrophic gut hormones such as gastrin, neurotensin, bombesin, and enteroglucagon. These enterotrophic responses are carried out by autocrine, paracrine, and systemic hormonal responses of the gut to luminal nutrients, which provide stimulus for gut structure and function. Examples of these effects include trophic effects on the stomach, duodenum, and possibly colon by gastrin. Neurotensin administered to rats stimulates mucosal growth and prevents jejunal atrophy produced by liquid elemental diets. Bombesin increases ileal and jejunal mucosal weight and stimulates pancreatic growth in rats fed elemental diets.

Avoidance of Total Parenteral Nutrition

Another reason for using enteral nutrition is to avoid the many side effects of TPN. Total parenteral nutrition, especially when given for prolonged periods, produces fatty liver, bone disease, catheter sepsis, and psychiatric disturbances. [*Editor's note*: I am not certain what is meant by "psychiatric disturbances," as we have not recognized this complication in our own patients.] These adverse effects are generally not associated with enteral nutrition. Additional factors support the direct provision of nutrients into the gut rather than intravenous feeding. First-pass processing of nutrients by the liver regulates plasma concentrations and the chemical form in which substrates are presented to target organs. Lipids, for example, are processed by the intestine into chylomicrons and subsequently into lipoproteins by the liver after enteral delivery. When lipid emul-

sions are delivered parenterally, abnormal plasma lipid profiles are detected.

Daily requirements for the enteral provision of nutrients, vitamins, and minerals are more clearly defined, especially in states of stress and disease, than in parenteral nutrition. Furthermore, enteral nutrition, calorie per calorie, is far cheaper to administer than parenteral nutrition.

Economics

In the era of cost containment in health care, attention has been directed toward the cost and cost-effectiveness of nutritional support provided by parenteral and enteral nutrition. The manufacturing costs for enteral nutrition are far less than for parenteral feeding; moreover, enteral nutrition may be more cost-effective than feeding oral diets to disabled or debilitated patients by hand. Because the administration of enteral nutrition does not require attention to aseptic technique for administration, additional cost benefit is derived [*Editor's note*: However, one must prevent overgrowth of bacteria in the feedings by refrigeration and not allowing feedings to remain hanging for more than 4–6 hours.]

Indications

General indications for enteral nutrition include the following: 1) the presence of protein energy malnutrition (arbitrarily defined as either the loss of 15% of usual body weight or a serum albumin level of less than 3.3 g/dl in the euvolemic state, or both), 2) a gastrointestinal tract that can be used safely, and 3) anticipated inadequate oral intake for at least 7 days. Safe usage of the gastrointestinal tract is possible in the absence of obstruction, severe intractable diarrhea, or massive hemorrhage. Hemodynamic instability is a further contraindication to enteral feeding. The anticipated duration of inadequate oral intake is based on judgment and experience.

Dietary Formulas

The large number of commercial enteral formulas currently available mandates a classification system to assist the clinician in selecting the proper formula for each patient. A practical classification system based on nutrient composition includes polymeric-balanced diets, "disease-specific" formulas, and modular supplements. A partial listing of available formulas is included in Table 4-1.

Polymeric Balanced Formulas

Polymeric formulas are "complete" balanced, isotonic diets that contain 100 percent of the recommended dietary allowance (RDA) for substrates, vitamins, and minerals when prescribed in recommended amounts. These formulas are palatable and therefore the first choice for oral supplementation or tube feeding when digestion and absorption are reasonably normal. The nitrogen source is an intact or partially hydrolyzed natural protein (e.g., egg, soy, lactalbumin), which requires the ability to digest protein in addition to carbohydrate and fat. The caloric density of these formulas is usually 1 kcal/ml, but can be as high as 1.5 to 2.0 kcal/ml. Calorie-dense formulas are reserved for patients with unusually high caloric requirements or fluid restrictions, and those in whom only limited feeding volumes are tolerated. As a group, the polymeric-balanced formulas are the least expensive, and the most frequently used. They are the formula of choice in approximately 90 percent of most surgical populations. The major disadvantage of polymeric-balanced formulas is their fixed nutrient composition; however, this can be altered with addition of modular supplements.

"Disease-Specific" Formulas

Disease-specific diets are modified to the nutrient deficits associated with certain pathologic conditions. Minimal digestion is required due to the predigested and "elemental" nature of the nutrients, which are almost completely absorbed. Crystalline amino acids provide the protein source; however, some pancreatic function is required for digestion of the carbohydrate component (oligosaccharides and disaccharides) and fat (up to 30% of which is provided as medium-chain triglycerides). Additionally, absorption of glucose, sodium, amino acids, fat, vitamins, and trace elements require intact mucosal transport systems. Unlike the polymeric-balanced diets, disease-specific diets are hyperosmolar, unpalatable, and expensive. In fact, they cost 3 to 10 times as much per calorie as the polymeric-balanced formulas. Rapid administration of these diets may produce diarrhea, and flavor supplementation is required for oral usage. Disease-specific diets may be indicated in states of absorptive insufficiency, such as chronic pancreatitis, short-bowel syndrome, and prolonged ileus, when polymeric diets are not tolerated. Controlled clinical trials are needed to evaluate their efficacy in these conditions.

Modular Supplements

Modular supplements contain single or multiple nutrients that can be added to

Table 4-1. Partial Listing of Commonly Used Commercial Enteral Feeding Formulas

Category	1.0 kcal/ml	1.5 kcal/ml	2.0 kcal/ml
POLYMERIC-BALANCED			
≤16% protein	Ensure, Resource Isocal, Osmolite, Nutren 1.0	Nutren 1.5, Ensure Plus, Resource Plus, Sustacal HC	Nutren 2.0, Isocal NCN, Magnacal
17–20% protein	Osmolite HN, Isocal HN, Ensure HN, Ultracal, Jevity	Ensure Plus HN	TwoCal HN
≤20% protein	Sustacal, Replete,	TraumaCal	
MODIFIED-CONVENTIONAL			
≤16% protein	Peptamen, Reabilan Vivinex Plus, Criticare HN		
17–20% protein	Vital HN, Reabilan HN, AlitraQ		
MODIFIED-DISEASE SPECIFIC (% PROTEIN)			
"Critical Care"	Impact (22%)	Perative (20%)	
"Renal"		Travasorb Renal (7%)	Nepro (14%) Suplena (6%) Amin-Aid (4%)
"Hepatic"	Travasorb Hepatic (11%) Hepatic-Aid (15%)		
"Pulmonary"		Pulmocare (17%) NutriVent (18%)	
"Glucose intolerance"	Glucerna (17%)		
MODULAR SUPPLEMENTS			
Protein	Propac, Casec, ProMod, Nutrisource Moducal,		
Carbohydrates	Polycose, Sumacal, Nutrisource Microlipid,		
Fat	MCT oil, Nutrisource		

"fixed ratio" diets without affecting the quantity of other nutrients. They are designed for patients whose dietary requirements lie outside the standard nutrient requirements. Commercially available modules include carbohydrate, fat, protein, mineral, electrolyte, and vitamin formulations.

Administration of Enteral Nutrition

Nutritional Assessment and Monitoring

Selection of patients who require enteral nutrition is based on body weight loss, anticipated duration of illness, and gastrointestinal function.

History and physical examination are the most important components of nutritional assessment. Body height and weight measurements provide an important baseline for nutritional repletion. Patients with a minimum of 15 percent loss (10% if severely stressed) of usual body weight are arbitrarily defined as malnourished and should receive some form of nutritional support. Biochemical indices in nutritional assessment include serum levels of albumin, transferrin, prealbumin, retinol-binding protein, and thyroxine-binding protein. Serum albumin alone has proven predictive value in chronic protein malnutrition and epidemiologic surveys. Serum albumin is an indicator of protein stores; however, it is a poor indicator of early protein malnutrition. This is because serum levels fall and recover slowly with flux in nutritional status. Additionally, the half-life of 20 days and large body pool of albumin account for the slow response to protein repletion. Falsely altered levels occur during volume overload, dehydration, or loss of capillary integrity. In general, serum albumin levels lower than 3 g/dl correlate with increased morbidity and mortality of hospitalized patients. Various degrees of protein depletion are reflected by albumin levels: mild depletion, 2.8 to 3.5 g/dl; moderate depletion, 2.1 to 2.7 g/dl; and severe depletion, less than 2.1 g/dl.

Nitrogen balance, the difference between nitrogen intake and nitrogen loss, reflects the degree of protein catabolism. In patients without severe diarrhea nitrogen is primarily lost in the urine, principally as urea. Therefore, measuring urinary urea nitrogen over a 24-hour period is an important determinant of nitrogen loss. The addition of 4 g nitrogen a day is often used as a clinical estimate of nonurea nitrogen losses (urine creatinine and ammonia, fecal and integumentary losses). Nitrogen intake is determined by dietary survey and determination of dietary intake.

Determination of Energy Requirements

Determination of caloric requirements is an integral component of nutritional support. It must first be clearly established whether the objective for nutritional support is either repletion or maintenance of lean body mass (fat-free energy-consuming tissue of the body). Patients who are critically ill have increased circulating levels of catabolic hormones, including cortisol, catecholamines, and glucagon. This hormonal milieu impairs nitrogen retention and inhibits anabolism; therefore, the caloric goal in these patients is to maintain and not replete lean body mass. Nutritional repletion occurs only in a hormonal environment, which supports an anabolic phase of recovery. Nutrient delivery cannot change a patient in the catabolic phase of illness into an anabolic state. In fact, excess delivery of nutrients in the catabolic phase of illness, especially in the presence of stress or sepsis, results in increased lipogenesis, leading to hepatic fat and glycogen deposition and a potentiation of the stress response. Thus, the caloric goal for the catabolic patient is maintenance of nutritional status. Primary treatment must be directed at the underlying cause of the catabolic state. When the catabolic state has been treated appropriately, the hormonal milieu supports anabolism and the goal for nutritional support is repletion of existing deficits.

Energy determination is based on age, gender, body build, activity level, and disease state. No single test measures the energy needs for all patients. Estimates for energy requirements are calculated by standard formulas or measured by indirect calorimetry. The formula most commonly used to predict resting metabolic expenditure (RME) is the Harris-Benedict equation:

RME male = $66 + 13W + 5H - 6.8A$

RME female = $655 + 9.6W + 1.8H - 4.7A$

RME = resting metabolic expenditure (kcal/day)

W = weight (kg)

H = height (cm)

A = age (years)

After determination of the RME, energy requirements are adjusted for physical activity and illness Table 4-2).

Determination of Protein Requirements

Protein requirements are influenced by energy intake, and depend on the nonprotein calorie-nitrogen ratio, which varies considerably in different clinical conditions. In the nonstressed patient, the optimal ratio of nonprotein calorie-nitrogen is 150:1. In critically ill patients, this ratio decreases to 100:1 because of requirements for synthesis of acute-phase proteins, and tissue repair. Precise levels of protein required for different levels of caloric intake have not been defined. However, practical guidelines have been created for initial protein and caloric regimen prescriptions. Adjustments of protein and calories should be made according to nitrogen balance studies and clinical course throughout nutritional support (Table 4-3).

Determination of Electrolyte and Micronutrient Requirements

Requirements for sodium, potassium, bicarbonate, chloride, magnesium, calcium, and phosphate are determined by baseline levels, calculated losses, and maintenance needs. (Rombeau, *Clin Nutr*, Vol II, 1988).

Table 4-2. Energy Requirement Factors for Hospitalized Patients

Clinical Conditions	Correct Factor (×RME)
Physical activity	
Confined to bed	1.2
Out of bed	1.3
Starvation	0.7
Fever	1.0 + 0.13 per C°
Elective surgery	1.0 − 1.2
Peritonitis	1.2 − 1.5
Soft-tissue trauma	1.1 − 1.3
Major sepsis	1.4 − 1.8

RME = resting metabolic expenditure.

Table 4-3. Protein Requirements and Nonprotein Calorie-Nitrogen Ratio in Hospitalized Patients

Clinical Conditions	N (g/kg/day)	NPC/N
Nonstress		
N maintenance	0.6–0.8	150:1
N repletion	1.0–1.2	150:1
Stress		
Active inflammation	1.2–1.5*	150:1
Major surgery	1.2–1.5	120:1
Sepsis	2.0–2.5	80:1

N (g/kg/day) = grams of nitrogen per kilogram of body weight per day; NPC/N = nonprotein calorie-nitrogen ratio.
*Add fecal losses.

Vitamins should be administered daily in quantities recommended by the Nutritional Advisory Group of the American Medical Association. Standard amounts of trace elements are included in most commercially available enteral formulas.

Monitoring

Patients who receive enteral nutrition require careful monitoring, which is best performed by a nutrition support team. A monitoring protocol may be helpful in institutions where physicians of variable levels of experience are responsible for writing patient orders.

Daily physical examination is essential for critically ill patients when dysfunction of the gastrointestinal tract may produce intolerance to enteral formulas. Intolerance is manifest as distention, diarrhea, nausea, and excessive gastric residuals. Nitrogen balance, body weight, and serum protein levels are monitored routinely and used in calculating nutrient requirements as discussed previously. Complementary use of TPN is often necessary to reach nutritional goals during the time interval required to reach total enteral nutrient goals. Detailed attention to metabolic status and fluid balance is also essential when treating critically ill patients. When standardized monitoring is followed, potential complications can be averted preemptively, often by simple maneuvers such as changing the dietary infusion rate, caloric density, or formulation (Table 4-4).

Enteral Access

Enteral nutrition can be administered by several routes depending on the anticipated duration of feeding and potential

Table 4-4. Standard Orders for Enteral Feeding

Feeding tube type and location of tip: _____

Check items to be completed:

_____ 1. Obtain chest x-ray after placement to confirm position.
_____ 2. Before feeding, confirm placement of tube by aspiration of gastric contents.
_____ 3. Elevate head to bed 30 degrees when feeding into the stomach.
_____ 4. Name of the formula _____
     a. Intermittent: Give _____ ml over 30 minutes every _____ hrs at _____ strength.
     b. Continuous: Give _____ ml per hour for _____ hrs at _____ strength.
_____ 5. Check for residual _____ hrs with gastric feeding.
     Return residual to stomach.
     Hold feedings for one hour if residual is greater than _____ ml and recheck in one hour.
     Notify physician if this occurs on two consecutive measurements of residual.
_____ 6. Weigh patient Monday and Thursday and record on chart.
_____ 7. Record intake and output daily.
     Chart volume of formula separately from water or other oral intake for each shift.
     Record number, volume, and consistency of bowel movements.
_____ 8. Change administration tubing and feeding bag daily.
_____ 9. Irrigate feeding tube with 20 ml water at the completion of each intermittent feeding, when tube is disconnected, following the delivery of medications and when the feeding is stopped for any reason.
_____ 10. Obtain complete blood count, complete serum chemistry profile, and total iron-binding capacity (transferrin) weekly.
_____ 11. Obtain basic chemistry profile every Monday and Thursday.
_____ 12. Begin 24-hr urine collection for urea nitrogen and creatinine at 7:00 AM on _____.
_____ 13. Notify physician for nausea, vomiting, severe diarrhea, or shortness of breath.

risk for aspiration. The oral route is preferred; however, it requires an alert patient with an intact gag reflex, who requires only supplementation with meals. For patients in whom the oral route is not possible, other methods for delivery of enteral nutrients include nasogastric tubes, nasoenteric tubes, gastrostomy, jejunostomy, and combined gastric-jejunal tubes.

Nasogastric tube or nasoenteric tube access is best used for patients who require short-term (arbitrarily defined as <4 weeks) enteral nutrition. The optimal tube types are composed of silicon or polyurethane and are soft, pliable, nonreactive, and well tolerated for 3 to 4 weeks. For this route of administration, patients must have intact gag reflexes and a competent lower esophageal sphincter. Ideal candidates include patients with poor oral intake such as secondary to cancer-induced anorexia. The stomach is the most physiologic and the preferred site of delivery; however, if gastroparesis exists or if the patient is at increased risk for aspiration, a nasoenteric tube should be advanced into the jejunum. The interventional radiologist or endoscopist is often helpful with tube placement into the jejunum.

Complications of placement of soft feeding tubes, although infrequent, include pneu-

mothorax, perforated viscus, pharyngeal tear, and perforated bronchus. Attention to proper tube placement techniques reduces these complications. A chest radiograph after tube placement is mandatory to confirm proper position before initiation of feedings with both nasogastric and nasoenteric tubes.

For patients who require long-term (greater than 4 weeks) of enteral nutrition, permanent access to the gastrointestinal tract through a tube enterostomy is the preferred method of delivery. Tube enterostomies are inserted with endoscopic assistance or by an open operative procedure. The most common sites for placement of permanent access include the stomach and jejunum.

Percutaneous Endoscopic Gastrostomy

The percutaneous endoscopic gastrostomy (PEG) has several advantages over open gastrostomy tube placement, including local anesthesia, avoidance of ileus, decreased procedure time, and absence of an incision. The speed, simplicity, safety, and low cost of PEG have made this technique the procedure of choice over surgical gastrostomy in most hospitals. Percutaneous

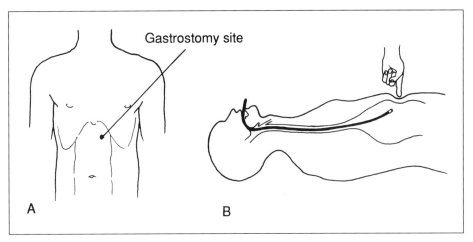

Fig. 4-1. PEG 1. A. Depicts correct PEG insertion site on the abdominal wall. B. The endoscopist observes "one-to-one" indentation of the stomach by the assistant's finger applied to the external abdominal wall.

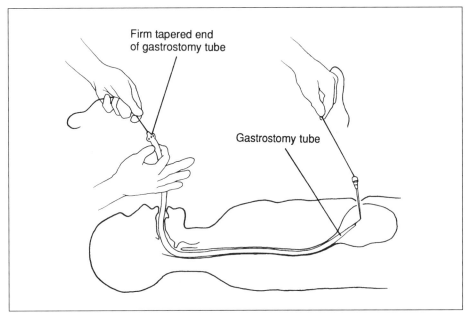

Fig. 4-2. PEG 3. The gastrostomy tube is secured to the guidestring and pulled through the oropharynx and out the abdominal wall. Depicted is the gastrostomy tube as it enters the stomach.

endoscopic gastrostomy is contraindicated in patients with strictures or obstructing lesions of the esophagus, and in those patients undergoing imminent abdominal surgery. Prior upper abdominal surgery is a relative contraindication for PEG. Either of the two basic PEG techniques, the standard technique with double endoscopy or the direct technique with single endoscopy, can be used. Both techniques require the patient to remain nil per os (NPO) for at least 8 hours before the procedure and are performed with the patient lying supine for the identification of abdominal landmarks. The PEG insertion site is in the left upper quadrant immediately below the costal margin to avoid injury to the transverse colon. In the pediatric patient, placement must accommodate for growth. If placed too close to the costal margin, the tube may erode into the ribs with dire consequences. After intravenous sedation and topical anesthesia of the pharynx, the gastroscope is passed into the stomach. The endoscope light must then be observed on the anterior abdominal wall for the procedure to continue. The stomach is then insufflated with air and kept distended throughout the procedure to appose the stomach and the anterior abdominal wall and displace the transverse colon inferiorly. The abdominal wall is cleaned antiseptically and the endoscopist observes for one-to-one variability of the gastric wall indentation by the operator's finger at the chosen insertion site. The two techniques for PEG placement diverge at this point (Fig. 4-1).

In the standard double endoscopy technique initially described by Ponsky and Garderer, the insertion site is anesthetized with 1% lidocaine solution and a 1-cm incision is made. A large-bore needle with inner stylet is inserted into the stomach (Fig. 4-2). The endoscopist confirms proper placement of the needle and the inner stylet is removed. The endoscopist then places a snare loosely over the end of the needle such that when a guidestring is inserted it can be tightly snared. The endoscope and ensnared guidestring are withdrawn, and the tapered end of the gastrostomy tube is threaded over the guidestring and pulled out through the anterior abdominal wall. The endoscope is then reinserted to verify that the tube abuts snugly to the gastric mucosa. The insufflated air is evacuated and the endoscope is withdrawn. The retention disk is placed over the tapered end of the gastrostomy tube and sutured to the skin. The tapered portion of the tube is cut and the tube fashioned to a universal adapter for gravity damage.

In the single endoscopy technique, also known as the Russel technique, the tube insertion site on the skin is infiltrated with 1% lidocaine solution and an 18-gauge needle is inserted into the stomach under endoscopic vision. A guidewire is then placed through the introducer needle and, once confirmed by the endoscopist, the needle is withdrawn (Fig. 4-3). The fascial opening is enlarged alongside the wire, and a No. 16 French dilator with a peelaway sheath is placed over the wire to enlarge the tract. The guidewire and dilator are removed, leaving only the sheath in the stomach lumen. A lubricated 12 or 14 Fr Foley catheter is placed through the sheath introducer and moved into position by the endoscope. The Foley balloon is inflated, pulled snugly against the abdominal wall, and the sheath is peeled away. The endoscopist confirms the correct position, and the catheter is sutured to the skin and dressed sterilely. The tube is then connected to a bag for gravity drainage.

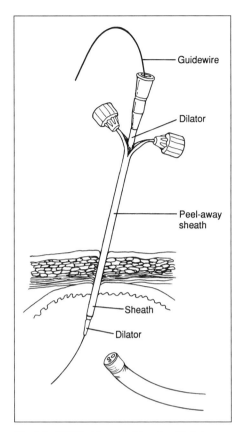

Fig. 4-3. PEG 2. After a stylet and guidestring are placed through the abdominal wall a peel away sheath and dilator are introduced under direct endoscopic vision to permit safe passage of a Foley catheter into the stomach.

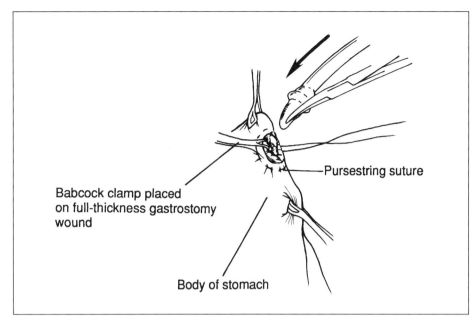

Fig. 4-4. Stamm gastrostomy. Babcock clamp placed in gastrostomy and gastrostomy tube insertion by extending the tip of the tube with a Kelly clamp.

Complications of PEG placement occur in between 1 and 7 percent of patients in most series, and include wound infections, gastrointestinal bleeding at the puncture site, premature dislodgment, and gastrocolonic fistula.

Infectious complications include cellulitis at the tube exit site, abscess at the abdominal wall, and leakage around the tube. Administration of intravenous antibiotics is often therapeutic; however, incision and drainage may be required. Necrotizing fasciitis has also been reported.

Gastrointestinal bleeding at the puncture site in the stomach or on the abdominal wall occurs very infrequently and is most often due to concomitant gastrointestinal lesions such as duodenal ulcer. This emphasizes the need for careful endoscopy at the time of tube placement.

Premature dislodgment of PEG tubes occurs most frequently in the neurologically impaired population. Following tube insertion, strong apposition between the stomach and abdominal wall occurs in approximately 2 weeks. Dislodgment before this time mandates nasogastric decompression and immediate water-soluble contrast radiographs to assess the presence of gastric leakage into the peritoneal cavity. If leakage is confirmed, the hole in the stomach should be closed operatively. If tube dislodgment occurs more than 2 weeks after insertion, the tube can be replaced percutaneously and a water-soluble contrast study must be performed through the tube to confirm placement.

The colon may be inadvertently entered when the tube is being placed through the abdominal wall before entering the stomach. This emphasizes the need for careful observation of one-to-one movement when the endoscopist visualizes the stomach wall indentation because of the assistant's digital compression on the abdominal wall. Insufflation of air into the stomach also displaces the colon inferiorly. Treatment of the fistula may require only tube removal or, if more severe, operative closure of the colonic injury.

Surgical Gastrostomy

Traditional surgical gastrostomy is the method of choice when PEG is not possible or is contraindicated. Surgical gastrostomy is performed by two common techniques: Stamm and Witzel.

Stamm gastrostomy is the easiest to perform. This technique is recommended when the patient is a poor operative risk, or the duration for anticipated tube feedings is relatively short. Mushroom-type, malecot, or Foley catheters can be used. The advantages are ease of placement and simplicity of removal.

An upper midline incision is made, the peritoneum is entered, and the stomach is brought into view by gentle traction on the greater omentum. [*Editor's note*: I prefer a short lateral (beyond the rectus) transverse incision, which is easily done under local anesthesia.] Two Babcock clamps are used to expose the anterior surface of the stomach near the greater curvature (Fig. 4-4). Two concentric pursestring sutures are placed in the seromuscular layer. The fascial layers of the abdominal wall are grasped with Kocher clamps and retracted medially, and a stab wound through the abdominal wall is made on the left side approximately 4 cm lateral to the incision and 2 cm inferior to the costal margin. The tube is then passed through the abdominal wall. Next, a stab wound is made in the center of the concentric pursestring sutures in the stomach wall and the gastrotomy is gently opened with a hemostat. The tube is placed into the stomach lumen through the gastrotomy and the pursestring sutures are tied. The tube is then gently retracted to appose the parietal peritoneum and the stomach wall, which is fixed around the tube with several interrupted sutures. Next, the tube is secured to the skin with nonabsorbable suture (Fig. 4-5).

Witzel gastrostomy differs from the Stamm technique only in that, before exiting the stomach, a seromuscular tunnel is created by making a 5- to 7-cm seromuscular incision laterally. The tube is then placed within the tunnel and either interrupted or continuous sutures are used to close the incision. The seromuscular tunnel minimizes the risk of leakage due to either gastric distention or tube removal. Tube replacement after dislodgment, however, is more difficult with this technique.

The complications following surgical gastrostomy occur in the range of 7 to 10 percent and can be divided into three groups: operative technique, stoma care, and tube related.

Complications due to operative technique include separation of the stomach from the abdominal wall. To prevent this complication, the stomach should be anchored to the parietal peritoneum around the tube before abdominal closure. Separation occurs following inadvertent tube removal and early reinsertion of the tube before there is firm adherence between the stomach and the parietal peritoneum. Tube replacement should be confirmed as discussed in the PEG section. Delayed recognition of this complication may result in severe peritonitis and death.

Wound infection is one of the most common complications and occurs with all types of tube enterostomies. Chronic bacterial overgrowth in the tube tract is the most common type of infection. Wound infection is usually limited to the skin and subcutaneous tissues, although full-thickness abdominal wall infections can occur.

Wound dehiscence, separation, and ventral hernia can occur similar to any laparotomy incision. These complications are often exacerbated by the poor nutritional status and debilitated nature of the patient. Minimizing incisional length, exiting the tube via a separate stab incision, and meticulous approximation of fascial edges help to decrease the incidence of these complications.

Internal tube migration producing gastric outlet obstruction is relatively common. Improper tube placement into the antrum, or internal migration, may result in pyloric obstruction by the balloon tip of a gastrostomy catheter. Leakage around the tube occurs more frequently when it is placed in this dependent position. Foley catheters migrate more commonly than tubes without balloons. Epigastric pain, leakage around the tube, or vomiting may signify tube migration. Simply pulling back the tube and resecuring the tube to the skin will alleviate these problems.

Skin irritation occurs frequently as a result of leakage of gastric contents and is compounded by the placement of occlusive dressings. The main cause of leak is pivoting of the tube at the exit site especially in children. An improperly large or stiff tube may also result in leakage. When identified the problem must be promptly addressed to subvert the spiral of skin excoriation and continued enlargement in stomal diameter. Limiting the use of the tube to water irrigation to maintain patency, avoiding occlusive dressings, and limiting tube motion may help close tract size and stop the leakage. Occlusive dressings should be avoided and exit sites should remain open and dry. Tube plugging occurs when irrigation after feeding is neglected or when the tube is used to deliver crushed medications. Forceful saline irrigation with a small-caliber syringe is often successful at unplugging the tube. The plugged tube should be changed when irrigation fails in a tube within a mature tract. Excessive granulation tissue at the tube exit site is a very common complication of gastrostomy and can be treated effectively by the application of silver nitrate.

Persistence of a gastrocutaneous fistula after intentional tube removal is uncommon. When gastrostomy tubes are removed the site usually closes within a few hours and almost always within a few days. If the tract persists after several weeks, operative closure is recommended.

Surgical Jejunostomy

Surgical jejunostomy is indicated for those patients at high risk for aspiration, or in whom the stomach cannot be used. Jejunostomies are also indicated as an adjunctive procedure when a prolonged postoperative delay in oral intake is anticipated. Examples of these conditions include hepatic, esophageal, or pancreatic operations

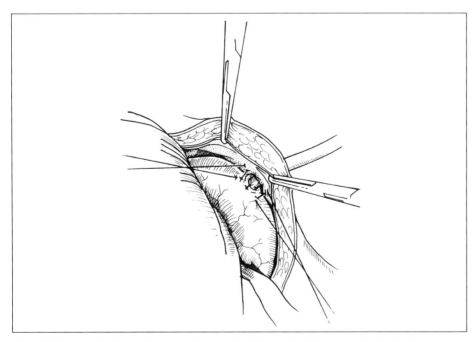

Fig. 4-5. Stamm gastrostomy. The stomach is sutured to the anterior abdominal wall with four interrupted sutures. All sutures are placed before tying and the most lateral suture is tied first.

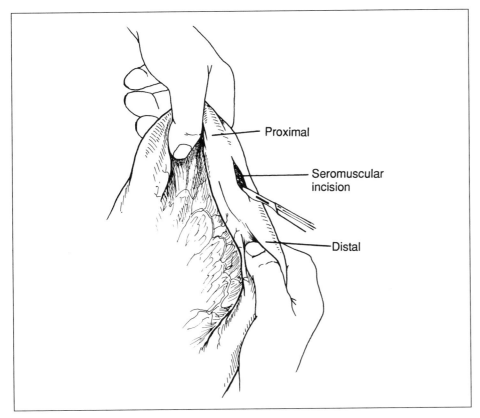

Fig. 4-6. Witzel jejunostomy. Jejunostomy site 20 cm distal to the ligament of Treitz.

when a postoperative catabolic state is anticipated. When feasible, adjunctive jejunostomy is recommended at the time of laparotomy for extensive abdominal trauma. Patients undergoing surgery for abdominal malignancy, who may require chemotherapy and radiation therapy, are additional candidates for surgical jejunostomy. Chemotherapy and radiation therapy produce nausea, anorexia, and vomiting, and jejunal feeding may help maintain the nutritional status of the patient.

Surgical techniques for jejunostomy placement include the Witzel and needle catheter jejunostomy methods.

Witzel jejunostomy utilizes a segment of jejunum 20 cm distal to the ligament of Tretiz (Fig. 4-6). This site permits simple apposition of the jejunum to the parietal surface of the anterior abdominal wall. After selecting the site for tube insertion, a small stab wound is made on the antimesenteric border of the jejunum and a medium red rubber tube is introduced distally for approximately 20 cm. A pursestring suture is placed around the tube at the jejunotomy (Fig. 4-7). A seromuscular incision is made proximally from the tube

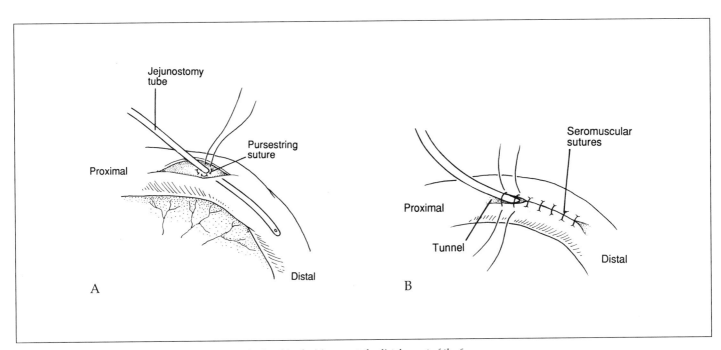

Fig. 4-7. Witzel jejunostomy. A. A pursestring suture is placed in the jejunum at the distal aspect of the 6-cm seromuscular incision and the tube is inserted. B. The muscularis and serosa are closed over the tube to create a tunnel.

for approximately 5 cm. The jejunostomy tube is then placed into the seromuscular tunnel, which is closed with interrupted silk sutures. The tube is brought out through a separate stab incision in the abdominal wall. The jejunum is positioned as a gentle curve and sutured to the anterior parietal peritoneum with several interrupted sutures around the catheter (Fig. 4-8).

Needle catheter jejunostomy is a simple and safe method for catheter placement and utilizes a technique analogous to the Seldinger technique for intravenous catheter placement. A needle similar to those used for central venous catheterization is placed in an oblique fashion through the antimesenteric wall of the jejunum 15 to 20 cm distal to the ligament of Treitz (Fig. 4-9). A 30- to 45-cm, 16-gauge polyvinyl catheter with a stylet is advanced into the lumen. The needle and stylet are withdrawn and the catheter is secured with a

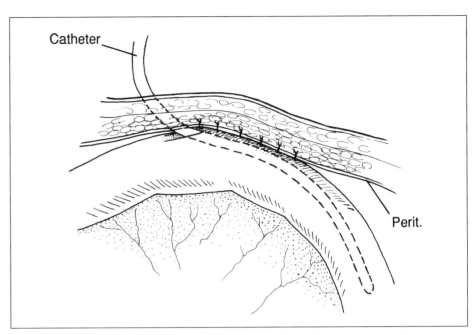

Fig. 4-8. Witzel jejunostomy. Attachment of jejunum with gentle curve to anterior parietal peritoneum to decrease the chance of volvulus.

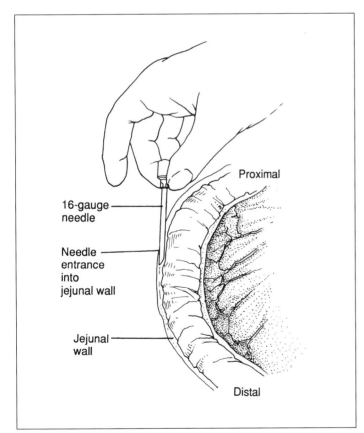

Fig. 4-9. Needle catheter jejunostomy. Needle catheter placed intramurally in the antimesenteric border of the jejunum.

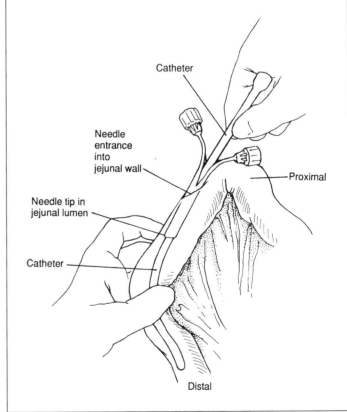

Fig. 4-10. Needle catheter jejunostomy. After dilatation, a peel-away sheath is placed over the guidewire and the catheter is placed through the sheath.

4-0 seromuscular pursestring suture (Fig. 4-10). A separate needle is then placed through a stab wound in the abdominal wall and the proximal segment of the catheter is threaded retrograde to exit the abdominal wall. The needle is removed, the catheter is secured to the skin, and the jejunum is sutured to the anterior parietal peritoneum as discussed previously. Water-soluble contrast studies are recommended before the initiation of feedings. A major side effect of needle catheter jejunostomy is frequent plugging of the tube. Laparoscopic techniques have now evolved to assist with jejunostomy placement. The safety of laparoscopic access compared to traditional open techniques awaits clinical trials.

Complications of jejunostomy placement are similar to those of gastrostomy. Inadvertent tube removal, infection, and leakage have been discussed previously. Volvulus may occur at the tube exit site. Using sufficient length of jejunum and securing the jejunal wall to the parietal peritoneum of the abdominal wall for a short distance help to minimize the risk.

Button Devices for Enterostomy

Button devices are simple skin-level, non-refluxing, synthetic conduits used for long-term enteral feedings in children and adults (Fig. 4-11). Buttons are placed through mature gastrostomy tracts provided they are placed at least 8 weeks postoperatively. Alternatively, buttons can be placed primarily as open operative

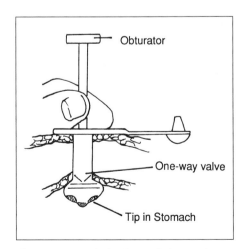

Fig. 4-11. Button device. Button devices can be used as alternatives in the stomach and jejunum.

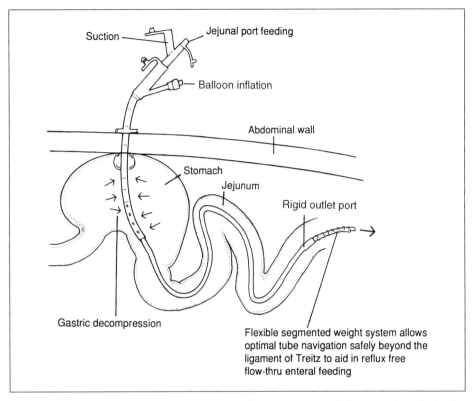

Fig. 4-12. Gastrostomy-jejunal catheter. G-J catheter with simultaneous gastric decompression and jejunal feeding. The separate portal of entry allows for jejunostomy tube replacement independent of the gastric tube.

procedures into the stomach and jejunum in much the same way as previously described for the Stamm gastrostomy. Purported advantages include fewer inadvertent tube dislodgments, decreased pivot motion, no external fixation sutures, and improved patient self-image. Removal and replacement of button devices can be performed as an office procedure, making them attractive alternatives for home patients.

Gastrostomy-Jejunal Tubes

Combined gastrostomy-jejunostomy (G-J) tubes have been devised for simultaneous jejunal feeding and gastric decompression. They are indicated in the malnourished patient who is at increased risk for aspiration. A stab gastrostomy near the greater curvature in the center of two concentric pursestring seromuscular sutures provides the tube entrance site. The jejunal portion of the catheter is grasped with ring forceps and placed through the pylorus and manipulated through the duodenum into the proximal jejunum. The gastrostomy portion of the catheter is then placed

into the gastrotomy. The pursestring sutures are secured around the tube on the stomach. The tube is withdrawn through an exit wound in the abdominal wall 4 cm lateral to the midline incision. The stomach is sutured to the posterior parietal peritoneum with suture (Fig. 4-12).

General Complications

General complications of enteral feeding are divided into four main categories: gastrointestinal, metabolic, infectious, and mechanical. Significant complications of enteral feeding occur infrequently; however, these are potentially lethal. The use of a standardized monitoring program is helpful to anticipate possible problems and implement actions when necessary.

Gastrointestinal

Diarrhea, defined as a daily stool output (or volume) of more than 200 g (or ml), is the most frequent complication of enteral nutrition, occurring in 10 to 20 percent of

Table 4-5. Causes of Diarrhea in Tube-Fed Patients

COMMON CAUSES UNRELATED TO TUBE FEEDING
Elixir medications containing sorbitol
Magnesium-containing antacids
Antibiotic-induced sterile gut
Pseudomembranous colitis

POSSIBLE CAUSES RELATED TO TUBE FEEDING
Inadequate fiber to form stool bulk
High fat content of formula (in presence of fat malabsorption syndrome)
Bacterial contamination of enteral products and delivery systems (causal association with diarrhea not documented)
Rapid advancement of rate (after GI tract is unused for prolonged periods)

UNLIKELY CAUSES RELATED TO TUBE FEEDING
Formula hypersomolality (proved not to be a cause of diarrhea)
Lactose (absent from nearly all enteral feeding formulas)

tube-fed patients. Possible causes are listed in Table 4-5.

Factors that have been suggested to cause diarrhea, but are not documented by controlled studies, include formula hyperosmolarity, lactose in the presence of relative lactase deficiency, and bacterial contamination of enteral products and delivery systems. Formula containers and administration tubing should be changed daily in order to avoid contamination. Formulas that contain high concentrations of fat may lead to steatorrhea in the presence of fat malabsorption. Examples include pancreatic exocrine insufficiency, extrahepatic biliary obstruction, ileectomy, or ileitis. Additional causes of diarrhea include antibiotics, magnesium-containing antacids, and hyperosmolar drug solutions including sorbitol-based elixirs. Recently clincians have become aware that many elixir medications contain substantial amounts (up to 65%) of sorbitol. All elixirs must therefore be considered as causes for diarrhea in tube-fed patients, and it is prudent to discontinue or change the route of administration to discern their role in the etiology of the diarrhea.

Treatment of the diarrhea is directed at the underlying cause. If the cause of the diarrhea cannot be identified, several therapeutic options are possible. Decreasing the rate of feeding may allow for intestinal adaptation if the gastrointestinal tract has not been used for extended periods of time (i.e., starvation and TPN-induced intestinal atrophy). A gradual increase in the rate of delivery can then be tried over a few days. TPN may be necessary to meet full nutrient requirements during this interval. Nonspecific antidiarrheal agents should be

used only cautiously. Supplementation of formulas with the fiber pectin may help solidify the stool and decrease transit time in patients not receiving broad-spectrum antibiotics. Most commercial formulas have soy polysaccharide as their fiber component and this has not been shown to reduce the incidence of diarrhea in critically ill patients.

Metabolic

Metabolic complications include hyperglycemia, fluid and electrolyte disorders, trace element deficiencies, vitamin K deficiency and abnormalities in protein tolerance.

Overhydration occurs in 20 to 25 percent of patients receiving enteral nutrition. Congestive heart failure and renal insufficiency aggravate this problem and impede its management. Decreasing the infusion rate or substituting a high-density caloric formula (i.e., 1.5–2.0 kcal/ml) is often therapeutic and diuretics are infrequently necessary for acute management. Although uncommon, hypertonic dehydration may occur in neurologically impaired patients receiving calorie-dense formulas, or in patients who are unable to communicate their thirst.

Hyperglycemia occurs in 10 to 30 percent of patients receiving enteral nutrition. Previously undiagnosed adult-onset diabetes mellitus may be discovered when high-caloric enteral diets are administered. Treatment of hyperglycemia involves decreasing the dietary flow rate if the patient is overfed or the administration of insulin, or both. The osmotic effects of hyperglycemia mandate close monitoring of the patient's volume status.

Most electrolyte and trace element abnormalities have been reported. Routine screening for these abnormalities allows early detection before clinical manifestations are apparent. Careful attention to electrolyte and trace element abnormalities is especially imperative for patients with renal, cardiac, or hepatic insufficiencies.

Infectious

Aspiration pneumonia is the most potentially lethal complication of enteral nutrition. Aspiration may be occult, without witnessed episodes of vomiting, and should be suspected with a new onset of tachycardia, fever, hypoxia, or acute changes in chest radiographs. The prevalence of aspiration varies from 1 to 44 percent depending on its definition. Nasogastrically fed patients appear to have a higher incidence of aspiration than do patients fed by gastrostomy or jejunostomy. A tracheostomy or an endotracheal tube substantially increases the risk of aspiration. Postpyloric positioning of nasoenteric tubes probably lowers the incidence of aspiration although there is no conclusive evidence to support this practice. Methods for detecting occult aspiration in tracheal aspirates include methylene blue dye placement in formula and monitoring glucose oxidant reagents strips. Preventive strategies include elevating the head of the bed 30 degrees, periodic measuring of gastric residuals, and gentle inflation of endotracheal tube cuffs. Obtaining a chest radiograph is mandatory before initiation of feedings in all patients who have nasogastric or nasoenteric tube placement.

Mechanical

Mechanical complications occur as a direct consequence of the feeding tube itself or its anatomic position. Nasoenteric tubes may cause nasopharyngeal erosions, discomfort, sinusitis, otitis media, gagging, esophagitis, esophageal reflux, tracheoesophageal fistulas, and rupture of esophageal varices. Feeding tubes frequently become clogged and can become knotted.

Clinical Trials

The benefit of providing nutritional support to selected cohorts of surgical patients versus traditional therapy with nil per os, nasogastric suction, and hypocaloric dextrose and electrolyte infusions has clearly been demonstrated. Several prospective, randomized clinical trials have compared the effects of total enteral nutrition (TEN) or TPN on postoperative clinical outcome. To correctly interpret the results of these clinical trials, it is important to recognize the many heterogeneous variables, including patient diagnoses, severity of illness, intercurrent surgery, dietary composition, dietary controls, amount of nutrients provided, and delivery methods.

Significant reduction in septic morbidity with TEN, when it is compared to TPN, has been demonstrated by several clinical trials. Seventy-five patients with an abdominal trauma index (ATI) greater than 15 and less than 40 were randomly assigned to receive TEN or TPN at initial laparotomy. Nutrient regimens were initiated within 12 hours postoperatively in both groups and isonitrogenous and isocaloric diets were administered. TEN was delivered via needle catheter jejunostomy. TEN patients developed 5 (17%) infections versus 11 (37%) in the TPN group ($P < 0.025$). Major septic morbidity included 1 abdominal abscess in the TEN group and 2 abdominal abscesses and 6 pneumonias in the TPN group. At a different institution, 98 patients with ATI greater than 15 were also randomized to receive either TEN or TPN. Patients receiving TEN had fewer septic complications, including pneumonias (11.8 vs 31% for TPN, $P < 0.02$), intraabdominal abscesses (1.9 vs 13.3% for TPN, $P < 0.04$), and line sepsis (1.9 vs 13.3% for TPN, $P < 0.04$) as well as significantly fewer infections per patient ($P < 0.05$). Furthermore, in a subset of the most severely injured, ATI greater than 40, there were significantly fewer infections per patient ($P = 0.03$) and fewer infections per infected patients ($P = 0.01$).

A meta-analysis combining eight prospective, randomized clinical trials confirmed the feasibility and decreased rate of septic complications in high-risk surgical patients who received early postoperative TEN when compared to those receiving TPN.

Many investigators have hypothesized that bacterial translocation from the gut may be responsible for systemic sepsis when gut function is impaired. Despite the compelling hypothesis, there is no conclusive evidence that bacterial translocation from the gut is the origin of the systemic

inflammatory response syndrome (SIRS). To address whether TEN could decrease the incidence of SIRS, a prospective randomized clinical trial assigned 66 critically ill patients to receive either TEN or TPN at the onset of hypermetabolism. No significant differences were found in multisystem organ failure or mortality between the two groups.

Conclusions from these trials include: 1) Postoperative sepsis, particularly pneumonia, is significantly reduced in patients with major abdominal trauma who receive TEN; however, whether these benefits are due to salutary effects of TEN or the absence of TPN and an indwelling central venous catheter is uncertain; 2) patients undergoing major general surgical operations have fewer infectious complications with postoperative TEN, versus TPN; and 3) early TEN does not reduce the incidence of SIRS in critically ill patients when compared to those receiving TPN. Regardless of the etiology by which enteral nutrients may enhance host immune function, the evidence for decreased septic morbidity establishes a clear rationale for their use in critically ill surgical patients. Finally, it cannot be overemphasized that if the gut can be used safely it is the preferred route for nutrient delivery to the malnourished surgical patient.

Future Directions

The growing knowledge of organ-specific nutrient requirements and the evolving understanding of the role of the hormonal milieu in nutrient metabolism will influence the composition of enteral nutrition in the future.

Glutamine

Increasing knowledge of the immunologic role of the gut and conditionally essential nutrients such as glutamine provides the rationale for disease-specific nutrient delivery. Glutamine is a nonessential amino acid characterized by the presence of two amino groups that provide the basis for its unique role as both a nitrogen acceptor and donor. Systemic glutamine is used as a metabolic fuel, and the majority of the nitrogenous end products appear as ammonia, alanine, and citrulline. Skeletal muscle is the primary site of glutamine synthesis and it contains levels 30 times higher than those of the systemic circula-

tion. In the small intestine, enterocytes preferentially extract glutamine over glucose, fatty acids, or ketone bodies. Investigations in many models show that glutamine is the principal oxidizable fuel for the small intestine and it is probably a conditionally essential nutrient during stress. Enterocytes have very active glutaminases that hydrolyze glutamine to glutamate and ammonia. Glutaminase activity and glutamine transport vary in different situations and glutaminase activity has recently been shown to be regulated by the presence of glucocorticoids in vitro. In critical illness selective uptake of glutamine by the intestine occurs at rates that exceed the ability of muscle to release glutamine stores. The net effect is decreased circulating glutamine concentrations, which remain low during recovery while other amino acid levels return to normal.

Few commercially available enteral formulas provide glutamine and, when present, the concentrations probably are insufficient to support intestinal mucosal growth. Most TPN formulas do not contain glutamine and this fuel deficit may play a role in TPN-induced intestinal atrophy. Experimentally, supplemented glutamine, whether provided enterally or parenterally, diminishes gut atrophy, and improves intestinal structure and function when compared to nonglutamine controls. [*Editor's note*: In our own studies, while enteral glutamine administration reproducibly increases gut mucosal thickness, protein, and DNA, we have been unable to find any effect of parenteral glutamine in any combination or permutations.]

Short-Chain Fatty Acids

In contrast to the enterocyte, colonocytes use *n*-butyrate, a short-chain fatty acid (SCFA), as the preferred oxidizable fuel, in deference to glucose, glutamine, or ketone bodies. Butyrate is not synthesized by the body, and, thus, it is available to the colon mucosa only as a result of bacterial fermentation of dietary polysaccharides in the colonic lumen. Butyrate and other SCFAs promote cell proliferation and growth in both the small bowel and colon. The suggested mechanisms for SCFA enterotrophic effects on the gastrointestinal tract include provision of energy substrate, stimulation of blood flow, production of exocrine pancreatic secretions, stimulation of the autonomic nervous system, and production of enterotrophic hormones.

Growth Factors

Growth hormone (GH), insulin-like growth factor–I (IGF-I), and epidermal growth factor (EGF) also are polypeptide hormones that are important mediators of enterocyte proliferation, replication, and differentiation.

Recombinant-manufactured growth hormone is available as an adjunct to specialized nutritional support. Several clinical trials of TPN have demonstrated significantly increased safety, efficacy, and improved nutrient utilization in those receiving growth hormone compared to standard parenteral feedings. In states of moderate surgical injury, such as postcholecystectomy, growth hormone preserved acute-phase protein synthesis, decreased wound infection, and decreased hospital stay. In a placebo-controlled double-blind study, hypocaloric parenteral nutrition produced improved nutrient utilization, significantly decreased the incidence of wound infections, and decreased hospital stay. [*Editor's note*: Laparoscopic cholecystectomy has rendered this moot. These studies should be repeated in other moderate-severity surgical procedures.] The role of growth hormone as an adjunct to enteral nutrient regimens is as yet undefined but holds great promise for the future.

Insulin-like growth factor–I is available to intestinal cells via the circulation and also through endogenous synthesis in the intestine. The actions of IGF-I are mediated by specific cell surface receptors, which are present in substantial quantities in small bowel and colonic mucosal cells. Intestinal cells also synthesize IGF-binding proteins, which are expressed on the cell surface and may stimulate or inhibit IGF-I action by modifying the availability of the hormone for interaction with its receptors. In experimental animal models of catabolic disease, increased intestinal cell growth in response to EGF and IGF-I infusion has been demonstrated. These responses of the intestinal mucosa to IGF-I and EGF infusion are not unexpected, since this tissue expresses IGF-I and EGF receptors and is sensitive to the effects of malnutrition and catabolic stress. IGF-I and EGF administration following small-bowel resection augments the adaptive increase in intestinal wet weight and cellularity in the remaining small bowel in rat models of intestinal resection. In summary, the production and metabolism of GH, IGF-I, and EGF are significantly altered in the presence of catabolic stress. The hormonal environment supports adaptive proliferative and functional responses in the intestine both as endogenously synthesized and exogenously administered growth factors.

Summary

The enterotrophic benefits, decreased cost, and ease of administration compared to TPN make enteral nutrition the preferred route for feeding malnourished surgical patients. Enteral access route depends on anticipated duration of feeding and aspiration risk. For short-term enteral access, nasogastric feedings are recommended and nasoenteric when aspiration risk is present. Long-term enteral access is provided by PEG or surgical gastrostomy; gastrostomy-jejunal tubes or surgical jejunostomy are used for those at risk for aspiration. Clinical trials of enteral feeding have demonstrated reduced septic morbidity in selected cohorts of surgical patients compared to parenteral feeding. Regardless of the mechanism, enteral nutrient delivery may enhance host immune function. The increasing knowledge of growth factors and their interactions with nutrient utilization provide exciting possibilities for the future. Delivery of enteral nutrients is best provided under the aegis of a nutritional support team. Adherence to the principle of dietary delivery and monitoring reduces complications and enhances patient outcome in selected patients.

Suggested Readings

American Society for Parenteral and Enteral Nutrition Cooperative Study Group. Guidelines for use of parenteral and enteral nutrition in adult and pediatric patients. *J Parent Enteral Nutr* 17:8SA, 1993.

Cerra FB, McPherson JP, Konstantinides, et al. Enteral nutrition does not prevent multiple organ failure syndrome (MOFS) after sepsis. *Surgery* 104:727, 1988.

Consensus Conference on Nutrition in the Critically Ill. *Chest* (in press).

Kudsk KA. Clinical applications of enteral nutrition. *Nutr Clin Prac* 9:165, 1994.

Kudsk KA, Croce MA, et al. Enteral versus parenteral feeding: Effects on septic morbidity after blunt and penetrating abdominal trauma. *Ann Surg* 215:511, 1991.

Lew JI, Rombeau JL. The Effects of Nutrients on the Intestinal Epithelium. In P Furst (ed), *New Strategies in Clinical Nutrition*. Munich: W. Zuckschwerdt Verlag, 1993. Pp 64–84.

Moore FA, Feliciano DV, Andrassy RJ, et al. Early enteral feeding, compared with parenteral, reduced postoperative septic complications. The result of a meta-analysis. *Ann Surg* 216:172, 1992.

Moore FA, Moore EM, et al. TEN versus TPN following major abdominal trauma-reduced septic morbidity. *J Trauma* 29:916, 1989.

Rombeau J. Indications for and Administration of Enteral and Parenteral Nutrition in Critically Ill Patients. In RW Carlson and MA Geheb, eds, *Principles of Practice of Medical Intensive Care*. Philadelphia: Saunders, 1993. Pp 1528–1551.

Rombeau JL, Rombeau JL, Rolandelli RH, Wilmore DW. Nutritional Support. In D Wilmore, *Care of the Surgical Patient*. New York: Scientific American Publishers, 1994. Pp 1–35. Enteral Nutrition. In *Cecil's Textbook of Medicine* (20th ed) (in press).

Rombeau JL, Caldwell MD, eds. *Clinical Nutrition: Enteral and Tube Feeding* (2nd ed). Philadelphia: Saunders, 1990.

Rombeau JL, Reilly KJ, Rolandelli RH. In Cummings, ed. *Physiological and Clinical Aspects of Short Chain Fatty Acids*. New York: Cambridge, 1995. Pp 401–426.

Rombeau JL, Caldwell MD, Forlaw L, Guenter PA, ed. *Atlas of Nutritional Support Techniques*. Boston/Toronto: Little, Brown, 1989.

Sarantos P, Abouhamze Z. Glucocorticoids regulate glutaminase gene expression in human intestinal epithelial cells. *J Surg Res* 57:227–231, 1994.

Vara-Thorbeck R, Guerrero JA, et al. Exogenous growth hormone: Effects on the catabolic response to surgically produced acute stress and on postoperative immune function. *World J Surg* 17:530–538, 1993.

Ziegler TR, Rombeau JL, et al. Recombinant human growth hormone enhances the metabolic efficacy of parenteral nutrition: A double-blind, randomized controlled study. *J Clin Endocrinol Metab* 74:865, 1992.

EDITOR'S COMMENT

Doctors Rombeau and Hamilton have produced an elegant but simply stated chapter concerning enteral feeding, which is now the preferred method of nutritional intervention. A common concern regarding enteral nutritional intervention is that in many circumstances one cannot deliver the entire nutritional supplement to the patient by the enteral route, and TPN must be utilized. Nonetheless, it is clear that there are benefits even to partial nutritional supplementation via the gut. Two different groups have recently come to this conclusion. Illig and associates (*JPEN* 17:25S, abstract 17, 1993) and Shou and colleagues *Am J Surg* 167:145, 1994) have both provided evidence that partial supplementation via intestine may provide immunologic benefits and also improve nitrogen balance with as few as 20 to 25 percent of the calories supplied enterally and the remainder supplied parenterally.

Doctor Rombeau and coworkers have correctly identified some of the controversies concerning the benefits of enteral nutrition in the posttraumatic patient. Enteral feeding, as opposed to parenteral feeding, has been shown to be most efficacious in burn and posttraumatic patients. There has been an unfortunate and automatic tendency to ascribe any benefits in outcome to enteral feeding, as opposed to TPN, to a decrease in bacterial translocation. As the authors correctly point out, this has never been demonstrated in any trial, and the role of bacterial translocation in the systemic inflammatory response syndrome has not been demonstrated despite multiple attempts to do so. One need only look to the other potential benefits of gut feeding, including improvement in hepatic protein synthesis, to name but one. Recent studies suggesting that the gut is a source, rather than only a target, of cytokines and other potentially immunologically active materials give another potential source of benefit even if bacterial translocation is not invoked.

The whole question of bacterial translocation needs to be re-examined in a dispassionate, unemotional fashion. Bacterial translocation is probably a normally occurring mechanism, perhaps for immunologic stimulation of gut-related immunologic tissue. The concept of bacterial translocation probably needs to be modified, as Alexander and colleagues have suggested (*Ann Surg* 56:530, 1994), to "bacterial clearance"; that is, of the bacteria that are translocated, how many of them escape destruction and therefore seed the portal system and other organs?

Be that as it may, Drs. Rombeau and Hamilton have made the case very well for the primacy of enteral feeding over parenteral feeding in today's environment. Cost-consciousness is another very good reason to use the enteral route first.

J.E.F.

5

Cardiovascular Monitoring and Support

Carmelo A. Milano   David C. Sabiston, Jr.

Cardiovascular monitoring provides important objective information that helps establish diagnoses and guide therapeutic interventions. Two general principles should be emphazied when interpreting this information: First, monitoring data supplements serial physical examination and must always be interpreted with the physical findings. Secondly, hemodynamic baselines vary greatly and trends in parameters are generally more useful than initial absolute values.

Invasive Monitoring
Continuous Arterial Pressure Monitoring

Intra-arterial pressures can be determined using fluid-filled catheters and more accurately reflect central or aortic pressure relative to measurements obtained using noninvasive methods. General indications for arterial catheterization and continuous monitoring include any patient with hemodynamic instability, or at risk for hemodynamic instability, and patients in whom frequent blood draws are required (e.g., those who need mechanical ventilation and frequent arterial blood gases). More specifically, patients who have undergone major cardiothoracic or vascular procedures should have arterial catheterization, as blood pressure fluctuations are common and may reflect bleeding at vascular anastomoses. In addition, continuous arterial pressure monitoring is useful following major general surgical procedures in patients with ischemic heart disease or congestive heart failure to allow for careful blood pressure control. Any patient who requires mechanical ventilation or

pharmacologic or mechanical cardiovascular support should have an arterial catheter and continuous pressure monitoring.

Arterial catharization is performed using a percutaneous Seldinger technique in which the catheter is placed over a finder needle that is introduced into the artery. After intra-arterial position is confirmed by arterial bleeding through the needle, the catheter is advanced into the artery over the needle, and the needle is then removed. The needle should be inserted straight in and withdrawn along the same course to prevent tearing or laceration of the artery. In addition a wire can be introduced through the needle into the artery and may help guide advancement of the catheter. While a local anesthetic can be used during insertion of the catheter, this can make the artery more difficult to palpate.

The preferred site for arterial catheterization is the radial artery at the wrist, since the artery is superficial, easily palpated, and of sufficient size in adults to allow placement of an 18- or 20-gauge catheter. Furthermore, the hand has a duel blood supply, reducing the risk of ischemia, and the site can be easily dressed and kept clean. While some still recommend the Allen test before radial artery catharization, Slogoff and associates prospectively evaluated 1699 patients and demonstrated that the Allen test result is not predictive of ischemic complications. Ejrup and associates found that a false-positive Allen test can be generated if the wrist is slightly hyperextended, and this probably represents its major limitation. If the radial artery site is not available then the next preferred site is the common femoral artery in the groin.

The femoral artery is easily cannulated and is not associated with a higher incidence of complications. The axillary artery can also be used; however, it is generally more difficult to cannulate and is associated with a higher incidence of local infections. The brachial artery site is generally avoided because thrombosis can lead to limb ischemia, and hematomas in this area can result in median nerve compression.

The most important complications of arterial catheterization is thrombosis and subsequent distal ischemia usually secondary to occlusion of the artery at the site of catheterization. Bedford showed that for radial artery cannulation the incidence of thrombosis was 11 percent when the vessel was cannulated for fewer than 4 days but rose to 29 percent in those cannulated for more than 4 days. In addition to the duration of cannulation, risk factors for thrombosis include larger catheters, smaller arteries (children or women), hypotension, use of vasoconstricting agents, and complicated insertion requiring multiple needle sticks. Although the incidence of thrombosis of the radial artery is high, significant distal ischemia occurs in fewer than 1 percent of patients. With a radial artery catheter in place, the hand must be inspected several times a day, and signs of ischemia warrant removal of the catheter. If signs of ischemia persist after removal, surgical exploration and possible thrombectomy should be undertaken within 6 hours.

Another important complication of arterial cannulation is infection. Maki and associates define local catheter infections as growth of more than 15 colonies on a blood agar plate inoculated with a segment of the removed catheter. Considering all radial artery catheters, the incidence of local wound infection is reported between 10 and 20 percent; the most important risk factors for the development of local infections are cutdown technique (9-fold increased risk) and duration of arterial cannulation. Despite this relatively high incidence of local infection, systemic infection or sepsis from arterial catheterization is rare (approximately 1%). Radial and femoral arterial line sites should be redressed using a sterile technique every 24 to 48 hours; these lines should be removed when there is evidence of local infection. If there is a question of local infection or secondary sepsis, the catheter can be exchanged over a wire and cultured to confirm infection; if the culture is positive the site should be changed. Norwood and associates (1991) found that, in a nonseptic patient with a clean site, routine changes of the site are not indicated.

Arterial catheters may function suboptimally for several reasons: The transducer can be placed incorrectly, air bubbles in the connecting tubing can lead to false reading, and, for radial artery catheters, bending of the wrist can kink the catheter and dampen the pressure reading. For these reasons, the system should be continually re-evaluated for problems, and noninvasive pressure measurements should be routinely obtained for comparison.

Central Venous Catheters

Central venous catheterization is typically achieved via the subclavian or the internal jugular vein; it provides access for volume infusion and for administration of inotropic and vasoactive agents. In addition, central venous pressure (CVP) may be monitored. CVP represents the right ventricular filling pressure and is an excellent parameter of right ventricular preload; normal CVP ranges from 0 to 7 mm Hg. The CVP, when combined with other data such as arterial blood pressure, heart rate, and urinary output, provides an estimation of intravascular volume status. Furthermore, CVP measurement can be very helpful in diagnosing specific conditions; for example, CVP measurement can distinguish between hypovolemic shock and cardiac tamponade following trauma. In many patients, however, CVP does not correlate well with the pulmonary artery wedge pressure (PAWP), which provides a better estimate of left ventricular preload. Right

ventricular dysfunction, right heart valvular disease, and pulmonary hypertension are conditions, for example, in which the CVP may be elevated despite normal or reduced left ventricular preload.

The Subclavian Vein Approach

The subclavian vein is the preferred site for central venous catheterization, as the landmarks are more distinct and long-term catheterization is more comfortable for the patient and easier to care for relative to venous sites in the neck. Furthermore, because the vessel adheres to adjacent ligaments, fascia, and periosteum, displacement and collapse do not occur even during severe hypovolemia. The subclavian vein begins lateral to the first rib and arches posterior to the clavicle and over the first rib just anterior to the site of the insertion of the anterior scalene muscle (Fig. 5-1). The subclavian vein is most easily accessed as it passes posterior to the clavicle and over the first rib. The external landmark for this site is the insertion of the lateral head of the sternocleidomastoid muscle or the clavicle. This site is also marked by the division of the medial and middle thirds of the clavicle. After the patient has been placed in slight Trendelenburg position, the skin and subcutaneous tissues are infiltrated with 1% lidocaine, and a 16-gauge needle is directed behind the clavicle at the previously described landmark. The needle is directed medially and cephalad in line with the deltopectoral groove toward a point approximately 2 to 3 cm above the jugular notch. Suction is applied with a syringe as the needle is advanced under the clavicle; return of venous blood indicates that the needle is in the subclavian vein. The needle can be advanced another 0.5 cm to ensure that the entire bevel is within the vessel; a wire is then threaded through the needle and the needle is removed. The entire wire should advance easily, and pain or resistance indicates misplacement and warrants removal of both the wire and the needle. When the needle is introduced under the clavicle, it is important that it remain parallel to the floor, avoiding a more posterior trajectory prevents injury to the lung. It is also important to pass the needle in and out along the same line, taking care to avoid turning the needle while it is inserted, which can cause laceration of the vein or artery. If the initial attempt fails to locate the vein, a slightly more cephalad trajectory is recommended since the vein

may be displaced cephalad as a result of hyperinflation of the lung. Once the wire is in place, a small skin incision is performed and a dilator passed over the wire to establish a subcutaneous tract; the dilator is then removed, a catheter is placed over the wire, and the wire is removed. The presence of a clavicular fracture, previous mastectomy, or local skin infection warrant use of the contralateral site. In general, the left site is preferred to the right since the left subclavian vein follows a straighter course, while the right subclavian vein turns more sharply upon entering the chest.

Internal Jugular Vein Approach

The internal jugular vein is also commonly used for central venous catheterization. While catheters in the neck are more uncomfortable for the patient and slightly more difficult to care for relative to the subclavian site, advantages include a reduced risk of pneumothorax and a straighter course to the right heart. The internal jugular vein lies slightly anterior and lateral to the common carotid artery in the lower third of the neck (Fig. 5-2). The patient is again placed in Trendelenburg position with the head turned slightly away from the side being approached. The primary landmark is the division of the medial (sternal) and lateral (clavicular) heads of the sternocleidomastoid muscle in the lower neck; a needle is introduced at this site and angled slightly inferior and toward the ipsilateral nipple avoiding the carotid artery, which lies more medially (see Fig. 5-2). A 20-gauge needle is initially used to locate the internal jugular vein and is then replaced with the larger 16-gauge needle through which the wire can be introduced. The smaller needle avoids more serious injury to the carotid artery, which can occasionally be inadvertently punctured. Once the wire has been introduced into the vein, the steps are similar to those for placement of a subclavian venous catheter. It is important to note that the internal jugular vein is a superficial structure (usually one 2.0–2.5 cm below the skin), and therefore it is not necessary to introduce the needle more deeply in the normal patient; deeper insertion increases the risk of pneumothorax and damage to other structures in the neck and is typically very painful for patients. The right internal jugular vein is the preferred side given the straight course to the brachiocephalic vein and superior vena cava.

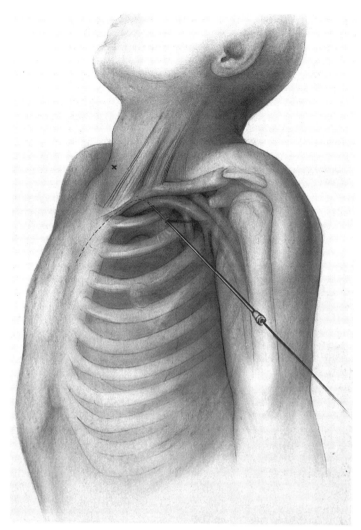

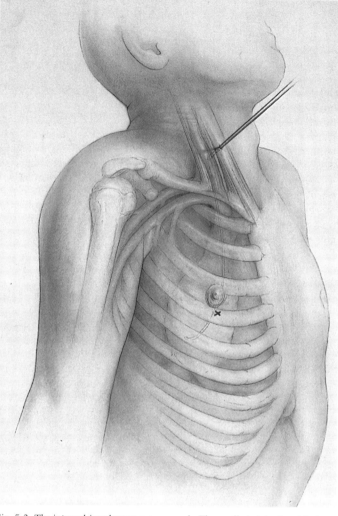

Fig. 5-1. The subclavian venous approach. The needle is introduced between the clavicle and the first rib as shown. The external landmark for the target subclavian vein puncture site is the clavicular head of the sternocleidomastoid muscle. The needle is directed cephalad and medial toward a point (X) located 2 to 3 cm above the jugular notch.

Fig. 5-2. The internal jugular venous approach. The needle is introduced just lateral to the carotid pulsation in the lower neck. The landmark for insertion of the needle is the union of the sternal and clavicular heads of the sterno-cleidomastoid. The needle is directed predominantly posterior and lateral toward the ipsilateral nipple (X).

Femoral Vein Approach

Femoral vein catheterization is infrequently employed since it requires that the patient remain flat at bed rest, and because some reports cite a higher incidence of catheter-related infection and association with venous thrombosis. Nevertheless, the site is easily accessible and the preferred site in special situations. For example trauma patients with cervical spine immobilization and patients with superior vena cava syndrome may require femoral venous catheterization. The femoral vein is approached several centimeters below the inguinal ligament; this location avoids both inadvertent intraperitoneal needle sticks and needle sticks to the deep femoral vein and greater saphenous vein, which are more inferior. The femoral vein lies just medial to the femoral artery, which usually can be easily palpated. If the artery cannot be palpated, the middle point of the inguinal ligament marks its location.

Complications of Central Venous Catheterization

Central venous catheterization may cause immediate or delayed complications. Immediate complications include arterial puncture and hematoma formation. If arterial puncture occurs the needle should be immediately removed and direct pressure applied. Rarely such injury may cause a pseudoaneurysm or an arteriovenous fistula may develop. The most important immediate complication of subclavian venous catheter placement is pneumothorax, which occurs in approximately 0.5 to 3 percent of patients. A chest radiograph should be obtained after either subclavian or internal jugular venous line placement and after any failed attempts. Small and asymptomatic pneumothoraces can be managed conservatively with administration of supplemental oxygen and a follow-up chest radiograph. Larger or symptomatic pneumothoraces warrant insertion of a chest tube or percutaneous catheter. In patients who require central venous catheterization, and who have a chest tube already in place for another condition, insertion should be performed on the side of the chest tube.

Other immediate complications include cardiac arrhythmias which result from the catheter or guidewire directly irritating the myocardium; treatment involves simply withdrawing the catheter. Air emboli may also occur, particularly in patients with very low central venous pressures. Covering the needle, capping the catheter, and flushing the catheter before insertion prevent this problem. Embolization of the guidewire or of catheter fragments has also been described; these can usually be retrieved noninvasively with a second catheter and fluoroscopic guidance. A variety of other rare immediate complications have been described, including cardiac puncture, hemothorax, mediastinal injury, thyroid injury, thoracic duct injury, and nerve injuries (phrenic nerve, brachial plexus, recurrent laryngeal nerve).

The most important delayed complication of central venous catheterization is infection. Bacterial skin flora adhere to catheters and propagate to where the catheter inserts into the vein; as bacterial counts rise either local or systemic infection may develop. Maki and associates define catheter-related infection as 15 colonies or more on a blood agar plate streaked with a catheter segment. Catheter-related infection predisposes to catheter-related septicemia, which is diagnosed by the isolation of the same organism from the catheter culture and from peripheral blood cultures. Catheter-related sepsis warrants removal of the catheter and treatment with intravenous antibiotics, and the incidence of catheter-related infection for central venous lines (e.g., triple-lumen catheters) is as high as 3.3 percent per day (Hampton and Sheretz), with the incidence of catheter-related sepsis ranging from 0.3 to 0.6 percent per day (Eyer et al, Norwood and Jenkins). Factors associated with a higher incidence of catheter-related infection and sepsis include increased age, impaired immune system function, the presence of remote infection, prolonged duration of site use, insertion requiring cutdown, and emergent insertion (Norwood et al, Norwood and Jenkins).

To avoid catheter-related sepsis certain guidelines should be followed: First, if a site is clearly purulent or tender then the site should be immediately changed. All catheters placed under emergent suboptimal conditions should undergo sterile guidewire exchange. Guidewire exchange is also indicated when there is clinical evidence of infection without a well-defined source (e.g., fever, leukocytosis, positive blood cultures, etc.). The old catheter is carefully removed from the sterile field and a 5-cm segment of both the tip and the subcutaneous portion are sent for culture. If the culture returns positive, the site should be changed. If the culture is negative the site is maintained with the new catheter. Sterile guidewire exchange serves as an important diagnostic technique and obviates the need for routine central venous catheter site changes (Norwood et al, Eyer et al).

[*Editor's note*: Catheter sepsis remains one of the most dreaded complications of parenteral nutrition and, except for the occasional misadventure, is the one most likely to result in mortality, particularly if fungemia is present. It is clear from a number of studies that bacterial catheter sepsis is related directly to the care that the catheters receive and the manipulation that they undergo. Thus, triple-lumen catheters have a much higher incidence than single-lumen catheters, as the authors document. In a classic study by Ryan and coworkers (*N Engl J Med* 290:757–761, 1974), catheters that were cared for had a much lower rate of sepsis than catheters in which technique was not observed.

The origin of bacterial catheter sepsis is from the skin. In a study from the University of Cincinnati, Bjornson and coworkers (*Surgery* 92:720–727, 1982) documented very nicely that if quantitative cultures of the catheter site were carried out, those catheters in which the skin culture concentration of bacteria was less than 10^3 were unlikely to develop catheter sepsis. However, those catheters in which the quantitative culture was higher than that figure were likely to develop sepsis. There was a gradient of colonization from the skin to the intradermal portion of the catheter to the intravascular portion.

The technique of changing catheters over a guidewire is theoretically not of value in preventing catheter sepsis. This is because the fibrin sleeve along the catheter is the area that really is infected in the bloodstream. However, it does appear as if changing the catheter over the guidewire obviates catheter sepsis most of the time. The reason for this may be that the sleeve that is attached to the catheter breaks off and embolizes in the bloodstream, and is dealt with by the usual body defenses.

If one does quantitative cultures and they show that the bacterial concentration around the catheter is 10^3 or greater, it is best that the catheter be removed and the site changed. Meticulous catheter care will prevent sepsis. *Candida* sepsis, however, appears to result from translocation through the gastrointestinal tract, as there was no relationship between *Candida* catheter sepsis and the skin cultures.

Pulmonary Artery Catheters

In 1970, HJC Swan and associates introduced catheterization of the right heart in humans, employing a flow-directed balloon-tipped catheter. The balloon-tipped

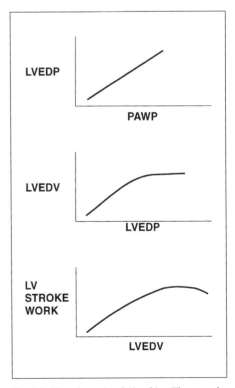

Fig. 5-3. Hemodynamic relationships. Three graphs illustrate the relationships between pulmonary artery wedge pressure (PAWP) and left ventricular end-diastolic pressure (LVEDP), LVEDP and left ventricle end-diastolic volume (LVEDV), and finally the Frank-Starling relationship between LVEDV and left ventricle (LV) stroke work.

catheter allowed for pulmonary artery occlusion pressure measurements, and, relative to previous catheters was faster, did not require fluoroscopy, and reduced the risk of cardiac puncture. Occlusion of a pulmonary artery generates a hydrostatic state across the pulmonary capillary bed to the left atrium, and the pressure at the catheter tip beyond the balloon (pulmonary artery wedge pressure) is therefore equal to left atrial pressure. Fitzpatrick and colleagues have confirmed this theoretical relationship by direct measurements in human subjects. Left atrial pressure approximates left ventricular end-diastolic pressure (LVEDP), which in turn relates to left ventricular end-diastolic volume (LVEDV) in a curvilinear fashion (Fig. 5-3). LVEDV describes preload and therefore relates via the Frank-Starling relationship to stroke work (Fig. 5-3).

Pulmonary artery (PA) catheters are commonly introduced via the subclavian vein or the internal jugular vein; the femoral vein can also be used in special situations. The most direct approach to the right heart is the right internal jugular vein. The central vein is typically catheterized with a No. 7 French introducer segment employing the techniques described earlier. A three- or four-port, 100-cm catheter that fits through the introducer is typically employed. Before introducing the PA catheter, all ports should be thoroughly flushed with sterile saline, the balloon test inflated, and the distal port of the catheter connected to a pressure transducer, which is displayed on a monitor. The pressure transducer is zeroed to the level of the left atrium, which is the midaxillary line at the

fourth intercostal space. A sterile sheath is usually placed over the PA catheter and connects to the introducer; this permits sterile manipulation of the catheter after the initial placement. The PA catheter is then introduced and advanced to 10 to 15 cm with the balloon deflated. Initially, small *a* and *v* waves as well as respiratory variations should be present in the pres-

sure tracing. Using a 1-ml syringe, the balloon is then inflated with 0.5 to 0.8 ml air (the balloon should not be inflated with fluid). As the catheter is advanced into the right ventricle (RV), RV systolic pressures appear, with diastolic pressures being equivalent to the central venous pressures; with further advancement, diastolic pressures abruptly rise and a pressure notch

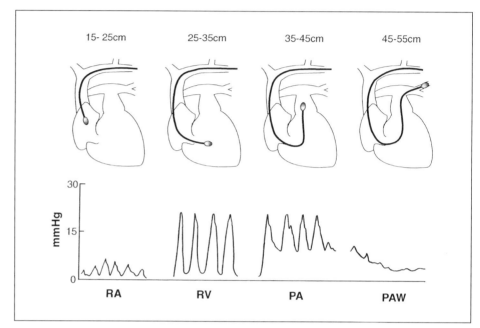

Fig. 5-4. Placement of pulmonary artery catheter. A balloon-tipped catheter is flow directed and courses from the left subclavian vein to the innominate vein to the superior vena cava. The catheter than passes though the right atrium and ventricle into the pulmonary artery and eventually wedges in a branch of the pulmonary artery. The approximate length of catheter inserted from the left subclavian position is shown above each of the four diagrams. Representative pressure tracings are shown below each of the four diagrams. (RA = right atrium; RV = right ventricle; PA = pulmonary artery; PAW = pulmonary artery wedge.)

Table 5-1. Hemodynamic Parameters

Parameter	Calculation	Normal Value
Central venous pressure (CVP)	—	0–7mm Hg
Pulmonary artery systolic pressure (PASP)	—	15–30mm Hg
Pulmonary artery diastolic pressure (PADP)	—	4–12mm Hg
Mean pulmonary artery pressure (MPAP)	—	9–16mm Hg
Pulmonary artery wedge pressure (PAWP)	—	2–12mm Hg
Cardiac output (CO)	—	4.0–8.0L/min
Mixed venous oxygen saturation ($S\bar{v}O_2$)	—	0.65–0.80 fraction
Cardiac index (CI)	CO/BSA	2.8–4.2L/min/m²
Systemic vascular resistance (SVR)	$\dfrac{(MAP - CVP)}{CO} \times 80$	900–1400 dyne × sec × cm^{-5}
Pulmonary vascular resistance (PVR)	$\dfrac{MPAP - PAWP}{CO} \times 80$	150–250 dyne × sec × cm^{-5}
O₂ delivery ($\dot{D}O_2$)	CO × SaO_2 × [Hgb] × 1.34	700–1400 ml/min
O₂ consumption ($\dot{V}O_2$)	CO × {($SaO_2 - S\bar{v}O_2$) × [Hgb] × 1.34}	180–280 ml/min

may be seen consistent with the catheter entering the pulmonary artery (Fig. 5-4). Further advancement results in PAWP, which typically is several mm Hg less than the pulmonary arterial diastolic pressure (see Fig. 5-4). The PAWP should continue to display ripples, which correspond to the cardiac cycle with some respiratory variation. At this point, deflation of the balloon should cause a return of the pulmonary artery pressure tracing. If the wedge pressure tracing remains even after deflation, the catheter may be "overwedged" and should be withdrawn slightly. Typically, 45 to 55 cm of catheter is introduced from the subclavian or internal jugular venous site to achieve adequate placement; this length is variable and depends on the size of the patient, the size of the right ventricle, and the starting site. Once the PA catheter has been properly positioned, a variety of hemodynamic parameters can be measured and calculated (Table 5-1).

Conditions in Which PAWP Does Not Reflect LV Preload

To ensure accurate PAWP readings, transducer calibration and placement must be correct, and the catheter must be devoid of air bubbles. PAWP should always be obtained from a hard copy or graphic display and not from the monitor. Furthermore, PAWP should be always measured at end expiration in the respiratory cycle; during end expiration for both spontaneously breathing and mechanically ventilated patients, intrathoracic pressure approaches atmospheric pressure and has minimal effect on PAWP.

Incorrect catheter position within the pulmonary arterial system can cause artifactual PAWP. West and associates described three lung zones based on the relationship of pulmonary arterial, alveolar, and pulmonary venous pressures (Fig. 5-5). In zones 1 and 2, alveolar pressure exceeds either pulmonary arterial or venous pressure; as a result, PAWP measures alveolar pressures rather than left atrial pressures. In zone 3 both pulmonary arterial and venous pressure exceed alveolar pressure, and therefore PAWP accurately measures left atrial pressure. Fortunately, the majority of blood flow occurs in zone 3, and therefore the flow-directed catheter is most likely to be positioned in this zone. Zone 3 typically lies in the most dependent region of the lung, and therefore in a supine patient, this would be the lung

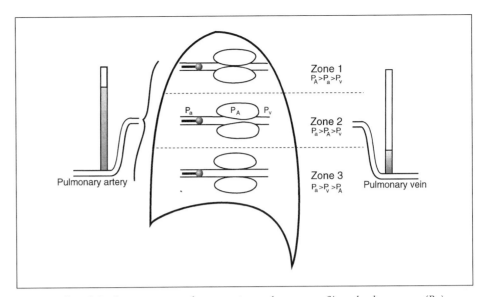

Fig. 5-5. Effect of alveolar pressure on pulmonary artery wedge pressure. Since alveolar pressure (P_A) exceeds either pulmonary artery pressure (P_a) in zone 1, and pulmonary venous pressure (P_v) in zone 2, catheter placement in either zones 1 or 2 results in artifactual pulmonary artery wedge pressure reflecting alveolar pressure. Only in zone 3 does an uninterrupted hydrostatic column of fluid exist between the catheter tip and the left atrium, and therefore pulmonary artery wedge pressure reflects left atrial pressure. (From JB West, CT Dollery, A Nuimark. Distribution of blood flow in isolated lung; relation to vascular and alveolar pressures. J Appl Physiol 19:713, 1964. Reproduced with permission.)

Table 5-2. Checklist for Determining Placement of Pulmonary Arterial Catheter

Test	Zone 3	Zone 1 or 2
Respiratory variations of PAWP	≤1/2 the change in airway pressure	>1/2 the change in airway pressure
PAWP contour	Cardiac ripple	Smooth
Catheter tip location on lateral CXR	Below LA level	Above LA level
PEEP reduction trial	Change in PAWP ≤1/2 PEEP reduction	Change in PAWP >1/2 PEEP reduction
Relationship of PADP, PAWP	PADP > PAWP	PADP ≤ PAWP

PAWP = pulmonary artery wedge pressure; LA = left atrium; PEEP = positive end-expiratory pressure; PADP = pulmonary artery diastolic pressure; CXR = chest x-ray.
Source: From JJ Marini. Obtaining meaningful data from the Swan-Ganz catheter. *Respir Care* 30:572, 1985. Reproduced with permission.

regions posterior to the left atrium. A variety of information is useful in determining whether the PA catheter is properly positioned in zone 3 (Marin) (Table 5-2); if it is not the catheter should be withdrawn and refloated. Of note is that conditions that increase alveolar pressure (e.g., mechanical ventilation) or decrease pulmonary arterial pressure (e.g., hypovolemia) increase the size of zones 1 and 2 and the chance for artifactual PAWP.

Diseases of the mitral valve may cause diastolic pressure gradients across the valve; therefore, in these conditions, while

PAWP may reflect left atrial pressure (LAP), it does not accurately reflect LVEDP or left ventricular preload. For example, with mitral stenosis, PAWP is significantly higher than LVEDP and inadequate LV preload may exist despite relatively high PAWP.

Another factor that affects the ability of PAWP to reflect LV preload is LV compliance. Left ventricular compliance is the inverse of chamber stiffness; Raper and Sibbald define it by the instantaneous relationship between the ventricular end-diastolic volume and pressure, and math-

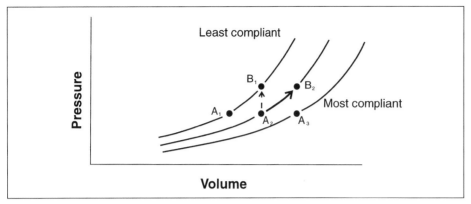

Fig. 5-6. Left ventricular compliance. Left ventricular diastolic pressure-volume curves are shown for three different states of left ventricular compliance. Compliance is the inverse of the instantaneous slope at a point on the curves ($\Delta v/\Delta p$). During diastole, as the ventricle fills, compliance progressively decreases ($A_2 \rightarrow B_2$). Left ventricular diastolic pressure may not reflect volume changes if there are simultaneous compliance changes ($A_1 \rightarrow A_2 \rightarrow A_3$). Conversely, changes in left ventricular diastolic pressure may represent changes in compliance and not changes in volume ($A_2 \rightarrow B_1$). (From R. Raper, WJ Sibbald. Misled by the wedge? The Swan-Ganz catheter and left ventricular preload. Chest 89:427, 1986. Reproduced with permission.)

ematically expressed it as the slope of the tangent to the diastolic volume-pressure curve (dv/dp). Without any change in the intrinsic properties of the ventricle, compliance decreases as LVEDV increases; however, both acute and chronic intrinsic myocardial changes can cause compliance changes. Therefore, in the absence of LVEDV changes, alterations in compliance result in change in LVEDP and PAWP (Fig. 5-6). Myocardial ischemia can acutely decrease LV compliance and raise PAWP in the absence of changes in LVEDV (preload). More chronically, LV hypertrophy also reduces LV compliance, and patients with aortic stenosis, for example, may require higher PAWP for adequate preload.

Another important consideration is that while PAWP estimates changes in LVEDP, changes in left ventricular end-diastolic, transmyocardial pressure more accurately reflect changes in end-diastolic volume. Stated differently it is the gradient between intraventricular and extraventricular pressure that determines ventricular volume. Often this distinction is not of clinical importance since extramyocardial or pericardial pressure is very low, and therefore transmyocardial pressure approximates intracavitary LVEDP, but there are important exceptions. For example, during pericardial tamponade, LVEDP and PAWP may be very high but because pericardial pressure is also increased, LVED transmyocardial pressure and LVEDV are low. A more common clinical situation in which intrathoracic and peri-

cardial pressures are increased is during mechanical ventilation and particularly with use of positive end-expiratory pressure (PEEP). This re-emphasizes the importance of obtaining PAWP readings at end expiration when changes induced by mechanical ventilation are minimized. The effects of PEEP on intrathoracic or percardial pressures, of course, are maintained throughout the respiratory cycle and depend on the pulmonary compliance. Momentary discontinuation of the PEEP has been advocated to exclude its effect on LVEDP and PAWP, but this maneuver may induce significant hypoxia and probably is not safe. Others have suggested that approximately half of the PEEP is transmitted to intrathoracic or pericardial pressure; therefore, Rapel and Sibbald suggest that simply subtracting half the PEEP from the PAWP may provide a more useful estimate of the true LVED transmyocardial pressure and therefore this calculation may be more helpful in estimating LVEDV.

While PAWP provides the best clinically available estimate of LV preload, the clinician must be aware of these limitations. Furthermore, it must be emphasized that trends in the PAWP or changes in response to treatment are more useful in assessing the adequacy of LV preload than is an isolated PAWP reading. Furthermore, the adequacy of LV preload is not as important as total oxygen delivery; therefore, PAWP and LV preload should

always be considered in view of the patient's total oxygen delivery, which is discussed below.

Measurement of Cardiac Output

Although determination of cardiac output (CO) by the method of dye dilution was described as early as the 1950s, by Fox and associates, determination by thermodilution using a flow-directed pulmonary artery catheter was first described in the early 1970s, by Ganz, Forrester, and co-workers. This advancement greatly simplified and popularized cardiac output measurement. Today, cardiac output is obtained on most critically ill surgical patients at the bedside. Cardiac output determination by the thermodilution method is an application of the indicator dilution principle in which the temperature of the blood is changed by the injection of a solution and the dissipation of the temperature change is measured. The dissipation of the temperature change is described by a plot of temperature versus time, and the area under this curve is inversely related to cardiac output (blood flow) by the Stewart-Hamilton indicator dilution equation (Ganz et al). Therefore, as cardiac output increases, the temperature change is more rapidly dissipated. Modern pulmonary artery catheters are equipped with a distal thermistor, which is positioned in the pulmonary artery, and a proximal port, which is 30 cm from the tip, lies in the right atrium, and is used for injection of a cooled saline bolus. The injectate is typically 10 ml of 5% dextrose in water, (D5W) and may be at room temperature or cooled in ice (volume and temperature are input into a bedside computer). The injection should be smooth and completed within 4 seconds; furthermore, the injection should be performed each time at the same point in the respiratory cycle. A temperature time curve is measured by the thermistor, and the computer determines the area under this curve and automatically calculates cardiac output in liters per minute. Three injections are typically performed in succession and an average CO is determined. Cardiac output determinations are incorrect if the injectate temperature or volume is incorrectly entered or if the proximal port is within the introducer sheath. The simultaneous central venous infusion of other fluids may also result in incorrect measurements. Finally, the presence of intracardiac shunts invalidates measurements.

Cardiac output is typically normalized to body surface area and expressed as cardiac index in liters/minute/meter^2 (liters/min/m^2). Average cardiac index for a normal adult is 3.5 liter/min/m^2 and ranges from 2.8 to 4.2 liters/min/m^2. Since cardiac index is a fundamental component of oxygen delivery, depressed cardiac index leads to suboptimal tissue oxygenation and anaerobic metabolism. Chatterjee and Matthay found that the clinician's ability to identify suboptimal cardiac output on the basis of the physical examination and noninvasive tests is poor, ranging from 44 to 51 percent. Invasive monitoring of cardiac output therefore allows for earlier determination of impaired cardiac output and earlier treatment. Cardiac output can be described as the production of stroke volume and heart rate; stroke volume, in turn, depends on ventricular preload, afterload, and the inotropic state of the ventricle. These four components must be individually assessed and modified to optimize cardiac output.

Mixed Venous
Oxygen Saturation

Pulmonary arterial catheters permit mixed venous blood sampling and determination of mixed venous oxygen saturation (SvO$_2$). Normal mixed venous oxygen saturation is about 80 percent, and assuming an arterial oxygen saturation of 100 percent, only 20 percent of the total delivered oxygen is consumed by the body under normal conditions. Stated differently a mixed venous oxygen saturation of 80 percent indicates that the ratio of total oxygen delivery to oxygen consumption is 5 to 1. A decrease in the mixed venous oxygen saturation to an abnormal value of 50 percent for example, indicates that oxygen delivery exceeds consumption by only a 2:1 ratio, and may further suggest that oxygen consumption has become dependent on oxygen delivery. This illustrates the utility of the mixed venous oxygen saturation as a warning signal indicating alteration in oxygen consumption-delivery ratio (Birman et al). A falling mixed venous oxygen saturation in a critically ill patient warrants careful evaluation of the patient's pulmonary and hemodynamic status.

Within the last decade, a new generation of pulmonary artery catheters have been developed with spectrophotometric oximeters built into the tip of the catheter. Nelson has shown mixed venous oxygen

saturation determined by oximetry to correlate closely with blood gas determinations. Pulmonary artery catheters with oximetry allow for continuous and more practical mixed venous oxygen saturation measurement.

Indications for PA Catheters

Pulmonary artery catheters are diagnostic devices and are placed to answer specific questions. They can help diagnose precise hemodynamic derangements, quantitate the severity of these derangements, and help document response to treatment. Clinical evidence of shock is perhaps the most common indication for PA catheter monitoring; PA catheters help determine the type of shock and guide treatment (Table 5-3). Hypovolemic shock, for example, is a state of reduced intravascular volume or reduced left ventricular preload. This is typically demonstrated by markedly reduced CVP and PAWP. Because of reduced preload, cardiac output is secondarily reduced. Conversely, with cardiogenic shock, cardiac dysfunction is the primary defect and may result from valvular disease, arrhythmias, ischemia, infarction, contusion, tamponade, or cardiomyopathy. In patients with cardiogenic shock, cardiac output is diminished despite increased CVP and PAWP. In both hypovolemic and cardiogenic shock, baroreceptors identify reduced arterial pressures, a reflex vasoconstriction is triggered, and systemic vascular resistance (SVR) is increased. In both conditions, mixed venous oxygen saturation is diminished since there is an imbalance between oxygen delivery and oxygen consumption.

Septic shock usually develops secondary to bacterial infections. Bacterial toxins

cause a dilation of peripheral vascular beds, shunting blood flow away from the coronary, cerebral, renal, and other central circulations. Cardiac output is secondarily increased, SVR decreased, and LV filling unchanged or decreased. Mixed venous oxygen saturation may rise reflecting peripheral shunting. Neurogenic shock similarly causes markedly decreased SVR from loss of autonomic innervation. Cardiac index may be normal or increased. Reflex tachycardia, which is commonly observed with septic shock, however, is typically not seen with neurogenic shock.

Other specific indications for PA catheters include perioperative myocardial infarction. In this setting, PA catheters help achieve adequate cardiac index while minimizing myocardial oxygen consumption. They are also helpful in distinguishing cardiogenic pulmonary edema from noncardiogenic pulmonary edema. Pulmonary artery catheters are routinely employed in cardiac surgery patients and in those undergoing major intrathoracic noncardiac or intra-abdominal surgery. Underlying cardiopulmonary disease is a relative indication for intraoperative and perioperative use of PA catheters during any major surgical procedure. Finally, although not widely practiced, prospective randomized studies have suggested that preoperative hemodynamic evaluation with PA catheters and "preoperative tuning" to predetermined hemodynamic levels is indicated for certain patient groups. In 100 high-risk surgical patients who underwent preoperative PA catheter insertion, Del Guercio and associates found that none of the patients had completely normal hemodynamics; a majority required intravascular volume and more than a third needed ad-

Table 5-3. Hemodynamics During Shock

Hemodynamic Status	HR	CO	CVP	PAWP	SVR
Hypovolemic shock	⇑	⇓	⇓	⇓	⇑
Cardiogenic shock (primary RV failure)	⇑	⇓	⇑	Normal	⇑
Cardiogenic shock (LV or biventricular failure)	⇑	⇓	⇑	⇑	⇑
Septic shock*	⇑	⇑	Normal or ⇓	Normal of ⇓	⇓
Neurogenic shock	Normal	Normal or ⇑	⇓	⇓	⇓

HR = heart rate; CO = cardiac output; CVP = central venous pressure; PAWP = pulmonary artery wedge pressure; SVR = systemic vascular resistance.
*Early septic shock is typically characterized by preserved ventricular function with increased CO and normal or reduced CVP and PAWP. Conversely, prolonged septic shock may result in impaired ventricular function with reduced cardiac output and increased CVP and PAWP.

ditional interventions. Berlauk and colleagues demonstrated that high-risk patients with peripheral vascular disease who underwent preoperative hemodynamic optimization with PA catheters had significantly fewer adverse intraoperative events, less postoperative cardiac morbidity, and reduced early graft failure; mortality was 2.2 percent for the group that underwent preoperative hemodynamic optimization, relative to 9.5 percent for the control group. In this study, patients in the test group were admitted to the SICU for approximately 24 hours before operation, and treated with fluids and inotropic or vasodilatory agents to achieve predetermined hemodynamic end points.

Oxygen Consumption and Delivery

While critically ill surgical patients have a variety of hemodynamic parameters measured or calculated, recent studies, such as that of Shoemaker, have suggested that determination of oxygen delivery and oxygen consumption is most useful for predicting outcome and guiding therapy. In addition, prospective randomized trials, such as that of Shoemaker and associates, on high-risk postoperative patients suggest that therapeutic interventions to maximize these parameters may improve morbidity and mortality.

Oxygen delivery ($\dot{D}O_2$) is the product of cardiac output and the arterial oxygen concentration (see Table 5-1). Considering a normal individual with a cardiac output of 5.5 liters per minute, a hemoglobin (Hgb) concentration of 13.7 g/dl, and an arterial oxygen saturation of 99 percent:

$$DO_2 = 5500 \text{ ml/min} \times (0.137 \text{ g/ml}$$
$$\times 1.34 \text{ ml O}_2/\text{g Hgb} \times 0.99)$$
$$\approx 1000 \text{ ml O}_2/\text{min}$$

The normal range for oxygen delivery is 700 to 1400 ml oxygen per minute. Oxygen consumptions ($\dot{V}O_2$) is a measure of total aerobic metabolism. Conditions in which oxygen consumption is increased include hyperthermia, states of increased catecholamines, and exercise; conversely, oxygen consumption is decreased during hypothermia, hypothyroidism, and paralysis. Oxygen consumption is the product of cardiac output and the difference between arterial and venous oxygen concentrations (see Table 5-1). Considering an individual with a cardiac output of 5.5 liters per min-

ute, a hemoglobin concentration of 13.7 g/dl, and arterial and mixed venous oxygen saturations of 99 and 79 percent, respectively:

$$\dot{V}O_2 = 5500 \text{ ml/min} \times [0.137 \text{ g Hgb/ml}$$
$$\times 1.34 \text{ ml O}_2/\text{g Hgb} \times (0.99 - 0.79)]$$
$$\approx 200 \text{ ml O}_2/\text{min}$$

Under normal conditions as mentioned earlier, oxygen delivery exceeds oxygen consumption by approximately fivefold. Furthermore, oxygen consumption is typically not altered by small changes in oxygen delivery; stated differently oxygen consumption is independent of changes in delivery. In conditions such as hypovolemic or cardiogenic shock, oxygen delivery becomes markedly compromised, and oxygen consumption becomes dependent on and limited by delivery. During septic shock, or following burn injury or major surgical procedures, total body oxygen requirement is increased dramatically and oxygen consumption rises. However, if parallel increases in oxygen delivery do not occur during these conditions, oxygen consumption is again limited, and true tissue oxygen requirements are not met. In general, an oxygen delivery to consumption ratio of approximately 4 to 5 and documentation that oxygen consumption is independent of delivery suggest that the patient's hemodynamic status has been maximized. Oxygen delivery can be maximized by increasing cardiac output, hemoglobin concentration, and arterial oxygen saturation. Two patient scenarios are shown (Fig. 5-7) in which clinical interventions are directed at improving the oxygen delivery to consumption ratio and achieving a state in which oxygen consumption becomes independent of delivery.

Complications of Pulmonary Artery Catheter

Infection is an important complication of PA catheterization. The incidence of positive catheter segment culture ranges from 5.8 to 33 percent (Norwood and associates [1991], Michel and colleagues, and Pinilla and coworkers). Pulmonary artery catheter infection has been strongly associated with the duration of placement and the presence of remote infection. The incidence of PA catheter–associated sepsis ranges from 0.8 to 2.7 percent, according to the same three studies. Guidelines for PA catheter management with regard to

infection are as follows: Obviously infected sites warrant site change, suspicion for catheter infection warrants guidewire exchange and catheter culture, and positive catheter culture in turn warrants a change in site. Routine site changes are probably of little benefit.

Another common complication of placement of PA catheters is arrhythmias. About half of all patients will have some ventricular arrhythmias with catheter insertion; and this usually occurs as the catheter tip passes through the right heart. Arrhythmias are most commonly premature ventricular beats or nonsustained ventricular tachycardia and resolve spontaneously. Sustained ventricular tachycardia can occur if the catheter tip is misplaced in the right ventricle and catheters can be accidentally pulled back with patient positioning or movement. Therefore continuous pressure transducing and periodic chest radiographs are necessary to maintain catheter position. If a patient with a PA catheter develops a ventricular arrhythmia, the position should be questioned and the catheter removed.

Conduction abnormalities may also occur, with new, sustained, right bundle branch block occurring in approximately 3 percent of patients with PA catheters (Sprung and colleagues). Typically this is of little clinical consequence and resolves spontaneously. However, in patients with preexisting left bundle branch block, a new right bundle branch block would result in complete heart block; therefore, some have advocated standby transvenous or transthoracic pacemaker equipment for such patients when PA catheters are placed (Sprung and colleagues).

Another important but rare complication of PA catheters is that of thromboembolism of the central veins, right heart, or pulmonary artery. Prospective autopsy studies of patients who have died with PA catheters in place, such as the study by Connors and colleagues, demonstrated a 53 percent incidence of thrombosis, with the superior vena cava being the most common site of thrombus. Furthermore, this study demonstrates a strong correlation between the duration of catheterization and the risk of thrombosis. This emphasizes the importance of removing PA catheters when they no longer provide useful data. The presence of thrombosis can be confirmed by contrast studies via

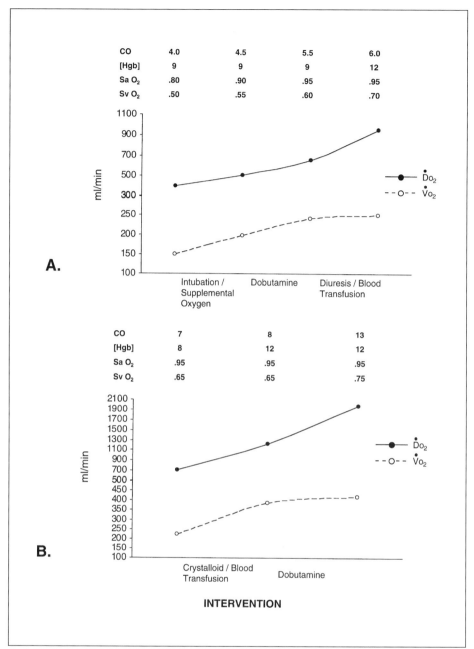

CO	4.0	4.5	5.5	6.0
[Hgb]	9	9	9	12
Sa O_2	.80	.90	.95	.95
Sv O_2	.50	.55	.60	.70

A.

Intubation / Supplemental Oxygen   Dobutamine   Diuresis / Blood Transfusion

CO	7	8	13
[Hgb]	8	12	12
Sa O_2	.95	.95	.95
Sv O_2	.65	.65	.75

B.

Crystalloid / Blood Transfusion   Dobutamine

INTERVENTION

Fig. 5-7. Illustrative cases of oxygen delivery and consumption relationships. Patient A developed congestive heart failure following a major surgical procedure. Subsequent therapeutic interventions improve both oxygen delivery ($\dot{D}O_2$) and consumption ($\dot{V}O_2$). In addition, the oxygen delivery:consumption ratio is enhanced following interventions and oxygen consumption becomes independent of delivery. Patient B developed septic shock following a major burn injury. Initial oxygen delivery and consumption are increased, reflecting this increased metabolic state; however, oxygen consumption is dependent and probably limited by delivery. Additional interventions achieve an improved oxygen delivery:consumption ratio and a state in which consumption is independent of delivery.

the proximal port. If thrombus is present, heparin anticoagulation is indicated.

A rare but devastating complication of pulmonary arterial catheterization is pulmonary artery perforation which has an incidence of 0.06 to 0.2 percent and an associated mortality as high as 65 percent (Kirton and colleagues). Barash and associates found that perforation may occur because of the following mechanisms: advancement of the catheter before balloon inflation, eccentric balloon inflation causing the tip to be directed through the side wall of the vessel, and finally balloon overinflation, causing disruption of the vessel. Therefore, the balloon should be tested for proper inflation prior to insertion, the catheter should never be advanced before inflation of the balloon, and the balloon should never be overinflated. Pulmonary artery perforation is usually accompanied by hemoptysis or hypotension and can be confirmed by wedge arteriography and bronchoscopy. Treatment of massive hemoptysis consists of isolation of the unaffected lung by selective endobronchial intubation. Pulmonary resection may be required. Risk factors for perforation include pulmonary hypertension, anticoagulation, and hypothermia. Survivors of an initial episode of pulmonary artery perforation frequently developed pulmonary artery pseudoaneurysms which are at risk for rupture and recurrent hemorrhage. Kirton and co-workers found transvenous catheter obliteration with coil embolization to be successful in management of pseudoaneurysm formation.

A final complication of pulmonary artery catheters is that of intraventricular knotting. This occurs more frequently when the right ventricle is dilated and when excessive catheter is introduced into the right ventricle. In general, no more than 10 cm of catheter should be introduced after the appearance of the right ventricular pressure tracing; failure of the PA pressure tracing to appear suggests an intraventricular catheter loop and warrants removal of the catheter. In more difficult patients with dilated right ventricles, fluoroscopy may be useful.

Noninvasive Monitoring

Continuous Cardiac Rate and Rhythm Monitoring

Although specific guidelines for the use of continuous ECG monitoring are not established, it is useful in a variety of settings, causes no additional risk for the patient, and should always precede more invasive monitoring. Continuous ECG monitoring permits identification of arrhythmias and is indicated for patients who are at increased risk, for example, patients with cardiac contusion, patients with underlying cardiac disease who have undergone major noncardiac procedures, and all patients who have undergone cardiac or pulmonary procedures. The presence of arrhythmias on continuous ECG monitor warrants a 12-lead ECG and an assessment of systemic perfusion.

Continuous ECG monitoring also permits closer evaluation of cardiac rate changes and is critical during anesthesia, during infusion of cardiovascular medications, and for patients who require fluid resuscitation. Tachycardia is an important manifestation of hypovolemia; however, changes in heart rate can be very nonspecific and may reflect level of sedation, pain, anxiety, body temperature, or respiratory status.

Urinary Output and Electrolytes

Renal function is commonly monitored in surgical patients since it reflects the adequacy of both renal and systemic arterial perfusion. Three important parameters that are frequently measured are urinary output, urinary sodium concentration, and the fractional excretion of sodium. Normal urinary output is generally greater than 0.5 ml/kg/hr for adults and greater than 1.0 ml/kg/hr for children. Urinary output below these limits suggests inadequate renal and systemic perfusion. Placement of a Foley catheter and hourly urinary output determination are helpful in a variety of situations, including intraoperatively when significant volume loss is anticipated, in patients with major trauma or burns, and for any patient in whom the status of intravascular volume is unclear. Diminished urinary output can be addressed with intravenous boluses of either crystalloid or colloid; improvement in urinary output in response to this treatment further confirms intravascular volume depletion. Despite the common use of urinary output as a measure of the intravascular volume status or systemic perfusion, many limitations must be realized. First, in patients with chronic renal insufficiency or renal artery stenosis, urinary output will not reflect renal or systemic perfusion. Furthermore, diuretics increase urinary output independent of renal perfusion and limit its usefulness. Intravenous contrast agents and hyperglycemia may affect an osmotic diuresis and similarly limit the usefulness of this parameter.

In patients with normal renal function, as renal perfusion decreases, sodium and water retention cause the production of a very concentrated urine with a low sodium concentration. Renal hypoperfusion and intravascular volume depletion are strongly suggested by a urinary osmolality greater than 500 mosm/kg and a urinary sodium concentration less than 20 meq per liter. These measurements combined with reduced urinary output suggest the need for further crystalloid or colloid infusion. In patients with reduced urine output, the fractional excretion of sodium (FE_{Na}%) is a reliable laboratory test for distinguishing renal hypoperfusion (a prerenal state) from acute tubular necrosis. This test can be performed by the simultaneous collection of urine and blood for measurement of creatinine and sodium.

$$FE_{Na}\% = [(U_{Na}/P_{Na})/(U_{Cr}/P_{Cr})] \times 100$$

A value less than 1 percent suggests renal hypoperfusion. In patients with acute tubular necrosis secondary to ischemia or nephrotoxic agents, reduced urine output is associated with an inappropriate increased urinary sodium concentration (>40 meq/liter) and a FE_{Na}% greater than 2.

Cardiovascular Support

A number of agents are available for modulating the cardiovascular system in critically ill patients. In general, these agents are employed to improve tissue oxygen delivery and restore a more favorable oxygen delivery-consumption relationship. More specifically, parenteral agents are available to provide positive inotropic effects, to increase vascular tone, and to reduce vascular tone. For the management of critically ill surgical patients, agents that are commonly employed for cardiovascular support have the following fundamental properties: parenteral administration, rapid onset of action, short half-life, and favorable side effect profiles. These agents are initiated only after proper hemodynamic monitoring has been established, which typically consists of at least a radial artery and pulmonary artery catheter. Furthermore, there should be specific therapeutic goals: for example, a target cardiac index, systemic arterial resistance, or mean arterial pressure. Generally, therapy is initiated at a dose below the expected required dose with subsequent upward titration to achieve the desired effect. Conversely, once hemodynamic stability has been achieved these agents are slowly weaned off while hemodynamic monitoring is continued.

Positive Inotropic Agents

Before positive inotropic agents are employed, optimal left ventricular preload must be established; this requires careful monitoring of changes in PAWP, cardiac index, and pulmonary status in response to volume infusion. Other considerations before initiation of an inotropic agent include normalization of body temperature, as hypothermia can significantly reduce the inotropic state. Arrhythmias must be controlled. Acidosis and electrolyte abnormalities that impair ventricular function must be corrected. Finally, agents that have negative inotropic effects, such as beta-adrenergic receptor (β-AR) antagonists and calcium channel blockers, should be promptly discontinued.

Ionized Calcium
Cardiac muscle function is dependent on intracellular calcium ions and in this regard ionized calcium is considered an inotropic agent. Normal ionized calcium levels are 1.00 to 1.25 mmole per liter. Several common events can lead to reduced ionized calcium levels, including large blood product transfusions containing citrate compounds that bind ionized calcium; administration of furosemide, which increases renal excretion; chronic renal failure; and recent cardiopulmonary bypass. Patients with impaired ventricular function should have ionized calcium levels normalized with infusions of calcium chloride or calcium gluconate. Drop and Scheidegger found that in this setting, intravenous calcium has several important effects, most importantly improved cardiac contractility and increased vascular tone. According to Zaloga and colleagues, when ionized calcium levels are normal, further calcium administration does not affect sustained increases in cardiac output or oxygen delivery. Therefore, patients with normal ionized calcium levels probably do not benefit from intravenous cal-

Table 5-4. Effects of Sympathomimetic Agents

Agent	Receptor Activation				Physiologic Effects				
	β_1	β_2	α	Dopamine	HR	CO	SVR	MAP	PAWP
Dobutamine, 2.5–10 μg/kg/min	+++	+	+	−	⇑	⇑⇑⇑	⇔	⇔	⇔⇓
Renal dose dopamine, 0.5–2 μg/kg/min	−	−	−	+++	⇔	⇔⇑	⇓	⇔	⇔
Dopamine, >5 μg/kg/min	+++	−	+++	+++	⇑	⇑⇑⇑	⇔⇑	⇑	⇔⇑
Low-dose epinephrine, <0.1 μg/kg/min	++	++	−	−	⇑	⇑	⇓	⇔	⇔⇓
Epinephrine, 0.1–0.3 μg/kg/min	+++	+++	+++	−	⇑	⇑⇑⇑	⇔⇑	⇑	⇑
Isoproterenol, 2–10 μg/min	+++	+++	−	−	⇑⇑	⇑⇑⇑	⇓⇓	⇓	⇓

Key: + = mildly activated; ++ = moderately activated; +++ = strongly activated; ⇑ = increased; ⇔ = unchanged; ⇓ = decreased.

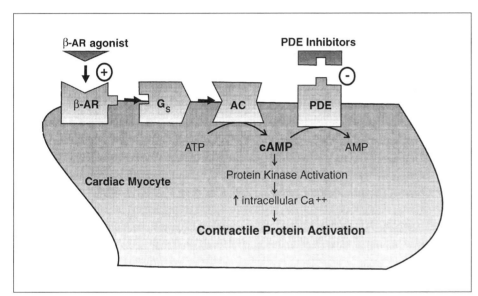

Fig. 5-8. Myocardial beta-adrenergic receptor system. An increased myocyte contractile state requires increased intracellular cAMP and calcium mobilization. Intracellular cAMP is increased by beta-adrenergic receptor (β-AR) agonists, which stimulate β-ARs, which in turn couple to and activate stimulatory guanosine triphosphate–binding protein (G_s) and subsequently activate adenylyl cyclase (AC). Phosphodiesterase (PDE) inhibitors also increase cAMP accumulation by reducing its degradation by phosphodiesterases (PDE).

cium treatment even though it may transiently increase arterial blood pressure.

Beta-Adrenergic Receptor Agonists

The most important positive inotropic agents act to increase myocardial intracellular cyclic adenosine monophosphate (cAMP) (Table 5-4). Beta-adrenergic receptor agonists bind myocardial β_1-ARs and β_2-ARs, which then couple to stimulatory guanine nucleotide-binding protein and activate the effector enzyme adenylyl cyclase; adenylyl cyclase in turn converts adenosine triphosphate (ATP) to cAMP which, through a biochemical cascade, enhances myocardial contractile protein interactions (Fig. 5-8).

Dobutamine. Dobutamine is a selective β_1-AR agonist. As such its primary effect is enhancement of ventricular function and increased stroke volume and cardiac output. While dobutamine generally increases heart rate, this effect is much less pronounced relative to nonselective β-AR agonists such as isoproterenol. This phenomenon may reflect the relative greater importance of β_2-ARs in modulating sinoatrial rate. Left ventricular end-diastolic pressure and PAWP generally decline with dobutamine infusions; coronary blood flow and myocardial oxygen consumption are usually increased.

Dobutamine has minimal effect on peripheral vascular resistance. It does not act on dopaminergic receptors and has small effects on peripheral vascular α_1 and β_2-ARs. Since stimulation of peripheral α_1-ARs mediates vasoconstriction while β_2-ARs effect vasodilatation, the net effect of dobutamine on systemic vascular resistance is minimal. If peripheral vasodilatation is desired to further enhance cardiac index, dobutamine can be combined with infusions of peripheral vasodilators such as nitroglycerin or nitroprusside. The addition of low-dose dopamine may be advocated to maximize renal perfusion.

The dose of dobutamine ranges from 2 to 20 μg/kg/min. It is specifically indicated for cardiogenic shock after acute myocardial infarction and after cardiac surgery (Diseva), and it can also be used in supporting cardiac function during septic shock. The most important complications of dobutamine are atrial and ventricular arrhythmias. Infusions can also produce mental status changes, presumably as a result of action of the drug on central nervous system β-ARs, but these effects are seldom limiting.

Dopamine is both a synthetic agent and an endogenous catecholamine. With low doses (<2μg/kg/min), it acts solely on dopaminergic receptors in the renal, mesenteric, coronary, and intracerebral vascular beds affecting vasodilatation. Goldberg and Rajifer demonstrated that low-dose dopamine convincingly augments renal blood flow in humans. Davis and associates have also shown it to increase urinary volume and decrease plasma renin activity in postoperative patients. Based on these data, low-dose dopamine is commonly employed, in surgical patients believed to be at increased risk for acute renal failure, for example, patients with renal artery stenosis, chronic renal insufficiency or sepsis, or patients who have undergone cardiopulmonary bypass or repair of abdominal aortic aneurysm.

At intermediate doses (2–5 μ/kg/min), dopamine begins to act on myocardial β_1-ARs, like dobutamine, to enhance LV function, increase stroke work, and increase cardiac output. At high doses (>5 μg/kg/min), dopamine also activates peripheral α_1-ARs with resultant peripheral vasoconstriction. While PAWP may actually decrease with low or intermediate doses of dopamine, high doses of dopamine usually lead to increased PAWP. Intermediate and high doses of dopamine are indicated for patients with cardiogenic shock following myocardial infarction or cardiopulmonary bypass. Studies have demonstrated that dopamine infusions, in experimental models of myocardial ischemia, can enhance myocardial blood flow in normal and mildly ischemic regions while not affecting perfusion of severely ischemic regions. The beneficial effect of this agent for ischemic LV dysfunction, however, may in some cases be limited by tachycardic responses, which reduce diastolic coronary perfusion. Intermediate and high doses of dopamine are also useful for supporting LV function following cardiac surgery, during sepsis, or in patients with chronic congestive heart failure. Dopamine has essentially replaced epinephrine and norepinephrine in these settings because, unlike these agents, it does not effect severe vasoconstriction of the renal, splanchnic, and peripheral beds. Furthermore, the vasoconstriction associated with high-dose dopamine can be reduced by simultaneous infusions of peripheral vasodilators such as nitroglycerin or nitroprusside.

Side effects of dopamine include arrhythmias, nausea, vomiting, and anxiety. High doses have been reported to effect peripheral limb ischemia, and extravasation into subcutaneous tissues can cause skin necrosis.

Epinephrine. Epinephrine is naturally secreted by the adrenal medulla and is the prototype catecholamine. It stimulates both α- and β-ARs. At low doses (<0.1 μg/kg/min), epinephrine activates predominantly β-ARs, which causes increased heart rate, increased contractility, and slightly decreased peripheral vascular resistance (secondary to activation of peripheral β_2-ARs). At higher doses of epinephrine (0.1–1.0 μg/kg/min), there is continued rise in heart rate and contractility due to stimulation of myocardial β-ARs, but peripheral vasoconstriction occurs as a result of activation of peripheral α-ARs, and arterial blood pressure rises. High-dose epinephrine can cause marked tachycardia and both atrial and ventricular arrhythmias. Its use is also limited by marked vasoconstriction of arterial beds, which can result in limb, mesenteric, and renal ischemia.

Indications for low-dose epinephrine include most causes of cardiogenic shock. Higher-dose epinephrine has more limited indications and should be used only when cardiogenic shock is accompanied by profound hypotension, for example, in patients after cardiac surgery with low cardiac index and persistent hypotension, or in patients with septic shock associated with cardiac dysfunction and hypotension. Intravenous, intracardiac, or intratracheal epinephrine bolus (1 mg) is indicated for cardiac arrest, and causes marked peripheral vasoconstriction, improving cerebral and coronary perfusion during CPR; in addition asystole may be converted to a sinus rhythm and myocardial contractility may be restored in cases of electromechanical dissociation.

Isoproterenol. Isoproterenol is a potent β-AR agonist. Infusions of isoproterenol cause tachycardia and increased myocardial contractility as well as peripheral vasodilatation and decreased SVR. Isoproterenol does not stimulate α-ARs. Use of isoproterenol for cardiogenic shock is limited by marked increases in heart rate, arrhythmias, and vasodilatation. Therefore, isoproterenol is indicated primarily for symptomatic sinus bradycardia and to help restore AV conduction during complete heart block. It has also been used to enhance heart rate in the denervated transplanted heart.

Phosphodiesterase Inhibitors

Myocardial cAMP is actively metabolized by cyclic nucleotide phosphodiesterases (PDEs) to adenosine monophosphate (AMP), which is inactive as a second messenger. Several fractions of phosphodiesterases have been described with the third fraction being most important in the myocardium for attenuating the cAMP response. Recently, specific inhibitors of type III phosphodiesterases have been developed as alternative inotropic agents; the primary mechanism for their positive inotropic effect is increased myocardial cAMP (see Fig. 5-8). In addition to this inotropic effect, these agents also effect vasodilatation by increasing cAMP and cyclic guanosine monophosphate (cGMP) metabolism in vascular smooth muscle; these second messengers are critical for triggering smooth-muscle relaxation.

Amrinone. Amrinone, which is the most widely used fraction III phosphodiesterase inhibitor, effects an increase in contractility, stroke volume, and cardiac output. Heart rate is minimally affected. Systemic and pulmonary vascular resistance typically are reduced with infusions of amrinone. Reflecting the minimal effect on heart rate and the reduction in vascular resistance, myocardial oxygen consumption is typically not affected by amrinone infusions despite the increased contractility. Therefore, it may be effective in myocardial dysfunction associated with infarction or ischemia.

Amrinone can be combined with dopamine, epinephrine, or norepinephrine infusions; these catecholamines stimulate myocardial cAMP production via the β-AR system and thereby act synergistically with amrinone to enhance contractility. In addition, these agents, by activation of peripheral α-ARs, can be used to offset amrinone-mediated vasodilatation, which would otherwise limit use of the agent in patients with hypotension and shock.

The elimination half-life of amrinone is 2.6 to 4.1 hours. A loading dose of 0.75 mg/kg over 2 to 3 minutes is required and can be repeated if no effect is observed. If given into the cardiopulmonary bypass circuit, a large loading dose of 1.5 to 2.0 mg/kg over 10 minutes is required. Following the loading dose, an infusion should be initiated at 5 to 20 μg/kg/min. Amrinone is indicated for essentially all forms of cardiogenic shock. It is typically added to more traditional β-AR agonists in refractory cases but can be used as a primary agent. It may be particularly helpful for patients with right ventricular dysfunction and increased pulmonary vascular resistance. Amrinone has also been employed during septic shock to help augment cardiac output, and in this setting addition of catecholamines with peripheral α-AR effects are again frequently required. Adverse reactions to amrinone include hypotension, supraventricular arrhythmias, and thrombocytopenia. Thrombocytopenia usually follows more chronic amrinone infusions, and recent studies in patients who received infusions for 24 hours after cardiac surgery identified no significant thrombocytopenia.

Milrinone. Milrinone is another fraction III PDE inhibitor available in the United States for parenteral administration and has been shown to have inotropic effects approximately 15 times more potent than those of amrinone. Hemodynamic effects parallel those of amrinone (Table 5-5) and include increased cardiac output, minimal heart rate effect, and reduced pulmonary and systemic vascular resistance. Milrinone, like amrinone, does not appear to increase myocardial oxygen consumption. Indications and usage for milrinone are similar to those listed for amrinone. The loading dose of milrinone is 50 μg/kg over 10 minutes followed by an infusion of 0.375 to 0.75 μg/kg/min. Side effects include fluid retention in 80 percent of patients, which frequently requires increased diuretics; diarrhea; and other mild gastrointestinal problems. Thrombocytopenia and arrhythmias are less common with milrinone than with amrinone.

Agents that Increase Vascular Tone

Agents with vasoconstricting effects are generally contraindicated in the management of shock since they may actually further impair oxygen delivery. In septic shock associated with severe hypotension, peripheral vasoconstriction may increase central pressures and improve coronary and cerebral blood flow; in this setting vasoconstrictor therapy may initially be appropriate while volume infusions are initiated. These agents should be discontinued as soon as volume infusions have stabilized or have corrected the hypotension. Other scenarios in which vasoconstrictors may be transiently helpful include neurogenic shock, hypotension associated with anesthesia, and hypotension associated with rapid warming. Again, these agents should be discontinued as soon as volume infusions have stabilized the arterial blood pressure.

Table 5-5. Hemodynamic Effects of Phosphodiesterase Inhibitors*

PDE Inhibitor	Change in Hemodynamics (%)					
	CI	PAWP	RAP	HR	MAP	SVR
Amrinone	+67	−36	−42	+3	−17	−48
Milrinone	+49	−31	−39	0	−13	−30

*Relative changes in cardiac index (CI), pulmonary artery wedge pressure (PAWP), right atrial pressure (RAP), heart rate (HR), mean arterial pressure (MAP), and systemic vascular resistance (SVR) in 10 patients treated with amrinone and 37 patients given milrinone at the University of California, San Francisco (all patients had congestive heart failure).
Source: From K Chatterjee. Digitalis, Catecholamines, and Other Positive Inotropic Agents. In WW Parmley, K Chatterjee (eds), *Cardiology*. Vol 1. *Physiology, Pharmacology and Diagnosis*. Philadelphia: Lippincott, 1993. Pp 1–58. Reproduced with permission.

Two potent vasoconstrictors are norepinephrine and phenylephrine. Norepinephrine is a potent α-AR and myocardial β_1-AR agonist; it does not activate peripheral β_2-ARs. In normal subjects, norepinephrine causes a marked increase in pulmonary and systemic vascular resistance and pulmonary systemic arterial pressures. These effects normally cause reduced perfusion; however, in patients with septic shock and profound hypotension, norepinephrine infusions may improve coronary, cerebral, and renal blood flow (Desjars et al, 1989; Meadows et al, 1988). Norepinephrine infusions should be initiated at very low doses, 0.025 to 0.1 μg/kg/min, and can be increased to a maximum of 1.0 to 1.5 μg/kg/min. Norepinephrine can cause arrhythmias and detrimental vasoconstriction and ischemia.

Phenylephrine. Phenylephrine is a pure α-AR agonist with no β-AR effect. Infusions cause marked increases in pulmonary and systemic vascular resistance. The limited indications are similar to those for norepinephrine. Phenylephrine is typically administered as an IV bolus while volume infusions are initiated; 0.5 mg can be initially administered IV over 2 to 3 minutes, and up to 5 mg can be given to achieve the desired effect.

Agents that Decrease Vascular Tone

Nitroglycerin and nitroprusside are parenteral vasodilators frequently employed in post operative management. Inhaled nitric oxide is an experimental agent that may provide selective pulmonary vascular dilatation. These three agents ultimately act within vascular smooth-muscle cells

(Fig. 5-9). Nitroglycerin is converted to nitric oxide via a dinitration process that requires sulfhydryl groups. Nitroprusside releases nitric oxide directly. Nitric oxide, through mechanisms that have not been completely elucidated, activates guanylate cyclase, with subsequent increases in smooth-muscle cGMP (see Fig. 5-9). cGMP, an important second messenger, activates protein kinase phosphorylation, resulting in reduced intracellular calcium and smooth-muscle relaxation.

Nitroglycerin. Nitroglycerin dilates the venous capacitance system, as well as effecting systemic arterial and arteriolar dilatation. By these mechanisms, it is a potent antihypertensive. In addition, these systemic effects cause reduced peripheral vascular resistance and enhanced cardiac output in patients with congestive heart failure. Nitroglycerin also effects coronary artery dilatation, reversal of coronary artery spasm, dilatation of stenotic coronary arterial segments, and improvement in collateral coronary flow. The combination of these systemic and coronary effects serves to ameliorate myocardial ischemia, which is the most common indication for this agent (Abrams, 1993).

Intravenous nitroglycerin should be initiated at a rate of 5 to 20 μg per minute and can be increased by 5 to 10 μg every 5 to 10 minutes until the desired effect is achieved. Topical nitroglycerin ointment (2%) can be applied as 0.5 to 2.0 inches every 6 hours. Specific indications for nitroglycerin include perioperative hypertension, myocardial ischemia, myocardial infarction, congestive heart failure without shock or hypotension, and pulmonary edema. Nitroglycerin is prophylactically employed during and after coronary ar-

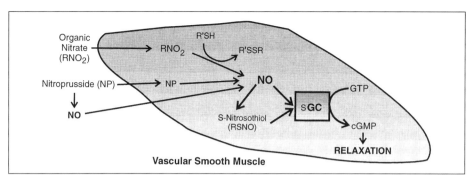

Fig. 5-9. Agents for vascular smooth-muscle relaxation. Illustrated is a current hypothesis for smooth-muscle relaxation in response to organic nitrates, nitroprusside, and inhaled nitric oxide (NO). Organic nitrates are converted to NO by a dinitration process that requires reduced sulfhydryl moieties (R'SH). Nitroprusside is more directly converted to NO. Nitric oxide acts within vascular smooth-muscle cells to directly or indirectly activate soluble guanylate cyclase (sGC). sGC converts guanosine triphosphate (GTP) to cyclic guanosine monophosphate, a second messenger, which in turn leads to relaxation. RSSR ≠ oxidized sulfhydryl moieties. (From J Abrams. Nitrates. In WW Parmley, K Chatterjee, eds, Cardiology. Vol 1. *Physiology, Pharmacology and Diagnosis.* Philadelphia: Lippincott, 1993. Pp 1–23. Reproduced with permission.)*

tery bypass surgery to prevent vasospasm of both the native coronary arteries and arterial grafts. Nitroglycerin is also prophylactically administered to patients undergoing peripheral vascular surgery who are at high risk for perioperative myocardial ischemia. In addition, it is typically part of the antihypertensive regimen during aortic cross clamping for abdominal aortic aneurysm surgery.

Common adverse effects of nitroglycerin are headache, reflex tachycardia, dizziness, and transient hypotension; less common effects include nausea and vomiting. Methemoglobin levels may become elevated in patients receiving enormous doses of intravenous nitroglycerin and may cause cyanosis.

Nitroprusside. Nitroprusside is a potent arteriolar dilator, and is essentially the first-choice parenteral agent for hypertension, but lacks many of the coronary vascular effects of nitroglycerin. Nitroprusside is commonly employed after cardiac or other major vascular surgery to control hypertension and reduce the risk of postoperative hemorrhage. Classic indications include hypertension following aortic valve replacement in patients with aortic stenosis, and for hypertension associated with aortic dissection. This agent is also important in reducing afterload and is commonly employed to maximize cardiac output in patients with congestive

heart failure or cardiogenic shock. In this setting, it is commonly combined with dopamine or dobutamine infusions.

The usual initial dose of nitroprusside is 0.5 μg/kg/min, which can be increased in increments of 0.25 to 1.0 μg/kg/min until the desired blood pressure is achieved. At doses above 5 μg/kg/min, addition of a second agent should be considered. The elimination half-life and the time to onset of effect are both about 2 to 3 minutes. The agent is administered via a central venous line, which should not be used for other infusions. Minimal extension tubing should be used between the pump and the port of the line to prevent accidental boluses and hypotension. Nitroprusside is metabolized by red blood cells and the liver to cyanide and thiocyanate, both of which are inhibitors of aerobic metabolism; cyanide toxicity is a rare but important side effect that limits the duration of nitroprusside use. This toxicity must be considered whenever high doses of this agent are used for greater than 24 hours and therefore alternative agents need to be initiated in these cases. Nitroprusside toxicity usually presents as an unexplained metabolic acidosis, an elevated serum lactate level, or an increased mixed venous oxygen saturation. Blood cyanide or thiocyanate levels confirm the diagnosis. Management of this toxicity includes immediate cessation of the infusion and administration of hydroxocobalamine, which complexes circulating cyanide.

Inhaled Nitric Oxide. A number of disease processes cause pulmonary arterial hypertension and an extensive experimental effort has been devoted to developing means of selectively producing pulmonary vasodilatation. Recent exciting studies employing inhaled nitric oxide have demonstrated selective vasodilatation of the pulmonary vascular bed. Nitric oxide directly activates smooth-muscle guanylate cyclase, resulting in increased cGMP and subsequent smooth-muscle relaxation. Inhaled nitric oxide appears to diffuse through the alveolar walls to affect the pulmonary vasculature; however, it is rapidly inactivated by hemoglobin on entering the bloodstream and therefore is not distributed to the systemic circulation. With this pattern of distribution and metabolism, its effect is confined to the pulmonary vascular bed.

Animal studies by Pearl, Frostell and colleagues (1991), and Fratacci and associates with different models of pulmonary hypertension have shown convincingly that inhaled nitric oxide at 5 to 80 ppm can induce rapid and reversible pulmonary vasodilatation. These initial studies have led to a variety of human studies. In normal human volunteers, inhaled nitric oxide had minimal effect on pulmonary vasculature, but Frostell and coworkers (1993) showed that in subjects exposed to hypoxia with secondary pulmonay hypertension, inhaled nitric oxide significantly reduced pulmonary hypertension with no effect on systemic arterial pressure or vascular resistance. Surprisingly, maximal effects in humans were seen with only 10 ppm, significantly less than required in animal studies. Inhaled nitric oxide has been employed to selectively reduce pulmonary artery pressure and pulmonary vascular resistance in patients with a variety of disease processes, including persistent pulmonary hypertension of the newborn, adult respiratory distress syndrome, and postcardiac and pulmonary transplantation pulmonary hypertension. In these patients, the reduced pulmonary hypertension is associated with improved oxygenation; this improvement in oxygenation occurs because inhaled nitric oxide is distributed to ventilated regions of the lung so that the associated vasodilatation improves blood flow to well-ventilated regions (Pearl, 1993).

Although the potential for nitric oxide to induce toxicity in injured lung has not been fully investigated, studies performed on normal animals have demonstrated no major adverse effects of nitric oxide with exposures up to 6 months (Pearl, 1993; Oda et al, 1976; Hugod, 1975). While inhaled nitric oxide must still be considered an experimental agent, current data suggest that it represents a powerful selective pulmonary vasodilator with relatively few side effects.

Suggested Reading

Abrams J. Nitrates. In WW Parmley, K Chatterjee, eds, *Cardiology*. Vol 1. *Physiology, Pharmacology and Diagnosis*. Philadelphia: Lippincott, 1993. Pp 1–23.

Band JD, Maki DG. Infections caused by arterial catheters used for hemodynamic monitoring. *Am J Med* 67:735, 1979.

Barash G, Nardi D, Hammond G, et al. Catheter-induced pulmonary artery perforation: mechanisms, management, and modifications. *J Thorac Cardiovasc Surg* 82:5, 1981.

Bedford RF. Long-term radial artery cannulation: Effects on subsequent vessel function. *Crit Care Med* 6:64, 1978.

Berlauk JF, Abrams, JH, Gilmour IJ, et al. Preoperative optimization of cardiovascular hemodynamics improves outcome in peripheral vascular surgery; a prospective randomized clinical trial. *Ann Surg* 214:289, 1991.

Bernard RW, Stahl WM. Subclavian vein catheterizations. A prospective study of non-infectious complications. *Ann Surg* 173:184, 1971.

Birman H, Haq A, Hew E, Aberman A. Continuous monitoring of mixed venous oxygen saturation in hemodynamically unstable patients. *Chest* 86:753, 1984.

Chatterjee K. Digitalis, Catecholamines, and Other Positive Inotropic Agents. In WW Parmley, K Chatterjee, eds, *Cardiology*. Vol 1. *Physiology, Pharmacology and Diagnosis*. Philadelphia: Lippincott, 1993. Pp 1–58.

Chatterjee K, Matthay M. Right-heart catheterization is a diagnostic procedure not a therapeutic intervention. *J Intensive Care Med* 6:101, 1991.

Christenson KH, Nerstrom B, Baden N. Complications of percutaneous catheterization of the subclavian vein in 129 cases. *Acta Chir Scand* 133:615, 1967.

Connors AF, Castele RJ, Farhat NZ, Tomashefski JF Jr. Complications of right heart catheterization, a prospective autopsy study. *Chest* 88:567, 1985.

Davis RF, Lappas DG, Kirklin JK, et al. Acute oliguria after cardiopulmonary bypass: Renal functional improvement with low dose dopamine infusions. *Crit Care Med* 10:852, 1982.

Del Guercio LRM, Savino JA, Morgan JC. Physiologic assessment of surgical diagnosis-related groups. *Ann Surg* 202:519, 1985.

Desjars P, Pinaud M, Bugnon D, et al. Norepinephrine therapy has no deleterious renal effects in human septic shock. *Crit Care Med* 17:426, 1989.

Diseva VJ. Pharmacologic support for postoperative low cardiac output. *Semin Thorac Cardiovasc Surg* 3:13, 1991.

Drop LJ, Scheidegger D. Plasma ionized calcium concentration: Important determinant of the hemodynamic responses to calcium infusion. *J Thorac Cardiovas Surg* 79:425, 1980.

Ejrup B, Fischer B, Wright IS. Clinical evaluation of blood flow to the hand; the false positive Allen test. *Circulation* 33:778, 1966.

Eyer S, Brummitt C, Crossley K, et al. Catheter-related sepsis: Prospective, randomized study of three methods of long-term catheter maintenance. *Crit Care Med* 18:1073, 1990.

Fitzpatrick GF, Hampson LG, Burgess JH. Bedside determination of left atrial pressure. *CMAJ* 106:1293, 1972.

Forrester JS, Ganz W, Diamond G, et al. Thermodilution cardiac output determination with a single flow-directed catheter. *Am Heart J* 83:306, 1972.

Fox IJ, Brooker LGS, Heseltine DW, et al. A tricarbocyanine dye for continous recording of dilution curves in whole blood independent of variations in blood oxygen saturation. *Mayo Clinic Proc* 32:478, 1957.

Fractacci MD, Frostell C, Chen TY, et al. Inhaled nitric oxide: A selective pulmonary vasodilator of heparin protamine vasoconstriction in sheep. *Anesthesiology* 75:990, 1991.

Frostell CG, Blomquist H, Hedenstierna G, et al. Inhaled nitric oxide selectively reverses human hypoxic pulmonary vasoconstriction without causing systemic vasodilation. *Anesthesiology* 78:427, 1993.

Frostell C, Fratacci MD, Wain JC, et al. Inhaled nitric oxide: A selective pulmonary vasodilator reversing hypoxic pulmonary vasoconstriction. *Circulation* 83:2038, 1991.

Ganz W, Donoso R, Marcus HS, et al. A new technique for measurement of cardiac output by thermodilution in man. *Am J Cardiol* 27: 392, 1971.

Goldberg LI, Rajifer SL. Dopamine receptors: Applications in clinical cardiology. *Circulation* 72:245, 1985.

Hampton AA, Sheretz RJ. Vascular access infections in hospitalized patients. *Surg Clin North Am* 68:57, 1988.

Hugod C. Effects of exposure to 43 ppm nitric oxide and 3.6 ppm nitrogen dioxide on rabbit lungs. *Int Arch Occup Environ Health* 42:159, 1975.

Kirton OC, Varon AJ, Henry RP, Civetta JM. Flow-directed, pulmonary artery catheter-induced pulmonary artery psuedoaneurysm: Urgent diagnosis and endovascular obliteration. *Crit Care Med* 20:1178, 1992.

Leroy O, Beuscart C, Sartre C, et al. Nosocomial infections associated with longterm artery cannulation. *Intensive Care Med* 15:241, 1989.

Maki DG, Weise CE, Sarafin HW. A semiquantitative culture method for identifying intravenous catheter related infection. *N Engl J Med* 296:1305, 1977.

Marini JJ. Obtaining meaningful data from the Swan-Ganz catheter. *Respir Care* 30:572, 1985.

Meadows D, Edward JD, Wilkins RG, et al. Reversal of intractable septic shock with norepinephrine therapy. *Crit Care Med* 16:663, 1988.

Michel L, Marsh HM, McMichan JC, et al. Infection of pulmonary artery catheters in critically ill patients. *JAMA* 245:1032, 1981.

Mojil R, Delaurentis D, Rosemund G. The infraclavicular venipuncture. *Arch Surg* 95:320, 1967.

Nelson LD. Continuous venous oximetry in surgical patients. *Ann Surg* 203:329, 1986.

Norwood S, Jenkins G. An evaluation of triple-lumen catheter infections using a guidewire exchange technique. *J Trauma* 30:706, 1990.

Norwood SH, Cormier B, McMahon NG, et al. Prospective study of catheter related infection during prolonged arterial catheterization. *Crit Care Med* 16:836, 1988.

Norwood S, Ruby A, Civetta J, Cortes V. Catheter-related infections and associated septicemia. *Chest* 99:968, 1991.

Oda H, Nogami H, Kusomoto S, et al. Long-term exposure to nitric oxide in mice. *J Jpn Soc Air Pollut* 11:150, 1976.

Pearl RG. Inhalted nitric oxide, the past, the present and the future. *Anesthesiology* 78:413, 1993.

Pinilla J, Ross DF, Martin T, Crump H. Study of the incidence of intravascular catheter infection and associated septicemia in critically ill patients. *Crit Care Med* 11:21, 1983.

Raper R, Sibbald WJ. Misled by the wedge? The Swan-Ganz catheter and left ventricular preload. *Chest* 89:427, 1986.

Shoemaker WC. Circulatory mechanisms of shock and their mediators. *Crit Care Med* 15:787, 1987.

Shoemaker WC, Appel PL, Kram HB, et al. Prospective trial of supernormal values of survivors as therapeutic goals in high risk surgical patients. *Chest* 94:1176, 1988.

Slogoff S, Keats AS, Arlund C. On the safety of radial artery cannulation. *Anesthesiology* 59:42, 1983.

Sprung CL, Elser B, Schein RMH, et al. Risk of right bundle branch block and complete heart block during pulmonary artery catheterization. *Crit Care Med* 17:1, 1989.

Swan HJC, Ganz W, Forrester J, et al. Catheterization of the heart in man with use of a flow-directed balloon-tipped catheter. *N Engl J Med* 283:447, 1970.

West JB, Dollery CT, Naimark A. Distribution of blood flow in isolated lung; relation to vascular and alevolar pressures. *J Appl Physiol* 19:713, 1964.

Zaloga GP, Prielipp RC, Butterworth JF, Royster RL. Pharmacologic cardiovascular support. *Crit Care Clinics* 9:335, 1993.

6

Respiratory Failure and Ventilatory Support

George F. Sheldon   Samir M. Fakhry   W. J. Messick

Respiratory failure can be defined as impairment in the ability of the respiratory system to maintain adequate oxygenation and carbon dioxide elimination. A variety of clinical conditions are associated with respiratory failure. These include neurologic and neuromuscular disorders, airway obstruction, pulmonary parenchymal disease, abnormalities of the chest wall, and pathology at the alveolar-capillary interface. Mechanical ventilation using a variety of positive-pressure techniques currently allows effective supportive therapy in the majority of patients with respiratory failure. This chapter provides a brief review of pulmonary physiology, an overview of respiratory failure, and a clinically oriented approach to mechanical ventilation. The common clinical signs of respiratory failure and the adult respiratory distress syndrome (ARDS) are discussed, along with adjunctive treatments (e.g., intubation, sedation, and muscle relaxants) for patients who require mechanical ventilation.

Pulmonary Physiology

Important functions of the pulmonary system include oxygenation and carbon dioxide (CO_2) elimination. Under most circumstances, carbon dioxide elimination is linearly related to minute ventilation, with other factors having little impact on the partial pressure of CO_2. Oxygenation is a more complex process that is dependent on several factors: the fractional inspired oxygen concentration (FIO_2), the degree of ventilation-perfusion mismatching ($\dot{V}/\dot{Q}$), and the diffusion of oxygen across the alveolar-capillary membrane. The oxygen tension in the alveolus (P_AO_2) is a function of FIO_2, barometric pressure (P_B), partial pressure of water vapor (P_{H_2O}), and alveolar carbon dioxide concentration (P_ACO_2), as shown in the modified alveolar gas equation (Table 6-1):

$$P_AO_2 = [(P_B - P_{H_2O}) \times FIO_2] - [P_ACO_2/0.8]$$

Since there is rapid equilibration between the two, it is possible to substitute $PaCO_2$ for P_ACO_2, thus simplifying the calculation of P_AO_2. Under normal circumstances in the patient breathing room air, P_AO_2 is 95 to 100 mm Hg, and PaO_2 is 85 to 90 mm Hg (Table 6-1).

The ability of oxygen to diffuse readily through the alveolar-capillary membrane, its high solubility in tissue, and the thin alveolar-capillary membrane are important for achieving optimal PaO_2. If the alveolar-capillary membrane is not normal, the gradient between the P_AO_2 and the PaO_2 will increase. The alveolar-arterial oxygen gradient (A-aDO_2) is normally 10 to 20 mm Hg and is increased when there is an obstacle to the diffusion of oxygen from the alveolus to the capillary lumen. As A-aDO_2 increases it indicates more serious dysfunction at the alveolar-capillary membrane. The A-aDO_2 gradient represents the sum total effect of many alveolar subunits throughout the lung and is therefore an average value. It is best determined by placing a patient on an FIO_2 of 1.0.

Ventilation-perfusion mismatching plays an important role in determining oxygenation. If a portion of the cardiac output is perfusing unventilated alveoli or bypassing the alveolar-capillary network altogether, this blood will remain unsaturated. This fraction is designated pulmonary shunt (Q_S/Q_T) and normally accounts for between 2 and 5 percent of the pulmonary blood flow. Cardiac output to the bronchial vessels makes up a significant portion of the physiologic shunt fraction. It should be noted that in the patient with high arterial oxygen saturation, increasing cardiac output or increasing the FIO_2 will generally result in no significant change in the shunt fraction. The shunted fraction of the cardiac output either bypasses the alveolar system completely, or else is perfusing unventilated alveoli and as such will remain unsaturated. Increases in cardiac output or FIO_2 will therefore not result in improvement of the saturation of this portion of the cardiac output. The overall effect is no net change in saturation in the left atrium. This is in contrast to other causes of hypoxemia and impaired saturation and can be used to distinguish between shunt and other causes of hypoxemia. The shunt fraction can be calculated as follows:

$$Q_S/Q_T = (C_cO_2 - C_aO_2)/(C_cO_2 - C_{mv}O_2)$$

where C_cO_2 is the oxygen content of pulmonary capillary blood, $C_{mv}O_2$ is the oxygen content of mixed venous blood, and C_aO_2 is the oxygen content of arterial blood. Oxygen saturation for the calculation of C_cO_2 is assumed to be that of fully saturated blood if the patient is receiving a high concentration of oxygen. In such cases it is most practical to assume that the blood in the pulmonary capillaries will be fully saturated, thus simplifying the determination of C_cO_2. Withdrawing a blood sample through the distal port of a pulmonary artery catheter with the balloon inflated provides an alternative way of measuring the saturation of pulmonary capillary blood. A shunt fraction of greater

Table 6-1. Pulmonary Variables

Abbreviation	Description	Derivation	Normal Value
PaO_2	Partial pressure of oxygen in arterial blood	Direct measurement	85–95 mm Hg (room air)
PAO_2	Partial pressure of oxygen in the alveolus	$[(P_B - P_{H_2O}) \times FIO_2] - PaCO_2/0.8$	98–100 mm Hg (room air), 630–670 mm Hg ($FIO_2 = 1.0$)
$PaCO_2$	Partial pressure of carbon dioxide in arterial blood	Direct measurement	35–45 mm Hg
$PACO_2$	Partial pressure of carbon dioxide in the alveolus	Direct measurement	40 mm Hg
$P_{mv}O_2$	Partial pressure of oxygen in mixed venous blood	Direct measurement	40–45 mm Hg
$P_{mv}CO_2$	Partial pressure of carbon dioxide in mixed venous blood	Direct measurement	45–50 mm Hg
A-aDO$_2$	Alveolar-arterial oxygen gradient	PAO_2-PaO_2	10–20 mm Hg (room air)
SaO_2	Oxygen saturation of arterial hemoglobin	Direct measurement	98% (room air)
$S_{mv}O_2$	Oxygen saturation of mixed venous hemoglobin	Direct measurement	75% (room air)
Q_s/Q_t	Shunt fraction	$\dfrac{C_cO_2 - C_aO_2}{C_cO_2 - C_{mv2}}$	5–8%
V_{min}	Minute ventilation	$V_T \times RR$	4–8 L/min
V_d	Dead space ventilation	$(PaCO_2 - PECO_2) \times V_T/PaCO_2$	
V_d/V_T	Efficiency rating	$(PaCO_2 - PECO_2)/PaCO_2$	
V_T	Tidal volume	Direct measurement	4–5 ml/kg
VC	Vital capacity	Direct measurement	65–75 ml/kg
FRC	Functional residual capacity	Direct measurement	2000–2500 ml
C_{dyn}	Dynamic compliance	Exp. $V_T/(PAP - PEEP)$	40–60-ml/cm H_2O
C_{stat}	Static compliance	Exp. $V_T/($plateau pressure $- PEEP)$	80–100 ml/cm H_2O

RR = respiratory rate; PECO$_2$ = partial pressure of expired CO$_2$; PAP = peak airway pressure; PEEP = positive end-expiratory pressure.

than 8 to 10 percent is considered abnormal.

The removal of carbon dioxide is dependent on adequate ventilation. Ventilation requires an unobstructed airway. Upper and lower airway abnormalities can substantially impair ventilation and thereby cause difficulty with both carbon dioxide removal and oxygenation. If anatomic airway obstruction is eliminated, the removal of carbon dioxide is dependent almost entirely on minute ventilation. Minute ventilation is the product of the patient's respiratory rate (RR) and tidal volume (V_T) and is normally 4 to 8 liters per minute. This includes dead space ventilation (V_d), approximately 150 ml at rest. The ratio of dead space ventilation to tidal volume is termed the efficiency rating (V_d/V_T) and quantitates the amount of air that does not take part in gas exchange.

The $PaCO_2$ plays an important role in regulating central respiratory drive. Carbon dioxide diffuses readily across the blood-brain barrier. An increase in the $PaCO_2$ will thus result in an increase in hydrogen ion concentration in cerebrospinal fluid (CSF). This increased acidity stimulates the respiratory centers, augmenting the activity of the muscles of respiration. Both the rate and the depth of respiration increase

with a subsequent rise in minute ventilation. Increasing minute ventilation increases the elimination of carbon dioxide, which tends to restore the $PaCO_2$ toward normal. The lowered $PaCO_2$ results in a return of CSF pH toward normal. The activity of the respiratory centers returns to its baseline level and minute ventilation will gradually normalize.

All exhaled carbon dioxide originates from the alveolus. Diffusion of carbon dioxide across the alveolar-capillary membrane is very rapid. Under basal conditions approximately 200 mls carbon dioxide is produced per minute as 250 mls oxygen is consumed per minute. The ratio of carbon dioxide production to oxygen consumption is defined as the respiratory quotient (RQ). It is dependent on the source and amount of calories consumed. When a standard diet is consumed, RQ is 0.8. In starvation or when the predominant fuel is fat, it falls to between 0.6 and 0.7. If lipogenesis is occurring, as is seen with overfeeding, with conversion of carbohydrate to fat, the RQ rises to between 1.0 and 1.2.

Carbon dioxide in blood exists either in the dissolved state, bound to hemoglobin in red cells, or in a state of equilibrium with bicarbonate. The majority of carbon dioxide transport in the blood occurs as bicarbonate and is governed by the reversible equation

$$HCO_3 \rightarrow + H^+ \rightarrow H_2CO_3 \rightarrow CO_2 + H_2O$$

As carbon dioxide is eliminated in the lung, the reaction is driven in the direction of carbon dioxide and water. In situations in which carbon dioxide elimination by the lung is impaired, the accumulation of carbon dioxide will drive the reaction back to the left, regenerating hydrogen ions and causing acidosis. The $PaCO_2$ reflects a balance between the production of carbon dioxide by the tissues and the elimination of carbon dioxide in the lung. Both factors must be considered in the interpretation of arterial blood gases (ABGs). In the majority of situations, the $PACO_2$ is equivalent to the $PaCO_2$. The equilibration of carbon dioxide in the pulmonary capillaries with carbon dioxide in the alveolus occurs almost instantaneously because of the high water solubility of carbon dioxide. Carbon dioxide elimination is therefore relatively unaffected by many of the conditions that impede oxygen transport from the alveolus to the blood.

Clinically relevant lung volumes and lung capacities are illustrated in Fig. 6-1. Tidal

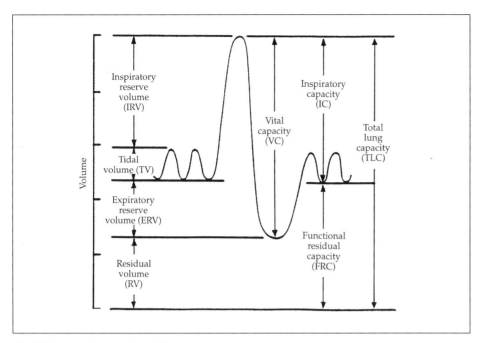

Fig. 6-1. Lung volumes and capacities.

volume (V_T) is defined as the volume of air exchanged by the lung during a normal inspiration following a normal expiration. Residual volume (RV) refers to the volume of air remaining in the lung after a maximal expiratory effort. The inspiratory reserve volume (IRV) is the difference between a maximal inspiratory effort and V_T. The expiratory reserve volume (ERV) represents the difference between a maximal expiratory effort and tidal volume. Total lung capacity (TLC) refers to the volume of air that is in the lung at the end of a maximal inspiratory effort. Vital capacity (VC) is the volume of air that results from a maximal inspiration following a maximal expiratory effort. The functional residual capacity (FRC) is the volume of air that remains in the lungs at the end of a normal tidal volume. Surgical procedures, anesthetics, and other commonly encountered clinical situations affect the FRC. Both prophylactic and therapeutic efforts are focused at maintaining or improving the FRC. Positive end-expiratory pressure (PEEP) increases FRC. Inspiratory capacity (IC) is the difference between TLC and FRC.

The degree to which the lung can be distended (its elasticity) can be quantitated by the measurement of compliance. Compliance is defined as the volume change that occurs with a unit pressure change:

Compliance
= change in volume/change in pressure

Total compliance includes compliance of both the chest wall and the lung. Compliance is divided into dynamic compliance and static compliance. Dynamic compliance is measured during air movement and in the ventilated patient is expressed as

Dynamic compliance
= expired tidal volume/(PAP − PEEP)

where PAP is peak airway pressure and PEEP is positive end-expiratory pressure. Dynamic compliance correlates with airway resistance. It is normally 40 to 60 ml/cm water. It is abnormally low in patients with mucous plugging and bronchospasm.

Static compliance is measured at the end of inspiration after air flow has ceased and the air within the lung has equilibrated. In the ventilated patient it is calculated as follows:

Static compliance = expired tidal volume/
(plateau pressure − PEEP)

Static compliance measures the elastic recoil of the lung and is normally 80 to 100 ml/cm water. It is useful in quantitating the degree of lung stiffness resulting from

conditions such as ARDS, cardiogenic pulmonary edema, tension pneumothorax, atelectasis, and pneumonia. Patients with severe ARDS have static compliance values of less than 20 ml/cm water. Patients with a static compliance of less than 50 ml/cm water have significant impairment of function that usually requires mechanical ventilation.

Respiratory Failure

Respiratory failure is a common reason for admission to a critical care unit. In the surgical patient, the need for mechanical ventilation is a frequent indication for critical care admission and many patients admitted to critical care units require mechanical ventilation at some time during their ICU stay. Advances in technology and clinical management have provided opportunities to support increasingly compromised patients with respiratory failure. An understanding of the pathophysiology of respiratory failure and the common clinical signs of respiratory dysfunction will enable surgeons to provide optimal care to patients with a variety of underlying conditions.

Diagnosis

The diagnosis of respiratory failure is generally made on the basis of clinical, laboratory, and radiologic observations. Respiratory failure is usually associated with a PaO_2 of less than 60 mm Hg and/or a $PaCO_2$ of greater than 50 mm Hg in a patient with previously normal ABGs. These somewhat arbitrary cutoffs are useful but relative. It is important to consider the impact of the fractional inspired oxygen concentration, the barometric pressure, the patient's age, underlying medical conditions, previous ABGs, and the time course preceding or surrounding the ABG determination. A variety of patients, especially those with chronic obstructive lung disease, may have a PaO_2 in the range of 50 to 60 mm Hg and a $PaCO_2$ of 50 mm Hg or greater without clinical evidence of respiratory distress. Although they may be considered to have a degree of respiratory failure, such patients clearly do not require acute interventions. Conversely, a patient who has a normal ABG but is expending more than 25 percent of his or her energy to do so, or a patient who progresses to acute deterioration of oxygenation and carbon dioxide elimination in association with respiratory distress, has acute progressive respiratory failure and requires acute interventions, including airway management and mechanical ventilation.

Classification

Respiratory failure can be classified, based on its duration, as either acute or chronic. Classifications based on the etiology of the respiratory failure have also been proposed. These include alveolar-capillary membrane dysfunction, hydrostatic pressure elevations, and mechanical/neurologic dysfunction. Of clinical relevance is a classification based on pathophysiology: hypoxemic versus hypoxemic/hypercapnic. In this classification, hypoxemia is common to both groups of patients, but the presence of hypercapnia distinguishes the two types: 1) Hypoxemia respiratory failure, also referred to as a type 1 or nonventilatory failure, is characterized by a PaO_2 of less than 60 mm Hg with a $PaCO_2$ of less than 40 mm Hg and a widened $A-aDO_2$ (alveolar-arterial/gradient), indicating the presence of substantial abnormalities of oxygen exchange at the alveolar-capillary membrane. 2) Hypoxic/hypercapnic respiratory failure, also known as type 2 or ventilatory failure, is characterized by a PaO_2 of less than 60 mm Hg with a $PaCO_2$ of greater than 50 mm Hg. Type 2 respiratory failure is generally more difficult to treat because of the added difficulty of maintaining an adequate minute ventilation.

Although the classification of respiratory failure into these subgroups has clinical utility, patients may change from one grouping to another as their disease progresses. In particular, patients with ARDS will generally have hypoxemic respiratory failure initially, with significant problems with oxygen exchange and little difficulty with carbon dioxide elimination. If their disease persists, they will gradually begin to have difficulties with carbon dioxide elimination and rising $PaCO_2$ levels in addition to the hypoxemia. In the patient with ARDS, this has unfavorable prognostic significance.

Perhaps the most clinically useful classification of respiratory failure requiring mechanical ventilation involves dividing patients into one of three major "etiologic" categories: 1) ARDS: patients with systemic inflammatory response syndrome (SIRS), sepsis, pneumonia, pancreatitis, pulmonary contusion, aspiration, and others; 2) hydrostatic pulmonary edema: patients with left heart failure or myocardial infarction; and 3) muscular and neurologic disorders: including patients with underlying disorders, severe malnutrition, postoperative pain, excessive sedation, or neuromuscular blockade.

In most patients in the surgical critical care setting at our institutions, severe respiratory failure is associated with ARDS. These patients have an underlying process that leads to respiratory failure (and other organ failure syndromes) that is manifest clinically as ARDS. Primary therapy is directed at the underlying disease process while the respiratory failure is managed supportively. In general, if the underlying disorder is either self-limited or responds to treatment promptly, the respiratory failure will ameliorate, and the patient can be successfully weaned from mechanical ventilation. Patients who continue to have evidence of ongoing systemic inflammation or infection and patients in whom the respiratory failure progresses from an acute hypoxemic form to a more chronic hypoxemic/hypercapnic form, have considerably poorer outcomes. Patients with preexisting medical conditions may also have their respiratory failure complicated by the development of hydrostatic pulmonary edema. In general, however, the use of invasive monitoring and judicious fluid management can limit the impact of hydrostatic factors. Patients with chronic obstructive lung disease and other chronic respiratory problems will also present challenges in management.

The Adult Respiratory Distress Syndrome

In 1967, Ashbaugh and colleagues described 12 patients with respiratory failure of varied etiologies characterized by dyspnea, tachypnea, hypoxemia, stiff lungs, and diffuse lung infiltrates on chest x-ray. This was subsequently termed the adult respiratory distress syndrome (ARDS). Numerous synonyms exist for ARDS, including shock lung, posttraumatic pulmonary insufficiency, Da Nang lung, wet lung, and progressive respiratory distress. ARDS currently affects an estimated 150,000 patients in the United States annually with a reported mortality of between 40 and 60 percent. High mortality has persisted for many years despite important advances in both the understanding and management of respiratory failure and ARDS.

The sepsis syndrome (also referred to as the systemic inflammatory response syndrome, SIRS) is the underlying process thought to be the cause of ARDS in approximately 80 percent of cases. Shock, pulmonary contusion, fat embolus syndrome, crush injury, inhalation of noxious substances (especially smoke inhalation), aspiration of gastric contents, pancreatitis, eclampsia, cardiopulmonary bypass, hemodialysis, and many other conditions have been associated with ARDS. The development of ARDS should prompt an aggressive search for a reversible etiology, especially a septic process.

The diagnosis of ARDS is generally made in the presence of the following:

1. A predisposing clinical condition that causes direct or indirect damage to the lung
2. Hypoxemia with a PaO_2 of less than 60 mm Hg with FIO_2 greater than 0.6; or a $PaO_2:FIO_2$ ratio of less than 250; and/or an A-a gradient of greater than 350
3. Respiratory distress with dyspnea and tachypnea
4. Diffuse bilateral pulmonary infiltrates
5. Stiff, heavy lungs (total static compliance <50 ml/cm water)
6. Noncardiogenic pulmonary edema (pulmonary capillary wedge pressure <20 mm Hg).

Several clinicopathologic phases have been identified in patients with ARDS. Initially, an exudative process lasting 2 to 3 days or longer develops. This phase is characterized by the development of marked fluid and protein leakage from the intravascular space through the damaged alveolar-capillary membrane into the pulmonary interstitium. The pulmonary lymphatics mobilize the fluid and protein from the interstitium initially but, as the volume of exudate increases, the pulmonary lymphatics are overwhelmed, and intra-alveolar edema ensues. During this phase, activated white cells, as well as inflammatory mediators, such as cytokines, prostaglandins, leukotrienes, vasoactive peptides, and platelet activating factor, are involved in the histopathologic response in the lung. Destruction of type I alveolar cells occurs and since these cells produce surfactant, surfactant production remains decreased within the affected alveoli in ARDS. The lung damage is not homogeneous and some areas of the lung will be relatively spared while others will undergo dramatic changes. This is reflected on the chest x-ray, as some areas of the lung appear to have significantly more congestion and intra-alveolar edema than others. If the process does not abate, ARDS enters the proliferative phase and the inflammatory response may subside. A cellular infiltrate appears with early organization of hyaline membranes within the lung. A small percentage of patients will go on to a chronic proliferative phase with progressive fibrosis of both the alveolar spaces and the small airways. These patients develop worsening compliance and increasingly larger dead space. Carbon dioxide elimination becomes a problem in these patients and a very large minute ventilation is required to prevent respiratory acidosis. In many patients entering the chronic proliferative stage, the initial inflammatory response has subsided and the inciting pathology may have been controlled. These patients, however, are at great risk for prolonged ventilator dependence and poor outcomes.

Treatment

Patients presenting with respiratory distress and a clinical history consistent with a diagnosis of ARDS are generally managed initially with supplemental oxygen. Attention should be directed at any underlying disorders that may be contributing to respiratory distress. It is especially important that in the older patient congestive heart failure or other causes of myocardial dysfunction be ruled out as a cause of worsening respiratory distress. In the setting of an inflammatory or septic process, and especially in the setting of shock, fluid resuscitation is ongoing and necessary. This may further complicate management of the respiratory dysfunction and invasive hemodynamic monitoring may be required to elucidate the nature of the underlying disorder. Once increased hydrostatic pressure from myocardial dysfunction has been ruled out as a cause of the respiratory distress, the patient should receive supportive measures as needed based on the underlying problem. In the absence of a clear infectious source, broad-spectrum antibiotic coverage is often initiated. Fluid resuscitation is required in most of these patients, especially those with resolving shock states or septic processes. Fluid resuscitation should be titrated to the usual end points of organ perfusion, including return of urine output, stabilization of vital signs, normal mental status, and resolution of acidosis. The use of crystalloids and blood products as needed is the standard approach. The use of colloids continues to be controversial and there are no definitive studies showing a major benefit from colloid infusion. Data exist suggesting that in the setting of ARDS, with injury at the alveolar-capillary membrane, protein leakage is pronounced and infusion of colloid will result in distribution of more proteinaceous substances into the interstitium, drawing water along with them. Similarly, the use of diuretics in a patient without *significant* elevation of the hydrostatic pressure (pulmonary capillary wedge pressure) is highly controversial. Once again, no definitive studies exist demonstrating a benefit to the use of diuretics in patients with established ARDS. It is clear, however, that diuresis with depletion of the intravascular compartment can worsen the patient's overall course, especially if the underlying etiology is sepsis, hemorrhage, or other hypovolemic problems.

Patients who do not respond to initial supportive measures, such as supplemental oxygen, fluid management, and treatment of the underlying disorder, will ultimately require mechanical ventilation. The currently available modes of mechanical ventilation require access to the airway via intubation and the application of positive-pressure breathing. These techniques are addressed in the subsequent portions of this text.

Management of the Patient with Respiratory Failure

The widespread use of mechanical ventilation can be traced to the poliomyelitis epidemics of the late 1940s and early 1950s. Anesthesiologists in Copenhagen began routinely intubating patients stricken with polio who appeared to be too weak to survive without ventilatory support. Due to the shortage of "iron lungs," the only means to ventilate patients at that time, these patients had to be intubated and ventilated manually. At the peak of the polio epidemic in 1952, the need for nurses and for manual ventilators (persons who could actually "bag" these patients) was so great that the Copenhagen medical school was closed and for that year 250 medical students were employed to "bag" the intubated patients. Ultimately, necessity gave rise to the invention of the Engstrom ventilator in Copenhagen that year, among the first positive-pressure ventilators. Routine intubation and positive-pressure mechanical ventilation, as well as other routine practices such as suctioning, were products of the response to the polio epidemics of the 1950s. Following the intervention of the first demand valve by Dr. Forrest Bird, also in 1952, mechanical ventilation became widely available in the United States. Since that time there have been many important advances in the field of mechanical ventilation, including the introduction of intermittent mandatory ventilation by Dr. Bird, the introduction and widespread use of PEEP, and the application of sophisticated technology, both in ventilators and in the monitoring devices used for patient care.

In the vast majority of patients who require mechanical ventilation, the initial step will be the establishment of an airway via tracheal intubation. This will allow the application of positive-pressure breathing. In most cases, sedation and occasionally neuromuscular blockade will also be required. We do not routinely advocate the use of neuromuscular blockers and prefer to use sedation with narcotics (primarily morphine) and benzodiazepines or sedative hypnotics (such as lorazepam or diazepam [Valium]). The management of the airway and the adjunctive use of sedation and paralysis are discussed below with a review of the various methods of mechanical ventilation.

Airway Management

Management of the airway consists of securing access to the airway by either intubation or surgical intervention in order to protect the air passages and deliver positive-pressure ventilation. Airway management in the emergency and intensive care settings can be lifesaving and professionals proficient in these skills should be available in settings of acute care.

Intubation may be needed for airway control, to increase oxygenation and to increase minute ventilation. "Airway control" is a very common indication for intubation and may be needed to relieve an obstructed airway, for control of secretions, or to prevent aspiration in a patient without an adequate cough or gag reflex. Oxygenation can be increased by maintaining adequate airway pressure using positive-pressure ventilation and PEEP in addition to delivering increased fractional inspired oxygen concentrations. Fractional inspired oxygen concentrations greater than 0.6 are very difficult to administer reliably without intubation in adults. Intubation allows delivery of adequate minute ventilation to those patients who can no longer exchange enough air to eliminate the carbon dioxide produced, either because of increased production, neuromuscular dysfunction (including excessive sedation), weakness, malnutrition, or other causes.

Although there are few absolute indications for intubation, progressive respiratory distress is generally accepted as a clinical trigger for securing the airway and instituting mechanical ventilation. Intubation should be strongly considered when any of the following conditions exist, especially in the presence of respiratory distress:

1. PaO_2 less than 50 mm Hg and/or $PaCO_2$ greater than 50 mm Hg
2. Respiratory rate greater than 30 per minute
3. Tidal volume less than 8 to 10 cc/kg
4. The patient is comatose, has a head injury, requires chemical paralysis, or has severe tracheal secretions.

Elective Intubation

Intubation is accomplished by either the orotracheal or the nasotracheal routes. Orotracheal intubation is generally preferred for most elective intubations. Elaboration on the technique required for orotracheal intubation is beyond the scope of this chapter; an outline is provided in Tables 6-2 and 6-3. Endotracheal tubes and suction catheters are selected based on the patient's age and size (Table 6-4). In general, most men require a size No. 8 French endotracheal tube and most women need a No. 7.5 Fr endotracheal tube for orotracheal intubation. A child's small finger approximates the size of the endotracheal tube needed for orotracheal intubation. Nasotracheal intubation can usually be accomplished with tubes that are one-half size smaller.

In an awake patient without injury or abnormalities of the nose or face, nasotracheal intubation can be employed. The patient's nose should be anesthetized with a topical spray such as Cetacaine. A vasoconstrictor, such as phenylephrine, can be used as well. Both the nares and the end of the tube should be liberally coated with viscous lidocaine. With the patient's head in a neutral position or perhaps slightly hyperextended, the tube is inserted in the nares and rotated as the tube is advanced gently toward the vocal cords. The tube should be advanced until the end is just above the cords as judged by breath sounds. On the next inspiration, the tube should be advanced through the cords. The patient will usually cough when placement is successful. If there is resistance, the tube should not be advanced, since it is probably lodged on the piriform sinus. In an unsuccessful placement of the endotracheal tube, there is an obvious lack of breath sounds and minimal chest excursions. If end-tidal carbon dioxide is monitored, it will be very low in case of improper placement (usually esophageal intubation).

Emergency Airway Management

In most cases the quickest and safest way to control the airways is to perform orotracheal intubation. In seriously compromised patients, no medications are required because hypoxia or shock, or both, has rendered the patient resistance free. However, a patient who appears moribund will occasionally awaken when a laryngoscope is inserted. These patients will require rapid-sequence induction during which drugs are administered sequentially without interposed ventilation and with application of cricoid pressure. This procedure is intended to accomplish rapid airway access for ventilation and oxygenation to protect vital organs, decrease the risk of aspiration, and facilitate rapid intubation in a compromised patient.

There is no role for nasotracheal intubation in the emergency setting. Although nasotracheal intubation has been touted for use in patients with possible cervical spine injuries, orotracheal intubation is generally associated with less disruption of cervical

Table 6-2. Technique for Orotracheal Intubation

Place patient on 100% oxygen
Assemble drugs and equipment
Clean and suction mouth
Place patient in proper position
Check endotracheal tube size and cuff
Insert stylet and lubricate tip of tube
Administer drugs (see Table 6-3)
Displace tongue
Lift jaw and tongue away at 45-degree angle to visualize cords
Use free hand to guide tube through cords
Remove stylet
Inflate cuff
Listen for breath sounds
Secure tube
Connect patient to ventilator
Mnemonic for intubations: **SOAP ME**
Suction
Oxygen
Airway equipment
Pharmacology (have drugs ready)
Monitoring
Equipment

Table 6-3. Suggested Pharmacologic Agents for Intubation

Oxygen
Thiopental (Pentothal), 1.5 mg/kg in an adult
or
Methohexital (Brevital), 1 mg/kg
Midazolam (Versed), 10 mg total in adult
Succinylcholine: 1.5 mg/kg in adult
                2 mg/kg in child <10 yr old
                3 mg/kg in newborn

Table 6-4. Choice of Endotracheal Tube According to Patient Size

Age	Endotracheal Tube (mm)[a]	Suction Tube Size (Fr)[b]
Premature	2.5	6
Newborn	3.0	6
6 mo	3.5	8
18 mo	4.0	8
3 yr	4.5	8
5 yr	5.0	10
6 yr	5.5	10
8 yr	6.0	10
12 yr	6.5	10
16 yr (small adult)	7.0	14
Most women	7.5	14
Most men	8.0	14
Large adult	9.0 or larger	16

[a]Size measured in internal diameter.
[b]Size in French No. R: 3.14 times outside diameter.

spine alignment while providing oxygen to the patient more rapidly. When an emergency airway is required and intubation cannot be obtained, then surgical access must be obtained.

Emergency Cricothyroidotomy

Emergency cricothyroidotomy is intended to provide emergency access to the airway in patients in whom intubation is either technically impossible or unsafe. A needle technique has been described in addition to the traditional surgical procedure.

A needle cricothyroidotomy involves placement of a large-bore 12- or 14-gauge needle into the cricothyroid membrane. If an angiocath is used, the catheter is advanced into the airway and the needle is withdrawn. A "Y" connector is then attached to the needle or catheter along with high-pressure tubing connected to a high-flow oxygen source. When a thumb is placed over the open end of the "Y" connector, oxygen flows into the tracheobronchial tree. Carbon dioxide is allowed to escape every 4 or 5 seconds by removing the occluding thumb. This technique is meant to provide oxygen therapy emergently for a short time (maximum about 20 minutes) until a more definitive airway can be secured.

The surgical technique begins with palpation and identification of the cricothyroid membrane between the lower border of the thyroid cartilage and the upper border of the cricoid cartilage. A local anesthetic such as 1% lidocaine is infiltrated into the skin. A horizontal (or sometimes vertical) incision is made in the overlying skin. A No. 11 blade is inserted into the cricothyroid membrane and the opening in the membrane is extended horizontally. The back of the knife handle or a hemostat is used to open the airway so that a No. 4 or 6 Shiley tracheostomy or an endotracheal tube can be inserted.

Elective Tracheostomy

The indications for tracheostomy are diverse and controversial. The authors have experienced complications from both tracheostomies and prolonged intubation. Generally, we recommend early tracheostomy (during the first 10–14 days) for patients who are expected to require prolonged intubation and mechanical ventilation. Tracheostomy can be performed at the bedside provided adequate lighting (such as a head lamp) and indi-

viduals experienced both in tracheostomy and in intubation (should this be required) are available. A folded towel placed horizontally under the patient's upper back will allow gentle hyperextension of the neck to improve exposure. After adequate anesthesia is established, a skin incision is made horizontally two fingerbreadths above the sternal notch overlying the second tracheal ring. Through the skin incision, a vertical dissection is made directly down to the trachea between the strap muscles. Often, the paired anterior jugular veins appear in the way and can be ligated if necessary. The trachea is exposed using the electrocautery device and the Kitner dissector ("peanut"). The thyroid can be retracted, but we frequently divide the isthmus between clamps to improve exposure. We use the electrocautery to aid in hemostasis. It is of paramount importance to stay midline as the dissection continues to avoid injuring the recurrent laryngeal nerve. We open the trachea with a knife using a distally based trap-door incision after scoring it with an electrocautery device. Two "stay" sutures are placed in the lateral aspects of the tracheal incision to provide access in case of tube dislodgment. A tracheal hook is then used to retract the proximal tracheal ring. The endotracheal tube cuff is then deflated and the tube withdrawn slowly under direct vision to just above the tracheal incision. A tracheostomy tube (cuffed Shiley No. 6 or 8) is advanced into the trachea and its cuff inflated. The patient is then ventilated through the tracheostomy and if no problems are apparent, the endotracheal tube is withdrawn. A chest radiograph is obtained to verify tube position and the status of the lung.

Percutaneous Tracheostomy

There are now several reports describing successful series of percutaneous tracheostomies. One reported advantage of this technique is the ability to avoid transport out of the ICU by performing the procedure at the bedside. We feel that percutaneous tracheostomy is most safely performed using bronchoscopic guidance to assure successful placement in the trachea. We advocate the routine use of bronchoscopy and have demonstrated a cost savings compared to open tracheostomy performed in the operating room with an anesthesiologist in attendance. Percutaneous tracheostomy should only be performed by surgeons skilled in the tech-

niques of surgical airway access. A variety of complications including death have been reported with percutaneous tracheostomies and the procedure should never be used for emergency airway access. The role of percutaneous tracheostomy has not yet been fully determined and we continue to encourage caution in its application.

Mechanical Ventilation

The iron lung used in the 1950s for patients with poliomyelitis in whom chest wall strength was inadequate for ventilation is an example of a negative-pressure ventilator. The iron lung was used primarily to increase ventilation and could not materially increase oxygenation. Most patients with respiratory failure require increases in oxygenation and modern ventilators are capable of providing both increased oxygenation and ventilation for a variety of indications (Table 6-5). Modern ventilators are generally positive-pressure ventilators and reduce the inspiratory work of breathing by inflating the lungs directly, delivering a volume-limited or a pressure-limited breath. Once a patient has an airway in place and the decision to use positive-pressure ventilator support is made, there are a variety of ventilators and modes from which to choose. The various modes and their relative advantages and disad-

Table 6-5. Indications for Mechanical Ventilation

I. Neuromuscular diseases
   A. Polio
   B. Guillain-Barré syndrome
   C. Succinylcholinesterase deficiency
   D. Spinal chord injury/paralysis
   E. Other neuromuscular disorders

II. Inadequate oxygenation
   A. Adult respiratory distress syndrome (ARDS)
      1. Pneumonia
   B. Sepsis
   C. Pulmonary contusion
   D. Pulmonary embolus
   E. Severe atelectasis with or without associated pneumonia

III. Inability to adequately ventilate and oxygenate
   A. Asthma
   B. Acute bronchospasm
   C. Chronic obstructive pulmonary disease with increased oxygen demand or increased requirement for CO_2 removal
   D. Increased oxygen demand and/or CO_2 production

---

vantages are listed in Table 6-6. The pressure, volume, and flow curves for various modes are illustrated in Fig. 6-2.

We initiate mechanical ventilation in the majority of patients using synchronized intermittent mandatory ventilation (SIMV). We begin with the following settings:

FIO_2 of 1.0

Tidal volume of 8 to 10 ml/kg and an SIMV rate of 10 to 12 to achieve a minute ventilation of 6 to 8 liters per minute

PEEP of 5 cm water

Accept the default settings for I:E ratio (usually 1:2 or 1:3)

Accept the default settings for inspiratory flow rate (approximately 600 ml/sec)

The settings for a 70-kg patient would then be: FIO_2 of 1.0, tidal volume of 700 ml, IMV rate of 10 breaths per minute, PEEP of 5 cm water, and I:E ratio of 1:2 to 1:3. We choose an FIO_2 of 1.0 to assure optimal ox-ygen saturation initially. We then wean as quickly as possible to an FIO_2 of 0.6 or less, maintaining an arterial oxygen saturation of 90 percent or greater. Older recommendations for tidal volumes in the range of 10 to 15 ml/kg were probably excessive and we generally attempt to deliver volumes of 8 to 10 ml/kg that are associated with peak pressures of less than 40 cm water. If the patient is not breathing spontaneously, the ventilator will deliver the set number of breaths. If the patient is breathing spontaneously ("overbreathing the ventilator"), the ventilator allows the spontaneous breaths and synchronizes the delivery of the machine breaths whenever possible to avoid "stacking." Stacking occurs when the machine breath is delivered to a patient who is in the process of taking a spontaneous breath, resulting in potentially deleterious overdistension of the lung. A critical pressure value slightly greater than the peak inspiratory pressure is selected to allow the breath to be released in the event of an excessive pressure rise. Modern ventilators also include

alarms for circuit disconnection from the patient and inability to deliver volumes, and other features to ensure patient safety. The SIMV mode is well suited to many surgical patients who require partial support in the sense that they are capable of taking some breaths but require significant assistance from the ventilator to attain their minute ventilation and oxygenation needs at an acceptable work of breathing (Table 6-7). As patients become stronger or more awake or their lung pathology ameliorates, the number of SIMV breaths delivered is decreased (in increments of 2–4) and ABGs are monitored. We convert patients to a continuous positive airway pressure (CPAP) mode once they reach an SIMV rate of four breaths per minute with an FIO_2 requirements of 0.5 or less. If they tolerate a CPAP level of 5 cm water, they are considered for extubation. Prolonged intervals on a low CPAP level or on a "T-piece" are generally avoided since the patient will often tire excessively from the resistance generated by the endotracheal tube and ventilatory circuit. A standard-

Table 6-6. Mechanical Ventilators

Ventilatory Mode	Full Support		Intermittent Support: Intermittent Mandatory Ventilation (IMV, SIMV)	Assisted Breathing	
	Continuous Mandatory Ventilation (CMV)	Pressure Control (PC)		Assist Control (A/C)	Pressure Support Ventilation (PSV)
Respiratory cycle determinants	Machine initiated	Machine initiated	Patient allowed spontaneous breaths and at regular preset intervals the ventilator delivers a preset volume[a]	Patient initiates breaths and receives preset volume (assist); otherwise ventilator delivers preset breaths (control)	Patient initiated; as inspiratory flow rate slows to 25% of peak flow rate, ventilator allows exhalation
	Volume limited	Pressure limited; time cycled	Volume limited; time cycled	Volume limited	Pressure limited, flow cycled
Patient comfort	Extremely uncomfortable (patient must be sedated +/− paralyzed)	Extremely uncomfortable (patient must be sedated +/− paralyzed)	Variable	Variable	Most comfortable as patient initiates breath, determines its duration and time of exhalation
Advantages	Ideal when full support required for compliant lungs	Lower peak pressures; possibly less risk of barotrauma	Useful for back-up ventilation during weaning; lower airway pressures with spontaneous breaths	Requires patient initiation of respiration otherwise no different from full support modes	Useful for weaning because of variable work load
Disadvantages	May result in barotrauma; lowers cardiac output	May result in inadequate gas exchange, e.g., mucous plugs will lower V_T[b]	Awake patients may "buck" ventilator	Easy to overventilate; barotrauma from high peak pressures	Inadequate V_T; mucous plugging[b]

V_T = tidal volume.

[a]In the synchronized IMV version, the ventilator will time the present machine breaths to occur when the patient initiates a breath. If a patient does not initiate a breath, the machine will deliver the present volume at preset intervals. Any breaths taken between the machine-initiated or assisted breaths will receive no inspiratory support.

[b]Mucous plugging results in inadequte support because the machine shuts off early when pressure limit is reached early from blocked airways.

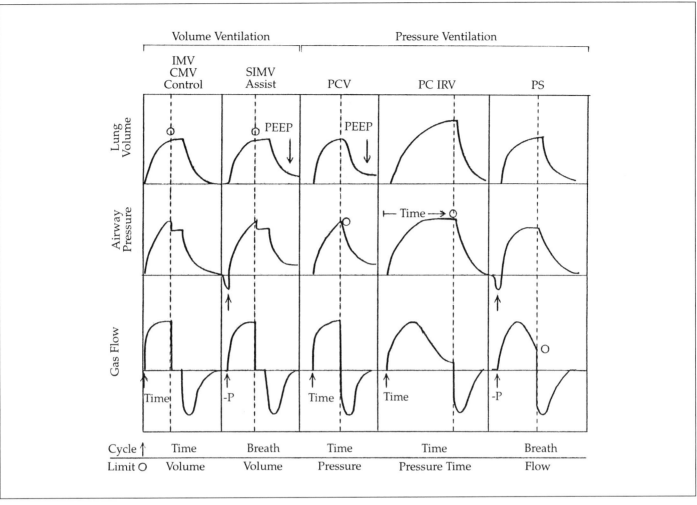

Fig. 6-2. Lung volume, airway pressure, gas flow, and inspiration-expiration (I:E) ratio during commonly used modes of mechanical ventilation. The event that starts the gas flow is in the cycle (↑), and the event that stops the gas flow is the limiting factor (O). The cessation of the gas flow is shown by the dotted lines separating inspiration from expiration. Time and negative pressure (−P) may be responsible for cycling or limiting gas flow, as indicated. PEEP is shown in two modes of ventilation as examples of the effect of that maneuver in elevating the baseline pressure tracing. IMV = intermittent mandatory ventilation; CMV = continuous mandatory ventilation; PCV = pressure control ventilation; PS = pressure support; SIMV = synchronized intermittent mandatory ventilation. (From RH Bartlett. Use of the mechanical ventilator. In DW Wilmore, LY Cheung, AH Harken, et al [eds]. Scientific American Surgery. Section II, Subsection 5. © 1995 Scientific American, Inc. All rights reserved.)

ized protocol for weaning a patient in stable condition without further acute lung pathology is presented in Table 6-8. Extubation criteria are presented in Table 6-9.

In most of our patients, we add pressure support ventilation (PSV) to patients on IMV. This is intended to assist spontaneous breaths and facilitate weaning. The use of PSV results in larger V_T and less work of breathing. This is accomplished by providing airflow in response to a pa-tient's negative inspiratory effort. The airflow is delivered to attain the preselected positive-pressure level, thus enhancing the patient effort. The ventilator monitors the patient's inspiratory flow rate and once it falls to 25 percent of the peak flow rate, the expiratory valve opens allowing passive exhalation. We titrate the level of pressure support to a V_T of 5 to 7 ml/kg (350–500 ml) and a normal respiratory rate (up to 30 breaths/minute). We wean patients on IMV and PSV as described previously and once the IMV is weaned, we begin weaning the PSV in increments of 2 to 5 until we reach a PSV level of 5 cm water.

Patients who have hypoxemia refractory to standard mechanical ventilation are treated with increasing levels of PEEP. Unfortunately, PEEP results in decreased cardiac output (by decreasing venous return to the heart) and can contribute to barotrauma. It is difficult to quantitate the barotrauma resulting from the use of PEEP

Table 6-7. Guidelines for Pulmonary Support in the Surgical Critical Care Unit

GOALS

Therapy should be directed toward specific physiologic end points in the context of overall patient care.

VENTILATION

Ventilation should be supported to assure that breathing pattern is comfortable, spontaneous ventilatory rate is generally less than 30, and $PaCO_2$ is generally between 35–50 and the resulting pH is 7.35–7.45. Ventilatory alkalosis/alkalemia should be avoided (except when intended to reduce cerebral blood flow or for permissive hypercapnia).

OXYGENATION

Oxygenation should be supported with supplemental oxygen and PEEP/CPAP to assure that arterial saturation (SaO_2) is greater than 0.90 by ABG (or > 0.92 by pulse oximetry) on an FIO_2 ≤ 0.50. A PaO_2 of 60–65 mm Hg is generally acceptable on a nontoxic (≤0.50) oxygen concentration. A saturation of 100% is not necessary and may be undesirable. ABGs are not needed after changes in FIO_2 when pulse oximetry is used.

GENERAL GUIDELINES

1. Lower FIO_2 to <0.6 to keep SaO_2 ≥ 92%.
2. Wean IMV to 2–4 breaths per minute.
3. Add PSV when needed for rate, comfort, tidal volume or $PaCO_2$.
4. Achieve comfortable spontaneous breathing on nontoxic FIO_2.
5. Avoid the use of 100% oxygen for more than a short time except in an arrest situation or for pretreatment for suctioning, airway procedures, transportation, etc.
6. Avoid PEEP/CPAP <5 cm H_2O.
7. Most patients need some inspiratory support while breathing through an endotracheal tube. Do not use prolonged (>1–2 hr) CPAP trials without IMV or PSV.
8. When patient is extubated avoid use of face tent except for specific indications (i.e., facial trauma). The delivered oxygen from these systems varies tremendously and causes unnecessary ordering of ABGs. Use a face mask at 40% O_2 (or less) and add a double flow system if adequate gas flow rates are not achieved during inspiration.

in critically ill patients since PEEP is often applied to patients who also have high peak inspiratory pressures and high mean airway pressures, both of which are more directly associated with barotrauma than PEEP. The level of PEEP is increased to allow the FIO_2 to be weaned to below 0.60 or until the cardiac output falls. The use of a pulmonary artery catheter can facilitate the monitoring of cardiac function especially the ventricular preload. As the PEEP is increased to 15 cm water or more, infusion of crystalloid to maintain adequate cardiac filling pressures is often necessary. Our primary goal in this setting is to ensure adequate tissue oxygen delivery and we routinely accept an arterial oxygen saturation of 90 percent (or a PaO_2 of 60 mm Hg). There is little advantage to PaO_2 much higher than 60 to 70 mm Hg in terms of tissue oxygen delivery, while the additional ventilator interventions to achieve an elevated PaO_2 will likely result in additional lung injury. We are less concerned with the $PaCO_2$ level as long as any increase is gradual. This is referred to as permissive hypercapnia. We do not aggressively treat the $PaCO_2$, even at the 50- to 60-mm Hg range, as long as the pH is in

the range of 7.30. Even lower pH levels and higher $PaCO_2$ levels have been shown to be acceptable as long as they are attained slowly. The kidneys compensate over several days by retaining bicarbonate and partially correcting the pH. If there is an acute drop in pH due to an acute change in $PaCO_2$, we adjust the ventilator by increasing the respiratory rate. Increasing the rate rather than the volume (or pressure setting in a pressure ventilator) probably results in less barotrauma.

The use of other modes of mechanical ventilation is dependent on the preferences and expertise of the physician. There are no randomized, controlled studies demonstrating the superiority of one mode over others for critically ill surgical patients. We have employed inverse ratio pressure-controlled ventilation (IR-PCV) for patients with severe respiratory failure and poorly compliant lungs who have been refractory to standard management with high FIO_2 and PEEP. In patients with an FIO_2 of 1.0 and high PEEP levels (15–20 cm H_2O or more) IR-PCV offers an alternative to higher levels of PEEP. By using PCV the peak pressure is limited to the

setting chosen on the ventilator. The mean airway pressure is likely to be the same or higher. By limiting the pressure delivered by the ventilator under PCV, the volume delivered to a very stiff lung will be small unless the inspiratory (I) time is extended with a resulting decrease in expiratory (E) time. We therefore employ inverse (I:E) ratios in the majority of patients who require PCV. The I:E ratio is usually set as 2:1 or 1:1, depending on the severity of hypoxemia. Although the ventilator limits the peak inspiratory pressure to the pressure setting used for PCV, the increase in mean airway pressure encountered with IR-PCV probably results in similar rates of barotrauma overall. It is important to note that employing IR-PVC results in significant shortening of the time available for exhalation. Since IR-PCV uses a prolonged I time, the E time will necessarily be shortened. Since PEEP has a similar effect on shortening of the E time, the combination of IR-PCV and high levels of PEEP can result in significant air trapping due to the very shortened E times. The possibility of barotrauma will then be increased. We therefore decrease the level of PEEP in order to prolong the expiratory interval.

Using IR-PCV we have been able to decrease the FIO_2 requirement in the majority of patients with severe respiratory failure for whom we have employed this technique. We therefore view IR-PCV as an alternative to standard therapy with SIMV and high PEEP that allows us to wean the FIO_2. It is likely that the associated barotrauma using IR-PCV is not significantly different from that encountered with standard ventilation and high levels of PEEP. To convert a patient on SIMV with high PEEP to IR-PCV:

Place the patient on FIO_2 of 1.0

Select a pressure setting to deliver the same volume as obtained with SIMV

Decrease the PEEP by 30 to 50 percent

Set the I:E ratio at either 1:1 or 2:1

Select the same rate as employed with SIMV

Monitor the patient's hemodynamic status and obtain ABG determination within 20 to 30 minutes of starting IR-PVC

Whereas volume modes such as SIMV are relatively easy to adjust by monitoring ABGs, ventilator changes with IR-PCV of-

Table 6-8. Standard Weaning Protocol

GOAL
To remove patient from ventilatory support for possible extubation

CANDIDATE GROUP
Routine postop patients with no complications, no shock, no sepsis, no gross compromise of lung function
Stable patients with no major ongoing illness that compromises level of consciousness, hemodynamics, or pulmonary function
Patients should be on ≤5 cm H_2O PEEP

PROTOCOL
Weaning from pulmonary support can be goal directed so that ventilation, oxygenation, and airway support can be weaned with relative independence.

Ventilation
Wean IMV 2–4 q1–2h to SaO_2 > 92% and RR < 30 (at IMV = 4, decrease IMV to 0)
Wean pressure support (PS) to 5 cm H_2O by 5 to maintain SaO_2 > 92%, RR < 30

Ventilation is weaned to achieve a comfortable breathing pattern at a spontaneous rate of < 30. Adequacy of ventilation is also assessed by measurement of ABGs. Generally, a $PaCO_2$ within 5–10 mm Hg of the patient's baseline value or a $PaCO_2$ of 35–50 with a pH of 7.30–7.45 is acceptable. IMV is the most commonly used method of ventilatory weaning, but pressure support ventilation (PSV) can be used in conjunction with or as an alternative to IMV.

Oxygenation
Wean FIO_2 by 10% q0.5–1h to FIO_2 of 40% keeping SaO_2 > 92%

Wean PEEP by 2–3 cm H_2O q4–6h to keep SaO_2 > 92% (generally not more than 10–12 cm H_2O q24 h)
FIO_2 should be reduced to 0.50 (always 0.60 or less) as quickly as tolerated. If the patient is on reverse I:E ratio ventilation and chemically paralyzed, an early priority is to normalize the reversed I:E ratio to at least 1:1 and then discontinue neuromuscular blockage. PEEP/CPAP should be weaned when the patient's overall condition has stabilized and he/she has been at his/her physiologic end point for a minimum of 12–24 h.

Arterial blood gases
Check ABGs at the start and completion of the weaning process
Obtain ABG prn SaO_2 < 90%, RR > 40 or < 6

Sedation orders
Hold all narcotics except MSO_4 0.5 mg/kg IV q2h prn pain
Hold all benzodiazepenes (Lorazepam, Valium, midazolam, Librium, etc.)

Call orders
Call physician for:
Acute hypotension   SBP < 90
Acute sustained hypoxia SaO_2 < 85%
Hypo- or hypercapnia, $PaCO_2$ < 25 or >50
HR < 60 or > 120
RR > 40 (not responsive to prescribed medications) or < 6
Acute rise in airway pressures
Increasing ventilatory requirements beyond starting values

Table 6-9. Extubation Criteria

After 1 hr on minimal ventilatory support (such as PEEP of 5 cm H_2O and PSV of 5 H_2O), check that the following apply:

1. Patient hemodynamically stable and breathing comfortably
2. Glasgow Coma Scale 14 or greater or patient is cooperative and responds to commands
3. Respiratory rate 10–25/min
4. Minimal ventilatory support settings
5. Pressure support ventilation (PSV) 5–8 cm H_2O or less
6. PEEP 5 cm H_2O or less
7. IMV 4 breaths per minute or less
8. Negative inspiratory force (NIF) better than −25 cm H_2O
9. Tidal volume > 5 cc/kg
10. Vital capacity > 10 cc/kg
11. Minute ventilation 6–8 liters per minute
12. Absence of excessive secretions requiring suctioning more often than q4 h

Before extubation, determine the reason for which the patient was intubated and any problems related to the intubation.

ten result in unpredictable ABG values. Oxygenation tends to be related to the mean airway pressure generated, the FIO_2 utilized, and the PEEP applied. The use of higher ratios such as 2:1 or 3:1 will often allow improved oxygenation but may result in decreased carbon dioxide elimination since the expiration interval is shortened, resulting in a smaller volume of effective gas exchange. Similarly, increasing the ventilator rate using IR-PCV results in shortened exhalation intervals with decreased effective gas exchange per breath and the possibility of higher $PaCO_2$ levels. This is in contrast to a volume mode such as SIMV in which an increase in the rate predictably results in a decrease of the $PaCO_2$ level. We therefore recommend that IR-PCV be used as a salvage mode of therapy in critical care units with the medical, nursing, and respiratory care resources necessary for this complicated ventilatory mode.

Sedation and Neuromuscular Blockage

Patients on mechanical ventilation generally require analgesics and sedatives. Our current preference is to use intravenous (IV) morphine as the analgesic and a moderately long-acting benzodiazepine such as lorazepam as a sedative. In the majority of patients who require narcotic analgesics for prolonged periods of time, we employ an IV morphine drip beginning at 2 to 5 mg per hour and gradually increase the dose until adequate analgesia is attained. We combine this with intermittent bolus dosing of lorazepam at 2 to 5 mg IV every 4 to 6 hours. This provides sedation and amnesia and potentiates the effect of the narcotic. Various agents available for analgesia and sedation are listed in Tables 6-10 through 6-12.

Using adequate doses of narcotics and benzodiazepines, we believe it is possible to ensure the comfort and safety of the vast majority of patients on mechanical ventilation. We do not believe that the use of neuromuscular blockade should be routine since there are no convincing data that they provide additional benefits to patients on mechanical ventilators over and above what is provided by adequate sedation. Neuromuscular blocking agents are indicated in some patients who are extremely difficult to control with narcotics and sedatives, including patients who require the use of uncomfortable modes of ventilation such as IR-PCV. Neuromuscular blocking agents may also be useful for the patient who is extremely agitated or uncooperative and in whom temporary paralysis will provide a therapeutic benefit in addition to ensuring the patient's safety and the safety of the caretakers. Use of neuromuscular blocking agents is associated with serious potential side effects, such as paralysis without adequate sedation, prolonged paralysis, and muscle weakness (especially in patients receiving corticosteroids or those with renal dysfunction) and the danger of apnea in case of accidental disconnection from the ventilator. We recommend the routine use of a twitch monitor to assess the depth of paralysis. Using the train-of-four technique, we administer neuromuscular blocking agents and allow the patient to maintain at least one or two twitches in response to the four sequential stimuli.

Table 6-10. Selected Narcotics Used in Mechanically Ventilated Patients

Drug	Dosage	Onset (min)	Duration of Action (hr)	Cardiovascular Effects	Respiratory Effects	Hospital Cost Comparison (Based on Relative Potency of 2 mg Morphine)	Comments
Morphine	2–10 mg IV q1–2h	3–5	2–3	Minimal depression in supine patient; infrequently associated with histamine release	Depression	$0.01	Orthostasis due to bradycardia, histamine release, decreased sympathetic tone, direct vascular effect
Meperidine (Demerol)	25–50 mg IV q2–4h	2–4 20–40	2–4	Depression	Potent depression	$0.02	Anticholinergic effects; mydriasis, dry mouth, tachycardia
Fentanyl	1–3 μg/kg IV	1	0.5	Minimal depression	Potent depression	$0.04	Quick onset, short duration

Table 6-11. Selected Sedatives Used in Mechanically Ventilated Patients

Drug	Dosage	Onset (min)	Half-life (hr)	Cardiovascular Effects	Respiratory Effects	Hospital Cost	Comments
Lorazepam	1–2 mg IV q10–15 min until sedated then 1–2 mg IV q2–6h	2–10	10–20	Minimal	Minimal	$9.23 per 2-mg vial (generic now available at less cost)	No active metabolites, moderate half-life
Midazolam	2–5 mg IV q1–2h; can be used as IV drip	1–5	1–12	Minimal depression	Depression	$59.43 for 50-mg vial	Expensive, short half-life but active metabolites prolong clinical effects
Diazepam	2.5–5 mg IV q5–15 min until sedated, then 2.5–10 mg IV q4–6h	1–5	24–50	Minimal depression	Depression	$0.34 for 10-mg vial	Long half-life and active metabolites; difficult to use IV drip (precipitate in fluid)
Haloperidol	2–5 mg IV q20–30 min until sedated	5–10	14	Minimal	Minimal	$0.49 for 5-mg vial	Inadequate sedation, neuroleptic malignant syndrome, and other CNS effects; monitor potassium and magnesium levels
Propofol	0.3 mg/kg/hr initially, increase up to 1–3 mg/kg/hr until sedated	1–2	24–48	Myocardial depression	Depression	$24.73 for 500-mg vial	Effective when patient resistant to other drugs; IV anesthetic; delivered in lipid vehicle

Patient Assessment

Regardless of the type of ventilator mode selected by the surgeon, an important aspect of ventilator management is assessing the patient as a whole. The clinician should observe the patient before checking the ventilator settings and laboratory values and determine whether the patient is agitated or comfortable on mechanical ventilation. When a patient is fighting or breathing asynchronously with the ventilator, clinicians sometimes inappropriately prescribe more sedation and more neuromuscular blocking agents. A more appropriate solution may be altering the ventilator or correcting some other aspect of the ventilator-patient relationship. Standard monitoring techniques for patients are outlined in Table 6-13.

A patient who is "fighting the ventilator" should be considered in respiratory distress until proven otherwise. Patients who are awake and cognizant but fighting the ventilator may benefit from reassurance and additional contact with their caregivers, including explanations regarding their illness and the ventilator. A variety of ventilator problems may contribute to patient distress. The FIO_2 should be checked as well as the adequacy of gas flow to match the patient's demands. A malfunctioning demand valve or a kink in the ventilator tubing or endotracheal tube should be considered. The patient should be disconnected from the ventilator and "bagged" with 100 percent oxygen. If immediate improvement occurs, then the ventilator may be the problem. A mucous plug in the airway can be treated by "bagging" and suctioning. A sudden change in respiratory status that does not resolve with these maneuvers should be evaluated and treated using the following suggested stepwise approach:

1. Observe the patient and assess for air hunger, particularly nasal flaring, acces-

Table 6-12. Selected Neuromuscular Blocking Agents Used in Mechanically Ventilated Patients

Drug	Dose	Elimination	Approximate Daily Charge for Equipotency* ($)	Advantages	Disadvantages
Pancuronium	Loading: 0.04–0.1 mg/kg IV Intermittent dosing: 0.1–0.2 mg/kg IV every 1–3 hr Continuous drip: 0.06–0.1 mg/kg/hr	Predominantly renal, 20% metabolized	18	Inexpensive May increase cardiac output	Tachycardia Slow onset
Vecuronium	Loading: 0.08–0.1 mg/kg IV Intermittent dosing: 0.1–0.2 mg/kg IV every 1–3 hr Continuous drip: 0.05–0.1 mg/kg/hr	80% hepatic metabolism and biliary excretion	225	Little or no hemodynamic effects Rapid onset	Expensive Most number of reported cases of prolonged weakness
Atracurium	Loading: 0.04–0.1 mg/kg IV Intermittent dosing: not recommended Continuous drip: 0.06–0.1 mg/kg/hr	Hoffman degradation (inactivated in plasma by spontaneous degradation and by the action of nonspecific blood esterases)	454	Hoffman degeneration No metabolites; drug of choice for patients with significant renal and hepatic dysfunction	Slow onset Very expensive

*Approximate daily charge from our institution, includes dispensing charge. Charges may vary by institution.

Table 6-13. Monitoring of Mechanically Ventilated Patients

Monitor/Laboratory Tests	Advantages	Disadvantages	Suggested Use
Pulse oximetry	Instantaneous readout of patient's current hemoglobin saturation with oxygen Noninvasive Reusable	Inaccurate with hypothermia, excess movement, or hypoperfusion (shock state) present	Routine use in ICU is advocated
ABG	Gives PCO_2 level, thus degree of ventilation, in addition to PO_2 and O_2 sats; pH reading reveals shock via degree of acidosis	Expense Often adds no information to pulse oximetry	Selectively Routine daily ABGs *not required* even if on mechanical ventilation
End-tidal CO_2	Helps in conjunction with emergency airway assessment, e.g., endotracheal tube is in place, *not* in esophagus Valuable as alarm in case of ventilator disconnection in paralyzed patient	Adds little in stable, routine patient Expense	Patients on NMB During intubation of trachea, during tracheostomy, while attempting a difficult wean.
Chest x-ray	Adds anatomic evidence to suspected diagnosis of pulmonary edema, ARDS, pneumothorax, pleural effusion, cardiomegaly, or pericardial effusion	Expense Radiation effect Adds only anatomic information, which lags behind physiologic changes Often does not influence what can already be determined by clinical exam	Selectively Daily use not necessary even in intubated patient
Pulmonary artery catheter	Effect of PEEP and positive-pressure ventilation on cardiac output can be determined Can use SvO_2 to monitor oxygen delivery, and relative effects of SaO_2 and PEEP on cardiac output and delivery can be assessed	Invasive Infectious complications Easily overused or left in too long No prospective studies have shown improved outcome in ventilated patients with use of pulmonary artery catheter	Rapid increase required for PEEP Hemodynamic instability Fluid balance in question, whether due to renal failure or other cause Any combination of above

NMBs = Neuromuscular blocking agents; SvO_2 = mixed venous oxygen saturation.

sory muscle use, or paradoxical breathing.

2. Obtain an ABG determination. Pending the results, assess monitored values. If oxygen saturation is less than 90 percent, increase FIO_2 to 1.0.

3. Treat hemodynamic instability as needed to ensure adequate tissue oxygen delivery.

4. Listen for breath sounds. If unilateral and time permits, obtain a portable chest radiograph to assess for pneumothorax. If unilateral and the patient's condition is very unstable, decompress the affected side of the chest with a needle or chest tube.

5. If the patient is hemodynamically stable, has acceptable oxygen saturation (and other ABG values as available), does not have a pneumothorax or mucous plugging, and continues to fight the ventilator, administer incremental doses of narcotics and benzodiazepines as needed. The ventilator settings may need to be adjusted as the patient's spontaneous respiratory effort decreases. Obtain a repeat ABG determination.

If a patient is on volume support mode, he or she may need to be switched to a pressure support mode. Also, the flow rate may be too slow. If a patient is on a T tube, the flow rate may need to be as high as 60 liters per minute to provide a rate sufficient to overcome resistance of the endotracheal tube and circuit. Often all that is required is for the therapist to ensure that the flow is sufficiently high so as to always exceed the negative inspiratory demand of the patient. A patient fighting the ventilator should be given more sedation only after the mode and flow rate have been adjusted appropriately and communication with the patient (if possible) is attempted.

Weaning and Extubation

The process of discontinuing ventilator support is commonly referred to as weaning. There is no consensus regarding the ideal method for weaning; however, it is generally believed that once a patient is recovering from the acute pathologic process that required mechanical ventilation (i.e., the patient's condition is no longer deteriorating), weaning should begin (see Table 6-8). If the patient is being slowly weaned, it is usually advisable to increase the patient's work of breathing gradually. It is important not to overdo this increase of work, because the work of breathing in

a patient who is struggling with ventilation can be as much as 50 percent of the total body energy expenditure. In a patient with marginal oxygen delivery, this can be tremendous. In a normal individual who is not on mechanical ventilation, the expenditure is only 2 to 3 percent. As a rule, the work of breathing should not increase more than 5 to 10 percent above baseline with each adjustment to the ventilator. If their work of breathing is not excessive and they are not tachypneic or in distress, then weaning is continued.

Although we do not commonly use them, many physicians advocate T-tube breathing trials. Physicians who routinely use T-tube trials suggest starting with 5-minute trials and eventually advancing to 15- to 30-minute trials as often as every 3 to 4 hours. If T-tube weaning is to be done, the flow rate should be high enough to meet the patient's needs. The suggested flow rate to maintain adequate flow is a value twice the patient's spontaneous minute ventilation.

Although we prefer pressure support weaning after the IMV has been weaned to 4 breaths per minute or less, there is no evidence to suggest that one maintenance or weaning method is superior to another. We believe, however, that it is counterproductive to make ventilator changes too quickly in a patient who has been chronically ventilated. Unlike the athlete who merely stops to rest after overexercising his or her muscles, a patient in whom diaphragmatic fatigue develops cannot rest without going on full ventilator support. A patient should be allowed to rest for several hours between drastic ventilator setting changes. We can be considerably more aggressive in "weaning" intubated patients who do not have underlying lung disease (see Table 6-8). We can be far more flexible in the patient who has recently been intubated. Every situation is different and patients should be evaluated individually.

Once a patient is weaned from mechanical ventilation, he or she is considered for extubation. We employ clinical judgment as the primary method for selecting patients for extubation since there is no single test or group of tests that reliably predicts which patient will be successfully extubated and which patient will fail extubation. We review traditional extubation parameters (see Table 6-9) and incorporate them into the decision-making process.

We believe that a patient's mental status and ability to respond to commands are vital to successful extubation and regard frequent suctioning for severe pulmonary secretions as a relative contraindication to extubation, especially in older and more debilitated patients.

Complications

Complications related to ventilators can be divided into the problems associated with intubation (Table 6-14), those related to the prolonged presence of the endotracheal tube (Table 6-15), and those associated with positive-pressure mechanical ventilation (Table 6-16).

Intubation is a critical time for any patient. Whether performed electively or in an emergency situation, it can result in a life-threatening event within seconds. Among the most serious complications associated with intubation is hypoxia from either poor technique, delay in securing the airway, or improper placement (e.g., esophageal intubation). Esophageal intubation is most easily recognized using capnography, a process to monitor the carbon dioxide return. The absence of carbon dioxide return or the absence of breath sounds is a sign that esophageal intubation has occurred and should prompt the removal of the tube and oxygenation by mask until reintubation can be done. It is our contention that the most skilled person available should perform emergency intubation.

Bleeding, usually from a laceration, can be caused by direct trauma from intubation. Blood in the mouth generally requires only suctioning and is usually self-limited. Since the priority is to provide oxygen to that patient, bleeding can be controlled after the airway has been secured.

Pharyngeal tears can occur from traumatic intubation but are rare. These generally require conservative management only. Esophageal tears can also occur, are usually very proximal, and will require surgical intervention if they are full thickness. Esophagoscopy, barium swallow, or both may be indicated to confirm an esophageal tear.

Aspiration is another dangerous complication associated with intubation. This complication may not be directly attributable to the technique of intubation but is often encountered with an obtunded pa-

Table 6-14. Complications of Mechanical Ventilation: Intubation

Complication	Diagnosis	Cause	Treatment
Hypoxia	Patient examination (cyanosis) Pulse oximeter <88% O_2 hemoglobin saturation	Traumatic intubation 1. Lack of preoxygenation 2. Esophageal intubation 3. Aspiration	Replace tube if incorrectyl placed; otherwise, if examination and chest x-ray confirms correct placement, simply provide adequate oxygenation
Bleeding	Blood present from mouth	Direct trauma in intubation	Leave endotracheal tube in place Check coagulation profile Suction as needed
Pharyngeal tear	Direct observation May be delayed	Trauma from intubation	Usually self-limited
Esophageal tear	Often delayed; if transmural and not recognized will result in signs of infection Endoscopy/swallow	Trauma from intubation	May require surgical intervention, drainage, and repair
Aspiration	Bronchoscopy, chest x-ray Pneumonia Underreported	Stomach not decompressed Not using Sellich (Sellick) maneuver* Drug sequence not effective Sometimes not preventable; occurs before intubation or simply cannot always be prevented	Immediate bronchoscopy and lavage Consider antibiotics if patient has already been in hospital >24 hr and/or Gram's stain shows dominant organism

*Compression of thyroid cartilage which effectively closes esophagus by pinching it between thyroid cartilage and cervical spine.

Table 6-15. Complications of Mechanical Ventilation: Indwelling Endotracheal Tube

Complication	Diagnosis	Cause	Treatment
Pneumonia	Examination—decreased breath sounds, rales Secretions/sputum Fever, CBC, sepsis Chest x-ray Bronchial alveolar lavage	Prolonged intubation Balloon cuff inflation not completed, allows entry into lungs, blocks effective coughing Suction trauma	Removal of endotracheal tube and off mechanical ventilation ASAP Antibiotics when bacteria identified Mobilize patient Suctioning and pulmonary toilet Avoid acid suppression in stomach
Subglottis stenosis	Usually not manifest until removal of tube	Endotracheal tube balloon cuff pressure too high Tracheostomy placed too high, at or above first tracheal ring Effects of excessive scarring Part of disease process especially with burns, inhalation injury	Reconstructive and/or laser surgery Prevention is best treatment
Tracheoinnominate fistula	Bright red blood from endotracheal tube	Erosion of trachea into innominate artery, cuff pressure too high	Surgery
Tracheoesophageal fistula	Inadequate oxygenation, excessive burping sounds, stomach distended with gas	Cuff pressure too high	Surgery, nasogastric decompression

tient who aspirates gastric contents soon after becoming unconscious or who has been ventilated emergently by mask without gastric decompression. The classic example is a head-injured patient. We recommend bronchoscopy if severe aspiration evidenced by severe hypoxemia occurs. The best treatment for aspiration is prevention. We recommend gastric decompression before intubation with an oral or nasogastric tube, if at all possible. The Sellick maneuver (firmly compressing the esophagus against the vertebral col-umn by cricoid pressure) is very effective in preventing aspiration during emergency intubation.

The most common complications of prolonged intubation and ventilation is pneumonia. Pneumonia is directy related to the duration of intubation. Patients who are treated with therapy to decrease gastric acidity (e.g., antacids or H_2 blockers) may have stomachs colonized with gram-negative bacteria. Regurgitant stomach contents travel up into the pharynx and back down to the vocal chords, which are held open by the endotracheal tube. Bacteria-laden mucus settles around the balloon and bacteria and mucus travel past the balloon and into the trachea and the pulmonary tree. Radiographic and radionuclide studies have shown that this process occurs almost daily in all intubated patients. The best treatment, besides good suction and vigorous pulmonary care, is to avoid overalkalinization of the stomach and to remove the endotracheal tube as soon as possible.

Table 6-16. Complications of Mechanical Ventilation: Positive-Pressure Mechanical Ventilation

Complication	Diagnosis	Cause	Treatment
Pneumothorax	Clinical unilateral breath sounds Respiratory distress Hypoxia Chest x-ray	Barotrauma from positive-pressure ventilation Rupture of alveolae through visceral pleura into pleural space Penetrating trauma, e.g., needle insertion directly into lung for central venous pressure line	Tube thoracostomy If on positive-pressure ventilation, peak inspiratory pressure can be lowered
Tension pneumothorax	Same as pneumothorax plus hemodynamic instability (acute)	Barotrauma, direct trauma Same as above with ball-valve effect	Immediate decompression with knife or needle (14 gauge) followed by tube thoracostomy Rx underlying cause
Subcutaneous emphysema	Crepitus on palpation of skin	Barotrauma	No specific Rx, follow carefully Rx underlying cause
Bronchopleural fistula	Continuous leak noted from chest tube, possible hypoxia	Same as above	Surgery if volume loss or hypoxia significant (discrepancy of >100 cc between inspired and exhaled volumes)
ARDS	Hypoxia Clinical respiratory distress Increased A-a gradient	Barotrauma or effect of high pressure on alveoli, bronchi, and trachea	Reduce pressure if at all possible
Low cardiac output Hypoperfusion	Signs of hypoperfusion (decreased urine output) Decreased SvO_2 if Swan-Ganz Shock	Lowering of venous return ? possible alteration of pump function of heart by alteration of ventricular walls	Decrease PEEP
Atelectasis, with or without hypoxemia	Respiratory distress Mucous plug Chest x-ray	Inadequate volume Uneven distribution of gas flow, e.g., endotracheal tube down right main stem bronchus clots, aspiration material	Reposition tube if required Pulmonary toilet Consider increasing mean airway pressure or PEEP Bronchodilators
Oxygen toxicity	Worsening hypoxemia or ARDS (no specific way to assess damage)	$FIO_2 > 0.60$ Free oxygen radicals	Decrease FIO_2 Increase PEEP

Many of the serious complications related to positive-pressure mechanical ventilation are the result of barotrauma and volutrauma. The most common such complication is pneumothorax. Barotrauma is excess pressure that damages alveolar lining cells and can cause rupture of the alveoli. If the alveoli rupture through the visceral pleura into the pleural space, a pneumothorax results. If the rupture extends along the subvisceral plane, the dissection will continue to the mediastinum and into the subcutaneous tissue, resulting in subcutaneous emphysema without a pneumothorax. We recommend that a chest tube be placed in a patient receiving positive-pressure ventilation who has a pneumothorax or subcutaneous emphysema. We do remove chest tubes in mechanically ventilated patients who no longer leak and have completely expanded lungs (clinically and by chest x-ray). Generally, chest tubes should be removed only when no demonstrable leak has occurred for at least 2 days and the lungs are expanded. All nonfunctioning chest tubes should be removed within 24 hours.

Tension pneumothorax may present as shock, absence of breath sounds, and jugular venous distention. Tension pneumothorax may mimic cardiac tamponade since the heart sounds are frequently diminished in both conditions. We recommend immediate decompression, preferably with a knife or a hemostat. A 14-gauge catheter inserted into the anterior chest wall can also be effective temporarily. Tube thoractostomy should be performed as quickly as possible after acute decompression. We recommend large-bore argyle tubes for this problem and avoid the use of collapsible tubes, such as red rubber catheters, or easily clogged tubes, such as central venous pressure (CVP) catheters.

Bronchopleural fistulas may result from barotrauma. If there is a large discrepancy between inhaled and exhaled volumes and there is difficulty maintaining adequate ventilation and oxygenation, surgical intervention may be warranted. In children, a noninvasive alternative to surgery is a bronchoscopic fibrin glue injection. After confirming cessation of the air leak by balloon occlusion of the subtended segment, the fibrin blue is inserted through the bronchoscope into the segment. Tetracycline sclerosis of the segments may also stop the leak and avoid thoracotomy.

Unusual Causes of Refractory Hypoxia

We have focused predominantly on parenchymal lung problems as the source of the hypoxia but decreased compliance can also come from extraneous sources. A typical example would be a patient who has a circumferential burn of the chest and mistakenly thought to have severe inhalation injury but in reality simply needs an expeditious truncal escharotomy.

Compromise of oxygenation and ventilation may occur as a result of abdominal compartment syndrome. Abdominal compartment syndrome typically is seen following significant intra-abdominal surgery after a catastrophe such as a ruptured abdominal aneurysm or massive trauma. The subsequent build-up of intra-abdominal pressure pushes the diaphragm upward, compromising pulmonary function and raising peak airway pressures. The intra-abdominal pressure can be measured through an indwelling bladder catheter. If other measures fail, decompression of the abdominal cavity by releasing the contents through a midline abdominal incision may allow adequate ventilation and oxygenation. A clear, sterile plastic bag or moistened gauze can be placed over the abdominal contents thus affording some protection.

Summary

Respiratory failure continues to be a significant problem in surgical critical care units. A large percentage of critically ill and severely injured patients will develop ARDS as part of the multiple organ failure syndrome. The care of these patients requires an understanding of the normal physiology of the lung and cardiovascular systems as well as a knowledge of the available technologies for supporting the patient who is unable to maintain adequate ventilation and oxygenation. Despite the seemingly endless array of mechanical ventilators and related devices, the fundamental concepts for support of the large majority of patients with respiratory dysfunction are within the grasp of the practicing surgeon. Patients with the most severe forms of respiratory failure will benefit from the presence on the surgical team of an expert in advanced ventilatory support. In the surgical critical care setting, pulmonary dysfunction is almost always the result of another underlying process. Mechanical ventilation in the surgical patient with respiratory failure will remain a supportive therapy and our attention should continue to be directed at treating the underlying disorder. The overriding principles are constant: to protect the airway, to prevent hypoxemia and ensure tissue oxygen delivery, and to protect the patient comfort and safety.

Suggested Reading

Ashbaugh DG, Bigelow DB, Petty TL, et al. Acute respiratory distress in adults. *Lancet* 2:319, 1967.

Bartlett RH. Use of the Mechanical Ventilator. In DW Wilmore, MF Brennan, AH Harken, et al (eds), *Care of the Surgical Patient*. Vol 1. Critical Care. New York: Scientific American, 1993. Pp 1–20.

Esteban A, Frutos F, Tobin M, et al. A comparison of four methods of weaning from mechanical ventilation. *N Engl J Med* 332:346, 1995.

Fakhry SM, Rutledge R. Monitoring. In JA Moylan (ed), *Surgical Critical Care*. St. Louis: Mosby-Year Book, 1994. Pp 73–100.

Marcy TW, Marini JJ. Inverse ratio ventilation in ARDS. *Chest* 100:494, 1991.

Sheldon GF, Messick WJ. Biology of Respiration and Ventilator Support. In JE Fischer (ed), *Surgical Basic Science. Editor: Josef E. Fischer*. St. Louis, Mosby-Year Book, 1993. Pp 205–223.

EDITOR'S COMMENT

This is a very good, common sense approach to ventilatory problems in patients. To be sure, each critical care unit and each critical care staff person develops his or her own techniques and truisms. There are a few here to which I would like to call attention because, although I am not a critical care specialist, I have treated enough sick patients to have observed some things in critical care that this chapter directly addresses and, that in my view, are quite correct.

Fighting the ventilator, as the authors correctly point out, is immediately taken as a sign of a disoriented patient who is out of touch. The authors' advice of assuming that the patient is, or feels, hypoxic is quite sound. Instead of sedating, paralyzing, or otherwise trying to overcome a strong-armed patient, a cooperative approach in trying to allay his or her fears, ascertaining what the problem is, and adjusting the ventilator to a comfort level is good advice well taken.

There is insufficient attention, in my view, to airway resistance in the management of patients on ventilators. All too often, one sees a very large patient with an inappropriately small orotracheal airway having difficulty in either ventilating or being weaned from the ventilator. Likewise, a trial of spontaneous ventilation with an orotracheal tube subjects the patient to fighting increased airway resistance when subjected to T-piece ventilation for a prolonged period of time. Here, I could not agree with the authors' advice more: Limit the amount of time that patients spend on T-piece ventilation, as they are likely to tire with an increased airway resistance and thus not be weaned when they could otherwise be easily weaned.

Every surgical resident and every surgeon should have the capacity to accurately intubate a patient. This is one of the techniques that surgical residents and all surgeons should have. There is nothing more terror-invoking in a surgeon than losing an airway. Some of the most sweat-provoking situations that I encounter are in patients who require intubation when something goes wrong with the airway so as to require tracheostomy. At the same time, it is important, but very difficult to remember, that one can take that extra second or two to clearly visualize what one is doing before intubating the patient. Emergency intubation is not the type of situation at which the third- or fourth-year student should have three of four passes before an expert establishes the airway. Under these circumstances, the most expert person in the room should wield the laryngoscope and the endotracheal tube. There is little room for error. The dangers of pharyngeal or other major laceration of the oropharyngeal structures, thus aspirating a good deal of blood, are stressed in the text.

Finally, the hypothetical construct concerning the adult respiratory stress syndrome and its etiology based on overwhelming of the pulmonary lymphatics is but one point of view. It is disappointing that, even with the prevalence of various cytokine antibodies, no form of therapy that utilizes anticytokine antibodies has thus far been effective. Perhaps the disease is too well established at the time that treatment is initiated to make any difference, but it certainly is strange that, despite all of the expensive biologic therapies available, no effect has been seen on the major killer of adult surgical patients, with a current mortality between 40 and 60 percent.

J.E.F.

7

Hemorrhagic Complications and Their Prevention: Blood Components and Their Use in Therapy

Anthony J. Comerota   Augustine R. Eze

Blood transfusion and blood component therapy are integral parts of current medical practice; however, the history is quite diverse and reflects the development and evolution of medical thought through the ages. The first documented blood transfusion occurred in the mid-seventeenth century and followed Harvey's description of the anatomy and physiology of the circulatory system. In 1818, James Blundell, a London obstetrician, revived interest in blood transfusion, but its general therapeutic use did not come for another 100 years. One of the pioneers in the United States was William Steward Halstead, who in 1881 transfused his sister with his own blood for treatment of postpartum hemorrhage. As he later stated, "This was taking a great risk, but she was so nearly moribund that I ventured it with prompt results."

The principal stumbling blocks that thwarted early progress were problems in immunologic compatibility, unavailability of anticoagulants, the lack of safe and aseptic techniques, and lack of practical methods of transfusion. Great strides in blood procurement and preservation have been made since the establishment of blood banks in 1937, just before World War II. However, with the increasing use of blood products, complications were observed including anaphylactic and hemolytic transfusion reactions, bleeding (typically disseminated intravascular coagulation), transmission of blood-borne diseases, and immunosuppression.

Components of Normal Hemostasis

Although a detailed account of normal hemostasis is well beyond the scope of this discussion, an overview that allows an appreciation of the potential pathophysiologic mechanisms that lead to disordered coagulation is worthwhile.

Hemostasis is the process by which blood is maintained in the fluid state under physiologic conditions but allows controlled clot formation to stop blood loss caused by blood vessel injury. Hemostasis involves four interconnected mechanisms: 1) vascular contraction; 2) formation of a hemostatic plug; 3) blood coagulation and fibrin formation; and 4) endogenous fibrinolysis.

When blood vessels are injured, the normal endothelial barrier is disrupted and blood is exposed to subendothelial substances that initiate coagulation. Blood vessel contraction occurs accompanying injury and is important in the early control of bleeding, especially when medium and small vessels are involved.

Upon exposure of subendothelial collagen, platelets bind von Willebrand factor (vWF), which stimulates adhesion, and subsequent binding of fibrinogen, which stimulates platelet aggregation. Protein cofactors such as factor V are secreted by platelets and assemble with other plasma factors on the platelet surface, leading to the formation of factor Va and the produc-

tion of thrombin. Through a positive feedback mechanism that converts factors V and VIII to activated cofactors, thrombin production is multiplied. Fibrin clot forms after thrombin cleaves fibrinogen, liberating fibrin monomers, which then undergo spontaneous polymerization. Subsequent fibrin cross-linking by factor XIIIa increases the stability of the clot, rendering it more resistant to fibrinolysis.

The coagulation process is modulated by antithrombotic compounds produced by endothelial cells, such as prostaglandin I_2, nitric oxide, thrombomodulin, and heparin. Other important regulators, which can be considered natural anticoagulants, include antithrombin III, C-1 inhibitor, alpha$_1$-antitrypsin, and activated proteins C and S.

Endothelial cells also produce plasminogen activators that convert plasminogen to plasmin, thereby stimulating fibrinolysis. This process serves to reduce clot burden and remodel thrombus. However, lysis is regulated by plasminogen activator inhibitors and antiplasmins. Therefore, clot formation and lysis are parts of the orderly formation of collagen and fibrous tissue and subsequent wound healing.

Types of Hemorrhagic Complications

The most important aspect of the management of bleeding complications is prevention of their occurrence. Central to this aim is an accurate personal and family history followed by a careful physical examination. Bleeding disorders can result from either a congenital or an acquired defect.

Congenital Bleeding Disorders

A deficiency state of each of the clotting factors has been described in the literature. However, disorders commonly encountered in the surgical patient will be discussed in this chapter.

Hemophilia A (Classic) and B (Christmas Disease)

Hemophilia A (classic) and B (Christmas disease) are two clinically indistinguishable disease entities that result from molecular defects in the genes that code for factors VIII and IX. Hemophilia A is caused by the absence or reduced activity of factor VIII, and hemophilia B is caused by the deficiency or reduced levels of factor IX. Both disorders are inherited as sex-linked recessive traits and hence are manifested in phenotypic males. Factor VIII deficiency accounts for 80 percent of instances of hemophilia. Patients with factor levels of less than 1 percent of normal are classified as having severe hemophilia. Patients with levels of 1 to 5 percent are considered moderate hemophiliacs, and patients with 5 to 50 percent levels are classified as mild hemophiliacs. Severe hemophiliacs have a lifelong bleeding disorder manifested by frequent spontaneous hemorrhages into joints, muscles, and soft tissues. Mild hemophiliacs may avoid spontaneous bleeding completely, and thereby escape diagnosis until late adulthood. The moderate hemophiliacs present with less frequent spontaneous hemorrhages, but are likely to bleed during surgical procedures. Unnecessary surgical procedures in hemophiliacs should be avoided, but required operations can be safely performed even in patients with less than 1 percent factor level, provided adequate preoperative treatment is initiated.

Treatment of Hemophilia A. The principal mode of treatment of hemophilia is replacement of the deficient factors with either factor concentrates or plasma fractions that contain sufficient factor levels. Factor VIII should be replaced to 80 to 100 percent (40–50 units/kg) of normal before major operations and maintained at 40 to 50 percent (20 units/kg every 8–12 h bolus) until wound healing is well advanced (7–21 days). Patients having minor operations, spontaneous muscle bleeds, or hemarthroses need replacement to about half the level required for patients having a major surgical procedure. The half-life of factor VIII is 8 to 12 hours. One unit of factor VIII activity is equivalent to the amount present in 1 ml of normal plasma.

Other therapeutic options available for factor replacement in hemophilia A are 1) DDAVP (1-desamino-8-D-arginine vasopressin), 2) cryoprecipitate, and 3) fresh frozen plasma (FFP). The infusion of DDAVP 0.3 μg per kg over 20 minutes causes release of factor VIII into the circulation resulting in two- to threefold increase in circulating factor VIII. A second infusion of DDAVP can be given the following day, but the response to this and subsequent infusions may be attenuated. Cryoprecipitate is obtained when blood plasma is frozen and thawed. The proteins that do not immediately redissolve include factor VIII (carried on vWF) and fibrinogen, which form a significant proportion of cryoprecipitate. For a 70-kg patient, complete correction of factor VIII activity level to 100 percent requires cryoprecipitate from 35 units of blood. This factor VIII is usually obtained from pools of plasma from numerous donors and is commercially processed to yield a stable lyophilized powder. The risk of transmission of blood-borne disease is therefore multiplied manyfold by the use of concentrates because of the large number of donors in the pool. In addition, inhibitors of factor VIII, characterized as antibodies of the gamma-G variety, appear in the serum of patients after multiple transfusions. FFP may be used. However, large volumes are required to achieve sufficient factor level, thereby limiting its use for only minor bleeds.

Treatment of Hemophilia B. The current treatment of factor IX deficiency is by replacement with factor IX concentrates. Christmas disease, like classic hemophilia, can exist in mild, moderate, or severe forms. The half-life of factor IX is about 24 hours, and replacement requires slightly lower plasma levels than classic hemophilia. Factor IX concentrates contain a thrombogenic material that may cause life-threatening thrombosis or consumptive coagulopathy if infused into a patient with liver disease or if administered by slow continuous infusion. Therefore factor IX should be given by bolus intravenous injection. Patients with cirrhosis should receive FFP to achieve adequate factor levels and avoid the use of concentrates. The thrombogenic effect of the concentrate can be reduced but not completely eliminated by mixing it with heparin. Approximately 10 percent of patients receiving factor IX develop antibodies, and in these patients it is advisable to avoid subsequent infusion whenever possible. If factor IX is required in these patients, its combination with cyclophosphamide might be effective.

von Willebrand Disease

von Willebrand disease is as common as classic hemophilia and is characterized by reduction in the level of factor VIII (procoagulant) activity. It is inherited as an autosomal dominant trait and patients characteristically have a prolonged bleeding time. Unlike classic hemophilia, in which factor VIII activity remains constant, the von Willebrand patient has variable levels of circulating factor VIII. The common form of the disease (type 1) gives rise to a rather mild but variable bleeding diathesis after a surgical procedure or trauma. Laboratory testing reveals a level of factor VIII–related antigen (factor VIII:Ag) that is disproportionately lower than that of factor VIII, and ristocetin fails to cause platelet aggregation in approximately 70 percent of patients. However, spontaneous joint or deep muscle bleeds do not occur. The etiology is partial lack of the multimeric protein (vWF) that mediates adherence of platelets to the edges of damaged blood vessels (disorders platelet adhesion).

Treatment of the disease in patients undergoing surgical procedures is by replacement with cryoprecipitate. High, purity concentrates of factor VIII lack the required VIIIR:wF (vWF). Replacement should begin a day prior to the surgical procedure, and aspirin should be avoided for 10 to 12 days before the day of operation. The dose of cryoprecipitate is 5 ml per kg (~50 units of factor VIII activity/kg). In patients with milder forms who are undergoing a minor operation, DDAVP may be used as previously described. This treatment increases factor levels two- to threefold and shortens the bleeding time.

Other Coagulation Disorders

As mentioned earlier, congenital defects have been described for each of the known clotting factors. In comparison to hemophilia and von Willebrand disease, these deficiencies are rare and may cause the patient little or no problem. Patients with afibrinogenemia may bleed, and treatment is by the use of cryoprecipitate or FFP. However, patients with only functional defects of fibrinogen that impair clotting may paradoxically have severe thrombotic tendency. Deficiency of factor XII leads to a marked prolongation of the partial thromboplastin time (PTT), but a bleeding diathesis is rare. The bleeding in patients with low levels of factors XI, X, VII, V, and II (prothrombin) does not correlate well with the factor level and is generally mild. Treatment of the various deficiencies can be achieved with the administration of FFP if bleeding problems occur during surgical procedures.

Congenital Platelet Disorders

The most common cause of bleeding in the surgical patient is related to either a qualitative or quantitative platelet disorder. This disorder may be congenital or acquired, but the latter is more frequently encountered. We have described von Willebrand disease, which is an inherited qualitative platelet disorder. Other congenital abnormalities are Glanzmann's thrombasthenia, Bernard–Soulier syndrome, and the storage pool defects.

Glanzmann's Thrombasthenia

Glanzmann's thrombasthenia is caused by an abnormality of platelet membrane glycoprotein (GP) IIb–IIIa. Although a rare disorder, the study of patients with this abnormality has contributed a great deal to our understanding of the normal events of primary hemostasis. The hallmark of Glanzmann's thrombasthenia is deficient platelet aggregation. Patients have a lifelong bleeding tendency because of a prolonged bleeding time, but a normal prothrombin time (PT) and PTT. It is inherited as an autosomal recessive trait, and symptoms occur only in patients who are homozygous for the gene. Epistaxis is the most common cause of severe bleeding in these patients and often is typically more severe in childhood. Spontaneous unprovoked bleeding is uncommon in Glanzmann's thrombasthenia, but purpura,

gingival hemorrhage, epistaxis, and menorrhagia are nearly constant features. Pregnancy and delivery represent particularly severe hemorrhagic risks. The most important aspects of management are to anticipate the risk and prevent bleeding with judicious use of platelet transfusion. Although DDAVP has been tried in some patients it is not generally effective. Severe hemorrhagic complications can occur, but the prognosis is excellent with careful supportive care.

Bernard–Soulier Syndrome

Bernard–Soulier syndrome results from the deficiency of the platelet membrane GPIb-IX complexes with a morphologically large spherical platelet. This defect causes abnormalities of platelet adhesion. The syndrome's clinical presentation and inheritance pattern are similar to those of Glanzmann's thrombasthenia. Again, treatment is largely by local control of hemostasis and judicious use of platelet transfusion.

Storage Pool Deficiency

As mentioned in the section on the formation of the platelet plug, complex interactions between platelets and the exposed subendothelial substances lead to the release of various granules and effector substances with the eventual formation of a platelet plug. A group of inherited disorders in which there are defective granules has been collectively referred to as storage pool deficiency (SPD). These disorders may be associated with other syndromes such as albinism or absent radii. Patients commonly present with mild bleeding tendency and easy bruising. Laboratory testing reveals an absence of the "second wave" of platelet aggregation. These disorders are very rare deficiencies and are managed with platelet transfusion.

Acquired Bleeding Disorders

Platelet Deficiency

As mentioned earlier, qualitative or quantitative abnormalities may lead to severe bleeding disorders. By far the most common is a quantitative platelet defect of thrombocytopenia. The clinical hallmark of thrombocytopenia from any cause is petechial hemorrhage (a nonblanching pinpoint rash) usually located on the extremities. It may be caused by a variety of diseases such as idiopathic thrombocyto-

penic purpura (ITP), systemic lupus erythematosus, hypersplenism or splenomegaly of sarcoid, Gaucher's disease, lymphoma, and thrombotic thrombocytopenic purpura (TTP). In these diseases, the marrow usually demonstrates a normal or increased number of megakaryocytes. By contrast, when thrombocytopenia occurs in patients with leukemia or uremia, there is a reduced number of megakaryocytes in the marrow. Patients with ITP are believed to have a disordered immune system, which causes platelets to be removed by the spleen. They frequently respond to a "burst" and "taper" corticosteroid therapy, followed (if necessary) by splenectomy.

TTP carries a high mortality. Unlike the patients with ITP who present with much less bleeding than would be expected on the basis of their low platelet count, patients with TTP have hemolytic anemia, fever, thrombocytopenia, bleeding, and multisystem disease. Renal failure is common and often resembles the hemolytic uremic syndrome. A trial of steroid therapy may be appropriate, but the results are not always predictable. Plasmapheresis occasionally has been effective.

Thrombocytopenia may occur acutely as a result of massive blood loss followed by replacement with stored blood. Massive transfusion is defined as transfusion of 10 units of PRBCs or replacement of more than one blood volume in 24 hours. In general, a platelet count of 60,000 is adequate for normal hemostasis, but if there is associated platelet dysfunction, correlation between platelet count and the extent of bleeding may be poor. Prophylactic platelet administration as a routine accompaniment to massive blood transfusion is not required. However, platelet transfusion is given based upon critically low platelet counts, the risk of bleeding, or ongoing blood loss.

Heparin administration has been associated with thrombocytopenia (heparin-induced thrombocytopenia [HIT]). Depending upon the threshold of definition, it occurs in 2 to 10 percent of patients treated with heparin, occurs most frequently with bovine than porcine heparin, and has also been observed with the new low–molecular weight heparin compounds. HIT follows prior exposure. Since heparin is ubiquitous in patients receiving medical care, it should be assumed that anyone who has been previously hospitalized has received heparin. HIT is caused by a heparin-dependent platelet antibody circulating in the patient's plasma, which triggers an antigen-antibody reaction on the platelet membrane resulting in platelet aggregation following exposure to heparin. A drop in platelet count to 50 percent or less from baseline or recurrent or unexplained thrombosis in patients receiving heparin should suggest HIT. The heparin should be discontinued with cautious protamine reversal, followed by the administration of low–molecular weight dextran and aspirin, and conversion to a warfarin compound if ongoing anticoagulation is indicated.

The diagnosis is confirmed by demonstrating at least 20 percent platelet aggregation within 15 minutes or 6 percent ^{14}C-serotonin release within 45 minutes when heparin is added to a mixture of donor platelets and the patient's platelet-poor plasma. However, these tests are not 100 percent sensitive, and therefore if clinical suspicion is high in the face of normal laboratory tests, patients should be treated as if they had HIT.

Qualitative platelet defects have been noted in patients with uremia, liver failure, acute ethanol ingestion, and use of aspirin and other drugs. Aspirin irreversibly inhibits the synthesis of prostaglandins by platelets, which reduces their ability to release their granular contents, resulting in slight prolongation of the bleeding time. Ticlopidine specifically inhibits platelet aggregation and also prolongs bleeding time. A variety of drugs such as dipyridamole, phenothiazines, penicillins, chelating agents, lidocaine, and cocaine have been described to affect platelet function. Despite these findings, there has been inadequate documentation that their effects are significant in clinical practice.

Clotting Factor Deficiency

In hospitalized patients, the combination of antibiotics and poor dietary intake regularly causes vitamin K deficiency. Generalized malnutrition also contributes to decreased synthesis of clotting factors by the liver. However, the most severe form of acquired bleeding disorder in the adult patient is the appearance of antibody to factor VIII in a previously normal person. The etiology of this disorder is unclear, but has been observed with the use of penicillins and in pregnancy. Patients present with severe deep muscle bleeds and ecchymoses. They have prolongation of their PTT, reduced factor VIII activity, and presence of factor VIII inhibitors. Immunosuppression may aid the disappearance of this inhibitor.

Certain diseases such as Waldenström's macroglobinemia and multiple myeloma, which are associated with the production of abnormal proteins, generally result in hemorrhagic complications when these proteins bind to platelets or clotting factors.

Disseminated Intravascular Coagulation

Disseminated intravascular coagulation (DIC) is a form of acquired hypofibrinogenemia. It is caused by the introduction of thromboplastic materials into the circulation. Because thromboplastin is found in most tissues, many disease processes may activate the coagulation system, leading to DIC.

When tissue thromboplastins are released into the circulation, blood coagulation is stimulated, which leads to significant thrombin production and fibrin generation. This change in turn activates the fibrinolytic system, which eventually leads to bleeding complications if the process continues, because of consumption of coagulation factors, depletion of fibrinogen, and ongoing plasmin activity. The fibrin degradation products produced by secondary fibrinolysis also have strong anticoagulant effects and further potentiate the bleeding diathesis. Clinically, the patient shows signs of diffuse bleeding with oozing from sites of vascular invasion and other surgical sites. The hemorrhagic complications of the perinatal period such as retained dead fetus, premature separation of placenta, and amniotic fluid embolus are caused by this pathologic mechanism. Other common causes of DIC are massive transfusions, hemolytic transfusion reaction, rickettsial infection, snakebite, shock, and extracorporeal circulation. There seems to be a synergy between shock and DIC. Certain disease states such as acute promyelocytic leukemia, widely metastatic adenocarcinoma, and aortic aneurysms with false channels also have been shown to lead to a chronic form of DIC.

Regardless of the etiology of DIC, the key to successful treatment remains in early recognition and treatment of the underlying disease. Although the diagnosis is largely made on clinical grounds, confirming laboratory tests include thrombocytopenia, hypofibrinogenemia, and elevation of the fibrin split products. The PT and PTT may also be prolonged. Intravenous fluids are frequently indicated as part of resuscitation. If bleeding is ongoing in severe DIC, patients are best managed by replacement of blood and deficient clotting factors using FFP, and occasionally cryoprecipitate. Platelet concentrates are infused for severe thrombocytopenia, while the precipitating cause of bleeding is eliminated.

Massive blood transfusion is frequently associated with hypothermia. Clotting factors are enzymes, and their activity is severely reduced at low temperatures. Hypothermic patients frequently have low-grade DIC, and warming of the core temperature near normothermia is important in the correction of the coagulopathy associated with massive transfusion.

The use of heparin for the treatment of DIC has been a topic of considerable debate. Most studies show that heparin is not helpful in acute forms of DIC. However, in chronic consumption coagulopathy, administration of heparin may be beneficial. If fibrinolysis continues after adequate heparinization, epsilonaminocaproic acid (EACA), 5 g loading dose and 1 g every hour, can be added to the regimen. However, use of EACA must be avoided if thrombosis is ongoing. In patients on the surgical services with DIC, we have not found the use of heparin or EACA necessary.

The most common form of acquired hypofibrinogenemia is DIC. Another rare form of acquired hypofibrinogenemia is primary hyperfibrinolysis. Primary hyperfibrinolysis is associated with conditions causing excessive fibrinolytic activation such as electric shock, extracorporeal circulation, acute hypoxemia, severe acidosis, and leukemia. Successful treatment of the underlying disorder usually results in a rapid spontaneous recovery. However, EACA is useful if the fibrinolytic state persists.

Hemorrhagic Disorders of the Vascular Wall

There are hemorrhagic disorders associated with intrinsic vascular wall abnormalities, which can be congenital or acquired. The serious forms are congenital and include Ehler–Danlos syndrome, pseudoxanthoma elasticum, Marfan's syndrome, osteogenesis imperfecta, hereditary hemorrhagic telangiectasia, and amyloidosis. Bleeding in these patients may be difficult to control. Elective surgical procedures should be avoided and in the Ehlers–Danlos patient; even arteriography is contraindicated. Invasive procedures can be fatal because of extreme friability of blood vessels resulting from disorders of connective tissue, which include abnormalities of collagen and fragmentation of elastic fibers. Successful treatment of bleeding disorders is most often associated with correction of deficient factors.

Blood Components and Their Use in Therapy

Blood can be described as the vehicular fluid that bathes all other organ systems. Its major function is the delivery of nutrients and oxygen to meet the body's metabolic demands and the removal of by-products of tissue metabolism. Blood is conveniently divided into the formed cellular elements and plasma. Red blood cells, with their oxygen-carrying capacity; white blood cells, which function in the body's defense mechanism; and platelets, which contribute to the hemostatic process, constitute the formed elements. The plasma component is the supernatant that remains after centrifuge fractionation of whole blood. When the clotting factors are removed from the plasma, the liquid phase is referred to as the serum. The plasma fraction also contains proteins and a number of other factors that affect cellular processes.

Blood components are used individually depending on the clinical situation. Products available from the American Association of Blood Banks include red cells, whole blood, FFP, single donor plasma, cryoprecipitated antihemophilic factor (AHF), platelet concentrates, and leukocyte concentrates. Albumin preparations of plasma protein fraction (PFF); 5% albumin; 25% albumin; antihemophilic factor; and concentrates of factors II, VII, VIII, IX are available in commercially produced off-the-shelf packages.

Whole blood is collected in citrate phosphate dextrose (CPD) or CP2D-adenine so-

lutions and stored between 1°C and 6°C. This solution permits the storage of blood for up to 35 days. About 70 percent of the transfused erythrocytes remain in the circulation and are viable 24 hours post-transfusion. During storage, however, banked blood undergoes several changes. These alterations include reduction in the intracellular red cell ATP and 2,3-diphosphoglycerate (2,3-DPG) concentration, which alters the rate of oxygen dissociation from hemoglobin and decreases the oxygen-transport function of blood. Banked blood is a poor source of platelets, since platelets do not survive after 24 hours of storage. In addition, the pH of blood decreases during storage, and the potassium concentration rises while the concentration of sodium remains essentially unchanged. Factor V and VIII levels are significantly reduced with storage.

Fresh whole blood refers to blood that is administered within 24 hours of its donation. It has the advantage of containing clotting factors and viable platelets. However, it is untested for HBsAg (hepatitis B), HTLV-III (AIDS), and syphilis. Potential hazards of the use of fresh whole blood are self-evident. Whole blood transfusion is no longer necessary in modern clinical practice since component therapy can be efficiently tailored to the patient's needs.

Red Blood Cells

The most common indication for blood transfusion in the surgical patient is hypovolemia caused by blood loss. However, assessment of the extent of hypovolemia that is tolerable or the level of the hemoglobin concentration necessary to supply sufficient oxygen to tissues has been debated since blood transfusion became common practice. In otherwise healthy individuals, about 40 percent of the blood volume, or 2 liters of blood, is lost before significant hypotension develops. Furthermore, measurements of hemoglobin or hematocrit in the face of acute blood loss may be misleading since the hematocrit may be relatively high in spite of a severely contracted blood volume. Therefore, with acute blood loss, clinical judgment is important in assessing the need for transfusion. In an attempt to clarify indications for red cell transfusion, some studies have introduced the concepts of minimally acceptable and optimal hemoglobin-hematocrit. Carrel and Lindberg have shown that isolated organs could survive and

grow in an extremely anemic environment (3 g/100 ml hemoglobin). However, most clinical studies have failed to define a hemoglobin-hematocrit level that is optimally tolerable. Thus, the decision to transfuse should be based on the patient's specific needs guided by the understanding that neither optimal nor minimally acceptable hemoglobin levels correlate well with the clinical symptoms of decreased oxygen delivery in every patient. However, it is clear that the past surgical practices of transfusing to a hemoglobin of 10 g per 100 ml in every patient should be abandoned. As a general recommendation, in patients who have normal preoperative blood values, an acute blood loss of up to 20 percent of the total blood volume (TBV) should be replaced with crystalloids. Blood loss of 50 percent TBV should be replaced with crystalloids, red cells, and albumin or plasma. Greater than 50 percent TBV blood loss should be replaced with FFP in addition to red cells and crystalloids.

Once the acute blood loss is controlled, the patient's clinical response to the ambient hemoglobin should guide the need for transfusion. As such, strict guidelines cannot be established. Patients with underlying cardiac or pulmonary disease do not tolerate anemia as well as patients with healthy hearts and lungs. Symptoms of excessive fatigue, angina, new ST–T changes on ECG, or other evidence of myocardial ischemia are indicators for RBC replacement. In patients who are tolerating their anemia, we withhold transfusion until their hematocrit (Hct) drops to 20 percent or less. However, if a patient faces a high likelihood of acute blood loss, we transfuse to a hematocrit equal to or more than 30 percent.

RBC transfusions are given with packed red cells, each unit having a volume of approximately 285 ml—200 ml of red blood cells and 85 ml of plasma, with a resultant Hct of 75 percent.

For patients for whom the need for transfusion can be anticipated, such as patients undergoing elective aortic aneurysm repair, autologous transfusion can be arranged. Patients routinely can predeposit 2 to 3 units of blood during the month before the planned operation. Using the predeposited blood in conjunction with salvaged, autotransfused blood during the operation, most patients can avoid the use of banked blood. We begin patients on iron supplementation (ferrous sulfate, 300 g tid) approximately six weeks before the planned procedure. The donation schedule is then based upon the number of units requested. Each unit is predeposited one week apart, and we prefer a period of at least 5 to 7 days from the last autologous deposit to the day of the planned procedure. If blood is deposited more than 35 days before the operation or if there is an unforeseen delay in the procedure, the autologous red blood cells can be frozen until the procedure is rescheduled.

Erythropoietin may have value in selected patients. However, it is currently limited to the treatment of anemia of chronic renal failure in patients requiring hemodialysis.

Fresh Frozen Plasma

FFP is separated from RBCs early after blood donation (within 6 h) and frozen. Since FFP contains anti-A and anti-B iso-agglutinins, ABO compatibility between donor and recipient is required. However, since FFP is essentially cell free, Rho (D) typing is not necessary. However, if the recipient is Rh negative, the use of Rh-negative plasma avoids the risk of sensitizing the recipient with Rh-positive red cells contaminating the donor plasma. FFP contains the essential clotting factors at about 1 unit per ml. Each 250 ml unit of FFP increases circulating fibrinogen by 25 mg per 100 ml. FFP is the source for replacement of necessary clotting factors, fibrinogen, antithrombin III, and proteins C and S in the majority of patients. However, the content of factors VIII and V in FFP gradually declines during the first several weeks of storage. We use FFP routinely in patients requiring rapid and large quantity blood replacement to replenish clotting factors and permit hemostasis.

FFP is the only agent currently available to treat bleeding episodes in patients with hereditary or acquired deficiencies of factor V, XI, or XIII (fibrin stabilizing factor). It is our first choice in the care of patients with severe hemorrhage whose hemostatic defect has not been clarified. Plasma is the preferred agent for treatment of deficiencies of the vitamin-K dependent factors, such as prothrombin, factor X, and factor VII. Vitamin-K dependent factors are preserved in non-frozen plasma. However, factor V is not.

We routinely use plasma to correct bleeding complications from the warfarin anti-coagulants or to rapidly reverse the effects of warfarin when invasive procedures are required. In these situations plasma provides the necessary clotting factors until the action of vitamin-K_1 is clinically apparent. We usually transfuse 2 to 4 units (500–1000 ml) acutely followed by 1 to 2 units every 12 hours until coagulation parameters are acceptably controlled.

We have also used FFP in patients requiring acute anticoagulation with heparin but who demonstrated "heparin resistance." Since anti-thrombin III is required for heparin to be effective, in deficient patients its replacement allows heparin to become rapidly effective.

Platelets

Platelets are obtained from the plasma fraction of whole blood. Since they survive poorly in stored blood, they are separated immediately upon donation and must be used within 72 hours, although earlier use improves their effectiveness. Only 40 percent of platelets are viable at 48 hours and 30 percent are at 72 hours.

Patients become sensitized to platelets, especially when receiving multiple transfusions from random donor platelets. Therefore, the life span of subsequently transfused platelets can be significantly decreased.

In general, the number of circulating platelets can be increased by 10,000 to 15,000 per unit of platelets, and it is customary to transfuse patients with 6 to 8 units at a time. However, in patients with hypersplenism or with platelet antibodies, the response to platelet infusion can be markedly reduced.

Platelet transfusion is improved with single donor platelets, in which a large number of platelets can be obtained from a single HLA-matched donor through plasmapheresis. However, the platelets must be used within 24 hours. In patients requiring multiple and ongoing platelet transfusions, the advantages of single donor platelets are evident.

If a patient's platelet count is equal to or more than 30,000 and the platelet function is normal, platelet transfusion is not indicated. However, when a patient's platelet count drops below 30,000, or if platelet function is altered, especially in the setting of recent operative wounds or ongoing blood loss, platelet transfusion is indicated.

Cryoprecipitate

Cryoprecipitate contains all of the plasma clotting factors, high levels of factor VIII, 200 to 250 g of fibrinogen, and fibronectin. Cryoprecipitate is a pooled plasma product; therefore the risk of blood-borne disease is multiplied by the number of donors from which the cryoprecipitate is pooled.

The indications for use are currently limited. We have restricted its use to patients suffering life-threatening bleeding complications associated with profound hypofibrinogenemia during thrombolytic therapy. With familiarity of the lytic agents, and the shift from streptokinase to urokinase and tissue plasminogen activator, bleeding complications have significantly diminished and severe hypofibrinogenemia is no longer observed. Currently, FFP provides the necessary clotting factors to essentially all surgical patients requiring replacement.

Cryoprecipitate has been used to treat the hematologic abnormalities of classic hemophilia and von Willebrand disease. It is an excellent source of fibrinogen for the treatment of patients with congenital or acquired hypofibrinogenemia or afibrinogenemia. A recommended treatment protocol for profound hypofibrinogenemia is one bag of cryoprecipitate initially for each two kg of body weight followed by one bag per 15 kg daily. If only replacement is required, without ongoing fibrinogen depletion (and normal production), the amount of cryoprecipitate required is substantially less. The benefit of cyroprecipitate may be in part caused by its content of fibronectin, especially in patients with DIC and amniotic fluid embolus.

Leukocytes

Patients who have bone marrow suppression caused by radiation or chemotherapy may require white cell transfusions. Therefore, granulocyte replacement is, for the most part, used by oncologists.

In order to obtain an adequate number of WBCs, 8 to 10 liters of whole blood is processed in approximately 2 hours from a single donor by a process called leukapheresis. This process allows the white cells (and platelets) to be harvested with the RBCs, and plasma is returned to the donor. Current methods yield approximately 2.0 to 4.0 × 10^{10} leukocytes, most of which are granulocytes.

Other Plasma Product Concentrates

The mainstay of therapy for replacement of deficient clotting factors is plasma; usually FFP is used in surgical patients. However, in patients with specific bleeding disorders, individual therapeutic agents may be indicated. We always rely upon the advice of our hematologic colleagues when treating these patients. Table 7-1 lists the available plasma product concentrates and their indications for use.

Complications of Blood Component Transfusion

There are three important complications associated with blood and component transfusion: 1) transfusion reactions; 2) disease transmission; and 3) immunomodulation.

Transfusion Reactions

When any untoward reaction occurs during or soon after a blood transfusion, a transfusion reaction must be assumed, and any remaining blood component discontinued. Although anaphylactic reactions are rare, they can be life-threatening. These reactions, which are caused by antibodies to IgA in patients with IgA deficiency who have become sensitized, occur early in the course of the transfusion, frequently after only a few milliliters have been infused. Patients frequently complain of nausea, vomiting, diarrhea, abdominal cramps, and hypotension. Fever is conspicuously absent. The rapid onset of gastrointestinal symptoms and the absence of a pyretic response characteristically distinguish an anaphylactic reaction from one caused by ABO incompatibility or sepsis. The diagnosis is made by measuring IgA levels in the patient. Subsequent transfusions, if required, should be obtained from IgA-free donors, from washed red blood cells, or from frozen red cells. If transfusion can be anticipated, ideally patients should predeposit their own blood.

Acute hemolytic reactions manifest as fevers, chills, back pain, chest pain, dyspnea, hypotension, and generalized oozing. If a patient is under general anesthesia, the most common signs are oozing from a previously dry operative field, cardiovascular instability, and hematuria. After stopping the transfusion, aggressive cardiovascular support is offered, with specific attention to avoiding acute renal failure and treating ongoing blood loss. The mismatched error is identified by sending the patient's blood sample to the blood bank for a Coombs test, and evaluation of plasma free hemoglobin. A urine sample should be tested for free hemoglobin. Once the cause for the incompatible blood is identified, transfusion with recrossmatched blood is safe.

Delayed transfusion reactions can occur days, weeks, or months following transfusion. A physician should have a high index of suspicion if evidence of a delayed hemolytic reaction occurs, with the gradual onset or recurrence of anemia, unexplained fever, and occasionally chemical (or rarely clinical) jaundice. These reactions occur when the patient has received a foreign antigen, and then has developed an antibody over the next several days, weeks, or months. If the antibody is formed while the inciting RBCs remain (antigen), a delayed hemolytic reaction results. The risk of sensitizing the recipient to a minor red cell antigen is approximately 1 percent per unit of blood transfused.

If a delayed transfusion reaction is suspected, a blood sample from the patient should be retyped and recrossmatched along with the initial blood specimen, antibody screens should be repeated, and direct and indirect Coombs tests should be performed along with total bilirubin and haptoglobin levels. Additional investigations may be required. If newly developed antibodies are detected, subsequent transfusion with washed RBCs may be required.

Disease Transmission

Although current methods of donor selection and blood testing are highly effective in minimizing the risk of transfusion-

Table 7-1. Plasma Product Concentrates and Their Indications for Use

Plasma Product	Indication
Factor VII	Congenital deficiency Reverse warfarin effect Severe liver disease
Factor VIII (lyophilized and recombinant products)	Congenital deficiency Hemophilia A von Willebrand's disease
Factor IX ("prothrombin complex" preparations)	Congenital deficiency Hemophilia B Reverse warfarin effect Congenital deficiency of factor II and X
Factor XI	Congenital deficiency
Factor XIII	Congenital deficiency Henoch-Schönlein's purpura
Gamma globulin	Immune thrombocytopenia purpura Passive prophylaxis Congenital agammaglobulinemias Other acquired immune disorders
Antithrombin III	Congenital deficiency Acquired deficiency states Possibly effective in liver transplantation and DIC
Protein C	Congenital deficiency
C1 esterase inhibitor	Hereditary angioedema
Alpha$_1$-antitrypsin	Hereditary deficiency emphysema cirrhosis
Fibronectin	Acquired deficiency states

transmitted disease, serious potential consequences continue to face patients receiving blood and its components. Many surgeons do not appreciate the problems of transfusions associated with hepatitis, AIDS, or HIV, since they do not see and treat the patients for these problems once they become evident.

The overall incidence of hepatitis associated with blood transfusion is unknown. Hepatitis B screening of donor blood is very effective. However, hepatitis C (non-A, non-B hepatitis) has become recognized with an alarmingly high frequently during the past decade. In patients followed by subsequent liver function studies, 10 percent were found to have hepatitis C and 1 percent hepatitis B in large multicenter prospective studies. Currently hepatitis C is the cause of 90 percent of transfusion-related hepatitis, with approximately 1 to 3 percent of patients infected progressing to fulminant, acute hepatitis associated with a 90 percent mortality. Progression to chronic hepatitis occurs in 40 to 50 percent of patients, which is associated with a 5 to 10 percent mortality. The current risk of hepatitis C transmission is substantially reduced because of the recent introduction of laboratory assays for surface and core-antigens of hepatitis C. Although we are confident that the risk of transfusion-associated hepatitis is substantially reduced, an accurate determination remains to be established. There are many parallels between HIV and AIDS and hepatitis in terms of transfusion-related disease transmission. We now have effective assays to detect HIV, and therefore the problem is substantially reduced. (The CDC has estimated that approximately 12,000 people in the United States have transfusion-acquired HIV.) Currently, the major problem with AIDS is the "window of infectivity," in which the donor has contracted and harbors the active virus but has not become HIV positive. While the risk of acquiring HIV from transfusion persists, it is low and has been estimated to be less than 1 in 20,000.

Immunomodulation

The evidence for an immunosuppressive effect of blood transfusion cannot be refuted. Both cellular and humoral factors appear to play a role. Macrophage function is altered after homologous blood transfusion, resulting in decreased migra-

tory capabilities. The strongest clinical support for an immunomodulatory effect of homologous blood transfusion has come from the work of Ahmed and Terasaki in 1974. They reported the enhancing effect of homologous blood transfusion in renal allograft recipients. Others have demonstrated an absolute decrease in T lymphocytes with reversal of normal helper-suppressor cell ratio after multiple transfusions. Tartter and colleagues studied prospectively the relationship between perioperative blood transfusion and postoperative infectious complications in 343 patients undergoing surgery for colorectal cancer. The incidence of infectious complications was 4 percent in nontransfused patients, compared with a 25 percent incidence in patients who received blood transfusions. Despite extensive laboratory investigational efforts, the mechanisms responsible for the immunomodulatory effects of blood transfusion have not been completely elucidated. In the transplant patient two major mechanisms seem to be responsible: 1) Induction of specific immune-responsiveness because of antigen sharing between transfused blood and the transplanted tissue; and, 2) The non-specific inhibition of the immune system. Depression of the natural killer cell (NK-cell) activity, changes in CD4-CD8 ratio, and decreased response of T cells to PHA and Con A have all been reported with blood transfusions.

These disturbances at the level of T cells and macrophages may well explain the increased susceptibility to postoperative bacterial infections in transfused patients. Given the dire consequences of infection in patients undergoing major surgical procedures, the potential for shortening survival in cancer patients, and the known risks of disease transmission, prudent surgical practice dictates the avoidance of homologous blood transfusion whenever possible.

Suggested Readings

Ahmed Z, Terasaki PI. Effect of transfusion in clinical transplants 1991. P Terasaki (ed). Los Angeles: UCLA Tissue Typing Laboratory, 1991. Pp. 305–312.

Barbara JA. Challenges in transfusion microbiology. *Trans Med Rev* 7:96, 1993.

Blumberg N. Transfusion-induced immunomodulation. *Trans Med Rev* 4(Supp 1):24, 1990.

Bucci E. Hemoglobin as oxygen carrier, Cell-free fluids. *MD Med J* 41:527, 1992.

Cameron CB. Perioperative management of patients with von Willebrand's disease. *Can J Anaesth* 37:341, 1990.

Chung M. Perioperative blood transfusion and outcome. *Br J Surg* 80:427, 1993.

Colman RW. Review of Normal Hemostasis. In AJ Comerota (ed), *Thrombolytic Therapy in Peripheral Vascular Disease*. Philadelphia: Lippincott, 1995.

Diamond LK. A History of Blood Transfusion. In MM Wintrobe (ed), *Blood, Pure and Eloquent*. New York: McGraw-Hill, 1980. Pp. 659–688.

Donald ME. Disorders of Hemostasis: Diagnosis and Treatment. In RD Liechty (ed), *Fundamentals of Surgery*. Philadelphia: Mosby, 1989.

Harrigan C, et al. Primary hemostasis after massive transfusion for injury. *Amer Surg* 48:393, 1982.

Humphrey PW, et al. Hemostatis and Thrombosis. In WS Moore (ed), *Vascular Surgery: A Comprehensive Review* (4th ed.) Philadelphia: Saunders, 1993.

Irving GA. Perioperative blood and blood component therapy. *Can J Anaesth* 39(10):1105, 1992.

Murphy MF. Clinical aspects of platelet transfusion. *Blood Coagul Fibrinolysis* 2:389, 1991.

Odling-Smee W. ABC of transfusion. Red cell substitutes. *Br Med J* 300:599, 1990.

Schwartz SJ, et al. Disorders of Surgical Bleeding. In SJ Schwartz (ed), *Principles of Surgery* (5th ed) New York: McGraw-Hill, 1991.

Spence RK. Transfusion and surgery. *Curr Prob Surg* 30:1101, 1993.

Tartter PI, Quintero S, Barron DM. Perioperative blood transfusion associated with infectious complications after colorectal cancer operations. *Am J Surg* 152:479, 1986.

White GC, et al. Approach to the Bleeding Patient. In RW Colman, et al (eds), *Hemostasis and Thrombosis: Basic Principles and Clinical Practice*, (3rd ed) Philadelphia: Lippincott, 1994.

EDITOR'S COMMENT

The practice of getting a PT and a PTT in most hospitals in the preoperative setting is becoming less and less defensible, especially after reading an excellent chapter such as that presented by Drs. Comerota and Eze. If one were to attempt to identify problems in patients about to undergo surgical procedures, one would, as Drs. Comerota and Eze state, take a very careful history and a family history, and then perhaps get a bleeding time and a clotting time. These steps might lead one to discover certain conditions that conceivably could cause intraoperative problems. However, we persist in getting PT and PTT.

It is also interesting that the mores with respect to transfusion have changed dramatically. Doctors Comerota and Eze will perhaps allow patients with a packed cell volume of 20 to tolerate their anemia, as will we. Ten years ago, this would have been considered below the standard of practice. Of course, as Drs. Comerota and Eze point out, it also depends on what the expectation for future blood loss may be.

The hesitation to transfuse is not only the result of transmittable diseases such as hepatitis, the rare and remote possibility of AIDS, and so forth but also of some of the more recent surgical literature in which immunosuppression is brought on by specific transfusion in transplantation patients, suggesting that both the rate of postoperative infection as well as the late recurrence in patients with neoplastic disease may be increased in patients receiving transfusions. More recent revisionist studies have suggested that this presumption is probably not correct: Patients who have undergone transfusion do not experience a higher rate of recurrence or a higher postoperative infection rate than patients who are not transfused. Nonetheless, caution should be the watchword, and unnecessary transfusion is to be avoided.

As an aside, while not documented, I believe that a reigning pope in the fourteenth century was the subject of the first rumored transfusion. An aged man, he attempted to restore his youth by obtaining the transfusion of blood from three young boys. All four died.

J. E. F.

8

Renal Function: The Pathophysiology of Renal Failure, Its Prevention, and Treatment

Frank B. Cerra   Catherine M. Wittgen

Acute renal failure (ARF) is a commonly used but poorly defined term in the surgical literature. Characterized by a decrease in glomerular filtration rate (GFR), retention of water, and inability to excrete nitrogenous metabolites, the syndrome presents to the clinician as an increase in blood urea nitrogen (BUN), increase in serum creatinine level, and oliguria. Once suspected, a careful history, physical examination, and laboratory evaluation should be performed (Fig. 8-1) to determine whether the ARF is caused by a reduction in renal blood flow (prerenal), intrinsic parenchymal damage (intrinsic renal), or obstruction to urine outflow (postrenal).

Incidence

Renal failure is, unfortunately, a frequent complication in the intensive care unit (ICU) patient. The reported incidence of 0.1 to 50 percent reflects the lack of a consistent definition as well as the many different types of patients included for review. As Hays and others have documented, approximately 5 percent of all patients admitted to the hospital will develop ARF. Despite recent advances in intraoperative monitoring and invasive hemodynamic monitoring, patients who have sustained trauma or are recovering from thoracic, cardiac, or vascular surgical procedures are most likely to develop ARF. This event significantly prolongs hospital stay and increases the risk of patient mortality (as high as 50% in some series) regardless of the underlying disease process.

Risk Factors

Identification of the patient who is at high risk to develop ARF allows the clinician to optimize the patient's volume status and to minimize nephrotoxic insults. What constitutes a risk factor is difficult to prove, however. Examination of existing series reveals poorly defined "abnormal" parameters, inconsistently applied statistical methods, and, consequently, an inability to perform a meaningful analysis of the existing data.

In a retrospective review of over 10,000 surgical patients, Novis and colleagues found an elevation in preoperative measures of renal function (serum creatinine, BUN, and creatinine clearance) to be associated with poor postoperative renal function. Advanced age and congestive

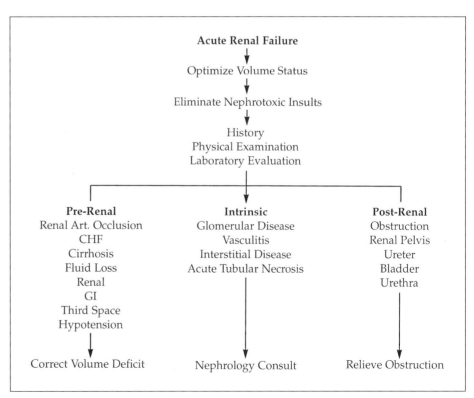

Acute Renal Failure
↓
Optimize Volume Status
↓
Eliminate Nephrotoxic Insults
↓
History
Physical Examination
Laboratory Evaluation

Pre-Renal	**Intrinsic**	**Post-Renal**
Renal Art. Occlusion	Glomerular Disease	Obstruction
CHF	Vasculitis	Renal Pelvis
Cirrhosis	Interstitial Disease	Ureter
Fluid Loss	Acute Tubular Necrosis	Bladder
Renal		Urethra
GI		
Third Space		
Hypotension		
↓	↓	↓
Correct Volume Deficit	Nephrology Consult	Relieve Obstruction

Fig. 8-1. Acute renal failure.

heart failure were also found to be associated with ARF in other series. Isolated reports have also noted an association of hypertension, diabetes mellitus, cancer, vascular disease, and cardiac surgical procedures with the development of postoperative renal failure. However, these findings were in small series and not consistently reported.

Reviews of series with more standardized preoperative evaluations (APACHE, Mortality Prediction Models, Acute Physiologic Score) have also been attempted but have encountered the same difficulties. Univariate analysis reveals hypovolemia, aminoglycoside use, congestive heart failure, and sepsis as being significant in the development of ARF. This analysis is in addition to findings from earlier regression analyses that identified the association of sepsis, hypertension, and advanced age with ARF.

Pathophysiology
Alterations in Renal Blood Flow

Since most cases of ARF in the surgical patient are caused by hypovolemia (prerenal) or ischemia (acute tubular necrosis [ATN]) an understanding of renal blood flow is essential. The kidneys receive approximately 20 percent of the cardiac output with 80 percent of total renal blood flow directed to the cortex and only 20 percent to the medulla. A number of intrinsic autoregulatory systems exist that further regulate this distribution.

One of these systems is the tubuloglomerular feedback mechanism in which excessive amounts of solute are prevented from being excreted by autoregulation of afferent and efferent arteriolar resistance. Another is the reduction in afferent arteriole blood flow after release of renin, aldosterone, or antidiuretic hormone (ADH). Sandin studied the renal tubular cell after a period of ischemia and found an altered pattern of metabolism, which produced increased amounts of adenosine, endothelin, and prostaglandin. Membrane defects that allowed these substances to pass out of the cell and act locally to augment vasoconstriction were also found. This change further reduced renal blood flow (and consequently oxygen) to the already ischemic organ.

Mechanisms of Cellular Damage

Most discussions of renal damage from ischemic insults concentrate on the effects observed in the proximal tubular cell, the best understood of all renal cell types. These cells are highly polarized structures joined by various tight junctions. This configuration maintains the electrical and concentration gradients established across apical and basal membranes. A complex internal cytoskeleton allows Na-K ATPase to remain on the basal membrane and the Na-H transport mechanism to remain apically oriented. Racusen has suggested that major alterations in this membrane conformation in viable cells may be responsible for the changes in urine composition observed in ATN.

These proximal tubular cells are capable of gluconeogenesis but have very limited glycolytic activity and only minimal energy stores. Their type of metabolism is very oxygen dependent, and they are thus highly susceptible to hypoxic damage. With ischemia, intracellular adenosine triphosphate (ATP) is depleted, and adenosine diphosphate (ADP) and phosphate diffuse out of the cell. The functional integrity of tight junctions, the microfilaments supporting cell structure, and the membrane's polarity are consequently unable to be maintained. Tubular cell transport is reduced, intracellular oxygen free radicals accumulate, mitochrondria malfunction, and phospholipases and peroxidases are activated. This series of events appears to be the final common pathway for renal tubular cell death from nephrotoxic agents as well.

With continued hypoxia, cells swell, portions of cell membranes slough, and some cells necrose. Damaged cells detach from their anatomic position, are shed into the tubular lumen, and combine with intraluminal proteins. Histologically this is seen as a low flattened tubular epithelium, tubular casts, and tubular obstruction. Why these cells do not remain anchored to the basement membrane is currently being investigated, but the effects are well documented. As summarized by Hays, urine (actually a filtrate of plasma with this degree of damage) accumulates proximally, intratubular pressure increases, and as a result the pressure gradient driving the GFR decreases. With already damaged

membranes and tight junctions, up to 50 percent of intratubular fluid can then leak back into the blood. This result is observed as a further decrease in the GFR.

Once cells are shed as casts, they are not replaced. For damaged cells, however, cellular repair begins almost immediately. The initial mechanism of recovery appears to be the reestablishment of membrane polarity with the ability to excrete or to conserve sodium and water. There is evidence that supports the role of the heat shock family of proteins in this process. They solubilize denatured proteins, degrade them, and then channel new proteins to their appropriate membrane-bound positions. Early response genes are induced. These genes are also currently being studied by Weinberg and many others for their role in epithelial growth and regeneration.

Types of Renal Failure
Prerenal Failure

As previously stated, most cases of renal dysfunction in surgical patients are caused by decreases in renal blood flow (prerenal). Induction of anesthesia, significant changes in circulating blood volume, and vasodilation secondary to sepsis in the perioperative period may be contributing factors. Clinically, the condition is associated with three characteristic changes in urine composition, as described by Kellerman.

Initially, both salt and water excretion are reduced. This reduction reflects the influence of aldosterone and vasopressin, which both increase in response to hypovolemia. These hormones cause a decrease in urine volume and a concomitant decrease in urine sodium (<20 meq/l). Urine osmolality generally increases (>450 mOsm/l) as does urine specific gravity (>1.020 mOsm/l).

Next, urea clearance declines. In the normal kidney, a variable amount of urea is passively reabsorbed from the tubules, and urea clearance is approximately 60 to 75 percent of creatinine clearance. It is not, therefore, an accurate estimate of the true GFR. The rate of tubular flow also appears to influence the amount of urea reabsorbed. At low urinary flow rates, more urea is reabsorbed and BUN concentration may increase without a significant change in serum creatinine. This change results in the increased ratio of BUN to creatinine that historically has been reported to be greater than 20 : 1 in low volume (prerenal) states. Other factors, such as increased endogenous or exogenous urea loads (i.e., catabolism, increased dietary protein, and gastrointestinal bleeding), may further increase this ratio.

The final change is a reduction in renal blood flow from persistent hypovolemia. This reduction causes a further decrease in the GFR. Adequate volume resuscitation and careful fluid management can largely eliminate this additional insult to already poorly functioning kidneys.

Intrinsic Renal Failure

Although a less common cause of renal failure in the perioperative period, acute exacerbations of occult intrinsic renal dysfunction do occur. Of instances of ARF in the adult hospitalized population, only 10 to 20 percent are from causes other than ATN. Faber and associates have noted a much lower incidence of ATN in outpatient as well as the pediatric populations in which renal failure presents more insidiously and other intrinsic causes account for over 50 percent of cases.

Once prerenal and postrenal causes have been eliminated, the suspicion of an intrinsic renal pathology can be confirmed with simple laboratory tests including urinalysis and calculation of the fractional excretion of sodium (FE_{Na}). Although not an extensive or exhaustive algorithm, there are four easily distinguishable categories of intrinsic renal disease that may present as ARF. The first, ATN, develops after ischemia or from systemic absorption or nephrotoxic drugs or chemicals (Table 8-1) and has been previously discussed.

Glomerulonephritis (GN), one of the major remaining types of intrinsic renal disease, is characterized by proteinuria, hematuria, and hypertension. Urinalysis usually reveals markedly abnormal sediment with many tubular cells and casts. Extreme proteinuria (nephrotic syndrome) is highly suggestive of membranoproliferative GN or systemic lupus erythematosus. Further aiding in the distinction of the many causes of GN, low complement levels suggest a postinfectious etiology. Sodium and water retention is typical, and FE_{Na} is usually low.

Table 8-1. Nephrotoxic Agents

Glycols
Organic solvents
Heavy metals
Insecticides
Hemoglobin
Myoglobin
Antibiotics
　Aminoglycosides
　Vancomycin
　Polymixins
　Bacitracin
Antifungals
　Amphotericin B
Chemotherapy
　Cisplatin
　Streptozotocin
　Methotrexate
　Interferon
Radiocontrast agents

Vasculitis, another major cause of intrinsic renal disease, can cause a number of functional defects depending on the location of the lesions. Small arteries are more commonly affected with scleroderma or polyarteritis nodosa, whereas capillaries are more commonly occluded in thrombocytopenic purpura or hemolytic uremic syndrome. The presence of generalized vasculitic symptoms can alert the clinician to this type of renal dysfunction.

Last, interstitial nephritis may occur after infections or treatment with certain medications. Clinically the condition presents as the sudden development of azotemia without any other systemic symptoms. Fever or rash occasionally occurs, and eosinophils may be observed in the urine sediment if urinalysis is performed early in the clinical course.

Diagnosis of these types of renal failure is usually confirmed with percutaneous biopsy. Specific treatment is then determined by the biopsy results and is beyond the scope of this chapter. The clinician searching for the etiology of uremia and a rising serum creatinine in the patient with ARF should be alerted to one of these possible diagnoses by the presence of hypertension, proteinuria, and an abnormal urinalysis. Prompt diagnostic evaluation should then be initiated with consultation from a nephrologist.

Postrenal Failure

Although a relatively uncommon cause of ARF, obstructive renal failure is an impor-

tant consideration in selected patients such as the pediatric or the elderly male population. Even in these patients, underlying renal damage and bilateral ureteral obstruction are usually present before significant abnormalities occur. Anuria alternating with periods of polyuria is characteristic of obstruction, although with partial ureteral obstruction, urine flow may appear normal. For patients with oliguria, placement of a Foley catheter or sterile irrigation of an existing catheter can effectively eliminate bladder outlet obstruction as a potential cause. For further evaluation, radiologic tests can define the site of abnormal or obstructed anatomy.

With incomplete obstruction, changes in renal function similar to those observed with hypovolemia may be seen. This effect is observed as a decrease in urine volume, increase in urine sodium, increase in BUN, and, if the obstruction persists, a decrease in GRF. With continued obstruction, renal vasoconstriction occurs and total renal blood flow decreases, which may then further worsen the renal function of an already obstructed kidney.

Clinical Course of Acute Renal Failure

The natural evolution of ARF has been divided into four phases by Finn: 1) the initial, 2) the oliguric, 3) the diuretic, and 4) the phase of functional recovery. Although not all of these phases may be observed in any single patient, knowledge of the natural progression of the syndrome can aid in its management.

Initial Phase

Beginning with the renal injury, the initial phase is characterized by a change in the composition of urine, which is initially seen as a decrease in urine urea and creatinine. Urine volume and sodium concentration may not be decreased, and normal salt and water balance may be maintained for a variable period of time (hours to days).

Oliguric Phase

The oliguric phase is characterized by a decrease in urine volume (<500 ml/day) for a variable period of time. Severe decreases in urine volume (<100 ml/day) suggest alternative diagnoses such as renal cortical necrosis or bilateral ureteral obstruction. Microscopic examination of the urine at this time reveals red blood cells, white blood cells, and tubular casts. A defect in the ability to excrete solute usually appears during this period as well.

Normal individuals excrete 0.5 to 1.0 mOsm per minute of solute in a variable amount of water while consuming a regular diet. The maximal concentration ability of the kidney is approximately 1400 mOsm per liter, so that all metabolized solute can be excreted in as little as 500 ml of urine per day. With a urine volume less than this, solute is retained intravascularly. Further contributing to this retention of solute is the damaged kidney's inability to maximally concentrate urine. In this setting of severe tubular dysfunction, the urine produced appears to be an ultrafiltrate or plasma.

There are a number of clinical measurements that can be performed to detect these concentrating defects in the tubular cell. Urine to plasma (U/P) ratios are commonly used. Normally the ratios of urea U/P range from 50:1 or 100:1. In ARF, as urea excretion decreases the ratio decreases to less than 10:1. This decrease is also reflected in the U/P osmolality ratio, in which a value less than 1.35 combined with an altered urea U/P ratio is suggestive of ARF.

These data should be interpreted cautiously in certain patient populations. The ability to concentrate urine decreases in the older patient without renal disease, and these calculated ratios may then be markedly inaccurate. Consequently, a number of indices have been proposed to aid in the diagnosis of ARF.

As a means to account for these baseline alterations in renal function, Espinel proposed the renal failure index (RFI) as an aid to diagnosis. The RFI is calculated by dividing the urine sodium (U_{Na}) concentration by an estimate of GFR ($U_{creatinine}/P_{creatinine}$). With ARF, U_{Na} concentration should increase because of tubular cell damage while the GFR decreases (RFI>5). In instances of prerenal azotemia, the urine sodium will be decreased while the GFR is unchanged (RFI<1).

In a similar fashion, the FE_{Na} has proved to be useful. To calculate this value, the amount of sodium excreted ($U_{Na} \times V$) is divided by the amount of sodium filtered ($P_{Na} \times GFR$). GFR is estimated by clearance of creatinine ($U_{creatinine}U/P_{creatinine}$) so that $FE_{Na} = U_{Na}V/(P_{Na} \times [U_{creatinine}V/P_{creatinine}]) \times 100 = (U_{Na} \times P_{creatinine})/(U_{creatinine} \times P_{Na}) \times 100$. As shown by the calculation, FE_{Na} is also based on an estimate of the patient's GFR and only differs from the RFI by the inclusion of the plasma sodium concentration. Generally a FE_{Na} greater than one is indicative of ARF while values less than one are highly suggestive or prerenal azotemia.

Occasionally the oliguric phase does not occur, and this is commonly referred to as nonoliguric or polyuric ARF. Solute excretion is still reduced because of the concentrating defect of the renal tubule even though urine output is maintained. Recovery from polyuric renal dysfunction appears to occur more frequently than from oliguric renal failure. This difference may be because kidneys that are not as severely damaged excrete more urine. It may also represent a true physiologic advantage of diuresis for the tubular cells since kidneys not obstructed by casts have a higher GFR.

Diuretic Phase

When oliguria occurs, it is followed by a period of diuresis with 100 to 200 ml per hour of urine excreted. Despite this increase in volume, though, the urine is still not of normal composition. Regenerating tubules are not capable of normal sodium and water reabsorption and remain largely unresponsive to endogenous and exogenously administered vasopressin. Excretion of urea and other nitrogenous metabolites remains decreased, and, consequently, urine osmolality remains low. Dialysis may still be required during this period to remove these metabolites. Electrolytes need to be monitored closely as does the patient's total volume status since both aggressive sodium and fluid replacement may be required. Hypotension as a result of hypovolemia is not uncommon in this period without use of the measures mentioned previously. Of all deaths occurring from ARF, Finn found nearly 25 percent occurring during this phase.

More commonly, however, the onset of diuresis is a gradual phenomenon with urine volumes increasing only 100 to 200 ml per day, and patient management is much less problematic. Slowly increasing urine volumes in these patients is characteristic of normalizing renal function. Once urine volume remains constant in this setting, the degree of recovery is virtually complete and further improvement should not be anticipated.

When polyuric renal failure occurs, urine volume is no longer a useful parameter to indicate improving renal function. Tubular cell regeneration can be observed clinically in these patients by changes in the composition of the urine (i.e., an increase in U_{urea}/P_{urea}, $U_{creatinine}/P_{creatinine}$, and a decrease in FE_{Na}).

Phase of Functional Recovery

After diuresis has occurred, BUN and serum creatinine levels slowly decline. As urea clearance approximates 60 to 75 percent of creatinine clearance, serum creatinine concentration will decrease first. In patients with an increased metabolic rate (catabolism) or increased nitrogenous loads, these expected changes can be quite delayed despite increased rates of clearance.

Whether any given patient can be expected to make a complete recovery appears to be influenced by a number of factors including the presence of other diseases, patient age, and the length of the oliguric phase. If clinical recovery occurs, it usually appears to be complete despite residual decreases in GFR, which are detected in 30 to 70 percent of patients. Patients may also have a deterioration in clinical status after the initial recovery with continued signs and symptoms of chronic renal failure. In addition, tubular defects may remain in patients who no longer require dialysis. These defects present to the clinician as a defect in the ability to concentrate urine maximally when the patient becomes dehydrated.

Diagnosis

Most difficulties in diagnosing ARF occur when attempting to distinguish prerenal azotemia from ATN. In a comprehensive review of the literature for the prediction and diagnosis of these two entities (Table 8-2), Kellen found urine volume and specific gravity to be neither predictive nor diagnostic of impending renal dysfunction. This finding is not unexpected since oliguria may be caused by increased levels of

Table 8-2. Common Diagnostic Tests
Performed in the ICU

BUN
Creatinine
Urinalysis
Urine sodium
Urine osmolality
Urine specific gravity
Fractional excretion of sodium (FE_{NA})
Renal failure index (RFI)
Creatinine clearance
Free water clearance

Table 8-3. Radiologic Evaluation of Renal
Dysfunction

Angiography
CT scan
Nuclear medicine scan
Ultrasound
IVP
Cystogram
Cystoscopy
Renal biopsy

renin, aldosterone, ADH, catecholamines, and hypovolemia regardless of the true GFR.

Urine osmolality was found to be helpful only at extreme values for distinguishing prerenal azotemia (>500 mOsm/l) from ATN (<350 mOsm/l) with a variable positive predictive value depending on the patient population studied. Unfortunately, with a large number of intermediate values being reported (350–500 mOsm/l), urine osmolality remained nondiagnostic in most instances. This failure most likely reflects the ability to detect only extensive tubular damage by this method.

Free water clearance ($U_{volume} - [(U_{volume} \times U_{osmolality})/P_{osmolality}]$) has also been shown to be of little diagnostic value. Like urine osmolality or specific gravity, free water clearance is subject to the same number of variables. It is also influenced by the age of the patient, serum protein and glucose levels, dextran, diuretics, antibiotics, contrast material, and hormonal imbalances that are independent of the GFR.

Both BUN and serum creatinine levels have also beeen found to be highly variable with poor diagnostic value. This finding may be secondary to the large degree of renal dysfunction required before alterations in these values are seen. Serum creatinine is also highly dependent on muscle

mass and inaccurately reflects renal function in a debilitated patient. Because of the higher metabolic rates caused by total parenteral nutrition, trauma or sepsis in the ICU patient (resulting in higher nitrogenous waste production), increases in BUN are unreliable.

Measurements of sodium excretion have been utilized in an attempt to assess tubular cell function, as previously mentioned in this chapter. Sodium excretion and reabsorption, however, is a complex process under the influences of aldosterone, ADH, diuretics, hydration status, and underlying diseases such as congestive heart failure and cirrhosis. Isolated urine sodium measurements have proven to be nonspecific in distinguishing prerenal azotemia from ATN. Much controversy exists regarding the sensitivity of FE_{Na} or the RFI in diagnosing these two processes. Both appear to be most clinically useful when calculated for patients with concomitant oliguria and, therefore, have poor predictive value for the future development of ARF.

Attempts have been made to obtain more accurate measurements of the GFR using radioisotope-labeled markers such as ^{99}Tc-DTPA or ^{51}Cr-EDTA. Unfortunately, their use in the ICU is not practical. The current gold standard in research, inulin clearance, also has limited applications since it requires intravenous infusion to a constant plasma level as well as accurately timed plasma and urine samples. Achieving a sufficient volume of urine for measurements may also be harmful to patients because of the large volume load required. Inulin analysis is also not routinely performed in most hospitals and results may not be accurate in patients with proximal tubular leak.

Creatinine clearance, the most useful value to measure clinically, is still not without potential sources of error. It is affected by alterations in creatinine production as previously mentioned, and there is also evidence that in instances of renal dysfunction, the intestine can also excrete up to 65 percent of this solute. Based on a 24-hour collection of urine, creatinine clearance may overestimate GFR by 10 to 20 percent, and this error may be propagated further by shortening the collection time to 2 to 4 hours and extrapolating the data.

Despite being known nephrotoxins, aminoglycosides can serve as a marker of re-

nal function for patients already receiving them since they are excreted by glomerular filtration. As shown by Robert and Zarowitz, timed serum levels can be used to calculate rate constants and provide an estimate of creatinine clearance.

For patients with suspected anatomic defects presenting as ARF, radiologic evaluation is indicated Table 8-3). If vascular insufficiency is suspected, angiography provides the most information. Renal excretion can be demonstrated by CT scan, nuclear medicine scan, or intravenous pyelogram (IVP). One should note, however, that with pre-existing renal dysfunction, the use of radiocontrast agents for angiography, CT scan, or IVP is not without the risk of additional tubular cell damage from these nephrotoxic agents. Ultrasound and CT scan both provide information on renal anatomy, whereas IVP, cystogram, or cystoscopy provide additional information on the condition of the ureters and bladder. Once a diagnosis of intrinsic renal disease is established, percutaneous renal biopsy by CT scan or ultrasound guidance can provide detailed information on the type of renal pathology present.

Treatment of Acute Renal Failure

The goals of care for the patient with ARF are deceptively simple. They are to minimize the extent of injury, to prevent the symptoms of uremia, and to promote rapid and complete recovery of renal function. The therapeutic options available to accomplish these goals are limited, however.

Diuretics

The use of diuretics in ARF remains controversial. Selected reports indicate that various agents may prevent ARF or reverse its natural course. Original studies investigating mannitol, an osmotic diuretic, found a number of theoretical benefits for its use in ARF, as documented in animal studies by Shilliday. Osmotic diuresis flushes tubular casts out of the lumen by increasing tubular flow. This change decreases intratubular pressure, increases intravascular pressure, and restores the GFR. This result has been confirmed by others who have documented an increase in renal blood flow (RBF) with mannitol use. Hypertonic solutions of mannitol have also been shown to reduce cell edema, cause plasma volume expansion, and reduce red blood cell aggregation in capillaries after ischemia. Mannitol can also decrease the rise in intramitochondrial calcium that occurs after ischemia and may inactivate oxygen free radicals.

Despite these apparent advantages, patient trials have shown less clinicial benefit. Most studies supporting the use of mannitol during cardiac or vascular surgical procedures were performed in the 1960s and, although diuresis is clearly documented, no significant improvement in renal function has ever been shown. Only one pediatric study after cardiopulmonary bypass demonstrated more rapid normalization of renal function when compared with controls. Treatment of rhabdomyolysis with mannitol has been based on an initial case report of seven patients who all received treatment, and none was managed with simple hydration. In addition, prospectively randomized studies have demonstrated any benefit in terms of increased urine output, increased creatinine clearance, or increased GFR for the oliguric patient with ARF.

The use of other diuretics such as ethacrynic acid, bumetanide, furosemide, and torosamide is also controversial. All these agents act by binding and inhibiting the Na/Cl/K transport on the luminal side of the thick ascending limb of Henle. As a result, intracellular chloride decreases, Na-K ATPase activity decreases on the basal lateral membrane, and the cells' energy expenditure and oxygen consumption decrease. Increased oxygen consumption may have some theoretical advantage in already ischemic cells by preserving ATP levels, maintaining cell structure, and thus increasing tubular flow. It may also inhibit chloride flux at the macula densa and inhibit tubuloglomerular feedback, thereby possibly decreasing renal vasoconstriction. These agents may also inhibit prostaglandin dehydrogenase, which causes increased levels of prostaglandin E_2 (PGE_2), a potent vasodilator. The total effect may be observed as an increase in renal blood flow.

Clinical trials have shown only greater ease of management for patients receiving these agents. By promoting polyuria, fluids and electrolytes are more easily regulated. Neither the creatinine clearance nor the GFR have been shown to improve. For patients who require dialysis and receive high-dose furosemide, the need for dialysis may be decreased but no effect on renal function has been observed.

Renal Vasodilators

Reducing renal blood flow has been shown to induce renal failure in many patients. Conversely, the reduction of renal vascular resistance has not been associated with any improvement in renal function after injury. Despite this, dopamine at 1.0 to 3.0 mcg/kg/minute has been commonly used in treatment of ARF. Its use in oliguric euvolemic ICU patients has been supported by documented increases in urine volume that fall when dopamine is stopped. Flancbaum and others have not noted any change in creatinine clearance, however. Other studies have documented maintenance of the GFR despite aortic cross clamping with dopamine use that is independent of its diuretic effect. Still others have shown that for patients who remain oliguric despite high-dose diuretics, dopamine may induce diuresis. For patients requiring dialysis, the combination of diuretics and dopamine decreases the need for dialysis but has not altered renal function or affected mortality. More recently, a randomized study by Duke and colleagues has confirmed the diuretic effect of dopamine without an increase in creatinine clearance. In contrast, when dobutamine is administered to this same group of patients, significant improvement in creatinine clearance without a significant change in urine output has been documented. This finding does not appear to be caused by simple improvement in cardiac output, since cardiac indices for both groups are statistically similar. Further research investigating the role of beta agonists in patients with ARF seems warranted.

Atrial Natriuretic Peptide

Atrial natriuretic peptide (ANP) is also under investigation for the treatment of ARF. Systemically administered, ANP lowers mean arterial pressure (MAP) while increasing GFR and sodium excretion. This increase in GFR appears to be caused by dilation of afferent arterioles and constriction of efferent arterioles. This change can be explained as partial inhibition of the tubuloglomerular feedback mechanism. In animal studies using ANP, Fischereder maintained renal function after ischemic insults and observed no decline in intracellular ATP levels. Like most studies with ANP, however, dopamine is simultaneously administered to maintain MAP during the infusion so results are difficult to analyze.

Patient trials have been limited and have shown minimal benefit. The severe hypotension associated with ANP use and its rapid degradation in vivo have limited trials to those patient with established renal failure. For this population studied by Shilliday, no change in GFR has been observed, but urine output and FE_{Na} have both been shown to increase.

Calcium Antagonists

Calcium antagonists are also being investigated for the treatment of ARF. Calcium, an intracellular ion of low cytosolic concentration, maintains its concentration gradient through the action of the Na-Ca exchange mechanism, the Ca-ATPase enzyme on the cell membrane, and the sequestration of the ion inside mitochondria and the endoplastic reticulum. With depolarization of the membrane after ischemia, these enzymes are no longer active, and intracellular concentrations rise. Prevention of this influx with calcium antagonists may provide a cytoprotective effect.

Increases in GFR without an increase in renal blood flow has also been documented with their use. This finding suggests an inhibition of vasoconstriction at the level of the afferent arteriole. Calcium antagonists have also been shown to increase natriuresis (independent of the reduction in MAP and diuresis), interfere with angiotensin II and alpha adrenergic-mediated vasoconstriction, and may decrease free radical formation. Epstein is currently investigating the renal protective effect of calcium antagonists when given to patients receiving radiocontrast agents, cyclosporin, aminoglycosides, or chemotherapy.

Cytoprotective Agents

Because of the devastating role of oxygen free radicals in cellular damage, xanthine oxidase inhibitors and free radical scavengers have been given to prevent the formation of reactive oxygen species and limit the formation of superoxide radicals and hydroxy compounds. Unfortunately, the most consistent improvement in post-ischemic renal function has been demonstrated when these compounds are given prior to the ischemic event. The role of peroxide scavengers such as glutathione and pyruvate is also being investigated in animal models.

The role of other agents such as ATPMgCl$_2$, thyroid hormone, endothelin antagonists, platelet-activating factor, PGE$_2$ analogues, and epidermal growth factor have all shown promise in animal models by their ability to attenuate the degree of renal failure. Definitive studies documenting consistent improvement in patients with ARF, however, have not been performed.

Nutrition and Metabolism

ARF usually occurs with other systemic illnesses. Metabolic alterations attributable to ARF are therefore difficult to isolate. However, the major goal in nutritional support is unchanged. Catabolism, defined as an increase in BUN greater than 28 mg/dl per day or a production of 25 g of urea per day, should be reduced. This reduction should be accomplished despite the global aberrations in protein, carbohydrate, and lipid metabolism, as well as the imbalances in the excretion of water, acids, and electrolytes.

In uremic patients with invasive hemodynamic monitoring, oxygen consumption has been shown to increase. This increase is probably a reflection of the underlying disease process since in animal models with isolated ARF, oxygen consumption and energy expenditure are usually decreased. Caloric requirements should therefore still be increased over basal energy expenditure for the patient with ARF since it rarely occurs as a single entity.

Negative nitrogen balance is common because of excessive protein catabolism from acidosis occurring with ARF. This condition presents as defective utilization of amino acids for protein synthesis by skeletal muscle, while clearance of amino acids is decreased as amino acids become concentrated in the liver. As a result, hepatic gluconeogenesis, ureagenesis, and acute phase reactant protein synthesis are increased.

Insulin resistance occurs and hyperglycemia with altered carbohydrate metabolism is common. Gluconeogenesis is increased despite high insulin levels because of the great number of amino acids released with protein catabolism, as previously mentioned.

The rate of protein catabolism can be decreased by the addition of as little as 100 g per day of carbohydrate in a nonstressed fasting patient. With an increased metabolic rate, carbohydrate needs should be calculated to provide 60 percent of the total calories required. The addition of insulin should be considered because of the pre-existing hyperglycemic state, and the use of hypertonic solution is advised to minimize volume overload.

Protein calories should be supplied to prevent net negative nitrogen balance. In a patient with isolated renal failure in the absence of a tissue injury who does not require dialysis, these needs are most often met by supplying 0.6 g per kg of body weight as protein. With hemodialysis, this supplementation should be increased to 1.0 g per kg, while in the setting of peritoneal dialysis, it can be increased to 1.5 g per kg. This change is to compensate for the protein losses in the effluent dialysate, which can range from 0.1 to 0.8 g per liter (20–60 g/day). Success of protein supplementation can then be quantified by measuring losses of nitrogen in the urine (and dialysate if the patient is receiving hemodialysis or peritoneal dialysis) against the change in total body urea nitrogen.

Lipolysis is also impaired in patients with ARF, and the concentration of plasma lipoproteins is markedly altered (increased VLDL, increased LDL, decreased HDL, and decreased cholesterol). Parenterally administered lipids also have a delayed elimination by greater than 50 percent regardless of the type supplied (long- or medium-chain triglycerides). Consequently nutritional support for these patients becomes somewhat more difficult. Fat requirements should still be calculated to supply 25 to 30 percent of total caloric intake, but serum triglyceride levels should be measured frequently.

Enteral intake during ARF is usually inadequate because of uremic symptoms (anorexia, nausea, and vomiting). A nutritional assessment performed in order to guide parenteral support is also difficult because of the volume overload, which dilutes plasma proteins and invalidates changes in patient weight as accurate nutritional parameters. In contrast, pre-albumin may be artificially elevated because of decreased renal clearance. Serum transferrin levels are generally used as the best indicator of adequate nutritional status in patients with ARF.

Nutritional support reduces morbidity and mortality in ARF. Both a greater extent of recovery and more rapid restoration of renal function have been observed, and these do not appear to be dependent on the protein composition of parenteral solutions (essential or nonessential amino acids) administered. Higher protein intakes have been shown to increase the need for dialysis, however, because of the greater volume of fluid administered and the greater rise in the serum BUN.

Nutritional support can also have a beneficial effect on the electrolyte management. The increased protein catabolism, as described in this chapter, causes muscle breakdown and release of potassium, phosphorus, magnesium, and urea. With adequate caloric intake, these ions can be transported intracellularly. With protein supplementation in mildly uremic patients, urea levels may actually decrease because of the decreased rate of catabolism.

Amino acids may also stimulate cellular repair and proliferation. Glycine and alanine have been shown by Weinberg to have major roles in maintaining tubular cell integrity. Specific combinations of amino acids have also been shown to produce vasodilation and increase the GFR in animal studies. Further investigations are continuing.

Electrolytes

In patients who develop ARF, significant changes in serum sodium, potassium, bicarbonate, phosphorus, and uric acid occur. As summarized by Dolson, sodium levels generally decrease, reflecting a total body increase in free water, while potassium levels increase, demonstrating the cellular reponse to acidosis and lack of renal excretion. Decreases in serum bicarbonate levels are common, which reflects the intravascular accumulation of phosphates, sulfates, and other organic acids and lack of hydrogen ion excretion by the tubular cells. Skeletal resistance to parathyroid hormone appears to develop, and decreases in 1,25-dihydroxycholecalciferol and calcium have been documented with concomitant phosphate level increases. Increased levels of uric acid also occur as a result of cellular destruction and metabolism of nuclear proteins. Despite lack of renal clearance, these levels are usually not exceedingly high because of the ability of intestinal bacteria to metabolize this substance.

Dialysis

Hemodialysis and peritoneal dialysis are important therapeutic options for patients with ARF. The development of continuous arteriovenous hemofiltration (CAVH) and continuous arteriovenous hemodiafiltration (CAVHD) further expand available treatment options. The choice of which treatment is the best modality for a given patient is a complicated one.

Peritoneal dialysis (PD) is widely available, simple to perform, and can easily correct volume overload. It can be used when there is a contraindication to central venous access and is able to be performed despite significant hypotension. Contraindications include a recent abdominal surgical procedure, open abdominal wounds, and the presence of peritonitis. PD also carries the risk of causing peritonitis and bowel perforation from catheter placement. Atelectasis and pneumonia can also develop as a consequence of the prolonged immobilization necessary for the procedure. It may be difficult to clear sufficient amounts of urea with this method, however, unless continuous PD is used.

Hemodialysis (HD) requires the presence of specially trained staff, intensive patient monitoring, some degree of patient anticoagulation, and placement of a large bore central venous catheter. These catheters may cause peripheral emboli, arterial thrombosis, or dissection. HD does, however, have the ability to remove large amounts of intravascular volume and to correct electrolyte abnormalities rapidly. It is also easily performed in patients who have contraindications to PD.

CAVH and CAVHD are options for patients who cannot tolerate conventional HD or PD. Both CAVH and CAVHD require an arterial and venous cannula, and

flow is dependent on the patient's arterial blood pressure. CAVHD uses dialysate for better clearance of urea and nitrogenous waste, whereas CAVH accomplishes ultrafiltration with simple diffusion. The major advantage is the rapid rate of ultrafiltration, which allows the removal of large amounts of fluid. With the addition of dialysate, the rate of urea clearance is significantly greater than that obtained with PD or HD.

With these general principles in mind, some specific indications merit consideration. Most surgical patients with ARF are hypermetabolic with high protein turnover and high BUN levels. It can be difficult to maintain BUN levels less than 100 mg per dl with standard intermittent HD. CAVH may also prove inadequate for these patients with the inability to clear large amounts of solute. PD is usually adequate therapy for children since the solute load is less (because of reduced patient size).

Volume excess is a more frequent indication for dialysis in the surgical patient with ARF than uremia. HD can achieve effective diuresis, but the patient is at risk of developing the disequilibrium syndrome since fluid is so rapidly removed during periods of HD. CAVH and CAVHD permit a slower and perhaps more effective means of diuresis with the ability to continually adjust the patient's volume status. This means does not appear to affect patient outcome, however. In the largest series comparing these modalities, Bellomo and Boyce found the patients receiving CAVH and CAVHD to have greater hemodynamic stability and lower BUN levels but no survival advantage when compared with patients receiving standard HD.

Institution of dialysis is indicated when patients have symptoms of uremia, BUN levels greater than 100 mg per dl, hyperkalemia, acidosis, fluid overload (unresponsive to diuretics), pericardial rub, or gastrointestinal hemorrhage attributable to uremia. Despite these indications, there is controversy concerning when to begin the procedure. This issue may be better understood when remembering that for the patient with end-stage renal disease, the goal is to maintain the patient off dialysis as long as possible. This goal is a direct contradiction to the therapeutic goal of treatment for ARF, which is to minimize

uremic complications. Supporting the need for early, aggressive dialysis is the evidence that early dialysis may actually improve survival.

Without obvious symptoms of uremia, the patient's volume status, BUN, serum electrolytes, and acid base balance, determine the frequency and duration of dialysis. Current recommendations are to dialyze to keep the BUN less than 100 mg per dl. For most patients with ARF, renal recovery occurs within four to six weeks and dialysis can then be terminated. If the need for dialysis persists beyond this period, chronic renal failure is assumed.

Outcome

When examining instances of ARF and predicting prognosis based on published data, one must remember ARF is not a disease but rather a syndrome from multiple causes and is heavily influenced by the mortality of the underlying disease. Recent studies have examined whether the need for dialysis influences patient survival, and this issue remains unresolved. In the reported multivariate analyses, risk factors such as hemodynamic instability, respiratory failure requiring mechanical ventilation, gastrointestinal dysfunction, sepsis, and congestive heart failure have been evaluated when occurring in patients requiring dialysis for ARF. Survival when all risk factors were present has been reported as only 6 percent. This finding is best interpreted as reflecting the influence of multiple system organ failure on the mortality from this syndrome.

Summary

ARF remains a frequently occurring serious complication for the hospitalized patient. Treatment should be focused on preventing its occurrence and minimizing its extent through careful patient monitoring and adequate hydration. The underlying cause should be eliminated as rapidly as possible, and the patient supported with the aggressive use of nutrition, fluids, pressors, and dialysis when necessary. The clinical application of growth factors, cytokine inhibitors, and oxygen-free radical scavengers to accelerate renal repair and to promote functional recovery remains an active area of investigation.

Suggested Readings

Abul-Ezz SR, Walker PD, Shah SV. Role of glutathione in an animal model of myoglobinuric acute renal failure. *Nat Acad Sci* 88:9833, 1991.

Bellomo R, Boyce N. Acute continuous hemodiafiltration: A prospective study of 110 patients and a review of the literature. *Am J Kidney Dis* 21:508, 1993.

Braam B, et al. Relevance of tubuloglomerular feedback mechanism in pathophysiology of acute renal failure. *J Am Soc Nephrol* 4:1257, 1993.

Brezis M, Epstein FH. Cellular mechanisms of acute ischemic injury in the kidney. *Annu Rev Med* 44:27, 1993.

Compher C, Mullen JL, Barker CF. Nutritional support in renal failure. *Surg Clin North Am* 71(3):597, 1991.

Dolson GM. Electrolyte abnormalities before and after the onset of acute renal failure. *Miner Electrolyte Metab* 17:133, 1991.

Druml W. Metabolic alterations in acute renal failure. Contrib Nephrol 98:59, 1992.

Duke GJ, Briedis JH, Weaver RA. Renal support in critically ill patients: low dose dopamine or low dose dobutamine? *Crit Care Med* 22:1919, 1994.

Epstein M. Calcium antagonist and the kidney: implications for renal protection. *Am J Hypertens* 6:251S, 1993.

Espinel CH. Diagnosis of acute and chronic renal failure. *Clin Lab Med* 13:89, 1993.

Faber M, et al. The differential diagnosis of acute renal failure. In JM Lazarus, BM Brenner (eds.) *Acute Renal Failure*. New York: Churchill-Livingstone 1993.

Finn WF. Diagnosis and management of acute tubular necrosis. *Med Clin North Am* 74:873, 1990.

Fischereder M, Trick W, Nath KA. Therapeutic strategies in the prevention of acute renal failure. *Sem Nephr* 14:41, 1994.

Flancbaum L, Choban P, Dasta J. Quantitative effect on low dose dopamine and urine output in oliguric surgical intensive care unit patients. *Crit Care Med* 20:S21, 1992.

Greene EL, Paller MS: Oxygen free radicals in acute renal failure. *Miner Electrolyte Metab* 17:124, 1991.

Hays S. Southwestern medical conference: ischemic acute renal failure. *Am J Med Sci* 304:93, 1992.

Humes DH. Potential molecular treatment for acute renal failure. *Cleve Clin J Med* 60:166, 1993.

Kellen M, et al. Predictive and diagnostic tests of renal failure: a review. *Anesth Analg* 78:134, 1994.

Kellerman PS. Perioperative care of the renal patient. *Arch Int Med* 154:1674, 1994.

Mehta RL. Therapeutic alternatives to renal replacement for critically ill patients in acute renal failure. *Sem Nephr* 14:64, 1994.

Narayanan S. Renal biochemistry and physiology: pathophysiology and analytical perspective. *Adv Clin Chem* 29:121, 1992.

Novis BK, et al. Association of perioperative risk factors with postoperative acute renal failure. *Anesth Analg* 78:143, 1994.

Racusen LC. Biology of disease: alterations in tubular epithelial cell adhesion and mechanisms of acute renal failure. *Lab Invest* 67:158, 1992.

Rahn KH. Acute disturbances of renal function. *Chest* 100:197s, 1991.

Rigden SP, Dillon MJ, Kind P. The beneficial effect of mannitol on postoperative renal function in children undergoing cardiopulmonary bypass surgery. *Clin Nephrol* 21:148, 1984.

Robert S, Zarowitz BJ. Is there a reliable index of glomerular filtration rate in critically ill patients? *DICP* 25:169, 1991.

Ron D, Taitelman V, Michaelson M. Prevention of acute renal failure in traumatic rhabdomyolysis. *Arch Int Med* 144:277, 1984.

Salahudeen AK, Clark EC, Nath KA. Hydrogen peroxide induced renal injury: a protective role for pyruvate in vitro and in vivo. *J Clin Invest* 88:1886, 1991.

Sandin R. Kidney function in shock. *Acta Anaesth Scand* 37:14, 1993.

Shilliday I, Allison MEM. Diuretics in acute renal failure. *Renal Failure* 16:3, 1994.

Stein JH. Acute renal failure: lessons from pathophysiology. *West J Med* 156:176, 1992.

Weinberg JM. The cell biology of ischemic renal injury. *Kidney Int* 39:475, 1991.

Weinberg JM. The effects of amino acids on ischemia and toxic injury to the kidney. Seminars in *Nephrology* 10:491, 1990.

9

Perioperative Antimicrobial Prophylaxis

Timothy D. Jacob   Richard L. Simmons

History and Epidemiology of Wound Infections

Elective surgery became possible in the nineteenth century in part because of increased success in the prevention of wound infections. This success was afforded by a better understanding of the cause of these infections. In 1546, the Italian physician Girolomo Fracastoro postulated that contagious diseases were caused by invisible organisms. In 1676, while attempting to refine the microscope, Antonj van Leeuwenhoek discovered microscopic organisms he termed "animalcules." Unfortunately, it was not until 1847 that Ignacz Semmelweis associated these organisms with infection. At the Allgemeines Krankenhaus of the University of Vienna, he made three observations related to puerperal fever: 1) the incidence was ten times higher on the ward attended by people performing daily autopsies (obstetricians and students) than on the ward attended by midwives; 2) the incidence was very low in mothers who gave birth at home; and 3) it was associated with serious injury to the cervix and uterus during childbirth. He postulated that "invisible cadaver particles" existed; he went on to produce infections in rabbits by injecting them with purulent discharge from cadavers. By washing his hands with chlorine after autopsies, he was able to decrease the mortality from puerperal fever from 18.3 percent to as low as 3.8 percent.

Because of the overwhelming mortality from wound infections, surgery in the mid-nineteenth century was limited to amputations for gangrene, incision of abscesses, and excision of infected cysts. Lister implemented a system of antisepsis because of his conviction that inflammation occurred only after an insult to normal tissue and Pasteur's germ theory that infection was caused by minute particles or germs on airborne dust. In 1870, Lister reported a decrease in mortality for amputation from 45.7 percent before antisepsis (1864–1866) to 15 percent with antiseptic technique (1867–1869). Armed with this success, he began to perform elective operations and ushered in a new era for surgery. The reasonable hypothesis was that the infection rate was proportional to the number of organisms to which the wound was exposed.

Refinements in antisepsis, such as steam sterilization used by Koch in 1882 and the rubber gloves introduced by Halstead in 1894, were implemented, but infections continued to be the major cause of operative morbidity and mortality. Site-specific infection rates ranged from as low as 5 percent for elective gastroduodenal operations to as high as 40 percent for colorectal operations and 49 percent for operations for upper gastrointestinal hemorrhage (Ta-

Table 9-1. Site-specific Infection Rates Without Antimicrobial Coverage

Site of Operation	Patients (No.)	Infected Wounds (No.)	Rate of Wound Infection (%)
Colorectal	1449	580	40
Appendix			
Normal	176	24	14
Inflamed	379	60	16
Gangrenous	149	83	56
Gastroduodenal, not specified	252	69	27
Duodenal ulcer			
Elective	165	8	5
Obstructed	50	8	16
Perforated	45	8	18
Gastric ulcer	66	15	23
Gastric tumor	61	19	31
Upper gastrointestinal hemorrhage	41	20	49
Cholecystectomy; risk factors			
Not specified	763	115	15
Present	97	20	30
Absent	81	10	13
Vascular	517	66	13
Head and neck	176	80	45

From Ludwig KA, Carlson MA, Condon RE. Prophylactic antibiotics in surgery. *Annu Rev Med* 44:385, 1993. Reproduced with permission, from the *Annual Review of Medicine*, Vol. 44, © 1993, by Annual Reviews Inc.

ble 9-1). In the 1950s, the National Research Council (NRC) attempted to stratify the risk of infection by classifying operative wounds in terms of the degree of expected bacterial contamination: 1) clean; 2) clean-contaminated; 3) contaminated; and 4) dirty and infected (Table 9-2). This classification has continued to have usefulness in the identification of risk factors for postoperative infections. In the 1970s, Cruse and Foord performed a long-term prospective study of 62,939 wounds at the Foothills Hospital in Calgary. They noted an overall infection rate of 4.7 percent (clean: 1.5%, clean-contaminated: 7.7%, contaminated: 15.2%, and dirty: 40%); wound infections added 10.1 days to the hospital stay. Other risk factors were found to play a role as well—a hexachlo-

Table 9-2. National Research Council's Classification of Operative Relation of Contamination and Increasing Risk of Infection

Clean
  Nontraumatic
  No inflammation encountered
  No break in technique
  Respiratory, alimentary, genitourinary tracts not entered
Clean-Contaminated
  Gastrointestinal or respiratory tract entered without significant spillage
  Appendectomy
  Oropharynx entered
  Vagina entered
  Genitourinary tract entered in absence of infected urine
  Biliary tract entered in absence of infected bile
  Minor break in technique
Contaminated
  Major break in technique
  Gross spillage from gastrointestinal tract
  Traumatic wound, fresh
  Entrance of genitourinary or biliary tract in presence of infected urine or bile
Dirty and infected
  Acute bacterial inflammation encountered, without pus
  Transection of "clean" tissue for the purpose of surgical access to a collection of pus
  Traumatic wound with retained devitalized tissue, foreign bodies, fecal contamination, or delayed treatment, or from dirty source

From Cruse PJE. Wound Infections: Epidemiology and Clinical Characteristics. In RJ Howard and RL Simmons (eds.), *Surgical Infectious Diseases* (2nd ed.). Norwalk: Appleton & Lange, 1988.

rophene shower reduced the infection rate after clean operations from 2.1 to 2.3 percent; shaving increased infection rates to 2.5 percent when compared with clipping the operative field (1.7%), or leaving it unshaven (0.9%); an incidental appendectomy during cholecystectomy decreased the infection rate to 4.5 from 1.4 percent. Other risk factors identified were prolonged preoperative stay (1 day: 1.2%; 1 week: 2.1%; >2 weeks: 3.4%), age greater than 66 years, use of electrocautery, diabetes mellitus, obesity, malnutrition, and the use of drains placed through the wound.

Based on these findings, surveillance programs were begun in the 1970s and 1980s to provide informational feedback to operating surgeons to encourage them to take steps to decrease their infection rates. In 1990, Olson and Lee reported a 10-year surveillance program, including 1032 wound infections in 40,915 operations, in which wound infection rates were decreased 38 to 56 percent with an estimated savings of $3 million.

Haley and colleagues were the first to utilize modern epidemiologic methods and multivariate statistical analyses to study the pathogenesis of operative wound infection. Carried out as part of the Center for Disease Control (CDC) Study on the Efficacy of Nosocomial Infection Control (SENIC), these studies analyzed multiple risk factors in 58,498 patients undergoing operations in 1970. An attempt was made to identify a simple index that would predict patients at high risk for wound infection. The validity of the index was prospectively tested on 59,352 patients undergoing surgical operations between 1975 and 1976. The index measured the risks in terms of both patient susceptibility and degree of wound contamination. Operations at high risk of infection proved to be procedures involving the abdomen, operations lasting greater than two hours, and procedures traditionally classified as either contaminated or dirty. Patients most susceptible to infection were identified as having more than three discharge diagnoses, aside from diagnoses reflecting surgical wound infections. By using these variables, they were able to identify 54 percent of the patients experiencing 90 percent of the complications. The result gave firm statistical support for the idea, now accepted, that certain patients were at high

risk for wound infection as a consequence of pre-existing or concurrent conditions. Thus, infection was not simply the result of excessive wound contamination or "poor" surgical technique.

In 1991, Culver and colleagues revised the SENIC risk index to include additional high risks: (1) a patient with an American Society of Anesthesiologists preoperative assessment score of 3, 4, or 5; (2) an operation classified as contaminated or dirty; and (3) an operation lasting longer than the seventy-fifth percentile for that given procedure. In 84,691 operations, 2376 surgical wound infections occurred. Patients with the same number of risk factors had roughly the same risk of wound infection irrespective of the NRC wound classification (0: 1.5%, 1: 2.9%, 2: 6.8%, and 3: 13%). The risk index also predicted which patients were at risk for postoperative infections remote from the wound, such as pneumonias and urinary tract infections. Furthermore, patients with a risk index of 1, 2, or 3 were more than twice as likely to develop a secondary bloodstream infection following a primary wound infection (0: 2.3%, 1: 5.2%, 2: 7.8%, and 3: 8.3%). This SENIC risk index is now thought to be a much better predictor than the traditional NRC wound classification.

Although these indices of risk were initially formulated to more clearly identify patients in whom surveillance might diminish the incidence of wound infection, they also became useful in identifying patients who would benefit most from the administration of prophylactic antibiotics. The economic factors have focused the need even more sharply. Postoperative wound sepsis continues to account for 14 percent of adverse events in hospitalized patients and 24 percent of an estimated 2 million annual nosocomial infections. As a consequence, antibiotics are now the most prescribed medications from hospital formularies, with prophylaxis accounting for 30 percent of these prescriptions.

In order to accurately assess the impact of surveillance and prophylactic antibiotic use on the incidence of surgical wound infection, the CDC has had to establish case definitions. As currently defined, surgical site infections (SSIs) are infections occurring within 30 days of operation if no prostheses or other foreign body was implanted. The period was extended to one year after operation if prostheses were used. SSIs are subclassified as superficial incisional SSI, deep incisional SSI, organ or space SSI, and SSIs involving more than one specific site. Detailed descriptions of these definitions may be found in Table 9-3.

Prophylaxis of Wound Infection

The establishment of a wound infection is dependent on the number and virulence of the bacteria inoculated and the resistance of traumatized host tissue. Host resistance to infection is the consequence not only of systemic factors but also of local factors. Many investigators have found that a smaller bacterial inoculum is required to produce an infection if even a single silk suture is used in the wound.

The traditional NRC wound classification adapted by the NRC stratifies patients based on the exposure of the wound to increasing concentrations of bacteria. Indeed, bacterial virulence is not a part of the system (Table 9-2). With a few exceptions, the etiologic microbes are exactly the ones one might expect to find inoculated into wounds at certain sites (Table 9-4). Thus, clean operations in which only the skin is broken result in infections caused by the organisms on the patient's skin (i.e., *Staphylococcus* species). Only rarely are hematogenous infections found at SSI. Conversely, SSI following operations during which a mucosal barrier was breached are caused by organisms that colonize that mucosal surface; such infections will generally contain many organisms, including both aerobic and anaerobic species.

The degree of contamination is only one factor in the pathogenesis of SSI. Extensive necrosis, fluid accumulation, hematoma formation, and fibrin deposition tend to isolate the inoculated bacteria from the inflammatory cells, so that phagocytic killing is impeded. In addition, damaged tissue provides a rich nutrient culture medium. In theory, premature or delayed administration of systemic prophylactic antibiotics will result in subeffective concentrations of drug within such damaged and poorly perfused tissue, allowing survival and proliferation of the bacteria. Similarly, the inability to deliver antibiotics to tissue underperfused because of shock,

Table 9-3. Centers for Disease Control Surgical Site Infection (SSI) Definitions

For surveillance classification purposes, SSIs are divided into *incisional SSIs* and *organ/space SSIs*. Incisional SSIs are further classified as involving only the skin and subcutaneous tissue (*superficial incisional SSIs*) or involving deep soft tissues (e.g., fascial and muscle layers) of the incision (*deep incisional SSIs*). Organ/space SSIs involve any part of the anatomy (organs or spaces) other than the incision opened or manipulated during the operative procedure.

Superficial Incisional SSI
Superficial incisional SSIs must meet the following criteria: infection occurs within 30 days after the operative procedure *and* involves only skin or subcutaneous tissue of the incision, *and* at least *one* of the following is present:
1. Purulent drainage from the superficial incision.
2. Organisms isolated from an aseptically obtained culture of fluid or tissue from the superficial incision.
3. At least one of the following signs or symptoms of infection—pain or tenderness, localized swelling, redness, or heat—*and* superficial incision is deliberately opened by surgeon, *unless* culture of incision is negative.
4. Diagnosis of superficial incisional SSI by the surgeon or attending physician.

The following are *not* reported as superficial incisional SSI: (1) stitch abscess (minimal inflammation and discharge confined to the points of suture penetration); (2) infection of an episiotomy or a neonate's circumcision site[a] (episiotomy and circumcision are not considered National Nosocomial Infection Surveillance System (NNISS) operative procedures, (3) infected burn wound[a], and (4) incisional SSI that extends into the fascial and muscle layers (see *Deep Incisional SSI*).

Deep Incisional SSI
Deep incisional SSIs must meet the following criteria: infection occurs within 30 days after the operative procedure if no implant[b] is left in place or within 1 year if implant is in place and the infection appears to be related to the operative procedure, *and* infection involves deep soft tissues (e.g., fascial and muscle layers) of the incision, *and* at least one of the following is present:
1. Purulent drainage from the deep incision but not from the organ/space component of the surgical site.
2. A deep incision spontaneously dehisces or is deliberately opened by a surgeon when the patient has at least one of the following signs or symptoms: fever (>30°C), localized pain, or tenderness, unless culture of the incision is negative.
3. An abscess or other evidence of infection involving the deep incision is found on direct examination, during reoperation, or by histopathologic or radiologic examination.
4. Diagnosis of a deep incisional SSI by a surgeon or attending physician.

Organ or Space SSI
An organ or space SSI involves any part of the anatomy other than the incision, opened or manipulated during the operative procedure. Specific sites are assigned to organ or space SSIs to identify the location of the infection. Organ or space SSIs must meet the following criteria: infection occurs within 30 days after the operative procedure if no implant is left in place or within 1 year if implant is in place and the infection appears to be related to the operative procedure *and* infection involves any part of the anatomy (e.g., organs or spaces) other than the incision opened or manipulated during the operative procedure, *and* at least *one* of the following is present:
1. Purulent drainage from a drain that is placed through a stab wound[c] into the organ or space.
2. Organisms isolated from an aseptically obtained culture of fluid or tissue in the organ or space.
3. An abscess or other evidence of infection involving the organ or space on direct examination, during reoperation, or by histopathologic or radiologic examination.
4. Diagnosis of an organ or space SSI by a surgeon or attending physician.

SSI Involving More Than One Specific Site
1. Infection that involves *both* superficial and deep incision sites is classified as deep incisional SSI.
2. Occasionally an organ or space infection drains through the incision. Such infection generally does not involve reoperation and is considered a complication of the incision. It is therefore classified as deep incisional SSI.

[a]Specific criteria are used for infected episiotomy and circumcision sites and for burn wounds.
[b]An implant is defined as a nonhuman-derived implantable foreign body (e.g., prosthetic heart valve, nonhuman vascular graft, mechanical heart, or hip prosthesis) that is permanently placed in a patient during operation.
[c]If the area around a stab wound becomes infected, it is not an SSI. It is considered a skin or soft-tissue infection, depending on its depth.
From Horan TC, et al. CDC definitions of nosocomial surgical site infections, 1992: a modification of CDC definitions of surgical wound infections. *Am J Infect Control* 20:271, 1992. Reproduced with permission.

Table 9-4. Pathogenic Bacteria
Commonly Found at Various Body Sites

Location	Pathogens
Nose	*Staphylococcus aureus*, pneumococci, meningococci
Upper respiratory	*Pneumococcus, H. influenzae*
Mouth/ pharynx	*Pneumococcus*, streptococci (χ, β), *E. coli, Bacteroides* oralis, *Bacteroides melaninogenicus, Fusobacterium*, peptostreptococci, *Actinomyces*
Colon	*E. coli, Klebsiella, Enterobacter, B. fragilis, Bacteroides* sp., peptostreptococci, clostridia
Biliary tract	*E. coli, Klebsiella, Proteus*, clostridia
Urinary tract	*E. coli, Klebsiella, Proteus, Enterobacter*
Skin	*Staphylococcus aureus, Staphylococcus epidermidis, Propionibacterium acnes*, diphtheroids
Vagina	Streptococci, staphylococci, *E. coli*, gonococcus, peptostreptococci, *Bacteroides* sp.

From Ludwig KA, Carlson MA, Condon RE. Prophylactic antibiotics in surgery. *Annu Rev Med* 44:385, 1993. Reproduced with permission.

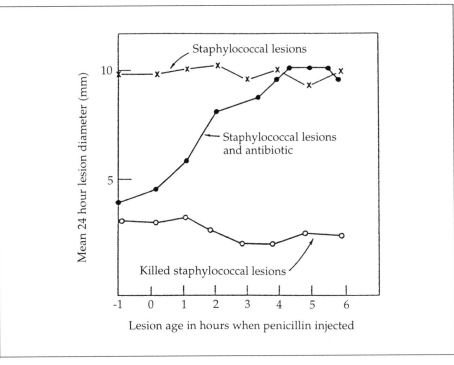

Fig. 9-1. Decreasing effect of penicillin on lesion diameter as lesion age on penicillin injection increases. (From Burke JF. The effective period of preventive antibiotic action in experimental incisions and dermal lesions. Surgery *50:161, 1961. Reproduced with permission.)*

hypoxia, or vasoconstriction renders systemic antibiotic prophylaxis less effective. In order to avoid these problems, rational prophylaxis is designed to deliver the antibiotic to undamaged tissue before contamination occurs. Systemic antibiotics should be administered immediately before the start of the procedure and adequate blood levels maintained until the end of the operation. Burke and colleagues first showed this critical relationship in a model in which bacteria were inoculated in the skin of guinea pigs. Penicillin given greater than three hours after inoculation provided no appreciable benefit; antibiotics were most effective when given before the inoculum with a diminishing response noted thereafter (Fig. 9-1).

Classen and Burke and colleagues later confirmed these findings in humans, prospectively evaluating 2847 patients undergoing clean or clean-contaminated procedures. Patients receiving preoperative or perioperative antibiotics had significantly fewer infections than patients receiving antibiotics either too early or postoperatively (pre: 0.6%, peri: 1.4%, early: 3.8%,

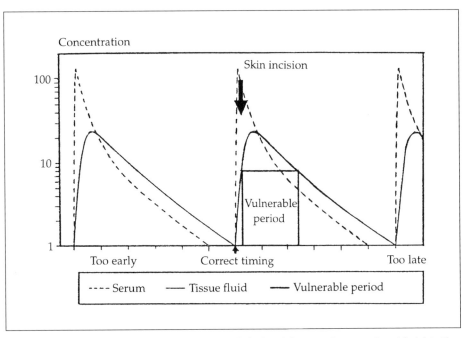

Fig. 9-2. The relation between timing of antibiotic prophylaxis and the start of an operation. Administration of the antibiotic needs to be properly timed so that effective serum and tissue concentrations are present during the vulnerable period when the wound is open and the tissues are subject to contamination. For antibiotics with a serum half-life of 1 to 4 hours, administration should occur as a bolus about 30 minutes before the skin incision, done most conveniently in conjunction with the induction of anesthesia. If given too early or too late, coverage during the vulnerable period will be inadequate. If the operation is longer than 4 hours, so that the vulnerable period is extended, the antibiotic should be redosed, with the second dose given 2 hours after the first dose. (From Wittmann DH, Condon RE. Prophylaxis of postoperative infections. Infection *19:S337, 1991. Reproduced with permission.)*

and late: 3.3%). When administered appropriately, antibiotics should be in serum and tissue fluid at adequate concentrations to prevent bacterial adherence to wounded tissue (Fig. 9-2).

Adequate prophylaxis can almost always be obtained with a single dose of antibiotics given during the induction of anesthesia. Whittmann and Condon summarized the results of 27 studies showing that single-dose prophylaxis was at least as good as, and frequently superior to, multiple-dose regimens. The level must be maintained, however, and if the level is permitted to fall, a higher rate of infection will be found. Prudent prophylaxis would be to redose patients during prolonged procedures (greater than double the half-life of the antibiotic), patients with a large blood loss, or patients requiring extracorporeal circulation (Fig. 9-3).

Traditionally, perioperative parenteral antibiotics have been used for prophylaxis against SSI because they allow the antibiotic to reach the tissue in adequate concentrations prior to incision. The bacteria are not able to adhere or to multiply, effectively stopping infection before its inception. Unfortunately, timing of administration is often incorrect. Classen and Burke and colleagues found that administration "on call to OR" often was much longer than anticipated and was associated with a much higher incidence of infection than when given in the operating room. They concluded that the most consistent timing was achieved with intravenous administration by the anesthetist just prior to induction of anesthesia (Fig. 9-4). This method is now accepted practice.

Patients in shock or who receive vasoconstricting agents are unlikely to have adequate tissue levels even if the antibiotics are administered in a timely fashion. Topical administration is a reasonable and cost-effective alternative to parenteral administration. Topical application consists of instilling antibiotic in the wound upon opening each tissue plane and at frequent intervals throughout the entire operation. It places control of the antibiotic administration in the hands of the surgeon, essentially eliminating timing errors. In many institutions this administration can be done directly through the surgical suite, eliminating pharmacy handling and infusion costs.

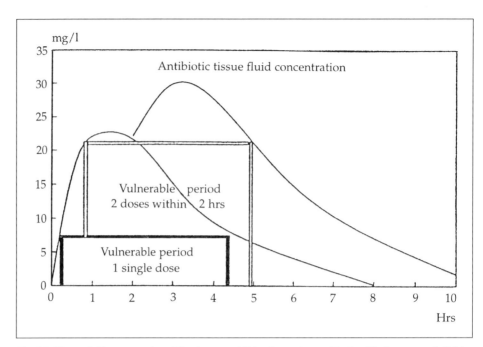

Fig. 9-3. Tissue fluid concentrations following two additive doses of an antibiotic with short serum half-life. The serum concentration is not shown. Note that the second dose is given 2 hours following the first dose to boost tissue concentrations. Maximal tissue saturation of an antibiotic with a half-life of approximately 1 hour is achieved and with most β-lactam antibiotics in the second hour following administration of a bolus injection. If the second dose of an antibiotic is given after 6 or 8 hours, most of the tissue compartment will be emptied and need to be refilled, and the high concentrations observed with a booster injection after 2 hours will not be attained. (From Wittmann DH, Condon RE. Prophylaxis of postoperative infections. Infection 19:S337, 1991. Reproduced with permission.)

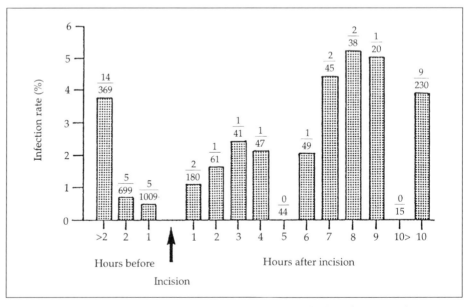

Fig. 9.4. Rates of surgical wound infection corresponding to the temporal relation between antibiotic administration and the start of surgery. The number of infections and the number of patients for each hourly interval appear as the numerator and denominator, respectively, of the fraction for that interval. The trend toward higher rates of infection for each hour that antibiotic administration was delayed after the surgical incision was significant (z score = 2.00; p < 0.05 by the Wilcoxon test). (From Classen DC, et al. The timing of prophylactic administration of antibiotics and the risk of surgical wound infection. N Engl J Med 326:281, 1992. Reprinted by permission of The New England Journal of Medicine © 1992, Massachusetts Medical Society.)

Table 9-5. Properties of an Ideal Topical
Antimicrobial Agent for Prophylaxis

Wide range of antimicrobial effect
Minimal local tissue irritation
Minimal systemic toxic effect
Minimal systemic absorption if toxicity is a
  hazard
Minimal allogenicity
Infrequent emergence of resistant microbial
  forms

From Malangoni MA. Chemoprophylaxis of Wound
Infections. In RJ Howard, RL Simmons (eds.), *Surgical
Infectious Diseases* (3rd ed.). Norwalk: Appleton &
Lange, 1995. p. 466. Reproduced with permission.

Topical administration is believed to be effective because it allows delivery of a highly concentrated antibiotic directly to the site of contamination. Malangoni recently reviewed this method. He points out the historical success of Jensen with topical sulfanilamide on open fractures (27% historical; 5% sulfanilamide) and the significant increase in survival of patients sustaining large burns with use of topical antibiotics. Multiple experimental studies have confirmed the effectiveness of this method in wounds potentially contaminated with almost any pyogenic organism because the concentrations of drug can be raised to very high levels, which tend to overcome resistant organisms.

Mora and Simmons reviewed the application of topical antibiotics in all types of surgical procedures and demonstrated significant improvement over placebo. Randomized clinical trials that accurately compare topical and parenteral antibiotics have not been done, but both are highly effective compared with the absence of any prophylaxis. Studies that add topical antibiotics to parenteral antibiotics do not show a significant difference except in experimental dirty wounds in which the combination may be of benefit. The properties of an ideal topical antimicrobial agent are listed in Table 9-5. In practice, a 0.1% solution of a first-generation cephalosporin is an excellent choice. This concentration will render almost all strains of pyogenic bacteria nonviable after 30 minutes. Aminoglycosides are frequently used, but they have two disadvantages—systemic absorption leads to toxicity, and anaerobes cannot be killed, regardless of concentrations.

All topically applied antibiotics will have some degree of systemic absorption, but in practice, systemic levels are too low to be responsible for their prophylactic effect. Indeed, a postulated advantage of topical prophylaxis is that systemic levels are so low that they are unlikely to alter endogenous flora on mucosal surfaces.

Complications

In selecting an antibiotic for prophylaxis, either parenteral or topical, the surgeon should choose the antibiotic that covers all of the expected bacterial flora and that has the lowest likelihood of toxicity. The most feared complications are anaphylaxis and death, which are most commonly associated with the beta-lactam antibiotics including the penicillins, cephalosporins, carbapenem, and monobactam. There is a 10 to 15 percent cross-reactivity between cephalosporins and penicillin, but there is no known cross-reactivity with aztreonam. Vancomycin occasionally produces red man syndrome—flushing, pruritus, chest pain, muscle spasm, and hypotension; this is not a true allergic reaction and does not require terminating the antibiotic, only decreasing the rate of administration and changing the mixing solution to normal saline. Of particular importance to surgeons is the knowledge that cephalosporins can occasionally cause hypoprothrombinemia and bleeding, but this result is unlikely with single-dose prophylaxis or topical application.

Nephrotoxicity and ototoxicity make aminoglycosides poor choices for prophylaxis. Furthermore, and more germane to perioperative use, is their ability to produce myoneural blockade and apnea when given concomitantly with muscle relaxants, particularly succinylcholine. A brief list of toxicities of commonly used antibiotics appears in Table 9-6.

Perhaps most dangerous, however, are the changes in patient and hospital bacterial flora that appear under the pressure of the heavy assault by antimicrobial agents in the environment. An increasing number of wound infections display multiply resistant organisms. Prophylactic antibiotics represent an important cause of this nosocomial antibiotic pressure. A recent survey by Widdison, Pope, and Brown demonstrated that greater than 90 percent of surgeons in the United Kingdom recom-

Table 9-6. Toxicities of Antibiotics Commonly Used for Prophylaxis

Antibiotic Class	Toxicity		
	Common	Occasional	Rare
Penicillins	Allergic reactions Rash Anaphylaxis Diarrhea	Hemolytic anemia Drug fever	Seizures Interstitial nephritis Electrolyte imbalance Marrow suppression
Cephalosporins	Thrombophlebitis Gastrointestinal symptoms	Allergic reactions Rash Serum sickness Anaphylaxis Drug Fever Coagulopathy Eosinophilia	Hemolytic anemia Pancytopenia Abnormal liver enzymes Interstitial nephritis Interstitial pneumonia Pseudomembranous colitis
Aminoglycosides	Nephrotoxicity Ototoxicity	Rash Nausea, vomiting	Myoneural blockade Apnea

Erythromycin		Gastrointestinal irritation
		Stomatitis
			Allergic reactions
			  Fever
			  Rash
			Colitis
			Coagulopathy

Clindamycin	Diarrhea Rash	Colitis Nausea, vomiting	Neutropenia
Vancomycin	Red man syndrome	Thrombophlebitis Chills and fever Ototoxicity	Nephrotoxicity Rash Neutropenia

From Page CP, et al. Antimicrobial prophylaxis for surgical wounds. Guidelines for clinical care. *Arch Surg* 128:79, 1993. Reproduced with permission. Copyright 1993, American Medical Association.

mend perioperative antibiotics in all clean-contaminated operations except noncardiac thoracic (63%). Olson and Lee reviewed a 10-year experience with 1032 wound infections in 40,915 operations and found that 32 to 64 percent of organisms cultured from the wounds were resistant to the prophylactic antibiotic used. Similarly, Garibaldi and colleagues found that 73 percent of bacteria cultured from postoperative wound infections were resistant to the antibiotic used for prophylaxis. In patients who did not receive perioperative antibiotics, only 11 percent had infecting organisms resistant to first- and second-generation cephalosporins. Furthermore, enterococci and *Pseudomonas aeruginosa* were grown almost exclusively from patients who received perioperative antibiotics. Finally, intraoperative cultures had a predictive value of only 32 percent with a false-positive rate of 82 percent, suggesting the organisms responsible for infection were not the predominant organism in the wound at the time of administration of the prophylactic antibiotic. These results are in synchrony with current paradigms of the pathogenesis of a wound infection. Polymicrobial contamination occurs whenever skin or mucosal barriers are breached. In the presence of prophylactic antibiotics, only the resistant organisms will survive. If the wound or the patient has compromised host defenses, the wound will become infected with the minor resistant subpopulations of bacteria even though the numbers of such organisms may be too few in the initial inoculum to be detected by clinical bacteriologic techniques.

Despite these findings, many surgeons believe that prophylaxis will not significantly change the hospital flora. Epidemiologists are not quite as confident. As pointed out earlier, 25 to 33 percent of all the antibiotics prescribed in a hospital are for prophylaxis. Only 27 percent of respondents in the United Kingdom survey recommended single-dose prophylaxis; the majority recommended at least a brief period of postoperative prophylaxis. More prolonged use is more likely to help select resistant organisms on the skin and mucosal surfaces, thereby increasing the risk of transmission of resistant organisms from patient-to-patient and to caregiver. Thus, it is not surprising that the organisms cultured from wound infections in patients receiving prophylactic antibiotics (*S. aureus:* 34%, enterococci: 17%, *E. coli:*

15%, *Enterobacter* sp.: 13%, and *Pseudomonas* sp.: 8%) are the same organisms that are responsible for all nosocomial infections caused by multiply resistant bacteria.

Of particular importance is the increasing incidence of methicillin-resistant *S. aureus* and *S. epidermidis* in wound infections after prophylaxis. This increase has been a particular problem in mediastinitis after sternotomies because such wounds are difficult to treat. The use of vancomycin to prevent and treat resistant staphylococci has been followed by the appearance of vancomycin-resistant *Enterococcus faecium* and the more common resistant *Enterococcus faecalis* species. Enterococcus infection after gastrointestinal perforation is particularly associated with cephalosporin therapy, and enterococcus is now the second most frequently reported cause of nosocomial infection. *Enterobacter* species has recently gained importance as a multiply resistant gram-negative nosocomial pathogen, similar to *Psuedomonas* sp. and *E. coli.* Candida is well established as a cause of superinfection, particularly in cases of intra-abdominal sepsis and perforation.

Pseudomembranous colitis, with its inherent morbidity and mortality, existed before antimicrobial prophylaxis but now is almost always associated with previous antibiotic use and the emergence of *Clostridium difficile.* Privitera and colleagues routinely tested patients undergoing elective procedures and receiving prophylaxis with either a cephalosporin, mezlocillin, or no antibiotic. Table 9-7 reveals that asymptomatic *C. difficile* was acquired more often in patients receiving broad-spectrum an-

tibiotics than in patients receiving narrow-spectrum agents and was not seen in patients undergoing elective operation without antibiotic prophylaxis. Yee and colleagues found 20 patients with *C. difficile*–associated disease following use of prophylactic antibiotics; 12 of these patients received antibiotics for less than 24 hours. The actual incidence of pseudomembranous colitis is not well established, however. Nevertheless, *C. difficile* is maintained within the hospitalized population—a situation partly caused by the "pressure" applied through the use of antibiotic prophylaxis.

Patient Selection

Who then should receive prophylactic antibiotics? Dirty wounds are considered infected and require antibiotic treatment, not prophylaxis. Contaminated wounds are at high risk for wound infection and warrant prophylaxis. Until recently, it was the consensus that clean-contaminated operations and clean operations in high-risk patients or patients requiring prostheses should be prophylaxed, but that clean operations in low-risk patients should not.

Clean Surgery

In 1990, Platt and colleagues published the results of a randomized, double-blinded trial of 1218 patients undergoing clean operations (606 breast, 612 hernia). The trial compared a single perioperative dose of cefonicid with placebo. They found 48 per-

Table 9-7. Incidence of *C. Difficile* and Cytotoxin
After Injection of a Single Dose of Different Antibiotics

Antibiotic	Number of Patients			
	Total	Evaluable	Colonized (%)	Toxin Positive (%)
Cefazolin	14	14	2 (14.3)	2 (14.3)
Cefoxitin	14	12	1 (8.3)	1 (8.3)
Cefotetan	21	20	4 (20.0)	4 (20.0)
Cefoperazone	17	16	7 (43.7)	4 (25.0)
Cefriaxone	12	12	3 (25.0)	3 (25.0)
All cephalosporins	78	74	17 (23.0)	14 (18.9)
Mezlocillin	30	30	1 (3.3)	1 (3.3)
All antibiotics	108	104	18 (17.3)	15 (14.4)
Controls	15	15	0	0

From Privitera G, et al. Prospective study of *Clostridium difficile* intestinal colonization and disease following single-dose antibiotic prophylaxis in surgery. *Antimicrob Agents Chemother* 35:208, 1991. Reproduced with permission.

cent fewer probable or definite postoperative infections, 51 percent fewer definite wound infections, 57 percent fewer wounds with purulent drainage, and 60 percent fewer urinary tract infections. *S. aureus* was the most common isolate (78%), but patients receiving cefonicid had 51 percent fewer *S. aureus* isolates. Prophylaxis was deemed cost-effective. Both breast and hernia surgical procedures appeared to benefit from administration of prophylactic cefonicid, but an inadequate number of patients were reported to find statistical significance when the analysis compared the results within the groups. Criticisms have also been raised about an inordinately high rate of infection in the placebo group. Data from other less-well-followed patient populations is frequently invoked. What Platt's study showed was that most wound complications, early and late, major and minor, were reduced by a single dose of prophylactic antibiotics directed primarily against skin pathogens. This result is what would be expected from the experimental data. However, the data is not strong enough to suggest that every hernia or breast biopsy is at risk for wound complications, only that prophylactic antibiotics will decrease the incidence.

In contrast, Gilbert and Felton found no significant difference with prophylactic antibiotics when they prospectively analyzed 2493 inguinal herniographies with and without mesh. Their data showed trends suggesting certain subgroups might benefit: patients greater than 60 years old, who accounted for 70 percent of all infections, and recurrent repairs with mesh (2.2 vs. 0.9%). They also concluded that wound infections could generally be treated conservatively and in no patient was removal of the mesh necessary. They concluded the expense of prophylactic antibiotics was not warranted in hernia repair.

Vascular Surgery

Because of the significant morbidity associated with wound infection and the potential for graft infection or mycotic aneursym formation, prophylactic antibiotics are generally recommended in vascular surgery despite relatively low incidences of infection (aortofemoral: 1 to 3%, femoral-popliteal: 2 to 4%, extra-anatomic: 1–

3%, and carotid and upper extremity: <1%). These rates are increased with subcutaneous routing, groin incisions, emergent procedures, early reoperation, and noninfectious early wound complications.

Most authors believe that the infecting organism enters the wound at the time of operation so that prosthetic grafts are contaminated at the time of insertion. Once the graft is incorporated and has an established pseudointima, it is relatively resistant to bacterial infection. The morbidity of limb loss and mortality of an infected prosthetic vascular graft indicate that prophylaxis is in order. There is no data in support of the idea that antibiotic prophylaxis should be prolonged beyond the immediate perioperative period. Hopkins' review discusses the benefits of topical or parenteral administration of antibiotics, citing Pitt and colleagues using cephradine (1977–1979—0/100 IV or topical; 3/59 IV and topical; 14/62 placebo), Hasselgren and colleagues using cefuroxime (1984—1 day 3.8%; 3 days 4.3%; placebo 16.7%), and Kaiser and colleagues using cefazolin 1 g IV on call to operating room and every 6 hours for 4 doses (placebo 6.8%; cefazolin 0.9%). In Kaiser's study, the benefit extended to all classes of severity of infection with no deep infections in the cefazolin group. Hopkins postulates that in vascular surgery, cost alone justifies prophylaxis even at an infection rate of 0.5 percent. Topical prophylaxis, by eliminating intravenous and pharmacy charges, would be less expensive and apparently no less effective.

Cardiothoracic Surgery

Evidence for use of prophylactic antibiotics in noncardiac thoracic operations is equivocal. Pulmonary and pleural infections are more morbid complications than wound infection, and most prophylactic regimens investigated have considered and directed their antibiotic selection toward these complications. Hopkins reviewed five studies addressing antibiotic use in pulmonary resection and found no clear benefit in reducing wound infection, but did see a nonsignificant trend toward benefit in overall infections. Fallon and Wears performed a meta-analysis of six clinical trials assessing routine prophylaxis for tube thoracostomies performed for trauma. Prophylactic antibiotics de-

creased the risk of empyema by a factor of five and had a significant effect on all infectious complications. First- or second-generation cephalosporins should be adequate even though a variety of gram-negative and gram-positive organisms must be considered.

Despite a low incidence of wound infection in cardiac operations, prophylactic antibiotics are used because of the significant morbidity and mortality of mediastinitis. Cephalosporins are usually used to cover the most common contaminants—*S. aureus* and *S. epidermidis*. Patients will require redosing during the procedure because of blood loss and dilution in the external bypass circuit. Many cardiac surgeons continue antibiotics after the perioperative period. LoCicero surveyed U.S. surgeons and found the majority administered antibiotics for at least 48 hours (1 day: 17.4%, 2 days: 54.6%, and 3 days: 16.7%). Still, other surgeons continue prophylaxis until drains and lines are removed. This prolonged administration has no proven benefit and may cause environmental pressure on cardiac wards, selecting out resistant organisms. Vancomycin prophylaxis, which has been shown to be more toxic than cephalosporin prophylaxis, may then be required in hospitals with high rates of methicillin-resistant *Staphylococcus aureus* (MRSA) and methicillin-resistant *Staphylococcus aureus* (MRSE) colonization and infection.

Head and Neck Surgery

Head and neck operations are either clean (not penetrating the mucosa) or clean-contaminated. In addition to normal skin flora, surgeons performing operations of the head and neck involving penetration of the mucosa must consider anaerobes and aerobic cocci of the oropharynx. Most infections are polymicrobial (88–96%) and have a high incidence of anaerobes. Patients at increased risk for these infections have higher staged tumors with positive lymph nodes, longer duration of surgery, preoperative radiation, and tracheostomies. A meta-analysis of major head and neck operations demonstrated a reduction in postoperative infections by 43 percent with perioperative antibiotics, and antibiotics effective against mouth anaerobes were superior to agents effective only against staphylococci (e.g., cefazolin alone). Gram-negative infections are not common after operations in this region. Perioperative prophylaxis with either clindamycin or a cephalosporin plus clindamycin is recommended for major reconstructions, maxillofacial fracture repair, orthognathic procedures, and craniofacial reconstructions. Topical antimicrobial irrigation of the operative field and mucosal surfaces has also been shown to be effective.

Esophageal and Gastric Surgery

The esophagus normally does not have a significant resident bacterial flora, but when diseased or obstructed it will become colonized with aerobic and anaerobic organisms from the oropharynx. Prophylaxis with a broad-spectrum cephalosporin is recommended at the time of operation. Technical factors plus the poor blood supply of the esophagus after dissection rather than the degree of bacterial colonization of the esophagus are believed to be the major causes of postoperative anastomotic leaks.

Like the esophagus, the stomach and proximal duodenum have a limited flora because the acid in the stomach functions to kill swallowed bacteria. Colonization with oral, skin, and coliform bacteria and candida occurs whenever gastric acidity is reduced by food, blood, antacids, or obstruction. Prophylaxis with single-dose cefazolin or another broad-spectrum cephalosporin is recommended, based on adequate concentrations being found in the blood, gastric mucosa, and subcutaneous tissue and on improved outcome in multiple clinical trials (Table 9-8). Patients undergoing morbid obesity operations may require a larger dose. Yeast become clinically significant only in aged patients or when large ulcerated tumors become infected. Candida found as the predominant flora after gastric perforation should be treated. When it is a minor component of a sparse flora after peptic perforation, it may be safely observed.

Biliary Surgery

The benefit of prophylactic antibiotics in biliary tract operations is well established.

Bactibilia is associated with a higher incidence of wound infection. Routine culturing of bile in noncomplicated cholecystectomies reveals 10 to 50 percent of these patients will have positive cultures. Common organisms grown from bile include *E. coli, Klebsiella, Enterococcus* sp., *Proteus*, and *Clostridia* sp. Patients with complicated disease, including cholecystitis, choledocholithiasis, common bile duct obstruction, and previous biliary tract surgery, and patients more than 70 years old are more likely to have positive cultures and are at high risk for postoperative wound infection. Chetlin and Elliott first showed benefit with the use of prophylactic intramuscular cephradine in these high-risk patients. The incidence of infection was decreased from 27 percent in the placebo group to 4 percent in the cephradine group. Even though 90 percent of the high-risk patients could be identified preoperatively, the high incidence of bactibilia in low-risk patients favors the use of single-dose prophylaxis in biliary tract operations. Table 9-9 summarizes the results of multiple studies using different antibi-

otics in biliary operations. Generally, 1 or 2 g of cefazolin prior to incision is adequate. Ongoing acute cholecystitis or cholangitis requires treatment, not prophylaxis.

Bowel Surgery

Operations on the small bowel carry a relatively low risk of infection, except when the bowel is obstructed or gangrenous. When obstructed, the small bowel becomes increasingly colonized with fecal organisms. A sixfold increase in septic complications is seen with simple decompression via an enterotomy. Therefore, use of a second-generation cephalosporin such as cefoxitin is recommended for prophylaxis. In instances of perforation or gangrene without gross perforation, the patient should be treated for peritonitis.

Appendectomy is performed under many different conditions under every NRC classification other than clean. It has varying incidences of infection: incidental ap-

Table 9-8. Antibiotic Prophylaxis in Gastroduodenal Operations

Prophylactic Agent(s)	Number of Studies	Number of Infections	Number of Operations	Rate of Infection (%)
Placebo	11	67	250	26.8
Penicillins	3	11	72	15.3
Cefuroxime	4	5	102	4.9
Aerobe/anaerobe combinations	4	16	378	4.2
Cephaloridine	2	2	54	3.7
Cefazolin or cefamandole	3	3	135	2.2

From Wittmann DH, Condon RE. Prophylaxis of postoperative infections. *Infection* 19:S337, 1991. Reproduced with permission.

Table 9-9. Antibiotic Prophylaxis in Biliary Operations

Prophylactic Agent	Number of Trials	Number of Patients	Infected Number	Infected Rate (%)
Cefotetan	1	90	13	14
Mezlocillin	2	359	24	7
Cefamandole	5	431	24	6
Gentamicin	2	202	11	5
Cefazolin	7	494	26	5
Cefonicid	2	99	4	4
Cefoxitin	2	92	3	3
Cefuroxime	5	353	10	3
Piperacillin	1	50	1	2
Cefotaxime	2	87	0	0

From Wittmann DH, Condon RE. Prophylaxis of postoperative infections. *Infection* 19:S337, 1991. Reproduced with permission.

pendectomy, 4 to 7 percent; appendicitis, 7 to 14 percent; gangrenous, 20 percent; perforated, 40 to 70 percent; and abscess, 94 percent. Perforated appendix and peri-appendiceal abscess are considered dirty and require treatment with antibiotics. Prophylactic antibiotics significantly decrease the rate of wound infection associated with nonperforated appendicitis or incidental appendectomy. Because enteric organisms, particularly *E. coli*, *Klebsiella*, *Enterobacter*, and *Bacteroides* sp. are commonly identified, use of a second-generation cephalosporin such as cefoxitin is most appropriate.

A surgical procedure on an unprepared colon is associated with one of the highest incidences of wound infection. Prophylaxis in elective cases requires mechanical removal of feculent material plus antimicrobial prophylaxis. Mechanical bowel preparation serves to eliminate the bulk stool but does not change the concentration of bacteria within the lumen; an infection rate of 35 to 45 percent was commonly reported for elective colonic resection, even after mechanical bowel preparation. Addition of three preoperative doses of neomycin and erythromycin base decreased this rate to 9 percent in a classic large Veterans' Administration cooperative study. Nichols has defined two separate colonic microflora, one related to the mucous lining and the other to the mucosa. He has pointed out that oral antibiotics are more effective when the antibiotics have anaerobic activity and that the quantity of micro-organisms is suppressed at the time of surgery. Studies have shown that significant intraluminal levels of neomycin and erythromycin and serum levels of erythromycin are present when the prep is performed properly. Theoretically, the intraluminal levels effectively decrease the quantity of bacteria in the mucin layer, whereas systemic levels are responsible for prophylaxis against the mucosa-related bacteria.

This finding has led many surgeons to add parenteral antibiotics to a mechanical prep and oral antibiotics. Use of parenteral antibiotics alone has proven beneficial in urgent operations on unprepared bowel or bowel mechanically cleansed on the table. Similarly, European surgeons had pioneered the use of mechanical bowel prep plus parenteral antibiotics without oral antibiotics. Success is dependent on choosing antibiotics with both anti-aerobic and anti-anaerobic activity. Effective regimens have included cefoxitin, cefotetan, metronidazole, or doxycycline alone or in combination with gentamicin. Thus, there is evidence that the benefit of systemic prophylaxis plus mechanical bowel prep is equivalent to the benefit of oral antibiotics and mechanical bowel prep. Figure 9-5 illustrates the results of Smith and colleagues comparing cultures in patients undergoing colon resections; maximal suppression was seen with the combination of mechanical prep plus oral and parenteral antibiotics. Clinical proof is not yet available that all three are necessary to significantly lower the wound complication rate. Table 9-10 lists Nichols' commonly used preoperative bowel preparations.

Obstetric and Gynecologic Surgery

Obstetric and gynecologic surgery has a relatively high incidence of infection and a large number of poorly constructed clinical trials. Cultures prior to infection are of little use because the large number of vaginal organisms make it difficult to distinguish pathogens from normal flora or contaminants (Table 9-11). Infections after hysterectomy can occur in the form of vaginal cuff cellulitis or abscess, parametrial

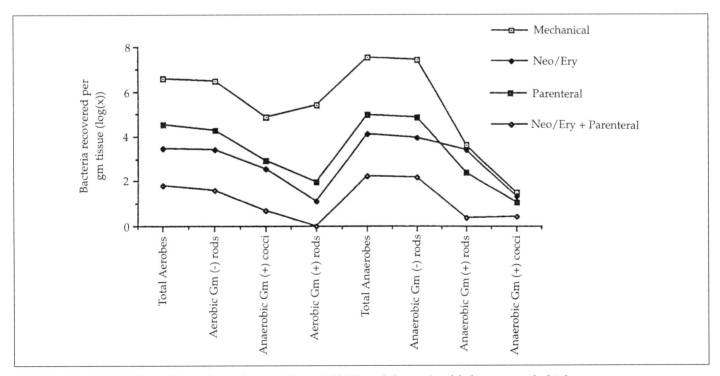

Fig. 9-5. Mucosal-associated bacterial counts (geometric means). (From Smith MB, et al. Suppression of the human mucosal-related colonic microflora with prophylactic parenteral and/or oral antibiotics. World J Surg *14:636, 1990. Reproduced with permission.)*

Table 9-10. Nichols' Approach to Preoperative Colon Preparation

SECOND DAY BEFORE SURGERY (AT HOME)

Dietary restriction: low-residue or liquid diet

Magnesium sulfate, 30 ml of a 50% solution (15 g) PO at 10 A.M., 2:00 P.M., and 6:00 P.M.

Enemas until clear in the evening

DAY OF HOSPITALIZATION (PREOPERATIVE DAY)

Admit in the morning

Clear liquid diet; IV fluids as needed

Magnesium sulfate in dosage as above at 10:00 A.M. and 2:00 P.M. *or*

Whole gut lavage with polyethylene glycol 1 L/hr for 2–4 hr until diarrhea effluent clear, before administration of oral antibiotic

No enemas

Neomycin and erythromycin base, 1 g each PO at 1:00 P.M., 2:00 P.M., and 11:00 P.M..

DAY OF SURGERY

Operation at 8:00 A.M.

Optional: One dose of antibiotic with aerobic-anaerobic activity given IV by anesthesia in the operation room just before incision

From Nichols RL. Rational Approach to the Use of Systemic Prophylactic Antibiotics in General Surgery. In RL Simmons, AO Udekwu (eds.), *Debates in Clinical Surgery.* Vol. 1. Chicago: Yearbook, 1990. Reproduced with permission.

Table 9-11. Potential Pathogens Recovered from Sites of Obstetric and Gynecologic Operations

Aerobic Bacteria	Anaerobic Bacteria
Gram-positive cocci	Gram-positive cocci
Enterococcus faecalis	*Peptostreptococcus* sp.
Streptococcus agalactiae	Gaffkya anaerobia
Streptococcus sp.	Gram-positive bacilli
Staphylococcus aureus	*Clostridium* sp.
Staphylococcus epidermidis	*Bifidobacterium* sp.
Gram-negative bacilli	Gram-negative cocci
Escherichia coli	*Veillonella parvula*
Enterobacter sp.	Gram-negative bacilli
Klebsiella sp.	*Bacteroides* sp.
Proteus sp.	*Bacteroides bivius*
Acinetobacter sp.	*Bacteroides fragilis*
Citrobacter sp.	*Bacteroides distasonis*
Pseudomonas sp.	*Bacteroides melaninogenicus*
Haemophilus influenzae	*Bacteroides ovatus*
Gram-positive bacilli	*Bacteroides thetaiotaomicron*
Diphtheroids	CDC GR 3452
	Fusobacterium sp.

From Hemsell DL. Prophylactic antibiotics in gynecologic and obstetric surgery. *Rev Infect Dis* 13:S821, 1991. Reproduced with permission.

phlegmon, pelvic abscess, and wound infection. Women undergoing vaginal hysterectomy are at higher risk than patients undergoing abdominal hysterectomy. Multiple studies have shown decreases in operative site infections with prophylactic antibiotics. Particular benefit has been seen in patients with low socioeconomic status, extremes of age, obesity, diabetes, preceding instrumentation, bacterial vaginosis, and trichomonal vaginitis. Present recommendations are for cefazolin IV unless a significant penicillin allergy is present, in which case either doxycycline or clindamycin may be substituted. Infections in cesarean section are caused by ascent of vaginal bacteria with labor, which is facilitated by membrane rupture. Recommendations are to administer 2 g of cefazolin or ampicillin after clamping and cutting of the umbilical cord. Failure may be predicted by culturing resistant organisms from the upper genital tract. A 50 to 70 percent reduction in wound infection and endometritis results from this prophylaxis. Topical antibiotic prophylaxis has been shown to be effective as well.

Common Misconceptions and Conclusions

Ehrenkranz recently analyzed common mistakes in the use of prophylactic antibiotics. Treatment with an antibiotic for ongoing infection does not eliminate the need for a perioperative dose of an antibiotic appropriate for the wound because insufficient concentrations may be achieved if a perioperative dose is not given. Prophylaxis for bacterial endocarditis is not the same as surgical prophylaxis; bacterial endocarditis prophylaxis requires postoperative dosing and often requires antibiotics that are different from the ones recommended for that particular wound. Tubes and lines are not an indication for continued administration of antibiotics in the name of prophylaxis. Reoperation through fresh wounds is considered a clean-contaminated operation and, because recent wounds are usually colonized, should be prophylaxed as such. Cultures may be required to facilitate adequate coverage.

Prophylactic antibiotics should be administered to all patients undergoing contaminated operations, clean-contaminated operations, and to patients undergoing clean operations who are at high risk, who are having a prosthesis inserted, or in whom the morbidity would be substantial. Table 9-12 lists recommendations for prophylactic antibiotics to prevent wound infection. The route of prophylaxis will depend on the level of contamination, the preference of the surgeon, and the reliability of the ancillary care. Both topical and parenteral administration have shown benefit in reducing wound infections when properly administered. Topical antibiotics trade diligence of the ancillary services for diligence of the surgeon. Topical antibiotics effectively decrease the bacterial flora of the wound fluid and superficial wound but do not provide the tissue levels that appropriately timed parenteral antibiotics provide. Therefore, they are effective only if they are constantly on the surface of the wound, ready to engage contaminating bacteria.

The key to successful prophylaxis is to choose an antibiotic that will cover the suspected pathogens and to be sure it is in the wound at the time of operation. Prophylaxis should be limited to perioperative administration only, with most procedures requiring a single preoperative dose or continuous administration if topical application is chosen. Prophylaxis is successful only if the benefits of decreased wound infection are not negated by complications caused by the administration. In this regard, the shortest course of prophylaxis possible will suffice. Finally, prophylactic antibiotics are not an excuse for poor technique. The words of

Table 9-12. Recommendations for Prophylactic Antibiotics to Prevent Wound Infection

Operation	Common Pathogens	Recommended Drugs	Dosage Before Operation
Clean			
Cardiac: prosthetic valve, coronary artery bypass, etc.	*S. aureus, S. epidermidis, Corynebacterium,* enteric gram-negative bacilli	Cefazolin or vancomycin	1 g IV 1 g IV
Neurosurgery: craniotomy	*S. aureus, S. epidermidis*	Cefazolin or vancomycin	1 g IV 1 g IV
Orthopedic: internal fracture fixation, prosthetic joint replacement	*S. aureus, S. epidermidis*	Cefazolin	1 g IV
Vascular: aortic surgery, prosthetic graft insertion, groin incision, amputation for ischemia	*S. aureus, S. epidermidis*	Cefazolin	1 g IV
Clean-Contaminated			
Appendectomy	Enteric gram-negative bacilli, anaerobes	Cefoxitin or cefotetan or cefmetazole	2 g IV 1–2 g IV 1 g IV
Biliary tract, hepatic, or pancreatic surgery	Enteric gram-negative bacilli, enterococci, *C. perfringens*	Cefazolin	1 g IV
Colorectal/distal ileum	Enteric gram-negative bacilli, anaerobes	Neomycin, erythromycin base or cefoxitin or cefotetan or cefmetazole	1 g each PO at 1, 2, 11 P.M. day before operation 2 g IV 1–2 g IV 1–2 g IV
Gastroduodenal; proximal small intestine—includes gastric bypass, gastrostomy	Enteric gram-negative bacilli, gram-positive cocci	Cefazolin	1 g IV
Head and neck—operations involving aerodigestive tract	*S. aureus,* streptococci anaerobes	Cefazolin or clindamycin	1 g IV 600 mg IV
Hysterectomy	Enteric gram-negative bacilli, anaerobes, group B streptococci, enterococci	Cefazolin	1 g IV
Cesarean section	Enteric gram-negative bacilli, anaerobes, group B streptococci, enterococci	Cefazolin	1 g IV after clamping of umbilical cord
Thoracic—pulmonary, esophageal surgery	*S. aureus,* anaerobes, streptococci, gram-negative enteric bacilli	Cefazolin	1 g IV
Urologic	Gram-negative enteric bacilli, enterococci	Cefazolin	1 g IV
Contaminated			
Penetrating trauma	Gram-negative enteric bacilli, anaerobes	Cefoxitin or cefotetan or cefmetazole	2 g IV 1–2 g IV 1–2 g IV
Blunt trauma	Gram-negative enteric bacilli	Cefazolin	1 g IV

From Malangoni MA. Chemoprophylaxis of Wound Infections. In RJ Howard, RL Simmons (eds.), *Surgical Infectious Diseases* (3rd ed.). Norwalk: Appleton & Lange, 1995. p. 477. Reproduced with permission.

Wangensteen remain true today: "Antibiotics may convert a third-class surgeon into a second-class surgeon, but never a second-class surgeon into a first-class surgeon."

Suggested Reading

Burke JF. The effective period of preventive antibiotic action in experimental incisions and dermal lesions. *Surgery* 50:161, 1961.

Chetlin SH, Elliott DW. Preoperative antibiotics in biliary surgery. *Arch Surg* 107:319, 1973.

Classen DC, et al. The timing of prophylactic administration of antibiotics and the risk of surgical wound infection. *N Engl J Med* 326:281, 1992.

Cruse PJE, Foord R. The epidemiology of wound infection. A 10-year prospective study of 62,939 wounds. *Surg Clin N Am* 60:27, 1980.

Culver DH, et al. Surgical wound infection rates by wound class, operative procedure, and patient risk index. *Am J Med* 91:152S, 1991.

Ehrenkranz NJ. Antimicrobial prophylaxis in surgery: mechanisms, misconceptions, and mischief. *Infect Control Hosp Epidemiol* 14:99, 1993.

Fallon WF Jr, Wears RL. Prophylactic antibiotics for the prevention of infectious complications including empyema following tube thoracostomy for trauma: results of meta-analysis. *J Trauma* 33:110, 1992.

Garibaldi RA, Cushing D, Lerer T. Risk factors for postoperative infections. *Am J Med* 91:158S, 1991.

Gilbert AI, Felton LL. Infection in inguinal hernia repair considering biomaterials and antibiotics. *Surg Gynecol Obstet* 177:126, 1993.

Haley RW, et al. Identifying patients at high risk of surgical wound infection. A simple multivariate index of patient susceptibility and wound contamination. *Am J Epidemiol* 121:206, 1985.

Hemsell DL. Prophylactic antibiotics in gynecologic and obstetric surgery. *Rev Infect Dis* 13:S821, 1991.

Hopkins CC. Antibiotic prophylaxis in clean surgery: peripheral vascular surgery, noncardiovascular thoracic surgery, herniorrhaphy, and mastectomy. *Rev Infect Dis* 13:S869, 1991.

LoCicero J III. Prophylactic antibiotic usage in cardiothoracic surgery. *Chest* 98:719, 1990.

Ludwig KA, Carlson MA, Condon RE. Prophylactic antibiotics in surgery. *Annu Rev Med* 44:385, 1993.

Olson MM, Lee JT. Continuous, 10-year wound infection surveillance. Results, advantages, and unanswered questions. *Arch Surg* 125:794, 1990.

Malangoni MA. Chemoprophylaxis of Wound Infections. In RJ Howard, RL Simmons (eds.), *Surgical Infectious Diseases* (3rd ed.) Norwalk: Appleton & Lange, 1995.

Mora E, Simmons RL. The Indiscriminant Use of Continuous Intraoperative Broad-Spectrum Topical Antibiotics for the Prevention of Wound Infection. In RL Simmons, AO Udekwu (eds.), *Debates in Clinical Surgery*, vol. 1, Chicago: Year Book, 1990.

Nichols RL. Rational Approach to the Use of Systemic Prophylactic Antibiotics in General Surgery. In RL Simmons, AO Udekwu (eds.), *Debates in Clinical Surgery*, Vol. 1, Chicago: Year Book, 1990.

Page CP, et al. Antimicrobial prophylaxis for surgical wounds. Guidelines for clinical care. *Arch Surg* 128:79, 1993.

Platt R, et al. Perioperative antibiotic prophylaxis for herniorrhaphy and breast surgery. *N Engl J Med* 322:153, 1990.

Privitera G, et al. Prospective study of *Clostridium difficile* intestinal colonization and disease following single-dose antibiotic prophylaxis in surgery. *Antimicrob Agents Chemother* 35:208, 1991.

Sheridan RL, Tompkins RG, Burke JF. Prophylactic antibiotics and their role in the prevention of surgical wound infection. *Adv Surg* 27:43, 1994.

Smith MB, et al. Suppression of the human mucosal-related colonic microflora with prophylactic parenteral and/or oral antibiotics. *World J Surg* 14:636, 1990.

Velanovich V. A meta-analysis of prophylactic antibiotics in head and neck surgery. *Plast Reconstruc Surg* 87:429, 1991.

Widdison AL, Pope NRJ, Brown EM. Survey of guidelines for antimicrobial prophylaxis in surgery. *J Hosp Infect* 25:199, 1993.

Wittmann DH, Condon RE. Prophylaxis of postoperative infections. *Infection* 19:S337, 1991.

Yee J, et al. *Clostridium difficile* disease in a department of surgery. The significance of prophylactic antibiotics. *Arch Surg* 126:241, 1991.

EDITOR'S COMMENT

Doctors Simmons, Wittmann, and Jacob have each contributed cogent comments on practices concerning the use of antibiotics and prophylaxis for operations as well as the treatment of peritonitis, one of the most serious life-threatening situations generally facing the surgical patient.

The chapter by Drs. Jacob and Simmons is a data-driven, calmly reasoned reflection of the current knowledge base in the area of surgical infection, and as such, in my view, gives most of the arguments concerning prophylaxis in surgery. A decade ago it was difficult if not impossible to argue that the use of a single dose of a relatively broad-spectrum cephalosporin should be given before clean cases, such as hernia or breast biopsies. Data that have accumulated over the past decade support the premise that in fact this practice is a useful and cost-effective way to deal with the bulk of clean elective cases that general surgeons perform, such as breast biopsies and herniorrhaphies. That this principle has not crept into the general practice is astounding to me, as there appear to be excellent data to support it.

Dr. Wittmann's techniques for dealing with abdominal infection are well founded on basic surgical principles. However, there are areas in which many individuals would not agree. Most of the data appear to support the concept that the outcome is better following a scheduled reexploration for situations such as Dr. Wittmann portrays. However, the data are not unanimous in supporting this approach. In my experience, in anastomosis or resection or closure of an enterotomy (which may be necessary but best avoided), it is absolutely essential to close the abdomen. If some type of artificial material is in any contact with the anastomosis, it will generally result in a gastrointestinal-cutaneous fistula. Under these circumstances, it is not often possible to close the abdomen, and some type of silastic, Goretex or Velcro-type of material must be used. It is far better to interpose some type of artificial material to have some cover (which may be opened and reopened) over the abdomen, rather than leave the abdomen totally open. Otherwise, a large hernia reults, which will be difficult to repair in the future if the patient survives. The likelihood of fistulization from intact bowel in an abdomen left entirely open with dressings placed directly on the bowel is very real and occurs with unfortunate regularity. Any ability to place some natural tissue or interpose it between either dressings or silastic or other material will decrease the fistula rate, which unfortunately is a very real complicating factor in these patients.

J.E.F.

SPECIAL COMMENT

NEWER METHODS OF OPERATIVE THERAPY FOR PERITONITIS

Impact of Operative Therapy on Mortality

The impact of operative management on the outcome of intra-abdominal infections including intra-abdominal abscess (so-called surgical peritonitis) becomes clearly visible when comparing mortality of nonoperative management with mortality of operative management. Before the beginning of this century, surgical techniques were not developed enough to allow for abdominal operations, and patients with suppurative peritonitis were treated conservatively, with an associated mortality of 90 percent. This outcome may be regarded as the natural course of the disease.

During the first decades of the twentieth century, the practice of medicine was advanced to a point that would allow for operative therapy of all patients suffering from peritonitis. Surgical principles were developed, and the therapeutic success was dramatic. Operative management reduced mortality from 90 percent to less than 50 percent.

The two surgical principles established during this period were formulated by Kirschner in 1926 and consisted of: 1) "plugging" the source of infection (generally an intestinal leak), and 2) purging bacteria, toxins and adjuvants.

These surgical principles became the gold standard of the operative management of intra-abdominal infections in subsequent decades during which, however, mortality did not substantially improve. Depending on the patient selection, reported mortality still ranged between 30 and 70 percent, stimulating further efforts toward improved management modalities.

The era of new operative concepts started in 1975 with the dissertation of Pujol from Paris University. He concluded that intra-abdominal infections too should be treated as any surgical infection, applying the classic treatment principles ("ibi pus, ubi evacua") and leaving the abdomen open. Subsequently, a series of authors published case series in which the abdomen was treated as an open wound, but results were inconclusive. These studies were uncontrolled and did not stratify severity of disease, making comparison with other methods impossible. Most studies, however, claim to use the newer approaches for patients who would have been otherwise abandoned for standard treatment. This finding leads one to conclude that the mortality reported represents a selection of the sickest patients and that mortality may have been higher if treated by standard methods.

In recent years, many papers have been published propagating a variety of other new operative approaches for the treatment of diffuse suppurative peritonitis. Most papers are anecdotal, making it difficult to assess whether the new methods represent any therapeutic improvement. In a few, patients have been stratified to allow for comparison. But comparison is difficult because methods vary from center to center and from strategy to strategy. For that purpose, the International Society of Surgery asked several experts in the field to convene at the International Surgical Week 1993 in Hong Kong to clarify ter-

minology. Four basically different methods have emerged:

1. Open abdomen/laparostomy (OPA)
2. Covered laparostomy (COLA)
3. Planned relaparotomy (PR)
4. Staged abdominal repair (STAR)

In addition to the classic surgical principles, the open abdomen techniques (OPA and COLA) avert deleterious effects of increased intra-abdominal pressure. Planned relaparotomies (PR) allow for control of surgical repair and purge as well as for early diagnosis and treatment of intra-abdominal complications. The STAR technique combines the advantage of both the open abdomen technique and planned relaparotomy but reduces the risk for some of the adverse effects associated with OPA, COLA, and PR such as incisional hernia and fistula formation.

Principles of Operative Management

Generally, treatment of acute suppurative peritonitis includes operative therapy, antimicrobial therapy, and supportive management of the systemic repercussions of infection. The operation remains the most important therapeutic modality. If it fails, all other measures will be unsuccessful and the patient will die.

Management principles of peritonitis are summarized in Table 9-13. While with standard operative management infectious material is prevented from leaking into the abdomen (**repair**) and pus, adjuvants, and bacteria are evacuated from the abdominal cavity (**purge**); the third (**decompress**) and fourth principles (**control**)

Table 9-13. Operative Principles and Various Procedures for Peritonitis

Principle 1: Repair
  Control the source of infection
Principle 2: Purge
  Evacuate bacterial inoculum, pus, and adjuvants (peritoneal "toilet")
Principle 3: Decompress
  Treat abdominal compartment syndrome
Principle 4: Control
  Prevent or treat persistent and recurrent infection or verify both *repair* and *purge*

are accomplished only with the more advanced operative techniques.

Principle 1. Terminate Infectious Material Leaking into the Abdomen (Repair)

Suppurative, secondary, peritonitis results from a focus from which infective material leaks into the abdominal cavity. **Principle 1** eliminates the source of infection; frequently it involves a simple procedure such as appendectomy or omentopexy for a perforated peptic ulcer. Occasionally, major resections to remove the infective focus are indicated, such as gastrectomy or colectomy, for perforated gastric carcinoma or colonic diverticulitis, respectively. Generally, the choice of procedure, and whether the ends of the bowel are anastomosed, exteriorized, or simply closed, depends on the anatomic source of infection, the degree of peritoneal inflammation and generalized septic response, and the patient's premorbid reserves. No formula is available, but the prevailing trend has been to minimize the immediate risk of complications by avoiding any intestinal suture lines in the presence of severe peritonitis.

Principle 2. Evacuate Bacteria, Pus, and Adjuvants from the Abdominal Cavity (Purge)

Infectious peritoneal fluid, pus, fibrin, necrotic tissue, and adjuvants either contain pathogenic bacteria or promote their growth. Pathologic peritoneal fluid may be serous, fibrinous, bilious, purulent, or feculent and should be removed. Necrotic peritoneal tissue should be debrided; an aggressive debridement should be avoided, however, to prevent excessive blood loss or bowel injury. All lavage or irrigation techniques are meant to help accomplish proper purge of the abdominal cavity. The addition of antibiotics to the fluid is not beneficial if the fluid is washed out immediately because pathogens, to be killed, require longer antibiotic exposure than that provided by simple irrigation. Systemic antibiotics provide more predictable concentrations in infected tissues and sustain predictable concentrations over the minimal bactericidal concentrations (MBC) for therapeutically adjustable periods.

Principle 3. Avoid Abdominal Compartment Syndrome (Decompress)

During acute peritonitis, the peritoneum and its submesothelial loose connective tissue may absorb more than 10 liters of inflammatory edema. Additionally, coexistent ileus and postresuscitation visceral and parietal edema may increase intra-abdominal pressure to levels producing a compartment syndrome. This result may impair cardiovascular, pulmonary, renal and hepatic functions as well as splanchnic blood flow and oxygenation. In some instances, closure of the abdominal wall fascia can be achieved only with enormous tension. Tension promotes further perfusion deficits and thus inhibits proper healing and antibacterial defenses. The standard operation does not address this issue, since the abdominal fascia is closed, often under extreme tension using retention sutures. Only with the open abdomen technique or with STAR can the abdominal compartment syndrome be avoided.

Principle 4. Control Repairs and Purge

With the standard operation there is no effective way to control whether an anastomosis heals, bowel segments remain viable, or new purulence forms within the abdominal cavity. These complications remain hidden and are usually diagnosed only once overt clinical symptoms appear. Additionally, the surgeon's bias toward his or her own complications tends to delay early detection of postoperative complications. It is more effective to plan a re-exploration when problems are suspected postoperatively, to ensure optimal healing, diagnose early bowel wall necroses, and evacuate newly formed pus. Bacteria grow quickly after irrigations of the abdominal cavity, and in 24 hours the same number of bacteria *is found* as before irrigation. This finding indicates that the abdominal cavity needs to be frequently re-explored until clean.

Operative Methods
Standard Operation: Repair and Purge

Principles 1 and **2** are affected. The intestinal leaks are managed as discussed above. The standard operation does not allow for intestinal anastomoses in the presence of established severe peritonitis, because local tissue repair processes are impaired and suture lines may leak as the edema abates. Purge is accomplished either by swabbing pus, bacteria, and adjuvants or by peritoneal irrigation. No irrigation fluid should remain in the abdomen before closure. The addition of antibiotic, although cosmetically appealing, is not beneficial when systemic antibiotics are given.

Additional purge methods may be used after termination of the standard operation. At the standard operation, multiple tube-drains are placed in the abdominal cavity to either continuously irrigate or to intermittently fill the abdomen and then drain it. These continuous postoperative irrigation procedures were popular in the early 1970s and 1980s, but their benefits were not proven in controlled studies. Sooner or later the irrigation fluid no longer irrigates the entire abdomen, because the healing process occludes most spaces and fluid flows from entry tube directly to the draining tube. Most surgeons have abandoned these labor intensive methods.

Open Abdomen/Open Laparostomy (OPA): Repair, Purge and Decompress

Open laparostomy is defined as a laparotomy without reapproximation and suture closure of the abdominal fascia and skin. In this method, the abdominal cavity is left open. Importantly, it counteracts deleterious rising of intra-abdominal pressure. The exposed intestines, however, perforate easily since augmented intraluminal pressure (ileus) is not counteracted by the abdominal wall. Also, definitive closure of the abdominal wall becomes impossible, since the abdominal wall fasciae retracts. Huge incisional hernias are the inevitable consequence and require secondary repair. Some surgeons combine the open-abdomen method with continuous postoperative abdominal lavage. The open-abdomen method has lost its popularity since surgeons realized its associated complications (i.e., formation of enteric fistulae and huge herniae).

Covered Laparostomy or Mesh Laparostomy: Repair, Purge and Decompress

Mesh laparostomy is defined as a laparotomy without reapproximation and suture closure of the abdominal fascia. The fascial gap is covered, however, with a mesh of Marlex, polyglycolic acid, or other material in order to protect the exposed viscera (Fig. 9-6). Some surgeons do not suture the fascia, but cover the intestines by suturing the skin. If there is too much skin tension, lateral abdominal relaxing incisions provide release. All these methods are consistently associated with large incisional hernias.

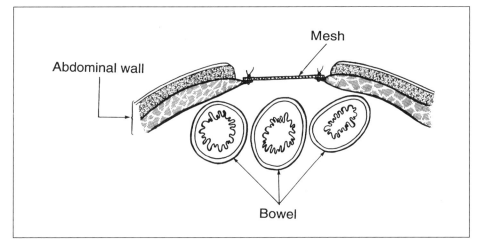

Fig. 9-6. Covered laparostomy: A mesh is sutured to fasciae to cover the gap that results from increased intra-abdominal pressure.

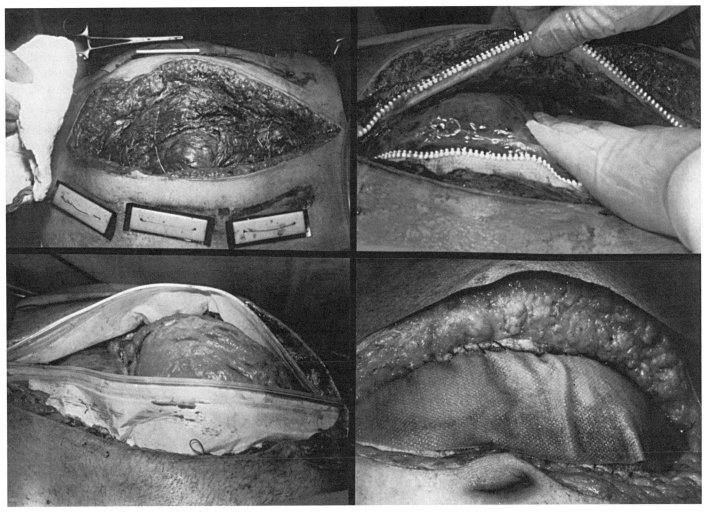

Fig. 9-7. Various devices used to temporarily close the abdominal wall following incision: Upper left: Retention sutures to temporarily close fascia to fascia; note the pressure necroses resulting from increased intra-abdominal pressure. Upper right: Use of a commercially available zipper. Lower left: Use of Ethizip, a zipper-like device that allows for closure with minimal tension: In this sample it has opened spontaneously due to increased pressure. Lower right: Artificial bur consisting of a Velcro-like material that covers the abdominal wall gap.

Planned Relaparotomy: Control

Another development of the open abdomen technique is the addition of planned relaparotomies. This approach involves "leaving the abdomen open" following the initial operation to allow for reexploration and irrigation, debridement or fistula closure, either in the operating room or in the intensive care unit. Reexploration intervals range from 12 to 48 hours and up to longer periods as the clinical situation mandates. Devices used to ease reexploration are depicted in Fig. 9-7, including the artificial bur that is used for STAR (lower right).

Staged Abdominal Repair: Repair, Purge, Decompress and Control

STAR is a series of abdominal operations with staged reapproximation and final suture closure of the abdominal fascia using an artificial bur. It is **planned** either before or during the first operation, called the INDEX STAR. The abdomen is closed temporarily, and controlled tension is exerted to the fascia, avoiding the consequences of increased intra-abdominal pressure. Relaparotomies are performed at 24-hour intervals in the operating room.

When STAR Is Indicated

STAR may be indicated in diffuse suppurative peritonitis, infected pancreatic necrosis, intestinal ischemia and trauma, when one or more of the following factors is present:

1. Critical patient condition precluding definitive repair
2. Excessive peritoneal and parietal edema (increased intra-abdominal pressure)
3. Massive abdominal wall loss
4. Impossible to eliminate or to control the source of infection
5. Incomplete debridement of necrotic tissue

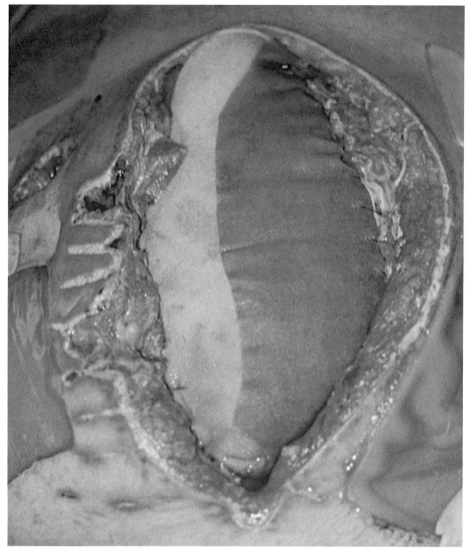

Fig. 9-8. Artificial bur in situ in a patient with diffuse peritonitis after an anastomotic leak of the sigmoid colon and multiple small-bowel perforations. The perforated small-bowel segment had been resected and the leak was closed. Note the bulging of the viscera against the bur. The two sheets are not fully approximated to adjust for increased pressure and at the same time exert some tension to the fasciae to prevent retraction.

slight tension is exerted to the attached fascia when the hooks are pressed into the loop sheet to effect closure (Fig. 9-9). An adhesive transparent dressing may be used to cover the wound from skin to skin, and to allow for suctioning leaking peritoneal fluid with a suction drain that is placed onto the wound above the burr sheets and underneath the adhesive dressing. With this method, protein losses can be easily measured and replaced. Measurement of intra-abdominal pressure, best by indirect intravesical method, may be used to adjust intra-abdominal pressure during temporary closure. As pressure decreases, the fascial edges may be reapproximated by pulling them together and trimming the superfluous part of the hook sheet (Fig. 9-9).

Operative Technique

The aim is to complete repair, debridement and purge; to check anastomotic healing; to diagnose complications early; and to treat and prevent abdominal compartment syndrome.

The operative strategy is outlined in the algorithm (Fig. 9-10). Upon recognition of an intra-abdominal problem that is difficult or impossible to manage with a single operation, the decision to proceed with STAR is made. A median or transverse incision is made as would be done for a standard operation. The infectious focus is removed or closed and peritoneal purge performed.

Surgical technique must be gentle to prevent bleeding or injury to the inflamed and friable bowel. If the patient's condition does not allow for extensive repair, necrotic bowel segments may be stapled off, resected, and the formation of anastomoses deferred to the next day when the patient's condition has stabilized.

If a problem that was recognized at the first operation persists or if new problems are encountered, further STARs are indicated. Complications such as hematomas, necrotic tissue, and leaking anastomoses are diagnosed and treated in a timely fashion. Leaks can be resutured. Anastomoses may heal better because perfusion is not compromised by increased intra-abdominal pressure. It is our impression that anastomoses could be sutured in the presence of established peritonitis and that healing

6. Uncertainty as to viability of bowel
7. Anastomosis or other repair needs reinspection
8. Uncontrolled bleeding (the need for packing).

Only about 10 to 15 percent of all patients with peritonitis meet these indications and thus may benefit from STAR.

Temporary Abdominal Closure Devices

For temporary abdominal closure the artificial bur has been shown to be most effective (Figs. 9-8 and 9-9). The bur consists of two polypropylene/nylon sheets that are armed with hooks and loops. The sheets adhere to each other like a bur adheres to fabric. The sheets, however, can be easily peeled off each other (Fig. 9-9). First, the sheet with the loops is sutured (with the loops facing outwards) to the fascia of one side of the wound. Second, the sheet with the hooks is sutured to the opposite fascial edge with a running 0 nonabsorbable suture. Third, the free end of the loop sheet is used to cover bowel and omentum and is pushed underneath the opposite edge of the abdominal wall. Fourth, the hook sheet is stretched, and

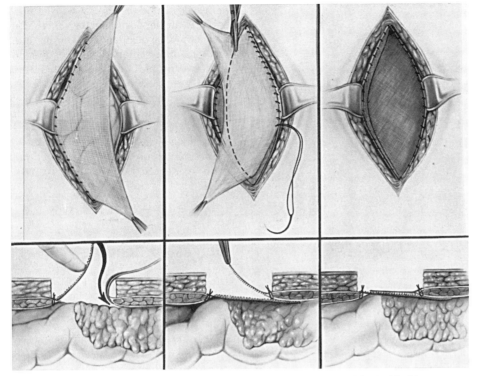

Fig. 9-9. Operative technique of using the artificial bur to temporarily close the abdominal incision.

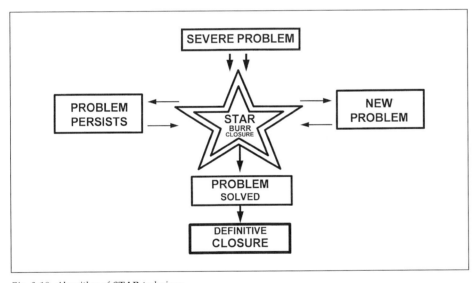

Fig. 9-10. Algorithm of **STAR** technique.

Table 9-14. Conditions Under Which the Abdomen Can Be Closed

Score predicted mortality <20%
No bowel persistent leak
Bowel continuity established
No healing problem expected
Debridement sufficient
Intra-abdominal pressure <15–20 mm Hg
    when fasciae are reapproximated

Final Closure

Once all problems are solved, the abdominal cavity can be formally closed (Table 9-14). During closure, some tension usually occurs but intra-abdominal pressure of up to 20 mm Hg is acceptable in hemodynamically stable patients. Established concepts of correct abdominal closure (suture length to wound length ratio greater than 3, and large fasciomuscular tissue bites) are as important as ever.

If more than five staged abdominal repairs have been performed, the presence of sufficient granulation tissue means that local host defenses are established in the subcutaneous wound to allow for primary skin closure.

Results

The value of STAR has never been subjected to a prospective randomized trial. A few recent retrospective or prospective, noncontrolled studies, failed to demonstrate the advantages of the open-planned reoperative methods versus the conventional closed abdomen techniques. In fact, the former were claimed to be associated with a higher rate of mechanical and infective postoperative complication. The methodology of these studies, however, was faulty and none used the methods of STAR described above. Conversely, our prospective but nonrandomized experience shows the STAR approach to be superior to conventional operative therapy when patients at equal mortality risk (as measured with the APACHE II scoring system) were compared (Figs. 9-11 and 9-12). In the survivors of STAR, primary wound healing was uncomplicated in 78 percent of patients, and fascial dehiscence developed in only 8 percent.

Unsolved Issues

It has been shown in trauma cases that repeated operations performed in patients in whom the cytokine-mediated inflammatory response is already "switched-on" by the traumatic event may act as a "second hit," escalating the systemic inflammatory response syndrome and precipitating multiorgan dysfunction. The "second hit" issue in the setup of reoperative therapy for peritonitis should be clarified: Does the interval of 24 hours between relaparotomies add wood to the inflammatory fire? A prospective, ran-

could be observed and corrected during subsequent STAR procedures. Consequently, colostomies may be avoided in favor of anastomoses.

Abdominal drainage, with its associated complications and the false sense of security it provides, is unnecessary during STAR procedures.

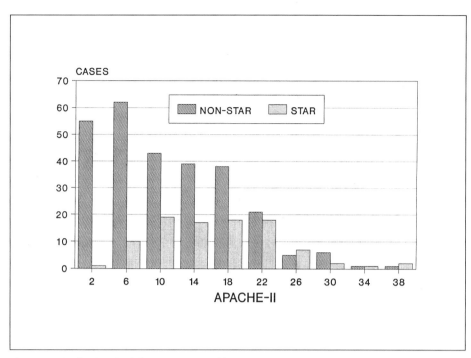

Fig. 9-11. Distribution of risk factors as measured by APACHE-II scores among patients treated by standard conventional operative management (n = 260) and STAR (n = 95).

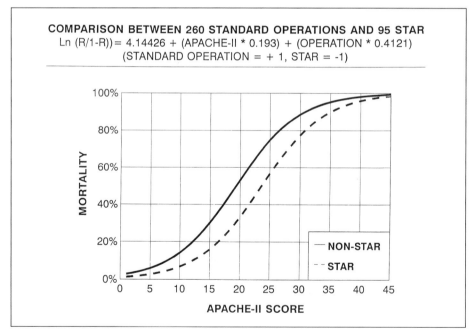

COMPARISON BETWEEN 260 STANDARD OPERATIONS AND 95 STAR

$$Ln\ (R/1\text{-}R)) = 4.14426 + (APACHE\text{-}II * 0.193) + (OPERATION * 0.4121)$$
$$(STANDARD\ OPERATION = +1,\ STAR = -1)$$

Fig. 9-12. Mortality of intra-abdominal infections for conventional operative management (non-STAR) and staged abdominal repair (STAR), and adjusted for risk factors (APACHE-II scores). The mortality curves were calculated using a logistic model yielding a significant difference at p = 0.018.

domized, multicenter study will be necessary to further document the value of the demanding, potentially harmful, and costly management modalities required to address principles 3 and 4 presented here. Meanwhile, from our experience, we believe these techniques to be beneficial if initiated early in well selected patients, for specific indications, and performed by a team of dedicated surgeons. Conversely, indiscriminate use, at inopportune times by inexperienced staff unfamiliar with the patient, is a formula for failure.

Dietmar H. Wittmann

Suggested Reading

Edmiston CE, et al. Fecal peritonitis: Microbial adherence to serosal mesothelium and resistance to peritoneal lavage. *World J Surg* 14:176, 1990.

Kirschner M. Die Behandlung der akuten eitrigen freien Bauchfellentzuendung. *Langenbecks Arch Chir* 142:52, 1926.

Levy E, et al. Septic necrosis of the midline wound in postoperative peritonitis. *Ann Surg* 207:470, 1988.

Pujol JP. La non fermature des incisions abdominales d'urgence. Techniques et résultes. Thesis, Paris, U.E.R. X Bichat, 1975.

Schein M, et al. The abdominal compartment syndrome: The physiological and clinical consequences of elevated intra-abdominal pressure. *J Am Coll Surg* 180:745, 1995.

Wittmann DH, et al. Laparostomy, open abdomen, etappenlavage, planned relaparotomy, and staged abdominal repair (STAR): Too many names for a new operative method. In TS Rüedi (ed.), *The State of the Art of Surgery* 1993/1994. Pratteln, Switzerland: International Society of Surgery, 1995.

Wittmann DH, et al. Staged abdominal repair compares favorably with conventional operative therapy for intra-abdominal infections when adjusting for prognostic factors with a conventional operative therapy for intra-abdominal infections when adjusting for prognostic factors with a logistic model. *Theor Surg* 9:201, 1994.

10

Multiple Organ Dysfunction Syndrome: Pathogenesis, Prevention, and Management

Charles J. Shanley   Robert H. Bartlett

Multiple organ dysfunction syndrome (MODS) remains one of the most important and challenging complications faced by surgeons today. Despite spectacular advances in life support technology, the mortality for this syndrome remains extraordinarily high (Sauaia et al, Meesters et al, St. John and Dorinsky, Beal and Cerra). The syndrome is characterized by the progressive functional deterioration of multiple interdependent organs after a major physiologic insult. MODS is a common, costly, and highly lethal complication in surgical patients and it is likely to remain an important problem for decades to come.

Terminology

The syndrome of progressive organ dysfunction in acutely ill patients was initially recognized when improvements in life support techniques allowed survival from lethal single organ failure (Deitch, 1993). Steady improvements in hemodynamic monitoring, resuscitation, renal replacement therapy, and pulmonary support have progressively increased survival from single organ failure in critically ill patients. For example, in a recent cohort study by Milberg and associates, the mortality for adult respiratory distress syndrome (ARDS) in septic patients decreased from 67 percent in 1990 to 40 percent in 1993. As a consequence of this progress, a subset of patients has emerged in whom progressive dysfunction in interdependent multiple organ systems develops, with a very high mortality. This syndrome has

been variously described as "progressive or sequential organ failure," "multiple organ failure," and "multiple systems organ failure" (Deitch, 1992). The term "failure" is no longer used because it suggests that organ function is either present or absent. The syndrome actually presents as a continuum of derangements in organ function that are usually progressive and are occasionally reversible. For this reason, "dysfunction" is a more accurate term to describe this condition because it reflects the dynamic nature of the physiologic changes that are encountered (Bone).

At first it may seem both superfluous and unnecessary to add yet another term (and another acronym) to the critical care lexicon. However, inaccurate terminology has resulted in a great deal of confusion, not only in terms of evaluating clinical risk factors and prognosis for MODS, but also with respect to disseminating and applying the results of basic science and clinical research on MODS (Bone). It is hoped that the current terminology, by emphasizing the dynamic and continuous nature of this process, will encourage early recognition of subtle changes in organ function in critically ill patients. In this manner, preventive and therapeutic interventions can be initiated when they have the best chance of being efficacious, that is, before the development of organ "failure."

MODS occurs in acutely ill patients after a variety of physiologic insults. Two distinct but not mutually exclusive clinical patterns of organ dysfunction are now recognized, "primary" and "secondary" (St. John and Dorinsky, Bone). Primary MODS

occurs early in the course of an acute illness and can be directly related to a well-defined insult. In this pattern, organ dysfunction may resolve, may progress rapidly to death, or may progress insidiously to "secondary" organ dysfunction (Fig. 10-1). In contrast to primary MODS, secondary MODS occurs later in the clinical course and is attributed to a generalized hormonal and inflammatory response that has become abnormally persistent and self-destructive. The clinical manifestations of this generalized response are now referred to as the systemic inflammatory response syndrome (SIRS) (Beal and Cerra, Bone, Rangel-Frausto et al).

SIRS is characterized by generalized activation of multiple inflammatory cascades in organs remote from the initial insult. According to Bone, a patient can be considered to have SIRS if he or she presents with two or more of the following clinical signs in the context of a major physiologic insult:

1. Temperature greater than 38°C or less than 36°C
2. Heart rate greater than 90 beats per minute
3. Tachypnea: respiratory rate greater than 20 per minute or $PaCO_2$ less than 32 mm Hg
4. White blood count greater than 12×10^9 cells/mm^3 or less than 4×10^9 cells/mm^3, or greater than 10 percent band forms

SIRS can develop in response to any sterile inflammatory process (i.e., pancreatitis, burn injury, anaphylaxis, etc.) or in re-

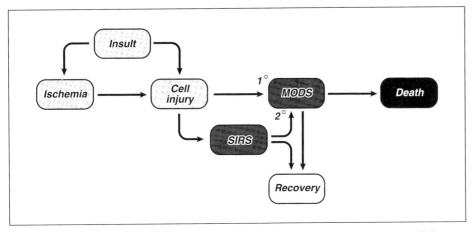

Fig. 10-1. *Theoretical pathogenesis of MODS. Any major physiologic insult can produce either cellular ischemia or injury. Primary MODS is directly attributable to the underlying insult whereas secondary MODS is the consequence of nonspecific activation of a generalized inflammatory response referred to as the systemic inflammatory response syndrome (SIRS).*

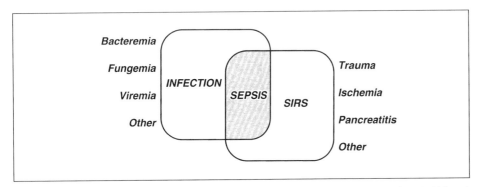

Fig. 10-2. *Theoretical relationship between infection, sepsis, and SIRS in the pathogenesis of SIRS. (Adapted from Bone RC. Multiple organ failure: Pathophysiology and potential future therapy.* Ann Surg *216:117–134, 1992.)*

Table 10-1. Diagnostic Criteria for Significant Organ Dysfunction

Organ System	Criteria
Pulmonary	Need for mechanical ventilation; $PaO_2:FIO_2$ ratio < 300 mm Hg for ≥ 24 hr
Cardiovascular	Need for inotropic drugs to maintain adequate tissue perfusion or CI < 2.5 L/min/m^2
Kidney	Creatinine > 3 mg/dl on 2 consecutive d or need for renal replacement therapy
Liver	Bilirubin > 3 mg/dl on 2 consecutive d or PT $> 1.5 \times$ control
Nutrition	10% reduction in lean body mass, albumin < 2.0 g/dl, or total lymphocyte count < 1000/mm^3
CNS	Glasgow Coma Scale < 10 without sedation
Coagulation	Platelet count $< 50,000$/mm^3; fibrinogen < 100 mg/dl or need for factor replacement
Host defenses	WBC < 1000/mm^3 or invasive infection including bacteremia

CNS = central nervous system; PT = prothrombin time; CI = cardiac index; PaO_2 = partial pressure of oxygen in arterial blood; FIO_2 = fraction of inspired oxygen; WBC = white blood cell count.

sponse to localized or systemic infection with a microorganism (Fig. 10-2). *Sepsis* is now defined as SIRS in association with a confirmed infectious process and is subcategorized as *severe sepsis* when patients manifest hypotension or signs of systemic hypoperfusion (i.e., lactic acidosis, oliguria, or altered mental status). According to Bone, *septic shock* refers to those patients with hypotension and signs of hypoperfusion despite adequate fluid resuscitation.

The natural history of SIRS was recently characterized by Rangel-Frausto and colleagues in a prospective cohort study of over 2000 critically ill patients. This study provides strong epidemiologic evidence of progression from SIRS to sepsis to severe sepsis to septic shock and ultimately to end-organ dysfunction and death. In this study, as patients progressed from SIRS to septic shock, mortality increased in a stepwise fashion from 7 to 46 percent. Furthermore, as patients progressed from SIRS to septic shock, the incidence of end-organ dysfunction increased in a similar fashion. These data suggest that development of SIRS in a critically ill or injured patient is a definite risk factor for MODS and death.

In this conceptual framework, *secondary MODS* can be defined as the presence of dysfunction in two or more organ systems in a patient with SIRS (see Fig. 10-1). At present, there are no standardized definitions of "significant" organ dysfunction. According to Bone, "dysfunction" can include complete organ failure requiring supportive or replacement therapy (i.e., respiratory failure requiring mechanical ventilation or renal failure requiring continuous hemofiltration or dialysis) or it may simply represent a biochemical abnormality that may or may not result in clinical findings (i.e., elevated serum creatinine or transaminases). In our intensive care unit, we use the diagnostic criteria outlined in Table 10-1 to identify patients with "significant" organ dysfunction. Although these criteria are somewhat arbitrary we have found them to be useful in identifying patients at increased risk for MODS and death. Similar criteria have been used in recent studies (Sauaia et al, Meesters et al, Proulx et al) to establish organ failure scoring systems in an attempt to identify patients at risk for MODS.

Epidemiology

As reported by Beal and Cerra, Deitch (1993), and Demling and colleagues (1993), MODS is currently the leading cause of death in the surgical intensive care unit. Mortality from MODS is most closely related to the number of dysfunctional organs (St. John and Dorinsky, Beal and Cerra, Deitch [1993], Bartlett et al, Knaus et al). In Bartlett and associates' prospective study of acute respiratory failure in 713 patients from 1976 to 1979, isolated respiratory failure had a mortality of 40 percent. However, as the number of dysfunctional organs increased from two to five, mortality increased progressively from 54 to 100 percent. A similar prospective study of 5677 critically ill patients reported by Knaus and coworkers in 1985 demonstrated that mortality from MODS depends not only on the number of failing organs but also on the duration of organ dysfunction. For example, when three or more organ systems show evidence of severe dysfunction for more than 3 consecutive days, mortality is almost universal. Finally, this study also demonstrated that advanced age and the presence of a serious premorbid illness significantly worsen the prognosis of MODS.

In most clinical series, organ dysfunction occurs in a predictable sequence beginning with the lungs. Acute lung injury (ALI) or ARDS is the most common form of organ dysfunction, and the lungs are usually the first organ system to become dysfunctional following a major physiologic insult (St. John and Dorinsky, Beal and Cerra, Deitch [1993], Bartlett et al, Knaus et al). Acute respiratory failure generally manifests between 24 and 72 hours after the initial insult; subsequently, according to Cipolle and colleagues, the liver, intestine, and kidneys become progressively dysfunctional. The precise sequence of organ dysfunction tends to vary according to the presence of preexistent disease and the nature of the primary insult. As reported by Beal and Cerra and by Cipolle and colleagues, death commonly occurs between 14 and 21 days after the initial insult.

MODS complicates a number of diverse conditions, including trauma, burns, sepsis, aspiration, transfusions, pancreatitis, and cardiopulmonary bypass. Deitch (1993) and Cipolle and colleagues found that the prevalence of this syndrome continues to increase as life support technology continues to improve. Furthermore, according to Beal and Cerra, established MODS prolongs hospital stay and significantly increases hospital costs. Consequently, a thorough knowledge of the pathogenesis, prevention, and treatment of MODS is essential for all surgeons.

Normal Response to Injury

Any major physiologic insult initiates a homeostatic *stress response* (Beal and Cerra, Demling et al [1993 and 1994], Cipolle et al). This response has hormonal, inflammatory, and immunologic components that have evolved primarily as self-protective mechanisms following major injury or infection. Among the changes that occur in response to any major insult are substantial increases in the levels of circulating *stress hormones*. The primary stress hormones are the catecholamines, cortisol, growth hormone, glucagon, and insulin. This hormonal response increases oxygen consumption, gluconeogenesis, and protein catabolism, and results in a hyperdynamic circulatory state.

A significant *inflammatory response* is also initiated that serves to prime the immune system to fight infection as well as to promote hemostasis and wound healing. The inflammatory response is mediated primarily by peptide cytokines, bioactive lipids, toxic oxygen metabolites, and neutrophil proteases. Initiation of the inflammatory response leads to systemic signs of inflammation including fever and leukocytosis. The clinical manifestations of this response are now referred to as the systemic inflammatory response syndrome (SIRS) (Beal and Cerra, Bone, Rangel-Frausto et al). Cipolle and colleagues found that this response normally peaks from 3 to 5 days after injury and has largely resolved by 7 to 10 days after the initial insult. In certain patients, however, SIRS persists and becomes greatly amplified, leading to dysfunction in multiple distant organs. Since the mediators that amplify this response are the same regardless of the underlying insult, it is not surprising that MODS is the final complication, leading to death for most critically ill patients.

Pathogenesis

Regardless of the underlying insult, the primary pathophysiologic abnormality in MODS is an abnormal, generalized, and persistent response to injury. The normal hormonal and inflammatory responses to injury are highly regulated and self-protective. MODS represents the unfortunate pathologic consequence when these responses become unregulated and self-destructive. When the normal response to injury becomes unregulated, abnormal activation of multiple inflammatory cascades leads to diffuse cellular injury and organ dysfunction. In addition, tissue oxygen demands increase significantly after a major insult or injury (Beal and Cerra, Demling et al [1993], Frankenfield et al, Bartlett et al); if oxygen delivery is inadequate to meet this increase in demand, diffuse cellular ischemia results. Ischemia exacerbates cellular injury and leads to further release of stress hormones and other inflammatory mediators. In this manner, a vicious circle is established that, if uncorrected, eventually leads to widespread organ damage, profound functional deterioration, and eventually death.

Oxygen Kinetics: The Relationship Between Oxygen Delivery and Oxygen Consumption

Significant structural and functional changes occur in all organs in patients with MODS. These changes significantly alter the normal relationship between oxygen delivery (DO_2) and oxygen consumption (VO_2) (St. John and Dorinsky, Beal and Cerra, Demling et al [1994], Russell and Phang). The primary pathologic changes are diffuse endothelial cell and parenchymal cell injury. Kreutzfelder and associates found that endothelial cell injury increases capillary permeability and leads to edema formation. In addition, endothelial cell injury may also lead to microvascular hemorrhage and thrombosis. These changes not only increase the distance for oxygen diffusion, but they also decrease the capillary surface area that is available for oxygen diffusion. To make matters worse, parenchymal cell injury may interfere directly with mitochondrial oxygen utilization. This is a particularly

Table 10-2. Oxygen Kinetics Formulas
and Definitions

FORMULAS

$CaO_2 = (Hgb \times SaO_2 \times 1.36) + (0.0031 \times PaO_2)$

$CvO_2 = (Hgb \times SvO_2 \times 1.36) + (0.0031 \times PvO_2)$

a-v $DO_2 = CaO_2 - CvO_2$

$O_2ER = $ a-v DO_2/CaO_2

$DO_2 = CI \times CaO_2$

*$VO_2 = CI \times $ (a-v DO_2) (Fick equation)

DEFINITIONS

CaO_2: arterial oxygen content (ml O_2/dl
   blood)

CvO_2: mixed-venous oxygen content
   (ml O_2/dl blood)

a-v DO_2: arteriovenous oxygen content
   difference (ml O_2/dl blood)

O_2ER: oxygen extraction ratio

DO_2: systemic oxygen delivery (dl O_2/
   m^2/min)

*VO_2: systemic oxygen consumption
   (dl/O_2/min)

Hgb = hemoglobin concentration (mg/dl
blood); SaO_2 = arterial oxyhemoglobin saturation; SvO_2 = mixed-venous oxyhemoglobin
saturation; PaO_2 = partial pressure of oxygen
in arterial blood (mm Hg); PvO_2 = partial pressure of oxygen in mixed-venous blood (mm
Hg); CI = cardiac index (dl/m^2/min).
*Use of the Fick equation to estimate VO_2 can
lead to spurious correlation between DO_2 and
VO_2 secondary to mathematical coupling of
shared variables (i.e., CI and CaO_2).
Adapted from CJ Shanley, RH Bartlett. The
Management of Acute Respiratory Failure. In
JM Daly [ed.], *Current Opinion in General Surgery.* Philadelphia: Current Science, 1995. Pp 7–
16.

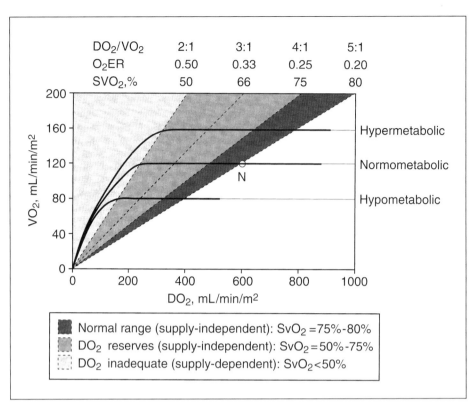

Fig. 10-3. *Theoretical relationship of systemic oxygen consumption (VO$_2$) to oxygen delivery (VO$_2$) at
several steady-state conditions of VO$_2$. DO$_2$/VO$_2$ ratios are represented by isobars corresponding to mixed-
venous saturation (SvO$_2$). For completeness, values for the oxygen extraction ratio (O$_2$ER) are shown as
well. Values assume 100 percent arterial saturation and no anatomic or functional arteriovenous shunting.
(Adapted from Shanley CJ, Bartlett RH. The Management of Acute Respiratory Failure. In JM Daly [ed.],*
Current Opinion in General Surgery. *Philadelphia: Current Science, 1995. Pp 7–16.)*

precarious situation because cellular oxygen demand is significantly increased. Peripheral ischemia may worsen tissue injury if oxygen delivery cannot increase
proportionally to meet the increased demands. For this reason, a clear understanding of the relationship between oxygen delivery and oxygen consumption is
essential to the intelligent management of
MODS. This relationship is most easily understood in terms of "global" or "systemic" oxygen kinetics (Table 10-2, Figs.
10-3 and 10-4); however, these principles
are readily applicable to individual organs
or cells.

Systemic
Oxygen Kinetics

According to Shanley and Bartlett, under
normal conditions, systemic DO_2 is ap-

proximately four to five times VO_2 (see
Fig. 10-3). Thus, 20 to 25 percent of the oxygen that is delivered to the tissues is extracted from arterial blood and the remainder returns to the heart in venous blood. If
arterial blood is 100 percent saturated, normal mixed-venous blood will be approximately 75 to 80 percent saturated. Acute
changes in either DO_2 or VO_2 result in corresponding changes in cardiac output in
order to maintain the normal DO_2/VO_2 ratio. If the DO_2/VO_2 ratio is persistently
less than 4:1, peripheral oxygen extraction
increases to maintain VO_2.

An increase in oxygen extraction increases
the difference between arterial and mixed-
venous blood oxygen content (a-v DO_2)
and decreases the saturation of venous
blood returning to the heart. For example,
if DO_2 decreases (or VO_2 increases) such
that the DO_2/VO_2 ratio is only 3:1,
roughly 33 percent of delivered oxygen

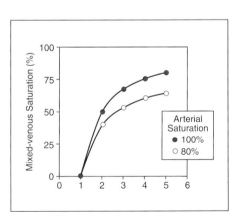

Fig. 10-4. *Theoretical relationship of mixed-venous
saturation (SvO$_2$) to the DO$_2$/VO$_2$ ratio under
varying conditions of arterial oxyhemoglobin
saturation. Notice that changes in the DO$_2$/VO$_2$
ratio produce corresponding changes in SvO$_2$;
however, when arterial saturation is reduced, the
mixed-venous saturation will be reduced
proportionately.*

will be consumed and mixed-venous oxygen saturation will fall to approximately 66 percent, assuming arterial blood is 100 percent saturated (see Fig. 10-3). If arterial blood is less than fully saturated, the difference between arterial and venous blood oxygen saturation determines the DO_2/VO_2 ratio. For example, if arterial blood is 80 percent saturated and mixed-venous blood is 64 percent saturated, the DO_2/VO_2 ratio will be 5:1.

Using this paradigm for systemic oxygen kinetics, it becomes clear that the status of the overall DO_2/VO_2 relationship is reflected most accurately in the amount of oxygen remaining in mixed-venous blood (Fig. 10-4). Because most of the oxygen in venous blood is bound to hemoglobin, mixed-venous saturation (SvO_2) is the best index of systemic oxygen kinetics. Conveniently, SvO_2 can be monitored continuously in the intensive care unit using a fiberoptic pulmonary artery catheter.

Under normal conditions, as DO_2 decreases, tissue oxygen extraction increases proportionately to maintain VO_2. Thus, VO_2 is normally independent of DO_2 (see Fig. 10-3). However, if DO_2 decreases below a "critical" threshold and oxygen extraction can no longer increase sufficiently to compensate, VO_2 will decrease. Thus, below this "critical" DO_2/VO_2 ratio, VO_2 becomes dependent on DO_2. Because increased extraction is no longer sufficient to maintain VO_2, anaerobic metabolism occurs and lactate levels increase. Clinically, the "critical" DO_2/VO_2 ratio is somewhere between 2:1 and 3:1. Thus, if arterial blood is fully saturated, a mixed-venous saturation that is consistently less than 50 percent is a harbinger that VO_2 is dependent on DO_2. If uncorrected, this situation will ultimately lead to severe lactic acidosis, hemodynamic instability, and death.

Controversy continues as to whether a state of "pathologic" dependence of VO_2 on DO_2 exists in patients at risk for MODS. Furthermore, it has been suggested that "pathologic" dependence may be a mechanism for the development of MODS (St. John and Dorinsky, Beal and Cerra, Demling et al [1993], Hanique et al). Carefully controlled laboratory investigation by Sinard and colleagues, Cilley and associates, and Hirschl clearly demonstrates that VO_2 is independent of DO_2 as long as the DO_2/VO_2 ratio exceeds approximately 2:1. Whenever the DO_2/VO_2 ratio falls below

this critical threshold, a "physiologic" state of DO_2 dependence occurs. This biphasic DO_2/VO_2 relationship exists at any steady-state level of VO_2 (see Fig. 10-3).

Proponents of the "pathologic" dependence theory hypothesize that a global defect in peripheral oxygen extraction exists in patients with sepsis, ARDS, and MODS (St. John and Dorinsky, Beal and Cerra, Russell and Phang, Pinsky). This "extraction defect" theoretically results in widespread tissue hypoxia and anaerobic metabolism. While this is an elegant hypothesis, most studies of DO_2 and VO_2 in ARDS or sepsis have used the same variables (i.e., cardiac output and oxygen content) to calculate both DO_2 and VO_2. Because of this flaw in experimental design, these studies are subject to mathematical coupling of shared measurement error which can result in an artifactual correlation between DO_2 and VO_2 (Russell and Phang, Hanique et al, Pinsky). Additionally, in every study in which DO_2 and VO_2 were measured independently to avoid mathematical coupling, VO_2 was not found to be dependent on DO_2 over a wide range of DO_2 values. By definition ischemia and cell injury occur whenever VO_2 is persistently DO_2 dependent, and therefore DO_2 dependence undoubtedly contributes to the pathogenesis of MODS. It has been our bias that VO_2 becomes dependent on DO_2 when the DO_2/VO_2 ratio remains persistently below 2:1. At present, continuous SvO_2 monitoring is the most effective way to continuously monitor this ratio.

It should be noted that this paradigm for systemic oxygen kinetics does not suggest that the "critical" DO_2 is the same for all organs (or patients). Clearly, the overall DO_2/VO_2 ratio is merely a weighted average of the DO_2/VO_2 ratios of all body cells and tissues. In fact, this paradigm assumes that in order to calculate the DO_2/VO_2 ratio, one must obtain paired, independently measured, values for both DO_2 and VO_2. The normal biphasic relationship between DO_2 and VO_2 suggests that VO_2 becomes dependent on DO_2 below a critical "threshold." It is therefore very possible, if not probable, that VO_2 becomes DO_2 dependent at higher levels of DO_2 in some individual organs (and patients) than it does in others. This is logically attributed to individual organ (and patient) variability with respect to VO_2 and DO_2. Furthermore, since metabolically active organs

(and patients) do not survive for long when VO_2 is dependent on DO_2, the existence of sustained DO_2 dependency may well be a moot point. At present, systemic oxygen kinetics can be continuously assessed using SvO_2 monitoring. One of the greatest challenges of the next decade will be to define organ-specific markers of function so that bedside information on both systemic and regional oxygen kinetics can be used to prevent failure of individual organs.

Inflammatory Response to Injury

When the inflammatory response is initiated, a wide variety of chemical mediators are released into the systemic circulation. The primary mediators of the inflammatory response are the proinflammatory peptides or cytokines, bioactive lipids including the eicosanoids and platelet activating factor (PAF), toxic oxygen metabolites, and neutrophil-derived tissue proteases.

Peptide Cytokines

Cytokines exert a broad range of biologic effects and are the central regulators of the host inflammatory response (Cipolle et al, Svoboda et al, Windsor et al, Baggiolini et al, Ferrante et al, Toledo-Pereyra and Suzuki, Strieter et al [1993, 1994], Nicod). Cytokine biology is an enormous field of basic science and clinical research and this discussion focuses on those mediators that have been clearly implicated in the pathogenesis of SIRS and MODS. The primary cytokine mediators of SIRS and MODS are tumor necrosis factor (TNF), interleukin-1 (IL-1), interleukin-6 (IL-6), and interleukin-8 (IL-8).

Tumor necrosis factor is clearly an important mediator in the inflammatory response. TNF is produced primarily by macrophages and blood mononuclear cells in response to a variety of stimuli. It appears that TNF is released very early in the inflammatory response; for example, when endotoxin is administered to experimental animals and human subjects, TNF levels increase markedly within minutes and return to baseline within several hours. Increased levels of TNF have been documented in a variety of conditions associated with the development of MODS, including trauma, burns, sepsis, and severe inflammation (i.e., pancreatitis). Thus, it appears that TNF is a central mediator in the pathogenesis of SIRS and MODS.

The systemic effects of TNF include hemodynamic instability, acute lung injury, and widespread organ damage. Tumor necrosis factor infusion in experimental animals and human volunteers produces a "shocklike" hemodynamic picture similar to that seen in severe sepsis and MODS. TNF administration also causes an acute pulmonary injury consisting of neutrophil sequestration, edema, and hemorrhage; this injury is analogous to that seen in ARDS. Finally, intravenous administration of TNF results in pathologic changes in a wide variety of distant organs analogous to those seen in MODS. These changes include hemorrhage, edema, and inflammatory cell infiltration and are seen in the liver, kidneys, and intestine. Thus, the systemic effects of TNF suggest that it plays a fundamental role in the pathogenesis of MODS.

Tumor necrosis factor also has a variety of effects at the cellular level that serve to amplify the inflammatory response. It stimulates the release of a variety of other proinflammatory cytokines and lipids that participate in the pathogenesis of MODS, including IL-1, IL-6, eicosanoids, and PAF. In addition, TNF upregulates the expression of adhesion molecules on the surface of endothelial cells and neutrophils; these adhesion molecules facilitate endothelial cell-neutrophil interaction. Furthermore, TNF enhances a number of neutrophil functions, including phagocytosis, degranulation, chemotaxis, and toxic free radical formation. Finally, TNF upregulates key enzymes in a variety of parallel inflammatory cascades, including phospholipase A_2, cyclooxygenase, and nitric oxide synthase. The net result of these cellular effects of TNF is endothelial cell injury, increased permeability, and edema formation. Thus, TNF amplifies the inflammatory response at multiple levels and is a primary mediator of MODS.

The central role of TNF in the pathogenesis of MODS is further emphasized by the ability of anti-TNF antibodies to significantly reduce organ injury and mortality in a variety of animal models of septic shock (St. John and Dorinsky [1993, 1994], Cipolle et al, Dauberschmidt et al). It is im-

portant to note, however, that these protective effects are limited to animals that receive the antibody before the dose of bacteria or endotoxin. This "pretreatment" effect probably explains the failure of anti-TNF antibodies to reduce overall mortality in human sepsis therapy trials to date.

Interleukin-1 (IL-1) is a polypeptide cytokine produced by a variety of cell types. It exists in two forms, IL-1α and IL-1β. Both forms of IL-1 have a variety of proinflammatory systemic and cellular effects (St. John and Dorinsky [1993, 1994], Cipolle et al, Svoboda et al, Fisher et al, Dinarello et al). Systemic effects include fever, hypotension, organ dysfunction, and shock. Cellular effects include increased release of other proinflammatory cytokines and lipids (TNF, IL-6, and PAF), endothelial cell activation, and increased adhesion molecule expression. Interleukin-1 levels peak several hours after an endotoxin challenge, which is significantly later than with TNF. However, as is the case with TNF, IL-1 administration results in an acute lung injury that is characterized by neutrophil sequestration, increased permeability edema, and hemorrhage. Furthermore, IL-1 administration leads to endothelial cell injury and increased vascular permeability in a variety of other organs, leading to generalized organ dysfunction and death. Finally, high doses of recombinant IL-1 receptor antagonist protein (IL-1ra) appear to block many of the adverse systemic and cellular effects of IL-1 in experimental animals (St. John and Dorinsky [1993, 1994], Cipolle et al, Fisher et al). However, as was the case with monoclonal antibodies to TNF, IL-1ra failed to reduce overall mortality in a large, double-blinded, prospective, randomized trial for the treatment of human sepsis.

Interleukin-6 (IL-6) is produced by macrophages and endothelial cells in response to injury. Interleukin-6 levels increase in response to other cytokines including TNF and IL-1. In addition, Cipolle and colleagues found that IL-6 levels are increased in patients with sepsis and MODS and may correlate better than TNF and IL-1 levels with mortality. It is not possible at this time to say whether increased IL-6 levels are the cause or the result of severe cellular injury. Trials are under way to investigate the role of both monoclonal antibodies to IL-6 and antagonists to the IL-6 receptor in the inflammatory response.

Interleukin-8 (IL-8) is a recently described (Marty et al, Feuerstein and Rabinovici, Leonard and Yoshimura, Baggiolini et al) cytokine produced by a variety of cell types with potent chemoattractant properties for neutrophils. IL-8 appears to play a significant role in neutrophil-mediated lung injury; however, the precise role of IL-8 in the development of MODS remains to be defined. Recently, increased levels of IL-8 have been documented in patients with sepsis and appeared to correlate with both the incidence of MODS and mortality. Given the central role of the neutrophil in tissue injury, it seems quite probable that IL-8 may play an important part in the pathogenesis of MODS. For a more extensive discussion of cytokines and other mediators, see Chap. 1.

Bioactive Lipids

A variety of bioactive lipids are involved in the inflammatory response. As described by Anderson and colleagues, phospholipase A_2 (PLA$_2$) represents a family of enzymes that regulate the inflammatory response through two separate but complementary pathways. One pathway involves the release of arachidonic acid from the cell membrane to form a series of bioactive lipids known collectively as the "eicosanoids." The term eicosanoid refers to the 20-carbon ("eicosa" = 20) fatty acid side chain of arachidonic acid. The second pathway is through the production of PAF, which has been implicated as an independent mediator of MODS.

Following injury, cell membrane–associated PLA$_2$ is stimulated through a G protein–dependent pathway to react with membrane phospholipids. Membrane phospholipids contain arachidonic acid, which is released by PLA$_2$. Arachidonic acid is then metabolized to form the eicosanoids by two major enzyme pathways—cyclooxygenase and lipoxygenase. Three groups of major eicosanoids are formed: the prostaglandins, thromboxanes, and leukotrienes (Cipolle et al, Gadaleta and Davis, Nuytinck et al).

Cyclooxygenase converts arachidonic acid to the prostaglandins, thromboxanes, and prostacyclin. Thromboxanes and prostacyclin are produced by platelets and endothelial cells, respectively. For the most part, these arachidonic acid metabolites have opposing hemodynamic and hematologic effects. For instance, thromboxane is a potent vasoconstrictor, it promotes platelet aggregation, and it increases neutrophil activation. In contrast, prostacyclin is a potent vasodilator, it inhibits platelet aggregation, and it inhibits neutrophil activation. The other major enzyme pathway for arachidonic acid metabolism is the lipoxygenase pathway. Gadaleta and Davis report that lipoxygenase converts arachidonic acid to the leukotrienes. Leukotrienes are vasoconstrictors, they also promote leukostasis and chemokinesis, and they stimulate release of toxic oxygen metabolites and neutrophil proteases. Thus, PLA$_2$ activation leads to the release of a variety of arachidonic acid derivatives, which can contribute to cellular injury and organ dysfunction.

Phospholipase A$_2$ also produces PAF by converting membrane phospholipid to inactive lyso-PAF. Lyso-PAF is subsequently acetylated to the active form of PAF. In contrast to the arachidonic acid metabolites, PAF activates macrophages, neutrophils, and platelets directly through specific cell surface receptors (Anderson et al [1991, 1994], Ou et al). When neutrophils are activated by PAF, they adhere to endothelial cells, perform chemotaxis, degranulate, and release toxic oxygen metabolites and proteases. PAF also increases neutrophil-endothelial cell interaction by increasing the expression of adhesion molecules on the surface of both endothelial cells and neutrophils. Furthermore, PAF causes macrophages to release cytokines and eicosanoids and it causes platelets to release histamine and serotonin. Thus, PLA$_2$ activation releases PAF from cell membranes, leading to nonspecific activation of a variety of inflammatory responses that can exacerbate tissue injury and lead to organ dysfunction.

Phospholipase A$_2$ is activated by several parallel mechanisms following injury. For instance, release of the proinflammatory cytokines (TNF and IL-1) activate PLA$_2$ and cause its release into the systemic circulation. Phospholipase A$_2$ is also activated by ischemia-reperfusion injury. In experimental animals, excessive levels of PLA$_2$ produce widespread organ injury resembling that seen in MODS. Furthermore, Uhl and colleagues documented PLA$_2$ release in a variety of the systemic inflammatory disorders that predispose to MODS, and PLA$_2$ levels appear to correlate with illness severity. Therefore, PLA$_2$ is activated by several parallel mechanisms following injury and appears to play a significant role in the pathogenesis of MODS.

Ischemia-Reperfusion Injury

Ischemia-reperfusion injury is an important mechanism of cell damage leading to MODS (Cipolle et al, Demling et al [1993], Yoshikawa et al). Regardless of the cause, cellular oxygen delivery decreases during ischemia. As a result of decreased oxygen delivery, less adenosine triphosphate (ATP) is produced and ATP is preferentially degraded to its purine bases. This leads to accumulation of hypoxanthine within the cell. Normally, hypoxanthine is converted by xanthine dehydrogenase first to xanthine and subsequently to uric acid. However, during ischemia, reduced cellular ATP levels also result in a loss of normal ion gradients and increased calcium flux into the cell. Increased intracellular calcium then activates proteases, which irreversibly convert xanthine dehydrogenase to xanthine oxidase.

Oxygen delivery increases during reperfusion, which increases intracellular oxygen. Xanthine oxidase also converts excess hypoxanthine to uric acid; however, in the process molecular oxygen is reduced to the superoxide anion (O_2^-). Superoxide anion produces a variety of other toxic oxygen metabolites, including hydrogen peroxide (H_2O_2), singlet oxygen (O_2), and the hydroxyl radical (OH). These toxic oxidant species initiate a variety of free radical reactions, the most harmful of which is peroxidation of fatty acids in the lipid bilayer, leading to cell membrane damage, diffuse capillary leak, and activation of a variety of inflammatory cascades.

Neutrophil-Endothelial Cell Interactions

Regardless of the underlying cause, cell injury releases a variety of activators that stimulate parallel humoral cascades (i.e., clotting, complement, fibrinolytic, kinin, etc.). Various polypeptide products of these reactions attract large numbers of neutrophils to the area of injury (Cipolle et al, Windsor et al, Toledo-Pereyra and Suzuki, Strieter et al [1990, 1993]). These mediators increase expression of adhesion molecules on the surface of both endothelial cells and neutrophils (Cipolle et al, St. John and Dorinsky [1993], Cowley et al, Law et al, St. John et al, Mileski et al). Endothelial cell adhesion molecules include intracellular adhesion molecule-1 (ICAM-1) and endothelial leukocyte adhesion molecule (ELAM). Neutrophils are also activated to express the neutrophil adherence receptor (CD-11/CD-18) on their cell surface. These adhesion molecules facilitate neutrophil-endothelial interaction, as well as neutrophil adherence, diapedesis, chemotaxis, and degranulation. This process ultimately results in the release of toxic oxygen metabolites as well as a variety of neutrophil-derived proteases that contribute to organ damage. Finally, in animal experiments, antibodies directed against the CD-18 portion of the leukocyte adherence receptor decreased organ injury following hemorrhagic shock (St. John and Dorinsky [1993, 1994], Mileski et al). Therefore, following injury, a variety of mechanisms serve to increase neutrophil and endothelial cell interaction and hence neutrophil-mediated tissue injury.

Windsor and colleagues found that, with respect to neutrophil-mediated oxidant injury, the membrane-bound enzyme, reduced nicotinamide adenine dinucleotide phosphate (NADPH) oxidase, catalyzes the formation of superoxide anion from molecular oxygen. These superoxide radicals are subsequently converted to hydrogen peroxide by superoxide dismutase. Hydrogen peroxide is then channeled into the production of the long-lived oxidant, hypochlorous acid, by the enzyme myeloperoxidase, which is released from the cytosolic granules of activated neutrophils. All of the oxidants formed by these reactions are unstable and highly reactive. They are capable of direct DNA damage that interferes with cellular metabolism, they can disrupt plasma membranes by the process of lipid peroxidation, and they can interfere with actin metabolism, leading to changes in endothelial cell shape. The end result is diffuse capillary leakage, cell death, and organ dysfunction. In recent experimental studies by Yoshikawa and associates, tissue levels of antioxidant enzymes were shown to be inversely related to susceptibility to organ damage following intravenous administration of endotoxin. Thus, neutrophil-derived oxidants appear to play a central role in the pathogenesis of MODS.

Damage to the vascular endothelium following injury also leads to the release of a variety of other ligands (i.e., tissue factor, plasminogen activator) that contact and activate proteases in the various humoral cascade systems responsible for hemostasis and wound healing. However, some of these system-specific proteases (i.e., kallikrein, plasmin, thrombin) also activate additional inflammatory cascades (i.e., kinin, complement, etc.), further amplifying the local inflammatory response. The end result of this activation process is increased neutrophil chemotaxis, sequestration, and activation, leading to the release of a variety of cytokines, eicosanoids, oxygen free radicals, and neutrophil-derived tissue proteases. Jochum and colleagues report that these proteases, especially neutrophil elastase and cathepsin B, appear to play a major role in the injury response, not only in terms of local tissue injury, but also in terms of propagation of the inflammatory response. In addition to local destruction of basement membrane and matrix proteins, these neutrophil proteases destroy important inhibitors for the system-specific proteinases and a variety of other plasma proteins. These inhibitors are crucial to tight control of the various inflammatory cascades. Furthermore, according to Windsor and colleagues (1993) and Jochum and associates, the timing of appearance and levels of these neutrophil proteases are highly predictive of the development of MODS. Thus, the extracellular release of neutrophil proteases, particularly PMN elastase, appears to play an important role in the pathogenesis of SIRS/MODS. Consequently, specific inhibitors of these proteases may have a therapeutic role in the prevention and treatment of MODS.

Endotoxin

Gram-negative bacterial sepsis is one of the most common predisposing factors for the development of SIRS/MODS (St. John and Dorinsky [1993, 1994], Beal and Cerra, Deitch, Demling et al [1993], Mileski et al). Endotoxin, a lipopolysaccharide derived from the cell wall of gram-negative bacteria, is an important mediator in the pathogenesis of MODS. Lipopolysaccharide (LPS) stimulates the inflammatory response at multiple levels and has been shown to release virtually all of the im-

portant mediators involved in the development of MODS. For example, low doses of endotoxin increase TNF levels within minutes in both experimental animals, as reported by Wakabayashi and colleagues, and human volunteers, as found by Michie and associates, suggesting that TNF plays an important early role in gram-negative sepsis. The central role of LPS in the pathogenesis of MODS is emphasized by the protective effect of monoclonal antibodies in LPS in animal models of bacterial sepsis (St. John and Dorinsky [1993, 1994], Cipolle et al). However, in prospective, randomized clinical trials, antibodies to LPS have thus far failed to increase overall survival or protect against the development of MODS. Subgroup analysis has suggested some benefits with severe sepsis and hemodynamic instability.

Nitric Oxide

Nitric oxide (NO) is an endogenous vasodilator produced by endothelial cells. It is derived from L-arginine and is important in maintaining vascular wall integrity. Cipolle and colleagues, and Demling and associates (1993), found that lipopolysaccharide increases endothelial NO release, suggesting that NO may be responsible for LPS-induced hypotension and vascular unresponsiveness in severe sepsis. The precise role of NO in the pathogenesis of MODS remains to be defined.

Role of the Gut

The gut appears to play a central role in the pathogenesis of MODS (Deitch, Corno, Pape et al, Kudsk, Mythen and Webb). The gut mucosa provides an important protective barrier to a wide variety of intraluminal bacteria and toxins. Loss of the integrity of this barrier leads to bacterial translocation and release of endotoxin. Bacterial translocation and endotoxemia lead to nonspecific activation of the inflammatory response and MODS. Furthermore, Moore and colleagues found that the gut appears to play a central role in priming circulating neutrophils, which are subsequently activated by endotoxin, setting the stage for neutrophil-mediated tissue injury and MODS.

It is becoming increasingly clear, as reported by Mythen and Webb, that is-

chemia of the gut mucosa is of fundamental importance to the pathogenesis of MODS. Splanchnic ischemia can occur whenever splanchnic DO_2 is inadequate relative to VO_2. A transient global decrease in DO_2 is common in patients at risk for MODS as a result of hypovolemia or cardiovascular dysfunction. Splanchnic vasoconstriction is the normal protective response to decreased systemic DO_2. This selective vasoconstriction occurs in order to protect the heart and brain; however, it is clear that decreases in systemic DO_2 lead to disproportionately larger decreases in splanchnic DO_2. For instance, a 15 percent reduction in circulating blood volume results in a 40 percent reduction in splanchnic blood volume despite a normal cardiac output and blood pressure. To add insult to injury, both gut mucosal and systemic VO_2 are increased in patients at risk for MODS. Thus, splanchnic DO_2 is disproportionately decreased at the same time that splanchnic demands for VO_2 are increased. This leads to gut mucosal ischemia, which can compromise the integrity of the mucosal barrier. A compromised mucosal barrier becomes "leaky" to bacteria and endotoxin. This sets the stage for bacterial translocation and, eventually, the development of MODS. Consequently, maintenance of this barrier is of central importance to the management of critically ill patients.

Prevention

Currently, other than supportive therapy for individual organ failure, there is no effective therapy for established MODS. Therefore, the only treatment for MODS is prevention. The priorities in managing patients at risk for MODS are to avoid ischemia by maintaining adequate oxygen delivery relative to metabolic needs, to avoid additional insults such as hypotension and infection, and to control any obvious sources of inflammation. In addition, it is necessary to provide adequate metabolic, nutritional, and occasionally mechanical support for dysfunctional organs until recovery occurs.

Recently, because of the central role of bacterial translocation in the pathogenesis of MODS, attention has focused on the use of selective gut decontamination as a means of prevention (St. John and Dorinsky, Beal and Cerra, Deitch, Reidy and Ramsay). Following injury, the oropharynx and upper gastrointestinal tract become rapidly colonized with a variety of pathogenic bacteria. The use of orally administered, nonabsorbable, antibiotics is postulated to reduce the risk of nosocomial pneumonia as well as gut-associated bacteremia. While this is an attractive hypothesis, prospective clinical trials have not demonstrated a significant reduction in overall mortality. On the other hand, selective gut contamination does appear to reduce the risk of ventilator-associated nosocomial pneumonia. To the extent that nosocomial pneumonia is an independent risk factor for MODS, selective gut decontamination may be a useful adjunct. For this reason, additional studies are needed to clearly define what role, if any, selective gut decontamination has in the prevention of MODS.

Finally, any approach to the prevention and management of MODS requires that attention be focused on controlling potential sources of inflammation. In surgical patients, this demands an aggressive approach toward early intervention in all aspects of the patient's care. There is no substitute for adequate resuscitation and appropriate physiologic monitoring. In addition, every effort must be made to ensure early definitive repair of injuries (i.e., fracture fixation), prompt excision of necrotic tissue, rapid control of peritoneal soilage, early abscess drainage, and aggressive treatment of nosocomial infection.

Management Principles

MODS is a syndrome of surgical progress and, as such, care of the patient with MODS is simply the care of the modern surgical patient. For this reason, the management of patients with MODS is the purview of all surgeons who wish to take complete responsibility for patient care. [*Editor's note:* Agreed!] To this end, I have purposefully avoided the term "intensivist" in this discussion because it implies that surgical "intensive" care is a responsibility that should be delegated rather than assumed as a matter of course. Prevention and management of MODS are nothing more than an exercise in applied surgical physiology. The major principles of the physiologic approach to the management of MODS used at the University of Michigan are briefly summarized here; for a more detailed discussion of these fascinating topics, the reader is referred to standard textbooks of "critical" care.

Oxygen Kinetics

While the DO_2/VO_2 debate wears on, it has become quite clear that efforts to "optimize" systemic DO_2 relative to VO_2 are clearly warranted in critically ill patients. Ischemia and cellular injury occur whenever DO_2 is persistently inadequate; therefore, a primary management goal for MODS must be to optimize the DO_2/VO_2 ratio. It should be noted that "optimizing" the DO_2/VO_2 ratio is quite different from blindly "maximizing" DO_2 (or VO_2) (Russell and Phang, Hanique et al, Pinsky, Barone). According to Shanley and Bartlett, any confusion regarding this management goal can be clarified if one realizes that a "normal" value for DO_2 may be profoundly "subnormal" if VO_2 is elevated, or "supranormal" if VO_2 is depressed (see Fig. 10-3). This pitfall can be completely avoided if one defines "optimal" DO_2 not as an arbitrary value but rather as that level of DO_2 that "optimizes" the DO_2/VO_2 ratio as reflected by the SvO_2.

The primary physiologic goal in the management of MODS must be to optimize SvO_2 and hence the DO_2/VO_2 ratio. It should be noted that this can be accomplished in a hypermetabolic patient by increasing DO_2 *or* by decreasing VO_2. Oxygen delivery can be increased by improving oxygenation, correcting anemia, and optimizing cardiac output. Oxygen consumption can be decreased by modifying those factors that tend to increase metabolic rate. This is accomplished by decreasing inflammatory stimuli (abscess drainage, wound debridement, fracture stabilization, treating infections), by decreasing stimuli for catecholamine release (adequate analgesia, sedation, preventing hypothermia, controlled beta blockade), by decreasing excessive skeletal muscle activity (sedation, paralysis), and by controlling severe hyperthermia (active cooling). In the modern management of MODS, all interventions are carefully and logically titrated to ensure an optimal DO_2/VO_2 ratio based on continuously measured SvO_2.

Metabolic and Nutritional Support

The role of adequate nutritional support in critically ill patients with MODS cannot be overemphasized (Deitch, Demling et al [1993], Bartlett et al, Kudsk, Frankenfield et al). Protein and energy requirements are continuous and essential to all body functions. In hypermetabolic, catabolic patients with MODS, energy and protein requirements are markedly increased (Beal and Cerra, Demling et al [1993], Cipolle et al, Bartlett et al). These requirements are met by endogenous sources in fasting or by exogenous treatment in the form of nutritional support. The consequences of failing to meet these requirements are progressive deterioration of organ function, impaired immunity, infection, and death. Therefore, avoidance of malnutrition is fundamental to the physiologic support of patients with MODS.

Whenever possible, nutritional support should be administered by an enteral route (Beal and Cerra, Demling et al [1993], Kudsk). Gut mucosal atrophy develops rapidly in the absence of enteral nutrients and early enteral nutrition is considered to be an effective way to preserve the gut mucosal barrier. To prevent or minimize the risk of aspiration in an obtunded patient, feedings should generally be administered distal to the pylorus. However, as a general rule, it is almost always possible to accomplish tube feedings with gastric infusion. If the patient will not tolerate total enteral nutritional support, partial enteral nutrition is recommended to maintain mucosal integrity. A number of studies, including those by Beal and Cerra, and by Demling and colleagues (1993), have clearly demonstrated that early enteral nutrition as opposed to early parenteral nutrition, or delaying enteral nutrition for 3 days, reduces the risk of MODS in acutely ill or injured surgical patients. Thus, enteral nutritional therapy should be initiated as soon as possible in the patient at risk for MODS. If enteral therapy is not possible, parenteral support should be used as needed to achieve positive caloric and nitrogen balance.

Any intelligent approach to nutritional support requires well-defined physiologic end points. Frankenfield and colleagues, and Bartlett and associates, found that, in a critically ill patient, the most accurate method of determining energy expenditure is indirect calorimetry. In this method, the amount of oxygen absorbed across the lungs is measured over a given period of time. Fick's axiom states that the amount of oxygen absorbed across the lungs is exactly equal to the amount of oxygen consumed in peripheral oxidative metabolism as long as the metabolic rate remains relatively constant. For the purposes of estimating nutritional requirements in mechanically ventilated surgical patients, this is almost always the case. Because the energy released during oxidation of various nutritional substrates is well known, oxygen consumption per minute can be mathematically converted to caloric requirements per hour or per day. In this manner, nutritional support can be tailored to ensure a positive caloric balance for any individual patient. Bartlett and coworkers have shown maintenance of a positive caloric balance to be independently predictive of survival in patients with MODS.

In patients with SIRS/MODS, significant alterations in intermediary metabolism occur as a direct result of the altered hormonal and inflammatory mileu (Beal and Cerra, Demling et al [1993], Bartlett et al). Glucose metabolism is altered in MODS and the use of glucose as an energy source is reduced when compared to simple starvation. Pyruvate dehydrogenase activity is also significantly reduced; excess pyruvate is subsequently converted to alanine and lactate, which are two of the principal substrates for hepatic gluconeogenesis. In addition, endogenous protein catabolism increases the amino acid load to the liver, which also increases gluconeogenesis. The net result is hyperglycemia, which is usually quite refractory to exogenous insulin.

The ultimate goal of nutritional support is to avoid an energy deficit and to minimize endogenous protein catabolism; overfeeding is potentially detrimental. Too many carbohydrate calories will promote hepatic lipogenesis. Increased lipogenesis leads to excessive carbon dioxide production, which increases requirements for mechanical ventilation. Similarly, overzealous administration of fat can lead to hypertriglyceridemia, hypoxemia, and immune problems. The physiologic approach to nutritional support is to provide sufficient calories to achieve a positive caloric balance. This goal is best achieved if calo-

ric support is administered based on daily energy balance studies using indirect calorimetry.

Protein metabolism is also significantly altered in SIRS/MODS (Beal and Cerra, Cipolle et al, Demling et al [1993], Bartlett et al). There is an impressive loss of lean body mass ("autocatabolism") as endogenous protein (i.e., skeletal muscle, intestinal viscera, and connective tissue) is consumed to meet energy requirements. This process releases large quantities of amino acids, which are used by the liver for gluconeogenesis. In skeletal muscle, branched-chain amino acids appear to be consumed as a primary energy source. Large amounts of glutamine are also released, providing a substrate for renal ammonia excretion as well as fuel for gut mucosal enterocytes and nucleotide synthesis. As a result of this increase in protein catabolism, urea production is markedly increased.

Urinary urea nitrogen constitutes approximately 85 percent of total nitrogen excretion. This allows urinary urea nitrogen to be used to measure nitrogen balance in critically ill patients. Currently, nitrogen balance can be measured directly using chemiluminescence techniques, as reported by Dechert and colleagues. From daily nitrogen balance data, protein catabolic rate as well as daily protein balance can be determined. In critically ill patients, nitrogen losses can exceed 15 to 20 g per day. Administration of exogenous protein and amino acids helps to preserve lean body mass, promote anabolism and wound healing, and increase immunity. Protein and amino acid supplementation is recommended in the critically ill patient with MODS based on daily nitrogen balance studies.

Currently, a variety of specially formulated amino acid solutions are available for use in critically ill patients. For the most part the data to support their use (and added expense) are quite limited, with perhaps two exceptions. Beal and Cerra, and Cipolle and colleagues, report that branched-chain amino acids (leucine, isoleucine, and valine) are the primary fuel consumed by catabolic skeletal muscle. By supplying this essential substrate, branched-chain amino acid formulations appear to promote nitrogen retention, decrease catabolism of endogenous protein,

and decrease ureagenesis. In addition, according to Demling and associates (1993), glutamine is the major fuel for gut mucosal enterocytes, and glutamine supplementation may promote maintenance of the gut mucosal barrier. Glutamine-enriched enteral and parenteral solutions are now available and may be useful in preserving gut mucosal integrity.

Pulmonary Dysfunction

Acute lung injury (ALI) and the adult respiratory distress syndrome (ARDS) are the sine qua non of MODS (St. John and Dorinsky [1994], Deitch, Bartlett et al, Cipolle et al, Demling et al). Studies exploring the biology of ARDS over the past two decades have contributed immensely to our understanding of the pathophysiologic mechanisms underlying all forms of organ injury. In patients at risk for MODS, pulmonary dysfunction usually precedes dysfunction in other organs and may be an initiating event in the development of SIRS/MODS. Evidence for a fundamental role for lung injury in the pathogenesis of MODS comes from the fact that a variety of diverse causes of "primary" lung injury are associated with the development of MODS (St. John and Dorinsky [1994], Beal and Cerra, Bartlett et al, Cipolle et al). These include pneumonia, aspiration, pulmonary contusion, inhalation injury, and near-drowning. Furthermore, "secondary" lung injury frequently occurs in association with a variety of diverse conditions that do not primarily affect the lung. These conditions include sepsis, acute pancreatitis, undrained abscess, multiple trauma, burns, cardiopulmonary bypass, prolonged hypotension, or under-resuscitation from any cause. Thus, a clear understanding of ALI/ARDS is fundamental to any discussion of SIRS/MODS.

It is instructive to review the pathophysiology of acute lung injury, not only because the pathologic changes that occur in the lung closely parallel the changes that occur in other organs, as reported by Kreuzfelder and colleagues, but also because these changes provide much of the rationale for a physiologic approach to the management of pulmonary and other organ dysfunction. Regardless of the initiating event, activated neutrophils and platelets adhere to the pulmonary capillary endothelium and release a variety of toxic substances. Multiple inflammatory cascades are activated, leading to diffuse endothelial cell injury and increased capillary permeability. The increase in capillary permeability leads to interstitial pulmonary edema, which gradually progresses to alveolar flooding and collapse. Endothelial cell injury also leads to microvascular hemorrhage and thrombosis, which further reduces the capillary surface area available for gas exchange. In addition to injury to the pulmonary endothelium, alveolar epithelial cells are also injured, which leads to loss of alveolar surfactant. Loss of surfactant, in turn, increases alveolar surface tension, which increases the tendency toward alveolar collapse. The end result is a diffuse loss of functional alveolar volume and a reduction in pulmonary compliance.

The primary gas exchange abnormality in ALI/ARDS is profound hypoxemia. Hypoxemia is the result of both ventilation-perfusion inequalities and physiologic shunt. Functional alveolar volume is markedly reduced in ARDS as a result of interstitial and alveolar pulmonary edema, which lead to alveolar collapse and flooding. For this reason, mixed-venous blood returning to the heart perfuses many alveoli, which are either poorly ventilated, collapsed, or flooded. This problem is compounded by the fact that most of the pulmonary blood flow is directed to the most dependent lung regions, which are also the most severely affected by interstitial and alveolar edema, flooding, and collapse. The end result is profound hypoxemia that is resistant to supplemental oxygen. Interestingly, CO_2 retention is almost never a problem in ALI because carbon dioxide is 20 times more diffusible than oxygen; therefore, even when the functional alveolar volume is markedly reduced, carbon dioxide clearance is usually more than adequate.

To make matters worse in patients with ALI, according to Beal and Cerra, the work of breathing increases substantially. This occurs because of the marked increase of pulmonary compliance due not only to a marked increase in extravascular lung water, but also to chest wall and diaphragmatic edema. In addition, systemic oxygen consumption (and carbon dioxide production) is markedly increased in ALI. This is particularly precarious because VO_2 (and VCO_2) are greatly increased; as a result, requirements for minute ventilation often exceed 15 to 20 liters per minute, which usually necessitates mechanical ventilation. Furthermore, systemic DO_2 is compromised secondary to hypoxemia. The end result is worsening peripheral ischemia that exacerbates organ injury. Therefore, the primary physiologic goal in the management of ARDS/MODS is to maintain adequate pulmonary gas exchange and systemic oxygen delivery.

From the standpoint of pulmonary gas exchange, the major pathophysiologic abnormality in ALI/ARDS is loss of functional alveolar volume with resultant hypoxemia and reduced lung compliance. The optimal approach to gas exchange support in ALI remains to be defined; however, most conventional techniques, as reported by Shanley and Bartlett, have employed some form of positive-pressure ventilation. In cases of severe respiratory insufficiency, high inspiratory pressures and volumes are often employed in an attempt to compensate for reduced lung efficiency. Unfortunately, these high pressures and volumes are directed toward the residual normal lung units, which are smaller but much more compliant. This leads to regional overdistention, which increases microvascular permeability and leads to mechanical disruption of the alveolar-capillary membrane. The resultant iatrogenic lung injury has been termed *barotrauma* or *volutrauma*. Completely safe tidal volumes and peak inspiratory pressures have not been identified; however, a common sense approach to positive-pressure ventilation is to manipulate tidal volume, inspiratory time, and inspiratory flow rate to keep the peak inspiratory pressure as low as possible, certainly less than 40 mm Hg.

Shanley and Bartlett found positive end-expiratory pressure (PEEP) to be a useful adjunct to improve oxygenation in ALI. PEEP prevents alveolar collapse, increases functional residual capacity, improves pulmonary compliance, and reduces physiologic shunt. However, it also increases mean intrathoracic pressure and reduces venous return. A reduction in venous return decreases systemic DO_2 by reducing cardiac output. Therefore, the level of PEEP should be physiologically titrated to maximize alveolar recruitment and oxygenation while simultaneously avoiding the adverse effects of PEEP on cardiac output. This physiologic goal is most readily accomplished if the optimal level of PEEP is defined as the level that optimizes the DO_2/VO_2 ratio. Consequently, PEEP is most logically titrated based on continuously measured SvO_2.

New approaches to mechanical ventilation in ALI, as described by Shanley and Bartlett and by Shapiro and Peruzzi, include the use of pressure-controlled inverse ratio ventilation (PC-IRV) and continuous positive airway pressure (CPAP). During PC-IRV, the inspiratory pressure is reduced and the inspiratory time is prolonged to more than half the respiratory cycle. By prolonging inspiration, PC-IRV allows more time for recruitment of collapsed alveoli and improves oxygenation at lower airway pressures. CPAP increases lung volumes during spontaneous breathing by maintaining increased airway pressure throughout the respiratory cycle. Increased airway pressure also reduces the work of breathing. Other ventilatory techniques include airway pressure release ventilation (APRV) and high-frequency jet ventilation (HFJV). The ultimate goal of these new techniques is to reduce the iatrogenic injury caused by high airway pressures and lung volumes. While there are a variety of theoretical advantages to these newer ventilatory techniques, at present it remains unproven that any of them has a clear-cut advantage over conventional mechanical ventilation that is carefully applied and physiologically directed.

Adjunctive treatment modalities in the management of acute lung injury include the use of prone positioning (by Lamm et al), permissive hypercapnia (by Dauberschmidt et al, Hickling et al, Reynolds et al, Bidani et al), efforts to decrease extravascular lung water, and avoidance of high inspired oxygen concentration. Prone positioning improves oxygenation by diverting pulmonary blood flow from the more collapsed posterior lung segments to the better inflated anterior ones. Permissive hypercapnia refers to the use of pressure-limited, low tidal volume ventilation to avoid iatrogenic lung injury. In this technique, arterial PCO_2 is permitted to increase and the resultant acidosis is treated pharmacologically. PEEP is then adjusted to maintain adequate oxygenation. In this manner, the deleterious effects of high airway pressures and volumes are avoided while adequate oxygen delivery is maintained. Efforts to decrease extravascular lung water include aggressive diuresis, fluid restriction, and even hemofiltration or dialysis. Reducing extravascular lung water improves gas exchange and pulmonary compliance and decreases requirements for mechanical ventilation. Finally, high concentrations of inspired oxygen are directly toxic to alveolar epithelial cells; in addition, they promote atelectasis by washing out alveolar nitrogen. Therefore, supplemental oxygen is administered to maximize arterial oxygen content rather than partial pressure. Because 99 percent of arterial oxygen is bound to hemoglobin, maintaining hemoglobin saturation is the critical factor. Adequate arterial hemoglobin saturation is obtained as long as the arterial PO_2 is greater than approximately 65 to 70 mm Hg. Oxygen content is also dependent on hemoglobin concentration, and transfusion is used to maintain hemoglobin concentration between 10 and 15 g/dl. The goal, as always, is to optimize the DO_2/VO_2 ratio based on continuously measured SvO_2.

Although mechanical ventilation and positive airway pressure appear to be lifesaving supportive maneuvers, evidence is rapidly accumulating that in some cases they may actually exacerbate lung injury. Because mechanical ventilation is only a supportive therapy, it is desirable that it not contribute to the ongoing pathophysiology of ALI/ARDS and hence SIRS/MODS. Unfortunately, those patients with the most severe forms of acute lung injury are the ones in whom the iatrogenic effects of mechanical ventilation may prove fatal. Bartlett believes that extracorporeal gas exchange may represent a superior life support technique in this group of patients. Extracorporeal life support (ECLS) refers to the use of prolonged extracorporeal circulation to provide temporary gas exchange or perfusion support for a period of days to weeks. At present the extremely high mortality of MODS precludes the use of ECLS as a routine pulmonary support technique for ALI in association with MODS. However, given the central role of acute lung injury in the pathogenesis of MODS, efforts to curtail iatrogenic pulmonary injury are clearly warranted. In the future, continued improvements in both the techniques of ECLS and the treatment strategies for MODS may witness increased application of ECLS for pulmonary support in this syndrome.

Renal Dysfunction

Acute oliguric or anuric renal failure in the context of MODS is a highly lethal event with a mortality of 50 to 90 percent (Frankenfield et al, Eliahou et al, Wardle, Cumming). From a physiologic standpoint, this is not surprising. The consequences of acute loss of kidney function in a patient who is hypermetabolic and catabolic with diffuse endothelial injury and "leaky" capillaries should be self-evident. In the absence of normal urine output, fluid overload develops rapidly, leading to acute increases in extravascular lung water that further impair pulmonary gas exchange. Worsening hypoxemia further compromises oxygen delivery, which exacerbates peripheral ischemia and organ injury.

In addition to these adverse pulmonary effects of hypervolemia, increased capillary permeability and edema in all organ systems significantly compromise function. This problem is exacerbated by compromised systemic oxygen delivery and impaired tissue gas exchange. In addition, hypermetabolism and protein catabolism lead to the rapid development of uremia and serious electrolyte abnormalities (particularly hyperkalemia). Finally, volume and solute restraints significantly compromise nutritional support. Malnutrition promotes autocatabolism, which significantly worsens uremia and electrolyte problems and also impairs host defenses. Consequently, the development of oliguric or anuric renal failure in the context of MODS is potentially a lethal event; as such, it must be recognized early and treated aggressively.

In patients with MODS, renal replacement therapy should be used aggressively for all patients with oliguric or anuric renal failure that persists despite adequate renal perfusion and a trial of loop diuretics, according to Mault and colleagues. Renal replacement therapy facilitates volume, electrolyte, and nutritional management. Adequate nutrition is absolutely essential in critically ill patients to minimize autocatabolism, to promote anabolism and facilitate wound healing, and to augment host defenses. Beal and Cerra, and Bartlett and associates, found that, in these pa-

tients, resting energy requirements are typically 50 percent above baseline levels and protein requirements are two to three times above baseline levels. Consequently, protein and calorie restriction is not only counterproductive, but is potentially detrimental.

It is clear that protein catabolism, urea generation, and hyperkalemia can be reduced by providing sufficient nonprotein calories to maintain a positive energy balance. Furthermore, it has been shown that nitrogen balance and possibly survival can be improved if protein intake is carefully supplemented based on protein balance studies. The advantage of essential amino acid formulations in patients with oliguric renal failure has yet to be conclusively demonstrated. [*Editor's Note:* I disagree. In the only study designed to show the advantage of essential amino acid solution, that advantage was conclusively demonstrated. (RM Abel et al. *N Engl J Med* 288:695, 1973.)] However, solutions that contain a high ratio of branched-chain amino acids may enhance positive nitrogen balance.

There are three primary forms of renal replacement therapy: intermittent hemodialysis, peritoneal dialysis, and continuous hemofiltration. Intermittent hemodialysis in the setting of MODS is associated with a high incidence of potentially lethal complications, including severe hypotension, hypoxemia, arrhythmias, and hemolysis, that severely limit its application. Peritoneal dialysis has several advantages including lack of the need for vascular access or anticoagulation and hemodynamic stability; however, risks of catheter infection and peritonitis significantly reduce the usefulness of this form of renal substitution in postoperative surgical patients.

Currently, the renal replacement therapy of choice for oliguric or anuric patients with MODS is continuous hemofiltration, according to Frankenfield and colleagues, and Mault and associates. This form of renal replacement is specifically intended for treatment of acute oliguric or anuric renal failure. Continuous arteriovenous hemofiltration (CAVH) is an extracorporeal ultrafiltration technique that facilitates removal of extracellular fluid and solutes (Fig. 10-5). Ultrafiltration is accomplished by creating a hydrostatic pressure gradient between indwelling vascular access catheters in the femoral artery and vein. A po-

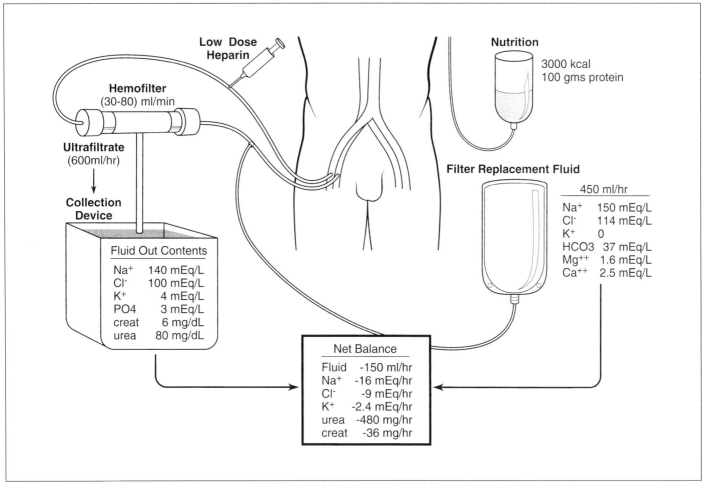

Fig. 10-5. Principles of continuous arteriovenous hemofiltration. Arterial blood is perfused through a hollow-fiber capillary membrane, producing an ultrafiltrate of plasma at a rate of 500 to 1000 ml per hour. Replacement fluid resembling extracellular fluid without the toxic solutes is infused at a rate sufficient to maintain the desired fluid balance. (Adapted from Mault JR, et al. Continuous arteriovenous filtration: An effective treatment for surgical acute renal failure. Surgery 101:478–484, 1987.)

rous, hollow-fiber, capillary membrane is used to filter off extracellular fluid and toxic solutes up to 10,000 daltons in size at a rate of 500 to 700 ml per hour. A replacement solution formulated to resemble extracellular fluid is simultaneously infused at a sufficient rate to achieve the desired hourly fluid balance. Overall fluid balance and serum electrolyte concentrations are easily titrated to any desired value by manipulating the composition of the replacement solution as well as the rate of fluid replacement.

Volume and solute clearance rates with CAVH are limited by the ultrafiltration/ replacement fluid exchange rate. Volume clearance, for all intents and purposes, is never a problem with hemofiltration; however, solute clearance can be enhanced by use of a dialysate bath. DiCarlo and

colleagues refer to this technique as CAVH-D (for "dialysis"). Continuous venovenous hemofiltration (CVVH) is an interesting variation on this theme in which venous blood is drained, perfused through a hemofilter using an extracorporeal blood pump, and subsequently returned to the venous circulation by means of a double-lumen venous access catheter similar to that used for acute hemodialysis. Another potentially useful therapeutic application of this technology is to covalently modify the filter fibers in order to selectively adsorb specific toxic mediators. A preliminary trial was conducted in which polymyxin B was covalently immobilized on the polystyrene fibers of a hemoperfusion column in order to bind endotoxin. Aoki and associates found endotoxin levels to be significantly reduced following 2 hours of this therapy, suggesting that this

type of modification may prove useful in the treatment of patients with sepsis and MODS.

In summary, continuous hemofiltration greatly simplifies management of oliguric or anuric patients with MODS. The ability to easily control fluid and electrolyte balance facilitates maintaining positive caloric balance; furthermore, positive nitrogen balance can be achieved by protein or amino acid supplementation without worsening uremia. Transfusion can be used liberally to optimize oxygen delivery while excess extravascular water is simultaneously removed. In addition, Vincent and Tielemans found that hemofiltration may remove toxic mediators, thus limiting the inflammatory response. All of these goals can be accomplished without the risk of exacerbating ischemia if they are directed by continuous SvO_2 monitoring. Thus, continuous hemofiltration should be used early and aggressively to facilitate volume, electrolyte, and nutritional management to oliguric or anuric patients with MODS.

Hepatic Dysfunction

At present, there is no readily available mechanical substitute for the failing liver. This is unfortunate given the central role of the liver in both normal homeostasis and the pathogenesis of MODS, as reported by Matuschak and colleagues. Before the advent of transplantation, the development of fulminant hepatic failure in the context of MODS was uniformly fatal. Recently, hepatic transplantation has been used successfully in a very small subset of noninfected patients with fulminant liver failure and MODS; however, the exceedingly high mortality of transplantation in this setting, the need for immunosuppressive drugs, and the scarcity of donor organs suggest that transplantation will never be a viable alternative for the vast majority of patients with acute liver failure and MODS. In the future, bioartificial liver substitutes or extracorporeally perfused donor livers may provide temporary hepatic support for patients in acute liver failure. At the present time, however, the manifestations of hepatic dysfunction (coagulopathy, hypoproteinemia, thrombocytopenia, ascites, encephalopathy) are treated symptomatically.

Specific Therapy

Immunotherapy

An explosion of recent advances in cellular and molecular biology have resulted in the development of a variety of novel immunologic approaches to MODS (St. John and Dorinsky, Beal and Cerra, Abraham and Raffin, Carson et al, Taylor et al, Mileski et al, Pizcueta and Luscinskas, van der Poll et al, Broaddus et al, Mulligan et al, Sekido et al). These approaches are targeted at a variety of the interdependent mediators of MODS. The site of action ranges from the initiators (i.e., LPS, tissue factor), to the various molecular mediators (i.e., TNF, IL-1, PAF), to the specific effector cells (i.e., the neutrophil CD-11/CD-18 receptor). Despite encouraging results in animal studies, the clinical results for these newer

therapies have been largely disappointing (Table 10-3). It appears that the protective effect provided by these agents is largely a "pretreatment" effect; that is, the agents are only effective if given before the injury or insult. This is not surprising when one considers the incredible complexity and redundancy of the inflammatory response. A useful analogy would be that by the time MODS is established, "the horse is out and running and the status of the barn door is of little consequence." On the other hand, this discrepancy between laboratory and clinical results suggests that outcomes may improve as our ability to identify patients earlier in the course of MODS gets better. In addition, these agents may have a synergistic effect if used together to inhibit the inflammatory response at multiple levels simultaneously. Finally, despite spectacular improvements in supportive therapy for MODS, overall mortality remains exceedingly high. Therefore, it is hoped that in the future novel cellular and molecular approaches will reduce mortality from MODS.

Other Agents

Theoretically, any agent that decreases the inflammatory response should decrease the risk of MODS. However, controlled trials using anti-inflammatory agents (i.e., steroids, prostaglandins, and cyclooxygenase inhibitor) have failed to show a reduction in either overall mortality or the incidence of MODS (St. John and Dorinsky [1994], Beal and Cerra, Demling et al [1993]). Similarly, given the central role of toxic oxygen species in the pathogenesis of MODS the use of antioxidants should re-

duce organ injury. However, clinical trials of free radical scavengers, such as allopurinol, iron chelators, and superoxide dismutase (SOD), have met with limited success (Beal and Cerra, Cipolle et al, Marzi et al). Thus, the use of specific therapeutic agents targeted at various aspects of the inflammatory response does not appear to have a significant impact on mortality when administered after MODS is established.

Conclusion

MODS is both the cause and the result of surgical progress. The past 20 years have witnessed tremendous advances both in terms of organ-based supportive therapy and in terms of our understanding of the basic cellular and molecular biology of the inflammatory response. Unfortunately, steady advances in organ-based supportive therapy have not resulted in a significant reduction in overall mortality from MODS. On the contrary, as life support technology has continued to improve, the prevalence of MODS has continued to increase. For this reason, MODS remains the most common cause of death in the surgical intensive care unit.

On the other hand, advances in cellular and molecular biology have made it possible to interrupt the inflammatory response at multiple levels, ranging from the initiating factors, to the various chemical mediators, to the specific effector cells. Early clinical results have been disappointing; however, this should not be taken as a justification for a nihilistic attitude to-

Table 10-3. Current Status of Molecular Approaches to Sepsis, ARDS, and MODS

Site of Action	Approach	Laboratory Studies: Efficacious?	Clinical Trials: Reduce Mortality?
LPS	MoAb	Yes	No
Tissue factor	MoAb	Yes	—
PAF	RA	Yes	No
TNF	MoAb	Yes	No
IL-1	RA	Yes	No
IL-6	MoAb	Yes	—
IL-8	MoAb	Yes	—
CD-11/CD-18	MoAb	Yes	Phase I

LPS = lipopolysaccharide; PAF = platelet activating factor; TNF = tumor necrosis factor; MoAb = monoclonal antibody; RA = receptor antagonist.
Adapted from St. John RC, Dorinsky PM. An overview of multiple organ dysfunction syndrome. *J Lab Clin Med* 124:478–483, 1994.

ward this problem. On the contrary, with respect to MODS, an important challenge for the future is to develop improved methods of accurately predicting in which patients this syndrome will develop (Sauaia et al, St. John and Dorinsky [1994], Cowley et al, Law et al, Rubin et al). In this manner, novel cellular and molecular approaches to therapy can be applied early in the course of critical illness, when they have the best chance of being effective.

Suggested Reading

Abraham E, Raffin TA. Sepsis therapy trials. Continued disappointment or reason for hope? (editorial; comment). *JAMA* 271:1876, 1994.

Anderson BO, Bensard DD, Harken AH. The role of platelet activating factor and its antagonists in shock, sepsis and multiple organ failure. *Surg Gynecol Obstet* 172:415, 1991.

Anderson BO, Moore, EE, Banerjee A. Phospholipase A_2 regulates critical inflammatory mediators of multiple organ failure. *J Surg Res* 56:199, 1994.

Aoki H, Kodama M, Tani T, Hanasawa K. Treatment of sepsis by extracorporeal elimination of endotoxin using polymyxin B–immobilized fiber. *Am J Surg* 167:412, 1994.

Baggiolini MB, Moser B, Clark-Lewis I. Interleukin-8 and related chemotactic cytokines. The Giles Filley Lecture. *Chest* 105:95S, 1994.

Baggiolini M, Walz A, Kunkel SL. Neutrophil-activating peptide-1/interleukin 8, a novel cytokine that activates neutrophils. *J Clin Invest* 84:1045, 1989.

Barone JE. Maximization of oxygen delivery: A plea for moderation. Part II. *J Trauma* 37:337, 1994.

Bartlett RH. Extracorporeal life support for cardiopulmonary failure. *Curr Probl Surg* 27:621, 1990.

Bartlett RH, Dechert RE, Mault JR, et al. Measurement of metabolism in multiple organ failure. *Surgery* 92:771, 1982.

Bartlett RH, Morris AH, Fairley HB, et al. A prospective study of acute hypoxic respiratory failure. *Chest* 89:684, 1986.

Beal AL, Cerra FB. Multiple organ failure syndrome in the 1990s. Systemic inflammatory response and organ dysfunction. *JAMA* 271:226, 1994.

Bidani A, Tzouanakis AE, Cardenas VJ Jr, Zwischenberger JB. Permissive hypercapnia in acute respiratory failure. *JAMA* 272:957, 1994.

Bone RC. American College of Chest Physicians/Society of Critical Care Medicine Consensus Conference: Definitions for sepsis and organ failure and guidelines for the use of innovative therapies in sepsis. *Crit Care Med* 20:864, 1992.

Broaddus VC, Boylan AM, Hoeffel JM, et al. Neutralization of IL-8 inhibits neutrophil influx in a rabbit model of endotoxin-induced pleurisy. *J Immunol* 152:2960, 1994.

Carson SD, Ross SE, Bach R, Guha A. An inhibitory monoclonal antibody against human tissue factor. *Blood* 70:490, 1987.

Cilley RE, Scharenberg AM, Bongiorno PF, et al. Low oxygen delivery produced by anemia, hypoxia, and low cardiac output. *J Surg Res* 51:425, 1991.

Cipolle MD, Pasquale MD, Cerra FB. Secondary organ dysfunction. From clinical perspectives to molecular mediators. *Crit Care Clin* 9:261, 1993.

Corno A, 1994. Role of the gut in the development of multiple organ dysfunction (letter; comment). *Ann Thorac Surg* 57:263, 1994.

Cowley HC, Heney D, Gearing AJ, et al. Increased circulating adhesion molecule concentrations in patients with the systemic inflammatory response syndrome: A prospective cohort study. *Crit Care Med* 22:651, 1994.

Cumming AD. Sepsis and acute renal failure. *Ren Fail* 16:169, 1994.

Dauberschmidt R, Mrochen H, Kuckelt W, et al. Increased oxygen affinity contributes to tissue hypoxia in critically ill patients with low oxygen delivery. *Adv Exp Med Biol* 345:781, 1994.

Dechert RE, Cerny JC, Bartlett RH. Measurement of elemental nitrogen by chemiluminescence: An evaluation of the Antek nitrogen analyzer system. *JPEN J Parenter Enteral Nutr* 14:195, 1990.

Deitch EA. Multiple organ failure: Pathophysiology and potential future therapy. *Ann Surg* 216:117, 1992.

Deitch EA. Multiple organ failure. *Adv Surg* 26:333, 1993.

Demling RH, Lalonde C, Ikegami K. Physiologic support of the septic patient. *Surg Clin North Am* 74:637, 1994.

Demling R, Lalonde C, Saldinger P, Knox J. Multiple organ dysfunction in the surgical patient: Pathophysiology, prevention, and treatment. *Curr Probl Surg* 30:348, 1993.

DiCarlo JV, Dudley TE, Sherbotie, JR, et al. Continuous arteriovenous hemofiltration/dialysis improves gas exchange in children with multiple system organ failure. *Crit Care Med* 18:822, 1990.

Dinarello CA. Interkeukin-1 and the pathogenesis of the acute-phase response. *N Engl J Med* 311:1413, 1984.

Eliahou HE, Ben-David A, Blau A. Recovery can be enhanced in acute renal failure of multisystem organ failure. *Contrib Nephrol* 106:59, 1994.

Ferrante A, Kowanko IC, Bates EJ. Mechanisms of host tissue damage by cytokine-activated neutrophils. *Immunol Ser* 57:499, 1992.

Feuerstein G, Rabinovici R. Importance of interleukin-8 and chemokines in organ injury and shock (editorial; comment). *Crit Care Med* 22:550, 1994.

Fisher CJ Jr, Dhainaut JF, Opal SM, et al. Recombinant human interleukin 1 receptor antagonist in the treatment of patients with sepsis syndrome. Results from a randomized, double-blind, placebo-controlled trial. Phase III rhIL-1ra Sepsis Syndrome Study Group. *JAMA* 271:1836, 1994.

Frankenfield DC, Reynolds HN, Wiles CE, et al. Urea removal during continuous hemodiafiltration. *Crit Care Med* 22:407, 1994.

Frankenfield DC, Wiles CE, Bagley S, Siegel JH. Relationships between resting and total energy expenditure in injured and septic patients. *Crit Care Med* 22:1796, 1994.

Gadaleta D, Davis JM. Pulmonary failure and the production of leukotrienes. *J Am Coll Surg* 178:309, 1994.

Hanique G, Dugernier T, Laterre PF, et al. Significance of pathologic oxygen supply dependency in critically ill patients: Comparison between measured and calculated methods. *Intensive Care Med* 20:12, 1994.

Hickling KG, Walsh J, Henderson S, Jackson R. Low mortality rate in adult respiratory distress syndrome using low-volume, pressure-limited ventilation with permissive hypercapnia: A prospective study. *Crit Care Med* 22:1568, 1994.

Hirschl RB, Heiss KF, Cilley RE, et al. Oxygen kinetics in experimental sepsis. *Surgery* 112:37, 1992.

Jochum M, Gippner-Steppert C, Machleidt W, Fritz H. The role of phagocyte proteinases and proteinase inhibitors in multiple organ failure. *Am J Respir Crit Care Med* 150:S123, 1994.

Knaus WA, Draper EA, Wagner DP, Zimmerman JE. Prognosis in acute organ-system failure. *Ann Surg* 202:685, 1985.

Kreuzfelder E, Joka T, Keinecke H, et al. Adult respiratory distress syndrome as a specific manifestation of a general permeability defect in trauma patients. *Am Rev Respir Dis* 137:95, 1988.

Kudsk KA. Gut mucosal nutritional support—enteral nutrition as primary therapy after multiple system trauma. *Gut* 35:S52, 1994.

Lamm WJ, Graham MM, Albert RK. Mechanism by which the prone position improves oxygenation in acute lung injury. *Am J Respir Crit Care Med* 150:184, 1994.

Law MM, Cryer HG, Abraham E. Elevated levels of soluble ICAM-1 correlate with the development of multiple organ failure in severely injured trauma patients (discussion). *J Trauma* 37:100, 1994.

Leonard EJ, Yoshimura T. Neutrophil attractant/activation protein-1 (NAP-1 [interleukin-8]). *Am J Respir Cell Mol Biol* 2:479, 1990.

Marty C, Misset B, Tamion F, et al. Circulating interleukin-8 concentrations in patients with multiple organ failure of septic and nonseptic origin. *Crit Care Med* 22:673, 1994.

Marzi, I, Buhren V, Schuttler A, Trentz O. Value of superoxide dismutase for prevention of multiple organ failure after multiple trauma. *J Trauma* 35:110, 1993.

Matuschak GM, Rinaldo JE. Organ interactions in the adult respiratory distress syndrome during sepsis. Role of the liver in host defense. *Chest* 94:400, 1988.

Mault, JR, Dechert RE, Lees P, et al. Continuous arteriovenous filtration: An effective treatment for surgical acute renal failure. *Surgery* 101:478, 1987.

Meesters RC, van der Graaf AV, Eikelboom BC. Ruptured aortic aneurysm: Early postoperative prediction of mortality using an organ system failure score. *Br J Surg* 81:512, 1994.

Michie HR, Manogue KR, Spriggs DR, et al. Detection of circulating tumor necrosis factor after endotoxin administration. *N Engl J Med* 318:1481, 1988.

Milberg JA, Davis DR, Steinberg KP, Hudson LD. Improved survival of patients with acute respiratory distress syndrome (ARDS): 1983–1993. *JAMA* 273:306, 1995.

Mileski WJ, Winn RK, Harlan JM, Rice CL. Transient inhibition of neutrophil adherence with the anti-CD18 monoclonal antibody 60.3 does not increase mortality rates in abdominal sepsis. *Surgery* 109:497, 1991.

Mileski WJ, Winn RK, Vedder NB. Inhibition of CD18-dependent neutrophil adherence reduces organ injury after hemorrhagic shock in primates. *Surgery* 108:206, 1990.

Moore EE, Moore FA, Francoise RJ, et al. The postischemic gut serves as a priming bed for circulating neutrophils that provoke multiple organ failure. *J Trauma* 37:881, 1994.

Mulligan MS, Jones ML, Bolanowski MA, et al. Inhibition of lung inflammatory reactions in rats by an anti-human IL-8 antibody. *J Immunol* 150:5585, 1993.

Mythen MG, Webb AR. Intra-operative gut mucosal hypoperfusion is associated with increased post-operative complications and cost. *Intensive Care Med* 20:99, 1994.

Mythen MG, Webb AR. The role of gut mucosal hypoperfusion in the pathogenesis of post-op-erative organ dysfunction. *Intensive Care Med* 20:203, 1994.

Nicod LP. Cytokines. 1. Overview. *Thorax* 48:660, 1993.

Nuytinck JK, Goris JA, Redl H, et al. Posttraumatic complications and inflammatory mediators. *Arch Surg* 121:886, 1986.

Ou MC, Kambayashi J, Kawasaki T, et al. Potential etiologic role of PAF in two major septic complications; disseminated intravascular coagulation and multiple organ failure. *Thromb Res* 73:227, 1994.

Pape HC, Dwenger A, Regel G, et al. Increased gut permeability after multiple trauma. *Br J Surg* 81:850, 1994.

Pinsky MR. Beyond global oxygen supply-demand relations: In search of measures of dysoxia. *Intensive Care Med* 20:1, 1994.

Pizcueta P, Luscinskas FW. Monoclonal antibody blockade of L-selectin inhibits mononuclear leukocyte recruitment to inflammatory sites in vivo. *Am J Pathol* 145:461, 1994.

Proulx F, Gauthier M, Nadeau D, et al. Timing and predictors of death in pediatric patients with multiple organ system failure. *Crit Care Med* 22:1025, 1994.

Rangel-Frausto MS, Pittet D, Costigan M, et al. The natural history of the systemic inflammatory response syndrome (SIRS). A prospective study. *JAMA* 273:117, 1995.

Reidy JJ, Ramsay G. Clinical trials of selective decontamination of the digestive tract: Review. *Crit Care Med* 18:1449, 1990.

Remick DG, Kunkel RG, Larrick JW, Kunkel SL. Acute in vivo effects of human recombinant tumor necrosis factor. *Lab Invest* 56:583, 1987.

Reynolds EM, Ryan DP, Doody DP. Permissive hypercapnia and pressure-controlled ventilation as treatment of severe adult respiratory distress syndrome in a pediatric burn patient [corrected and republished article originally printed in *Crit Care Med* 21:468–471, 1993]. *Crit Care Med* 21:944, 1993.

Rubin DB, Wiener-Kronish JP, Murray JF, et al. Elevated von Willebrand factor antigen is an early plasma predictor of acute lung injury in nonpulmonary sepsis syndrome. *J Clin Invest* 86:474, 1990.

Russell JA, Phang PT. The oxygen delivery/consumption controversy. Approaches to management of the critically ill. *Am J Respir Crit Care Med* 149:533, 1994.

Sauaia A, Moore FA, Moore EE, et al. Early predictors of postinjury multiple organ failure. *Arch Surg* 129:39, 1994.

Sekido N, Mukaida N, Harada A. Prevention of lung reperfusion injury in rabbits by a monoclonal antibody against interleukin-8. *Nature* 365:654, 1993.

Shanley CJ, Bartlett RH. The Management of Acute Respiratory Failure. In *Current Opinion in General Surgery. 1994.* pp. 7–16, 1995.

Shapiro BA, Peruzzi WT. Changing practices in ventilator management: A review of the literature and suggested clinical correlations. *Surgery* 117:121, 1995.

Sinard JM, Vyas D, Hultquist K, et al. Effects of moderate hypothermia on O_2 consumption at various O_2 deliveries in a sheep model. *J Appl Physiol* 72:2428, 1992.

St. John RC, Dorinsky PM. Immunologic therapy for ARDS, septic shock, and multiple-organ failure. *Chest* 103:932, 1993.

St. John RC, Dorinsky PM. An overview of multiple organ dysfunction syndrome. *J Lab Clin Med* 124:478, 1994.

St. John RC, Mizer LA, Kindt GC, et al. Acid aspiration-induced acute lung injury causes leukocyte-dependent systemic organ injury. *J Appl Physiol* 74:1994, 1993.

Strieter RM, Lukacs NW, Standiford TJ, Kunkel SL. Cytokines. 2. Cytokines and lung inflammation: Mechanisms of neutrophil recruitment to the lung. *Thorax* 48:765, 1993.

Strieter RM, Koch AE, Antony VB, et al. The immunopathology of chemotactic cytokines: The role of interleukin-8 and monocyte chemoattractant protein-1. *J Lab Clin Med* 123:183, 1994.

Strieter RM, Lynch JP, Basha MA, et al. Host responses in mediating sepsis and adult respiratory distress syndrome. *Semin Respir Infect* 5:233, 1990.

Svoboda P, Kantorova I, Ochmann J. Dynamics of interleukin 1, 2, and 6 and tumor necrosis factor alpha in multiple trauma patients. *J Trauma* 36:336, 1994.

Taylor FB Jr, Chang A, Ruf W, et al. Lethal E. coli septic shock is prevented by blocking tissue factor with monoclonal antibody. *Circ Shock* 33:127, 1991.

Toledo-Pereyra LH, Suzuki S. Neutrophils, cytokines, and adhesion molecules in hepatic ischemia and reperfusion injury. *J Am Coll Surg* 179:758, 1994.

Tracey KJ, Beutler B, Lowry SF, et al. Shock and tissue injury induced by recombinant human cachectin. *Science* 234:470, 1986.

Uhl W, Beger HG, Hoffmann G, et al. A multi-center study of phospholipase A_2 in patients in intensive care units. *J Am Coll Surg* 180:323, 1995.

van der Poll T, Levi M, Hack CE, et al. Elimination of interleukin 6 attenuates coagulation activation in experimental endotoxemia in chimpanzees. *J Exp Med* 179:1253, 1994.

van der Poll T, Levi M, van Deventer SJ, et al. Differential effects of anti-tumor necrosis factor monoclonal antibodies on systemic inflammatory responses in experimental endotoxemia in chimpanzees. *Blood* 83:446, 1994.

Vincent JL, Tielemans C. Continuous hemofiltration in severe sepsis: Is it beneficial? *J Crit Care* 10:27, 1995.

Wakabayashi G, Gelfand GA, Jung WK, et al. *Staphylococcus epidermidis* induces complement activation, tumor necrosis factor and interleukin-1, a shock-like state and tissue injury in rabbits without endotoxemia. Comparison to *Escherichia coli. J Clin Invest* 87:1925, 1991.

Wardle EN. Acute renal failure and multiorgan failure. *Nephron* 66:380, 1994.

Windsor AC, Mullen PG, Fowler AA, Sugerman HJ. Role of the neutrophil in adult respiratory distress syndrome. *Br J Surg* 80:10, 1993.

Yoshikawa T, Takano H, Takahashi S, et al. Changes in tissue antioxidant enzyme activities and lipid peroxides in endotoxin-induced multiple organ failure. *Circ Shock* 42:53, 1994.

EDITOR'S COMMENT

I offer just two brief comments on two theoretical issues that are central to this fine chapter. The role of cytokines in the systemic inflammatory response syndrome is central to the issue. Are cytokines paracrine, autocrine, or neurocrine? Do concentrations of these substances in the blood indicate that they have escaped and that these are always damaging, or is there an endocrine function to cytokines that are released into the bloodstream? On this philosophical issue really hangs the whole concept of whether or not one should use cytokine antibodies. If blood cytokines have an endocrine function, one should not block the cytokines. If, on the other hand, as preliminary data suggest, the levels of IL-6 (acknowledgedly a paracrine functional cytokine) correlate with death—the higher the IL-6 level, the more likely the patient is to die—then it is entirely appropriate to use a cytokine antibody.

Disturbing to me, at least, is the frequent equation of multiple organ dysfunction syndrome, bacterial translocation, and the causative nature of bacterial translocation for the multiple organ dysfunction syndrome. This hypothesis is far from proven. Indeed, the authors acknowledge that intestinal sterilization (sometimes with polymyxin B costing over $1000 per day) has failed to reveal any evidence of benefit, except for decreases in nosocomial pneumonias, but no change in outcome. It would be appropriate to point out that 22 studies have now investigated the possibility that intestinal sterilization improves outcome with multiple organ dysfunction syndrome, without beneficial effect. Thus, if anything, it is highly unlikely that bacterial translocation is the cause of multiple organ dysfunction syndrome, as numerous others in this volume have pointed out. There is a form of death in patients who are terribly ill, in which they lose absolutely all gut integrity approximately 48 hours before they die. In this syndrome, patients manifest random bacteremias for which there are no foci. That is a far cry from the situation of most patients with the multiple organ dysfunction syndrome.

J.E.F.

11

Management of the Complications of Immunosuppression

John F. Valente   J. Wesley Alexander

Impaired immunologic function may be the result of a variety of factors in the surgical patient and can be classified as primary (as in the immunodeficiency syndromes) or acquired. Acquired immunodeficiency can occur in patients as a result of disease, such as cancer, injury, or malnutrition, or as a result of therapy, such as irradiation or the administration of immunosuppressive drugs. Many other scenarios of acquired immunosuppression in surgical patients exist (Table 11-1). All such forms of immunosuppression lead to an increased risk of infection, malignancy, or impaired wound healing and predispose the patient to a number of disorders and complications. Several of these factors are often present in a single patient and combine to increase the immunosuppressive effects and risk of subsequent complications. We will attempt to further outline four of the common settings of acquired immunosuppression (cancer, radiation, transplantation, and malnutrition) in sur-

Table 11-1. Common States of Acquired Immunodeficiency in Surgical Patients

Transplantation/drugs	Cancer
Trauma	Anesthesia
Transfusion	Chemotherapy
Advanced age	Diabetes
Chronic infection	Radiation
Viral infection	Drug abuse
Burn injury	Alcohol abuse
Renal failure	Hepatic failure
Splenectomy	Malnutrition

gical patients and discuss the related morbidity along with some strategies for management of these common problems. The combination of underlying disease and pharmacologic therapy results in a profound state of immunosuppression in transplant and cancer patients, who suffer the broadest range of complications. Exposure to ionizing radiation can result in a spectrum of destructive effects, ranging from local intestinal barrier dysfunction to the severe multisystem syndromes seen with whole-body exposure. Malnutrition is perhaps the most common state of acquired immunosuppression in surgical (and other) patients and has a significant impact on hospital morbidity.

Indeed, surgery and anesthesia themselves are immunosuppressive. It is important to remember that recovery of immune function will follow the correction of inflammatory disorders, and in this regard surgical intervention is a positive immunomodulator. Thus, the combination of surgical intervention, pathology, and associated immunosuppressive conditions places the chances for a positive outcome in the balance. Strict attention to meticulous surgical technique, along with the application of the recently appreciated immunoenhancing effects of pharmacologic nutrients, allows for a positive outcome in most cases. This chapter starts with a review of the general mechanisms of immunosuppression and their effects, and then proceeds to specific examples of management strategies for these conditions in surgical patients.

Mechanisms of Immunodeficiency and Their Sequelae

Both specific (antibody) and nonspecific (complement and other serum proteins) deficiencies of humoral immunity may exist. Syndromes associated with an immunoglobulin A (IgA) or immunoglobulin M (IgM) deficiency are usually manifested by recurrent bacterial infections, especially with encapsulated organisms (pneumococci, *Haemophilus influenzae*). Long-term IgA deficiency can also be associated with an increased risk of esophageal and pulmonary cancers. Hypogammaglobulinemia is associated with recurrent staphylococcal (including methicillin-resistant *Staphylococcus aureus*) and encapsulated organism infections. Sinopulmonary infections, meningitis, cellulitis, and bacteremia are also common. *Haemophilus influenzae* epiglottitis is a particularly life-threatening condition in these patients and is not limited to children. Lymphoma, leukemia, and gastric cancer are also seen in patients with long-standing hypogammaglobulinemia. Patients with deficiencies in complement proteins are at risk for recurrent infection (meningococci, pneumococci, *H. influenzae*, and staphylococci) and have an increased risk of death from sepsis. Complement deficiencies have been associated with rheumatologic diseases and a variety of bacterial infections.

Outside the realm of iatrogenic immunosuppression, isolated T-cell deficiency syndromes are rare. Fungal and viral infections are common manifestations of T-cell immunodeficiency. Defects in natural killer cell activity may also exist and are associated with increased risk of viral infection. Combined cellular and humoral immunodeficiency can result in severe, often life-threatening, infection with *Candida*, cytomegalovirus (CMV), *Pneumocystis carinii*, or other opportunistic organisms. Defects in T-cell receptor (TCR) function are associated with abnormal cytokine production and a variable severity of resulting infections. Thymomas can be associated with acquired hypogammaglobulinemia and some patients have deficient T-cell immunity as well. Recurrent infection can be a presenting sign of thymoma in some patients. Patients with combined immunodeficiency are unable to attack/reject foreign immunocompetent cells and thus are at risk of graft-versus-host disease (GVHD). Patients with reduced leukocyte adhesion molecule function are at risk for recurrent bacterial infection, are unable to form significant exudates/inflammatory responses, and have abnormal antibody responses to infection. Combined disorders can be expected to have adverse effects on wound healing as well.

Phagocytic dysfunction can be due to a number of defects in enzymatic function, adhesion molecules, chemotaxis, complement, and tuftsin deficiency (in splenectomized patients). Simple acquired granulocytopenia, due to bone marrow suppressive drugs, is the most common defect, however. Recurrent gram-negative or gram-positive bacterial infections and fungal infections can occur in these patients.

Perhaps the most nonspecific aspect of the immune system is the mucocutaneous barrier. A number of local and systemic bacterial, fungal, and viral infections occur with barrier function disruption. Percutaneous tubes, drains, burns, and vascular access catheters all create a breach in the skin, while ischemia, ulcerations, local infections, chemotherapeutic agents, irradiation, and malnutrition result in disruption of mucosal barriers. The microbiology of these infections depends upon the particular barrier at fault (i.e., gut vs skin) and the local colonization pattern. Bacterial or fungal translocation across certain dysfunctional barriers can result in a severe systemic inflammatory response syndrome associated with multiple systems organ failure.

States of Acquired Immunodeficiency in Surgical Patients

Immunosuppressive Therapy and Transplantation

One of the most significant states of immunosuppression seen in surgical patients is that associated with immunosuppressive drug therapy after transplantation. Both T-cell signaling and immune system proliferative responses are routinely impeded and a state of predominantly T-cell and nonspecific immunosuppression exists. Thus, increased susceptibility to bacterial infection, recurrent opportunistic infections, impaired wound healing, and increased risk of malignancy are all seen. The signs and symptoms of infection are often blunted or absent, making diagnosis difficult.

Barrier function in transplanted bowel (including the duodenal segment associated with a pancreatic allograft) can be expected to be poor initially. Phagocytosis of transplanted hepatic reticuloendothelial cells may undergo a transient period of dysfunction as well. A host of pharmacologic side effects of immunosuppressive agents used in transplantation exist. Many result in compounded effects on host defense (bone marrow suppression, hepatotoxicity, renal failure, etc.). Periods of intensive drug therapy around episodes of rejection result in higher risks of infection and a greater cumulative risk of certain malignancies.

Cancer and Cancer Chemotherapy

Malignancy can be both a cause and a result of immunosuppression. Advanced cancer is associated with defects in both T- and B-cell function. Peripheral blood lymphocytes from these patients are unable to develop into fully effective lymphokine activated killer cells. Although somewhat inconsistently observed, impaired production of interleukin-1 (IL-1), interleukin-2 (IL-2), and other cytokines as well as their receptors is seen in cancer patients. A number of immunosuppressive tumor-derived factors including transforming growth factor-β (TGFβ) have been described. Acquired anergy to delayed-type hypersensitivity (DTH) tests is well known and associated with an increased risk of infection. Multiple myeloma, lymphomas, and chronic lymphocytic leukemia are associated with immunoglobulin deficiencies and recurrent encapsulated bacterial infections as well as gram-negative infections. Hodgkin's disease, acute lymphocytic leukemia, lymphomas, and metastatic solid tumors generate cell-mediated immune dysfunction and result in opportunistic infections: *Pneumocystis*, *Toxoplasma*, *Nocardia*, *Mycobacteria*, viruses, and fungi. The acute-phase proteins produced by the liver in septic cancer patients depress lymphocyte proliferative responses.

The use of chemotherapeutic agents is an obvious source of immunosuppression in cancer patients. Bone marrow toxicity with acquired granulocytopenia is an extremely common complication of myelotoxic chemotherapy. The use of parenteral narcotics for the management of pain is often an integral part of patient management but may inhibit natural killer cell function and antibody-dependent cell cytotoxicity. The presence of other factors in patients with cancer (i.e., percutaneous catheters, drains, local erosive effects of solid tumor growth, malnutrition, transfusion, etc.) is the rule rather than the exception. The developmet of secondary tumors as a consequence of cancer treatment is an increasingly important aspect of oncologic management. As an example, the incidence of leukemia following chemotherapy for breast or ovarian cancer is 1.5 and 5 percent, respectively.

Radiation Therapy and Toxic Exposure

Radiation toxicity is a well-known phenomenon. Whole-body irradiation is associated with bone marrow depression and pancytopenia resulting in profound immunosuppression. Local effects of irradiation depend greatly upon the specific tissue or organ involved. Immediate destruction of immune system cells, general hypocellularity, and scar formation are some characteristics of local tissue injury due to radiation. Irradiated bowel acutely looses barrier function as DNA injury translates into reduced mitotic activity and denudation of mucosal lining. Progression to vascular and ultimately transmural damage results in poor motility and bacterial overgrowth in chronic radiation enteritis.

The effects of radiation on the immune system are many. The most radiosensitive cells are lymphocytes, many of which are killed immediately (making radiation an adjunct to immunosuppressive and rejection treatment protocols in transplantation). The humoral arm of the immune system is more radiosensitive than the cellular arm, and activated cells are less sensitive than nonactivated cells. Following antigen presentation, proliferating lymphocytes become highly radiosensitive, while those past the point of cellular division are much more resistant. Lymphocyte subset populations may be permanently altered following radiation exposure, a finding discovered in atomic bomb survivors. Another major mechanism of radiation-induced injury involves damage to DNA, especially in its relation to tumorigenesis. Following pelvic radiation for benign or malignant disease in women, prolonged but stable chromosomal aberrations are identified and associated with a twofold increase in leukemia rates.

Nutritional Deficiency

While brief periods of starvation (probably less than 24–48 hours) may be immunostimulatory and even protective against infection, prolonged starvation or shorter periods of starvation associated with injury will result in adverse immune system effects. Malnutrition results in both B-cell and T-cell deficits (the T-cell depression is more severe), with reduced immunoglobulin secretion and response to T-cell mitogens. Macrophage functions are decreased in protein-calorie malnutrition (PCM). Alterations in neutrophil chemotaxis and reduction in complement levels also occur, depending on the level of protein deficiency. An increased susceptibility to bacterial infection and reduced wound healing ability is well recognized in malnutrition.

The routine application of advanced parenteral nutritional support fails to provide consistent benefits. Intravenous lipids have been correlated with decreased phagocytosis, decreased immunoglobulin

synthesis, some endothelial demargination of white cells with impaired leukocyte chemotaxis, profound (>75%) inhibition of lymphoproliferative response to specific antigens, and an inconsistently observed depression in reticuloendothelial function with impaired bacterial clearance. The use of omega-6 fatty acids inhibits antibody formation, natural killer cell activity, and cytokine release, while the use of omega-3 fatty acids (as in fish oil–based supplements) results in immunoenhancement and decreased thromboxane, prostaglandin, and monokine release. Dietary supplementation of arginine, glutamine, ribonucleic acids, and omega-3 essential fatty acids is associated with improved survival in sepsis models, a fact taken advantage of in some commercially available enteral nutrition formulas. Dietary route is also important. Survival increases when malnutrition is reversed, but the enteral route is clearly superior (resulting in a halving of septic complications) compared to parenteral refeeding, even when parenteral formulas are used enterally. The mortality is at least doubled when protein-malnourished patients become septic.

Implications of Immunosuppression

Many of the necessary steps in the complex process of wound healing require the interaction of various immune system cells and the elaboration of cytokines and growth factors. The suppression of white cell function associated with steroids, the loss of protein integrity associated with malnutrition or cancer, and the local destructive effects of radiation all contribute to delays in wound healing. Chemotherapeutic agents present risk associated with resultant myelosuppression, and elective surgical procedures should be timed well before or after neutrophil count nadirs. A recent review of postoperative complications after chemotherapy use shows that the majority of wound dehiscences and GI complications happen within one month of therapy and advise delay in elective surgical procedures.

The principal teleologic function of the immune system can be considered that of protection from infection. The presence of viral and opportunistic infections in cancer and transplant patients associated with impaired cellular immunity is well known.

Fungal and aggressive bacterial infections are a principal cause of morbidity and mortality in radiation exposure and malnutrition.

The recently recognized immunosurveillance functions of the immune system can be significantly impaired. Viral-mediated skin and mesenchymal tumors are signifciantly more common in transplant recipients. The formation of secondary cancers due to the dissimilating effects of radiation therapy and chemotherapy for cancer is also well documented. Furthermore, the presence of these tumors in an already immunocompromised patient results in a more aggressive course. When possible (as in transplant patients) a reduction of immunosuppression may be all that is necessary for tumor regression (as in posttransplant lymphoproliferative disorders).

A number of systemic syndromes associated with immunosuppression and its complications can present management challenges to physicians. Protein-calorie malnutrition, cytokine release syndromes, tumor lysis syndromes, combined radiation injuries, and so forth, all present in association with underlying immunosuppression in these patients. Although quite variable in pathophysiology and management, these syndromes all have several things in common: increased risk of infection and sepsis, increased length of hospital stay and cost, and increased rates of morbidity and mortality.

Management of Specific Complications
Transplantation

Wounds and Surgical Technique
All transplant patients share two things in common: a combination of varying degrees of iatrogenic and underlying immunosuppression, and some baseline organ dysfunction. Renal, liver, cardiac, and pulmonary failure are all associated with some degree of malnutrition, microcirculatory derangements, and impaired wound healing. Perhaps even more significant are the combined effects of long-standing diabetes in pancreas transplant recipients. Immunosuppressive agents, especially steroids, result in poor wound healing as well. The demands for meticulous surgical technique and attention to

wound healing factors are evident and necessary to prevent postoperative infection.

The principles of wound closure help to illustrate the surgical approach to these obstacles. Suture selection should take into account the prolonged delay in wound healing. Skin closure with nonabsorbable suture such as Prolene is preferred and removal should be delayed for a minimum of 2 weeks. Application of a sterile tape reinforcement is routinely performed at time of suture removal. The subcutaneous tissues are routinely closed to eradicate dead space and avoid fluid collection, which can result in infection or wound breakdown. The placement of subcutaneous sutures must include both the wound margins and the surface of the underlying fascia to achieve complete eradication of dead space while avoiding strangulation and ischemia of tissue, thereby defeating the purpose of this layer closure. The appropriately placed subcutaneous layer affords an improved closure that outweighs the small effect of tissue ischemia produced in the relatively small amount of subcutaneous tissue involved in this suture line. A nonabsorbable, continuous running suture is preferable for this purpose. Fascial closure must always be with nonabsorbable suture with anatomic reapproximation of all layers. Selection of running versus interrupted technique is preferred and size 0 or No. 1 or 2, depending on patient size and the layer being closed, Prolene or Novafil is used for fascial closures.

The same general principles of wound closure apply to all internal procedures as well. Reliance on nonabsorbable sutures with a close interrupted or running technique and anatomic approximation of all layers are important. Longer-lasting suture materials should be used where absorbable suture is employed (i.e., bladder or common bile duct). We do not favor the use of stapling devices except in areas of minimal distention (as in the end of a Roux en Y limb for biliary drainage or in the lateral closure of the duodenal segment of a pancreatic allograft). Even in these cases, however, complete reinforcement with a second layer of nonabsorbable or slowly absorbing monofilament suture is required. Inner layers for bowel anastomosis and biliary or ureteral anastomoses are performed with Maxon, to take advantage of a longer-lasting absorbable suture. In multilayer bladder closures or tunneled ureteroneocystostomies, chromic gut sutures are acceptable. Where significant adverse factors exist, two-layered techniques are preferred, such as in the allograft to jejunal anastomosis for diversion to enteric drainage of a pancreatic transplant.

Infections

Over 80 percent of transplant recipients will experience at least one episode of infection. The profound state of immunosuppression required to prevent allograft rejection results in susceptibility to a number of opportunistic pathogens, including *P. carinii*, cytomegalovirus, and various fungi. Previously encountered infectious agents, such as *Varicella zoster*, herpes simplex virus (HSV), CMV, Epstein-Barr virus (EBV), mycobacteria, and granuloma-associated infections, may reactivate. Transplant patients are also at least equal risk to contract bacterial infections. Predisposing factors are frequent (drugs, diabetes, debilitated states) and portals of entry for infectious agents are many (central venous access catheters, drains, transplanted tissue, etc.). A pretransplant evaluation should include viral screens for CMV, EBV, varicella zoster virus (VZV), human immunodeficiency virus (HIV) and HSV as well as hepatitis A, B, and C. A nasal swab for methicillin-resistant staphylococcus, or purified protein derivative (PPD) skin test, and a rapid plasma reagin (RPR) test should also be done. Pretransplant vaccinations for hepatitis B and pneumococcus should be administered. Following transplantation, prophylaxis with antiviral, antifungal, and anti-*Pneumocystis* therapy is often needed (Table 11-2). It should be remembered that even patients well out from their transplant procedure require such prophylaxis (along with ulcer prophylaxis) if antirejection therapy is initiated.

Given the high incidence and mortality of posttransplant infections, an infection evaluation should be included in the initial management of nearly any ill transplant patient. A gastrointestinal bleed may be due to CMV ulcers or colitis, substernal chest pain may be due to viral or fungal esophagitis, and *Pneumocystis* may masquerade as acute congestive heart failure.

The initial management of a transplant patient depends somewhat on presenting signs and symptoms, if any. Simple fever should be managed with full cultures (urine, sputum, blood, pharyngeal, and, if indicated, bile or cerebrospinal fluid) for viral, aerobic, and anaerobic bacterial and fungal organisms. A chest x-ray, serum viral markers, and evaluation for potential rejection (including biopsy if indicated) should be included. In patients who have undergone a renal transplant, an ultrasound is helpful, while those who have just had a pancreas or liver transplant may

Table 11-2. Prophylactic Therapeutics in the Transplant Recipient

Infection	Patient Characteristic	Treatment
Wound infection	Kidney recipients	Cephazolin or nafcillin × 2 doses
	Liver recipients	Ampicillin/sulbactam × 5 d
	Kidney/pancreas recipients	Imipenem/vancomycin × 5 d
CMV	During antilymphocyte Rx	Ganciclovir × 3 wk
	Routine	Acyclovir
Pneumocystis	Routine	Trimethoprim-sulfamethoxazole or
	Sulfa allergic	pentamidine q mo
HSV	All positive recipients	Acyclovir
EBV	Donor pos., recipient neg. (combination)	? CMV immune globulin or acyclovir
Fungal	Kidney recipients	Nystatin or clotrimazole (Mycelex)
	Liver/pancreas recipients	with or without fluconazole
DVT	All patients	Compression boots
	Liver recipients	Subcutaneous heparin q8h
Stress GIB	All patients	Antacids/H₂ blocker

Key: CMV = cytomegalovirus; HSV = herpes simplex virus; EBV = Epstein-Barr virus; DVT = deep venous thrombosis; GIB = Gastrointestinal bleeding *or* stress-related gastrointestinal bleeding.

harbor asymptomatic intra-abdominal infections, and CT scans are often indicated. Pulmonary infections frequently demand immediate bronchoscopy, which may require ICU monitoring and intubation. Broad-spectrum antibiotics, including coverage for CMV, *Pneumocystis*, and *Legionella*, can be later tapered to appropriate coverage for the cultured organism. Biliary and urinary tract infections can be especially life threatening if associated with obstructing lesions and appropriate imaging studies and decompression are essential. Central nervous system infections are often associated with headache, lethargy, mild photophobia, or mental status changes but complaints and signs may be quite minimal and are easily overlooked. Head CT scan followed by lumbar puncture for routine studies including India ink stains and cryptococcal antigen are helpful. The monoclonal antibody, OKT3, can cause a sterile meningeal irritation and should be suspected when a predominantly lymphocytic infiltrate exists, all cultures are negative, meningeal inflammation is not present on CT, and the patient has received OKT3 within the last 6 weeks. Situations in which the inciting organism cannot be detected but clinical improvement is seen with antibiotic therapy should be treated with at least a 7-day course.

Tumorigenesis

De novo cancers arise in roughly 6 percent of all organ transplant recipients. Men and women are affected equally. The most common types of malignancies seen are skin and lip tumors and non-Hodgkin's lymphomas. Advances in immunosuppressive therapy (polyclonal antilymphocyte globulin, OKT3, and perhaps tacrolimus) have resulted in a trend toward an increased incidence and earlier presentation of lymphoproliferative diseases including lymphoma in transplant patients (Table 11-3). Soft-tissue tumors (especially Kaposi's sarcoma), renal carcinomas, gynecologic tumors, and hepatomas are also much more prevalent in transplant patients than in the general population (Table 11-4). Sarcomas, renal tumors, and hepatobiliary tumors are managed as in the general population. In management of skin tumors, local destruction (surgical, radiation, freezing, etc.) is necessary, while in premalignant skin lesions, topical therapy with tretinoin or 5-fluorouracil is recommended.

Table 11-3. Spectrum of Posttransplant Lymphoproliferative Disease

Presentation	Typical Age (Yr)	Time of Onset	Therapy	Comment
Classic mononucleosis	<40	Any (naive pt exposed to EBV)	ACV	Rare
B-cell hyperplasia	<40	<1 yr post TXP	ACV/GCV	Benign condition
Polyclonal B-cell lymphoma	<40	<1 yr post TXP	ACV/GCV/IFN-α, reduce immunosuppression	Can progress
Monoclonal B-cell lymphoma	>40	>1 yr post TXP	Withdraw immunosuppression, chemotherapy, radiation, surgery	Unresponsive to therapy

TXP = posttransplant; ACV = acyclovir; GCV = ganciclovir; IFN-α = interferon-alpha; EBV = Epstein-Barr virus.

Table 11-4. Reported Malignancies in Transplant Patients[a]

Site/Type of Malignancy	Adult Recipients (No.)	Pediatric Recipients (No.)	Patients with a History of Cancers Before Transplantation No.	Patients with a History of Cancers Before Transplantation Percent Recurrence after Immunosuppression
Skin/lips	2897	68	91	60%
Lymphoma	1276	167	31	10%
Lung	428	0		[b]
Uterus	319	8	19	11%
Kaposi's sarcoma	311	8		[b]
Colorectal	280	0	40	20%
Kidney	265	5	59	0% Incidental
			171	30% Symptomatic
Breast	246	2	66	24%
Head/neck	223	7		[b]
Genitalia	200	13		[b]
Bladder	175	2	43	26%
Leukemia	149	6		[b]
Hepatobiliary tumor	135	10		[b]
Prostate	112	0	22	23%
Thyroid	99	9	41	7%
Stomach	91	1		[b]
Sarcomas	90	11	14	28%
Testicular tumor	69	3	35	3%
Ovary	57	5		[b]

[a]Data from Cincinnati Transplant Tumor Registry: 7393 cancers in 6934 transplant recipients reported as of 1994.
[b]No patients with history of this tumor reported with subsequent transplant.

Posttransplant lymphoproliferative disorders represent a spectrum of conditions, ranging from active EBV infection with B-cell hyperplasia, through polyclonal B-cell tumors, to aggressive monoclonal lymphomas. The diagnosis can be made by biopsy of lesions, along with serum protein electrophoresis, measurement of quantitative serum immunoglobulins, cytogenetic studies, and immunoglobulin gene rearrangement studies. Incidence correlates with total immunosuppressive therapy and therefore also with the number of treated rejection episodes. Treatment with OKT3 is implicated as a risk factor but most likely is due to its overall potency and incorporation in rejection treatment protocols rather than to a specific drug action. Presenting symptoms relate to the location of the tumor. Involvement of the transplanted organ, regional lymph nodes, or multiple sites is common. The brain is disproportionately involved in transplant patients (one-fourth of cases) and may be the only site of tumor. Masses in lymph-bearing areas (i.e., tonsils), milky-appearing fluid collections in the chest or abdomen, unusual lymphocytic infiltrates seen on allograft biopsy, protein-losing enteropathy, or any new soft-tissue tumor seen after the transplant should be evaluated as a possible posttransplant lymphoproliferative lesion. Treatment depends on cell types and degree of malignant conversion. Initial therapy with reduction in immunosuppression alone is necessary and often all that is needed. Antiviral therapy for polyclonal tumors with ganciclovir or IV acyclovir (preferred) is initiated, and chemotherapy, radiation, interferon, and immune globulin therapy can be added as indicated. Advanced, monoclonal tumors are often unresponsive to treatment.

Systemic Syndromes

Bone Demineralization. Osteoporosis is a common finding in posttransplant recipients. The bone loss is associated with the use of steroids, often in combination with renal failure and secondary hyperparathyroidism, resulting in either a local bone destruction (e.g., aseptic necrosis of the femoral head) or a generalized reduction in bone density. The measurement of bone density on radiograph, or more accurately with nuclear imaging techniques, allows for assessment of the degree of demineralization. Reversal of demineralization is difficult and limiting further bone loss with calcium supplementation, vitamin D, or occasionally calcitonin is important. Vertebral compression and long-bone fractures can be quite disabling and difficult to treat. A functioning kidney is one major step toward control of calcium balance and bone integrity. Serious consideration for combined liver/kidney or heart/kidney transplantation is indicated when irreversible renal failure is already present or highly likely after the transplant in patients with liver or cardiac disease who are undergoing transplant evaluation. Attention to endocrine abnormalities is important. Almost all patients receiving dialysis have some degree of secondary hyperparathyroidism, but severe forms should be addressed before renal transplantation. The presence of pathologic fractures, advanced demineralization, calciphylaxis, and marked elevations in serum parathyroid hormone levels despite medical management are indications for pretransplant parathyroidectomy. Onset of tertiary hyperparathyroidism, renal calcifications or urinary stones, depression, or persistent hypercalcemia are possible posttransplant indications, but these problems should be avoided by aggressive pretransplant evaluation and treatment. Aluminum toxicity in patients undergoing dialysis may result in significant demineralization and anemia causing apparent hyperparathyroidism and should be ruled out in dialysis-dependent patients, as parathyroidectomy does not result in full improvement in these cases.

Bone Marrow Suppression. Several commonly used drugs, including azathioprine, cyclophosphamide, ganciclovir, and trimethoprim-sulfamethoxazole (TMP-SX), may result in significant bone marrow suppression in the transplant patient. Other drugs in combination with ganciclovir may be further myelosuppressive. Dose limitation, or drug elimination in the case of cyclophosphamide or azathioprine, may be needed. Folinic acid and dose reduction with TMP-SX toxicity can be employed. The use of G-CSF at 300 units subcutaneously each day the white blood cell count remains below 3.0 is often helpful. Cytomegalovirus infection itself may be myelosuppressive. In both liver and kidney transplant patients, prior hypersplenism may persist for several weeks after transplant. Antilymphocyte therapy with ATGAM may be associated with thrombocytopenia or leukopenia (less common) and require subsequent dose limitations or cessation of therapy. Any patient with a documented presence of bone marrow suppression before transplant should undergo careful evaluation, including a bone marrow biopsy to rule out any myelodysplastic syndromes.

Cytokine Release Syndrome (CRS). The CRS can be defined as the systemic responses to inflammation mediated by cytokine release. Thus, in the transplant patient, etiologies include not only fungal, bacterial, and viral infections, but especially the systemic responses to OKT3 and polyclonal antilymphocyte sera. These agents cause the release of tumor necrosis factor, interleukin-6, platelet activating factor, and a number of other cytokines. Severity depends on the degree of systemic inflammation generated. In OKT3 induced CRS, the highest degree of CD3$^+$ cell destruction occurs with the first one or two doses/days of therapy. Once CD3$^+$ cells are eliminated, further cell lysis and activation with attendant TNF release are minimal. The remainder of the OKT3 course simply keeps those cell lines in check. Treatment of CRS includes all the conventional measures of critical care support, while carefully avoiding overaggressive fluid administration. The prevention of severe side effects with OKT3 can be achieved with the use of glucocorticoids (e.g., methylprednisolone), diphenhydramine, acetaminophen, and indomethacin 30 to 60 minutes before the dose. Steroid administration both 1 and 6 hours before OKT3 dosing may be beneficial. Pentoxifylline may also be helpful in two respects. It limits TNF secretion in response to OKT3 and also suppresses intracellular adhesion molecule (ICAM) expression, reducing leukocyte binding to pulmonary endothelium, possibly reducing the white cell contribution to the onset of adult respiratory distress syndrome (ARDS).

Graft-Versus-Host Disease (GVHD). The characteristic findings of cutaneous (maculopapular rash) and gastrointestinal lesions due to immunocompetent attack from donor cells are rare in solid organ transplant recipients. Liver transplantation, blood product transfusion, and bone marrow transfusion can all result in a small rate of GVHD. The presence of generally histoincompatible cells with a similar antigen between donor and recipient to allow presentation of recipient antigens and recognition by donor cells is a key factor, for instance, where no recipient to donor antigen mismatch occurs, but the recipient has an antigen not present on donor cells. The management is somewhat challenging, especially in acute and hyperacute cases where mortality is nearly uniform. High-dose steroids often help, while the role of cyclosporine is purely preventive and has no use in established GVHD apart from baseline immunosuppressive therapy. The differential diagnosis must include a variety of viral and fungal infections as well as posttransplant lymphoproliferative disease, depending on the presenting symptoms and findings. Excessive recipient immunosuppression is often present and susceptibility to infection is increased. Therapy should therefore include prophylactic antibiotics and surveillance cultures.

Drug-Related Side Effects

Adverse reactions and expected toxicities of immunosuppressive drugs are commonly seen in transplant patients. The recognition of these problems and their initial management is an important aspect of the care of transplant recipients with which all surgeons who might care for these patients should be familiar. The essential details of recognition and management are outlined in Table 11-5.

Cancer and Cancer Chemotherapy

Wounds and Surgical Technique

Wound problems are common in patients with advanced cancer. The general principles of surgical wound management remain the same as for transplant patients, with some added points. The use of non-braided cutaneous sutures to secure venous catheters and drains is preferred. Every attempt at primary wound closure should be made, as rates of secondary healing are slow and a long-standing open wound in a patient with end-stage cancer impairs the quality of time remaining for the patient. Timing of surgical treatment well away from chemotherapeutic administration is unnecessary except to avoid an elective procedure during a period of leukopenia. Double-layer, or closed single-layer, hand-sewn intestinal anastomoses are preferred. Fascial closure with running, nonabsorbable heavy suture is appropriate. Retention sutures are not used primarily and such closures should be especially avoided in patients with significant amounts of ascites or in those receiving peritoneal dialysis, as leaks along the suture tracts become persistent and problematic. Plastic closures with regional flaps or extensive regional undermining are sometimes necessary, but should be avoided when adverse factors, such as severe malnutrition, residual local tumor, or renal failure, are present. The use of subcuticular skin closures is appropriate only for nonadvanced or benign tumors in areas of good blood supply or where cosmesis (i.e., in the face) is an acceptable concern.

Infections

Infection in the cancer patient is an important cause of morbidity and mortality. The febrile granulocytopenic patient repre-

Table 11-5. Management of Immunosuppressive Drug Complications

Drug	Complication	Management
Steroids	Hypertension	Na restriction, furosemide antihypertensives
	Glucose intolerance	Diet, hypoglycemics, insulin
	Hyperlipidemia	Diet, exercise, lipid-lowering agents
	Osteoporosis	Calcium, vitamin D, check bone density
	Weight gain	Diet, exercise, dose reduction
	Poor wound healing	Diet, dose reduction
	Cataracts	Dose reduction, surgery
	Growth retardation	Alternate-day dosing, dose reduction
Cyclosporin A	Hypertension	Na restrict, Ca channel blocker
	Hyperuricemia	Diet, allopurinol, probenecid, colchicine
	Hyperkalemia	Furosemide, potassium-binding resins, diet
	Hyperlipidemia	Diet, HMG-CoA inhibitors
	Neurotoxicity	Avoid hypomagnesemia, correct electrolytes, avoid IV form
	Hypertrichosis	Avoid similar drug tox (i.e., minoxidil)
	Gingival hyperplasia	Oral hygiene, oral surgery, avoid agents with similar toxicity
	Hepatotoxicity	Dose reduction
	Nephrotoxicity	Ca^{2+} channel blockers, fish oil capsules, pentoxifylline, avoid other drugs with like toxicity; conversion to tacrolimus
Azathioprine	Myelosuppression	Lower dose, G-CSF, stop drug
	Hepatotoxicity	Lower dose, stop drug, change to cyclophosphamide, 50–100/d
	Alopecia, tumor, GI disturbance	Lower dose or stop drug
Cyclophosphamide	Myelosuppression	Lower doses, G-CSF, stop drug
	Hemorrhagic cystitis	Stop drug, local measures
	Alopecia, tumor, GI disturbance	Lower dose or stop drug
OKT3	Infection	Prophylaxis for CMV/fungi
	Cytokine release syndrome (CRS)	Premedicate: acetaminophen, indomethacin, pentoxifylline, steroids, diphenylpyraline
	Pulmonary edema, low BP (severe CRS)	Respiratory support, furosemide, CVVH, pressors, ATGAM initially for 1–2 doses
	Antibody formation	Cyclophosphamide or azathioprine during OKT3
ATGAM	Infection	Prophylaxis for CMV/fungi
	Anaphylaxis	Predose skin test, steroids, antihistamines, epinephrine
	Platelet, WBC antibodies	Decrease dose, new batch
	Fever, chills, pain	Slow infusion rate, lower dose

G-CSF = granulocyte colony stimulating factor, 300 μg SQ qd; CVVH = continuous venovenous hemofiltration.

sents a particularly dangerous situation. Aggressive and early antibiotic management, protective isolation, nutritional support, careful physical examination supplemented by radiologic testing (chest x-ray and CT when needed), and meticulous attention to obtaining reliable cultures (e.g., bronchoscopically directed pulmonary cultures) are all essential. Consideration of antibiotic coverage for opportunistic organisms, such as *Nocardia, Listeria, Legionella, Salmonella, Cryptococcus, Candida, As-*

pergillus, and other fungi, is important. Culture results may be delayed, and where infection is likely and the antibiotic regimen is benign, empiric therapy should be started.

The attention to specific nutritional needs in patients with cancer may help to reverse the immunosuppressed state in these individuals and thus reduce the severity and incidence of infections. The enteral supplementation of arginine was evaluated in a blinded, randomized, prospective fashion in 30 malnourished patients with GI malignancies who were undergoing resection. Achievement of positive nitrogen balance, improvement in T-cell responses, and an increase in CD4 expression were seen only in the arginine-supplemented patients. In a study by Daly and colleagues, a commercially available diet containing arginine, RNA, and omega-3 fatty acids (Impact, Sandoz Nutrition, Minneapolis, MN) has been compared to a standard enteral diet (Osmolite HN, Ross Laboratories, Columbus, OH) in patients with upper gastrointestinal malignancies who were undergoing resection. An increase in mean nitrogen balance (15.6 vs 9.0 g/dalton) with a reduction in wound infection rates (11 vs 37%) and hospital stay (15.8 vs 20.2 days) was seen in patients receiving Impact. [Editor's Note: This study was not isonitrogenous and the results might be attributed to increased nitrogen administration in the Impact group. Subsequent studies are isonitrogenous and have achieved the same result.]

The underlying anorexia and weight loss seen in cancer represent a significant obstacle generated by the combined effects of drug toxicities, tumor burden, and cytokine (i.e., TNF) release. These symptoms, along with weakness, anemia, and progressive loss of protein and fat stores, define the cancer cachexia syndrome and result in increased risk of infection and death. Furthermore, the resultant organ dysfunction leads to poor drug clearance/metabolism and to further increased complication rates from chemotherapeutic agents. Both cannabinoids and progestational agents (i.e., megestrol acetate in doses up to 800 mg/day) are shown to be helpful in reversing the anorexia of malignancy. Megestrol acetate has surprisingly few side effects and has proven efficacy in randomized prospective trials.

Cancer Recurrence and Secondary Tumors

Adverse immunologic factors, such as acquired immunodeficiency states, blood transfusions, malnutrition, and so forth, can be expected to increase the rate of tumor recurrence. Interestingly, the presence of predisposing genetic and immune actors may result in the occurrence of several primary tumors of different cell line origins in the same patient (Table 11-6). Adverse immune factors may also play a role in the formation of secondary tumors. Such tumors arise in patients as a result of chemotherapy or especially radiation therapy. Often these secondary malignancies are hematologic, and directly related to prior cancer treatment. In as many as one in six patients treated for Hodgkin's disease, a second cancer will develop within 15 years. Bladder cancer due to cyclophosphamide (Cytoxan) therapy is seen in both cancer and transplant patients. Urinary excretion of the drug results in local irritative effects, hemorrhagic cystitis, and a tendency toward cancer formation.

Drug-Related Side Effects

The vast array of chemotherapeutic agents available are all noted for some degree of toxicity. The majority of chemotherapeutic agents have some degree of myelosuppression as an important side effect. Several other notable effects of particular importance include 1) an increased pulmonary sensitivity to oxygen toxicity after bleomycin exposure, 2) the well-known cardiac effects of doxorubicin hydrochloride (Adriamycin), and 3) the renal toxicities of cisplatin-based regimens. Some of the common toxicities from chemotherapeutic agents are shown in Table 11-7.

Table 11-6. Risk of Secondary Leukemia Following Cancer Treatment

Primary Malignancy	Risk (%age)
Ovarian cancer	5–11, associated with alkylating agents
Non-Hodgkin's lymphoma	8
Lung cancer (non small cell)	44
Lung cancer (small cell)	25
Breast cancer	1.5

Other Common Secondary Malignancies

Leukemia	Soft-tissue sarcoma
Non-Hodgkin's lymphoma	Breast cancer
Lung cancer	Thyroid cancer
Gastric cancer	Bladder cancer
Melanoma	Bone sarcoma

Table 11-7. Common Toxicities of Chemotherapeutic Agents

Drug Class	Agent	Toxicity	WBC Nadir	WBC Recovery
Alkylating agents	Cytoxan	MS, cystitis	8–15 d	17–28 d
	Melphalan	MS	5 d, 3 wk	>6 wk
	Lomustine	MS	15 d, 6 wk	7–8 wk
	Carmustine	MS	5–6 wk	6–8 wk
	Cisplatin	Renal	18–23 d	13–62 d
	Thiotepa	MS	10–14 d	>30 d
Antimetabolic agents	Cytarabine	MS	7–9, 15–24 d	34 d
	5-Fluorouracil	MS	9–14 d	Rapid 24–48 hr
	6-Mercaptopurine	MS	1–2 wk	Dose dependent
	Methotrexate	MS, D, GI perforation	4–7 d 7–13 d	Dose dependent
Antitumor antibiotics	Actinomycin	MS, GI	1–7 d	14–21 d
	Bleomycin	P, Mc	N/A	N/A
	Doxorubicin	MS, GI	10–14 d	21 d
	Mitomycin-C	MS	6 wk	Severe
Alkaloids	Vinblastine	MS	4–10 d	7–14 d
	Vincristine	Neuro, MS	Mild 2–4 d	<7 d
	Etoposide	MS	7–14 d	20 d
Other agents	Dacarbazine	GI, MS	2–4 wk	Variable
	Procarbazine	MS	2–8 wk	Variable

MS = myelosuppression; P = pulmonary; GI = gastrointestinal; Mc = mucocutaneous; D = dermatologic.

Table 11-8. Management of Chemotherapy Toxicities

Complication	Management
Myelosuppression	G-CSF
Impaired wound healing	Arginine, vitamin A, C
Gut toxicities	Glutamine, GM-CSF
Bladder toxicity (cyclophosphamide)	Mesna (Na$^+$–2-mercaptoethanesulfonate)

Management of some of the complications of chemotherapy are shown in Table 11-8.

Radiation Therapy and Toxic Exposure

Wound Management and Surgical Concerns

The general surgeon is most familiar with the effects of radiation as it applies to postradiation intestinal injury. All body tissues have some degree of radiation tolerance, which, when exceeded, results in significant local damage and impaired wound healing. Avoidance of surgical incisions in radiated fields/areas of skin, if possible, is helpful. Intestinal anastomosis in extensively damaged bowel should be avoided, and side-to-side bypass is preferred to resection of such segments, especially when extensive adhesions are present or complete resection is impossible. Fascial closure is performed as in cancer patients while skin closure can be problematic. Reliance on monofilament, nonabsorbable suture is best. When dealing with radiation-induced intestinal injury, it should be remembered that the severity and extent of damage are often greater than anticipated.

Tumorigenesis

The specific tumor-inducing effects of ionizing radiation are well known and the management of these tumors is often challenging. Age is a major factor, as most malignancy risks escalate with radiation exposure earlier in life. Most well known are the thyroid malignancies, and postradiation solid tumors are now surpassing the incidence of hematologic cancers among secondary malignancies (e.g., this population has a more than 4-fold increase in the incidence of breast cancer, rising to a 10-fold increase in women who survive longer than 15–20 years). Differentiation of de novo malignancies versus recurrent malignancies in radiated fields (recurrent tumors are most common) remains less important than the realization that new nodules or any painful lesion is cancer until proven otherwise, as such determinations must be made to allow appropriate treatment planning.

Infections

Intestinal radiation injury may cause destruction of the gut mucosal barrier. Following sufficient ionizing radiation to generate DNA damage in the crypt cells, mucosal regeneration fails and gaps in the cellular lining form coalescing ulcers and areas of mucosal denudation that place the patient at risk for opportunistic infection. These local infections can play a role in the progression of the subsequent vascular changes and result in bowel wall necrosis/fibrosis and increased symptomatology. Irradiated bowel presents an inefficient barrier to bacterial and fungal translocation, predominantly gram-negative rods. Intestinal decontamination with oral antibiotics such as trimethoprim-sulfamethoxazole has met with variable success in prevention of infections. The use of ciprofloxacin may result in improved efficacy in prevention of bacterial infection.

Total Body Irradiation

The most severe immunosuppressive effects of radiation exposure are seen in nuclear or industrial accident cases. A well-described body of information also is available from the study of post–atomic bomb sequelae in Japan. A number of considerations exist, but the management of these patients is interesting and includes strict attention to monitoring of bone marrow suppression, infection control and prevention measures, broad-spectrum antibiotic coverage, conservative management of most wounds, fungal prophylaxis, and the full gamut of nutritional and immune support measures mentioned elsewhere.

Malnutrition

Wounds and Surgical Implications

The significant surgical risks presented by the malnourished patient are well known. Impaired wound healing, higher rates of respiratory failure, infection, and decreased survival are all familiar problems. At any time, up to 10 percent of patients on a general surgical service are severely malnourished. These rates increase to 40 percent when intensive care, multiple trauma, or end-stage cancer patients are considered. The indigent, elderly, alcoholics, heavy smokers, and diabetics are also populations at increased risk. Many patients acquire protein-calorie malnutrition during their hospital course as a consequence of inadequate supplementation and hypercatabolism. Severely malnourished surgical patients have an in-hospital mortality of well-nourished age-matched control subjects. Complications related to malnutrition in all patients are principally those of infection (fatal and nonfatal sepsis, intra-abdominal abscess, wound infection) and impaired wound healing (wound dehiscence and anastomotic breakdown). In general, severely malnourished patients have complication rates that exceed 50 percent, while well-nourished patients suffer these complications very infrequently (<2%). The management of specific wound problems should include a search for nutritional deficiencies and their immediate correction. The immunosuppressive effects of severe malnutrition require a similar approach to tissue approximation and suture selection as mentioned for chemically immunosuppressed patients. Anorexia in patients who are receiving chemotherapy often compounds this immunosuppressed state because of malnutrition.

Infections

Impairment of host resistance to infection is a well-known sequela of severe malnutrition. Diminished mucosal barrier function may also play a role. The institution of at least low-volume enteral nutrition, "feeding the gut," is of significant importance. Strict attention to sterility in handling central venous access catheters is key. Unusual opportunistic pathogens are less common than typical nosocomial bacterial and fungal infections but the mortality of these infections is increased. Reactivation of prior mycobacterial, fungal, or viral infections, such as tuberculosis, histoplasmosis, or varicella-zoster (shingles), can be seen. Prolonged antibiotic management is often necessary and occasionally ineffective until nutritional parameters are improved.

Systemic Syndromes

The systemic effects of severe nutritional depletion are easily recognized in terms of weight loss, muscle wasting, impaired physical activity, anorexia, and so forth. The differentiation between standard protein-calorie malnutrition and PCM with hypoalbuminemia reveals that only the hypoalbuminemic patients are at increased risk of death and sepsis. It is difficult, however, to show an advantage with albumin replenishment unless albumin levels are extremely low (<2 g/dl). This is possibly due to the implied hepatic reprioritization toward acute-phase protein synthesis as a response to systemic inflammatory cytokines in these hypoalbuminemic patients.

Nutritional Immunosuppression

The restoration of caloric supply is essential in malnourished patients, but the route and composition of nutritional support will have profound effects on immune system function. The increased susceptibility of parenterally fed patients to septicemia, especially candidemia, is well recognized. Neutrophil and lymphocyte function as well as serum microbicidal activity are depressed in parenterally fed patients. Enteral alimentation through support of the gut immune system (including mucosal barrier function) reverses these defects. The type of diet plays a role, as complex diets are often better absorbed, while elemental diets are potentially immunosuppressive. The utilization of these nutritional concepts (provision of specific nutritional supplements, some in pharmacologic proportions, via the enteral route) has already been shown in prospective studies to decrease the incidence of sepsis and length of hospital stay (Table 11-9). The use of biologic response modifiers as adjuncts to nutritional immune support is under ongoing study.

As noted above, selected nutrients have pharmacologic effects on both specific and nonspecific immune defenses. Among the nutrients shown to have pharmacologic effects are the omega-3 fatty acids, glutamine, arginine, and vitamins A, C, and E. Among these, vitamins A and C, along with arginine, can have positive and independent effects on wound healing. Glutamine and vitamin A may have specific effects on gut mucosal barrier preservation and healing of intestinal injury or anastomoses. Again it is the enteral route of administration of glutamine that will have the best results.

The use of parenteral nutrition is not to be condemned, however. Many surgical patients cannot be alimented for at least brief periods of time. When preoperative enteral feeding has been held for more than 3 to 5 days in severely malnourished patients, perioperative parenteral nutrition has proven benefits. In this setting, parenteral nutrition should be started immediately and continued until the enteral route is available and able to support the caloric needs of the patient. A brief period of overlap while enteral nutrition is increased and total parenteral nutrition (TPN) is phased out can be expected. It must be emphasized, however, that enteral nutrition can be given in the vast majority of patients with added effect.

Surgical Complications

Surgical conditions in the immunosuppressed patient include those that occur in the general population, some special and relatively rare conditions (spontaneous splenic rupture), and a large number of difficult and unusual presentations of common problems. Signs and symptoms of inflammation are often masked and the formation of pus/infiltrates is depressed in granulocytopenic patients. Incision of "abscesses" may yield only serosanguineous, turbid fluid with few white cells, as local pus formation and inflammatory thrombosis of small regional vessels may not be possible. Progression of disease when focal inflammation is absent can be quite impressive. Acute conditions such as diverticulitis or acalculous cholecystitis may progress to small-vessel erosion and present with hemoperitoneum or hemobilia. The effects of malnutrition, lack of enteral supplementation, granulocytopenia, corticosteroids, and radiation result in mucosal barrier dysfunction, intestinal thinning and dilatation, and reduced regional immune defenses. These patients are at increased risk for spontaneous focal intestinal damage/necrosis and perforation.

The preoperative preparation for these patients is usually straightforward. Broad-spectrum antibiotic coverage where contamination is suspected can consist of ampicillin-sulbactam or imipenem-cilastatin if *Pseudomonas* is suspected. The use of vancomycin for nosocomial or device-related infections can be altered as soon as culture results allow. Aminoglycosides are best avoided in the acute setting if the patient is receiving other nephrotoxic drugs (such as cyclosporin, tacrolimus, or amphotericin). Intraoperative irrigation with cefazolin or kanamycin is performed and amphotericin irrigation is used for reoperations or where GI perforations exist. Any patient receiving broad-spectrum antibiotics should also be placed on antifungal therapy. We prefer fluconazole for this purpose. The addition of antiviral therapy, preoperative steroids, and granulocyte

Table 11-9. Immunoenhancement via Enteral Nutrition: Prospective Trials

Study	Subjects	No. of Patients	Total Infections	Length of Stay (d)
Alexander and Gottschlich (1990)	Pediatric burn pts	33 (C)	37	1.21/% BSA burn
		17 (S)	7	0.83/% BSA burn
Daly et al (1992)	Adult GI surgery pts	41 (C)	15	20.2 +/− 9.4
		36 (S)	4	15.8 +/− 5.1
Moore et al (1994)	Adult major trauma	47 (C)	11.0	17.2
		51 (S)	0	14.6

C = control; S = subjects; BSA = body surface area.

colony stimulating factor (G-CSF) depends on the individual patient.

The stomach should be emptied in diabetics or those with gastroparesis. Nasogastric decompression and removal of residual oral contrast should be performed immediately after a preoperative CT scan. A preoperative coagulation profile is drawn and appropriate blood products ordered. We often use cryoprecipitate for the temporary compensation of "uremic" platelet dysfunction. If a fresh incision or implantable device is to be used, skin preparation with iodine, alcohol, or Duraprep, followed by adhesive iodine-impregnated barrier coverage, is used. Intraoperative pneumatic compression stockings are used in most cases.

Acute Abdomen

The acute abdomen is not uncommon in immunosuppressed patients, occurring in 4 percent of all patients with leukemia. The immunocompromised patient with acute abdominal pain presents a significant challenge to the surgical consultant. A broad range of potential conditions may result in acute abdominal pain, some related to the underlying immunosuppression (viral enteritis, neutropenic colitis, gastrointestinal lymphoma, pneumatosis intestinalis), and others to specific surgical concerns in the patient population (allograft pancreatitis, spontaneous bacterial peritonitis, obstructing carcinoma), while some conditions are those that are possible in any patient (gastrointestinal perforations, appendicitis, cholecystitis, pancreatitis, etc.). The workup is made more difficult by the frequent lack of significant inflammatory responses and localized findings in the immunosuppressed patient. Initial evaluation, along with a complete physical examination, must include full laboratory investigation, plain films of the chest and abdomen, ECG, urinalysis, blood cultures, viral serologies when appropriate, and abdominal CT scan if any doubt regarding the diagnosis exists. When noninvasive evaluation fails to make the diagnosis, exploratory laparotomy is indicated.

Anorectal Disease

The development of subcutaneous perirectal abscess formation in patients with malignant disease is common and inversely related to the granulocyte count. Patients often present with fever or septicemia or perianal pain or tenderness (which may be mild), and later develop signs of local irritation. Early antibiotics to cover gram negatives, anaerobes, and enterococcus should be started and tapered, according to results of intraoperative cultures. Local incision and drainage are all that are needed unless a fistula is discovered (found in up to 50%). Fistula tracts are laid open and wet-to-dry dressings are started. Healing rates are also dependent on granulocyte count, and G-CSF should be considered in neutropenic patients with signs of septicemia.

Neutropenic Enterocolitis

"Typhlitis" is a well-known complication of neutropenia, seen most often in patients with hematologic malignancies (2–3% of cases). Presenting signs of granulocytopenia, fever, right lower quadrant tenderness, rebound, bloody stools, vomiting, and, rarely, a palpable mass are helpful but nonspecific. Radiologic findings on plain film and barium enema are also nonspecific and consistent with signs of cecal inflammation. On CT scan, the cecum and right colon will be fluid filled and have a thickened wall, while the appendix, if seen, appears normal. Pneumatosis limited to the cecum and ascending colon may be seen on plain film or CT scan. This is a necrotizing process with bowel wall edema, mucosal ulcerations, localized hemorrhage and infiltrate, and eventual progression to perforation. Diminished intestinal motility with localized ileocecal bacterial overgrowth may be one underlying factor in the pathogenesis. Specific chemotherapeutic agents have been implicated including vincristine and cytarabine, but a wide variety of agents were used in the reported cases. Chemotherapy induction with resultant granulocytopenia is clearly the greatest risk factor. Support with intravenous fluids, antibiotics, and G-CSF should be followed rapidly by immediate exploration, as nonoperative management results in assured mortality. The diseased bowel is resected and, in the absence of gross perforation and peritoneal contamination, a primary ileocolic anastomosis is performed using an inner layer of 4-0 Maxon and an outer layer of 3-0 Prolene. Otherwise, an end ileostomy with mucous fistula is selected.

Gastrointestinal Perforation

Both colonic and small-bowel perforations have been described and occur in 1 to 2 percent of patients following transplantation. Complicated gastroduodenal ulceration is seen in over 6 percent of patients. Focal intestinal ischemia, often without underlying vascular thrombosis, appears to be an underlying cause. These small lesions heal poorly (especially in association with steroid administration) and subsequently can perforate. Most patients suffer from some degree of abdominal distention and pain around the time of perforation. Corticosteroids are of great significance in apparent spontaneous intestinal perforation. Predisposition to diverticular and gastroduodenal perforations in patients receiving steroids is well known. We favor a simplified approach to upper GI perforations, with control of hemorrhage, local excision with primary closure of perforations, and reliance on steroid reduction and medical management for prevention of recurrence. All focal ulcerations, regardless of appearance, are cultured for CMV and *Campylobacter pylori*. Small-bowel perforations are so often associated with local pathology that segmental resection and primary anastomosis are required. Colonic perforations are treated by resection and end colostomy, with Hartmann's procedure for left-sided lesions and mucous fistula for more proximal procedures. Subsequent colostomy takedown is performed after a minimum of 2 months' wait and after steroid reduction if possible. Recent rejection episodes with ongoing steroid taper preclude elective colostomy takedown. We attempt to avoid high-output small-bowel ostomies because of difficulties in immunosuppressive medication, fluid balance, and nutritional management. It should be noted that these problems are not a contraindication to ileostomy, when needed.

Fecal impaction is another cause of intestinal perforation in posttransplant patients. Narcotics and aluminum-based antacid therapy, steroid use, preexisting diverticular disease, and constipation are all risk factors. Strict attention to avoidance of posttransplant constipation is key. Once the diagnosis of fecal impaction is made, discontinuation of narcotic analgesics, disimpaction, and aggressive use of stool softeners are started. The progression to perforation is rare, but results in a need for colonic resection, Hartmann's procedure, and end colostomy. The occurrence of colonic pseudoobstruction (Ogilvie's syndrome) is common in these patients. Diagnosis can be made on plain abdominal films and an aggressive approach to colonoscopic decompression (when cecal diameter reaches 12 cm) is standard. Prophylactic antibiotic coverage should be administered before colonoscopy in immunosuppressed patients. The use of surgical decompression by tube cecostomy or colostomy is also an option if endoscopic management fails. Resection of the right colon is occasionally required.

Postsplenectomy Infection

The immune functions of the spleen including mechanical filtration and mediator generation (complement, tuftsin, IgM) combine with the anatomic features of the spleen to allow the effective removal of encapsulated and other bacteria and possibly some protozoa including *Babesia microti* and *Plasmodium* species. The asplenic state is associated with a higher mortality during infection with these organisms. The occurrence of overwhelming postsplenectomy infection (OPSI) is highest in children, with a rate of one fatality per 300 to 350 years of patient follow-up. Adult rates are half those of children and decrease with age. Triple immunization with *H. influenzae b,* meningococcal serogroup C, and pneumococcal vaccines is safe and can greatly reduce, but not eliminate, OPSI. The use of prophylactic penicillin is indicated in children, but no compelling evidence exists for antibiotic prophylaxis in adults.

The treatment of serious infections in asplenic patients requires an aggressive approach with immediate hospitalization. OPSI is associated with all of the end-stage manifestations of septic shock, and tertiary critical care support is necessary.

Pancreatitis

Pancreatitis following transplantation, drug administration, hypercalcemia, or infection is frequently mild and self-limited. Severe cases and fatalities have been described, however, and early reports of posttransplant pancreatitis document high (50%) mortality and complication rates.

The usual conservative measures often suffice, with steroid reduction, conversion to brief parenteral nutrition, and intravenous medications including antibiotic coverage. Progression to hemorrhagic pancreatitis or pancreatic necrosis and abscess formation is uncommon, but seen even with some cases of drug-induced pancreatitis. Once fungal or bacterial infection is documented, either by blood culture or direct CT-guided aspiration, aggressive surgical debridement and large-bore irrigation/suction drainage with soft multi-channel drains are performed. Mesenteric vasodilatory doses of dopamine are employed. Strict intensive care management is instituted and complications, such as ARDS, renal impairment, and hepatic dysfunction, are managed in standard fashion. Overall, the etiology of pancreatitis posttransplant is multifactorial and the outcome is usually good.

Pneumatosis Intestinalis

Often a benign condition, the presence of intramural intestinal air is seen in cases of chronic obstructive pulmonary disease (COPD), posttransplant, in intestinal obstruction, and in ileus, among others. The presence of an active tissue-invasive GI infection is believed to predispose to pneumatosis intestinalis in transplant recipients. The intestinal tract is usually not ischemic. A benign abdominal examination is required for conservative management, which consists of broad-spectrum intravenous antibiotics (including ganciclovir) and parenteral nutrition. Serial abdominal films and examinations must be instituted. Even free air in the setting of benign abdominal examination can be observed. However, given the tendency of immunosuppressive medications to mask the inflammation and symptoms of peritonitis, even slight signs of inflammation, ischemia, or septicemia require immediate surgical intervention. Continued observation until the pneumatosis radiographically resolves is required and usually takes less than a week.

Biliary Tract Pathology

The incidence of biliary tract pathology is similar to that of the general population. Hepatotoxicity is seen with several chemotherapeutic and immunosuppressive agents. Cyclosporin is associated with an increased incidence of biliary calculous

disease. The diagnosis of biliary colic or simple acute cholecystitis is not different in this patient population and should be treated by laparoscopic cholecystectomy after appropriate preparation. The tendency toward acalculous or gangrenous cholecystitis is higher than in the general population, however. Hypoalbuminemic patients may have pericholecystic fluid or gallbladder wall thickening due to tissue edema, making these findings less helpful. The presence of a nonfunctioning gallbladder on nuclear scan is usually sufficient evidence to raise the suspicion of gallbladder pathology. The laparoscopic approach is taken initially, but due to advanced progression of disease, the rate of conversion to an open procedure will be higher. Great care must be taken to avoid ductal injury, as many of these patients cannot tolerate subsequent biliary reconstruction. Intraoperative cholangiograms are always performed but postoperative endoscopic retrograde cholangiopancreatography (ERCP) is still occasionally required to evaluate abnormal liver function tests.

Solid Organ Abscesses

Opportunistic infections of the liver and spleen are seen often in immunocompromised patients. Predisposing factors include neutropenia, recent chemotherapy, steroids, prolonged use of broad-spectrum antibiotics, and preexisting GI candidiasis. Localization of opportunistic infection in the liver parenchyma occurs in a variety of settings, including hematologic and other malignancies, aplastic anemia, transplant, agammaglobulinemia, and AIDS. Hepatic candidiasis is especially well described in cancer patients. Liver function tests are usually elevated, especially the alkaline phosphatase. Biopsy shows candidal elements, microabscesses, or granulomas in 75 percent of patients while blood cultures are routinely negative. Diffuse, small abscesses may be seen on ultrasound and progression to involvement of the biliary tree has been described. Associated involvement of the kidney, spleen, heart, lung, or GI tract occurs in more than half of the reported cases. Treatment for candidal abscess is with prolonged amphotericin (>2-g course) and 5-flucytosine. Larger hepatic collections can be drained percutaneously under ultrasound guidance. Splenic abscesses can also be drained percutaneously (often a preference in children) or treated by splenectomy. Despite aggressive and early treatment, mortality approaches 50 percent in adult patients, and untreated mortality is 100 percent. Other pathogens are treated similarly, with specific antibiotics and drainage when indicated.

Pulmonary Mycoses

Opportunistic pulmonary fungal infections tend to occur in neutropenic cancer and transplant patients and are often difficult to treat. *Aspergillus, Zygomycetes, Mucor*, and *Cryptoccocus* are the more common localizing pulmonary infections seen. Systemic therapy with amphotericin before or after operation and regional pulmonary resection are indicated. Preoperative chest CT is helpful and evidence of angioinvasion is a poor prognostic sign. Early mortality averages 30 percent despite aggressive antibiotic and resectional therapy. A standard surgical approach is used and complete resection is the underlying principle. Chest tube drainage is continued until fluid accumulation is minimal, to prevent fungal empyema. Chest wall involvement requires extended resection.

Conclusion

Acquired states of immunosuppression are common in surgical patients. The presence of multiple factors, such as malnutrition, cancer, blood transfusion, radiation, anesthesia, and drug-induced myelosuppression, often coexist, resulting in cumulative effects. Indeed, an isolated etiology of immunosuppression most often exists in transplant recipients, in whom drug-induced effects are the principal factor. The complications associated with these varied immunosuppressive conditions are quite similar and include impaired wound healing, opportunistic infection, and secondary tumors. The general supportive mea-

sures, perhaps the most specific being nutritional immunomodulation, are again the same for each group. Transplant patients have one significant advantage over other immunosuppressed patients in that their medication doses can often be reduced or withdrawn to result in improved immune function.

Suggested Reading

Alexander JW. Immunoenhancement via enteral nutrition. *Arch Surg* 128:1242, 1993.

Daly JM, Leberman MD, Goldfine J, et al. Enteral nutrition with supplemental arginine, RNA, and omega-3 fatty acids in patients after operation: Immunologic, metabolic and clinical outcome. *Surgery* 112:56, 1992.

Detsky AS, Baker JP, O'Rourke K, et al. Predicting nutrition-associated complications for patients undergoing gastrointestinal surgery. *JPEN* 11:440, 1987.

Ferguson A. Immunological functions of the gut in relation to nutritional state and mode of delivery of nutrients. *Gut* 1 (Suppl):S10, 1994.

Fryer JP, Granger DK, Leventhal JR, et al. Steroid-related complications in the cyclosporin era. *Clin Transplant* 8:224, 1994.

Hanto DW. Classification of Epstein-Barr virus–associated posttransplant lymphoproliferative diseases. *Ann Rev Med* 46:381, 1995.

Kahan BD, Flechner SM, Lorber MI, et al. Complications of cyclosporin-prednisone immunosuppression in 402 renal allograft recipients exclusively followed at a single center for from one to five years. *Transplantation* 43:197, 1987.

Meakins JL. Surgeons, surgery and immunomodulation. *Arch Surg* 126:494, 1991.

Rigotti P, Van Buren CT, Payne W, et al. Gastrointestinal perforations in renal transplant recipients immunosuppressed with cyclosporin. *World J Surg* 10:137, 1986.

Rossi SJ, Schroeder TJ, Hariharan S, First MR. Prevention and management of the adverse effects associated with immunosuppressive therapy. *Drug Safety* 9:104, 1993.

Windsor JA. Underweight patients and the risks of major surgery. *World J Surg* 17:165, 1993.

Yee J, Cristou NV. Perioperative care of the immunocompromised patient. *World J Surg* 17:207, 1993.

EDITOR'S COMMENT

Doctors Valente and Alexander have contributed an excellent chapter, and have emphasized the fact that the individuals they care for are extremely difficult patients. Here again, nutritional depletion places the patient at major risk. Doctor Alexander refers to his own findings in the laboratory that, at least during the first 24 to 48 hours of acute sepsis, protein deprivation may be helpful and result in a lower mortality.

Technically, I have only one quibble with all of the excellent suggestions following surgical technique, and that is the use of subcuticular closures in patients who are nutritionally depleted. I don't believe that I have used the skin suture in the past 26 years, and I have operated on all sorts of patients at terrible risk. I believe that the incidence of complications is lower. At present, I use a No. 5-0 polydioxanone (PDS) suture for subcuticular closure, which seems to give excellent results. In normally nourished patients in whom cosmesis is required, pull-out 3-0 nylons are utilized and the sutures are pulled out in 4 days. In both of these closures, Steri-Strips are used to reinforce the suture line.

Many of the lessons that are learned from immunocompromised patients in transplantation operations can be transposed to the general population with malignancy or severe infection. These are lessons well learned and should be taken seriously. J.E.F.

TWO

BASIC SURGICAL SKILLS: NEW AND EMERGING TECHNOLOGY

12

Abdominal Wall Incisions and Repair

Israel Penn

The most important factors in the choice of an abdominal incision are the anticipated intra-abdominal pathology, the contemplated operative procedure, and the general condition and build of the patient. The type of incision used should fulfill three requirements:

1. *Adequate Exposure.* It must provide ready and direct access to the diseased or injured area and give sufficient room for the required procedure to be performed. Exposure of the operative site can be greatly enhanced by proper positioning of the patient, efficient illumination, and proper positioning of retractors and packs.
2. *Extensibility.* If the extent of the operation requires greater exposure than originally anticipated, the incision should be conveniently extended upward or downward, medially or laterally. Any extension should limit or avoid sacrifice of nerves that supply the abdominal musculature.
3. *Security.* Closure of the wound must be reliable and secure and ideally should leave the abdominal wall as strong as it was preoperatively.

An incision should be so placed that it will not interfere with future stages of planned surgery. It should be placed to avoid or incorporate, as indicated, any existing sinuses, fistulas, colostomies, and so forth. Any error, such as a poorly placed incision, unsatisfactory methods of closure, or inappropriate selection of sutures, can lead to complications, including hematoma, stitch abscess, infection, complete wound dehiscence, an incisional hernia, or an unsightly scar.

Types of Incisions (Fig. 12-1)

1. *Vertical.* These can be midline or paramedian. They can be supra- or infra-umbilical and, if necessary, for example, for extensive intra-abdominal trauma can be extended upward to the xiphoid and downward to the symphysis pubis.
2. *Transverse or oblique.* The best examples are Kocher's subcostal incision for cholecystectomy, McBurney's incision for appendectomy, Pfannenstiel's incision for gynecologic surgery, and a transverse or oblique lateral incision for exposure of the colon.
3. *Retroperitoneal and extraperitoneal approaches.*
4. *Thoracoabdominal.* This gives excellent exposure of upper abdominal organs by connecting the pleural and peritoneal cavities into a single space.

Choice of Incision

Choice of incision often varies with the surgeon's individual experience and preference and will depend on the organ(s) that need to be exposed, whether rapid access is needed as for hemorrhage, the habitus of the patient, the degree of obesity, and the presence of previous abdominal incisions.

Many surgeons prefer oblique or transverse incisions since the pull of the lateral abdominal muscles is in line with or roughly parallel to the incisions, and there is much less tension on the edges than with vertical incisions, so that the wounds are stronger and less liable to dehiscence or herniation. However, these incisions are somewhat more time-consuming than a midline approach, as, also, is the paramedian incision.

In emergency operations, for example, for intra-abdominal hemorrhage, the midline

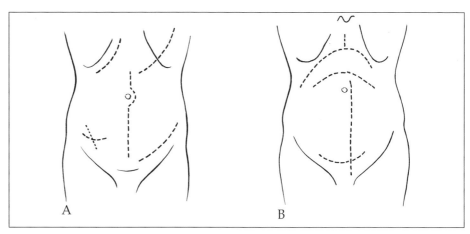

Fig. 12-1. Common types of vertical, transverse, and oblique incisions including thoracoabdominal incision.

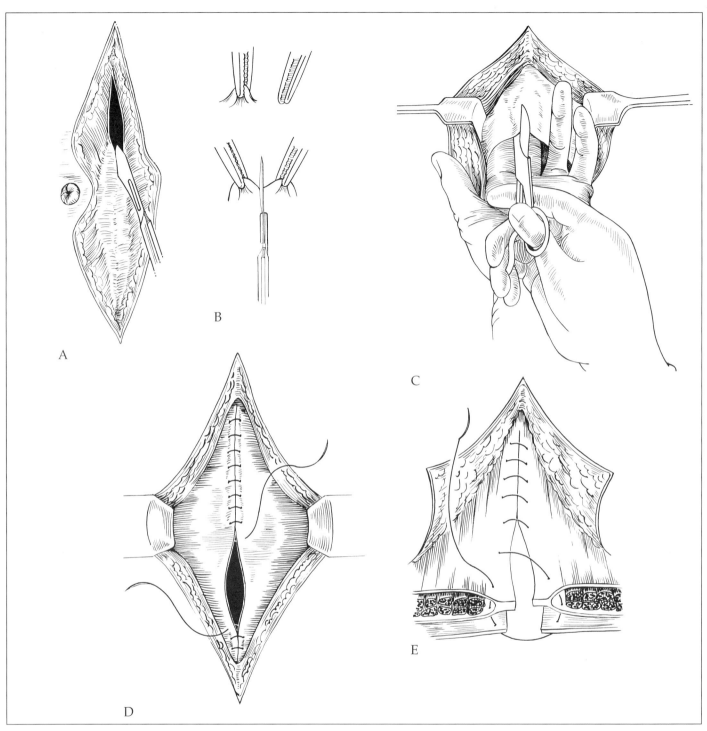

Fig. 12-2. A. Midline incision curving around the umbilicus. The peritoneum is being opened in the upper part of the incision. B. Peritoneal fold being opened. This technique avoids injury to underlying viscera. C. Peritoneum is opened with scissors. The surgeon's fingers are interposed between the scissors and the underlying viscera. D. Closure of the linea alba by two continuous sutures starting from the upper and lower ends. E. Closure of linea alba and peritoneum as one layer. Inclusion of the peritoneum is not essential to obtain good wound healing.

approach gives the most rapid access and, if necessary, can be quickly extended from the xiphoid to the symphysis pubis. One also prefers an upper midline incision in a thin patient with a narrow subcostal angle, but in an obese patient with a wide subcostal angle, an oblique subcostal incision gives excellent exposure of the biliary system or spleen.

For appendectomy, McBurney's muscle-splitting incision is excellent and can be easily extended medially or laterally if greater exposure is required. If an ileostomy or colostomy is to be part of the operative procedure, the main incision should be kept as far from the stoma as possible, using either a midline incision or a paramedian approach on the contralateral side to the planned stoma.

When reoperating on an abdomen one should, if possible, enter through the previous incision, particularly if it entails excision of an ugly scar or repair of an incisional hernia. When operating through a previous scar one should be on the lookout for adhesions to it of bowel or omentum. One should try to avoid making a fresh incision closely parallel to a previous scar, as it may cut off the blood supply to the tissue between the incisions, leading to necrosis of the skin bridge.

Vertical Incisions

Midline Incisions
The midline incision is the simplest approach. It offers adequate exposure to any part of the abdominal cavity. When speed is essential, it is the incision of choice, as it is easy to make and to repair. It is almost bloodless, no muscle fibers are divided, and no nerves are injured. It can be extended upward and downward the full length of the abdomen by curving the skin incision around the umbilicus (Fig. 12-2A). The incision is deepened through skin, subcutaneous fat, linea alba, properitoneal fat, and peritoneum. Properitoneal fat is abundant in obese individuals. If the falciform ligament interferes with exposure of the upper abdomen, it should be clamped, divided, and ligated. Upper midline incisions provide good exposure for most operations on the esophageal hiatus, abdominal esophagus (and vagus nerves), stomach, duodenum, gallbladder, pancreas, and spleen. Lower midline incisions provide good exposure for most opera-

tions on the lower abdominal and pelvic organs.

When making lower abdominal incisions, one should enter the peritoneum near the umbilicus to avoid injury to the bladder. Care must be exercised in opening the peritoneum to avoid injury to an underlying bowel loop, particularly when the bowel is distended. A safe method is to pick up a fold of peritoneum with forceps, palpate it to ensure that no other structure has been caught up with it, clamp it with two hemostats placed slightly apart, and then carefully incise the raised fold with a scalpel (Fig. 12-2B). The small opening is enlarged to admit two fingers, which are used to protect the underlying viscera, while the peritoneum is opened through the length of the incision (Fig. 12-2C). When operating through a previous scar one must beware of underlying adhesions. If possible the incision should extend a little beyond the previous scar so that the peritoneum can be opened away from any adhesions. Once the peritoneum has been opened, its edges are held up with

Kocher's clamps so that the attachments of adhesions can be seen and carefully divided under direct vision.

Paramedian Incisions
This vertical incision is made 2.5 to 5.0 cm from the midline (Fig. 12-3A). It is deepened through the subcutaneous fat to the anterior rectus sheath, which is opened for the whole length of the wound (Fig. 12-3B). The medial portion of the sheath is then dissected off the muscle to the midline. This dissection is more difficult in the upper abdomen because of the tendinous attachments of the rectus muscle to the anterior sheath. These are located just below the xiphoid, at the umbilicus, and midway between these two points. Segmental vessels are encountered when freeing the tendinous intersections and need to be electrocoagulated. Once the muscle is free anteriorly and medially, it can be retracted laterally since it is not adherent to the posterior sheath. The posterior sheath and the peritoneum are then incised vertically for the whole length of and in line with the skin incision. The lower rectus sheath dif-

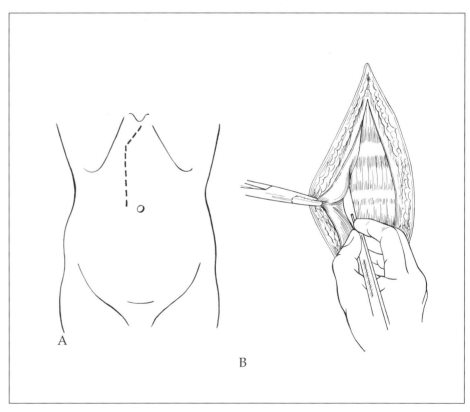

Fig. 12-3. A. Upper abdominal paramedian incision. The upper part of the skin incision is curved toward the midline to avoid crossing the costal margin. B. The anterior rectus sheath is being freed from the rectus muscle, which will be retracted laterally to expose the posterior rectus sheath and peritoneum.

fers from the upper in two respects: The posterior layer is largely absent below the semilunar line of Douglas and the inferior epigastric vessels need to be divided and ligated as they run across the lower part of the incision.

The paramedian incision avoids injury to nerves, limits trauma to the rectus muscle, allows an anatomic and secure closure, and permits good restoration of function. If necessary, it can be extended from the pubis to the xiphoid, by sloping the upper end of the incision medially toward the bone. When placed on the appropriate side it can be employed satisfactorily for any intra-abdominal surgery. The theoretical advantage of this incision is that, when repaired, the rectus muscle resumes its original place and splints the incisions in the anterior and posterior sheath and should diminish the risk of wound dehiscence and incisional hernia. Many surgeons see little advantage of paramedian over midline incisions and avoid using them because they are more time consuming.

Vertical Muscle-Splitting Incisions
This incision is performed in the same way as the paramedian incision, except that the rectus muscle is split longitudinally in its medial third, after which the posterior rectus sheath and peritoneum are opened in the same line. The incision can be quickly made and repaired. It is very satisfactory when a limited incision is needed, for example, for placement of a Tenckhoff peritoneal dialysis catheter. However, an extensive incision should be avoided because it results in more injury to nerve and muscle, and in more bleeding, than the midline or paramedian incision. If more than two nerves are sacrificed there will be weakness of the corresponding area of the abdominal wall postoperatively. The incision's main value is in reopening the scar of a previous paramedian incision, when it is very difficult to dissect the rectus muscle from scar tissue in its sheath, and a muscle split is therefore preferable.

Transverse or Oblique Incisions

There are many varieties of transverse or oblique incisions (see Fig. 12-1). Transverse incisions may be truly horizontal or may curve to varying degrees. Similarly, oblique incisions may be straight or curved and may vary considerably in angle. The incision may be limited to the oblique muscles or may involve division of part of one rectus muscle, or even the entire width of both recti.

Transverse or oblique incisions mostly follow Langer's lines and give good cosmetic results. Any nerve damage that occurs is usually limited to one, or rarely two, nerves. In general, transverse or oblique incisions give limited exposure if disease is found in both the upper and lower abdomen, except possibly in a short individual with a wide abdomen and a wide costal margin. In such a patient a long, transverse supraumbilical incision gives satisfactory exposure for most intra-abdominal surgery with the exception of the pelvis.

The transverse tendinous inscriptions attach the rectus muscle to the anterior rectus sheath, thereby keeping it from retracting significantly when it is incised. However, tendinous inscriptions do not occur below the umbilicus, and there may be some retraction of the incised rectus muscle in that area unless it is sutured to the anterior sheath. One should avoid making a transverse incision close to the symphysis pubis, since if a hernia develops, sufficient fascia must be available along the lower margin of the wound to permit satisfactory repair.

Kocher's Subcostal Incision
Frequently, a right subcostal incision is used for open operations on the gallbladder and bile ducts, particularly in obese or muscular individuals with wide subcostal angles (Figs. 12-1 and 12-4). A left-sided incision is used mainly for elective splenectomy. A bilateral subcostal incision provides excellent exposure of the upper abdomen. It is useful for performing total abdominal gastrectomy in an obese individual, for anterior exposure of both adrenal glands, for some major liver resections, and in hepatic transplantation.

The standard subcostal incision starts in the midline 2.5 to 5.0 cm below the xiphoid

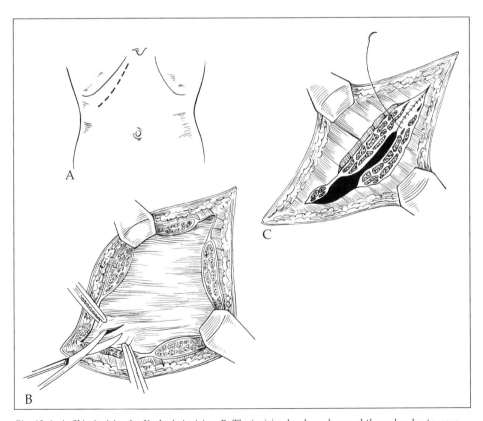

Fig. 12-4. A. Skin incision for Kocher's incision. B. The incision has been deepened through subcutaneous fat, anterior rectus sheath, and muscle. The posterior rectus sheath and peritoneum are being opened. Note lateral abdominal muscles divided in lateral part of incision. C. Closure of posterior rectus sheath and peritoneum as one layer starting in the medial corner.

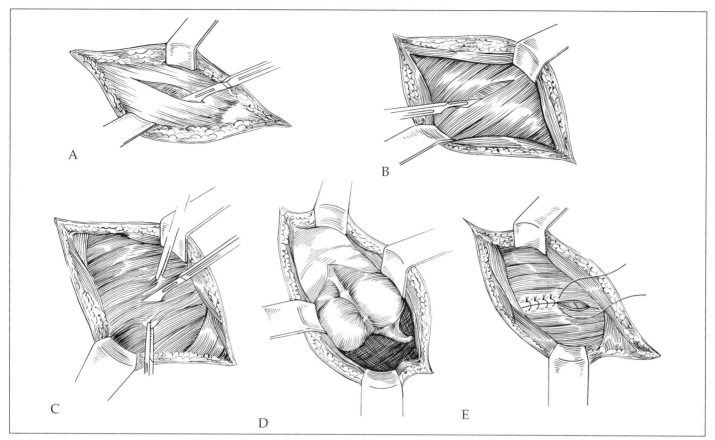

Fig. 12-5. Modified McBurney's incision. A. After the skin and subcutaneous tissues have been opened transversely, the external oblique muscle and aponeurosis is opened in the direction of its fibers. B. Shows opening of the internal oblique muscle in the direction of its fibers. C. The transversus abdominis muscle is split in the direction of its fibers. D. The peritoneum has been opened to expose the cecum and appendix. E. After the peritoneum is closed each muscle layer is separately repaired.

and extends downward and laterally approximately 2.5 cm below the costal margin for a variable distance, depending on the build of the patient (Fig. 12-4A). If the liver is enlarged, the incision may have to be placed at a lower level. The incision should not be made too close to the costal margin since, if a hernia develops, enough abdominal wall must be available at the upper margin to permit a satisfactory repair. After the anterior rectus sheath is incised, the rectus muscle is divided along the length of the wound, using electrocoagulation to control branches of the superior epigastric artery. The lateral abdominal muscles can be divided in an outward direction for a short distance. Although the eighth intercostal nerve is almost invariably divided, care must be taken to preserve the ninth nerve to prevent weakening of the abdominal musculature. The incision is then deepened to open the peritoneum (Fig. 12-4B). Although the rectus

muscle is divided, this results in no weakening of the abdominal muscles, provided that the anterior and posterior sheaths are repaired, because the incision passes between adjacent nerves without injuring them. As the muscle has a segmental nerve supply, there is no risk that a transverse or slightly oblique division of it will deprive its distal part of its innervation. Healing of the incision simply results in an iatrogenically produced additional fibrous inscription in the muscle.

McBurney's Incision

This incision is used for open appendectomy or for performing a cecostomy. The position and length of the incision will depend on the suspected location of the appendix and the degree of obesity of the abdominal wall. A useful clue is palpation of the abdomen once the patient is anesthetized. A mass may be felt and the incision should be made over it. If nothing is pal-

pated, the incision is centered at McBurney's point at the junction of the middle and outer third of a line between the umbilicus and anterosuperior iliac spine. The skin incision is placed transversely to obtain a cosmetically satisfying scar. The oblique incision originally described by McBurney has largely been abandoned because it leaves an obvious scar (see Fig. 12-1).

After the skin and subcutaneous tissues are divided, the external oblique muscle is divided in the direction of its fibers to expose the internal oblique muscle (Fig. 12-5A). Its overlying fascia is opened so that the muscle can be split in the direction of its fibers, usually adjacent to the lateral border of the rectus sheath (Fig. 12-5B). The underlying transversus abdominis is similarly opened in the direction of its fibers, exposing the peritoneum (Fig. 12-5C). A small opening is then made in the

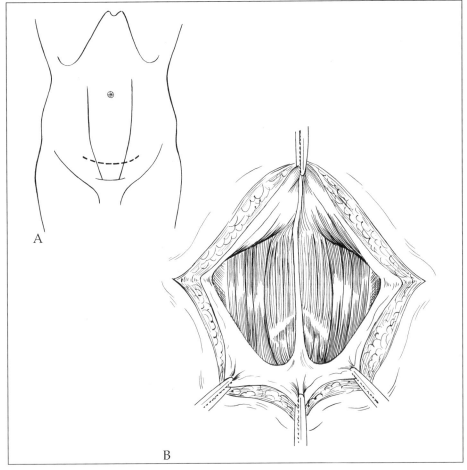

Fig. 12-6. A. Pfannenstiel's incision. Curved transverse skin incision in the interspinous crease. B. Both anterior rectus sheaths are divided in the line of the incision, and then freed upward and downward from the underlying muscle. Note the small pyramidalis muscles to either side of the midline in the lower part of the incision.

peritoneum and enlarged as much as is necessary to expose the appendix and adjacent portion of the cecum (Fig. 12-5D). If further exposure is necessary, the wound is easily enlarged by opening the anterior rectus sheath, retracting the muscle medially, and extending the peritoneal opening medially into the posterior rectus sheath and underlying peritoneum.

If the wound needs to be enlarged laterally, this can be accomplished by a combination of splitting and dividing the three lateral abdominal muscles. The extended McBurney's incision can be used to perform a right hemicolectomy in suitable individuals. A similar incision on the left side can be used for performing a sigmoid colostomy or sigmoid colectomy in suitable subjects.

Pfannenstiel's Incision

This incision is frequently used for gynecologic procedures or, in the male, for extraperitoneal retropubic prostatectomy. The skin incision is placed in the curved interspinous crease with its center located about 5 cm above the symphysis pubis (Fig. 12-6A). Both anterior rectus sheaths are exposed and divided for the entire length of the wound. Hemostats are used to elevate the divided upper and lower edges of the sheaths, which are then freed widely from the underlying rectus muscles upward almost to the umbilicus and downward to the symphysis (Fig. 12-6B). The rectus muscles are then retracted laterally and the peritoneum opened vertically in the midline, taking care not to injure the bladder at the lower end of the

wound. The exposure obtained is rather limited and the incision should not be used when a procedure outside the pelvis may be necessary. The incision, being in a skin crease, leaves a barely noticeable scar, which, in any case, is hidden by the pubic hair.

Retroperitoneal and Extraperitoneal Approaches

Such approaches decrease the handling of intra-abdominal viscera and limit postoperative bleeding and urinary extravasation to the retroperitoneal area. Bleeding is much more likely to be tamponaded here than when it occurs in the general peritoneal cavity. Infections are more frequently localized here than in the abdomen and are more readily drained. The limited retraction and displacement of viscera with retroperitoneal operations reduce postoperative ileus.

These incisions can be used for operations on the kidney; ureter; adrenal glands; bladder; splenic artery and vein; distal pancreas; groin hernias; vena cava; abdominal aorta; common, internal, and external iliac vessels; and lumbar sympathetic chain. Three commonly used retroperitoneal incisions include the retroperitoneal approach to the lumbar area, to the adrenal glands, and to the iliac fossa.

Retroperitoneal Approach to the Lumbar Area

This incision is most frequently used for nephrectomy, aortic surgery, lumbar sympathectomy, or ureterolithotomy. For operation on the right side, the patient is positioned in the supine position with the right side elevated approximately 30 to 45 degrees and with the right knee and hip flexed. The incision begins at the level of the umbilicus at the margin of the lateral rectus sheath and is extended into the flank toward the twelfth rib for 12 to 20 cm (Fig. 12-7A). If necessary a portion of the rib is resected, taking care not to injure the underlying pleura. The skin and subcutaneous tissues are dissected free from the underlying fascia; the external and internal abdominal obliques and transverse abdominis muscles are opened in line with

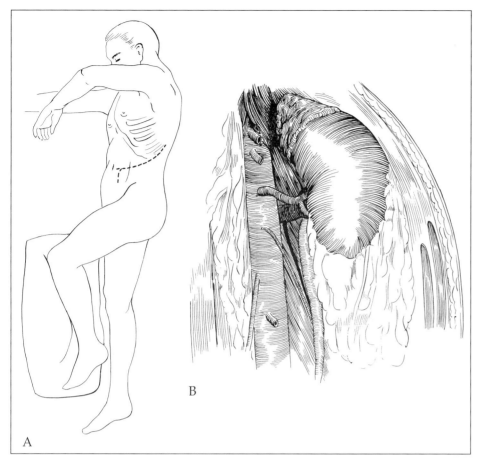

Fig. 12-7. A. Left retroperitoneal approach to the lumbar area. If necessary the incision can be extended downward along the rectus sheath to obtain additional exposure. B. The peritoneum has been retracted forward with the adrenal gland, kidney, and ureter to expose the aorta. Origins of the celiac, superior mesenteric, left renal, and inferior mesenteric arteries are shown.

their fibers. Exposure is facilitated by undermining each layer. When the retroperitoneal space is entered, the peritoneum and retroperitoneal fat are dissected forward (anteriorly) by blunt dissection with fingers and sponge sticks. Care must be taken *not* to dissect behind the psoas muscle. This common mistake may make an otherwise easy dissection confusing and difficult. By continuing this forward displacement, the sympathetic nervous system, ureter, and lower pole of the kidney are easily identified (Fig. 12-7B). On the right, the vena cava is exposed and, on the left, the aorta. If the peritoneum is inadvertently opened, it is closed immediately with a continuous absorbable suture. At the conclusion of the operation, the retroperitoneal fat and viscera fall back into place and the muscle layers are repaired with continuous sutures.

Retroperitoneal Approach to the Adrenal Glands

This is the preferred approach except in patients with pheochromocytomas (who should be explored transabdominally), or in those who have large adrenal tumors, especially if malignancy is suspected.

With the posterior approach, there is little danger of inadvertent injury to the viscera or spleen because dissection is carried out entirely in the retroperitoneal space. Isolation and ligation of the right adrenal vein at its junction with the vena cava, a maneuver that is perhaps the most dangerous step in performing adrenalectomy, is facilitated. Postoperative ileus is rare. Moreover, patients have less pain and fewer pulmonary complications than those who have undergone adrenalectomy via the transabdominal approach, and their overall hospital stay is shorter.

The patient is placed in the prone jackknife position to eliminate the lumbar lordosis. The incision is made in a curvilinear fashion from the tenth rib (three fingerbreadths lateral to the midline) toward the iliac crest (four fingerbreadths lateral to the midline) (Fig. 12-8A). It is deepened through subcutaneous fat, the posterior layer of the lumbodorsal fascia, and the fibers of the latissimus dorsi muscle, which take origin from it. This exposes the erector spinae muscle, which is retracted medially toward the spine to reveal the glistening middle layer of the lumbodorsal fascia and the twelfth rib. The quadratus lumborum muscle, which is directly subjacent, is visible through the lumbodorsal fascia. Several vessels and nerves penetrate the fascia to enter the erector spinae muscle. These are secured between clamps, divided, and ligated. Using the electrocautery, the attachments of the erector spinae to the twelfth rib are divided, and the rib is then resected subperiosteally, taking care not to injure the underlying pleura (Fig. 12-8B). The middle layer of the lumbodorsal fascia is then incised longitudinally along the lateral margin of the quadratus lumborum muscle to expose Gerota's fascia, which invests the kidney and perirenal fat. The subcostal vessels are now visible directly below and parallel to the bed of the resected twelfth rib. The subcostal nerve usually lies about 1.5 cm below the vessels. The subcostal vessels are clamped, divided, and ligated while the subcostal nerve is gently retracted downward.

The insertion of posterior fibers of the diaphragm into the periosteum of the twelfth rib is identified. The glistening pleura is directly above. With hyperinflation, the lower margin of the lung comes into view. The diaphragmatic attachment is divided while the pleura is gently pushed out of the way (Fig. 12-8C). Should the pleural cavity be inadvertently entered, the resultant pneumothorax is easily dealt with during closure. A large-bore catheter is left in the pleural space and brought out through the wound. The fascial layers are closed snugly around the catheter. Just before closure of the skin, the lungs are hyperinflated to evacuate all air from the pleural cavity, and the catheter is quickly removed at the height of positive-pressure inspiration.

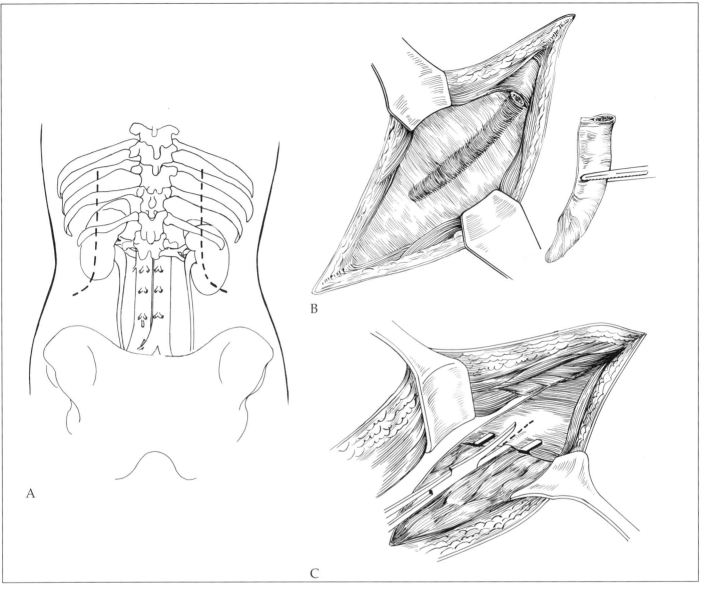

Fig. 12-8. A. J-shaped incision over the lower ribs. B. Subperiosteal resection of the twelfth rib. C. The diaphragmatic attachment to the periosteum of the twelfth rib is divided, taking care not to injure the underlying pleura.

Retroperitoneal Approach to the Iliac Fossa

This incision gives exposure to the distal ureter, bladder, common iliac, hypogastric, and external iliac vessels. It is frequently used for transplantation of the kidney into the iliac fossa and for surgery on the iliac arteries. The incision extends from 2 cm above the anterosuperior iliac spine to just lateral to the symphysis pubis (Fig. 12-9A). It can be extended cephalad as far as the costal margin, if desired. The external oblique, internal oblique, and transversus abdominis muscle and transversalis fascia are divided in line with the skin incision. The external and internal inguinal rings are not seen, as they lie distal to the lower edge of the incision. On entering the retroperitoneal area, the retroperitoneal fat and peritoneum are bluntly dissected upward and medially and maintained there by retractors. This incision gives excellent exposure of the iliac fossa (Fig. 12-9B). Closure of the various layers is accomplished by either absorbable or nonabsorbable, continuous or interrupted, sutures on each muscular and fascial layer. If the peritoneum is inadvertently opened during the exposure, it should be closed immediately.

Thoracoabdominal Incision

The incision provides excellent exposure by converting the pleural and peritoneal cavities into a single space. This incision, appropriately placed on the right or left, is indicated for lesions of the lower esophagus or cardia of the stomach, or both, for

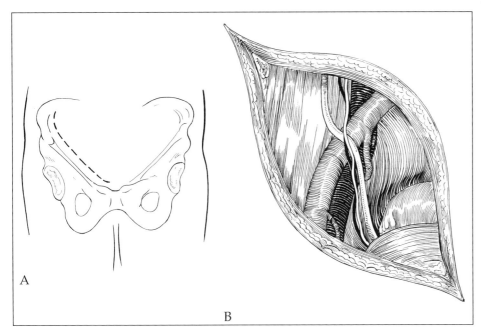

Fig. 12-9. A. Skin incision. B. The peritoneum is retracted medially and upward to expose the iliac vessels, ureter, and bladder.

some resections of the right lobe of the liver, for some portacaval shunts, for large adherent spleens, and for other large upper abdominal masses, mostly involving the kidneys or adrenals. Abdominal aortic aneurysms that extend above the renal vessels can be exposed by a long, combined incision that extends into the lower abdomen, but a retroperitoneal approach is preferred. When an operation can be safely accomplished via an abdominal approach, this is preferable, as it is associated with less morbidity than the thoracoabdominal incision. Pain from division of the costal arch or from an injury to an intercostal nerve is among the problems that should be avoided, if possible.

The patient is placed in the "corkscrew" position. The thorax is placed in the lateral position while the abdomen is tilted about 45 degrees to the horizontal by means of sandbags (Fig. 12-10A). This position allows maximal access to both the abdomen and the thoracic cavity. In patients with carcinoma of the lower esophagus or of the stomach, it may be advisable to complete the abdominal part of the incision first to determine resectability before extending the incision into the chest. Preferably, a subcostal upper abdominal incision is used, which continues directly into the thoracic part of the incision. Alternatively,

a midline or left paramedian incision is used, and then its upper end is angled obliquely into the eighth intercostal space. It is not necessary to resect a rib, as the intercostal approach gives satisfactory exposure and has less morbidity than rib resection. The eighth intercostal space is easily identified, as it lies immediately below the inferior angle of the scapula.

Once the abdomen is opened, the thoracic incision is deepened through the latissimus dorsi, serratus anterior, and external oblique muscles. The intercostal muscles of the eighth interspace are incised to open the pleural cavity, after which the costal margin is divided. A short segment of costal cartilage should be removed, as this facilitates later closure of the chest. A self-retaining chest retractor is inserted and slowly opened to widely separate the intercostal space (see Fig. 12-10B). The diaphragm is split radially with ligation and division of phrenic vessels. The diaphragmatic incision is usually made in the direction of the esophageal hiatus (see Fig. 12-10C), but it can be directed further posteriorly for operations on the kidney or adrenal gland. If the contemplated operation does not require an incision down to the esophageal hiatus, the diaphragm should be divided in a semicircular manner about 2 to 3 cm from its attachment to

the chest wall (Fig. 12-10D). This leaves only a small area of permanently paralyzed diaphragm. After completion of the operative procedure, a chest tube to drain the pleural cavity is brought out through a separate stab incision. The diaphragm is then repaired with nonabsorbable sutures. Paracostal sutures are passed around the ribs, and the costal arch is stabilized by passing one or two heavy sutures through the divided cartilaginous ends of the ribs with a strong cutting-edged needle. This is followed by closure of the chest muscles in layers with chromic catgut, polyglycolic acid, or polypropylene. The abdominal wall is then repaired in layers.

Repair of Abdominal Incisions

I prefer to close a midline incision with two No. 1 continuous polypropylene sutures starting at either end (see Figs. 12-2D, E). Because of the bulky knot that occurs I make every effort to bury it. Wide bites must be taken, a minimum of a centimeter from the wound edge, and placed at approximately 1-cm intervals, incorporating all layers of the abdominal wall, except for skin and subcutaneous fat. The skin is then closed with a continuous No. 5-0 nylon suture or with interrupted sutures or staples.

It is not necessary to close the peritoneum, particularly in severely distended individuals, in whom it may tear easily. Studies have shown that laparotomy wounds heal just as well whether or not the peritoneum is closed.

One should always avoid bringing drains or ostomies out of the main abdominal incision, as they tend to weaken it and predispose to infection.

I never use tension sutures through all the layers of the abdominal wall, as they are painful and many leave ugly scars. Furthermore, there is no evidence that they reduce the risk of dehiscence or of incisional hernia. In difficult abdominal closures, I use several widely spaced, buried interrupted sutures to reinforce the closure, which is done with a continuous suture. In cases of abdominal dehiscence, I prefer to close the abdomen with deep bites of buried figure-of-8 sutures. The skin and subcutaneous tissues are left open in all cases in which sepsis is encountered. If such a

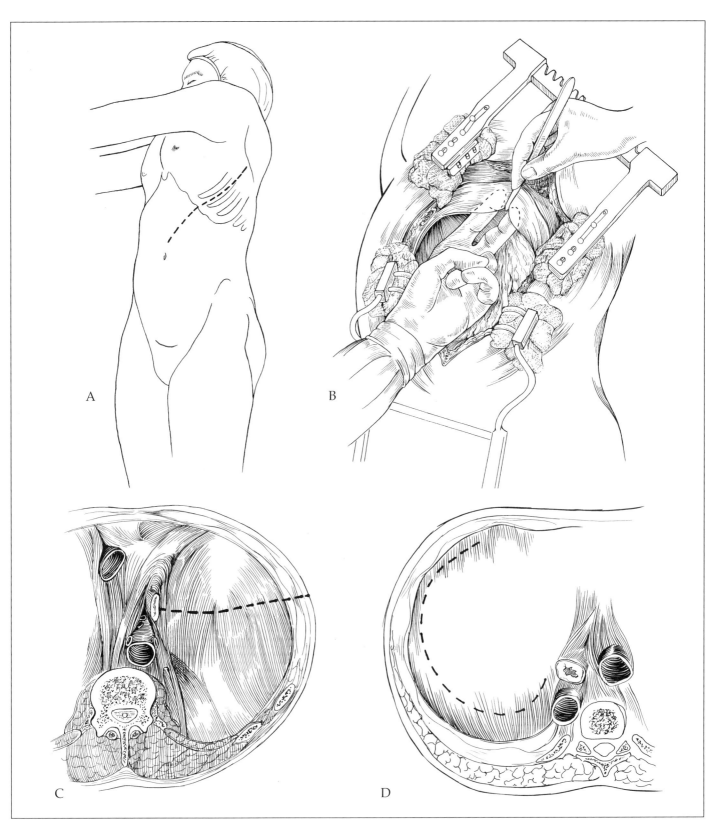

Fig. 12-10. A. Shows patient placed in the "corkscrew" position and the thoracoabdominal skin incision. B. A self-retaining retractor is placed to open the eighth intercostal space. The abdominal muscles have been divided in the line of the skin incision and the peritoneal cavity is being opened. C. Radial incision of the diaphragm extending to the esophageal hiatus. D. Semicircular incision of diaphragm. This preserves phrenic innervation to most of the diaphragm.

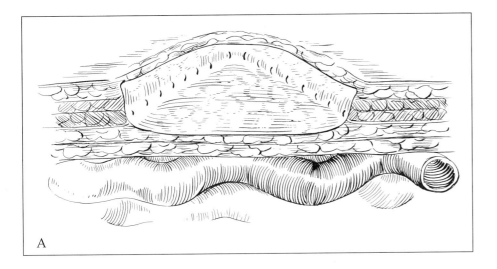

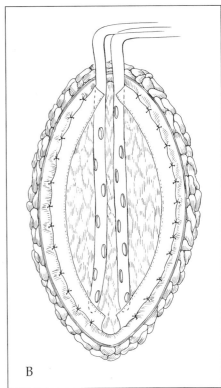

Fig. 12-11. A. Prosthetic mesh sewn to edges of linea alba. The omentum is interposed between the prosthesis and the intestines. B. Suction drains placed anterior to mesh to remove exudate.

wound appears to be clean a few days later, the skin edges are coapted either with sutures, or preferably, with Steri-Strips.

I prefer a two-layer closure of the divided deeper structures in Kocher's incision, closing the posterior rectus sheath and peritoneum with a continuous suture (see Fig. 12-4C) and the anterior rectus sheath with a separate suture. For McBurney's incisions, I prefer to close each layer, including the peritoneum, separately, using long-acting absorbable sutures, such as polydioxanone (PDS), polygalactic acid (Vicryl), or polyglycolic acid (Dexon).

In patients in whom repeat laparotomies are likely to be necessary, for example, for pancreatic sepsis, experience has shown that repeated opening and suture of an incision often leads to fascial necrosis and necrotizing infection. For these cases I prefer to place a prosthesis such as Marlex mesh or a Silastic sheet (Fig. 12-11A). Suction drains are placed across the mesh to remove exudate during the first 48 hours (Fig. 12-11B). Re-explorations are performed through an incision in the prosthesis, permitting maintenance of abdominal wall integrity. Temporary use of a pros-

thesis is also indicated in occasional patients in whom the bowel has become grossly edematous, preventing safe closure of the abdomen using the patient's own tissues. As the edema subsides, daily pleating of the mesh can be undertaken, until it can finally be removed and delayed primary fascial closure can be performed.

In cases in which acute abdominal wall defects have occurred from trauma or necrotizing fascial infection, a multistaged repair is required. First a prosthesis is placed to retain the abdominal viscera in position. Once granulation tissue has formed, about 2 to 3 weeks later, the prosthesis is removed. Several days later a split-thickness skin graft is applied to the granulation tissue. Six to twelve months later definitive reconstruction of the incisional hernia is undertaken.

Suggested Reading

Cooper P. Abdominal Incisions and Exploration. In P Cooper (ed), *The Craft of Surgery*. Boston: Little, Brown, 1964. Pp 823–834.

Edis AJ. Posterior Adrenalectomy. In RA Malt (ed), *Surgical Techniques Illustrated: A Compara-tive Atlas*. Philadelphia: Ardmore Medical Books, 1985. Pp 682–687.

Ellis H. Abdominal Wall: Incisions and Closures. In SI Schwartz, H Ellis (eds), *Maingot's Abdominal Operations* (9th ed). Norwalk, CT: Appleton & Lange, 1989. Pp 179–193.

Ellis H, Bucknall TE, Cox PJ. Abdominal incisions and their closure. *Curr Probl Surg* 22:1, 1985.

Fabian TC, Croce MA, Pritchard FE, et al. Planned ventral hernia. Staged management for acute abdominal wall defects. *Ann Surg* 219:643, 1994.

Gardner GP, Josephs LG, Rosca M, et al. The retroperitoneal incision. An evaluation of postoperative flank "bulge." *Arch Surg* 129:753, 1994.

Greene MA, Mullins RJ, Malangoni MA, et al. Laparotomy wound closure with absorbable polyglycolic acid mesh. *Surg Gynecol Obstet* 176:213, 1993.

Hedderich GS, Wexler MJ, McLean APH, et al. The septic abdomen: Open management with Marlex mesh with a zipper. *Surgery* 99:399, 1986.

Israelson LA, Jonsson T. Closure of midline laparotomy incisions with polydioxanone and nylon: The importance of suture technique. *Br J Surg* 81:1606, 1994.

Poole GV Jr. Mechanical factors in abdominal wound closure: Prevention of fascial dehiscence. *Surgery* 97:631, 1985.

Richards PC, Balch CM, Aldrete JS. Abdominal wound closure: A randomized prospective study of 571 patients comparing continuous vs interrupted suture techniques. *Ann Surg* 197:238, 1983.

Shepard AD, Scott GR, Mackey WC, et al. Retroperitoneal approach to high risk abdominal aortic aneurysms. *Arch Surg* 121:444, 1986.

Weichert RF III, Drapanas T. Abdominal Wall and Peritoneum. In PE Nora (ed), *Operative Surgery. Principles and Techniques.* Philadelphia: Lea & Febiger, 1974. Pp 343–377.

Williams GM, Ricotta J, Zinner M, et al. The extended retroperitoneal approach for treatment of extensive atherosclerosis of the aorta and renal vessels. *Surgery* 88:846, 1980.

Zollinger RM Jr, Zollinger RM. *Atlas of Surgical Operations* (7th ed). New York: McGraw-Hill, 1993. Pp 22–29.

EDITOR'S COMMENT

Abdominal wall incisions remain one of the more controversial issues in abdominal surgery, with one's training and experience largely determining the choice of direction in making the incision, as well as the technique to be employed in closing the incision. Any incision is useless if it does not provide optimal exposure to the organ(s) upon which the operation must be carried out, but there are many areas, especially in the central abdomen, where the incision can and should be tailored to the patient's body habitus, the nature of the disease process (clean vs septic), and the patient's nutritional status. A muscle-splitting incision is always used when one expects to drain an abscess or other collection of purulent material. McBurney's incision, usually with the Rockey-Davis skin modification, has long been the standard for appendectomy, but excision of Meckel's diverticulum or localized lesions, even in the pelvis, can be dealt with through an appropriately placed muscle-splitting incision.

The transverse abdominal incision, or one of its modifications, specifically subcostal or oblique in the lower abdomen and pelvis, is embraced by some experienced surgeons whenever possible, and avoided by other, equally experienced individuals.

This issue can be resolved if one keeps in mind that the predominant direction of abdominal wall fascial fibers is essentially transverse; minimal damage is caused to these fibers when the incision follows the direction of the fibers, whereas vertical incisions transect all fascial layers of the abdominal wall throughout the entire length, and the closure of the vertical incision has the marked disadvantage of sutures being placed parallel to the fascial fibers. When the suture is tied, especially in obese patients or those with abdominal distention, there is a considerable tendency for these sutures to "tear out" or loosen because the suture is pulling "with the grain." On the other hand, when transverse incisions are closed, stitches are placed and tied "against the grain" and the very strong fascial fibers are encompassed by those sutures and have considerably greater holding power. It is noteworthy that vertical incisions have at least three to five times the incisional hernia incidence as do transverse incisions.

Doctor Penn's fine description of abdominal incisions includes Pfannenstiel's incision, which is an interesting modification of both vertical and transverse incisions. In actuality, as he accurately describes, the fascial incision is transverse through the anterior rectus sheaths, whereas the peritoneal incision is vertical. Whether there is any real advantage to the vertical peritoneal extension is difficult to say, and most general surgeons would probably prefer a transverse incision continued through all layers of the abdominal wall when performing pelvic or low abdominal surgery. In addition, the extraperitoneal approach described and frequently used for aortic or caval exposure is essentially a modification of the transverse, since much of the incision is made with separation, rather than cuttting, of fascial and muscle fibers.

The author makes an excellent point when describing re-entry into a previously operated on abdomen. If the initial incision was vertical, I vastly prefer to reoperate through a transverse or oblique incision, if that approach is compatible with the operative goal and the organ to be approached. The repair is stronger, entry into the abdomen is facilitated by having "virginal" tissue on both sides of the incision, and the closure is far more secure than the closing of a previous vertical incision. On the other hand, when reoperating a patient

who has had a transverse incision done previously, I prefer to re-enter the transverse incision, extending it 1 to 2 inches beyond the original incision at one end or the other so that the entry is through previously unviolated tissue. Under any circumstances, one must assiduously avoid a second incision parallel to a previous incision, especially if the initial incision was made within 6 to 12 months of the second operation. Hernias often occur when such parallel incisions are closer than 5 cm from each other, and the skin slough may lead to serious or necrotizing infection.

When making vertical or transverse incisions in the lower anterior abdominal wall, it is possible for the unwary surgeon to enter the bladder; this is an especially important problem in older patients, who tend to have dilated bladders. When doing a vertical incision, the anterior fascial incision can go directly to the os pubis, but the posterior incision through properitoneal fat and peritoneum should be angled laterally to avoid the midline bladder structure. Likewise, one should carefully explore the properitoneal fat, if it is abundant, with blunt dissection in order to determine that the edge of the bladder is not in the line of incision. Transverse incisions placed very low for low pelvic surgery can also cause bladder injury.

The bilateral subcostal incision has proved to be a superior operative approach to organs that lie above the umbilicus. Unless the patient is thin with a narrow costal margin, the approach to the pancreas, for example, is always best done through a long left subcostal (Kocher's) incision with a somewhat shorter right-sided extension, an "arrowhead" incision. If the pancreatic lesion is very large, it is possible to provide added exposure by a vertical midline extension upward alongside the xiphoid.

Method of closure for abdominal wall incisions provokes as much difference of opinion as does the direction of the incision, and the numerous possibilities for closure, including continuous versus interrupted sutures, one layer versus two layers, absorbable versus nonabsorbable sutures, and full-thickness or "mass" closure with intra-abdominal sepsis, remain open questions. I only use absorbable suture material in muscle-splitting incisions in which there has been pus or an acutely inflamed organ in the field, for example, appendectomy through a Rockey-Davis incision. However, new long-acting absorbable sutures, specifically PDS, have proved to be excellent suture materials for abdominal wall closure, since the duration of maintenance of tensile strength is substantially longer than with other absorbable sutures. With transverse incisions, unless pus or fecal content has been present in the operative field, I often use continuous nonabsorbable suture material, polypropylene being the most useful, and use a continuous suture on the posterior fascia and peritoneum, and either a continuous or interrupted suture on the anterior fascia, if the incision is infraumbilical. It is probably not important whether one uses continuous or interrupted sutures, unless there has been gross contamination of the wound, in which case I feel more comfortable with the interrupted suture technique. I often close both anterior and posterior fascia layers as one, but then believe it important to use interrupted, heavy (No. 0 or 1) sutures for secure closure.

In terms of wound closure, one of the most trying circumstances is when the patient has "abdominal hypertension" from sepsis, massive tissue trauma, major fluid resuscitation preoperatively and in the operating room, or excessive bowel distension, especially with edema and intestinal obstruction. The attempts to close by any conventional means are often frustrated by weakness of the tissue, especially in the elderly, and closure may be more harmful than not. It is in these circumstances that a mesh closure is particularly useful, in addition to those mentioned by the author for patients who are to be reoperated. The use of polygalactic acid (Vicryl) mesh has been a significant advance in dealing with such abdominal wall closures. The mesh can be placed precisely as described by Dr. Penn, but has the great advantage of being soft and slightly yielding, and there is no tendency for abrasion or damage to the intestinal wall from the Vicryl mesh. Likewise, if the mesh is allowed to remain in place, and the intra-abdominal sepsis is controlled, the mesh actually becomes incorporated into the granulation tissue that results, allowing closure of the wound with split-thickness skin grafts. Obviously, this mesh will be absorbed, so that a ventral hernia will inevitably result and require closure at a later point.

Overall, abdominal wall incisions that are closed and in which necrotic tissue does not remain in the abdominal wall, especially those in which intra-abdominal sepsis requires that the skin be left open (which we prefer), are expected to heal in the vast majority of instances, and hernia formation will be minimized. However, if the wound becomes infected, the sequelae inevitably include a high incidence of herniation at best, and frank wound dehiscence or evisceration at worst.

R.J.B.

13

Stapling Techniques in Operations on the Gastrointestinal Tract

Felicien M. Steichen

Mechanical sutures and stapling instruments, initially considered to be a technical curiosity, have now been accepted as an established technique equal to manually placed sutures in all types of operations on the gastrointestinal tract. Although the use of staples has changed some aspects of surgical technique that had been "consecrated" by experience and predictable results, stapling has not changed the indications for a given operative procedure to cure or palliate a well-defined pathologic condition. Similarly, staples have not altered necessary perioperative measures, designed to monitor and suport all vital functions and to achieve success for a given surgical approach. However, because stapling techniques facilitate the reconstructive phase of an operation, especially in the creation of substitute organs after a long and arduous extirpative procedure for cancer, it is possible to avoid two-stage operations, previously indicated for technical reasons. One instance would be the construction of replacement organs after total esophagectomy, gastrectomy, or colectomy.

Time-honored steps in surgical technique known to be safe, reliable, and reproducible by master surgeons and their students alike have been modified progressively by stapling techniques as these techniques passed experimental scrutiny and entered the field of expanding, creative, often original clinical applications. These modifications include everting suture lines with mucosa-to-mucosa healing, known to be safe since the work of Travers in 1812. Linear duodenal, gastric, intestinal, and bronchial closures without reinforcing or covering the staple lines are the well-established examples of this change. The only "routine" oversewing of a staple line at present takes place when the GIA staples are used on both gastric walls for the formation of a gastric tube.

Overlapping of staple lines facilitates desirable features, such as closing the open end of a functional end-to-end anastomosis and enlarging the anastomotic cross section of this anastomosis. The acceptance of overlapping staple lines has led to a wide variety of clinical applications of this new technical principle. The intersecting of staple lines, first used in the two-stage reconstruction of colorectal continuity based on the Hartmann procedure, was soon introduced by Knight and associates as a primary procedure in the same area.

The technical innovation has been expanded to operations in which the intersection of a linear staple line by a circular staple line and in fact the intersection of a circular staple line by a linear line can be used to great advantage in the overall planning and execution of a given operation. End-to-end (manual and mechanical) anastomoses may result in a modest to moderate narrowing of the anastomotic cross section. With functional end-to-end anastomosis by the GIA–TA instruments, the anastomotic cross section can be greatly enlarged depending on whether the open end of the GIA lines is closed in an O or a V shape.

The use of stapling instruments has also rendered reconstruction easier in areas of difficult access, such as above and below the clavicle, above and below the diaphragm, and deep in a narrow pelvis. In such situations the anastomosis first–resection second sequence allows one to maintain the specimen temporarily in place and to provide gentle traction in the dissection and subsequent reconstruction of visceral continuity. This approach, first described as a new concept by Welter for Billroth II gastrectomy, has been used serendipitously in other anastomotic areas.

Operations on the Esophagus

For malignant lesions of the upper and middle third of the thoracic esophagus without metastatic spread below the diaphragm, the entire thoracic esophagus and the esophagogastric junction are excised by an abdominal, transhiatal approach or through separate midline laparotomy and anterolateral right thoracotomy incisions. More recently, whenever possible, this method has been replaced by right thoracoscopic esophageal mobilization. The choice among the three approaches depends on the level of tumor staging, technical feasibility, general condition of a given patient, and aim of the operation in achieving cure or palliation. If a transhiatal route or thoracoscopic mobilization is elected, the anastomosis between the esophagus and the substitute organ takes place in the neck, whereas with a combined abdominal and open thoracic approach, the anastomosis may take place high in the right chest or in the neck. This anastomosis is easier to construct in the neck, where disruption is of a lesser consequence.

For the replacement of the entire esophagus, we prefer the reverse or isoperistaltic tube made from the greater curvature of the intact stomach. This slender tube occupies a minimal volume in the mediastinum, resembles the original esophagus anatomically and functionally, and is usually free of food and gastric juice regurgitation. Gastric tubes do not fill with air, food, and fluid in their passage through the chest, as the entirely transposed stomach often does.

Of all the available esophageal substitutes, gastric tubes are blessed by the most reliable vascular supply and they are easily advanced high up into the chest or into the neck. The reverse greater curvature tube is used for the replacement of the excised esophagus, leaving a remnant of stomach in the abdomen. The isoperistaltic greater curvature tubes (Postlethwait) without resection of either esophagus or stomach is preferred for palliative bypass of the esophagus, since this tube allows for continued drainage of the esophagus distal to the tumor into the antrum via the lesser curvature, and from there through the pylorus into the duodenum.

On rare occasions, greater length than either the reverse or full-length isoperistaltic tube can provide is required in the reconstruction of the alimentary canal, such as after a pharyngolaryngoesophagectomy for extensive cancers in the pharyngolaryngeal or cervical esophagus area. In such patients we have used the extended reverse gastric tube that includes the pylorus and most of the first portion of the duodenum. Gastroduodenal continuity is reestablished by a Billroth I gastroduodenostomy.

At times the stomach or a tube fashioned from the stomach cannot or should not be used because of a previous gastrectomy, a caustic burn of the stomach, or advanced mucosal lesions of severe gastroesophageal reflux disease in the remaining proximal esophagus to avoid direct gastric and esophageal contact. In such cases a carefully prepared colon segment from either the right or left colon or the transverse colon can provide satisfactory esophageal replacement. Staple techniques are also used to close the neck of a cervical Zenker's diverticulum or of a lower esophageal epiphrenic diverticulum.

Reversed Greater Curvature Gastric Tube for Esophageal Replacement

The vascular supply to the gastroepiploic arcade is based on the left gastroepiploic vessels (Fig. 13-1A). A splenectomy is

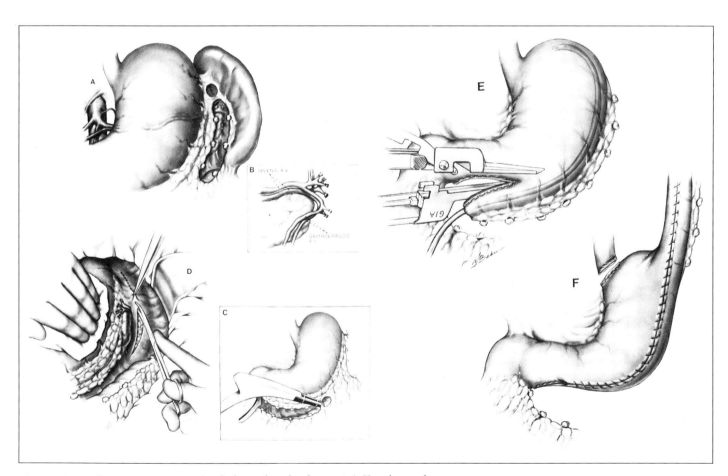

Fig. 13-1. Reversed greater curvature gastric tube for esophageal replacement. A. Vascular supply. B. Ligation of splenic vessels. C. Ligation and division of gastrocolic omentum. D. Mobilization of pancreas. E. Bougie in place to guide the stapler. F. Completed reversed tube. (From Steichen FM. The creation of autologous substitute organs. Am J Surg 134:659, 1977.)

always indicated to facilitate mobility of the gastric tube and to improve arterial blood flow and venous drainage.

In favorable situations, the dissection of the esophagus takes place through a transhiatal or thoracoscopic approach. In patients with tumors invading the entire esophageal wall or extending beyond it, the dissection is accomplished through an anterolateral right thoracotomy. The original esophagus is then pulled upward through the previously performed neck incision and the attached gastric tube follows the esophagus into the posterior mediastinum and the base of the neck. Great care is taken to keep the vascular arcades on the left side of the patient, so that the long GIA staple line ascends with a gentle curve from left to right. After transection of the cervical esophagus, the proximal anastomosis between the gastric tube and the esophagus is hand sewn.

After complete mobilization of the spleen, the splenic vessels are ligated close to the hilus and splenic capsule to preserve the left gastroepiploic artery, vein, and arcade (Fig. 13-1B). The short gastric vessels supplying the fundus of the stomach are also preserved.

The gastrocolic omentum is serially ligated and divided peripheral to the gastroepiploic arcade (Fig. 13-1C). A ''bare'' space separating the left and right gastroepiploic arcades is often encountered at the level of the mid-greater curvature. However, intramural anastomoses and vascular connections are of sufficient size to ensure blood flow throughout the entire greater curvature tube even after the right gastroepiploic artery has been tied and transected.

At this point, the stomach is retracted forward, and the peritoneal attachments to the left and deep to the tail of the pancreas are incised (Fig. 13-1D). The tail of the pancreas together with the splenic vessels and the posterior wall of the stomach are then elevated from left to right to the level of the aorta. This maneuver increases the mobility of the junction of the gastric tube with the remainder of the body of the stomach.

Through a small incision at a right angle to the long axis of the greater curvature and 2 to 3 cm proximal to the pylorus, a No. 38 French bougie is passed along the greater curvature and kept in place to serve as a guide for serial applications of the GIA instrument (Fig. 13-1E).

The reversed greater curvature tube is accomplished by five to six applications of the GIA instrument. The staple lines are oversewn (the only ''routine'' exception to the general rule) as a precaution to reinforce the short-limbed GIA staples placed on the double thickness of the gastric wall. The esophagogastric junction is transected between two applications of the TA 55 instrument.

The reversed tube (Fig. 13-1F) is then attached to the abdominal end of the previously dissected and liberated esophagus and pulled up into the mediastinum and the neck, as the liberated esophagus is removed through the neck incision.

Isoperistaltic Greater Curvature Tube for Esophageal Replacement After Esophagogastrectomy

After mobilization of the middle and lower thoracic esophagus as well as of the gastroesophageal junction, the gastroepiploid arcade is prepared (see Fig. 13-1C), based this time on the right gastroepiploic vessels. The final specimen is composed of the esophagus, the entire lesser curvature, and the fundus of the stomach (Fig. 13-2A).

The distal transection of the specimen and the construction of the isoperistaltic greater curvature tube are performed simultaneously by serial applications of the GIA instrument (Fig. 13-2B). In patients with cancer of the gastroesophageal junction, a large segment of the proximal stomach is excised; therefore, only a short gastric tube is feasible. This tube reaches comfortably into the apex of the right chest cavity.

If the tumor is in the lower third of the esophagus, less proximal stomach need be excised and a longer and broader isoperistaltic tube is possible, comprising most or all of the greater curvature up to and including the fundus. This type of tube can be anastomosed to the esophagus at the apex of the chest cavity, but it also reaches comfortably into the base of the neck, like the reversed gastric tube in Fig. 13-1.

A Kocher maneuver is then performed, as is a pyloromyotomy or pyloroplasty. Through a transverse gastrotomy in the body of the remaining isoperistaltic tube, the EEA instrument is advanced without the anvil. The central rod is pushed through the proximal tip of the gastric tube and a pursestring suture is placed around the central rod. The anvil is now attached to the central rod, and the entire EEA instrument is used to advance the gastric tube from the abdomen through the enlarged hiatus into the right chest (Fig. 13-2C). A pursestring suture is applied to the esophageal circumference.

The anvil is advanced into the esophageal lumen, the pursestring is tied, and the end-to-end anastomosis is performed between the esophagus and gastric tube (Fig. 13-2D).

After removal of the EEA instrument, the anastomotic doughnuts and the anastomosis itself are examined for completeness. If possible, the anastomosis is wrapped by excess greater omentum. The EEA introduction site, located below the diaphragm, is used for a gastrostomy if possible. The longitudinal pyloroplasty incision is closed transversely with a TA-55 staple line (Fig. 13-2E).

Operations on the Lower Esophagus and the Gastroesophageal Junction

Operations at and around the gastroesophageal junction require special consideration for anatomic and physiologic reasons. Because a tumor-free segment of proximal stomach in operations for malignant disease is needed, esophagogastric resections have to include most or all of the lesser curvature with the corresponding lymph nodes, all the lymphatic drainage of the celiac area as well as the tail of the pancreas and the hilus of the spleen, often including those two organs in the resection. If the operation is indicated in the treatment and prevention of a physiologic disturbance such as gastroesophageal reflux and its complications, direct contact between esophageal and gastric mucosa should be avoided.

We favor esophageal and proximal gastric resection that includes all the lesser curvature of the stomach and the corresponding lymphatic drainage for all pa-

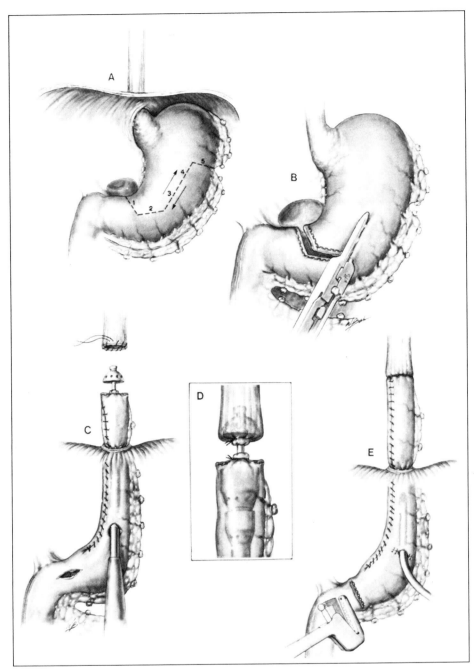

Fig. 13-2. Isoperistaltic greater curvature tube for esophageal replacement after esophagogastrectomy. A. Outline of specimen. B. Transection of specimen and construction of tube. C. Gastric tube being advanced through the hiatus into the right chest. D. Body of EEA instrument in the gastric tube and anvil in the esophagus just before anastomosis is made. E. Completed isoperistaltic tube. (From Ravitch MM, Steichen FM. Principles and Practice of Surgical Stapling. Chicago: Year Book, 1987.)

vature tube such as is illustrated in Fig. 13-2. In patients with carcinoma of the lower esophagus, a relatively smaller portion of proximal stomach must be resected to allow the construction of a greater curvature tube involving most of the curvature, which then comfortably reaches into the neck if necessary. This method allows the surgeon the choice to proceed with the esophageal dissection either through a transhiatal approach or through a separate right anterolateral thoracotomy, in which case the anastomosis can be accomplished high in the apex of the right chest.

In patients with cancers at the gastroesophageal junction or in the proximal stomach, a relatively larger portion of stomach should be resected, making only a shorter isoperistaltic gastric tube available for reconstruction. This tube always reaches comfortably into the upper right hemithorax. For patients with extensive proximal gastric cancers or multiple cancers, we prefer total gastrectomy and replacement of the stomach with a jejunal reservoir.

For patients suffering from gastroesophageal reflux without stricture or shortening of the esophagus, we perform a standard Nissen procedure through an abdominal approach. If the reflux is complicated by a stricture that can be dilated pre- and intraoperatively and the esophagus is shortened, we perform a Collis gastroplasty followed by a Nissen fundoplication usually performed through a left lower thoracic approach. However, in elderly patients, who often have long-standing esophageal reflux and repeated pulmonary aspirations with resultant fibrosis and diminished pulmonary function, a thoracic approach would represent an intolerable burden on the respiratory and cardiovascular systems. In such patients, who often have a critical need for help, the Collis–Nissen procedure can be performed through a laparotomy with the help of stapling instruments using the intersection of circular and linear staple lines.

Finally, if continued gastroesophageal reflux has led to a tight fibrous stenosis that cannot be dilated in a patient in whom the gastroesophageal complex has been destroyed over the years, interposition of a segment of transverse colon is our preferred operation. With the use of the colon, the esophageal mucosa is most effectively separated and protected from regurgitation and reflux of gastric acid juice and

tients with carcinoma of the lower esophagus, the gastroesophageal junction, and the proximal stomach. Resection of the tail of the pancreas and of the spleen may be added to this operation if lymph nodes in these areas are found to contain tumor on frozen section or are suspicious. These organs should be removed based on the judgment of the operating surgeon.

Continuity between the esophagus and the residual stomach is established by the construction of an isoperistaltic greater cur-

bile. Although the colonic mucosa in this new position is not entirely resistant to the effects of contact with acid and biliary secretions, ulcerations of the colon occur much less frequently than if a jejunal bypass had been used, especially if stasis within the stomach is alleviated by a satisfactory pyloric drainage procedure.

Abdominal Collis–Nissen Operation for Gastroesophageal Reflux with Stricture and Shortening of the Esophagus

The esophageal stricture is dilated pre- and intraoperatively (Fig. 13-3A). If the stricture cannot be dilated, a colonic interposition is indicated (see Fig. 13-4).

Approximately 5 to 6 cm below the angle of His and somewhat to the left of a line prolonging the angle of His inferiorly, stab wounds surrounded by pursestring sutures are made in the anterior and posterior walls of the stomach. These wounds are large enough only to accept the central rod of the EEA-21 or EEA-25 instrument (Fig. 13-3B).

The central rod of the circular EEA instrument is passed through the stab wounds; the pursestring sutures are tightened; and the anvil is fastened to the central rod behind the stomach. The stapler is activated (Fig. 13-3C), and a buttonhole is made in the anterior and posterior gastric walls.

Through the stapled gastric buttonhole the GIA instrument is placed upward, holding both gastric walls within its arms in a line extending from the buttonhole to the left of the angle of His (Fig. 13-3D). In patients with a shortened esophagus, the gastroesophageal junction is contained in the lower mediastinum, so that the slender arms of the instrument can be advanced up into the mediastinum.

After the GIA instrument is activated, the Collis gastric tube is formed and separated from the remaining fundus (Fig. 13-3E). The GIA suture lines both on the tube and on the fundic flap are enforced with a running suture of absorbable material.

The fundic flap is wrapped around the gastric tube and sutured to the left of it

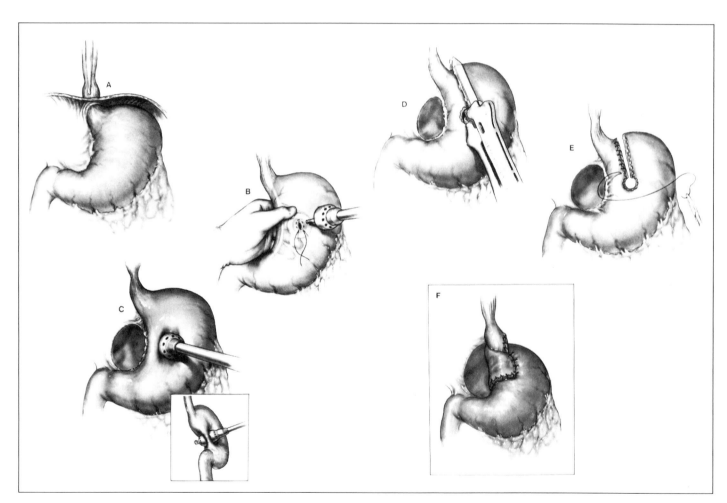

Fig. 13-3. Abdominal Collis–Nissen operation for gastroesophageal reflux with stricture and shortening of the esophagus. A. Dilation of esophageal stricture. B. Stab wounds in the gastric wall. C. Stapler in the stomach making a buttonhole. D. Position of the GIA stapler. E. Collis gastric tube. F. Fundic flap wrapped around gastric tube. (From Steichen FM. Abdominal approach to the Collis gastroplasty and Nissen fundoplication. Surg Gynecol Obstet 162:272, 1986. By permission of Surgery, Gynecology & Obstetrics.)

onto the gastric body, forming the new fundus (Fig. 13-3F). A complete fundoplication of the gastroplasty tube is thus obtained.

Coloplasty for Replacement of the Gastroesophageal Junction and the Entire Esophagus

Colonic interposition using the transverse colon is usually chosen to replace the distal esophagus and the gastroesophageal junction after excision of benign strictures. The transverse colon is based on the middle colic vessels, and the marginal vessels are ligated and transected at both the hepatic and splenic flexures. The transverse colon segment is then delineated by stapling and dividing the intestine at or near the flexures with the GIA instrument (Fig. 13-4A). The length of transverse colon obtained for the interposition should vary with the distance required to bridge the gap between the esophagus and proximal stomach without tension. The transverse colon is used in an isoperistaltic manner.

Alternatively, and depending on the vascular anatomy, a segment of distal transverse colon with the splenic flexure may be based on the left colic artery to advance the colon into the chest in an isoperistaltic manner. In this situation the middle colic vessels are ligated and transected near the superior mesenteric vessels, and the marginal arcade is ligated and divided at the level of the respective transection and stapling with the GIA instrument.

The lower esophagus and the esophagogastric junction are dissected through a separate left lateral thoracotomy. The fundus of the stomach is then doubly stapled and divided through the midline laparotomy. The colon is advanced into the posterior mediastinum alongside the esophagus, and a bayonet anastomosis is performed by inserting the GIA limbs into corresponding colic and esophageal openings (Fig. 13-4B). The site of anastomosis on the esophagus is well proximal to the area of stricture and inflammation. An even greater margin is required if the operation is done for a localized tumor.

The side-to-side anastomosis is greatly facilitated by gentle traction on the fundic portion of the specimen.

A somewhat oblique placement of the TA-55 instrument across the entire esophagus and the now common GIA opening completes the anastomosis, and the specimen is resected distal to the TA instrument (Fig. 13-4C). This technique illustrates the sequential anastomosis (anastomose-réséction intégrée) made possible by the use of the GIA–TA technique at various levels of the alimentary tract.

Alternatively, an end-to-end esophagocolostomy can be performed with the EEA instrument placed through the opened distal colonic segment, advanced from the abdomen into the chest (Fig. 13-4D). The anastomosis is a classic one with purse-string sutures on both esophageal and colonic ends.

The colonic segment is anastomosed to the stomach in an end-to-side manner by inserting the GIA instrument through a cutaway corner of the colonic staple line and through a stab wound in the stomach. After this anastomosis, the now common GIA opening is closed with the TA-55 instrument in an everted manner (Fig. 13-4E).

For replacement of the entire thoracic esophagus with an esophagocolic anastomosis in the neck, a long segment of transverse colon, usually including the splenic flexure, may be used. More often, we prefer either the ascending colon, including the hepatic flexure, or the distal transverse and descending colon. It must be understood that the vascular supply to the left side of the colon is more constant and reliable than the marginal arcades to the right side of the colon. This advantage is counterbalanced by the fact that raising the ascending colon is somewhat easier technically than liberating the distal transverse and the descending colon.

The final decision as to which side to use can be made by preoperative arteriography and intraoperative examination of the vascular arcades and continuity of marginal vessels between the territories of the right, middle, and left colic arteries. The importance and patency of the inferior mesenteric artery should be established in instances in which the left colon is used in an isoperistaltic manner.

For coloplasty using the right colon, the ileocecal and right colic vessels are tied

and divided manually or with the LDS instrument after their temporary occlusion (15–20 minutes) with small vascular clamps to ascertain intraoperatively the integrity of the middle colic vessels and the continuity of the right marginal arcade with the middle colic vessels. The GIA instrument is used to transect and close the terminal ileum as well as the colon at the hepatic flexure (Fig. 13-4F). The segment for coloplasty is then advanced through a retrosternal tunnel or through the posterior mediastinum into the neck in an isoperistaltic manner. Anastomosis in the abdomen is shown in Fig. 13-4E and in the neck in Fig. 13-4H–J.

The left colon can be used in an antiperistaltic manner, basing the vascular supply on the middle colic vessels (Fig. 13-4G). In this situation a temporary (15–20 minutes) occlusion of the left colic vessels near their origin determines the safety and reliability of the vessels and marginal arcade chosen for support of this segment of the left colon. Alternatively, and if the left side of the colon is advanced into the neck in an isoperistaltic manner, the vascular supply can be based on the left colic vessels. In this situation the middle colic vessels are temporarily occluded close to their origin from the superior mesenteric artery. If the vascular supply is found to be adequate, the middle colic vessels are tied and transected at the level of the temporary occlusion, and the marginal vessels of Drummond are interrupted distal to the two branches of the left colic artery and proximal to the first branch of the inferior mesenteric artery proper.

In any event, the colon is again transected and stapled by the GIA instrument at the sites that delineate the coloplasty segment.

Regardless of the segment of colon chosen, intestinal continuity between the terminal ileum and the transverse colon or between the right and left colon is established by functional end-to-end anastomosis as in Fig. 13-10 or by EEA. The instrument is illustrated in Figure 13-11.

The colon is brought up into the neck through a retrosternal or posterior mediastinal approach and is placed alongside the cervical esophagus as shown here for the cecum.

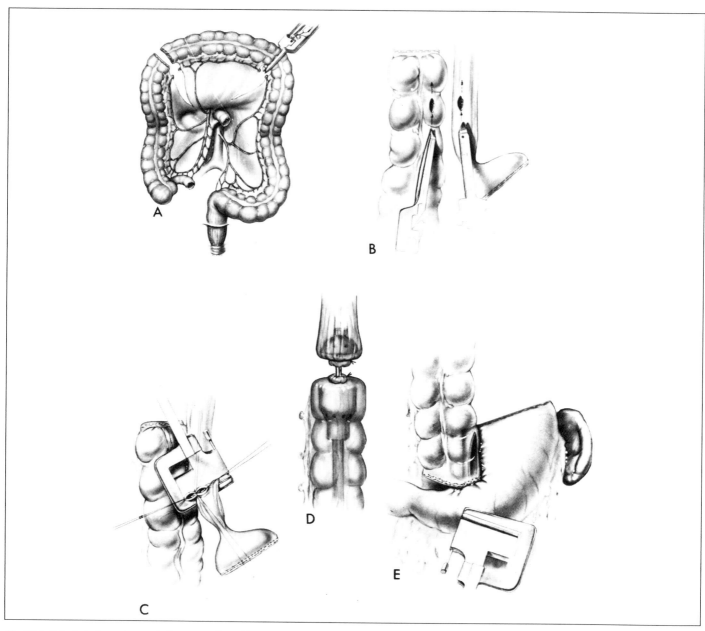

Fig. 13-4. Coloplasty for replacement of gastroesophageal junction and entire esophagus. A. Transverse colon stapled and divided. B. GIA stapler limbs in the esophageal and colic openings. C. Oblique placement of the TA-55 stapler across the esophagus and common GIA openings. D. Alternative approach using the EEA stapler. E. Completed anastomosis of colon to stomach.

Through stab wounds in the cecum (or blind end of a left colonic segment) and the cervical esophagus, the arms of the GIA instrument are placed cephalad and a side-to-side anastomosis is performed (Fig. 13-4H). Again, this maneuver is greatly facilitated by keeping gentle traction on the specimen, still in continuity with the cervical esophagus distal to the GIA anastomosis.

After the GIA instrument is withdrawn, the TA-55 stapler is used to close in a linear everting manner the entire lumen of the cervical esophagus as well as the now common GIA opening (Fig. 13-4I). The esophagus is then transected caudad to the TA instrument. This procedure results once more in a sequential anastomosis, first-resection second-technical mode.

A pyloroplasty or a pyloromyotomy is added. If the pyloroplasty is of the Heineke–Mikulicz type, the TA-55 stapler may be used to close the longitudinal incision transversely. The completed reconstruction (Fig. 13-4J) results in 13 suture lines and anastomoses, including reconstruction of intestinal continuity by functional end-to-end anastomosis.

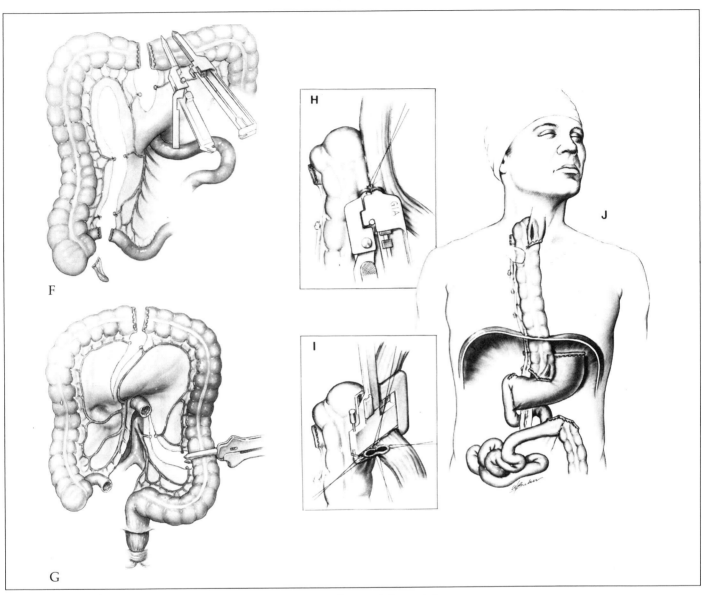

Fig. 13-4 (Continued) F. GIA stapler used to transect the colon at the hepatic flexure and the terminal ileum. G. Use of the left colon (alternate method). H. Anastomosis of esophagus to colon in the neck. I. Closure of the lumen of the cervical esophagus and the GIA opening. J. Completed reconstruction. (From Steichen FM, Ravitch MM. Stapling in Surgery. *Chicago: Year Book, 1984.)*

Operations on the Stomach and the Duodenum

Distal gastrectomy, with or without truncal vagotomy in the treatment of antral and duodenal ulcer disease, is now reserved to a limited group of patients who suffer from complications refractory to treatments with H_2-blockers. Because of this change, the previously well-established guidelines of using a Billroth I reconstruction after gastric resection for gastric ulcer and a Billroth II reconstruction after duodenal ulcer have somewhat merged, provided the gastric resection and, if needed, the vagectomy eliminate acid gastric secretions. Reconstruction of gastroduodenal or gastrojejunal continuity depends therefore on the anatomic condition of the tissues used for anastomosis. With a healthy duodenum we prefer the Billroth I reconstruction using the triple-stapled anastomosis as illustrated in Fig. 13-5, A through E. In all other instances, especially if the indication for operation was a malignant lesion of the antrum, a Billroth-II-type reconstruction with the GIA–TA instrument is used.

After total gastrectomy for extensive cancers at either end of the stomach, or for multiple cancers or a larger cancer of the body of the stomach, the preferred method

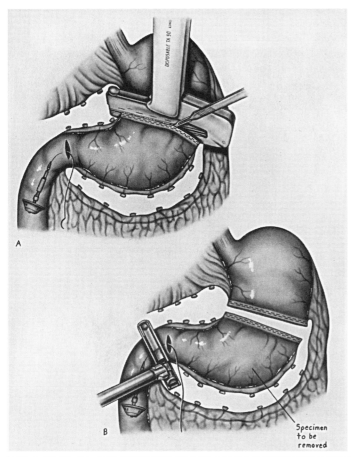

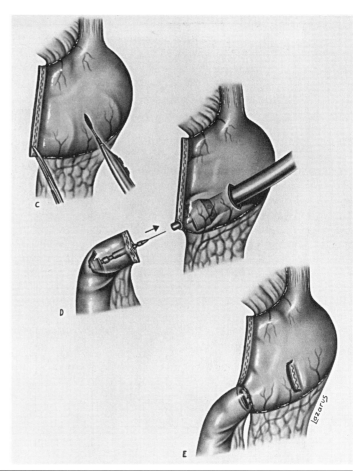

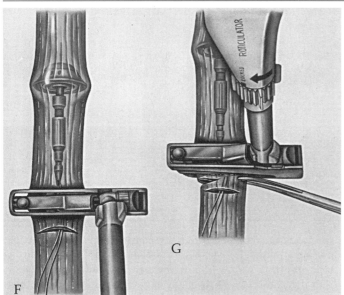

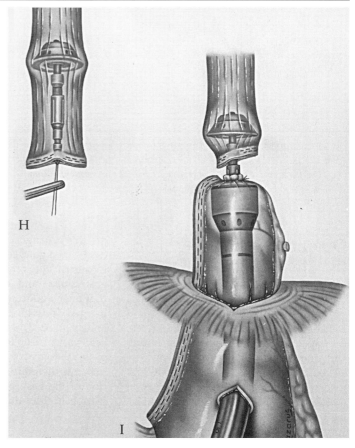

Fig. 13-5. Distal gastrectomy with Billroth I reconstruction using the triple-stapled anastomosis. A. Transection of proximal stomach between two TA-90 staple lines and placement of EEA anvil into duodenum. B. Closure of duodenum. C. Creation of openings for EEA cartridge placement. D. Mating of cartridge and anvil. E. Completed anastomosis. Gastric stab wound closed with linear stapler. Proximal gastrectomy and esophagogastrostomy using the triple-stapled anastomosis.

F. Placement of anvil and ''leash'' and esophageal closure. G. Transection of esophagus leaving the leash intact. H. Pulling the anvil shaft through esophageal closure. I. Mating of anvil and EEA cartridge prior to end-to-end esophagogastrostomy.

jejunal reservoir.* Our second choice is the Hunt–Lawrence gastric substitute.

Only in patients who could not tolerate even the relatively short additional time for the construction of a jejunal reservoir do we use a jejunal loop interposed between the esophagus and duodenum or the esophagus and the duodenojejunal segment through Roux-en-Y anastomosis.

In patients who require a gastrojejunostomy, the anastomosis should be placed on the posterior wall of the stomach close to the pylorus in a retrocolic position. If such a drainage procedure is considered a palliative measure, for example, in a patient with inoperable distal carcinoma, the stomach proximal to the tumor should be transected between two lines of TA-90 staples and a classic gastroenterostomy constructed, rather than an anterior, antecolic gastroenterostomy high on the greater curvature. This type of gastroenterostomy with the stomach in continuity results in malfunction and repeated vomiting.

Distal Gastrectomy with Billroth I Reconstruction (Using the Triple-Stapled Anastomosis)

After complete liberation of the greater and lesser curvatures, including portions of fat, omentum, and lymph node–bearing areas as required by a given lesion, the TA-90 instrument is placed twice at the selected site of transection. The specimen is separated from the remaining stomach between the two staple lines, along the inferior edge of the TA-90 stapler, used proximally after the specimen closure had been done distally first. A proximal duodenotomy is performed, and the anvil of the appropriately sized EEA instrument is ad-

*The modification of the Paulino gastric substitute (Roux-en-Y jejunal pouch) with the added digestive "round about" to facilitate the merging and mixing of food, duodeno-pancreatic juices, and bile, is the result of personal communications with the creator of this concept, Dr. Slobodan Konjovic, Department of Surgery, Klinikum Niederberg, Velbert, Germany. Dr. S. Konjovic has placed the gastric substitute between esophagus and duodenum, as an interposition graft, with excellent operative outcomes and long-term functional results in over 50 patients. Joining his original concept to Paulino's innovative modification of the Roux-en-Y principle results in a technically easier jejunal pouch construction with similar functional results. (See Fig. 13-8.)

vanced into the lumen of the duodenum. The tip of the anvil shaft is held with a heavy prolene suture ("leash"), left dangling through the middle of the duodenotomy (Fig. 13-5A).

The proximal duodenum is closed transversely, with the linear stapler distal to the duodenotomy, and the prolene leash is allowed to exit through the center of the staple line (Fig. 13-5B). Using the proximal edge of the stapler as a guide, the duodenum is transected between duodenotomy and stapler, taking great care to preserve the prolene leash.

Next a gastrotomy for the placement of the EEA cartridge is performed along the greater curvature, approximately 5 cm proximal to the gastric closure. The corner of this closure, at the greater curvature, is excised (Fig. 13-5C).

The EEA cartridge is then placed into the gastric lumen and its hollow central rod is advanced through the excised corner of the TA-90 staple line. By pulling at the prolene leash, the pointed anvil shaft is drawn through the duodenal staple line and the flat surface of the anvil is held against the inside of the duodenal closure. Anvil shaft and cartridge rod are mated after removal of the prolene leash (Fig. 13-5D).

End-to-end circular anastomosis is performed through two staple lines.

With the anastomosis accomplished, the EEA instrument is removed. The gastric stab wound is closed in an everting manner with the TA-55 stapler (Fig. 13-5E).

Proximal Gastrectomy and Esophogogastrostomy (Using the Triple-Stapled Anastomosis)

In patients requiring a distal resection of the esophagus and partial, proximal gastrectomy, the triple-stapled technique can be used. This technique allows the entire operation to take place through an abdominal approach, with a safe, relatively high anastomosis in the posterior mediastinum.

After dissection and liberation of the future specimen, a transverse esophagotomy is performed, at a safe proximal distance from the lesion. The anvil and shaft held

by a prolene leash are advanced through the esophageal opening into the proximal lumen of the esophagus. The esophagus is closed, distal to the tip of the anvil shaft and proximal to the esophagotomy. The prolene leash is let out through the center of this TA-55 closure (Fig. 13-5F).

By using the roticulator, it is possible to advance the instrument into the mediastinum and then elevate its shaft to provide better visibility. The esophagus is transected along the distal edge of the TA-55 roticulator, by leaving the prolene leash intact (Fig. 13-5G).

Next, the pointed tip of the anvil rod is drawn through the staple line by pulling on the prolene leash (Fig. 13-5H).

The specimen is resected in the abdomen after closure of the stomach with the TA-90 stapler at the elected distal site of transection. With the EEA cartridge placed inside the stomach through an appropriate stab wound, the remaining distal stomach is elongated along the greater curvature, as it is carried by the EEA instrument into the lower mediastinum, to meet the anvil. The anvil shaft and hollow cartridge rod are mated and anastomosis is performed as in Fig. 13-5E. The linear staple lines are slightly rotated in opposing directions to avoid their direct overlapping (Fig. 13-5I).

Distal Gastrectomy and Billroth II Reconstruction

The omental vessels are stapled and divided with the ligating, dividing stapler (LDS) instrument (Fig. 13-6A). With each application, this instrument fires two staples and divides the tissue between them. The extent to which omentum, fat, and node-bearing tissue is removed depends on the type of tumor spread and local metastatic involvement.

After the segment of stomach to be removed is liberated completely, the duodenum is closed with a TA-55 instrument and transected between this instrument and a Payr clamp. Similarly, the proximal stomach is closed with a TA-90 instrument and is transected between it and a long Payr clamp (Fig. 13-6B).

A gastroenterostomy is performed on the posterior wall of the stomach. Through a

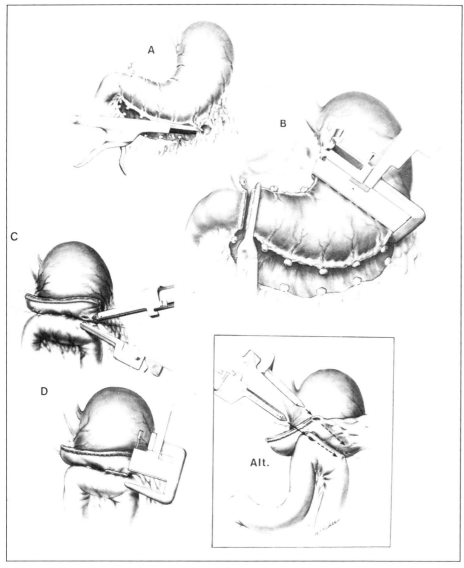

Fig. 13-6. Distal gastrectomy and Billroth II reconstruction. A. Omental vessels stapled and divided with LDS instrument. B. Stomach being transected and closed with TA-90 stapler proximally and TA-55 distally. C. Gastroenterostomy with GIA stapler. D. Closure of GIA orifice with TA stapler. Inset: Alternative method of anastomosis.

Posterior Retrocolic Gastroenterostomy

The posterior wall of the stomach close to the pylorus is drawn through an avascular rent in the mesocolon (Fig. 13-7A).

The edges of the rent in the transverse mesocolon are sutured to the stomach. The stomach and proximal loop of jejunum, usually 8 to 10 cm beyond the ligament of Treitz, are held together with stay sutures. The forks of the GIA stapler are placed through stab wounds made in the posterior wall of the stomach and in the antimesenteric wall of the jejunum (Fig. 13-7B). The instrument is activated and a side-to-side anastomosis performed. After the GIA instrument has been removed, the anastomosis is inspected to ensure hemostasis. Occasional bleeders are sutured or cauterized.

The edges of the now single GIA opening are closed with the TA instrument, and the excess tissue beyond the TA jaws is excised (Fig. 13-7C).

Jejunal Reservoir as Gastric Substitute After Total Gastrectomy

After total gastrectomy we leave the lumen of the esophageal end open and close the duodenal stump with an everting linear staple line. The jejunum is then transected and closed on both sides with the GIA instrument, approximately 25 cm distal to the ligament of Treitz.

The distal jejunal end is brought up to the esophagus and the continuity of the alimentary tract is reestablished using the EEA instrument placed through the opened end of the distal jejunal loop. The segment of distal jejunum to the left of the projected anastomosis measures approximately 15 cm. To accomplish this anastomosis, a pursestring suture is placed in an over-and-over configuration at the esophageal end. The EEA instrument is advanced into the lumen of the curved jejunal loop without the anvil, and the central rod is brought out through a stab wound in the antimesenteric vortex of the jejunum, approximately 15 cm beyond its open end. A pursestring suture is placed around the central rod. The anvil is advanced into the esophageal lumen and the previously placed pursestring suture is

stab wound at the greater curvature, about 2 cm proximal to the gastric closure, and stab wound in the antimesenteric wall of the proximal jejunum, a side-to-side anastomosis is performed with the GIA instrument parallel to the gastric staple line. After the GIA instrument is removed, the anastomotic staple lines are inspected for bleeding. An occasional pumping vessel may be clamped and ligated or may be treated by thermocautery.

After the GIA instrument has been removed and the anastomosis inspected, the

now common GIA opening is closed in a V shape as shown in Fig. 13-10.

Alternatively, the axis of the gastroenterostomy can be placed along the greater curvature of the stomach, through the excised corner of the gastric staple line at the greater curvature (Fig. 13-6, inset). In this anastomotic technique, again, the common GIA staple line is closed with the TA instrument (Fig. 13-6D) in a V shape after inspection and hemostasis, if necessary, have been accomplished.

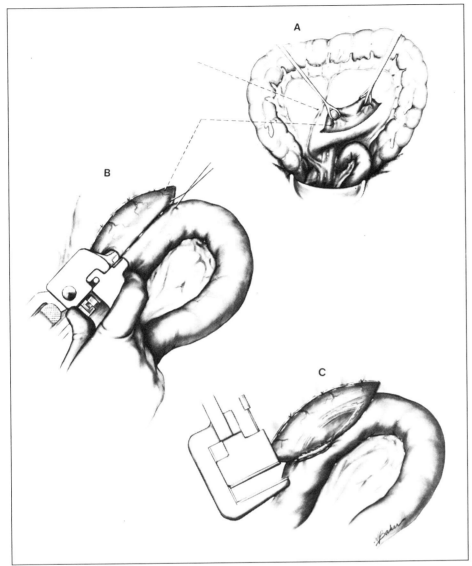

Fig. 13-7. Posterior retrocolic gastroenterostomy. A. Gastric wall brought through rent in mesocolon. B. Forks of GIA stapler through posterior wall of stomach and antimesenteric wall of jejunum. C. Edges of GIA opening closed with TA stapler. (From Ravitch MM, Steichen FM. Technics of staple suturing in the gastrointestinal tract. Ann Surg 175:815, 1972.)

tied. The anvil shaft and cartridge rod are mated, the instrument is closed, and anastomosis performed (Fig. 13-8A). Alternatively, the technique shown in Fig. 13-5F–I, can be used.

After anastomosis, the open end of the redundant jejunal loop is closed with a linear stapler, and the excess tissue beyond this closure is excised (Fig. 13-8B).

A jejunal collar, as described by H. W. Schreiber, is then performed around the esophagojejunostomy to serve a reinforcement and antireflux function. To avoid obstruction at the level of the plication and tension with narrowing of the anastomosis, various configurations have to be tried before the first suture is placed. After a satisfactory shape of the collar has been formed, the first suture is placed from left to center to right, so as to place the collar closure in front of the anastomosis and avoid acute kinking of the jejunal lumen to the left of the esophagojejunostomy. In practical terms this means that the first bite is taken into the upper border of the encircling jejunal loop and sufficiently to the left of the esophagus and the end-to-side anastomosis, in order to avoid acute angulation at this level. The second bite is taken into the anterior aspect of the esophageal wall, 1 to 2 cm above the anastomosis. The third bite is taken into the anterior wall of the upper border of the jejunal loop closure (Fig. 13-8C).

After this first, critical suture has been placed and tied, the collar is closed anteriorly with interrupted sutures that extend from the left, plicated segment of jejunum to the right, closed end of jejunum, by invaginating this closure. Furthermore, the collar is anchored superiorly to the anterior esophageal wall and inferiorly to the descending, distal jejunum (not shown in the drawing) with individual sutures (Fig. 13-8D).

Next the Roux-en-Y principle as described by Paulino, enhanced by Konjovic's concept of slowing the passage of foodstuffs and extending their exposure to duodeno-pancreatic-biliary secretions, is used to create a jejunal pouch. Twenty cm of the duodenojejunal segment is placed in an antiperistaltic fashion alongside the distal jejunum, starting at 45 cm caudad to the esophagojejunostomy (Fig. 13-8E).

Two pouches are then created, one proximally and one distally, by anastomosing both ends of the duodenojejunal segment to the apposed loop of distal jejunum with the GIA-60 in a side-to-side manner (Fig. 13-8F).

The segments of proximal and distal jejunum between the two pouches are left intact. In this fashion the result is a proximal 6 cm jejunal pouch, with transit into two separate 8-cm jejunal segments, followed by a second caudad jejunal pouch (Fig. 13-8G).

The GIA introduction sites are closed transversely with the TA-55 roticulator (Fig. 13-8H), proximally and distally.

The passage of foodstuffs and mixture with digestive upper intestinal juices are enhanced by the circulation and recirculation of food and digestive secretions. This "brassage" has been clearly demonstrated by timed barium meals and tagged food particles (Fig. 13-8I).

Our preferred mode of anastomosis within the peritoneal cavity is a functional end-to-end anastomosis rather than an end-to-end anastomosis with an EEA instrument, for which a second intestinal opening is re-

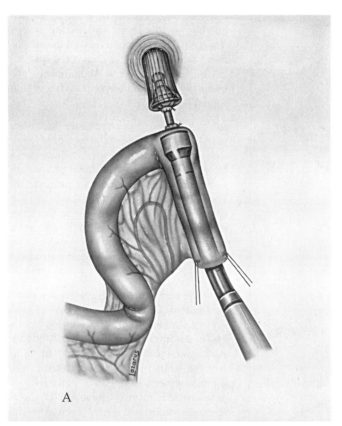

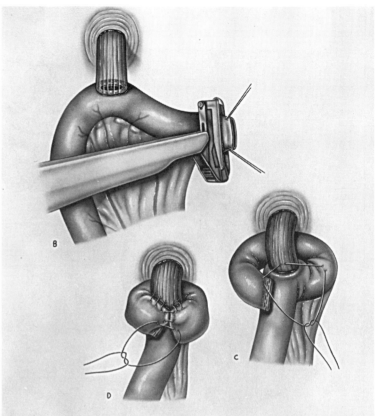

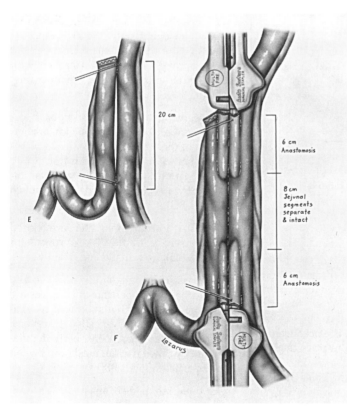

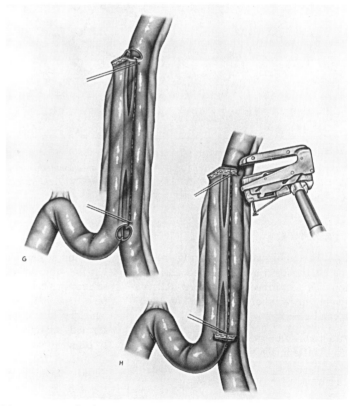

Fig. 13-8. Paulino–Konjovic jejunal reservoir after total gastrectomy. A. Esophagojejunostomy to redundant loop of distal jejunum. B. Linear, transverse closure of redundant jejunum. C. Outline and tailoring of jejunal wrap. D. Completion of jejunal collar. E. Outline of antiperistaltic-isoperistaltic jejunal reservoir. F. Construction of jejunal "round about." G. Final aspect of Paulino–Konjovic reservoir. H. Transverse linear closures of GIA introduction sites.

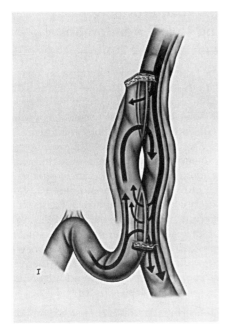

Fig. 13-8. (Continued) I. Merging, mixing, and circulation of food and digestive secretions.

quired to place the instrument within the intestinal lumen. We reserve the use of the EEA instrument for placement through a natural orifice or through an opening in the intestinal lumen made anyway in the course of the operation; this opening can then be closed with a linear stapler.

Whenever the anatomic and pathologic situation allows, the sequential anastomosis first-resection second technique of enteroenterostomy as shown in Fig. 13-9 is used.

This procedure has the advantages of closing the functional end-to-end anastomosis in a V shape and exposing the peritoneal cavity to a minimum of possible contamination from the intestine. Even when the resection of the specimen takes place first, we close the GIA opening of the functional end-to-end anastomosis in a V shape to separate the GIA linear anastomosing lines.

Enteroenterostomy

The sequential anastomosis first-resection second technique (Fig. 13-9) requires first the mobilization of the intestine to be resected, followed by a side-to-side anastomosis with a GIA instrument in healthy tissue proximal and distal to the lesion.

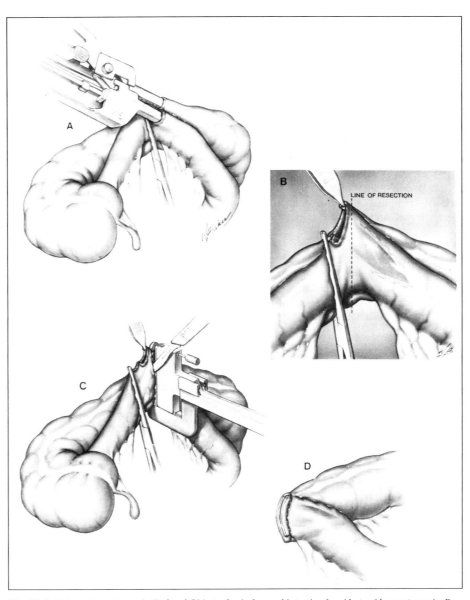

Fig. 13-9. Enteroenterostomy. A. Forks of GIA stapler in loops of intestine for side-to-side anastomosis. B. Outline of healthy tissue. C. Excision peripheral to TA stapler. D. Finished anastomosis. (From Ravitch MM, Steichen FM. In R Maingot [ed.], Abdominal Operations [7th ed.]. Norwalk, Connecticut: Appleton-Century-Crofts, 1979.)

When the linear TA stapler is placed to close the now common GIA opening and to delineate and staple the lines of resection, the excision of the specimen becomes a part of the anastomosis and is performed after the anastomosis has been accomplished. The final result is the same as the one obtained with the anatomic side-to-side and functional end-to-end anastomosis shown in Fig. 13-10.

The sequential anastomosis first-resection second technique may be done with the specimen in continuity as shown here in Fig. 13-9 or with the specimen stapled and transected at the level of resection opposite the planned, integrated anastomosis–resection. In both modes the specimen is used to exert gentle traction and to facilitate the anastomosis as shown in Figs. 13-4 and 13-9.

In an ileocolectomy, the terminal ileum and right colon are liberated from their vascular supply together with the corresponding right mesocolon. The antimesenteric borders are matched at the level of the planned anastomosis, identified by the junctions of viable and nonviable intestine. A clamp or stay suture is used on the specimen side to immobilize the intestinal loops. The GIA forks are placed through paired openings on the antimesenteric borders of the viable loops, and a side-to-side anastomosis is performed (Fig. 13-9A).

After the GIA staple lines are completed and inspected, the terminal closure of both the GIA opening and the intestinal lumina is outlined in healthy tissue (Fig. 13-9B).

The TA-55 instrument is then placed across the two loops of intestine to exclude the GIA opening, and the specimen is excised peripheral to the TA instrument (Fig. 13-9C). This technique greatly reduces the period of open intestines and hence reduces the likelihood of contamination.

The final result is a functional end-to-end anastomosis with the TA staple line holding the GIA staple lines in a V shape, which increases the anastomotic surface almost threefold.

Enteroenterostomy: Anatomic Side-to-Side and Functional End-to-End Anastomosis

The functional end-to-end enteroenterostomy is most often performed with ends of intestine that have been stapled and closed earlier in the procedure. In this technique as originally performed (Fig. 13-10A), excision of the antimesenteric corners of the intestinal closures, as in Fig. 13-10B, was followed by placement of the GIA forks, as in Fig. 13-10C. After removal of the GIA instrument, the remaining terminal opening was then closed transversely with the TA stapler, in the same axis as the original intestinal closures, resulting in an oval-shaped anastomosis with juxtaposition of GIA staple lines at the apex and bottom of the oval. With this technique some rare stenoses and even strictures were reported, presumably because of secondary healing of the live anastomotic walls from one GIA staple line across the transection to the opposite line. To prevent this phenomenon, the V configuration of the functional end-to-end anastomosis was found

to represent an ideal solution as shown in Fig. 13-10G through I. This technique is accomplished most easily if the intestinal loops are left open at the time of resection.

If the ends of intestine have been stapled and closed earlier in the procedure, the steps in Fig. 13-10B through F are helpful.

With this method, after the GIA instrument is activated and removed, the anastomosis made lies in a transverse axis that forms a 45-degree angle with the transverse axis of the two loops of intestine. Two stay sutures are then placed, one in each lateral angle of the common GIA opening. By pulling the stay sutures apart, this opening is straightened into the same transverse axis as the intestinal loops. This results in a moderate V formation of the GIA staple lines, separating both lines at the terminal, temporary opening of the anastomosis (Fig. 13-10D).

The common GIA opening is now closed transversely with the TA instrument (Fig. 13-10E), maintaining the moderate V formation.

The final result obtained with a narrow V configuration (Fig. 13-10F) increases the anastomotic surface, albeit not to the same extreme degree as the open V mode does.

Figure 13-10G through I shows the steps for anastomosis of ends of intestine not stapled earlier in the operation. In Fig. 13-10G, the GIA anastomosis has been performed through the open ends of both loops of intestines. The GIA staple lines are held apart in an open V with stay sutures. The common GIA opening, constituting the entire circumference of both loops of intestine, is then closed in a terminal manner with the transverse placement of a TA-55 instrument (Fig. 13-10H). Again, care is taken to incorporate the entire circumference of this opening into the jaws of the TA instrument. The excess tissue is excised.

A wide V-shaped anastomosis is thus obtained (Fig. 13-10I), resulting in an almost threefold increase in anastomotic surface compared with the original, oval configuration of the functional end-to-end anastomosis. This particular mode is best used if the loops of intestine to be anastomosed are left open as shown.

Enteroenterostomy: End-to-End Anastomosis with an EEA Stapler

The functional end-to-end anastomosis with the GIA–TA technique illustrates one of the original examples of an everting staple line, healing across from one intestinal wall to the other without reinforcing or serosa-to-serosa sutures. If, however, a true end-to-end anastomosis with invagination of the intestinal ends is preferred, the EEA instrument should be used, with the knowledge that the size of the stapling instrument and hence the size of the anastomotic surface is decided by the smaller intestinal lumen if there is discrepancy in the widths of the lumina. Use of the EEA instrument necessitates an additional enterotomy and staple closure.

Pursestring sutures are placed in both ends of the intestine. This step can be achieved by an over-and-over whipstitch or by the use of a special pursestring instrument (Fig. 13-11A). An enterotomy is performed in the intestinal loop best suited technically for the placement of the EEA instrument. If there is intestinal discrepancy, the larger loop is usually preferred. The pursestring suture on the cartridge side is closed after the anvil has been separated from the cartridge by turning the wingnut of the instrument counterclockwise.

The anvil is advanced into the opposite intestinal lumen and the pursestring suture is tied. Placement of the anvil is facilitated by holding the intestinal lumen open with Allis clamps or with stay sutures (Fig. 13-11B).

The second pursestring suture is tied, and the intestinal ends containing the anvil on one side and the staple cartridge on the other are approximated by turning the wingnut of the instrument clockwise (Fig. 13-11C).

After the instrument is activated, a circular, inverting anastomosis is achieved. The anvil and cartridge are again separated from each other, and the instrument is disengaged from the anastomosis (Fig. 13-11D). This maneuver is facilitated by using a stay suture on the antimesenteric border of the anastomosis and elevating the intestinal loops so as to slip the anvil through the anastomosis with minimal trauma.

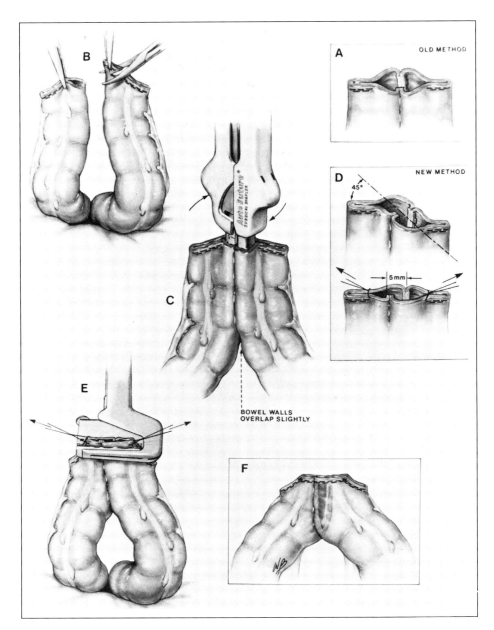

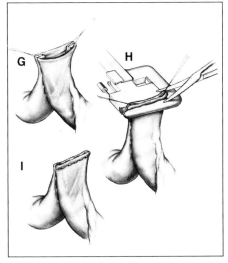

Fig. 13-10. Enteroenterostomy by anatomic side-to-side and functional end-to-end anastomoses. A. Original method. B. The antimesenteric borders of the previously stapled and closed ends of intestine are excised. C. The GIA stapler is placed with one arm into each intestinal opening. As the stapler is closed, the antimesenteric borders of the intestine are slightly rotated to form overlapping walls, which now touch each other beyond the exact antimesenteric border on one side and short of this border on the opposite side. D. New method of anastomosis. E. Closure of common GIA opening. F. Completed anastomosis in a narrow **V**. G. Staple lines of open ends of intestine held apart with stay sutures. H. Closure of ends with TA-55 stapler. I. Completed anastomosis. (From Steichen FM, Ravitch MM. Mechanical sutures in operations on the small intestine. In RL Nelson, LM Nyhus [eds.], Surgery of the Small Intestine. Norwalk, Connecticut: Appleton & Lange, 1987.)

After removal of the EEA instrument from the intestinal lumen, the placement enterotomy is closed transversely with an everting TA staple line (Fig. 13-11E). Surgeons who cannot accept everting closures may complete this step of the procedure manually with inverting sutures.

Operations on the Rectosigmoid Colon

Whereas the EEA instrument has extended the use of stapling to lower colorectal anastomoses and in fact improved the fea-

sibility and safety of these anastomoses, reconstruction of intestinal continuity between the proximal colon and the midrectum can also be easily achieved with a bayonet anastomosis using GIA–TA staplers. This technique was used in this area long before the EEA stapler became available. If the lesion for which this operation takes place is located in the lower sigmoid colon or the high rectum, this approach permits a satisfactory reconstruction without putting a patient in a modified lithotomy position. After healing takes place, this anastomosis straightens out, and endoscopic examinations reveal only minimal, if any, cul-de-sacs.

For lower anterior resection with an anastomosis deep in the pelvis, we have come to rely entirely on the use of an EEA instrument introduced through the anus with the patient in the lithotomy position.

Since most often it is difficult to place a pursestring suture on the rectal stump (unless it is done through an anterior perineal incision as advocated by Welter), and since there is often a discrepancy between the size of the rectal lumen and the size of the lumen of the proximal colon, we now routinely make a linear closure of the rectal stump with a TA-55 roticulator. By using the triple TA–EEA technique of intersec-

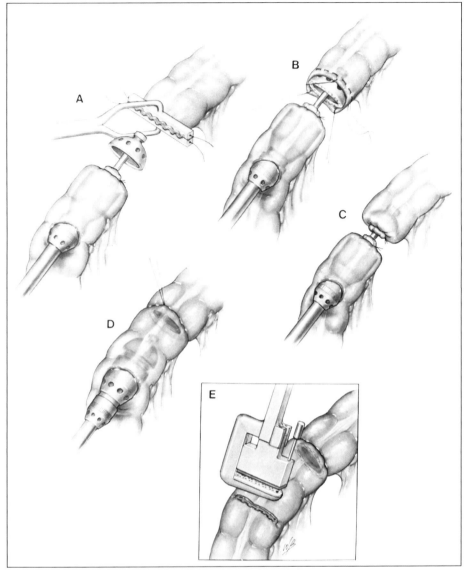

Fig. 13-11. Enteroenterostomy by end-to-end anastomosis with an EEA stapler. EEA stapler through one end of intestine and special pursestring on the other end. B. Anvil advanced into opposite end of intestine. C. Both pursestrings tied and ends of intestine approximated. D. Stapler being disengaged from anastomosis. E. Transverse everting closure of placement enterotomy. (From Steichen FM, Ravitch MM. Stapling in Surgery. *Chicago: Year Book, 1984.*)

tion of two linear closures by the circular EEA instrument for colorectal anastomosis, we safely extend the lower margins of resection and anastomosis in patients with carcinoma of the midrectum.

Rectosigmoid Resection and GIA Functional End-to-End Anastomosis

This technique is particularly suited for an anastomosis of the descending colon to the upper rectum. The operation is performed entirely through an intraperitoneal approach.

The intestine is divided at the appropriate proximal level (Fig. 13-12A), using either a GIA instrument or the edge of the TA instrument. For most procedures of this type, the splenic flexure must be mobilized for the descending colon to reach the proximal rectum. Proximal and distal levels of transection are selected on the basis of pathologic findings and viability of the bowel ends after interruption of the vascular supply to the specimen (Fig. 13-12A).

Following rectosigmoid resection, the rectal stump and descending colon are joined side-by-side in a shotgun fashion. The antimesocolic corners of the stapled-closed bowel ends are excised, and the linear anastomosing instrument is placed with one arm into each bowel lumen. The instrument halves are matched, and the stapling-cutting mechanism is activated, creating a linear side-to-side anastomosis corresponding to the length of the arms of the chosen instrument (Fig. 13-12B).

After removal of the instrument, the staple lines are examined, deficiencies are corrected, and the now single bowel opening, held up by stay sutures, is closed transversely with a linear stapler. Excess tissue is excised using the free edge of the instrument as a guide (Fig. 13-12C).

For this linear closure, the staple lines are held apart at the open end of the anastomosis, and the resulting functional end-to-end configuration ensures a V-shape that can be narrow or wide according to the surgeon's preference. As the anastomosis heals, it will espouse the tubular shape of the host bowel ends, without narrowing or kinking, making follow-up flexible and rigid endoscopy possible (Fig. 13-12D).

Anterior Resection and Low Colorectal Anastomosis (Triple-Staple Technique)

After complete dissection as indicated by the pathologic findings, the rectum is closed temporarily below the tumor and irrigated transanally with povidone iodine solution or distilled water (Fig. 13-13A).

The rectum is closed permanently distal to the temporary closure and transected on the specimen side, using the edge of the stapler as a guide. Proximally the sigmoid is disconnected from the specimen and its lumen is closed temporarily with a soft bowel clamp. It will be reopened at the transection site to place the anvil and rod inside the colon (Fig. 13-13B).

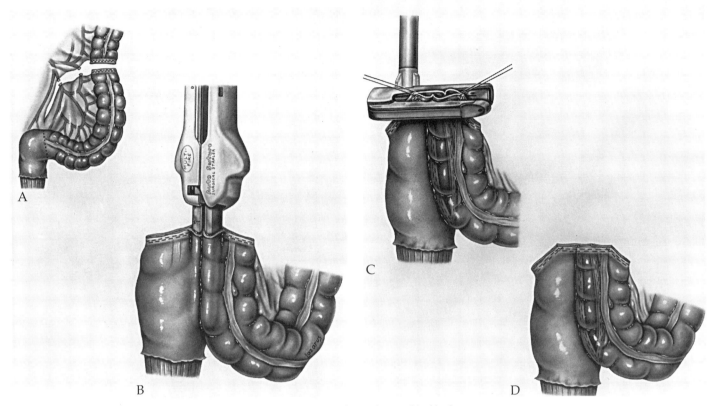

Fig. 13-12. *Rectosigmoid resection and functional end-to-end anastomosis. A. The specimen and its blood supply are separated from remaining blood supply. B. Rectum and colon are joined in shotgun fashion, and side-to-side GIA anastomosis is performed. C. GIA opening closed transversely with linear stapler. D. Final, functional end-to-end shape of anastomosis (From Steichen FM et al.* Perspectives in Colon and Rectal Surgery. *St. Louis: Quality Medical Publishers, 1992.)*

Before introducing the anvil, intraluminal debris or small fecal remnants are aspirated, and, if necessary, the bowel is carefully irrigated with povidone iodine solution. Gloves, irrigation-suction catheters, and protective drapes are changed, and the anvil and rod are advanced entirely into the bowel lumen (Fig. 13-13C).

After placing the entire anvil-rod assembly into the sigmoid colon, the open lumen is closed in the direction of the mesocolon with the linear stapler (Fig. 13-13D). A small incision is made with the scissors into the middle portion of this linear closure. The rod of the anvil is advanced through this opening (Fig. 13-13E).

The CEEA instrument, carrying the cartridge and the recessed trocar, is introduced transanally into the rectal stump. The trocar is advanced through the previously incised center of the transverse rectal staple line and removed as the hollow

shaft of the cartridge emerges beyond the linear rectal closure. The anvil rod and hollow instrument shaft are mated (Fig. 13-13F).

The instrument is closed, compressing the transverse linear rectal closure and the anterior-posterior linear colon closure between anvil and cartridge. As the instrument handles are compressed, the circular anastomosing staple rows intersect with the linear staple lines, which are transected by the circular knife, one at a time, at 12, 3, 6, and 9 o'clock (Fig. 13-13G).

Following completion of the anastomosis, the circular instrument is disengaged, and the anastomotic integrity is examined by the usual means. The triple-staple technique is useful if there is disparity in caliber between the rectum and proximal colon. For a bulky rectum, only a flat anastomotic surface corresponding to the colon

circumference is used with this approach (Fig. 13-12H).

Double Staple Technique in Colorectal Anastomosis (Second-Stage Hartmann Procedure)

With the availability of the EEA instrument, it soon became apparent that reestablishment of intestinal continuity after a Hartmann procedure was greatly facilitated. What was at times a difficult dissection of the rectal stump was made easy by introducing the EEA cartridge without the anvil into the rectum and pushing against the blind end of the rectal pouch to facilitate identification from above. At this point only enough rectal pouch need be liberated from surrounding structures, especially the bladder, to permit the central rod to be advanced through a stab wound

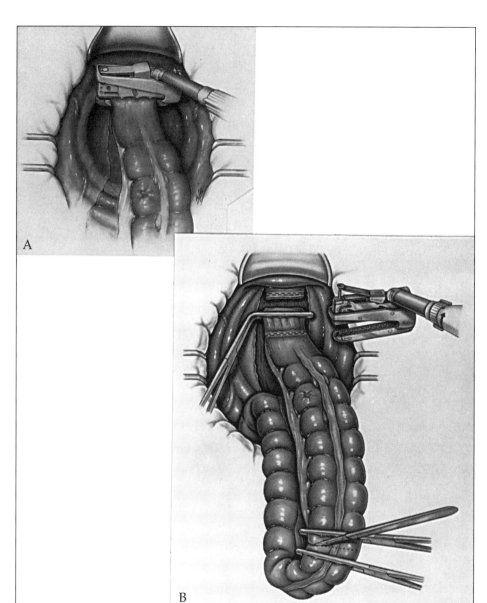

Fig. 13-13. Anterior resection and triple-stapled colorectal anastomosis. A. Preliminary closure of rectum and transanal irrigation and cleaning. B. Definitive closure of rectal stump. Proximal transection of sigmoid colon. C. Placement of anvil into proximal sigmoid colon. D. Linear staple closure of sigmoid colon. E. Incision into center of linear sigmoid closure. F. Mating of anvil shaft and cartridge hollow rod. G. End-to-end anastomosis. H. Final aspect of colorectal anastomosis (From Steichen FM, et al. Perspectives in Colon and Rectal Surgery. *St. Louis: Quality, Medical Publishers, 1992.)*

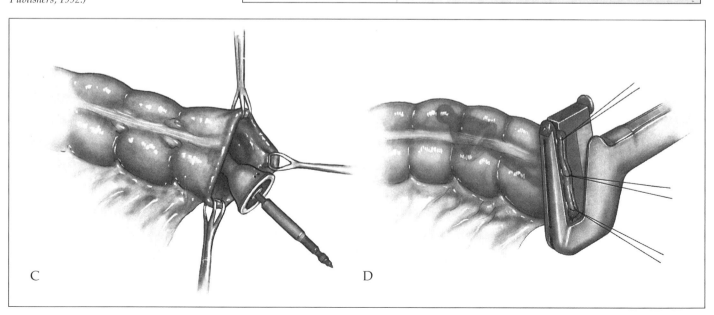

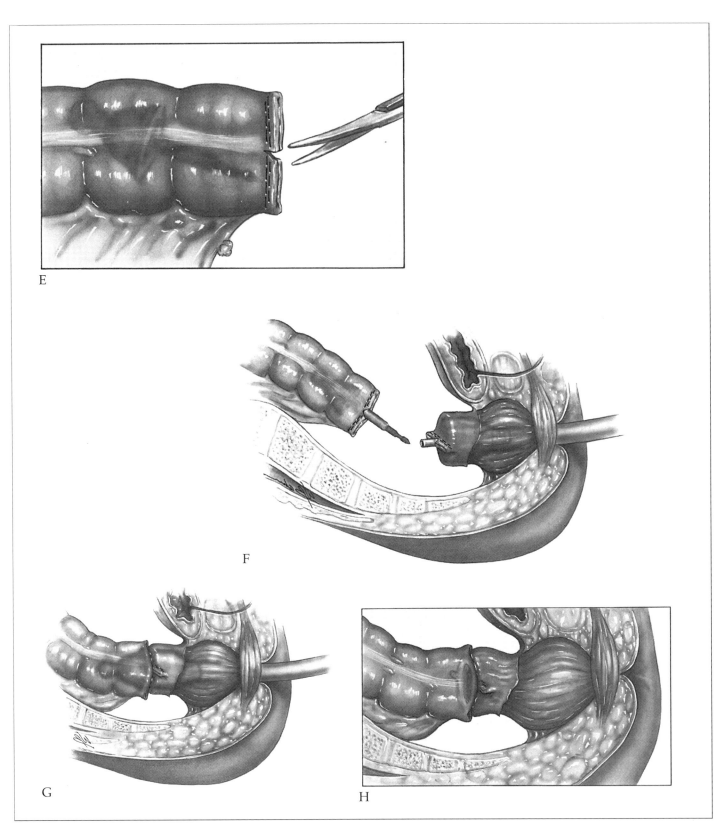

E

F

G

H

Fig. 13-13. (Continued)

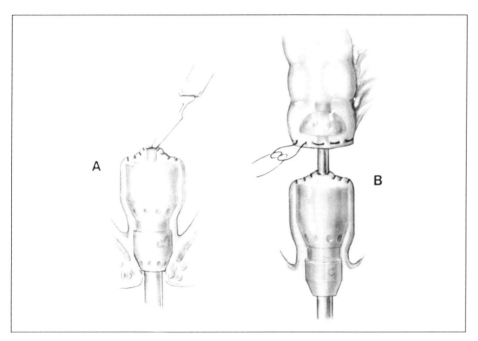

Fig. 13-14. Double-staple technique in colorectal anastomosis (second-stage Hartmann procedure). A. EEA stapler cartridge in rectum. B. Anvil in proximal colon. Anvil and cartridge are joined and anastomosis is performed.

in the fibrous tissue surrounding the previous rectal closure (Fig. 13-14A) and to prevent the inclusion of any other organs in the future anastomosis.

After the central rod has been advanced, the anvil is placed into the pursestringed proximal colon, and the anvil shaft and hollow cartridge rod are joined (Fig. 13-14B). The pursestring suture is tied and the anastomosis performed as in Fig. 13-13F through H. This technique can also be performed primarily, in one stage, as first demonstrated by Knight and Griffen.

Bricker–Johnston Sigmoid Colon Graft for Repair of Postradiation Rectovaginal Fistula and Stricture

In women with radical hysterectomy for cancer, followed by radiation, who have developed a rectovaginal fistula, but are cured of their disease, the Bricker–Johnston sigmoid colon graft will give an anatomically reconstructed ano-rectal-vaginal area with normal evacuation and control of bowel movements. The surgical task is formidable and can be satisfactorily accomplished in three stages, with the use of staplers. The operative procedure represents a showcase for various concepts made possible by mechanical sutures: eversion, overlapping, crossing, and transection of various staple lines by others.

The rectovaginal fistula is shown approximately 4 cm above the anterior anal mucocutaneous junction (Fig. 13-15A).

A Hartmann procedure is performed first at the level of the junction between descending colon and sigmoid colon. The closed sigmoid end is tagged to the undersurface of the abdominal wall, along the inferior edge of the descending end–colostomy, to make identification and dissection of the colostomy and blind sigmoid loop easier during the second-stage procedure. The mesosigmoid is incised to the division of the inferior mesenteric artery, separating left colic and sigmoid vessels, to prepare for the second stage and improve the individual vascular supply to each colon segment (Fig. 13-15B, C).

The second stage is accomplished as soon as the perineum is clean and dry. The Hartmann procedure is taken down and the descending end–colostomy is separated from the blind sigmoid closure and the descending mesocolon from the mesosigmoid along the incision performed during the first stage. Great care is taken to preserve the sigmoid vessels on the side of the future pedicle graft. The descending colon is now supplied and drained by the left colic, and marginal vessels of Drummond.

The length of sigmoid colon necessary to reach the fistula is measured. The apex of the arch formed by the posterior rectosigmoid and the anterior onlay graft of mid and proximal sigmoid colon is incised through its antemesosigmoid wall for the late placement of the CEEA instrument, without anvil (Fig. 13-15D).

The posterior vaginal wall is elevated from the rectum and incised above and on both sides of the fistula. The vaginal cuff is pulled anteriorly and the fibrous rim of the fistula—consisting of attenuated vaginal and rectal walls—is exposed. No pursestring suture is necessary (Fig. 13-15E).

The central rod of the CEEA instrument is advanced through the linear closure of the proximal sigmoid colon, and the instrument is used to guide the sigmoid graft deep into the pelvis, anterior to the rectum. The hollow central rod of the CEEA is then advanced through the fistula into the rectum and is joined by the shaft of the anvil, advanced transanally. The transanal advancement of the anvil is facilitated by holding the anus open with short retractors and avoiding the inclusion of anal mucosa into the anastomosis as the anvil is closed against the cartridge. Similarly, at this point care is taken to position the lower rim of the anvil at or above the pectinate line and to avoid taking a bite out of the sphincter muscles anteriorly. The instrument is closed and activated, anastomosing the proximal sigmoid circumference to the anterior soft wall of the rectum. The fibrous scarred rim of the fistula consisting of posterior vaginal and anterior rectal walls, is excised while this anastomosis takes place (Fig. 13-15F).

The CEEA 28 or 31 instrument is then advanced through the anus and rectum to accomplish circular anastomosis between the apex of the arch formed by the rectum and turned down sigmoid colon and the completely mobilized descending colon above this (Fig. 13-15G).

Finally, a long side-to-side rectosigmoid-ostomy is achieved with a GIA 80 or 90 instrument, by placing one arm of the instrument transanally into the rectum and the other arm through the anus and previous fistula (now end-to-end rectosigmoidostomy), into the sigmoid colon. Care is taken to rotate the sigmoid to displace the mesosigmoid to the left and keep it out of the anastomosis. This linear side-to-side anastomosis opens the rectosigmoid spur and creates a large rectal pouch (Fig. 13-15F).

The posterior vaginal opening is sutured to the anterior sigmoid wall to cover the lower CEEA rectosigmoid anastomosis (previous fistula site) as best possible. A portion of the posterior vaginal wall will by necessity be formed by the lower most semi-circumference of this anastomosis, but healing has not been impaired (Fig. 13-15I, K).

To protect the repair, the proximal descending colon is provided with a side-to-side colocolostomy whose open common stoma is brought out onto the skin for temporary diverson as a vented colocolostomy. The abdomen is then closed (Fig. 13-15J).

The third stage is accomplished approximately 6 to 12 weeks later. Under local anesthesia and on an ambulatory basis, the narrowed stoma of the colocolostomy is dissected free down to the peritoneum. The double barrel stoma is then closed extraperitoneally with a linear stapler and the skin approximated over this staple line (Fig. 13-15L–O).

Suggested Readings

Gavriliu D. Aspects of esophageal surgery. *Curr Prob Surg* 1975.

Knight CD, Griffen FD. Techniques of low rectal reconstruction. *Curr Prob Surg* 20:391, 1984.

Kremer K, et al. Chirurgische Operations lehre: ösophagus, magen, duodenum. New York: G. Thieme Verlag, Stuttgart, 1987.

Paulino F, Roselli A. Carcinoma of the stomach. *Curr Prob Surg* 12, 1973.

Ravitch MM, Steichen FM. *Principles and Practice of Surgical Stapling.* Chicago: Year Book, 1987.

Steichen FM. Varieties of stapled anastomoses of the esophagus. *Surg Clin North Am* 64:481, 1984.

Steichen FM, Ravitch MM. *Stapling in Surgery.* Chicago: Year Book, 1984.

Steichen FM, Iraci JC, Loubeau JM. Varieties of stapled transabdominal colorectal anastomoses. *Perspect Colon Rectal Surg* 5:65, 1992.

Steichen FM, Loubeau JM, Iraci JC. Varieties of stapled transanal colorectal anastomoses. *Perspect Colon Rectal Surg* 5:199, 1992.

Steichen FM, et al. Bricker–Johnston sigmoid colon graft for repair of postradiation rectovaginal fistula and strictures performed with mechanical sutures. *Dis Colon Rectum* 35:599, 1992.

Ulrich B. Klammernahttechnik. *Chir Gastroenterologie.* Hameln: Verlag, 1986.

Ulrich B, Winter J. Klammernahttechnik *Thorax und Abdomen.* Stuttgart: Verlag, 1986.

Welter R, Patel J. *Chirurgie Mécanique Digestive.* Paris: Masson, 1985.

EDITOR'S COMMENT

Doctor Steichen has been one of the most important individuals to bring forth stapling techniques as the standard for performing operations on the gastrointestinal tract. He and Ravitch essentially adapted European technology, primarily developed in the former Soviet Union, to introduce the entire concept of stapling the gastrointestinal tract. The technological advances in this almost universally adopted modification of hand-sewn anastomoses has been nothing less than spectacular in the past 15 years and has extended to many areas outside the alimentary tract.

Even more important, new operations are based on the opportunity to join segments of intestine in almost inaccessible areas, the most impressive of which is in the mid and distal rectum, where the EEA staplers have made anastomosis to the distal and terminal rectum a standard procedure, saving patients ileostomy or colostomy on a permanent basis, and allowing the creation of various conduits and storage pouches.

Surgeons vary considerably in their faith in suture lines, and it is only fair to point out that oversewing of a staple line with permanent suture material may not be necessary in some circumstances, but adds considerable confidence in the procedure under circumstances in which the intestinal wall is extremely edematous, inflamed, thickened, or when the intestine itself is substantially dilated and perhaps thinned out, as with distal obstruction. The placing of a row of interrupted permanent sutures, or even a continuous suture line, is perhaps analogous to the "belt and suspenders" attitude that characterizes some surgeons, perhaps the ones with some innate skepticism of all mechanical devices, but certainly does not hurt the innate integrity or quality of the staple anastomosis. Oversewing the staple line of the diseased duodenum that harbors a peptic ulcer, for example, may not be necessary in Billroth II gastrectomy but does relieve the anxieties about healing that frequently exist.

Esophageal surgery has, without question, been revolutionized by the use of staplers, and almost no surgeons operate on the esophagus without using the stapler device at some stage of the resection or closure. Furthermore, as laparoscopic surgery has become more commonplace and has been extended to operations on the intestinal tract, staplers have become critically important in dealing with the mesentery, in mobilization of various segments of the upper and lower gastrointestinal tract, and in dealing with a variety of unexpected or untoward circumstances that would not be possible without the truly remarkable instruments that have been developed for laparoscopic use.

Nevertheless, there remain certain areas in which purists question the use of the stapler. Hand-sewn closure of the neck of a Zenker's diverticulum, requiring very few sutures and allowing for a precise identification of the layers of the esophagus with a hand-sewn closure, still has great attraction. Likewise, removing a Meckel's diverticulum with a broad base can certainly be done with a stapler, but in such a short procedure there is a temptation to use the hand-sewn technique, perhaps simply to be sure that it does not disappear from the armamentarium of the well-trained and well-rounded surgeon.

There has been a major departure from hand-sewn gastrointestinal anastomotic techniques in favor of what usually proves to be a faster method of reestablishing intestinal continuity. Nevertheless, mechanical instruments are occasionally subject to failure, and the surgeon may be forced to resort to hand-sewn techniques and must be trained and prepared to do so. It is always of interest to see a surgeon in training who is adept at the various applications of staplers, but who is somewhat less efficient at performing a classic hand-sewn

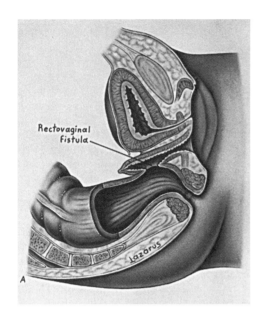

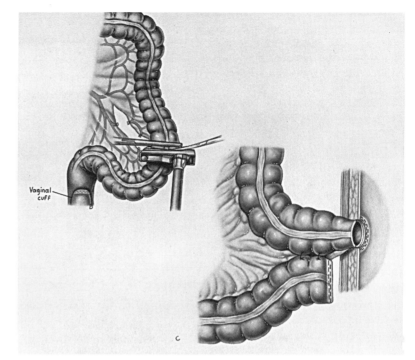

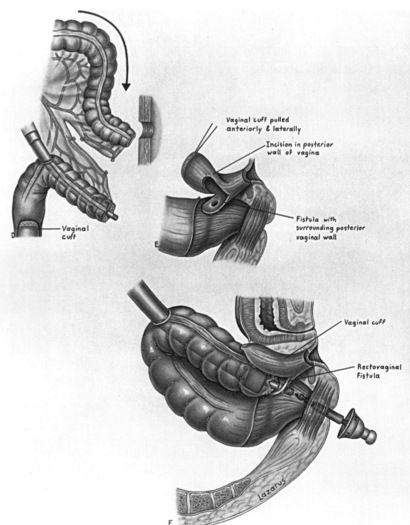

Fig. 13-15. Repair of rectovaginal fistula.
A. Rectovaginal fistula proximal to anal canal.
B, C. First stage: Hartmann procedure. D–K.
Second stage: D. Dismantling of Hartmann
procedure and preparation of sigmoid colon graft.
E. Dissection of fistula and elevation of vaginal
stump. F. End-to-end, transfistula and transanal
sigmoid-rectal anastomosis.

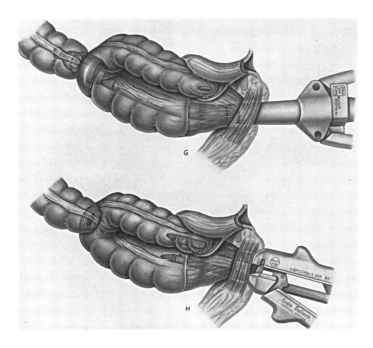

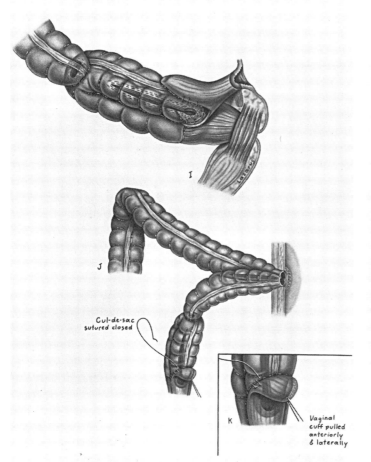

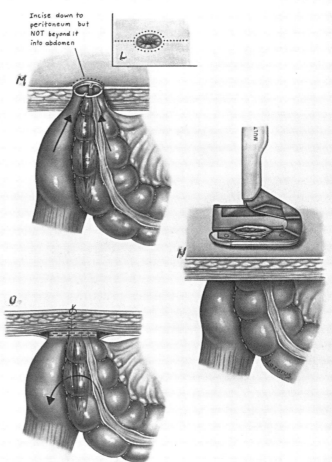

Fig. 13-15. (Continued) G. Reconstruction of continuity by colocolostomy at apex of pouch. I. Completed repair of rectovaginal fistula with sigmoid colon graft. J. Double barrel, vented colostomy proximal to repair. K. Vaginal stump sutured to colon graft. L–O. Third stage: Closure of vented, double barrel, side-to-side colocolostomy under local anesthesia (From Steichen FM et al. Dis Colon Rectum 35: 1992.)

anastomosis. For that reason, sewing a normal common bile duct to a loop of jejunum or a pancreas to an intestinal segment in complex procedures in and around the pancreatobiliary system still requires manual and judgment skills that the routine use of staplers tends to erode. For all of us who are active surgeons, in training or beyond, it is imperative that we maintain all our skills and not allow some to deteriorate in favor of adopting new skills with more initial appeal to the possible detriment of dealing with the technical challenge in the long run.

R.J.B.

14

Intraoperative Ultrasound: A Surgical Tool of Great Versatility

Junji Machi   Bernard Sigel

It is more than 15 years since high-resolution real-time B-mode ultrasound was first introduced in the operating theater as intraoperative ultrasound (IOUS). The feasibility of this imaging tool has since been demonstrated in a variety of surgical fields including general surgery, neurosurgery, and cardiovascular surgery. In spite of its numerous benefits, it is our impression that IOUS has not yet been used as effectively and widely as it could or should be. This underuse is caused by the unavailability of special equipment in the operating room, and the lack of sufficient awareness of the potential benefits and current ease of application of IOUS.

We have performed IOUS in approximately 2800 operations and have identified indications, benefits, and limitations. Our major applications of IOUS have been in hepatobiliary, pancreatic, and vascular surgery. In this chapter, we review the indications, advantages, and limits of IOUS but mostly consider technical issues. These issues are considered in terms of instrumentation, scanning techniques, scanning of specific organs, intraoperative ultrasound guidance, and laparoscopic ultrasound scanning of bile ducts.

Indications

The indications for IOUS are multiple, and we have classified them into four general categories: 1) acquisition of new information, 2) complement to or replacement for conventional operative roentgenography, 3) confirmation of successful completion of

operation, and 4) guidance of surgical procedures.

Acquisition of new information that is not obtained by preoperative studies or intraoperative exploration includes new diagnosis of diseases, localization or exclusion of previously suspected lesions, and acquisition of other anatomic information. IOUS helps to assess the extent of tumor spread (tumor staging). For example, vascular invasion and lymph node and liver metastasis of hepatobiliary and pancreatic carcinoma can be diagnosed more accurately with IOUS than by preoperative methods. IOUS has changed previously planned surgical procedures for hepatic tumors in 30 to 50 percent of operations. When used as a screening procedure, IOUS has detected occult liver metastases from colorectal carcinoma in 5 to 10 percent of operations. Precise localization of nonpalpable lesions such as hepatic malignancies, liver cysts and abscesses, intrahepatic stones, pancreatic cysts, and dilated pancreatic ducts is possible. For example, as many as 40 percent of hepatocellular carcinomas in cirrhotic livers are not palpable during operation but can be localized by IOUS. IOUS is now regarded as one of the best means to localize islet cell tumors or parathyroid tumors. In addition to diagnosing focal lesions, important anatomic structures (e. g., portal vein and common duct) can be identified prior to extensive dissection. By providing new imaging information early during operation, IOUS facilitates the selection of the most appropriate surgical operation.

IOUS is useful as a complement to or replacement for operative roentgenogram studies. In comparison with operative cholangiography during open cholecystectomy, IOUS has demonstrated equal or superior accuracy in diagnosing bile duct stones. During open biliary operations, IOUS can replace traditional operative cholangiography as a routine screening test, and cholangiography can be reserved for selective application when IOUS results are inconclusive. Laparoscopic ultrasound can completely examine the biliary tract, but further evaluation is required to fully assess its potential.

Confirmation of successful completion of the operation includes both the assessment of adequate tissue resection or calculus and foreign body extraction and discovery of technical problems. During peripheral vascular surgery, IOUS has been as accurate as operative arteriography in detecting vascular defects, such as intimal flaps, strictures, and thrombi. Therefore, IOUS can be used as a completion examination immediately after vascular reconstructions. During carotid endarterectomy, IOUS is a preferable method because the risk of operative roentgenogram contrast arteriography is avoided. For confirmation of completion of the operation, IOUS can also be used after removal of biliary or renal calculi, extraction of foreign bodies, and extirpation of tumors in solid organs (e. g., liver and brain).

Ultrasound guidance of various manipulations during operations has the advantage of real-time imaging without using ionizing radiation. Surgical procedures assisted by ultrasound guidance are intraoperative needle or probe placement and tissue dissection. IOUS–guided needle or probe placement is performed for fluid aspiration (e. g., aspiration of cysts), injection of contrast agents, catheter introduction, biopsy, and probe placement for nonresectional treatment of tumors (e. g., cryosurgery or electrocoagulation of tumors). IOUS–guided tissue dissection is performed for the purpose of incision or resection of organs and extraction of calculi or foreign bodies. IOUS guidance avoids blind procedures, and permits biopsy and resection of deep-seated nonpalpable tumors using less dissection. In addition, new surgical techniques, such as IOUS–guided systematic subsegmentectomy of the liver, have been made possible.

Advantages and Limits

Although inspection and palpation by surgeons are the most important means of directing surgical procedures, intraoperative imaging provides additional useful information. IOUS is a relatively new modality compared with intraoperative roentgenography (e. g., cholangiography), which is already established as a standard method. However, IOUS has the advantages of safety, speed, accuracy, more imaging information, wider applicability, and ability to guide procedures.

IOUS is inherently safer than contrast roentgenography because, unlike contrast roentgenography, it does not require cannulation, contrast injection, and radiation. Therefore, IOUS can be used repeatedly as necessary during the course of an operation. Once learned, the scanning technique is relatively simple, and the results of scanning are obtained immediately on real-time images. IOUS can be performed in a short period of time. For example, biliary or carotid IOUS or IOUS scanning of liver metastasis is completed within 5 minutes. Even detailed evaluation of hepatobiliary or pancreatic cancer requires about 10 minutes. IOUS usually reduces operating time when used to assist excisional operations.

IOUS is highly accurate compared with preoperative imaging studies or even with surgical exploration of deeper lesions or structures. Hepatic and endocrine tumors are more accurately detected with IOUS than with percutaneous ultrasound and computed tomography. Vascular tumor invasion (e. g., portal vein invasion by pancreatic cancer) and the size of lymph nodes is more precisely assessed. IOUS provides multiplanar images from multiple angles in real time, thus offering more imaging views than operative roentgenography. IOUS is applicable to hepatobiliary, pancreatic, endocrine, cardiovascular, neurosurgical, gastrointestinal, urological, thoracic, and gynecologic operations. IOUS has been useful in evaluating vascular anastomoses in transplants.

Color Doppler imaging (CDI), which displays blood flow in real-time color on B-mode gray scale images, has recently been introduced during operations. This modality seems to enhance the efficacy of IOUS during general and cardiovascular surgery by offering blood flow information in addition to anatomic information. Intraoperative CDI can detect and localize smaller vessels and can more promptly distinguish them from ductal structures and tissue spaces than can conventional B-mode ultrasound. During vascular surgery, CDI improves detection and evaluation of various types of vascular defects.

With rapid expansion of laparoscopic procedures, new laparoscopic ultrasound equipment has become available recently. Preliminary results have shown the feasibility of this technique, and complete examination of the bile duct can be performed in a relatively short time (<10 minutes) during laparoscopic cholecystectomy. Although technically more demanding, evaluation of the liver, pancreas, and other abdominal organs is possible with laparoscopic ultrasound. One disadvantage of laparoscopic procedures is the inability of surgeons to perform palpation of organs to assess deep-seated structures or lesions. Thus, laparoscopic ultrasound has the potential to become a valuable adjunct during laparoscopic operations, although further assessment of this modality is needed.

IOUS has certain limits and disadvantages. A limitation of IOUS, which is actually a limitation of all ultrasound imaging using hand-held transducers, is operator dependency. Just as in physical examination, ultrasound examination results are related to the operator's experience and diligence. There is a limitation in the detectability of small tumors. Tumors less than 3 to 5 mm in size cannot be delineated even with high-resolution IOUS. IOUS displays smaller fields of view than operative roentgenography. Diagnosis and localization of fistulae are limited. Special transducers that are small and customized to fit in the operative field are required for IOUS scanning. The learning process for IOUS by surgeons is relatively slow, because of unfamiliarity with performance and interpretation of ultrasound. These limitations are outweighed by the multiple advantages of IOUS. The issue of a slow learning curve will be solved by surgeons' recognition of the benefits of IOUS, which should provide sufficient motivation to acquire the needed skills.

Instrumentation

The standard intruments used for most clinical ultrasonography are a scanner, a hand-held probe containing an ultrasound transmitting and receiving transducer(s), a monitor screen, and a recorder. The basic ultrasound system used in IOUS is the small parts scanner. Small parts scanners function at higher frequencies (5–10 MHz) than body scanners. Ultrasound at higher frequencies penetrates less deeply, but provides images of greater resolution. This difference is a favorable trade-off for IOUS because penetrating the body wall is not an issue. B-mode ultrasound instruments that provide two-dimensional images in real-time or color Doppler scanners that add blood flow information to the B-mode displays are used in IOUS. With a 7.5-MHz transducer, the sound penetration depth is 6 to 8 cm. Because IOUS scanning is performed directly on the organs or target lesions, the sound penetration of this depth is usually sufficient. With high-frequency ultrasound, small lesions such as 1-mm calculi, 1- to 2-mm vascular defects, and 3- to 5-mm tumors can be delineated. Differences in these limits are related to the amount of contrast between the object of interest and the surrounding tissue or medium. For example, a 1-mm calculus is very distinct because of its extreme echogenicity and shadowing. A small arterial intimal slap is clearly detected in a hypoechogenic vascular lumen. Tumors, on the other hand, display lesser differences in the gray scale from surrounding tissue.

The essential features of IOUS probes are their size and shape. A small size probe with a flexible cable that can be manipulated in the narrow operative field is required. There are two basic shapes of IOUS probes: flat probes configured into T or I shapes and cylindrical probes (Fig. 14-1). Flat probes usually consist of a series of small transducers arranged in a linear array and incorporated in a "pad" set at the end or the side of the probe. Thus, they have a side- or end-viewing capacity. The most commonly used flat T- or I-probes are side-viewing. The span of tissue in contact with linear-array transducers is usually 3 to 6 cm. This 3- to 6-cm contact distance is displayed on the ultrasound monitor screen as the footprint of the transducer. Cylindrical probes often have flattened sides to achieve greater slimness and have an end-viewing imaging capability. Cylindrical probes produce fan-shaped sector images. Consequently, they have narrower footprints than flat probes. The flat probes with the larger footprints are particularly suitable for scanning large organs with a relatively flat surface such as the liver, pancreas, and kidney. The side-viewing flat probes are ideal for the IOUS examination of the liver because an end-viewing probe cannot be easily positioned between the liver and the diaphragm or the anterior abdominal wall. The cylindrical sector probes are especially useful for the scanning of small areas situated deeply in the operative field such as the extrahepatic biliary tract, spinal cord, and peripheral vessels.

Several manufacturers have developed laparoscopic ultrasound probes. These are 10 mm in diameter and approximately 50 cm in length, with most transducers functioning at 7.5-MHz frequency. The majority of the current probes have side-mounted transducers near the tip of a rigid shaft. Some probes are flexible, which facilitates the intracorporeal scanning of organs from various directions.

Scanning Techniques

Our purpose is to provide a brief overview of how to acquire and develop basic ultrasound scanning techniques that can be used during a surgical procedure. For more detailed information, further review of specific fields of interest is recommended. The overview of scanning techniques will consider the following: probe-image orientation, preparation and deployment of instruments, transducer placement, and scanning maneuvers.

Probe-Image Orientation

Interpretation of a two-dimensional real-time ultrasound image requires familiarity with how the position of the transducer relates to the image on the monitor screen. Transducers display images in a scan plane. First, the location of the transducer in the scan plane must be known. Usually it is either at the left-hand edge or the top of the monitor screen. A second requirement is to relate regions of interest in the scan plane to the position of the transducer in the image. The transducer must have operator eye-hand coordination in order to understand where a particular anatomic region is represented on the screen. To acquire this type of orientation, the surgeon who is not familiar with the transducer and scan display on the monitor is well advised to take a few minutes to scan with the transducer in a small basin of water. A metal instrument (e. g., hemostat) should then be placed in the water bath in front of the transducer and moved. The metal instrument is readily recognized on the monitor screen by its echogenic appearance and associated shadowing. The movement of a metal target in the scanning plane quickly enables the operator to realize how structures in the monitor image are related to the transducer.

It is helpful for a surgeon starting IOUS to practice ultrasound scanning without using operating time. This practice can be done in a simple manner by placing a surgical specimen (e. g., an excised gallbladder) or a surgical instrument in a water-filled receptacle and by scanning it from different positions and directions, while operating the ultrasound equipment and observing the monitor screen. This practice will help the surgeon learn image orientation of a target in relation to the position of the probe and interpretation of images. Practice with percutaneous ultrasound examination (e. g., scanning of the liver and gallbladder) may also be helpful. Collaboration with radiologists is important; however, we believe that surgeons should eventually perform IOUS and have radiologists function as consultants. This situation would be consistent with the precedent of having surgeons perform most intraoperative radiographic imaging (e. g., cholangiography and arteriography). In various surgical procedures, it would be particularly important for the surgeon to perform the IOUS guidance.

Preparations and Deployment of Instruments

Usually the person performing the scan should be in the surgeon's position. The monitor screen and operative field should be easily viewed with minimal change-of-gaze movement. It is important to set up instruments and place a sterile probe in the operative field before intraoperative scanning to minimize the use of operating time solely for preparation.

IOUS can be performed at any time during the operation. We usually insert the probe in a "dry field" for optimal visual placement, and then add saline for acoustic coupling. The field may have sufficient fluid accumulation already to obviate the need for saline. We almost never use coupling gel that is commonly used in surface scanning. Early in the course of the operation, IOUS is used to obtain new information, which may determine the approach or the type of procedure to be performed. For example, immediately after laparotomy for intra-abdominal malignancy, following exploratory inspection and palpation, IOUS can be conducted to evaluate the liver and lymph nodes as well as the primary lesion. IOUS at this time, which may require about 10 minutes, helps early intraoperative decision making and often decreases operating time. IOUS can be used during the surgical procedure for guidance. After finishing a procedure but prior to closure, completion IOUS examination can be performed to look for problems that still may be corrected. For example, technical misadventures in vascular reconstructions (e. g., intimal flaps) or incomplete tumor extirpation from a solid organ (e. g., brain and liver) can be recognized. Therefore, it may be useful to keep the IOUS equipment available and the probe sterile until closure so that IOUS scanning can be repeated whenever indicated.

Transducer Placement and Movement

Ultrasound scanning is a two-step process: probe placement and probe movement. Knowledge of the exact position of the transducer and how its movements are depicted on the monitor is critical to good ultrasound imaging. This importance is why we often place the probe in a dry field for visual orientation before adding saline,

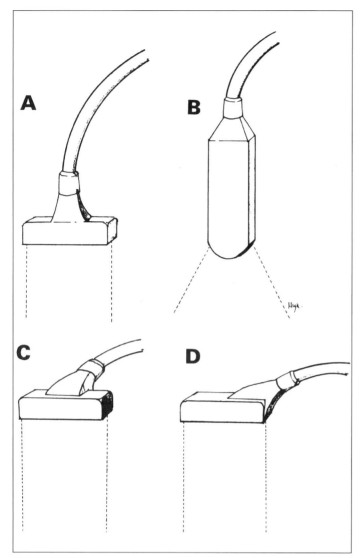

Fig. 14-1. Different types of intraoperative ultrasound probes. A. Linear-array, flat T-shaped, end-viewing. B. Sector, cylindrical, end-viewing. C. Linear array, flat T-shaped, side-viewing. D. Linear array, flat I-shaped, side-viewing. (From Machi J. Operative Ultrasonography. Tokyo: Life Science Ltd, 1987. Reproduced with permission.)

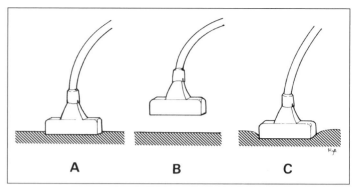

Fig. 14-2. Basic scanning positions of the probe in relation to the surface of the tissue or organ. A. Contact scanning. B. Probe-standoff scanning. C. Compression scanning. (From Machi J. Operative Ultrasonography. Tokyo: Life Science Ltd, 1987. Reproduced with permission.)

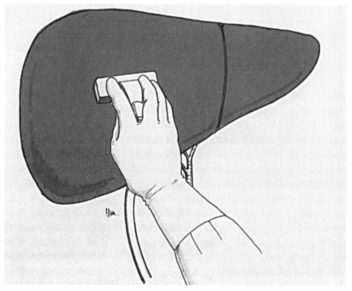

Fig. 14-3. Contact scanning of the liver using a flat T-shaped side-viewing probe. This probe is placed in contact with the anterior-superior surface of the liver. The T-shaped side-viewing probe has been most frequently used for scanning of abdominal organs including the liver and pancreas. (From Machi J. Operative Ultrasonography. Tokyo: Life Science Ltd, 1987. Reproduced with permission.)

which may obscure the probe-tissue contact. Practice prior to scanning in an operative field will enhance the surgeon's understanding of movement.

Various techniques can be performed to facilitate IOUS scanning and to obtain the best imaging information. Two basic transducer placement techniques of IOUS are contact scanning and probe-standoff scanning. In contact scanning the probe is placed in direct contact with the tissue or organ, whereas in probe-standoff scanning the probe is positioned 1 to 2 cm away from the surface of the structure (Fig. 14-2). Transducers are usually focused. The image between the transducer and the focal distance is the near field. The image beyond the focal distance is the far field. A common focal distance for a 7.5-MHz transducer is 1 to 2 cm from the transducer membrane. The sharpest images are obtained at the focal distance. We try to position the transducer to place the region of interest at the focal distance or the far field just beyond the focal zone. Because the ultrasound resolution in the near field is low, placement of the region of interest in the near field should be avoided.

The size of the target organ and the distance from the probe to the area of interest in the organ determines which scanning technique should be used. Usually, contact scanning is used for examination of the interior of the liver, kidney, or pancreas (Fig.

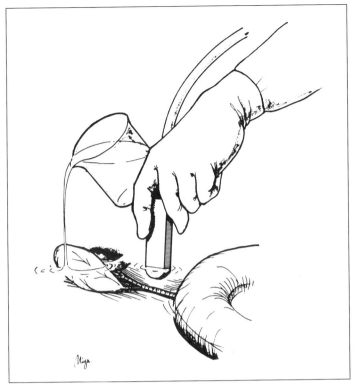

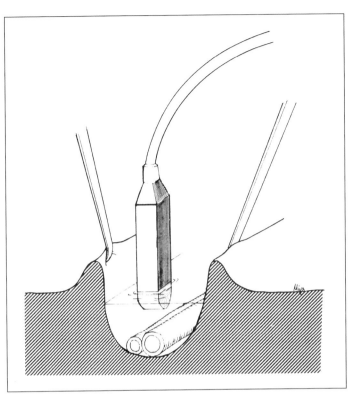

Fig. 14-4. Probe-standoff scanning of the extrahepatic bile duct using a cylindrical end-viewing probe. Note the space between the probe head and the bile duct. Saline solution is being poured to obtain acoustic coupling. (From Machi J. Operative Ultrasonography. Tokyo: Life Science Ltd, 1987. Reproduced with permission.)

Fig. 14-5. Upward retraction of skin flaps for probe-standoff to scan peripheral blood vessels. Flap retraction permits probe stand-off in superficial operative fields. (From Machi J. Operative Ultrasonography. Tokyo: Life Science Ltd, 1987. Reproduced with permission.)

14-3). However, when the surface or the superficial area of the organs needs to be examined, probe-standoff scanning should be used. For examination of relatively small structures such as the extrahepatic bile ducts and the peripheral blood vessels, probe-standoff technique is particularly important (Fig. 14-4). In probe-standoff scanning, acoustic coupling is obtained between the tissue and probe by filling the operative field with saline until the transducer surface of the probe is immersed beneath the solution (Fig. 14-4). During laparotomy, it is easy to keep saline in the abdominal cavity. When the target structures are not easily submerged (e. g., during peripheral vascular surgery), the edges of the wound can be retracted upwardly to introduce a sufficient amount of saline (Fig. 14-5). The probe-standoff with saline immersion technique is a unique IOUS method that is not commonly used in percutaneous ultrasound. This technique permits placement of the target at the appropriate focal distance and also prevents

inadvertent compression of structures by the probe. One additional useful technique is compression scanning, in which the tissue is compressed intentionally by the probe (Fig. 14-2). This technique helps to eliminate air between the transducer and the tissue. Also, air in the gastrointestinal tract lumen that overlies a region of interest can be displaced by compression. This approach is especially effective when air in the duodenum obscures the distal common bile duct. Compression is also used to distinguish arteries from veins, which are more easily compressed.

The second step of the scanning process is movement of the probe in the surgical field. For a thorough examination, the target lesion or organ should be scanned from various positions and directions in a systematic manner. In general, it is important to use longitudinal, transverse, and (at times) oblique scan paths. Scan paths are the direction of the moving transducer in relation to the longest axis of the organ or

tissue being examined. Longitudinal scanning provides scan planes parallel to the long axis of the structure being examined (e. g., body, extremity, or organ). Transverse scanning is at right angles to the long axis and provides additional information (Fig. 14-6). Oblique scanning obtains scan planes that are intermediate in position between longitudinal and transverse scan planes. For larger organs such as the liver and pancreas, combinations of longitudinal, transverse, and oblique scanning are used to systematically examine the entire organ (Figs. 14-7 and 14-8).

Scanning Maneuvers

Scanning maneuvers are the ways that a probe is manipulated during its movement. The use of different scanning maneuvers is essential for complete IOUS examination. There are three basic scanning maneuvers of the probe: lateral movement, rotation, and angulation. In lateral movement scanning, the probe slides

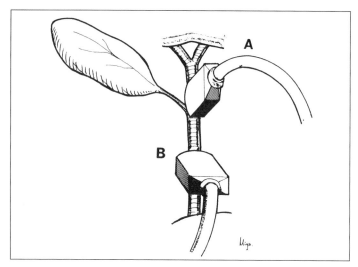

Fig. 14-6. Longitudinal and transverse scanning of the extrahepatic bile duct. A. In longitudinal scanning, the scan path is along the long axis of the bile duct. B. In transverse scanning, the scan path is at a right angle to the bile duct. (From Machi J. Operative Ultrasonography. Tokyo: Life Science Ltd, 1987. Reproduced with permission.)

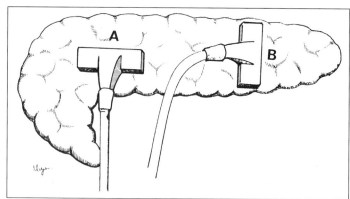

Fig. 14-8. Longitudinal and transverse scanning of the pancreas with a T-shaped side-viewing probe. A. In longitudinal scanning, the scan path is along the course of the main pancreatic duct. B. In transverse scanning, the scan path is at a right angle to the pancreatic duct. (From Machi J. Operative Ultrasonography. Tokyo: Life Science Ltd, 1987. Reproduced with permission.)

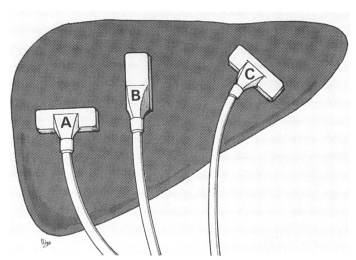

Fig. 14-7. A. Transverse scanning of the liver with a T-shaped probe. B. Longitudinal scanning with an I-shaped probe. C. Oblique scanning with a T-shaped probe. (From Machi J. Operative Ultrasonography. Tokyo: Life Science Ltd, 1987. Reproduced with permission.)

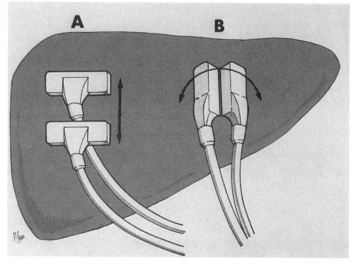

Fig. 14-9. Probe maneuvers during scanning of the liver using flat probes. A. Lateral movement with a T-shaped probe. This maneuver is most frequently used to examine the entire liver. B. Angulation along the transverse path with an I-shaped probe. (From Machi J. Operative Ultrasonography. Tokyo: Life Science Ltd, 1987.)

across the superficial surface of the target while the probe-to-surface geometry is maintained. An example is to slide the probe in contact with the surface of the liver (Fig. 14-9). Lateral movement can be along longitudinal or transverse scan paths of the target (Fig. 14-10). Figures 14-9 and 14-10 also illustrate lateral and angulation scanning maneuvers performed with flat and cylindrical probes. Lateral movement is usually the best maneuver to scan the entire organ in a systematic fashion. In rotation scanning, the probe is rotated (clockwise or counter clockwise) at the same location while the region of interest is maintained in the image the entire time of scanning. With this maneuver, lesions or structures are visualized continually from longitudinal to oblique to transverse views or vice versa. In angulation scanning, the probe head (transducer surface) is kept in place while the shaft of the probe is swung to different positions. This maneuver provides multiple scan planes while the probe head is in a relatively stationary location (Fig. 14-9). The sweep of the angle can be along either the longitudinal or the transverse path. This maneuver is particular useful in a deep narrow operative field where angulation scanning

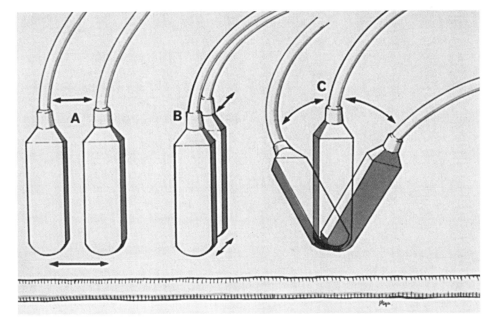

Fig. 14-10. Probe maneuvers during scanning of a peripheral blood vessel using a cylindrical probe. A. Lateral movement along a longitudinal scan path. B. Lateral movement along a transverse scan path. C. Angulation movement with minimal transducer head motion. (From Machi J. Operative Ultrasonography. Tokyo: Life Science Ltd, 1987. Reproduced with permission.)

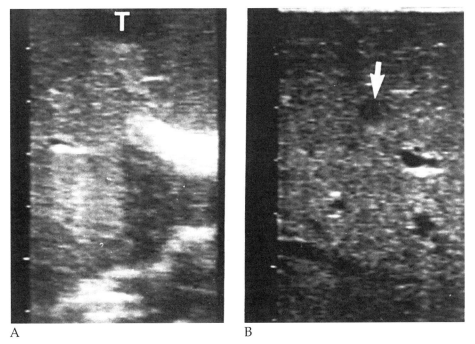

A   B

Fig. 14-11. An occult liver metastasis from a colon cancer. Preoperative computed tomography was negative for metastasis. Another metastatic tumor was visible and palpable. A. The visible and palpable tumor (T), 17 mm in size, is located at the surface of the medial segment of the left lobe. B. In addition, IOUS detected a 4-mm occult tumor (arrow) in the anterior-inferior segment of the right lobe. This was 2 cm from the liver surface.

is usually performed with a cylindrical probe (see Fig. 14-10). Usually, combinations of these three scanning maneuvers are performed simultaneously.

Scanning of the Specific Organs

The liver is best scanned with the side-viewing linear-array flat T- or I-shaped probes. The probe is passed over the liver surface under the anterior abdominal wall or the diaphragm. In the majority of operations, the entire liver is visualized by scanning from the anterior-superior surface of the liver (see Fig. 14-3). Scanning from the inferior surface may be needed at times for examination of the posterior segment of the right lobe. Intrahepatic vessels are scanned using lateral, rotational, and at times minimal angulation maneuvers. The right and left portal veins are followed from the hilum to the peripheral branches. Intrahepatic bile ducts and hepatic arteries are followed in a similar manner. The three main hepatic veins are then identified and followed from their confluence with the vena cava and tracked back into the liver. Hepatic veins are easily distinguished from portal vein branches because they do not show a double-layered or thickened wall. The reason for this appearance is the lack of investment of hepatic veins by Glisson's capsule. Identification of each of the intrahepatic portal and hepatic veins is essential to determine the segmental or subsegmental location of lesions. Following visualization of the blood vessels of the liver, scanning of the right and left lobes is performed to systematically examine the entire liver. This examination is accomplished by lateral scan maneuvers that encompass the entire liver (Fig. 14-9). The systematic examination of the entire liver should be thorough to screen for occult lesions. Figure 14-11 shows an occult tumor diagnosed by IOUS, but not discovered by preoperative studies or by palpation at exploration.

The extrahepatic bile duct is best scanned with the end-viewing cylindrical sector probe, although the flat probe may be used when the operative field is wide and sufficient space is available. Probe-standoff scanning is critical for the exposed or superficially situated bile ducts. The supra-duodenal portion of the bile duct is first visualized longitudinally, as the probe is

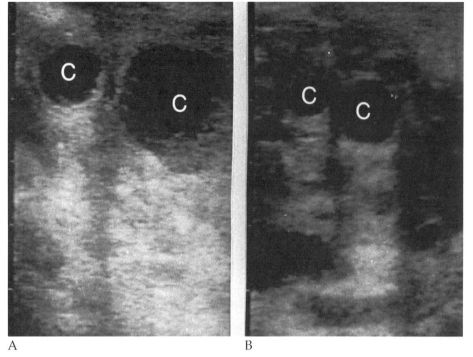

A   B

Fig. 14-12. Small pancreatic pseudocysts. A. During an operation for chronic pancreatitis, two preoperatively known pseudocysts in the pancreatic head were readily localized by IOUS. B. In addition, two small pseudocysts (C), 8 mm and 4 mm in size, were found in the pancreatic body only by IOUS.

moved from the hepatic hilum to the duodenum (see Fig. 14-4). The retroduodenal and intrapancreatic portions are then scanned through the duodenum, occasionally with gentle compression. The extrahepatic bile duct is also examined transversely (see Fig. 14-6), which displays the portal vein and hepatic artery.

The pancreas is best scanned with a flat probe after the exposure of the anterior surface of the pancreas following entrance into the lesser sac. However, the pancreas can also be visualized through the stomach, omentum, or mesocolon. If the operative field is limited, the cylindrical probe is useful. Viewing the pancreas through other structures is most often needed in the presence of adhesions or peritonitis. Both contact and probe-standoff techniques should be used to completely examine the superficial and deep portions of the pancreas. The entire pancreas is imaged using longitudinal and transverse scanning (see Fig. 14-8). The pancreatic head and the uncinate process can be scanned together with the examination of the intrapancreatic bile duct. The main

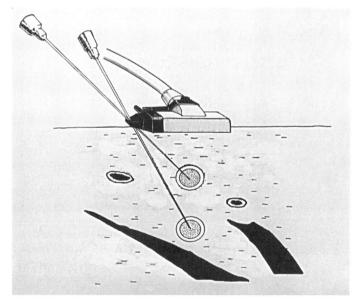

Fig. 14-13. IOUS–guided needle placement to the targets within liver parenchyma using the needle-guide probe-adapter. (From Machi J. Operative Ultrasonography. Tokyo: Life Science Ltd, 1987. Reproduced with permission.)

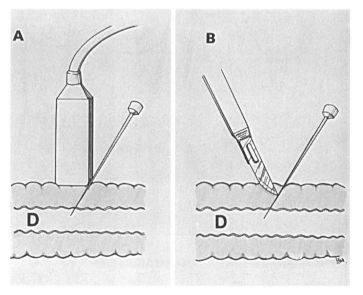

Fig. 14-14. IOUS–guided pancreatotomy for opening the pancreatic duct using needle guidance. A. The pancreatic duct (D) is localized by IOUS. An exploratory needle is inserted into the pancreas under ultrasound guidance. B. An incision is performed along the needle to open the pancreatic duct (D) at its center. (From Machi J, et al. Ultrasound-guided pancreatotomy for opening the pancreatic duct. Surg Gynecol Obstet 173:59, 1991. Reproduced with permission.)

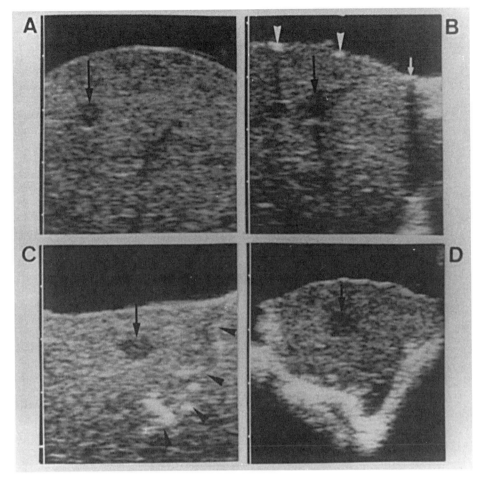

Fig. 14-15. *IOUS–guided resection of a nonpalpable tumor. A. A 5-mm nonpalpable hepatocellular carcinoma (black arrow) in a cirrhotic liver is localized in the anterior-inferior segment of the right lobe by IOUS. B. Markings are made on the liver surface using electrocautery. Two white arrowheads indicate the location of the tumor. A white arrow indicates the starting point of hepatic transection. C. The hepatic transection plane is delineated as an echogenic line (black arrowheads), which shows the relation of the transection line to the tumor. D. The resected specimen containing the tumor is scanned in the water bath to confirm adequacy of resection. (From Machi J.* Operative Ultrasonography. *Tokyo: Life Science Ltd, 1987. Reproduced with permission.)*

pancreatic duct, even when normal size, can be visualized best by scanning from the head to the tail of the pancreas. Figure 14-12 shows small pancreatic pseudocysts detected by IOUS.

Intraoperative Ultrasound Guidance

IOUS is used to guide needle or probe placement into solid organs for biopsy or other purposes. An adapter attachable to a probe for needle guidance is often available. The needle-guide adapter may be re-

quired to place a needle into very deep-seated lesions (Fig. 14-13). However, in most instances, IOUS–guided needle placement can be conducted in a free-hand manner. A needle is inserted from the lateral aspect of the probe into tissue so that the needle shaft is visualized while the needle is advanced. Motion of a needle facilitates the localization of the tip in the image.

IOUS guidance assists tissue dissection by helping to place a needle into a region of interest. For example, finding and opening the pancreatic duct during an operation for chronic pancreatitis is performed by

IOUS–guided insertion of a needle into the duct, followed by incision along the needle track (Fig. 14-14). During resection through solid organs, the plane of transection can be demonstrated as an echogenic line on ultrasound images. Figure 14-15 shows IOUS–guided resection of a nonpalpable hepatic tumor.

Laparoscopic Ultrasound Scanning of Bile Ducts

We have developed a dual scanning technique using a rigid side-viewing laparoscopic ultrasound probe for the complete examination of the extrahepatic bile ducts during laparoscopic cholecystectomy. This technique entails transverse scanning of the ducts via the subxiphoid trocar and longitudinal scanning of the ducts via the umbilical trocar. First, the probe is introduced into the peritoneal cavity through the subxiphoid port under laparoscopic observation and is positioned perpendicular and lateral to the edge of the hepatoduodenal ligament (Fig. 14-16). This placement produces a transverse section of the bile duct, portal vein, and hepatic artery. The probe is then moved along the long axis of the bile duct. Small rotational movements with the probe are also used to scan the ductal system not in direct contact with the probe. Figure 14-17 shows a small calculus detected in the common bile duct during laparoscopic cholecystectomy. After transverse scanning of the bile ducts through the subxiphoid port, the probe is inserted through the umbilical port, and is placed parallel and anterior to the hepatoduodenal ligament (Fig. 14-18). This step provides longitudinal sections of the bile duct and associated vascular structures. The probe is moved along the duct from the hepatic hilum to the duodenum. To examine the intrahepatic bile ducts, the probe is positioned atop the liver surface above the hilum. In our preliminary experience with the rigid laparoscopic ultrasound probe, scanning of the entire liver and pancreas was possible using subxiphoid and umbilical ports.

Flexible laparoscopic probes are becoming available. Such probes may simplify examination of the bile ducts by permitting complete examination with a single insertion of the laparoscopic transducer.

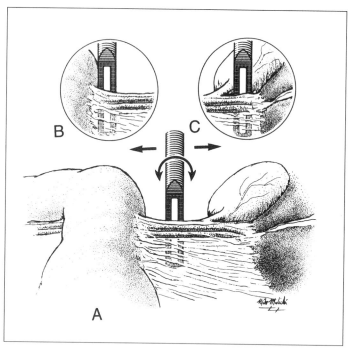

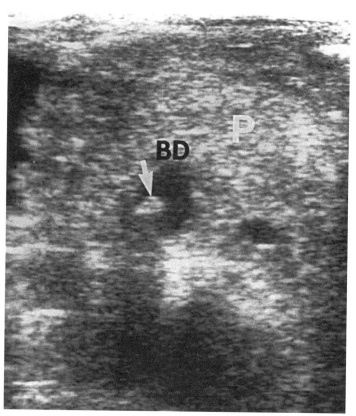

Fig. 14-16. Transverse scanning of the bile duct via the subxiphoid trocar during laparoscopic ultrasound. A. The laparoscopic ultrasound probe is positioned lateral to the hepatoduodenal ligament inferior to the cystic-hepatic duct junction. B. The probe is moved inferior to the duodenum. C. The probe is positioned superiorly to the cystic-hepatic duct junction if space permits. (From Machi J, et al. Technique of ultrasound examination during laparoscopic cholecystectomy. Surg Endosc 7:544, 1993. Reproduced with permission.)

Fig. 14-17. A 3-mm calculus (arrow) detected in the intrapancreatic portion of the common bile duct (BD) by laparoscopic ultrasound during laparoscopic cholecystectomy. P is the pancreatic head.

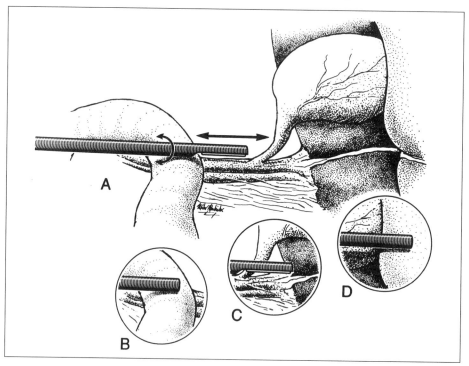

Fig. 14-18. Longitudinal scanning of the bile duct via the umbilical trocar during laparoscopic ultrasound. A. The laparoscopic ultrasound probe is positioned anterior to the hepatoduodenal ligament. B. The probe is moved across the duodenum. C. The probe is moved toward the hepatic hilum. D. The probe is placed on the surface of the liver to scan the intrahepatic bile ducts. (From Machi J, et al. Technique of ultrasound examination during laparoscopic cholecystectomy. Surg Endosc 7:544, 1993. Reproduced with permission.)

Suggested Reading

Bismuth H, Castaing D, Garden OJ. The use of operative ultrasound in surgery of primary liver tumor. *World J Surg* 11:610, 1987.

Gozzetti G, et al. Intraoperative ultrasonography in surgery for liver tumors. *Surgery* 99:523, 1986.

Jakimowicz JJ, et al. Comparison of operative ultrasonography and radiography in screening of common bile duct for calculi. *World J Surg* 11:628, 1987.

Machi J, et al. Accuracy of intraoperative ultrasonography in diagnosing liver metastasis from colorectal cancer: Evaluation with postoperative follow-up results. *World J Surg* 15:551, 1991.

Machi J, Sigel B. Intraoperative ultrasonography. *Radiol Clin NA* 30:1085, 1992.

Machi J, et al. Operative ultrasonography during hepatobiliary and pancreatic surgery. *World J Surg* 17:640, 1993.

Machi J, et al. Technique of ultrasound examination during laparoscopic cholecystectomy. *Surg Endosc* 7:544, 1993.

Makuuchi M, et al. The use of operative ultrasound as an aid to liver resection in patients with hepatocellular carcinoma. *World J Surg* 11:615, 1987.

Norton JA, et al. Localization of an occult insulinoma by operative ultrasound. *Surgery* 97:381, 1985.

Sigel B. Operative Ultrasonography (2nd ed). New York: Raven, 1988.

Sigel B, et al. Operative ultrasonic imaging of vascular defects. *Semin Ultrasound CT MR* 6:85, 1985.

Sigel B, et al. Comparative accuracy of operative ultrasound and cholangiography in detecting common bile duct calculi. *Surgery* 94:715, 1983.

Smith SJ, et al. Intraoperative sonography of the pancreas. *AJR* 144:557, 1985.

EDITOR'S COMMENT

Intraoperative ultrasound (IOUS) performed by surgeons has not increased in popularity as was predicted in the early 1980s, primarily because of the cost of the equipment and, perhaps even more important, the reluctance of radiologists to share the technology and credentialing of surgeons for this extremely important intraoperative technical advance. There are precious few radiologists who are interested in coming to the operating room and in participating actively in IOUS despite its obvious superior imaging precision as compared with transcutaneous techniques. It is truly incumbent on surgeons to aggressively pursue the acquisition of a dedicated instrument for the operating room in any institution in which the volume of surgery on the liver, biliary tract, pancreas, kidney, and other solid viscera is substantial. It is very difficult to operate on patients in most instances with pancreatitis, acute or chronic, without having such an instrument available, and its use in the search for endocrine-producing tumors in various locations, including the pancreas, the parathyroid, and elsewhere has been well documented.

When the instrument is brought to the operating room from the ultrasound suite, and a cooperative radiologist is willing to accompany the instrument, it has been estimated that 25 to 30 scanning experiences (in a similar number of patients) will afford the surgeon the expertise required to gain confidence in interpreting the findings. Of great benefit is the advent of the color ultrasound unit, which visualizes moving fluid (blood) by showing red and blue hues. The scanning techniques outlined by the authors are straightforward. Photographs of interesting images are important to obtain, are part of the technology of the instrument, and enter the patient's permanent record.

Areas in which scanning is quite different are primarily the ones in which there is a hollow viscus in front of the target organ to be examined. The duodenum, for example, makes the distal common bile duct (in the retroduodenal position) more difficult to assess with ultrasound. On the other hand, the "flattening out" techniques, which the authors describe can be helpful, and lesions, calculi, or significant narrowing can be detected. Very much analogous to the use of intrarectal ultrasound to assess the prostate and lesions of the rectum, and similarly analogous to vaginal ultrasound, the use of intraoperative ultrasound is a skill that surgeons can and should acquire, taking every opportunity to hone those skills in the operating room and in the radiology suite, assuming a cooperative colleague at that location.

R.J.B.

15

Electrocautery, Argon Beam Coagulation, Cryotherapy, and Other Hemostatic and Tissue Ablative Instruments

Fabrizio Michelassi   Roger D. Hurst

Electrocautery

Electrocautery uses electrical energy as a means to generate heat for tissue cauterization. The heat so generated results in either tissue vaporization as with a cutting current or tissue desiccation and small vessel occlusion as seen with the coagulation current. The practice of electrosurgery is not new and dates back to the 1920s. Although it has taken many years for its routine use to be accepted among general surgeons, it is now considered an indispensable part of operating room equipment. Virtually all surgeons in the industrialized world use the electrocautery as a standard surgical tool. In spite of its widespread use, surprisingly few are familiar with how this device works and many are not aware of its potential hazards. In order for the surgeon to use this technology safely and efficiently, a basic understanding of the concepts behind this device is necessary.

Physicians and scientists have been experimenting with the application of electrical current in living tissues since the latter part of the sixteenth century. However, it was not until the 1890s when d'Arsonal, experimenting with the physiological effects of high-frequency alternating currents, laid the groundwork for the beginning of electrosurgery. Working with crude spark generators d'Arsonal, discovered that oscillating currents with extremely high frequencies, above 10,000 Hz,

were not capable of neuromuscular stimulation as seen with lower frequency currents or with direct currents. In 1908 Lee deForest developed a high-frequency generator capable of delivering an easily controlled cutting current that would make clean incisions with little bleeding. In spite of the significance of these discoveries, the clinical application of these initial devices was very limited. With deForest's electrosurgical unit, vacuum tubes were used to generate the high-frequency currents necessary for effective electrosurgery without neuromuscular depolarization. The major disadvantage of this device was the great expense; the vacuum tubes were costly and frequently required replacement. The cost issue was overcome with the introduction of spark-gap generators. W. T. Bovie, a Ph.D. in physiology, developed a low-cost spark-gap generator while working in Boston. In 1926 a demonstration of Bovie's device was seen by the eminent neurosurgeon, Harvey Cushing, who realized this technology could revolutionize neurosurgery.

Although today's electrosurgical units rely on solid state circuitry rather than spark-gap electrodes or vacuum tubes, the current frequency and waveforms are essentially the same as the ones generated by the original Bovie. Harvey Cushing's endorsement of electrosurgery and its profound effects on neurosurgery as a whole did not result in instantaneous acceptance among general surgeons. Before the development of nonflammable inhalation an-

esthetics in the 1950s, the use of electrosurgery posed a very serious risk of fire and explosion. In addition to the safety risks, there was general concern over the effects of thermally injured tissue and its consequences on wound healing and infection. With time, however, these concerns were overcome and electrosurgery is now considered one of the most essential tools available to the general surgeon.

Principles of Operation

Key to the principles of operation with electrosurgery is the phenomenon that high-frequency oscillating currents do not depolarize excitable membranes. Currents greater than 10,000 Hz do not cause convulsive muscle contractions of nerve stimulation as they pass from the active electrode to the grounding pad. When low-frequency current passes through muscle, most of the fibers depolarize, resulting in muscular contraction, and nerves are stimulated, resulting in the unpleasant sensation of an electrical shock. These undesirable effects are avoided by using extremely high-frequency currents. Most electrosurgical units operate in a radiowave frequency range of 500,000 Hz to 3 mHz. Although the phenomenon is not entirely understood, excitable membranes are not depolarized by such currents. Occasionally, however, sparks of current at the contact site can give rise to signal degeneration and demodulation that results in localized depolarization. It is this demodulation that results in localized contraction when muscle itself comes into direct contact with the active electrode.

The electrical surgical unit is an electrical generator that requires a closed circuit through the patient in order to operate. To complete the electrical circuit through the tissues there are two electrodes that come into contact with the patient. The current enters the patient through what is referred to as the active electrode and exits the patient through the return electrode (Fig. 15-1). In monopolar electrocautery, the handheld tip is the active electrode, and the grounding pad acts as the return electrode. In bipolar electrocautery, both the active and return electrodes are present in the handheld instrument with one tip of the bipolar forceps acting as the active electrode and the other tip the return electrode.

The amount of electrical energy released by a specific current is dependent on the resistance of the medium through which the current is flowing. Resistance is directly proportional to the length of the conductor and inversely proportional to the cross-sectional area. The active electrode is designed so that the point of contact with the tissues has a very small surface area and, hence, a very high electrical resistance at the point of contact between the active electrode and the tissues, allowing for high energy release at this point of high resistance. As the current spreads out from the point of contact through the body, it is conducted over a much greater surface area, reducing the effective resistance and current density so that no significant energy release in heating occurs beyond the area of contact. The current harmlessly exits the body through a return electrode that is designed to have a large surface area with high conductivity and low resistance. Improper placement or malfunction of the return electrode may result in conduction of current over a small surface area, resulting in a point of high resistance and high energy release, thus placing the patient at risk for a burn at the return electrode site.

The effect of electrical current on tissue is dependent on the power of the current and the waveform that is generated. Doubling the current output quadruples the power delivered to the tissues. Although increasing power means more cutting or coagulation effect, it also means more heat transfer to the tissues. The heat produced by the electrocautery is proportional to the power of the current, multiplied by the length of time the current is delivered. Therefore, to avoid excessive heat production and resulting tissue damage, it is important to avoid excessive power or prolonged contact with the cautery. The power of the cautery should be set at the lowest possible setting to produce the desired effect of either cutting or cauterization. If the power is too high, it will result in excessive tissue destruction. If it is too low, prolonged contact time will be necessary, which will cause heating of surrounding tissues.

It is an empirical finding that a high-frequency current with a sinusoidal waveform results in a pure cutting effect (Fig. 15-2). The sinusoidal cutting current results in very high energy transfers over a small surface area. Temperatures at the point of contact with the tissues have been measured at over 600° C. This high temperature results in instant tissue vaporization and pyrolysis. Although the cutting waveform is highly effective for focal tissue vaporization, it has virtually no desiccating or coagulation effect. The coagulation mode is produced by a series of dampened sinusoidal waves that are produced in rapid bursts (Fig. 15-3). Such a waveform is effective at coagulation, but has very limited cutting capabilities. The coagulation waveform requires less energy than cutting and results in desiccation and destruction of surrounding tissues. Desiccation occurs as water evaporates from the cells and a coagulum of dried, shriveled, cellular debris forms as tissues boil in their own fluids and surrounding lymph. The associated heat transfer results in a shrinkage of small blood vessels and occlusion of the lumen by the coagulum of the contracted tissue and thrombosis.

A combination of both cutting and coagulation effects is possible with a current that is a blend of the pure sinusoidal cutting current and the periodic dampened coagulation current. The relative cutting versus coagulation effect can be varied by altering the blended waveform. The waveform with very little dampening that closely resembles a pure cutting current will have more cutting effect than coagulation effect, whereas a current at a higher degree of dampening will have more coagulation effect with little ability to cut. Most of the electrical surgical units available today can generate an adjustable graded blend between pure cutting and pure coagulation currents.

Monopolar Electrocautery

Monopolar electrocautery uses a handheld active electrode and a distantly placed large surface area return electrode or

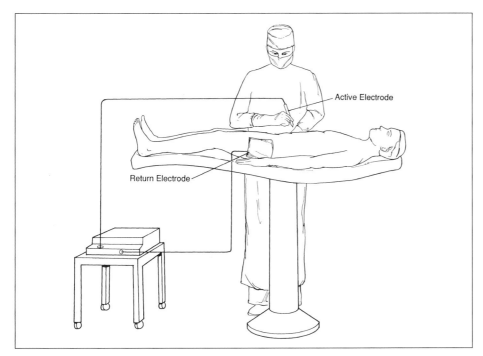

Fig. 15-1. Active and return electrodes for monopolar electrocautery.

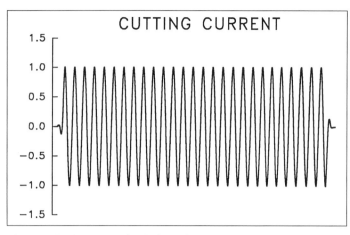

Fig. 15-2. Cutting current electrical waveform.

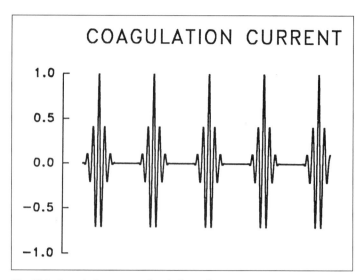

Fig. 15-3. Coagulation current electrical waveform.

grounding pad. Control switches to activate either the cutting or coagulation currents are located on the hand piece and can be activated through the use of a foot pedal. The active electrode should be held in the surgeon's dominant hand, like a pencil, with the index finger positioned over the control switch. The flat blade tip can be rotated for convenient alignment. If foot pedal controls are used, it is important that the surgeon holding the cautery hand piece also controls the foot pedal (Tate's rule). If an assistant operates the foot pedals while the operating surgeon holds the active electrode, miscommunication and risk of inappropriate current application and injury to the patient may occur.

The monopolar electrocautery can be used with either the cutting or coagulation modes. Each of these two currents has its own specific advantages as well as disadvantages.

Cutting Current
The cutting current allows for precise and accurate control when making incisions into tissue. Unlike the steel scalpel, which has a lot of drag, the cutting electrocautery can incise tissue with little resistance and is therefore particularly useful in making curved or circular incisions. Cutting current is particularly good at incising through relatively avascular tissue. The cutting currents on most modern electrosurgical units do have a small degree of coagulation effect, and tiny blood vessels will often be sealed at the time of incision.

Cutting currents are most efficiently delivered through a needlepoint electrode, and it is important to use only the tip of the electrode rather than the side or the shaft of the electrode. It must be remembered that the cutting effect of the electrosurgical unit is generated by the electrical current, not by the pressure of the electrode against the tissues. There should be virtually no resistance to the movement of the tip of the electrode to the tissue. If resistance is encountered one must be sure that the active electrode is clean, that only the tip of the electrode is in contact with the tissue, and that the power is at an adequately high setting. We find the cutting current to be particularly useful for dissecting along fine tissue planes. This current is distinct from the coagulation current, which desiccates surrounding tissues and tends to fuse tissue planes.

We do not use the electrocautery cutting current to incise skin that is intended for primary closure. We prefer instead to cut the epidermis and superficial dermis with a steel scalpel and then use the electrocautery cutting current to cut through the deep dermis. When used in this fashion, the cutting current will incise the deep dermis while at the same time sealing many of the smaller vessels supplying the skin at the level of the deep dermis. In situations in which primary closure of the skin is not anticipated, for instance for drainage of subcutaneous or perirectal abscesses, incising the epidermis with the monopolar cutting current works well.

Coagulation Current
The coagulation current is used to achieve hemostasis or to dissect with hemostasis. Hemostasis can be obtained either by **obliterative coagulation** or **coaptive coagulation.** Obliterative coagulation is achieved by direct contact between the active electrode and the bleeding points within the tissue. Desiccation of the surrounding tissue results in shrinkage of the vessel wall and occlusion of the lumen by coagulum and thrombosis formation. The technique of obliterative coagulation by direct contact is best suited for vessels less than 0.5 mm in size. For larger vessels, 0.5 to 1.5 mm, the coaptive technique of hemostasis can be used. The coaptive technique of hemostasis is achieved by mechanically apposing the edges of the vessels with a hemostat or forceps and applying the current to the instrument (Fig. 15-4). This step results in the sealing shut of the vessel at the point where the walls of the vessel are apposed by the forceps and formation of coagulum and thrombosis in proximity to the sealed vessel. The coaptive technique is performed by simply grasping the bleeding vessel with the forceps and then applying the coagulation current by contacting the active electrode to the metal forceps. When using the cautery as a dissecting tool, the coaptive technique can be applied to cauterize vessels prior to transection by grasping the vessel with a forceps, applying the coagulation current, and then dividing the vessel by direct contact of the cautery electrode at the point where the vessel sidewalls have

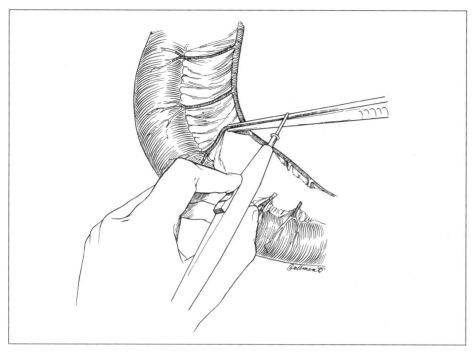

Fig. 15-4. Technique for operative coagulation of small vessels with the monopolar electrocautery.

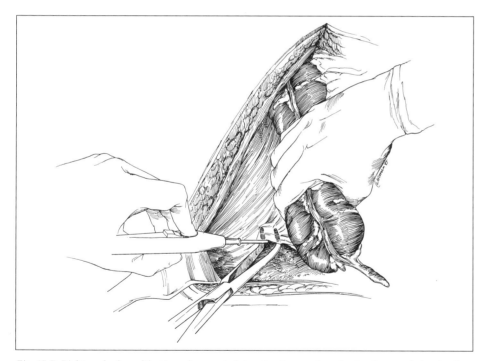

Fig. 15-5. Right-angle clamp lifts tissue from underlying structures and applies tension-countertension for division with coagulation current.

rather than a metal tip, which is likely to short circuit the current. The coagulation current results in the rapid buildup of char deposits on the active electrode. To ensure efficient operation of the cautery, the tip should be frequently cleaned by abrading deposits from the active electrode.

In addition to hemostasis, the coagulation current is useful as an aid to dissection. The destructive nature of this desiccating current can be used to divide tissue. It is important to remember, however, that if the coagulation current is to be used to incise tissue, it is critical that tension and counter-tension be applied to the tissue, otherwise separation will not occur, resulting in excessive thermal injury to surrounding tissues. Conversely, excessive tension and counter-tension separates the tissue too quickly, not allowing for sufficient contact with the coagulation current to seal small bleeders. We find the coagulation current particularly helpful in dividing such tissues as subcutaneous fat and muscle. If appropriate tension is maintained on these tissues, cautery will divide them quite easily while at the same time sealing all vessels and keeping blood loss to a minimum.

A common technique that we find particularly useful is the use of the electrocautery in the dissection of tissue with the aid of a right-angle clamp. For example, while incising the peritoneal reflections to mobilize the right or left colon, we dissect and lift up the peritoneum with the right-angle clamp while the first assistant cauterizes and divides the tissue with the electrocautery (Fig. 15-5). The right-angle clamp separates the peritoneum from surrounding critical structures and maintains some degree of tension of the tissue so that it can be divided with the coagulation current. When larger visible vessels are encountered using this right-angle technique, the vessels are grasped with the forceps and coagulated using the coaptive technique prior to division.

Using a combination of the previously described techniques, it is possible to perform most major intra-abdominal operations with minimal blood loss. It is important to remember to take full advantage of both the cutting and coagulation modes of the electrocautery, but that with the monopolar cautery, tissue injury can extend for some distance away from the

been previously coapted. When using the monopolar electrocautery to achieve hemostasis, it is important to remember that the electrical current will diffuse throughout any conductor of electricity including blood. Therefore, it is imperative that the field in general be dry at the time of application of the current.

If suction is necessary to maintain a dry field at the time of cauterization, it is best to use a nonconductive plastic suction tip

point of contact. For this reason, the electrocautery should not be used with direct contact onto a hollow viscus because this may lead to perforation. In addition, electrocautery should not be used in close proximity to a major blood vessel since this may lead to vessel wall injury and excessive bleeding.

Bipolar Electrocautery

With the bipolar cautery both the active and the return electrodes are located at the tip of the handheld unit. The coagulation current is focused on the tissue that is grasped by the tips of the bipolar forceps. Electrical heat energy is concentrated between the two electrodes and does not dissipate throughout the tissues. For this reason, the bipolar cautery has the advantage of causing less thermal injury to surrounding tissues than monopolar electrocautery (Fig. 15-6). Additionally, because the active electrode is not located at a distant site, there is less risk of burn injury. Bipolar cautery does not interfere with ECG monitors or pacemaker function. Another advantage is that the bipolar cautery can be used in wet fields. The bipolar cautery uses only a coagulation current and has no cutting or dissecting capabilities (Table 15-1).

The bipolar cautery is excellent for obtaining hemostasis in areas that may be in close proximity to delicate structures. Its use in neurosurgical procedures is indispensable. It is also valuable in head and neck surgery where monopolar cautery runs the risk of injury to fine nerve structures.

The bipolar cautery seals vessels by a coaptive technique. Vessels that are actively bleeding or are to be divided are grasped by the bipolar forceps. The coagulation current seals the walls of the vessels with the formation of coagulum. The unit is activated either by a foot pedal or by a switch located at the base of the bipolar forceps. The hand switch is activated automatically when the tips of the forceps are brought to within 1 to 2 mm of each other (Fig. 15-7). Care must be taken not to allow the tips of the bipolar forceps to come into direct contact with each other, because this contact will create a short circuit and coagulation will not occur. The tissue should be lightly grasped to allow a 1- to 2-mm gap between the electrode tips. Coagulation with the bipolar forceps tends to be a self-limiting process since desiccation of tissue between the points will ultimately prevent further flow of current. For

efficient use of the bipolar forceps, the tips must be free from the buildup of charcoal and coagulum. Therefore, frequent cleansing of the tips is required.

Potential Hazards and Precautions

Mishaps and injuries caused by use of the electrocautery are uncommon; however, when they do occur they can often be severe or even fatal (Table 15-2). Use of the electrocautery is so common that its routine use can lead to complacency regarding safety issues. Only through a complete understanding of the potential hazards and constant vigilance can injuries be avoided. It should be emphasized that it is ultimately the responsibility of the operating surgeon to see that every reasonable precaution is taken to protect both the patient and the operating team (Table 15-3).

Table 15-1. Comparison of Mono- Versus Bipolar Electrocautery

	Advantage	Disadvantage
Monopolar	Ease of use Cutting and coagulation currents Dissecting capabilities	Larger volume of tissue injured Can interfere with pacemakers Requires distant return electrode
Bipolar	Small volume of tissue injured Less risk of burn injury Safe with pacemakers Effective in wet fields	More skill required Coagulation current only No dissecting capabilities

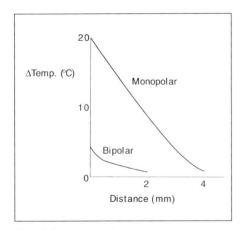

Fig. 15-6. Increase in tissue temperature as a function of distance from the active electrode.

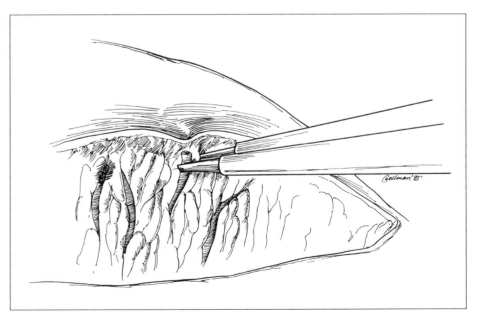

Fig. 15-7. Coaptive coagulation with the bipolar electrocautery.

Table 15-2. Potential Hazards of Electrosurgery

1. Electrical burns
   Active electrode injuries
   Return electrode injuries
   Current diversion injuries
     Coupled current diversion
     Uncoupled current diversion
2. Flame burns and explosion hazards
   Flammable anesthetics
   Flammable solvents
   Flammable drapes
   Flammable intestinal gas
3. Interference with electrical equipment
   Pacemakers
   ECG monitors
4. Smoke inhalation

Table 15-3. Safety Precautions with Electrosurgery

1. Do not use with flammable anesthetics.
2. Do not use near oxygen source.
3. Dry all ETOH and other flammable solutions.
4. Store hand piece in plastic holster when not in use.
5. Always use return electrode monitoring with monopolar cautery.
6. Use only number 1–rated fire retardant drapes.
7. Use lowest current setting necessary to deliver desired effect.
8. Do not use cautery blade as a retractor or blunt dissector.
9. Keep tip clean.
10. Respond immediately to inappropriate sounding of the cautery tone.
11. Follow Tate's rule.
12. Use short burst to avoid interference with ECG and pacemakers.
13. Do not coil cautery cord around metal instruments.
14. Wrap foot pedal in plastic.
15. Use proper procedure for grounding pad placement.
16. Use suction to remove smoke.

Electrical burns can occur at the grounding pad or at the active electrode. Electrical injuries result from either direct current flow or by coupled and uncoupled current diversion. Flame burns can also occur if combustible materials are ignited by the electrical spark.

Return Electrode Injuries

Return electrode injuries were once quite common. Poor electrical contact between the patient and the grounding pad can lead to areas of high resistance and impedance, resulting in energy discharge and injury. Fortunately, return electrode injuries have been significantly diminished with a recent innovation in the design of the electrosurgical generators. Modern units are equipped with return electrode monitoring (REM), a process that constantly monitors the efficiency of the contact between the patient and the gounding pad. If the REM circuitry depicts a poor contact with the patient the unit automatically shuts down and an alarm sounds. REM represents the standard for electrosurgical units, and generators that lack this capability should not be used. Even with the safeguard of REM, it is important to use good technique in placing the return electrode. Grounding pads should be placed on a broad patch of skin that is both clean and dry. Additionally, the grounding pad should be placed in a location that is unlikely to be exposed to moisture during the operation.

Active Electrode Injuries

Burns at the active electrode often occur with accidental activation of the unit. The most effective way of preventing these injuries is to store the pencil unit in an insulated plastic quiver when not in use. Covering the operative field with an adhesive plastic drape can also prevent active electrode injuries. It is important that the volume of the activation alarm or tone of the electrosurgical unit be set high enough to be easily heard by the surgeon who must be ready to act reflexively if the unit is unintentionally activated. When using the monopolar cautery the surgeon must take care that the uninsulated portion of the active electrode comes into contact only with the tissue that is to be coagulated. This precaution is particularly important when working in a deep cavity through a small skin incision where the base of the cautery blade can easily contact the skin edge if care is not taken.

Coupled Current Diversion

Coupling of current occurs when the active electrode comes into contact with a conductor of electricity. For instance, this phenomenon occurs intentionally when a forceps is used to coapt a vessel while the current is applied to the forceps. When coupling occurs unintentionally, injuries often occur. The surgeon should always be aware of the possibility of current arcing or direct contact with metal that is within the operative field. Coupling injuries are a particular concern during laparoscopic surgery in which conductive instruments are often held in close proximity to each other and during which high density of smoke can lead to current arcing. It should be noted that coupling is not limited to current diversion to instruments and retractors, but may also occur with staples, clips, guidewires, and metal sutures. Any metal located within the operative field can be a potential route for current diversion with potential injury to the tissues as well as the metal devices themselves.

Uncoupled Current Diversion

Uncoupled diversion of current is a peculiar phenomenon that can occur with high-frequency oscillating currents. Unlike direct current, alternating currents can travel across electrical capacitors. Oscillating currents can traverse thin insulators as long as the electrical conductivity is sufficient on either side of the insulator. Unintended diversion of current through a capacitor is referred to as an uncoupled current. This diversion most often occurs when the surgeon or first assistant holds the forceps for coaptive coagulation and feels an electrical shock as the current is delivered to the forceps. This shock can occur without a hole in the glove. Perspiration underneath the glove can increase the conductivity of the surgeon's hand to such a degree that the oscillating current traverses the capacitor that consists of the forceps and the hand separated by the thin insulator of the glove. This uncoupling phenomenon can also occur during laparoscopic surgery in which long metallic instruments covered by a thin plastic insulation can produce uncoupled currents with structures that come into contact with the plastic sheath.

Flame Injuries

Flame injuries are the most feared of electrosurgical complications. Fire in the operating room almost always results in sifnificant injury and puts the lives of the patient and the operating personnel in jeopardy. Flammable anesthetics are rarely, if ever, used in operating rooms. Needless to say, electrocautery should not be used in the presence of flammable anesthetics. (Flammable anesthetics are not used in the operating room, but are still occasionally used in the laboratory. When operating on animals always confirm that nonflammable agents and noncombustible drapes are being used prior to using electrocautery.) Flammable solvents such as alcohol and tinctures are commonly used in the operating room. Care must be taken to ensure that such solutions are completely dried before turning on the power to the electrosurgical unit. Flame injuries can also occur if cloth or paper drapes ignite from an electrical spark. All surgical drapes and gowns should be made of fire-retardant material with a "class one" fire rating.

Even materials that are fire resistant can ignite in the presence of high concentrations of oxygen. Fires resulting from the use of electrocautery in the presence of high oxygen tensions typically occur during minor head and neck procedures when the patient is given supplemental oxygen by mask or nasal cannula. Carelessness under such conditions has led to explosive fires with devastating injuries and even death. *Never use the electrocautery near a source of oxygen.*

Intestinal Gas Explosions

A potentially explosive mixture of hydrogen, methane, and oxygen can be present within the unprepped colon. Fortunately, ignition of flammable bowel gas by the electrocautery is uncommon, but the risk exists and fatalities have been reported. To prevent such accidents, the bowel should be mechanically prepped prior to any procedure that may result in the exposure of the electrocautery to bowel gas. Furthermore, mannitol- or sorbitol-containing bowel cleansing preparations that may promote methane production should be avoided.

Interference with Pacemakers

Great caution should be exercised when using monopolar electrocautery in patients with internal cardiac pacemakers (Table 15-4). Although most pacemakers made today contain safety devices that protect the unit from low-grade electrical interference, monopolar cautery, under certain circumstances, can result in the loss of the pacemaker's programmed settings. Under such circumstances, most pacemakers will pace at a preprogrammed back-up mode, usually VOO. However, there is great variation between differing makes and models of pacemaker units, and it is best to consult an expert in pacemaker programming prior to surgery. Direct contact

Table 15-4. Perioperative Management of Patients with Pacemakers

Preoperative
  Identify make and model of pacemaker
  Determine reset mode, program, thresholds, and battery status
  Deactivate rate responsiveness and magnet-initiated threshold testing
  Consider programming to asynchronous (VOO) or triggered mode (VVT) for pacemaker-dependent patients
Intraoperative
  Use bipolar cautery when possible
  Have personnel with programming expertise present in OR
  Ensure that pacemaker is accessible to programmer
  Use magnet with caution (may cause reprogramming in some units)
  Set to VVT if necessary
  Place return electrode so that main current flow does not pass through thorax
  Use short bursts
  If reset mode is hemodynamically unstable, reprogram pacemaker
  Do not use cautery in close proximity to pacemaker or its leads
  Use pulse oximeter to monitor heart rate
Postoperatively
  Check pacemaker program, thresholds, and battery status
  Reprogram as needed
  Replace pacemaker as needed

between the active electrode of the monopolar cautery and the metallic casing of the pacemaker often results in the destruction of the pacemaker unit. In patients with pacemakers, we prefer to rely on a bipolar cautery. If monopolar cautery is to be used in patients with pacemakers, it is best to set the cautery to the lowest effective setting, place the grounding pad far from the thorax, use short bursts of current, and have the necessary equipment and expertise in the operating room to reprogram the pacemaker should it be necessary.

Electrocautery Smoke

Recently, there have been some concerns expressed over the potential hazards of inhaling the smoke generated by the electrocautery. Components of the electrocautery smoke have been shown to be mutagenic to bacteria in high concentration. While components of electrocautery smoke can be mutagenic, they have not yet been shown to be carcinogenic. Concerns have also risen over the possible aerosolization of viral particles, especially during the

cauterization of viral lesions such as condylomata. The hazards of electrocautery smoke, if any, are not known. However, as a precaution, it is our practice to use a standard surgical suction device to clear smoke from the surgical field. Not only does this lessen the amount of smoke inhaled by the operative team, but it also helps clear the view of the surgeon. When cauterizing viral lesions, we recommend the use of specialized filter masks to help filter out aerosolized particles.

Argon Beam Coagulation

Like the standard electrocautery units, the argon beam coagulator uses high-frequency oscillating current to generate coagulating heat. The argon beam coagulator differs from standard electrocautery in that it uses a spray of ionized argon gas as the active electrode rather than a metallic blade. This spray allows even, efficient, and broad application of the coagulating current to the tissues. The argon beam coagulator consists of a current generator, a grounding pad, and a handheld active electrode. The device is activated by a foot pedal that initiates the flow of pressurized ion gas through the end of the handheld unit. Once a solid column of gas connects the handheld active electrode to the patient, the electrical current arcs across the argon gas to the tissues. The type of current used with the argon beam coagulator is almost identical to the type used with standard electrocautery. To use the argon beam coagulator, the handheld unit is held like a pencil with the end directly pointed at the tissue from a distance of 1 to 2 cm. The foot pedal is activated by the same person holding the active electrode (Tate's rule). A jet of argon gas is emitted from the end of the handheld unit, completing the circuit between the argon beam coagulator and the patient. The cautery current is delivered to the surface of the tissue in contact with the argon stream (Fig. 15-8).

To cauterize large surface areas, the unit can be used like a paintbrush using slow small strokes across the tissues. The power settings on most units range from 0 to 150 watts. As with the standard electrocautery, conduction is dependent on many factors, including the conductivity of the tissue. Therefore, we recommend starting with a relatively low power setting of 50 to 60

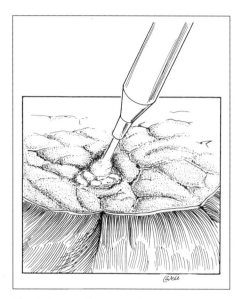

Fig. 15-8. Argon beam coagulator.

watts and increasing as necessary. Because of its efficiency in coagulating large irregular surfaces, the argon beam coagulator is ideal for obtaining hemostasis along the cut surface of the liver following hepatic resection. The argon beam coagulator can also be helpful in controlling bleeding from minor splenic trauma or other oozing surfaces. It has also been used as a means of tumor debulking by fulgurating metastatic ovarian carcinoma. The argon beam coagulator offers some advantages over conventional electrocautery in that with the argon beam coagulator there is no physical contact between the active electrode and the tissues. This lack of physical contact means that no adhesion of the active electrode to the tissues occurs, which allows for improved eschar integrity. In addition, there is no need to clean the char from the instrument. The flow of argon gas blows the blood and secretions away from the solid tissue to be coagulated, allowing for effective and efficient coagulation of tissue surfaces that are actively oozing, and less smoke is generated than with conventional electrocautery.

The argon beam coagulator has some disadvantages: its lack of precision and its expenses both with the unit itself as well as the consumable argon gas. In addition, although the argon beam coagulator is excellent at standard coagulation function, it has no coaptive capabilities and is very limited as a dissecting tool. Because the argon beam coagulator is essentially a monopolar electrocautery device, all pre-

cautions applicable to monopolar cautery should apply to the argon beam coagulator. Because of the risk of possible injury, we avoid the use of the argon beam coagulator in close proximity to delicate structures such as intestines, major vascular structures, ureters, and bile ducts. With the argon beam coagulator's relative lack of precision, special precautions should be taken to avoid current diversion through metallic instruments or retractors. Inadvertent activation of the pedal can result in significant injury and fire, and so the argon beam coagulator should always be stored in a plastic holster when not in use.

Cryotherapy

Cryotherapy is a technique of in situ tissue ablation that uses freezing temperatures to cause cell death. Cryotherapy has been used to treat a variety of benign and malignant lesions. For several decades, in situ destruction of tumor by cryotherapy has been used for cutaneous lesions. More recently, this mode of therapy has been applied to tumors of the head and neck, cervix, rectum, prostate, breast, and liver. Initially the technology consisted of the simple direct application of liquid nitrogen to surface lesions with a cotton swab. As advances in technology allow for the controlled delivery of liquid nitrogen and other cryogens deep into tissues, the applications of cryotherapy are expanding. Today sophisticated cryoprobes are available for the delivery of extremely low temperatures by means of pressurized liquid nitrogen. The probes come in varying sizes with differing capabilities. The delivery systems are complex, and their use requires personnel with special expertise in their operation and maintenance.

Although this technology is new and to a degree still unproven, ultrasound-assisted cryotherapy appears to have great promise in the treatment of liver tumors. In situ cryodestruction of tumor is best applied to unresectable or multiple liver metastases from colorectal cancer, where complete tumor ablation may lead to improved long-term survival.

Cryotherapy causes tumor destruction and cell death by a combination of several possible mechanisms. These mechanisms include cold shock injury, reduction of cell volume by osmotic dehydration, denatur-

ation of vital cellular enzymes, perforation of cell membranes by intracellular ice crystals, and destruction of tumor microvasculature. To ensure complete cell death, temperatures in the tissue should be lowered to below −35° C, maintained in the frozen state for at least 3 minutes, and then slowly thawed. The thawing cycle is particularly important, because too rapid or too slow thawing will allow survival of a portion of the tumor cells. For this reason, at least two freeze-thaw cycles should be applied to each tumor to ensure complete cellular destruction.

Before performing cryoablation therapy on liver lesions, the surgeon must have a thorough knowledge of the three-dimensional segmental anatomy of the liver. Additionally, the surgeon must have extensive experience with performing and interpreting hepatic ultrasonography (see Chap. 14).

Cryoablation of Liver Tumor

Patients undergoing cryoablation of liver tumors should be placed on a circulating heating pad. We use the Barir Hugger, a warmed air flow heating device to maintain normothermia. Core temperature should be monitored by either an esophageal temperature probe, or by the temperature probe of a Swan-Ganz catheter for patients requiring pulmonary artery pressure monitoring. An initial subcostal incision is made to explore the abdomen and determine the presence of extrahepatic disease. If none is found, the incision is enlarged to a bilateral subcostal incision with or without upper midline extension. The liver is fully mobilized by taking down the coronary and triangular ligaments of the liver. The liver is thoroughly palpated and then examined with real-time ultrasound using a 7.5-mHz linear array transducer. If the lesion or lesions can be resected with a 1-cm margin, these lesions should be surgically removed either by wedge resection or standard anatomic partial hepatectomy. Cryotherapy is reserved for unresectable lesions.

Once a tumor is identified for cryoablation, the lesion and surrounding parenchyma are closely examined with the ultrasound, and proximity to vascular structures is noted. The surrounding organs and the diaphragm should be packed away from the liver with dry laparotomy packs as a precaution against accidental injury from the freezing process. An 18-gauge needle is then introduced into the liver under ultrasound guidance. The needle is directed to avoid vascular structures. If a single cryoprobe is used, the top of the needle is placed directly into the lesion (Fig. 15-9A). If the lesion is large, and multiple probes are to be used, the needle is placed near the periphery of the lesion. A guidewire is then threaded through the needle so that the tip of the wire is seen by ultrasound to be curling out the end of the needle (Fig. 15-9B). The wire is then held in place and the needle is removed. A pointed obturator with an overlying sheath is then threaded over the guidewire and positioned at the end of the wire (Fig. 15-9C). The guidewire and obturator are removed, leaving behind the plastic sheath. The cryoprobe is then introduced into the tunnel of the sheath so that the tip of the probe lies at the end of the sheath (Fig. 15-9D). The sheath is retracted approximately 2 cm to expose the tip of the probe to the tumor (Fig. 15-E). If multiple probes are to be used to freeze the same lesion, the temperature of the probe should be turned down to −100° C before placing the other probes. This step makes

the probe stick in place and prevents dislodgement during the placement of additional probes. Once all the probes are placed, the freezing process is begun with the pumping of liquid nitrogen to achieve a probe temperature of −160°C to −180°C.

Creation of the ice ball is monitored with the ultrasound transducer. By ultrasound, the ice ball appears as a dark, well delineated hypoechoic area usually with posterior acoustic shadowing. The ultrasound is used to determine the extent of freezing, which should proceed at least 1 cm beyond the ultrasonic border of the tumor. Once tumor freezing with the minimum 1 cm of surrounding tissue has been achieved, the probe's nitrogen supply is turned off, and the liver is allowed to completely thaw. Each freeze-thaw cycle take about 20 minutes to complete. The freezing process is then repeated for a total of two complete freeze-thaw cycles. Prior to completion of the second thaw cycle, the probe and sheath are removed and a rolled piece of gelfoam is packed into the frozen tract to prevent bleeding once the area has completely thawed. Additional lesions are sequentially treated in the same manner. It is possible to freeze up to four lesions at one session with this method.

The freeze-thaw processes lead to liquefying necrosis of the tumor and surrounding liver parenchyma. With time, significant scar formation occurs in the area of cryoablation. This scar tissue can be difficult to discern from tumor by CT scan. Therefore, we routinely obtain an abdominal CT scan 2 to 3 months after cryoablation, as a baseline study to use as a comparison with subsequent diagnostic scans.

Precautions

It is very important that the cryoprobes are properly maintained. The extremes in temperatures can lead to metal fatigue of the delicate cryoprobe tips, which cause leakage of liquid nitrogen. With a volume ratio of liquid to gaseous nitrogen of 1:680, the spillage of even a small amount of liquid nitrogen can theoretically result in the risk of significant air embolism. Hence, it is important to visually examine the probes before and after each pair of freeze-thaw cycles.

When liver tissue freezes, it becomes very brittle and easily fractures. Cracks that occur in frozen liver can often lead to troublesome bleeding once the tissue has thawed. Therefore, it is important to protect the frozen liver from blunt trauma caused by impact with instruments or retractors.

The freezing process not only destroys tumor and liver parenchyma but can also injure bile ducts, and persistent bile leaks have been reported. Because of the concern over injury to major bile ducts, we do not use cryotherapy to treat lesions that are in close proximity to the portahepatis. Unlike bile ducts, large blood vessels are relatively protected from the effects of cryotherapy. This protection results from the flow-assisted thermal conduction by the warm blood that prevents freezing of the vessels. This thermal conduction protects the vessels, but it may also protect tumor cells that may be close to the vessel. For this reason, we are concerned about the effectiveness of cryotherapy for lesions located near large vessels. To help overcome this we often inject 100% ethanol into the tissues that lie between the tumor and a nearby vessel. The absolute alcohol is cytotoxic and will help kill tumor cells that may escape the effects of the cryoprobe. The injection is accomplished with a thin

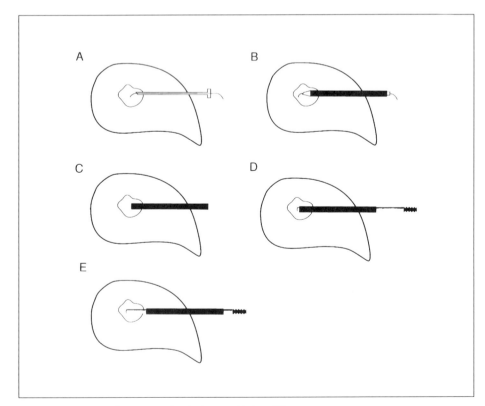

Fig. 15-9. Techniques for position of probe for cyroablation of liver tumor.

spinal needle directed to the appropriate area under ultrasound guidance.

Although hypothermia is not a common problem with cryotherapy of liver lesions, it is important to monitor core temperatures during and immediately after the procedure and treat hypothermia should it occur.

With the treatment of large or multiple lesions, a substantial amount of liver parenchymal necrosis occurs. In the immediate postoperative period, the patient should be monitored for hyperkalemia and myoglobinuria. Because of the risk of renal tubular necrosis secondary to myoglobinuria, urine pH should be maintained above 7 with intravenous sodium bicarbonate for as long as the urine shows myoglobin. The generation of necrotic liver tissue can also lead to intrahepatic abscess formation. This complication is fortunately not common and can often be managed with percutaneous drainage when it does occur. However, because of concerns over bacterial seeding of necrotic hepatic tissue, we do not perform hepatic cryoablation at the same time as resection of the primary colon tumor.

Infrared Coagulator

The infrared coagulator generates coagulation heat energy by infrared irradiation. The infrared coagulator consists of a transformer unit with a foot pedal switch and a handheld wand. The wand is a round metallic cylinder that generates the infrared light that emanates through the crystal lens at the end of the wand. The heat energy produced by the infrared irradiation causes rapid heating of the tissues in contact with the crystal, and this heating results in desiccation and coagulation.

The infrared coagulator is most useful for coagulating oozing tissue surfaces such as the cut edge of the liver following hepatic resection. The flat crystal is pressed against the tissue in a manner such that little or no light can escape from the end of the wand. The foot pedal is then pressed to activate the wand and generate the infrared irradiation. Approximately 1 to 2 seconds of exposure is usually sufficient to result in tissue coagulation and hemostasis, which are signified by the boiling of fluids at the edge of the crystal and the generation of a small amount of smoke. It

is important that the wand not be pulled away from the tissue until the infrared generation has ceased. After each application, the end of the wand should be wiped with a moist sponge to cool the crystal and to remove char from the tip. The infrared coagulator is an effective device for coagulating oozing surfaces and has the advantage of not requiring electrical current to pass through the patient. Hence, the infrared coagulator does not interfere with ECG monitoring or pacemaker function.

Ultrasonic Dissector

The ultrasonic dissector is a surgical tool that uses high-frequency mechanical vibrations to fragment tissue. Developed in the late 1960s, this technology was originally applied to ophthalmic surgery, but has gained wide use in neurosurgery, hepatobiliary surgery, and oncologic cytoreductive surgery. The ultrasonic dissector system consists of a rather bulky hand piece connected to a function control console that is controlled by a standard foot pedal. The end of the handheld unit consists of a metal contact probe that vibrates at a frequency between 20,000 and 40,000 times per second. Because this vibration frequency is above the audible range, it is referred to as ultrasonic. No audible sound or electromagnetic radiation is emitted and the vibrating tip must be in direct contact with the tissues to bring about its effect. The vibrations are generated by transducers that rely on piezoelectric crystals or magnetostrictive laminations to convert electrical energy into mechanical vibrations.

The ultrasonic dissector fragments tissue by contact with high water content cells. The vibrations generate vapor pockets within the cells that lead to cellular disruption and fragmentation. While fragmenting high water content cells, the dissector does not readily disrupt collagen-rich tissue such as blood vessels and ducts. Hence, the device can divide parenchymal tissue while leaving blood vessels intact so that they can be individually ligated prior to division.

The coils within the handheld unit can generate a significant amount of heat, and most units are equipped with an internal cooling system that is pumped to the

handheld unit. Additionally, the tip itself is automatically irrigated to wash away cellular debris and to cool the contact element. To remove the cellular debris and irrigation fluid, a suction port is located at the tip of the instrument. Ultrasonic vibration, irrigation, and aspiration are all simultaneously activated by compression of the foot pedal. Adjustable power to the ultrasonic dissector is usually calibrated from 0 to 100 percent of full capacity. Some units are also equipped with monopolar electrocautery capabilities, with the cauterizing current emanating from the dissector tip and activated by a separate switch on the handheld unit.

The most common general surgical application of the ultrasonic dissector is for the division of the liver parenchyma during hepatic resection. To accomplish this division, the liver is first examined and mobilized in the standard fashion. Vascular and hilar ductal structures are dissected and ligated as appropriate. The ultrasonic dissector is set at 50 to 60 percent power for a normal liver and approximately 80 percent for a cirrhotic liver. The foot pedal is compressed and the tip of the unit is lightly pressed against the tissue to be divided. Short linear strokes are used to cut through the parenchyma. Even though the ultrasonic dissector is equipped with suction, standard conventional suction is also used to clear blood and fluid from the area of dissection. When small vessels and ducts are encountered, we coagulate them with standard electrocautery using the coaptive technique described earlier. The cauterized structures are then divided with scissors. Large vessels and ducts are cleared of parenchyma by the ultrasonic dissector and then ligated before division (Fig. 15-10). Oozing from the cut surface of the liver is periodically controlled with compression, the electrocautery, or the argon beam coagulator. In addition to dividing liver tissue, the ultrasonic dissector can be used to incise other solid organs such as the spleen, kidney, and brain.

In addition to its use as a dissecting tool, the ultrasonic dissector can be used as a means of tissue ablation. It has been extensively applied in cytoreductive surgery in the treatment of metastatic ovarian cancer. Ovarian epithelial cancers tend to have a high water content with very little fibrous stroma, hence, these tissues readily fragment with the ultrasonic dissector. When

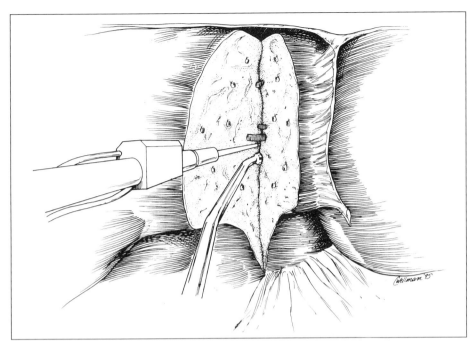

Fig. 15-10. Division of liver parenchyma with the ultrasonic dissector.

the ultrasonic dissector is used for this purpose, it is important to be aware that tumor infiltration can involve full thickness penetration of hollow or tubular structures such as intestine, bladder, and blood vessels. Therefore, it is important that the surgeon be prepared to deal with possible perforation of these structures. With this in mind, we always order complete mechanical bowel cleansing with prophylactic intravenous antibiotics for patients undergoing cytoreductive surgery. Additionally, prior to applying the ultrasonic dissector to a tumor that is in close proximity to major vascular structures, it is advisable to first gain proximal and distal control of the vessel.

The ultrasonic dissector is a convenient way of dividing solid organ parenchyma with little blood loss. When used appropriately, this device is relatively safe and mishaps are infrequent. The ultrasonic dissector has some disadvantages: its high cost, the bulkiness of the unit itself, and it has not been demonstrated to be consistently superior to standard dissecting techniques. For most routine liver resections, we use a combination of electrocautery and finger fracture technique for noncirrhotic livers and reserve the ultrasonic dissector for patients with mild to moderate cirrhosis.

Suggested Reading

Barold SS, et al. Interference in Cardiac Pacemakers: Exogenous Sources. In N El-Sherif, P Samet (eds), *Cardiac Pacing and Electrophysiology* (3rd ed). Philadelphia: Saunders, 1991.

Cushing H. Electrosurgery as an aid to the removal of intracranial tumors. *Surg Gynecol Obstet* 47:751, 1928.

Glover JL, Bendick PJ, Link WJ. The use of thermal knives in surgery: Electrosurgery lasers, plasma scalpel. *Curr Probl Surg* 15:1, 1978.

Huff T, Brand E. Pseudomyxoma peritonei: treatment with the argon beam coagulator. *Obstet Gynecol* 80:569, 1992.

Nduka CC, Super PA, Monson JRT, and Darzi AW. Cause and prevention of electrosurgical injuries in laparoscopy. *J Amer Coll Surg* 197:161, 1994.

Putman CW. Techniques of ultrasonic dissection in resection of the liver. *Surg Gynecol Obstet* 157:474, 1993.

Ravikumar TS, et al. Hepatic cryosurgery with intraoperative ultrasound monitoring for metastatic colon carcinoma. *Arch Surg* 122:463, 1987.

Ravikumar TS, Steele GD. Hepatic cryosurgery. *Surg Clin North Am* 69(2):433, 1989.

Rubinsky B, et al. The process of freezing and the mechanism of damage during hepatic cryosurgery. *Cryobiology* 27:85, 1990.

EDITOR'S COMMENT

The authors have performed a real service in illuminating an area of surgical instrumentation that is almost universally used but is often poorly understood by surgeons. Electrocautery has become an instrument that virtually every operation requires. Its use saves operative time and eliminates the need for meticulous ligation of multiple bleeders. Electrocautery has made ligation of small soft-tissue bleeders a thing of the past. Many surgeons abandon the scalpel once the dissection is carried below the dermis, and the resulting conservation of blood, saving of time, and demonstrated quality of wound healing more than justify the confidence placed in this device.

Nevertheless, for reasons well outlined in this chapter, electrocautery must be treated with respect, and a basic understanding of the technique is mandatory. All surgeons have had experience with unplanned tissue injury, usually not serious but annoying, when the cautery blade inadvertently touches the skin of the incision or soft tissue adjacent to that which is to be cauterized. Critical points made by the authors are that proper use of the instrument requires lower amounts of current, rather than higher; that contact time between the activated cautery tip and the tissue should be as short as possible; and that the heat produced can spread to surrounding tissues with substantial potential for damage. The use of monopolar cautery in laparoscopic surgery is of growing concern; there is an expanding body of evidence that the almost excessive amount of cautery required to dissect tissues when the monopolar cautery is used can, and occasionally does, injure the common hepatic duct, resulting in devascularization and stricture or even perforation of the duct.

Although not always practical, the bipolar cautery current instrument is an attractive alternative. This device has recently been adapted for laparoscopic surgery, and it has a highly desirable quality: only the area between the two electrodes can be affected by the heat-producing current. In addition, it has no effect on pacemakers or monitoring devices. Another benefit is that its use makes it extremely unlikely that tissue adjacent to the shaft of the instrument will be burned; the shaft is well insulated. The trade off is that the amount of current, or heat, delivered to the end of the instrument and the tissue is not as effective as the amount delivered by the monopolar cautery. Dissection of tissues such as the gallbladder bed or the lateral attachments of the colon is substantially slower than with the monopolar cautery device.

Of great concern is the use of monopolar cautery in the presence of high oxygen concentrations in or near the operative field. A recent experience with a colleague cauterizing lesions on the neck and shoulder in a healthy patient who was being given oxygen for no apparent reason demonstrated the hazards of the monopolar cautery most dramatically; there was a layering of oxygen under the drapes, a sudden flash of flame, and the patient's face and neck were burned, although superficially. A second episode occurred in which a patient was undergoing tracheostomy to replace an endotracheal tube and maintain the airway, and the surgeon elected to open the trachea with cautery through which oxygen at approximately 60 percent concentration was flowing. A significant flash flame occurred, which surprisingly did more damage to the operating surgeon than to the patient. Such incidents are not cited to fault the technique, but rather the understanding and judgment of the operator, who must realize the potential for catastrophic events if appropriate precautions are not taken.

One of the more troubling aspects of the use of electrocautery is the situation in which one is operating on a patient whose tissues harbor a potentially serious or lethal virus. Viruses are protein moieties that theoretically are vaporizable, although the significance of that has yet to be definitively determined. In fact, procedures as simple as cauterization of anal condylomata share with lasers the potential for transmission of disease to operating room personnel. Whether that potential is real is not known, nor is the need to evacuate smoke from lasers and electrocautery proven, although it would seem wise to use a smoke evacuator until definitive data do appear concerning the real risks of virus vaporization.

The other coagulant-dissecting instruments mentioned by the authors have proven to be of extraordinary benefit in management of lesions in solid viscera, such as splenic and hepatic trauma; injuries and tumors of the kidney; as well as elective resection of metastases to the liver and other tissues. In particular, the argon beam coagulator has been of great benefit in centers in which many patients with trauma are treated. This instrument has added substantially to the trauma surgeons' armamentarium. Once the operator no longer has the tendency to touch the tip of the coagulator to the tissue and learns to rely on the argon beam, the efficiency and performance of this instrument are substantial. Cryotherapy for tumors has been applied in a number of ways, by far the most sophisticated of which is the current cryotherapy probe described here. Although the results have been interesting, there is no uniformity of opinion about the overall effectiveness of this particular modality, and its use has largely been limited to larger cancer centers in which very specific clinical criteria have been applied.

R.J.B.

16

Upper and Lower Gastrointestinal Endoscopy

Jeffrey L. Ponsky

The introduction of flexible fiberoptic endoscopes over three decades ago began an era in which physicians and surgeons could reliably, safely, and comfortably inspect the interior of the upper and lower gastrointestinal tract. They were soon able to photographically record the findings and deliver therapy. Today, with marked improvements in instrumentation and technique, flexible endoscopy remains the mainstay of diagnosis and therapy of a host of conditions affecting the gastrointestinal system.

Indications for Digestive Endoscopy

Endoscopy of the esophagus can be prompted by complaints of dysphagia, odynophagia, or persistent unremitting pyrosis. Suspected foreign body impaction, an abnormal barium roentgenogram, and gastrointestinal bleeding also are indications for endoscopic examination. Although originally carried out as an isolated procedure, endoscopic inspection of the esophagus is usually performed with investigation of the stomach and duodenum, a procedure known as esophagogastroduodenoscopy. Additional indications for upper endoscopy include the necessity for establishment of gastric access for feeding, persistent vomiting, unremitting epigastric pain, gastric polyposis, and surveillance for neoplasia in patients with conditions predisposing to malignancy such as Barrett's esophagus, gastric ulcer, pernicious anemia, and previous gastrectomy. Suspected pancreatic or biliary disease will often prompt the performance of endoscopic retrograde cholangiopancrea-

tography (ERCP). In most instances, the modern endoscopist is prepared to deliver therapy during the same procedure in which the diagnosis is established. Therapy may include removal of foreign bodies, dilation of strictures, laser ablation of tumors, sclerotherapy or ligation of varices, control of hemorrhage, placement of feeding tubes, polypectomy, and insertion of biliary or pancreatic duct stents.

Common indications for colonoscopy include suspected colorectal polyps or cancer, diagnosis of infectious or inflammatory colitis, surveillance for dysplasia or carcinoma in patients with ulcerative colitis, and lower gastrointestinal bleeding. Additional indications may include foreign body retrieval and colonic decompression.

Instrumentation

Fiberoptic technology enabled the development of flexible gastrointestinal endoscopes, and fiberoptic endoscopes have, until recently, been the mainstay of modern gastrointestinal endoscopy. Recent developments in digital camera technology have allowed the integration of the two modalities so that modern video endoscopes deliver light by fiberoptic bundle, but transmit the endoscopic image by digital signal to a processor and video screen. The latter allows for a larger, brighter image, which can be easily recorded and electronically enhanced, if necessary. A large variety of endoscopes are available for diagnostic and specialized therapeutic purposes in adults and children. These endoscopes include small-caliber gastroscopes and colonoscopes for pediatric use,

large- and double-channel scopes for therapeutic applications, side-viewing instruments for cannulation of the ampulla of Vater, mother-daughter scope combinations for complex biliary and pancreatic ductoscopy, and long slender enteroscopes for small-bowel examination.

Technique of Esophagogastroduodenoscopy

The patient is prepared for upper endoscopy by ensuring that the stomach is empty. This process usually involves a 4- to 6-hour fast or, in urgent cases, gastric lavage. The patient is positioned with the left side down, and sedation is administered intravenously while vital signs and blood oxygen saturations are monitored. Topical posterior pharyngeal anesthesia is also useful. The endoscope can be introduced by digital palpation, with the endoscopist's finger(s) being used to guide the scope, or by advancement under direct vision (Fig. 16-1). The latter is the safest approach and can be more comfortable for the patient. It can also prevent inadvertent introduction of the instrument into a Zenker's diverticulum.

Once the endoscope is in the esophageal lumen, air is insufflated. A long view of the esophagus should be obtained and its mucosa inspected. Peristalsis should be noted, and evidence of inflammation or Barrett's epithelium sought. Interruptions in the normal mucosa by inflammation or suspected neoplasm should be assessed by cytologic brushing and biopsy. A hiatal hernia will appear as a saccular portion of

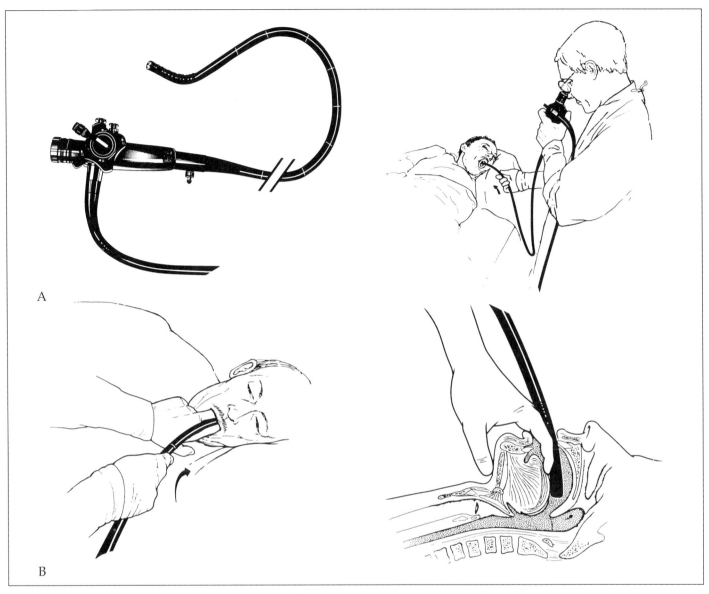

Fig. 16-1. A. The gastroscope can be introduced under direct vision. This method is best for observing the uppermost esophagus. B. The scope can be introducd by digital guidance, using the endoscopist's fingers to depress the tongue and center the instrument. (From Ponsky JL. Atlas of Surgical Endoscopy. *St. Louis: Mosby, 1992. Reproduced with permission.)*

gastric mucosa above the pinching action of the diaphragm. Normally, the esophagus turns slightly to the left as it traverses the diaphragm and enters the abdomen. The esophagogastric junction is noted by the z line, an irregular junction of the orange columnar gastric mucosa with the pale pink squamous mucosa of the esophagus (Fig. 16-2).

The stomach should be fully inflated with air. Any redundancy in the scope should be reduced and the parietes carefully observed. With the instrument in the gastric body, the stomach's posterior wall is at the 3 o'clock position, the lesser curvature at the 12 o'clock position, the anterior wall at the 9 o'clock position, and the greater curvature at the 6 o'clock position (Fig. 16-3). Small movements of the control knobs will direct the tip of the scope in any desired direction. Noted abnormalities can include ulcerations, gastritis, vascular lesions, neoplasia, or extrinsic impressions on the gastric wall. The location of such extrinsic impression can indicate the probable source. For example, a large impression on the posterior wall of the stomach,

noted at the 3 o'clock position, can indicate a pancreatic mass, such as a pseudocyst or tumor.

As the endoscope is advanced toward the gastric antrum, the incisura angularis will be noted on the lesser curvature. It is a smooth curved arch dividing the gastric body from the antrum. Marked elevation of the instrument's tip and a small turn to the left while the scope is positioned at the gastric angle will usually permit a retroflexed view of the gastric cardia and fundus (Fig. 16-4). This maneuver is critical to

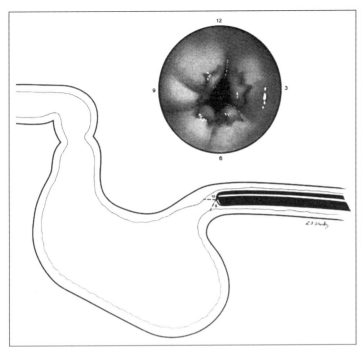

Fig. 16-2. The z line appears at the esophagogastric junction. It represents the change from the squamous esophageal mucosa to the columnar epithelium of the stomach. (From Ponsky JL. Atlas of Surgical Endoscopy. St. Louis: Mosby, 1992. Reproduced with permission.)

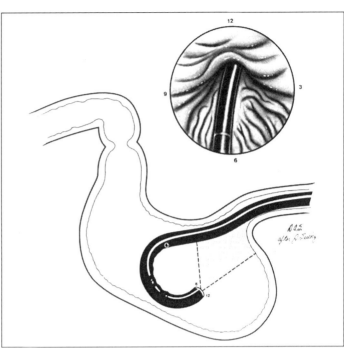

Fig. 16-4. A retroflexed view can be easily accomplished and permits inspection of the cardia and fundus. (From Ponsky JL. Atlas of Surgical Endoscopy. St. Louis: Mosby, 1992. Reproduced with permission.)

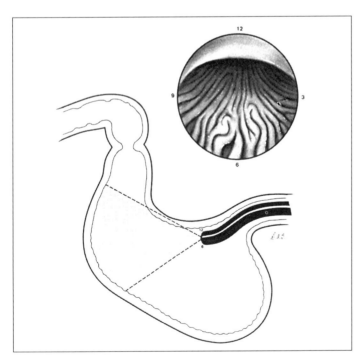

Fig. 16-3. In the body of the stomach, with the patient in the left lateral decubitus position, the lesser curvature is at the 12 o'clock position, the posterior gastric wall at 3 o'clock, the anterior wall at 9 o'clock, and the greater curvature at the 6 o'clock position. The gastric angle, separating the gastric body from the antrum, is seen as a smooth arch along the lesser curvature. (From Ponsky JL. Atlas of Surgical Endoscopy. St. Louis: Mosby, 1992. Reproduced with permission.)

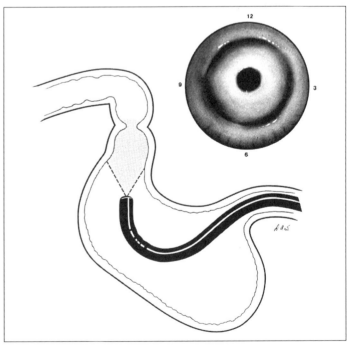

Fig. 16-5. The antrum has few rugal folds. The pylorus is typically round and can be observed to open and close. (From Ponsky JL. Atlas of Surgical Endoscopy. St. Louis: Mosby, 1992. Reproduced with permission.)

the complete examination of the stomach and allows careful assessment of the cardia, fundus, and the lesser curvature.

The normal large rugal folds noted on the greater curvature of the stomach's body disappear as the antrum is entered. The tip of the scope is elevated to permit its advancement toward the pylorus. Small circular motions of the scope's tip will allow visualization of the entire antrum. The pylorus is normally round and can be observed to open and close (Fig. 16-5). Irregularities of the pyloric shape might hint at past or present ulceration. While keeping the pyloric orifice directly in the center of view, the scope is advanced, with gentle pressure and slight insufflation of air, into the duodenal bulb. The bulb has no folds and is a frequent site of inflammation and ulceration. Small motions of the instrument's tip help reveal the more obscure corners of the bulb where ulcers may be hidden (Fig. 16-6). Once inspection of the bulb is complete, the scope is advanced into the descending duodenum. This step usually requires a somewhat blind maneuver. The scope's tip is turned to the right as the shaft of the instrument is also rotated to the right. The tip is first moved

upward and then down. This move turns the instrument posterior and then downward into the retroperitoneal, second portion of the duodenum. Once the lumen of the descending duodenum is in view, slight pressure can be applied to the shaft of the scope to introduce it further. If resistance is encountered, the scope is pulled back and straightened. This maneuver usually results in further advancement of the endoscope into the duodenum as the redundant gastric loop is reduced. The scope is then withdrawn while close attention is addressed to the mucosal detail. The small intestine is noted by the semicircular folds, which are the hallmark of its architecture. The ampulla of Vater can be seen in profile at the 9 o'clock position in the descending duodenum (Fig. 16-7). Its orifice is usually difficult to observe with the end-viewing panendoscope used for this examination. The accessory papilla, the orifice of Santorini's duct can sometimes be observed slightly proximal to the ampulla of Vater in the 1 o'clock position. The instrument is pulled back, with the endoscopist slowly manipulating the controls to again survey the walls of the duodenum, stomach, and esophagus. As a final maneuver prior to removing the endoscope,

the tip of the instrument can be directed slightly upward and to the left just after exiting the cricopharyngeus region. This step brings the vocal cords into view and permits a rapid assessment of this area.

Therapeutic Interventions During Upper Endoscopy

The ability to deliver endoscopic therapy has increased greatly in recent years as technologies permit treatment at a distance through the working channel of the endoscope. These applications include the ability to coagulate bleeding lesions with monopolar or bipolar probes, or to inject them with long needle injection catheters. Esophageal varices can be treated with injection sclerotherapy or rubber band ligation, controlling hemorrhage and eventually obliterating the large venous trunks. Small-caliber, hydrostatic balloons can be introduced through the endoscope to dilate esophageal, anastomotic, and pyloric strictures, and laser energy can be directed through the scope to debulk obstructing

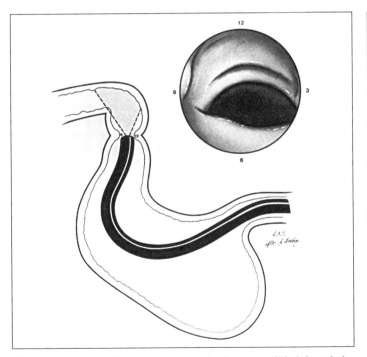

Fig. 16-6. Inspection of the duodenal bulb is often best accomplished through the pylorus or with the scope's tip in the pyloric channel. The superior duodenal fold marks the downward turn of the second portion of the duodenum. (From Ponsky JL. Atlas of Surgical Endoscopy. St. Louis: Mosby, 1992. Reproduced with permission.)

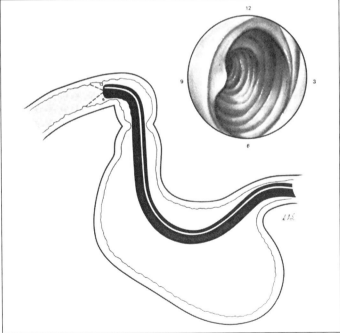

Fig. 16-7. Once in the descending duodenum, the scope is pulled back and straightened. The ampulla of Vater can be seen in profile at the 9 o'clock position on the medial duodenal wall. (From Ponsky JL. Atlas of Surgical Endoscopy. St. Louis: Mosby, 1992. Reproduced with permission.)

esophageal tumors or to treat vascular lesions of the stomach. Gastric polyps are excised using wire snares with electrocautery, and a myriad of tools are available for the endoscopic removal of foreign bodies. Additionally, the endoscope has been used to direct the placement of gastrostomy tubes used for feeding or gastric decompression.

ERCP involves the use of a side-viewing duodenoscope to visualize and cannulate the ampulla of Vater. This technique is an extension of routine upper endoscopy, but it requires more training and experience to become proficient. While providing useful diagnostic information regarding the status of the biliary and pancreatic ductal systems, the therapeutic extensions of this method have been exciting, including removal of common duct stones, stenting of malignant biliary obstruction, and management of biliary leaks after laparoscopic cholecystectomy.

Technique of Colonoscopy

For effective examination of the colon, proper cleansing must be accomplished before the procedure. This process can involve a mechanical preparation including up to 48 hours of a clear liquid diet before the procedure, accompanied by cathartics such as citrate of magnesia and enemas just before starting the procedure. Alternatively, hypertonic lavage-type preparations, usually containing polyethylene glycol, can be used to purge the colonic contents in approximately 4 hours. The latter approach is highly effective and widely used, although somewhat distasteful to the patient.

The left lateral decubitus position is used to begin the procedure, although it is common to turn the patient occasionally during the course of the procedure to facilitate passage of the instrument through tortuous areas. A careful digital rectal examination should precede introduction of the scope in order to dilate the rectum as well as to ensure that no low-lying lesions are overlooked. The colonoscope is positioned in the rectal vault and inserted proximally by a combination of maneuvers, which include manipulation of the endoscope tip with the control knobs, advancement and torsion of the instrument shaft, repeated hooking of the scope's tip around colonic folds and withdrawal to remove redundant coils in the shaft, and repeated suctioning (Fig. 16-8). Although early descriptions of the technique involve fluoroscopy to assess the position of the instrument, it is rarely used today.

The colonoscope should be advanced only when the lumen ahead is visible. Blind insertion of the scope in hopes that it will slide by is dangerous and can cause perforation. Although the latter method is oc-

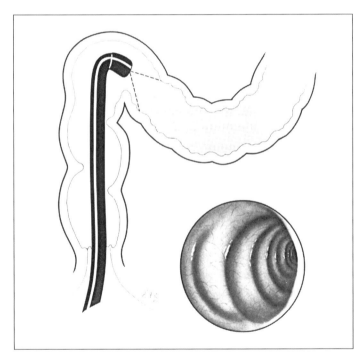

Fig. 16-8. After insertion into the rectal vault, the colonoscope is inserted under direct vision. (From Ponsky JL. Atlas of Surgical Endoscopy. *St. Louis: Mosby, 1992. Reproduced with permission.)*

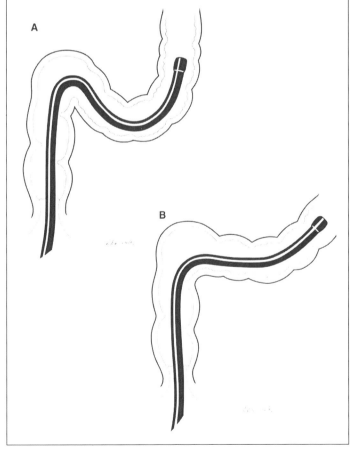

Fig. 16-9. Hooking the tip of the scope around folds and pulling back often permits advancement through tortuous colonic turns. (From Ponsky JL. Atlas of Surgical Endoscopy. *St. Louis: Mosby, 1992. Reproduced with permission.)*

casionally used by experts in difficult circumstances, it remains risky and should be used sparingly. When the lumen is visible ahead, the scope can be inserted further. If the lumen disappears, it is most effective to pull the shaft back slightly and inflate it a bit, and then reassess the position of the lumen. These repeated pull-backs and advancements can be accomplished quite rapidly and facilitate insertion of the instrument through difficult areas (Fig. 16-9). At times, in spite of visible lumen ahead, insertion of the scope's shaft does not result in advancement of the tip. Further introduction of the scope usually causes the patient discomfort as a large sigmoid colon loop is formed, stretching the mesentery. In such situations, it can be useful to have an assistant apply some pressure to, or lift, the left side of the abdomen. This step stiffens the sigmoid loop and allows advancement of the scope. Alternatively, the patient's position can be changed to alter the position of the colonic loops. Placing the patient in the supine position while trying to proceed through a difficult sigmoid colonic segment is often effective.

Even when direct pressure continues to result in advancement of the scope's tip, it is useful to remove redundant loops occasionally by stopping, hooking the tip, and pulling back in an effort to telescope the colon onto the scope's shaft and remove redundant loops (Fig. 16-10). This maneuver is best accomplished after entering the transverse colon and turning downward into the right colon. In fact, pulling back on the shaft can actually produce significant advancement of the scope's tip. Finally, the application of suction, while the instrument is positioned in the center of the colonic lumen, often draws the colon up onto the scope. The latter technique can be particularly useful in intubating the final several centimeters of the cecum.

After insertion to the cecum, the instrument is slowly withdrawn while the tip position is slightly adjusted to ensure complete visualization to the colonic parietes. The anatomic appearance of the various areas of the colonic interior helps the endoscopist define the location of the endoscope's tip and the location of any pathology encountered. The cecum demonstrates an arching convergence of the colonic tenia (often described as the "Mercedes' sign"), and the appendiceal orifice can

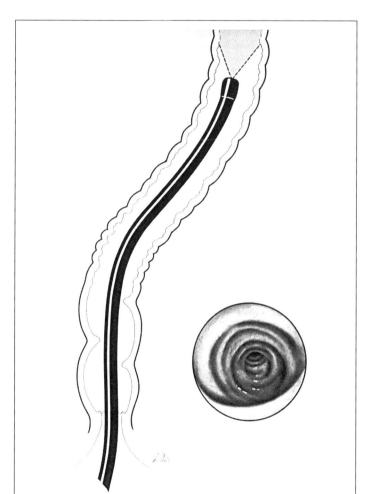

Fig. 16-10. Multiple sequences of hooking and pulling back should result in straightening of the colonic loops and telescoping of the colonic segments onto the scope. (From Ponsky JL. Atlas of Surgical Endoscopy. St. Louis: Mosby, 1992. Reproduced with permission.)

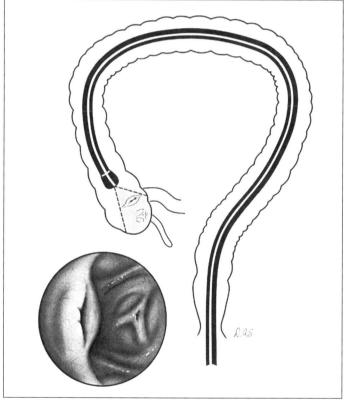

Fig. 16-11. The cecum can be recognized by the confluence of the colonic tenia (the "Mercedes' sign") and the profile of the ileocecal valve. (From Ponsky JL. Atlas of Surgical Endoscopy. St. Louis: Mosby, 1992. Reproduced with permission.)

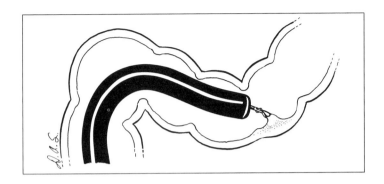

Fig. 16-12. A hot biopsy forceps permits sampling of small lesions with their simultaneous destruction. Care must be taken to avoid excessive application of current with subsequent transmural injury.

usually be defined. Just slightly above (distal) this area is the ileocecal valve, appearing as a slightly thickened fold, occasionally yellow in hue secondary to some lipomatous infiltration (Fig. 16-11). The hepatic flexure transmits the bluish cast of the liver adjacent to it. Triangular folds are the distinguishing anatomic feature of the transverse colon, and long segments of the lumen can be viewed at one time. Care should be taken to look behind large folds for lesions, such as small neoplasms, which may be hidden behind them.

As the scope is withdrawn from the transverse colon past the splenic flexure, the sharp turns can hinder complete examination of the lumen, and reinsertion past this point several times may be necessary to accomplish satisfactory examination of the area. The descending colon usually ap-

A.

B.

C.

D.

Fig. 16-13. A. Pedunculated polyps are surrounded by a polypectomy snare. B. The snare is tightened at the junction of the stalk and the polyp head. C. Coagulation current is then used to transect the stalk. D. The head is retrieved for pathologic examination.

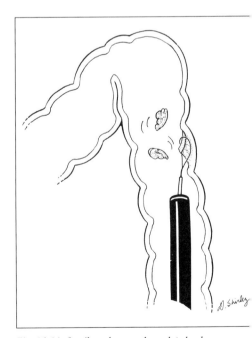

Fig. 16-14. Sessile or large pedunculated polyps can require piecemeal excision. All fragments should be retrieved for pathologic examination.

pears as a long straight tube with little haustration, and the endoscopist will recognize entry into the sigmoid colon when the lumen turns frequently and folds become eccentric. Finally, the endoscopist will note that the rectum displays prominent vasculature and a widened lumen.

Once the colonoscope has been withdrawn to the level of the rectal columns, a retroflexed view of the rectal vault is usually performed to ensure that lesions just adjacent to the anal opening are not overlooked. The retroflexion is accomplished by directing the tip of the instrument severely upward while rotating the shaft of the scope to the left and inserting it further. Should the patient experience pain with this maneuver, the scope should be withdrawn and the procedure restarted. Satisfactory retroflexion is recognized by visualization of the scope entering the rectum, with the dentate line clearly visible. In this position, the scope is brought closer to the dentate line by withdrawing the shaft. Rotation of the shaft permits full examination of the rectal vault. Finally, the scope is straightened, air is suctioned from the colonic lumen, and the scope is removed.

Therapy During Colonoscopy

The most frequent interventions performed at colonoscopy are biopsy and polypectomy. Biopsy forceps can be passed through the working channel of the colonoscope to sample tissue. Areas of suspected neoplasia, dysplasia, or inflammation are sampled. Insulated forceps with large jaws permit simultaneous biopsy and thermal destruction of small lesions (Fig. 16-12). Coagulation current is used in small bursts to accomplish this step, while care is taken that excessive energy, which might cause a transmural burn, is not applied.

Polypectomy is the most common therapeutic application of colonoscopy. Techniques have been well described and involve the encirclement of polypoid tissue with a wire loop, subsequent tightening of the loop, and application of coagulation current to effect separation of the tissue (Fig. 16-13). Small or pedunculated polyps are removed with one application of the snare loop, whereas larger or sessile lesions usually require piecemeal excision.

Samples are retrieved with suction or baskets and sent for pathologic examination (Fig. 16-14). Additional therapeutic interventions through the colonoscope include laser ablation of tumors and vascular malformations, colonic decompression, and detorsion of volvulus.

Summary

Digestive endoscopy has evolved from an interesting diagnostic curiosity to a major therapeutic modality in the approach to gastrointestinal disease. Techniques and technology continue to proliferate, expanding the opportunities for minimally invasive therapy, and benefiting patients. Surgeons must be introduced to these methods early in their training, and gastrointestinal surgeons should become proficient in their performance. The lines of traditional surgery and minimally invasive therapy have become increasingly blurred as surgeons incorporate the techniques of digestive endoscopy into their delivery of patient care.

Suggested Reading

Cotton PB, Williams CB. *Practical Gastrointestinal Endoscopy* (3rd ed). Oxford: Blackwell, 1990.

Guillem J, et al. The impact of colonoscopy on the early detection of colonic neoplasms in patients with rectal bleeding. *Ann Surg* 206:606, 1987.

Ponsky JL. *Atlas of Surgical Endoscopy*. St. Louis: Mosby, 1992.

Schrock T. Colon and rectum: Diagnostic techniques. In R Condon (ed), *Shackelford's Surgery of the Alimentary Tract, Volume 4: Colon and Anorectum* (3rd ed.), Philadelphia: Saunders, 1991.

Schuman BM, Sugawa C. Diagnostic endoscopy of upper gastrointestinal bleeding. In C Sugawa, BM Schuman, CE Lucas, (eds.), *Gastrointestinal Bleeding*. New York: Igaku-Schoin, 1992.

Shinya H. *Colonoscopy: Diagnosis and Treatment of Colonic Diseases*. Tokyo: Igaku-Shoin, 1982.

Winawer S, Schottenfeld D, Flehinger B. Colorectal cancer screening. *J Natl Cancer Inst* 83:243, 1991.

EDITOR'S COMMENT

Upper and lower gastrointestinal endoscopes have become the most important instruments available for diagnosis, and sometimes treatment, of lesions of the upper and lower gastrointestinal tract. Our reliance on these diagnostic interventions has become so great that the surgeon who does not perform endoscopy should observe all endoscopic procedures in order to see firsthand what is a remarkable display of the nature and extent of the disease process to be treated surgically. Citable examples include inflammatory bowel disease, small neoplasia of both upper and lower intestinal tract, vascular anomalies of the stomach or colon, and numerous other lesions. Training programs should provide the opportunity for surgical trainees to learn these techniques. Modern technology and the video monitor can illuminate the precise pathology.

Enteroscopy of the small intestine will be possible in many institutions in the near future. The very long slender enteroscope is not yet as accurate or precise a localizer of a disease process as is the upper gastrointestinal endoscope or the colonoscope, but constant improvements in the available technology will undoubtedly change that circumstance. Hypotonic duodenography and radiographic contrast studies of the small intestine are easier to do, but they are limited to lesions that alter the outline of the intestine. The enteroscope can uncover mucosal variations; inflammation; and small, multiple tumors that the radiologist is seldom able to firmly identify.

Limitations of endoscopic procedures still exist. Lower gastrointestinal hemorrhage is discouraging to the endoscopist, since it is almost impossible to keep the lens clear of tarlike blood mixed with stool. In addition, it is unusual for colonoscopy to give the endoscopist a precise view of the bleeding lesion during an acute and significant bleed. However, once the bleeding has stopped, viewing lesions that are present becomes a far more practical matter and is generally widely accomplished. Upper gastrointestinal hemorrhage is much easier to diagnose and often treat through the endoscope since the blood is fluid, and even clotted blood can be irrigated out of the stomach and duodenum to provide accurate and helpful information concerning the source of the bleed.

The incidence of complications of lower gastrointestinal endoscopy has diminished steadily in the past decade, with the overall incidence of significant complications of perforation or hemorrhage from colonoscopy (from polypectomy or biopsy) in the range of 0.1 to 0.15 percent. The exact incidence of significant complications of upper GI endoscopy, such as perforation of the esophagus, pneumoperitoneum, or bleeding from excision of a lesion of the upper gastrointestinal tract is probably of the same magnitude. The more invasive and somewhat more hazardous therapeutic interventions, such as papillotomy and pancreatic duct cannulation during ERCP have substantially higher complication rates, with significant bleeding from the papillotomy at approximately 0.5 percent and pancreatitis following pancreatography at 2 to 4 percent.

Nevertheless, the diagnostic information that has become available to the pancreatobiliary surgeon in the past few years has made us totally reliant on the truly remarkable amount of information that we can obtain in both benign and malignant disease of the pancreatobiliary apparatus.

R.J.B.

17

Basic Techniques of Diagnostic and Therapeutic Minimally Invasive Surgery (Laparoscopy, Thoracoscopy)

Abe Fingerhut Bertrand Millat

We will treat herein only those operations that in our opinion may have a real place in the armamentarium of the general surgeon performing video-assisted laparoscopic and thoracoscopic surgery. These include operations for which the advantages are obvious (if not overwhelming, and still never formally proved), such as cholecystectomy, but also operations that we believe should or are becoming the gold standard, such as surgery of the common bile duct, surgical repair of gastroesophageal reflux disease (GERD), and Heller's myotomy, and, last, procedures that have not been proved to be any better than traditional, open surgery, but for which evidence is accumulating and the advantages or disadvantages will soon be known, such as inguinal hernia repair.

We will not deal with appendectomy, intestinal obstruction, colonic, or gastric (ulcer) surgery. We do not believe that appendectomy should be performed laparoscopically as such, not that it seems difficult or dangerous to do so, but because, in the male patient at least, laparoscopic appendectomy has no proven advantage over open appendectomy and costs much more. Because of the high rate of appendectomies with removal of "normal" appendices for gynecologic diseases in the young premenopausal female, diagnostic laparoscopy may well be the first step in the presence of lower right quadrant abdominal pain associated with guarding, fever over 38°C, and WBC over 10,000/mm³. Laparoscopy allows adequate pelvic exploration that would oth-

erwise be impossible through a small gridiron incision. Once the diagnosis is made, appendectomy can then be performed either laparoscopic or open. According to randomized published trials, the rate of incisional infection may be lower but the rate of deep abscess is higher. There is no proven advantage, however, between laparoscopic and open appendectomy. The diagnosis and the treatment of acute intestinal obstruction are difficult laparoscopically. Laparoscopic surgery has not been proved to be of any real interest in this setting, and the conversion and complication rates are high. Laparoscopic colonic surgery has not been shown to be more effective than open surgery, whether for carcinoma or benign disease. Moreover, it is associated with much more morbidity (over 30%) and higher costs. Colonic surgery should be performed only in controlled studies, particularly in the case of carcinoma.

Elective surgery for duodenal ulcer is rarely performed in 1995. Perforated duodenal ulcer has been treated laparoscopically, the usual treatment being closure of the perforation either by simple suture or reinforced by omental patch (*Current Opinion in Surgery*). At least two controlled trials have shown, however, that definitive (open) surgery (truncal vagotomy) for duodenal ulcer perforation provides better long-term results. It is not known whether Taylor's posterior truncal vagotomy and anterior seromyotomy, the operation most often performed under videolaparoscopy, provides similar results in this setting.

Laparoscopy and thoracoscopy are being reported with increased frequency in the trauma setting. In our opinion, both are of limited value and need to be evaluated further before they can be advocated for widespread use. Clinical signs and hemodynamic status are the priority decision strong points as to whether or not to perform surgical exploration. According to several authors, diagnostic laparoscopy may be indicated in certain hemodynamically stable patients with positive diagnostic peritoneal lavage to eliminate a nonbleeding lesion and avoid a nontherapeutic laparotomy. Hospital stay for nonoperative surveillance may then be shorter. Therapeutic laparoscopic procedures should remain the exception in trauma. Thoracoscopic repair of stab wounds to the diaphragm, on the other hand, seems interesting and will be described.

Video-assisted thoracoscopic surgery is emerging as a widely used technique for treatment of pneumothorax and will be addressed. Other thoracoscopic procedures are not covered here.

Much has been written about the potential benefits of laparoscopy and thoracoscopy in diagnostic evaluation for carcinoma. These procedures are straightforward, provided that visualization is adequate for tissue retrieval for pathology. In association with other diagnostic procedures including laparoscopic sonography, direct vision of the abdominal cavity and its contents may help to define the stage of disease and to determine the proper strategy for abdominal or thoracic carcinoma. A theoretical advantage is the diagnosis of unsuspected carcinomatosis precluding unnecessary laparotomy. On the other hand, port implants of carcinoma have been noted in cases considered for curative resection, and, in our opinion, video-assisted staging has not yet been sufficiently evaluated or standardized.

General Considerations

The prerequisites for laparoscopic surgery as regards the profile of the patient include careful assessment of the risk of cardiac compromise when the abdomen is inflated under pressure with carbon dioxide as the preload is decreased and the afterload increased. The respiratory compromise is usually less of a problem. Bleeding disorders have to be taken into consideration. Last, but not least, it must be remembered that conversion to open surgery is always a possibility so that the candidate for laparoscopic surgery should be a potential candidate for open surgery as well. As such, the patient should always be prepped and draped so that conversion to open surgery can be made without delay.

Spontaneous micturition before anesthesia avoids the need for bladder catheterization, and antibiotic prophylaxis is routinely administered. The patient is (most often) under general anesthesia.

Patient Position and Draping; Surgeon's Position

For most supracolonic procedures in France, the surgeon usually stands between the legs of the patient, who is placed in the lithotomy position, whereas in the United States, the surgeon usually stands on the left (or right) according to the procedure. When the procedure is in the lower part of the abdomen, the patient is positioned supine with the arms adducted, allowing the surgeon and assistant(s) to stand at the patient's upper torso and neck. The television monitor is placed opposite the surgeon, and should always be in the general direction of the *instruments*. An additional monitor for the assistant is especially useful when the assistant stands opposite the surgeon.

The *pneumo peritoneum* is established by insertion of a Veress needle, either in the midline, near the umbilicus, or, in patients with a previous midline incision, in one of the hypochondria. Typically, the Veress needle is inserted below the umbilicus (no need to incise the skin), with the skin held up by the left hand (on the left) of the surgeon and the right hand (on the right) of the assistant. With experience, the surgeon recognizes the typical "click" of the spring mechanism, indicating that the needle point has entered the peritoneum. Classically, a syringe containing a few milliliters of saline is attached to the Luer lock and injected; then the aspirate is assessed for blood and urine or fecal matter. In the absence of any of these, the laparoscopic procedure can proceed. It is important to observe the pressure gauge closely. A low- or negative-pressure reading usually means that the needle is within the abdominal wall. Intra-abdominal pressure should not be allowed to increase more than 2 to 4 mm Hg per liter of carbon dioxide insufflated. Manual precussion of the prehepatic region is an easy way to monitor the correct progress of the pneumoperitoneum.

Trocars are inserted after an adequate skin incision, not too small if burning of the skin margins is to be avoided, and not too wide, in order to preclude leakage of the pneumoperitoneum. Once the pneumoperitoneum is satisfactorily created, the first blunt-nosed trocar can be inserted blindly (closed technique) if the abdomen has not yet been violated by previous surgery. The other trocars are always inserted under direct intra-abdominal vision. Particular attention must be paid to the abdominal volume foreseen once the pneumoperitoneum is achieved and to the thickness of the abdominal wall for choosing the proper sites of trocar placement. In obese patients the classic umbilicus site for the laparoscope is, in fact, rarely the best choice. Generally speaking, the thicker the abdominal wall, the closer the port should be to the operation field. The thickness of the abdominal wall can limit the maneuverability of instruments within the abdomen. Accordingly, it may be necessary to modify the site of trocars, as well as to change the placement of the optical device during operation.

Most of the disposable and some of the reusable trocars are provided with a so-called safety system, the aim of which is to

prevent underlying visceral wounds. Attention must be paid to the fact that this system is *not* 100 percent foolproof. Catastrophic injuries to major vessels have been described associated with "vigorous" introduction of trocars in patients with a thin abdominal wall (children and the elderly, for instance). One must remember that the aortic bifurcation is located vertically just beneath the umbilicus. To minimize the risk of puncture, the right- (left) handed surgeon should place him- or herself on the left (right) of the patient and introduce the first (blind) trocar at a 45-degree angle toward the pelvis. The "force" with which the trocar is inserted must be incremented progressively and controlled.

Intraoperative adhesions secondary to previous surgery may restrict indications for laparoscopic surgery. Complications such as perforation of bowel and injury to blood vessels during placement of trocars have been reported when adhesions attach the viscera or omentum to the anterior abdominal wall. If the patient has already had a previous midline incision, the Veress needle should be inserted in an unviolated part of the abdomen (hypochondrium or iliac fossa). If this does not work, a 10-mm blunt-nosed trocar should be inserted with the open technique or with the Visiport (USS) or Optiview (Ethicon), also in an unviolated area. Once the trocar has been inserted, a small volume of carbon dioxide is inflated. When 5 to 8 mm Hg pressure is reached, the feasibility of inserting the other trocars and of the procedure itself is re-evaluated. In the case of digital exploration of the port hole, it may be necessary to insert a pursestring in the skin around the trocar to ensure airtightness.

A reusable Veress needle is highly recommended in all procedures to curtail costs of laparoscopic surgery. As stated, the safety system must be checked routinely before each use.

Normally, a pneumoperitoneum pressure of 12 to 14 mm Hg is necessary to adequately view the peritoneal cavity. In certain operations, the pressure can be lowered to 10 mm Hg after the initial exploration. Several "gasless" apparatuses are currently available, but have not been adopted by all because proper exposure is still less than ideal. These apparatuses can be indicated in patients with cardiac compromise.

All trocar wounds of 10 mm or more are routinely closed with a Vicryl (Ethicon) suture (Vicryl, 0.13-mm round ½ circle needle). The skin is closed either with skin staples (USS) or fast absorbable Vicryl.

Simple Cholecystectomy

Though laparoscopic cholescystectomy (LC) was first performed by E. Mühe in Germany and then by Ph. Mouret in France, F. Dubois and J. Perissat were the first to publish their cases of successful LC. Through fierce industry-driven competition and patients' preference for minimal invasive procedures, widely diffused through the media, LC was universally adopted and rapidly became the "gold standard" for symptomatic cholelithiasis even before randomized trials could be performed.

Indications

The indications for LC in itself should be no different from those for traditional cholecystectomy. In view of its advantages, LC is indicated in documented, symptomatic cholelithiasis, and more rarely in asymptomatic cholelithiasis as in porcelain gallbladder (because of the risk of cancer), or immunosuppression. Absolute contraindications include patients unfit for general anesthesia, with known gallbladder carcinoma, and with uncorrected coagulopathy. Relative contraindications include obstructive lung disease, morbid obesity, and cirrhosis with portal hypertension. Pregnancy is a relative contraindication, but as gynecologists have been performing laparoscopic procedures for many years, this has recently been questioned. Patients with acute cholecystitis, empyema with or without peritonitis, cholecystoenteric fistulas, and previous upper abdominal surgery are undergoing laparoscopic procedures more and more often as experience with these entities increases but the conversion rates remain high. LC can be combined with other laparoscopic procedures, as desired.

Insertion of Trocars

A pneumo peritoneum is created through the reusable Veress needle inserted just below the umbilicus (Fig. 17-1). A 10- to 12-mm quarter-moon infraumbilical incision allows introduction of the first (same diameter) trocar, through which the optical device is inserted. A second 10- to 12-mm trocar is inserted 1 to 2 cm to the left of the midline, halfway between the first trocar and the xiphoid under direct vision. Likewise, a 5-mm trocar is then introduced 2 cm caudad and 2 cm medial to the anterior and superior iliac spine.

Ordinarily, one of the authors (AF) uses the (original) three-trocar technique. A fourth trocar, inserted near the xiphoid and used to retract the liver, is often used.

No matter how many trocars are inserted and whatever the technique performed, a pair of (small-toothed) grasping forceps is inserted through the right iliac port and picks up the fundus and then the infundibulum (sometimes after maneuvering with a second instrument in another port). We believe that it is best to pull the gallbladder to the right (flag technique) with these forceps rather than vertically (US technique), thus exposing Calot's triangle (Fig. 17-2).

Dissection is begun close to the gallbladder, with tissues being lysed and pushed from right to left with a blunt dissector, forceps, or closed scissors. Before visualization of Calot's triangle, coagulation

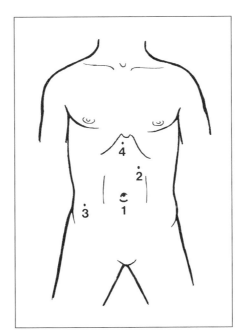

Fig. 17-1. Trocars are placed as seen on a line running from the extremity of the 12th rib on the left to the extremity of the 8th or 9th rib on the right. The line should be higher in a patient who is obese.

should be avoided. Although many prefer to use bipolar as compared with monopolar coagulation here, we choose to see all the structures first and then only to use (monopolar) coagulation sparingly.

The peritoneum covering the cystic duct is then opened *both on the anterior and posterior aspects* (the so-called flag technique). This "opens" the triangle of Calot and facilitates the identification of its boundaries. As soon as the duct becomes apparent, the dissecting scissors can be gently pushed through Calot's triangle and the cystic duct dissected free for 1.0 to 1.5 cm. The cystic artery usually is obvious, running parallel to the cystic duct, and should ideally be identified and dissected free at this time, but not ligated or clipped before complete identification of all anatomic structures in the area. Complementary information is obtained through intraoperative cholangiograms, performed routinely in our practice. The cystic duct is then clipped near the gallbladder with cholangiography (Fig. 17-3).

Intraoperative Cholangiogram

Performance of intraoperative cholangiography (IOC) during laparoscopy is controversial. According to the positive predictive values of biochemical tests and ultrasound findings used preoperatively to detect common bile duct (CBD) stones, nearly half of patients thus selected undergo useless but also potentially harmful preoperative investigations, that is, echoendoscopy or endoscopic retrograde cholangiography (ERC), or both. Overall, one out of three CBD stones will not be suspected preoperatively. The false-negative rate in patients with successful catheterization and failure rates of preoperative ERC are in the range of 3 to 5 percent. Eleven to 35 percent of patients with preoperative endoscopic sphincterotomy (ES) have residual stones at the time of IOC. If IOC is performed selectively in patients with ultrasonographic dilated CBD (diameter > 6 mm), CBD stones may be overlooked in 2 percent of patients, that is, in 13 to 20 percent of patients with CBD stones (the prevalence being between 10 and 15%). In our opinion, and to those who firmly believe that detection and extraction of all CBD stones, whether symptomatic or not, are essential to correct surgical treatment of biliary lithiasis, routine

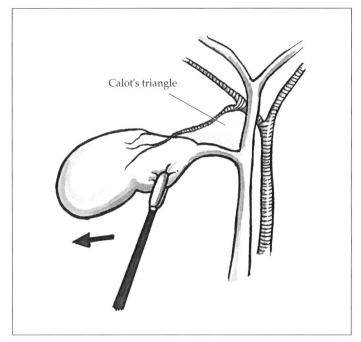

Fig. 17-2. The infundibulum of the gallbladder is grasped and pulled to the right exposing Calot's triangle.

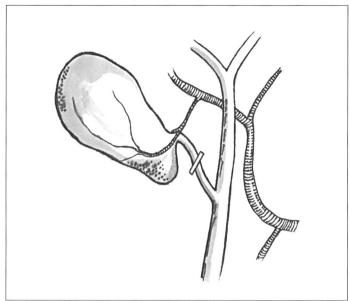

Fig. 17-3. The cystic duct is clipped near the gallbladder after dissection of the immediate area.

IOC seems unavoidable. In terms of cost-effectiveness, if IOC is performed routinely, patients fit for surgery and scheduled for LC do not need other costly preoperative investigations for detection of CBD stones.

Another (controversial) point of interest is that IOC may minimize the potential for CBD injuries by clarifying uncertain anatomy, and indicate without any delay whether an iatrogenic injury has occurred, provided that a complete intrahepatic cholangiogram is obtained.

Feasibility rates of IOC during LC are probably influenced more by the willingness to perform IOC than by whether or not it is possible to do so. If, however, the catheter does not enter the cystic duct easily, maneuvers have been described to attain success, although caution is advised not to force the passage in order to avoid perforation of the main bile duct or its junction. The time required for IOC ranges between 5 and 15 minutes. Several techniques have been described, some requiring special and expensive instruments. The two techniques outlined herein have been validated by several hundred IOCs performed routinely with over 99 percent feasibility.

One technique consists of catheterization of the cystic duct with a No. 4 French catheter placed through an Ohlsen cholangio-clamp inserted through the right lateral subcostal port (Fig. 17-4). This clamp has a channel, allowing easy introduction of the catheter, and with jaws that, when closed over the incision in the cystic duct, secure the catheter and prevent leakage of contrast medium. The following technical points are associated with the success of IOC. First, catheterization of the cystic duct is easier when the incision is performed with scissors introduced previously through the right lateral subcostal port (same trocar as that used for the cholangioclamp). In the three-trocar technique, the same scissors used for dissection are used to open the cystic duct laterally, through the left port. Second, although initial dissection and control of the cystic duct near Hartmann's pouch are often advocated, careful dissection of the duct until reaching the junction with the CBD will make it easier to cannulate. Spiral valves, a small diameter, and the length of the cystic duct are definite obstacles to successful IOC. When the end of the catheter reaches the CBD, spontaneous reflux of bile through the catheter previously filled with contrast medium is an indication that quality IOC can be expected.

Third, the ideal direction of the cholangio-clamp is perpendicular to the cystic duct. Two to 3 cm of catheter should be left free at the opening of the channel of the cholangioclamp, and the extremity of the catheter is held and introduced into the cystic duct with another forceps passed through the left port while Hartmann's pouch is held with the jaws of the cholangioclamp itself. Once the catheter is introduced, it is secured to the cystic duct with the clamp and filling of the CBD can begin. The laparoscope is withdrawn from the fluoroscopic field of vision and a smooth palpator is inserted into the left lateral port for further maneuvers. Although radiographic techniques can be adapted according to available resources, a C-arm screening apparatus using an image magnifier with hard-copy capability has definite advantages. Our personal technique consists of gentle compression of the CBD under real-time fluoroscopy with an atraumatic instrument (palpator). Gentle compression associated with initial injection of 2 to 3 ml contrast medium allows thin-layer visualization and detection of small filling defects along with the ability to discriminate false-positive images due to air bubbles. Free flow of contrast material into the duodenum must be obtained, eventually with magnified visualization of Oddi's

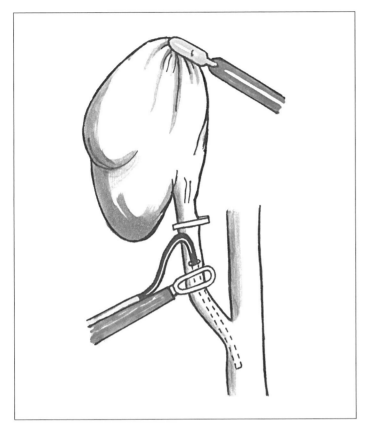

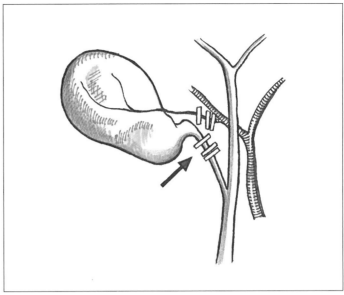

Fig. 17-5. The cystic duct is doubly clipped proximally and divided, followed by the cystic artery.

Fig. 17-4. Intraoperative cholangiogram (IOC). A catheter is introduced into the cystic duct via an Ohlsen Cholangioclamp.

sphincter, obtained with high-resolution apparatuses. Compression of the CBD with the palpator makes it easier to fill the intrahepatic bile ducts; Trendelenburg's position or intravenous morphine sulfate administration, or both, are of little, if any, use to this end. Filling of the entire bile duct during IOC is mandatory for a clear-cut definition of anatomy and detection of biliary ducts at risk for injury due to anatomic variations. In this view, full knowledge of the frequent variations from normal biliary anatomy is mandatory when performing any hepatobiliary procedure, even the simplest LC.

A less expensive alternative to the cholangioclamp is the use of a hollow gasketed needle introduced electively under the right subcostal margin, directly through the skin. The same No. 4 Fr cholangiocatheter can be used and the rest of the procedure is similar. When using this technique, attention must be paid to the site of introduction of the needle, which is chosen according to the anatomy of the hepatoduodenal ligament and the orientation of the cystic duct, visualized while the index finger palpates the potential landmarks on the skin. When the needle is introduced into the abdominal cavity, the opening in the cystic duct is "presented" for catheterization, according to the axis of the needle, with a forceps grasping Hartmann's pouch. When the extremity of the catheter reaches the CBD and provided the injection pressure of contrast is moderate, anchoring the catheter in place with a clip placed across the duct is not required and bile or contrast medium leakage seldom occurs.

Usually, the cystic duct stump is doubly clipped (Fig. 17-5). If an internal drainage is indicated, absorbable suture material is used to secure the drain. We prefer the Escat or the Pedinielli drains. We avoid the Endoloop material, which in our opinion is reabsorbed much too quickly. We usually secure the drain with Vicryl sutures.

The cystic artery can now be divided between two clips. We always place at least two clips on the proximal artery (and cystic duct stump) before division. The peritoneum behind the artery should be opened adequately before division, to be sure that the right hepatic artery is not at risk, which will usually open the plane of dissection of the gallbladder. With traction on the gallbladder to the right and slightly cephalad, the areolar tissues between the two layers of peritoneum spreading out from the liver to cover the anterior and posterior aspects of the gallbladder are identified. With the scissors and coagulation, the space between the gallbladder bed and the gallbladder is progressively opened and the gallbladder is dissected free. We always insert the gallbladder into a plastic sac before extraction. Extraction is made through the left paramedian 10- to 12-mm port (two strong fascia layers) and never on the midline. No abdominal drainage is needed. Wound closure follows the protocol outlined previously.

Particular Situations and Special Tricks and Hints

Certain anatomic variations and pathologic states can influence the ease with which cholecystectomy is performed.

Simple adhesions between the gallbladder and the duodenum/colon/stomach are usually avascular and can easily be taken down by ordinary dissection. Care must be taken not to coagulate near the hollow viscus. Adhesions with the liver must be freed with caution, avoiding laceration of the capsule, which will cause troublesome bleeding. Adhesions on the upper surface of the liver, with the abdominal wall or the diaphragm, or both, need not be taken down routinely.

A short cystic duct may be a threat to lateral impingement on the common bile duct. It is essential to identify the cysticobiliary confluence anatomically and through intraoperative cholangiograms before any ligation is performed. It is best to suture-ligate the short cystic stump rather than to place two clips, risking lateral clipping of the common bile duct. Furthermore, this condition, more than any other, should preclude the use of electrocautery in the area. The best way of avoiding injury to the common bile duct is to adequately visualize both edges of the duct before clipping. The very rare cholecystocholedochal, cholecystoduodenal, or cholecystocolonic fistula is usually suspected when dense adhesions are noted. Operative cholangiograms can occasionally define the fistula. Although attempts at laparoscopic repair have been reported, conversion is usually indicated.

Occasionally the cystic duct is wider than the length of the available clips (11 mm). In this case, we always prefer to suture-ligate the cystic remnant rather than to use two staggered clips.

Routine intraoperative cholangiograms will on occasion demonstrate anatomic variations such as an aberrant bile duct. Only those that drain into the vesicular bed can, if unrecognized and not selectively ligated, give rise to postoperative bile collection.

A difficult extraction may be due to a large stone, retained bile in the closed gallbladder, or a thickened or fragile gallbladder wall. In any case, the gallbladder should be placed in a sac before extraction. The large stone can be fragmented once a forceps can be introduced into the open end of the sac outside the abdomen. Retained bile can be suctioned out in a similar manner. If this is not sufficient, the orifice should be enlarged (and closed), avoiding the forceful extraction. If the sac is pulled on too hard, the sac will burst, dispersing bile and stones in the wound and in the abdominal cavity.

Perforation of the gallbladder during dissection or extraction is not a reason to convert routinely. The only adverse consequence to perforated gallbladders is an operation that takes longer. Spilled stones are occasionally difficult to retrieve. Every effort must be made to retrieve the pigmented variety, which is known to harbor bacteria and lead to potential infectious complications.

The retracted and/or scleroatrophic gallbladder may be difficult to dissect and especially to isolate from the liver. If mucosa is left behind, it is best to coagulate it.

Carcinoma is rarely recognized before pathology examination. In any case, and even though this is not sufficient to prevent port seeding, the gallbladder should be placed routinely in a plastic sac before removal from the abdomen.

If a lateral rent is found (or made) in the main bile duct, it is imperative to recognize and treat it immediately. In most instances, immediate conversion to insert a T tube is required. Laparoscopic insertion of a T tube requires experience and mastery of laparoscopic skills. A completion cholangiogram should be obtained in all cases before one leaves the abdomen to make sure that no leak is present and that the drain is correctly positioned.

When dissecting the gallbladder free from the liver, care must be exercised to start the dissection *near* the gallbladder, staying away from the ducts and liver. Once the space is found, delicate traction on the gallbladder, to the right and above, avoids tearing the liver capsule or detachment of the gallbladder bed (especially in acute cholecystitis), both of which may be troublesome sources of bleeding.

If unexpected bleeding occurs during dissection of the cystic artery before the artery can be adequately clipped, calm is a prerequisite to proper control of the situation. It must be remembered that aspiration of the blood will aggravate matters, as the pneumoperitoneum will disappear, and bleeding will continue while one waits for the pneumoperitoneum to refill. High flow irrigation is the proper means of quickly seeing the source of bleeding, which should be grasped with a forceps on the left and then clipped under direct vision.

Direct clipping within the structures of Calot's triangle is *very dangerous* and *must be avoided* at all costs. If simple grasping and rapid clipping of the source of bleeding are not achieved, a wide and atraumatic forceps should be placed on the source of bleeding and rapid conversion done. Also, when unexpected bleeding is encountered during dissection of the gallbladder from the liver, the same maneuvers can be accomplished as long as traction is exercised on the gallbladder. If the gallbladder has already been freed, then a forceps must grasp the bleeder before clipping in order to avoid aggravating the situation.

Acute cholecystitis can singularly complicate the performance of LC. The rate of conversion and of injury to the main bile duct are probably highest in this setting. When any doubt exists as to anatomy, a complete cholangiogram must be obtained *before* division or ligation of any sort. Particular attention should be paid to the dissection of the cystic artery, which may be adherent to the inflamed infundibulum. In the case of acute cholecystitis, provided that operation is performed within the first 24 to 48 hours, edema may actually improve dissection.

Hydrops and *empyema* are two pathologic conditions that may occasionally, but not always, increase difficulty in dissection. In order to avoid laceration of the gallbladder and spillage of bile and stones, it is usually best to puncture the gallbladder directly, void it of all bile, and then place a clamp over the hole.

Bile should be retrieved for culture in all situations.

Common Bile Duct Exploration Under Laparoscopy

Whenever stones are demonstrated during routine laparoscopic IOC, laparoscopic extraction of stones should be attempted. In case of failure of laparoscopic extraction, we prefer to convert to open common bile duct (CBD) exploration, rather than to rely on a potentially successful postoperative extraction with endoscopic sphincterotomy. Patients with suspected CBD stones are routinely informed preoperatively of an eventual open conversion.

Although most technical procedures used for laparoscopic CBD exploration are similar to those performed during open surgery, laparoscopic surgery precludes helpful, normal manual manipulations, duodenum mobilization, and palpation. Whenever CBD exploration is required, our basic technique includes insertion of an additional trocar close to the right subcostal margin. The exact location of this trocar is determined by laparoscopic visualization in order to provide the best angle for insertion of the choledochoscope and instruments. The other trocars (3 or 4) are the same as for cholecystectomy. The position of both the patient and surgeon are also the same.

According to anatomic conditions, a percutaneous stitch to suspend the liver at the level of the round ligament can advantageously replace the infraxiphoid trocar. On the other hand, an additional trocar for insertion of a duodenal retractor lateral to the right rectus muscle is occasionally required for adequate anterior CBD wall exposure. A 0-degree laparoscope is currently used.

The transcystic approach is preferred whenever possible, according to the size of the stones and the cystic duct diameter, respectively. A nondilated CBD is a further indication for the transcystic approach. Careful balloon dilatation of the cystic duct according to the size of the largest stone to be removed may increase the success rate of the transcystic approach. Difficulties in adequate closure due to extreme thinness of the cystic duct wall or even disruption at the cysticocholedochal junction are, however, severe misadventures. We prefer discontinuation of the transcystic maneuvers in favor of choledochotomy whenever easy extraction is not achieved.

During the laparoscopic transcystic approach the CBD should be considered as a closed system. Fluoroscopic visualization provides valuable information for the surgeon. A No. 4 Fr Dormia basket inserted through the right subcostal port is the major tool for stone extraction. The same maneuvers described for cholangiography (smooth instrument inserted in the left trocar) may facilitate stone mobilization and entrapment of the stones in the basket, while preventing stone migration to the upper bile ducts. Re-injection of contrast medium is sometimes required during the extraction maneuvers. Whenever necessary and if the caliber of the cystic duct

permits, choledochoscopy is performed through the cystic duct. A small flexible choledochoscope (3 mm) has been proposed for transcystic CBD exploration, but due to its small caliber, this apparatus is diagnostic rather than therapeutic. In the case of residual stones during choledochoscopy, extraction under direct visualization with a wire basket inserted through the operating channel should be attempted. When choledochoscopy is performed through the cystic duct, angulation at the choledochal junction usually precludes the 180-degree rotation required for exploration toward the hepatic ducts. A completion cholangiogram is mandatory followed by proper closure of the cystic duct with metallic or Absolock absorbable clips (Ethicon-Endosurgery). External biliary drainage through the cystic duct is seldom necessary.

When the stone size is not consistent with retrieval through the cystic duct, we proceed with laparoscopic choledochotomy and endoscopic stone extraction through the choledochotomy. This procedure requires some experience with laparoscopic surgery, including endosuturing techniques. The anterior wall of the supraduodenal CBD wall is exposed and incised with scissors, according to the size of the largest stone to be extracted. Classically, a horizontal incision is preferred when the CBD diameter is small. Prompt and sharp opening of the duct sometimes allows stones to evacuate spontaneously, because of the pressure gradient in the CBD created by cholangiography.

Once the choledochotomy is performed, the CBD is no longer a closed system, and the usual open manipulations to facilitate CBD endoscopic exploration are indeed impossible. To provide adequate irrigation for the proper distention and exploration of the ducts, a special pressure irrigation system is required. As the same instrument channel is used for the advancement of the Dormia or balloon catheters and irrigation, the resistance to irrigation created by the narrow channel reduces the possibilities for adequate simultaneous observation and coordinated manipulation in extracting calculi. To overcome this inconvenience the basket wire or balloon catheter can be inserted along the choledochoscope instead of inside the instrument channel. Due to the fact that the tip of the scope can be moved in only one plane, a second assistant is needed to apply rota-

tional forces for adequate exposure. The same assistant has to advance the basket or balloon catheter, while the other provides permanent exposure of the CBD opening with the laparoscope. To enable this teamwork, additional videoequipment with a second camera attached to the eyepiece of the endoscope is very helpful. Extreme care in handling, maintenance, and operation must be exercised because these fiberoptic instruments are fragile and expensive. The fiberoptic choledochoscope should never be inserted directly through a trocar to avoid possible damage to the external sheath of the instrument. The choledochoscope is first placed in a reducer and they are introduced together into the trocar. Any internal manipulation of the instrument with metallic grasping forceps is proscribed. The distal end of the reducer containing the choledochoscope must reach the opening of the CBD. The flexible instrument is then pushed inside the CBD with proper deflection of the tip, and there is no need to grasp the scope. Gallstones are identified and may be free floating. They sometimes evacuate spontaneously on withdrawal of the endoscope because of the irrigation. In the case of floating stones, the Dormia basket or balloon catheter should be positioned beyond the stone to be retrieved under direct vision. The basket is then opened carefully and both the basket and the endoscope are moved together until the stone(s) is entrapped. The endoscope and the basket are then withdrawn together. Repeated endoscopic examinations are necessary to make sure that complete stone evacuation is achieved. The distal and proximal portions of the biliary tree are both inspected easily through choledochotomy. Passing the instrument through the papilla into the duodenum to make sure that the distal end is cleared is useless and inadvisable. The stones are placed inside an Endopouch (Ethicon Endosurgery) or Endocatch (USS) for later removal with the gallbladder.

Most often after clearing the biliary system, a T tube is placed and sewn in place. The latex T tube is modified by removing the distal half of the circumference and shortening the limbs of the horizontal bar. The entire drain is then placed in the abdominal cavity. The long (vertical) limb will be withdrawn with the subcostal trocar at the end of the operation. For insertion of the trimmed limbs in the CBD, it is easier to slip both limbs upward into the choledochotomy while grasping the T junction and then setting the T tube in correct position while pulling carefully on the long limb of the T tube rather than to try to insert the proximal and distal limbs separately. When the choledochotomy is vertical, the T junction is placed at the upper end of the choledochotomy and repair of the CBD is commenced just below the T-tube in the CBD incision, using 5/0 continuous or absorbable sutures. An alternative method is to close the choledochotomy primarily. In that case, a completion cholangiogram through the cystic duct is mandatory, allowing confirmation of an entirely stone-free duct and demonstration of adequate tightness of closure.

Unorthodox techniques, according to available resources, can sometimes be employed. The traditional rigid choledochoscope or rigid stone forceps, or both, have been used successfully for CBD exploration and stone extraction. In this case the rigid instruments are best inserted through the infraxiphoid skin orifice, after removal of the trocar sheath. Similarly, use of the rigid irrigation device, introduced into the choledochotomy, may facilitate spontaneous stone fragment evacuation, providing that the opening is large enough to allow free flow of the fluid on each side of the cannula.

The operation is usually terminated by suction drainage inserted through the right lateral trocar orifice, and placed under direct vision in the infrahepatic area posterior to the hepatoduodenal ligament.

Closure is as mentioned previously for cholecystectomy.

Cholangiograms are obtained through the T tube on the fifth postoperative day and, when normal, the tube should be clamped closed 24 hours later. It is removed on the 21st day in the outpatient department.

Laparoscopic Inguinal Hernia Repair

We will the describe the two most widely used techniques of laparoscopic inguinal hernia repair. Both make use of a preperitoneal mesh, which is inserted either through the *transperitoneal* or the *extraperitoneal* routes. The theoretical problems that surround the question of laparoscopic in-guinal hernia repair are multiple. In favor of the procedure are the minimal invasive character (less skin incision) and "tensionless" hernia repair, as in the open techniques that make use of prostheses, thus theoretically reducing postoperative pain and increasing the possibilities of early return to normal activities, and the risk of tearing of strongly approximated tissues. On the other hand, the procedure still requires general anesthesia in the large majority of cases, incurs the use of expensive resources not required by conventional herniorrhaphy, and cannot be used to perform simple repair for types I or II hernia (Nyhus). In addition, there is the problem of inserting a foreign body, which might not be necessary. The mesh is the only solution irrespective of the parietal defect. Although many studies are currently being undertaken, and some have shown that postoperative pain is lessened, there are not any that have definitely proved that the long-term recurrence rate is less or at least equivalent to that of the gold standard, that is, the open Shouldice repair. Laparoscopic hernia repair is regarded by many surgeons as an excellent indication for recurrent hernia, avoiding dissection of scarred tissues with the ever present risk of injury to the testicular vessels. Even in the case of previous open repair with mesh, repeat repair through the laparoscopic route is practically always possible. Most surgeons performing laparoscopic hernia repair have adopted the transabdominal preperitoneal approach.

Laparoscopic Hernia Repair: The Transabdominal Approach

The bladder must be empty (see below). The abdomen is prepared and draped in a standard fashion. A single video monitor

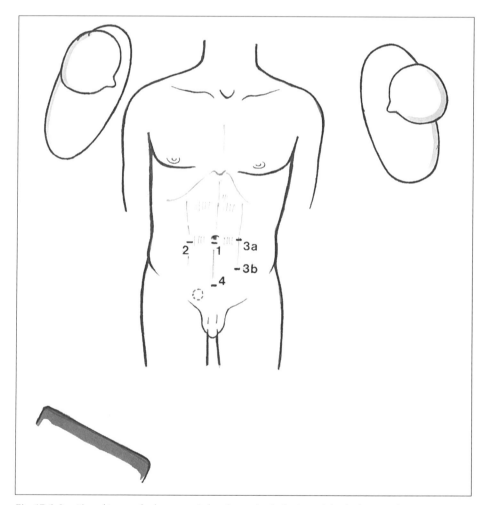

Fig. 17-6. Location of trocars for laparoscopic hernia repair via the transabdominal approach.

is placed at the foot of the operating table. The pneumoperitoneum is established via an umbilical incision using a reusable Veress needle and the abdominal cavity is inflated to a pressure of 15 mm Hg. Simultaneous monitoring of abdominal pressure, inflow rate, and disappearance of hepatic dullness is mandatory during inflation.

A 10-mm safety disposable or reusable trocar is inserted through the umbilical incision (Fig. 17-6). A 0-degree video laparoscope is routinely used. A steep Trendelenburg's position and elevation of the ipsilateral side are helpful, allowing the intestines to slide away from the pelvis. Exploratory laparoscopy allows determination of the type of hernia or hernia defects, along with anatomic landmarks (Fig. 17-7), including the external iliac and inferior epigastric vessels, the pubic tubercle and umbilical fold, the vas deferens and testicular blood vessels, or the round ligament in females. Accessory trocars are placed under direct vision. Left and right ports are located lateral to the rectus sheath. The 10-mm port ipsilateral to the hernia is inserted at the transverse umbilical level (Fig. 17-6[2]). A 10-mm contralateral port is placed at the same level in the case of bilateral hernia (Fig. 17-6[3a]), or a 5-mm port somewhat lower in the case of unilateral hernia (Fig. 17-6[3b]). In the case of bilateral hernia, a midline suprapubic 5-mm accessory port is sometimes useful, particularly in obese patients (Fig. 17-6[4]).

Regardless of the type of defect, a peritoneal incision is made beginning laterally at the level of the anterior and superior iliac spine, extending medially to the ipsilateral umbilical ligament, remaining close to the internal ring. Division of the umbilical ligament is seldom required (i.e., heavy adipose deposits or large direct hernia defect). In this case, care must be taken to avoid injury to the bladder. The posterior peritoneal flap is elevated first and Cooper's ligament is exposed medially. The peritoneal sac is dissected in continuity with the posterior flap and completely freed from the inguinal canal, cord structures, vas deferens, and iliac vessels. Indirect hernia sacs are always dissected and excised irrespective of their size. When a sliding hernia is present, the hollow viscus is dissected free from all peritoneal attachments before the sac is dissected. In females, the round lig-

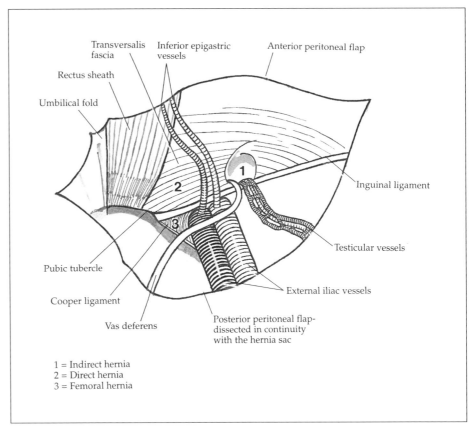

Fig. 17-7. Anatomic landmarks and hernial defects: (1) the location of an indirect hernia, (2) the location of a direct hernia, and (3) the location of a femoral hernia.

ament is ligated and divided at the internal inguinal ring. The anterior leaf of the peritoneum is then elevated, thus exposing the inferior epigastric vessels, the transversalis fascia, the inguinal ligament, the conjoined tendon, and the pubic tubercle. In view of facilitating peritoneal re-approximation over the mesh, it is strongly recommended to keep the anterior flap as large as possible. There usually is no problem in obtaining a large posterior flap. Dissection is considered complete when clear identification of both the anatomic landmarks and hernia defects is consistent with secure and wide covering by the prosthetic mesh.

A 10- × 14-cm polypropylene mesh (Prolene, Ethicon Endosurgery) is introduced through the 10-mm port using a strong grasping instrument inserted through the contralateral port and exteriorized in a retrograde fashion. The posterior edge of the mesh is positioned along Cooper's ligament, over the iliac vessels and laterally along the iliopubic tract. The mesh is unrolled, and pushed up ("uprolled"), posi-

tioned along the transversalis fascia, the transversus abdominis arch, and the conjoined tendon. Provided the mesh is large enough to cover the hernia defects with sufficient margins, it need not be stapled (avoiding further increased costs). In the case of a large direct hernia defect, stapling the mesh along Cooper's ligament, the rectus sheath, and the conjoined tendon to the level of the inferior epigastric vessels avoids potential repeat herniation medially to an unattached mesh. Stapling the posterior edge of the mesh or laterally to the inferior epigastric vessels, however, should be avoided if neurovascular injury is to be avoided. As was mentioned previously, to preclude herniation of other nearby sites, the mesh must cover all the potential abdominal wall defects, fascia transversalis, femoral canal, and internal inguinal ring at the end of the operation.

Once the mesh has been correctly placed, the pneumoperitoneum is reduced to 8 mm Hg, allowing easier re-approximation of the peritoneal flaps. Perfect re-approximation is mandatory to avoid potential repeat herniation through peritoneal defects and intestinal incarceration. In this respect, a continuous absorbable suture seems more secure than stapler re-approximation.

In the case of bilateral hernia, two prostheses can be used and placed separately. A large 13- × 25-cm single mesh covering both sides and passing anterior to the bladder, however, seems to be the most effective procedure. In this case, stapling (increased expense) is useless.

When repair is completed, the instruments and trocars are removed with the deflation of the pneumoperitoneum. Closure of trocar wounds is as outlined previously. In the case of bladder catheterization, the Foley catheter is removed at the end of the procedure.

Laparoscopic Hernia Repair: The Extraperitoneal Approach

Laparoscopic extraperitoneal hernia repair offers several theoretical advantages over the transperitoneal route, including less postoperative pain (strictly tensionless mesh); no peritoneal aggression, and therefore no risk of postoperative complications such as incarceration, with consequent or independent obstruction or intra-abdominal injuries; and no automatic conversion to open or transperitoneal repair necessary if a peritoneal tear occurs, as the insufflation pressure can be kept low. The operative field is the space between the peritoneum and the fascia transversalis and this constitutes one of the disadvantages, as this space is limited. Another disadvantage is that it is more difficult to highly ligate the indirect sac without opening it to ensure that no visceral structures are present before closure.

Indications

Once hernia repair with prosthetic mesh is decided upon and if there are no further contraindications to general anesthesia (generally necessary for this technique), this technique can be used for all types of inguinal hernia. Relative contraindications to the extraperitoneal route are previous scarring due to appendectomy. Absolute contraindications include previous transvesical operation, vascular prostheses, and radiation therapy.

Technique

The patient is placed supine, legs apart, prepped, and draped. The operator is on the left to begin and operates on the side opposite the hernia repair. The first assistant is opposite the operator. The television monitor is placed at the foot of the patient. Because of the limited space, a 30-degree laparoscope is helpful. *A 2-cm horizontal incision* is made approximately 1 cm below the umbilicus. Small retractors are introduced laterally and pull the skin and subcutaneous tissues caudad. The extraperitoneal fatty plane is reached by cutting through the fascia, slightly to the side. (This avoids opening the peritoneum and makes it easier to find the correct plane of dissection).

A 10- to 12-mm trocar is introduced. The optical device is then introduced and pushed until it reaches the retropubic spine. Dissection is pursued with the forceps. No coagulation is necessary. Dissection of the preperitoneal space can also be accomplished with the balloon (inflated with air or water) dissector (Origin) but this is not indispensable and increases costs. If only one side is to be repaired, the surgeon should place the entire palm of one of his or her hands on the side of the rectus muscle that does *not* require operation, in order to leave the subperitoneal space intact on that side. A second 5-mm trocar is inserted in the midline if a bilat-

eral repair is envisioned, and on the opposite side if only one side is to be repaired, at middistance between the initial incision and the pubis. This second trocar is useful in the dissection and should be inserted quickly after the first for dissection (if the balloon dissector is not being used to dissect; i.e., the optical device should not be used to dissect the extraperitoneal space, but just to reach the pubis on the midline). The extraperitoneal space can now be insufflated to 8 mm Hg. The dissection is initiated *lateral* to the epigastric vessels in order to visualize the lateral area that can be seen by transillumination. The dissection should be pursued until Douglas' arcuate line is reached.

The skin is then incised 2 cm above the iliac crest, behind the anterior and superior iliac spine, in order to introduce *by hand* a 12-mm trocar, *without forcing (because the vessels are just behind)*. All three trocars should be placed with the screw device, in order to work with a maximum of the trocar outside the patient (*space is short!*). The fatty tissues should be dissected with two atraumatic forceps, separating the peritoneum from the vessels laterally and the vas deferens medially (Fig. 17-8). Next, a (clawed) forceps is introduced from medial to lateral behind the cord and is pushed all the way out of the lateral trocar.

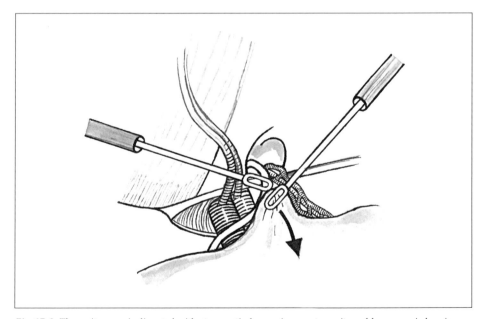

Fig. 17-8. The peritoneum is dissected with atraumatic forceps in an extraperitoneal laparoscopic hernia repair.

A 14- × 10-cm mesh (minimum) is then rolled up and grasped, and introduced into the preperitoneal space. As the cord structures have been freed, the mesh is placed on the hernia area, making sure that all possible defects have been largely covered. If the dimensions of the mesh are chosen correctly, no stapling is necessary. One should verify that the mesh remains in place on release of the pneumopreperitoneum. Another (more expensive but very convenient) solution is to use a special mesh preslitted for the cord (Parietex). The mesh is prepared by tightening the two extremities of the strings, which allows it to be inserted easily into the trocar. The threads at one of the extremities of the mesh are then cut off and the extremity is entered into the extraperitoneal space first. The mesh is placed with the precut slit edge up and is placed behind the cord. The mesh is introduced until the slit is exactly behind the cord and then the (clawed) forceps is raised vertically in order the unroll the mesh conveniently. The remaining threads are then pulled out. The mesh regains its initial (curved) shape in the dissected space. The slit should be clipped together behind the cord. If the mesh is not large enough or if the Parietex model is used, a US Surgical, 4-mm, 0-degree stapler (ref 174027) is passed through the 12-mm trocar.

Two staples are placed on (the upper margin of) Cooper's ligament and two further staples on the deep aspect of the rectus muscle sheath; last, the mesh is stapled to itself around the cord. The mesh *should not be stapled laterally* in order to avoid injury to the nerves. Closure follows the same protocol as above. No drainage is necessary. The patient is allowed to sit up, eat, and ambulate on the evening of surgery.

Particular Situations and Special Tricks and Hints

When a tear in the peritoneum does occur, the pneumoperitoneum can reduce the already small working space. One solution is to repair the defect with a running suture. Another is to insert a Veress needle or 5 mm trocar into the abdominal cavity, which is left open in order to let the gas escape.

Bleeding in the field of dissection can be avoided, even without having to use electrocautery, provided that the correct plane is used and that dissection is performed slowly and carefully. In the case of injury to the epigastric vessels, it is possible to secure the vessel above and below the injury with percutaneous sutures, passed through skin under visual control. An unnoticed or neglected injury, even if the bleeding seems to be contained, will inevitably result in postoperative hematoma. In this event, nothing should be done if infection does not occur. Aspiration is not very useful, as the blood clots are difficult to evaluate.

One fairly frequent incident is the occurrence of postoperative seroma. Collection of serosanquinous fluid in the canal previously occupied by the hernia will occur and is often viewed by both the surgeon and the patient as an immediate recurrence. This collection usually disappears spontaneously within 2 to 3 weeks. Although some have advocated routine closure of the deep inguinal ring or of the wall defect in direct hernia, and others prefer incomplete resection of the indirect sac, no real preventive measures seem possible. Ultrasonic investigation is sometimes the only sure way to exclude recurrence and to reassure both the surgeon and the patient. Percutaneous puncture should be avoided because of the possibility of infecting the underlying prosthesis, and because recurrence of seroma usually occurs.

Antireflux Surgery

Although medical therapy has been advocated to relieve GERD, a definite trend toward surgical repair of the incompetent cardia has been seen with the advent of minimally invasive surgery. After a correctly performed antireflux procedure, the patient should no longer require either medication, postural, or dietetic therapy. The principles of correct antireflux surgery are known and must be respected laparoscopically. The gastroesophageal junction should be placed in its normal intra-abdominal position, the lower esophagus effectively anchored intra-abdominally, and an *effective* and *durable* antireflux mechanism (Nissen 360-degree gastric fundic wrap or Belsey Mark IV) fashioned.

Indications

Primarily, these are patients with endoscopically proven esophagitis, disabling heartburn, or persistent or recurrent symptoms while under medical therapy; reflux coughing (chronic aspiration); esophageal stricture; and/or pH-metric–proven acid reflux who are considered for antireflux surgery. Manometric studies are useful when esophageal disease or gastric causes of reflux have to be eliminated. Patients with Barrett's columnar-lined esophagus associated with reflux, even if uncomplicated by esophagitis, ulceration, and/or stricture, should have the option of definitive surgical therapy. Patients undergoing cure for large paraesophageal (rolling) hernia, even if the esophagogastric junction is correctly positioned, should have an associated antireflux procedure because of the potential gastroesophageal incompetence that results from dissection and reduction of the hernia. Last, an antireflux procedure is recommended when the repair of achalasia is performed.

Indications for Laparoscopic Repair

It has now been amply shown that laparoscopic repair of GERD can be accomplished with the same techniques and with the same results as in open surgery. The procedure is, however, difficult and full of traps, which must be avoided at all costs if surgery of a nonmalignant, functional disorder is to be indicated rather than long-term medication. Laparoscopic repair of large rolling hernia and of achalasia are treated elsewhere. As stated, an antireflux procedure should be added and can be accomplished under laparoscopic control.

Principles for Restoration of the Competent Cardia

As indicated elsewhere in this text (see de Meester), the technique of antireflux mechanism repair should 1) permanently restore at least 1.5 to 2.0 cm of abdominal esophagus but we recommend 4 to 6 cm; 2) construct a conduit that ensures the transmission of intra-abdominal pressure changes around the abdominal esophagus, preventing postoperative adhesions and scarring; 3) permanently increase the resting distal esophageal sphincter pressure as in the Nissen or the Belsey Mark IV repair; and 4) use only the fundus of the stomach to construct the wrap and avoid damage to the vagus nerves.

Technique

The patient is placed supine, the legs spread apart (French position) and draped. The monitor is usually placed behind the patient's left or right shoulder. The operator is between the legs of the patient, the first assistant is on the left cephalad, and the second assistant is either on the right or also on the left, but caudad. It is essential that the operation table be in the anti-Trendelenburg's position and slightly rolled to the right.

The carboperitoneum is initiated through a Veress needle placed just under or above the umbilicus. An insufflation pressure of 13 to 15 mm Hg is used to start but can be reduced to 10 to 12 mm Hg after the crura have been identified. Four 10- to 12-mm trocars are placed, equidistant from the anterior projection of the esophagogastric junction (Fig. 17-9), all above the umbilicus. A fifth 5-mm trocar is placed as cephalad as possible, near the xiphoid, more or less to the left or to the right, according to the size of the left liver, and is used to retract the left liver lobe. (Either the aspiration/irrigation device or one of the commercially available winged retractor devices can be used.) One author (BM) uses the most lateral right trocar to grasp the center of the diaphragm with forceps lifting the left lobe of the liver out of the operative field. The distance between the sites of introduction of the trocars must be re-evaluated once the abdomen is inflated to make sure that the instruments will be able to reach the hiatal area with ease. We usually ask the anesthesiologist to introduce an ordinary nasogastric tube into the stomach.

The operation commences by pulling gently on the anterior aspect of the stomach, or using the fat pad near the esophagogastric junction, in order to visualize the esophagus (Fig. 17-10). Usually, a fat pad can be identified to the right of the esophagus and grasped with the leftmost forceps. Otherwise, the stomach itself, and never the esophagus, should be grasped. Traction to the left allows identification of the pars flaccida. A word of caution is necessry, however, as inadvertent or excessive traction will result in (sometimes unapparent but irreversible) injury to the esophagus. The pars flaccida is opened with coagulator scissors and the right crus is identified and followed downward until

the left crus is reached (Fig. 17-11). These structures are left posteriorly as dissection progresses. To avoid injuring the esophagus or the mediastinum inadvertently while looking for the correct plane of dis-

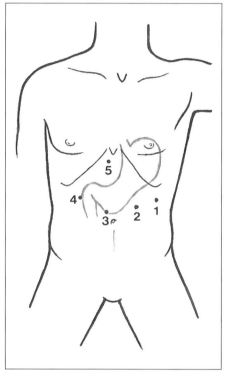

Fig. 17-9. Location of trocars for laparoscopic antireflux surgery.

section, we recommend following the crus rather than the esophagus. The right crus is first identified *cephalad*, and then dissected *caudad* while the left crus is dissected from *caudad* to *cephalad*. The phrenoesophageal ligament and then the gastrophrenic ligament must be identified and divided.

Once a passage is identified behind the esophagus, a curved (or right-angled) forceps is passed from right to left under the esophagus, in order to bring an umbilical tape (or Penrose sling) behind the esophagus (Fig. 17-12). The best angle of "attack" is from the extreme left- or righthand trocar. Dissection of the esophagus is pursued until 4 to 6 cm of abdominal esophagus has been freed and reduced into the abdomen. Excessive traction must be avoided at all costs. The right vagus nerve is left on the esophagus as it lies, as a recent controlled study showed that motor function was undisturbed whether or not the vagus nerve was dissected free. What ·is most important is not to include it in any ties.

Once the esophagus is freed and the crura clearly identified, we prefer to mobilize the fundus *before* suturing the crura. Either the fundus is already redundant, or most often, a few short gastric vessels must be divided to do so. It should be emphasized that the wrap must be "floppy" if excessive postoperative dysphagia is to be

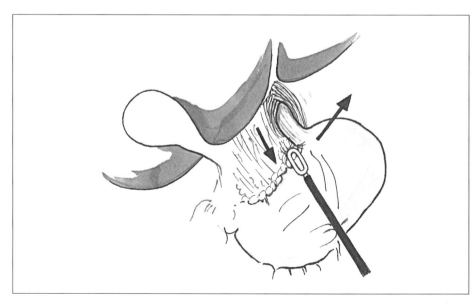

Fig. 17-10. The stomach is pulled down to visualize the esophagus and then to the left to identify the pars flaccida.

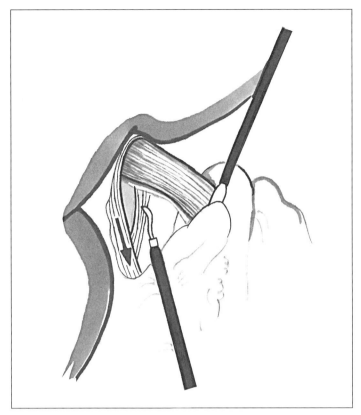

Fig. 17-11. *The pars flaccida is opened and the right and left crura of the diaphragm are identified.*

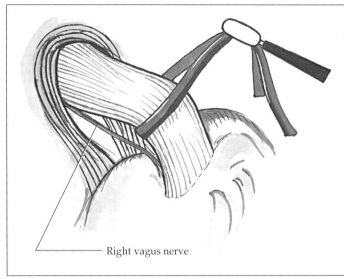

— Right vagus nerve

Fig. 17-12. *An umbilical tape is brought under the esophagus excluding the right vagus nerve, which is dissected free.*

avoided. This is probably more true in laparoscopic than in open GERD surgery, because of the lack of adequate tension evaluation. When dividing the short gastrics, we recommend starting in a relatively avascular area of the gastrosplenic ligament, which is thin and becomes transparent when held taut between two graspers. A hole is made and the vessels are identified, completely and clearly skeletonized, and then doubly clipped. Only one to three vessels should be divided initially. This is usually largely adequate. The hooked stapler (Ethicon or Origin) is very helpful for this. The short vessels are divided from caudad to the esophageal junction distant from the spleen. It is important to mobilize the fundus completely at this stage, before suturing the crura together. The esophagofundic junction (the angle of His) should be clearly visualized. This usually means pulling the stomach (or esophagus by the Penrose sling or umbilical tape) far to the right or changing the optical device to the left of the midline, or both (Fig. 17-13). The mobilized fundus should come around behind the esophagus *without any*

undue tension (Fig. 17-14). This can be evaluated by letting the fundus go once it has been pulled to the right of the esophagus and lifting the esophagus up with the umbilical tape. The fundus should remain behind the esophagus and not spring back to the left. If this is not the case, one should make sure that the posterior attachments between the esophagus and proximal stomach have been adequately divided, and, if this does not suffice, one should go back to the short vessels and divide them from cephalad to caudad until the fundus can be fully mobilized and remains spontaneously behind the esophagus as described. It may sometimes be easier to identify and divide the higher short vessels from behind rather than from above, that is, by lifting the esophagus anteriorly and working from the right to left on the gastrophrenic ligament and then the vessels. Once the fundus has been adequately mobilized, the nasogastric tube is replced by a large Faucher tube (at least No. 40 Fr) and, the crura are sutured. Whether the vagus nerve is left outside or within the wrap, care must be exercised to clearly

identify it and to leave it outside the sutures. We always tie our knots intracorporally. The two flaps can be sutured either with the same suture material or, as in our most recent cases, with the new Endostitch machine made by US Surgical.

In any case, we always suture the valve to the esophagus to avoid the slipping mechanism (Fig. 17-15). Our technique consists of suturing the uppermost part of the two flaps together, with the needle biting into the esophagus as high as possible. The first knot is tied and the free slip is left long (2–3 cm). A running suture is then made between the two flaps and the anterior aspect of the esophagus from cephalad to caudad. Once the desired length is attained, the same running suture purchases the flaps only from caudad to cephalad and then is tied to the slip left long. This should be done without any undue tension. Care must be exercised, of course, not to be penetrating. The antireflux wrap is made as long as desired (minimum 1.5–2 cm, but 4 cm is best) and its length can be measured with an instrument such as the right-an-

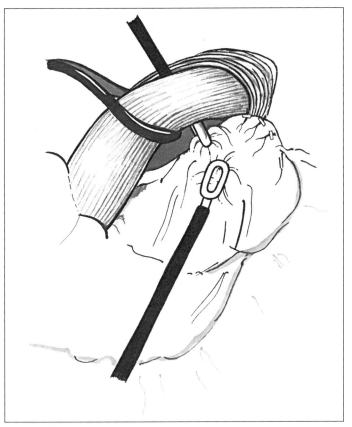

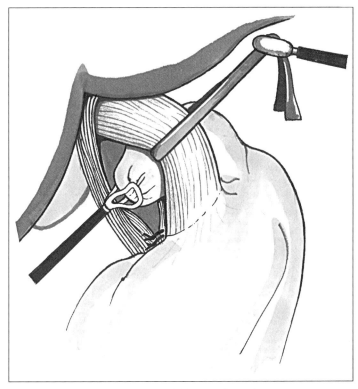

Fig. 17-13. *The fundus of the stomach is mobilized by dividing the short gastric arteries.*

Fig. 17-14. *The mobilized fundus is pulled under the esophagus.*

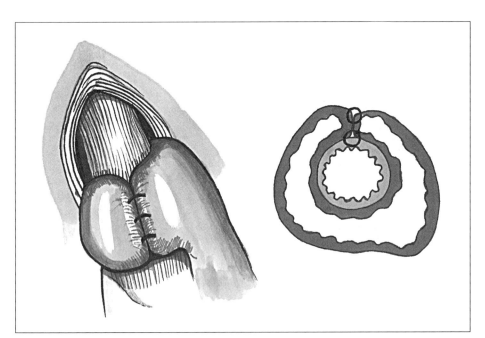

Fig. 17-15. *The two flaps of the valve are sutured to the esophagus and then to each other with a running suture.*

gled clamp (the length of the jaws is known or can be measured beforehand). One of the authors (AF) prefers to suture the crura together in all cases. If it is not possible to suture the crura together conveniently without tearing, two to three sutures are placed on the posterior aspect of the wrap, securing it to the right crus. The Faucher tube is removed (and no further nasogastric tubes are needed). Before closing, we check that there is no oozing or injury to the liver or stomach, and then we inject anesthesia as described previously. No drainage is necessary. The trocar orifices are checked for bleeding and closed as indicated above.

Particular Situations and Special Tricks and Hints

Adequate identification of the angle of His with resection of fatty deposits is essential to ensure that the fundic flaps turn around the abdominal portion of the esophagus and not the upper part of the stomach, responsible for severe postoperative dysphagia or recurrence of heartburn. In the case of large, sliding hernias, one of the authors (BM) advocates placing a continuous suture starting at the angle of His and running cephalad, purchasing the left margin of the esophagus to the adjacent gastric fundus to further preclude the "slipped Nissen" complication.

One particular intraoperative problem is perforation of the esophagus during dissection. As was mentioned previously, initial dissection close to the crura, rather than directly on the esophagus, and from cephalad to caudad and then caudad to cephalad, is recommended to avoid injury of the esophagus. In experienced hands, perforation of the esophagus has been successfully repaired laparoscopically (it is necessary to purchase both the *mucosa* and the muscular layers, and to cover the opening with the wrap). However, when in doubt, it is best to open to make sure that the repair is complete. Do not hesitate to inject air or methylene blue through the nasogastric tube and observe the area of dissection carefully under videoscopic control.

As the dissection might open the mediastinum to the pneumoperitoneum, the patient may experience desaturation or pneumothorax, or both. If this does occur, rather than converting routinely, it is possible to shut the pneumoperitoneum down completely, and, whenever indicated, to insert a needle into the pleural cavity involved. Once the wrap is ready, it can be used to close off the hiatal aperture. Even in the case of pleural violation, a needle rather than a drain tube is usually sufficient to decompress the pleural space.

If a hematoma is created when the wrap is sutured, the tie can be held taut for a couple of seconds, until it no longer spreads.

Excessive traction on the esophagus must be avoided at all costs because, as tactile evaluation is lacking, rupture of the vagal nerves, potentially responsible for postoperative diarrhea or gastroparesis, or both, or even of the esophagus, can occur.

All intracorporeal knots must be *tied* and not just clipped. Clips slip.

Paraesophageal or rolling hernia accounts for fewer than 10 percent of all hiatal hernias. It may be associated with sliding hernia or be an isolated condition. This type of her-nia can also be treated by laparoscopic dissection. The dissection of the sac is facilitated by the high pressure due to the carboperitoneum. It is most important to close the crura and to secure the stomach either to the crura or to the posterior rectus sheath (anterior gastropexy). Although the gastroesophageal junction functions theoretically in a normal fashion in pure paraesophageal hernia, an antireflux (Nissen) procedure is generally recommended because of the usual destruction of the hiatal area and the resulting incompetence after reduction of the paraesophageal hernia.

Achalasia is a neuromuscular disorder associating hypertrophy and esophageal dilatation. Although many patients are treated with success by forceful bouginage or pneumatic dilatation, some, especially those with wide dilatation, have recurrent symptoms after dilatation, or it becomes impossible to perform bouginage without risking perforation. While bouginage has been successful in mild achalasia, this condition is best treated by Heller's extramucosal cardiomyotomy. This operation can be accomplished under videolaparoscopy. The ports and trocar setup are similar to those used for GERD repair. Dissection should be performed exactly as in open surgery, that is, dissecting carefully with scissors to find the correct plane between the mucosa and the muscular layers. Care must be exercised to divide *all* the muscular fibers lest dysphagia persist. The length of the incision must be long (10 cm is an ideal) and above all must extend at least one centimeter below the gastroesophageal junction over the stomach. The highest collateral of the left gastric artery is a good landmark. Electrocautery (bipolar) should be used sparingly, if at all. We strongly recommend some form of testing for airtightness at the end of the operation to make sure that the mucosa is intact. Some authors recommend using intraoperative fiber endoscopy. We prefer to inject air or methylene blue through a nasogastric tube placed under direct visual (laparoscopic) control. The operation is usually completed by a preventive antireflux procedure, generally an anterior wrap (Dor) or 270-degree wrap (Lind), conceived either as a reinforcement of the mural defect or in order to maintain the separation of the serosal margins. One of us (BM) recommends making only the right half (posterior) of the antireflux procedure, thus maintaining the serosal gap. The Nissen repair is not recommended because the esophagus is aperistaltic, and this can lead to persistent obstruction.

Thoracic Procedures

Pleurectomy for Pneumothorax

It has long been established that recurrent (two or more), complicated (tension pneumothorax or persistent air leaks) spontaneous pneumothorax and the risk of bilateral pneumothorax should be treated surgically. The question of the best way to treat pneumothorax remains open, but most authors agree that parietal pleurectomy (associated with removal of the causative blebs) offers the best long-term results. In spite of the absence of controlled trials to prove its superiority, our personal opinion tends toward *apical pleurectomy* rather than simple talcum poudrage or irritation of the parietal pleura, which are associated with 2 to 8 percent and 2 to 5 percent of recurrence, respectively. The advantages of video-assisted pleurectomy include rapid and full postoperative expansion of the lung with minimal trauma to the chest, less postoperative pain leading to low morbidity and short hospital stay, the same rate of recurrence as in open thoracotomy, and complete visualization of the pleural cavity, as well as adequate assessment and treatment of the causative lesion.

Under general anesthesia, the patient is placed in a standard lateral thoracotomy position with the upper extremity cradled in an armrest. The surgeon places him- or herself in direct line of sight with the monitor. Two pliable, short, 5-mm silicon ports especially conceived for thoracoscopic surgery are inserted on the anterior and posterior axillary lines in the sixth costal interspaces. A 10- to 12-mm similarly short port is inserted on the midaxillary line in the eighth or ninth costal interspaces, creating a triangle. Most often this is used for the camera. We tend to incise the skin and muscle and open the pleura by pushing the index finger into the pleural cavity, precluding injury of the adherent lung. Selective intubation with a double-lumen endotracheal tube allows deflation of the ipsilateral lung but there is no need to insufflate the pleural cavity. The pleura is incised along a half circle on the sixth rib from a point lateral to the mammary artery anteriorly to a point lateral to the sympathetic chain posteriorly in the costovertebral sulcus. A vertical, vault-shaped incision is then made in the pleura from one end to the other of the initial incision at right angles from the first. The pleura is grasped with forceps inserted through one of the 5-mm ports, while a blunt instrument peels the pleura of the thoracic wall until the entire area is cleared of pleura. Occasional bleeders are coagulated, but care must be exercised to stay away from the intercostal bundle, the brachial plexus, and the major vessels.

The resection of blebs (located in more than 90% of cases in the apex) can take place either before or after the pleurectomy. This requires inserting another 10- to 12-mm port, usually in the most advantageous (anterior or posterior) 5-mm port already created. The optical device and the linear stapler are placed to correctly identify, isolate, and remove the bleb by cross-stapling. The pleural cavity is then filled with 200 to 300 ml saline and the lung is reinflated in order to detect any persistent leaks. Two drains are left in the pleural cavity through the 5-mm ports, one placed anteriorly, the other posteriorly, as in traditional thoracic surgery. The trocar orifices are checked for bleeding and, after injection of a mixture of 20 ml saline, 20 ml of 2% lignocaine containing 1 in 80,000 adrenaline, and 20 ml of 0.5% bupivacaine into the skin incisions, the skin is closed either with staples (USS) or fast absorbable Ethicon sutures. The drains are removed on day 2 or 3, once the lung is fully expanded; then the patient can be discharged.

Thoracoscopy is an excellent modality for creating pleurodesis using talc insufflation in intractable thoracic infusion. The trocars are inserted as for pneumothorax.

Laparoscopy and Thoracoscopy for Trauma

Diagnostic laparoscopy is being used with increasing frequency in trauma centers, in order to increase diagnostic accuracy with respect to peritoneal lavage (which does not allow identification of the type of lesion, whether it is actively bleeding, or the organ involved), to evaluate peritoneal violation in certain penetrating wounds, and to reduce the 10 to 25 percent rate of nontherapeutic laparotomy associated with positive findings on diagnostic lavage. Diagnostic peritoneal lavage usually misses retroperitoneal bleeding and diaphragmatic injury. Although computed tomography may help identify retroperitoneal injuries and the exact nature of solid organ injuries, it does not pick up diaphragmatic, hollow viscus, and mesenteric injuries, and does not distinguish between actively bleeding or stable lesions. Diagnostic laparoscopy is being used more and more often with local anesthesia, with a special 5-mm videoscope. We cannot, however, recommend many therapeutic procedures other than coagulation, which should still be considered as occasionally possible without risk, because they are highly debatable in their indications, and they should be performed with extreme circumspection. The pitfalls of diagnostic laparoscopy in the trauma setting include the difficulty in running and adequately visualizing the small intestines, and adequate assessment of the spleen (the 30-degree scope is indicated here) and of the pancreas. Furthermore, the risk of gas embolism in the case of venous injury is not known. Hemorrhage can rapidly become an obstacle to adequate vision, and this is definitely a limiting factor. Last, in the case of diaphragmatic injury, one should be aware of the possibility of creating a tension pneumothorax. The placement of the ports is variable but should include the four quarters of the abdomen to obtain adequate visualization of the entire cavity. Diagnostic laparoscopy should be considered in the hemodynamically stable patient only, with a penetrating wound and without parietal signs of hollow viscus injury, and used to rule out peritoneal violation. In all other cases, when a doubt exists as to intra-abdominal injury, we prefer to perform laparotomy.

Thoracoscopy in penetrating trauma allows visualization and suture of diaphragmatic rents. Indications are difficult to evaluate at this stage, but the technique should probably be restricted to those patients with penetrating trauma to the chest 1) sustained less than 24 hours before admission; 2) below the fourth intercostal space (ICS) anteriorly, sixth ICS laterally, and eighth ICS posteriorly, and hemodynamically stable (sustained systolic blood pressure > 90 mm Hg); and 3) in whom the chest tube drains less than 1.5 liters initially and less than 500 liters per hour for 2 consecutive hours, or both.

The patient can be placed in a half lateral decubitus position, allowing draping that is consistent with thoracoscopic maneuvers and then laparotomy only by changing the lateral rotation of the table. The trocars should be placed in a triangular fashion according to the rent and the best angle of attack. Usually this means inserting a 10-mm trocar in the third interspace in the midaxillary line and two others, usually one 10 mm in front and a 5-mm trocar behind, in the fifth or sixth interspace. The operator stands at the head of the patient, with the monitor on the opposite side, toward the feet of the patient. The use of standard suture material or the recently available Endostitch (USS) is obviously easier on the convex aspect of the diaphragm. The suture is straightforward and does not offer any major difficulties. The pleural cavity is drained for 24 to 48 hours at the most. Of course, the proper treatment for the abdominal side of the diaphragmatic wound (laparoscopy first? or rather laparotomy?) must be carefully evaluated.

Suggested Reading

Association Universitaire de Recherche en Chirurgie: Lenriot JP, Le Néel JC, Hay JM, et al. Cholangio-pancréatographie rétrograde et sphinctérotomie endoscopique pour lithiase biliaire. Evaluation prospective en milieu chirurgical. *Gastroenterol Clin Biol* 17:244, 1993.

Barkun JS, Barkun AN, Sampalis JS, et al. Randomized controlled trail of laparoscopic *versus* mini-cholecystectomy. *Lancet* 340:1116, 1992.

Barkun JS, Fried GM, Barkun AN, et al. Cholecystectomy without operative cholangiography. Implications for common bile duct injury and retained common bile duct stones. *Ann Surg* 218:371, 1993.

Bittner HB, Meyers WC, Brazer SR, Pappas TN. Laparoscopic Nissen fundoplication: Operative results and short term follow-up. *Am J Surg* 167:193, 1994.

Boulay J, Schellenberg R, Brady PG. Role of ERCP and therapeutic biliary endoscopy in association with laparoscopic cholecystectomy. *Am J Gastroenterol* 87:837, 1992.

Cadière GB, Houben JJ, Bruyens J, et al. Laparoscopic Nissen fundoplication: Technique and preliminary results. *Br J Surg* 81:400, 1994.

Collard JM, de Gheldere CA, de Kock M, et al. Laparoscopic antireflux surgery. What is real progress? *Ann Surg* 220:146, 1994.

Consensus Conference Moderators: A Paul (Germany), A Fingerhut (France). Panelists: B Millat (France), V Schumpelick (Germany), JL Dulucq (France), J Himpens (Belgium), E Laporte (Spain), L Nyhus (US), C Klaiber (Switzerland), J Mouiel (France), P Go (The Netherlands), JH Alexandre (France). Madrid: EAES Congress, September 15–17, 1994.

Cotton PB. Endoscopic management of bile duct stones: Apples and oranges. *Gut* 25:587, 1984.

Cuschieri A, Hunter J, Wolfe B, Swanstrom L. Multicenter prospective phase II evaluation of laparoscopic anti-reflux surgery: A preliminary report. *Surg Endosc* 7:505, 1993.

Dallemagne B, Weerts JM, Jehaes C, et al. Laparoscopic Nissen fundoplication: Preliminary report. *Surg Laparosc Endosc* 3:138, 1991.

Deluz A, Millat B, Fingerhut A. Laparoscopic management of choledocholithiasis. Kyoto: World Congress of Endoscopic Surgery, June 1994.

Deziel DJ, Millikan KW, Economou SG, et al. Complications of laparoscopic cholecystectomy: A national survey of 4,292 hospitals and an analysis of 77,604 cases. *Am J Surg* 165:9, 1993.

Fernandez-del Castillo C, Warshaw AL. Pancreatic carcinoma. *Curr Op Gastroenterol* 10:507, 1994.

Filipi CJ, Fitzgibbons RJ, Salerno GM, Hart RO. Laparoscopic herniorrhaphy. *Surg Clin North Am* 72:1109, 1992.

Fingerhut A, Lointier P, Millat B, et al. Laparoscopic assisted colonic resection: Feasibility and safety. The French experience. *Endosc Surg.*

Fitzgibbons R, Annibali R, Litke B, et al. A multicenter trial on laparoscopic hernia repair: Preliminary results (abstract). *Surg Endosc* 7:115, 1993.

Flowers JL, Zucker KA, Graham SM, et al. Laparoscopic cholangiography. Results and indications. *Ann Surg* 215:209, 1992.

Franklin M. Is laparoscopic colon resection feasible? (abstract). *Minimally Invasive Therapy* I(Suppl 1):85, 1992.

Frazee RC, Roberts J, Symmonds R, et al. Combined laparoscopic and endoscopic management of cholelithiasis and choledocholithiasis. *Am J Surg* 166:702, 1993.

Frazer RA, Hotz SB, Hurtig JB, et al. The prevalence and impact of pain after day-care tubal ligation surgery. *Pain* 30:189, 1989.

Geis WP, Malago M. Laparoscopic bilateral inguinal herniorrhaphies: Use of a single giant preperitoneal mesh patch. *Am J Surg* 60:558, 1994.

Geis WP, Crafton WB, Novak MJ, Malago M. Laparoscopic herniorrhaphy: Results and technical aspects in 450 consecutive procedures. *Surgery* 114:765, 1993.

Grace PA, Qureshi A, Burke P, et al. Selective cholangiography in laparoscopic cholecystectomy. *Br J Surg* 80:244, 1993.

Graham SM, Flowers JL, Scott TR, et al. Laparoscopic cholecystectomy and common bile duct stones. The utility of planned perioperative endoscopic retrograde cholangiography and sphincterotomy: Experience with 63 patients. *Ann Surg* 218:61, 1993.

Grand L, Toledo-Pimentel V, Manterola C, et al. Value of Nissen fundoplication in patients with gastro-oesophageal reflux judged by long term symptom control. *Br J Surg* 81:548, 1994.

Gold BS, Katz DS, Lecky JH, Neuhaus JM. Unanticipated admission to the hospital following ambulatory surgery. *JAMA* 262:3008, 1989.

Guillou PJ. Laparoscopic surgery for diseases of the colon and rectum quo vadis? *Surg Endosc* 8:669, 1994.

Hauer-Jensen M, Karesen R, Nygaard K, et al. Predictive ability of choledocholithiasis indicators. A prospective evaluation. *Ann Surg* 202:64, 1985.

Hay JM, Lacaine F, Kohlman G, Fingerhut A. Immediate definitive surgery for perforated duodenal ulcer does not increase operative mortality: A prospective controlled trial. *World J Surg* 12:705, 1988.

Hinder RA, Filipi CJ, Wetscher G, et al. Laparoscopic Nissen fundoplication is an effective treatment for gastroesophageal reflux disease. *Ann Surg* 220:472, 1994.

Jamieson GG, Warson DI, Britten-Jones R, et al. Laparoscopic Nissen fundoplication. *Ann Surg* 220:137, 1994.

Keane FBV, Tanner WA, Gillen P. Operative cholangiography and laparoscopic bile duct exploration. *Br J Surg* 80:957, 1993.

Lichtenstein IL, Shulman AG, Amid PK, Montilor MM. The tension free hernioplasty. *Am J Surg* 157:188, 1989.

Lillemoe KD, Yeo CJ, Talamini MA, et al. Selective cholangiography. Current role in laparoscopic cholecystectomy. *Ann Surg* 215:669, 1992.

McKernan JB, Wolfe BM, MacFayden BV. Laparoscopic repair of duodenal ulcer and gastroesophageal reflux. Laparoscopy for the general surgeon. *Surg Clin North Am* 72:1153, 1992.

McMahon AJ, Baxter JN, O'Dwyer PJ. Preventing complications of laparoscopy. *Br J Surg* 80:1593, 1993.

Miles RH, Carballo RE, Prinz RA, et al. Laparoscopy: The preferred method of cholecystectomy in the morbidly obese. *Surgery* 112:818, 1992.

Millat B, Fingerhut A, Deleuze A, et al. Laparoscopic treatment of choledocolithiasis: A prospective evaluation in 121 consecutive unselected patients. *Br J Surg.*

Milsom JW, Iavery IC, Church JM, et al. Use of laparoscopic techniques in colorectal surgery. Preliminary study. *Dis Colon Rectum* 37:215, 1994.

Monson JRT, Darzi A, Carey PDD, Guillou PJ. Prospective evaluation of laparoscopic-assisted colectomy in an unselected group of patients. *Lancet* 340:831, 1992.

Muhe E. Long-term follow-up after laparoscopic cholecystectomy. *Endoscopy* 24:754, 1992.

Narchi P, Benhamou D, Fernandez H. Intraperitoneal local anaesthetic for shoulder pain after day-case laparoscopy. *Lancet* 338:1569, 1991.

Neoptolemos JP, Carr-Locke DL, Fossard DP. Prospective randomised study of preoperative endoscopic sphincterotomy versus surgery alone for common bile duct stones. *Br Med J* 294:470, 1987.

Neoptolemos JP, Shaw DE, Carr-Locke DL. A multivariate analysis of preoperative risk factors in patients with common bile duct stones. Implications for treatment. *Ann Surg* 209:157, 1989.

Oschner MG, Lowery RC, Frankel HL, Champion HR. Thoracoscopy: Technical details and application. *Trauma Q* 10:301, 1994.

Oschner MG, Rozycki GS, Lucente F, et al. Prospective evaluation of thoracoscopy for diagnosing diaphragmatic injury in thoracoabdominal trauma: A preliminary report. *J Trauma* 34:704, 1993.

O'Rourke NA, Heald RJ. Laparoscopic surgery for colorectal cancer. *Br J Surg* 80:1229, 1993.

Pace BW, Cosgrove J, Breuer B, Margolis IB. Intraoperative cholangiography revisited. *Arch Surg* 127:448, 1992.

Pappas TN. Laparoscopic colectomy—the innovation continues. *Ann Surg* 216:701, 1992.

Peacock EE. Here we are: behind again! (editorial). *Am J Surg* 157:187, 1989.

Peillon CP, Manouvrier JL, Labreche J, et al. Should the vagus nerves be isolated from the fundoplication wrap? *Arch Surg* 129:814, 1994.

Phillips EH, Carroll BJ, Pearlstein R, et al. Laparoscopic choledochoscopy and extraction of common bile duct stones. *World J Surg* 17:22, 1993.

Phillips EH, Franklin M, Cartoll BJ, et al. Laparoscopic colectomy. *Ann Surg* 216:703, 1992.

Pope CE. Acid-reflux disorders. *N Engl J Med* 331:656, 1994.

Prasad A, Foley RJE. Laparoscopic management of cholecystocolic fistula. *Br J Surg* 81:1789, 1994.

Rattner DW, Ferguson C, Warshaw AL. Factors associated with successful laparoscopic cholecystectomy for acute cholecystitis. *Ann Surg* 217:675, 1993.

Reddick EJ, Olsend DO. Laparoscopic laser cholecystectomy: A comparison with mini-laparotomy cholecystectomy. *Surg Endosc* 3:131, 1989.

Richter JE. Surgery for reflux disease—reflections of a gastroenterologist. *N Engl J Med* 326:825, 1992.

Rosenblum M, Weller RS, Conrard PL, et al. Ibuprofen provides longer lasting analgesia than fentanyl after laparoscopic surgery. *Anesth Analg* 73:255, 1991.

Rutkow IM. Laparoscopic hernia repair. The socioeconomic tyranny of surgical technology. *Arch Surg* 127:1271, 1992.

Saltzstein EC, Peacock JB, Thomas MD. Preoperative bilirubin, alkaline phosphatase and amylase levels as predictors of common duct stones. *Surg Gynecol Obstet* 154:381, 1982.

Schwab G, Pointner R, Wetscher G, et al. Treatment of calculi of the common bile duct. *Surg Gynecol Obstet* 175:115, 1992.

Seid AS. Significance of groin nerve anatomy for laparoscopic hernia repair (abstract). *Surg Endosc* 7:115, 1993.

Shulman AG, Amid PK, Lichtenstein IL. The safety of mesh repair for primary inguinal hernias: Results of 3019 operations from five diverse surgical sources. *Am Surg* 58:255, 1992.

Southern Surgeons Club. A prospective analysis of 1518 laparoscopic cholecystectomies. *N Engl J Med* 324:1073, 1991.

Spechler SJ, Department of Veterans Affairs Gastroesophageal Reflux Disease Study Group. Comparison of medical and surgical therapy for complicated gastroesophageal reflux disease in veterans. *N Engl J Med* 326:786, 1992.

Stain SC, Cohen H, Tsuishoysha M, Donovan AJ. Choledocholithiasis. Endoscopic sphincterotomy or common bile duct exploration. *Ann Surg* 213:627, 1991.

Stiegmann GV, Goff JS, Mansour A, et al. Precholecystectomy endoscopic cholangiography and stone removal is not superior to cholecystectomy, cholangiography and common duct exploration. *Am J Surg* 163:227, 1992.

Stoker DL, Spiegelhalter DJ, Singh R, Wellwood JM. Laparoscopic versus open inguinal hernia repair: randomized prospective trial. *Lancet* 343:1243, 1994.

Swanstrom L, Wayne R. Spectrum of gastrointestinal symptoms after laparoscopic fundoplication. *Am J Surg* 167:538, 1994.

Tate JJT, Kwok S, Dawson JW, et al. Prospective comparison of laparoscopic and conventional anterior resection. *Br J Surg* 80:1396, 1993.

Wexner SD, Cohen SM, Johansen OB, et al. Laparoscopic colorectal surgery: A prospective assessment and current perspective. *Br J Surg* 80:1602, 1993.

Widdison AL, Longstaff AJ, Armstrong CP. Combined laparoscopic and endoscopic treatment of gallstones and bile duct stones: A prospective study. *Br J Surg* 81:595, 1994.

EDITOR'S COMMENT

This chapter by Professors Fingerhut and Millat is a very well-reasoned, conservative, and guarded approach to laparoscopy that is well worthwhile when considering this new technique. They emphasize utility, cost, and efficacy, which are always valid measures of new surgical procedures. It is of interest that individuals such as Professors Fingerhut and Millat, who have played a major role in the development of this technique, do not believe that laparoscopic appendectomy is indicated, except perhaps rarely (see Chap. 135 by Dr. Fitzgibbons for a slightly different point of view), and are very tentative about colonic surgery and duodenal ulcer. With respect to colonic surgery, trocar port recurrence, which in some series is as high as 7 percent and seems to be related to the pressure within the peritoneal cavity, bringing about implantation of tumor cells in the ports experimentally, is a major problem for patients with carcinoma of the colon since it may compromise patients who should be cured. With respect to duodenal ulcer, especially perforated duodenal ulcer, parietal cell vagotomy as definitive therapy is a technique that I prefer, and I use Graham patch, not imbrication of the perforation, to definitively treat duodenal ulcer. Our own experience with trauma, as well as that of others (and we are doing a number of studies, as are others), suggests that the number of missed injuries, including those to the mesentery, the bowel, and especially the ureter, is substantial, thus clouding the question of whether laparoscopy should be used in trauma except as part of a study.

I have a number of comments concerning the techniques outlined. The controversy over intraoperative cholangiography recalls the controversy concerning routine cholangiography in the early 1960s. The number of retained stones appears to be not too terribly different. However, if one thinks of costs, it seems unreasonable for patients undergoing laparoscopic cholecystectomy to undergo prior endoscopic retrograde cholangiopancreatography (ERCP) since the physician charges for ERCP approximate those of laparoscopic cholecystectomy, and the hospital costs of the procedure itself approximate those of the operating room. It would be much more efficacious for surgeons to become expert at extracting common duct stones either laparoscopically or, under the same anesthetic, by performing procedures at the lower end of the common duct. The current health care system as it is evolving in the United States will reward that approach and make prior or subsequent ERCP a procedure gone begging, since no patients will be available for it on an economic basis. Carrying out cholangiography under fluoroscopy is an essential part of the procedure, and the availability of fluoroscopy is essential if one is to extract common duct stones such as the authors propose.

Carcinoma of the gallbladder is usually not discovered until the specimens are analyzed. Wedge resection is totally without efficacy as far as survival, and even right hepatic lobectomy yields limited survival in most series. Thus, the argument concerning carcinoma of the gallbladder and laparoscopic cholecystectomy is not germane. On the other hand, the question of whether carcinoma of the gallbladder can be effectively removed because of seeding of the ports is a real one, especially since it does not appear to be the colonic cells from the tumor itself when they are removed that seed, but rather the insufflation that appears to be the guilty party, at least thus far experimentally.

Finally, the authors give superb advice concerning bleeding during laparoscopic cholecystectomy. If there is a single aspect of this chapter that makes it worthwhile, it is the admonition that one does not blindly clip, but that one grasps and controls and then secures the bleeding. It is essential that individuals do not lose their equanimity while this is going on, and the authors' advice is excellent.

The authors are ever so mindful of the controversies concerning *hernia*. The questions in my mind are the violation of basic surgical principles in inserting a foreign body when no such foreign body is necessary. Postoperative neuritis is referred to repeatedly in the text. What is of interest is the absence of staples from the transabdominal, intraperitoneal approach to hernias, something about which many American laparoscopic surgeons would probably disagree.

There is little question that the use of *antireflux procedures* has increased since laparoscopic and minimally invasive repair has become popular. It is particularly unfortunate that the number of open procedures has decreased to the extent that it may be difficult to accomplish a proper randomized prospective trial. This is particularly important for Barrett's esophagus since it is controversial as to whether Barrett's esophagus will regress even with conventional repairs for which the efficacy has been tested. In my view, it is essential that, before the adoption of further laparoscopic procedures, there be some measure of efficacy that will validate their continued usage. Failure to do so, in view of the expense, will probably act negatively toward these procedures in the long run.

J.E.F.

18

Flaps and Other Reconstructive Techniques

Luis O. Vasconez   Jae-Wook Oh

During the last two decades, plastic surgery has made remarkable advances in reconstructive techniques. The muscle flap, the musculocutaneous flap, the fasciocutaneous flap, and the free flap using microvascular anastomosis have become routine procedures in reconstruction. Numerous muscle and musculocutaneous flaps, including the latissimus dorsi, the pectoralis major, the rectus abdominis from the abdomen, and the gracilis and tensor fascia lata from the lower extremity have provided durable coverage and volume effect to fill dead space. These enable the reconstructive surgeon to solve such difficult problems as mastectomy defects, abdominal wall defects, pelvic defects after abdominoperineal resection, radiation ulcers, and chest wall defects after cardiac surgery. The development of microvascular surgery provides the free flap as an elegant method of tissue movement without any restriction by pedicle; thus, it has been possible to transfer compound tissue from the donor site to the defect of most topographic regions of the body in a one-stage procedure. The introduction of the fasciocutaneous flap, such as the scapular flap, subscapular flap, radial forearm flap, and medial and lateral thigh flap, provides a good opportunity to treat the defects in the head and neck, and upper and lower extremities.

Today, many kinds of defects that were unsolved or challenging problems in general surgery have been successfully reconstructed; adequate margin resections maximize the chance of cure or palliation in cancer surgery, and extensive removal of contaminated tissue or debridement offers the best chance of successful wound healing in treatment of traumatic defects or radiation ulcers. Moreover, aesthetic and functional restoration have been possible by using the variety of available techniques and considerable refinements in flap surgery. In this chapter, these typical defects, such as postradiation ulcer, mastectomy defect, abdominal wall defect, pelvic defect after abdominoperineal resection, wounds in the immunosuppressed posttransplant patient, and their reconstructive techniques are introduced.

Treatment of Postradiation Ulcer

Radiation therapy is used as a definitive or important adjuvant modality in the treatment of cancer. Although current radiation delivery techniques have been improved to avoid most acute radiation complications, the problems of late complications have not been solved. Similarly, modern techniques try to avoid damage to the overlying skin, but we do see skin ulcerations and complications. The late complications of radiation therapy are from obliterative endarteritis, which impairs local circulation and produces tissue ischemia. There is also considerable fibrosis in the wound due to proliferation of fibroblasts. Even minor trauma to the radiated area of the skin is often followed by infection, thus resulting in a chronic ulceration. Just as important, if one is to make an incision in a postradiation area, that wound will not heal and will promptly reopen, necessitating reconstructive treatment, as is outlined below. The distribution of postradiation ulcer is related to the sites of tumors that are treated by radiation combined with different types of surgery. Therefore, the

common sites of radionecrosis are the oral cavity, chest wall, lumbar region, and sacrum. The symptoms and signs are similar to those of other ulcers, but the unrelenting pain is characteristic. The question frequently comes up, particularly in postradiation ulcers of the chest, of whether they represent pure traumatic ulcerations or tumor recurrence. This distinction is immaterial because the treatment is going to be the same, and consequently in our practice biopsy of the ulcer is not necessary. More often than not, if a biopsy is performed, the pathologist will indicate, "Chronic ulceration, tumor cannot be ruled out," which is not helpful. Local therapy for these postradiation wounds is of little benefit except for the control of the superficial bacterial infection, which can be done with the use of topical antibacterials, such as silver sulfadiazine or Betadine.

The principle of treatment for postradiation ulcers consists of very wide excision of the ulceration, which should include removal of *all* of the portal of radiation. By this we mean that we should remove all of the adjacent tissue that has been damaged by the radiation. The postradiation skin is determined by the hyperpigmentation of the area as well as the lack of skin appendages, telangiectasia, and woody induration of the overlying skin. If underlying bones, such as ribs, have also been exposed to radiation, they should also be removed in one stage. Following this extensive debridement, the defect should be covered immediately by a muscle or musculocutaneous flap or, if that is not appropriate, by omentum. We recommend that surgical debridement and wound coverage be performed simultaneously. Otherwise, the debrided wound tends to enlarge because the radiated wound does not contract or granulate.

Treatment of Sacral Ulcer with Gluteus Maximus Myocutaneous Flap

Postradiation sacral ulcer usually results from pelvic irradiation after surgical treatment of uterine cancer. A very large sacral defect is usually left after wide excision of the radiated tissue. Several types of gluteal flaps have been used to cover the sacral wound, but these flaps have the potential for impairment of muscle function. Maintaining the function of the gluteus maximus muscle is important in ambulatory patients. The "sliding gluteus maximus myocutaneous flap" is used to cover the postradiation ulcer in the sacrum. After design of a V-shaped incision, the skin island is made on the gluteus maximus muscle (Fig. 18-1A). The surrounding buttock skin is elevated from the muscle. The gluteal muscle is freed and elevated from its origin. The elevation is started from the inferior border of the muscle. The periosteal origin on the lower sacrum and coccyx is elevated and the fibers on the sacrotuberous ligament are detached; blunt dissection is continued until the inferior gluteal neurovascular pedicle is reached. The elevation of the superior border of the muscle is started and dissection is continued bluntly until the piriformis muscle and the superior gluteal vessels are identified. After elevation of all areas of the muscular origin, the muscle is attached only to the inserting fibers of the iliotibial tract and the femur (Fig. 18-1B). For larger defects, bilateral elevation of flaps is necessary and sometimes muscular insertion on the fascia superior to the greater trochanter may be released. The muscles are sutured to each other over the sacrum. The skin is closed in a V-Y advancement manner (Fig. 18-1C) and large suction drains are placed.

Reconstruction of the Breast

The objective of breast reconstruction is to obtain an aesthetically acceptable and symmetrical breast using a safe and relatively simple procedure. The methods for breast reconstruction include reconstruction with implants, autogenous tissue reconstruction, and autogenous tissue plus a permanent implant. The use of implants for breast reconstruction can be subdivided into three categories: submuscular implant insertion, tissue expansion with subsequent permanent implant, and permanent expander prosthesis. Autogenous tissue reconstruction is usually performed using the TRAM flap as a pedicle flap or free flap. The gluteus maximus myocutaneous flap and the lateral thigh flap can be transferred to the breast as a free flap. In the breast reconstruction with autogenous tissue plus a permanent implant, the latissimus dorsi myocutaneous flap is used as autogenous tissue and it is usually necessary to use an implant to provide the breast mound.

Timing of the breast reconstruction is an important consideration when the patient is seen before definitive local treatment. Although controversy still exists within the surgical community and specific standards encompassing all situations for all patients simply cannot be made, there is a trend toward immediate breast reconstruction, and a growing number of women are requesting this immediate procedure. Whether reconstruction is immediate or delayed, the breast reconstruction is a part of total care of breast cancer, and therefore it is important for the reconstructive surgeon to have a close relationship with members of the breast management team, especially with the oncologic surgeon, in planning the procedures of mastectomy and reconstruction.

Immediate Postmastectomy Breast Reconstruction

Virtually any patient can be considered a candidate for immediate breast reconstruction based on the stage of her disease. Especially when the woman with early breast cancer does not want to live even a short time with a mastectomy defect, this procedure of reconstruction is an acceptable approach. It is a single-stage procedure that encompasses mastectomy and reconstruction and is associated with a psychological advantage, but it requires a long operative time, and blood transfusion is usually necessary in the autogenous tissue technique. The incidence of wound complications is relatively high and some patients seem disappointed with the reconstructed breast because they have not had the opportunity to experience the mastectomy deformity. All the methods of breast reconstruction can be used for immediate breast reconstruction.

Reconstruction with Permanent Expander Prosthesis

Recently, the use of a permanent expander prosthesis has become more popular when nonautogenous breast reconstruction is planned. This type of expander has a valve apparatus that can be removed under local anesthesia once the desired breast volume has been reached. The expander is inserted in one of two ways: the serratus anterior method or the pectoralis major and subcutaneous lower dissection (Fig. 18-2A). In the serratus anterior method, the dissection of the pocket commences through a vertical incision into the serratus anterior, 4 cm lateral to the pectoralis major. This method, although bloodier, has the advantage of providing total muscle cover for the expander. One should always be careful to place the expander low enough. In pectoralis major and subcutaneous lower dissection, the muscle is retracted or occasionally split in the line of its fibers and the submuscular pocket is created. In each method, the injection portal is brought to lie in a subcutaneous position, where it is easily palpable and accessible for percutaneous injection, as well as subsequent easy removal. After dissection of a large, low pocket, the expander implant is inserted and the tubing is connected with the injection portal after proper shortening (Fig. 18-2B). A separate pocket is dissected subcutaneously to house the injection portal away from the expander. Suggested locations for the injection portal are the midaxillary line, the lateral costal margin, or, rarely, the midsternum. After closure of all the wounds, the expander is inflated percutaneously through the injection portal with 100 to 150 ml saline (Fig. 18-2C). This maneuver flattens the expander and avoids wrinkles or folds, assures that the portal is not upside down, and creates a small breast mound. After 1 or 2 weeks, an average of 50 ml saline is injected with 23- or 25-gauge needles every week. When the desired inflated size is achieved the injection portal is removed under local anesthesia. It usually takes 6 to 8 weeks.

Reconstruction with TRAM Flap

Abdominal tissue provides a sufficient and satisfactory source for reconstruction of a mastectomy defect, allowing reconstruc-

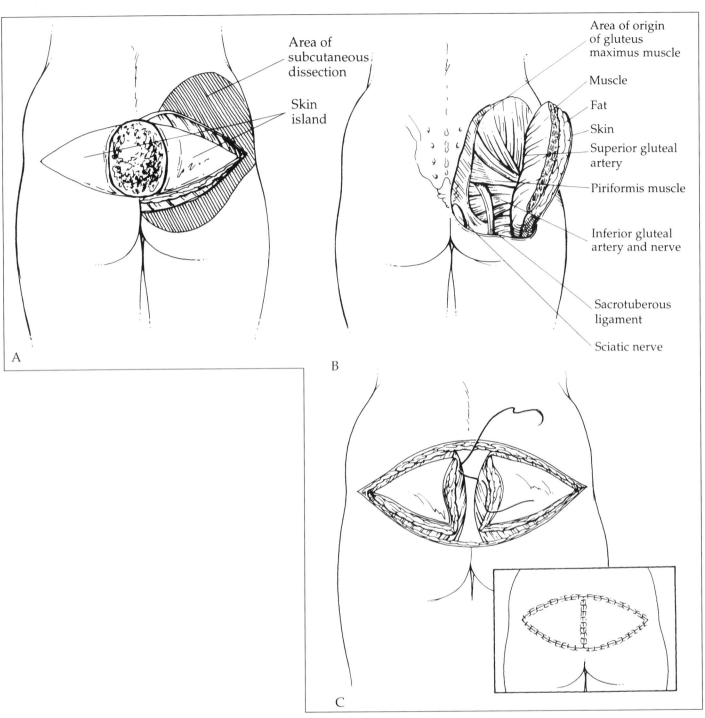

Fig. 18-1. *The use of the sliding gluteus maximus myocutaneous flap. A. The design of a bilateral V-shaped incision. The skin island overlies the gluteus maximus muscle. The surrounding buttock skin is elevated from the muscle. B. The relationship of the gluteal pedicles, piriformis muscle, sciatic nerve, and gluteus maximus muscle. The entire gluteal muscle origin is freed except for the inserting fibers of the iliotibial tract and the femur. C. The gluteus muscles are sutured to each other in the midline. The skin is closed in a V-Y advancement manner. (From OM Ramirez, JC Orlando, DJ Hurwitz. The sliding gluteus maximus myocutaneous flap.* Plast Reconstr Surg *74:68, 1984. Reproduced with permission.)*

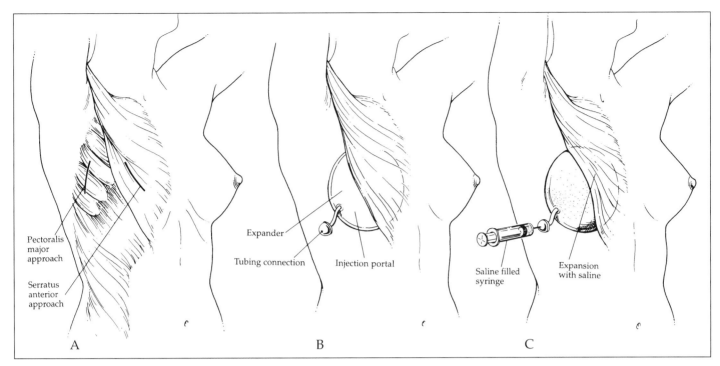

Fig. 18-2. Reconstruction of the breast with permanent expander prosthesis. A. The expander is inserted in one of two ways: the serratus anterior approach or the pectoralis major approach. B. The implant is inserted and the tubing is connected with the injection portal. C. After closure of all wounds, the expander is inflated percutaneously through the injection portal with saline. (From LO Vasconez, M Lejour, M Gamboa-Bobadilla. Atlas of Breast Reconstruction. *Philadelphia: Lippincott, 1991. Chap. 2. Reproduced with permission.)*

tion of the breast without the use of an implant, and it does not create distortion and asymmetry of the donor site as does the gluteal free flap. Therefore, the TRAM flap is useful for the patient who is unwilling to have a reconstruction with implant or who has had complications with it such as recurrent capsular contracture. Moreover, the patient has the effect of an aesthetic abdominoplasty. When it is selected by an experienced surgeon, the TRAM flap can be transferred as a free flap for immediate breast reconstruction. For a unilateral immediate breast reconstruction, a single-pedicled contralateral TRAM flap is used in the majority of patients. This flap is the procedure of choice for reconstruction when the cancer has recurred or when complications have developed after radiation therapy.

The flap is designed with the upper incision just above the umbilicus. The lower incision is made as for an aesthetic abdominoplasty. Using the principle of triangulation, which places two sutures in the midline, one above the xiphoid and the second at the pubis, the flap is outlined symmetrically on both sides (Fig. 18-3A). The umbilicus is first circumscribed com-

pletely. The stalk of the umbilicus is then dissected down to the fascia. The upper incision of the design is made deep to Scarpa's fascia. The upper abdominal flap is elevated to the costal margin and xiphoid superficial to the anterior rectus sheath. As a teaching guide, the flap has been divided into four zones (Fig. 18-3B). The segment of anterior rectus sheath is marked and incised, 3 to 4 cm in width, to include the two rows of perforators from the costal margin to the upper level of the abdominal flap. The lower incision is made down to the anterior rectus sheath and the external oblique fascia. The random side of the flap is elevated above the rectus fascia to approximately 1 cm beyond the midline (Fig. 3C). The flap on the pedicle side is elevated to the point where the lateral fascial incision was made above the flap; then the lateral edge of the fascia is divided (Fig. 18-3D). The medial division of the fascia is done approximately 1 cm from the midline using the superior fascia incision as a guide. From the level of the lowest perforator, division of the fascia is tapered into a triangular shape near the pubis. Once the fascia is divided, the rectus muscle is elevated bluntly; then the deep inferior epigastric vessels are identified to enter the

undersurface of the muscle and are divided between suture ligatures. The muscle should be transected just below the semicircular line, preserving the remaining distal muscle to cover the weakened area and, thus, avoiding a lower abdominal bulge. The flap is then dissected superiorly to the costal margin by freeing the muscle from the posterior rectus sheath and dividing the segmental intercostal vessels and nerves. A subcutaneous tunnel is created over the sternum to connect the abdominal dissection with the mastectomy defect. The flap is then delivered through the dissected subcutaneous tunnel into the mastectomy defect (Fig. 18-3E). Zone IV and a portion of zone II are immediately discarded. Zone III, which is usually hanging down along the anterior axillary line, is to be deepithelialized and tucked under. When the appropriate modeling has been accomplished, the patient is placed in a sitting position so that the final adjustment can be made, comparing with the contralateral breast. During the time a team of surgeons is molding and closing the breast, another team proceeds with the abdominal closure. The upper border of the transected rectus muscle and the remnant of the anterior rectus sheath are sutured to

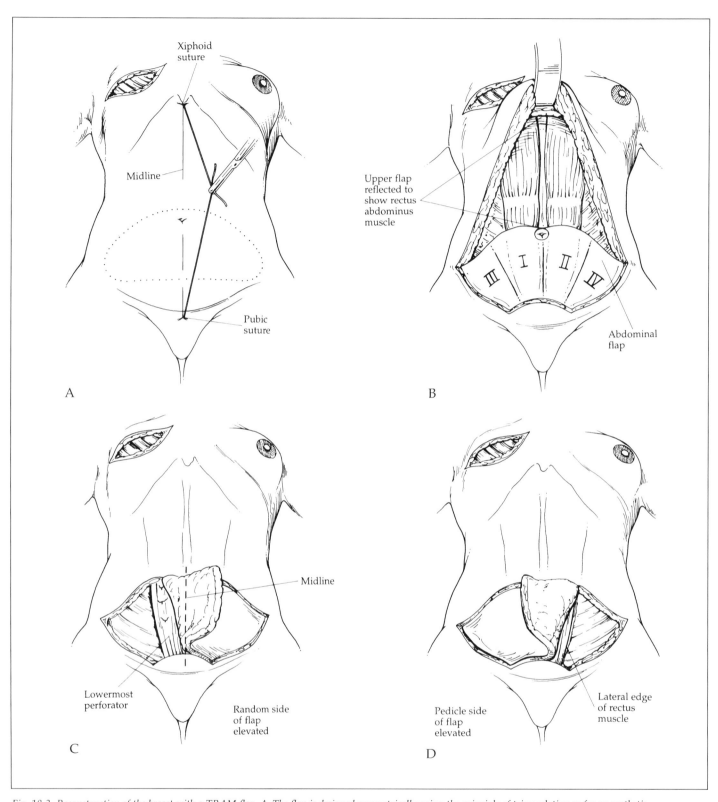

Fig. 18-3. Reconstruction of the breast with a TRAM flap. A. The flap is designed symmetrically using the principle of triangulation as for an aesthetic abdominoplasty. B. The upper abdominal flap is elevated to the costal margin and xiphoid, superficial to the anterior rectus sheath. C. The random-side flap is elevated above the rectus fascia to approximately 1 cm beyond the midline. D. The pedicle-side flap is elevated to the point where the lateral fascial incision was made above the flap.

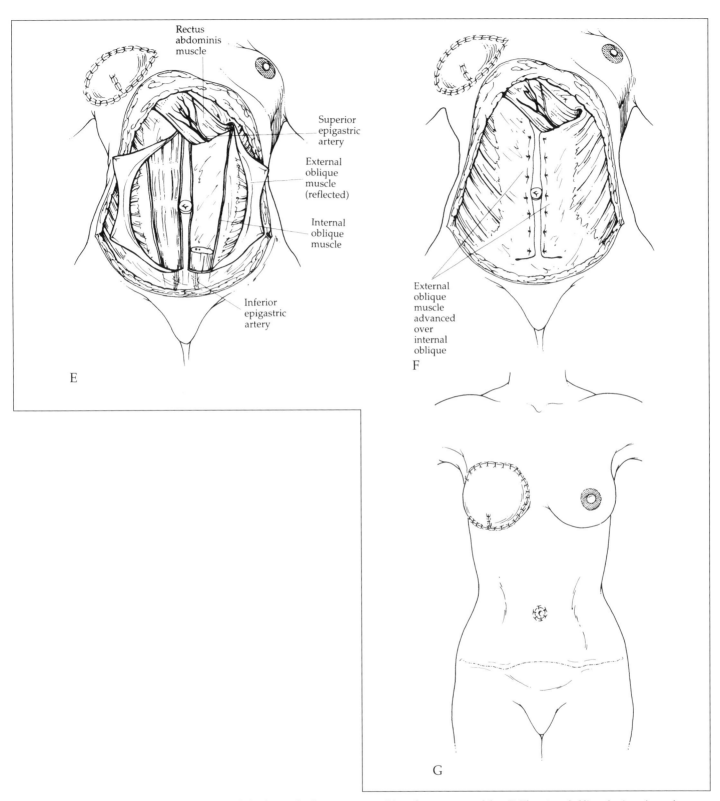

Fig. 18-3 (Continued) E. The flap is delivered through the dissected subcutaneous tunnel into the mastectomy defect. F. The external oblique fascia and muscle are dissected from the internal oblique muscle and are sutured to the midline rectus sheath separately in a layered closure. G. The umbilicus is reconstructed at a new position and the abdominal closure is completed. (From LO Vasconez, M Lejour, M Gamboa-Bobadilla. Atlas of Breast Reconstruction. Chap. 4. Philadelphia: Lippincott, 1991.)

18. Flaps and Other Reconstructive Techniques   **279**

the level of semicircular line selectively. The external oblique fascia and muscle are dissected from those of the internal oblique and are sutured to the midline rectus sheath separately in a layered closure (Fig. 18-3F). The umbilicus is reconstructed at a new position. The table is flexed and abdominal closure is completed (Fig. 18-3G). Suction drains are used in both the breast and the abdomen.

Reconstruction of Postlumpectomy Breast Defects

The surgery for early breast cancer has changed remarkably in the last few decades with the trend toward breast conservation, so that the breast conservation and skin-sparing mastectomy technique is becoming a treatment of choice for some patients with early breast cancer. Although a number of controversies surround selection of patients, radiation technique, and adjuvant therapy, lumpectomy and radiation therapy represent the best treatment for early breast cancer. Therefore, recent areas of concern for the reconstructive surgeon are postlumpectomy and radiation breast deformities. These deformities vary according to the size and shape of the breast, the location of the tumor, and the surgical techniques, and therefore they have to be individualized and assessed carefully. Reconstruction of these defects is very difficult and there are no patterns to follow. The most common deformity is an asymmetry between two breasts. When the asymmetry is slight, minor touch up such as mastopexy or reduction of the normal breast can provide cosmetic improvement in most cases. In contrast, for the patient with considerable radiation damage or recurrent breast carcinoma, or both, total mastectomy and reconstruction with a TRAM flap are recommended. Most of the postlumpectomy defects with depression can be corrected satisfactorily with latissimus dorsi muscle or musculocutaneous flap. The muscle flap is advisable when the deformity is relatively mild or when one needs to cover an implant. The deepithelialized latissimus dorsi myocutaneous flap is a good choice for volume replacement, especially for the subclavicular hollow defect, and the musculocutaneous flap is recommended when nipple-areola position changes because of the skin defect. Sometimes these defects are repaired with local glandular flap or mastopexy of the

affected breast and mastopexy on the contralateral breast to have symmetry.

Reconstruction of Postlumpectomy Defect with Latissimus Dorsi Flap

The latissimus dorsi muscle is thin and a certain amount of atrophy can be expected when it is transferred. It can supply well-vascularized tissue with skin coverage, however, and when volume replacement is needed, it can be used as a deepithelialized flap or as a muscle flap with implant. To harvest the latissimus dorsi myocutaneous flap, the upper border of the skin island is designed a little lower than the upper limit of the patient's brassiere with the patient in a standing position (Fig. 18-4A). The patient is placed on the operating table in a semilateral position, exposing the entire operative field, including back and both breasts. Skin incisions are made and the surrounding skin is elevated. After the surrounding skin flap is elevated, the

muscle is dissected from the superior border bluntly with the finger and the muscle and skin island are elevated in a bloodless field. As the dissection proceeds, the anterior border of the muscle is identified. The muscle is then divided along its tendinous origin near the midline. A transverse cut is made from the anterior border of the muscle to join the vertical cut along the midline of the back, freeing the unit from its medial, posterior, and inferior attachments. The dissection continues superiorly toward the insertion of the muscle and its vascular pedicle. When the thoracodorsal vessels are identified, the dissection continues toward the insertion of the muscle so that every attachment is freed, and the whole unit can be moved as a pendulum on a relatively narrow pivot point. After the recipient site is prepared, the flap is transposed through a high tunnel (Fig. 18-4B). The skin island is adjusted and positioned with temporary staples to orient and tailor it accordingly; then final closure is performed with subcutaneous sutures of

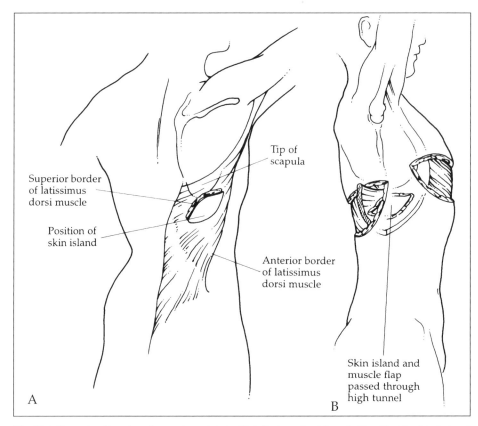

Fig. 18-4. Reconstruction of postlumpectomy defect with latissimus dorsi flap. A. The skin island is designed a little lower than the upper limit of the patient's brassiere with the patient in standing position. B. After complete dissection of the flap, it is transposed to the recipient breast defect through a subcutaneous tunnel. (From LO Vasconez, M Lejour, M Gamboa-Bobadilla. Atlas of Breast Reconstruction. Philadelphia: Lippincott, 1991. Chap. 3. Reproduced with permission.)

fine nylon. The donor site is closed in layers and at least one or two suction catheters are placed through separate stab wounds.

Reconstruction of the Abdominal Wall

Acquired defects of the abdominal wall can result from trauma, infection, resection of tumor, therapeutic radiation, and postoperative incisional hernia. Many methods have been introduced to repair these defects. The most desirable way to close the abdominal defect is simple approximation of the wound margin without tension. The majority of defects can be repaired by this method and, if necessary, undermining of the various components of abdominal wall will allow primary closure of very large defects, which was thought to require a distant flap. When direct closure is not possible, the reconstruction becomes a challenging surgical problem.

These defects of the abdominal wall may be partial thickness or full thickness. The former require reconstruction of the investing fascia or soft-tissue coverage alone and the latter need reconstruction of all layers. In most types of hernias, the defect exists in the transversalis fascial layer and repair is essential to establish abdominal wall integrity. The defect in soft-tissue coverage can result from infection, trauma, or resection of tumor. Before making the decision to use a specific reconstructive technique, one should consider not only the thickness of the defect but also other existing conditions, such as the age, health status, and body habitus of the patient; the size and location of the defect; and the availability of local and distant tissue.

Recently, the procedures of choice for reconstruction of large abdominal defect have been pedicled flaps from the thigh, the tensor fascia lata, and the rectus femoris. These muscle flaps can bring the fascia lata to the defect. The fascia lata is strong enough to re-establish abdominal integrity. When this vascularized fascia is not able to be used or the defect is too large to be covered, synthetic material should be utilized to restore the fascial layer. A variety of synthetic materials have been used, such as tantalum, Nylon, Orlon, Teflon, Dacron, Prolene, and Marlex. Among these materials, Marlex has become one of the most popular synthetics. Marlex mesh is strong and resists infection because of its uniform molecular structure, and is infiltrated with fibrous tissue, which allows the ingrowth of granulation tissue. Recently, Gore-tex (PTFE) has been advertised to have less bacterial adherence and to produce fewer adhesions. In severely injured or contaminated wounds or when the patient's condition is not stable, the emergency use of more complex procedures such as distant musculocutaneous flaps is unwise. In such situations, the preferred initial management may be the use of synthetic mesh and frequent dressing changes. When a clean granulating surface is established through the mesh, a split-thickness skin graft is applied as an intermediate stage. The skin graft placed on the synthetic material should be replaced with durable tissue flap later.

Reconstruction of the Abdominal Defect with the Tensor Fascia Lata Flap

The tensor fascia lata (TFL) myocutaneous flap is a good choice for most reconstructive surgeons to close a lower abdominal wall defect. This flap contains fascia lata, which is strong enough to re-establish abdominal wall integrity, and therefore it can be used for reconstruction of the full-thickness abdominal wall defect. Because the skin territory is innervated by two sensory nerves, the lateral cutaneous branch of the twelfth thoracic nerve and the lateral cutaneous nerve of the thigh, this flap can be transferred as a sensate unit. The flap elevation is designed on the anterolateral thigh. The flap is based on the transverse branch of the lateral circumflex femoral artery, which enters the deep surface of the muscle approximately 8 to 10 cm below the anterosuperior iliac spine (Fig. 18-5). The skin territory lies between two vertical lines dropped from the anterosuperior iliac spine and the greater trochanter to the knee. For larger fascial defects, the fascia lata of the whole lateral thigh can be raised with the tensor fascia lata muscle (TFLM) as an extended unit. Elevation of the flap proceeds proximally from the distal border in the plane between the fascia lata and vastus lateralis. When the deep surface of the TFLM is identified, dissection continues deep to the muscle avoiding the major pedicle. After complete dissection, the skin incision is completed and the flap can be rotated nearly 180 degrees for coverage of

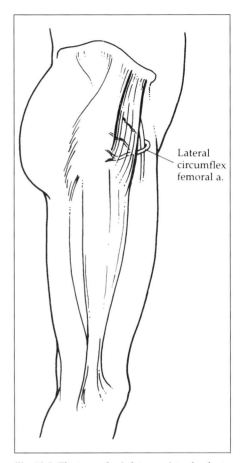

Lateral circumflex femoral a.

Fig. 18-5. The tensor fascia lata consists of a short muscle body and a long fascial component. It is most useful for coverage of wounds in the region of the trochanter and has also been used for reconstruction of lower abdominal and groin defects. (From LO Vasconez, JB McCraw, AG Camargos. Muscle, musculocutaneous and fasciocutaneous flaps. In JW Smith and SJ Aston [eds], Grabb and Smith's Plastic Surgery *(4th ed). Boston: Little, Brown, 1991. P 1130. Reproduced with permission.)*

the abdominal wall (Fig. 18-6). The fascia lata is sutured into the muscle and fascial margin of the abdominal defect and then the skin is closed. In most cases, the donor site can be closed directly when the width is less than 8 cm.

Reconstruction with the Rectus Femoris Flap

The rectus femoris muscle or musculocutaneous flap is reliable and is handy to use to cover the abdominal wall defect. Its arc of rotation is more advantageous because it pivots in the midthigh, as opposed to the lateral thigh for the TFL flap. This muscle flap provides well-vascularized tissue and

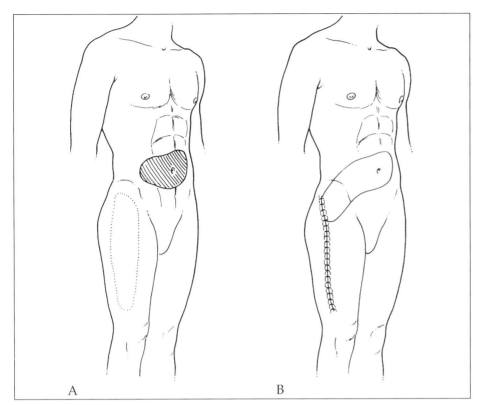

A   B

Fig. 18-6. Reconstruction of the abdominal wall with a tensor fascia lata (TFL) flap. A. Outline of flap and abdominal wall defect. B. Transposed island flap and donor area closed directly. (From SJ Mathes, F Nahai. Clinical Atlas of Muscle and Musculocutaneous Flap. *St. Louis: Mosby, 1982. P 377. Reproduced with permission.)*

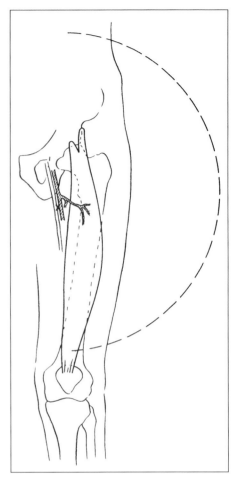

Fig. 18-7. The rectus femoris muscle with its blood supply from the descending branch of the lateral femoral circumflex artery located approximately 8 cm below the inguinal ligament. (From WY Hoffman and G Trengove-Jones. The rectus femoris flap. In B Strauch, LO Vasconez, EH Hall-Findly [eds], Encyclopedia of Flaps. *Vol. 3. Boston: Little, Brown, 1990. P 1409. Reproduced with permission.)*

is preferred for defects with chronic infection that result from trauma or radionecrosis, particularly over the pubis. The rectus femoris muscle flap can be elevated with fascia lata of the lateral thigh to provide a large cover for muscular and fascial defects of the abdominal wall. This is an important muscle, but the potential for impairment of knee extension can be minimized by suturing the distal tendon to the midline vastus intermedius fascia or by re-approximation of the vastus medialis and the vastus lateralis muscle in the midline of the thigh. The rectus femoris muscle always reliably reaches the lower abdomen, but its upward mobilization is somewhat limited due to its lower level of entry of the dominant vascular pedicle; therefore, it cannot reach the upper abdomen except in thinner patients. The dominant vascular supply is from the descending branch of the lateral femoral circumflex artery located in the superior one-third of the muscle, approximately 8 cm below the level of the inguinal ligament (Fig. 18-7). The anterior third of the thigh skin can be elevated with the muscle. The overlying

skin is innervated by the anterior femoral cutaneous nerve, which can be used to create a neurosensory flap. A branch of the femoral nerve to the muscle should be saved to provide ueural support and preserve muscle mass across the abdominal defect. The skin island is designed directly over the muscle at the anterior third of the thigh (Fig. 18-8B). The incision is made and the distal muscle is identified and then divided, as it becomes tendinous just above the knee. The flap is elevated from the distal border; then submuscular dissection is continued until the sartorius muscle is identified. At this level, the dominant pedicle is shown deep to the muscle. After complete dissection, the flap is transferred to cover the defect (Fig. 18-8C). If the donor site is less than 8 cm in width, it can be closed directly (Fig. 18-8D).

Other Flaps

The rectus abdominis myocutaneous flap can be elevated to cover the unilateral defect of the abdominal wall. This flap can be based on the superior or inferior epigastric

artery depending on the defect. During the elevation of the flap, this muscle is denervated and cannot support the integrity of the abdominal wall; therefore, the integrity of the fascial support must be preserved. The extended latissimus dorsi flap is a large single unit that includes the latissimus dorsi muscle, with its lumbodorsal fascia and also pregluteal fascia as the extended part. Therefore, the use of this flap in selected patients is warranted where other methods of reconstruction are contraindicated or impossible. The external oblique myocutaneous flap can be transposed superiorly or inferiorly and the gracilis myocutaneous flap is able to reach the lower abdomen, but these flaps have a

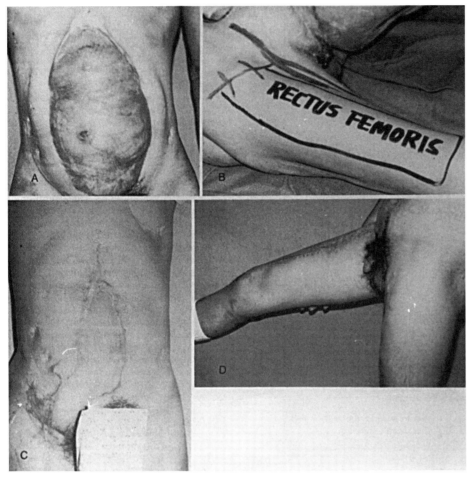

Fig. 18-8. Reconstruction of the abdominal wall with a rectus femoris flap. A. Abdominal wall defect to be covered with myocutaneous flap. B. Rectus femoris flap outlined on anterior thigh. C. Flap in place with repair of abdominal wall defect. D. Flexon of hip with extension of knee reversed and primary closure of wound.

limited arc of rotation. The axial groin flap can be used selectively for soft-tissue defects that do not require fascial reconstruction. Omentum can be used to provide blood supply to support a skin graft, but its use usually requires synthetic mesh for structural support. When these techniques are inadequate or cannot be used to cover the defect, free flaps, such as latissimus dorsi or tensor fascia lata myocutaneous flap, is rarely indicated.

Reconstruction of the Pelvis Following Abdominoperineal Resection

After total pelvic exenteration and abdominoperineal surgery, massive defects in the

pelvis, perineum, and groin are created. The extirpative surgery on this area is often complicated by radiation therapy, urinary and fecal contamination, and fistulization. Moreover, vital structures such as femoral vessels are occasionally exposed as a result of groin dissection in this region. Traditional methods, including skin graft, local skin flap, and distant tubed flap for tissue coverage and reconstruction in this area require multiple procedures, with incomplete or inadequate results leading to a prolonged length of recovery. The muscle and musculocutaneous flaps offer a blood supply based out of the field of radiation therapy with a volume effect to obliterate massive dead space in the pelvis and lead to early rehabilitation of patients through a one-stage immediate reconstruction. These flaps have their own advantages and disadvantages, which are related to their technical complexity, the

requirement of the recipient site, and the potential morbidity of the donor site; therefore, it is important to select the flap of choice in various situations.

Reconstruction of the Vagina

Immediate vaginal reconstruction is highly recommended. If reconstruction is delayed, the dissection of the space for the new vaginal cavity is very difficult due to adhesions between the bowel and the adjacent pelvic structures. Many methods have been proposed to reconstruct the vagina after extirpative surgery or radiation. The medial thigh fasciocutaneous flap can be elevated independently and used to reconstruct vagina and perineum without gracilis muscle, but this flap has some problems in infected and irradiated wounds. The pudendal-thigh flap was introduced to repair the vaginal defect after total pelvic exenteration for malignancy, but this flap is not indicated in patients with squamous cell carcinoma of the vulva or lower third of the vagina because there is a high likelihood of lymphatic spread to the groin. The perineal artery axial flap was used to reconstruct the vagina, but it will not cover a major defect. The gracilis myocutaneous flap or the inferiorly based rectus abdominis myocutaneous flap is generally used in the reconstruction of vagina and pelvic defects at the same time. These two flaps provide bulk, which is important to obliterate the pelvic dead space. The transverse or vertical rectus abdominis myocutaneous flap is suitable to fill the massive dead space during low and high pelvic reconstruction because of its dependability, large size, and versatility of design, but it requires laparotomy for inset of the flap into the lower region of the pelvis.

The flap of choice for vaginal reconstruction after total pelvic exenteration is a gracilis myocutaneous flap. This muscle is totally expendable from a functional standpoint. For total vaginal reconstruction with lower pelvic defect, this flap is used bilaterally. The patient is placed in a modified lithotomy position. For the orientation of the flap design, a straight line is drawn on the skin between the easily palpated adductor longus tendon at the pubic tubercle and the semitendinosus tendon at the knee. The gracilis muscle and its cutaneous portion lie posterior to

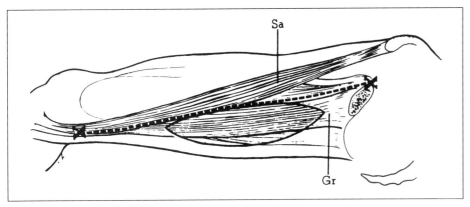

Fig. 18-9. The design of the gracilis myocutaneous flap. A straight line is drawn between the adductor longus tendon at the pubic tubercle (X) and the tendon of the semitendinosus at the knee (X). The gracilis muscle and its cutaneous portion lies posterior to this line. Sa = sartorius; Gr = gracilis. (From FR Hecker. Gracilis musculocutaneous and muscle flap. Clin Plast Surg 7:32, 1980. Reproduced with permission.)

this line (Fig. 18-9). The maximum size of the skin island can be about 8 cm in width and 22 cm in length and usually does not extend into the distal third of the thigh. Through a small incision on this line, the gracilis tendon is found just above the knee, lying between the sartorius fibers anteriorly and the semimembranosus fascial expansion posteriorly. After circumferential dissection, this tendon is retracted to palpate the muscle, and the correct orientation of the skin island is outlined over the muscle. Once the skin island is outlined, the skin incision is deepened to the fascial level and dissection proceeds in the avascular plane between the adductor longus and the gracilis. The distal minor pedicles are divided as they are encountered. The dominant pedicle, the medial circumflex femoral artery, is identified at a point about 8 cm distal to the pubic tubercle. The gracilis muscle is dissected posteriorly by dividing the semimembranosus fascia. The

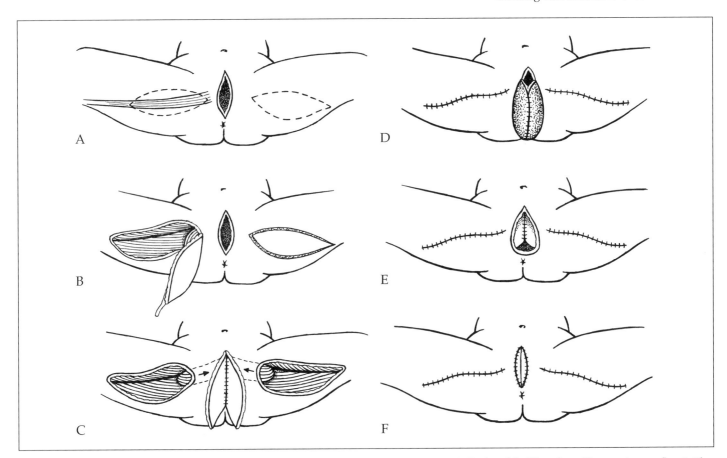

Fig. 18-10. Reconstruction of the vagina with gracilis myocutaneous flap after total pelvic exenteration. A. Design of the bilateral gracilis myocutaneous flap. B. The muscle is divided at the distal insertion and the skin island is elevated. C. The flaps are rotated posteriorly and passed through the subcutaneous tunnel. D. Bilateral skin islands are sutured into a pouch-like configuration with the skin-side facing internally. E. Reconstructed vaginal pouch is rotated into the pelvic defect. F. Skin edges are sutured to labial skin and a new vagina is constructed. (From SJ Mathes and F Nahai. Clinical Applications for Muscle and Musculocutaneous Flaps. St. Louis: Mosby, 1990. P 411. Reproduced with permission.)

muscle is then divided at its distal insertion and the flap is transposed (Fig. 18-10B). Division of the proximal origin is unnecessary. For a greater arc of rotation, the major pedicle can be dissected or mobilized by retracting the adductor longus. A wide subcutaneous tunnel is made under the skin bridge between the thigh incision and the vaginal defect. Dissection and mobilization of the pedicles are advised to avoid tension. The flap is rotated posteriorly and passed beneath this skin bridge. The same procedure is done on the other thigh. The left thigh flap is rotated clockwise, and the right thigh flap is rotated counterclockwise around its vascular pedicle (Fig. 18-10C).

After removal of the excess skin and fat, the bilateral skin islands are sutured into a pouchlike configuration, with the skin side facing internally (Fig. 18-10D). The new vaginal pouch is rotated caudally into the pelvic defect (Fig. 18-10E). The tendinous ends are then anchored to the presacral fascia to avoid postoperative prolapse. The distal ends of the flaps become the apex of the vagina, and the proximal ends become the vaginal introitus. Skin edges are sutured to the labial skin to complete single-stage vaginal reconstruction (Fig. 18-10F).

Reconstruction of the Perineum

Several flaps can be used to cover perineal defects. These are the gracilis, the tensor fascia lata, the rectus femoris, the gluteus maximus and rectus abdominis myocutaneous flap, the medial thigh fasciocutaneous flap, and the gluteal thigh flap. Among these flaps, the gluteal thigh flap and the gracilis myocutaneous flap are preferable for perineal reconstruction. The gluteal thigh flap may measure up to about 34 cm in length and 15 cm in width, when centered over its axial vessel, the descending branch of the inferior gluteal artery. This flap can be transposed with the gluteus maximus muscle as a compound musculocutaneous flap or as a fasciocutaneous flap (Fig. 18-11). The patient is placed in the prone position. The flap is designed over the central axis of its neurovascular pedicle, which is located midway between the greater trochanter and the ischial tuberosity and is perpendicular to the gluteal crease (Fig. 18-12A). An in-

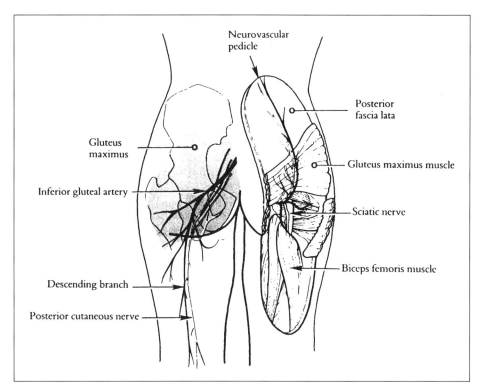

Fig. 18-11. The anatomy of the gluteal thigh flap. The inferior gluteal artery comes from the sciatic foramen beneath the piriformis and courses under the gluteus maximus muscle. It then continues down the midline of the posterior thigh. Just medial to the artery, the posterior femoral cutaneous nerve is usually found. (From RJ Walton, DJ Hurwitz, and J Bunkis. Gluteal thigh flap for reconstruction of perineal defect. In B Strauch, LO Vasconez, and EH Hall-Findly [eds], Encyclopedia of Flaps. Vol. 3. Boston: Little, Brown, 1990. P 1456. Reproduced with permission.)

cision is made along the inferior margin of the flap through the deep fascia. Careful identification of the posterior femoral cutaneous nerve is important to determine the level of dissection. Just lateral to the nerve, the inferior gluteal vessels are usually found encased in fat. The vessels and nerve are divided and freed from the underlying muscles. During elevation of the flap, one must include the deep fascia in order to incorporate the neurovascular pedicle in the flap. When the inferior margin of the gluteus maximus muscle is reached, several large femoral perforators should be divided if they interfere with transposition of the flap. If more length is needed, the gluteus maximus muscle can be split and the neurovascular pedicle included as the proximal base of the flap, so that the flap can reach the perineum and the pelvic cavity medially, the greater trochanter laterally, and the sacrum and the anterosuperior iliac spine superiorly (Fig. 18-12B). Large branches from the sciatic nerve should be preserved in ambulatory

patients. When the inferior gluteal vessels are not palpable, even using an island flap, it is important to preserve the deep fascia and to incorporate the overlying subcutaneous tissue and a portion of the gluteus maximus muscle as a composite pedicle. The flap is then transferred to the recipient defect.

Reconstruction of the Groin

Many flaps are available for the coverage of soft-tissue defects in the groin. The rectus femoris flap and the vastus lateralis flap are large and reliable units, but their use in ambulatory patients may lead to difficulties in moving the hip and knee. The gracilis myocutaneous flap is not the choice for groin coverage because the distal third of the flap is not reliable, which is essential to cover groin defects. The contralateral groin flap, the omentum, or the free flap is rarely indicated. For groin defects with an exposed vascular prosthesis,

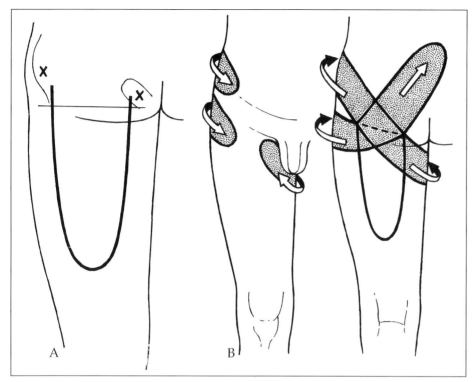

Fig. 18-12. A. The gluteal thigh flap is designed over the central axis, which is midway between the greater trochanter and the ischial tuberosity and perpendicular to the gluteal crease. B. The flap can reach the perineum and pelvic cavity medially, greater trochanter laterally, and sacrum and anterosuperior iliac spine superiorly. (From DJ Hurwitz, WM Swartz, SJ Mathes. The gluteal thigh flap: a reliable, sensate flap for the closure of buttock and perineal wounds. Plast Reconstr Surg 68:521, 1981. Reproduced with

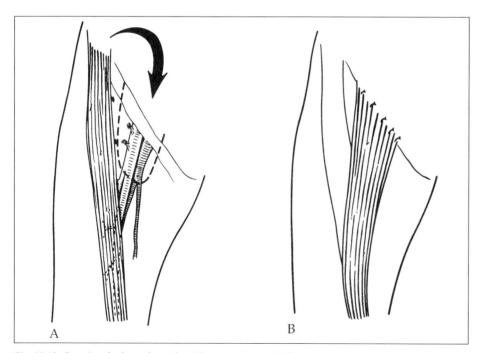

Fig. 18-13. Covering the femoral vessels with a sartorius muscle flap transposition. A. Exposed femoral vessels. B. Transposed sartorius covers vessels. (From SJ Mathes and F Nahai. Clinical Applications for Muscle and Musculocutaneous Flaps. St. Louis: Mosby, 1982. P 419. Reproduced with permission.)

direct coverage with muscle is preferred. Therefore, when the exposed area is not large, the sartorius flap is the flap of choice to cover the exposed femoral vessels or vascular prosthesis. Through a transverse groin incision, the muscle that is most superficial is identified. The upper one or two pedicles are ligated and the muscle origin from the anterosuperior iliac spine is divided; then the muscle is transposed medially into the groin (Fig. 18-13). For the large groin defect, particularly after groin dissection for lymphadenectomy, the tensor fascia lata flap is the first choice. After extirpative surgery for vulvar carcinoma with bilateral groin metastasis, extensive groin and vulvar defects remain. A bilateral extended TFL flap is most useful to reconstruct these defects at the same time. The procedure for flap elevation has been described previously. The lateral circumflex femoral artery comes from the profunda femoral artery between the vastus lateralis muscle and rectus femoris muscle at a level approximately 8 to 10 cm from the anterosuperior iliac spine. After dissection of this pedicle, the skin incision is completed and the flap is elevated as an island flap for transposition. After the flap is transferred to the groin and vulvar defect, the skin is closed and the donor defects can be closed primarily. An inferiorly based rectus abdominis myocutaneous flap is also useful in large groin defects, especially when the femoral vessel or vascular prosthesis is exposed.

Treatment of Wounds in the Immunosuppressed Posttransplant Patient

Organ transplantation increased remarkably in frequency in the past few years. Advances in immunosuppression as well as early recognition and intervention in organ rejection have resulted in more successful transplants. Wound complications do occur in a small number of patients who present challenging problems to the transplant and reconstructive surgeons.

The immunosuppressed patient has delayed healing and there is an impairment of the microbial defense mechanism, making wound infection and wound dehiscence important complications in the transplant patient. The contributing factors include the malnourished state of the patient with an underlying disease, such as diabetes, chronic renal failure, or chronic hepatic insufficiency, and the presence of foreign bodies, including catheters, prosthetic materials, and so forth. It is also important to note that the usual inflammatory signs of an infected wound are masked in the immunosuppressed patient, particularly if the patient is receiving corticosteroids. Consequently, the redness, swelling, and tenderness that are usually present in an infected wound are delayed in their appearance in immunosuppressed patients, requiring constant vigilance on the part of the physician to allow early diagnosis. Wound dehiscence, isolated or in combination with abdominal infection, is seen in immunosuppressed patients, particularly in those receiving corticosteroids. If they occur in post–heart transplant patients, it requires immediate debridement and coverage with adjacent muscle flaps or with omentum. In patients who have had pancreas transplants, when the anastomosis to the bladder has broken down, acute necrosis and digestion of the abdominal wall can be seen due to the leakage of pancreatic enzymes.

To treat wound infection in a transplant patient, wide debridement and adequate drainage are important. Appropriate antibiotic therapy and frequent dressing changes with povidone-iodine solution are recommended. Granulation tissue develops very slowly, if at all, in the immunosuppressed patient and because of that, skin grafts take poorly for the coverage of those wounds. It is preferable, if the wound is clean, that a debridement of the edges be done and a secondary closure with permanent sutures of nylon be attempted. When the infection is severe or necrotizing fasciitis has developed, wide debridement and radical excision of the infected area, including the undermined portion of the deep fascia, are essential. Excisional defects in these cases can be temporarily covered with a skin graft or the use of prosthetic mesh, such as polypropylene, to be followed by definitive coverage with adjacent musculocutaneous flaps, as described in the section on reconstruction of the abdominal wall. Careful consultation with a transplant surgeon is essential so that the immunosuppression can be minimized while the infection is being controlled.

Dehiscence of the Mediastinal Wound Following a Heart Transplant

Mediastinal wound dehiscence or infection is more likely to occur in patients who have undergone second or third heart transplant procedures, largely due to bleeding, or re-entry into the mediastinum. If the mediastinal instability is recognized early, we favor immediate intervention, which usually consists of debridement of the wound, including the removal of the mediastinal wires and part of the sternum, and coverage with adjacent pectoralis major muscles if they will cover most of the exposed heart, and often with the addition of the rectus abdominis muscle. If the latter muscle is considered essential for coverage of the transplanted heart, we prefer to use the omentum, which can be harvested by extending the midsternotomy incision down to the abdomen, freeing the omentum from the transverse colon and along the greater curvature of the stomach, pivoting it on the right gastroepiploic vessels. The omentum is passed through a rent in the diaphragm or at the subcutaneous tissue level to cover the transplanted heart. We then approximate only the pectoralis major muscles as well as the overlying skin. We do not favor the rewiring of the sternum once instability has been discovered because we believe that it is very likely to fail, as it did the first time.

Abdominal Wound Necrosis Following Leak of Pancreatic Anastomosis

This is a rare occurrence and, when it happens, it can produce a considerable amount of necrosis of the abdominal wall, which needs to be debrided. The judgment of the transplant surgeon is respected concerning whether the transplant needs to be resutured, and, if this is done, the suture line should be reinforced, probably by wrapping it with omentum or with a portion of the rectus abdominis muscle based on the deep inferior epigastric vessels. The abdominal debridement must be thorough and it is followed by frequent moist dressing changes until the wound appears to be relatively clean and under control. In this case, we favor the use of meshed split-thickness skin grafts. The skin graft take may not be 100 percent but will certainly facilitate further management and more definitive treatment of the wound, which will consist of rotation of a musculocutaneous flap. In this case, we favor the rectus femoris, which will reach the wound without difficulty and allows for primary closure of the secondary defect in the anterior thigh (see Fig. 18-8).

Suggested Reading

Fisher JC. Complications in Radiation Therapy. In NG Georgiade, GS Georgiade, R Riefkoh, WJ Barwide (eds), *Essentials of Plastic, Maxillofacial and Reconstructive Surgery.* Baltimore: Williams & Wilkins, 1987. Pp 1120–1126.

Goldman, MH, Rose RC. Complications of Immunosuppression. In LJ Greenfield (ed), *Complications in Surgery and Trauma.* Philadelphia: Lippincott, 1990. Pp 216–230.

Grotting JC, Carriquiry C, Vasconez LO. Abdomen. In MJ Jurkiewicz, TJ Krizek, SJ Mathes, S Aryan (eds), *Plastic Surgery. Principles and Practice.* St. Louis: Mosby, 1990. Pp 1139–1167.

Hecker FR. Gracilis myocutaneous and muscle flap. *Clin Plast Surg* 7:27, 1980.

Hoffman WY, Trengove-Jones G. The Rectus Femoris Flap. In B Strauch, LO Vasconez, EH Hall-Findly (eds), *Encyclopedia of Flaps.* Vol 3. Boston: Little, Brown, 1990. Pp 1408–1409.

Hurwitz DJ, Swartz WM, Mathes SJ. The gluteal thigh flap: A reliable, sensate flap for the closure of buttock and perineal wounds. *Plast Reconstr Surg* 68:521, 1981.

Mathes SJ, Hurwitz DJ. Repair of chronic radiation wound of the pelvis. *World J Surg* 10:269, 1986.

Mathes SJ, Nahai F. Clinical applications for muscle and musculocutaneous flaps. St. Louis: Mosby, 1982. Pp 364–425.

McCraw JB, Horton CE, Horton CE Jr. Basic Techniques in Genital Reconstructive Surgery. In JG McCarthy (ed), *Plastic Surgery.* Vol 6. Philadelphia: Saunders, 1990. Pp 4121–4152.

McDowell F. Introduction, flap refinements; logs into harpsichords. *Clin Plast Surg* 17:xiii, 1990.

Petit J, Rietjens M. Deformities After Conservative Breast Cancer Treatment. In RB Noone (ed), *Plastic and Reconstructive Surgery of the Breast.* Philadelphia: Decker, 1991. Pp 455–466.

Ramirez OM, Orlando JC, Hurwitz DJ. The sliding gluteus maximus myocutaneous flap; its relevance in ambulatory patients. *Plast Reconstr Surg* 74:68, 1984.

Vasconez LO, Lejour M, Gamboa-Bobadilla M. *Atlas of Breast Reconstruction.* Philadelphia: Lippincott, 1991.

Vasconez LO, McCraw JB, Camargos AG. Musculocutaneous and Fasciocutaneous Flaps. In JW Smith, SJ Aston (eds), *Grabb and Smith's Plastic Surgery* (4th ed). Boston: Little, Brown, 1991. Pp 1113–1141.

Walton RL, Hurwitz DJ, Bunkis J. Gluteal Thigh Flap for Reconstruction of Perineal Defects. In B Strauch, LO Vasconez, EH Hall-Findly (eds), *Encyclopedia of Flaps.* Vol 3. Boston: Little, Brown, 1990. Pp 1455–1461.

EDITOR'S COMMENT

The role of reconstructive plastic surgical techniques in managing problems concurrent with or resulting from surgical treatment of tumors, infections, decubitus ulcers, and other conditions, which the general surgeon creates or encounters, has increased remarkably as plastic surgeons have developed ingenious techniques for transfer of viable, vascularized, and innervated tissues. For the surgeon who does a substantial number of surgical breast procedures for cancer, immediate reconstruction of the excised area, or of the entire breast when it is removed, has sometimes been a source of great satisfaction and relief to the patient. This prevents the perception of disfigurement that women with breast cancer often experience. Reconstruction of numerous sites of extensive tissue loss has added enormously to the quality of the result of major extirpative procedures in various parts of the body, and Dr. Vasconez and colleagues have been pioneer innovators in this important contribution to patient welfare.

Repair of decubitus ulcer was one of the earliest lesions for which the plastic surgeon was called on to provide flap coverage, and substantial success was achieved in managing what formerly was often a fatal complication for a bedridden patient, with extensive infection, including osteomyelitis, as the terminal event, since these wounds can and did serve as an entry point for highly pathogenic bacteria in debilitated patients. The problem has hardly been eliminated, but for younger patients, the quality of the tissues used to reconstruct is often good enough to permit prolonged periods free of the terrible defects over bone that were so commonly a cause of morbidity and death in the past.

In patients with abdominal wall defects, often following trauma or operations to correct major intra-abdominal sepsis, and particularly when large volumes of fluid have been given to resuscitate the patient, abdominal hypertension is a serious concern. Under these circumstances, it is often not possible to close the abdomen without seriously impairing the excursion of the diaphragm and ventilation as well as putting enormous pressure on the venous drainage of the intra-abdominal gastrointestinal tract. A number of operative strategies are available to overcome this circumstance, ranging from simply closing the skin over the defect and leaving the fascia and peritoneum wide open, to doing relaxing incisions of both fascia and skin well away from the wound, closing the primary wound and skin grafting the resulting defect; more recently, mesh of some type has been used, including Marlex, PTFE and, most recently, Vicryl mesh. This is used to close the peritoneofascial defect, and the skin is left open, allowing the wound to granulate through the mesh. There is a significant hazard of placing Marlex, or even PTFE mesh in the wound, the former because of its tendency to abrade and ultimately erode the bowel and lead to intestinal fistulas, the latter because the mesh is not permeable to fluid and there is a lack of drainage through the mesh, allowing fluid to accumulate below it and to become infected. The Vicryl mesh, although it is a temporary expedient, has the advantage of being porous, allowing fluid to drain through it and permitting granulation tissue from the bowel surface to replace the mesh, over a period of weeks. Its physical qualities do not encourage infection to develop in or around the mesh and has made it most valuable in our hands. If, after 7 to 14 days, the abdominal hypertension subsides and the abdominal wall is loose, the Vicryl mesh can be excised and the wound closed by retention sutures. If, however, the distention persists, the mesh will ultimately become incorporated into the granulating surface, as indicated. Some weeks later, definitive closure of the abdominal wall can be accomplished by primary closure, if possible, or by the use of one of the several flaps that the authors have detailed.

R.J.B.

THREE

HEAD AND NECK

I

Lesions of the Parotid and Other Salivary Glands

Anatomy of the Parotid Gland, Submandibular Triangle, and Floor of the Mouth

Aaron Ruhalter

Anatomy of the Parotid Gland

The parotid gland is the largest of the paired salivary glands. The gland is wedged into the parotid space.

Parotid Space

The parotid space has a skeletal background created by the ramus of the mandible anteriorly, the styloid process medially, the mastoid process posteriorly, and the external acoustic meatus and the posterior part of the temporomandibular joint posterosuperiorly (Fig. 19-1). A soft-tissue background is created by the muscles that are attached to these bony landmarks—the masseter, medial pterygoid, and temporalis muscles on the mandible; the stylohyoid, styloglossus, and stylopharyngeus muscles arising from the styloid process of the temporal bone; and the sternocleidomastoid and digastric muscles related to the mastoid process and the lateral portion of the posterior occipital line.

Parotid Gland

The superficial surface of the parotid gland is triangular in shape, with the apex pointing inferiorly (Fig. 19-2). The deep surface of the gland is wedged into this parotid space, and presents anteromedial and posteromedial surfaces. The gland frequently extends beyond the limits of the parotid space. Glandular tissue may extend from the anterosuperior edge of the superficial surface, creating what is called the facial process, and is superior to the parotid duct. The extension of glandular tissue

may be separate from the main portion of the gland. This isolated segment of gland (accessory parotid) has a duct that empties into the main duct. There are frequently extensions from the deep surface of the

gland toward the pharynx or the medial pterygoid muscle.

The parotid gland is somewhat artificially divided into two lobes by the facial nerve

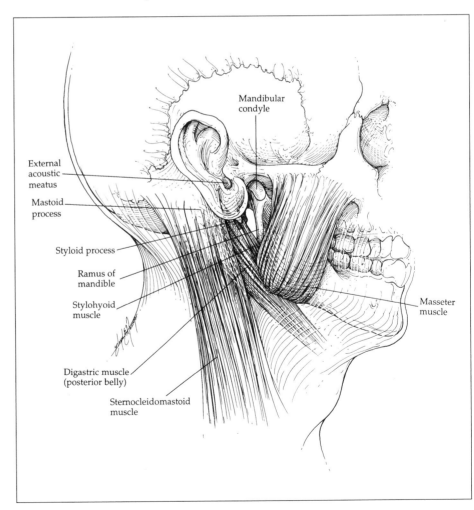

External acoustic meatus

Mastoid process

Styloid process

Ramus of mandible

Stylohyoid muscle

Digastric muscle (posterior belly)

Sternocleidomastoid muscle

Mandibular condyle

Masseter muscle

Fig. 19-1. Parotid bed.

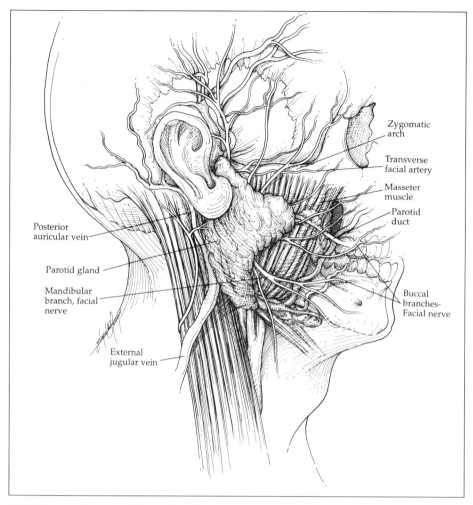

Fig. 19-2. *Superficial view of the parotid region.*

Labels on figure:
- Zygomatic arch
- Transverse facial artery
- Masseter muscle
- Parotid duct
- Buccal branches-Facial nerve
- Posterior auricular vein
- Parotid gland
- Mandibular branch, facial nerve
- External jugular vein

---

as it passes through. Endofacial (deep) and exofacial (superficial) portions are created. There are, however, multiple communications between the lobes, created by bridges of glandular tissue. A large area of communication, referred to as the isthmus, is related to the proximal part of the intraparotid portion of the facial nerve.

The parotid duct is about 2 inches in length, and lies on the superficial surface of the masseter muscle, about 1 cm below the zygomatic arch. The transverse facial artery is interposed between the duct and the arch, while the buccal branches of the facial nerve can be found inferior and superior to the duct. When this conduit reaches the anterior margin of the masseter muscle, it turns sharply, penetrates the buccinator muscle, and ends in the vestibule of the oral cavity opposite the upper second molar tooth.

Fascial Relations

The gland is encased by a split in the investing layer of the deep cervical fascia. The deep layer passes superiorly and attaches to the base of the skull. A portion of this fascia between the tip of the styloid process and the angle of the mandible is thickened, creating the stylomandibular ligament. This ligament supports the temporomandibular joint and separates the parotid gland from the submandibular gland. The superficial layer of this fascial split is much thicker, invests the masseter muscle, and attaches to the zygomatic arch. Its thickness and unyielding nature are responsible for the severe pain that results from enlargement of the gland.

Neurovascular Relations

Neurovascular structures pass through the parenchyma of the gland, and can conven-

iently be described in layers or planes. From deep to superficial, there are arterial, venous, and nervous layers.

Arterial Plane

The arterial layer includes the *external carotid artery*, which enters the parotid space after passing deep to the posterior belly of the digastric muscle (Fig. 19-3). At this point the external carotid artery gives rise to the *posterior auricular artery*, which gives off a *stylohyoid branch* that enters the stylomastoid foramen. This blood vessel is usually superficial to the facial nerve trunk as it exits from the skull by way of this same foramen. The posterior auricular artery then continues posteriorly, running under cover of, and parallel to, the superior edge of the posterior belly of the digastric muscle. It should be noted that this muscle passes superficial to and protects almost all of the structures passing between the submandibular triangle superiorly and the carotid triangle inferiorly. This includes the *internal jugular* vein and the *internal carotid artery* in the carotid sheath, the last four cranial nerves, and the external carotid artery. However, the *retromandibular vein* or its branches, the *cervical branch of the facial nerve*, and the *greater auricular nerve* pass superficial to the posterior belly of the digastric muscle.

The external carotid artery then pierces the medial surface of the parotid gland, and when it reaches the neck of the condylar process of the mandible it ends by giving rise to the *maxillary artery* and the superficial temporal artery. The maxillary artery passes medial to the condylar process of the mandible and enters the infratemporal fossa. The superficial temporal artery continues superiorly, accompanied by *superficial temporal veins*. The *transverse facial artery*, which arises from the proximal part of the superficial temporal artery, courses just superior to the parotid duct. The superficial temporal artery then enters the temporal region after passing between the external acoustic meatus and the temporomandibular joint. Accompanying these vascular structures at this level is the auriculotemporal nerve, which arises from the mandibular branch of the trigeminal nerve in the roof of the infratemporal fossa. It provides sensory innervation to the external acoustic meatus, external surface of the tympanic membrane, temporomandibular joint, and cutaneous sen-

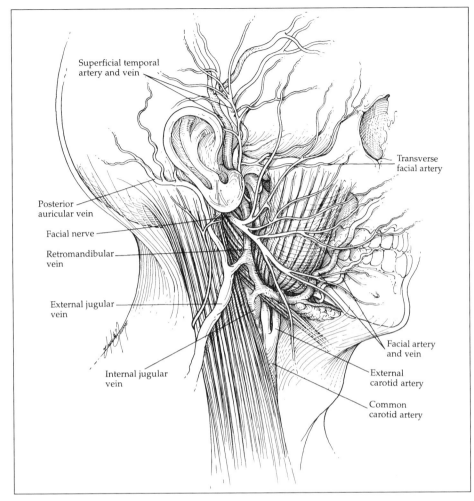

Superficial temporal artery and vein

Transverse facial artery

Posterior auricular vein

Facial nerve

Retromandibular vein

External jugular vein

Internal jugular vein

Facial artery and vein

External carotid artery

Common carotid artery

Fig. 19-3. Vascular background.

Nerve Plane

The nervous plane is created by the facial nerve and its branches (Fig. 19-4). The *facial nerve* (VIIth cranial nerve) exits from the skull through the stylomastoid foramen. At this point it is found with the stylomastoid branch of the posterior auricular artery, which enters the foramen and supplies the mucosa of the tympanic cavity, the mastoid cells, and the semicircular canals. The artery is usually superficial to the facial nerve. After emerging from the foramen, two branches arise from the facial nerve before it enters the parotid gland—the *posterior auricular nerve*, providing innervation to the posterior auricular muscles, and the intrinsic muscles of the auricle. The second branch, arising from the extraparotid portion of the facial nerve, provides motor innervation to the posterior belly of the digastric and stylohyoid muscles. This portion of the nerve, about one centimeter in length, then penetrates the posteromedial surface of the parotid gland. This nerve trunk passes forward in the glandular parenchyma for a distance of about one centimeter or less, then divides into two branches—a larger *temporofacial branch*, which creates *temporal* and *zygomatic* nerves, and a smaller *cervicofacial branch*, which gives rise to *buccal, marginal mandibular, and cervical nerves*. An isthmus of glandular tissue separates the temporofacial branch from the cervicofacial branch.

sory innervation to the auricle and temporal scalp region.

Venous Plane

The venous plane is superficial to the arterial plane (see Fig. 19-3). It includes the *retromandibular vein* and/or its branches. The retromandibular vein is created by the union of the superficial temporal and maxillary veins. The maxillary vein is formed by the union of veins that are part of a large plexus of veins surrounding the lateral pterygoid muscle. This venous plexus communicates with veins of the face as well as with the cavernous sinus within the skull. The parotid veins also communicate with the pterygoid venous plexus. This pterygoid venous plexus in turn represents a potential pathway for the spread of superficial cutaneous infections to the cavernous sinus. This is a potentially lethal condition.

The retromandibular vein passes inferiorly through the substance of the parotid gland, and is found between the branches of the facial nerve and the arterial layer. The retromandibular vein terminates at the lower edge of the gland by giving off anterior and posterior branches. The posterior branch joins with the *posterior auricular vein* to form the *external jugular vein*, which continues inferiorly, superficial to the posterior belly of the digastric muscle, then passes obliquely across the sternocleidomastoid muscle. It is frequently found just anterior to the great auricular nerve, which is on its way to the skin overlying the parotid gland. The anterior branch of the retromandibular vein unites with the anterior facial vein, forming the common facial vein. This passes inferiorly, superficial to the digastric muscle, to empty into the internal jugular vein.

The facial nerve provides motor innervation to the muscles of facial expression. The platysma is included in this category of muscle. The nerve branches, as they pass through the parotid gland, divide it into two portions. The part of the gland that is superficial to the nerves is referred to as the superficial (exofacial) lobe, and the portion of the gland that is internal to the nerve layer is referred to as the deep (endofacial) lobe. There are multiple communications between the nerve branches as they pass through the gland. The zygomatic and temporal nerves are frequently multiple, while the mandibular and cervical branches are often single. The cervical and mandibular branches can extend below the mandible, while the cervical branch passes superficial to the posterior belly of the digastric muscle. The nerves become more superficial as they pass distally.

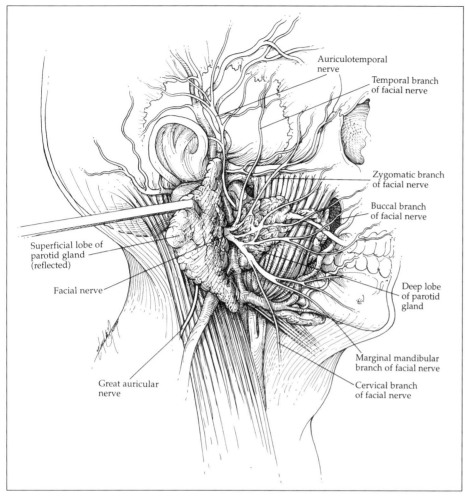

Fig. 19-4. Nervous plane.

Nervous Innervation

The parotid gland receives postganglionic sympathetic fibers from a plexus of nerves that travel with the external carotid artery. Secretomotor postganglionic parasympathetic fibers reach the infratemporal fossa by way of the lesser petrosal nerve, synapse in the otic ganglion, and then travel to the parotid gland by way of the auriculotemporal nerve.

Lymphatic Drainage

The lymphatic drainage of the parotid gland is related to two systems (see Figs. 25-10, 25-11). Superficial nodes in the superficial fascia (preauricular) drain into the superficial system of cervical nodes. These are related to the external jugular vein, and pass to the supraclavicular nodes in the

posterior triangle. The second set of nodes is found within the fascial covering of the parotid gland. These nodes drain into the deep cervical nodes and the jugular chain.

Anatomic Aids

It is possible to find the main trunk of the facial nerve by tracing one of its branches proximally. The mandibular and cervical branches are more frequently used because they are often single and more convenient to find.

The parotid duct is about one centimeter inferior to the lower edge of the zygomatic arch. The pathway of the duct can be recreated by a line between the lower end of the tragus of the ear and the commissure of the mouth.

Two nerves may be found with the superficial temporal vessels. The auriculotemporal nerve is posterior, while the temporal branches of the facial nerve lie anterior to these vessels.

The *great auricular nerve* is frequently found posterior to the external jugular vein. This nerve and vein travel together until the inferior edge of the parotid gland is reached. The nerve passes to the subcutaneous tissues superficial to the gland, providing sensory innervation to the skin overlying the parotid gland. The remainder of the face receives its sensory innervation only from the trigeminal nerve. The vein is seen to emerge from the substance of the gland.

The *external carotid artery* is related to the medial boundary of the parotid space. The *internal carotid artery* is slightly deeper. The two vessels should not be confused. It must be remembered that the internal carotid artery does not have any branches in the neck. Separating the external carotid artery from the internal carotid artery are the styloid process or stylohyoid ligament, the stylopharyngeus muscle, and the glossopharyngeal nerve.

The stylohyoid muscle and the posterior belly of the digastric muscle diverge at their points of attachment to the skull. The main trunk of the facial nerve passes through this interval.

At the junction of the cartilaginous portion with the osseous portion of the auditory canal, there is frequently a downward projection of cartilage that points to the main trunk of the facial nerve.

When the external jugular vein is traced superiorly to its parent structure, the retromandibular vein, it will lead to the interval between the superficial and deep lobes of the parotid gland. It is also a means of locating the cervical or mandibular branches of the facial nerve, since they pass superficial to the vein.

The stylomastoid branch of the posterior auricular artery enters the stylomastoid foramen and is superficial to the facial nerve trunk.

The internal jugular vein may be in contact with the deep surface of the gland.

Anatomy of the Submandibular Triangle

The submandibular triangle is part of the anterior triangle of the neck, and is suprahyoid in position. It is sometimes referred to as the digastric, or submaxillary triangle.

Muscular Boundaries

The muscular boundaries of the submandibular triangle are the *posterior belly of the digastric* and *stylohyoid muscles* posteriorly, and the *anterior belly of the digastric muscle* anteriorly (Fig. 19-5). The inferior margin of the body of the mandible creates a superior boundary to this triangular area. The digastric muscle attaches posterosuperiorly to the *mastoid process* of the temporal bone, posterior to the stylohyoid muscle, which arises from the posterolateral surface of the styloid process. The two muscles quickly approach each other and remain in intimate contact down to the region of the hyoid bone, where an intermediate tendon of this double-bellied muscle is found. This tendon passes through a split in the tendon of insertion of the stylohyoid muscle. The intermediate tendon is bound to the hyoid bone by a fascial thickening. The anterior belly then passes superomedially and ends by attaching to the internal aspect of the mandible near the midline. The digastric muscle elevates the hyoid bone and assists in depression of the mandible. The posterior belly of the digastric and the stylohyoid muscles are innervated by the facial nerve, and the anterior belly of the digastric muscle is innervated by the mylohyoid nerve branch of the inferior alveolar nerve. This latter nerve is a branch of the posterior division of the mandibular nerve.

Muscular Floor

The muscular floor of the submandibular triangle consists of four muscles (see Fig. 19-5). The direction of the muscular fibers of each of the muscles is characteristic and allows for recognition of the boundaries between neighboring muscles. These muscles do not lie in the same plane. The anterior muscles are more superficial than those posterior, which creates a steplike pattern to this muscular floor of the sub-

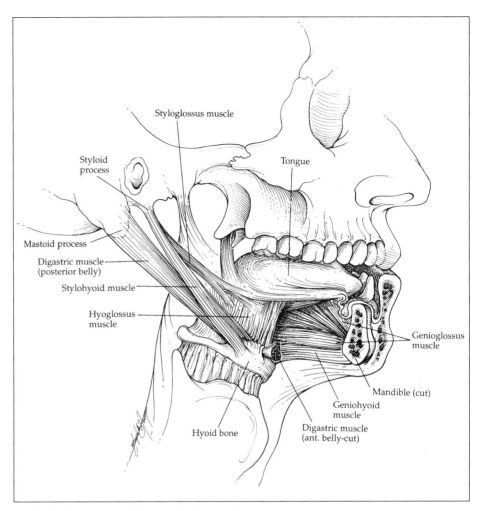

Fig. 19-5. Musculoskeletal background and floor of the mouth.

Labels in figure: Styloglossus muscle; Styloid process; Tongue; Mastoid process; Digastric muscle (posterior belly); Stylohyoid muscle; Hyoglossus muscle; Genioglossus muscle; Mandible (cut); Geniohyoid muscle; Digastric muscle (ant. belly-cut); Hyoid bone

mandibular triangle. Passing from anterior to posterior, one encounters *the mylohyoid* and then the *hyoglossus* muscles. The inferior portion of the *superior constrictor* muscle, and the superior portion of the *middle constrictor* muscle, complete the floor of the submandibular triangle.

The mylohyoid muscle (Fig. 19-6) is the most anterior and superficial of the muscles creating the floor of the mouth. It arises from the inner aspect of the mandible, and the two halves pass inferomedially where the majority of the fibers insert into a midline fibrous raphe extending from the midportion of the mandible to the center of the body of the hyoid bone. The more posterior fibers insert into the body of the hyoid bone. The two halves of the muscle create a floor for the oral cavity. The mylohyoid muscle presents a posterior free edge. When this muscle contracts, it will raise the floor of the mouth, causing

elevation and posterior displacement of the tongue. This is an integral part of the swallowing mechanism.

The hyoglossus is a quadrangular-shaped muscle that arises from the entire length of the greater horn of the hyoid bone. It passes superiorly and attaches to the lateral surface of the tongue. Its deep relations include the *stylohyoid ligament, glossopharyngeal nerve,* and *lingual artery.* Passing superficial to the hyoglossus muscle are the *lingual nerve,* the *hypoglossal nerve* and its *two venae comitantes,* and the *submandibular duct.* Those structures that are superficial to the hyoglossus muscle will become deep relations of the mylohyoid muscle when they reach the free posterior edge of the mylohyoid muscle and then travel in the interval between these muscles. The hypoglossal nerve innervates the hyoglossus muscle and the other extrinsic tongue muscles, as well as

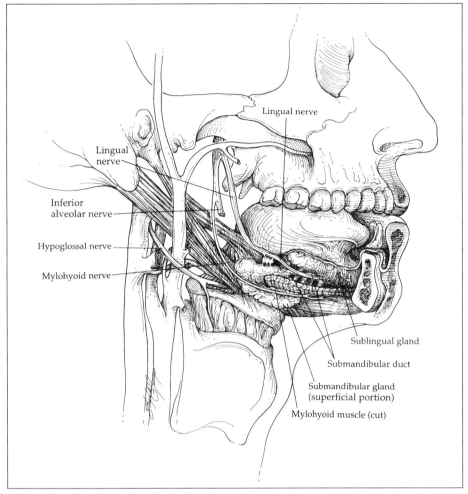

Lingual nerve

Lingual nerve

Inferior alveolar nerve

Hypoglossal nerve

Mylohyoid nerve

Sublingual gland

Submandibular duct

Submandibular gland (superficial portion)

Mylohyoid muscle (cut)

Fig. 19-6. Submandibular triangle and floor of the mouth. This figure illustrates nerve contents, superficial, and deep portions of the submandibular gland.

all of the intrinsic muscles of the tongue. The mylohyoid muscle and the anterior belly of the digastric muscle are innervated by the mylohyoid nerve, which arises from the inferior alveolar branch of the mandibular nerve.

Fascial Coverings

A fascial roof and carpet are created by the investing layer of the deep cervical fascia when it splits to invest the submandibular gland. The superficial layer attaches to the inferior edge of the mandible, while the deep layer attaches to the inner aspect of the mandible, just below the attachment of the mylohyoid muscle.

Contents of the Submandibular Triangle

Submandibular Gland

The submandibular gland is the main content of this triangle (see Fig. 19-6). It actu-

ally overflows and extends beyond its boundaries. The gland wraps itself around the posterior free edge of the mylohyoid muscle. This creates a superficial lobe that lies on the external surface of the mylohyoid, and a smaller deep lobe that lies internal to the mylohyoid muscle. The duct of the gland passes medial to the deep lobe and ends in the floor of the mouth at a small elevation just lateral to the frenulum. The *lingual nerve* at first is superior to the duct as they both pass superficial to the hyoglossus muscle. The hypoglossal nerve is at a more inferior level.

Neurovascular Structures

The structures that are superficial to the submandibular gland include the cervical branch of the facial nerve, and the distal ends of the anterior facial vein and anterior branch of the retromandibular (posterior facial) vein (Fig. 19-7). These veins unite in the tissues overlying the submandibular

triangle, creating the *common facial vein*, which passes inferiorly to empty into the internal jugular vein. Occasionally, the mandibular branch of the facial nerve will descend below the inferior edge of the mandible, and can be injured when incisions are made in this area.

Structures in the submandibular triangle found between the submandibular gland and the mylohyoid muscle include the facial artery and the mylohyoid nerve and vessels. The facial artery is the most superior of the vessels that arise from the anteromedial surface of the external carotid artery. It begins in the carotid triangle, just superior to the tip of the greater cornu of the hyoid bone, passes deep to the posterior belly of the digastric muscle, and enters the submandibular triangle. It passes superiorly and reaches a point well above and medial to the lower edge of the body of the mandible. It then passes over the superior and lateral surfaces of the gland, and is adherent to these surfaces. It now arches superiorly in contact with the external surface of the mandible, creating a groove just anterior to the insertion of the masseter muscle. It gives a *submental branch* that runs along the inferior surface of the mandible in contact with the upper surface of the gland.

Appearing at the anterior edge of the gland are the mylohyoid nerve and vessels. The nerve arises from the inferior alveolar branch of the mandibular nerve. Neurovascular structures are found deep to the submandibular gland, but on the other side of (deep to) the mylohyoid muscle. They are located in the interval between the hyoglossus and mylohyoid muscles, and are responsible for tongue function and nutrition.

The *lingual nerve*, a branch of the mandibular nerve, passes through the interval until it reaches the anterior margin of the hyoglossus muscle. It then turns medially, after looping around the submandibular duct, and penetrates the tongue. It provides general sensation for the anterior two-thirds of the tongue.

The chorda tympani (arising from the facial nerve) joins the lingual nerve in the upper part of the infratemporal fossa. It carries taste fibers from the tongue and brings preganglionic parasympathetic fibers to the submandibular ganglion. This ganglion is attached to the lingual nerve and is the site of synapse for these pregan-

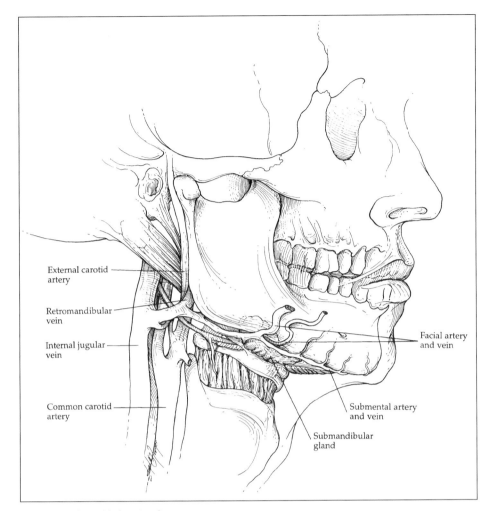

Fig. 19-7. Submandibular triangle.

glionic fibers. Postganglionic secretomotor fibers then pass to the sublingual and submandibular glands. The hypoglossal nerve and lingual veins are also seen in this region. Accompanying these neurovascular structures is the submandibular (Wharton's) duct. The deep lobe of the submandibular gland is also found internal to the mylohyoid muscle.

Lymphatic Drainage

The lymphatics of the submandibular gland are found within its parenchyma, whereas other lymph nodes are outside the fascial covering of the gland (see Figs. 25-10, 25-11). The lymphatics of the mandibular region can be divided into horizontal and vertical systems. The horizontal chain runs along the mandible from the parotid gland to the midline, receiving afferent channels from the ipsilateral face and oral cavity. The lymphatics of the sub-mental triangle also drain into this horizontal system. From this submandibular collecting area, vertical channels pass to the system of nodes related to the internal jugular vein (deep cervical nodes). Other vertical channels pass into the posterior triangle to the superficial posterior cervical system (found with the external jugular vein) and the deep posterior cervical system (found with the spinal accessory nerve). There are named lymph nodes in the internal jugular channels, which are found where double-bellied muscles pass superficial to the internal jugular vein (i.e., jugulodigastric and jugulomylohyoid).

Anatomic Aids

The mandibular and cervical branches of the facial nerve may extend below the lower edge of the mandible. All other structures of concern lie deep to the posterior belly of the digastric muscle. Inci-sions can be made down to this muscle with little fear of injuring any vital neurovascular structures.

The fascial coverings of the submandibular gland are less adherent to the gland surface than are the coverings of the parotid gland. This allows for easier enucleation of the submandibular gland.

The facial artery is very adherent to the internal and superior surfaces of the gland, and frequently must be removed with the gland after proximal and distal control is obtained.

The hyoglossus muscle is an anatomic landmark. It is superficial to the glossopharyngeal nerve and the lingual artery, but is found internal to the lingual and hypoglossal nerves, the submandibular duct, and a deep process of the submandibular gland. The lingual veins are also superficial to this muscle, and are closely related to the hypoglossal nerve.

The lingual nerve is superior to the deep process of the submandibular gland and its duct before forming a loop around the duct by passing lateral and then inferior to it prior to penetrating the framework of the tongue. The hypoglossal nerve and its venae comitantes are inferior to the duct.

The hypoglossal nerve crosses the internal and external carotid arteries superficially. The glossopharyngeal nerve, the pharyngeal nerves arising from the vagus, and the stylopharyngeus muscle pass between these same arteries, while the superior laryngeal nerve (arising from the vagus nerve near the base of the skull) passes deep to those arteries.

Small nerve branches arise from the lingual nerve and submandibular ganglion, which enter the submandibular gland. These must be transected during excision of the gland in order to prevent avulsion injuries to the lingual nerve.

Anatomy of the Floor of the Mouth

The mylohyoid muscle is the anatomic structure that separates the oral cavity from the neck, and thereby creates the floor of the mouth. The attachments of this muscle have been mentioned previously. The hyoglossus muscle contributes a posterolateral boundary to this separation be-

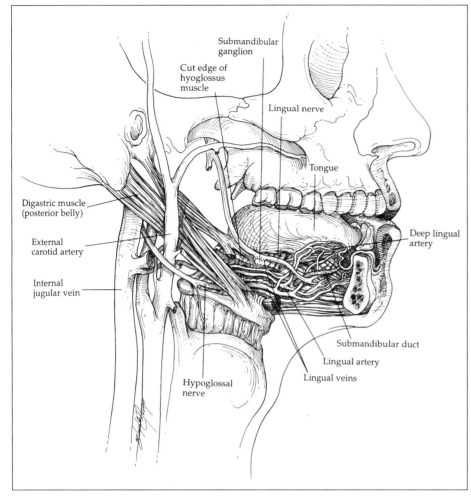

Fig. 19-8. Submandibular triangle and floor of the mouth (deep structures).

tween the floor of the mouth and the submandibular triangle (part of the anterior neck). The floor of the mouth can also be defined as the area between the tongue and its lateral mucosal reflections, and the mylohyoid muscle.

The Tongue

The tongue is a massive muscular structure that faces the oral cavity and the pharynx (see Figs. 19-5 and 19-6). It is attached to the floor of the mouth, the mandible, and the hyoid bone.

Extrinsic Muscles

The extrinsic muscles of the tongue include the genioglossus, hyoglossus, styloglossus, and palatoglossus. The genioglossus muscle arises from the genial tubercles found on the internal aspect of the midportion of the mandible and passes to most of the dorsum of the tongue. The hyoglossus arises from the hyoid bone, passes superiorly, and attaches to the lateral aspect of the tongue. The styloglossus muscle arises from the tip of the styloid process and the proximal part of the stylohyoid ligament. Its fibers pass anteroinferiorly and attach to the lateral surface of the tongue, where they interdigitate with the fibers of the hyoglossus muscle.

Intrinsic Muscles

The intrinsic muscles of the tongue consist of longitudinal, horizontal, and vertical fibers that create an interlocking network.

Movements

Because of the extensive interdigitation of the muscles of the tongue, a wide variety of movements are possible. In addition, the mylohyoid muscle will be displaced by movements of the hyoid bone. These movements are created by contraction of the suprahyoid and infrahyoid muscle groups. The mandible can be depressed by contraction of the mylohyoid, stylohyoid, digastric, and geniohyoid muscles if the hyoid bone is fixed in position by contraction of the infrahyoid musculature.

Innervation

All of the intrinsic and extrinsic muscles of the tongue receive their innervation from the hypoglossal nerve. The one exception is the palatoglossus muscle, which is innervated by the pharyngeal plexus of nerves. Sensory innervation of the anterior portion of the floor of the mouth is provided by the lingual nerve. Traveling with this nerve are fibers of the chorda tympani (VIIth), which provides taste sensation for the anterior portion of the tongue, and preganglionic secretomotor fibers on their way to synapse in the submandibular ganglion before proceeding to the submandibular and sublingual glands. Sensation and taste for the posterior one-third of the tongue are provided by the glossopharyngeal nerve.

Vascular Supply

The vascular supply to the tongue is provided by the lingual artery, which arises from the external carotid artery in the carotid triangle, passes into the submandibular triangle, and enters the region of the floor of the mouth after passing deep to the hyoglossus muscle. It gives a sublingual branch and then, as the deep lingual artery, passes to the apex of the tongue just lateral to the midline. There is little communication across the midline between the left and right deep lingual vessels.

Contents of the Floor of the Mouth

Geniohyoid Muscle

The geniohyoid muscle originates just below the origin of the genioglossus and passes anteroinferiorly to attach to the body of the hyoid bone. The left and right parts of this muscle lie side by side. When they contract, the hyoid bone is displaced anteriorly and superiorly.

Salivary Glands and Their Ducts

The sublingual gland is found in the floor of the mouth, between the geniohyoid muscle and the mandible (see Fig. 19-6). It is the smallest of the three paired salivary glands, and frequently has two systems of ducts. One is composed of multiple ductules, which empty directly into the floor of the mouth. The second system consists of a duct (or ducts) of varying size emptying into the larger submandibular duct. In this same area is found the deep process of the submandibular gland and its duct. This deep process may be of significant size, and may appear to blend in with the sublingual gland. The submandibular duct, lingual nerve and veins, and hypoglossal nerve are medial to the sublingual gland. There is anatomic flow between the submandibular triangle and the floor of the mouth (sublingual space), which allows for passage of the contents of one area into the domain of the other.

Lymphatic Drainage

The lymphatic drainage of the floor of the mouth is complex (see Figs. 25-10, 25-11). Lesions from the central part of the floor of the mouth and the tip of the tongue can drain into submandibular glands on either side, or drain directly into submental nodes, and then into submandibular nodes (horizontal system). The drainage is then directed primarily toward the deep cervical system, which is associated with the vertical system of lymphatics found with the internal jugular vein. There may be some spread to the superficial posterior cervical system in the posterior triangle, which is found with the external jugular vein. The lymph drainage from the posterior part of the tongue is directly into the deep cervical nodes of either or both sides.

Anatomic Aids

There is little communication across the midline of the tongue between the deep lingual arteries. This will limit blood loss at the time of hemiglossectomy.

Suggested Reading

Arnold M. *Reconstructive Anatomy* (1st ed). Philadelphia: Saunders, 1968.

Delmas A. *Atlas Aide-Memoire d'Anatomie* (Rouviere). Paris: Masson, 1991.

Hollinshead WH. *Anatomy for Surgeons* (2nd ed). New York: Harper and Row, 1971.

20

The Parotid Gland

Ronald H. Spiro

The earliest references to "para-auricular swellings," as the Greeks called them, described the findings associated with calculi and inflammation. It was not until the mid-seventeenth century that the anatomy of the parotid glands and the role of the main parotid ducts were appreciated. Interestingly, Niels Stensen, in 1660, identified the duct that bears his name during dissection of a sheep's head but apparently never fully appreciated the connection between the duct and the parotid gland.

Between 1650 and 1750, salivary gland surgery was limited to the treatment of ranulas and oral calculi. The concept of parotidectomy for the treatment of a tumor has been attributed to Betrandi (1802). Initially, surgeons were concerned primarily about hemorrhage and patients were inevitably left with major disfiguration if they were fortunate enough to survive a parotid resection.

By the mid-nineteenth century, focus had shifted to facial nerve anatomy and techniques that would provide access for resection with nerve preservation. Most physicians are aware that the first operation to employ ether inhalation anesthesia was a parotid tumor resection performed by Dr. John C. Warren in Boston in 1846. The first total parotidectomy with facial nerve preservation is said to have been accomplished by Codreanu, a Romanian, in 1892.

During the early years of this century, many authors verified that removal of parotid gland tumors was possible with facial nerve preservation. Blair, Sistrunk, and others attempted to systematize the surgical approach to the facial nerve. The first attempts at facial nerve grafting date from the early 1950s.

In addition to the unique anatomic problem posed by the course of the facial nerve through the parenchyma of the gland, parotid tumors are a special challenge to surgeons because of the diversity of histologic subtypes and the remarkable variation in clinical behavior that they display. Small benign tumors are quite indistinguishable from their malignant counterparts, but even if their benign nature can be established with reasonable certainty, few patients will be happy with the disfiguration of an enlarging benign tumor, which is the usual outcome when "watchful waiting" is selected, rather than surgery.

Experienced clinicians agree that resection is indicated for all patients in whom a parotid mass develops unless medical problems preclude general anesthesia. Although this presentation is focused exclusively on parotidectomy for tumor resection, it should be remembered that gland excision is also occasionally indicated when symptomatic, recurrent chronic parotitis proves refractory to conservative measures.

Clinical Presentation

Tumors of the parotid gland account for fewer than 4 percent of head and neck neoplasms, about 20 percent of which are malignant. Estimates of parotid gland carcinoma incidence in the United States range from 1 to 2 per 100,000. Aside from the relationship between salivary gland neoplasms and prior radiation therapy, there is very little solid information about potential risk factors.

Although parotid gland tumors can occur at any age and have no gender predilec-tion, certain histologic subtypes are more common in some age groups. Primary squamous carcinoma, for example, almost invariably afflicts older patients, while the most common malignant tumor in the young patient is low-grade mucoepidermoid carcinoma. An asymptomatic swelling is the usual complaint, and the fact that the lump has been present for years is no guarantee that the lesion is benign. About 10 percent of parotid tumors arise below the facial nerve in the so-called deep lobe. Deep parotid origin will be appreciated preoperatively in the relative few who present with a parapharyngeal mass, which medially displaces the tonsil or soft palate. The fact that a tumor is deep to the nerve but lateral to the mandible will seldom be recognized until the time of operation.

Patient Evaluation

Any painless swelling near the ear is best assumed to be a parotid gland neoplasm until proved otherwise. When dealing with a small, typical parotid tumor, many experienced surgeons will make a diagnosis and proceed with resection without performing additional diagnostic tests. Although numerous authors assert that fine-needle aspiration biopsy (FNAB) and imaging studies (CT or MRI) are important, if not essential, prerequisites, the information derived is unlikely to influence management in the setting just described. In fact, the treatment is usually the same whether a small tumor is benign or malignant.

When the tumor is larger, parapharyngeal, or closely related to the main trunk of the

Table 20-1. WHO Classification of Salivary Gland Tumors

Benign	Malignant
Pleomorphic adenoma	Acinic cell carcinoma
Myoepithelioma	Mucoepidermoid carcinoma
Basal cell adenoma	Adenoid cystic carcinoma
Warthin's tumor	Polymorphous low-grade adenocarcinoma
Oncocytoma	Epithelial-myoepithelial carcinoma
Canalicular adenoma	Basal cell adenocarcinoma
Sebaceous adenoma	Sebaceous carcinoma
Ductal papilloma	Papillary cystadenocarcinoma
Inverted ductal papilloma	Mucinous adenocarcinoma
Sialadenoma papilliferum	Oncocytic carcinoma
Cystadenoma	Salivary duct carcinoma
Papillary cystadenoma	Adenocarcinoma
Mucinous cystadenoma	Malignant myoepithelioma
Benign lymphoepithelial lesion	Carcinoma in pleomorphic adenoma
Salivary cysts	Squamous cell carcinoma
	Small-cell carcinoma
	Undifferentiated carcinoma

Table 20-2. Histologic Classification*

Tumor	No. of Patients	Percent
BENIGN		
Pleomorphic adenoma	1274	45.4
Warthin's tumor	183	6.4
Benign cyst	29	1.0
Lymphoepithelial lesion	17	0.6
Oncocytoma	20	0.7
Monomorphic adenoma	6	0.2
MALIGNANT		
Mucoepidermoid carcinoma	439	15.7
Adenoid cystic carcinoma	281	10.0
Adenocarcinoma	225	8.0
Malignant mixed tumor	161	5.7
Acinic cell carcinoma	84	3.0
Epidermoid carcinoma	53	1.9
Other (anaplastic et al)	35	1.3
Total	2807	100.0

*A cumulative 35-year Memorial Hospital experience pooling all salivary sites.

Table 20-3. Distribution of Parotid Tumor Types*

Tumor	No. of Patients	Percent
BENIGN	1342	68.2
MALIGNANT		
Mucoepidermoid carcinoma	272	13.8
Malignant mixed tumor	107	5.5
Acinic cell carcinoma	75	3.8
Adenocarcinoma	62	3.2
Adenoid cystic carcinoma	54	2.8
Epidermoid carcinoma	45	2.3
Anaplastic carcinoma and others	8	0.4

*Summary of a 35-year Memorial Hospital experience with 1965 parotid gland tumors.

facial nerve, a histologic diagnosis by FNAB may facilitate treatment. Moreover, imaging in such patients can define extraglandular spread, the extent of parapharyngeal disease, and the status of the cervical lymph nodes. Cost considerations require that each patient be individualized. Unless dental artifact or contrast allergy precludes adequate imaging, or true coronal or sagittal views are required, CT, rather than MRI, will suffice in most instances.

Classification and Stage

The current World Health Organization (WHO) classification lists a bewildering variety of tumors that can arise in the parotid gland, the precise identification of which can be a challenge even to the most experienced pathologists (Table 20-1). It is also worth remembering that grading of malignant tumors is not always possible or consistently reproducible. Detailed discussion of the spectrum of histologic diagnoses is beyond the scope of this presentation.

We find that the original classification proposed years ago by Foote and Frazell still serves most of our clinical needs and is certainly much easier to use (Table 20-2). Delineation of uncommon and unique subtypes may be of considerable interest to the pathologist, but has limited value for the surgeon. Based on a sizable parotidectomy experience, the incidence of the var-

ious tumor subtypes treated at a major referral center is given in Table 20-3.

More important for clinicians is an appreciation that the stage of a malignant parotid gland tumor seems to be more significant than its histologic appearance. The clinical staging system formulated by the American Joint Committee in 1978 has grown more complex with each revision, but it is essential for treatment planning and assessment of results. Low stage (I, II) currently includes tumors up to 6 cm if there is no clinically obvious local extension to adjacent tissues, as well as tumors 4 cm or less with local extension. For the purpose of this discussion, high stage (III, IV) refers to tumors 4 to 6 cm in size with local extension, tumors more than 6 cm in greatest dimension with or without local extension, and any size tumor associated with obvious nodal metastases (N+).

One unique problem concerns the rare patient with adenoid cystic carcinoma who presents initially with a chest radiograph consistent with metastatic disease. With any other tumor type, stage IV disease with distant metastasis would be considered a nonsurgical problem. Argument can be made for parotidectomy in this setting in carefully selected patients with adenoid cystic carcinoma because some can live more than a decade with very slowly progressive, asymptomatic pulmonary metastases. In such patients, effective surgical treatment that achieves local tumor control may afford significant palliation.

Neck Dissection and Adjunctive Therapy

Neck dissection is performed when nodes are clinically positive. This is usually a comprehensive operation resecting all nodal levels, but modification may be feasible when the metastasis is solitary and adjacent to the tail of the gland. With the exception of high-grade mucoepidermoid and anaplastic carcinomas, occult node involvement is uncommon and there is no compelling indication for elective lymph-adenectomy.

Adjunctive radiation therapy should be considered after resection of high-stage carcinomas or when there is concern about the adequacy of resection margins. Evidence suggests that this can significantly reduce locoregional recurrence. Unfortunately, no single chemotherapeutic agents or drug combinations have proved consistently effective in patients with parotid carcinomas. For this reason, neither neoadjuvant nor maintenance chemotherapy can be justified as part of the initial therapy unless the patient is involved in an ongoing clinical trial.

Surgical Technique

Oral endotracheal anesthesia is employed with the patient in the supine position. The head is extended by elevating the shoulders and rotated to the opposite side. Draping the head separately from the body and incorporating the endotracheal tube within the head drape allows free movement of the head without having to worry about the airway. Transparent plastic is used for the final layer, exposing the eye, cheek, and mouth on the operative side, as well as the endotracheal tube and its connections. Muscle relaxants are not employed.

The skin incision starts anterior to the ear just above the tragus. It is carried inferiorly to the level of the lobule, and then angled posteriorly under the lobule and directed anteriorly for a suitable distance in the upper neck. This part of the incision should correspond to the mentum-to-mastoid incision used for elevation of a lower cheek flap (Fig. 20-1). The dotted lines indicate the potential extensions of the typical pa-rotidectomy incision anteriorly, in the rare instances when a mandibulotomy may be necessary for resection of a deep tumor, or superiorly and anteriorly when exposing a lesion arising in accessory parotid tissue.

Incision is made through skin and subcutaneous tissue, developing the plane between the cartilaginous external canal and the posterior aspect of the gland. A suture through the subcutaneous tissue is used to retract the ear and facilitate exposure. The sternomastoid muscle is identified and its anterior border exposed as the tail of the gland is reflected away from it (Fig. 20-2). No attempt is made to preserve the greater auricular nerve unless its course takes it close to the mastoid process. Dissection continues in this plane, severing attachments to the mastoid, until the posterior belly of the digastric muscle is visualized below the digastric groove. The anterior flap is elevated in the plane of the parotid

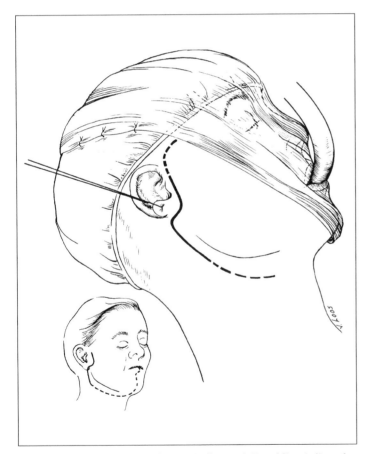

Fig. 20-1. The incision for parotidectomy is illustrated. Dotted lines indicate the superior and anterior extensions, which may be required in special situations. A clear plastic drape allows visualization of facial movement and keeps the airway connections in view. Inset shows the incision required for the rare instance when resection of a large deep lobe tumor requires a mandibulotomy approach.

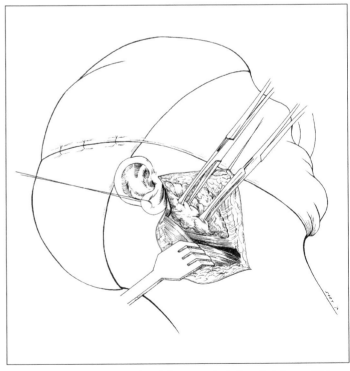

Fig. 20-2. After incision is made and flaps are raised, the tail of the parotid is reflected off the sternomastoid muscle and the plane between the cartilaginous canal and the gland is developed to allow for identification of the superior border of the digastric muscle as it passes into its sulcus in the mastoid.

capsule, remembering that the terminal branches of the facial nerve are at risk if the dissection is carried past the anterior border of the gland.

The facial nerve is identified shortly after its emergence from the stylomastoid foramen. A variety of landmarks have been described that facilitate the exposure of the main trunk, such as the cartilaginous "pointer" of the external canal and the tympanomastoid sulcus. If the volar aspect of the fifth finger is placed deeply on the junction of cartilaginous and bony external auditory canal and wedged against the bone cephalad, the main trunk will be found below the inferior border of the finger and a few millimeters above the exposed superior border of the posterior belly of the digastric muscle as it enters its groove in the mastoid bone (Fig. 20-3).

Good traction on the reflected parotid tissue is essential, as a clamp is used to elevate and incise the overlying tissue in layers. Meticulous hemostasis and good illumination are most important at this point. A small arterial branch often located just lateral to the nerve must be identified and ligated. With careful layer-by-layer dissection and a solid knowledge of the anatomy, a nerve stimulator is unnecessary. Some twitching of the facial muscles due to mechanical stimulation of the facial nerve is likely in the nonparalyzed patient, which can be of assistance in the dissection.

On occasion, exposure of the main trunk is complicated by the presence of a sizable tumor directly overlying it. Removal of the mastoid tip may help, but it is important not to persist when there is serious risk of capsular rupture and tumor spillage. In this situation, it makes more sense to identify one of the peripheral branches of the facial nerve and work from anterior to posterior until the main trunk is isolated. This tends to be a more tedious dissection that carries a higher risk of injury to small nerve branches, which is why the posterior approach to the nerve is preferred.

The most demanding and time-consuming part of the operation involves the identification and preservation of all branches of the facial nerve as the tumor, surrounded by the normal, superficial portion of the gland, is removed. The bifurcation of the upper and lower divisions is first identified by gentle clamp dissection in the areolar plane directly over the nerve as appropriate traction is maintained. Clean removal of parotid tissue lateral to the nerve branches requires that the dissection must proceed from the periphery toward the center of the gland. As the temporalis and ramus marginalis branches are cleared, it must be remembered that these peripheral branches of the facial nerve are least likely to recover when injured (Fig. 20-4). Nerve injury can result from desiccation, as well as from mechanical trauma, which is easily avoided if moist sponges are used during the dissection.

What should be done when the facial nerve trunk or its branches are intimately related to the tumor? From the historic perspective, radical parotidectomy with facial nerve sacrifice was advocated years ago in patients with carcinoma with minimal regard for the extent of the tumor or

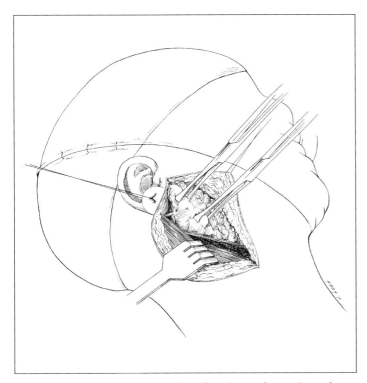

Fig. 20-3. With gentle layer-by-layer clamp dissection, good retraction, and careful attention to hemostasis, the main trunk of the facial nerve is identified shortly after its emergence from the stylomastoid foramen.

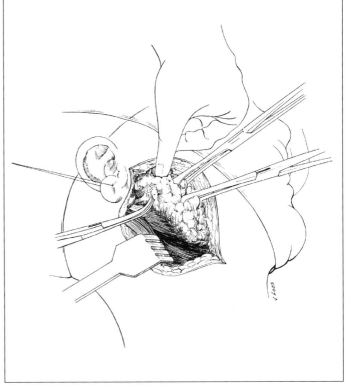

Fig. 20-4. Working from the periphery toward the isthmus, each branch of the facial nerve is identified and separated from the overlying lateral portion of the gland.

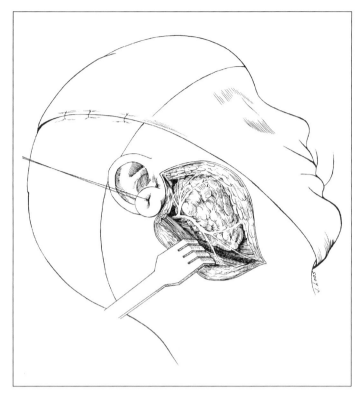

Fig. 20-5. *After the lateral portion of the gland has been removed, all nerve branches should be exposed. If a clean dissection has been performed, at least a portion of the masseter muscle should be in view. Stensen's duct is transected and ligated anteriorly.*

its relationship to the nerve. More recently, it has been appreciated that the nerve can usually be spared when it is not directly involved. At least part of this conservatism relates to the enhanced local control achieved by adjunctive, postoperative radiotherapy when margins are close.

Unfortunately, it may be difficult to distinguish between tumor adherence and direct involvement of the nerve. Persistence with facial nerve dissection in this setting may be reasonable when prior FNAB has yielded a benign diagnosis. This is one argument in favor of preoperative needle biopsy when the tumor location suggests that facial nerve exposure is likely to be tedious.

With or without a histologic diagnosis, it is important that surgeons not be carried away by the current zeal for nerve preservation. Those who might consider piecemeal tumor excision in order to preserve a nerve branch that should be sacrificed should remember one of the basic principles in surgical oncology: Even the best postoperative radiotherapy is no substi-

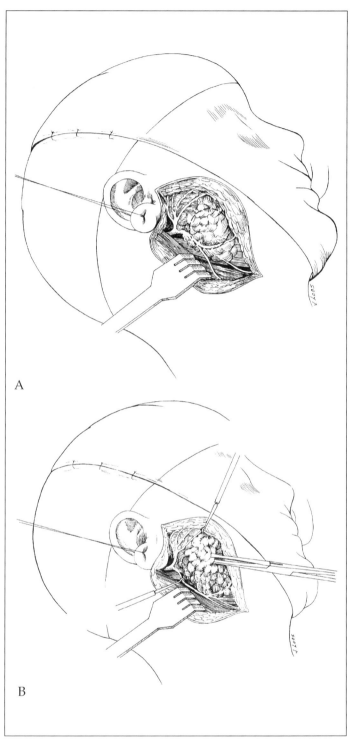

A

B

Fig. 20-6. *A. About 10 percent of parotid tumors are found to lie deep to the plane of the nerve. B. Most of these are lateral to the mandible and can be removed after superficial parotidectomy by gentle elevation and retraction of the overlying facial nerve branches.*

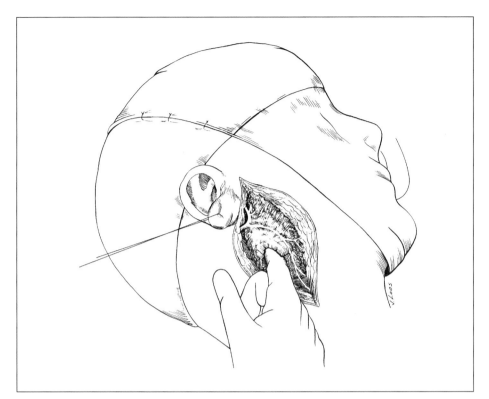

Fig. 20-7. *Deep tumors that involve the retromandibular portion of the gland can usually be removed by a transcervical approach. At least the lowest branches of the facial nerve must be exposed so they can be carefully retracted and spared as the parapharyngeal extension of the tumor is mobilized and delivered by finger dissection.*

tute for adequate, en bloc resection. Preoperative discussion with the patient must deal with the possibility of a facial nerve deficit, and nerve grafting. The patient needs to be aware that in rare instances it may be wiser to sacrifice a nerve branch than to risk seeding of the wound, even if the tumor proves to be benign.

With the specimen removed, the integrity of the facial nerve is carefully checked as the wound is copiously irrigated with sterile water (Fig. 20-5). A single suction drain is brought out through a separate stab wound and fine sutures are used for a layered closure. For the first 24 hours, a pressure dressing is used. The suction drain can usually be removed in a day or two and skin sutures are generally removed by the sixth postoperative day. It is worth remembering that it is best to assess facial nerve function as soon as the patient awakes from anesthesia. Although minor weakness can progress to major dysfunction within a few hours, presumably due to swelling, the patient can be reassured that return to at least the immediate postoperative status is certain.

Deep Tumors

At times, what starts out as a routine subtotal parotidectomy proves otherwise when a tumor that seemed superficial to the nerve is found to lie deep to the main trunk or one of its branches (Fig. 20-6A). In this situation, all major nerve branches should be fully exposed before tumor removal is attempted. The latter is accomplished by elevation and retraction of the overlying nerves. Whether the tumor is below the main trunk, or smaller distal branches, it can usually be removed after nerve displacement inferiorly, or superiorly. When a deep tumor involves the isthmus, excision is usually achieved by retracting the upper division superiorly and lower division inferiorly (Fig. 20-6B). Nerve injury due to stretching is common in this situation, and the most gentle nerve retraction is likely to be provided by the surgeon rather than by his or her assistant.

Retromandibular parotid gland tumors merit special consideration. As a rule, deep parotid gland origin is suspected clinically. Treatment planning is facilitated

when a histologic diagnosis can be achieved via FNAB, and an appropriate imaging study is usually indicated in order to confirm parotid origin and to be sure that the extent of the lesion is not underestimated.

Almost all retromandibular tumors can be resected through a transcervical approach. The conventional parotidectomy incision is extended more anteriorly than usual. The key lies in exposure of the main facial trunk and its lowest branch so that they are in view at all times. Complete removal of the lateral portion of the gland is not essential, but may prove helpful in some situations.

Entry into the retromandibular space is achieved by finger dissection just above the posterior belly of the digastric muscle (Fig. 20-7). With larger tumors, this access can be enhanced by removal of the submandibular gland, division of the posterior belly of the digastric, and/or anterior displacement of the mandible. Essentially, the tumor is enucleated using blunt finger dissection. Occasionally, this can be facilitated by transection of the styloid process near its base.

The limitations of the transcervical approach to the retromandibular portion of the parotid gland are obvious to all who have performed this operation. Exposure is usually less than adequate, and there is a risk of significant hemorrhage. More importantly, finger dissection does not allow for tumor excision with an adequate margin of normal tissue. The incidence and distribution of malignant tumor types is the same as that encountered in more superficial parotid tumors, and our experience has been that local control and survival have also been similar. Nevertheless, it seems clear that postoperative irradiation is indicated after resection of malignant retromandibular tumors because tumor margins are almost invariably minimal.

On rare occasion, retropharyngeal tumors reach a size that precludes resection transcervically. Our preference in this situation calls for paramedian, rather than lateral, mandibulotomy. Exposure is similar through both methods, but the obvious disadvantage of the lateral approach is that it places an osteotomy directly in the center of a subsequent irradiation field if the tumor proves to be malignant (Fig. 20-8A). In questionable situations, it may be

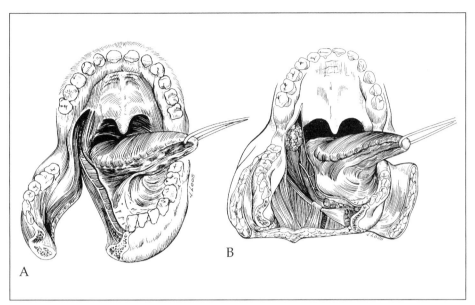

Fig. 20-8. *In rare instances, retromandibular deep parotid tumors are too large or inaccessible for transcervical removal. In that case, the incision is extended anteriorly over the mentum and a paramedian mandibulotomy is performed. The lingual nerve can usually be preserved as the paralingual extension is carried across the anterior pillar superiorly onto the hard palate. Although this provides direct access to the parapharyngeal space and greatly facilitates resection, excision margins are still unlikely to be generous. Osteotomy repair can be accomplished either with miniplate or wire fixation. A. A lateral mandibulotomy. B. A paramedian mandibulotomy, the preferred technique.*

appropriate to start with an attempt at transcervical resection. If the access proves inadequate, it is better to stop and extend the incision anteriorly for a mandibulotomy rather than risk rupture of the capsule with tumor spillage.

The paramedian mandibulotomy performed in this setting is identical to that used for resection of certain oral or oropharyngeal tumors. The difference is that the paralingual extension is carried posteriorly up the anterior tonsillar pillar onto the palate. This opens the parapharyngeal space widely, allowing for direct tumor access (Fig. 20-8B). The bone cut should be angled if the osteotomy is to be repaired with wire. If miniplates are preferred, a simple transverse cut will suffice. These patients will require a tracheostomy and tube feeding for about a week. Despite the better access provided by this open approach, tumor margins are unlikely to be generous.

Radical Parotidectomy

For an encouraging variety of reasons, we now see fewer patients with far-advanced, parotid gland carcinomas. When such is the case, however, the surgeon and the patient must both be prepared for an extended parotidectomy, which may involve resection of overlying skin, adjacent mandible and soft tissue, temporal bone, and/or a portion of the adjacent external ear. The facial nerve is almost invariably sacrificed in such patients, and free tissue transfer may be necessary for repair.

When tumor extends to the stylomastoid foramen, which is not unusual with advanced disease, some surgeons unroof the facial nerve within the temporal bone in order to perform a free graft. Following radical resection with nerve transection at the skull base, the advisability of partial temporal bone resection to facilitate a graft is questionable in patients with high-stage tumors. The prognosis is so poor and the importance of local tumor control is so overriding that it may be unwise to increase the risk of complications by a more complex operation, which may delay the all-important postoperative radiotherapy.

Suggested Reading

Armstrong JG, Harrison LB, Spiro RH, et al. Malignant tumors of major salivary gland origin, a matched-pair analysis of the role of combined surgery and postoperative radiotherapy. *Arch Otolaryngol Head Neck Surg* 116:290–293, 1990.

Attie JN, Sciubba JJ. Tumors of major and minor salivary glands, clinical and pathologic features. *Curr Probl Surg* Feb 1981. Pp. 68–155.

Conley J. *Salivary Glands and the Facial Nerve.* Stuttgart: Georg Thieme, 1975.

Foote FW Jr, Frazell EL. *Tumors of the Major Salivary Glands. Cancer* 6:1065–1133, 1953.

Johnson FE, Spiro RH. Tumors arising in accessory parotid tissue. *Am J Surg* 138:576, 1979.

McNaney D, McNeese M, Guillamondegui OM, et al. Postoperative irradiation in malignant epithelial tumors of the parotid. *Int J Radiat Oncol Biol Phys* 9:1289, 1983.

Nigro MF Jr, Spiro RH. Deep lobe parotid tumors. *Am J Surg* 134:523, 1977.

Rankow RM, Polayes IM. *Diseases of the Salivary Glands.* Philadelphia: Saunders, 1976.

Seifert G, Sobin LH. The World Health Organization's Histological Classification of Salivary Gland Tumors. *Cancer* 70:379, 1992.

Spiro RH, Huvos AG, Strong EW. Carcinoma of the parotid gland, a clinicopathologic study of 288 primary cases. *Am J Surg* 130:452, 1975.

Spiro RH, Armstrong J, Harrison L, et al. Carcinoma of major salivary glands. *Arch Otolaryngol Head Neck Surg* 115:316, 1989.

EDITOR'S COMMENT

Doctor Spiro has given us an excellent account of salivary gland tumors and his approach to them. The no-nonsense approach to dividing the classification of salivary gland tumors into benign and malignant, according to the Memorial Sloan-Kettering Cancer Center experience, probably has real merit since trying to decide the pathology of a parotid gland tumor has been the happy hunting ground of pathologists for many years. While intellectually interesting, what one really needs to know is how aggressive to be in the treatment of a patient with a salivary gland tumor.

Doctor Spiro's technique follows the time-honored approach of identifying and carefully preserving the facial nerve, and not sacrificing it except in situations in which one is absolutely certain that the sacrifice will aid the result. The protection of the ramus mandibularis by tying off the facial vein and including the ramus mandibularis in the subcutaneous flap, which others have advocated, is not mentioned, but is undoubtedly part of Dr. Spiro's approach. It probably is so second nature in all incisions of this type that it is not believed to be especially important to mention.

The evolution of parotid gland surgery, even including such benign lesions as pleomorphic adenoma, has been toward prevention of recurrence. The long-term life history of patients with pleomorphic adenomas is such that one can expect survival in 95 to 98 percent of them over 10 years. This, however, is not the issue. The issue is whether the patient is free of recurrence. A good case in support of identification of the facial nerve and complete resection of the superficial parotid rather than enucleation is that of Phillips and Olsen (*Ann Otol Rhinol Laryngol* 104:100, 1995). In this study, 126 patients with recurrent pleomorphic adenoma of the parotid gland treated at the Mayo Clinic from 1965 to 1985 were reviewed. While malignant disease occurred in a low 7.1 percent of patients, tumor recurrence was 32.5 percent after one operation, but only 7.1 percent after two operations and 1.6 percent

after three operations. After all surgical procedures, partial facial nerve paralysis was noted in 13.5 percent and total facial nerve paralysis in 5.5 percent of patients. Thus, they conclude that an aggressive surgical approach could result in good tumor eradication with low morbidity.

A surprising dissent from the aggressive surgical point of view was recently published by Liu and associates from Princess Margaret Hospital in Toronto (*Head Neck* 17:177, 1995), in which a surprising number of patients (55 of 76) underwent enucleation of pleomorphic adenoma with postoperative radiotherapy. Postoperative radiotherapy was particularly important for patients with recurrent disease. Thirty-two of the 76 patients underwent enucleation alone and were followed by x-ray radiation for reasons that included the presence of recurrent disease, microscopic residual disease, gross residual disease, tumor spill, and so forth. The 10-year probability of remaining relapse free was 55 percent of the entire population, while survival was in the 95 to 100 percent range.

Control of recurrent disease was achieved in 13 of 16 patients who had postoperative radiotherapy, while recurrence developed in 16 of 17 who were not irradiated; 9 of these were subsequently treated with postoperative radiotherapy, with control of recurrence achieved in 8. Thus, there appears to be some advantage to aggressive surgical therapy with nerve preservation, although in the hands of the Princess Margaret Hospital group, transient facial paralysis developed in 5 of 16 patients (31%) following a third operation, one (6%) of which was total.

Taking all of these bewildering statistics together, it appears that an aggressive surgical approach, rather than postoperative radiotherapy, offers the best chance of controlling recurrence. Radiotherapy should be reserved for patients in whom the nerve is involved microscopically, in which case it probably can be sterilized with postoperative radiotherapy, although this is not certain.

J.E.F.

21

Operations on the Submandibular and Sublingual Glands

Joseph N. Attie   *James Sciubba*

Anatomy of the Submandibular and Sublingual Glands

The submandibular region consists of a triangle formed by the lower border of the mandible and the anterior and posterior bellies of the digastric muscle (Fig. 21-1A). The roof of the triangle is a well-defined fascial sheath formed by the continuation of the investing layer of the deep cervical fascia, which split to envelop the submandibular salivary gland. The floor of the triangle is composed of the mylohyoid, hyoglossus, and styloglossus muscles, going from anterior to posterior. The styloglossus muscle parallels the posterior belly of the digastric muscle.

The triangle contains the submandibular salivary gland and a group of lymph nodes lying along the horizontal ramus of the mandible and flanking the facial artery and the anterior facial vein. The submandibular gland occupies the major portion of the triangle. It is a lobulated gland, yellowish tan in color, soft, and measuring 4 × 3 × 2 cm. In contrast to the parotid gland, no lymph nodes are located within the substance of the submandibular salivary gland. The mandibular branch of the facial nerve courses parallel to the horizontal ramus of the mandible just deep to the deep fascia. It passes between the nodes superficial to the facial vessels, just below or just above the mandibular border. It may divide early into two or more fine nerve branches, making it vulnerable to injury. The hypoglossal nerve passes into the triangle deep to the posterior belly

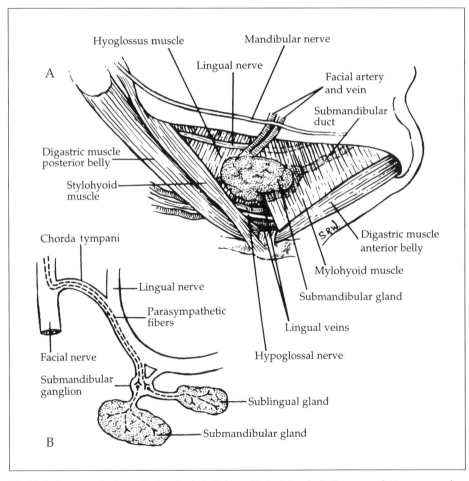

Fig. 21-1. Anatomy of submandibular gland. A. Submandibular triangle. B. Parasympathetic nerve supply of submandibular gland.

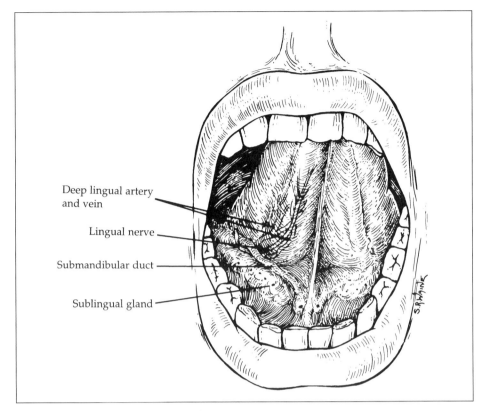

Deep lingual artery
and vein

Lingual nerve

Submandibular duct

Sublingual gland

Fig. 21-2. Anatomy of the floor of the mouth.

The sublingual gland is a thin elongated structure lying beneath the mucosa of the floor of the mouth just lateral to the midline, contiguous with the submandibular duct (Fig. 21-2). It lies on the styloglossus and hyoglossus muscles and further forward on the genioglossus muscle. Approximately 12 tiny ducts (the ducts of Rivinus) open directly into the mucosa of the floor of the mouth. Occasionally, several of the ducts unite to form a larger duct (Bartholin's duct), which joins the submandibular duct near the papilla to empty with it into the floor of the mouth.

Histologically, the submandibular and sublingual glands consist of lobules separated by connective tissue septa. The ducts form a treelike pattern; the finest branches are the intercalated ducts that empty into striated ducts and then into the excretory duct. The mucous and serous acini are located terminally at the ends of the intercalated ducts.

The six major salivary glands develop embryologically as ectodermal buds arising from the lining of the stomodeum subsequent to invagination into the adjacent mesenchyme. Cytodifferentiation and morphogenesis lead to the fundamental organization of salivary tissue into a precise pattern relating to its ultimate function. The acini are composed of pyramidal secretory cells surrounding a small central lumen. All acini are surrounded by a basal lamina separating the acinar cells from the connective tissue stroma. At the epithelial side of the basal lamina lie the myoepithelial cells, flattened cells of probable epithelial origin that contract to cause the release of salivary secretion into the intercalated duct system.

The daily volume of saliva is 1000 to 1500 ml, of which approximately 90 percent is from parotid and submandibular glands, 5 percent from sublingual, and 5 percent from minor salivary glands. With minimal stimulation (at rest), the submandibular gland secretes twice as much saliva as the parotid, whereas with maximal stimulation the parotid secretes about two-thirds of the salivary flow. Salivary components aid deglutition, maintain mucosal integrity, aid in remineralization of teeth, help mediate taste, and contain an array of antimicrobial components, including lysozyme, thiocyanate, lactoferrin, lactoperoxidase, immunoglobulin, and electrolytes.

of the digastric and the styloglossus muscles coursing superficial to the hyoglossus muscle, where it is usually accompanied by two facial veins to run deep to the mylohyoid muscle, terminating in and supplying the muscles of the tongue. The lingual artery is not found within the triangle; it lies deep to the hyoglossus muscle.

Further superiorly, lying on the floor of the triangle, the lingual nerve courses forward at or slightly above the level of the mandibular border. The submandibular ganglion lies between the lingual nerve and the submandibular gland, and is connected to the two structures via rami communicantes, usually two in number.

An extension of the submandibular gland passes anteriorly deep to the mylohyoid muscle. From the anterior tip of the gland arises the submandibular (Wharton's) duct, which courses anteriorly toward the floor of the mouth to terminate at an orifice on a papilla near the midline. The submandibular duct passes on the lateral surfaces of the hyoglossus and genioglossus muscles, lying below the lingual nerve. The lingual nerve descends anteriorly and crosses lateral to the duct; further anteri-

orly, the duct lies medial and adjacent to the sublingual gland. The lingual nerve passes below the duct and then crosses medial to it, thus making almost a complete loop around the duct.

The posterior border of the submandibular gland is adjacent to the tail of the parotid gland and is separated from it by the sphenomandibular ligament. The facial artery passes across the posterosuperior portion of the submandibular gland, forming a deep groove in the gland and giving off two or more arterial branches to the gland. In resecting the salivary gland, the segment of the facial artery attached to it can be excised or the branches ligated and divided and the artery preserved.

The lingual nerve provides sensory and taste fibers to the tongue and also contains parasympathetic fibers that control salivary secretion of both the submandibular and sublingual glands. The preganglionic parasympathetic fibers originate in the glossopharyngeal (IXth) nerve intracranially, join the facial nerve, then the chorda tympani, and from there join the lingual nerve (Fig. 21-1B). Sympathetic fibers reach the salivary glands by way of other nerves and vessels.

Secretory activity of the major salivary glands results from stimulation of parasympathetic nerve fibers. Parasympathetic innervation of the submandibular and sublingual glands occurs via the superior salivary nucleus by way of the nervus intermedius and the chorda tympani. The submandibular ganglion is the synapse site at the distal portion of the chorda tympani. The sympathetic innervation of the salivary glands has its primary effect on the vascular elements, which subsequently influence secretion.

Submandibular Sialolithiasis

Calcific concretions occur in the ducts of major or minor salivary glands. Calculi occur 10 to 12 times more frequently in the submandibular duct than in the parotid duct. There are several reasons for the prevalence of submandibular calculi: 1) The saliva produced by the submandibular gland is more alkaline than that of the parotid and has a greater concentration of calcium and phosphate salts; 2) the secretion of the submandibular gland contains more mucus, making it more viscous with a greater tendency for stasis to occur; and 3) Wharton's duct is longer than Stensen's and runs an uphill course to its termination, favoring stagnation of its contents. Submandibular calculi have a nidus of concentrated mucoid molecules around which calcium and other salts precipitate. The most common site of submandibular calculi is the posterior border of the mylohyoid muscle, where the duct makes a 90-degree turn around the muscle.

Submandibular stones can be solitary or multiple, and are sometimes bilateral. They are usually spherical or cylindrical in shape but are sometimes faceted when multiple. They vary in size from 1 to 2 mm to 2 to 3 cm. The smaller calculi tend to occur in the distal duct close to the orifice; calculi 4 to 5 mm in size are found in the middle third of the duct, while larger stones are near the hilum of the gland or even within the gland.

The evolution of calculi in the submandibular duct differs from that in the parotid duct. In the submandibular duct, the calculus causes obstruction, which results in inflammation of the gland. In the parotid, inflammation of the gland precedes and usually causes the formation of stones; the matrix of parotid calculi reveals desquamated epithelial cells, debris, and inflammatory cells indicating an inflammatory cause.

The clinical picture in submandibular sialolithiasis varies. Ductal or intraglandular calculi may be found incidentally on routine x-ray study or on palpation through the floor of the mouth with no symptoms. Most frequently there is partial obstruction of the duct with intermittent attacks of pain and swelling of the submandibular gland after eating, with resolution a few hours or sometimes a day or two later. Attacks are more likely to occur following ingestion of sour or bitter food, or with decreased liquid intake. In such cases, applying pressure on the gland produces thick, gelatinous material through the orifice of the duct. If the calculus completely obstructs the duct, an acute suppurative process in the duct and gland may result. Severe pain and swelling may occur, often with systemic symptoms of fever and malaise. The floor of the mouth mucosa is edematous and tender, making palpation of the calculus difficult.

The diagnosis of submandibular calculi is often made on clinical grounds, with the stone being palpable in the floor of the mouth. Calculi in the anterior two-thirds of the duct can be demonstrated by occlusal dental radiographs. Stones in the hilum of the gland are better seen in oblique external radiographs. Computed tomography scans are more accurate, revealing single or multiple calculi in the gland and duct. The use of sialography to demonstrate calculi or other abnormalities has been almost completely discontinued. Aside from the fact that accurate diagnosis can be made with plain films or CT scans, there is potential harm in using sialography: The valve action of the orifice can be damaged, stones in the duct can be displaced to a different position in the duct or into the gland, and a partial obstruction can be converted to a complete one.

Treatment of Submandibular Calculi

During the acute phase of obstruction, considerable inflammation and swelling in the floor of the mouth usually occur, in addition to swelling of the submandibular gland. As a result, it may be impossible to palpate the calculus through the mucosa. Increased fluid intake and antibiotics will hasten resolution of the acute situation. No attempt to remove the calculus at this stage is advisable. Occasionally, pus forms in the duct or gland, or both, distal to the obstruction. Gentle insertion of a fine lacrimal probe through the orifice of the duct to a point distal to the calculus may release the purulent material.

Sialodocholithotomy can be performed if the calculus is palpable in the floor of the mouth. Calculi may occur in three general locations in the course of the duct; the technique of removal is different in each instance. If the calculus is small (1–3 mm) and lies close to the orifice of the duct, a small incision is made immediately over the stone, using topical anesthesia, and the calculus is forced through the wound by the tip of the No. 11 scalpel blade or by a small clamp (Fig. 21-3A). The backed-up secretions are expressed by pressure on the gland. The wound is left open.

Larger calculi (4–10 mm) often lodge in the middle third of the duct, where they may be impacted. In this location, the duct lies immediately beneath the mucosa. A local anesthetic is injected over the region of the calculus, and a longitudinal incision is made in the mucous membrane. A suture is placed around the duct proximal to the calculus and pulled up gently to partially occlude the duct and prevent the stone from falling back into the gland (Fig. 21-3B). The incision is deepened into the duct and the calculus removed; this can be accomplished with a clamp, a toothed forceps, or a stone extraction forceps (e.g., Randall forceps). No attempt is made to close the wound.

Calculi in the hilar region of the gland at the junction with the proximal end of the duct are palpable in the floor of the mouth at the level of the last lower molars. These calculi range from 1 to 3 cm in size and may be multiple. They lie deeper than more anterior calculi. The duct in this area is crossed by the lingual nerve, and exposure of the duct may be difficult. General anesthesia via nasal intubation allows adequate exposure by retraction of the tongue medially and, after incising the mucosa, retraction of the lingual nerve laterally. A longitudinal incision is then made in the duct and the stone extracted, again using a clamp or the extraction forceps (Fig. 21-3C). Because a longer incision is used, the wound is partially closed with a few sutures of chromic catgut.

Very tiny calculi sometimes present at the orifice of the duct and extrude after gentle pressure proximally. Larger calculi usually cannot be extruded through a dilated orifice; they should not be removed by incising and enlarging the duct orifice, as this can destroy the valvular mechanism and result in stricture.

Recurrent calculi or calculi within the submandibular gland often cause repeated attacks of submandibular swelling or chronic inflammation and fibrosis with permanent enlargement of the salivary gland. The treatment in such cases is resection of the submandibular gland and duct through a cervical incision.

Ranula

Obstruction of one or more of the sublingual ducts results in a mucous retention cyst known as a ranula. It can be caused by trauma or by precipitation of calcium salts into tiny sialoliths. It is uncommon and occurs at all ages. The cyst is usually situated in the floor of the mouth superficial to the mylohyoid muscle beneath the thinned-out overlying mucosa below the tongue, which may be pushed up by the lesion (Fig. 21-4A). It has a bluish hue and resembles a frog's belly, from which its name, "ranula," is derived. At times the cyst ruptures spontaneously but reforms after a symptom-free interval. When very large it insinuates itself through the mylohyoid into the submandibular triangle as an external swelling, known as "plunging ranula." It can be differentiated from cystic hygroma in that it does not empty on pressure or increase in size after a Valsalva maneuver.

Treatment

Generally asymptomatic, ranulas can be left untreated. When large or troublesome, they can be treated by marsupialization. The roof of the cyst with overlying mucosa is excised, a small gauze packing is inserted, and the edges of the open trough are attached to the adjacent mucosa with absorbable sutures, leaving the floor and sides of the ranula open to the oral cavity (Fig. 21-4B). Smaller cysts or large ones that recur after marsupialization are treated by resection of the sublingual gland. A longitudinal incision is made over the cyst and sublingual gland, and

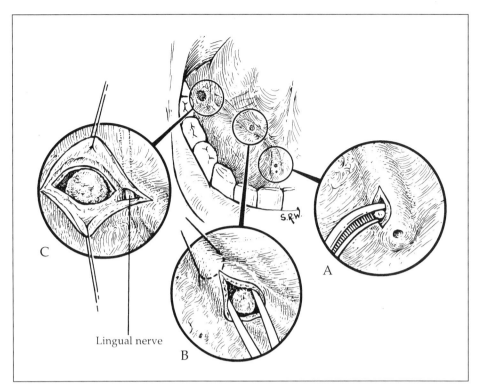

Fig. 21-3. Calculi in submandibular duct. A. Removal of small calculus in distal duct. B. Removal of calculus in midduct. C. Removal of calculus in proximal duct.

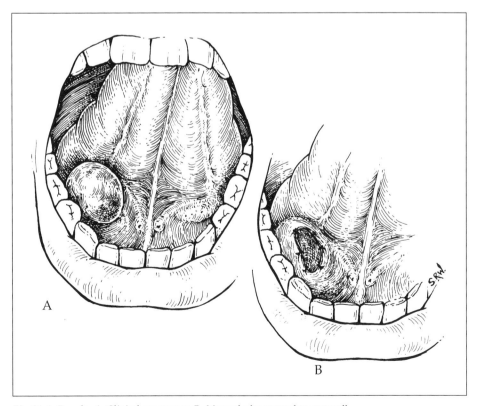

Fig. 21-4. Ranula. A. Clinical appearance. B. Mucosal edge sutured to cyst wall.

the mucosa is elevated as a flap. The sublingual gland is exposed in its entire length along the medial aspect of the submandibular duct (Fig. 21-5). The duct is preserved by carefully dissecting the sublingual gland by blunt dissection, preserving the duct. A tiny cannula can be inserted into the duct to facilitate the dissection. The mucosa is resutured with absorbable sutures.

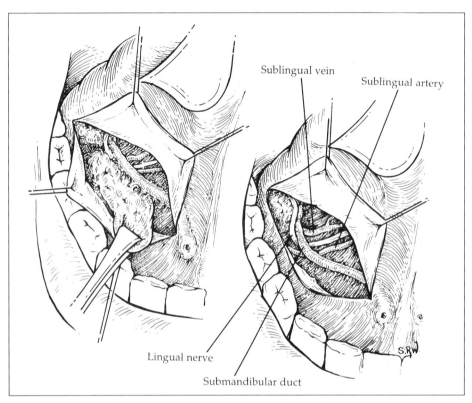

Fig. 21-5. Excision of sublingual gland.

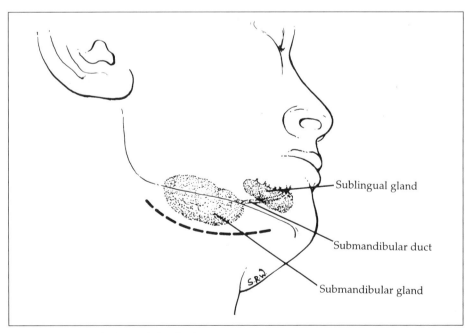

Fig. 21-6. Resection of submandibular gland: incision.

Sialadenitis

Acute sialadenitis of the submandibular gland is rare and usually due to duct obstruction. Recurrent sialadenitis often results in chronic enlargement of the gland, which becomes hard and difficult to differentiate from salivary gland neoplasm. Needle aspiration biopsy may not be conclusive. In such instances, resection of the submandibular gland is performed. The submandibular gland may be involved as part of Sjögren's syndrome or may form a benign lymphoepithelial lesion either as a localized tumor-like formation or a diffuse involvement of the salivary gland. Sjögren's syndrome may involve both submandibular glands and one or both parotid glands. Resection of such submandibular glands is performed because of difficulty in differentiating them from neoplastic glands and because occasionally the lymphoid elements of the lesion proceed to malignant lymphoma.

Tumors of Submandibular Salivary Glands

For every 100 tumors of the parotid, there are approximately 10 tumors in the submandibular glands, 10 tumors in the minor salivary glands, and 1 tumor in the sublingual gland. Whereas 15 percent of parotid tumors are malignant, 50 percent of submandibular tumors are malignant. Survival rates for neoplasms of the submandibular glands are poorer than those for the parotid glands.

The most common benign tumor of the submandibular gland is the pleomorphic adenoma (mixed tumor). Papillary cystadenoma lymphomatosum (Warthin's tumor) is rare in this location, since intraglandular lymph nodes are not found in the submandibular gland. Benign cysts and oncocytomas are extremely rare in the submandibular gland. Benign neoplasms of the submandibular and sublingual glands are twice as common in females as in males, whereas malignant tumors are more common in males.

Adenoid cystic carcinoma is the most commonly occurring cancer in the submandibular and sublingual glands, followed by mucoepidermoid carcinoma, undifferentiated carcinoma, squamous cell carcinoma, malignant mixed tumor, and adenocarcinoma, in order of frequency. The clinical stage of the disease is of more prognostic importance than the histologic appearance of the tumor. Adenoid cystic carcinoma, although slow growing, exhibits infiltrative behavior early, with a propensity toward spread along nerves, resulting in frequent recurrences and a generally poor prognosis.

Clinical Picture

A submandibular neoplasm generally presents as a painless mass in the submandibular triangle. It is usually firm and well circumscribed, and can be palpated through the skin or through the mucosa of the floor of the mouth. The rate of growth is variable and usually slow except in high-grade malignancies. Invasion of adjacent structures occurs with progression of the cancer: mandibular nerve involvement causes paresis of the lower lip, lingual nerve invasion results in numbness of the side of the tongue, and invasion of the hypoglossal nerve results in hemiparalysis of the tongue. The muscles of the submandibular triangle may be invaded and, rarely, the mandible is involved. High-grade cancers may metastasize to regional lymph nodes.

Differentiation from submandibular lymphadenopathy and inflammatory conditions of the submandibular gland may be difficult. Computed tomography scans or magnetic resonance images (MRI) are of help in distinguishing submandibular tumors from enlarged lymph nodes or from lesions deep to the gland, such as muscle tumors or tumors of nerve origin. Fine-needle aspiration is often diagnostic. Sialography is of little help and has practically been abandoned in the study of submandibular neoplasms.

Submandibular Gland Resection

Indications for Surgery

The removal of the submandibular salivary gland is most often performed for salivary gland neoplasms. Less frequently, sialadenectomy is indicated for acute or chronic sialadenitis with or without calculi. In the majority of cases, a diagnosis has been made by fine-needle biopsy. If the tentative diagnosis is a benign tumor

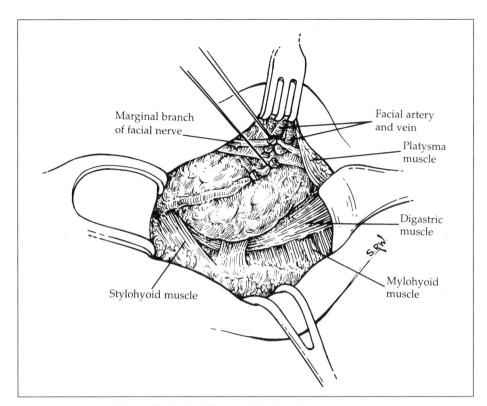

Fig. 21-7. Resection of submandibular gland: ligation of facial vessels.

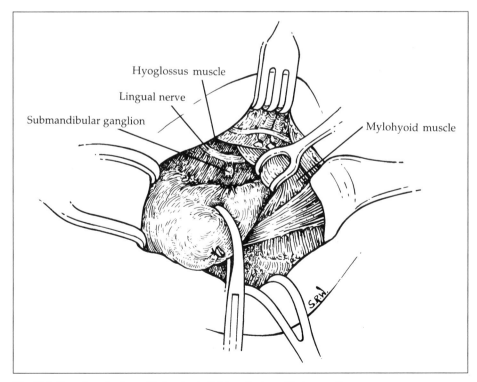

Fig. 21-8. Resection of submandibular gland: division of submandibular ganglion.

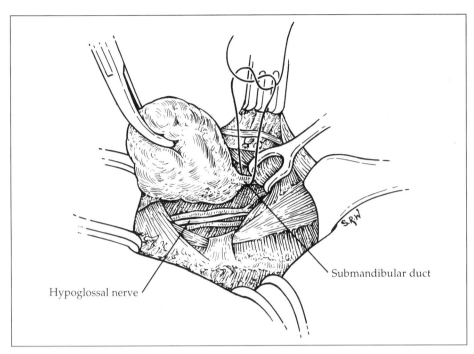

Fig. 21-9. *Resection of submandibular gland: division of submandibular duct.*

Hypoglossal nerve

Submandibular duct

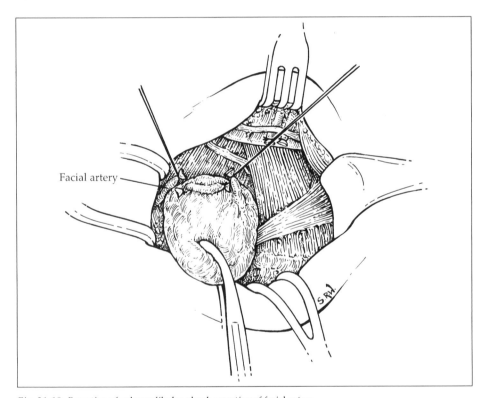

Fig. 21-10. *Resection of submandibular gland: resection of facial artery.*

Facial artery

section in patients with primary tumors in the tongue, cheek, floor of the mouth, lip, skin of the face, and parotid gland.

Technique

A transverse incision is made below and parallel to the lower border of the mandible (Fig. 21-6). To avoid injury to the marginal mandibular branch of the facial nerve, the incision should be made 1 to 2 cm below the mandible. Skin flaps including the platysma muscle are developed a short distance above the mandibular border and inferiorly to the hyoid bone. Hemostasis is controlled with cautery. The rest of the dissection is done by spreading a fine mosquito clamp to develop a plane, and dividing the tissues with cautery. Blunt dissection transversely parallel to the course of the mandibular nerve isolates and preserves the nerve. The facial artery and vein passing deep to the nerve are doubly ligated with 3-0 chromic catgut inferior to the nerve and divided between the ligatures (Fig. 21-7).

In cases of salivary gland cancer, the nodes along the mandibular border are carefully separated from the marginal mandibular nerve and from the facial vessels, and are left attached to the submandibular gland to be resected with it en bloc. In benign cases, the lymph nodes are not removed; the dense fascia covering the submandibular triangle is divided at its mandibular attachment to free the superior border of the submandibular gland. By lifting the inferior border of the submandibular gland, the underlying anterior and posterior bellies of the digastric muscle are exposed and the submandibular triangle is entered. Retraction of the mylohyoid muscle anteriorly permits exposure of the contents of the triangle. By pulling inferiorly on the submandibular gland, the lingual nerve is brought into view with the intervening submandibular ganglion and its rami communicantes (Fig. 21-8). The ganglion is transected with cautery, allowing the lingual nerve to retract to safety beneath the mandible. The submandibular gland is then pulled posteriorly, bringing the submandibular (Wharton's) duct, an anterior extension of the submandibular gland, and the posterior portion of the sublingual gland into view. In the floor of the triangle, lying on the hyoglossus muscle, the hypoglossal (XIIth) nerve, usually with two accompanying lingual veins, is visualized and not disturbed. The submandibular

or an inflammatory process, resection of the gland without removal of the lymph nodes in the submandibular triangle is performed. If the diagnosis is that of a malignant tumor, it is necessary to resect the regional nodes with the salivary gland (su-

prahyoid neck dissection); if nodes are involved by carcinoma, some form of radical neck dissection should be done as well. The submandibular gland and the contents of the submandibular triangle are also resected as part of radical neck dis-

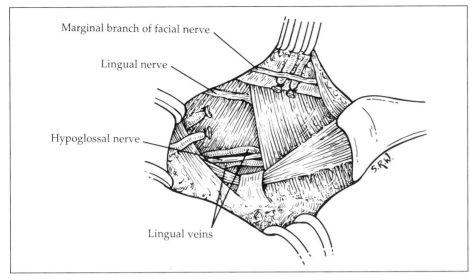

Fig. 21-11. *Resection of submandibular gland: wound after removal of submandibular gland.*

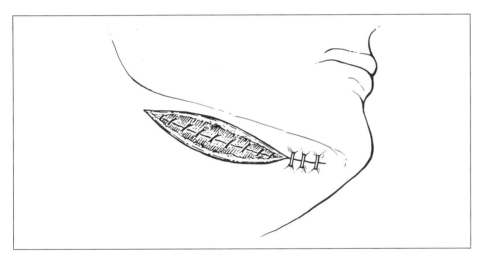

Fig. 21-12. *Resection of submandibular gland: wound closure.*

duct is doubly ligated as far anteriorly as possible with 2-0 chromic catgut and divided (Fig. 21-9). Some sublingual salivary glandular tissue adherent to the duct is resected with the duct. It is not necessary to resect the entire sublingual gland unless it is invaded by malignant tumor.

The submandibular gland is attached only by the facial artery, which courses along the gland's posterosuperior margin. If the artery can be separated from the salivary gland, the small branches entering the gland are doubly ligated with 3-0 chromic catgut and divided, and the artery is preserved. If the artery is intimately adherent to the gland, it is transected between ligatures as it enters and emerges from the gland, and the arterial segment is removed

with the submandibular gland (Fig. 21-10). In cases of carcinoma of the submandibular gland, the lymph nodes of the upper jugular chain are exposed and, if enlarged or suspicious, one or more are removed for pathologic study; if there is involvement by metastatic carcinoma, a radical neck dissection is completed at the same or a subsequent operation. If the diagnosis is carcinoma (other than the low-grade mucoepidermoid type), surgery is followed by a course of postoperative radiation therapy.

Hemostasis is secured with cautery. The anatomy of the empty triangle is seen in Fig. 21-11. The wound is closed without drainage, using 3-0 catgut sutures in the platysma and staples in the skin (Fig. 21-

12). The staples are removed in 24 hours and replaced by Steri-Strip dressing to maintain wound apposition. The patient is discharged 24 hours after operation.

Complications following submandibular gland resection are rare. Occasional seromas are easily aspirated with a fine-gauge needle. Trauma to the mandibular branch of the facial nerve gives rise to transient weakness or paresis of the lower lip.

Neoplastic Invasion of the Submandibular Duct

Benign primary tumors in the submandibular duct are rare. Primary cancers of the duct can be mucoepidermoid, squamous cell, or adenocarcinomas. Involvement of the submandibular duct by adjacent malignant tumors, such as squamous cell carcinomas of the mucosa of the floor of the mouth or cancers that arise in the sublingual or minor salivary glands, can occur in any part of the duct. The treatment of small malignant lesions or benign tumors involving the distal portion of the submandibular duct can be treated by wide excision of the tumor with the distal portion of the duct, followed by reimplantation of the divided end of the duct into the mucosa of the floor of the mouth. To reimplant the duct, the cut end is cut at an angle to increase its diameter. A small circular incision is made in the floor of the mouth posterior to the mucosal defect. Four or five sutures of 5-0 chromic catgut are placed circumferentially, approximating the duct to the mucosal opening. No stent is necessary; prompt drainage of saliva usually occurs through the new orifice.

Suggested Reading

Attie JN, Sciubba J. Tumors of major and minor salivary glands. *Curr Probl Surg* 13:65, 1981.

Batsakis JG. Neoplasms of the minor and lesser salivary glands. *Surg Gynecol Obstet* 135:289, 1972.

Baurmash HD. Marsupialization for treatment of oral ranula. *J Oral Maxillofac Surg* 50:1274, 1992.

Chisholm DM, Mason DK. *Salivary Glands in Health and Disease.* Philadelphia: Saunders, 1975.

Johns ME. Salivary gland tumors: Anatomy and embryology. *Otolaryngol Clin North Am* 10:261, 1977.

Quick CA, Lowell SH. Ranula and the sublingual salivary glands. *Arch Otolaryngol* 103:397, 1977.

Rankow RM, Polayes IM. *Diseases of the Salivary Glands*. Philadelphia: Saunders, 1976.

Spiro RH, Hajdu SI, Strong EW. Tumors of the submandibular gland. *Am J Surg* 132:463, 1976.

Thawley SE. *Comprehensive Management of Head and Neck Tumors*. Philadelphia: Saunders, 1987.

Young JA, VanLennep EW. *The Morphology of Salivary Glands*. New York: Academic, 1978.

EDITOR'S COMMENT

Doctors Attie and Sciubba have given us an excellent chapter on the rare but troublesome tumors of the sublingual and submandibular glands. These are comparatively rare tumors as compared to the much more common parotid tumors, but can be just as lethal in the case of malignant disease. The origin of malignant tumors is thought to be reserve cells located in the intercalated and excretory ducts, with acinar cells playing little or no role in the process. Recently, Bassett and coworkers (*J Otolaryngol* 24:184, 1995) utilized a postirradiated submandibular gland to study salivary gland tumorigenesis. In contrast to the commonly accepted hypothesis, they found that acinar cells were involved by using the marker for proliferating cell nuclear antigen as a marker for cycling cells. Thus, they reasoned that the common hypothesis for tumorigenesis was not valid, and that acinar cells needed to be considered as cells of origin for salivary gland tumors.

Yoshimura and colleagues (*J Oral Maxillofac Surg* 53:280, 1995) compared three methods used in the treatment of plunging ranula, including excision of the ranula, marsupialization, and removal of the sublingual gland combined with excision of the ranula. Recurrence rates for the first two methods were 25 and 36 percent, respectively, whereas no recurrences occurred following excision of the sublingual gland together with the mucocele. The results suggest that it may be worthwhile to consider more radical forms of therapy initially, and certainly when ranulas recur.

J.E.F.

II

The Mouth, Tongue, and Lips

22

Surgical Anatomy of the Tongue and Lips

Jack L. Gluckman   Lyon L. Gleich

Anatomically, the tongue and lips are considered part of the oral cavity, and are essential structures for effective deglutition, speech, and even adequate mastication. While this chapter is specifically directed to the lips and tongue, it is obviously impossible to discuss their form and function in isolation, and at least a rudimentary appreciation of their relationship to the rest of the oral cavity as a whole is necessary.

The oral cavity by definition extends from the vermilion border of the lips to the oropharyngeal isthmus, which is formed by the junction of the palate, the tonsillar pillars, and the junction of the anterior two-thirds and base of the tongue. The hard palate and maxillary alveolar ridges superiorly, and the mandible anterolaterally, form the rigid bony boundaries of the oral cavity, with the tongue, floor of the mouth, buccal mucosa, and lips comprising the mobile portion. Patently, any disease process or surgical procedure that impacts either the rigid bony structures or the mobile soft tissues will have a significant effect on the function of the oral cavity.

An understanding of the basic embryology is necessary for a better appreciation of the complex anatomy of the oral cavity. A number of structures develop around the primitive oral cavity (stomodeum) and evolve into the walls and contents of the oral cavity. These include

1. The frontonasal process, which projects down from the cranium, forming the nose, nasal septum, philtrum of the upper lip, and premaxilla
2. The maxillary processes on either side, which fuse with the frontonasal process; these form the cheeks, upper lip (except for the philtrum), palate, and superior alveolar ridges exclusive of the premaxilla
3. The mandibular processes, which meet in the midline, forming the mandible and lower lips

Abnormalities in this complicated developmental process can result in a myriad of deformities, for example, cleft lip and palate, inclusion dermoids, macrostomia, and microstomia.

The oral cavity is lined by nonkeratinizing squamous epithelium of varying thickness, for example, thinnest on the floor of the mouth and ventral surface of the tongue, and thickest on the dorsum of the tongue. Throughout the oral cavity a large number of submucosal minor salivary glands can be identified (Fordyce spots). These become more visible with age. The larger salivary glands drain into the oral cavity; for example, the submandibular duct (Wharton's duct), which drains the submandibular and sublingual glands, opens into the floor of the mouth on either side of the frenulum, and the parotid duct (Stensen's duct), which drains the parotid gland, opens into the buccal mucosa at the level of the upper second molar.

The floor of the mouth is comprised of a mobile muscular sling from the mandible to the hyoid bone that supports the tongue. Lip and cheek support and motion are provided by the facial musculature. Synchronous function of all these muscles is essential to maintaining the integrity of the oral cavity, and this is provided by the trigeminal, facial, and hypoglossal nerves, which provide motor innervation to these muscles. The mandibular division of the trigeminal nerve supplies the four paired muscles of mastication, that is, the masseter, temporal, and internal and external pterygoid muscles. The facial nerve supplies the facial musculature. The hypoglossal nerve innervates all the tongue muscles. In addition, the trigeminal nerve provides general sensory innervation to the oral cavity via its maxillary and mandibular divisions, and this, too, is vital to achieve a coordinated functioning oral cavity.

The blood supply to the oral cavity is supplied by branches of the external carotid system via the facial, lingual, and internal maxillary branches. Venous drainage parallels the arterial supply and enters the jugular venous system.

The lymphatic supply to the oral cavity is extremely rich, in general draining in a sequential manner to first-echelon nodes in the submental, submandibular, and parotid areas, and subsequently to the jugular chain of nodes. Drainage to the contralateral nodes can and does occur, and structures in the posterior oral cavity and oropharynx can spread to the retropharyngeal nodes.

Tongue

The tongue is a vital structure, essential for initiating the first phase of swallowing, moving food in the oral cavity to permit adequate mastication, and, of course, for articulation. It is small wonder, therefore, that any abnormality of the tongue, either due to disease or surgery, will cause the patient significant dysfunction. It can quite easily be appreciated how severe a punishment the medieval practice of amputation of the tongue could be for the unfortunate victim. By definition the anterior two-thirds of the tongue should be regarded as part of the oral cavity while the base is part of the oropharynx.

Embryology

Tongue development commences at the end of the fourth week with a midline mass (the tuberculum impar) that develops immediately anterior to the thyroid anlage. Paired lingual swellings from the ventral aspect of the first branchial arch then surround this structure anteriorly and laterally and fuse in the midline to form the anterior two-thirds (oral portion) of the tongue. The area of fusion of these lingual swellings is the septum linguae. The hypobranchial eminence from the ventral aspect of the third and fourth arches forms the posterior third (oropharyngeal portion) of the tongue. The division between the anterior and posterior tongue is the sulcus terminalis just posterior to the circumvallate papillae. Therefore, the sensory nerve supply to the anterior two-thirds of the tongue is the trigeminal nerve, reinforced by the chorda tympani, and to the tongue base is the glossopharyngeal nerve, reinforced by the vagus. The tongue muscles are derived from the occipital myotomes, which migrate forward, dragging their nerve supply (XIIth) with them.

General Structure

As was already stated, the tongue consists of a mobile anterior two-thirds and a relatively immobile base. The junction is marked by a V-shaped groove on the dorsal surface, the sulcus terminalis. At the apex of this is the foramen cecum, the site of the embryologic origin of the thyroid gland. The circumvallate papillae are aligned immediately anterior to the sulcus terminalis. The midline lingual septum, which corresponds to the junction of the lingual swellings, separates the two halves of the tongue and may be apparent on the dorsum. The frenulum, a thin mucosal fold, is evident in the midline on the ventral surface of the tongue.

Mucosa

The dorsal surface of the tongue consists of thick, stratified squamous epithelium characterized by thin filiform papillae in the anterior two-thirds (Fig. 22-1). Larger fungiform, foliate, and vallate papillae are interspersed between them and all these

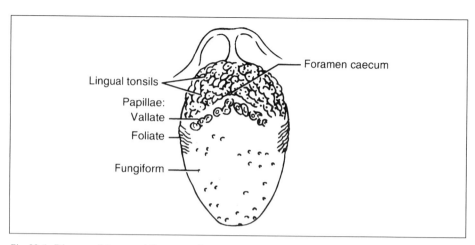

Fig. 22-1. *Diagram of dorsum of the tongue demonstrating topographic landmarks.*

contain taste buds. The circumvallate papillae are arranged in a V just anterior to the sulcus terminalis and the foliate papillae are prominent on the lateral aspect of the tongue. Both these papillae are often misdiagnosed by patients and physicians alike as early tumors because of their prominence. The posterior third has no papillae, but is covered with lymphoid tissue (the lingual tonsils) that, with the faucial tonsils and adenoids, make up "the lymphoid ring of Waldeyer." These lingual tonsils can be quite prominent and asymmetrical, mimicking the presence of a tumor. Normal lingual tonsils are usually soft to palpation. They can become chronically infected (lingual tonsillitis) and, of course, lymphoma may arise in these structures. The filiform papillae occasionally become denuded in isolated patches for no apparent reason, causing great consternation to the patient, but this is of little clinical significance ("geographic tongue"). There are numerous mucous and serous glands in the tongue that can be the source of retention cysts, which may present as submucosal masses.

Musculature

The bulk of the tongue is formed largely by the *intrinsic* muscle fibers, which are separated in the midline by the septum linguae. These muscles are arranged in longitudinal, transverse, and vertical groups, and alter the shape of the tongue. They interact with the *extrinsic* tongue musculature, which move the tongue as a whole. These extrinsic muscles originate from the mandible (the genioglossus, which protrudes the tongue), the styloid process (the styloglossus, which retracts the tongue),

the hyoid bone (the hyoglossus, which depresses the tongue), and the palate (the palatoglossus, which closes the oropharyngeal isthmus, but does not affect the tongue movement directly) (Fig. 22-2). The genioglossus forms a fanlike structure that sagittally inserts into the anterior and posterior tongue and even some fibers into the hyoid bone. The hyoglossus extends from the hyoid bone superiorly into the substance of the tongue, where its fibers intermingle with the styloglossus and the intrinsic musculature. The styloglossus arises from the styloid process, spreading out to the lateral aspect of the tongue (where its action is to raise the edges of the anterior tongue) and also to the substance of the tongue, where it interdigitates with the hyoglossus and retracts the tongue.

The complex interaction between all these muscles permits the marvelous array of movement needed for the tongue to perform its wide range of functions. It is for this reason that any attempt at meaningful reconstruction of a functioning tongue after total glossectomy continues to confound us in spite of new and creative reinnervation and revascularization techniques.

Nerve Supply

The hypoglossal nerve supplies all the intrinsic and extrinsic tongue muscles, with the exception of the palatoglossus, which is supplied by the vagus via the pharyngeal plexus. General sensation in the tongue parallels its embryologic development, with the anterior two-thirds being supplied by the nerve of the first pharyngeal arch, that is, the lingual nerve, a

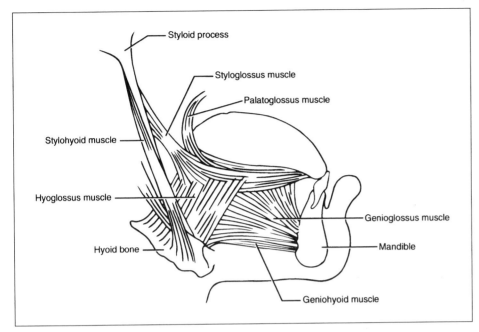

Fig. 22-2. Extrinsic musculature of the tongue.

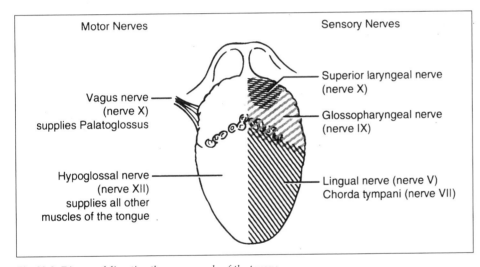

Fig. 22-3. Diagram delineating the nerve supply of the tongue.

branch of the mandibular division of the trigeminal nerve. This nerve also transmits the taste fibers from the geniculate ganglion via the chorda tympani (VIIth). The base of the tongue is supplied via the nerve of the third pharyngeal arch, the glossopharyngeal nerve, for both taste and general sensation. A few fibers of the superior laryngeal nerve, a branch of the vagus, may also supply the base of the tongue (Fig. 22-3).

An appreciation of the course of the lingual and hypoglossal nerves in the neck is important to avoid injury to these nerves during neck operations. The lingual nerve is closely related to the submandibular duct in the submandibular triangle and must be identified and dissected free from the duct when performing a submandibular gland excision. The hypoglossal nerve is likewise at risk during upper neck dissections. It runs under the posterior belly of the digastric muscle accompanied by the vena comitans nervi hypoglossi, which are branches of the lingual veins and, if not ligated, become an irritating source of bleeding during the procedure. Attempts at blindly clamping these vessels can result in inadvertent nerve injury.

Vascular Supply

The rich arterial supply to the tongue is derived from the lingual artery bilaterally, which supplies the floor of the mouth and posterior tongue before entering the anterior tongue. This vessel has a number of named branches, that is, the dorsal lingual to the base of the tongue and the sublingual and deep lingual to the anterior tongue. Correlating with embryologic development, there is minimal flow across the midline raphe, which is a relatively avascular plane, although it does anastomose with the end branches of its counterpart at the tip of the tongue. In the substance of the tongue, it runs together with the lingual vein and the lingual nerve. The base of the tongue is also supplied by branches of the ascending pharyngeal artery.

The venous drainage of the tongue is via the lingual veins, which either enter the internal jugular vein directly or via the facial veins. The deep lingual veins run with the branches of the lingual artery in the substance of the tongue. The ranine veins (vena comitans nervi hypoglossi) accompany the hypoglossal nerve along its course. The rich blood supply of the tongue renders it very vascular during surgery. For this reason, the use of a bovie for resection of lesions of the tongue is ideal. Before closure of the defect, meticulous hemostasis is necessary to avoid the possibility of hematoma formation, which can spread interstitially between the muscle fibers and prove refractory to evacuation.

Lymphatics

The anterior tongue is drained by marginal and central lymphatic vessels. The marginal vessels drain from the lateral tongue into the submandibular and upper deep cervical nodes or directly into the middle deep cervical nodes, while the central vessels drain the medial tongue to the submental and then upper and middle deep cervical nodes. Drainage is then to the lower deep cervical nodes secondarily. Normal lymphatic drainage from the lateral margins has little spread to the contralateral side; however, the tongue base and tip, which are drained by the central vessels, can spread to the contralateral side. Since the base of the tongue develops embryologically as a single structure, it has a rich lymphatic communication between the two sides. Metastases from tumors in the tongue base, therefore, occur early and bilaterally to the upper deep cervical nodes primarily, but also can metastasize to the retropharyngeal nodes.

It should be appreciated that while lymphatic metastases from the tongue usually follow a sequential pattern, that is, first to submental and submandibular nodes and then to deep cervical nodes, "skip" metastases can occur, with spread directly to upper and middle deep cervical nodes and rarely even to lower deep cervical nodes without involving the primary-echelon nodes. This knowledge is important in selecting the appropriate neck dissection for cancer of the tongue. In general it is better to perform a complete neck dissection that encompasses all nodal groups rather than the increasingly popular selective neck dissection, unless the surgeon is extremely experienced and well versed in the vagaries of lymphatic spread of cancer of the tongue.

Lips

The lips provide the gateway to the oral cavity and adequate function is essential not only for aesthetic appearance, but also for the integrity of the oral cavity as a whole. Any disease process or surgical procedure that interferes with the function of this extraordinary complex structure can result in drooling, dysarthria, and, of course, a readily apparent cosmetic deformity. The lips can best be appreciated as a mobile sphincter with its delicate movement governed by a complex series of muscles suspended between relatively fixed bony structures, that is, the mandible and maxilla. The circumferential orbicularis oris maintains the competency of the sphincteric function, while the depressors and elevators change the overall position of the lips on the face as well as the changes that are essential for facial expression.

Embryology

While of little practical value to the surgeon, it should be appreciated that there is some controversy as to the exact mechanism of embryologic development of the lips; however, the classic viewpoint describes the upper lips as being formed by the fusion of the lateral maxillary pro-

cesses with the midline frontonasal process. The result of these three processes fusing is the creation of a vertical groove in the midline, the philtrum, which, by virtue of its characteristic curvature, is referred to as Cupid's bow. Failure of fusion of the maxillary processes is thought to result in a wide variety of different types of cleft lips and palates. The lower lip is formed by fusion of the mandibular processes in the midline. Macrostomia and microstomia can result from abnormalities in this development.

Mucosa

The vermilion border, or red margin, of the lip is the portion that is visible when the lip is pursed. This mucosa is dry and orthokeratotic without adnexa. The junction of the vermilion border with the keratinizing adnexal skin is a readily visible line. The site at which the lips make contact with each other is the "wet line." Posterior to this, the epithelium changes from the orthokeratotic vermilion border to a moist, thinner, parakeratotic epithelium that is confluent with the oral mucosa. This mucosa is loosely attached, and can easily be elevated as a separate layer. These topographic features are important, as repair of even the simplest lacerations necessitates careful reapproximation of the mucocutaneous junction since any malalignment will be clearly visible. The labial submucosa contains a large number of minor salivary glands, which are a common site for retention cysts.

Musculature

The orbicularis oris is the most important muscle, essential for the integrity of the sphincteric action of the lips (Fig. 22-4).

Whether it truly anatomically encircles the lip in a complete sphincteric manner or, more likely, is a continuation of the various elevators and depressors, with crisscrossing and interdigitating fibers, is unclear and probably of no real practical importance. What is known is that it effectively functions as a sphincter, arising directly or indirectly via the various surrounding muscles from the maxilla and mandible, and inserts into the skin and mucosa of the lips. The orbicularis oris purses the lips, retracts them against the teeth, and draws in the commissures. The depressors of the lips (depressor anguli oris, depressor labii inferioris, mentalis) depress the angles of the lips and protract the lower lips. The elevators (risorius, zygomaticus major and minor, and the levator group of muscles) all elevate various parts of the lips. It should be appreciated that these muscles are so interdigitated that it is essential to normal function that they all function in unison.

Nerve Supply

Motor supply to the lip musculature is via the mandibular and buccal branches of the facial nerve, which innervate the lip depressors and levators, respectively.

Sensation to the lower lip is provided by the mental nerve, a branch of the mandibular division of the trigeminal nerve, which enters the mandible as the inferior alveolar nerve, and exits at the mental foramen. The upper lip is innervated by the infraorbital nerve from the maxillary division.

Preservation of the nerve supply to the lip musculature is obviously essential, with damage to even a small branch having potentially serious effects on function and

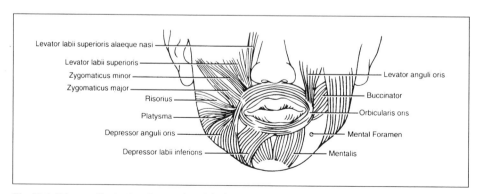

Fig. 22-4. Diagram illustrating the muscles of the lips.

aesthetics (see Fig. 23-1). For example, injury to the mandibular division of the facial nerve can cause significant cosmetic deformity and a tendency to bite the lower lip when chewing, as well as mild drooling.

Vascular Supply

The superior and inferior labial arteries arise from the facial artery, traveling in a plane that is close to the mucosa and between the fibers of the orbicularis oris before anastomosing with the vessel from the contralateral side (see Fig. 23-1). Occasionally there may be two separate inferior labial arteries. The labial veins drain into the anterior facial vein and thence to the jugular system. The rich blood supply of the lips permits the design of various "lip-switch" flaps, which can have an extremely narrow pedicle based on the labial artery alone, with excellent survival.

Lymphatics

The lower lip drains initially to the submental and submandibular nodes via a medial lymphatic trunk that drains the mid-third to the submental nodes, and a lateral lymphatic trunk that drains the lateral third into the submandibular nodes (see Fig. 25-11). There are numerous lymphatic anastomoses across the midline and, therefore, central cancers may metastasize bilaterally. Lymphatics may also enter the mental foramen, with spread of cancer into the mandible itself.

The upper lip drains to the preauricular, infraparotid, submandibular, and submental nodes. Cancers of the upper lip appear to have a higher incidence of lymphatic metastases and all these nodal groups will have to be addressed in treating these cancers.

Suggested Reading

Davies J, Duckert L. *Embryology and Anatomy of the Head, Neck, Face, Palate, Nose and Paranasal Sinuses*. In M Paparella, D Shumrick, J Gluckman, W Meyerhoff (eds), *Otolaryngology*. Chap 3, Vol 1. Philadelphia: Saunders, 1991.

Hollingshead WH. *Anatomy for Surgeons. The Head and Neck* (3rd ed). Philadelphia: Lippincott, 1982.

23

Lip Reconstruction

Maurice J. Jurkiewicz   *Glyn Jones*

Appropriate reconstruction of acquired defects of the lips involves re-creating a functional, competent stoma with acceptable appearance. Achieving these goals requires a detailed understanding of the anatomy, physiology, and aesthetics of the normal lip.

Anatomy

The upper and lower lips consist of the circumoral orbicularis oris muscle, lined internally with oral mucosa and externally with lip and cheek skin. The lip margins are covered with vermilion lining, consisting of an internal wet vermilion and an external dry vermilion. These components contribute both to the appearance of the lips and to their function. Wet vermilion lies in contact with the teeth during speech and facial animation while dry vermilion provides a resilient external colored surface to the lips that does not dry out and crust on exposure. The upper lip contour is broken up by the formation of Cupid's bow centrally, formed by the heaping up of lateral columns of the orbicularis muscle on either side of the central philtrum dimple. The upper and lower lips converge in a complex interweaving of the orbicularis muscles at the oral commissures (Fig. 23-1). The relationship between the orbicularis muscles and the other radial muscles of facial expression provide distinctive anatomic features for both facial expression and the maintenance of oral competence.

Blood supply to the lips is derived from the superior and inferior labial branches of the facial vessels. These arteries anastomose with the lateral nasal arteries to communicate with the infraorbital and oph-thalmic vessels, and via the septal artery to communicate with the sphenopalatine arteries. The inferior labial artery anastomoses with the submental, lingual, and inferior alveolar vessels.

Motor innervation of the upper lip is derived from the buccal branch of the facial nerve while the lower lip is innervated by the mandibular branch. Additional animation of the mouth is provided by the elevator and depressor muscles of facial expression, also supplied by the facial nerves. Sensory innervation is supplied by the intraorbital and inferior alveolar nerves.

Lymphatic drainage of the lip parallels vascular supply. The upper lip, oral commissures, and lateral segments of the lower lip drain primarily to the submandibular nodes and thence to the jugulodigastric nodes. The central portion of the lower lip drains into the submental lymph nodes. Some lip lymphatic flow appears to drain to the preauricular nodes, as evidenced by the pattern of lymph node involvement in metastatic carcinoma of the lip.

Physiology

Lip function involves both competence of the oral stoma and an ability to articulate. Implicit in both functions is provision of adequate lip seal during animation of the orbicularis muscle. Failure to achieve lip seal during eating results in leakage of liquids as well as solids with embarrassing drooling; inability to seal during speech results in distortion when pronouncing labial consonants. Reconstruction should provide innervated muscle and sensate skin and mucosa with a deep labial sulcus to achieve these goals. In addition, microstomia should be avoided; many of these patients wear dentures and a small oral commissure can render denture use impossible. It is imperative that any reconstructive procedure should aim to re-create oral competence.

Pathobiology

Cancers of the lip are usually well differentiated and 95 to 98 percent arise from the dry vermilion lining. These tumors are less aggressive than intraoral squamous carcinomas but more aggressive than squamous carcinomas of the skin. Basal cell cancers are seen more often on the upper lip; keratoacanthomas, melanomas, and minor salivary gland tumors occur very infrequently. Leukoplakia is associated with lip carcinoma in a high percentage of patients and carcinoma in situ is a common accompaniment in these lesions.

Lymph node metastases occur in 2 to 5 percent of small, well-differentiated tumors. In the uncommon, poorly differentiated tumors, or in lesions over 3 cm in diameter, the incidence of regional nodal spread rises to 20 to 30 percent. Fortunately, lymphatic spread from the lip progresses in an orderly anatomic progression and lymph node spread is usually easily detected clinically. Although upper tumors were thought to have a greater metastatic potential than lower lip tumors, they have subsequently been shown to have similar stage distributions and cure rates. Five-year survival for stages I and II tumors is 90 and 85 percent, respectively, while it is 40 percent for stage III tumors.

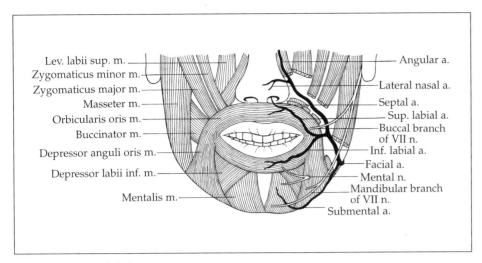

Lev. labii sup. m.
Zygomaticus minor m.
Zygomaticus major m.
Masseter m.
Orbicularis oris m.
Buccinator m.
Depressor anguli oris m.
Depressor labii inf. m.
Mentalis m.

Angular a.
Lateral nasal a.
Septal a.
Sup. labial a.
Buccal branch of VII n.
Inf. labial a.
Facial a.
Mental n.
Mandibular branch of VII n.
Submental a.

Fig. 23-1. Anatomy of the lips.

Surgical Principles

Surgical excision remains the treatment modality of choice for lip carcinoma, providing simplicity of management for early lesions and more reliable control of extensive tumors than radiotherapy. Surgery should aim primarily at tumor extirpation followed by careful attention to function and form.

- Tumor resection: Complete local excision of tumor bulk must be achieved with or without regional node dissection.
- Function: Oral continence and adequate speech should be preserved at all costs. This includes provision of innervated orbicularis oris, mucosal and vermilion reconstruction, adequate labial sulcus depth, and stomal size. Facial animation should be maintained.
- Form: Restitution of lip contour should be achieved with a full-bodied vermilion, contiguous white roll, adequate horizontal width of the lower lip, a normal Cupid's bow, and preservation of the philtrum in the upper lip.

Tumor Resection Margins

Surgical excision margins range from 5 mm for small lesions to approximately 1 cm for larger tumors. Frozen section histologic evaluation at the time of surgery is strongly recommended before a major lip reconstruction is undertaken. Up to 5 percent of patients with lip cancer present with hypesthesia of the lower lip, mandating a frozen section biopsy of the affected mental nerve. Perineural invasion of the mental nerve is an indication for a hemimandibulectomy. Tumor adhesion to the mandible requires either a marginal or full-thickness mandibulectomy at the tumor site.

Management of the Neck

A clinically negative neck in the presence of a tumor smaller than 3 cm requires no further intervention. In poorly differentiated tumors larger than 3 cm, upper nodal dissection for staging is advised. In patients with regional metastases, neck dissection should be performed with preservation of the spinal accessory if this nerve is free of adherent tumor. Preservation of the marginal mandibular branch of the facial nerve is mandatory to maintain lower lip function. Postoperative radiotherapy is advisable in patients with regional nodal spread in order to reduce locoregional control. If a nodal dissection is required for upper lip cancer, it should be done in conjunction with a superficial parotidectomy in order to clear preauricular nodes. Leukoplakia of the lip is an indication for concomitant lip shave in the setting of preexisting lip carcinoma and should be strongly advised in patients who have on-going outdoor exposure to sunlight or who are deemed unreliable for follow-up.

Trauma

Lip trauma commonly accompanies facial injury, particularly in vehicular accidents and blunt facial assault. Both of these mechanisms result in a crushing type of injury with a tendency for the injured lip to burst open yielding ragged lacerations. Tooth impact further lacerates the wet vermilion and lining mucosa and may produce through-and-through bite wounds. These internal lip lacerations should be carefully sought for, as they may be extensive and their extent is often grossly underestimated. They are also a site for hidden foreign bodies including fragments of teeth and bone from maxillary and dentoalveolar fractures.

It is uncommon for lip lacerations to result in tissue loss. Ragged lacerations can result in severe distortion of the lips with the appearance of tissue loss, but simple restoration of displaced tissue usually reveals a fairly normal lip contour that can be treated with careful suturing (Fig. 23-2). This should commence internally with repair of the mucosa, followed by muscle repair and finally meticulous suturing of the skin and vermilion. The most critical suture in repair of the external portion of the lip is the accurate alignment stitch within the white roll at the junction of the dry vermilion and lip skin. Failure to correctly place this suture can result in malalignment of the lip, with a grossly distorted final appearance. Once the white roll is repaired, the remainder of the lip can be sutured safely.

In rare situations, true partial or full-thickness lip loss occurs. Human bites tend to produce significant tissue loss and a heavily contaminated wound. Fortunately, most tissue losses tend to be fairly limited and can often be treated by converting the wound to a well-excised wedge or W excision, as illustrated later in the text, with primary closure. Human bites require broad-spectrum antibiotic coverage and may need delayed closure. Significant tissue loss should be treated by skin-to-mucosa suturing followed by elective reconstruction using the most appropriate technique once a healed, stable wound has been achieved.

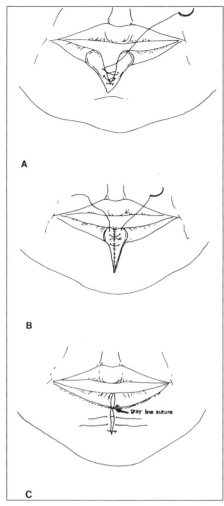

Fig. 23-2. Suturing a simple lip laceration. A. Repair of the lip mucosa commencing at the labial sulcus. B. Intermuscular suture. C. Skin closure commencing with the initial gray line suture for correct orientation.

Electrical Burns

Electrical burns of the mouth are usually found in young children who accidentally chew electrical cables. Typically, the burn involves either the commissure or the central lip and is almost always full thickness in depth. Usually these injuries heal well with simple wound cleaning and debridement as needed but scarring can be a major problem. Central lip burns tend to contract with recruitment of the adjacent lip tissue, healing with a notch that can then be excised using the W excision. Commissural burns are the most difficult wounds to manage and can result in severe distortion and stenosis if mismanaged. During heal-

ing, lip stenting may be necessary to limit stenosis but the splints are difficult to keep in place. Subsequent commissurotomy is usually required and a number of techniques are illustrated at the end of this chapter.

Approaches to Lip Reconstruction

Lip reconstruction techniques may involve simple procedures to correct essentially cosmetic defects, such as lip notching, to complex procedures designed to reconstruct part or all of the lip. Simple lip reconstructions involve either shield or W excisions with primary closure. Larger defects may require surgical manipulation of adjacent tissues in an effort to reconstruct important anatomic landmarks and maintain function. These latter procedures can be divided into four categories:

1. Averaging procedures with local transposition flaps, for example, an Abbé-Estlander flap
2. Lip tissue redistribution of innervated orbicularis oris, for example, a Karapandzic flap
3. Cheek advancement techniques, for example, the Bernard-Burow technique
4. Distant tissue transfer techniques, for example, a deltopectoral flap or free tissue transfer, all of which suffer from a lack of innervated functional potential

These techniques can be divided into several categories:

- Lip shave
- Reconstruction of defects of one-third of the lower lip
- Reconstruction of defects of two-thirds of the lower lip
- Reconstruction of defects of the entire lower lip
- Upper lip reconstruction
- Ancillary corrective procedures

Surgical Techniques for Lip Reconstruction

Lip Shave

Lip shave is the treatment of choice for leukoplakia whether in isolation or in conjunction with lip carcinoma. The specimen

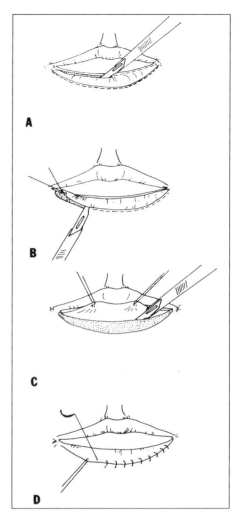

Fig. 23-3. Lip shave. A/B. Excision of vermilion border of the lip. C. Elevation and undermining of the intraoral lip mucosa. D. Advancement and suture of lip mucosa to resurface the denuded lip musculature.

should be carefully tagged with orientation sutures for pathologic reference, as it may harbor invasive carcinoma requiring further excision. Accompanying diagrams are useful for the pathologist. The technique involves simple resection of the involved vermilion from the underlying orbicularis muscle with advancement of the internal labial mucosa onto the lip margin. Some authorities believe that the appearance of the lip is improved by beveling the mucosal flap from superficial to deep in order to provide for easier advancement (Fig. 23-3). Undermining the wet vermilion is not necessary to facilitate advancement and can invite bleeding and hematoma formation.

Reconstruction of Less than One-third of the Lip

Fortunately, most lip cancers are less than 2 cm in diameter at presentation. Resection of one-third or less of the lip provides adequate margins and good function and form due to recruitment of adjacent lip tissue. There is some degree of cross innervation from the contralateral side in laterally based excisions, resulting in good preservation of lip motor function. In addition, reinnervation across the scar also occurs to some extent. Wedge excisions should be performed in one of two ways to prevent notching of the lip secondary to vertical scar contracture:

- Shield excision (Fig. 23-4). This design allows for a wider margin of excision and greater vertical height of the lateral and medial walls of the wound. Subsequent closure produces a fuller, natural height to the lip.
- W excision (Fig. 23-5). In larger tumors, a shield design may not allow adequate central projection and lip height. Incorporation of a W into the design greatly facilitates closure and a normal contour.

Reconstruction of One-third to Two-thirds Lip Defects

Defects of 3 to 5 cm in width require tissue transfer techniques. The use of innervated flaps wherever possible maintains function. Included in this section, we will discuss the Abbé and Estlander techniques, which, although not neurotized, often develop some cross innervation, and can provide excellent function and cosmesis.

- Step excision (Fig. 23-6). This procedure is a logical progression from the W excision. The stepladder design recruits sensate, vascularized tissue from below and vermilion advancement reconstitutes the vermilion border. The scars are well hidden in the labiomental fold and vertical advancement maintains the height of the gingivolabial sulcus. The procedure becomes limited by the availability of vermilion.
- Myocutaneous transposition flaps (Estlander and Abbé) (Fig. 23-7). These flaps rely on a two-staged transfer based ini-

tially on a pedicled blood supply from the superior labial artery. At the initial procedure, a template of the defect is marked on the appropriate donor site on the upper lip. The flap should never be greater than one-third the width of the upper lip. The upper lip flap is raised, with great care being taken to preserve the posterior 5 to 8 mm of lip muscle and labial mucosa, within which lie the superior labial vessels. The flap is turned down into the defect and sutured in place. Ten to 14 days later, the pedicle is divided and the free edge of the flap is trimmed and sewn down into the lower lip to complete the transfer. The major disadvantage of these flaps is that they are not innervated and can lead to drooling if large segments are transposed; some cross innervation tends to develop over 6 to 12 months and this can allevi-

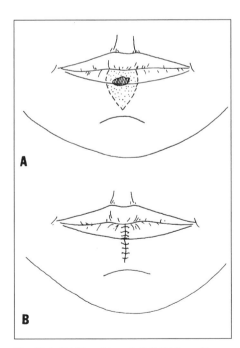

Fig. 23-4. Shield excision. A. Full-thickness lip excision using shield pattern. B. Layered closure of lip with central lengthening produced by approximation of the curved margins of the shield pattern.

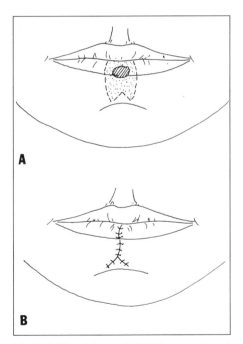

Fig. 23-5. W excision. A. Full-thickness excision of lip with inferior W-plasty; the apex of the W should lie equidistant from the tumor as the lateral resection margins. Lateral extension may be required to facilitate closure of a wide defect but care should be taken to preserve the mental nerves. B. Closure in layers with the base of the scar close to the labiomental fold.

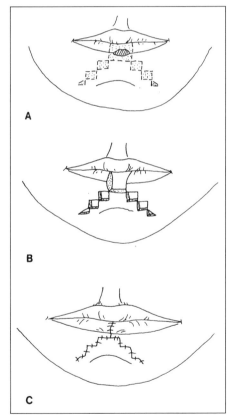

Fig. 23-6. Step excision. A. Rectangular excision of the lesion is followed by two- to four-step excisions, none of which should cross the labiomental fold. Each step is 10 mm horizontally and 8 mm vertically, allowing a minimum of 2-cm advancement to reduce the surgical defect. B. Flaps are mobilized at the periosteal level to facilitate movement. C. Three-layer flap closure.

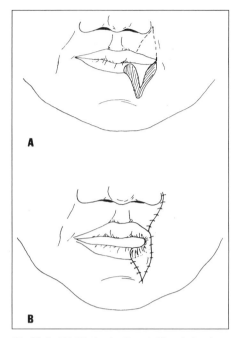

Fig. 23-7. Abbé-Estlander flap. A. Flap design for a peripheral tumor. Flap position is dependent on the position of the excisional defect. B. The flap rotated into the lower lip defect; note the distortion of the commissure, which can be corrected secondarily. When used for more central defects, the vascular pedicle will require division at 3 weeks.

ate the problem. Central lower lip defects should not be treated by medial advancement of the remaining lower lip and an upper lip Abbé-Estlander, as this denervates half of the upper lip and two-thirds of the lower lip.

Reconstruction of Defects of More than Two-thirds of the Lip

The following techniques are useful for defects that involve 70 to 90 percent of the lower lip but can also be used in lesser excisions and have the advantage of incorporating innervation for function.

- Karapandzic flap (Fig. 23-8). This flap is a useful technique for up to 75 percent lower lip loss, resulting in a functional, aesthetically acceptable reconstruction that is quick and simple to perform. The orbicularis muscle fibers are mobilized from the surrounding radial muscles with their blood supply and innervation intact. The lip is then redistributed and sutured. The larger the defect, the more likelihood there is that microstomia may result but this only tends to occur with

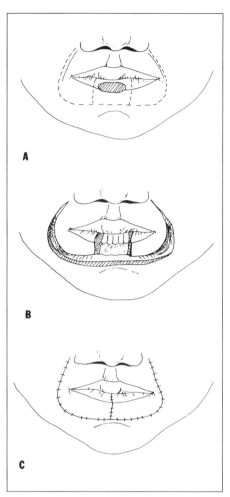

Fig. 23-8. Karapandzic flap. A. Preoperative skin markings for central tumor excision. B. Skin and subcutaneous fat are incised sharply; fat is gently dissected off muscles to expose orbicularis. (b) Orbicularis oris, together with its nerve supply, is carefully dissected and left attached to underlying mucosa. C. Mucosa, orbicularis, and skin are then advanced into the defect and sutured. Nasolabial incisions are closed after appropriate dog-ear corrections are performed proximally at the alar bases.

massive defects. The functional results are good and revision is rarely required. The flap should be used with caution in patients who have large defects of the lower lip with a very thick, prominent upper lip, as the discrepancy in lip thickness can be alarming. A major advantage is the ease with which natural commissures reform without requiring surgical intervention.

- Bromley-Freeman modification of the Bernard-Burow repair (Fig. 23-9). This repair is based on the principle of sliding innervated cheek flaps into the defect,

with Burow's triangles being excised along the nasolabial and labiomental folds. The horizontal incisions extending into the cheek divide orbicularis but preserve continuity of buccinator and its nerve supply. The Burow's triangles alleviate tension considerably and ultimately contribute quite significantly to a tension-free aesthetic lip closure. The mucosal incisions are less extensive than the cutaneous ones. The vermilion border is recreated by either vermilion advancement or preferably by a tongue flap, which can be divided in 10 to 14 days. The Bromley-Freeman variant of this procedure maintains the integrity of the orbicularis and recreates a modiolus.

Total Lower Lip Reconstruction

- Sliding cheek advancement flap (Fig. 23-10). This procedure provides some innervated cheek musculature and is particularly useful when commissure resection is performed concomitantly. This is achieved at the expense of lengthy scars crossing the cheek from the preauricular area. Vermilion reconstruction may require a tongue flap.
- Fujimori gate flap (Fig. 23-11). The modified version of this flap is shown and relies on transposition of large, vascularized nasolabial flaps based inferiorly. One skin island carries innervated muscle and a paddle of cheek mucosa for lip lining and vermilion reconstruction while the other contains only skin and subcutaneous tissue for the inferior portion of the lip below the labial sulcus. Fujimori's original description utilized simple transposition flaps with intact skin at their bases while the newer modification converts these to bilateral island flaps, allowing easier rotation into the lower lip defect and more aesthetic closure of the donor sites. The major disadvantage is unilateral upper lip paralysis on the side from which the full-thickness flap is harvested, resulting in some degree of distortion of the upper lip during animation. This improves with time but may not resolve completely.

Upper Lip Reconstruction

Upper lip tumors constitute only 2 percent of all lip carcinomas. The principles of repair are identical to those of the lower lip.

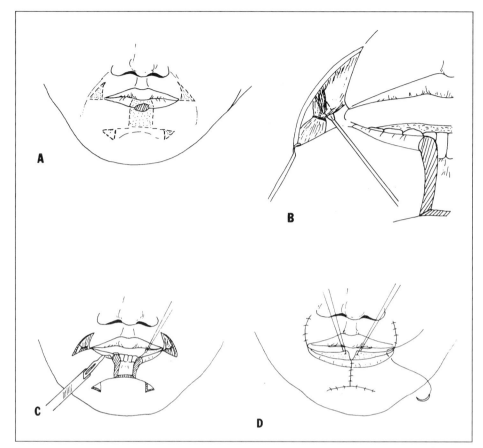

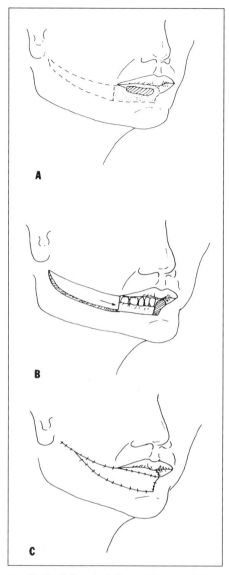

Fig. 23-9. Bromley-Freeman modification of the Bernard-Burow repair. A. Skin incisions for a central tumor excision. B. Dissection of the orbicularis from the mucosa with redefinition of the modiolus raphe at an appropriate new level to compensate for the commissural distortion that would otherwise accompany skin flap advancement. Suturing of the modiolus is performed with either nylon or polyglycolic sutures. C. Mucosal and vermilion mobilization to provide lip lining. D. Layered closure with suturing of vermilion-mucosal flaps to provide lip resurfacing.

Fig. 23-10. Sliding cheek flap. A. Tumor excision and planned triangular flap extending close to the earlobe. B. Dissection is carried down to muscle, preserving facial vessels and nerve branches. Facial muscles are then bluntly split to allow advancement, keeping mucosa intact. C. Three-layer closure using advanced excess mucosa to provide lip lining.

The exception is that the upper lip is more forgiving of the use of denervated flaps than is the lower lip but poor function can still result as a consequence. Every effort should be made to preserve muscle function.

Defects of Less than One-third of the Upper Lip

• Wedge excision. Most lesions can be treated with wedge excisions as in the lower lip, incorporating a W if necessary. A particular problem, which is fortunately rare, is the management of a central carcinoma in the philtrum. This can be excised as a wedge but advancement of the tissue at the nasal base may require the use of perialar wedge excisions, as shown in Fig. 23-13. Another alternative is the use of an Abbé cross lip flap from the lower lip to reconstruct the philtrum (Fig. 23-12).

• Perialar crescentic advancement flap (Fig. 23-13). This procedure is extremely useful for defects at the alar base but can be of value in providing tissue mobility for excisions extending up to the alar base from the lateral lip. The scar is neatly concealed in the nasolabial fold and provides outstanding cosmetic results.

Defects Greater than One-third of the Upper Lip

Larger defects require the use of imported tissue in the form of either Abbé-Estlander flaps or Karapandzic-type procedures. The Bernard-Burow technique is also useful.

Massive Defects and the Role of Distant Tissue

Wherever possible, local or adjacent tissue should be used for lip reconstruction. Dis-

tant pedicled options center on the delto-pectoral flap described by Bakamjian but suffer from the disadvantages of poor color match and lack of muscle function causing intractable drooling. The advent of free tissue transfer provides for a wider choice of distant tissue options but they suffer the same disadvantages. The radial forearm flap can be transferred with the tendon of palmaris longus incorporated as a static sling but this tends to stretch and

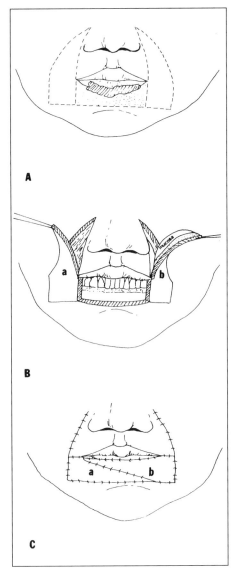

Fig. 23-11. Fujimori gate flap. A. Resection of almost the entire lower lip with planned large nasolabial flaps. B. Flap "a" consists of skin and subcutaneous fat, incorporating the nasolabial branch of the facial vessels. Flap "b" consists of skin, fat, muscle, and a paddle of cheek and lip mucosa, taking care to preserve the parotid duct orifice. C. Flap "a" is transposed onto the chin while flap "b" is transposed to create the bulk of the free edge of the lower lip lined with mucosa carried on its internal surface.

a drooling, atonic lip remains. In upper lip defects in men, a free temporal scalp flap can provide aesthetically acceptable cover with a mustache if desired, but again, the problem of lining and muscle tone is not overcome. In general, distant tissue should be avoided if at all possible.

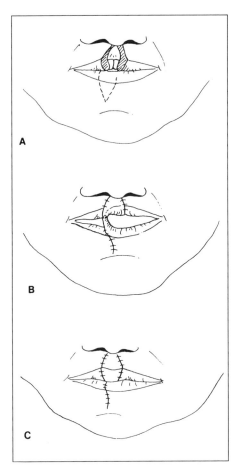

Fig. 23-12. Cross lip flap. A. For central upper lip defects, an Abbé flap identical to that used for correcting severe cleft lip deformities is designed. The flap is transposed and sutured into the defect (B) and is divided at 2 to 3 weeks and inset (C).

Ancillary Procedures

- Skin grafts and local skin flaps. For cutaneous defects close to the vermilion border, skin grafts may have a place provided that they are performed in cosmetic units so as to offset the color mismatch that may arise. Suitable donor sites include pre- and postauricular skin and lower neck skin. Local flaps include the wide variety of geometric flaps described. Nasolabial flaps are useful, as are the rhombic (Limberg) and slide-swing flaps.
- Notch lip correction. This unsightly deformity occurs after either vertical scar contracture or irradiation. The defect is amenable to improvement by muscle imbrication and is avoided by the use of the shield or W excision.

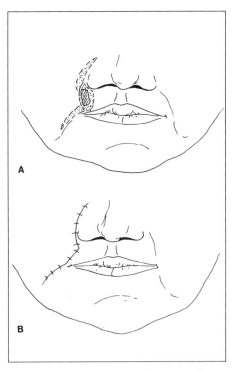

Fig. 23-13. Perialar crescentic advancement flap. A. Design shown for lateral upper lip excision with accompanying skin excisions to allow advancement. B. Completed advancement with scar camouflaged in the nasolabial fold.

- Cupid's bow (Fig. 23-14). Cupid's bow can be simulated by excising skin in an arch above the vermilion and then advancing the vermilion border into the defect.
- Vermilion tongue graft (Fig. 23-15). A lack of mucosa or vermilion can be filled by a tongue flap graft. This two-stage procedure can give adequate results and provide a full appearance to the vermilion. The patient should be warned that the lip will initially appear rough but the mucosa gradually smoothes out with time.
- Commissural reconstruction (Fig. 23-16). Commissural definition may be lost in a number of the previously described procedures. This structure can be reproduced with the use of simple local flaps without further affecting lip function, but their lack of success in reconstructing a clearly defined commissure can be disappointing.

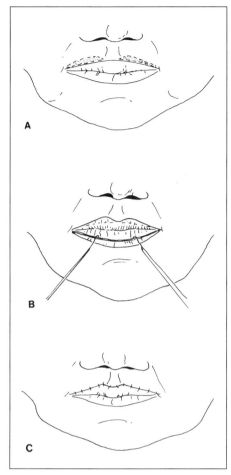

Fig. 23-14. Cupid's bow simulation. A. Upper lip skin immediately adjacent to the vermilion is excised to the desired new level. B. Vermilion of the upper lip is elevated from the free border of the lip. C. Vermilion is advanced into the new position and sutured in place.

Suggested Reading

Abbé R. A new plastic operation for the relief of deformity due to double harelip. *Med Rec* 53:477, 1898.

Bailey B. Management of carcinoma of the lip. *Laryngoscope* 87:250, 1977.

Burow A. Zur blepharoplastik. *Monatsschr Med Augenheilkd Chir* 1:57, 1838.

Bernard C. Cancer de la lèvre inférieure opéré par un procédé nouveau. *Bull Soc Chir Paris* 3:357, 1853.

Estlander JA. Eine methode aus der einen Lippe substanzverluste der anderen zu ersetzen. *Arch Klin Chir* 14:622, 1872.

Freeman BS. Myoplastic modification of the Bernard cheiloplasty. *Plast Reconstr Surg* 21:453, 1958.

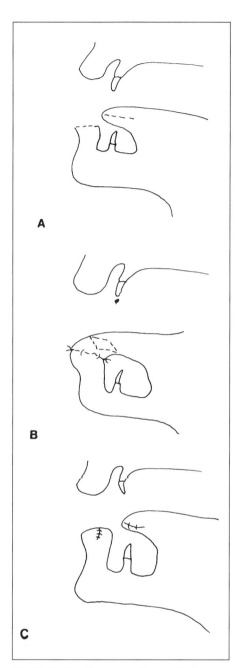

Fig. 23-15. Vermilion tongue flap. A. The free border of the tongue is incised transversely and sutured to the denuded surface of the lower lip. B. Two to three weeks later, a diamond-shaped excision of tongue is performed at an appropriate level to allow long enough flaps of tongue mucosa to close both the lip and the tongue donor site. C. Suturing of both sets of flaps with catgut.

Gillies HD. *Plastic Surgery of the Face.* Oxford, England: Oxford Medical Publications, 1920.

Gullane PJ, Martin GF. Minor and major lip reconstruction. *J Otolaryngol* 12:75, 1983.

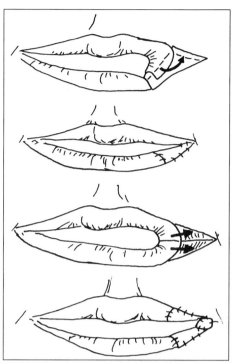

Fig. 23-16. Commissural reconstruction. Two types of commissure reconstruction are shown. The upper procedure uses dry vermilion from the distorted commissure as a flap to resurface the upper lip into the commissure, with lip mucosal advancement onto the lower lip. The lower procedure utilizes equal sharing of commissural vermilion between the two lips, with a mucosal triangular flap advancement into the commissural angle.

Hendricks JL, Mendelson BC, Woods JE. Invasive carcinoma of the lower lip. *Surg Clin North Am* 57:837, 1977.

Jabaley ME, Clement RL, Orcutt TW. Myocutaneous flaps in lip reconstruction: Application of the Karapandzic principle. *Plast Reconstr Surg* 59:680, 1977.

Jackson IT. *Local Flaps in Head and Neck Reconstruction.* St. Louis: Mosby, 1985.

Johanson B, Aspelund E, Breine U, Holmstrom H. Surgical treatment of non-traumatic lower lip lesions with special reference to the step technique: A follow-up on 149 patients. *Scand J Plast Reconstr Surg* 8:232, 1974.

Karapandzic M. Reconstruction of lip defects by local arterial flaps. *Br J Plast Surg* 27:93, 1974.

Lore ES, Kaufman S, Grabau JC, Popovic DN. Surgical management and epidemiology of lip cancer. *Otolaryngol Clin North Am* 12:81, 1979.

McHugh M. Reconstruction of the lower lip using a neurovascular island flap. *Br J Plast Reconstr Surg* 30:316, 1977.

Smith JW. The anatomical and physiologic acclimatisation of tissue transplanted by the lip switch technique. *Plast Reconstr Surg* 26:40, 1960.

EDITOR'S COMMENT

The lips and the circumoral area are such a major part of facial expression that it is difficult to imagine a cosmetic problem that is more oppressive than neoplasms and other injuries to the lip area. The necessity for providing an adequate Cupid's bow when possible, and an accurate reconstruction of the junction between the lip and the skin, as well as the fullness of the lips, cannot be better stated than Drs. Jurkiewicz and Jones have done.

The sophistication of the techniques is not surprising, as these practices have been evolving since before the turn of the century. The emphasis is on innervation, blood supply, and function to prevent drooling, and a number of techniques have been portrayed, the intent of which is not only to restore function but also to restore cosmesis.

Other techniques have been put forth in massively destructive lesions, especially those of the upper lip. Jacob (*Aust NZ J Surg* 65:251, 1995) has proposed a primary reconstruction of the upper lip with a hair-bearing portion of the scalp. The bilateral pedicle flap is based on the posterior branch of the superficial temporal artery and is swung down in visor fashion over the entire upper lip, with the pedicles on either side left intact. Since the flap is hair bearing, the patient, in cases described by Jacob of male patients, would support a mustache. The mustache, however, provides good cover for an otherwise mutilating deformity and the inability to reconstruct the vermilion border. After the blood supply to the graft has been established in 2 to 3 weeks, the bridges are divided and returned to the scalp. A good cosmetic result is pictured in the two cases described by Jacob.

A more common problem is the lack of bulk and a deficiency in the free border of the lip, which is the final result of secondary cleft lip deformities. This free border usually consists of the orbicularis oris marginalis muscle and its overlying subcutaneous tissue, mucosa, and vermilion. A temporoparietal fascial flap has been proposed by Chen and associates (*Plast Reconstr Surg* 95:781, 1995) to increase the fullness of the free border of the lip when there is a shortage of subcutaneous tissue or orbicularis oris marginalis muscle. They propose this as an alternative to more complicated procedures such as an Abbé flap or a tongue flap. Twenty cases were reported in the above-mentioned paper, which seemed to give quite reasonable results from the pictures provided.

The importance of the lips to the appearance and self-esteem of an individual cannot be overstated. This excellent chapter by Drs. Jurkiewicz and Jones illustrates the meticulous approach and the concepts applied to these difficult cases.

J.E.F.

24

Hemiglossectomy, Excision of the Floor of the Mouth, and Mandibular Resection for Oral Cancer

Donald G. McQuarrie

New cancers of the tongue and mouth develop in approximately 18,000 people a year. Approximately 5000 persons die of oral cancer each year. Tobacco-induced oral cancer is much less frequent than tobacco-induced lung cancer (15:1). Easier detection and more effective treatments give oral cancers a higher survival rate than lung cancer. Early detection is the key to an effective cure of oral cancer with minimal disability. Early oral cancers should have a 5-year tumor-free survival rate exceeding 80 percent. Unfortunately, approximately 75 percent of lesions are diagnosed as a tumor of stage T2 (>2 cm in largest diameter) or larger, with frequent involvement of cervical lymphatics. About 15 percent of the time, the first presenting symptom is a large metastatic node in the neck.

Oral cancer is not uniformly distributed throughout the oral cavity. Figure 24-1 shows the areas of increased vulnerability. Oral cancer may appear as an area that is reddened and rough, whitened, or mixed red-white plaque. Malignancy should be the foremost suspicion when one is confronted with an oral lesion that has persisted over 2 weeks in a heavy smoker, anyone using smokeless tobacco, an elderly person, an alcoholic, or a patient with poor oral hygiene.

After a diagnosis of oral cancer is confirmed by a biopsy, a spectrum of therapies is needed to cover the various stages of the disease. A surgeon needs to enlist the constructive advice and therapeutic contributions of radiation oncologists, medical on-

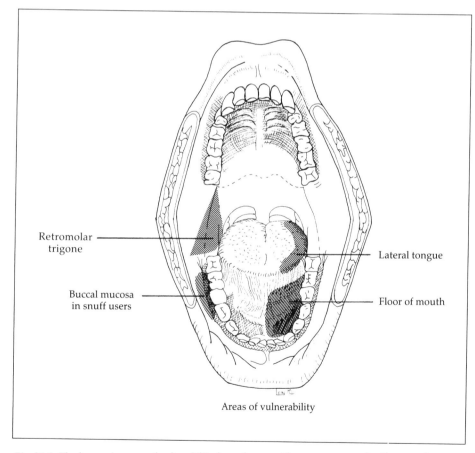

Fig. 24-1. The four major areas of vulnerability for oral cancer. The areas correspond with areas where tobacco exposure is greatest with puddling of saliva, direct contact, or turbulent impingement. (From DG McQuarrie et al. Head and Neck Cancer: Clinical Decisions and Management Principles. *Chicago: Year Book, 1986. Reproduced with permission.)*

cologists, speech therapists, oral surgeons, and prosthetists—all of whom work together in a multidisciplinary program coordinated for each patient.

Good therapeutic decisions require accurate knowledge of tumor size, degree of invasion, estimates of involvement of cervical nodes, and a search for distant metastases or a synchronous second oroairway primary lesion. With this knowledge, one can stage the cancer in one of the TNM categories outlined in Table 24-1. Accurate staging is essential for planning the therapy. After staging, one must weigh the occupational requirements of the patient, status of general health, and life-style (e.g., reliable, chemically dependent, or derelict). After adequate discussion and con-

sultation with radiologic and oncologic coworkers, one must have a careful informed-consent discussion with the patient, describing the best estimates of the options.

Several basic truths have to be faced. First, inadequate "try-a-little" therapy does no good. Each desperate attempt at salvage has a minimal yield of less than 20 percent, despite "chirurgical heroics" or "roentgen magic." It is not fair to a patient to withhold a full curative effort with surgery, irradiation, or combined therapy for some minimal cosmetic benefit.

Second, all attempts at treating oral cancer trade disability for disease. The changes brought about by an operation are immediately obvious. Radiation therapy, when given at the full dose required to cure an oral cancer, produces definitive changes that progress with time, causing progressive obliteration of arterial structures, poor-to-absent tissue healing, xerostomia, changes in taste, or occasional necrosis of soft tissue and bone. Teeth can be preserved in very few patients who undergo irradiation. Preservation requires perfect dentition, no significant dental restorations, and precise habits of an oral hygiene program.

Even though treatment frequently exacts a burdensome toll of facial changes and oral disability in an attempt at a cure, the deformity and disability are *much less* than the agony, misery, and disability of untreated disease or therapeutic failure.

Third, contemporary care of oral cancer necessitates that surgical rehabilitative measures are a planned component of the initial treatment effort. The panoply of options for immediate replacement of soft tissue and bone means that few patients need to endure long periods of waiting before arduous multistep reconstructive procedures are started. Only resection of the most advanced cancers results in a patient who is crippled beyond the ability to converse intelligibly or swallow.

In the following discussion, I discuss some of the common "workhorse" surgical therapies and reconstructions with the reader's understanding that there is a richer repertoire of options to be applied. Most of the therapies and reconstructions I discuss are modest variations of the procedures.

I do not discuss the treatment of the cervical lymphatics with technical detail be-

cause neck dissection is discussed in Chapter 27. For most early anteriorly situated oral cancers, the spinal accessory chain of nodes is rarely involved and the neck dissection can be modified to carefully spare the nerve, thus avoiding the major disability of the classic neck dissection (i.e., loss of trapezius muscle function). One can consider a modified neck dissection if (1) the neck is staged N0 and there are no large or suspicious nodes encountered in the upper jugular area, (2) the only palpably involved node is well anterior to the spinal accessory nerve, and (3) the lesion is not deeply invasive at the tonsillar fossa area.

Smaller T1 Oral Cancers

The first and most important distinction in selecting treatments involves further subclassification of T1 lesions into lesions that are thin (<1–1.5 mm maximum thickness) and lesions that are more deeply invasive. Occasionally the lesion is thin, pliant, and has a histology somewhere between severe dysplasia and minimally invasive cancer, with only one or two microscopic areas where the lamina propria is broken with invasive cancer. A wide (1.5-cm margin), deep excisional biopsy may be the only treatment required. The dimensions are shown in Fig. 24-2A through D for the tongue and Fig. 24-2E for the floor of the mouth. Because some cancers of the floor of the mouth involve the submental and submandibular salivary gland ductal systems, it may be necessary to perform a suprahyoid dissection to prevent severe sialadenitis in the postoperative period. For patients who have some other end-stage disease (e.g., cirrhosis, cardiac failure, emphysema), one can consider cryosurgical ablation or laser excision of a thin, localized, minimally invasive lesion. If one extends the indications for local excision to include thicker, more invasive small lesions, then the local recurrence rate increases to more than 20 percent and metastases subsequently appear in the neck in more than one-third of patients. The 5-year survival rate falls from an achievable 80 to 85 percent to 60 to 65 percent. When one waits until clearly palpable nodes are present in the neck before doing a neck dissection, then many such necks are really at stage N2, in which a salvage neck dis-

Table 24-1. American Joint Committee on Cancer Staging—Oral Cancer

PRIMARY TUMOR (T)

T0 No evidence of primary tumor

Tis Carcinoma in situ

T1 Greatest diameter of primary tumor 2 cm or less

T2 Greatest diameter of primary tumor >2 cm, but not >4 cm

T3 Greatest diameter of primary tumor >4 cm

T4 Massive tumor >4 cm in diameter with deep invasion to involve cortical bone, antrum, pterygoid muscles, base of tongue, skin of neck

LYMPH NODES (N)*

N0 No clinically positive node

N1 Single clinically positive ipsilateral node 3 cm or less in diameter

N2 Single clinically positive ipsilateral node >3 cm, but not >6 cm in diameter, or multiple clinically positive ipsilateral or contralateral nodes, none >6 cm in diameter

  N2a Single clinically positive ipsilateral node >3 cm, but not >6 cm in diameter

  N2b Multiple clinically positive ipsilateral nodes, none >6 cm in diameter

  N2c Metastases in bilateral or contralateral nodes, none >6 cm in greatest dimension

N3 Metastases in one or more nodes >6 cm in greatest dimension

DISTANT METASTASIS (M)

M0 No (known) distant metastasis

M1 Distant metastasis present

*Same definitions to be used if postsurgical treatment–pathologic staging is used.

Source: Adapted from OH Beahrs, et al (eds.). *Manual for Staging of Cancer.* 4th ed. Philadelphia: Lippincott, 1992.

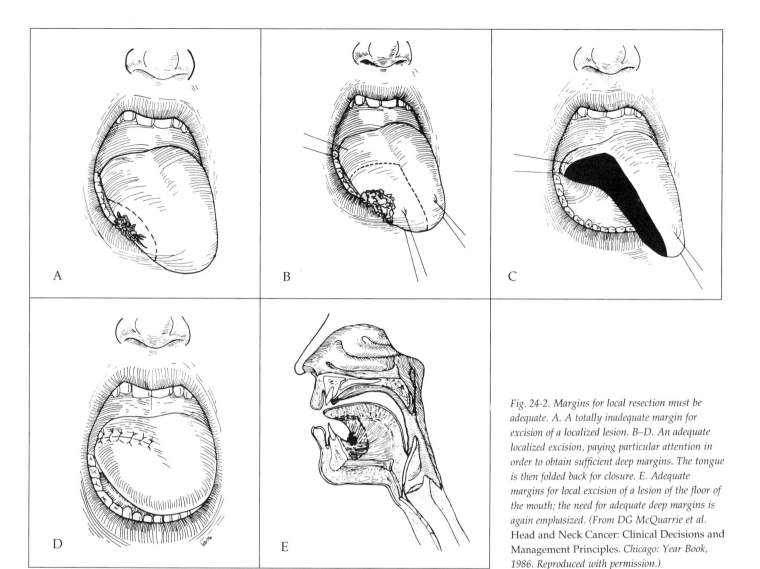

Fig. 24-2. Margins for local resection must be adequate. A. A totally inadequate margin for excision of a localized lesion. B–D. An adequate localized excision, paying particular attention in order to obtain sufficient deep margins. The tongue is then folded back for closure. E. Adequate margins for local excision of a lesion of the floor of the mouth; the need for adequate deep margins is again emphasized. (From DG McQuarrie et al. Head and Neck Cancer: Clinical Decisions and Management Principles. *Chicago: Year Book, 1986. Reproduced with permission.*)

section has a much lower rate of effectiveness (≤30% 5-year survivors).

Smaller oral cancers (stage T1) that are clearly invasive, thicker, and more nodular need effective treatment of the local lesion and the cervical lymphatics. More than 25 percent of patients already have palpable cervical metastases. Although no nodes are palpable, physical examination is notoriously inaccurate and has a high false-negative rate.

Invasive lesions require treatment of cervical lymphatics. A cervical lymphadenectomy is not radical. It has a low added mortality (<0.5%). It has a high yield of nonpalpable microscopically involved nodes. The result is proven long-term survival.

Effective surgical treatment of stage T1 lesions results in a high, 5-year disease-free survival rate (>80%). Furthermore, when the cancer is detected and treated early, tissue loss is minimal, oral function is good, and cosmetic appearance is excellent, especially if a pull-through-type procedure can be done with a hockey-stick cervical incision and an oral route for resection, avoiding incisions on the front of the face. This approach for the tongue is illustrated in Figs. 24-3 and 24-4. The field of resection can be extended to cover a tongue lesion extending onto the floor of the mouth. Similarly, appropriate margins of tongue can be included when a cancer of the floor of the mouth extends to the underside of the tongue. The extent of oral resection is shown in Figs. 24-3 and 24-4. If the invasive cancer is close to the midline, one

should consider treating the contralateral side of the neck by a modified lymphadenectomy or by irradiation.

When a stage T1 oral lesion is located away from the mandible, when there are no detectably involved cervical lymph nodes, and when a reliable patient has occupational requirements for impeccable speech or unblemished appearance, then irradiation of both the primary site and cervical areas may be recommended. This recommendation carries the provisos that follow-up treatment is precise and that any reappearance of cancer is promptly and widely excised. For smaller oral lesions (primarily of the tongue), the survival results of irradiation plus surgical salvage are approximately equivalent to rates of primary surgical treatment only. On the

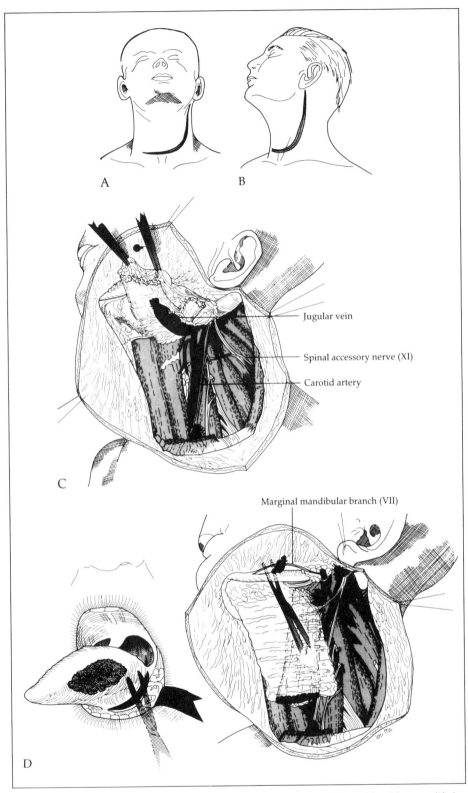

Fig. 24-3. Pull-through procedure for hemiglossectomy. A. Curved utility incision used for either a modified neck dissection (sparing the spinal accessory nerve) or a standard neck dissection (B) if upper jugular nodes are involved. C. Lateral dissection into the mouth. D. Tongue is freed laterally by dissection from both the mouth and the neck. (From DG McQuarrie. Cancer of the tongue. Selecting appropriate therapy. Curr Prob Surg *23:562, 1986. Reproduced with permission.)*

positive side, a certain proportion of patients (approximately 60%) require no subsequent resection of functioning oral structures. On the negative side, patients who require salvage-type operations usually need more extensive resection with increased complication risk and with fewer reconstructive or rehabilitative options because of impaired healing as a result of full-dose irradiation therapy.

Moderately Sized or Aggressively Invasive Oral Cancers

More than 75 percent of oral cancers are stage T2 or higher when diagnosed. Moderate extension of an oral cancer within the restricted confines of the mouth poses many problems for effective curative treatment and functional reconstruction. A number of simpler guidelines have been helpful for treatment planning:

1. Try to achieve a 2- to 2.5-cm gross margin around the tumor with the tissue in an unstretched state. Patients with resection margins that are initially positive on frozen section and then re-resected and rendered negative by the end of the procedure have a higher rate of local recurrence.
2. If there is not at least 1 to 1.5 cm of pliant tissue between an oral tumor and the mandible, strongly consider a marginal resection of the mandible in the area. If the tumor is abutting the mandible but not directly invading it, a marginal resection is required.
3. If the tumor directly invades the mandible, resect the involved area of the mandible with a 2.5-cm margin from any roentgenographically involved bone. A large resection of the anterior arch then requires some means of mandibular reconstruction in order to support the functioning remnant of tongue.
4. Malignant squamous cell cancer in the mouth is unpredictable in the direction of its growth and extension. There are no barriers to direct growth or lymphatic metastases across the midline. Resection margins should not be compromised just because the midline has been reached. Adequate margins must be confirmed by gross and frozen section studies.

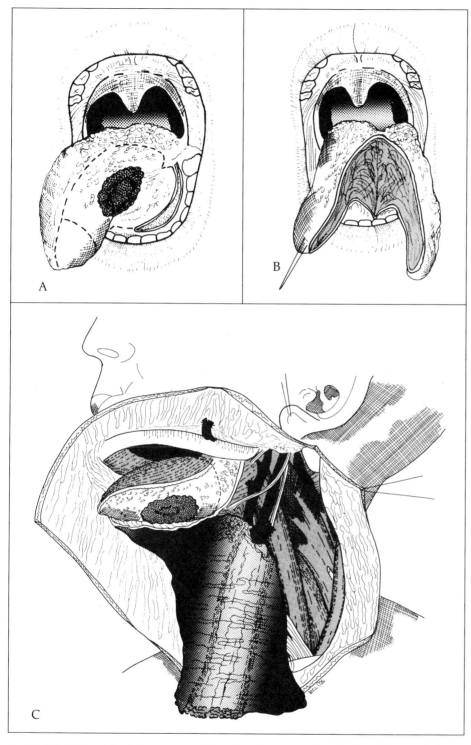

Fig. 24-4. Pull-through hemiglossectomy. A. Intraoral incisions are continued to the midline or onto the underside of the tongue. B. Tongue is divided down the midline. This frees the tongue so the specimen can be tipped laterally under the mandible and delivered into the neck, where the posterior division can be made under direct vision. C. Lingual vessels that are encountered can be seen and ligated without difficulty. After good hemostasis, the oral closure is accomplished by sewing the cut edge of the tongue to the alveolar mucosa. (From DG McQuarrie. Cancer of the tongue. Selecting appropriate therapy. Curr Prob Surg *23:562, 1986. Reproduced with permission.)*

5. Make reconstruction a planned component of the resection. Primary reconstruction at the time of resection is easier and provides the patient with the best functional results. Late multistep procedures take 3 to 8 operations and 100 to 200 days to complete.

6. Larger oral resections require good full-thickness oral lining. If a large resection removes more than 10 to 12 cm² of oral surface area, secure primary closure can rarely be achieved. If primary closure is initially accomplished under tension, an orocutaneous fistula is liable to develop. Furthermore, tight displacement of pliant tissues into a rigid oral closure impairs the mobility of the tongue and mouth, thus increasing difficulty with speech and swallowing. Installation of a flap clearly improves oral function and reduces risk. Modern techniques have provided many reliable flaps. These flaps include the Bakamjian cervical flaps, deltopectoral myocutaneous flaps, and free flaps from several sites.

7. When reconstructive techniques are used, it is wise to choose simple over complex, local over distant flaps, and direct over free microvascular transfer.

8. The incision and resection lines must be carefully planned to provide for reconstructive options. The plan must also allow for the worst-case scenario, in which the resection must be extended or in which the primary reconstructive option meets with early failure.

As one approaches the larger cancers, the cervical lymphadenectomy is done first. The neck dissection is completed to the lower border of the mandible. The sternocleidomastoid muscle and the jugular vein are divided. This step leaves the neck specimen pedicled on the inner border of the mandible. At about the level of the hyoid bone, it is necessary to decide the limits of the oral dissection. As the dissection is carried cephalad, a cone of resected tissue must be developed in order to ensure adequate deep margins. For most cancers of the floor of the mouth and the tongue, the resection includes all or part of the geniohyoid, digastric, and myelohyoid muscles. The submaxillary and submental glands are resected. The lingual nerve is generally sacrificed. If the lesion is anterior in the floor of the mouth, the hypoglossal nerve is identified and followed forward. Usually every structure superficial to the hypoglossal nerve is included in the specimen. With this much of the dissection done, it is necessary to begin the oral resection by developing appropriate cheek flaps.

The lower lip is divided in the midline. The incision is then made through the midline or around the soft tissue of the chin, depending on the prominence or configuration of the chin. The cheek flaps on one or both sides are extended back in the buccal sulcus. If a marginal resection of the internal mandible is planned, the external periosteum must be carefully preserved along with about 1 mm of soft tissue. As the flaps are made, care is taken to ensure adequate margins, if needed. If a marginal mandibulectomy is to be done, I prefer the technique shown in Fig. 24-5. This technique preserves the lower, outer cortical bone. Cuts with a longer high-speed side-cutting burr are a little more complex but give a better margin of resection. Postoperatively, the bone configuration provides a better platform for restorative dentures. After the bone cuts are freed, the specimen is outlined in the mouth with adequate incisional borders. By working from the neck and intraorally, the specimen is resected. If the hypoglossal nerve is to be preserved, it must be kept in sight during the final resective phase. A concomitant hemiglossectomy is frequently required to ensure adequate tissue margins. Large, anterior, midline cancers of the floor of the mouth can require an anterior one-third glossectomy (Fig. 24-6).

If the arch of the mandible is preserved or reconstructed, the pectoralis major myocutaneous flap is too bulky for the confined space, especially if the patient is well nourished. Larger defects require a thin, pliant oral lining from some site. A cervical flap (Bakamjian type) or a free radial artery–based forearm flap facilitates subsequent function and rehabilitation. Currently, the radial artery microvascular free full-thickness flap is the preferred option.

With large invasive anterior oral cancers that are deeply invading bone near the midline of the mandible, much of the anterior arch has to be resected. Free bone grafts spanning more than 6 to 8 cm have a high failure rate, even with good soft-tissue coverage. Because of this problem I

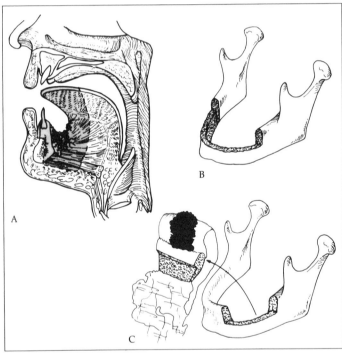

Fig. 24-5. Marginal mandibular resection for a tumor of the floor of the mouth or a cancer of the tongue adjacent to but not invading the mandible. A. Cross-section showing the depth of resection to ensure adequate margins. B. Bone cuts made for a resection of the midline floor of the mouth. This approach spares the outer lower cortex. To preserve bone viability, one must keep the overlying periosteum intact. C. When tongue lesions invade laterally to the mandible, a block of bone can be removed, thus preserving a good supporting lateral strut. (From DG McQuarrie et al. Head and Neck Cancer: Clinical Decisions and Management Principles. Chicago: Year Book, 1986. Reproduced with permission.)

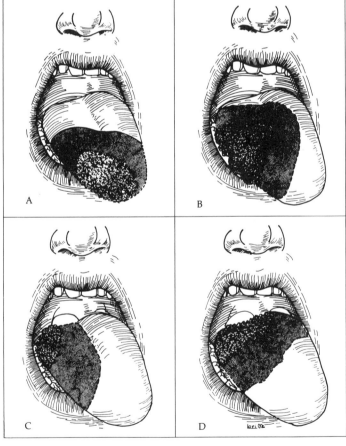

Fig. 24-6. Nonstandard resection lines may be required to ensure adequate margins around larger oral cancers. One should not be hesitant to use diagonal resections (A) or go across the midline (B). Although the tongue tip in (C) will be denervated, it will provide some pliant oral lining. If the hypoglossal nerve on one side can be preserved in a large resection (D), the reconstruction with a pliant flap will result in adequate tongue function for intelligible speech and deglutition. (From DG McQuarrie. Cancer of the tongue. Selecting appropriate therapy. Curr Prob Surg 23:562, 1986. Reproduced with permission.)

Fig. 24-7. Reconstruction of a large defect in the anterior arch of the mandible by using sliding myo-osseous advancement of a segment of mandible. A. Lateral view. The masseter and pterygoid muscles are freed in the upper portions. The posterior attachments of the mandible are divided. Care is taken to preserve muscle attachments as shown in B, medial view, and C, lateral view. D. A horizontal osteotomy is made to allow the inferior segment to move forward. The principle is that of a swing advancement of the lower vascularized segment. E. An oscillating saw is used for the osteotomy. (From DG McQuarrie et al. Head and Neck Cancer: Clinical Decisions and Management Principles. *Chicago: Year Book, 1986. Reproduced with permission.)*

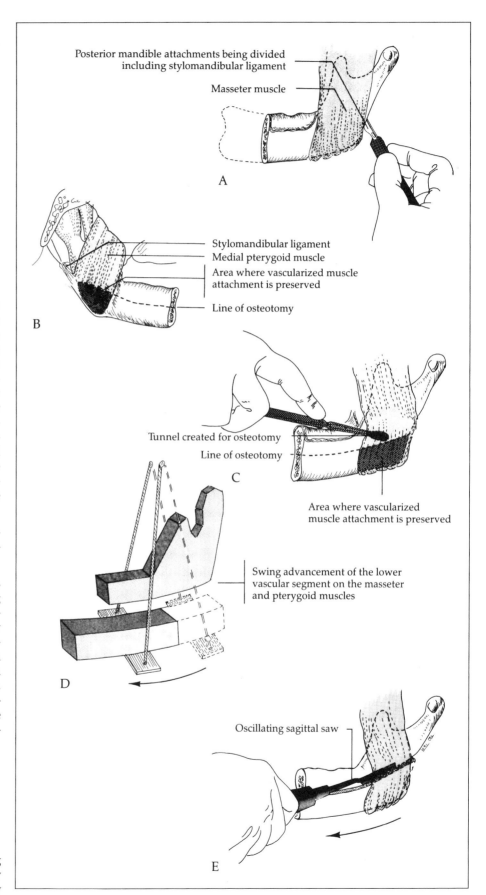

use a sliding myo-osseous graft as shown in Figs. 24-7 and 24-8. Alternatively, other surgeons have used vascularized bone grafts of rib, iliac crest, radius, or the fibula as a myo-osseous–cutaneous graft or as a vascularized free flap. Microvascular connection of free complex tissue grafts is now quite reliable in experienced hands. Our group prefers fibular bone transfer because there is more bone with less deformity. Because a skin paddle transferred with the fibula is not reliable, fibular bone graft to the mandible is frequently combined with radial forearm soft tissue mouth lining or external coverage.

All viable bone transfers need secure fixation with modern bendable or miniplating systems.

With any technique, oral function takes precedence over cosmesis. The remaining tongue needs the support of bone reconstruction, a prosthesis, or a temporary wire bridge. The pliant oral lining and external tissues need to be abundant enough for safe, secure, tight closure with enough redundancy to maintain tongue mobility. Occasionally it is better to accept a shortened mandibular contour than to bring the chin too far forward, creating a large nonfunctional salivary sump.

Cancers of the Alveolar Ridge and Retromolar Trigone

The studies of early cancers by Mashberg suggest that squamous cell cancer usually arises in one of the areas of vulnerability

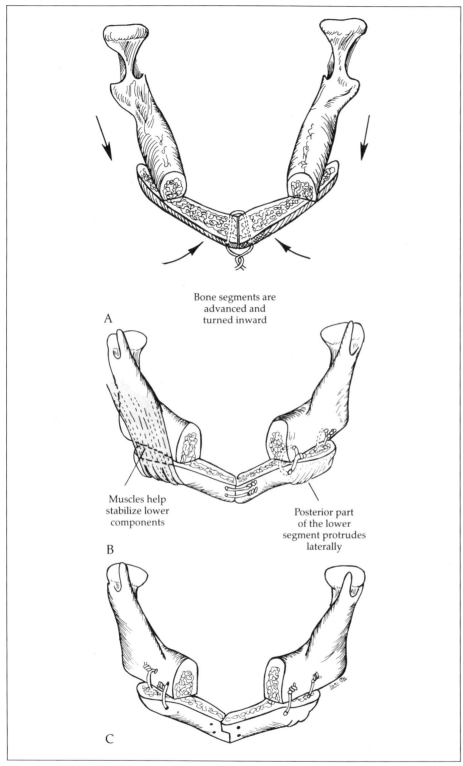

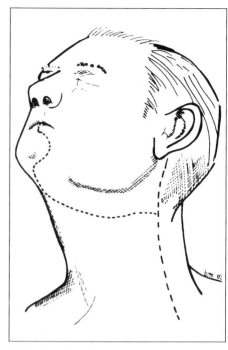

Fig. 24-9. Preferred incision for a composite resection. There is a gentle curvature around the chin. The horizontal incision is made 2 to 3 finger breadths below the mandible. The transverse incision meets posterior to the carotid. The incision crosses the carotid artery at only one point. Note (1) vertical limb posterior to carotid artery, (2) incisions meet at right angle, and (3) gentle curve of horizontal incision. (From DG McQuarrie et al. Head and Neck Cancer: Clinical Decisions and Management Principles. Chicago: Year Book, 1986. Reproduced with permission.)

Fig. 24-8. Sliding myo-osseous mandibular advancement. A. The mobilized segments are moved forward, rotated inward, and secured with wire. Clinically, this maneuver results in a secure arch that supports the remaining tongue. B. The shorter mandible does result in some overbite, but because the remaining tongue is not overextended to a normal mandibular contour, the oral function is good. C. For best stability, the midline junction should be mortised and carefully fitted. Wires in the midline (not shown) should be crossed. (From DG McQuarrie et al. Head and Neck Cancer: Clinical Decisions and Management Principles. Chicago: Year Book, 1986. Reproduced with permission.)

(particularly the retromolar trigone) and then secondarily involves the mandible. To the contrary, I occasionally see primary squamous cell cancer strictly confined to the periodontic gingiva in patients with abysmal dentition. Essentially, they have a few snags in a field of tumor. These tumors are deeply invasive and spread axially in the mandibular cancellous bone and along the alveolar nerve. In this instance, it is important to obtain good bony margins and to resect the perineural tissues well above where the nerve enters the posterior mandible.

Tumors that arise in the area of the retromolar trigone are particularly troublesome. They are usually large when recognized. Bone is generally contiguous or invaded over a sizeable area. The tongue, tonsil, pharyngeal pillars, and even soft palate are areas of spread. Many times it is impossible to assign a true site of origin.

For small cancers in the area that are not directly invading bone a marginal resection of bone can be designed to give adequate distance from the cancer and to preserve the lower part of the mandible.

The surgical approach to the more posterior parts of the oral cavity demands broad exposure. The appropriate cervical lymphadenectomy is done to the level of the mandible. A lateral cheek flap is turned (Figs. 24-9 and 24-10), taking care to maintain adequate margins as the cancer-bearing area is approached. When the mandible is to be preserved and only a posterior marginal resection done, it is difficult to gain exposure for the intraoral resection unless the mandible is sectioned as shown in Fig. 24-11. The mandible can then be securely approximated at the end of the procedure. With larger invasive cancers, the mandible is resected as shown in Figs. 24-10 and 24-12. With shifts in location of cuts, this approach is applicable to many large oral cancers. Almost always, additional tissue must be brought into the area by either a local Bakamjian-type flap (Fig. 24-13) or by a deltopectoral myocutaneous flap (Fig. 24-14). A major advantage to the frequent use of flaps is that the surgeon is free to resect the tumor with adequate margins. The cure does not have to be compromised by worry about closure of the wound or not having good tissue coverage of the carotid artery. With the added bulk and pliancy of the flap, oral function is good and the cosmetic results are acceptable. If one attempts a tenuous primary closure without additional flap tissue, breakdown is frequent, the posterior pharynx is constricted, the tongue is immobilized and poorly functioning, and there is a conspicuous hollow in the side of the cheek. If the anterior 3 to 4 cm of mandibular arch is preserved, the tongue is functional. If teeth remain, a specially made occlusion appliance aligns the remaining teeth despite the absence of the posterior mandible and much of the vertical ramus.

Larger Oral Cancers
Combined Therapeutic Programs

The treatment of early oral cancers is best described as unimodal. After a consultation, either surgical excision or irradiation is selected as the primary therapy based on

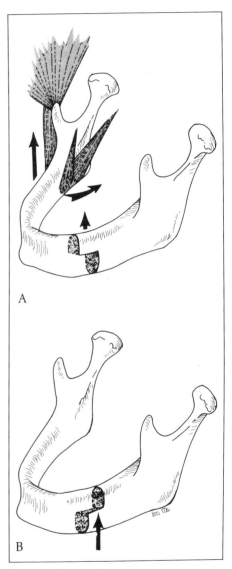

Fig. 24-11. If a mandibular resection is not required, many posteriorly situated lesions need an osteotomy to gain adequate exposure for resection. A. Forces normally exerted on the mandible. If the mandible is sectioned, then the muscular forces tend to disrupt the junction. B. The step osteotomy takes advantage of natural tensions to secure the junction. (From DG McQuarrie. Cancer of the tongue. Selecting appropriate therapy. Curr Prob Surg 23:(8)562, 1986. Reproduced with permission.)

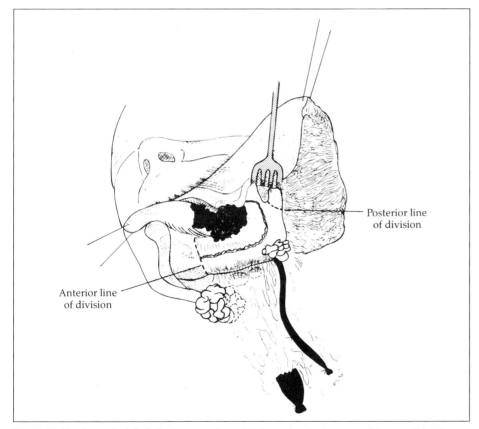

Posterior line of division

Anterior line of division

Fig. 24-10. Development of cheek flap to expose the oral lesion and posterior ramus of the mandible. The masseter muscle is elevated with the flap protecting the parotid gland and the facial nerve. The proposed bone cuts for this lesion are shown as dotted lines. (From DG McQuarrie et al. Head and Neck Cancer: Clinical Decisions and Management Principles. Chicago: Year Book, 1986. Reproduced with permission.)

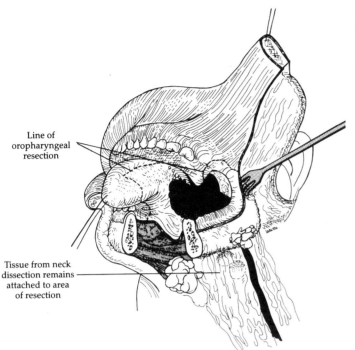

Line of
oropharyngeal
resection

Tissue from neck
dissection remains
attached to area
of resection

Fig. 24-12. Resection of posterior oral lesion. With the mandible divided, the lesion is better exposed. If the mandible is to be sacrificed, section of the ascending ramus (as shown in Fig. 24-10) and division of the attachments of the temporalis muscle allow the mandibular segment to be rotated outward, giving much better exposure than illustrated here for resection of the base of the tongue and the lateral pharyngeal wall. (From DG McQuarrie et al. Head and Neck Cancer: Clinical Decisions and Management Principles. Chicago: Year Book, 1986. Reproduced with permission.)

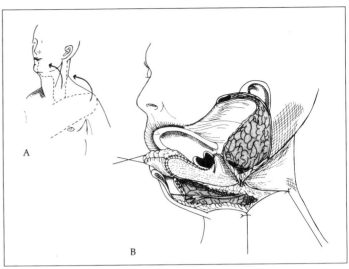

A

B

Fig. 24-13. Bakamjian cervical flap with a medially based pectoral flap to cover the defect. A. The general design of the two flaps. B. The cervical flap incorporates the platysma. It is a tubed "skin-side-in" flap for a short distance and then it is folded outward for oral lining. The cheek flap then covers the nonepithelialized surface. Careful attention must be paid to the achievement of secure closure at all three-sided junctions of flap and mucosa. The deltopectoral flap is brought up to cover the lateral neck. The deltopectoral donor site is covered with split-thickness skin. This flap is used when the mandible or a portion of the mandible has remained. Because an epithelialized communication is made into the mouth, it requires an easy second-stage closure under local anesthesia 4 to 6 weeks later. (From DG McQuarrie et al. Head and Neck Cancer: Clinical Decisions and Management Principles. Chicago: Year Book, 1986. Reproduced with permission.)

lesion size, nodal status, patient condition, patient reliability, occupational requirements, and local skills and resources. Repeat surgical excision or irradiation is reserved for surgical failures, and surgical excision is done for irradiation failures. No center would recommend adjuvant therapies for a stage T1 or T2 cancer that is node-negative by pathologic staging. Since the likelihood of long-term disease-free survival drops precipitously when the tumor is massive or multiple-node metastases are present, it is in this advanced-stage disease that combined therapies have been tried. Unfortunately, patient study groups are quite heterogeneous, subject to selection bias, and confounded by wide variation in population characteristics in different centers. Firm conclusions cannot be made.

Adjuvant Irradiation

The Radiation Therapy Oncology Group (RTOG) did two definitive studies that showed that there was no difference be-

tween pre- and postoperative adjuvant irradiation for treatment of advanced oral and supraglottic cancers. Because there were considerably fewer complications in the postoperative period, most radiation therapists recommend postoperative adjuvant irradiation if it is used in advanced disease. The question not answered by the RTOG study was whether there would be an increase in survival time of patients who received adjuvant irradiation over patients who did not. There was no unirradiated control group. I reviewed a large number of studies in other publications and can only give my impression from the aggregate of poor data.

First, adjuvant postoperative irradiation should probably be reserved for patients with massive invasive cancers or patients with more than two nodes that are positive or a large node (>3 cm) that has likely breeched its capsule. Second, adjuvant postoperative irradiation probably delays the appearance of metastases so that short-term survival data (2–3 years) will be deceptively optimistic. Third, any increment in survival rate that is gained from post-

operative adjuvant irradiation is probably quite modest at a 5-year follow-up period. Benefits, if present, probably do not exceed much more than a 10 to 15 percent increment in 5-year survival rates while producing permanent radiation changes. In practice, I discuss the risks, morbidity, and modest benefits with patients and offer patients with massive aggressive cancers or with stage N2 or a higher stage disease the option of adjuvant postsurgical irradiation.

Adjuvant Chemotherapy

Presently there is no clear-cut evidence that adjuvant chemotherapy for advanced oral cancer has any long-term (5-year) survival benefit, despite increasing frequency of transient partial and complete responses to multidrug regimens. A 1990 review done by Vokes and Weichselbaum analyzed randomized trials of concomitant chemotherapy-radiotherapy. In 3 of 5

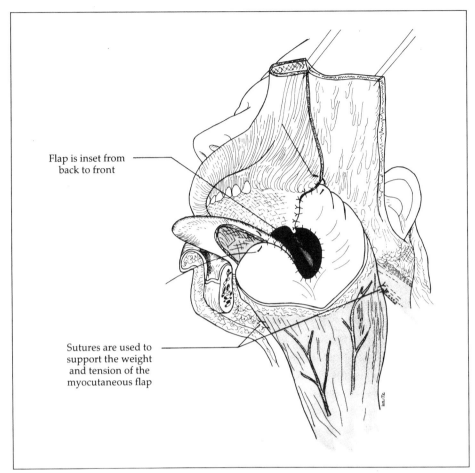

Flap is inset from back to front

Sutures are used to support the weight and tension of the myocutaneous flap

Fig. 24-14. Use of a pectoralis major myocutaneous flap for oral closure. This illustration shows a fair-sized full-thickness flap carried on the vascularized pectoralis muscle. Because of its weight, it has supporting sutures. The flap is then sutured into position. This flap is somewhat thick and bulky, making it difficult to use if the arch of the mandible is preserved. (From DG McQuarrie et al. Head and Neck Cancer: Clinical Decisions and Management Principles. *Chicago: Year Book, 1986. Reproduced with permission.)*

trials, disease-free survival rates reached statistical significance but the differences were very small with significant therapeutic complications. "Since the differences were small and the overall survival was poor, none of these concomitant programs have been adopted as a standard therapy" (Vokes and Weichselbaum). A few patients may have their disease converted from unresectable to resectable status after marked shrinkage of the primary tumor. A well-done protocol by the Eastern Cooperative Oncology Group enrolled 462 patients. There were three arms: (1) resection plus irradiation, (2) induction chemotherapy plus surgical excision plus irradiation, and (3) induction chemotherapy plus surgical excision plus irradiation plus maintenance chemotherapy. All three protocols had statistically similar survival rates after 2 years of follow-up study. Al-

most any major hospital or cancer treatment center can enter patients into sanctioned protocols. For the present, adjuvant chemotherapy should be reserved for administration within sanctioned clinical trials.

Suggested Reading

Ariyan S, Cuono CB. Use of the pectoralis major myocutaneous flap for reconstruction of large cervical, facial, or cranial defects. *Am J Surg* 140:503, 1980.

Bakamjian VY, Long M, Rigg B. Experience with the medially based deltopectoral flap in reconstructive surgery of the head and neck. *Br J Surg* 24:174, 1971.

Larson DL. Management of complications of radiotherapy of the head and neck. *Surg Clin North Am* 66:169, 1986.

Lydiatt DD, Markin RS, Willimas SM, et al. Computed tomography and magnetic resonance imaging of cervical metastasis. *Otolaryngol Head Neck Surg* 101:422, 1989.

Mashberg A. Erythroplasia vs. leukoplasia in the diagnosis of early oral squamous carcinoma. *N Engl J Med* 297:109, 1977.

McQuarrie DG. Cancer of the tongue: Selecting appropriate therapy. *Curr Probl Surg* 23:562, 1986.

McQuarrie DG, Adams GL, Shons AR, Browne GA. *Head and Neck Cancer: Clinical Decisions and Management Principles.* Chicago: Year Book, 1986.

O'Reilly BJ, Leung A, Greco A. Magnetic resonance imaging in head and neck cancer. *Clin Otolaryngol* 14:67, 1989.

Snow JB, Belber RD, Kramer S, et al. Randomized pre-operative and post-operative radiation therapy for patients with carcinoma of the head and neck: Preliminary report. *Laryngoscope* 90:930, 1980.

Spiro RH, Huvos AG, Wong GY, et al. Predictive value of tumor thickness in squamous carcinoma confined to the tongue and floor of the mouth. *Am J Surg* 152:345, 1986.

Tannock IF, Browman G. Lack of evidence for a role of chemotherapy in the routine management of locally advanced head and neck cancer. *J Clin Oncol* 4:1121, 1986.

Vokes EE, Weichselbaum RR. Review Article: Concomitant Chemoradiotherapy. Rational and clinical experience in patients with solid tumors. *J Clin Oncol* 8:911, 1990.

EDITOR'S COMMENT

Doctor McQuarrie has modified his previous chapter to incorporate some of the newer techniques that have been used in contemporary head and neck surgery, including some of the forearm free flaps as well as microvascular bone grafts, of which he prefers the fibula.

There are several underlying principles that all authorities in head and neck cancer seem to proscribe to:

1. The initial treatment, as in any other cancer, is the patient's best chance for survival.
2. Initial attempts that are too conservative done in the interests of better cosmesis ultimately backfire. The patient must later undergo a more destructive and

probably not curative resection in an effort to salvage the situation.

3. The rates of long-term survival following salvage surgery and adjunctive therapy are relatively low, in the 20 to 30 percent range.

4. Doctor McQuarrie argues for early aggressiveness in the nodal dissection, again pointing out that although nodes can be clinically negative, this finding can be deceptive. The appearance of positive nodes after an interval, even in a compliant and reliable patient, often puts the patient into a category of disease that is relatively unfavorable as compared, for example, with early nodal dissection in a patient with clinically negative nodes. This stance is admittedly controversial, but if one reads the literature in a certain way, it is difficult to explain the salvage of 15 to 30 percent in patients who have clinically negative nodes and later have some microscopically positive nodes.

5. All authorities, including Dr. Benjamin Rush, the author of Chapter 27, agree that the node that is larger than 3 cm and can breach the capsule is particularly dangerous to long-term survival and should be aggressively treated with postoperative radiation therapy.

6. Doctor McQuarrie emphasizes the importance of the spread along the neurovascular bundles from the teeth and the necessity for frequent nerve sacrifice, a point of view that is supported by Lydiatt (*Head & Neck* 17:247, 1995).

The issue of pre- or postoperative radiation therapy remains controversial. Fein and coworkers (*Head & Neck* 16:358, 1994) compared a relatively small group of patients with carcinoma of the oral tongue treated between 1964 and 1990. Before 1985, primary radiation therapy with or without neck dissection was used in 105 patients, and after 1985, surgery was the principal mode in 65 patients. The groups are small, and it is not possible to draw many conclusions. However, local control rates were improved for T3 and T4 lesions in patients treated surgically. There was no difference between T1 and T2 patients, but again the groups (18 versus 17 and 48 versus 19) are probably too small to draw conclusions. Complication rates were of course higher in the radiation group with the T3 and T4 lesions. The entire study is rendered suspect because the patients with radiation therapy were primarily treated before 1985 and the surgical patients after 1985. The data in that paper do not seem to support the conclusions for surgical treatment for T1 and T2 lesions with the addition of postoperative twice-daily radiation therapy in selected situations.

J.E.F.

III

Lesions of the Neck

25

Anatomy of the Neck: Anterior and Lateral Triangles

Jack L. Gluckman   Lyon L. Gleich

No matter how experienced the surgeon, one never ceases to be amazed by the complexity of the anatomy of the neck. A clear understanding of this anatomy is essential to appreciate the symptomatology caused by diseases in this area and to facilitate surgical procedures. Entire books have been dedicated to this area of the body, but we will attempt to emphasize only the anatomic aspects that are relevant to the practicing surgeon.

Anatomic Landmarks

Before discussing the detailed anatomy of the neck, it is necessary to review the basic surface landmarks that should be identified before commencing any neck operation. These landmarks should be used in planning the surgical incisions (Fig. 25-1).

In the upper neck, three bony structures can be palpated: the *mastoid tip* just posterior to the ear lobe, the *transverse process of the atlas* (C1) just inferior and anterior to the mastoid tip, and the *angle of the mandible*. The transverse process of the atlas is of particular importance because it is often misinterpreted by both patients and physicians as a pathologic mass in the neck. It is also an important landmark to the upper end of the jugular vein. The sternocleidomastoid muscle (SCM) can easily be seen extending from the clavicle and manubrium to the mastoid, particularly if the patient's head is rotated to the opposite side. A skin incision along the anterior aspect of this muscle is commonly used for surgical procedures on the carotid artery and in neck trauma. The angle of the man-

dible should be palpated, as should the inferior aspect of the ramus of the mandible.

In the midline, the notched upper surface of the *thyroid cartilage* is readily visible, particularly in males. Superior to the thyroid cartilage is the hyoid bone, which is separated from the thyroid cartilage by the thyrohyoid membrane. The *greater horn of the hyoid bone* can be easily palpated and is often misinterpreted as a pathologic mass. Below the thyroid cartilage, the *cricoid cartilage* can be palpated separated by the cricothyroid membrane. Other than the cricothryoid vessels, this membrane is devoid of any vital structures and is the site of immediate entry into the airway during an acute emergency (cricothyroidotomy).

The *clavicle*, which forms the lower border of the neck, should also be palpated and marked prior to a neck dissection. Re-

peated palpation of the *suprasternal notch* can be necessary during a tracheostomy to confirm that the surgeon is operating in the midline.

Skin

The skin and subcutaneous tissues of the neck are thin and quite flexible. The platysma, which lies almost immediately subcutaneously, is usually incorporated in any skin flaps that are elevated. However, it is not present in the midline or posteriorly. The blood supply of the neck skin is from superiorly and inferiorly, principally from the facial artery.

Neck incisions, which are planned to provide adequate exposure, need to ensure the vascular supply of the skin flaps, particularly in the previously irradiated neck

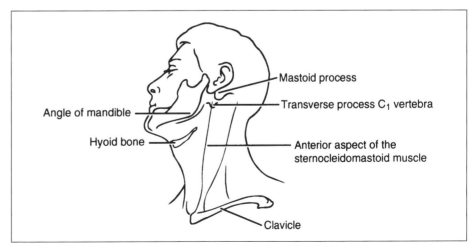

Fig. 25-1. Surface landmarks of the neck that are helpful in designing appropriate neck incisions.

where the blood supply is tenuous. In addition, cosmesis should be considered and incisions should be made in the horizontally oriented relaxed skin tension lines. Elevation of flaps with the underlying platysma muscle maximizes the vascular supply to the flaps. Because the platysma is not present posteriorly, these flaps have a more tenuous blood supply, and therefore, large posterior flaps should be avoided.

The issues involved in determining the types of incisions used and flap design involve balancing adequate exposure, cosmesis, and flap viability (Fig. 25-2). The MacFee incision, which uses parallel horizontal incisions to avoid a trifurcation, provides excellent cosmesis and flap viability but limits visualization. The Schobinger and Conley incisions, which use a horizontal incision and a posteriorly placed vertical incision to provide excellent exposure, optimize flap viability by the posterior placement of the vertical incision. The long anterior flap is viable be-cause of the incorporation of the platysma. The choice of flap is ultimately dictated by the areas to be optimally exposed and the experience of the surgeon.

Muscles

Muscles and triangles of the neck are shown in Fig. 25-3. The *platysma* arises from the clavicle and upper thorax and ascends superiorly and slightly anteriorly to pass over the mandible, where the fibers blend with the facial muscles and superficial musculocutaneous aponeurotic system. The platysma is innervated by the cervical branch of the facial nerve. The facial artery is the major blood supply of the platysma and the overlying skin. A platysma muscle flap has been described for reconstruction of the oral cavity. However, it is somewhat tenuous and has never really gained acceptance. In general, most neck flaps are elevated in the subplatysmal layer.

The *SCM* arises from the sternum and clavicle inferiorly, and inserts into the mastoid and skin superiorly. It is innervated by the accessory nerve and cervical nerves. The vascular supply of the SCM is from the occipital, superior thyroid, and transverse cervical arteries. This muscle divides the neck into anterior and posterior triangles and covers the carotid sheath. During a radical neck dissection the SCM is routinely sacrificed; however, it is preserved in many of the modified and selective neck dissections. A flap consisting of the SCM together with overlying skin can be used for reconstruction of the oral cavity based either superiorly or inferiorly. However, with increasing mobilization of this muscle the blood supply to the cutaneous portion of the flap can be compromised with unpredictable survival, but the underlying muscle always remains viable. Therefore, care should be taken to suture the muscle as well as the overlying skin to the edges of the reconstructed defect to prevent fistula formation.

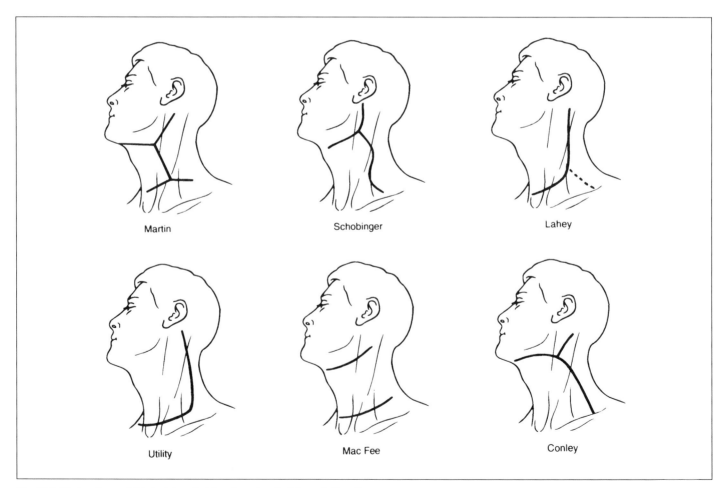

Martin

Schobinger

Lahey

Utility

Mac Fee

Conley

Fig. 25-2. Various types of skin incisions that have been described for neck dissections.

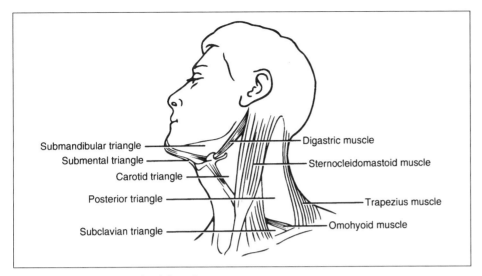

Fig. 25-3. Muscles and triangles of the neck.

The *trapezius* muscle forms the posterior border of the posterior triangle of the neck. It is innervated by the accessory nerve, with varying contributions from the cervical nerves. Therefore, even after the division of the accessory nerve, the function of the muscle can still be preserved. The trapezius muscle can be used together with a portion of the scapula as an osteomyocutaneous flap if the transverse cervical artery is preserved during the neck dissection.

The *omohyoid* muscle extends from the hyoid bone to the superior border of the scapula with an intervening tendon overlying the carotid sheath. This muscle is part of the strap muscles and therefore is innervated by the cervical plexus via the ansa cervicalis. This muscle works in unison with the other strap muscles—the sternohyoid, sternothyroid, and thyrohyoid muscles—to change the position of the larynx.

The *digastric* muscle extends from the mastoid process to the anterior mandible with an intervening tendon attached to the hyoid bone. The anterior belly then crosses the mylohyoid muscle to its insertion in the mandible. The posterior belly of the digastric is an important landmark when performing upper neck surgical procedures. Its mastoid attachment is a guide to the facial nerve during parotidectomy, and the posterior belly itself is a guide to the hypoglossal nerve, which lies just beneath it. During a radical neck dissection, it is a landmark for identification of the upper end of the internal jugular vein, which lies

just beneath it. The *stylohyoid* muscle, which arises from the styloid process, descends parallel to the posterior belly of the digastric muscle and inserts into the hyoid bone. Both the posterior belly of the digastric muscle and the stylohyoid muscle are innervated by the facial nerve. The *mylohyoid* muscle runs from the hyoid to the mandible and forms a mobile sling for the tongue and floor of mouth. The anterior belly of the digastric and the mylohyoid are innervated by the mylohyoid nerve, which is a branch of the mandibular division of the trigeminal nerve.

The *scalene* muscles form the floor of the posterior triangle of the neck. The anterior scalene muscle is separated from the middle scalene muscle by the brachial plexus and subclavian artery. The phrenic nerve descends on the surface of the anterior scalene muscle. Inferiorly, the anterior scalene muscle is crossed by the subclavian vein. It is important to preserve the fascia overlying the scalenes during a neck dissection to ensure protection of these vital structures.

Fascia

The *superficial fascia* of the neck is similar to the superficial fascia throughout the rest of the body in that it lies just below the dermis. However, in the neck it splits to enclose the platysma muscle.

The *deep cervical fascia* consists of three distinct layers (Fig. 25-4): 1) The *superficial layer* attaches to the vertebral spinous pro-

cesses and ligamentum nuchae posteriorly; the zygomatic arch, mastoid process, external occipital protuberance, and superior nuchal line superiorly; and the scapula, clavicle, and sternum inferiorly. It surrounds the neck. It splits to enclose the SCM, trapezius, strap muscles, muscles of mastication, and the major salivary glands. 2) A *middle layer* (visceral or pretracheal fascia) separates from the superficial layer of the deep cervical fascia and encloses the thyroid, trachea, esophagus, and constrictor muscles. 3) The *deep layer* of the deep cervical fascia arises from the transverse and spinous process of the cervical vertebrae and from the ligamentum nuchae. This layer surrounds the scalene muscles and fuses in the midline over the prevertebral muscles. This fascia forms the floor of the posterior triangle of the neck. In the midline, it splits into an anterior alar fascia and a posterior prevertebral fascia.

The *carotid sheath* is formed by coalescence of all the layers of the deep cervical fascia. It encloses the carotid artery, internal jugular vein, and vagus nerve.

Fascial Spaces

The fascial layers delineate potential spaces throughout the neck. Knowledge of these spaces is particularly important in treating neck space infections.

The *submandibular space* is contained by the oral mucous membrane superiorly and the superficial layers of the deep cervical fascia inferiorly. Therefore, it is limited inferiorly by the hyoid bone, anteriorly by the mandible, and posteriorly by the tongue musculature. The mylohyoid muscle divides the submandibular space into a superior *sublingual space* and an inferior *submaxillary space*, which communicate. The submandibular gland occupies both spaces, and the sublingual space contains the sublingual gland, the submandibular duct, and the hypoglossal nerve. The submaxillary space is further subdivided by the anterior belly of the digastric muscle into a midline *submental compartment* and a lateral *submaxillary compartment*. All these compartments freely communicate with each other and across the midline into the spaces in the contralateral neck, thereby permitting rapid spread of infection across the neck. Infection of this space is known as Ludwig's angina, which requires urgent incision and drainage be-

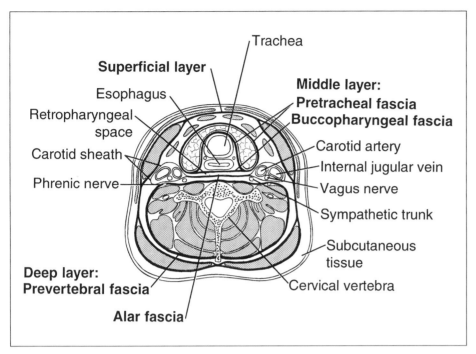

Fig. 25-4. Cross-section of the neck demonstrating the fascial layers.

In the figure:
- Trachea
- **Superficial layer**
- Esophagus
- Retropharyngeal space
- Carotid sheath
- Phrenic nerve
- **Middle layer: Pretracheal fascia Buccopharyngeal fascia**
- Carotid artery
- Internal jugular vein
- Vagus nerve
- Sympathetic trunk
- Subcutaneous tissue
- Cervical vertebra
- **Deep layer: Prevertebral fascia**
- **Alar fascia**

Arteries

The arteries of the neck are shown in Fig. 25-5. The carotid sheath contains the carotid artery system medially and the internal jugular vein laterally with the vagus nerve lying between the vessels. The *common carotid artery* arises from the innominate artery on the right and from the aorta on the left. It ascends in the carotid sheath and then bifurcates at the level of the thyrohyoid membrane. At the carotid bifurcation is a pressure receptor, the carotid sinus, and a chemoreceptor, the carotid body. Both receptors are innervated by a branch of the glossopharyngeal nerve.

Following the bifurcation, the *internal carotid artery* runs posterolaterally to the external carotid artery to the carotid canal at the base of the skull. As it ascends it is crossed by the hypoglossal nerve, the posterior belly of the digastric, and by the muscles that originate from the styloid process.

The *external carotid artery* exits the carotid sheath and passes superiorly terminating at the superficial temporal and internal maxillary arteries. The *ascending pharyngeal artery* arises from the deep surface of the external carotid artery to supply the pharynx and palate. This vessel can rarely be the source of a posterior epistaxis and can need to be embolized or ligated as part of the treatment of this condition. The first anterior branch of the external carotid artery is the *superior thyroid artery*, which runs with the superior laryngeal nerve and supplies the thyroid gland, larynx, SCM, and strap muscles. During a thyroidectomy, the artery should be divided close to the gland to avoid injury to this nerve.

The *lingual artery* passes deep to the digastric and stylohyoid muscles to supply the tongue. The *facial artery* (external maxillary artery) arises from the external carotid artery anteriorly near the angle of the mandible. It courses deep to the digastric muscle and either passes through the submandibular gland or is closely related to it. It then crosses the mandible to supply the facial skin and muscles. This vessel needs to be identified and ligated early in the procedure during a submandibular gland excision.

The *occipital artery* arises posteriorly at approximately the level of the facial artery. It crosses superficial to the internal carotid

cause the floor of the mouth and tongue can be elevated and displaced posteriorly by abscess formation, leading to airway compromise.

The *masticator space* is enclosed by the superficial layer of the deep cervical fascia as it surrounds the masseter, ptyergoid, and temporalis muscles. Infection in this space is often preceded by a dental abscess, and can present as a mass posterior to the ramus of the mandible. The *parotid* space encloses the parotid gland and is formed by the superficial layer of the deep cervical fascia encircling the gland. Acute parotitis with abscess formation can therefore be extremely painful and proper drainage can require incision not only superficially but also on the under surface of the parotid gland.

The *parapharyngeal space* is an inverted pyramid with its base superiorly at the base of the skull and its apex at the hyoid bone. It is bound medially by the pharyngeal fascia along the lateral pharyngeal wall. Its lateral border is the superficial layer of the deep cervical fascia overlying the mandible, internal pterygoid muscle, and parotid gland. The styloid process divides the parapharyngeal space into anterior and posterior compartments. The carotid sheath is contained in the posterior compartment. The parapharyngeal space com-municates anteriorly, around the submandibular gland, with the submandibular space, posterolaterally with the parotid space, laterally with the masticator space, posteriorly with the carotid sheath, and posteromedially with the retropharyngeal space. Therefore, it is particularly important in the spread of cervical infections.

The *peritonsillar space* is located between the tonsillar capsule and the pharyngeal fascia. An abscess in this space (peritonsillar abscess, quinsy) is treated by transoral incision and drainage. If left untreated, it can rupture into the parapharyngeal space.

The *retropharyngeal space* is the most anterior of the midline spaces that involve the entire length of the neck. It lies between the posterior pharyngeal wall and the alar fascia and laterally communicates with the parapharyngeal space. The retropharyngeal space extends inferiorly to the tracheal bifurcation in the chest. Posterior to the retropharyngeal space, deep to the alar fascia, is the *prevertebral space*, which extends the length of the vertebral column. Any infection that has progressed to involve the spaces posterior to the pharynx needs urgent drainage to prevent the spread of infection into the mediastinum and beyond.

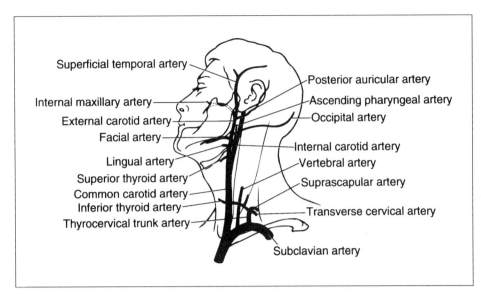

Fig. 25-5. Arteries of the neck.

artery, internal jugular vein, and hypoglossal nerve. The *posterior auricular artery* arises from the positive aspect of the external carotid artery. It supplies the parotid gland, auricle, mastoid, tympanic cavity, and scalp. A branch from this artery, the stylomastoid artery, is closely related to the facial nerve and causes troublesome bleeding during parotidectomy.

The terminal branches of the external carotid artery are the superficial temporal artery and internal maxillary artery. The *superficial temporal artery* continues superiorly and supplies the scalp and forehead. The *internal maxillary artery* passes anteriorly, deep to the ramus of the mandible, where it divides into its many branches in the pterygomaxillary fissure. It is this vessel and its branches that are the cause of most refractory cases of epistaxis. It can be approached via the maxillary antrum to gain control during severe epistaxis.

In the supraclavicular area, the *thyrocervical trunk*, which arises from the subclavian artery, branches into the inferior thyroid, transverse cervical, and suprascapular arteries. The *inferior thyroid artery* courses anteriorly, deep to the carotid artery, to reach the thyroid gland. This vessel must be carefully ligated during thyroidectomy, because it can retract out of the field behind the carotid artery. The *suprascapular artery* runs across the posterior triangle, superficial to the prevertebral fascia, and accompanied by the *transverse cervical artery*, which runs parallel to it. The transverse cervical artery supplies the middle and lateral portions of the trapezius muscle. Care must be taken to preserve this artery when using the trapezius osteomyoocutaneous flap for mandible and floor of the mouth reconstruction.

Veins

The veins of the neck (Fig. 25-6) are variable in configuration and have multiple anastomoses. The *external jugular vein* is formed by the union of the posterior branch of the retromandibular vein and posterior auricular vein. It runs vertically on the superficial surface of the SCM and empties into the subclavian vein in the subclavicular area. The external jugular vein can anastomose with the internal jugular vein. The *anterior jugular vein* originates from multiple submental veins and descends superficial to the strap muscles to empty into the external jugular or subclavian veins. It does communicate with its counterpart on the opposite side of the neck.

The *internal jugular vein* is a continuation of the sigmoid sinus at the jugular foramen. It is then joined by the facial vein, formed from the union of the anterior and posterior facial veins, at the level of the hyoid bone. As the internal jugular vein continues inferiorly, the superior thyroid, pharyngeal, lingual, and middle thyroid veins all enter it. During a radical neck dissection, the internal jugular vein must be ligated and divided both inferiorly and superiorly. It is important to double tie and suture ligate the lower end to prevent accidental loss of control and hemorrhage. Because of its close relationship to the vagus nerve, care must be taken not to include this nerve in the ligature.

The internal jugular vein joins the subclavian vein to form the innominate vein. At this junction, the thoracic duct on the left and right lymphatic duct enter.

Nerves

The nerves of the neck are shown in Fig. 25-7.

The *marginal mandibular branch of the facial nerve* can descend into the upper neck below the lower border of the mandible, as it passes forward to innervate the orbicularis oris and depressor anguli muscles. To avoid inadvertently damaging this nerve, neck incisions are not made within 2 cm of the lower border of the mandible, and as the upper flap is elevated, the nerve should be identified. However, the best technique to prevent injury to the nerve is to ligate the facial vein deep to the superficial layer of the deep cervical fascia over the submandibular gland and elevate the flap in a plane deep to this fascia using the superior stump of the vein as a guide. The nerve always lies superficial to this plane and therefore is always protected.

The *spinal accessory nerve* exits the skull at the jugular foramen between the internal jugular vein and internal carotid artery. In most instances, it then crosses the internal jugular vein, passing either through or deep to the SCM, and then descending through the posterior triangle to innervate the trapezius muscle. The path of the accessory nerve in the posterior triangle is extremely superficial, running between the superficial and the deep layers of the deep cervical fascia without any overlying muscle coverage. Therefore, it can be easily damaged during elevation of the posterior flap or even during a posterior cervical lymph node biopsy. The best technique to identify the accessory nerve in the posterior triangle is to identify *Erb's point*, where the *great auricular nerve* crosses the posterior border of the SCM. The spinal accessory nerve emerges from the SCM 2 cm superior to Erb's point.

The *hypoglossal nerve* emerges from the hypoglossal canal and passes into the neck

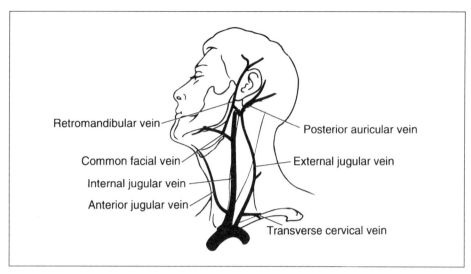

Fig. 25-6. Veins of the neck.

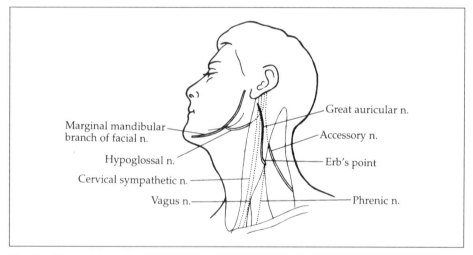

Fig. 25-7. Nerves of the neck.

between the internal jugular vein and internal carotid artery. It then passes forward, crossing the lateral surface of the internal and external carotid arteries. It lies deep to the posterior belly of the digastric muscle throughout its course, lying on the surface of the hyoglossus muscle, inferior to the submandibular gland and deep to the mylohyoid muscle. The nerve gives small branches to the extrinsic tongue musculature and then enters the substance of the tongue to innervate the intrinsic musculature. During neck dissection it is very important to identify and protect this nerve. One technique is to identify the ansa hypoglossi (contributions from the upper cervical nerves, which join the ansa cervicalis) and follow it superiorly. Another is to isolate it posterior to the carotid

and follow it anteriorly. A third technique is to identify it below and deep to the posterior belly of the digastric.

The *vagus nerve* exits at the jugular foramen and descends in the neck posteromedial to the internal jugular vein. The *pharyngeal branch* descends between the internal and external carotid arteries and joins with the pharyngeal branch of the glossopharyngeal nerve to form the pharyngeal plexus. This plexus constitutes the motor supply to the pharynx. Therefore, high vagal injury can result in significant dysphagia. The *superior laryngeal nerve* runs with the superior thyroid artery and gives off an external branch, which is the motor nerve to the cricothyroid muscle, and an internal branch, which enters the

larynx via the thyrohyoid membrane and supplies sensation to the supraglottis and glottis.

The *recurrent laryngeal nerve* is a branch of the vagus that ascends in the neck after arising in the mediastinum. The right nerve loops posteriorly around the subclavian artery before ascending, while the left nerve arises at the level of the aortic arch, looping around the ligamentum arteriosum. The recurrent laryngeal nerves then ascend in or near the tracheoesophageal groove supplying the trachea and esophagus. The recurrent laryngeal nerves enter the larynx at the cricothyroid membrane. The recurrent nerves innervate all the intrinsic muscles of the larynx and provide sensation to the subglottis and portions of the glottis. The easiest technique to identify this nerve during thyroidectomy is to trace the inferior thyroid artery medially. The nerve has a variable relationship to this artery, usually running deep to it, but occasionally it is superficial and rarely intertwines between its branches. Do remember that occasionally the right recurrent nerve may be noncurrent, coming off the vagus directly.

The *cervical sympathetic trunk* consists of the ascending preganglionic sympathetic fibers from the upper thoracic nerves. It lies posterior and medial to the carotid artery. There are multiple ganglia, the largest being the stellate, or inferior cervical ganglion, and the superior cervical ganglion. Injury to this trunk, resulting in Horner's syndrome of ptosis, myosis, and facial anhydrosis, can occur during neck dissection when dissection is inadvertently continued deep to the carotid artery.

The *phrenic nerve* arises from C3–C5 and descends on the surface of the anterior scalene muscle deep to the prevertebral fascia. Damage to this nerve results in paralysis of the hemidiaphragm. Therefore, the deep layer of the deep cervical fascia should be preserved intact in a neck dissection to prevent damage to this nerve.

Lymphatics

The neck contains one-third of all the lymph nodes in the body. Knowledge of the intricate lymphatic drainage patterns and sites of the various nodes is useful in predicting the site of primary cancer when cervical metastases are present as well as in planning treatment of the neck when dealing with an upper aerodigestive tract cancer. The nodes of the neck can best be thought of as occurring in the following groups.

Occipital Nodes

Occipital nodes are divided into a superficial and a deep group (Fig. 25-8). The *superficial* group consists of two to five nodes that are located between the SCM and trapezius muscle at the apex of the posterior triangle. They are superficial to the splenius muscle and just deep to the superficial investing fascia. The *deep* group of one to three occipital nodes is located deep to the splenius muscle and follows the course of the occipital artery. The superficial nodes drain the occipital scalp and posterior portion of the neck and then drain into the deeper group as well as into the upper spinal accessory nodes. In addition, the deep group of nodes drains the deep muscular layers of the neck in the occipital region.

Postauricular Nodes

The postauricular nodes vary from one to four in number and are situated over the dense fibrous portion of the anterior border of the SCM overlying the mastoid bone (Fig. 25-8). They drain the posterior parietal region of the scalp as well as the skin of the mastoid region and posterior auricle. The efferent vessels drain into the infra-auricular parotid nodes and also into the internal jugular and spinal accessory

nodes. These nodes must be included in any dissection for cancer of the posterior scalp.

Parotid Nodes

The parotid nodes are divided into an extraglandular and an intraglandular group. The *extraglandular* group is further divided into *preauricular* and *infra-auricular* nodes. They drain the lateral and frontal aspects of the scalp as well as the anterior portion of the auricle, the external auditory canal, the lateral aspect of the face, and the buccal mucosa of the oral cavity (Fig. 25-9). The *intraglandular* nodes drain the same regions and are also connected with the extraglandular nodes. Embryologically, the lymphatic system develops before the parotid gland, which surrounds the nodes as it develops. The efferent vessels of both groups then drain into the internal jugular or external jugular chain of lymph nodes. There can be up to 20 parotid lymph nodes. Anterior scalp, temporal bone, and buccal mucosal cancers must all have these nodes addressed in the appropriate situation, usually necessitating a parotidectomy, to obtain adequate clearance.

Submandibular Nodes

The submandibular lymph nodes are divided into five groups: 1) preglandular, 2) postglandular, 3) prevascular, 4) postvascular, and 5) intracapsular (Fig. 25-10).

The preglandular and prevascular groups are located anterior to the submandibular gland and facial artery, respectively,

whereas the postglandular and postvascular groups are posterior to these structures. The submandibular gland differs from the parotid gland in that there are no true intraglandular nodes; however, an occasional node located inside the capsule of the gland has been identified. The submandibular nodes drain the ipsilateral lower and upper lip, cheek, nose, mucosa of the nasal fossa, medial canthus, anterior gingiva, anterior tonsillar pillar, soft palate, anterior two-thirds of the tongue, and submandibular salivary gland (Fig. 25-11). The efferent lymph vessels empty into the internal jugular group of nodes in the subdigastric region. However, an accessory route exists from the preglandular and prevascular nodes into the deep internal jugular nodes via a lymphatic vessel running along the posterior edge of the omohyoid muscle. This route explains the multiple-level involvement often noted with lesions of the anterior oral cavity.

Submental Nodes

There are usually two to eight nodes in the submental node group (Fig. 25-10). They are located in the soft tissue of the submental triangle between the platysma and mylohyoid muscles. They drain the mentum, the middle 60 to 70 percent of the lower lip, the anterior gingiva, and the anterior one-third of the tongue. The efferent vessels usually drain into the ipsilateral and contralateral preglandular and prevascular submandibular nodes or into the internal jugular group via a lymphatic vessel following the hypoglossal nerve.

Sublingual Nodes

The sublingual nodes are located along the collecting trunk of the tongue and sublingual gland. They drain the anterior floor of the mouth and ventral surface of the tongue. They subsequently drain into the submandibular group of nodes, or they can follow the hypoglossal nerve or lingual artery and empty directly into the internal jugular group by passing behind the stylohyoid and digastric muscles or even enter the jugular chain lower down.

It should be appreciated from the preceding discussion that the lymphatic vessels from the submental, submandibular, and sublingual regions do not have a simple drainage pattern and can empty into the internal jugular system at multiple levels.

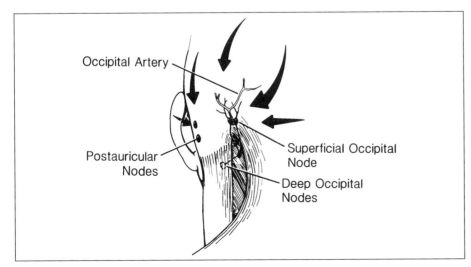

Fig. 25-8. Occipital and postauricular nodes.

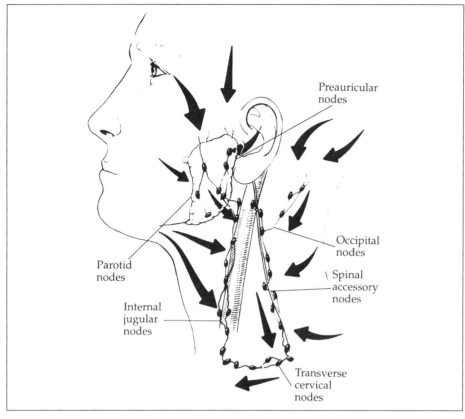

Fig. 25-9. Drainage pattern to the lateral deep cervical node group including the parotid nodes.

Retropharyngeal Nodes

The retropharyngeal nodes are divided into a lateral and a medial group (Fig. 25-11). The *lateral* group consists of one to three nodes, which are located at the level of the atlas, in close relationship to the internal carotid artery and can extend to the base of the skull. The *medial* group is located near the midline and is more inferior. These nodes are more numerous and can extend inferiorly down to the level of the postcricoid area. Both groups are located between the pharynx and prevertebral fascia. They drain the posterior region of the nasal cavity, sphenoid sinus, ethmoid sinus, hard and soft palate, nasopharynx, and posterior pharyngeal wall to the level of the cricoid. The efferents drain into the upper internal jugular group. The management of these nodes must be considered when dealing with malignancies in any of the drainage areas mentioned, particularly oropharyngeal and hypopharyngeal cancers. They are not included in a routine neck dissection and must be actively sought and removed.

Anterior Cervical Nodes

The anterior cervical nodes are divided into two groups: 1) the anterior jugular chain and 2) the juxtavisceral chain.

The *anterior jugular* chain follows the anterior jugular vein and is located superficial to the strap muscles. Although the nodes are not consistently present, the col-

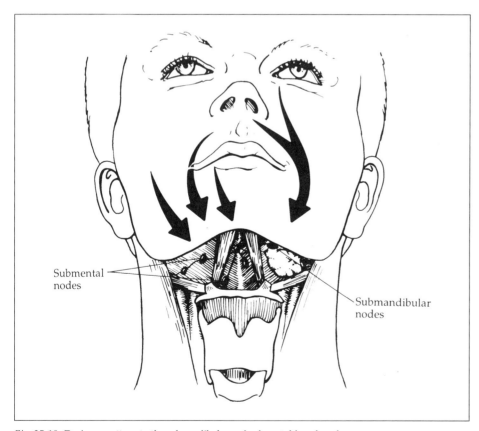

Fig. 25-10. Drainage pattern to the submandibular and submental lymph nodes.

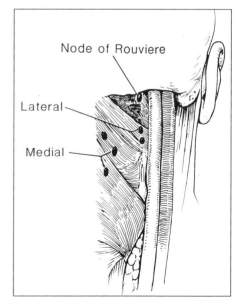

Fig. 25-11. Retropharyngeal nodes.

lecting vessels are always present. They drain the skin and muscles of the anterior portion of the neck, and the efferent vessels empty into the lower internal jugular nodes. The *juxtavisceral* chain is separated into the prelaryngeal, prethyroid, pretracheal, and paratracheal nodes (Fig. 25-12). The *prelaryngeal* nodes are located over the thyrohyoid membrane. The *upper* nodes drain primarily the supraglottic larynx, whereas the *lower* nodes drain the infraglottic larynx, the thyroid isthmus, and the anteromedial aspects of the thyroid lobes. The single lymph node overlying the thyroid cartilage is often referred to as the Delphian node. The *pretracheal group* consists of nodes lying between the isthmus of the thyroid gland down to the innominate vein. They are continuous with the pretracheal lymph nodes of the anterior superior mediastinum. They vary from 2 to 12 in number and drain the region of the thyroid gland and trachea, as well as receive vessels from the prelaryngeal group. The efferent vessels empty into the paratracheal chain and into the internal jugular group. They also communicate with the anterior superior mediastinal nodes.

The *paratracheal* group is often referred to as the recurrent nerve chain because the nodes characteristically follow this nerve.

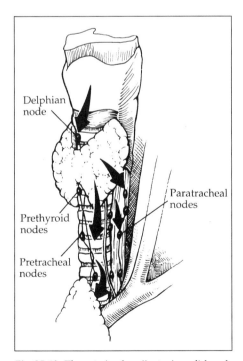

Fig. 25-12. The anterior deep (juxtavisceral) lymph node chain with arrows indicating the drainage pattern.

They drain the lateral aspects of the thyroid lobes, the parathyroid glands, the posterior infraglottic region of the larynx, the trachea, and the esophagus. They also receive vessels from the pretracheal and retropharyngeal lymph nodes. The efferent vessels drain into the lower jugular nodes or the lower jugular–subclavian vein junction. There can also be communication with the anterior superior mediastinal nodes.

These nodes are frequently forgotten during neck dissection for cancer and must be actively sought and dissected. In addition, it is important to remember that in the anterior portion of the neck there is no division in the midline between the lymphatics, with cancer easily spreading to the contralateral side.

Lateral Cervical Nodes

The lateral cervical nodes are divided into a superficial and a deep group (see Fig. 25-9). The superficial group follows the external jugular vein and drains into either the internal jugular or the transverse cervical nodes of the deep group. The deep group consists of the spinal accessory chain, the transverse cervical chain, and the internal jugular chain.

These nodes form a triangle, with the base formed by the transverse cervical group, the posterior limb by the spinal accessory group, and the anterior limb by the internal jugular group. The *spinal accessory* chain follows the course of the spinal accessory nerve and can consist of up to 20 nodes. These nodes normally receive drainage from the occipital, postauricular, and suprascapular nodes, as well as from the posterior part of the scalp, the supraspinous fossa, the nape of the neck, the lateral aspect of the neck, and the shoulder. The upper nodes of this group intermingle with the upper internal jugular chain nodes. These junctional nodes drain a large portion of the upper aerodigestive tract. The *transverse cervical* group follows the transverse cervical vessels and consists of up to 12 nodes. The medial nodes of this chain overlie the scalene muscles (the scalene nodes). These nodes receive drainage from the spinal accessory group and the transverse cervical group, as well as the collecting trunks from the skin of the upper chest and lower lateral neck. The most medial nodes also intermingle with the lower internal jugular nodes. The *internal*

jugular chain consists of a large system of nodes covering the anterior and lateral aspects of the internal jugular vein and extending from beneath the digastric muscle superiorly to the junction of the internal jugular vein and subclavian vein inferiorly. These nodes have been arbitrarily divided into an upper, a middle, and a lower group. There can be as many as 30 nodes in this chain. The final efferent vessels from this chain empty into the venous system via the thoracic duct on the left and multiple lymphatic channels on the right. This group of nodes drains all the previously discussed groups. In addition, this chain can receive direct input from the entire nasal fossa, the pharynx, tonsils, external and middle ear, eustachian tube, tongue, hard and soft palates, hypopharynx, major salivary glands, and thyroid and parathyroid glands.

As is apparent, this lateral cervical group of nodes constitutes a major and important aspect of lymphatic drainage in the head and neck and must be addressed in most cervical lymphadenectomies for cancer of the upper aerodigestive tract.

Although these patterns of drainage are fairly consistent, alteration can occur with malignant involvement or after radiation therapy. In these situations, rerouting can occur, and metastases can arise in unusual sites. Metastases have also been shown to skip first echelon nodes and present in

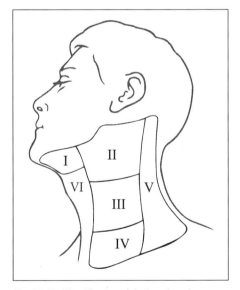

Fig. 25-13. Classification of the lymph nodes according to level. This scheme is an arbitrary clinical classification to aid the clinician in comparing various types of lymph node dissections.

lower jugular nodes even under usual circumstances.

The lymph nodes of the neck have clinically been classified into six levels (Fig. 25-13). Level I is above the posterior digastric muscle and contains the submental and submandibular nodes. Level II includes the upper deep cervical nodes. Level III includes the middle deep cervical nodes. Level IV contains the lower deep cervical nodes. Level V includes the posterior triangle nodes. Level VI includes the anterior cervical node group.

The classic radical neck dissection was originally described to ensure removal en bloc of all the cervical lymphatics of the neck. Modified neck dissections have been designed to preserve select structures normally removed in the radical dissection, while at the same time removing all the nodal groups. These structures include the accessory nerve, the SCM, and internal jugular vein. Modified neck dissections should be performed only by surgeons experienced in these techniques, since an incomplete dissection can lead to failure to remove all the cancer-bearing nodes.

Selective neck dissections have been developed to remove only the levels at greatest risk of metastatic disease. These dissections should be used only in very carefully selected situations by experienced surgeons who clearly understand the disease process.

Suggested Reading

Brown DF, Richtsmeier WJ. *Infections of the Fascial Spaces of the Head and Neck*. 2nd ed. Alexandria, VA: American Academy of Otolaryngology—Head and Neck Surgery Foundation, Inc., 1987.

Hollinshead WH. *Anatomy for Surgeons—The Head and Neck*. 3rd ed. Philadelphia: Lippincott, 1982.

Jones KR. Anatomy of the Neck. In Shockley WW, Pillsbury HC (eds.). *The Neck. Diagnosis and Surgery*. St. Louis: Mosby, 1994.

Rabuzzi DD, Johnson JT, Weissman JL. *Diagnosis and Management of Deep Neck Infections*. 3rd ed. Alexandria, VA: American Academy of Otolaryngology—Head and Neck Surgery Foundation, Inc., 1993.

Robbins KT. *Neck Dissection Classification and TNM Staging of Head and Neck Cancer*. Alexandria, VA: American Academy of Otolaryngology—Head and Neck Surgery Foundation, Inc., 1991.

Savoury LW, Gluckman JL. Cervical Metastases. In Paparella M, Shumrick DA, Gluckman JL, et al (eds.). *Otolaryngology*. 3rd ed, Vol. III. Philadelphia: Saunders, 1991.

26

Diagnostic Approach to Neck Masses

Mimis Cohen   Rudolph F. Dolezal   H. Wayne Slone   Dimitrios G. Spigos

Neck masses, solitary or multiple, are caused by a variety of medical conditions. They represent a wide spectrum of abnormalities ranging from isolated enlargement of an underlying anatomic structure, to a tumor metastasis, or manifestation of a generalized systemic disease.

Several classifications have been proposed to facilitate a comprehensive differential diagnosis of neck masses. In general, however, these masses can be classified into three categories: congenital and developmental, inflammatory and neoplastic, and benign or malignant (Table 26-1).

A careful history and physical examination are of paramount importance in the evaluation of cervical masses. The age group of the patient should be taken into consideration and is an important factor in the differential diagnosis. In children and adolescents, there is a significantly higher incidence of masses of inflammatory or congenital origin. Malignant lesions are relatively rare in this age group. After the age of 40, unless proven otherwise, a mass in the neck should be considered to be a primary or metastatic cancer from the head and neck area, or even a metastasis from a primary tumor originating from a site below the clavicles.

The location and characteristics of the mass can also indicate enlargement of an underlying structure, such as the thyroid gland, or can be characteristic of an embryonal remnant, such as a branchial cleft cyst located in the upper and middle neck along the anterior border of the sternocleidomastoid muscle, or a thyroglossal duct cyst located in the midline of the upper neck. If the neck mass is caused by a metastatic tumor, then the group of involved neck nodes can provide a clue about the location of the primary tumor. Approximately 30 percent of all lymph nodes in the body are found in the cervical area and the lymphatic drainage to the neck from the head and neck area is highly predictable. Thus, the location of a cervical mass can be helpful in search for the primary site of the malignancy (Fig. 26-1).

A detailed history provides considerable information. A history of recent dental treatment can provide a clue for a subsequent inflammatory reaction in the neck. Exposure to household pets, such as cats or parrots, can direct a search for cat-scratch fever or toxoplasmosis; exposure to radiation or radiation therapy for benign diseases, such as facial acne, can be responsible for the development of thyroid cancer several years or even decades later. The use of tobacco and alcohol are well-known contributing factors to the development of oropharyngeal or laryngeal carcinomas, and a high incidence of carcinoma of the maxillary sinuses has been reported in workers in the chromium and nickel industries.

Tuberculosis caused by typical or atypical bacterial strains and infections resulting from HIV have significantly increased during the last decade and should also be taken into consideration in the differential diagnosis of neck masses.

The timing of onset of the symptoms and the physical characteristics of a mass are also helpful in the diagnosis. Firm, painful neck masses of short duration tend to be of inflammatory origin. An existing lesion that is unchanged for a long period can be of congenital origin or can be a benign tumor, whereas rapidly enlarging masses are often malignant. Nontender, matted, rubbery nodes are consistent with Hodgkin's disease and other lymphoproliferative disorders.

Another presenting symptom of head and neck tumors is pain. The pain can be caused by local irritation, such as an intraoral ulceration, or can be referred from another area. Thus, persistent otalgia without evidence of external or middle ear disease can represent the first sign of an intraoral malignant tumor, referred through connections between the lingual and auriculotemporal nerves. The presence of other coexisting physical signs indicative of neoplastic disease in the head and neck such as dysphagia, hoarseness, persistent cough, hemoptysis, changes in hearing or smell, nasal obstruction, and specific cranial nerve dysfunction, including hypesthesia in the distribution of the branches of the trigeminal nerve should also be evaluated, when appropriate, during the head and neck examination.

Physical Examination

A physical examination is the single most important diagnostic step in the evaluation of a cervical mass. The physician should undertake a thorough examination of the entire head and neck area to establish a correct diagnosis and prescribe the appropriate treatment, particularly when a malignancy is suspected. The skin of the face and scalp should be inspected carefully for the presence of ulcerations, nodules, and pigmented or other suspicious lesions. Examination of the nasal airway with a nasal speculum can reveal evidence of epithelial discontinuity or the presence of a mass. Persistent epistaxis can be the presenting symptom of neoplasms of the nose or paranasal sinuses, and an examination of the ear canal can reveal the presence of a neoplastic skin lesion.

A complete intraoral evaluation using a bright light source should include direct inspection and mirror examination of the entire oral cavity, including the lips, nasopharynx, hypopharynx, and larynx. The vocal cords should be visualized and their mobility inspected. Palpation of the oral cavity and its contents with a bimanual examination of the floor of the mouth should follow. Any suspicious lesion, ulcerative or nodular, should undergo a biopsy. In the presence of a large ulceration, it is imperative to obtain biopsy specimens from the periphery of the lesion, because it is likely that the center of an ulcerated mass has undergone necrosis, and a biopsy from this area will not provide an accurate diagnosis. Panendoscopy should be routinely performed at the completion of the physical examination whether or not a primary source has been found, because of the multifocal presentation and high incidence of a second primary squamous cell carcinoma in the aerodigestive tract. Panendoscopy, including nasopharyngoscopy, direct laryngoscopy, esophagoscopy, and bronchoscopy, can provide the surgeon with important additional information about the extent of the tumor and thus assist in the organization of a treatment plan.

Diagnostic Tests

In a number of instances, despite a thorough physical examination, the physician is unable to establish a firm diagnosis, and additional tests are required. Blood tests, immunologic and serologic evaluations, and cultures with sensitivity tests can confirm the diagnosis of a number of infections and neoplastic diseases. An increased number of monocytes and a positive monospot test are pathognomonic of infectious mononucleosis. A positive purified protein–derivative (PPD) skin test indicates exposure to mycobacterial infection, whereas a positive Kveim test is pathognomonic of sarcoidosis. In the presence of thyroid gland enlargement, specific tests for thyroid function are required. High-serum titers for Epstein–Barr virus, anticapsid antibodies, and serum immunoglobulin A (IgA) have a high correlation with the presence of a nasopharyngeal carcinoma.

Fine-Needle Aspiration Biopsy

Fine-needle aspiration biopsy, although extremely useful for the diagnosis of neck masses, has only recently received proper attention. It is a simple, safe, and cost-effective procedure with minimal risk for complications or seeding of tumor cells in the needle tract. The technique provides quick, useful information to clinicians and has become the standard of care for the evaluation and management of thyroid nodules, parotid gland enlargements, and differentiation between cystic and solid neck masses (Figs. 26-2 and 26-3).

The surgeon can gain early information about the exact nature of the mass and plan the treatment or operation accordingly. Furthermore, in patients with lymphomas and masses of infectious origin, confirmation of the diagnosis with fine-needle aspiration biopsy will prevent the need for panendoscopy and the subsequent additional cost and patient inconvenience.

Metastatic neck masses can be accurately diagnosed with fine-needle aspiration biopsy. The presence of Reed–Sternberg cells in the aspirate is indicative of Hodgkin's disease. The usefulness of fine-needle aspiration biopsy in the diagnosis of other lymphomas lies in the confirming involvement of nodal groups that appear clinically suspicious, demonstrating recurrence or extension to new groups of lymph nodes during or after therapy, and separating lymphomas from lymphadenitis, particularly in the head and neck area.

Although positive findings on a fine-needle aspiration biopsy confirm the diagnosis, negative findings do not preclude the possibility of malignancy. In fact, the major criticism regarding the use of fine-needle aspiration biopsy in establishing a preoperative diagnosis has been the number of false-negative results obtained.

A prerequisite for a high rate of success with fine-needle aspiration biopsy is the cooperation of an experienced cytopathologist. With increased experience, the incidence of false-negative results in the head and neck area has been estimated to be as low as 7 percent, and it is believed that with further experience, the accuracy of this test will be further improved.

To avoid any delay in treatment when negative results of a fine-needle aspiration biopsy do not correlate with the clinical evaluation or do not answer all diagnostic questions, the surgeon should repeat the

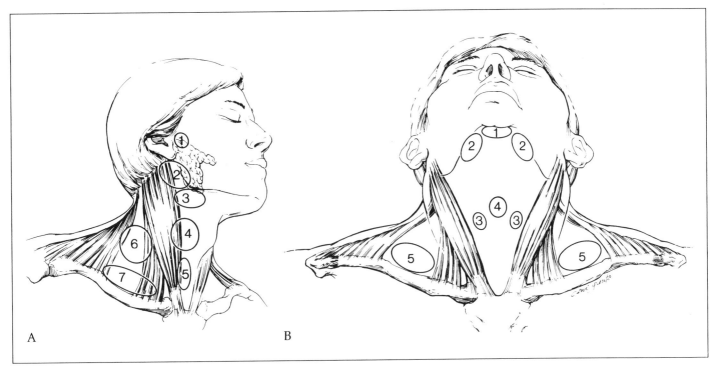

Fig. 26-1. *The primary lymphatic drainage to the neck is highly predictable. The location of the neck mass is a useful guide for investigating the location of the primary tumor. A. 1 = Preauricular nodes: scalp, parotid gland, face, ears. 2 = Upper deep and posterior cervical nodes: maxillary sinus, nasopharynx, oropharynx. 3 = Superior deep jugular nodes: paranasal sinus, nasopharynx, oropharynx, oral cavity, hypopharynx, base of tongue, supraglottic larynx. 4 = Deep midjugular nodes: hypopharynx, larynx, thyroid. 5 = Lower deep jugular nodes: thyroid, larynx, cervical esophagus. 6 = Spinal accessory nodes: posterior scalp, paranasal sinuses, nasopharynx, oropharynx. 7 = Supraclavicular nodes: infraclavicular primary tumors. B. 1 = Submental nodes: lower lip, anterior floor of mouth, tip of tongue. 2 = Submandibular nodes: upper and lower lip, anterior floor of mouth, skin of the midface. 3 = Paratracheal nodes: larynx, hypopharynx, cervical esophagus, trachea, thyroid gland. 4 = Prelaryngeal or Delphian nodes: larynx, thyroid. 5 = Supraclavicular nodes: infraclavicular primary tumors.*

biopsy or proceed with other diagnostic tests, including an open biopsy.

Biopsy

Early excisional or incisional biopsy of a neck mass to establish tissue diagnosis, although tempting, is strongly discouraged and should be avoided until full clinical, laboratory, and radiologic evaluations of the mass are completed.

When the nature of the mass remains uncertain despite thorough clinical and laboratory evaluations, the surgeon should proceed with a biopsy. The incisions for an open biopsy should be planned within the lines of a potential future radical neck dissection and, if the frozen section from the specimen reveals a squamous cell carcinoma or melanoma, the surgeon should be prepared to perform an immediate neck dissection. If the frozen section reveals a

lymphoproliferative disorder or an adenocarcinoma, the wound should be closed and the patient should undergo further work-up and staging prior to definitive treatment.

Therefore, it is imperative that the patient is thoroughly informed prior to any biopsy, and consent should be given not only for this procedure but also for a potential neck dissection.

Imaging for Cervical Masses

Computed tomography (CT) and magnetic resonance imaging (MRI) are the best imaging modalities available to evaluate neck masses. Rarely ultrasound and digital subtraction angiography are also used. Although CT is the most established imaging technique, MRI is being used with increasing frequency. The choice of CT

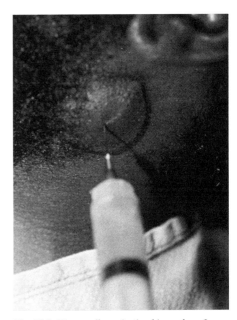

Fig. 26-2. *Fine-needle aspiration biopsy for a 2-cm lesion in the upper neck.*

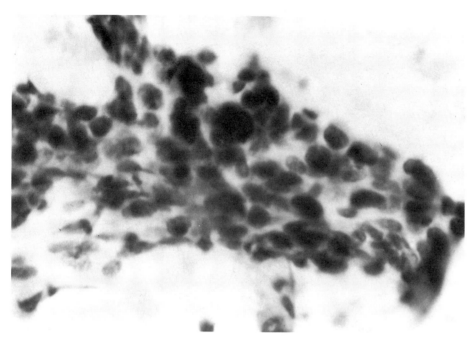

Fig. 26-3. Fine-needle aspiration biopsy of a neck mass, without gross clinical evidence of a primary tumor, demonstrating metastatic squamous cell carcinoma. Papanicolaou stain × 400. (Courtesy of Dr. Kent N. Nowels, Department of Pathology, University of Illinois, Chicago.)

versus MRI often depends on the availability, expertise, and experience of the radiologist, as well as the quality of the CT and MRI equipment. MRI could eventually exceed all advantages of CT with continued development of millisecond imaging techniques, magnetization transfer analysis, spectroscopy, and lymph node–seeking contrast agents.

Table 26-2 lists the main advantages of CT and MRI when these modalities are compared.

Computed tomography is the technique of choice for a solitary neck mass in most instances, mainly because its ability to characterize the mass is similar to MRI's ability and it is a less costly examination. Ultrasonography has a limited role in evaluation of a neck mass, but it may be useful when the mass is in the thyroid or related to the vasculature.

Benign tumors of the neck are usually homogeneous in attenuation and signal intensity on CT and MRI, respectively. With CT, these solid tumors have similar attenuation to muscle, whereas cystic tumors are lower in attenuation, similar to cerebrospinal fluid. Solid benign tumors are usually homogeneous and intermediate in signal intensity on T1-weighted MRI. The signal intensity usually increases on T2-

Table 26-2. Main Advantages of CI and MRI

CT
Fast acquisition time
Lower rate of claustrophobia
Less expensive
More sensitive in detecting calcifications, bone destruction
No absolute contraindications (cardiac pacemaker and cerebral aneurysm clip are absolute contraindications for MRI)

MRI
Iodinated contrast not necessary
No radiation exposure
Multiplanar capability
No beam hardening artifacts from mandible, shoulders, dental amalgam
Better soft tissue contrast

weighted MRI. Exceptions to this appearance are fatty tumors such as lipomas, which are high signal on T1-weighted images and lower signal on T2-weighted images (Fig. 26-4). Cystic tumors are low in signal intensity on T1-weighted MRI and high in signal intensity on T2-weighted MRI. Both MRI and CT show benign neoplasms as well circumscribed masses with preserved surrounding fascial planes. Malignant tumors are most often poorly circumscribed masses with loss of definition of surrounding fascial planes. These tumors are usually heterogeneous in atten-

uation on CT and in signal intensity on MRI. Cystic and necrotic areas within the tumor are low attenuation on CT, low signal on T1-weighted MRI, and high signal on T2-weighted MRI. The solid portion of both benign and malignant tumors can be enhanced with intravenous contrast. These imaging features can help characterize a mass as more likely benign or malignant, but most of the time no pathognomonic signs exist.

Congenital masses of the neck, which are most often cystic, are usually equally well characterized by CT and MRI (Fig. 26-5). The multiplanar capability of MRI is often useful in depicting craniocaudal extent of the mass (e. g., suprahyoid thyroglossal duct cyst) and masses that are often transpatial (e. g., cystic hygroma).

Inflammatory masses are usually equally well visualized with either CT or MRI. Both modalities can easily distinguish between cellulitis and abscess. Intravenous contrast should be used with both of these techniques to define the full extent of the infectious process. In addition, imaging should extend through the superior mediastinum because inflammatory processes can extend along fascial planes to this region. Calcifications are often seen with granulomatous lymphadenopathy (e. g., tuberculosis), and CT is most sensitive for detecting this associated finding.

Computed tomography with intravenous contrast remains the study of choice for evaluating inflammatory masses within the head and neck area because of its ability to identify associated calculus disease and mandibular or maxillary osteomyelitis. Abscesses are seen as low-density masses with peripheral rim enhancement (Fig. 26-6). Associated manifestations that can be seen include enlargement of the adjacent muscles (myositis), thickening of the overlying skin, abnormal increased attenuation of the subcutaneous fat, and enhancement of the fascial planes (cellulitis). Panorex film of the mandible is useful when a tooth infection is a possible source of the neck infection. The role of plain film radiography is otherwise limited in the evaluation of a neck mass.

When a mass is superficial within the parotid gland by palpation, superficial parotidectomy is often performed without imaging. However, when the mass is deeper or malignant, then CT or MRI should be used to determine deep tissue

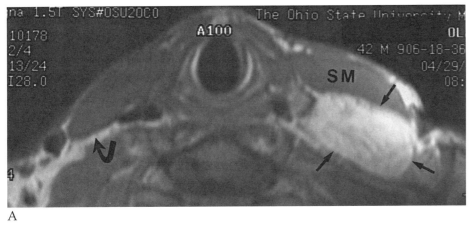
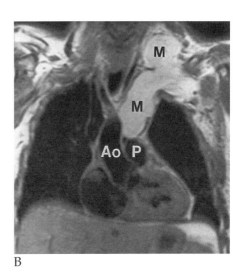

A

B

Fig. 26-4. Lipoma. A. Axial T1-weighted MR image at the level of the cricoid cartilage demonstrates oval shaped, well-circumscribed mass (arrows) within the left posterior cervical space displacing the sternocleidomastoid muscle (SM) anteriorly. Signal characteristics parallel the characteristics of fat. Normal fat on the opposite side is labeled for comparison (curved arrow) B. Coronal T1-weighted MR image through the lower neck and chest more clearly shows the full extent of the mass (M). The mass can be seen extending into the left pulmonary apex and mediastinum down to the level of the aortopulmonary window. This image demonstrates the multiplanar capability of MRI. Ao = aorta; P = pulmonary artery.

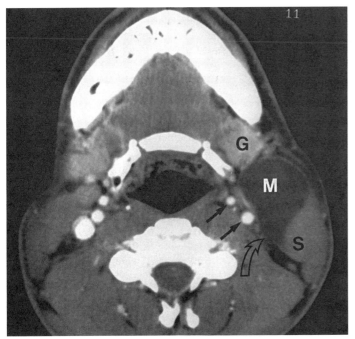

Fig. 26-5. Branchial cleft cyst. Axial CT image at the level of the hyoid bone shows a well-circumscribed homogeneous low-density mass (M) posterolateral to the submandibular gland (G), anteromedial to the sternocleidomastoid muscle (S) and lateral to the external and internal carotid arteries (arrow). A small portion of the cyst can be seen herniating into the posterior cervical space (curved open arrow). The location and appearance are characteristic of second branchial cleft cyst.

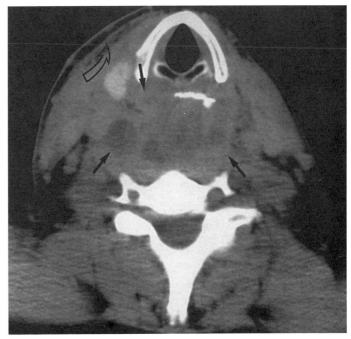

Fig. 26-6. Abscess. Axial CT image at the level of the thyroid cartilage visualizes a large mixed attenuation mass (arrows) centered in the posterior visceral space, with extension into more superficial structures bilaterally. Thickening of fascial planes and hazy appearance of surrounding fat suggest an inflammatory process. Note the thickened platysma muscle on the right (curved open arrow) caused by extension of inflammatory process. This mass represented an abscess in a patient with recent Zenker's diverticulum resection.

extent. MRI is more effective at assessing perineural spread of tumors that have this tendency (e. g., adenoid cystic carcinoma).

Thyroid masses can be well characterized with ultrasound when small and not extending outside the gland. Larger masses are probably best evaluated with CT. This modality is most useful in demonstrating extension into the superior mediastinum (e. g., multinodular goiter), detecting associated calcification, and determining displacement of surrounding structures such as the vessels and the airway. No imaging technique can distinguish a benign thyroid mass from a malignant one.

Either CT or MRI can be used in the diagnosis and staging of squamous cell carcinoma of the oral cavity, pharynx, and larynx (Fig. 26-7). It should be emphasized that MRI and CT do not detect the majority of mucosal lesions in the early stages, but they are most useful in assessing deep tissue extent and lymph node metastases. Other indications for use of CT or MRI include assessment for tumor recurrence, re-

sponse to chemotherapy or radiation therapy, and the instance of unknown primary with squamous cell carcinoma found within a neck lymph node. In all these instances, the scan should extend from the skull base to the clavicles. MRI is better for assessment of these tumors near the skull base (e.g., nasopharyngeal carcinoma), because of the multiplanar capability with greater sensitivity in detecting intracranial extension. With oropharyngeal carcinoma, MRI is more effective in assessing perineural spread. MRI is preferred by many in staging oropharyngeal carcinoma because it is less affected by dental amalgam artifact and compared with CT, it is more sensitive to the true extent of the tumor. However, CT is more sensitive to bone destruction, and therefore these examinations are often complementary.

When a patient presents with squamous cell carcinoma of unknown primary by lymph node biopsy, then a neck CT or MRI from the skull base to the clavicles should be performed. Specific areas that should be

examined closely for primary tumor include the lateral pharyngeal recess, the inferior recess of the pyriform sinus, and the faucial and lingual tonsillar crypts. These areas are the most common sites for a ''hidden'' primary unknown by clinical examination. The imaging examination can also be used to evaluate the extent of the lymphadenopathy for the purpose of staging.

Laryngoceles can be well visualized with either MRI or CT (Fig. 26-7). When the laryngocele is of the mixed type, coronal MRI can optimally demonstrate its relationship to the thyrohyoid membrane, through which it herniates. A laryngocele occurring in an adult patient who smokes should prompt a search for an occult squamous cell carcinoma of the airway as a cause of this lesion. Zenker's diverticulum of the upper esophagus can appear as an oval mass within the posterior visceral space on CT and MRI, but it is usually diagnosed with barium esophagography.

Glomus jugulare, glomus vagale, and carotid body glomus tumors arise from the paraganglionic cells. These lesions show diffuse enhancement on CT and MRI because of their vascular nature (Fig. 26-8). Glomus tumors can cause erosion of the bones of the base of the skull, especially the jugular fossa. Angiography plays a significant role in the diagnosis and management of these lesions. Glomus tumors are very vascular, receiving their blood supply from branches of the external carotid artery and occasionally from the vertebral artery and thyrocervical trunk. Transcatheter therapeutic embolization is commonly performed preoperatively.

Carotid body tumors produce tumor stain and splaying of the external and internal carotid arteries (wine glass sign, a finding better appreciated on the lateral view).

Juvenile angiofibroma is the most common benign tumor of the nasopharynx in adolescents. It affects young males who complain of nasal obstruction and epistaxis. Computed tomography is used to identify the extent of tumor and associated body deformities. Selective carotid angiography demonstrates the characteristic findings of a vascular tumor (i. e., tumor blush) and identifies the tumor's blood supply. Such information is necessary when surgical extirpation or more commonly therapeutic embolization is considered.

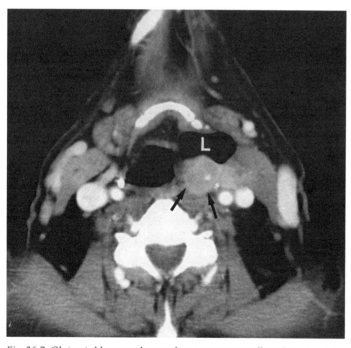

Fig. 26-7. Obstructed laryngocele secondary to squamous cell carcinoma. Axial CT image at the level of the thyrohyoid membrane shows heterogeneous mass (arrows) in the left pyriform sinus representing the carcinoma. Air collection (L), located anterior to this mass, can be seen extending through the region of the thyrohyoid membrane into the more superficial structures of the left neck. This mass represents a mixed (internal and external) type of laryngocele secondary to obstruction of the left laryngeal ventricle by the tumor. More inferior images (not shown) showed extension of the carcinoma into the supraglottic region, which was the cause of the obstructed laryngocele.

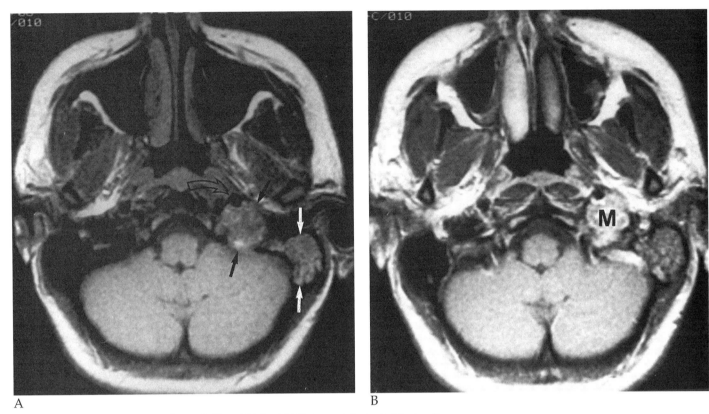

A

B

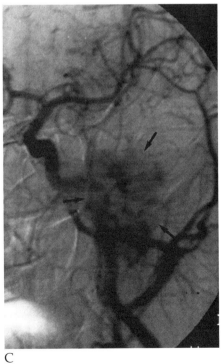

C

Fig. 26-8. Glomus jugulare paraganglioma. A. T1-weighted axial MR image at the level of the jugular foramen demonstrates a heterogeneous mass (straight black arrows) centered in the region of the left jugular foramen, which results in mild anterior displacement of the left internal carotid artery (curved open arrow). Incidental note is made of left mastoid air cell disease (white arrows). B. The mass (M) shows diffuse enhancement after administration of intravenous gadolinium. C. Oblique digital subtraction angiogram, after left common carotid artery contrast injection, demonstrates dense tumor blush (arrows), in the region of the left jugular fossa, characteristic of a glomus tumor.

Congenital Anomalies of the Neck

Branchial cleft cysts, sinuses, and fistulas are the most common congenital anomalies seen in the lateral neck. Almost 90 percent of these congenital anomalies derive from the second branchial cleft, and 6 to 8 percent derive from the first branchial cleft. Anomalies of the third and fourth branchial clefts are quite rare.

Branchial remnants might be present at birth, but most cystic sinuses or fistulas appear before age 10. Some can also present during the second or third decade of life. These anomalies can be found anywhere from the preauricular area to the lower middle third of the neck along the anterior border of the sternocleidomastoid muscle.

These cysts present as soft, nontender, mobile masses without adherence to the overlying skin, unless complicated by an infection. When a sinus tract is present, a clear fluid might drain from it. Branchial cleft fistulas primarily derive from the second arch. The external opening is found in the lateral neck below the level of the hyoid bone, whereas the internal opening is usually found in the region of the tonsillar fossa. The fistulous tract passes between the internal and external carotids and laterally to the glossopharyngeal and hypoglossal nerves.

The presence of a sinus tract or fistula confirms the diagnosis, whereas in their absence, the differential diagnosis of a lateral neck mass should include benign lymphadenopathy, lymphomas, lipomas, lymphangiomas, hemangiomas, or other unusual lesions. The diagnosis is primarily based on the clinical evaluation of the mass and further diagnostic tests are seldom necessary in uncomplicated cases (Fig. 26-9).

Thyroglossal Duct Cysts

Thyroglossal duct cysts are embryologic remnants of the thyroid gland and can be found in the midline of the neck anywhere from the area of the isthmus of the thyroid gland to the foramen cecum at the base of the tongue. If not complicated by an infection or rupture, these cysts present as soft nontender, mobile masses with smooth contour, without adherence to the overlying skin. In contrast to other midline masses, thyroglossal duct cysts ascend with swallowing or protrusion of the

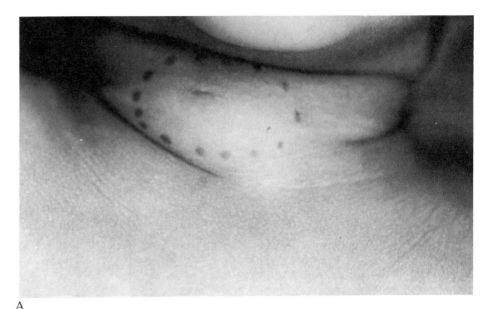

A

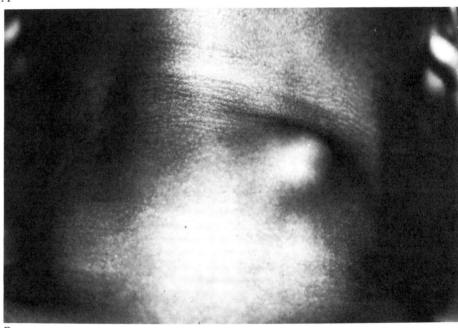

B

Fig. 26-9. A. Typical appearance of branchial cleft cyst in the lateral neck with a draining sinus at the center. B. Infected branchial cleft cyst at the anterior border of the sternocleidomastoid muscle, which appeared spontaneously after an upper respiratory infection.

tongue, because of the connection with the hyoid bone and less commonly with the foramen cecum at the base of the tongue. The cyst is seldom present at birth but is usually identified within the first few years of life. The presence of a sinus is unusual unless a previous incomplete excision of the cyst was performed or an infection of the cyst resulted in a spontaneous drainage. A sinus tract might extend to the hyoid bone or occasionally to the foramen cecum. The differential diagnosis

includes epidermoid or dermoid cyst, enlarged lymph nodes, cystic hygroma, or even an enlarged pyramidal lobe of the thyroid. The diagnosis is based primarily on clinical evaluation. Ultrasound evaluation might be of some assistance, but aspiration of the cyst is seldom necessary to confirm the diagnosis.

It is prudent to remember that a midline mass might represent an ectopic thyroid gland and possibly the patient's only func-

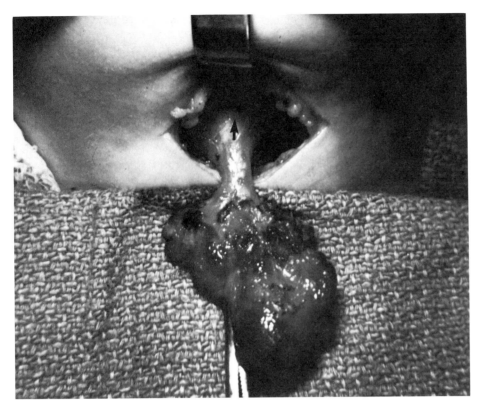

Fig. 26-10. Intraoperative view of a dissected thyroglossal duct cyst demonstrating the connection of the cyst with the hyoid bone and the base of the tongue (arrow).

tioning thyroid tissue. In fact, the incidence of ectopic thyroid tissue in midline masses has been reported to be as high as 1 in every 75 midline neck masses, occurring most frequently in females. For this reason, caution must be exercised before an operation because of the possibility of removing the patient's only functioning thyroid tissue. In some instances, it is advisable to perform thyroid scans preoperatively for females who do not have a history of inflammation or fluctuation in size of a midline mass (Fig. 26-10).

Dermoid Cysts

A dermoid cyst is usually a midline mass that is present at birth. It is derived from remnants of epithelial cells and can contain skin, skin appendages, hair, and desquamated epithelium. The mass can be found anywhere from the floor of the mouth to the upper neck. Frequently the cyst is located in the submental region, where it is found above or between the mylohyoid muscles; thus, bimanual palpation of the floor of the mouth is necessary for accurate evaluation of these masses. Dermoid cysts are generally soft, painless masses that do not follow the movements of the tongue. Surgical removal is the treatment of choice.

Inflammatory Lesions

Acute Infections

Neck masses of inflammatory origin are by far the most common cervical masses seen in children and young adults. They are usually multiple, unilateral or bilateral, firm, mobile, and tender on examination. Associated symptoms and signs of an acute infection such as malaise, fever, and chills are also present.

Because the source of infection lies within the head and neck area, a complete examination of this area is needed to reveal the diagnosis and appropriate therapy.

Advanced or neglected infections, however, might extend into the various neck spaces. The most common sources of infection are dental disease, extension from tonsillitis and other oropharyngeal infections, intravenous drug use, and infections caused by central lines. Deep neck infections might present as diffuse neck tenderness, dysphagia, hoarseness, trismus, pain on neck extension, and upper airway ob-

struction. The diagnosis is based on the history and clinical evaluation. Nodes are usually multiple, unilateral or bilateral, firm, mobile, and tender on examination. Associated symptoms and signs of an acute infection such as malaise, fever, and chills are also present. Because the source of infection often lies within the head and neck, a complete examination of this area is needed to reveal the diagnosis and to prescribe appropriate therapy. A complete blood count as well as cultures from the area of infection, such as the tonsils, should be obtained to direct the course of treatment. Viral infections usually subside spontaneously without antibiotic treatment, whereas infections of bacterial origin generally respond well to the appropriate antibiotic therapy. With proper treatment, the inflammatory processes generally resolve within a few days.

Fine-needle aspiration yields purulent material for culture and sensitivity. Appropriate roentgenography to reveal the extent of the abscess are necessary in most advanced situations prior to drainage.

The differential diagnosis of an infection should include other infectious processes presenting with enlarged nodes. Infectious mononucleosis is commonly seen in puberty and early adulthood and presents with enlarged, bilateral, tender lymph nodes and general malaise. Immunologic tests, such as monospot, and heterophile titers are helpful in confirming the diagnosis.

Ludwig's angina is a potentially life-threatening condition in the head and neck area. It is usually caused by an extension of a dental infection to the submental and submandibular space. Because the floor of the mouth is also involved, there is a significant amount of discomfort even with slight tongue movement. Swelling of the floor of the mouth becomes life-threatening when the tongue is pushed upward and posteriorly, resulting in upper airway obstruction. The diagnosis is based on the history and clinical evaluation, and urgent surgical treatment in combination with appropriate antibiotic therapy is indicated.

Chronic Infections

Several chronic infections present with unilateral or bilateral cervical adenitis. Tuberculosis has been under control for several years in the United States. However, its incidence has been rising, primarily because of the influx of immigrants from Third World countries and the increased number of patients with AIDS.

Tuberculosis caused by *Mycobacterium tuberculosis* is common among adults, whereas children are affected more often with atypical bacteria. Patients present with painless, unilateral or bilateral masses and have a history of generalized malaise, weight loss, fever, night sweats, and cough. The masses are firm and consist of a conglomerate of nodes located primarily in the posterior triangle. Cold abscesses can be found in the advanced stages. A chest x-ray might reveal pulmonary tuberculosis, and gastric washing might demonstrate the presence of *Mycobacterium*. A positive tuberculin test might confirm the diagnosis.

Atypical acid fast tuberculosis has a different presentation. The affected nodes are generally unilateral. There may be a sinus or spontaneous drainage to the skin surface. The nodes are discrete rather than conglomerate masses of lymph nodes as seen in infection with typical myobacterial strains. In contrast to acute cervical adenitis, symptoms of infection such as pain and fever are absent. The PPD test is negative and only skin testing with antigens from atypical strains produce positive reactions.

Actinomycosis is relatively rare. Infected patients present with hard tissue and swelling of the neck without involvement of the neck nodes. Intraoral involvement is also common. The overlying neck skin is discolored, and frequently multiple abscesses and fistulas are present.

Diagnosis is based on the identification of the causative organism (*Actinomycosis israeli*) in the drainage or pus from the sinus tract.

Neoplasms

Neoplasms of the neck can derive from:

1. Proliferation of local tissues and present as tumors of epidermal, adipose, vascular, lymphatics, neural, or skeletal muscle origin
2. Enlargement of local structures such as the thyroid, parathyroid, or salivary glands
3. Lymphoproliferative disorders and
4. Metastatic disease from squamous cell or other carcinomas.

Enlargement of the thyroid gland represents approximately 50 percent of all neck masses, and it is easily diagnosed clinically because of its location in the lower neck. Tumors of various tissue origins represent a small and heterogeneous group of neck masses. Only the most common masses will be presented.

Benign Tumors and Epidermal and Sebaceous Cysts

Cysts are relatively common masses. They grow slowly, mostly in a superficial portion, and are painless unless complicated by an infection. The presence of a pore and adherence to the overlying skin are helpful for the diagnosis.

Lipomas

These lesions present as painless swelling of various sizes in different areas of the neck. The adipose tissue is encapsulated, and if completely excised, the incidence of recurrence is negligible (Fig. 26-11). Lipomas are relatively rare in the neck. They

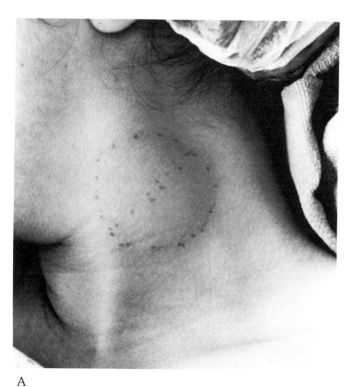

A

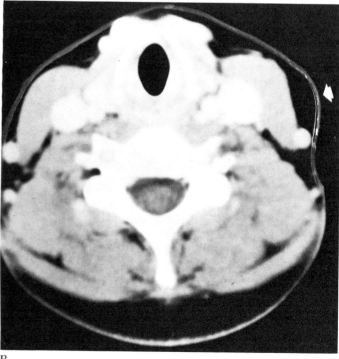

B

Fig. 26-11. A. Lateral neck mass that is soft, painless, slow growing, mobile, and without involvement of the overlying skin or underlying soft tissues. B. Computed tomography (CT) scan demonstrating a hypodense area (arrow) with Hounsfield numbers equal to adipose tissue, accurately demonstrating preoperatively the presence of a lipoma.

are primarily diagnosed with a biopsy, and radical excision is the treatment of choice. Liposarcomas are relatively rare in the neck. They are primarily diagnosed with a biopsy and radical excision is the preferred treatment.

Paragangliomas

Paraganglionic cells originate from the neural crest and migrate in close association with the autonomic ganglion cells. In the head and neck, paragangliomas are found mainly in the carotid body of the jugular bulb, whereas a smaller number originate from the vagus and other cranial or sympathetic nerves.

These tumors are generally benign neoplasms that present as painless masses in the lateral neck. The location of the mass depends on its origin. Because they usually originate from the carotid bifurcation, most paragangliomas present in the upper neck along the anterior border of the sternocleidomastoid muscle. They are firm, nontender masses that move in a lateral rather than vertical direction, occasionally transmitting an arterial pulse. Jugular paragangliomas present high in the neck, and the ones originating from cranial nerves or the sympathetic chain might be found anywhere in the neck or upper mediastinum. Associated symptoms and signs vary with the location and include headaches and dizziness, dysphagia, Horner's syndrome when the sympathetic chain is involved, and hoarseness when the vagus nerve is involved. These tumors are extremely vascular and present with a characteristic vascular blush on arteriographic studies. Therefore, arteriography is the procedure of choice in the investigation of pulsatile masses of the neck and any other mass presenting with signs or symptoms of a paraganglioma. Computed tomography is most helpful in the preoperative evaluation of vagal body tumors and other paragangliomas originating from cranial nerves, because it provides information about possible extension of the lesion to the base of the skull. A small number of paragangliomas secrete catecholamines, and additional preoperative endocrine studies might also be required to determine the level of catecholamines and their metabolites in the blood or urine.

Cystic Hygromas

Cystic hygromas (lymphangiomas) are benign tumors of lymphatic origin. Approximately 50 percent of them are present at birth and most of the remainder present by age 2. Clinically, these tumors are irregular, soft, nontender masses of variable sizes that are usually found in the posterior cervical triangle and the supraclavicular area. The lesion can be confined to the neck or extend to the face or even into the mediastinum. Sudden enlargement of these masses is caused primarily by intracystic hemorrhage or infection. The diagnosis of a cystic hygroma is based primarily on clinical evaluation of the mass. Aspiration of fluid to establish a diagnosis is unnecessary, but a plain roentgenogram of the chest is helpful and advisable preoperatively to demonstrate possible extension of the mass into the chest (Fig. 26-12).

Tumors of the Thyroid and Salivary Glands

Benign masses of the neck can be caused by enlargement of local structures or the presence of benign tumors such as lipomas, epidermal cysts, and other miscellaneous benign tumors (Fig. 26-13). Enlargement of the thyroid gland represents approximately 50 percent of all neck masses and is easily diagnosed because of its location in the lower neck. Of interest in the differential diagnosis of neck masses

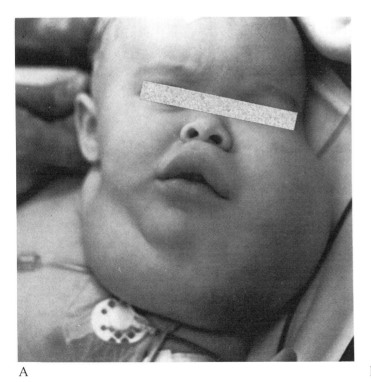
A

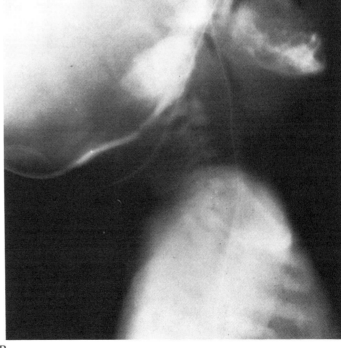
B

Fig. 26-12. A. Cystic hygroma occupying the neck and lower face, which was present at birth. B. Lateral roentgenogram delineating a cystic hygroma and demonstrating no extension into the mediastinum.

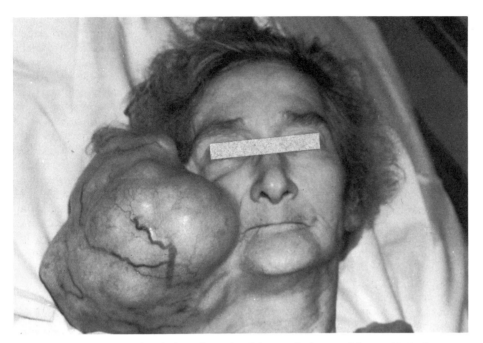

Fig. 26-13. Large mass occupying the lower face and neck from a mixed tumor of the parotid gland.

is the presence of aberrant thyroid tissue. This ectopic tissue can undergo slow enlargement. It presents as a mass at the base of the tongue (lingual thyroid) or anywhere in the midline of the upper neck. It is firm and painless and moves with swallowing and tongue protrusion. Airway obstruction and dysphagia might be present with large masses. A thyroid scan is useful in the preoperative evaluation of the mass to determine the presence of functional thyroid tissue. Thyroid function studies should also be performed preoperatively to detect borderline hypothyroid conditions resulting from suppression of the thyroid gland by functioning aberrant thyroid tissue.

Parotid gland tumors might present as a lump in the upper neck, since the tail of the parotid gland lies over the angle of the mandible. Thus upper neck masses should be carefully evaluated and their connection with the parotid gland considered. Benign tumors of the parotid gland usually present as painless, slow-growing masses of variable size without adherence to the overlying skin (Fig. 26-13). Most tumors of the parotid gland are benign pleomorphic adenomas (mixed tumors). Warthin's tumors are commonly seen in the tail of the parotid gland and have a high bilateral incidence. The most common parotid tumors in children are hemangiomas, followed by pleomorphic adenomas. Infiltration of the

overlying skin and weakness or paralysis of the main trunk or branches of the facial nerve are indicative of malignancy. There is approximately a 30-percent incidence of deep lobe involvement, primarily with parotid carcinomas. Therefore, intraoral examination should be included in the evaluation of every parotid gland mass.

Evaluation by CT with or without enhancement by sialography is seldom necessary. Fine-needle aspiration biopsy has become an important additional tool for the evaluation of parotid masses. The final diagnosis, however, is usually attained by exploration of the parotid gland, a superficial parotidectomy, and microscopic examinations of the specimen.

Enlargement in the area of the submandibular gland can be caused by infection and benign or malignant tumors. Inflammatory swelling of the gland in the acute phase presents with the characteristic signs of infection, such as tenderness, swelling, redness, and possible purulent drainage from the duct. If the swelling is caused by obstruction of the duct from a calculus, it can be readily demonstrated with a dental occlusion roentgenogram. Submandibular gland tumors, in contrast to parotid tumors, have a high incidence of malignancy, approaching 50 percent. Tumors of the submandibular gland present as painless, slow-growing swellings

without adherence to the overlying skin. Because of their location, tumors of the submandibular gland should be evaluated by a bimanual examination. The differential diagnosis of these masses should also include lymphomas and enlarged lymph nodes of infectious origin or metastatic cancer from the head and neck.

Malignant Tumors

Most malignant neck masses are metastatic from primary carcinomas of the head and neck or infraclavicular organs. However, several malignant tumors, such as thyroid cancers, cancers of the parotid and submandibular glands, tumors of lymphatic or neural origin, and tumors of the soft tissues of the neck, arise from primary sites within the neck.

Persistent nontender neck masses in patients over age 40 should be considered malignant unless proved otherwise. These masses might be the only initial presentation of a malignant tumor of the head and neck or of a malignant tumor originating from an organ below the clavicles. With a thorough history and physical examination, 90 percent of primary tumors can be identified and a firm diagnosis established. Lymphatic drainage to the neck is

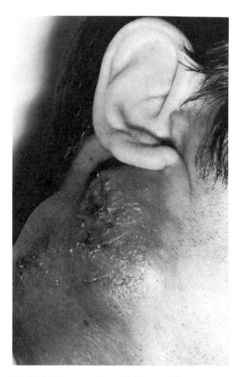

Fig. 26-14. Large malignant abscess of the upper neck from a metastatic cancer of the nasopharynx.

highly predictable, and the location of the neck mass, without immediate evidence of a primary tumor, can direct the physician to the appropriate investigation (Fig. 26-14).

The submental nodes receive primary drainage from the lower lip, the chin, the anterior third of the tongue, and the anterior floor of the mouth. The submandibular nodes receive primary drainage from both the upper and lower lips and anterior floor of the mouth. The upper jugular lymph nodes receive drainage primarily from the tonsillar fossa, tonsils, soft palate, base of the tongue, and pyriform sinuses (see Fig. 26-1). The middle deep jugular nodes receive primary drainage from the larynx and the lower pyriform sinuses, whereas the inferior deep jugular nodes receive primary drainage from the thyroid, cervical esophagus, and trachea. The spinal accessory group of lymph nodes receives primary drainage from the posterior scalp, neck, nasopharynx, oropharynx, and paranasal sinuses, whereas the supraclavicular nodes commonly represent sites of metastasis from infraclavicular tumors (Fig. 26-15). The various nodal groups in the neck also receive secondary drainage from other areas of the head and neck, and to facilitate diagnosis the examining physician should be aware of this pattern during clinical evaluation.

In 5 percent of malignancies, patients present with cervical metastatic disease from a tumor of unknown origin. If the primary source of malignancy has not been identified despite an extensive clinical evaluation, further investigation is needed. This investigation includes an evaluation under anesthesia and multiple blind biopsies from areas potentially involved with tumor, such as the nasopharynx, pyriform sinuses, and the base of the tongue. Further studies, if necessary, should include an extensive clinical and roentgenographic evaluation of potential sources of primary tumors located below the clavicles (i. e., lung, stomach, kidney, breasts, and gonads). (See Table 26-1.) As a last resort, a biopsy of a neck mass should be undertaken to confirm a diagnosis and facilitate the decision for surgical or medical management.

Lymphomas

Hodgkin's Disease

Hodgkin's disease is a lymphoproliferative disorder with a bimodal age distribution: The early incidence is between ages 10 and 13; late incidence is seen in patients over age 55. The disease is mainly confined to the lymph nodes, and extranodal involvement is rare. In the head and neck, nontender, matted, rubbery nodes that are clustered together are found primarily in the posterior triangle of the neck. Enlargement of other lymph nodes such as axillary and inguinal nodes might also be present. Accompanying symptoms include unexplained persistent fever, weight loss, pruritus, and night sweats. The presence of these symptoms has important prognostic and therapeutic implications.

The erythrocyte sedimentation rate is often elevated in Hodgkin's disease, and abnormal renal and liver functions might demonstrate extension of the disease to these organs.

Fine-needle aspiration biopsy provides valuable information in distinguishing a lymphoma from other malignancies. The presence of Reed–Sternberg cells is pathognomonic for Hodgkin's disease, but a negative biopsy does not preclude the presence of a malignancy. An open biopsy of an appropriate neck node can assist in the diagnosis. The entire lymph node should be removed along with its capsule and submitted fresh to the pathologist for microscopic and immunologic studies.

Extensive roentgenographic evaluation with CT of the neck, chest, and abdomen is also necessary, along with a bone marrow biopsy and laparotomy to assist in the staging of the disease and development of the most appropriate treatment plan.

Non-Hodgkin's Lymphoma

Non-Hodgkin's lymphoma represents 2 percent of all malignant tumors. There is a steady increase in the incidence of non-Hodgkin's lymphomas from childhood to late adulthood, with the exception of Burkitt's lymphoma, which is primarily seen in Africa and usually affects young patients. Non-Hodgkin's lymphoma is characterized by nodal and extranodal involvement, particularly in the area of Waldeyer's ring and the nasopharynx. As with Hodgkin's disease, accompanying symptoms might be present and an extensive evaluation is necessary not only for staging but also for establishing a baseline of various criteria for future evaluation of the progress of the disease.

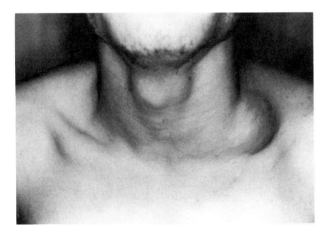

Fig. 26-15. Supraclavicular node presenting as an initial sign of a carcinoma of the ipsilateral lung.

Suggested Readings

Anzai Y, Blackwell KE, Hirschowitz SL, et al. Initial clinical experience with dextran-coated superparamagnetic iron oxide for detection of lymph node metastases in patients with head and neck cancer. *Radiology* 192:709, 1994.

Cates GA. *Current Therapy in Otolaryngology—Head and Neck Surgery.* Toronto: Decker, 1990.

Cummings CW, Krause CJ, Schuller DE, et al (eds.). *Otolaryngology—Head and Neck Surgery.* St. Louis: Mosby, 1986.

Gonjalez CF, Doan HT, Han SS, Filippe GJ. Extracranial vascular angiography. *Radiol Clin North Am* 22:239, 1984.

Harnesberger HR (ed.). *Handbook of Head and Neck Imaging.* 2nd ed. St. Louis: Mosby, 1995.

Jesse RH. Management of the suspicious cervical lymph node. *Postgrad Med* 48:1446, 1972.

Knight PJ, Hamound AB, Vassy LE. The diagnosis and treatment of midline neck masses in children. *Surgery* 93:603, 1983.

Lindberg R. Distribution of cervical lymph node metastases from squamous cell carcinoma of the upper respiratory and digestive tracts. *Cancer* 29:1446, 1972.

Mafee MF, Rasouli F, Spigos DG, et al. Magnetic resonance imaging in the diagnosis of non-squamous cell tumors of the head and neck. *Otolaryngol Clin North Am* 19:523, 1986.

McQuarrie DG, Adams GL, Shons AR, et al (eds.). *Head and Neck Cancer: Clinical Decisions and Management Principles.* Chicago: Year Book, 1986.

Naumann HH. *Differential Diagnosis in Otolinolaryngeloge,* Stuttgart: Thieme, 1993.

Shockley WN, Pillsbury HC III. *The Neck: Diagnosis and Surgery.* St. Louis: Mosby, 1994.

Som PM, Bergeron RT (eds.) *Head and Neck Imaging.* 2nd ed. St. Louis: Mosby, 1991.

Sonnino RE, Spigland N, Laberge J-M, et al. Unusual patterns of congenital neck masses in children. *J Pediatr Surg* 24:966, 1989.

Thawley SE, Panje WP, Batsakis JG, et al (eds.). *Comprehensive Management of Head and Neck Tumors.* Philadelphia: Saunders, 1987.

Yousem DM, Montone KT, Sheppard LM, et al. Head and neck neoplasms: magnetization transfer analysis. *Radiology* 192:703, 1994.

EDITOR'S COMMENT

Doctor Cohen and coauthors have provided a complete look at the various lesions within the head and neck area, with a varied diagnostic approach. Fine-needle aspiration biopsy is of course a technique coming into its own, and as increased expertise has been gained with the technique, the number of false-negatives and false-positives has diminished. There is a certain amount of redundancy in this chapter and some of the other chapters on the head and neck, but that is to be expected in a volume of this nature. In the area of the thyroglossal cyst, for example, Dr. Cohen as well as Dr. Altman in Chapter 28 are concerned that the thyroglossal duct cyst can harbor the only thyroid remnant that the patient has. In the comment on Chapter 28, the utility of ultrasound as opposed to thyroid scan is emphasized.

A principal problem in malignant disease is the invasion of the carotid artery. Yousem and coworkers (*Radiology* 195:715, 1995) attempted to predict the invasion of the carotid artery by head and neck masses by using MRI with T1-weighted, T2-weighted, and gadolinium-enhanced T1-weighted images. The criteria of nonresectability was assumed to be more than 270 degrees of circumferential involvement of the carotid artery. Sensitivity of this technique was 100 percent, specificity was 88 percent, and accuracy was 91 percent. Accuracy was 100 percent for squamous cell carcinomas. Thus, if one is confronted with an MRI that suggests that there is encasement of the carotid artery for more than 270 degrees' circumference, one should assume that the lesion is inoperable unless the carotid artery is replaced.

J.E.F.

27

Radical Neck Dissections

Benjamin F. Rush, Jr.

The classic radical neck dissection as we know it today was introduced in 1906 by George Washington Crile of the Cleveland Clinic. The operation was designed to remove lymph nodes potentially involved by cancer from all areas and triangles of the neck anterior to the trapezius muscles. The procedure was developed primarily for metastatic carcinoma from lesions involving the mucosa of the upper aerodigestive tract. It was also used for malignant tumors of the thyroid and melanomas of the skin of the head and neck. In the era in which the operation was introduced, mortality and morbidity from operations for cancer of the head and neck were usually so great that the choice of therapy for primary lesions in this area was radiation therapy. It was generally recognized that radiation therapy was much more successful in the treatment of primary mucosal lesions than in the treatment of lymph nodes, and very often patients would have the primary lesion treated by radiation therapy and concurrent cervical lymph nodes would be untreated until it became clear that the primary lesion had been eradicated by radiation. At that point, a radical neck dissection would be done to remove the involved lymph nodes. Frequently during this period of waiting, the nodes progressed and became inoperable even though the primary lesion was controlled. Immediately following World War II, a number of technical innovations made operating on primary lesions in the mucosa of the aerodigestive tract much more feasible and successful. These innovations were the introduction of antibiotics, the ready availability of blood transfusion, and the more widespread use of endotracheal intubation. With these tools, Hayes Martin of the Memorial Center for Cancer in New York and Grant Ward from the Johns Hopkins Hospital in Baltimore began to devise combined procedures whereby the local lesion could be removed together with a radical neck dissection. These procedures were much more effective than the older techniques of radiation with 250 kv x-ray and delayed operation. The number of radical neck dissections done either alone or together as combined procedures increased markedly during the 1950s and 1960s.

One of the older indications for a neck dissection, Hodgkin's lymphoma, was no longer a factor. It was thought that this lymphoma was a lesion that arose systemically and could not be cured by eradicating any specific area of tumor. In the 1950s, Daniel Slaughter of Chicago was able to show that for early Hodgkin's disease, especially involving nodes of the upper neck, a radical neck dissection cured a significant number of patients. This finding led to the understanding that the lesion truly did begin in a specific site and spread from that site into adjacent lymph-bearing area. The older technique of using small but not curative doses of radiation therapy to control lymph node beds was abandoned, and high-dose radiation was introduced to treat the various stages of Hodgkin's lymphoma. This treatment proved highly effective both alone and subsequently with the use of chemotherapy. Radical neck dissection for this disease was thus abandoned.

Another historic indication for the use of radical neck dissection was during the era of unpasteurized milk in the early part of the century. Unpasteurized milk could cause tuberculosis, which involved the lymph nodes of the neck (scrofula). These nodes often coalesced into a thick mat of scarred tissue with multiple fistulae draining from the core of nodes onto the skin of the neck, a highly distressing situation. At times the only way in which this mass of tissue could be effectively removed was by radical neck dissection. Radical neck dissection in this setting was extremely difficult and much more difficult than for malignant disease. Fortunately, the introduction of pasteurized milk has almost eradicated this disease in the United States. However, in this era of AIDS-related and antibody-resistant tuberculosis we might see it again.

Radical neck dissection has faded from the skills of many general surgeons as otolaryngology has taken over more and more of the operations in the head and neck. My bias is that unless general surgeons have maintained skill in this operation, then they should not perform surgical procedures on the thyroid or melanomas in this area.

Indication

Some of the indications for radical neck dissection have been mentioned above. The marriage of radiation therapy and operation in the treatment of the more advanced lesions of the head and neck (stages III and IV) has led to a number of other indications. Many head and neck surgeons believe that nonpalpable lymph nodes in the head and neck are more likely to contain "micrometastases" if they contain cancer, and that such lesions are curable with radiation therapy alone. Surgical procedures should be used to concentrate on control of the primary lesion, sparing the patient the necessity of having a neck dissection. Palpable lymph nodes in the presence of malignant disease should always be removed by operation, if resectable. When patients have had preoperative radiation therapy and enlarged lymph nodes have disappeared, subsequent radical neck dissection is still required. Although micrometastases in lymph nodes can be eradicated in the majority of instances, this is not true when gross disease is or has been present. At times preoperative radiation therapy is mandatory before radical neck dissection can be done, since lymph nodes can be fixed and deemed unresectable. This situation can be changed in some cases by preoperative radiation that "downstages" the lesion.

Modified Radical Neck Dissection

The definition of what constitutes a modified neck dissection has been confusing and extremely variable. Shah and Anderson have attempted to standardize the approach to this question by defining the five nodal levels in the neck, with Level I being in the submaxillary area, Level II including the upper third of the sternocleidomastoid, Level III being the middle third of the sternocleidomastoid, Level IV being the lower third of the sternocleidomastoid, and Level V being the posterior triangle of the neck. They have also identified the three major elements that are sometimes saved in the modified radical neck dissection: the sternocleidomastoid muscle, the spinal accessory nerve, and the internal jugular vein. By defining the number of structures saved and the number of lymph node beds removed, an orderly pattern of lymph node dissection can be defined.

For instance, for metastatic, differentiated thyroid carcinoma they recommend what they call modified radical neck dissection III, in which they would remove lymph nodes at all levels but save the sternocleidomastoid, the inferior jugular vein, and the spinal accessory nerve. Table 27-1 is based on a large review of the literature and summarizes their conclusions in terms of the type of neck dissection and indications. In addition, the thickness of the oral lesion dictates whether or not the lymph nodes in the neck need to be removed. Very thin lesions, even though they cover a substantial area, which might even class them as T3 (more than 4 cm), are at very little risk for metastasis if they are less than 1.5 mm in thickness. On the other hand, if the lesions are 1.6 mm or thicker anywhere in the anterior oral cavity, a suprahyoid neck dissection should be carried out and the nodes examined for the presence of metastases. Another alternative would be to automatically radiate the neck in all such patients for lesions thicker than 1.5 mm.

Advice to Patients

There are a number of morbidities that can result from a routine radical neck dissection, which should be discussed with every patient prior to operation. Some of these conditions are avoidable and some are not. The ramus mandibularis is a tiny branch and even if identified and held out of the way during the operation, it can occasionally suffer transient or permanent damage. This damage results in paralysis of half of the lower lip on the side of the lesion. Patients will have difficulty in whistling or pursing their lips. When the mouth is open wide it will form a C rather than an O. There is a tendency at first to drool on the side of the lesion, although this usually disappears as the tone of the lip gradually improves. Another deficiency, which is unavoidable, is the total loss of sensation in the skin of the neck, ear, and shoulder as the result of turning the flaps and the sectioning of cutaneous nerves. The patient usually complains that the skin in the area feels like wood. Usually the patient can be reassured that sen-

Table 27-1. Summary of Neck Dissection Types and Indications

Type of Neck Dissection	Nodal Levels Dissected	Structures Preserved	Indications
RND	1–5	None	Metastatic tumor from any primary site where SAN is involved or encased by tumor and cannot be dissected free, or in presence of previous radiotherapy or surgery in the neck
MRND I	1–5	SAN	Metastatic carcinoma, any site except differentiated thyroid cancer, SAN free of disease
MRND III	1–5	SCM IJV SAN	Metastatic differentiated thyroid carcinoma
Supraomohyoid neck dissection	1–3	SCM IJV SAN	Elective neck dissection in cases of squamous carcinoma of the oral cavity and oropharynx (include level 4) and malignant melanoma with primary site anterior to ear (include parotidectomy for facial and scalp lesions)
Lateral (jugular) neck dissection	2–4	SCM IJV SAN	Elective neck dissection for squamous carcinoma of the hypopharynx and larynx
Posterolateral neck dissection	2–5	SCM IJV SAN	Elective neck dissection for malignant melanoma of the posterior scalp and neck

Key: SAN = spinal accessory nerve; SCM = sternocleidomastoid; IJV = internal jugular vein.
Source: JP Shah and PE Anderson. The impact of patterns of nodal metastasis on modifications of neck dissection. *Ann Surg Oncol* 1:521, 1994.

sation will gradually return around the edges of the flap, although there will always remain a central area that is completely numb.

If the spinal accessory nerve is resected, there will be a "dropped" shoulder on the side of resection. The extent of the drop and how painful to the patient is quite variable and probably depends partly on the strength of the levator scapulae muscle, which takes over the function of the paralyzed trapezius. The spinal accessory nerve is so long that sometimes dissecting it out completely, even though it has been preserved, results in loss of some or all function. The surgeon cannot totally guarantee that the nerve will function following neck dissection. Dropped shoulder is one of the most annoying of the various problems following neck dissection. The patient should be prepared for it and instructed as to how to put the shoulder at rest by supporting the elbow by various strategies whenever possible. In our litigious society, all these points should be explained to the patient and advice should be documented in the physician's record.

Anesthesia

Modern anesthesia has been one of the keystones that permitted extensive head and neck surgery, including radical neck dissection. If the patient has had tracheostomy before the operation, selection of a position in which the anesthesiologist and the equipment are out of the way of the operating team is quite simple. The endotracheal connections can be led down and across the chest and the anesthesiologist situated below the armpit. This positioning leaves the patient's shoulders, neck, and head exposed to the operating team, and they can be positioned around the head with the surgeon on one side, first assistant on the other, and a second assistant standing at the head of the table behind the patient's head. If the patient needs oral or nasal intubation, the convenient location of the operating team promptly clashes with the area in which the anesthesiologist sits, which is usually at the head of the table. Fortunately, today's techniques for monitoring the patient have made it possible for the anesthesiologist to back away from the field far enough so that all members of team can

stand in their most convenient position. If necessary, arterial pressure can be monitored with the use of a A-line so that it is unnecessary for the anesthesiologist to feel, for the patient's pulse.

It is extremely important that muscle paralysis *not* be used during the operation. If this step is required in the course of intubation and will make it more convenient for the anesthesiologist, that is permissible as long as the agent is promptly reversed after intubation has been completed. The reason for this restriction is that the location and testing of nerves are a very important part of this procedure and from time to time a surgeon might want to estimate the viability of the spinal accessory, the hypoglossal, and the phrenic nerve or occasionally others.

Positioning the Patient

A position that exaggerates the space between the clavicle and the mandible is preferable. This position is usually achieved by putting a roll beneath the shoulders and dropping the head of the table slightly to place the neck in extension with the patient supine. Some warn against the use of the semi-sitting (Fowler's) or the reverse Trendelenburg position, indicating that either can create a negative pressure in the veins of the neck, which could cause an air embolism. This result can be a complication of an exaggerated upright position, but in moderate reverse Trendelenburg position, which I have used for the last thirty years, I have never found any morbidity as a result of the position. Occasionally a few bubbles may be seen in the venous distribution of the neck, but these are negligible and apparently of no physiologic importance. The advantage of the position is that it reduces venous bleeding.

Incision

The original incision for radical neck dissection recommended by Crile was a T incision with a cross arm just below the mandible and the vertical part of the T straight down the neck. Martin, a major pioneer of head and neck surgery, preferred a so-called double Y incision with a triangle at the top of the neck and a triangle at the

bottom of the neck connected by a relatively short vertical incision. A number of other complex incisions were recommended and all had the advantage of excellent exposure. Because of the excellent blood supply, incisions of the neck usually have negligible infection and usually heal with a good cosmetic result, even though the skin tension lines (Langer's) are violated. Now that preoperative radiation is frequently used, complex incisions that bring together many small points are likely to develop a necrosis at the tips. This necrosis sometimes leads to a gradual separation of wound edges. Wound dehiscence in the neck is almost as catastrophic as wound dehiscence in the abdomen. The flaps retract widely and the carotid as well as the pharyngeal and laryngeal structures are exposed. If there are any suture lines within the pharynx or larynx, they are subject to fistula formation. An exposed carotid artery can breakdown and hemorrhage. These devastating problems can usually be avoided by the use of simpler incisions that do not include small pointed flaps (Fig. 27-1).

We adopted an L, or hockey stick, incision in our clinic. This incision has the disadvantage that the distance from the supraclavicular area to the submental triangle is considerable. However, by extending the lower end of the incision slightly into the opposite neck and using good retraction, the skin of the neck will stretch enough so that the margin of the incision from the level of the supraclavicular area can be drawn all the way up to the tip of the chin, and the entire neck can be exposed. The only exception to the use of this incision is when the lip must be split to enter the oral cavity for a combined procedure. The other simple incision in the neck is that of McFee, which involves two parallel incisions. Through the lower incision the lower half of the neck can be dissected, and through the upper incision the remainder of the neck is dissected. In addition, the upper incision can be extended to pass up through the midline of the lip so that a flap consisting of the lip and cheek can be reflected to expose the oral cavity. If the procedure in the oral cavity that is being combined with a neck dissection is not too extensive, the L shape previously described can be used and the oral cavity entered from the neck, usually by way of the digastric and submental triangles. Le-

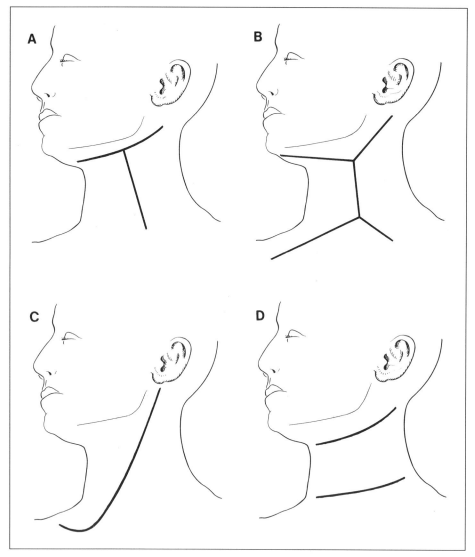

Fig. 27-1. A sampling of the main neck incisions used for radical neck operations. A. Crile. B. Martin. C. Hockey stick. D. McFee.

sions of the floor of the mouth and tongue can easily be approached in this fashion. This method has the advantage of avoiding incisions on the face. Even though splitting the lip does not produce an overwhelming deformity, nonetheless, it is noticeable and I believe most patients would prefer to avoid it.

Hemostases

The neck is blessed with a superabundance of blood vessels, which contribute to rapid healing and low incidence of infection. However, they make it somewhat problematic for surgeons to operate in this

area. There is an increasing use of the bovie to control bleeding, and there are some head and neck surgeons who are trained to use the bovie effectively. By doing so, they can reduce blood loss to less than 100 cc during a radical neck dissection. However, it should be possible to do any radical neck dissection without the necessity of a blood transfusion and with maximum losses of no more than 400 or 500 cc of blood even without the use of a bovie. I strongly believe that surgeons in training for head and neck surgery should operate without excessive use of the bovie in their initial operations, if only because it helps them to learn where the bovie is unnecessary. The neck has many planes

and spaces, which if taken advantage of will reduce the amount of bleeding enormously. It takes greater skill to operate with a bovie and at the same time avoid serious injury to nerves, which can often be unintentionally stunned or killed by propagation of bovie current through the tissues. Once one knows precisely where to look for these structures, the use of a bovie becomes considerably safer.

Development of the Neck Flaps

I use a hockey stick incision for most of my operations. I can gain access to the posterior oral cavity easily through this incision and exposure of the anterior oral cavity can be obtained by extending the incision to the opposite side of the neck and actually drawing the entire flap up over the jaw like a veil. In terms of a radical neck dissection, all the various areas that should be encompassed by the operation can be reached through this incision. After inscribing my intended line of incision with a marking pencil, the assistant and the surgeon keep firm pressure on the wound edges while an incision is made down through the skin, subcutaneous fat, platysma muscle, and subplatysmal fat. Some have described the platysma as a "fat sandwich" with a layer of fat on either side of the muscle. The incision extends from 2 to 3 cm beyond the midline to a point in the posterior triangle, about two finger breaths above the clavicle and from there curves upward to run parallel with the anterior border of the trapezius muscle to the tip of the mastoid. Bleeding is controlled by finger pressure on the edges of the wound while the bovie can be used to touch bleeding points. Alternatively, multiple small clamps can be used to clamp the bleeders. These clamps then act as tractors in the course of the subsequent reflection of the flap. The only major bleeders that require ligation at this point are the external jugular vein, which arises as the midpoint of the sternocleidomastoid muscle, and the anterior jugular vein, which can be found just medial to the anterior border of the sternocleidomastoid muscle in the lower neck. Both of these vessels lie just beneath the platysma, and if the platysma is divided lightly at these points the vessels will be exposed and can be clamped, ligated, and divided. This dissection of the flap is then carried up the neck. I prefer to leave the superficial cervical fascia on the flap. The flap is comparable to the anterior abdominal wall in abdominal surgery, and obviously loss of the flap is a serious problem that substantially increases morbidity and mortality in the head and neck patient. This plane has the advantage of being almost bloodless so that the dissection can be done using Metzanbaum dissection scissors. This advantage exists particularly for the sternocleidomastoid, and dissection can be done there. In order for the flap to be turned upward, prolongations from the superficial cervical fascia down into the neck, anterior and posterior to the sternocleidomastoid, muscle must be divided. These prolongations of fascia contain the major bleeders in this area so the division should be done either with a bovie or with clamps at hand. Using this approach, the flap can be fairly quickly stripped away from the underlying structures. I usually carry the dissection up to the angle of the mandible. Dissection should be carried out posteriorly as high as the mastoid, and the flap should be turned a centimeter or so above the lower edge of the horizontal ramus of the mandible and carried forward to the midline of the chin. A major concern at this point in the dissection is for the ramus mandibularis. This branch of the seventh nerve emerges from behind the tail of the parotid in the neck and usually crosses the facial vein and artery 2 to 3 cm below the facial notch in the mandible. It lies beneath the platysma, so as the platysma is turned one should be careful not to damage it in the course of the platysmal dissection. One of the small technical details introduced by Hayes Martin was to ligate the facial vein below the point where the ramus mandibularis crosses the vessel. The vein is then turned upward over the ramus and sutured to the flap, pulling the nerve out of the neck and out of harm's way during the rest of the dissection (Fig. 27-2).

It is clear that almost the entire flap that is developed in this approach is anterior and superior. There is a small 2- to 3-cm inferior component, which is easily undermined down to the clavicle and a very small posterior component, which is dissected under the skin posteriorly to the anterior border of the sternocleidomastoid.

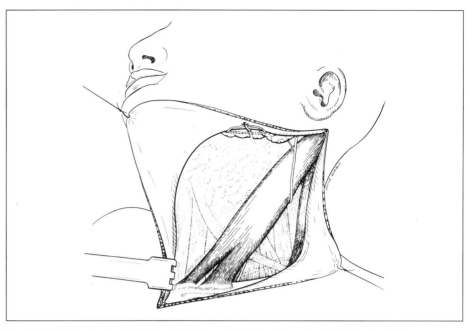

Fig. 27-2. Initial reflection of the flaps of a hockey stick incision. Note that the facial vein has been transected and tacked to the flap, elevating the remus mandibularis of the facial nerve away from the field.

Development of the Posterior Triangle

Unroofing the posterior triangle by turning the flaps reveals a space bound by muscle and filled with fatty areolar of tissue. It is the surgeon's aim to free this fatty areolar triangle from the floor and edges of this space.

I begin my dissection posteriorly by spreading the fat away from the trapezius muscle superiorly where it crosses under the sternocleidomastoid. There is a layer of fascia over the muscle. If this layer can be opened, a finger can be inserted under the fascial layer and slid down along the anterior edge of the trapezius. If this fascia is then incised, it will loosen up most of the lateral portion of the contents of the triangle. In the lower third of the trapezius, the spinal accessory nerve becomes quite superficial so that it is important to incise the fascia of the trapezius along its external edge. Careful dissection along the internal edge reveals the spinal accessory nerve. Stimulation of this nerve with a nerve stimulator results in a violent shrug of the shoulder and affords clear differentiation from the sensory branches of the cervical plexus, which pass down and laterally

over the posterior triangle. The contents of the triangle can now be swept forward across the floor of the triangle. A number of vessels lie in the lower portion of the triangle and more or less parallel the clavicle. Two of these are the transverse cervical artery and vein, which supply blood to the lower portion to the trapezius. Under some circumstances, this vascular pedicle is preserved in order to use the lower portion of the trapezius as a myocutaneous flap. In ordinary circumstances, however, these vessels are sacrificed. Even lower in the neck are the transverse scapular artery and vein, which lie at the level of the clavicle. As these various vessels are divided laterally and the specimen is reflected medially, numerous, small cutaneous nerves will be seen running anterior to the clavicle. Any nerve in this location is clearly sensory and must be divided in order to reflect the contents of the triangle. As the dissection moves from lateral to medial, there is sequential exposure of the levator scapula, the posterior scalene, the middle scalene, and finally the lateral border of the anterior scalene muscle. If the sternocleidomastoid is then elevated with a retractor, visualization of the anterior border of the anterior scalene can be carried medially all the way to the carotid sheath. The phrenic nerve can be looked

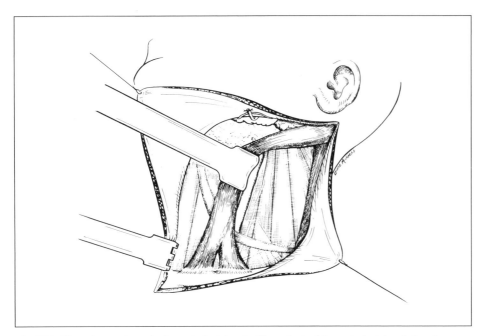

Fig. 27-3. *Dissection continues in the posterior triangle. The contents of the posterior triangle have been removed, and the sternocleidomastoid muscle is retracted medially to show the anterior scalene muscle with the overlying phrenic nerve.*

for at this point and will be found turning around the lateral edge of the anterior scalene muscle and running from lateral to medial across the belly of the muscle (Fig. 27-3). It is the only structure in the neck that runs from lateral to medial rather than from medial to lateral or up and down. As the lower third of the triangle is dissected medially and elevated, the brachial plexus can be seen emerging from between the anterior and middle scalene muscles. It is covered by a translucent layer of deep cervical fascia sometimes called the "safety layer." If left intact, it protects against injury to the plexus. The posterior belly of the omohyoid will be seen in the lower third of the space passing from the scapula to a sling situated on the fascia of the strap muscles at their lateral border. This point is approximately 4 cm above the sternoclavicular joint. The omohyoid is transected at the level of the trapezius and reflected medially with the rest of the specimen. At this point, the dissection of the posterior triangle is complete.

Ligation of the Jugular Vein

A Kelly clamp is slipped under the belly of the sternocleidomastoid approximately 1 cm above its insertion to the clavicle and sternum. The muscle is then transected on the clamp using the cutting current of a bovie. An important structure encountered at this point is the thyrocervical trunk, which lies under the clavicular portion of the sternocleidomastoid. The transverse cervical branch of this artery has probably already been ligated in the course of dissecting the lateral triangle. The subscapular branch might have been encountered laterally and, if not, can be left alone. The third branch of the inferior thyroid artery might be in the way of the resection. If so, it can be ligated at this time. The carotid sheath lies immediately below the small triangular space that separates the sternal and clavicular heads of the sternocleidomastoid inferiorly. The carotid sheath can be opened at this point, revealing the jugular vein and the more medial and posterior carotid artery. The clamp should be gently placed between the carotid artery and jugular vein and spread to reveal the vagus nerve, which lies just deep to these two structures and between them. Once the vagus nerve has been identified, Kelly clamps can be placed on the jugular vein. As a matter of safety, two clamps are placed below and one above. The vein is divided between the upper and middle clamp and a 2–0 silk

tie is used to doubly ligate the proximal stump of the jugular vein and a single tie is used to ligate the distal stump. There are two important points to note during this portion of the procedure: 1) sometimes there is a small tributary of the jugular vein that leads medially and can be 2 to 4 cm above the clavicle. This tributary should be ligated and divided before the jugular vein is divided. 2) On the left side, the thoracic dust arises from the mediastinum and crosses behind the carotid artery and jugular vein to enter the venous system at the junction of the jugular and subclavian vein. This structure is translucent and in the fasting patient can be almost invisible. Often the first evidence of its presence is the appearance of small to large amounts of yellow fluid accumulating in the wound. This structure should be carefully looked for and since it is so often injured in the course of the dissection, should be ligated when found. Remember that when the duct is observed in the neck it is running from above and down: the upper end of the ligated duct is the end from which the lymph is coming. Very often as soon as the duct is ligated it will distend with straw-colored fluid, confirming its identity.

Reflecting the Sternocleidomastoid

The next step in the operation is to reflect the contents of the posterior triangle and the attached sternocleidomastoid up the neck to the origins of the muscle (Fig. 27-4). The muscle is freed anteriomedially by clearing the anterior belly of the omohyoid from its underlaying structures up to the level of the hyoid where it is transected. Finger dissection underneath the muscle reveals a muscular aponeurotic tunnel. The lateral border of the muscle is held down by an attachment between the superficial and deep cervical fascia, which forms a firm lateral wall of this space all the way to the base of the skull. Medially, there is a similar attachment to the carotid sheath. The lateral cervical fascia can be divided with impunity since it contains no important structures. This division will allow the surgeon to turn up the lateral edge of the sternocleidomastoid to better observe the length of the jugular vein as it lies in the carotid sheath. By dissecting

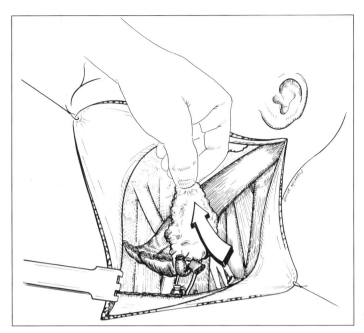

Fig. 27-4. Transection of the sternocleidomastoid muscle and the underlying jugular vein. Note double ligature on jugular stump. The omohyoid muscle has also been transected. The contents of the posterior triangle are shown here being pulled upward.

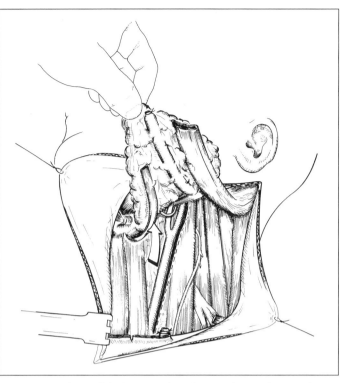

Fig. 27-5. Completion of the dissection along the carotid artery elevating the associated lymphoareolar tissue, muscle, and vein. The dotted line marks the course of the vagus nerve, which helps to guide this portion of the dissection.

along the vagus nerve, the carotid sheath can be divided and the sternocleidomastoid muscle elevated throughout most of its length (Fig. 27-5).

At the junction of the medial and upper third of the neck, the dissection will be held back by branches of the cervical plexus as they enter the posterior triangle, which is being reflected with the rest of the specimen. These branches were originally divided at the level of the clavicle. They must now be divided again to continue to reflect this specimen upward. Since the phrenic nerve also springs from the same plexus, surgeons sometimes have difficulty differentiating the sensory nerves from the phrenic. Remember that the phrenic nerve runs downward and medially, while the sensory branches run into the specimen. It can quickly be determined which nerves need to be divided. As soon as the sensory nerves are divided, the entire specimen is loosened and substantial progress is made in the upward dissection. Dissection continues superiorly and posteriorly until the mastoid is reached. At this point, the sternocleidomastoid muscle can be detached from the mastoid. As this

transection is carried forward, the posterior belly of the digastric muscle is found. At this point, the jugular vein passes upward to the base of the skull. The specimen can be loosened anteriorly by carrying the dissection upward 1 or 2 cm above the carotid bulb. Here, the hypoglossal nerve will be seen descending between the internal and external carotid arteries and crossing the external carotid. Dissecting anteriorly along this nerve, the tendon of the digastric muscle will be identified since the nerve passes beneath it. The common facial vein will also be encountered passing over the nerve. This vein can be divided and ligated.

As mentioned previously, the posterior belly of the digastric lies over the upper end of the jugular vein. Some surgeons prefer to remove this muscle as part of the specimen and others simply reflect it to reveal the jugular vein as it enters the base of the skull. The vein is double ligated and transected. At this point, the anterior triangle is the only portion of the dissection that has not been completed. Cervical fascia along the horizontal ramus of the mandible can be incised (if this was not done

when the flaps were originally dissected). There are usually a number of small bleeders at this point that must be controlled. The fatty areolar tissue in the submental area is dissected from medial to lateral. At the point where the submental contents are attached to the submaxillary gland, the anterior edge of the submaxillary gland is reflected from the lateral border of the digastric muscle exposing the underlying mylohyoid. The mylohyoid muscle is retracted medially to demonstrate the deep portion of the submaxillary gland (Fig. 27-6). The gland is retracted downward at this point. The chorda tympani entering the gland will be seen attached to the lingual nerve, which is pulled down in a V by the traction. The chorda tympani is clamped, tied, and divided, permitting the lingual nerve to retract behind the lower edge of the mandible and the submaxillary gland to be drawn down even further. Wharton's duct will be seen running anteriorly beneath the mylohyoid and parallel by the hypoglossal nerve, which lies deeper in the triangle. Wharton's duct is divided and tied, and the final attachments of the submaxillary gland are divided freeing the entire radical neck dissection specimen. The specimen consists of the posterior triangle, sternocleidomastoid muscle, and jugular vein together with the associated fat and lymphoareolar tissue in which the jugular lymph nodes are buried, the lymphoareolar tissue of the submental area, and the submaxillary gland.

Closure of the Neck

The operative wound is thoroughly irrigated with warm saline and any residual bleeders are clamped and tied or touched with a bovie. The neck flaps are now ready for closure (Figs. 27-7 and 27-8). I like to place a row of sutures connecting the platysma muscle to the strap muscles medially to the carotid artery and a second row lateral to the carotid artery suturing the flap to the anterior scalene. This step forms a tunnel for the carotid artery. In combined operations in which the mouth or pharynx has been entered, this tunnel protects the carotid if the suture line to the aerodigestive tract breaks, down draining saliva into the neck. Even if a fistula is not a concern, this technique divides the neck into smaller compartments, which prevents large seroma from forming. These seroma would cause the flap to "float" and not adhere to the underlying structures during healing. A Jackson–Pratt drain is placed anterior to the artery (Fig. 27-9). A second drain is placed in the space posterior to the artery. I prefer to place these drains on wall suction for the first 24 hours. Further closure of the flaps is done with interrupted 4–0 silk in the platysma muscle, followed by closure of the skin with staples.

Postoperative Care

This operation involves superficial tissues; major body cavities have not been entered. Patients tolerate this type of procedure remarkably well. The patient can begin on a liquid diet on the night of the operation and begin a regular diet the following day,

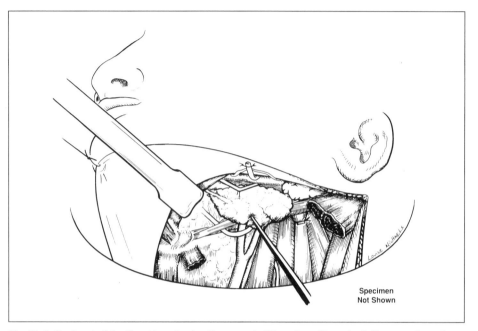

Fig. 27-6. Final part of the dissection, showing the removal of the submaxillary gland. Downward traction on the gland and retraction of the mylohyoid muscle reveal the chorda tympani and lingual nerve above the gland.

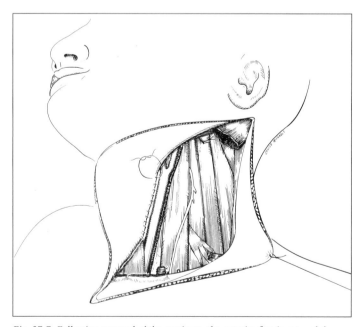

Fig. 27-7. Following removal of the specimen, the anterior flap is sutured down along the carotid artery to form an anterior compartment.

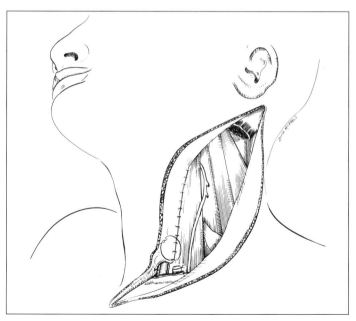

Fig. 27-8. Closure is continued by a second suture line posterior to the carotid artery to form a compartment guarding the carotid.

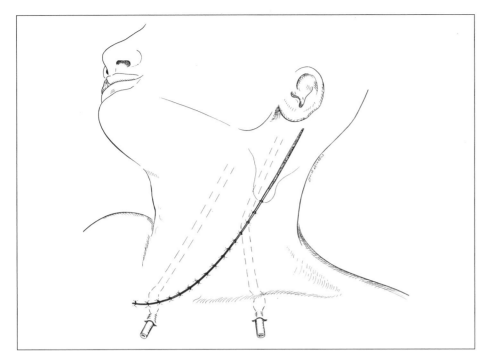

Fig. 27-9. Final closure of the skin. The anterior and posterior compartments formed by the sutures along the carotid artery are drained separately by suction drains.

to these structures is usually rare. If an attempt is being made to save the spinal accessory nerve, the nerve is most at risk at the point at which it is most superficial to the skin flaps in the lower third of the trapezius. Great care must be exercised to avoid the nerve at this point. The long length of the nerve that must be dissected out along the posterior triangle and the upper portion of the sternocleidomastoid sometimes leads to a permanent loss of function. This complication can exist because of damage to the blood supply even when the nerve is intact at the end of the operation.

Summary

Radical neck dissection is an operation dealing with an area packed closely with anatomic structures. Fortunately, the anatomy is dependable and anomalies are rare. By following the course of some of these structures, other important structures are revealed. I like to say all you have to do is "cut on the dotted line."

A summary of the structures that will lead on to each step of the operation are

1. Posterior triangle
   A. Anterior border of the trapezius muscle leads to the vagus nerve.
   B. Anterior surface of the anterior scalene muscle reveals to the phrenic nerve.
   C. Lower one-third of the anterior scalene muscle leads to the brachial plexus.
2. Structures below the sternocleidomastoid muscle
   A. Vagus nerve after division of sternocleidomastoid muscle and jugular vein dissect along nerve to release entire sternocleidomastoid muscle, jugular vein, and associated lymph nodes. Above carotid bulb, the hypoglossal nerve appears.
   B. Hypoglossal nerve leads to facial vein and digastric tendon.
3. Anterior triangle
   A. Anterior belly of the omohyoid muscle describes medial limit of dissection to level of the hyoid bone.
   B. Hypoglossal nerve leads under the digastric tendon to deep lobe of submaxillary gland and Wharton's duct.
   C. Mylohyoid muscle when retracted reveals deep lobe of submaxillary

assuming that there has been no associated operations in the mouth or pharynx. The patient can ambulate immediately with full toilet privileges. Depending on the amount of drainage from the suction drains, they can usually be removed by the third or fourth day and the patient can be discharged on the fifth or sixth day for follow up as an outpatient.

Complications

Mortality following radical neck dissection unaccompanied by any other procedure is no more than 1 percent. If there has been no prior radiation therapy, the plentiful blood supply to the neck makes wound healing excellent and infection rare. Sometimes seromas accumulate beneath the skin flap, preventing their adherence to the underlying structures. This complication can be avoided by suturing down the flaps as described under closure of the wound above. Overly enthusiastic dissection below the trapezius and clavicle into areas that are beyond the normal drainage basin of the aerodigestive tract not only adds nothing to the curative value of the procedure but also creates additional spaces where the overlying skin flaps are not

sucked down by suction drainage, which leads to persisting fluid collection.

Seromas can be treated by aspiration and a pressure dressing over the flap. If such an attempt fails, the best result will be obtained from draining this seroma either by opening a portion of the incision or by adding a counterincision and allowing the flaps to collapse onto the underlying surface.

A fairly annoying and sometimes serious complication is a chylous fistula in the left neck, caused by the failure to ligate the thoracic duct after it has been divided. Enzymes in the chylous fluid can damage the surrounding tissue and even create difficulties with a carotid blowout if the fistula is allowed to continue over a long period of time. Although these fistulas sometimes seal spontaneously, the quickest solution is to re-explore the wound and ligate the site of lymphatic fluid loss. Damage to nerves in the course of the dissection is another complication. Fortunately, this is relatively uncommon, except for the ramus mandibularis which, as described previously, should be looked for carefully and protected. Although there is the potential for injury to the vagus, hypoglossal, phrenic, and the sympathetic trunk, injury

gland, Wharton's duct, and hypoglossal nerve.

D. Submaxillary gland when retracted downward reveals lingual nerve and chorda tympani.

Suggested Reading

Crile G. Excision of cancer of the head and neck with special reference to the plan of dissection based on 132 operations. *JAMA* 47:780, 1906.

Martin H. Neck dissection. *Cancer* 4:441, 1951.

Shah JP, Anderson PE. The impact of patterns of nodal metastasis on modifications of neck dissection. *Ann Surg Oncol* 1:521, 1994.

Slaughter DP. Current concepts in cancer. 2. Hodgkin disease: Radical surgery. *JAMA* 191:26, 1965.

Ward G, Hendrick J. *The Diagnosis and Treatment of Tumors of the Head and Neck.* Williams & Wilkins, Baltimore: 1950.

EDITOR'S COMMENT

Doctor Rush has presented the classic radical neck dissection in which the internal jugular vein and sternocleidomastoid muscle are sacrificed. However, he does make a plea and provides a technique for the salvage and sparing of the spinal accessory motor nerve (nerve XI). As in most studies of malignant disease, there are revisionist attitudes toward the completeness of radical dissections. One of the most frequent revisionist areas is the use of a modified or functional radical neck dissection, and the arguments for and against. The central issue for the control of carcinomas of the head and neck is the control of disease in the neck. The presence of metastatic nodes from oral cancer results in decreased survival by approximately 50 percent. There are other means of controlling disease in the neck, but most head and neck surgeons choose radical neck dissections since there is some quoted evidence that radiation to positive lymph nodes of the neck does leave viable disease. In addition to this evidence, there is the widely quoted and generally agreed to fact that even in patients with oral cancer with clinically negative nodes, radical neck dissection reveals that 30 percent of the patients have occult micrometastases. There is also some evidence, although this is widely disputed, that radical neck dissections in patients with clinically negative nodes who have positive micrometastases might result in improved survival. However, the contrary argument is that in patients with clinically negative nodes, who might have micrometastases, it is not necessary to sacrifice these major structures since this does not adversely affect the outcome.

The standard radical neck dissection as described by Crile and popularized by Martin has, one must agree, until recently been the standard treatment for palpable or potential surgical metastases from head and neck cancer. Recurrence of disease varies according to the bulk of disease present, ranging from less than 10 percent in the N_0 neck to greater than 70 percent with multiple positive nodes of various levels (Strong EW, *Surg Clin N Amer* 49:271, 1969). Thus, the introduction of pre- or postoperative radiation, either before or after radical neck dissection, has reduced the incidence of recurrence by at least 50 percent (Goffinet DR, et al., *Arch Otolaryngol* 110:736, 1984; Vikram B, et al., *Head & Neck Surg* 6:724, 1984). Since it might not make any difference whether radiation is done pre- or postoperatively, most surgeons prefer to give postoperative radiation since it makes dissection easier and minimizes complications.

The thickness of the lesion within the oral cavity correlates with occult metastasis, with only 7.5 percent of lesions less than 2 mm thick having occult metastases, 26 percent of lesions 2 to 8 mm, and 41 percent of lesions greater than 8 mm (Spiro RH, et al., *Am J Surg* 152:345, 1986). In addition, an appreciation for the various zones of the neck and the likelihood of nodal metastasis, given the location of the original lesion, has also gained popularity. Preoperative imaging with CT has not caught on as proposed by some and is not widely practiced.

One can therefore make an argument for sparing the spinal accessory motor nerve when there is little disease in the posterior triangle or sparing the internal jugular vein, the sternocleidomastoid, or both, depending on circumstances. Nodes that are greater than 3 cm often burst a capsule and attach to surrounding structures, making sparing of the internal jugular vein and the sternocleidomastoid theoretically unwelcome.

Given the complexity of the anatomy, one could argue that only surgeons practiced in radical neck dissection should perform the operation. The functional radical neck dissection, developed by Bocca, seems to have little role in patients with oral cancer. In patients with clinically N_0 neck, one can safely preserve the sternocleidomastoid, the internal jugular vein, and the spinal accessory motor nerve, but then it is not usually necessary to dissect all five nodal levels. However, in patients with nodal positive necks, it can be unwise to preserve the sternocleidomastoid and the internal jugular vein, since the incidence of local recurrence is very high (Bocca E, et al., *Laryngoscope* 94:942, 1984).

J.E.F.

28

Congenital Lesions: Thyroglossal Duct Cysts and Branchial Cleft Anomalies

R. Peter Altman   Daniel H. Hechtman

Thyroglossal duct cysts and branchial cleft malformations are clinical manifestations of anomalous migration of the thyroid gland or resorption of the branchial apparatus in utero. These lesions are usually identified during the evaluation of a patient with a new or recurrent neck mass or an epidermal pit, particularly in the pediatric age group. Early diagnosis and surgical excision reduce the chance of infection and enhance the likelihood of a successful outcome.

Thyroglossal Duct Cyst

Thyroglossal duct cysts are a frequent cause of anterior midline neck masses in the first decade of life. More than 25 percent present before the age of 5 and 40 percent by the age of 10. Interestingly, thyroglossal duct cysts appear at a constant rate of almost 10 percent per decade in the ensuing years.

Embryology

An appreciation of the embryology of the thyroid gland is important for an understanding of the surgical approach to excision of thyroglossal duct cysts. During the third week of gestation, an epithelial thickening develops at the tuberculum impar on the anterior pharyngeal wall. This thickening, the median thyroid anlage, divides into a bilobed structure representing the developing thyroid gland. Rostral growth of the embryo results in caudal displacement of the median thyroid anlage with persistence of a median stalk stretching to the tuberculum impar. Canalization

of the median stalk produces the thyroglossal duct, which typically courses ventral to the hyoid anlage, but can pass through or dorsal to it. In the fifth week of gestation, the duct degenerates and is resorbed. Secretion by epithelium-lined remnants of the duct can lead to thyroglossal duct cyst formation. The stimulus for secretion by these remnants is unknown but can occur at any time, accounting for the delayed appearance of these cysts in later life.

Clinical Presentation and Evaluation

A thyroglossal duct cyst is usually diagnosed on routine physical examination or during evaluation of a suddenly appearing, unsightly, or inflamed midline neck mass. The cyst is located within 2 cm of the midline and typically overlies the hyoid bone, although it can be found anywhere along the course of the thyroglossal duct (Fig. 28-1). Unless infected, the cyst is smooth and mobile without communication with the overlying skin. A sinus tract can occur following spontaneous drainage or incision of an infected cyst.

Routine examination requires nothing more than a careful history and physical examination. A typically positioned mass that rises in the neck with swallowing or protrusion of the tongue is diagnostic. If the mass is atypical in location or examination is hampered by inflammation, ultrasound is helpful. Confirmation of the thyroid in its normal location by palpation or demonstration by ultrasound is important. Dermoid cysts are occasionally iden-

tified at a surgical procedure or pathologically following excision of a presumed thyroglossal duct cyst. The former can usually be distinguished intraoperatively by the finding of thick, white, sebaceous contents.

An operation is scheduled at the earliest convenience to avoid the morbidity of intervening infection. If infection is present, the operation is deferred until the inflammatory process is fully resolved. Incision and drainage are rarely required.

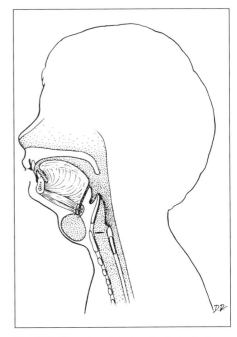

Fig. 28-1. Thyroglossal duct cyst anterior to the hyoid bone with the thyroglossal duct tract passing through the hyoid bone and extending to the foramen cecum.

Surgical Technique

The contemporary approach to excision of thyroglossal duct cysts is attributed to Sistrunk, for whom the procedure is named. He incorporated resection of the central hyoid bone and the tract extending to the foramen cecum with excision of the cyst. This maneuver reduced the incidence of recurrence to less than 5 percent from the 25 percent recurrence rate for cystectomy alone.

Under general endotracheal anesthesia, the patient is positioned with the neck extended using a roll beneath the shoulders. A transverse skin incision is made, centered around the midline, and extended 0.5 cm to each side of the mass (Fig. 28-2A). After division of the subcutaneous fat and platysma muscle, the cyst is identified and the surrounding tissues are circumferentially dissected from its surface. A typical thyroglossal duct cyst is thin-walled and contains translucent fluid unless infected or previously drained. A solid mass should prompt identification of the thyroid to avoid excision of a partially descended gland. A nontranslucent cyst is aspirated to identify a dermoid cyst, which appropriately is excised without the adjacent hyoid bone.

Unless recently inflamed, the cyst can be mobilized circumferentially by applying traction to the loosely adherent surrounding tissues. The cyst should not be grasped directly because dissection is facilitated by avoiding entry into the cyst. If the cyst wall is inadvertently violated, the collapsed cyst is held with a fine Allis clamp for the remainder of the procedure.

The hyoid bone is palpated lateral to the cyst. Using cautery, the sternohyoid and thyrohyoid strap muscles are divided at their points of insertion along the inferior aspect of the hyoid bone. Dissection is then performed circumferentially around the hyoid, inserting a short right-angle clamp posterior to the ramus of the bone approximately 0.75 cm lateral to its midpoint. The bone is divided with bone shears or cautery depending on the stage of ossification (Fig. 28-2B). Sufficient hyoid must be resected to ensure adequate excision of thyroglossal duct remnants (Fig. 28-3).

The geniohyoid and mylohyoid muscles are incised and subsequently divided from the superodorsal aspect of the hyoid bone leaving a 0.5-cm stalk of tissue with the thyroglossal duct at its center. The stalk is dissected to the foramen cecum at the base of the tongue where it is suture-ligated with an absorbable suture and divided (Fig. 28-4). It is not advisable to skeletonize the tract as it courses cephalad. Rather, the investing connective tissue should be resected with that of the rostral tract. This technique ensures that duplicate, branching, or multiple tract remnants will not be left behind, thus minimizing the risk of recurrent neck infection postoperatively. When inflammation is present at the time of the operation, the procedure is more difficult and the likelihood of recurrence greater. A wider dissection is performed encompassing all of the inflamed tissues.

It has been suggested that dissection of the tract and its ligation at the foramen cecum can be facilitated by the application of digital pressure to the base of the tongue by the anesthesiologist. In our opinion, this maneuver is of minimal usefulness and we do not incorporate it into the procedure.

Meticulous hemostasis is obtained with electrocautery and local anesthetic is infiltrated into the skin and subcutaneous tissues. The edges of the hyoid bone are not approximated and a drain is not routinely inserted. In situations in which the cyst was infected before excision, it is advisable to leave a small drain overnight, particularly if the cyst was entered during the mobilization and dissection. The platysma muscle and skin are closed in layers with absorbable suture, and an occlusive dressing is applied. Following extubation and recovery from anesthesia, the patient is discharged.

Complications and Recurrence

The most potentially dangerous complication following thyroglossal duct excision is postoperative wound hemorrhage with resultant airway compression. Careful hemostasis, not routine drainage of the wound, is the optimal approach to avoiding this uncommon complication. Wound

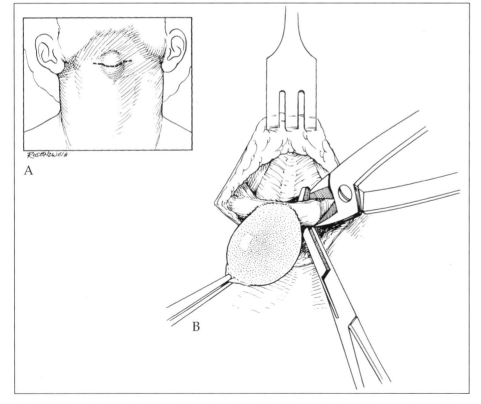

Fig. 28-2. Thyroglossal duct cyst—technique of excision. A. Incision is placed over the presenting cyst. No skin is excised. B. The thyroglossal duct cyst has been dissected from surrounding tissues. The hyoid is exposed after division of the sternohyoid and thyrohyoid muscles at insertion. The bone is encircled with a short right-angle clamp 1.0 cm from its midpoint where it is divided with a bone cutter or cautery.

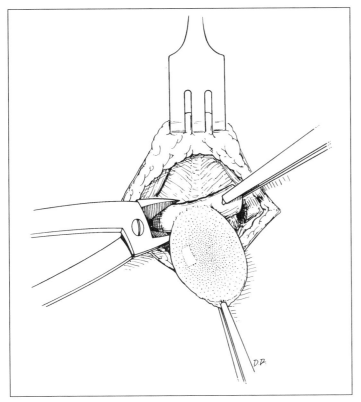

Fig. 28-3. Traction on the divided hyoid facilitates exposure and division of the opposite ramus.

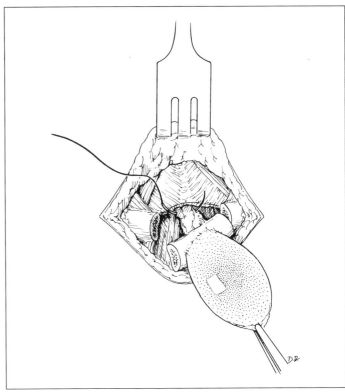

Fig. 28-4. Dissection proceeds cephalad to the foramen cecum where the tract and investing tissues are suture-ligated.

infections are infrequent and respond to treatment with oral antibiotics.

Recurrence following thyroglossal duct cyst excision occurs in approximately 5 percent of patients, typically within 1 year of the procedure. Inflammation of the anterior neck associated with localized swelling or a draining sinus tract is the characteristic presentation. Recurrence is usually attributed to inadequate excision of thyroglossal duct remnants. Recurrence can be caused by distortion of the tissues by inflammation or inadequate resection of the hyoid bone or the central stalk leading to the foramen cecum. The presence of multiple tracts can also lead to recurrent disease. Rupture of the cyst at the time of excision has similarly been associated with an increased incidence of recurrence.

Patients typically present with recurrent infection in the upper neck. Antibiotics are administered and continued until inflammation has resolved. The previous operative report is always reviewed to determine whether the excision was adequate, particularly resection of the central hyoid bone. A reoperation is performed through the same incision. Fibrotic and inflamed tissues, the central hyoid bone, and the midline geniohyoid muscle are widely excised.

Branchial Cleft Anomalies

Branchial cleft anomalies comprise a heterogeneous group of congenital malformations derived from incomplete in utero resorption of the pharyngeal clefts and pouches. Fistulas, cysts, sinus tracts, and cartilaginous remnants of the first and second branchial clefts are the most common clinical manifestations. These anomalies are excised to prevent the morbidity of subsequent infection.

Embryology

During the third to fifth gestational week, the primitive pharynx develops four pairs of endodermally lined pouches along its inner walls as an equal number of ectodermally lined clefts form on the surface of the embryo. These pouches and clefts approximate each other, creating intervening mesodermal arches. Proliferation of the mesoderm later in gestation obliterates the epithelial outpouchings, with the exception of the first branchial cleft and pouch, which develop as the auditory canal, tympanic membrane, and middle ear. Persistence of a branchial cleft or pouch results in a cervical anomaly located along the anterior border of the sternocleidomastoid muscle from the tragus of the ear to the clavicle.

Clinical Presentation and Evaluation

The branchial cleft anomalies include sinuses, with openings on the skin or into the pharynx, fistulas, with communications between the skin and the pharynx, or cysts, without extension to either surface. The second cleft and pouch account for greater than 90 percent of anomalies with the remainder originating from the first and, less frequently, the third and fourth branchial structures.

An external sinus or fistula presents with intermittent drainage from a skin ostium located in the midneck along the anterior border of the sternocleidomastoid muscle. These anomalies are less common than cysts, present in the first decade of life, are bilateral in 20 percent of cases, and have a slight female preponderance. The diagnosis is apparent on examination and further roentgenographic evaluation is usually unnecessary. Internal sinuses drain into the tonsillar fossa and present as a mass or inclusion cyst when the draining tract becomes obstructed.

Branchial cysts appear after the first decade of life and are located higher in the neck than the external ostia of sinuses and fistulas. A cyst is identified as a palpable mass at the level of the carotid bifurcation. These lesions can be confused with and should be distinguished from cystic hygromas, hemangiomas, lymphadenopathy, and particularly, lymphatic or metastatic tumors. Ultrasonography differentiates solid and cystic masses and is the only imaging study routinely performed. Further diagnostic studies with CT, MRI, or fine-needle aspiration biopsy might be indicated, particularly for solid masses.

Patients with evidence of infection are treated with an antibiotic until the inflammatory process has fully resolved. At times, incision and drainage are necessary. Unlike thyroglossal duct cysts, however, branchial cleft anomalies are related anatomically to nerves and vessels, which are vulnerable to injury during drainage procedures. To ensure safety, adequate sedation or general anesthesia is advised.

When sinus tracts or fistulas are identified in neonates, excision is delayed until 6 months of age to allow for growth, and consequently, an easier dissection. In older children surgical procedures are scheduled conveniently to minimize the risk of intervening infection.

Anatomy

Knowledge of the regional anatomy is important to avoid injury to adjacent structures and to predict the course of a sinus tract or fistula. Second branchial cleft sinuses and fistulas have an external ostium located along the anterior border of the sternocleidomastoid muscle at the junction of its middle and lower thirds (Fig. 28-5). As the tract passes in a cephalad direction, it courses between the internal and external carotid arteries and over the hypoglossal and glossopharyngeal nerves. A fistula or an internal sinus then passes medially entering the pharynx in the tonsillar fossa. Cysts occur anywhere along this tract but

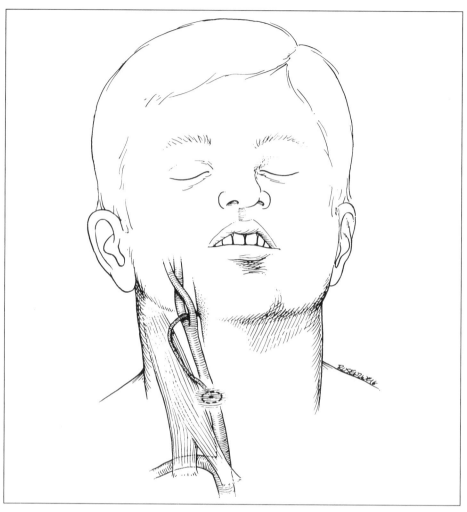

Fig. 28-5. Course of a second branchial cleft fistula. The external ostium is at the anterior border of the sternocleidomastoid muscle. The fistula passes between the internal and external carotid arteries and enters the pharynx at the tonsillar fossa.

are found most frequently below the level of the hyoid bone, lateral to the carotid artery (Fig. 28-6).

Much less common are first branchial cleft anomalies, which are separated into two distinct entities. Type 1 sinuses or cysts are identified around the inferior half of the concha of the ear. A tract, if present, parallels but does not penetrate the auditory meatus. Type 2 anomalies are located in the anterior neck above the level of the hyoid bone. Tracts pass posteriorly, superficial to the angle of the mandible, ending in or adjacent to the auditory meatus. The course of the tract is through the parotid gland with a variable relationship to the facial nerve.

A third branchial cleft sinus or fistula has a skin pit similar in location to second cleft anomalies. The tract, however, passes between the glossopharyngeal and hypoglossal nerves, courses posterior to the carotid vessels, and penetrates the thyrohyoid membrane to enter the pyriform sinus. Fourth branchial cleft anomalies are not clinically relevant.

Surgical Technique

Although branchial anomalies can originate from any of the four clefts, those arising from the second cleft are of primary importance. Therefore, the following discussion will emphasize the excision of these anomalies.

Previous inflammation complicates excision of branchial cleft anomalies. Adherence to the principles of careful dissection and identification of tissue planes are important in avoiding injury to adjacent structures and in performing an adequate

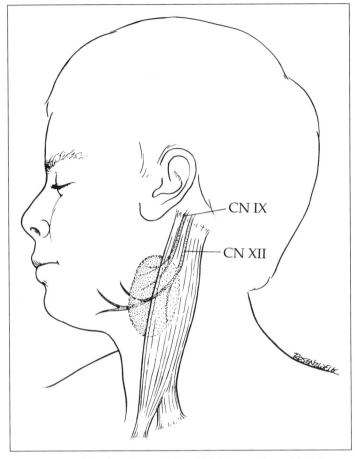

Fig. 28-6. *Typical location of a second branchial cleft cyst. The cyst is at the level of the carotid bifurcation. No external opening is present. Note the relationship to regional nerves.*

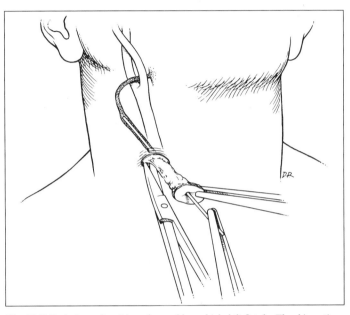

Fig. 28-7. *Technique of excision of second branchial cleft fistula. The skin ostium is incorporated in the elliptical incision. Note the lacrimal duct probe in the tract to facilitate its dissection.*

resection. Definitive procedures are best delayed until inflammation has fully resolved.

Under general endotracheal anesthesia, the patient is positioned with the neck extended using a roll beneath the shoulders. A skin opening, if present, is probed with a fine lacrimal duct probe to identify the course and length of the tract. This step is a delicate maneuver requiring care to avoid penetrating the tract wall into adjacent tissues. We specifically recommend against the use of methylene blue to identify the tract. Extravasation of dye is almost inevitable and leads to confusion. A transverse elliptical skin incision is made encompassing the skin ostium, and the underlying subcutaneous fat is sharply dissected onto the tract with tenotomy scissors (Fig. 28-7). This method permits a more precise dissection than electrocautery. Skin hooks or fine rake retractors are placed in the wound, and the skin ellipse is grasped with a clamp to provide tension

on the tract during dissection. Dissection is greatly facilitated by the previously placed fine probe. The tract is mobilized in a posterocephalad direction in a plane directly on its wall (Fig. 28-8). The carotid vessels and cranial nerves are never specifically visualized as the tract is dissected and excised.

If the sinus tract or fistula is long, exposure is eventually limited by the depth of the wound as dissection extends cephalad. Dissection should not be performed through an inadequate incision. To avoid tearing the tract and performing an incomplete incision and to enhance the dissection while maintaining a cosmetically acceptable appearance, the tip of a fine clamp is passed along the course of the dissection and palpated 2 to 3 cm above the initial incision. A transverse counter or "stepladder" incision is made over the clamp through which the previously dissected tract is passed (Fig. 28-8). The distal tract and skin ostium are now delivered

through the cephalad counter incision (Fig. 28-9). Further dissection is continued until the tract ends, either blindly or in the tonsillar fossa (Fig. 28-10). The base of the tract is suture-ligated with an absorbable suture, and the tract is excised. The small transverse incisions are closed in layers with approximation of the platysma and dermis. Local anesthetic is infiltrated into the skin prior to closure, and occlusive dressings are applied. Following extubation and recovery from anesthesia, the patient is discharged.

Occasionally, a small cyst containing a cartilaginous remnant, typically identified along the anterior border of the sternocleidomastoid muscle, is encountered. Invariably these lesions are localized and are not associated with a cephalad sinus tract. It is neither necessary nor advisable to attempt probing the cyst in an attempt to identify a tract. Excision of the local lesion is curative.

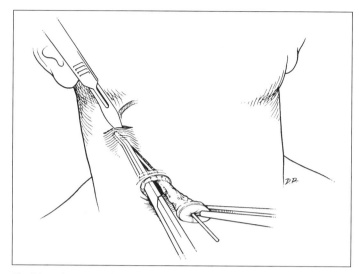

Fig. 28-8. *The extent of the tract eventually limits the dissection. A clamp is passed along the dissected tract to guide the performance of a counter or "stepladder" incision.*

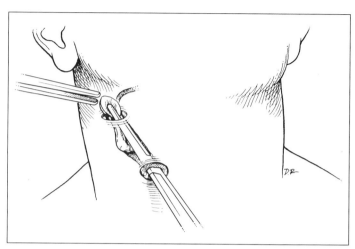

Fig. 28-9. *The previously mobilized tract is passed from the original incision to the counter incision.*

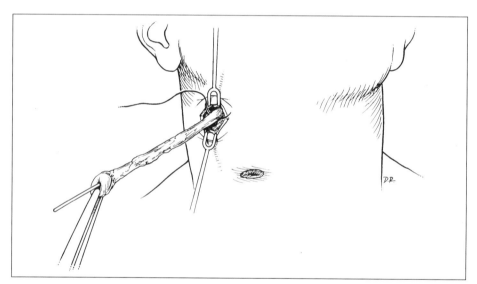

Fig. 28-10. *This maneuver facilitates further dissection of the tract in a superomedial direction to its termination at the tonsillar fossa where it is suture-ligated and divided.*

Branchial cleft cysts are of variable size and have no associated skin opening. These cysts are removed through an incision centered in a skin crease over the mass and carried down through the platysma. Cautery facilitates this dissection. The cyst is located deep to the sternocleidomastoid muscle, which is reflected laterally. Dissection onto the cyst wall is crucial to safe excision and is performed by spreading and retracting the surrounding tissues to avoid injuring adjacent nerves and vessels displaced by the mass. The plane immediately adjacent to the cyst is identified and developed circumferen-

tially. Dissection is hampered by decompression of the cyst, which should be avoided. Occasionally, a tract can be identified on the medial aspect of the cyst, which continues to the tonsillar fossa. This tract represents an internal sinus that has become obstructed, resulting in the formation of an inclusion cyst. The tract is suture-ligated at its base and divided. Drainage of the wound is unnecessary.

Resection of first branchial cleft anomalies requires a more extensive procedure involving exposure and preservation of the facial nerve. Accurate preoperative diag-

nosis is important to approach and safely resect these lesions.

Complications and Recurrence

Morbidity is attributable to injury of adjacent structures at the time of the surgical procedure or to incomplete excision of the branchial cleft anomaly. The incidence of these complications is magnified by inflammation occurring before or at the time of surgical excision. Recurrence is rare unless there has been prior infection. However, recurrence exceeds 20 percent when infection has preceded excision. For these reasons, excision is indicated once a branchial cleft anomaly has been diagnosed.

Suggested Reading

Bennett KG, Organ CH Jr, Williams GR. Is the treatment for thyroglossal duct cysts too extensive? *Am J Surg* 152:602, 1986.

Burge D, Middleton A. Persistent pharyngeal pouch derivatives in the neonate. *J Pediatr Surg* 18:230, 1983.

Ein SH, Shandling B, Stephens CA, et al. The problem of recurrent thyroglossal duct remnants. *J Pediatr Surg* 19:437, 1984.

Freidberg J. Pharyngeal cleft sinuses and cysts, and other benign neck lesions. *Ped Clin North Am* 36:1451, 1989.

Hoffman MA, Schuster SR. Thyroglossal duct remnants in infants and children: Reevaluation of histopathology and methods of resection. *Ann Otol Rhinol Laryngol* 97:483, 1988.

Mickel RA, Calcaterra TC. Management of recurrent thyroglossal duct cysts. *Arch Otol* 109:34, 1983.

Moore KL, Persaud TVN, Shiota K. *Color Atlas of Clinical Embryology*, Philadelphia: Saunders, 1994.

Roback SA, Telander RL. Thyroglossal duct cysts and branchial cleft anomalies. *Sem Pediatr Surg* 3:142, 1994.

Sistrunk WE. The surgical management of cysts of the thyroglossal tract. *Ann Surg* 71:121, 1920.

Sistrunk WE. Technique of removal of cysts of the thyroglossal tract. *Surg Gynecol Obstet* 46:109, 1928.

Skandalakis JE, Gray SW, Todd NW. Pharynx and its derivatives. In Skandalakis JE, Gray SW (eds.). *Embryology for Surgeons*. 2nd ed. Baltimore: Williams & Wilkins, 1994.

Telander RL, Filston HC. Review of head and neck lesions of infancy and childhood. *Surg Clin North Am* 72:1429, 1992.

EDITOR'S COMMENT

Doctors Altman and Hechtman have provided a standard and concise appreciation of thyroglossal ducts and cysts as well as branchial cleft anomalies. The critical issue concerning a thyroglossal duct cyst is of course whether it contains the only thyroid tissue that the patient has. Accidental excision of the ectopic thyroid, which is the patient's only functioning thyroid tissue, will result in hypothyroidism. Preoperative thyroid scintigraphy has been proposed as being necessary in patients with presumed thyroglossal duct cysts to document a normal thyroid. Ultrasound, however, can be almost as accurate and is considerably less invasive. A recent study by Lin-Dunham and associates (*Am J Radiol* 164:1489, 1995) in 30 patients demonstrated sonographically normal thyroid glands in all patients. Only three patients had preoperative radionuclide thyroid scans that were normal. They conclude that routine thyroid scintigraphy is not necessary.

As with all cysts, it is only a matter of time before the routine operation and excision of cysts are challenged in favor of radiographically-guided pigtail catheter aspiration and ablation. Fukumata and associates (*Ann Plast Surg* 33:615, 1994) treated six patients with Baker's cyst, three with branchial cleft cysts, and two with thyroglossal duct cysts by percutaneous aspiration and absolute ethanol sclerotherapy using a 7Fr pigtail catheter. Presclerosing cystography was performed to confirm that the lesion was monocystic and that it did not have a communication with a hollow viscus. There was but one recurrence, that of a Baker's cyst, in a relatively short follow-up of 25 months. This type of approach, which follows the aspiration approach to other surgically drained or excised cysts such as pseudocysts, was inevitable given the outstanding ability of roentgenography to identify and accurately aspirate cysts. It would seem that the dangers of this approach, and the 10-percent recurrence rate as opposed to almost no recurrences of cysts (following surgery), plus the possibility of missing a communication and injecting absolute alcohol into the pharynx or tonsillar fossa, for example, suggest at least to me that this technique will not become popular. However, one must be aware of the fact that this is being proposed.

A final comment, perhaps more generic, concerns the latter type of incisions in the excision of the branchial cleft cyst. The authors inject local anesthesia before closing. It has been my experience with relatively short incisions that a mixture of short- and long-acting local anesthetics before the incision, even if the patient is asleep, plus a subcuticular closure and thus the absence of skin sutures, are perhaps the two most important aspects to avoiding postoperative pain. The anesthesia literature is quite replete with references to the fact that preincision injection of local anesthesia is far superior to postincision of local anesthesia in minimizing inflammation, decreasing the release of cytokines, and other accompaniments of the trauma of operation. These two small incisions should require very little pain medication if these two tenets are followed.

J.E.F.

Vascular and Lymphatic Anomalies of Childhood

Robert M. Arensman   Mindy B. Statter

Hemangioma
Classification and Pathology

In the past, the understanding of vascular birthmarks was difficult because of the confusing and often contradictory nomenclature used to describe vascular anomalies. However, in 1982, a biologic classification of vascular anomalies of infancy and childhood, based on physical findings, natural history, and cellular kinetics, was introduced. According to this biologic classification, there are two major categories of pediatric vascular birthmarks: hemangiomas and vascular malformations (Table 29-1). Hemangiomas demonstrate endothelial hyperplasia and increased numbers of mast cells. Multilaminated basement membranes are the ultrastructural hallmark that persist throughout the life cycle of the tumor. It is clinically useful to cate-

Table 29-1. Biologic Classification of Cutaneous and Soft Tissue Vascular Lesions

Hemangioma	Malformation
Proliferative phase	Capillary: CM
Involutive phase	Lymphatic: LM
	Venous: VM
	Arterial: AM
	Combined: CLM, CVM, LVM, AVM

Key: CM = capillary malformation; LM = lymphatic malformation; VM = venous malformation; AM = arterial malformation; CLM = capillary lymphatic malformation; CVM = capillary venous malformation; LVM = lymphatic venous malformation; AVM = arteriovenous malformation.

gorize hemangiomas as being in either the proliferative phase or the involuting phase. However, vascular malformations are errors of vascular morphogenesis with normal endothelial turnover and normal numbers of mast cells. Malformations are subcategorized as either slow flow (capillary, venous, lymphatic) or fast flow (arterial).

Clinical Course

Hemangioma is the most common tumor of infancy. The incidence is 1 to 2 percent in neonates and 12 percent by the age of 1 year. There is an increased incidence (23%) in premature infants with a birth weight less than 1000 g. Hemangiomas occur more frequently in women than men, in a ratio of 3:1. Most hemangiomas (60%) occur around the head and neck (Figs. 29-1 and 29-2), 25 percent are located on the trunk, and 15 percent on the extremities. The majority of these lesions present singularly; however, 20 percent of affected infants have multiple tumors that may manifest in any body site. Infants with multiple cutaneous lesions represent the group at higher risk to harbor visceral hemangiomas.

Hemangioma's hallmark is rapid growth during the infantile period. The proliferative phase begins in the first few weeks after birth and lasts approximately 6 to 10 months. After 6 to 10 months of age, the hemangioma's growth rate generally becomes proportionate to the growth rate of the child, and the involuting phase begins. Complete resolution of a hemangioma occurs in 50 percent of lesions by the age of

5 years, 70 percent by 7 years, with the remaining lesions continuing to regress until 10 to 12 years (Fig. 29-1). The rate of regression is not influenced by or related to site, size, or appearance. Normal skin is restored in 50 percent of patients. After involution, the skin can exhibit minor atrophy, a fibrofatty residuum, wrinkling (like crepe paper), telangiectasias, yellowish hypoelastic patches, or scars where previous ulceration occurred during proliferation.

In contrast, vascular malformations, by definition, are present at birth but might not manifest until childhood, adolescence, or sometimes adulthood. They have no predilection for either sex. They generally grow commensurately with the child but can suddenly expand because of trauma, infection, or hormonal modulation.

Most hemangiomas are accurately diagnosed by history and physical examination. Hemangioma is fibrofatty in consistency, and its blood cannot be evacuated completely by compression. If imaging is indicated, ultrasound, with color flow Doppler, is the most cost effective (Fig. 29-2). Although useful in differentiating slow-flow vascular malformations (venous and lymphatic), this modality cannot always distinguish lesions with high-flow characteristics (proliferating hemangioma versus arterial malformation).

Early experience with magnetic resonance imaging (MRI) suggests it might be the study of choice, demonstrating both the extent of involvement within tissue planes and rheologic characteristics. Computed tomography (CT) is useful in defining spa-

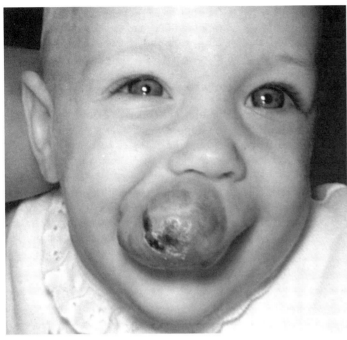

Fig. 29-1. *Hemangioma of the upper lip showing signs of early involution. No pharmacologic treatment was necessary.*

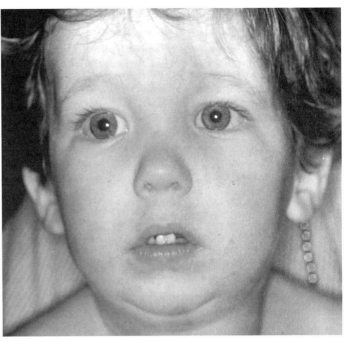

Fig. 29-2. *This cervical mass had a bluish tinge; ultrasound examination confirmed the diagnosis of hemangioma.*

tial relationships of vascular anomalies and alterations in skeletal structures but cannot quantitate blood flow. A proliferative hemangioma appears as a well-circumscribed tumor with homogeneous parenchymatous density and intense enhancement. An involuting hemangioma appears heterogeneous with distinct lobular architecture and large draining veins in the center and the periphery. Vascular malformations present as tissue heterogeneity on CT. Lymphangiomas, as discussed later, appear as nonenhancing low-density multiloculated cysts with enhancing septa. Angiography is rarely necessary for diagnostic purposes.

The Kasabach–Merritt syndrome is a coagulopathy characterized by profound thrombocytopenia caused by platelet trapping in large or disseminated hemangiomas. This syndrome usually presents in the neonate. In contrast, a true coagulopathy can occur in an older patient with a large or extensive venous malformation. Stasis within dilated ectatic venous channels precipitates the coagulopathy.

Proliferating hemangiomas must be distinguished from pyogenic granulomas. The term *pyogenic granuloma* is a misnomer in that these lesions are neither infection-induced nor granulomatous. Unlike hemangiomas, which are more common in fe-

males, males are more commonly affected with pyogenic granulomas, generally on the scalp and face but at any skin site. These lesions typically begin as solitary red papules that can assume a pedunculated appearance as they grow rapidly on a small pedicle. Histologically, pyogenic granulomas demonstrate a lobular arrangement of capillaries. The proliferating hemangiomas, as previously mentioned, lack this lobular pattern. Proliferating hemangiomas have an increased number of mast cells, a finding not present in pyogenic granulomas. Both pyogenic granulomas and hemangiomas can occur early in infancy as rapidly growing masses. Bleeding is very common with pyogenic granulomas and can be severe and unresponsive to pressure or cautery. Significant bleeding is rare with proliferative hemangiomas, occurring mainly with deep ulceration or in association with Kasabach–Merritt syndrome. The natural history of pyogenic granulomas is not one of spontaneous involution; surgical excision is the treatment of choice.

Treatment

The majority of hemangiomas require no treatment since only 10 percent become problematic. Generally these problems result from ulceration or bleeding. Ulcer-

ation occurs in 5 percent of lesions, most commonly the ones located on the lips and anogenital areas (Fig. 29-1). Ulceration can result in secondary infection and destruction of soft tissue and cartilage. Treatment consists of cleansing, daily application of topical antibiotics, and with associated cellulitis, systemic antibiotics. An ulcerated hemangioma should heal within a few weeks by epithelialization.

Localized bleeding is rare, except where ulceration is present. Bleeding from punctate areas is usually controlled by applying continuous pressure for 10 minutes. Repeated bleeding requires evaluation for coagulopathy. Generalized bleeding with petechiae, ecchymoses, intralesional hemorrhage, or internal bleeding suggests the Kasabach–Merritt syndrome. Mortality is 30 to 40 percent in this setting despite therapy. High-output congestive heart failure can occur in the presence of multiple cutaneous and visceral lesions or with a large cutaneous tumor without visceral involvement.

Pharmacologic therapy is indicated for lesions with major ulceration; recurrent infection; distortion and deformation of soft tissues; obstruction of visual, auditory, respiratory, or gustatory function; or life-threatening complications such as bleeding and congestive heart failure.

Systemic corticosteroids are the mainstay of current medical therapy for problematic hemangiomas. Prednisone or prednisolone is given at a dose of 2 to 3 mg/kg/day orally for 2 to 3 weeks. A positive response to therapy includes softening of the lesion, lightening of the color, and slowing of growth within 7 to 10 days of initiating therapy. If there is a response, the full dosage should be given for 4 to 6 weeks and then tapered. If rebound growth occurs, a higher dose of steroids is given for 2 weeks before tapering. Steroids should not be continued once involution starts. The response to systemic steroids varies from a dramatic response in 30 percent, where within 2 to 3 weeks the hemangioma stops growing and begins to shrink and appear pale; to an equivocal response in 40 percent; and a complete failure to respond in 30 percent.

Intralesional steroids can be considered for small, localized hemangiomas. One to three injections are generally given at 4- to 6-week intervals. A long-acting steroid (e. g., triamcinolone) can be combined with a short-acting steroid (e. g., cortisone acetate). The response rate for intralesional steroids is similar to the response rate for systemic steroids. Adverse effects of steroid therapy include adrenal suppression, growth retardation, and immunosuppression, but are all uncommon because of the short duration of therapy. Intralesional steroids can also cause local problems such as subcutaneous fat atrophy or necrosis, depigmentation, and blindness caused by embolization of particles in the suspension.

The mechanism of action of steroids is unclear. Angiostatic steroids are a class of compounds that inhibits angiogenesis in the presence of a nonanticoagulant heparin fragment. Tetrahydrocortisol, a major metabolite of cortisol, is the most potent of the naturally occurring angiostatic steroids. This class of compounds induces capillary basement membrane dissolution only within growing capillaries.

The concept of angiogenic diseases, nonneoplastic diseases in which the principal feature is pathologic growth of capillary blood vessels, was introduced by Folkman and Klagsbrun in 1987. Subsequently, studies of vascular growth regulation led to the discovery of angiogenic factors. These factors act directly on vascular endothelial cells to stimulate migration or mitosis, or indirectly by mobilizing and activating host cells such as macrophages to release endothelial growth factors. Immunohistochemical studies demonstrated high expression of basic fibroblast growth factor (bFGF) in both the proliferating and involuting phases of hemangiomas. High levels of bFGF have been demonstrated in the urine of infants and children with hemangiomas. Urinary bFGF levels are currently being used as a marker in the management of hemangiomas with interferon; it has been noted that infants and children with high levels of urinary bFGF have a more favorable response to interferon alfa-2a therapy.

Corticosteroid-resistant hemangiomas with associated life-threatening complications (Kasabach–Merritt syndrome) should be treated with interferon alfa-2a. Other potential indications for interferon include conditions that involve the destruction of vital organs or structures and conditions that result in disfigurement, disability, or potential amputation. Inteferon's possible mechanisms of action include: 1) inhibiting the proliferation and migration of endothelial cells; 2) inhibiting the effects of endothelial cell or fibroblast growth factors; 3) decreasing fibroblast and smooth-muscle cell proliferation and collagen synthesis; or 4) enhancing the production of endothelial prostacyclin.

Less conventional modalities such as tranexamic acid and ϵ-aminocaproic acid have been used for steroid-resistant hemangiomas. Both are fibrinolytic inhibitors that exert their effect through inhibition of plasminogen activator, plasmin, and inhibition of tumor vessel proliferation.

The emergence of laser technology and specifically that of pulsed yellow light has added another potential modality for the management of hemangiomas. However, current laser technology does not yet have a well-defined role in the routine management of hemangiomas. Yellow light is selectively absorbed by hemoglobin. The only other competing chromophore is melanin. Two pulsed yellow light lasers are currently used: copper vapor laser and flashlamp pumped-dye laser. Pulsed light has two advantages: 1) the high-peak power will result in more efficient absorption by the chromophore (hemoglobin), and 2) the time between pulses allows thermal cooling of the chromophore and reduces the extent of heat transmission to the surrounding tissues. These two properties act synergistically in allowing selective photocoagulation of vascular tissue. Clinical experience has shown that the flashlamp pumped-dye laser is superior in treating superficial small-vessel disease; the copper vapor laser is more effective in treating large-vessel disease.

Treatment outcomes are dependent on the stage of the life cycle of the hemangioma (proliferative vs. involuting). Laser treatment is most effective in the stage of early proliferation. Once the lesion has become established, laser photocoagulation becomes ineffective because of the thickness of the subcutaneous component and the fact that the lesion is composed of tubules of plump endothelial cells with very small lumens and less target chromophore. In instances of extensive cutaneous and subcutaneous hemangiomas undergoing early involution, preoperative laser photocoagulation can be useful. Surgical resection is performed at least 6 weeks later. Since the laser therapy allows elevation of skin flaps in a less vascular plane, hemostasis and primary closure are facilitated. During late involution, laser photocoagulation is useful only in dealing with residual telangiectasia.

Hemangioma of the head and neck can cause obstruction of the visual, auditory, or respiratory system. Orbital lesions can cause proptosis with corneal exposure, strabismus and amblyopia, optic atrophy, and bony malformation. Ophthalmologic consultation is mandatory for every orbitopalpebral hemangioma. Lesions near the parotid can compress the external auditory canal, resulting in conductive hearing loss.

Subglottic hemangiomas can compromise the airway. These lesions typically precipitate biphasic stridor at 6 to 8 weeks of age. Approximately half of the infants with subglottic hemangioma also have cervicofacial cutaneous hemangiomas. Subglottic hemangiomas have a mortality of 40 to 70 percent if simply observed. Therapeutic measures are directed as maintaining the airway while minimizing long-term sequelae. Tracheotomy can secure the airway. However, tracheotomy alone has been associated with a mortality as high as 45 percent. The conventional treatment for airway hemangioma is either corticosteroids or destruction with the carbon dioxide laser since open surgical excision of isolated subglottic hemangioma can be associated with postoperative scarring and subglottic stenosis. Interferon alfa-2a has been used successfully in life-threatening airway hemangiomas unresponsive to conventional treatment and can be the treatment of choice in a rapidly expanding hemangioma when urine examination reveals an elevated bFGF, a marker that suggests favorable response.

Some cranial and cervical hemangiomas are now detected on antenatal ultrasound for evaluation of maternal polyhydramnios. Since obstruction of the hypopharynx by a cervical hemangioma can complicate establishing an airway immediately postnatally, orotracheal intubation can be attempted as an adjunct to cesarean section with the placental and umbilical cord circulation maintained to avoid potential hypoxia. If this procedure is unsuccessful, the umbilical cord can be divided and a surgical airway established.

Surgical resection of a hemangioma is rarely indicated in infancy. Indications for excision include obstruction of the visual axis; obstruction of luminal structures; uncontrollable ulceration, hemorrhage, or infection; life-threatening hemangiomas unresponsive to medical therapy; lesions demonstrating atypical growth suggesting an alternative diagnosis; and small or pedunculated lesions that can be excised without cosmetic or functional risk.

Whatever action is used should not result in a worse outcome than one seen with natural involution. If surgical excision is required, to avoid the psychosocial consequences of a readily visible hemangioma the operation should be done during the preschool period when the child is beginning to develop a defined body or facial image. After involution is complete, residual, redundant, or fibrofatty tissue can require resection. A protrusive hemangioma often causes a tissue expansion effect making skin excision possible without distorting normal anatomic lines or contour.

Lymphangioma
Classification and Pathology

Lymphatic malformations are benign tumors of the lymphatic system that consist of localized or generalized anomalous lymphatic channels and cysts. They can occur in any lymphatic bed and in order of decreasing frequency commonly occur in the cervicofacial region, axilla, thorax, and extremities. There are two morphologic types, macrocystic and microcystic, which are often combined. Macrocystic lymphatic malformations are large, soft, smooth, translucent masses under normal or bluish skin. Microcystic lymphatic malformations are clear, tiny cutaneous vesicles that permeate the skin and muscles. These vesicles are often firm and give the impression of a brawny edema. Congenital abnormalities of the lymphatic system have been classified on a pathologic basis (Table 29-2). Although lymphangioma has been described as a primary dysplastic process and lymphangiectasia as a secondary dilatation of preexisting normally developed lymph vessels, the distinction is not always clear. A clinical classification based on the presentation of the conditions has been suggested in order to guide diagnosis and management (Table 29-3).

Clinical Course

Approximately 65 percent of lymphangiomas are apparent at birth, and 90 percent appear by the second year of life. The size of lymphatic malformations often expands because of intralesional hemorrhage, cellulitis, or increasing fluid accumulation. This increasing fluid is noted with viral or bacterial infections. Pure lymphatic mal-formations or combined lymphaticovenous malformations, such as Klippel–Trenaunay syndrome, can be associated with soft-tissue hypertrophy and skeletal overgrowth. Disfigurement is the principal reason patients seek medical attention. Spontaneous regression is rare. Malignant degeneration is unlikely.

Treatment

Lymphatic malformations that obstruct the aerodigestive tract can require aspiration, incision and drainage, tracheostomy, or feeding tube placement. Aspiration or incision and drainage play a role in emergency decompression but are not considered definitive treatment. Surgical excision is indicated for lesions that interfere with function, cause major cosmetic distortion, or become easily infected. Complete resection is the goal of surgical therapy but because of the tendency to infiltrate and surround adjacent tissues and major structures, resection of a lymphangioma is often incomplete. Because these lesions are not malignant, most pediatric surgeons agree that an extensive resection with sacrifice of vital structures is not warranted. Drains do not diminish the incidence of seromas. Nonsurgical therapies have included intralesional injection of bleomycin, OK-432, fibrin adhesive, and Ethibloc, a derivative of maize. All yield marginal results at least, and resection remains the mainstay of treatment.

Table 29-2. Pathologic Classification of Abnormalities of the Lymphatic System

Lymphangiomas
  Lymphangioma simplex
  Cavernous lymphangioma
  Cystic lymphangioma or cystic hygroma
  Lymphangiosarcoma
Lymphangiomatosis
  Multifocal, isolated to one organ system
  Generalized, involving different organ systems
Lymphangiectasia
  Isolated to a specific system
  Generalized
Mixed vascular lymphatic angiomas
Lymphedema
Combinations of lymphatic and other tissues
  Lymphangiomyoma
  Lymphangiomyomatosis
  Lymphangiolipoma

Table 29-3. Clinical Classification of Congenital Abnormalities of the Lymphatic System

Masses
Bone lesions
  Single
  Generalized
Presentations caused by a single abnormal function of the lymphatics
  Lymphedema
  Ascites or pleural effusions
  Respiratory distress
  Edema and hypoproteinemia
Presentations caused by a combination of abnormal functions of the lymphatics
Associated abnormalities
  Lymphopenia
  Hypogammaglobulinemia
  Impaired splenic function
  Abnormalities in hemostasis and coagulation
Symptoms related to mixed angiomatosis

Cystic Hygroma
Clinical Course

Cystic hygromas are macrocystic lymphangiomas of the neonatal period that classically appear in the cervical, axillary, and inguinal areas. These lesions are dysplasias that arise from the sequestration of lymphatic tissue that fails to communicate with the lymphatic tree. A cystic hygroma is not produced by the mere enlargement of a few congenitally sequestered endothelial-lined lymphatic spaces; active growth of the endothelium results in the invasive process that characterizes the lesion. Grossly, the lesions are multilobular, multilocular cystic masses composed of many individual cysts varying in size. The mass is often associated with groups of enlarged lymph glands. Microscopically, the cyst walls consist of a single layer of flattened endothelium. Neonatal lymphangiomas, more commonly called cystic hygromas, are present in 50 to 60 percent of infants at birth, and at least 90 percent are present by the end of the second year of life. Cystic hygromas occur equally in males and females, except for inguinal hygromas, which are five times as numerous in males.

Cystic hygromas are becoming more commonly diagnosed on prenatal ultrasounds.

Widely disparate prognoses accompany cystic hygromas. In most surgical series, a cystic hygroma is an isolated lesion with an excellent prognosis following surgical excision. Reports in the obstetric and genetic literature indicate that there is often an association of cystic hygromas with Turner's syndrome or other chromosomal defects and that the outcome is almost universally fatal. The presence of a nuchal cystic hygroma in a first-trimester fetus indicates an increased incidence of autosomal aneuploidy, most commonly Turner's syndrome, trisomy 13, trisomy 18, and trisomy 21. Cystic hygromas in fetuses with normal karyotypes are likely to be associated with Noonan's syndrome, Robert's syndrome, or polysplenia syndrome. It is likely that many cystic hygromas associated with both Turner's and Noonan's syndromes regress; this regression might explain the webbed neck seen in children with these conditions.

Cystic hygromas presenting late in gestation tend to be more anterolateral and are not generally associated with hydrops or other anomalies. Patients should be advised about the prognosis according to category: 1) first-trimester diagnosis with karyotypic abnormality—59 percent chance of poor outcome; 2) first-trimester diagnosis without karyotypic abnormality—89 percent chance of reaching viability; however, dysmorphic sequelae occur in 20 percent; 3) second- and early third-trimester diagnosis (before 30 weeks)—guarded; and 4) third-trimester diagnosis after 30 weeks' gestation—good.

These masses are soft, often compressible, sometimes poorly defined, and can be seen in almost any part of the body but are most commonly found in the head, neck, abdomen, and axilla. Three-quarters of cystic hygromas are seen in the neck (Figs. 29-3 and 29-4), and 20 percent are observed in the axillary region (Fig. 29-5). The remaining 5 percent are distributed around the body in the mediastinum, retroperitoneum, and groin. The majority of cystic hygromas affecting the neck occur in the posterior triangle, occasionally communicating beneath the clavicle with an axillary hygroma. Some occur in the anterior triangle, are often associated with intraoral lymphangiomas, and are the ones most prone to cause pharyngeal compression and interference with the airway. Of all cervical hygromas, 2 to 3 percent are associated with extensions into the mediastinum that can extend to the diaphragm (Fig. 29-6). All patients with cervical cystic hygromas should have a preoperative chest x-ray to determine the presence or absence of mediastinal involvement. Chy-

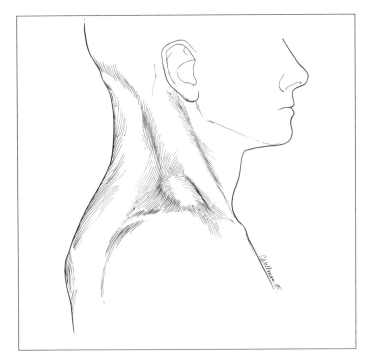

Fig. 29-3. Typical presentation of a posterior cervical cystic hygroma.

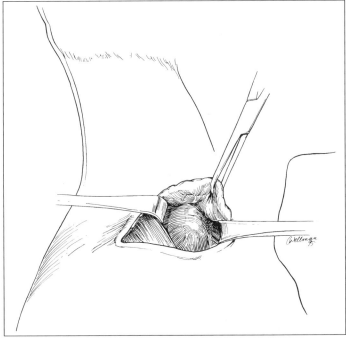

Fig. 29-4. Cystic hygroma with intracystic hemorrhage.

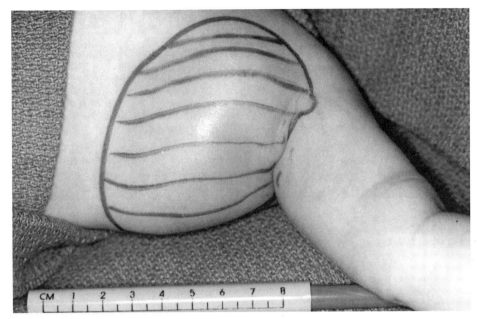

Fig. 29-5. Typical presentation of an axillary cystic hygroma.

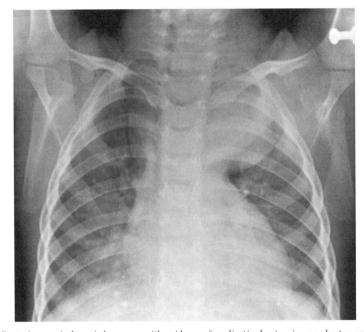

Fig. 29-6. Posterior cervical cystic hygroma with evidence of mediastinal extension on chest x-ray.

attributed to cyst size and site with extension into the floor of the mouth, epiglottis, or mediastinum.

Treatment

Excision is the treatment of choice and the only effective available treatment. Generally, operative treatment is indicated whenever one of these lesions is encountered, because of the risks of spontaneous infection, progressive growth leading to substantial disfigurement with extension into uninvolved areas, and the possibility of airway obstruction and dysphagia. Cystic hygromas of the neck are best removed through a simple transverse cervical incision. Axillary hygromas can be approached through an incision in an axillary crease. The pectoralis major muscle can be retracted; it is not necessary to divide it. For cervical hygromas that extend into the axilla, the infant is draped with the side elevated and the arm draped into the field. The cervical portion is dissected until the hygroma is seen to pass below the clavicle. The axillary portion is then dissected out through a transverse axillary incision. Cervicomediastinal hygromas are approached through a standard transverse cervical incision. If the hygroma cannot be reached from this approach, an upper sternal split can be performed to allow complete excision in continuity. Parotid hygromas do not involve the gland itself; therefore, a formal parotidectomy is not indicated. A cystic hygroma is not a malignant neoplasm and normal structures should not be sacrificed in the course of the operation. Postoperative complications include infection, Horner's syndrome, recurrent laryngeal nerve palsy, and damage to the spinal accessory and marginal mandibular nerves. A recurrence rate of 10 percent can be expected as a result of incomplete excision.

Lymphangioma of the Tongue

Lymphangiomas of the tongue are also a subset of lymphatic malformations seen in the newborn. Lymphangiomas of the tongue are the most common nonsyndromic cause of macroglossia in infancy. The lymphagiomatous tissue can extend into the floor of the mouth and bilaterally to the submandibular area. The posterior

lothorax and chylopericardium have been complications of cervicomediastinal hygroma. Cystic hygromas of the parotid region are not of the gland itself and are to be distinguished from hemangiomas of the parotid.

The presenting complaint of most patients is a soft mass in the posterior triangle of the neck. It is easily transilluminated unless intracyst hemorrhage has occurred. The characteristic location and consistency of these lesions allow easy differentiation from other cervical masses. Branchial cleft cysts probably represent the most likely diagnostic alternative. Except for their visible presence, hygromas usually cause no symptoms. Dyspnea and dysphagia can be

half of the tongue is rarely involved. Macroscopically, the tongue has a granular appearance with multiple vesicles present on the major portion of the distal surface. Occasionally, there is bleeding into these vesicles from trauma.

Microscopically, there are cystic endothelial-lined spaces containing blood and lymph in the epithelial, subepithelial, and muscular tissue. Atrophy of the striated tongue musculature can occur. After birth, the tongue can enlarge from inflammation caused by trauma and upper respiratory tract infection. The enlarged tongue usually protrudes through the lips and becomes cracked and dry causing further infection and bleeding. Repeated episodes of inflammation caused by trauma and infection lead to fibrosis. This condition leads to further dilatation of lymphatic channels and permanent enlargement of the tongue. Deformity of the mandible is often produced by pressure from the mass of lymphangiomatous tissue in the tongue and the floor of the mouth.

Treatment

The most effective treatment is a surgical procedure, which should be performed during the first year of life. Surgical excision should restore adequate breathing and swallowing; leave a tongue capable of normal speech, taste, sensation, and orofacial development; and achieve a good cosmetic result. To achieve these goals, marginal V-shaped wedge resections can be performed. Surface carbon dioxide laser photocoagulation can be used for follow-up therapy. Lymphangiomatous extensions into the floor of the mouth and submental and submandibular areas can be resected during secondary procedures.

Suggested Reading

Balakrishnan A, Bailey CM. Lymphangioma of the tongue. A review of pathogenesis, treatment and the use of surface laser photocoagulation. *J Laryngol Otol* 105:924, 1991.

Enjolras O, Mulliken JB. The current management of vascular birthmarks. *Pediatric Dermatology* 10:311, 1993.

Ezekowitz RAB, Mulliken JB, Folkman J. Interferon alfa-2a therapy for life-threatening hemangiomas of infancy. *N Engl J Med* 326:1456, 1992.

Fishman SJ, Mulliken JB. Hemangiomas and vascular malformations of infancy and childhood. *Pediatr Clin North Am* 40:1177, 1993.

Folkman J, Klagsbrun. Angiogenic factors. *Science* 235:442, 1987.

Hancock BJ, St-Vil D, Luks FI, et al. Complications of lymphangiomas in children. *J Pediatr Surg* 27:220, 1992.

Langer JC, Fitzgerald PG, Desa D, et al. Cervical cystic hygroma in the fetus: clinical spectrum and outcome. *J Pediatr Surg* 25:58, 1990.

Ravitch M, Rush B. Cystic Hygroma. In Welch KJ, Randolph JG, Ravitch MM, et al (eds). *Pediatric Surgery*. Chicago: Yearbook, 1986.

Skandalakis JE, Gray SW, Ricketts RR. The Lymphatic System. In Skandalakis JE, Gray SW (eds). *Embryology for Surgeons*. Baltimore: Williams & Wilkins, 1994.

Takahashi K, Mulliken JB, Kozakewich HPW, et al. Cellular markers that distinguish the phases of hemangioma during infancy and childhood. *J Clin Invest* 93:2357, 1994.

Waner M, Suen JY, Dinehart S: Treatment of hemangiomas of the head and neck. *Laryngoscope* 102:1123, 1992.

White CW. Treatment of hemangiomatosis with recombinant interferon-α alfa. *Sem Hematol* 27:15, 1990.

EDITOR'S COMMENT

This chapter by Drs. Arensman and Statta stresses the differences between hemangiomas and arterial malformations. For individuals such as myself, who continually get into difficulty by confusing the two, the following table from Bartels and Horsch (*Angiology* 46:191, 1995) is very useful. This table distinguishing features of hemangiomas and arterial venous malformations is derived by Bartels and Horsch from Mulliken and Glowacki (*Plast Reconstr Surg* 69:412, 1982). It summarizes the critical aspects of management and the fact that if a lesion can be identified as a hemangioma, then it is likely to involute and does not require surgical therapy. It might, however, require steroid therapy.

Distinguishing Features of Hemangiomas and Arteriovenous Malformations

HEMANGIOMA	ARTERIOVENOUS MALFORMATIONS
Neoplasm	Congenital abnormality
30% present at birth	90% present at birth
Proliferative phase: 1 year	
Female:male = 5:1	Female:male = 1:1
Endothelial proliferation	No cellular proliferation
Growth in tissue culture	No growth in tissue culture
Cellulare stroma	
Increased mast cells	No mast cells
Spontaneous involution in 95% by age 7	No spontaneous involution
No treatment required in vast majority	Treatment sometimes necessary

The reasons for such involution and a possible means of providing evaluation were recently proposed by Takahashi and coworkers (*J Clin Invest* 93:2357, 1994). Immunohistochemical analysis of nine independent markers was carried out. In the proliferating phase, there was a high expression of proliferating cell nuclear antigen, vascular endothelial growth factor, and type IV collagenase. While there was a high expression of the basic fibroblast growth factor (bFGF) in urokinase both in the proliferating and involuting phases, there was coexpression of bFGF in endothelial phenotypic markers, CD31, and von Willebrand factor in the proliferating phase. The involuting phase is explained by elevated expression of the tissue inhibitor of the metalloproteinase, TIMP-1, an inhibitor of new blood vessel formation. This tissue inhibitor was expressed only in the involuting phase. The authors suggest that such immunohistochemical markers might be used in diagnosis and to plan different forms of therapy, depending on the identification of the lesion, when the lesion is difficult to identify by other means. This might be a reasonable proposal.

J.E.F.

30

Carotid Body Tumors

Wesley S. Moore   Michael D. Colburn

The only known pathologic condition associated with the carotid body is a carotid body tumor. Nonetheless, even today in the final years of the twentieth century, these lesions, which were first described by Marchand in 1891, remain a topic surrounded by considerable misunderstanding and confusion. Much of this misconception can undoubtedly be traced to the lack of established data related to the histologic origin, biologic behavior, and incidence of malignancy associated with carotid body tumors. As one might predict, this situation has generated considerable controversy regarding the appropriate management of these lesions.

Carotid body tumors are uncommon neoplasms. Unfortunately their exact incidence remains unknown. In 1971, approximately 500 cases had been recorded in the world literature, and by the early 1980s this figure had doubled to just over 1000. Like most other types of benign and malignant neoplasms, the precise etiology of carotid body tumors is not known. Also, as it frequently the case with other endocrine tumors, these lesions are recognized to occur in two distinct forms: sporadic and familial. The sporadic form is more common although the familial pattern has been recognized by some authors in as many as 10 percent of cases. A review of familial cases of cervical paragangliomas suggests an autosomal dominant inheritance pattern. In addition to genetic predisposition, chronic hypoxia has also been implicated as a possible factor that may contribute to the appearance of these neoplasms. It has been long appreciated that chronic hypoxia is associated with enlargement of the carotid body in some patients. Although these changes are usually not classified as tumors, histologic examina-

tion of carotid body tissue from these patients does frequently reveal marked cellular hyperplasia. This observation, combined with epidemiologic data that suggest an increased incidence of carotid body neoplasms occurring in individuals who live at high elevations, has led some investigators to implicate prolonged hypoxemia as a possible etiologic factor related to the development of these uncommon tumors.

This chapter reviews our current practice for the treatment of patients with carotid body tumors. Because many of these management principles are based on an understanding of the pathology and biologic behavior of these lesions, we have included a summary of the current understanding of these important topics. With an appreciation of these principles, and the use of operative techniques developed from them, one should be able to safely manage even the most challenging carotid body lesions. Alternatively, inadequately planned neck explorations in improperly prepared patients, or biopsies of seemingly unimpressive neck masses, will often result in disastrous consequences. Even when the presence of a carotid bifurcation paraganglioma is correctly diagnosed preoperatively, resection of this lesion can be a humbling experience even for the most experienced surgeons.

Pathology

The normal carotid body is an ovoid nodule, measuring approximately 0.5 × 0.5 cm, that is located along the posterior surface of the carotid bifurcation. This structure represents the largest mass of che-

moreceptive tissue found anywhere in the body. The blood supply to the carotid body is usually derived from branches of the external carotid artery and the venous return occurs through tributaries of the lingual and laryngopharyngeal veins. The innervation is exclusively sensory. Small nerve fibers arising from the carotid body join the larger glossopharyngeal nerve before entering the cranium through the jugular foramen. Stimuli that evoke a response by the chemoreceptor cells include increases in either the plasma carbon dioxide tension or blood temperature, or a decrease in the plasma pH or arterial oxygen tension. Once activated, the stimulation of carotic body chemoreceptors causes several physiologic responses, including increased minute volume ventilation, increased pulse rate, and an elevation of the mean systemic blood pressure. Embryologically, the carotid body derives elements from both neural crest ectoderm and mesodermal tissue originating from the third branchial arch. The neural crest ectoderm differentiates into chemoreceptor cells that migrate in close association with the autonomic ganglion cells, and are therefore frequently referred to as paraganglioma cells. The mesodermal tissue develops into a highly vascular fibrosis stroma that both supports and nurtures these clusters of chemoreceptor cells.

Carotid body tumors are neoplastic growths that arise from these chemoreceptive structures. The morphologic appearance of carotid body tumors closely resembles that of normal carotid body tissue. Grossly the tumor is reddish-brown and highly vascular. Microscopically, one sees chemoreceptor cells embedded in a fibrous stroma situated adjacent to abundant capillaries. Overall, the lesions have a very well-differentiated benign appearance. Degenerative malignant characteristics, such as unusual nuclear forms, increased mitotic activity, and vascular invasion, are only very rarely seen. Historically, there has been considerable confusion regarding the terminology and classification of these tumors. The term *glomus tumor* is a misnomer and was introduced based on the mistaken impression that these highly vascular tumors were in fact a form of neurovascular arteriovenous malformation. In 1950, because these tumors are comprised of cells with both chemoreceptor and secretory function, Mulligan introduced the term *chemodectoma* to describe these lesions. Advanced immunohistochemical studies have subsequently suggested that carotid body tumors are capable of synthesizing numerous different neuroendocrine substances. Secretory granules containing a wide variety of neuropeptides, and several enzymes involved in the cytoplasmic synthesis of catecholamines, have all been demonstrated. For unclear reasons, however, patients with carotid body tumors almost never manifest any clinical evidence of excessive endocrine hormone secretion. Since it is believed that these tumors arise embryologically from epithelioid cells of the neural crest that have migrated with neural tissue adjacent to the autonomic ganglion, they have also been referred to as *paragangliomas*. Paragangliomas actually comprise a family of neoplastic tumors that can occur anywhere along the autonomic ganglion chain from the organ of Zuckerkandl to the glomus intravagale. Classically, paragangliomas arising in the adrenal medulla secrete high levels of catecholamines and usually stain positive for chromaffin. Interestingly, despite having been found to contain granules rich in catecholamines within their cytoplasm, using sophisticated staining techniques, carotid body tumors are most commonly nonfunctional and classically stain negative for chromaffin.

Grossly, these tumors are highly vascular and often invade the adventitia of the adjacent carotid vessels. The tumors grow slowly, beginning along the posterior aspect of the carotid bifurcation. As they enlarge, they typically gradually widen the angle between the internal and external carotid arteries. Frequently, when carotid body tumors grow very large, they encase the main trunk and proximal tributaries of the external carotid artery. Without expla-

nation, however, they only very rarely do the same to the internal carotid vessel. This phenomenon may be related to the origin of the blood supply to the tumor from branches of the external carotid artery. Nonetheless, it is a consistent feature found in large carotid body tumors and has important ramifications related to the strategy for resection, which is discussed in more detail in a later section.

Although most carotid body tumors are considered benign lesions, malignancy does occur. Unfortunately, it is generally accepted that the biologic behavior of a given carotid body tumor cannot be predicted based solely on the histologic appearance of the resected specimen. Benign-appearing tumors are quite capable of both locally aggressive growth and nodal and distant metastatic spread. Adherence to vascular and neurologic structures is well known and even extension through the base of the skull into the cranium has been described. Therefore, as is the case with many other neuroendocrine tumors, malignancy is determined by how the lesion behaves clinically. This is quite different from most other types of cancers, in which histologic appearance remains the primary criterion for identification of malignancy.

Clinical Presentation

By far the most common presentation of a carotid body tumor is that of an incidentally noted asymptomatic neck mass. The lesion typically causes no pain and is located just below the angle of the mandible. Usually the tumors grow very slowly over several years; however, more rapidly growing lesions are occasionally encountered. Most carotid body tumors are diagnosed in the third or fourth decade, but they have been reported in both younger and older patients. No gender predominance has yet been established. When the tumor occurs in a familial pattern of inheritance, there is up to a 30 percent incidence of bilateral tumors, as opposed to 2 to 20 percent in nonfamilial cases.

Occasionally when a carotid body tumor becomes very large, compression or local invasion of adjacent structures can lead to a variety of different symptoms. Local discomfort, such as pain, fullness, and numbness, is not uncommon. In this situation, some patients may complain of difficulty in swallowing, hoarseness, and chronic

cough due to compression of the airway or involvement of adjacent cranial nerves.

Despite the fact that carotid body tumors are frequently classified as neuroendocrine neoplasms, clinical evidence of any endocrine imbalance resulting from secretory function of these lesions is almost never encountered. Interestingly, however, the histologic machinery to do so is apparently present. As was mentioned previously, careful ultrastructural and immunohistochemical examination of these tumors has revealed that carotid body tumors are capable of producing secretory granules containing a large variety of catecholamines. Nevertheless, "functional" cervical paragangliomas are exceedingly rare. Only very rarely will a case be reported describing a patient who suffers from both hypertension and a concomitant neck mass in whom the hypertension resolves following resection of the associated carotid body tumor. The assumption, although not proven, is that the hypertension in these cases occurs on the basis of excessive "tumor-related" catecholamine secretion.

On examination these lesions are often described as painless fixed masses located at the angle of the jaw. In fact, more careful examination will usually demonstrate that, although movement is limited longitudinally, the tumor can readily be moved in a lateral direction. This is an important feature of the physical examination and helps establish an association of the mass with the longitudinally running neurovascular structures. Typically, the mass will be firm, smooth, and lobulated. Frequently transmission of the carotid pulsation will be appreciated during palpation. Furthermore, in approximately 30 to 40 percent of patients, an audible bruit will be present over the tumor. Locally aggressive tumors may invade or compress adjacent cranial nerves. In fact, careful examination yields clinical evidence of nerve dysfunction in approximately 10 percent of patients who present with carotid body tumors. Most commonly the hypoglossal or vagal nerves are affected but laryngeal nerve involvement and Horner's syndrome have also occasionally been reported. Very large tumors can extend into the base of the skull or present as a bulge in the lateral wall of the oropharynx with deviation of the soft palate. Ischemic cerebrovascular symptoms rarely, if ever, occur. Patients with carotid body tumors who also present with transient or permanent ischemic events are usually found to have concomitant carotid bifurcation atheroma or another unrelated cause to account for the cerebrovascular systems.

The differential diagnosis of a patient who presents with an enlarging neck mass is extensive. Congenital lesions such as branchial cleft abnormalities, hygromas, and vascular malformations should all be considered. Chronic lymphadenitis, reactive lymphadenopathy, and other inflammatory reactions must also be excluded. Many other benign and malignant neoplastic processes, such as lipomas, neurofibromas, salivary gland and parotid tumors, metastatic head and neck cancers, leukemias, and lymphomas, can also present in this way. Vascular abnormalities such as carotid aneurysms, coils, and kinks should also not be overlooked. A thorough history and physical exam combined with carefully selected diagnostic studies can usually distinguish these other pathologies and successfully identify most cervical paragangliomas. Clearly, however, this orderly work-up is critical as the appropriate treatment for many of these lesions varies greatly.

Natural History and Indications for Surgery

Once identified, all carotid body tumors should be removed. Although these lesions are slow-growing neoplasms with a relatively low risk of malignancy, small tumors are easier to excise and eventually most, if not all, will progress and become locally invasive. These tumors continue to grow and, in time, extension to the base of the skull or involvement of cranial nerves may complicate their management. In addition, the threat of distant metastases, although low, is real. Despite being categorized as generally benign, malignant transformation of carotid body tumors has been reported. The exact incidence of malignancy is difficult to quantitate and depends on the definition of the term used. Unfortunately, the biologic behavior and malignant potential of a given carotid body tumor cannot be predicted by histologic examination. Rather, malignant potential is identified by clinical behavior. If strict criteria of regional lymph node or distant metastatic spread are used, the incidence of metastatic spread from carotid

body tumors would be quite low, although it is definitely not zero. Some reports have suggested that the true incidence of distant metastases in untreated lesions approaches 10 percent. However, locally aggressive growth patterns of carotid body tumors are not at all uncommon and certainly lesions that invade adjacent structures can be considered at least potentially malignant. Consequently, most authorities consider all cervical paragangliomas capable of malignant behavior. Death from carotid body tumors does occur, and not always from metastatic disease. Relentless local growth of these lesions can cause death by airway compression, cranial neuropathies, or intracranial extension. Also, regional lymph node and distant metastases, which are exceedingly rare at presentation, can occur years after the primary tumor has been resected. It should also be mentioned that, because of this low risk of malignancy, a case can be made against operative treatment in the very high-risk or elderly surgical patient who presents with a small, asymptomatic carotid body tumor. In most cases, however, in view of the natural history of progressive enlargement, frequent local invasion, and the small but unpredictable risk of distant metastases, most surgeons recommend surgical resection once the diagnosis of a carotid body tumor has been established.

Preoperative Evaluation

The preoperative evaluation of patients being considered for resection of a carotid body tumor is very important and should be directed to address several questions. What is the overall general medical condition of the patient? Are other cervical paragangliomas present? What is the anatomic extent of the lesion under investigation? Is there any cranial nerve involvement detectable preoperatively? Is there any evidence of endocrine dysfunction or hormonal imbalance? As always, each patient should undergo a thorough history and important risk factors should be identified. Likewise, the physical examination should be complete, with particular emphasis on the neurologic and cerebrovascular systems. Clearly an asymptomatic elderly patient who is considered to be a poor operative risk may not be well served by a potentially hazardous resection of what is most commonly a benign neo-

plasm. Likewise, the presence of multiple lesions or extension of a tumor into the base of the skull would obviously influence the operative approach. Involvement of cranial nerves suggests at least a locally aggressive tumor, and documentation of these deficits preoperatively is obviously very important. Several imaging techniques are now available to both diagnose and characterize carotid body tumors. As is frequently the case, each of these modalities has specific strengths and weaknesses that should be carefully considered.

The preoperative evaluation of patients with carotid body tumors has traditionally relied on the results of selective carotid angiography. This is largely due to the unmatched demonstration of anatomic detail in a familiar format that is easily interpreted by most clinicians. The carotid bifurcation is particularly easy to demonstrate with this examination. Information regarding the overall size, proximal and distal extent, and degree of vascularity of the lesion can usually be easily assessed (Fig. 30-1). Information regarding the major arterial blood supply to the tumor is also obtained. Infrequently, an unusual tumor blood supply from an aberrant ascending cervical or vertebral artery branch will be identified, which can be very important information preoperatively. Another advantage of angiography is its ability to evaluate the entire distribution of the brachiocephalic and cerebrovascular tree including the origin of the vessels as they arise from the aortic arch and the intracranial portion of the branch vessels. This is important because angiography is an extremely sensitive method of identifying cervical paragangliomas and allows the surgeon to easily detect occult nonpalpable synchronous or contralateral tumors. Also, angiography can occasionally suggest malignancy by demonstrating encasement of the carotid vessels. Rarely, this may alert the surgeon to the presence of extensive internal carotid involvement and allow planning, preoperatively, for the possible need for a vascular reconstruction. Lastly, by imaging the lumen of the carotid vessels, any atheromatous plaques or significant ulcerations can be documented. Kinks, coils, aneurysms, and the presence of any other unsuspected anatomic variations are also all easily identified with this technique. Intracranial pathology that may influence management decisions include arteriovenous malfor-

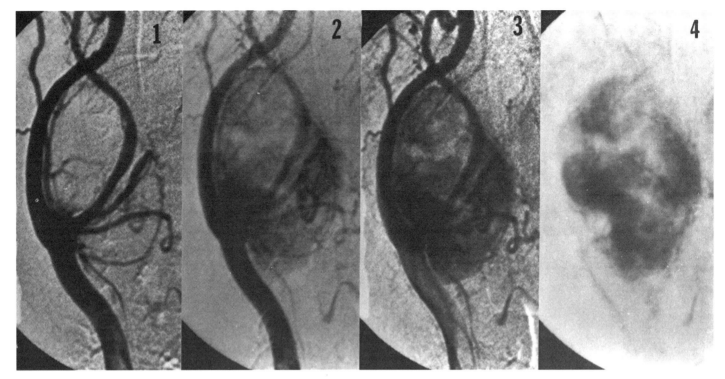

Fig. 30-1. *Typical angiographic appearance of a carotid body tumor. Initial injection view (1) demonstrates the characteristic "splaying" of the carotid bifurcation. Subsequent delayed views (2, 3, 4) show the anatomic extent of lesion and the degree of vascularity.*

mations, cerebral aneurysms, and significant siphon stenoses. Finally, some authors have reported the use of preoperative embolization as an adjunct before the resection of particularly large or highly vascular carotid body tumors. As such, although we have not found this necessary (and consider it potentially hazardous), one might qualify the ability to consider this treatment option as another potential advantage to support the use of angiography during the preoperative evaluation of these patients.

Unfortunately, the risks associated with cerebral angiography are numerous. First, this technique is an invasive procedure that requires arterial access, and wound complications are therefore not infrequent. Hematoma formation, acute arterial dissection, false aneurysms, and distal embolization have all been reported. The incidence of these complications has not been documented consistently; however, they probably occur in between 1 and 2 percent of cases. Second, catheter manipulation within the carotid artery can lead to serious complications as a result of either dissection or embolization. In one review of over 5000 cerebral angiographic procedures, the overall risk of neurologic

sequelae was 0.9 percent, with 0.06 percent of patients suffering a permanent stroke. Others have placed the risk of neurologic events and stroke at 2.6 and 0.6 percent, respectively. Although most of these reviews include patients being evaluated for atherosclerotic vascular disease and not carotid body tumors, it is probably accurate to estimate that, during cerebral angiography, the risk of a neurologic event is approximately 1 percent. Finally, the contrast injected during angiography can induce allergic reactions, renal failure, and alterations in the coagulation system. Allergic reactions range from mild rashes and gastrointestinal upset to life-threatening hypotension, bronchospasm, pulmonary edema, and cardiac arrhythmias. The risk of contrast reactions in all types of angiographic studies varies between 2 and 8 percent. For cerebral examinations, it is in the lower range, with a rate of approximately 2 percent. In high-risk patients with antecedent renal disease, the risk of acute renal failure following the administration of contrast can be as high as 40 percent, with over 8 percent of patients requiring permanent dialysis. Finally, depending on the institution, the cost of angiography is as high as $5000 per procedure.

In summary, angiography has long been considered the "gold standard" for the evaluation of patients with carotid body tumors. Indeed, some surgeons consider this examination mandatory before performing a resection of this neoplasm. However, as described, this imaging technique is not without risks, and with the emergence of newer noninvasive imaging modalities, others have questioned whether this study is really necessary in all cases. Also, because the morbidity of any preoperative examination must be added to the overall risk associated with the surgical intervention, methods of safely treating these generally benign tumors without routine angiography are even more desirable. These forces have led several investigators to attempt to gain experience managing these lesions without the benefit of angiographic data.

Duplex scanning has emerged as an accurate noninvasive method of evaluating patients with carotid body tumors. In terms of technical performance, it clearly has several advantages over angiography. The examination is noninvasive and involves little or no patient discomfort. In contrast to the multiple wound and contrast-related problems associated with angiog-

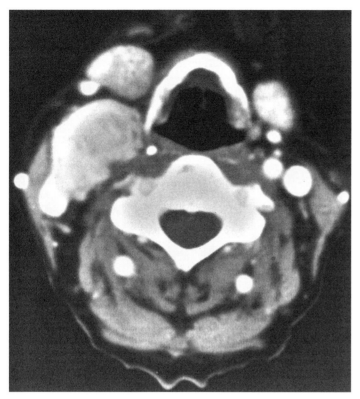

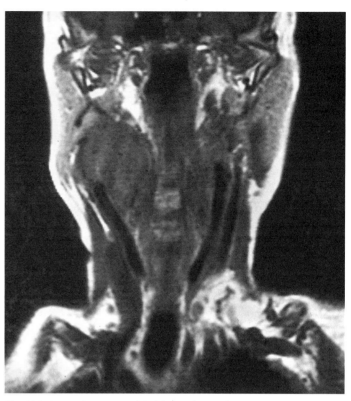

Fig. 30-2. Computed tomographic (CT) scan demonstrating large carotid body tumor with probable encasement of the external carotid artery.

Fig. 30-3. Magnetic resonance (MR) image showing large right-sided carotid body tumor.

raphy, duplex scanning is essentially without risk. The anatomic detail, while not as good as with angiography, is quite satisfactory. The tumor can be localized to the carotid bifurcation and, with the addition of color-flow technology, an estimate of the vascularity of the lesion can be obtained. Also, as with angiography, tumor size can be estimated and the bifurcation screened for evidence of tumor encasement or concomitant atherosclerotic disease. Finally, most hospitals charge approximately $300 to $400 for a duplex scan, or roughly one-tenth the cost of a cerebral angiogram.

The major limitation of duplex scanning is its inability to clearly image either the proximal or very distal areas within the neck. Both proximal and distal extensions of very large lesions will be poorly visualized. Also, any significant intracranial component to a tumor will invariably go unrecognized. In addition, this study is not as sensitive for very small lesions and, when compared to angiography, small occult tumors may not be readily identified. Likewise, potentially helpful detail such as the presence of an important aberrant blood vessel is unlikely to be obtained dur-

ing duplex scanning. Lastly, and perhaps most importantly, the reliability of any duplex study greatly depends on the individual performing the examination, and results obtained by different operators vary greatly.

When more information is required, both computed tomography (CT) and magnetic resonance (MR) scanning are useful techniques. Both tests can be extremely helpful, particularly in very large tumors or when multiple lesions are suspected (Figs. 30-2 and 30-3). Unlike with duplex scanning, large lesions can be defined even in the proximal or distal portions of the neck. Also, both studies can reveal tumor encasement of the vascular structures or invasion of an aggressive lesion into the base of the skull. Magnetic resonance images have the additional advantage of being able to be analyzed by software that reconstructs angiographic detail. These MR angiograms have gained popularity by virtue of their ability to noninvasively depict the cerebral vessels in a format similar to that of conventional arteriography. Whether these images possess enough accuracy to safely plan carotid body resec-

tions and replace conventional angiography remains unproven.

To summarize, the duplex scan is an accurate, noninvasive imaging technique that is useful for screening patients with neck masses. It can most often establish an association between the mass and the carotid bifurcation but frequently cannot provide enough anatomic detail to establish the diagnosis of a carotid body tumor or safely plan for its resection. Traditionally, most surgeons have used cerebral angiography to accomplish these goals; however, there is no question that arteriography exposes patients to an increased risk that must be added to the operative morbidity when calculating the overall risk of surgical therapy. Experience with CT and MR scanning is growing and both will undoubtedly have important future roles in the management of these patients.

Surgical Management

In experienced hands, the removal of a carotid body tumor can be accomplished with very low morbidity and mortality. However, several important operative principles must be appreciated to consistently achieve these results. It cannot be overemphasized that carotid body tumors are, as a rule, extremely vascular lesions. In fact, one can safely say that an inexperienced surgeon who does not appreciate this characteristic, and fails to plan his or her operative approach accordingly, will not soon forget the experience.

The senior author's technique for safe resection of even very large carotid body tumors is based on several observations. First, the majority of the blood supply to carotid body tumors arises from a rich matrix of small vessels that surround the bifurcation in a periadventitial plane and originate mostly from small branches of the external carotid artery. Second, perhaps because of this blood supply pattern, very large carotid body tumors frequently completely encase the external carotid artery but only rarely do the same to the internal. Third, all but the very smallest tumors will frequently distort the normal anatomy and often displace important cranial nerves away from their usual location. Lastly, it is critical to always bear in mind the relative importance of the internal carotid circulation compared to the external and its branches.

Together, these observations have influenced an operative approach that combines isolation and protection of the internal carotid system with the safe and bloodless resection of these highly vascular lesions. To avoid several unnecessary complications during the resection, it is extremely important to minimize bleeding during the dissection. Excessive hemorrhage will not infrequently persuade the inexperienced surgeon to attempt ill-advised maneuvers in order to control the bleeding. Unfortunately, these maneuvers are commonly the cause of postoperative cranial nerve injuries and strokes. Also, excessive bleeding can occasionally lead to unnecessary transfusions along with their well-known associated complications. Using the operative approach described below, the senior author has not recently had to administer blood products to a patient undergoing resection of even the largest of carotid body tumors.

Preoperative Embolization

One recent advance, which can aid in the management of very large and hypervascular carotid body tumors, is preoperative selective arterial embolization. Using a percutaneous catheter technique, the external carotid artery is selectively catheterized. Thrombogenic particles, such as Gelfoam or coils, are introduced into the large nutrient vessels that feed the tumor. This technique has been shown to be effective and can greatly facilitate the resection of very vascular tumors that would otherwise have been extremely difficult to approach safely. As we mentioned previously, we have not found this technique to be necessary in the majority of patients and have serious concerns about its safety. However, it is an available treatment adjunct and we recognize that certain individuals have acquired sufficient experience to perform this procedure with relatively low morbidity.

Anesthesia

Both local and general anesthesia are accepted techniques for this type of surgery. Local techniques usually include a regional cervical block in combination with direct skin infiltration of anesthetic agents. Regional cervical block is easily accomplished by infiltrating the cervical plexus with a mixture of 1% lidocaine (Xylocaine) and 0.5% bupivacaine hydrochloride (Marcaine). Rapid skin anesthesia with a prolonged duration can also be obtained by this combination. Subcutaneous injections, as well as deep injections along the posterior border of the sternocleidomastoid muscle to anesthetize the superficial nerves of the cervical plexus, complete the local block. Occasionally, additional injections within the carotid sheath may be required.

The advantages of local anesthesia are related to the avoidance of the cerebral and myocardial depressant effects of general anesthesia. The improved tolerance of the elderly or cardiac-impaired patient to local anesthesia allows for a safer operation in these high-risk individuals. Most surgeons, however, prefer general anesthesia for patients undergoing resection of carotid body tumors. It provides a more controlled operative setting including excellent airway control and less movement in the operative field.

Cerebral Monitoring and Protection

Because reconstruction, or at least temporary occlusion, of the internal carotid artery is occasionally necessary during resection of a carotid body tumor, we believe that some method of both cerebral monitoring and protection should always be utilized during resection of these lesions. Several techniques are available to monitor cerebral perfusion during carotid surgery. These include measurement of distal internal carotid artery back pressure, continuous scalp-recorded electroencephalographic (EEG) monitoring, and direct observation and continuous assessment of the awake patient. In general, although a conscious patient is a very sensitive intraoperative indicator of adequate cerebral blood flow, as was already mentioned, we prefer general anesthesia for operations on the carotid artery. At the University of California at Los Angeles (UCLA), our practice has been to utilize brain-mapping technology in conjunction with continuous scalp-recorded EEG in all patients undergoing carotid surgery. This technique utilizes several scalp electrodes normally placed over the distribution of the middle cerebral artery. The EEG is recorded continuously throughout the operation and represents the summation of cortical neuron postsynaptic potentials located beneath each electrode. The newer-generation machines equipped with brain-mapping capabilities utilize multiple electrodes and color output displays to divide each hemisphere into smaller monitoring parcels and therefore detect more focal abnormalities. Changes in the recorded EEG strongly correlate with alterations in cerebral blood flow. Cortical ischemia is detected by a reduction in the recorded wave amplitude or frequency. In those instances when carotid clamping produces measured cerebral ischemic changes, cerebral protection (using an internal carotid artery shunt) can then be employed.

As was mentioned previously, an alternative method of determining when cerebral protection is necessary is the internal carotid artery back pressure measurement. Using this technique, the adequacy of collateral blood flow to the ipsilateral hemisphere during proximal artery occlusion is determined by measurement of the back pressure. A 22-gauge needle is bent 2 cm from the tip, to an angle of 45 degrees, and connected to an arterial pressure transducer. The needle is inserted into the common carotid artery with the angulated tip lying longitudinally in the lumen and directed toward the bifurcation. First, an open carotid artery pressure is measured, and it should be compared to the peripheral radial artery catheter or cuff pressure to ensure that the carotid pressure transducer is functioning correctly. Then, with the external and proximal common carotid arteries temporarily occluded, the internal carotid artery back pressure is recorded. Although no precise consensus has been reached, most authorities define the range of 30 to 50 mm Hg as the pressure below which cerebral protection is mandatory. If this is the case, the clamps on the external and proximal common carotid arteries are removed and preparations are made for use of an internal bypass shunt.

Whichever method of cerebral monitoring is used, once it is determined that cerebral perfusion is inadequate during carotid cross-clamping, the ipsilateral cerebral cortex must be protected by insertion of a temporary internal bypass shunt. Safe placement of a carotid artery shunt requires an appreciation of several principles. Most importantly, full exposure of all three major carotid vessels is mandatory. This allows complete proximal common carotid control and full appreciation of the distal extent of any concomitant atherosclerotic disease in both the internal and external carotid arteries. With the internal and external carotid arteries controlled, the common carotid is occluded proximally with a soft clamp. The arteriotomy in the common carotid vessel should be placed comfortably away from the proximal extent of the tumor. The distal internal carotid is allowed to back bleed and an internal shunt with an appropriate diameter is gently inserted. We prefer to use the Javid shunt; however, other types are available. The shunt is flushed, clamped, and subsequently inserted into the common carotid artery proximally. Snares (Rumel tourniquets) are used to secure the shunt, and the occluding clamp on the common carotid is removed. Thus, in the final configuration, the shunt is in place with only a single occluding clamp in its midportion. One should remove this clamp slowly, watching carefully for air or debris, which may be visible through the proximal portion of the shunt. Once the shunt is in place and cerebral protection accomplished, attention can be directed toward resection of the tumor. If reconstruction of the internal carotid becomes necessary, it is possible to maintain cerebral perfusion at all times by performing a by-pass over the shunt while it remains in situ. Following completion of the procedure, the shunt is clamped and removed, and the carotid vessels are flushed beginning distally, as always. The arteriotomy closure is then completed, with the vessels temporarily occluded. Alternatively, a Satinsky partially occluding clamp can be used to maintain anterograde flow while the arteriotomy is being repaired.

Exposure

The patient should be positioned supine on the operating table and the head rotated away from the operative side. The head of the table is raised 10 to 15 degrees, which reduces venous pressure and minimizes incisional blood loss. Depending on individual differences in body habitus, the neck can be extended by the placement of a small towel roll beneath the shoulders.

A longitudinal incision is made that follows the anterior border of the sternocleidomastoid muscle (Fig. 30-4). The approximate position of the carotid bifurcation can often be determined by palpation of the lesion or from the preoperative diagnostic studies. Ideally, the incision should be centered longitudinally so that the bifurcation is below the midpoint. When necessary for additional exposure, this incision can be continued down to the sternal notch, and cephalad to the mastoid process. The plane of dissection remains along the anterior border of the sternocleidomastoid until the belly of this muscle can be reflected off the carotid sheath. Often the posterior tail of the parotid gland is encountered at this level and when this occurs further dissection is required. The gland should be mobilized and reflected anteriorly rather than divided. Transecting the gland can cause excessive bleeding and occasionally lead to a salivary fistula. Once the carotid sheath is visualized, it should be opened along the anterior border of the jugular vein, which can usually be easily identified through the sheath. The jugular vein is mobilized completely and any large branches identified. The common facial vein is a broad-based tributary that commonly joins the jugular vein just above the carotid bifurcation. This vein provides a useful marker for the location of the carotid bifurcation and, once identified, it should be divided between ligatures. Particularly in high bifurcations, the hypoglossal nerve can also be located deep to the facial vein and care must be taken to avoid inadvertent injury to this structure.

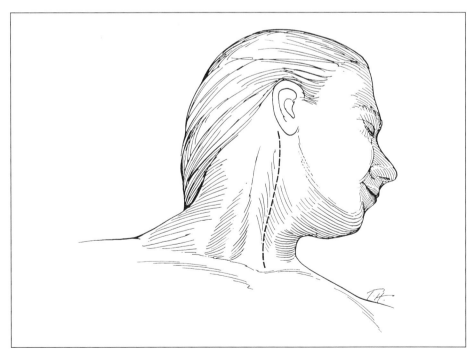

Fig. 30-4. Location of the incision along the anterior border of the sternocleidomastoid muscle with the head rotated away from the operative side. For additional cephalad exposure, the incision can be curved posteriorly and extended across the mastoid process behind the ear.

After the facial vein is divided, the jugular vein can be reflected laterally, providing exposure of the carotid vessels (Fig. 30-5). The vagus nerve, which is ordinarily posterior, can be located anywhere within the carotid sheath. Therefore, in each case, its course must be identified and protected to avoid injury. The laryngeal nerves, which are usually recurrent, can arise directly off the vagus and cross anterior to the carotid artery at this level where it enters the vocal musculature. When not recognized, division of this nerve will lead to vocal paralysis. It should also be mentioned that, although this anomaly is more common on the left side, its presence has also been described on the right.

Once the sheath has been entered and all pertinent structures identified and protected, the common carotid artery is sufficiently mobilized proximally to allow complete delineation of the extent of disease, and to provide sufficient length in case a bypass shunt is required. Next, the bifurcation and external and internal carotid arteries are mobilized in a similar fashion. Reflex bradycardia can occur during manipulation of the carotid bulb as a result of stimulation of the carotid body. This can be prevented, or reversed when necessary, by a local injection of an anesthetic agent to block the nerves that arise from the carotid body. The external and internal carotid arteries must be mobilized for a sufficient length to clearly identify the distal extent of the tumor. The hypoglossal nerve must be carefully identified, particularly when the internal carotid artery is mobilized.

Extended Exposure Techniques

When one encounters a very large tumor that extends up toward the base of the skull, or when a particular patient's carotid artery bifurcates high in the neck, it may be necessary to obtain additional exposure in the superior aspect of the incision. Several techniques have been described to increase exposure in this area, and surgeons performing carotid surgery should be familiar with these maneuvers. The simplest and most important technique is to extend the skin incision completely across the mastoid process behind the ear. This allows additional mobilization of the sternocleidomastoid muscle up to its tendinous insertion. The spinal accessory nerve enters the muscle at this level and must be preserved. When additional exposure is necessary, the posterior belly of the digastric muscle can be detached from its origin, the mastoid process. The digastric muscle consists of two muscle bellies united by a rounded tendon. The posterior belly arises from the mastoid process and the anterior portion inserts on the mandibular symphysis. It is helpful to appreciate the superficial anatomic position of the posterior digastric muscle when dissecting in this area. All important neurovascular structures lie deep to the digastric at this level. Only the external jugular vein, and branches of the facial and great auricular nerves, pass superficial to the posterior belly of the digastric. Below the muscle, particular care must be taken to avoid injury to the hypoglossal and spinal accessory nerves as well as the facial branch of the external carotid artery. In addition, it should be mentioned that the stylohyoid muscle can also be divided. This muscle stretches between the styloid process and the hyoid bone, and its removal, along with that of the styloid process, can provide additional exposure of the distal internal carotid artery at the base of the skull. When the tumor extends very high, it is possible to gain additional exposure by anteriorly subluxating the condylar process of the mandible. The displaced mandible can be secured in place with wires. This maneuver alters the geometry at the base of the skull by turning a triangular space into a rectangle, thereby enlarging the operative field. Lastly, techniques by which the ramus of the mandible is divided have also been described. This is an involved procedure that greatly complicates the postoperative course of these patients. Fortunately, in our experience, we have never found this maneuver necessary.

Resection of the Tumor

After completion of the exposure, the initial dissection is directed toward the proximal common and distal carotid branches, staying away initially from the area of the carotid bifurcation. Control of the common, internal, and external carotid arteries should be obtained before dissection of the tumor. Very small tumors can be approached directly and a periadventitial dissection plane can usually be developed. However, as was mentioned earlier, these lesions are typically extremely vascular and, especially in large adherent tumors,

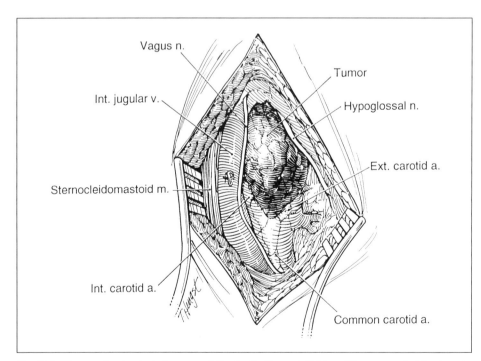

Fig. 30-5. Diagram showing typical exposure following ligation and division of the common facial vein and lateral retraction of the sternocleidomastoid muscle and jugular vein.

the correct plane for safe dissection is often difficult to locate adjacent to the bifurcation. Therefore, we suggest placing a vessel loop on the proximal common carotid artery, as well as on both the internal and external carotid vessels distal to the tumor, before beginning the resection. Our first concern during the dissection is to resect the tumor away from the internal branch of the carotid artery and preserve normal intracranial perfusion. Thus, after control has been achieved with vessel loops, the extensive periadventitial matrix of small vessels is ligated with fine suture, beginning at a convenient spot along the common carotid proximal to the lesion (Fig. 30-6). This dissection is continued distally, following the course of the internal carotid artery along a longitudinal plane located 180 degrees opposite the takeoff of the external carotid branch (Fig. 30-7). Since carotid body tumors frequently grow around the external carotid while pushing away the internal, beginning the dissection in a plane opposite the origin of the external is the safest technique for isolating and separating the tumor from the cerebral cir-

culation. Once the periadventitial vessels have all been divided to a point beyond the distal extent of the tumor, the dissection is directed proximally toward the bifurcation along the inner surface of the internal carotid (Fig. 30-8). At this point, the tumor is carefully separated from the bifurcation. Nutrient vessels supplying the tumor are often encountered in this location and should be ligated. When the tumor is very large or particularly adherent, division of the origin of the external carotid artery can be a useful maneuver. This allows rotational mobilization of the lesion and, because feeding vessels often arise from branches of the external carotid, can reduce blood loss (Fig. 30-9). Otherwise, it is usually possible to meticulously dissect the carotid body tumor away from the external carotid and its branches, ligating each nutrient tumor vessel as it is encountered (Fig. 30-10). Rarely, resection of the tumor cannot be accomplished without complete removal of the carotid bifurcation. This situation is almost always indicative of malignancy. When necessary, vascular reconstruction can be accomplished

by the placement of an interposition graft. We prefer to repair the carotid using a prosthetic bypass graft. Others have advocated the use of autologous vein for these reconstructions.

Wound Closure

Closure of the incision following a carotid body tumor resection should be meticulous and adhere to all of the basic principles of surgery. The wound should be irrigated generously with warm saline solution and perfect hemostasis assured. The platysma is reapproximated with a running suture and the skin is closed with either subcuticular sutures or stainless steel staples. We only very rarely place a drain but, should this option be selected, it should be a closed suction drain system that is placed beneath the platysmal layer and brought out through a separate stab wound. Lastly, a sterile dressing is applied and the patient observed carefully while awakening from anesthesia.

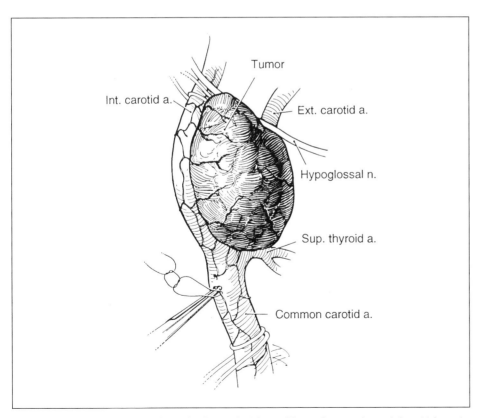

Fig. 30-6. After obtaining proximal and distal control with vessel loops, the extensive periadventitial matrix of small tumor feeding vessels is ligated with fine suture, beginning along the proximal common carotid artery in an area located 180 degrees opposite the takeoff of the external carotid.

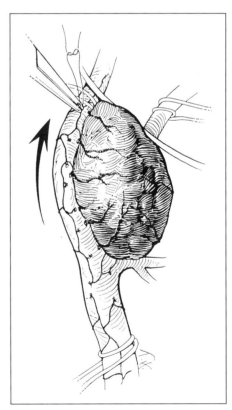

Fig. 30-7. The dissection is continued cephalad, following the course of the internal carotid artery, again staying in a periadventitial longitudinal plane located 180 degrees opposite the origin of the external carotid artery.

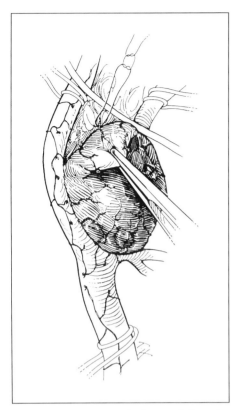

Fig. 30-8. Once the tumor feeding vessels located along the internal carotid have all been divided to a point beyond the distal extent of the tumor, the dissection is continued proximally toward the bifurcation along the inner surface of the internal carotid.

Postoperative Care

Immediately after the patient awakens from anesthesia, a preliminary neurologic assessment should be made. Subsequently, the patient is transferred to the recovery room, followed by the intensive care unit, for careful monitoring during the first 24 hours after surgery. Particular attention should be made to frequently assess the systemic blood pressure and neurologic function during this period. In addition, careful wound observation is essential to detect the formation of a hematoma, which can threaten the patient's airway. After 24 hours the closed suction drain, if placed, can be removed and the patient returned to the general hospital ward. Most patients undergoing carotid surgery are admitted to the hospital the morning of operation and are discharged home on the second or third postoperative day. Before discharge, the skin staples are replaced with adhesive Steri-Strips and an appointment is made for the patient to re-

turn within 2 to 3 weeks for the first postoperative visit.

Radiation Therapy

For completeness a comment regarding the use of radiation therapy, either as an adjunct or as a primary therapeutic option in the treatment of carotid body tumors, is appropriate. Traditionally, the statement has been made that cervical paragangliomas are not radiosensitive lesions. Unfortunately, very few clinicians have acquired a sufficient experience to make sound conclusions regarding the efficacy of this treatment modality in this setting. Most often radiation is reserved for bulky, inoperable, or recurrent tumors, which may account for the disappointing reported results. There are in fact a number of sporadic reports in the literature indicating successful control of carotid body tumors by radiotherapy. Long-term follow-up for most of these anecdotal cases is currently not available. We admit little experience with this method of treating these tumors and, due to the safety and excellent documented long-term success, continue to recommend surgical resection for the majority of our patients. We acknowledge, however, that in poor surgical candidates with aggressive symptomatic lesions, radiotherapy may have a role in the management of carotid body tumors. Clearly this form of treatment requires further investigation.

Complications

An uncomplicated resection of a carotid body tumor is an extremely well-tolerated operation. The tissue trauma and operative blood loss are normally minimal and patients are routinely discharged from the hospital on the second or third postoperative day. For this reason, perioperative complications are particularly discouraging and must be avoided at all costs. Operative intervention, particularly in the setting of a histologically benign neoplasm, will only continue to be justified by keeping the operative morbidity and mortality of the procedure to a minimum.

Of course, technical errors that occur during any operative procedure are preventable. As was mentioned earlier, one major cause of technical complications occurring

during the resection of carotid body tumors is inadequate hemostasis. Clamping of incompletely identified structures or the temporary occlusion of major cerebrovascular vessels can lead to cranial nerve or neurologic injuries.

As was described previously, several peripheral nerves must be identified and protected during exposure of the carotid bifurcation. The frequency of injury to these structures is difficult to quantitate but it is probably in the range of 1 to 15 percent. This difference is due, at least in part, to the variable expertise of the individual making the assessment. It must also be remembered that many cranial nerve deficits are related to tumor involvement and not caused intraoperatively. Once again, the importance of carefully examining these structures preoperatively cannot be overemphasized. Nonetheless, at least half of all postoperative cranial nerve injuries go unnoticed by both the surgeon and the patient. The remainder are usually either very obvious or otherwise only identified following a detailed examination. Most of these injuries, fortunately, are not permanent. It should be acknowledged, however, that all cranial nerve injuries that occur during carotid surgery can be prevented if surgeons become familiar with the normal and possible abnormal anatomic neurovascular relationships and carefully protect these structures during the procedure.

Results

Today, results following resections for carotid body tumors are excellent. However, this has not always been the case. Early series from the 1950s consistently reported a mortality of 5 to 15 percent of patients, cranial nerve injuries in 30 to 40 percent, and significant cerebrovascular complications in as many as 10 to 20 percent. Advances in preoperative diagnosis and localization, intraoperative anesthetic and surgical management, and postoperative care have all contributed to a significant decrease in these complication rates. Today, in experienced hands, a perioperative mortality of less than 0.5 percent, essentially no significant cerebrovascular sequelae, and a cranial nerve injury or other minor complication rate of no higher than 5 percent can be expected.

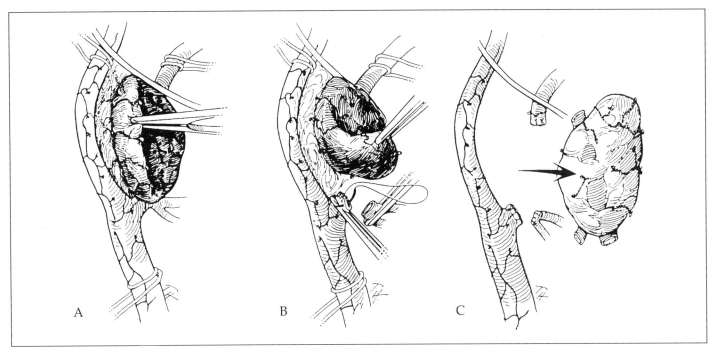

Fig. 30-9. When the tumor is very large or particularly adherent, division of the origin of the external carotid artery can be a useful maneuver. Following detachment of the tumor from the internal carotid artery, the tumor is carefully separated from the bifurcation (A). Next the origin of the external carotid is clamped and divided (B). This allows rotational mobilization of the lesion and ligation of nutrient tumor vessels, which are often encountered posteriorly in this location. Finally, division of the superior thyroid and distal external carotid artery (or its branches) allows for the safe removal of the carotid body lesion (C).

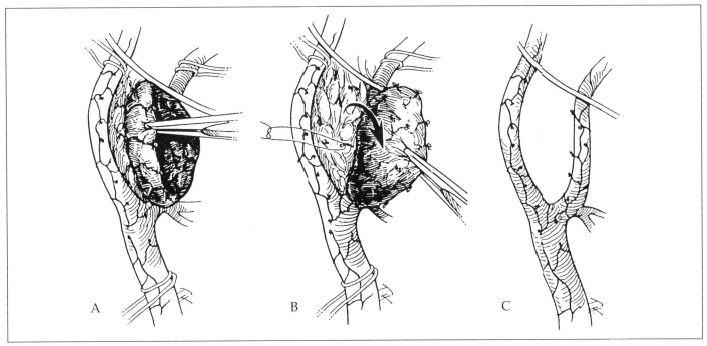

Fig. 30-10. Alternatively, with careful dissection, it is frequently possible to remove the carotid body tumor without sacrificing the external carotid artery or any of its main branches. Once again, the tumor is carefully separated from the bifurcation (A). Again, by rotating the lesion along the axis of the external carotid, nutrient vessels supplying the tumor posteriorly can usually be ligated easily (B). Finally, the carotid body tumor is meticulously dissected free, leaving the carotid bifurcation intact (C).

Suggested Reading

Bernard RP. Carotid body tumors. *Am J Surg* 163:494, 1992.

Grufferman S, Gillamn MW, Pasternak RL, et al. Familial carotid body tumors. Case report and epidemiologic review. *Cancer* 46:2116, 1980.

Hallett JW, Nora JD, Hollier LH, et al. Trends in neurovascular complications of surgical management for carotid body and cervical paragangliomas: A fifty-year experience with 153 tumors. *J Vasc Surg* 7:284, 1988.

Kraus DH, Sterman BM, Hakaim AG, et al. Carotid body tumors. *Arch Otolaryngol Head Neck Surg* 116:1384, 1990.

LaMuraglia GM, Fabian RL, Brewster DC, et al. The current surgical management of carotid body paragangliomas. *J Vasc Surg* 15:1038, 1992.

McCabe DP, Vaccaro PS, James AG. Treatment of carotid body tumors. *J Cardiovasc Surg* 31:356, 1990.

Nora JD, Hallett JW, O'Brien PC, et al. Surgical resection of carotid body tumors: Long-term survival, recurrence, and metastasis. *Mayo Clin Proc* 63:348, 1988.

Rabl H, Friehs, I, Gutschi S, et al. Diagnosis and treatment of carotid body tumors. *Thorac Cardiovasc Surg* 41:340, 1993.

Sanghvi VD, Chandawarkar RY. Carotid body tumors. *J Surg Oncol* 54:190, 1993.

Smith LL, Ajalat GM. Tumors of the carotid body: Diagnosis, prognosis, and surgical management. In WS Moore (ed), *Surgery for Cerebrovascular Disease*. New York: Churchill Livingstone, 1987. Pp 579–588.

Wax MK, Briant TDR. Carotid body tumors: A review. *J Otolaryngol* 21:277, 1992.

Worsey MJ, Laborde AL, Bower T, et al. An evaluation of color duplex scanning in the primary diagnosis and management of carotid body tumors. *Ann Vasc Surg* 6:90, 1992.

EDITOR'S COMMENT

This excellent account of the ability to remove carotid body tumors, as well as the discussion concerning the embryology and function, is indicative of a master vascular surgeon who has been there. This is not child's play, as the authors indicate. Doctor Moore is well known for his writings on carotid body tumors. The careful preparation, meticulous dissection, and testing for continued cerebral profusion when the common carotid artery can be clamped, by back pressure and the use of a Javid shunt, are all important aspects of the dissection.

In prior decades, removal of a carotid body tumor resulted in significant mortality, a fairly high occurrence of stroke rate, and neurologic damage, as the authors have indicated. A recent review of 1181 published cases treated through surgical resection reveals a continuing high surgical mortality and complication rate; 3.2 percent of patients undergoing surgical intervention died. Aphagia and hemiplegia occurred in 6.3 percent of the patients.

More importantly, the internal carotid artery was injured in 23.2 percent of the cases and the cranial nerve in 22 percent. Amazingly, arteriography was used in only 52 percent of the cases, but was diagnostic in all instances. A review of the central nervous system complications and deaths revealed that all of the complications and all but one death occurred in the subgroup of patients with an injured internal carotid artery and that many of those whose arteries were injured did not have preoperative assessment with angiography. The majority of the injuries were repaired intraoperatively through simple arteriography, with 3.2 percent neurologic sequelae. In 32 percent of the cases of arterial injury, the internal carotid artery was ligated, with a 66 percent prevalence of stroke and a 46 percent mortality. As Dr. Moore would agree, this should almost never happen and is the result of lack of angiographic appreciation of the extent of the tumor and of what one is dealing with. One cannot disagree with the conclusion of Drs. Moore and Colburn: "Today, in experienced hands, a perioperative mortality of less than 0.5 percent, essentially no significant cerebrovascular sequelae, and a cranial nerve injury or other minor complication rate of no higher than 5 percent can be expected." In order to achieve this paradigm, preoperative evaluation, including arteriography, duplex evaluation, and MRI, and careful perioperative preparation and meticulous intraoperative technique are essential.

J.E.F.

IV
Larynx and Trachea

31

Resection of the Larynx and the Pharynx for Cancer

Kerry D. Olsen   Lawrence W. DeSanto

The larynx is a complex neuromuscular system of fixed and mobile cartilages that serve to separate the digestive and respiratory tracts. Phonation is an adaptive function of the larynx. Cancers of the larynx are relatively common; in North America, more than 10,000 new patients with laryngeal cancer are treated each year.

Some parts of the larynx are not required for continued function of the valve. The concept of a simplified larynx as the end result of cancer treatment requires a precise definition of the various tumors. One can no longer think in general terms of cancer of the larynx or even in terms of cancer of its major divisions. A precise, three-dimensional definition of the lesion and a clear understanding of the biologic potential of each growth are essential for treatment planning.

The TNM (tumor, nodes, metastasis) classification system is designed for end-stage reporting; its use for treatment planning appears attractive but is not satisfactory. The TNM system preceded many of the ongoing refinements in operations on parts of the larynx for cancer and the expanding concept of the simplified larynx. There are certain principles that are more useful in treatment planning than the TNM classification system alone. The first principle is that treatment planning requires a precise definition of the tumor.

The major subdivisions of the larynx are the glottic, supraglottic, and subglottic areas (Fig. 31-1). Each subdivision has its characteristic cancers (Figs. 31-2, 31-3, and

31-4).A fourth type of laryngeal cancer is transglottic cancer, which overlaps two or more of the traditional areas (Fig. 31-5).

Glottic Cancer

The glottic area is that portion of the larynx defined by the paired vocal folds and the anterior junction of these folds—the anterior commissure. The vertical dimension of the glottic area can be considered to ex-

tend from the midportion of the ventricle above to the upper border of the cricoid cartilage below. Posteriorly, the glottis extends at least to the vocal process of the arytenoid cartilage.

In our practice, glottic cancers are the most frequently seen cancers within the larynx. Of 1112 cancers of the larynx reviewed during a 12-year period ending in 1975, 832 were glottic. All were squamous cell carcinomas.

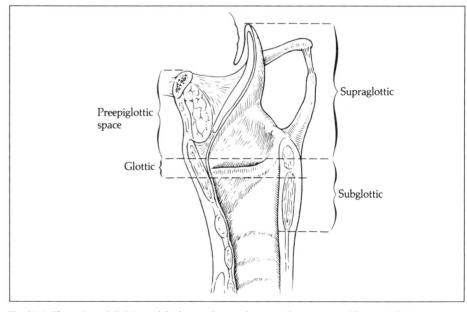

Fig. 31-1. The major subdivisions of the larynx that can be seen at laryngoscopy. The preepiglottic space cannot be evaluated topographically, but it is a major consideration in treating cancers of the larynx. The preepiglottic space is that area anterior to the epiglottis bordered by the hyoid bone, thyrohyoid membrane, and superior rim of the thyroid cartilage. Supraglottic cancer has direct access to this space through preformed foramina in the epiglottis. (From LW DeSanto, BW Pearson. Initial treatment of laryngeal cancer: Principles of selection. Minn Med 64:691, 1981. With permission.)

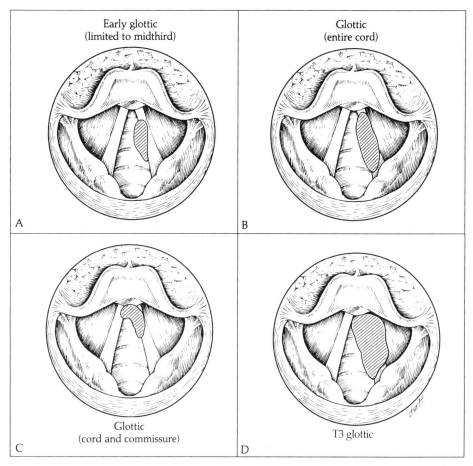

Early glottic (limited to midthird)	Glottic (entire cord)
A	B
Glottic (cord and commissure)	T3 glottic
C	D

Fig. 31-2. Representative laryngoscopic views of invasive glottic cancers in a range of severity from early lesions to moderately advanced growths. All are lesions for which partial operation is possible. A. Lesion can be removed endoscopically if it can be totally exposed; otherwise, laryngofissure with cordectomy is appropriate. B. Lesion extends from front to back on the mobile cord. This growth is too extensive for endoscopic treatment but is ideal for laryngofissure and cordectomy. C. Lesion involves the anterior commissure and one cord. This lesion is best managed by the frontolateral variation of the partial vertical operations. D. Lesion is bulky and invasive but limited to the cordal area on one side. Laryngofissure with cordectomy may not be sufficient, and total laryngectomy may be too radical. If the thyroid cartilage is not invaded by cancer, hemilaryngectomy may be suitable. Intraoperative advice from the surgical pathologist is important.

It is both important and possible for glottic cancers to be diagnosed early because their presenting symptom of hoarseness is well recognized as a danger sign of cancer. Cancers no bigger than a microbiopsy forceps on the free edge of the vocal cord alter the voice. At this early stage, most glottic cancers can be successfully treated.

In Situ Cancer and Other Epithelial Changes

Whether cancer arises from normal epithelium or from benign but unhealthy and histologically abnormal epithelium is a debated question. A plethora of descriptive terms is used in discussions of epithelial changes on the vocal cords that are not actually invasive cancer. Some of these terms are *leukoplakia, atypia, keratosis, pachydermia, epithelial hyperplasia,* and *cancer in situ.* These histologic conditions cannot be differentiated visually at laryngoscopy. The descriptive term used is of little importance if each lesion is treated appropriately by removal at laryngoscopy. Each of these changes indicates an unhealthy epithelium, but the words used by the pathologist tell nothing of the ultimate threat to the larynx.

A consensus seems to exist that carcinoma in situ of the larynx is a more serious prob-

lem than keratosis, atypia, or so-called leukoplakia. This is not a completely rational consensus. To begin with, not all pathologists agree on what is carcinoma in situ and what is epithelial atypia. The two probably merge into one another as a spectrum of severity, and the point at which one change of epithelium begins and the other ends is a matter for individual judgment. There is uncertainty as to whether or not in situ cancer evolves inevitably into frank invasive carcinoma. It probably does. If it does, invasive cancer develops over months or even years but certainly not in days or weeks.

In situ cancer of the glottic larynx is best treated endoscopically by removing the diseased epithelium. More aggressive treatment, such as radiation or partial laryngectomy, is rarely necessary. Extensive carcinoma in situ or microinvasive carcinoma that involves the anterior commissure area or wide regions of the subglottic larynx can be treated endoscopically. However, recurrence in this region or extensive disease that cannot be visualized or removed endoscopically can be treated with radiation therapy. Patients must be encouraged to stop smoking, and frequent observation of the larynx is essential. Most of the in situ cancers are small and can be removed endoscopically. At the Mayo Clinic, more than 200 patients have been treated for early lesions labeled as in situ cancer by the pathologist. There have been few recurrences, and the need for further treatment after careful removal at laryngoscopy has been infrequent.

Invasive Glottic Cancer

An early glottic cancer is a lesion of the true vocal cord and anterior commissure that has not invaded the cord sufficiently to limit vocal cord motion. Vocal cord mobility is the single most important factor in the staging and treatment of glottic cancers. A patient with cancer of the glottic larynx who has normal cord mobility is usually a candidate for endoscopic removal or a partial laryngeal operation. This operation preserves all the glottic functions. Whether a patient is treated surgically, however, depends on other factors besides the cancer, such as the patient's age, general health, and preference; the importance of voice quality to the patient; and his or her availability and reliability for follow-up care. Most patients with la-

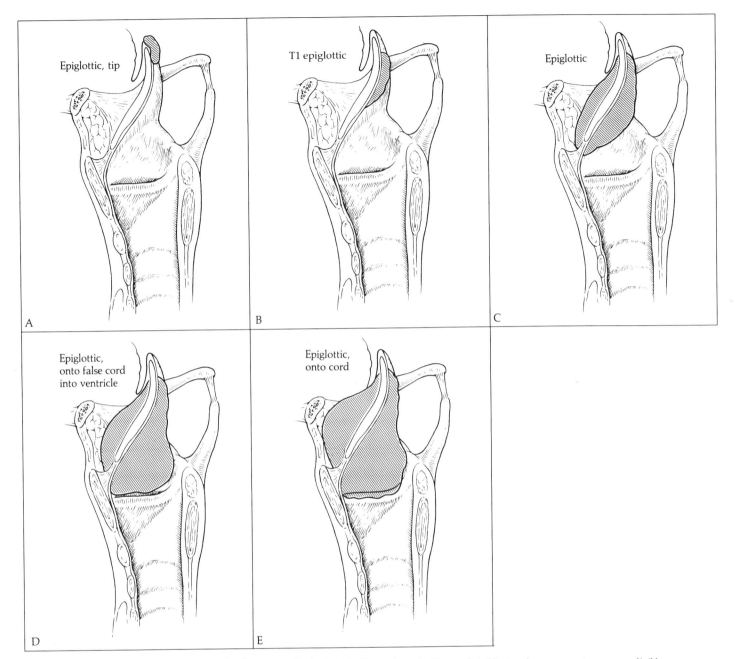

Fig. 31-3. The range of supraglottic cancers. A. Small tumor at tip of epiglottis. Cancer is rarely diagnosed at this stage because symptoms are negligible or overlooked. When the lesion is diagnosed, it may be possible simply to amputate the epiglottic tip transorally using the suspension laryngoscope. B and C. Typical early epiglottic cancers. Although they may involve aryepiglottic folds, false vocal cords, and preepiglottic space, tumors of this dimension are suitable for supraglottic partial operation. D. The largest supraglottic cancer that can be managed safely by supraglottic partial operation. This tumor is almost to the cordal level, and its suitability for excision is ultimately determined at operation with frozen section guidance. Lower margins of a few millimeters are safe if they can be established during an operation. E. When the lesion extends downward onto the vocal cords, total laryngectomy is the safest operation.

ryngeal cancer are men; at our last review, 97 percent of the patients with early glottic cancers were men. Not surprisingly, as the incidence of smoking has risen dramatically in women, a marked increase in the number of female patients with cancer of the larynx is now occurring.

The continuing debate on the subject of radiation versus surgical therapy for early glottic cancers revolves mostly around the issue of voice quality. Most physicians involved in the selection of treatment for patients with early glottic cancers recognize that only minor differences exist in patient

survival rates between these two treatments. These differences may relate more to the subtleties of patient selection and data analysis than to intrinsic differences in their potential for eliminating disease. Because the issue of living or dying is not really a consideration in patients with

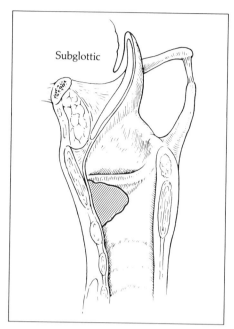

Fig. 31-4. Subglottic cancer. This type is rare; only about 5 percent of cancers of the larynx originate in the subglottic area. Diagnosis is often delayed, and laryngectomy is almost always necessary.

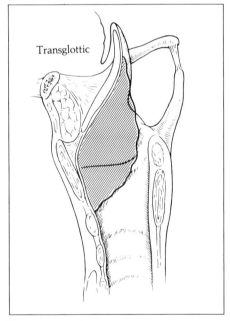

Fig. 31-5. Transglottic cancer. This type is usually large, involves all areas of the larynx, and requires laryngectomy.

early cancers, survivorship numbers alone are not adequate in the selection of therapy.

If it were simply acknowledged that either radiation skillfully delivered or a laryngeal operation skillfully performed is appro-

priate to eliminate early glottic cancers, then the debate would end. The treatment choice would become the patient's choice and not the clinician's. The issue is an attitudinal one, and most patients, given an objective appraisal of the options, make a thoughtful and appropriate choice. Surgical intervention alters the voice, but it can be done quickly and safely, whereas radiation, if successful, leaves most patients with an unaltered voice. Radiation takes longer, and the outcome is not known as early as it is with surgical treatment, for which the margins can be determined by the pathologist in the operating room.

Radiation for early growths might be considered excessive treatment for young patients with cancer of the glottic larynx. Radiation is usually considered a one-time treatment. If one recognizes the field nature of cancer, the use of radiation early in life may be untimely because of the risk of another upper-airway cancer.

These issues, rather than the question of living and dying, are the important factors in the choice of treatment of early glottic cancers.

Endoscopic Removal of Early Glottic Cancer

Early cancers of the glottic larynx have been successfully managed endoscopically since the report by Lynch in 1920. He described the successful treatment of nine cases managed by the transoral route. In 1973, Lilly and DeSanto presented their results of a large series of invasive and in situ T1 glottic cancers that were managed via the endoscopic route. Strong and others have shown increasing success using the carbon dioxide laser to treat early glottic cancer. In situ tumors or small, midcord lesions that are superficially invasive can be easily managed endoscopically as a simple outpatient procedure. These lesions can be effectively eradicated via the use of microlaryngoscopy instrumentation or a laser.

For large, invasive tumors that are limited to the mobile vocal cord and do not extend to the anterior commissure area, an endoscopic cordectomy can be performed. The lesion must be able to be completely visualized via a laryngoscope and there should be no extension to the subglottic area, ventricle, or false cord. Individual exceptions, however, do occur when there is coexisting in situ or very superficial inva-

sion at the anterior commissure area or onto the opposite cord that can also be managed endoscopically.

In general, invasive cancer at the anterior commissure area cannot be predictably managed by the endoscopic approach. The depth of invasion and ability to obtain free surgical margins are difficult. In the absence of anterior commissure invasion, large invasive tumors can be effectively eradicated via an endoscopic cordectomy.

For endoscopic procedures, we have not discerned any special advantage with the use of conventional microsurgical instruments, the cautery, or the laser. One report of 34 patients who underwent endoscopic cordectomy found local recurrence in 4 individuals (11.8%). These 4 patients were all successfully managed with further operation, 1 with a laryngofissure-cordectomy, 2 with a second endoscopic procedure, and the last patient with a total laryngectomy. No patient had recurrence after the first salvage operation and no patient died of known laryngeal cancer. The vocal quality after endoscopic cordectomy is acceptable and generally improved compared to the dysphonia caused by their tumor. The defect is allowed to heal secondarily and the amount of scarring often approximates the appearance of a normal vocal cord.

Although some surgeons now aggressively treat invasive laryngeal cancer at the anterior commissure area with laser ablation, we believe that invasive squamous cell carcinoma of the anterior commissure area is a contraindication to the endoscopic approach. At the anterior commissure area, only 2 to 3 mm separates cordal tissue from the underlying cartilage, and a T1 cancer can rapidly become a T4 lesion. The finding of invasive cancer extending to the anterior commissure area is the main indication for our current use of an open or partial vertical operation for early glottic cancer.

Partial Vertical Operation for Early Glottic Cancer

Laryngofissure with a cordectomy is the keystone procedure from which all other partial vertical operations evolve. Cordectomy via laryngofissure is not often performed but is utilized for a large bulky carcinoma with obvious deep extension on a mobile vocal cord when the anterior commissure area is not involved with invasive cancer. A secondary reason for performing a cordectomy via laryngofissure may be the inability to adequately visualize a tumor for an endoscopic procedure. The tumor can extend beneath the vocal cord but not for a distance greater than 5 mm. The tumor can extend onto the vocal process but should not involve the body of the arytenoid. The capability to have frozen section evaluation for margins is necessary for all laryngeal surgical procedures (see Fig. 31-2A and B).

Technique

1. The skin incision can be either vertical or horizontal (Fig. 31-6A). We prefer a horizontal incision slightly higher than that used in thyroidectomy. After the skin flap (including the platysma muscle) is elevated to the level of the hyoid bone, a tracheotomy is placed and the anesthesia tube and anesthetic equipment are repositioned to the side of the patient opposite the surgeon. The anesthesia tube and equipment should be readied early in the procedure, before the team begins the operation.

2. After the strap muscles are retracted laterally, an incision is made into the airway lumen through the cricothyroid membrane (Fig. 31-6B).

3. The thyroid cartilage is cut vertically from the thyroid notch above to the cricothyroid ligament below (Fig. 31-6C). An oscillating saw is used because the thyroid cartilage usually is partially ossified. The saw cut should extend through the full thickness of the cartilage. This can be detected by a distinct "pop" as the last bit of cartilage is divided.

   The cartilage cut can vary slightly from one side or the other from the midline, depending on the position of the growth. If the growth clearly is away from the anterior extremity of the cord, the precise midline cut is appropriate. If the lesion approaches the anterior end of the cord, the cut through the cartilage should be moved off to the opposite side by a few millimeters. The cartilage cut should be made at a right angle to the thyroid cartilage regardless of its position. If the cut is angled, the cord that remains can be filleted lengthwise by the oscillating saw.

4. The mucous membrane of the subglottic larynx and the anterior commissure is incised (Fig. 31-6D) by placing hooks into the opening that has been made through the cricothyroid membrane and gently retracting them laterally through the opening. By careful incision of the tense mucosa vertically and upward, one can gradually widen the fissure and eventually view directly the undersurface of both cords and their junction at the anterior commissure. The upward incision continues through the commissure or the front portion of the uninvolved cord. Farther upward passage of the knife and progressive upward repositioning of the hooks allow the larynx to open similarly to the opening of a book. Both cords can then be directly visualized (Fig. 31-6E).

5. A plane is easily dissected between the internal perichondrium of the thyroid cartilage and the thyroarytenoid (vocalis) muscle (Fig. 31-6F). Under direct vision, mucosal cuts are then made around the cord and the tumor. We prefer to make these cuts with a needle-tipped electrocoagulation current. The cord and an appropriate margin of normal mucosa above and below can be dissected off the cartilage (Fig. 31-6G). Often an artery is divided at this time, resulting in brisk bleeding, but this bleeding is best ignored for a few seconds while the scissors pass behind the specimen and the specimen is snipped off. This scissors cut usually passes through the vocal process of the arytenoid cartilage in the simple cordectomy (Fig. 31-6H). The bleeding in the bed of the specimen can then be electrocoagulated easily.

   Some authors recommend a mucosal closure of the raw area after removing the specimen. We prefer to leave this area open (Fig. 31-6I). A scar that is eventually epithelialized fills the gap. Sometimes, after a year or more, the epithelialized scar has the appearance of and moves like a normal vocal cord; even an experienced eye has difficulty at laryngoscopy in detecting the difference between the side that was operated on and the one that was not. We believe that leaving a raw bed to scar and epithelialize facilitates a vocal quality superior to that achieved after the various cordal reconstruction procedures. We have not noticed a serious vocal handicap after this operation, and most patients are content with their voices.

6. The final phase is to pull the epiglottis gently forward with a single stitch through the base and attach this stitch to the thyroid cartilage (Fig. 31-6J). A few stitches through the external perichondrium of the thyroid cartilage close the thyrotomy (Fig. 31-6K).

We usually leave a non-cuff tracheostomy for a few days. A feeding tube can be placed through the nose for 2 or 3 days to facilitate nutrition.

Results and Complications. A review of the results in a series of 182 patients treated by this operation at the Mayo Clinic up to 1974 showed that four patients (2%) had recurrence of their cancer of the larynx, three (1.6%) of these died of laryngeal cancer, and three patients lost their larynx eventually (one of these patients died). The mean length of hospitalization was 6 days, with a range of 3 to 16 days. Complications that increased the hospital stay were lung atelectasis, severe subcutaneous emphysema of the neck and face, and bleeding from the tracheostomy site or within the larynx. No deaths were attributed to surgical complications. Late complications included delayed wound healing and cartilage sequestration in two patients and laryngeal stenosis in two others. Each of these four patients had had previous radiation treatment. One patient acquired a laryngeal web that required retreatment. Granulation tissue was noted in 20 patients at the 3- and 4-month follow-up visits, and laryngoscopy was done on each to evaluate for recurrent residual tumor.

Frontolateral Partial Laryngectomy (Partial Vertical Laryngectomy)

The most common open operation for early glottic carcinoma is performed for cancer that involves the anterior commissure region. Removal of a portion of the thyroid cartilage adjacent to the location of the cancer is the best way to ensure a safe anterior surgical margin. The amount of cartilage removed depends on the tumor's extent, but is less than half of the thyroid cartilage that is removed in a hemilaryngectomy. A frontolateral partial laryngectomy can be performed for cancers that involve one vocal cord and cross the midline to involve as much as the anterior third of the opposite cord. Again, the tumor should not involve the body of the arytenoid, the subglottic larynx, or the false vocal cord.

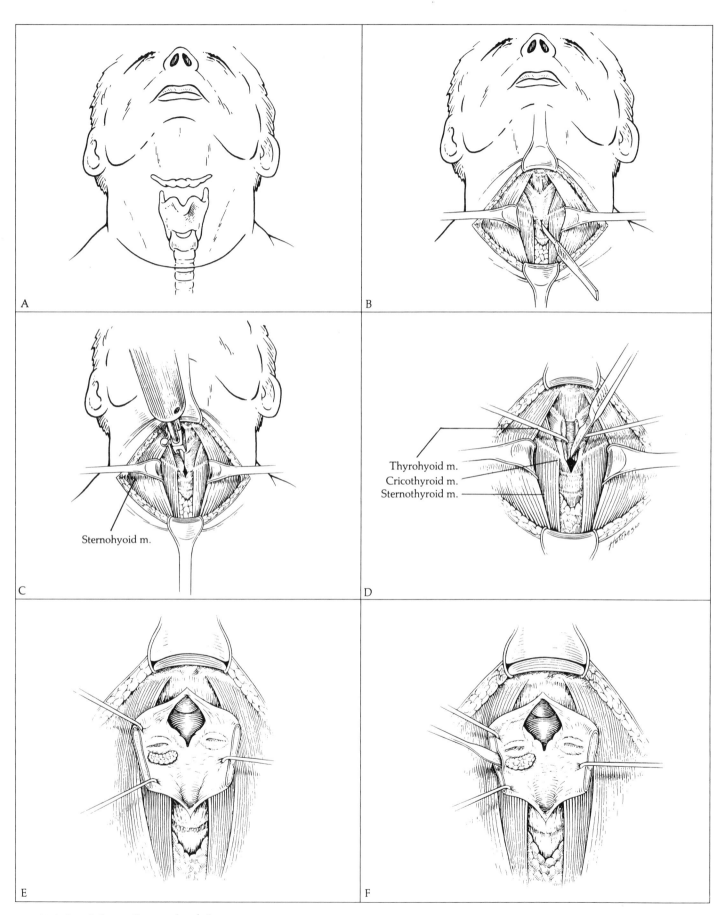

Fig. 31-6. *Steps in laryngofissure and cordectomy.*

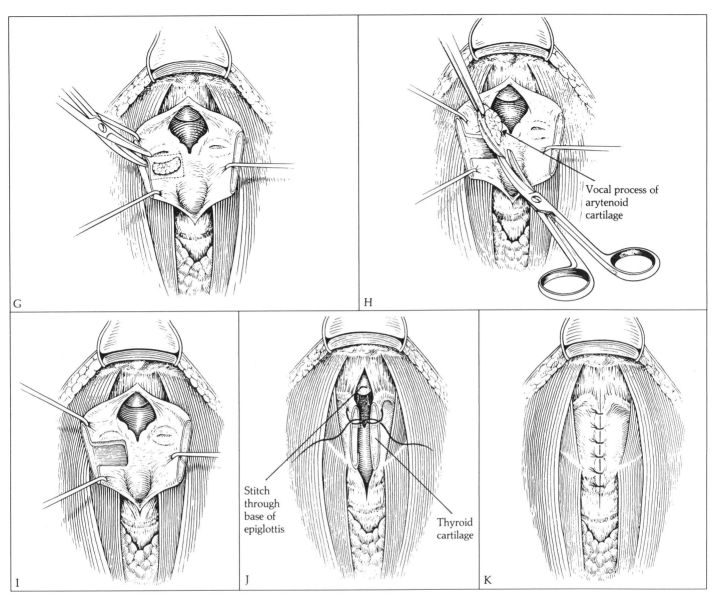

Fig. 31-6 (Continued)

The initial steps of the operation are identical to those described in laryngofissure and cordectomy. During the initial exposure, the delphian lymph node should always be sent to the pathology laboratory for histologic study. Metastasis to the delphian lymph node is associated with an increased risk of ipsilateral cervical node metastasis, and a modified neck dissection is done when metastasis to the delphian node is discovered. After the thyroid cartilage is exposed, a cartilage cut is made approximately one centimeter from the midline on the side opposite the cancer (Fig. 31-7A). An elevator is used to raise the anterior thyroid perichondrium back to the midportion of the thyroid ala on the tumor side. This perichondrium is often

helpful in later wound closure. Under direct vision, the cricothyroid membrane is entered and soft tissue excised superiorly through the cartilage cut. The vocal cord is divided under direct vision from below beyond the cancer's extent. A second cartilage cut is now made on the side of the tumor (see Fig. 31-7B). The amount of cartilage removed depends on the tumor's size but one-third of the thyroid ala is generally removed. The cartilage segment is grasped with a forceps and the laryngeal musculature and soft tissues are dissected from the posterior thyroid perichondrium back to the level of the arytenoid (see Fig. 31-7C). Cuts are then made in the subglottic area beneath the tumor and through the false cord (see Fig. 31-7D). The posterior

incision is made under direct vision with Panzer scissors. The specimen is then sent to pathology for frozen section study. Margins can also be taken from the patient if concern is raised about the tumor's extent.

After pathologic confirmation of free surgical margins is obtained, a feeding tube is inserted and hemostasis secured. The contralateral true and false cords are reattached to the external or internal thyroid perichondrium and the ipsilateral false cord is sutured anteriorly (see Fig. 31-7E). A suture is placed to reattach the base to the epiglottis, superiorly to the hyoid bone. The cricothyroid membrane and preepiglottic tissues are sutured and the perichondrium flap re-approximated. The

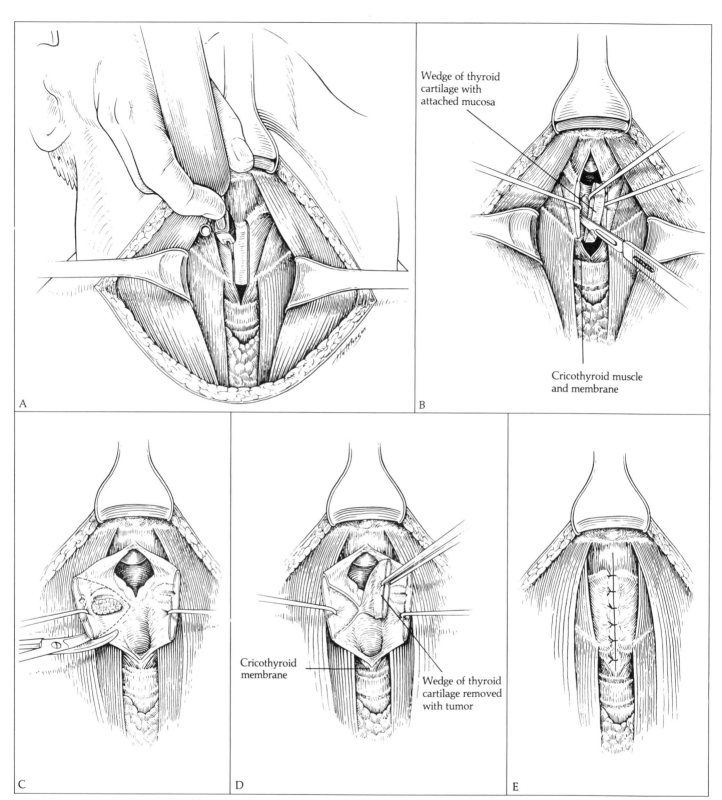

Fig. 31-7. Steps in a fronterolateral partial laryngectomy.

Wedge of thyroid cartilage with attached mucosa

Cricothyroid muscle and membrane

Cricothyroid membrane

Wedge of thyroid cartilage removed with tumor

final closure proceeds as in the laryngofissure-cordectomy operation.

Open laryngeal procedures continue to be a versatile and efficacious way of managing a wide spectrum of large T1 glottic carcinomas. A recent review from our institution of 82 patients undergoing a frontolateral partial vertical laryngectomy found 8 with recurrent tumor. For the entire group of patients who had open operations, the probability of survival at 3 and 5 years was 91 and 84 percent, respectively. The probability of remaining free of local recurrence at 3 and 5 years after operation was 94 and 93 percent, respectively. In our entire updated series of open operations, no patients have died of local recurrence. Only 6 percent of patients needed laryngectomy for salvage.

Anterior Commissure Procedure

The anterior commissure operation, a variation of the laryngofissure operation, is designed for the removal of cordal cancers that involve the anterior commissure region alone (see Fig. 31-2C). With this technique, up to the anterior half of each vocal cord can be removed. The procedure allows removal of the thyroid cartilage anterior to the anterior commissure tendon and whatever cordal substance is required by the lesion.

Technique

1. Anesthesia is delivered as in the laryngofissure operation. An endotracheal tube is inserted, and after the patient is asleep, prepared, and draped, it is followed by a tracheostomy. Skin incisions can be vertical or in the midline, or a horizontal collar-type incision can be made.
2. After the larynx is skeletonized, as in the laryngofissure operation, cartilage cuts are made to the left and right of the midline of the thyroid cartilage (see Fig. 31-8A). The exact position of each cartilage cut varies, depending on the precise location of the cancer and its relation to the anterior commissure. The cuts through cartilage are made down to but not through the soft tissues within the larynx. The soft tissues within the larynx are then dissected away from the internal perichondrium of the thyroid cartilage. The larynx is entered through the cricothyroid membrane, and one divides the laryngeal mucosa by working upward and joining the cartilage cuts with the mucosal cuts in the larynx. The cancer, surrounding normal tissue, and anterior wedge of the thyroid cartilage are excised under direct vision (Fig. 31-8B). After the resection we place a keel made of silicone rubber or polytetrafluoroethylene (PTFE) between the raw edges of the cut vocal cord to prevent scarring between these cords and to preserve as much of the anteroposterior dimension as possible (Fig. 31-8C–E).

Closure is accomplished by approximating the thyroid cartilage on each side by placing a few sutures through the external perichondrium.

Hemilaryngectomy

Hemilaryngectomy, a variation of the laryngofissure operation, is the ultimate extension of the partial vertical operations that avert permanent tracheostomy. This operation is suitable in carefully selected patients who have glottic cancers that have progressed to partial or complete fixation of vocal cord mobility. This fixation must be caused by tumor bulk and muscle invasion of the cord rather than by tumor invasion into the thyroid cartilage or vocal cord (see Fig. 31-2D). Fixation from downward extension into the subglottic larynx or from tumor that has actually infiltrated the recurrent laryngeal nerve is not safely managed by hemilaryngectomy. A safe hemilaryngectomy requires the active help of a surgical pathologist skilled in the interpretation of fresh frozen section preparations. Whether or not the operation can be performed on a tumor that is suitable for hemilaryngectomy must be decided in the operating room after direct exposure of the growth and with the help of a pathologist. There is no roentgenographic substitute for direct vision of the tumor and the guidance of the pathologist. The literature on laryngeal surgery suggests that some indirect techniques can replace the pathologist, but these techniques are less useful. Hemilaryngectomy and its variations are also useful for the rare invasive tumors that extend posteriorly to involve the body of the arytenoid.

Hemilaryngectomy allows removal of the entire vertical half of the larynx from the superior rim of the cricoid cartilage below to the epiglottis and aryepiglottic fold above.

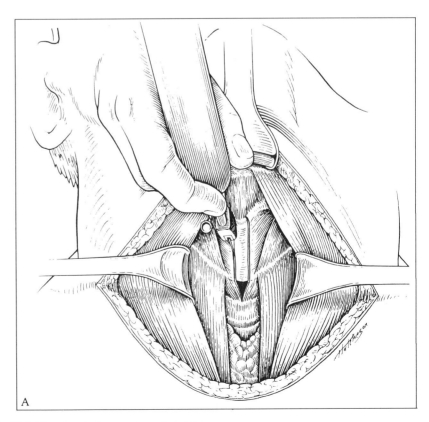

Fig. 31-8. Steps in anterior commissure technique.

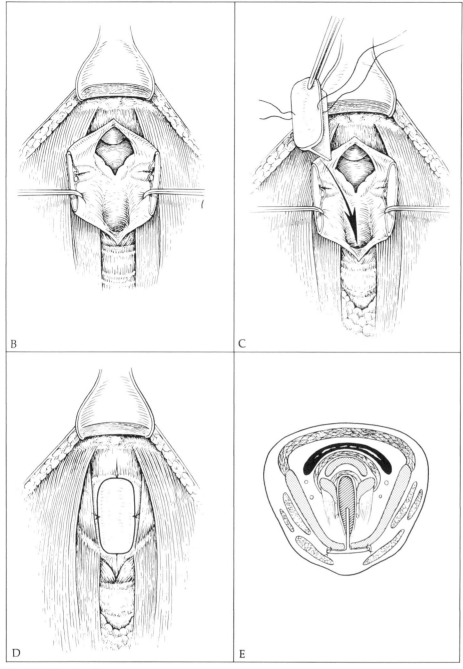

B

C

D

E

Fig. 31-8 (Continued)

The technique of hemilaryngectomy is similar to that of the frontal lateral operation, except that the posterior cartilage cut on the side of the tumor is placed as near as possible to the posterior edge of the thyroid lamina. The cartilage cut is vertical on the affected side. All the thyroid cartilage and soft tissue are then excised, leaving only the external perichondrium of the thyroid cartilage, which is used to close the lumen by sutures to the opposite side.

Technique

1. After thyroid cartilage is exposed as in cordectomy, the external perichondrium of the thyroid cartilage on the side of the lesion is elevated off the cartilage. If cancer shows through the cartilage, the hemilaryngectomy is terminated and a laryngectomy is performed (Fig. 31-9A).

2. Vertical cartilage cuts are made near the midline and a few millimeters from the posterior edge of the thyroid cartilage (Fig. 31-9B and C).

3. Mucosal cuts are made through or behind the arytenoid cartilage, and the entire hemilarynx is removed, preserving only the external perichondrium of the thyroid cartilage on the side of the tumor (Fig. 31-9D).

4. Closure is accomplished by suturing the external perichondrium to its original position (Fig. 31-9E).

Multiple techniques have been described to reconstruct the laryngeal lumen after hemilaryngectomy. These techniques use muscle pedicles from the strap muscles, the epiglottic cartilage, mucosal flaps, and free skin grafts. We simply close the larynx by placing a bipedicle strap muscle flap and covering this with the external perichondrium of the thyroid cartilage. Glottic cancers with vocal cord fixation are rarely suitable for hemilaryngectomy. We use this operation primarily for glottic cancers with impaired mobility or with extension onto the body of the arytenoid. At no time in the surgical treatment of laryngeal cancer, with perhaps the exception of the supraglottic partial operation and cordectomy, are surgical margins of a few millimeters between the cancer and normal tissue acceptable.

Supraglottic Cancers
The Supraglottic Partial Operation

Supraglottic cancers arise from the epiglottis, the aryepiglottic folds, and the false vocal cords. Supraglottic cancers that have not advanced beyond the midventricle on the surface and do not extend below the surface to the level of the vocal cord are suitable for partial supraglottic laryngectomy. This operation preserves functioning vocal cords and a glottic sphincter that serves for breathing, talking, and swallowing. Because the number of submucosal lymphatic vessels decreases as one approaches the anterior commissure, partial resection of the larynx is possible. Supraglottic cancers remain confined within the larynx above the cords for a period, which allows partial operation if the diagnosis is made before the cords are involved. Anterior extension of cancer is less restrained. Cancers can advance through preformed

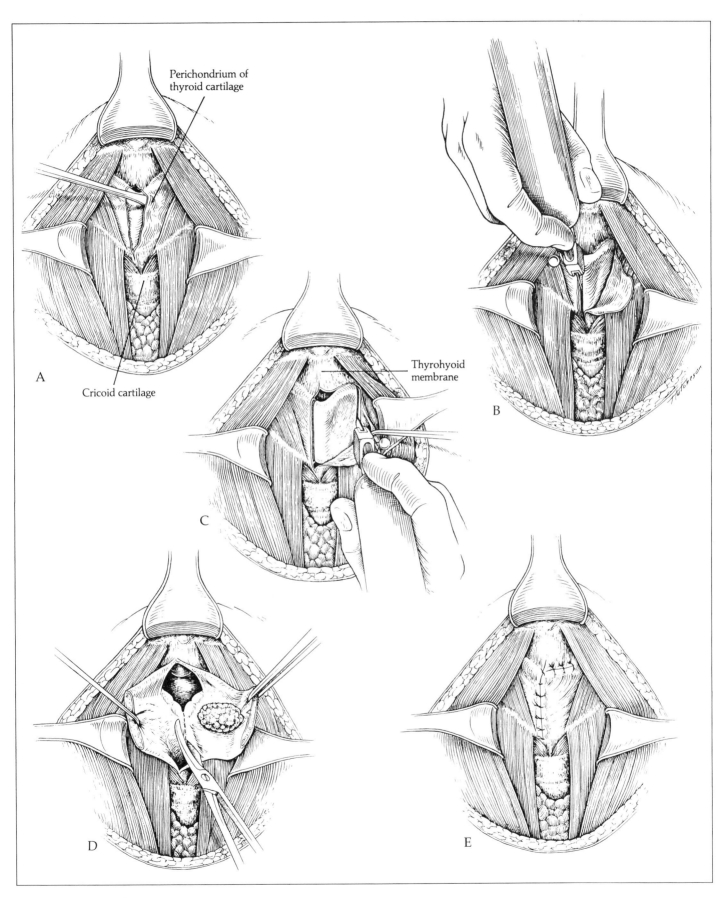

Fig. 31-9. Steps in hemilaryngectomy.

Perichondrium of thyroid cartilage

Cricoid cartilage

Thyrohyoid membrane

A

B

C

D

E

foramina in the epiglottic cartilage and grow into the so-called preepiglottic space. This space is below the hyoid bone, above the rim of the thyroid cartilage, and behind the thyrohyoid membrane (see Fig. 31-1). The supraglottic partial laryngectomy is an operation for cancer that encompasses the preepiglottic space and all the supraglottic structures down to the vocal cord and the arytenoid cartilage. Tumor margins of several millimeters at the cordal level are tolerable for biologic reasons, with the guidance of the surgical pathologist.

Tumors suitable for this operation are those confined to the epiglottis, aryepiglottic folds, false vocal cords, and various combinations of these sites. The key requirement is vocal cord mobility (see Fig. 31-3A through D).

Although the laryngologic literature describes special roentgenographic and laboratory tests used in the planning of supraglottic laryngectomy, only two requirements are essential: The tumor must be suitable for the operation and the patient must be capable of tolerating the operation.

A suitable tumor is one that does not fix the vocal cords. This is determined by looking at the larynx with the laryngeal mirror or flexible laryngoscope, or both, and listening to the patient's voice. If the vocal cords appear to be mobile and the voice is not hoarse in the glottic sense, the tumor is suitable for a partial operation. Not all patients with such tumors, however, are candidates for partial operations.

The patient factor is probably more important in this situation than in any other head and neck operation. The demands on the patient during convalescence after supraglottic partial laryngectomy are strenuous. Both airway and digestive functions are served by a common tract. The patient coughs and aspirates, and strong lungs with reasonable pulmonary function are required to survive.

Although debilitated patients cannot predictably tolerate the supraglottic operation, they usually can tolerate a laryngectomy, in which breathing and swallowing are distinctly separated. Much is written about special roentgenographic and pulmonary function tests. These are helpful but not as helpful as clinical judgment.

Computed tomography and MR evaluations of the larynx are often helpful in assessing the extent of a supraglottic carcinoma. The existing staging system for supraglottic tumors includes invasion of the preepiglottic space and cordal fixation as requirements for a T3 supraglottic tumor. Likewise, invasion of the thyroid cartilage is, by definition, a T4 tumor. Preoperative imaging studies, therefore, are used in clinical staging. It has been stated that involvement of the preepiglottic space makes a lesion less likely to be curable by radiation therapy. The presence or absence of involvement of the preepiglottic space on imaging studies, however, does not change the ability to perform a supraglottic laryngectomy, as this space is removed by the operation. In actuality, pathologic involvement of the preepiglottic space is often seen when imaging studies are normal. Pulmonary function tests are usually obtained preoperatively. An FEV$_1$ of less than 40 percent of predicted value is indicative of significant pulmonary compromise, and factors such as age, patient motivation, and detailed history and experience are necessary to recommend a supraglottic laryngectomy in these patients.

The final decision as to the feasibility of a supraglottic partial laryngectomy is made in the operating room when the surgeon looks directly at the tumor and its proximity to the true vocal cords and consults with the surgical pathologist. If the tumor extends to or below the level of the anterior commissure, total laryngectomy or near-total laryngectomy is required. If extension into the paraglottic space is seen pathologically, total laryngectomy may be necessary. The surgeon and the patient need to be prepared for this contingency.

Technique

1. Except in the presence of a bulky tumor in which endotracheal intubation is risky and tracheotomy as a preliminary procedure is safer, anesthesia is rendered using an endotracheal tube. With the patient's neck extended, a curtain incision is made from the contralateral lower end of the sternocleidomastoid muscle across to the ipsilateral sternocleidomastoid muscle and then up and laterally to the mastoid tip (Fig. 31-10A). A complete neck dissection on the side of the lesion or of palpable metastases is done on all patients except

those with small lesions near the epiglottic tip. The neck dissection is preceded by a low tracheostomy and repositioning of the anesthesia equipment. The neck flap includes the platysma muscle.

2. The infrahyoid muscles are detached from the hyoid bone and preserved. Usually, both lobes of the thyroid gland are preserved.

   The suprahyoid muscles are detached from the hyoid bone down to the vallecula. An incision is then made along the superior rim of the thyroid cartilage through the external perichondrium of the cartilage. The perichondrium is elevated off the thyroid cartilage past the midportion of this cartilage (Fig. 31-10B).

   This dissection is best done with a blunt cottonoid dissector and forceps, with care taken to elevate a full thickness of perichondrium. If at this point the tumor is seen within the underlying thyroid cartilage, the procedure must proceed to total laryngectomy. This is rare.

3. With the oscillating saw, cuts are made through the thyroid cartilage, beginning at the superior horn of one side, angling down to the center of the midline and then back up to the superior horn of the other side (Fig. 31-10C). The cut should go completely through the cartilage to the soft tissue of the endolarynx. Bleeding at this point is safely ignored. The hyoid bone is divided lateral to the lesser horn on both sides (Fig. 31-10D).

4. The constrictor muscles are freed from the thyroid cartilage laterally, and the pharynx is entered through the part of the piriform recess (sinus) that is most distant from the tumor. By placing a large retractor into the pharynx and retracting upward, the surgeon can advance the pharyngeal mucosal cuts upward toward the tongue base and then across the tongue base to separate the larynx from the tongue. The hyoid bone and preepiglottic space are part of the specimen (Fig. 31-10E).

5. It is very important that the critical internal mucosal cuts are done only after the pharyngeal and laryngeal reflexes are completely eliminated by the anesthetist. The first internal mucosal cut is down the aryepiglottic fold most distant from the tumor. The cut is carried down to the ventricle and forward to the anterior commissure. A scissors can

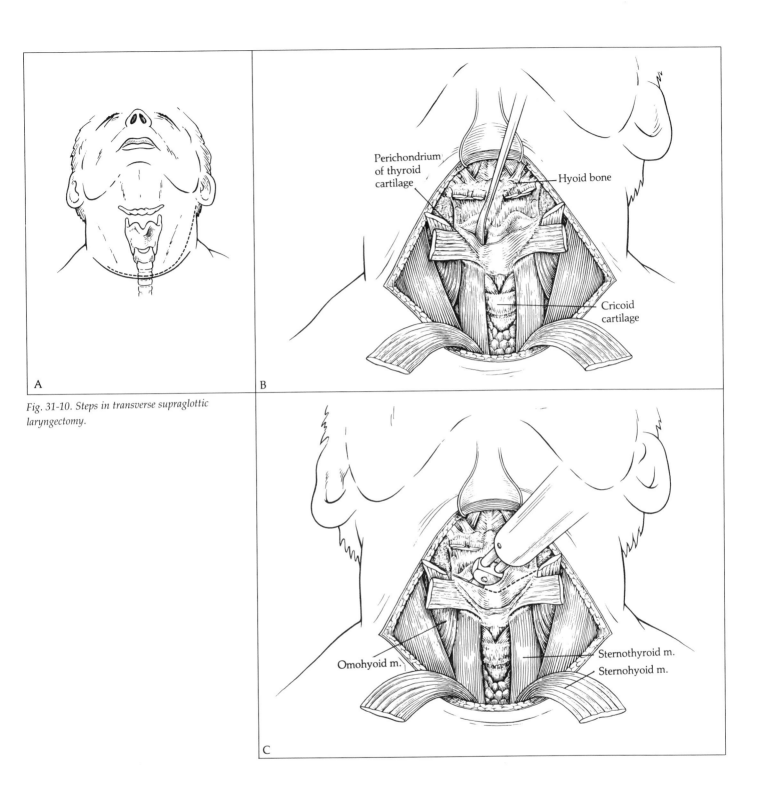

Fig. 31-10. Steps in transverse supraglottic
laryngectomy.

then be placed with one blade in the inside mucosal cut and the other blade
through the cartilage cut on that side;
with gradual closure of the scissors, the
cuts are joined and the larynx is opened
(like a book) away from the tumor. This
gives direct exposure to the growth. A

mucosal cut around the tumor can then
be made under direct vision, and the
supraglottic structures are removed
(Fig. 31-10F).
6. Some surgeons cover the raw surface of
the arytenoid cartilages or aryepiglottic
folds, although we do not.

A myotomy of the cricopharyngeal muscle
is done before closure. This is believed to
help ease the beginning of swallowing.
The surgeon accomplishes the myotomy
by placing a finger through the esophageal
introitus and dividing the cricopharyngeal
muscle completely from top to bottom. If

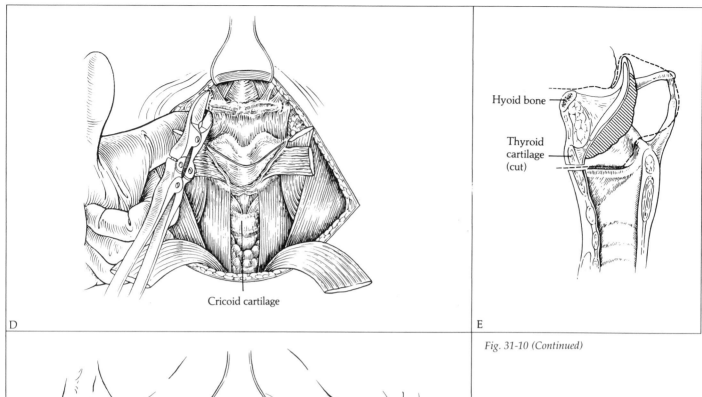

Cricoid cartilage

D

Hyoid bone

Thyroid cartilage (cut)

E

Fig. 31-10 (Continued)

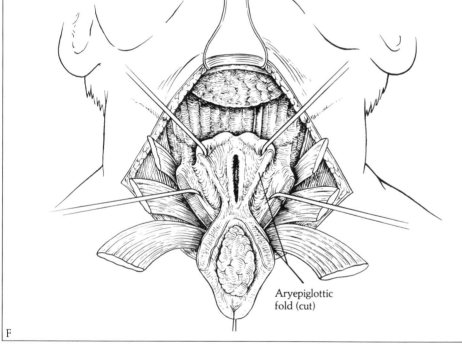

Aryepiglottic fold (cut)

F

the myotomy is done as far posterior as possible, damage to the recurrent laryngeal nerve is unlikely.

No mucosal closure is attempted. A stitch between the pharyngeal mucosa and the tongue base on each side helps identify the corners. Further attempts to approximate pharyngeal mucosa to the tongue base narrow the gullet and compromise swallowing. A closure that does not narrow the pharynx is vital. Closure involves approximating the preserved and previously elevated external perichondrium of the thyroid cartilage to the tongue base. Ten to twelve large sutures (00 black silk) are placed through the external perichondrium of the thyroid cartilage and then through the substance of the tongue base. Large deep bites are taken into the tongue base. The sutures are not tied until all are in place (Fig. 31-10G).

A helpful modification is to pull the larynx forward and tilt the anterior commissure upward by a suspension suture. This is a single, large, absorbable stitch placed around the anterior midcricoid and then to the soft tissue or even bone of the mandible in the anterior midline (Fig. 31-10H). By tightening this suture, the large pharyngeal gap is narrowed and the previously placed black silk sutures can be tied with lessened tension. Perichondrial clo-

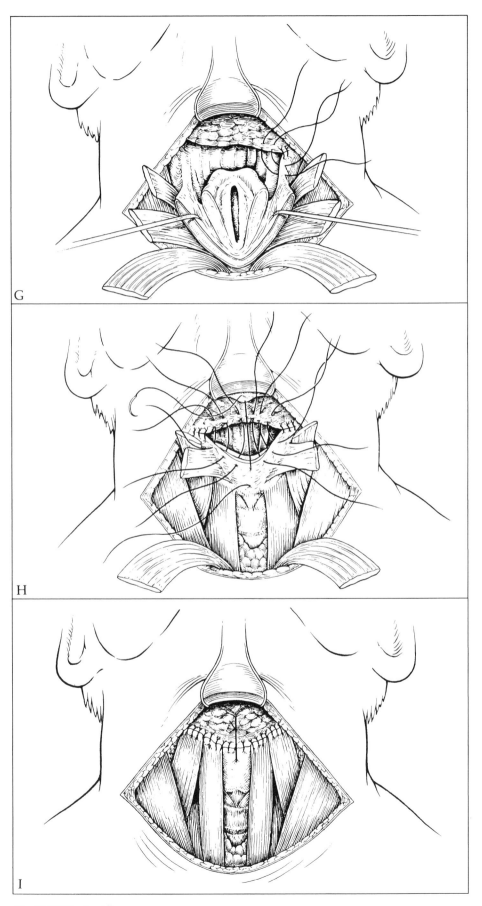

G

H

I

sure at the tongue base appears to be the key to successful swallowing. Attempts at mucosal closure narrow the pharynx and make eventual swallowing less likely.

Bits and pieces of strap muscle and cervical fascia can be sewn together to support the primary closure. These extra sutures do not add much strength and probably are redundant, but they tidy up the area before skin closure (Fig. 31-10I).

Postoperative Care

The patient is returned to his or her room with a nasogastric tube held in place by a suture into the membranous nasal septum. A cuffed tracheotomy tube is also in place. The large suction tube drains are positioned under the neck flaps before skin closure.

All dressings are removed the morning after the operation. Suction tubes are removed when they no longer are draining, usually in 3 or 4 days. The cuffed tracheotomy is replaced by a No. 4 or 5 metal tube about 2 days after the early postoperative period.

The change from a cuffed to a plain metal tube helps determine when the tracheotomy tube can be removed. The metal tube is removed as soon as it can be corked for 24 hours without resulting in stridor, usually on the sixth or seventh postoperative day.

Eating is tried on the tenth day if all has gone well. Few patients simply sit down and start eating the first time food is placed before them. Usually, they cough, retch, and become terribly discouraged. Considerable time is spent before the operation and during the postoperative hospital period preparing patients for swallowing. They are encouraged to practice swallowing saliva after the fifth or sixth day. They are prepared for disappointment when first attempting to eat, and it is suggested to them that they may go home with the nasogastric tube in place.

If swallowing cannot be mastered but all other problems are under control, we encourage patients to go home with the feeding tube in place. The many commercially available tube feedings assure good nutrition. Blender diet recipes are provided, and all patients are well trained in tube feedings by the tenth or eleventh postoperative day.

Fig. 31-10 (Continued)

A certain amount of strength and confidence is required of the patient before easy swallowing evolves, and neither is easy to acquire in the hospital. After 10 days to 2 weeks away from the hospital, most patients can swallow without difficulty. A few patients require a longer time, and some never swallow adequately. In a group of more than 200 patients who have had supraglottic partial laryngectomies, we have performed two permanent gastrostomies.

The Neck in Supraglottic Cancer

Local control of supraglottic cancer by supraglottic laryngectomy is predictable. A local recurrence rate of 1.5 percent with the supraglottic operation is possible to obtain with rigid adherence to surgical principles, by not attempting to accomplish more in the operation than feasible (i.e., not extending the operation to resect cancers that have fixed a vocal cord), and by depending on the help of a skilled surgical pathologist. The oncologic problem is the control of cervical metastases.

The supraglottic lesions, unlike those at the glottic level, can metastasize to either side of the neck because the supraglottic larynx is a midline structure. Approximately 50 percent of patients with supraglottic cancer have cervical metastases. There is not general agreement regarding the best treatment for the cervical nodes.

Four clinical conditions are generally seen with supraglottic cancer as they relate to cervical metastases: Metastatic lesions are not palpable; large, palpable neck nodes exist on the side ipsilateral to the cancer; large, palpable neck nodes exist on the side contralateral to the cancer; and large, palpable neck nodes exist on both sides of the neck.

Principles that should be adhered to in regard to cervical lymph nodes are 1) the probability of metastatic disease in the neck is high, even when nodes are not palpable; 2) if one side of the neck contains metastatic disease, there is no reason to assume the other side does not; 3) the only way to know the true status of the neck is by microscopic study of the nodes; and 4) a neck dissection performed in the absence of palpable disease that is free of metastases gives valuable information to the surgeon and patient—the concept of the staging neck dissection.

Applying these principles to the four clinical settings, we manage the neck in the following manner.

1. For a midline T1 supraglottic tumor, when the neck is clinically normal, we do a modified or select neck dissection on one side. The pathologist studies the resected specimen while the supraglottic partial operation is performed. If there is no microscopic disease, no further resection is required. These patients do well, and there is no need for further adjunctive therapy. If the lesion is a T2 or T3 supraglottic tumor, bilateral modified or functional select neck dissections are always performed in the presence of a clinically negative neck.
2. When there is palpable cancer on one side, we do a complete neck dissection on the side of the palpable disease and a functional neck dissection on the clinically normal contralateral side.
3. The same approach is used as in setting 2, except that the functional neck dissection and complete neck dissection are reversed as to the side.
4. When there is palpable disease in both sides of the neck, the only rational approach is bilateral complete neck dissection. This is done all in the same session if the patient's condition permits. Usually, the patient's condition does permit such a procedure because patients at poor risk should not have supraglottic partial laryngectomies.

Radiation to a clinically normal neck is a controversial issue. The question often asked is, Which unnecessary treatment is the least harmful and most valuable? The morbidity of single neck dissection is negligible, and the information acquired regarding the true status of the neck is well worth the time, effort, and morbidity involved. Single neck dissection or even bilateral neck dissection with the preservation of one jugular vein is far less stressful and causes fewer long-term problems than does radiation to the full neck after surgical intervention. After a supraglottic laryngectomy, radiation therapy is generally utilized for the high-risk neck. In this scenario, it is necessary to maintain a tracheotomy tube in position, even if corked, during radiation therapy due to the possibility of significant edema and airway compromise to the patient who had undergone a supraglottic laryngectomy, bilateral neck dissections, and then a course of postoperative radiation therapy.

Total Laryngectomy for Glottic and Supraglottic Cancers

Total laryngectomy is still an appropriate operation for cancer. In properly selected patients, laryngectomy allows quick treatment, gets the patient out of the hospital safely, has few local recurrences, and ultimately leaves many patients satisfied and cured. The problems with total laryngectomy are clear. The airway and digestive pathway are separated, and a permanent tracheostomy is required. Some form of speech rehabilitation is needed. Nevertheless, total laryngectomy is not a concession of failure but an acceptance of the reality of late diagnosis. Laryngectomy is also required for many tumors and for those that have fixed the glottic larynx. A near-total laryngectomy is a new option for many T3 glottic carcinomas unless there is tumor involvement of either the interarytenoid area or most of the opposite cord or subglottic airway. Laryngectomy or near-total laryngectomy is also used in poor-risk patients with supraglottic cancers that otherwise would be suitable for partial laryngectomy. The use of radiation therapy and chemotherapy has been recently popularized as an alternative to total laryngectomy for tumors with cordal fixation. The long-term efficacy of this approach in a broad-based representative series of patients, however, has still not definitively shown that survival is not adversely impacted by this treatment approach. We currently are not recommending chemotherapy and radiation therapy as an alternative form of treatment for T3 and T4 glottic cancer.

Technique

1. After the neck is prepared and draped, a low collar incision is made. If intubation has been performed, the endotracheal tube is replaced by a flexible cuff tube that is inserted into a low tracheostomy. If the neck dissection is included, the incision is extended obliquely up the mastoid tip on the side of the neck dissection (Fig. 31-11A and B).

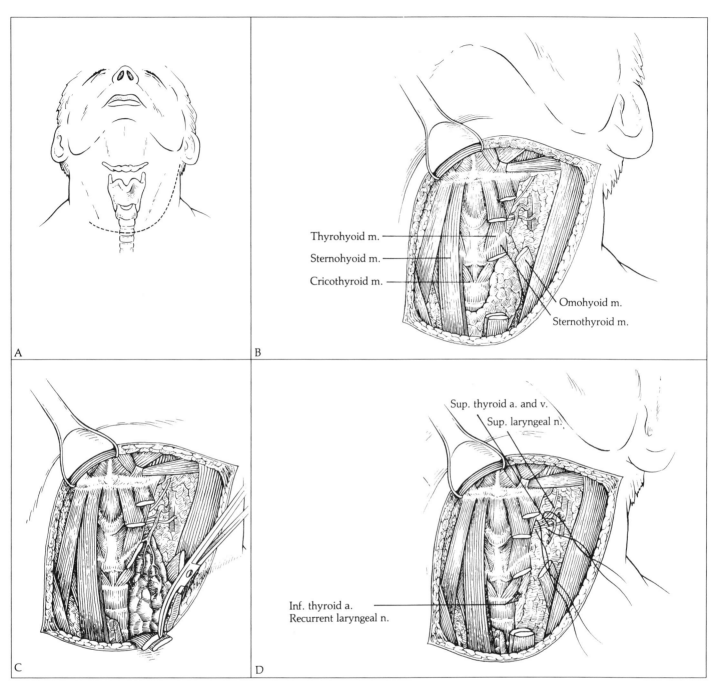

Fig. 31-11. Steps in total laryngectomy.

The indications for neck dissection depend on the clinical setting, as noted in the discussion of supraglottic partial resection. A functional neck dissection is generally performed for a glottic cancer with cordal fixation, even if the neck is clinically negative. Although the probability of pathologic metastasis is low, the morbidity of a functional neck dissection is minimal. With transglottic tumors, bilateral neck dissections should

be strongly considered, as described in the discussion of supraglottic cancer. In this setting, the probability of pathologic metastasis is less than in supraglottic cancer, and a staging neck dissection is not performed.

2. The strap muscles in the neck (the sternohyoid, sternothyroid, and omohyoid) are divided as low as possible (Fig. 31-11B). The isthmus of the thyroid gland is divided and ligated, and the

thyroid halves are mobilized off the trachea. The lobe on the side of the lesion in glottic and subglottic cancer is included in the resection. This is accomplished by clamping the paratracheal tissues, ligating the inferior thyroid artery, and dividing the recurrent laryngeal nerve. The trachea is then laid bare to the esophageal muscle (Fig. 31-11C).

3. The suprahyoid muscles are separated from the superior rim of the hyoid

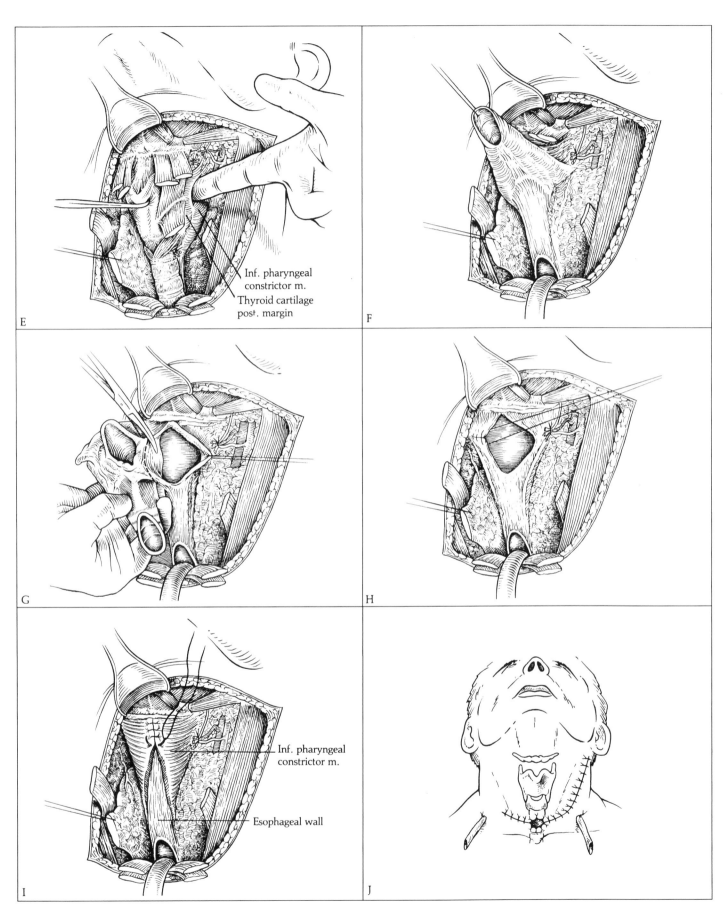

E

Inf. pharyngeal
constrictor m.
Thyroid cartilage
post. margin

F

G

H

Inf. pharyngeal
constrictor m.

Esophageal wall

I

J

Fig. 31-11 (Continued)

bone. By cutting as close to the bone as possible, bleeding is lessened and the hypoglossal nerves can be avoided. By placing a clamp on the most posterior end of the hyoid bone, scissors can be slipped behind the bone, and the hyoid can be completely separated from its upper attachments on both sides.

The superior laryngeal bundle of artery, vein, and nerve is then isolated just below the end of the hyoid bone and is clamped, divided, and tied (Fig. 31-11D).

The insertions of the inferior constrictor muscles are freed from the posterior aspect of the thyroid lamina with a knife. This maneuver can be done easily by placing a laryngeal hook behind the upper end of the thyroid cartilage and rotating the larynx away from the surgeon. These constrictors are free on both sides (Fig. 31-11E).

4. The trachea is then sectioned obliquely upward from front to back. This beveling, which extends over two, three, or four tracheal rings, permits a wide caudal tracheal stump, which produces a large tracheostoma. The back wall of the trachea is then divided, and the trachea is separated from the cervical esophagus by sharp dissection. Usually there is brisk bleeding, but these vessels are easily controlled by electrocoagulation (Fig. 31-11F).

5. The pharynx is entered as far from the tumor as possible. If the tumor is a supraglottic cancer, the pharynx is entered in the piriform recess. If the tumor is in the piriform recess or at the level of the glottis, the pharynx is entered in the vallecula. By placing a large retractor such as a Deaver into the pharynx, the entire larynx and hyoid bone are progressively separated from the pharyngeal mucosa and removed (Fig. 31-11G).

6. After the wound is thoroughly irrigated with sterile water and adequate margins are assured by inspection and consultation with the pathologists, the pharynx is closed. A feeding tube is inserted through the nose and passed through the esophagus into the stomach.

7. The pharyngostoma can be closed with a running suture or by interrupted single sutures. We prefer interrupted sutures of 000 chromic material. A T-shaped closure is usual. The vertical limb of the T begins at the esophagus and works up the midportion to the tongue base. The second, or horizontal, limb begins at the lateral junction of the tongue base and the pharynx on both sides, is carried to the middle, and is joined near the vertical closure. A second layer of interrupted chromic sutures is placed over these sutures for reinforcement. The constrictor muscles are usually no longer reapproximated to allow for later use of a tracheoesophageal puncture device for voice rehabilitation. It is important that a complete pharyngeal myotomy is done at the time of the laryngectomy (Fig. 31-11H and I).

8. The final step is to construct a permanent tracheostoma. The caudal lip of the previously beveled tracheostoma is first sutured to the skin over the jugular notch with interrupted absorbable sutures. The cephalad portion is then attached to the midline of the collar flap (Fig. 31-11J). It is usual to excise a semicircular portion of the skin to open the tracheostoma further. A wide-open tracheostoma can be assured by cutting the tracheal stump on each side and interdigitating a "V" of skin into the gap created in the trachea. The neck skin is then closed in layers over two large Hemovac suction catheters. A non-cuffed, large metal tracheostomy tube is inserted. If a large tracheotomy has been fashioned and there is no need for postoperative radiation therapy, before the pharyngeal closure, a tracheoesophageal puncture device can be placed into position. A long-term device, such as a Groningen or Provox prosthesis, is selected. In all other cases, if there is concern about the stoma or the need for radiation therapy, a tracheoesophageal puncture device is not considered until final healing is complete and the stoma is mature.

Postoperative Care

The postoperative convalescence after laryngectomy is seldom difficult. Nasogastric feedings are started on the second day, Hemovac suction catheters are removed on the third or fourth day, and the sutures are removed on the sixth or seventh day. Instruction on tracheostomy care begins as soon as the Hemovac catheters are removed. Speech therapy begins with a consultative session before the operation. Early in the convalescence following the laryngectomy, generally on the third or fourth day, the patient is given an electric larynx and instructed in its use. Multiple instruction periods continue until the patient is dismissed from the hospital.

Laryngectomy and Pseudoglottic Reconstruction

A long-held goal of laryngeal surgeons has been to reconstruct a vocal apparatus after total laryngectomy. Any connection between the trachea and esophagus after laryngectomy can produce speech. Many ingenious techniques to connect the trachea to the esophagus have been devised. However, problems have plagued all of the so-called fistula operations, especially food and saliva contamination of the trachea and stenosis and closure of the fistula. These procedures have been abandoned by our group. In our practice, however, many patients have an artificial valve inserted between the tracheal stoma and the neogullet after total laryngectomy. The concept of the available valves (Singer, Panje) is that they permit air to pass from the trachea to the neogullet but do not allow food or liquid to pass in the opposite direction. These devices are successful in many but not all patients. Stomal shape and size or patients' degree of manual dexterity may not permit the successful closure of the stoma necessary to force air into the prosthesis and permit speech.

Near-Total Laryngectomy

Since the first edition of this book, the need for total laryngectomy has been decreased dramatically. The reason for this is the better understanding of the place for the near-total operation and the experience gained that makes this a predictable procedure. The patients who undergo total laryngectomy in our practice today are either those in whom radiation failed, the rare patients with primary subglottic cancer, patients with transglottic cancer with considerable subglottic extension, patients with extensive laryngeal cancer involving both vocal cords, individuals with tumor extension into the interarytenoid area, or those with postcricoid hypopharyngeal malignancies.

The concept of near-total laryngectomy is a logical extension of the conservation operation based on a firm infrastructure of whole laryngeal section studies. Total laryngectomy has been used for certain laryngeal and pharyngeal cancers, not because the entire larynx must be removed for oncologic safety but rather to separate the airway and the upper digestive system. There is only so much larynx that can be sacrificed if the patient is to be able to continue to swallow and breathe through the remaining passages. Traditional conservation operations have defined those limits. Supraglottic, partial laryngectomy, and partial vertical laryngectomies (laryngofissure and cordectomy and hemilaryngectomy) are designed to safely resect stages I and II laryngeal cancers and yet maintain oral and nasal pulmonary continuity and a lung-powered glottic voice without a permanent tracheostomy.

Since the time of the first laryngectomy, it has been known that any connection between the trachea and the neogullet after laryngectomy permits lung-powered laryngeal speech. The laryngologist's quest has been to discover how to make the connection precisely so that speech can be produced without aspiration using pulmonary air pressure. The problem has been that most connections that are large enough to permit speech are also large enough to allow aspiration and pulmonary soilage. Connections too small to permit aspiration often are too tight to allow speech. The near-total concept recognizes that if one studies the patient and the tumor carefully, an intermediate operation between a conventional conservation operation and total laryngectomy can be used with oncologic safety. This operation provides a valve-tissue connection between the airway and gullet that can be used for speech. The connection is too small for breathing, so a permanent tracheostomy is the price paid for late diagnosis. In other words, parts of the larynx that would otherwise be discarded to accommodate the separation of breathing from swallowing are used instead to accommodate speech.

This concept was developed by Pearson and has been used by our group in selected patients since 1979. In that time interval, more than 200 patients have been so treated and the place for the near-total operation has been clarified.

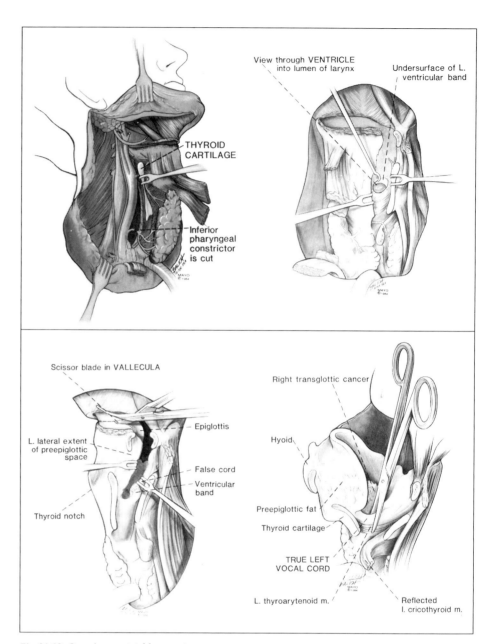

Fig. 31-12. Steps in near-total laryngectomy.

Patient Selection

Stage III Glottic Carcinoma

Stage III glottic carcinoma implies vocal cord fixation on one side of the larynx. The traditional surgical treatment has been laryngectomy. Paraglottic space invasion by T3 vocal cord cancers necessitates removal of the cricoid cartilage to ensure oncologic safety. Removal of the cricoid has been synonymous in the past with total laryngectomy. Radiation therapy has been abandoned by our group for this stage of disease because of the predictably high failure rates, because of the unacceptably large percentage of patients who require salvage operations, because of too many complications, and because of a higher death rate than from surgical therapy alone. We now believe that the near-total option is ideal for this group of patients. It settles the problem quickly, has few local recurrences, and is cost-effective compared with radiation therapy for cure with surgical intervention reserved for salvage. The usual stage III glottic cancer has a portion of the contralateral hemilarynx that is free of cancer. Rather than being dis-

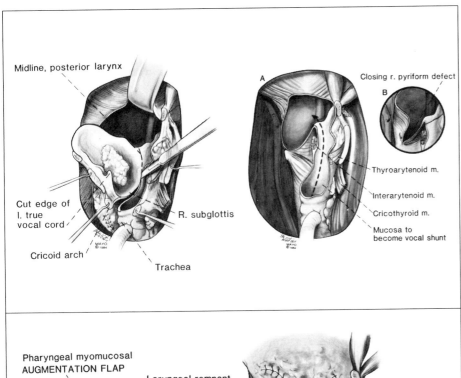

Midline, posterior larynx

Cut edge of
l. true
vocal cord

Cricoid arch

Trachea

R. subglottis

Closing r. pyriform defect

A

B

Thyroarytenoid m.

Interarytenoid m.

Cricothyroid m.

Mucosa to
become vocal shunt

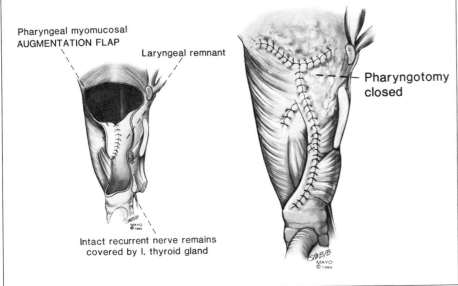

Pharyngeal myomucosal
AUGMENTATION FLAP

Laryngeal remnant

Pharyngotomy
closed

Intact recurrent nerve remains
covered by l. thyroid gland

Fig. 31-12 (Continued)

carded, this tissue is used to construct a dynamic valve that protects the airway during swallowing and still permits speech. The only oncologic contraindications to the near-total option for stage III glottic carcinoma are posterior or interarytenoid extension, tumor involvement of both vocal cords, considerable subglottic extension, or prior radiation therapy.

Supraglottic Cancer
Most patients with stages I and II supraglottic cancers can be treated surgically by supraglottic partial laryngectomy. However, some of these patients cannot tolerate the postoperative stress intrinsic to a supraglottic laryngectomy. This may be because of advanced age or poor pulmonary function. The near-total option is an ideal compromise for this subgroup because of its physiologic and oncologic safety. The availability of a procedure in between has been a great step forward in the treatment of laryngeal cancer for these patients. Likewise, many stage III supraglottic cancers for which the traditional treatment has

been total laryngectomy can now be treated using the near-total option. As described for stage III glottic cancers, usually a portion of the uninvolved larynx can be safely used for neoglottic reconstruction. In addition, supraglottic tumors that extend to involve a portion of the anterior vocal cords and yet retain vocal cord mobility, that is, T2 lesions, can be effectively managed with a near-total laryngectomy.

Technique

1. If it is assumed that the patient has a transglottic T3 carcinoma involving the right side of the larynx, then preliminary laryngoscopy has shown that the posterior portion of the left true cord is not involved with tumor. A low tracheotomy is first done beneath the third tracheal ring. A complete neck dissection is usually performed on the right side, and the right side of the larynx is mobilized exactly as one would do in a total laryngectomy procedure (Fig. 31-12A).

2. The strap muscles are reflected laterally off the left side of the larynx, and the midportion of the left thyroid cartilage is removed (Fig. 31-12B). The thyroarytenoid muscle is now visible, and entering the larynx above the midportion of this muscle allows access to the ventricle. Cuts are now made up through the left false cord and across the vallecula (Fig. 31-12C).

3. Under direct vision, the left cord is divided where it is free of tumor, and this cut is continued anteriorly across the cricoid cartilage (Fig. 31-12D). The posterior cricoid and interarytenoid muscles are divided, allowing the specimen to open completely. The pharyngeal mucosa on the right side is divided and the specimen removed (Fig. 31-12E).

4. The remaining structures include a continuous strip of mucosa from the trachea to the pharynx with an arytenoid and portion of the left cord with some of its intrinsic musculature and nervous innervation (left recurrent laryngeal nerve) (Fig. 31-12F).

5. A portion of the remaining cricoid cartilage is removed submucosally to allow tubing of the fistula. The fistula is closed around a No. 12 or 14 red rubber catheter. If there is not enough mucosa at the level of the arytenoid cartilage to permit closure, a small flap of pharynx

can be used to augment the fistula (Fig. 31-12G).

6. The red rubber catheter is removed and the pharynx is closed in layers over a feeding tube (Fig. 31-12H). A permanent tracheostomy is made from the skin to the side of the trachea.

Cancer of the Hypopharynx

Early symptoms of cancer of the hypopharynx, unlike those of cancer of the larynx, are few because lesions in the location do not interfere with breathing, swallowing, or talking until they are large and far advanced. Survival statistics are poor, as compared with those for cancer of the larynx, because of the advanced stage of the primary tumor on initial presentation and the incidence of cervical metastasis.

The hypopharynx is the lower subdivision of the pharynx, extending from the level of the epiglottic tip to the lower border of the cricoid cartilage. It is composed of three parts: the piriform recess, the postcricoid structures, and the posterior pharyngeal wall. The piriform recess is bounded above by the glossoepiglottic fold, inferiorly by the apex of the piriform recess at the entrance to the cervical esophagus, laterally by the thyroid cartilage, and medially by the aryepiglottic folds. Posteriorly, the piriform sinus is limited by the posterior pharyngeal wall. The anatomic division is a vertical line at the level of the arytenoid cartilage and its midposition.

The postcricoid region is the posterior surface of the larynx behind and below the arytenoid cartilages. These anatomic boundaries merge imperceptibly as do cancers in this region. The site of origin of hypopharyngeal cancer is difficult to define unless cancer is seen early.

The treatment of hypopharyngeal cancer is intimately related to that of laryngeal cancer, because laryngeal structures are medial and anterior to the pharynx and no barrier prevents pharyngeal cancers from spreading into the larynx. At the time of diagnosis, most pharyngeal cancers involve the larynx. The surgical treatment of laryngeal cancer is therefore inescapably entwined with that of pharyngeal cancer.

The diagnosis of hypopharyngeal cancer requires the laryngeal mirror for surface examination and the hand for palpating the neck for nodes suspected of metastasis. Generally, the data required for treatment planning are obtained by these means.

Flexible esophagoscopy should be performed preoperatively for all cases of hypopharyngeal carcinoma. The incidence of esophageal second primaries is higher with hypopharyngeal carcinoma, and the discovery of an occult esophageal cancer is essential in accurate preoperative assessment. Appropriate therapy in these cases may be esophagectomy, laryngectomy, and pharyngectomy with gastric pull-up reconstruction. Esophagoscopy can also evaluate the inferior extent of a hypopharyngeal carcinoma and evaluate involvement of the esophageal introitus. Computed tomography scans may provide additional information about the extent of a large, obstructing hypopharyngeal carcinoma. When performed, the scan should extend into the mediastinum to evaluate the mediastinal nodes. Treatment planning is done primarily in the examination room with a mirror, flexible scope, manual examination, and information gained from esophagoscopy and CT imaging. Direct laryngoscopy for examination and biopsy only supplements office planning, and this is usually done at the time of definitive surgical treatment. Most of these cancers are squamous cell epitheliomas.

The observations needed for treatment planning include the presence or absence of laryngeal involvement and assessment of the mobility of the vocal cords; the extent of mucosal involvement on the posterior wall of the pharynx, because this is a basic consideration in planning for the contingency of total pharyngeal reconstruction; and the pooling of mucus in the pharynx. The last observation is suggestive of cervical esophageal extension or obstruction of the introitus of the cervical esophagus.

Treatment Planning

The planning of initial surgical therapy requires judgment regarding involvement of the larynx and the nodes of the ipsilateral and contralateral sides of the neck and a decision regarding the need for and type of pharyngeal reconstruction as well as the role of combined therapy.

The free edge of the aryepiglottic fold separates the piriform sinus, the most frequent site of hypopharyngeal cancer, from the intrinsic larynx. Whether a glottic valve can be preserved despite sacrifice of a portion of the larynx along with the involved pharynx depends on the extent of laryngeal involvement. The usual guideline for partial resection of the larynx along with the piriform recess is laryngeal fixation. A mobile vocal fold, absence of thyroid cartilage invasion, and freedom from downward extension to the apex of the piriform recess are the factors that often permit a safe partial laryngopharyngectomy. Whether this operation can succeed depends further on the overall health and stamina of the patient.

Because nearly two thirds of patients have either clinical or microscopic evidence of cervical metastases, a unilateral neck dissection generally is part of the definitive operation.

Partial Pharyngectomy

For rare, small, posterior pharyngeal wall carcinomas or lateral pharyngeal wall piriform sinus carcinomas, these tumors can be removed with preservation of all laryngeal function. The pharynx is opened generally via a transhyoid pharyngotomy and, under direct vision, the lesions are excised. Confirmation is made of free surgical margins and the pharynx is closed directly. For the posterior pharyngeal wall lesions, depending on the size of the defect, the area can be left open to heal secondarily or a split-thickness skin graft can be placed into the wall. For the lateral pharyngeal lesions, the edges of the wound can be approximated directly. It is unusual to find tumors at an early enough stage in this location to be treated in the above manner.

Total Laryngectomy– Partial Pharyngectomy

Total laryngectomy–partial pharyngectomy differs in only a limited way from simple total laryngectomy. The steps are identical up to the point of entering the pharynx. The pharynx should be entered at the vallecula to obtain direct vision of the lesion. Mucosal incisions then extend down the pharynx opposite the cancer, with preservation of all possible mucosa. By rolling the larynx away from oneself, as in the opening of a book, one can view the pharynx directly. Mucosal cuts are made down the midpharynx, far from the cancer, and the larynx and pharynx are delivered to the pathologist. Careful visual appraisal of the remaining mucosa for foci of abnormal epithelium is essential. Laryngeal cancer is a field disease, and occasionally isolated foci of early invasive or in situ carcinoma can be seen and destroyed under direct vision with electrocautery. Closure is the same as in total laryngectomy, except that the uninvolved pharynx is rotated around a feeding tube. The near-total laryngectomy procedure can now be used for many piriform sinus carcinomas that do not extend into the interarytenoid area.

Partial Laryngopharyngectomy

Partial laryngopharyngectomy is suitable for carefully selected patients who have tumors of the high/medial piriform sinus that do not reach the apex of the piriform recess or impair cordal mobility. Invasion of the thyroid cartilage precludes the operation.

The basic procedure is a variation of the supraglottic partial laryngectomy, and all steps up to the cartilage cuts are the same as in that procedure. Neck dissection is a part of this operation because of the high frequency of cervical metastasis.

Technique

1. Unlike the cartilage cuts of the partial supraglottic operation, the cartilage cuts here extend from the superior horn of the thyroid cartilage on the contralateral side to the inferior horn on the affected side (Fig. 31-13A).
2. The pharynx is entered at the vallecula, above the hyoid bone, after the suprahyoid muscles are separated from the hyoid bone. Mucosal cuts are made down the contralateral aryepiglottic fold to the ventricle. The cartilage and mucosal cuts are joined, and the larynx is opened to expose the opposite cord and pharynx. Mucosal cuts are then made around the pharyngeal lesion and joined to the cartilage, and the specimen is removed (Fig. 31-13B).
3. The closure, including the cricopharyngeal myotomy, is the same as in the supraglottic partial operation.

Total Laryngopharyngectomy

Extensive carcinomas of the posterior pharyngeal wall, circumferential tumors of the

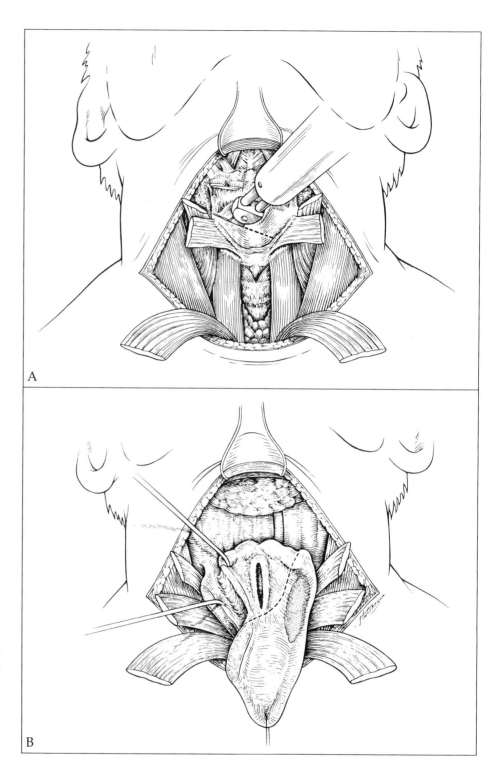

Fig. 31-13. Steps in partial laryngopharyngectomy.

postcricoid area and pharynx, or piriform sinus cancers that extend down into the cervical esophagus are treated by total pharyngectomy and cervical esophagectomy. The survival rates for this disease are low and the frequency of distant metastasis and uncontrolled regional metastasis is high. There is a legitimate philosophical question as to whether advanced pharyngeal cancers are a surgical disease.

The problem with the disease is not controlling the primary tumor. Total pharyngectomy in properly selected patients can

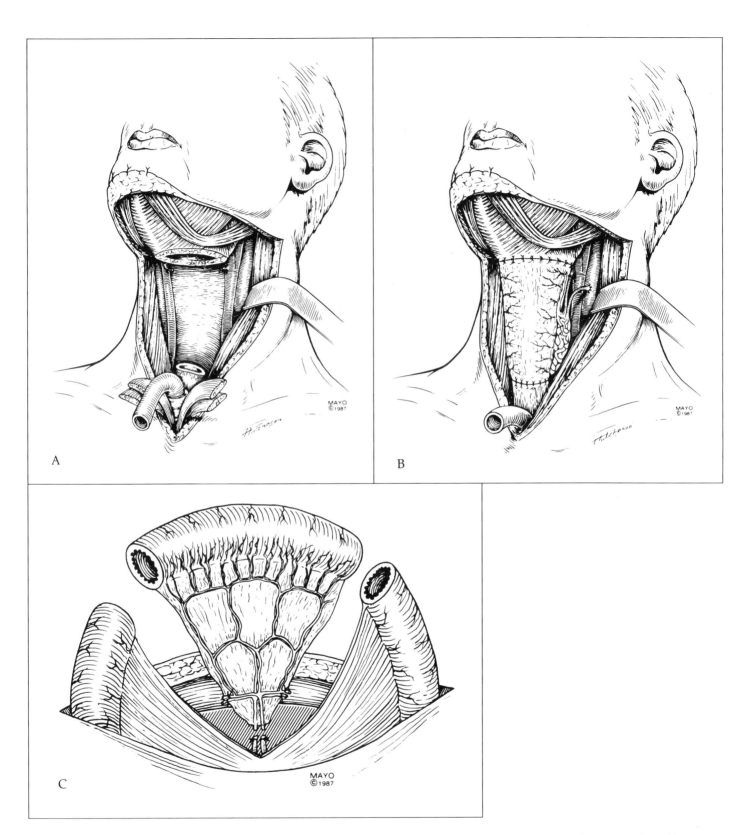

Fig. 31-14. *Jejunal reconstruction in total laryngectomy–pharyngectomy. A. Circumferential defect of the pharyngectomy. B. Jejunal segment in place with venous and arterial anastomosis. C. Appropriate length of jejunal segment isolated.*

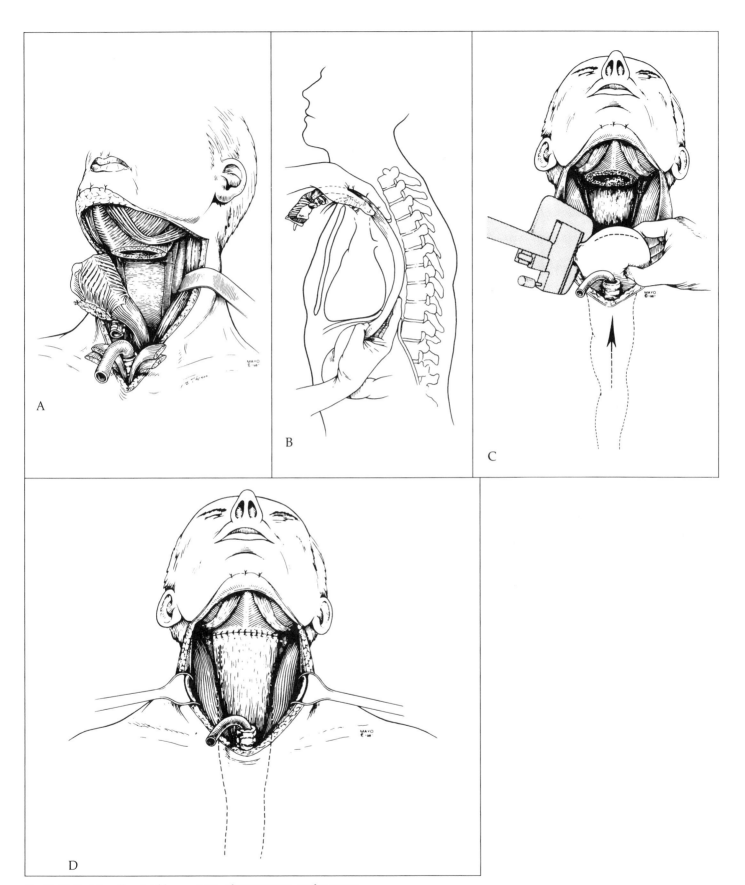

Fig. 31-15. Gastric pull-up total laryngectomy–pharyngectomy–esophagectomy.

be effective. Local failure is likely when tumor extends to the level of the palate and uvula or invades deeply into the parapharyngeal soft tissues, constrictor muscles, or pterygoid muscles. Multicentricity is also a problem, and one reason some believe that partial esophagectomy is inappropriate and total pharyngoesophagectomy is better for local control.

Our perception of the oncologic problem is that distant and uncontrolled regional disease, not local control, is the major cause of failure. Of 18 patients, 10 died of distant metastasis and 4 of local regional failure. This dismal result caused considerable suspicion about whether surgical therapy is appropriate for cure. Nevertheless, patients present themselves with obstructed swallowing and no clear indication that treatment is not possible. Radiation therapy fails, the patients present with localized disease, and surgeons are forced to substitute hope for reality.

Technique

1. The technique of total pharyngolaryngoesophagectomy is relatively simple. One or both sides of the neck are dissected using either complete or modified neck dissections, depending on the clinical findings. Both sides of the neck should be dissected if there is disease in either side because this disease is a midline cancer and potentially metastatic to both sides of the neck. In many instances total thyroidectomy or at least unilateral lobectomy is needed, and careful cleanout of the lower midneck, paratracheal region, and upper mediastinum is done.

2. After the neck excision is finished, dissection between prevertebral fascia and the pharyngoesophagus determines whether tumor has extended through the posterior wall of the gullet and into the prevertebral space. Prevertebral fascial invasion is an ominous finding.

3. The pharynx is entered anteriorly, usually through the vallecula. A circumferential cut is made, freeing the larynx, pharynx, and esophagus above. This maneuver allows extra distal margins by extracting more cervical esophagus from the thoracic outlet. The esophagus is divided below and the entire block is delivered (Fig. 31-14A). Our team approach allows the reconstructive team access to the abdomen during the neck

procedure. In this way, time delay is less in that a jejunal segment has been harvested and the abdomen closed by the time the neck work is finished (Fig. 31-14B).

In the course of the neck dissection, appropriate vessels are freed up. The arteries used are the lingual, superior thyroid, or the main trunk of the external carotid. Ideally, the common facial vein is used for the venous anastomosis from the jejunal segment.

4. Microvascular anastomosis of these large vessels is easily and predictably performed. The jejunum is then anastomosed to the esophagus and oropharynx (Fig. 31-14C).

5. If the extent of the cancer necessitates removal of the esophagus at a low level that does not permit a safe anastomosis between jejunum and esophagus, an alternative reconstructive method must be used. The extent usually can be determined preoperatively by endoscopy and a roentgenogram of the esophagus. In these situations, a gastric pull-up is used to reconstruct the pharynx. The stomach and esophagus are mobilized and the entire esophagus is removed with the specimen (Fig. 31-15A and B). The esophagus is amputated from the stomach and the site closed with staples. The fundus of the stomach is opened and anastomosed to the oropharynx (Fig. 31-15C and D). We have also used the near-total option for vocal rehabilitation with total pharyngoesophagectomy and reconstruction with regional flaps and visceral interposition.

Suggested Reading

Boca E, Pignataro O, Oldini C. Supraglottic laryngectomy: 30 years of experience. *Ann Otol Rhinol Laryngol* 92:14, 1983.

Carpenter RJ, III, DeSanto LW. Cancer of the hypopharynx. *Surg Clin North Am* 57:723, 1977.

DeSanto LW. T$_3$ glottic cancer. Options and consequences of the options. *Laryngoscope* 94:1311, 1984.

DeSanto LW. Cancer of the surpaglottic larynx: A review of 260 patients. *Otolaryngol Head Neck Surg* 6:705, 1985.

DeSanto LW, Devine KD, Lillie JC. Cancers of the larynx: Glottic cancer. *Surg Clin North Am* 57:611, 1977.

DeSanto LW, Lillie JC, Devine KD. Cancers of the larynx: Supraglottic cancer. *Surg Clin North Am* 57:505, 1977.

Devine KD. Laryngectomy: Vicissitudes in the development of a good operation. *Arch Otolaryngol* 78:816, 1963.

Dumich PS, Pearson BW, Weiland LH. Suitability of near-total laryngopharyngectomy in pyriform carcinoma. *Arch Otolaryngol* 110:664, 1984.

Komorn RM, Vocal rehabilitation in the laryngectomized patient with a tracheoesophageal shunt. *Ann Otol Rhinol Laryngol* 83:445, 1974.

Myssiorek D, Vanbutas A, Abramson AL. Carcinoma in situ of the glottic larynx. *Laryngoscope* 104:463–467, 1994.

Neel HB, III, Devine KD, and DeSanto LW. Laryngofissure and cordectomy for early cordal carcinoma: Outcome in 182 patients. *Otolaryngol Head Neck Surg* 88:79, 1980.

Olsen KD, Thomas JV, Desanto LW, Suman VJ. Indications and results of cordectomy for early glottic carcinoma. *Otolaryngol Head Neck Surg* 108:277–282, 1993.

Pearson BW. Near Total Laryngectomy. In CE Silver (ed), *Atlas of Head and Neck Surgery*. New York: Churchill Livingstone, 1986.

Pearson BW, Woods RD, II, Hartman DE. Extended hemilaryngectomy for T$_3$ glottic carcinoma with preservation of speech and swallowing. *Laryngoscope* 90:1950, 1980.

Steiner W. Results of curative laser microsurgery of laryngeal carcinomas. *Am J Otolaryngol* 14:116–121, 1993.

Thomas JV, Olsen KD, Neel HB, et al. Early glottic carcinoma treated with open laryngeal procedures. *Arch Otolaryngol Head Neck Surg* 120:264–268, 1994.

Thomas JV, Olsen KD, Neel HB, et al. Recurrences after endoscopic management of early (T1) glottic carcinoma. *Laryngscope* 104:1099–1104, 1994.

Zeitels SM, Koufman JA, Davis RK, Vaughan CW. Endoscopic treatment of supraglottic and hypopharynx cancer. *Laryngoscope* 104:71–78, 1994.

EDITOR'S NOTE

Doctors Olsen and DeSanto have presented an excellent chapter on the functional preservation of speech and, secondarily, swallowing following ablative operations for laryngeal and oropharyngeal cancer. As they correctly point out, the issue here is only partially that of function; it is also the ablation of the cancer and local control of the disease. Pfister and associates (*J Clin Oncol* 13:671–680, 1995), in an effort at organ function preservation in patients with advanced oropharyngeal cancer, utilized induction chemotherapy based on three cycles of cisplatin followed by external beam radiation with or without interstitial implant. Neck dissection and surgery to the primary tumor site were reserved for patients with less than a partial response after chemotherapy. Postoperative radiotherapy was also recommended. Overall median survival and failure-free survival rates at 5 years were 41 percent. Unfortunately, chemotherapy toxicity certainly contributed to the deaths of two patients and was suspect in two others. Forty-two percent of the patients experienced local control without any surgery. The downside of this therapy is that of the patients who survived, their speech was subjectively described as "always understandable"—hardly a ringing endorsement.

The use of a nasoduodenal feeding tube initially and preoperatively has not been emphasized by the authors. Since local complications may result in long-term inanition in these patients, it is probably best to treat these patients by placing a nasoduodenal tube preoperatively. A No. 10 or 12 French tube placed under fluoroscopy and not in the stomach will enable adequate feeding from the first postoperative day and thus avoid a period of inanition on top of a major operative procedure. Of course, if the pharynx is being violated, it is probably not good to have a nasoduodenal tube in place. However, this can be manipulated in the stomach at the time of operation and then, if required, manipulated into the duodenum subsequently. The role of nutrition in head and neck cancers is probably not given as much weight as it should, although many surgeons who specialize in the head and neck have long been aware of the need for permanent nutrition-utilizing gastrostomies. Percutaneous endoscopic gastrostomy is a useful adjunct that has been utilized extensively in our institution in conjunction with the head and neck cancer patient. There use of a No. 10 or 12 nasoduodenal tube allows one a great deal of latitude as far as the type of food that can be used, and should not be neglected.

J.E.F.

32

Resection and Reconstruction of the Trachea

Douglas J. Mathisen   Hermes Grillo

The indications for tracheal reconstructive operations are 1) primary tumors, principally adenoid cystic and squamous cell carcinoma, and a wide variety of malignant, low-grade malignant, and benign tumors; 2) secondary tumors, chiefly thyroid carcinoma, bronchogenic, and, rarely, esophageal carcinoma; 3) postintubation lesions, including cuff and stomal stenoses, malacia, tracheoesophageal fistula, and brachiocephalic arterial fistula, plus proximal stenosis including the subglottic larynx; and 4) stenosis of many causes, including trauma, prior operations, tuberculosis, amyloidosis, relapsing polychondritis, congenital malformation, mediastinal fibrosis, idiopathic stenosis, and Wegener's granulomatosis.

Preoperative Preparation

The lesions are best defined by standard roentgenograms, including anteroposterior filtered views to show the entire upper airway; lateral cervical views; oblique views; tomograms as necessary for detail, especially at the carina; and fluoroscopy for vocal cord function and malacia. Computed tomography (CT) adds data about mediastinal invasion by tumors. It is as important to know the extent of uninvolved airway left for reconstruction as it is to define the lesion itself.

Bronchoscopy is essential but can often be deferred to the time of resection unless the problem is unusually complicated. Rigid instruments used with general anesthesia provide better visualization of detail, superior biopsy specimens, and the potential

for airway management and improvement. Care must be exercised when using flexible bronchoscopy in the outpatient setting to evaluate tracheal stenosis for fear of precipitating airway obstruction.

Emergency tracheal resection is now rarely done. Critical obstruction can be relieved by dilation under anesthesia of benign stenosis with rigid pediatric bronchoscopes and dilators, and by coring out obstructing tumor with a rigid bronchoscope and biopsy forceps. Laser techniques have little use. Once the acute obstruction is relieved, careful diagnostic studies and examinations can be performed.

Patients must be in optimal condition to ensure the best chance for success. Those with postobstructive pneumonia or active mucosal inflammation, or those who are receiving high-dose steroids, should be dilated and the conditions allowed to subside. Repeated dilations may be necessary in some circumstances. Patients should no longer require mechanical ventilation. If it is decided that tracheostomy must be reinserted, it is mandatory to place the tracheostomy tube through the most damaged portion of the tracheal stenosis to preserve the maximal amount of normal trachea for subsequent reconstruction.

Surgical Technique
Basic Principles

Although not all problems have been solved, the last 25 years have seen the development of standard and dependable methods for reconstruction of the trachea. Because few patients with lesions requiring such operations are likely to be seen by

one thoracic surgeon, it is important that close attention be paid both to basic principles and to the special techniques of this type of operation. The rates of failure and complications in tracheal surgery remain unacceptably high when these operations are performed by surgeons who only occasionally operate on the airway.

Close attention to the basic principles of reconstruction will avoid many serious complications, which seem to occur frequently.

1. The trachea that is to remain in the patient must not be devascularized. Extensive circumferential dissection of the trachea should not extend beyond the levels of resection. Preferably, no more than 1–2 cm of trachea should be circumferentially freed from lateral attachments beyond the line of resection.
2. Approximation must be performed without excessive tension. Levels of tension in grams beyond which dehiscence can be expected to occur have been measured precisely in the laboratory. Skilled surgeons, however, know whether they are attempting to pull the ends of the trachea together under excessive tension. Surgeons who operate on the trachea must be familiar with all available techniques for mobilization of the trachea in order to lessen this tension. They must also make a mature judgment in advance of resection on whether sufficient trachea will be left to perform a safe anastomosis.
3. Precise anastomotic technique is required. Lines of resection should be cut cleanly. Fine absorbable suture material must be used. We use 4-0 polyglycolic

acid polymer (Vicryl) sutures for all anastomoses in adults; 5-0 polyglycolic acid polymer is used in small children. Stay sutures are 2-0 polyglycolic acid polymer and are usually left in place to reduce anastomotic tension.

4. Second-layer coverage of all intrathoracic anastomoses is required, especially after carinal reconstruction when the pulmonary artery is adjacent. The anastomosis should be airtight when tested under saline solution before application of the second-layer closure.

5. The airway reconstruction should function satisfactorily at the conclusion of the operation. It should not require internal stenting or protection by tracheostomies above, below, or through the anastomosis. If the anastomosis is not adequate at the conclusion of the operation, it is not likely that it will be so later on, even if stented. An exception to this general rule follows repair of a traumatically divided cervical trachea where both recurrent laryngeal nerves have been defunctioned, leading to an inadequate glottic aperture. In such a patient a tracheostomy is necessary well below the anastomosis in order to provide an adequate airway until the glottis can be repaired later. A second exception may be some patients with subglottic intralaryngeal stenosis.

Anesthesia

Most tracheal reconstructive procedures are performed under spontaneous ventilation, although assistance is given during the intrathoracic portions of these procedures as needed. Prolonged paralysis of respiration is avoided, since it is desirable that the patient resume spontaneous respiration postoperatively without the need for ventilatory support. We generally use halothane or ethrane. After the trachea has been divided either by the anterior or the intrathoracic approach, a sterile, flexible endotracheal tube with attached connecting tubing is introduced into the distal trachea for maintenance of ventilation. In carinal resection ventilation is usually maintained through the opposite (usually the left) lung after resection of the carina. With experience the use of such tubes is not cumbersome. The alternative of high-frequency ventilation through a catheter also works well and is used preferentially in special instances. While cardiopul-monary bypass can be used for simple tracheal operations—in which it is not needed—it produces hazards when it is used in complicated operations, since extensive manipulation of the lung while heparin is being used can lead to intrapulmonary hemorrhage.

Anterior Approach

The anterior approach to the trachea is used for most benign strictures of the trachea, even at the supracarinal level, and also for tumors of the upper and middle trachea. A low collar incision is used, and the upper flap is elevated to a point above the cricoid cartilage if there is no laryngeal involvement (Fig. 32-1). The lower flap is carried to the sternal notch. The anterior surface of the trachea is exposed. In postintubation stricture with prior or existing tracheostomies, or when prior operative procedures have been performed, dissection may be difficult and tedious. The strap muscles are generally elevated. The thyroid isthmus is dissected away from the trachea and retracted laterally with sutures. The important principle is to keep dissection close to the trachea so that the operator does not injure the recurrent laryngeal nerves while working laterally around the area of maximum disease, where there is maximum scar tissue and inflammation. No effort is made to expose the nerves in instances of inflammation, since this would likely lead to their injury. Circumferential dissection is carried only a short distance above and below the lesion to preserve the lateral blood supply of the proximal and distal trachea. The anterior surface of the trachea below is freed bluntly as far as the carina to provide mobility.

With tumors, dissection is not carried as close to the trachea as it is for other lesions. When the operation is for a tumor, the recurrent laryngeal nerves are identified distal to the lesion and followed to the area around the lesion to provide a greater margin around the tumor. If the nerve is involved, it must be sacrificed. At least one recurrent laryngeal nerve should be preserved. Adjacent tissue sometimes has to be taken with the specimen to provide adequate margins. This may include a lobe of the thyroid gland or part of the esophageal wall. Adjacent lymph glands should be removed with the specimen, but it is impossible to perform an extensive medi-astinal node dissection without possible injury to the blood supply of the residual trachea.

In an upper-tracheal lesion, dissection is carried first circumferentially around the trachea inferior to the lesion. This dissection is performed immediately below the lesion in order not to free excess trachea. Moreover, if the back wall of the trachea were entered unintentionally during dissection, entry would be adjacent to the lesion and would not injure the tracheal wall that is to remain.

Traction sutures (00 polyglycolic acid polymer) are placed at the midlateral position of the trachea on both sides through the full thickness of the tracheal wall and at least a centimeter below the projected level of division. The trachea is divided and the oral endotracheal tube is withdrawn above the lesion. The distal trachea is intubated across the operative field with a flexible endotracheal tube and sterile anesthesia tubing. An assistant holds this tube in position easily by arrangement of the lateral traction sutures, which can be drawn on to pull the distal trachea away from the field of dissection. The specimen is grasped with forceps and elevated. This makes dissection of benign stenosis from the esophagus much easier. It also gives access to tumors that have a posterior extension. If the esophageal wall is involved, either the muscular portion can be resected or the muscular and mucosal layers taken. The esophageal wall is closed with two layers of interrupted sutures, which provide a conduit both for saliva and for liquid feedings. This narrowed esophagus can be dilated later, although frequently it dilates itself with the passage of food by a process of intussusceptive growth.

Lateral traction sutures are placed on either side of the trachea proximal to the level of upper transection, and the specimen is removed. In upper-tracheal stenoses or tumors, this means that the lateral traction sutures are frequently placed in the substance of the larynx. If the division is very high, a catheter is usually sutured to the end of the peroral endotracheal tube so that it can be withdrawn out of the larynx to remove its bulk. The catheter remains as an aid for replacement of the endotracheal tube later in the operation.

In low lesions, division of trachea is usually done above the lesion so that the le-

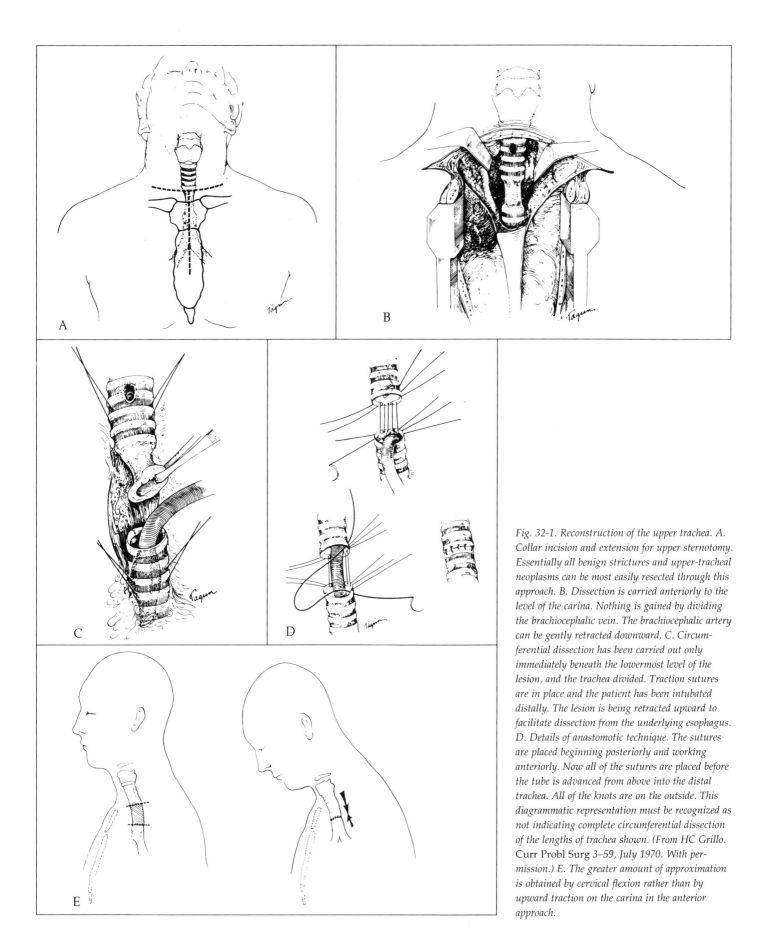

Fig. 32-1. Reconstruction of the upper trachea. A. Collar incision and extension for upper sternotomy. Essentially all benign strictures and upper-tracheal neoplasms can be most easily resected through this approach. B. Dissection is carried anteriorly to the level of the carina. Nothing is gained by dividing the brachiocephalic vein. The brachiocephalic artery can be gently retracted downward. C. Circumferential dissection has been carried out only immediately beneath the lowermost level of the lesion, and the trachea divided. Traction sutures are in place and the patient has been intubated distally. The lesion is being retracted upward to facilitate dissection from the underlying esophagus. D. Details of anastomotic technique. The sutures are placed beginning posteriorly and working anteriorly. Now all of the sutures are placed before the tube is advanced from above into the distal trachea. All of the knots are on the outside. This diagrammatic representation must be recognized as not indicating complete circumferential dissection of the lengths of trachea shown. (From HC Grillo. Curr Probl Surg 3–59, July 1970. With permission.) E. The greater amount of approximation is obtained by cervical flexion rather than by upward traction on the carina in the anterior approach.

sion itself serves as a handle to facilitate distal dissection. When the specimen has been fully dissected, distal traction sutures are placed and the specimen is divided inferiorly. If the lesion is a tight stenosis, it is dilated under direct vision and the anesthesia tube is placed through the stenosis.

The surgeon and assistant now pull the lateral traction sutures together on either side while the anesthetist flexes the patient's neck. This maneuver determines whether the ends can be approximated without excessive tension. If the ends can be approximated, the neck is allowed to fall back into extension and the anastomosis is begun. If tension is excessive, a suprahyoid laryngeal release is done. While it is possible to elevate the major skin flap to the level of the hyoid bone, we find it more cosmetic and convenient to make a second transverse incision directly over the hyoid bone to perform suprahyoid laryngeal release. We have noted fewer early postoperative difficulties with deglutition and aspiration when this procedure is elected in preference to thyrohyoid release. After completion of the release, the upper incision should be closed with appropriate drainage since it becomes inaccessible when the neck is flexed later.

Anastomosis is performed with interrupted 4-0 polyglycolic acid polymer sutures placed approximately 4 mm back from the cut edge of the trachea and about 4 mm distant from each other. The sutures are placed so that the knots can be tied outside the lumen. We prefer to place all sutures before completing the anastomosis. We begin with the most posterior suture in the membranous wall in the midline, placing each successive suture until the lateral traction suture is reached on that side. This step is repeated on the opposite side to the level of the opposite lateral traction suture. These sutures are individually clipped with a hemostat and then further clipped with a second hemostat to the drapes in an orderly manner. The most posterior suture is clipped cephalad and each successive one follows. The sutures are tied in the opposite order in which they are placed. Care must be taken not to confuse the placement of the sutures. The sutures anterior to the lateral traction sutures are next placed and these are fanned out on the operative drapes over the chest.

The divided distal trachea is suctioned frequently to prevent blood from seeping past the occluding cuff, which can possibly lead to postoperative atelectasis and a need for ventilation. After all sutures are placed, the tracheobronchial tree is suctioned thoroughly, the distal endotracheal tube is removed, and the endotracheal tube from above is passed into the distal trachea. The patient's neck is flexed, supported by blankets beneath the head. The lateral traction sutures are next tied on either side simultaneously by the surgeon and the assistant so that the ends are approximated. This permits the anastomotic sutures to be tied without tension.

The anterior sutures between the two lateral traction sutures are tied first. The excess of each suture is cut after tying. One lateral traction suture is gently pulled to one side by the assistant, and the surgeon proceeds to tie the sutures posterior to the traction suture down to the posterior midline in order. Each is cut after being tied. This procedure is repeated on the opposite side. The anastomosis is now complete. It can be tested for adequacy under saline solution. If the anastomosis is distal to the occluding cuff, the anesthetist can provide 30 cm of pressure to test the anastomosis. If the anastomosis is proximal, it is impossible to occlude the airway easily, and instead the cuff of the endotracheal tube is deflated and the anesthetist provides 30 cm of pressure. Gas escapes through the larynx, but at that pressure it demonstrates leaks under saline solution.

We leave the traction sutures in place even though they penetrate the wall of the trachea. We have observed no difficulty with absorbable sutures. The thyroid isthmus can be reapproximated and the strap muscles sutured over the trachea. A second layer is not necessary over cervical and mediastinal tracheal anastomoses. If the brachiocephalic artery lies directly over the anastomosis, it is not usually necessary to interpose tissue unless the artery has been dissected free in the original exposure. We avoid baring the artery. Dissection is carried out on the surface of the trachea rather than on the surface of the artery. This approach avoids the postoperative hemorrhage that has been reported so often after this type of operation. In reoperations in which the artery is necessarily exposed or in tumors in which the arterial surface has been exposed, tissue

should be interposed between the anastomosis and the artery. Thymus or one of the strap muscles is sutured between the two structures.

Transthoracic Approach

The transthoracic approach is used for tumors of the lower trachea as well as the carina (Fig. 32-2). We prefer a posterolateral right thoracotomy entering the chest through the fourth interspace. The azygos vein is divided, the pleura opened, and the trachea exposed. The vagus nerve is divided as it crosses obliquely over the trachea. If the dissection is carried high in the chest, care must be taken not to injure the right recurrent laryngeal nerve as it loops back around the subclavian artery. In dissection of the lower trachea, care must be taken not to injure the left recurrent nerve as it passes on the other side of the trachea over the aortic surface. The principles of resection are the same as in the upper trachea. If the distal trachea is resected, crossfield intubation is generally done through the lower trachea into the left main bronchus. This has the added advantage of collapsing the right lung. High-frequency ventilation can also be used. If intubation is used and partial pressure of oxygen (PO_2) begins to fall, a shielded vascular clamp can be placed on the right pulmonary artery to eliminate shunting through the unventilated lung. This is rarely necessary. An alternative is to continue high-frequency ventilation in that lung also, since this does not massively inflate the lung.

If it appears that there will be excessive tension when the ends are drawn together despite cervical flexion by the anesthetist during the tentative approximation, intrathoracic intrapericardial mobilization should be used (Fig. 32-3). If this measure is certain to be required, it is easier to do it before resection of the tracheal lesion. The inferior pulmonary ligament is divided. A U-shaped incision is made in the pericardium just below and around the lower portion of the inferior pulmonary vein, the structure that most ties the hilus down. Often this degree of release is all that is required to provide sufficient upward movement of the hilus for anastomosis. If upward movement is not adequate, complete circumferential division of the pericardium around the hilus of the right lung can be performed. When the

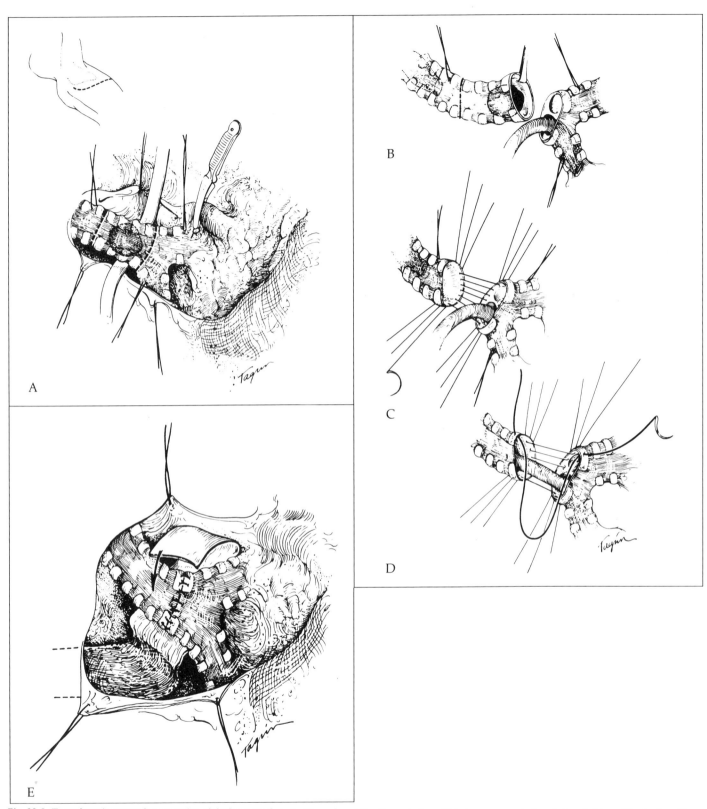

Fig. 32-2. Transthoracic approach to resection of the lower trachea. A. As much mobilization as is thought to be necessary is done before division of the trachea. The drawing shows the placement of a clamp on the pulmonary artery, but clamps are not placed routinely. Proximal and distal traction sutures are placed as in the cervical procedure. B. The trachea has been divided just above the carina and the left main bronchus has been intubated. C. Detail of anastomotic suture placement. D. The tube from above is advanced distally and the balance of the sutures placed. E. Once the anastomosis has been demonstrated to be airtight, a pedicled pleural flap or pericardial fat pad is placed over the anastomosis for security. (From HC Grillo. Curr Probl Surg 3–59, July 1970. With permission.)

pericardium is so divided, we attempt to save the pedicle of vessels and lymphatics in the posterior hilus by looping a tape around them. Salvage of these lymphatics may be important for the early postoperative function of that lung. It is important to remember that the neck should be flexed during the anastomosis, since this delivers a considerable amount of cervical trachea into the mediastinum. Laryngeal release does not help free the trachea for distal or carinal reconstruction.

After the reconstruction is completed and tested under saline solution, second-layer closure is made with a broad-based pleural flap or pedicled pericardial fat carried in a circular manner around the anastomosis and sutured into place.

The distal trachea can also be approached through a median sternotomy using Perelman's variation of the Abruzzini incision, exposing the lower trachea and carina between the aorta and vena cava, retracting the pulmonary artery and the brachiocephalic artery. The pericardium is opened front and back. It is not a truly adequate incision for difficult or larger tumors, especially those that might involve the esophagus posteriorly. The exposure is inadequate for complex anastomoses such as many for carinal reconstruction. It has the advantage, however, of allowing bilateral intrapericardial release should this be needed. In complex procedures, such as operations for large tumors of the middle and lower trachea, we have sometimes used a "trap-door" incision, which consists of a collar incision and median sternotomy that angles to open the right fourth interspace. This incision provides access to the entire airway from the hyoid bone to the carina. In such circumstances hyoid release and intrapericardial release may both be necessary.

Carinal Reconstruction

Our preferred approach for resection and reconstruction of the carina is right thoracotomy. Anesthesia and dissection are carried out as described earlier. The origin of the left main bronchus is easily accessible through the right hemithorax. The anatomic method of reconstruction is determined by the extent of the tumor and the amount of tissue removed. In a few instances it is possible to suture the medial walls of the right and left main bronchi together to form a new carina, anastomosing

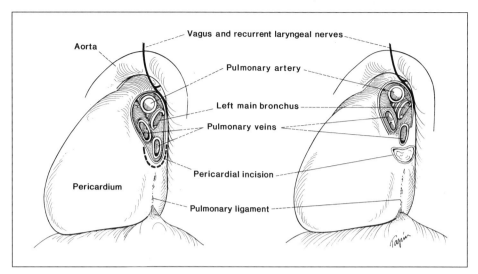

Fig. 32-3. The left-side intrapericardial hilar release technique, showing the U-shaped pericardial incision, which allows 1 to 2 cm of upward hilar mobility to facilitate the creation of a tension-free anastomosis.

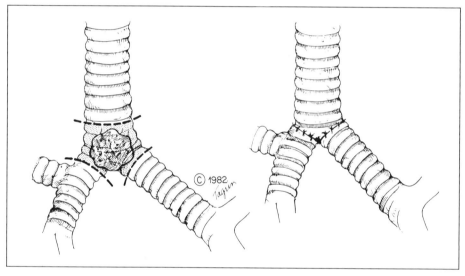

Fig. 32-4. Resection with restitution of the carina. This technique is applicable only for small, centrally placed tumors. (From The Society of Thoracic Surgeons Ann Thorac Surg 34:356, 1982. With permission.)

this to the distal trachea (Fig. 32-4). This procedure is rarely possible because fixing the right and left main bronchi together below the level of the aortic arch prevents upward movement. All the length necessary has to come from cervical flexion with downward devolvement of the trachea.

When more trachea has to be removed, we usually anastomose the trachea end to end to the left main bronchus (Fig. 32-5). The right main bronchus is elevated and sutured into a side opening made in the trachea 0.5 to 1 cm above the end-to-end anastomosis. An ovoid opening is made in the lateral cartilaginous wall so that carti-

lage is all the way around the margin of the anastomosis. The anastomosis must be done with precision. Pericardial mobilization is often necessary to permit elevation of the right main bronchus.

If a greater amount of trachea has to be sacrificed, the trachea and left main bronchus will not reach one another. Under these circumstances, with full intrapericardial mobilization, the right main bronchus is elevated to the stump of the trachea and an end-to-end anastomosis is made. The end of the left main bronchus is anastomosed to an opening in the medial wall of the bronchus intermedius (Fig. 32-6).

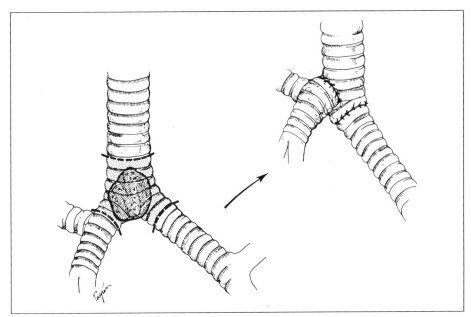

Fig. 32-5. Carinal reconstruction after resection. The trachea is anastomosed end to end to the left main bronchus and the right bronchus placed into the lateral wall of the trachea above the first anastomosis. (From The Society of Thoracic Surgeons Ann Thorac Surg *26:112, 1978. With permission.)*

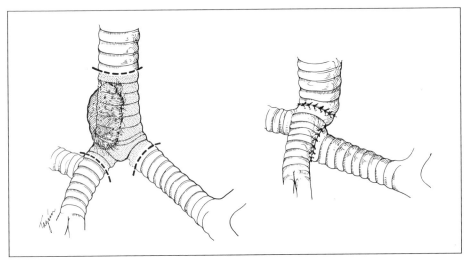

Fig. 32-6. More extensive tracheal resection, with advance of the right main bronchus to the end of the trachea and implantation of the left main bronchus into the bronchus intermedius. (From The Society of Thoracic Surgeons Ann Thorac Surg *34:356, 1982. With permission.)*

If the right upper lobe also has been sacrificed because of extension of tumor or in localized bronchogenic carcinoma of the right upper lobe extending to the carina, the bronchus intermedius or lower-lobe bronchus can be anastomosed to the trachea end to end (Fig. 32-7), or to the left main bronchus if it fails to reach the trachea.

In a number of patients who had prior left pneumonectomies and who required ca-

rinal resection for residual or recurrent tumor, resection has been done through the right chest, with care taken to maintain ventilation in the right lung, the surgeon retracting the lung gently to provide access to the carina without collapsing the lung (Fig. 32-8).

In a small number of patients, the approach has been made from the left side when a tumor involves a large length of left main bronchus but a small portion of

the carina. In this situation the left lung cannot be salvaged by any current technique. Tapes are placed around the base of the trachea and the right main bronchus to gain enough access to excise the carina and left lung, and a direct end-to-end anastomosis of trachea to right main bronchus is done from the left side. We have tried dividing intercostal vessels and approaching the carina from the left posterior aspect to the aortic arch, but this has not proved to be of much help.

An unsatisfactorily solved problem is how to approach a tumor involving a large amount of carina and a long segment of left main bronchus. If the approach is through the right chest alone, the tumor can be excised and the left main bronchus stapled off from the right side. Perelman proposed this procedure along with ligation of the left pulmonary artery to avoid shunting in the nonfunctional left lung. A left pneumonectomy can be done later. Another approach is bilateral thoracotomy. In patients who have satisfactory respiratory reserve, the approach has been through a bilateral anterior thoracotomy crossing the sternum in the fourth interspace. This approach provides excellent exposure for the resection, the right-sided anastomosis of the right main bronchus to the trachea, and the left pneumonectomy. However, it places demands on the patient's physiology and requires postoperative ventilation for some time. An alternative is a median sternotomy, which allows access for left pneumonectomy.

All suture lines are covered with flaps in carinal reconstructions. If a patient needs postoperative ventilation, as some may because of the extent of the procedure, safe ventilation can be accomplished with the cuff placed well above the anastomosis. The anastomosis can tolerate gas pressures but should not have a foreign body resting against it, which may cause inflammatory injury. If secretions cannot be cleared by physiotherapy, flexible bronchoscopy can be used freely.

Partial Laryngeal and Tracheal Resection

Postintubation or idiopathic benign strictures or neoplasms, primary or secondary, may involve the lower portion of the larynx as well as the upper trachea. In such circumstances it is possible after careful assessment of the extent of the disease to salvage a functional larynx. The problem is different in inflammatory lesions and in neoplastic lesions.

Laryngotracheal Resection in Benign Stenosis

If a subglottic intralaryngeal stenosis stops short of the vocal cords so that there is a space beneath the cords to which the trachea can be sutured, it is possible to correct many of these lesions and yet salvage recurrent laryngeal nerve function. The lower anterior portion of the larynx involved by the stenosis is resected with the specimen. The line of resection begins inferior to the lower border of the midline of the thyroid cartilage (Fig. 32-9). The vocal cords are just above this level. The line of resection sweeps laterally downward on either side through the cricothyroid membrane in general in the line of the inferior margin of the thyroid cartilage. It then transects the lateral laminae of the cricoid cartilage on either side and next angles posteriorly just below the inferior margin of the posterior plate of the cricoid cartilage. Dissection must be made with extreme care and must be very close to the cricoid cartilage to avoid injury to the recurrent laryngeal nerves, which enter the larynx medial to the inferior cornua of the thyroid cartilage.

If the intralaryngeal portion of the stenosis is entirely anterior, as it often is in stomal lesions due either to cricothyroidotomy or erosion by a high tracheostomy, the posterior mucosa overlying the posterior plate of the cricoid cartilage may be intact. If, on the other hand, the stenosis is circumferential, as occurs from pressure due to a large endotracheal tube, then the scar that overlies the posterior plate must also be removed. The scar is removed by excising it down to the surface of the posterior cricoid plate leaving cartilage intact. The upper line of mucosal division may lie just below the arytenoid cartilages. It is necessary to resurface this bared cartilage.

Distally, the line of resection of the trachea is beveled backward along the thickness of just one cartilage so that a prow is formed. Posteriorly, the membranous wall can be transected horizontally if a mucosal flap is not needed to resurface the posterior plate of the cartilage. If the posterior plate has been bared by removal of scar, a broad-based flap of membranous wall is preserved, as indicated in Fig. 32-9.

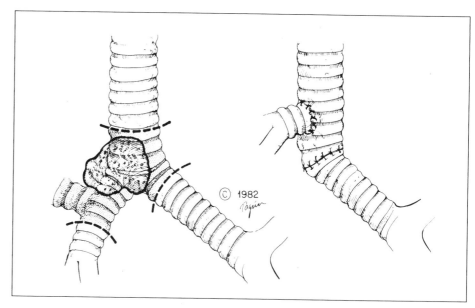

Fig. 32-7. Carinal resection with right upper lobectomy. With mobilization, the bronchus intermedius is advanced to the side of the trachea and implanted above the anastomosis of the trachea and the left main bronchus. If it fails to reach the trachea, it is implanted into the side of the left main bronchus. (From The Society of Thoracic Surgeons Ann Thorac Surg *34:356, 1982. With permission.)*

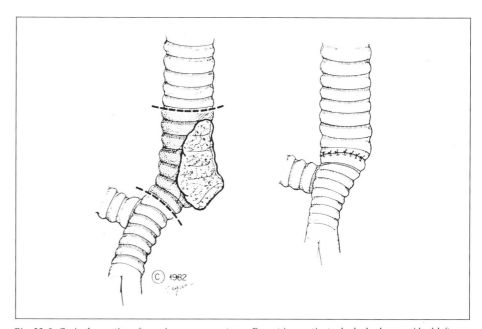

Fig. 32-8. Carinal resection after prior pneumonectomy. Except in a patient who had a long residual left main bronchial stump, these procedures were carried out through the right hemithorax. (From The Society of Thoracic Surgeons Ann Thorac Surg *34:356, 1982. With permission.)*

Where there is no posterior flap to be inserted, anastomosis is done in the conventional manner. Where there is a flap, we first place four sutures from the inferior margin of the posterior cricoid plate to a point about 5 mm down on the back of the membranous wall of the trachea so that the flap is free to cover over the bared cartilage inside. These sutures are carefully marked but not tied. After this step, all of the posterior anastomotic mucosal sutures are placed from in front from the margin

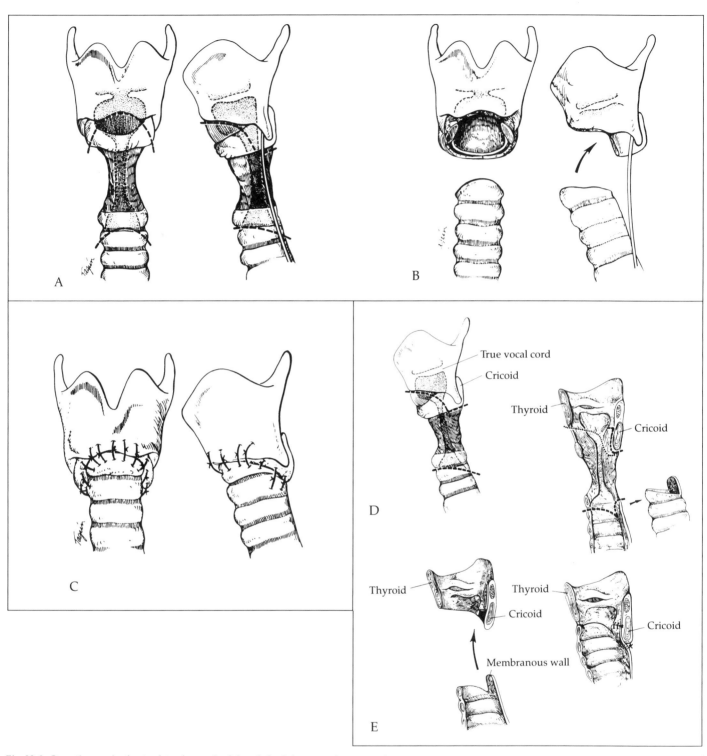

Fig. 32-9. Operative repair of anterolateral stenosis of the subglottic larynx and upper trachea. A. Anteroposterior and lateral views showing the extent of disease and the ultimate lines of transection. B. Larynx and trachea after removal of the specimen. Recurrent nerves have been left intact. The mucous membrane of the larynx has been transected sharply at the same level of division as the cartilage. C. Anteroposterior and lateral views of reconstruction. D. Resection and reconstruction of circumferential stenosis of the subglottic larynx and upper trachea. The external line of cartilaginous division of both the larynx and trachea is the same as in anterolateral stenosis. Interior view of the larynx and trachea demonstrates modifications necessary when stenosis involves mucosa and submucosa just in front of the posterior cricoid plate. Superior dotted line indicates external cartilaginous division of the larynx. Dashed line against the anterior wall of the cricoid plate indicates that the mucosa with its scarring will be cut back to within a short distance of the arytenoid cartilages, if necessary. Inferiorly, the posterior membranous wall has been retained as a broad-based flap. E. Resected specimen, leaving bare the area of the intraluminal portion of the lower part of the cricoid posterior lamina. The flap of the membranous wall of the trachea is fitted into the defect to provide complete mucosal coverage shown at the right. The mucosa of the larynx has been anastomosed to the mucosa of the membranous wall of the trachea. External to the lumen, connective tissue of the membranous wall has been fixed with four sutures to the inferior margin of the cricoid cartilage to assure that the flap stays firmly applied to the surface. (From The Society of Thoracic Surgeons Ann Thorac Surg 33:3, 1982. With permission.)

of the membranous wall flap to the mucosa within the posterior wall of the larynx. These sutures are placed so that the knots lie outside the lumen. The first few lateral anastomotic sutures, which go through the full thickness of the cartilage and mucosa of the trachea as well as the mucosa and some of the cartilage of the lateral laminae of the cricoid, are placed. The lateral traction sutures are tied. The first four fixing sutures are tied and cut. The mucosal sutures inside the larynx are tied with the larynx open so that the surgeon's finger can go into the larynx. After the posterior mucosal flap has been sutured into place, the balance of the lateral and anterior anastomotic sutures are placed in the usual manner, and tying is continued.

In some patients with inflammatory disease, a considerable amount of submucosal thickening and edema remains in the subglottic larynx all the way to the undersurface of the vocal cords. Therefore, reconstruction has to accept a narrowed airway. If the airway is inadequate after the reconstruction because of edema, a small, uncuffed endotracheal tube is placed well below the anastomosis for a number of days. If there is still airway obstruction after the tube is removed, a small tracheostomy is placed in a previously marked area well below the anastomosis. With time the edema usually regresses and the tracheostomy tube is removed.

Laryngotracheal Resection for Tumor

Occasionally, a high primary tumor, such as adenoid cystic carcinoma, or a secondary tumor, such as differentiated but invasive thyroid carcinoma, involves the lower larynx. Often one recurrent laryngeal nerve is already paralyzed. The line of resection is tailored to the particular tumor (Fig. 32-10). On the involved side this line may lie beneath the vocal cord. The amount of cricoid cartilage that has been resected anteriorly and posteriorly varies. The recurrent laryngeal nerve on the opposite side must remain functional. On the uninvolved side the resection line is just below the lower margin of the cricoid cartilage. Completeness of resection is checked by frozen sections. The line of tracheal resection is made to correspond to the line of laryngeal division so that the two can be mortised together. A protecting

tracheostomy is usually not necessary in these patients.

Tracheoesophageal Fistula

Tracheoesophageal fistulas often result from erosion by tracheostomy tubes or endotracheal tube cuffs pressing against an inlying hard nasogastric tube. The common wall of the trachea and esophagus is destroyed between the two foreign bodies (Fig. 32-11A). Usually there is also circumferential injury to the trachea caused by the pressure of the cuff. Weaning from a ventilator is accomplished by removing any foreign body from the esophagus, us-

ing as low a pressure seal of the trachea as possible and preferably putting the seal below the fistula. A gastrostomy is done to prevent reflux through the fistula, and a feeding jejunostomy placed. When the patient has been weaned from ventilation, a single-stage operation is done by the anterior approach. The injured tracheal segment is resected along with the esophageal fistula (Fig. 32-11B). The esophagus is closed in two layers with fine interrupted sutures (Fig. 32-11C). A strap muscle, usually the sternohyoid muscle, is pedicled downward and sutured over the esophageal closure to interpose healthy tissue between the esophageal closure and the tra-

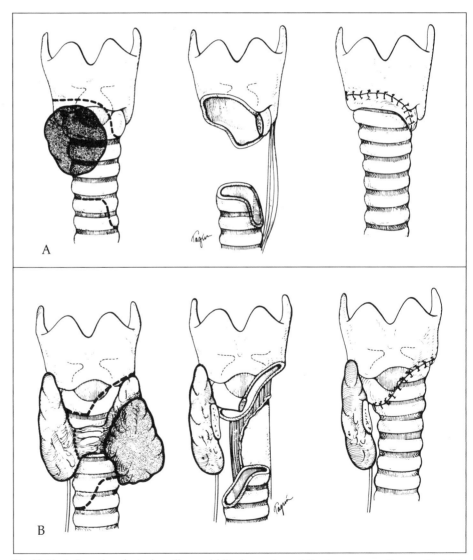

Fig. 32-10. A. Resection of mixed papillary and follicular carcinoma following recurrence 2 years after total thyroidectomy. B. Mixed papillary and follicular carcinoma, not previously treated, managed by complex resection, including removal of the anterolateral muscular wall of the esophagus. (From The Society of Thoracic Surgeons Ann Thorac Surg *42:287, 1986. With permission.)*

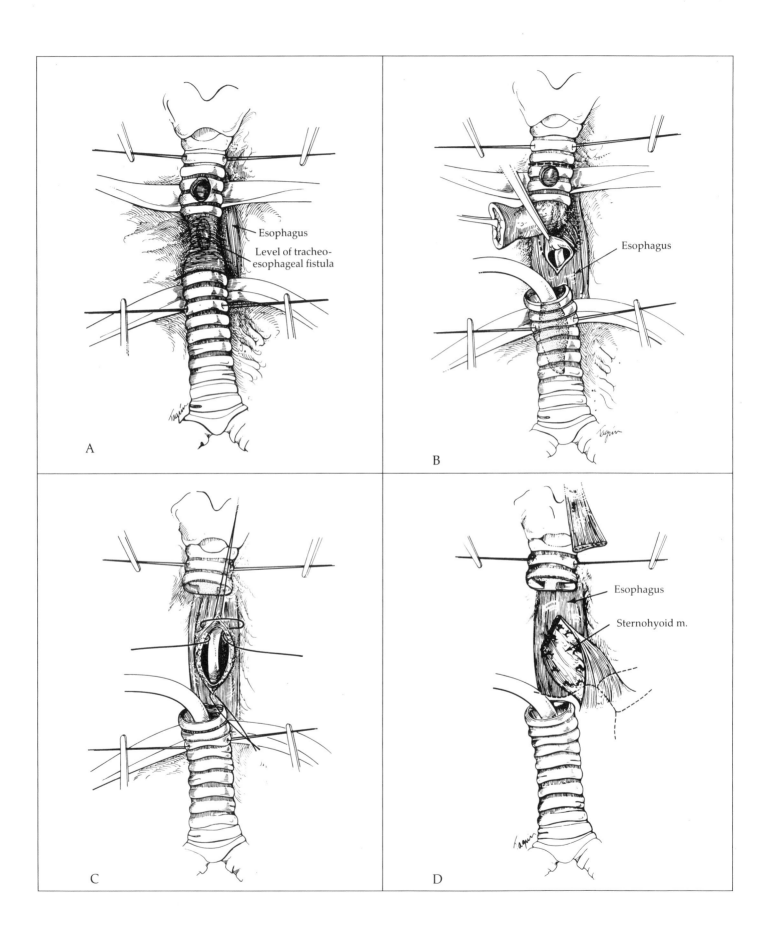

A

Esophagus

Level of tracheo-
esophageal fistula

B

Esophagus

C

D

Esophagus

Sternohyoid m.

cheal anastomosis (Fig. 32-11D). The anastomosis of the trachea is done in the usual manner. Interposition of tissue prevents recurrent fistulas.

Laryngotracheal Trauma

After the diagnosis is made, control of the airway is critical. If there is any doubt about the status of the airway, emergency tracheostomy should be performed. Repeated attempts at oral intubation should be avoided for fear of loss of the airway altogether. Examination of the traumatized airway is best done in the operating room with a flexible bronchoscope over which an endotracheal tube has been placed. This allows inspection of the airway and placement of an endotracheal tube if necessary. If difficulty is encountered, an *emergency tracheostomy* should be performed.

Patients should be scrupulously examined for associated injuries, such as laryngeal, vascular, esophageal, and spine injuries. The presence of these injuries may influence management of the airway injury.

Simple lacerations should be repaired by interrupted, simple sutures of 4-0 polyglycolic acid sutures (Vicryl). Complex injuries require individual solutions. Placing a tracheostomy through damaged trachea to secure the airway with repair of associated injuries may be appropriate in some cases. It should be stressed that all viable trachea should be preserved for further reconstruction. Concomitant esophageal injuries should be repaired in two layers and covered by a pedicled strap muscle to separate the esophageal and tracheal suture lines (Fig. 32-12). Laryngeal injuries are best managed in conjunction with an otolaryngologist and often require a protect-

ing tracheostomy. Complete transections of the airway almost always have damage to one or both laryngeal nerves. A protecting tracheostomy is needed after repair of such injuries because of the risk of adduction of the vocal cords.

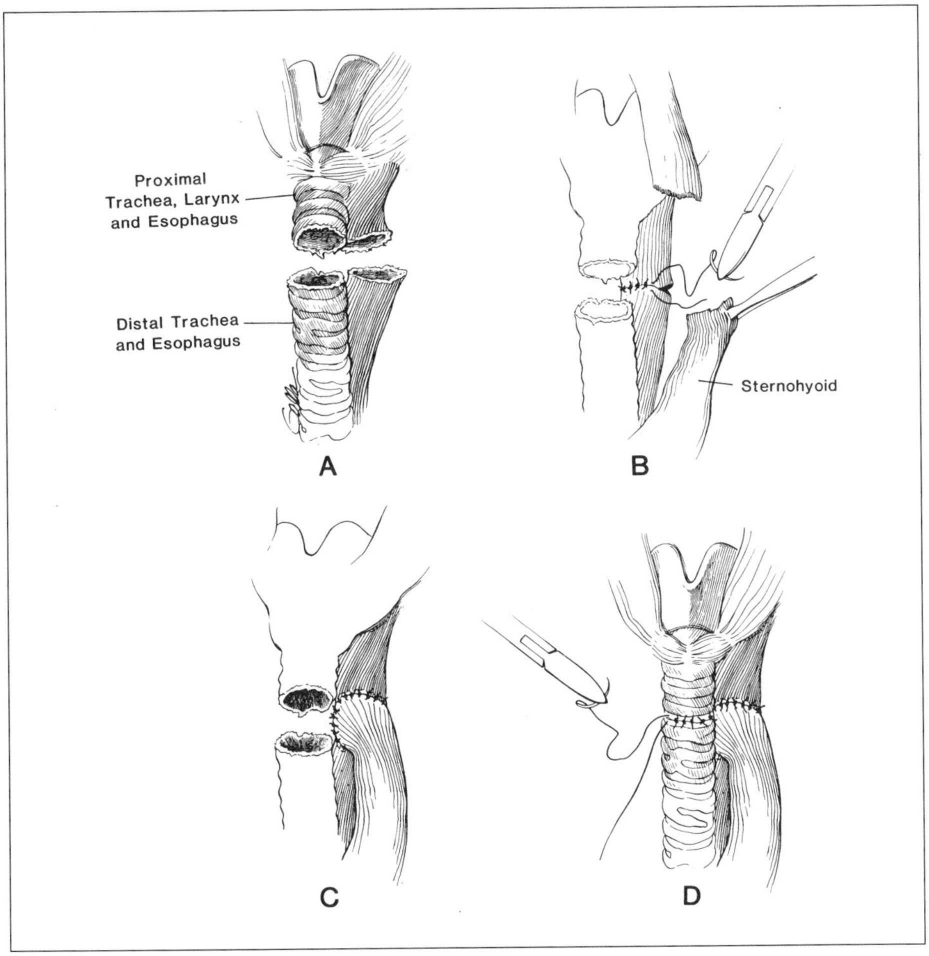

Pediatric Tracheal Stenosis

Tracheal stenosis in children is an uncommon problem. When present, if the child is of sufficient size, resection and end-to-end anastomosis is the procedure of choice for correction. If the child is deemed too small, a tracheostomy or T tube is preferable until the child attains sufficient size. Congenital tracheal stenosis is even more uncommon. Short-segment tracheal stenosis is best managed by resection and end-to-end anastomosis. If long-segment stenosis exists and respiratory distress develops, two main options are available. One option involves incising the stenosis (O-rings) and inserting a pedicled pericardial patch. The second method, described by Goldstraw and recently by Grillo, has been dubbed "slide tracheoplasty." It involves dividing the stenosis at its midpoint. The anterior surface is incised in the distal segment and posterior surface in the proximal segment (Fig. 32-13). The proximal and distal segments slide over one another and then an anastomosis is performed, as described for tracheal reconstruction.

Subtotal Tracheal Resection

We do not recommend the use of tracheal prostheses or staged tracheal reconstructions using skin tubes or other tissues. While successes have been seen with both techniques, the numbers of complications and hazards are so great that these procedures seem unjustified. It is extraordinarily rare for a benign stenosis to require a resection that cannot be managed by primary reconstruction unless it is in a patient who has had an inappropriate tracheal operation previously. In such situations a safely placed silicone tracheal T tube performs the same function as a silicone prosthesis placed surgically with considerably more hazard. Adenoid cystic carcinoma involving great lengths of the trachea would provide an indication for a prosthesis were a safe one available. At present we advise full-dose radiation therapy for such patients.

Fig. 32-12. A. View of transected trachea and esophagus. B. Esophagus closed in two layers. C. Strap muscle interposed between the esophageal and tracheal suture line. D. Completed repair.

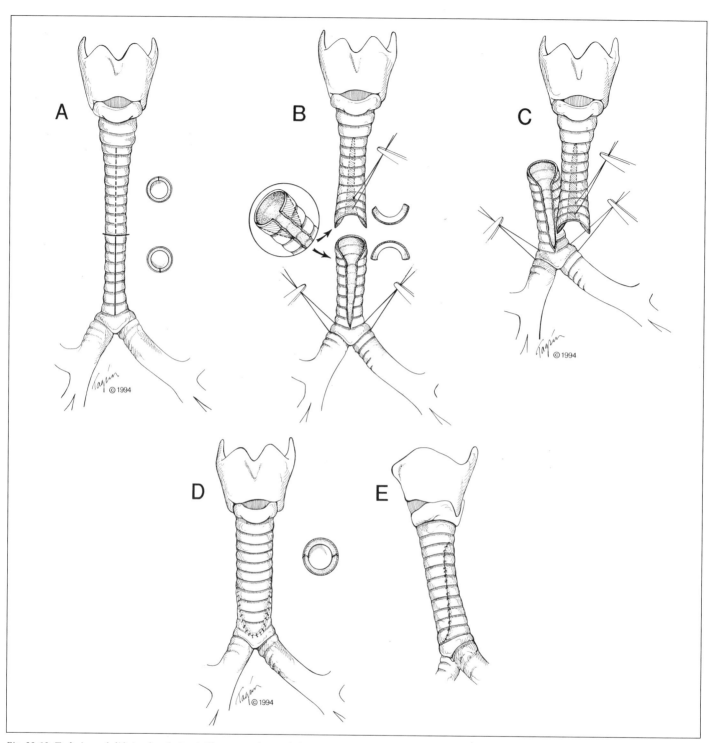

Fig. 32-13. Technique of slide tracheoplasty. A. The extent of stenosis is precisely identified. The stenotic segment is divided transversely in its midpoint following circumferential dissection at that locus only. The upper stenotic segment is incised vertically posteriorly and the lower segment anteriorly for the full length of stenosis. B. The right-angled corners produced by these divisions are trimmed above and below. A stay suture near the tip of the superior flap is helpful, as are traction sutures at the tracheobronchial angles or main bronchi below. Minimal dissection of lateral blood supply is performed. C. The two ends are slid together after placement of individual anastomotic sutures around the entire oblique circumference of the tracheoplasty. D and E. The circumference is doubled, resulting in quadrupled cross-sectional area.

Suggested Reading

Grillo HC. Slide tracheoplasty for long-segment congenital tracheal stenosis. *Ann Thorac Surg* 58:613, 1994.

Grillo HC. Carinal reconstruction. *Ann Thorac Surg* 34:356–373, 1982.

Grillo HC. Slide tracheoplasty for long segment congenital stenosis. *Ann Thorac Surg* 58:613–621, 1994.

Grillo HC, Mathisen DJ, Wain JC. Laryngotracheal resection and reconstruction for subglottic stenosis. *Ann Thorac Surg* 53:54–63, 1992.

Grillo HC, Zannini P, Michelassi F. Complications of tracheal reconstruction: Incidence, treatment, and prevention. *J Thorac Cardiovasc Surg* 91:322–328, 1986.

Grillo HC, Suen HC, Mathisen DJ, Wain JC. Resectional management of thyroid carcinoma invading the airway. *Ann Thorac Surg* 54:3–10, 1992.

Grillo HC, Donahue D, Mathisen DJ, et al. Postintubation tracheal stenosis: Results of surgical treatment. *J Thorac Cardiovasc Surg* 109:486, 1995.

Mathisen DJ, Grillo HC. Laryngotracheal trauma. *Ann Thorac Surg* 43:254–262, 1987.

Mathisen DJ, Grillo HC, Wain JC, Hilgenberg AD. Management of acquired nonmalignant tracheoesophageal fistula. *Ann Thorac Surg* 52:759–765, 1991.

Montgomery WW. The surgical management of supraglottic and subglottic stenosis. *Ann Otol Rhinol Laryngol* 77:534, 1968.

Salassa JR, Pearson BW, Payne WS. Gross and microscopical blood supply of the trachea. *Ann Thorac Surg* 24:100, 1977.

Tsang V, Murday A, Gilbe C, Goldstraw P. Slide tracheoplasty for congenital funnel-shaped stenosis. *Ann Thorac Surg* 48:632, 1989.

Wilson RS. Anesthetic Management of Tracheal Reconstruction. In HC Grillo, H Eschapasse (eds), *International Trends in General Thoracic Surgery*. Vol II. Philadelphia: Saunders, 1987. Pp 3–12.

EDITOR'S COMMENT

In this chapter Drs. Mathisen and Grillo have extended some of the techniques that Dr. Grillo pioneered in tracheal resection and reanastomosis for benign and malignant tumors and after cuff and other injuries following prolonged ventilation. Particularly imaginative, and a new addition to this volume, is slide tracheoplasty, in which an otherwise unresectable and unreconstructable long stenotic segment is opened anteriorly and posteriorly and reanastomosed. Since mobility of the upper and lower trachea of up to 6 cm presumably can be achieved by neck flexion, mobilization of the right hilum, and opening of the pericardium, presumably even a long segment of stenosis such as described in Fig. 32-13 is reparable.

This chapter is an excellent example of how the occasional operator would probably be best off, if possible, in stabilizing the patient's condition and referring the patient to surgeons who perform these techniques on a regular basis. As such, the general surgeon would hardly have occasion to utilize the techniques described in tracheal reconstruction. However, it is possible that one may have the opportunity to use the techniques that are so well described in surgery of the thyroid when one unexpectedly encounters ingrowth into the anterior surface of the trachea, and occasionally in the resection of esophageal carcinoma, in which the preoperative evaluation should reveal invasion of the left main stem bronchus or the trachea, or both. In these unfortunate circumstances, the techniques described herein would be quite useful.

In the posttraumatic situation, it may be difficult to stabilize the condition of the patient so that the patient can be transferred elsewhere, and it is the responsibility of the trauma surgeon or the general surgeon, or both, to deal with major disruptions of the trachea-bronchial tree without benefit of outside help. In our increasingly missile-prone society, suspicion of a bullet wound of the carina or trachea should be entertained whenever a bullet appears to traverse the neck or superior mediastinum. A bronchoscope is the first line of diagnosis. However, air in the subcutaneous tissues of the neck or the upper mediastinum should suggest that a tracheal injury is present. While some have suggested that small, opposed, nondisplaced wounds of the trachea can be managed by endotracheal intubation and ventilation for 4 to 5 days, this is somewhat less satisfying than identification of the rent in the trachea and careful reapproximation.

The collar incision provides excellent exposure of the cervical trachea and of the upper thoracic trachea. In the trauma situation, the sternal split can provide additional mobilization. Teeing off the sternal split into the right fourth or fifth intercostal space, as in the old trap-door incision, may provide additional mobilization, but most thoracic surgeons prefer a separate fourth or fifth intercostal space incision. A vascularized pleural flap or interposition of various strap or other muscles is useful, particularly if the patient has an injury to another main structure such as an artery or the esophagus, or both.

Wounds of the more distal bronchial tree usually manifest themselves as persistent air leaks through the thoracostomy tube and mediastinum emphysema. One should particularly suspect a bronchial injury when one cannot keep up with the leakage of air through two or more tube thoracostomies. Emergency bronchoscopy must be carried out. Under these circumstances, the wounds are generally 12 to 24 hours old and a good deal of inflammation is present around the wounds, making repair difficult. The interposition and reinforcement of suture lines carried out with meticulous technique after debriding the edges is essential if healing is to occur.

Others have advocated manubrial resection in dealing with tracheal tumors, most often for the ability to bring out an end tracheostomy, but at times in trying to obtain adequate margins of a tracheal tumor that has invaded the posterior manubrium (Howard and Haribhakti, *J Laryngol Otol* 108:230, 1994).

Two additional issues deserve mention. The first is that of a prosthesis. It is highly unlikely that any plastic prosthesis (mesh with lining, etc.) is going to be acceptable. Consequently, some laboratories have begun to experiment with tracheal transplantation. Since the vessels are very small, one requires the entire area to be transplanted and this has its limitations, especially if one bases the transplant on the carotid artery and the common venous trunk or superior vena cava. Lenot and his coworkers (*Transplant Proc* 27:1684, 1995) described a vascularized tracheal autograft. This is perhaps a somewhat wild idea, but suggests the way into replacement of trachea in a situation in which too much of the trachea has been lost.

Finally, another absolutely insane idea is the possibility of taking out the heart and putting the patient on perfusion, and then replacing the heart, in situations in which the patient has bilateral carinal disease and one needs to work in an unobstructed field. Since this has been done in the liver for bench surgery and certainly is routinely performed in difficult renal situations—for example, a tumor in a single kidney that requires segmental resection—it is appropriate to ask whether this has any merit at all. The problems of heparinization and other difficulties in having functional lungs after heparinization and cardiovascular bypass are real, but perhaps this idea should be considered.

Despite such philosophical musings, tracheal surgery has come a long way. Operations that were once fraught with danger now appear to be almost routine in the proper hands.

J.E.F.

V

Trauma to the Face and Neck

33

Evaluation and Repair of Common Facial Injuries

Henry W. Neale   W. John Kitzmiller

The management of trauma remains fundamental in surgical training and practice. Successful outcome depends on a team approach. The trauma surgeon becomes the primary care physician for the seriously injured individual. This chapter focuses on evaluation and repair of common facial injuries. Facial trauma occurs in a wide spectrum of severity and affects all age groups. Trauma patients may have preexisting conditions that will affect treatment and outcome. Often, soft-tissue injuries can be easily managed by the well-trained general surgeon by adherence to fundamentals of wound care. More complex injuries require a cooperative effort of the trauma surgeon and consultants in neurosurgery, otolaryngology, ophthalmology, oral surgery, and plastic surgery.

In this chapter, aspects of the history and physical examination that dictate special management of common facial injuries are emphasized, and the indications for radiologic examinations are discussed. A preferred approach to treatment of soft-tissue injuries is comprehensively detailed. This discussion includes choice and application of local anesthetics, wound preparation and debridement, the role of antibiotics, the technique of wound closure, and scar management. Recognition of injuries to the nasal lacrimal system, Stensen's duct, and the facial nerve is emphasized. A description of physical findings indicative of facial skeletal injury is detailed. These more complex injuries are routinely managed by the specialist. General considerations and operative approaches to these problems are described.

Initial Evaluation

Implicit in the initial evaluation of facial injuries are the principles advocated by the advanced trauma life support course of the American College of Surgeons. Assessment of airway, breathing, and circulation in the primary survey remains paramount. The detailed assessment of facial injuries is performed in the secondary survey. This chapter focuses on diagnosis and management of common facial injuries after the basic life support maneuvers have been performed.

Knowledge of the details of the traumatic episode is a tremendous aid in focusing further diagnostic and therapeutic measures. The mechanism of injury and the elapsed time until presentation should be noted. Sources of history besides the patient include witnesses of the accident, family members, and emergency medical staff. It is important to ascertain whether or not the patient is under the influence of intoxicating substances. Appropriate toxicology screens should be ordered if there is a reasonable level of suspicion. Alteration of visual acuity, dental occlusion, hearing, or nasal airway should be elicited. The past medical history and current medications should be recorded. The immunization status with particular regard to tetanus prophylaxis is important to document.

Management of facial injury is incomplete without an assessment of the cervical spine. Two to four percent of patients with facial fractures have concomitant cervical

spine injuries. Conditions such as rheumatoid arthritis and osteoporosis increase the likelihood of cervical spine injury after relatively minor trauma. Any history of posttraumatic neck pain or alteration in peripheral motor or sensory function merits further investigation before operative treatment of facial injuries.

Physical examination should include a notation of all lacerations, abrasions, ecchymoses, and external stigmata of trauma. Ideally, photographs of significant wounds should be taken in the emergency department. A second choice would be to make simple sketches of the wounds as part of the initial record.

Bleeding from the scalp and facial lacerations may be significant and can result in hypovolemic shock if they are not addressed. In almost every case, bleeding can be controlled by local pressure while the remainder of the primary and secondary trauma survey is completed. The level of consciousness should be succinctly recorded according to the Glasgow Coma Scale (Table 33-1).

Examination of the eye and appropriate ophthalmologic consultation when indicated is an important aspect of treatment of facial injuries. In the conscious patient, documentation of the visual acuity in each eye with the use of a pocket-sized visual acuity chart is important. An assessment should be made of pupil size, shape, symmetry, and reaction to pen light illumination. One should determine the presence or absence of blood in the anterior cham-

Table 33-1. The Glasgow Coma Scale

Eyes open	Never	1
	To pain	2
	To verbal stimuli	3
	Spontaneously	4
Best verbal response	No response	1
	Incomprehensible sounds	2
	Inappropriate words	3
	Disoriented and converses	4
	Oriented and converses	5
Best motor response	No response	1
	Extension (*decerebrate* rigidity)	2
	Flexion abnormal (decorticate rigidity)	3
	Flexion withdrawal	4
	Localized pain	5
	Obeys	6
	Total	3–15

From Oreskovich MR, Carrico CJ. Trauma: Management of the Acutely Injured Patient. In DC Sabiston (ed). *Textbook of Surgery* (13th ed.). Philadelphia: Saunders, 1986. P 324. Reproduced with permission.

ber of the eye and the presence of a red retinal reflex on funduscopic examination. Alteration of visual acuity, a history that suggests globe penetration, blood in the anterior chamber, and loss of red reflex are indications for emergency ophthalmologic consultation. A ruptured globe may be very apparent on physical examination if there is alteration of the shape of the pupil, loss of visual acuity, and loss of intraocular pressure. The findings are not always so obvious. If a penetrating injury to the globe is suspected, ophthalmologic consultation is mandatory.

Nasal fractures are very common. They are identified on physical examination by instability and crepitance on palpation of the nasal bridge. This is usually accompanied by significant tenderness, swelling, and ecchymosis that may involve the periorbital area. Key determinations are the presence or absence of a septal hematoma or cerebrospinal fluid (CSF) rhinorrhea. An untreated nasal septal hematoma can result in avascular necrosis or infection of the cartilaginous septum. This, in turn, can result in loss of nasal support and eventual nasal collapse. This troubling sequence of events can be prevented by early recognition of a nasal septal hematoma and establishment of adequate drainage. A septal hematoma is usually recognized by the

bulging of the nasal mucosa on intranasal inspection. A septal hematoma can be easily evacuated in the emergency department. After application of a topical hemostatic agent such as phenylephrine (Neo-Synephrine) or topical cocaine, an incision is made in the dependent area of the septum. The hematoma is evacuated and the nose is packed.

Cerebrospinal fluid rhinorrhea reflects a basilar skull fracture and a dural tear in the area of the cribriform plate. Suspected CSF leaks warrant neurosurgical consultation. Cerebrospinal fluid rhinorrhea often does not become apparent immediately after the accident. It may present 12 to 24 hours after the accident as a watery nasal discharge. The use of nasal airways and nasal intubation should be avoided in these patients under these circumstances.

Nasal hemorrhage after facial trauma is almost always self-limiting. If hemorrhage is uncontrolled by local pressure for 10 minutes, a complete intranasal examination should be performed by a specialist. In the hemodynamically stable patient, this can be performed in the emergency room. Intranasal examination requires the use of a head light and vasoconstriction of the nasal mucosa. A nasal speculum is used to visualize the nasal cavity. Mucosal lacerations are loosely approximated with chromic sutures and bleeding points can be coagulated. Anterior nasal packing with ¼-inch Vaseline gauze is usually sufficient. If anterior packing is insufficient to control bleeding, posterior nasal packing is indicated. One method of posterior nasal packing is with Foley catheters. After an airway is secured, the catheters are inserted through the nares and passed into the posterior nasal pharynx. The balloons are inflated and then the nose is packed anteriorly. These maneuvers should control virtually any nasal hemorrhage. Posttraumatic refractory nasal hemorrhage is most common after high-energy impact injuries with an associated coagulopathy. Once the coagulopathy is corrected, the packing can be removed or changed after 48 to 72 hours.

Examination of the oral cavity includes inspection of the dentition and a search for intraoral lacerations or ecchymoses. Missing teeth may have been aspirated or may be embedded in local soft tissue. They

should be searched for on plain chest x-ray and during wound debridement. Any alteration in the occlusion suggests a mandibular or maxillary fracture. Mandibular fractures that involve major segments of the anterior mandible may result in airway compromise. These patients should be watched closely. A secure airway is of paramount importance. Patients may require intubation or tracheotomy, or both, with early fixation of their fractures as the safest course of management. The edentulous osteopenic mandible and maxilla are very prone to fracture under relatively low-energy conditions.

The ear is often involved in facial injuries. Careful inspection of the tympanic membrane may disclose blood in the middle ear. Cerebrospinal fluid otorrhea and blood in the middle ear are signs of basilar skull fracture and warrant close clinical observation. The external ear is quite susceptible to trauma. Fortunately the collateral circulation around the ear is excellent and complex lacerations often heal well after adequate debridement and loose reapproximation. A hematoma may collect under the perichondrium of the ear after blunt trauma—for example, wrestling. If untreated, necrosis or infection of the cartilage can occur, with eventual major necrosis of the cartilaginous framework and distortion of the ear. Such a hematoma is recognized by swelling and loss of normal landmarks. Treatment involves prompt drainage of the hematoma and application of a gentle pressure dressing with close subsequent follow-up to ensure adequate drainage.

A complete physical examination of the head and neck after trauma should include bimanual palpation of the facial skeleton for the diagnosis of fractures and dislocations. The surgeon should carefully palpate for discontinuity in the facial skeleton that may indicate acute fractures. Discontinuities are most typically found along the nasal bridge, infraorbital rim, and zygomatic arch. Maxillary fractures are recognized by bimanual palpation of the upper alveolar ridge with the head stabilized (Fig. 33-1). Mandibular fractures can be identified by palpation of the mandibular contour in an effort to assess instability and deformity. Malocclusion can be a symptom of either maxillary or mandibular fracture.

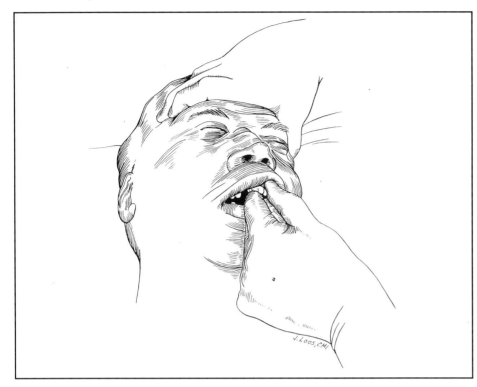

Fig. 33-1. Bimanual palpation of the facial skeleton for the diagnosis of midface fractures.

Radiologic Evaluation

Anteroposterior (AP) and lateral x-rays of the cervical spine with an odontoid view are important early radiologic studies in patients with injuries of the head and neck area. Abnormalities or questionable findings should be reviewed with a radiologist and a neurosurgeon.

Facial x-rays are obtained electively, depending on the findings of physical examination. Routine radiologic documentation is not necessary for the diagnosis or management of nasal fractures. The reverse Water's view is probably the most helpful plain film view for diagnosis of zygomaticomaxillary complex fractures (Fig. 33-2).

A cranial/caudal view or "bucket handle view" will show excellent detail of the zygomatic arch. Plain films of the mandible are quite helpful for diagnosis and management of a suspected mandibular fracture. A panorex examination is helpful for those injuries involving the mandible and maxilla. This examination can give detailed information about the nature of the dentition and dental roots. Panorex ex-

amination requires that a patient have a cleared cervical spine and be able to sit up in the examining chair. This study is occasionally not feasible acutely in patients with multiple trauma.

The indications for facial CT scan evaluation continue to evolve. At present, facial CT scans are indicated for the diagnosis and management of complex facial skeletal injuries. Injuries that involve the frontal bone and frontal sinus merit CT examination for diagnosis of intracranial pathology and to determine the degree of injury to the posterior table of the frontal sinus. A comminuted posterior frontal sinus fracture likely has an accompanying dural tear. Operative repair of this problem should be planned as a cooperative effort of the neurosurgery and plastic surgery departments. Significant comminution of the anterior table of the frontal sinus suggests the need for bone graft reconstruction. The potential need for bone grafting should be discussed with the patient and his/her family in the preoperative period. Significant disruption in the area of the nasoorbital ethmoid complex results from high-energy injuries. A precise diagnosis on physical examination alone may be dif-

ficult because of massive facial swelling. Computed tomographic examination of this area provides reliable information that may dictate a coronal incision for optimal exposure of this area as well as for a bone graft donor site.

Computed tomographic examination of the midface provides valuable information about orbital floor injuries. The degree of comminution and the size of the orbital floor defect often cannot be determined by plain films alone. To prevent late complications of enophthalmos and facial asymmetry, early diagnosis and the reduction of orbital floor and zygomaticomaxillary complex fractures are indicated. Axial CT cross sections give important information about the degree of displacement of zygomatic fractures. Critical information about the structure of the zygomatic arch posteriorly is readily available from this study. Comminuted fractures that involve the posterior arch of the zygoma may require a coronal incision for reduction and fixation. If there is significant comminution of the orbital floor with a resultant defect of 2 cm^2 or greater, significant enophthalmos can result. Accurate information about the bony continuity of the orbital floor can be obtained by coronal CT cuts.

Injuries of the lower third of the face are usually well detailed without the aid of CT scans. Mandibular fractures can be easily diagnosed by plain films and panorex. Injuries that involve the condyle with displacement of the condyle into the middle cranial fossa may be best visualized by coronal CT examination.

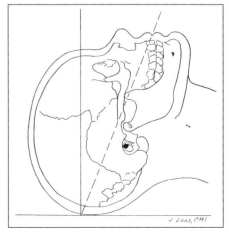

Fig. 33-2. Positioning for the reverse Waters' view.

Computed tomographic scanning has become a standard diagnostic test for major facial skeletal injuries. Computed tomographic findings are often influential in the decision for or against operative intervention. Computed tomographic scans provide important information that may dictate the operative approach and the need for acute bone grafting.

Treatment of Soft-Tissue Injuries

After completion of the primary and secondary surveys, soft-tissue injuries of the face can be definitively treated. If the patient has no other significant injuries, these can be surgically treated in the emergency unit. Alternatively, soft-tissue repair can be done in the operating room while the patient is undergoing definitive treatment for other injuries. Operating room treatment of isolated soft-tissue injuries of the face is indicated in the presence of severe contamination, airway compromise, or hemorrhage that is not easily controlled. Children or uncooperative patients may require general anesthesia for operative treatment for lesser injuries. The surgical goal is to remove devitalized tissue and debris and to evacuate any hematoma. The wound is then accurately reapproximated to obliterate dead space and restore normal anatomic landmarks without tension.

Anesthesia

Local anesthesia is used in virtually every case. Local anesthesia with epinephrine 1 : 200,000 provides excellent anesthesia and aids with hemostasis. Several aspects of the application of anesthesia merit further discussion. It is best to choose one local anesthetic with which to become very familiar. As a routine, the local anesthetic is neutralized with sodium bicarbonate to lessen the pain of injection. Bicarbonate solution 8% is combined with local anesthetic in a 1 : 4 ratio immediately before injection. Topical application of local anesthesia to the laceration may provide a level of analgesia that will allow subsequent injection with a minimum of discomfort. Nerve blocks of the supraorbital, supratrochlear, infraorbital, or mental areas are quite helpful and easily performed (Fig. 33-3). Local anesthetic, 2 ml, is injected into the appropriate location and 5

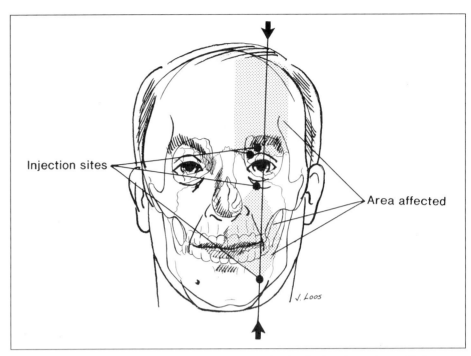

Fig. 33-3. Sites for injection and affected areas for supraorbital, infraorbital, and mental nerve blocks.

to 7 minutes are allowed for the anesthetic to take effect. Ideally, local anesthetic should be injected before wound preparation. Nerve blocks limit the amount of local anesthesia that is necessary for analgesia and allow reapproximation with minimal distortion of anatomic landmarks. A ring block provides excellent anesthesia for treatment of external auricular injuries. The vermilion border of the lip should be tattooed with methylene blue on a No. 25-gauge needle before injection of local anesthetic or application of topical vasoconstrictive agents in this area so that valuable anatomic landmarks are not lost.

Tetracaine adrenaline cocaine (TAC) is quite useful for anesthesia when treating small lacerations that do not involve mucosal surfaces in children or fearful patients. Two milliliters of solution is adsorbed onto a cotton ball and applied topically for 15 minutes. The agent may provide enough analgesia and vasoconstriction for surgical repair without injection. Frequently supplemental injection is necessary.

Conscious sedation can be safely administered in the emergency unit when necessary. In a study of over 2000 patients, intravenous fentanyl (Sublimaze) was given to children undergoing repair of injuries in

the emergency department. No serious adverse sequelae occurred (Billmire et al, *Trauma* 25:1079, 1985). Conscious sedation is particularly helpful for lacerations about the oral cavity in the child. Naloxone should be available before the procedure is begun. One should be aware of the side effects of Sublimaze—respiratory depression and chest wall rigidity. The Sublimaze should be reversed immediately if these side effects are recognized. Table 33-2 lists maximum doses of common local anesthetics.

Wound Preparation

After an adequate level of anesthesia is obtained, the wound is thoroughly irrigated with saline solution and all debris is removed. All clearly nonviable tissue is sharply debrided. If the patient has a full-thickness laceration of the lip or cheek, the oral mucosa should be reapproximated at this time with absorbable sutures. The field is then prepared with PhisoHex or povidone-iodine (Betadine) solution with care to protect the eyes. Direct scrubbing of the wound with antiseptic solution is avoided. Chlorhexidine gluconate (Hibiclens) is avoided in the head and neck areas because it can cause severe conjunctivitis.

A minimum of scalp is shaved in the immediate proximity of the laceration. Eyebrows are never shaved because they are valuable anatomic landmarks. Drapes are applied to create a clean surgical field. The entire face is exposed to allow better visualization of landmarks and alleviate patient anxiety. The wounds are thoroughly irrigated once again. Examination and removal of any remaining debris are facilitated with the use of magnifying loupes of 2.5 power or greater. Macerated or nonviable tissue edges are freshened. Any marginally viable flaps of tissue are preserved. Lacerations are usually closed in two layers. One layer consists of buried absorbable suture. The skin is closed with monofilament nylon. If there is significant dead space, a portion of the wound is left open and a small rubber band or Penrose drain is left in a dependent position. The drain is removed within 24 to 48 hours. Animal and human bite wounds are managed in a similar fashion. Although animal and human bite wounds are generally not closed elsewhere on the body, bite wounds of the face can be closed primarily. As a routine, antibiotics are not necessary for simple lacerations of the face. Parenteral antibiotics are recommended before debridement of complex soft-tissue wounds or bite wounds. A 5-day course of a first-generation cephalosporin or its equivalent is prescribed after closure of bite wounds. Tetanus prophylaxis is given according to the guidelines of the American College of Surgeons (see Table 33-3).

Puncture wounds are managed by thorough irrigation and debridement. Little or no closure of the surface wound is performed to provide adequate drainage.

Black powder injuries and traumatic tattooing represent a special case of facial injury that demands unique treatment. In this injury, a myriad of tiny foreign bodies are embedded at various levels within or just below the skin. If untreated, this will result in permanent deformity. To minimize deformity, debridement in the operating room is recommended. The black powder or small foreign bodies can be removed by extraction with the aid of magnification. This process can be assisted with dermabrasion or laser vaporization, or both.

Local wound care for facial gunshot wounds is determined by the nature of the

Table 33-2. Maximum Dose of Common Local Anesthetics

Generic Name	Trade Name	Maximum Dose (mg)*	Onset	Duration (mm/hr)
Lidocaine	Xylocaine	300 (400)	Rapid	60–120 min
Mepivacaine	Carbocaine	200 (300)	Rapid	90–180 min
Bupivacaine	Marcaine	175 (250)	Slow	4–8 hr
Procaine	Novocain	500 (600)	Slow	30–45 min
Tetracaine	Pontocaine or Cetacaine	100 topical	Slow	3–10 hr
Cocaine	Cocaine	150–200	Slow	1–2 hr

*Figures in ( ) are maximum dosage when epinephrine is added to solution.
From PL Kelton, Jr. Local Anesthetics. *Selected Readings in Plastic Surgery*. Oct 1988. P 10. University of Texas Southwestern Medical Center/Baylor University Medical Center. Dallas, TX and the Plastic Surgery Educational Foundation.

Table 33-3. Recommendations of Committee on Trauma, American College of Surgeons, for Tetanus Prophylaxis

I. Previously immunized individuals
  A. When the attending physician has determined that the patient has previously been fully immunized and the last dose of toxoid was given within 10 years
    1. For non–tetanus-prone wounds, no booster of toxoid is indicated
    2. For tetanus-prone wounds and more than 5 years have elapsed since the last dose, give 0.5 ml adsorbed toxoid. If excessive prior toxoid injections have been given, this can be omitted.
  B. When the patient has had two or more prior injections of toxoid and received the last dose more than 10 years previously, give 0.5 ml absorbed toxoid to both tetanus-prone and non–tetanus-prone wounds. Passive immunization is not considered necessary.

II. Individuals *not* adequately immunized
  A. When the patient has received only one or no prior injections of toxoid or the immunization history is unknown
    1. For non–tetanus-prone wounds
      a. Give 0.5 ml absorbed toxoid
    2. For tetanus-prone wounds
      a. Give 0.5 ml absorbed toxoid
      b. Give 250 units (or more) of human toxin-antitoxin
      c. Consider providing antibiotics

From The Committee on Trauma of the American College of Surgeons. A guide to prophylaxis against tetanus in wound management. *Bulletin American College of Surgeons* 69(July), 1979. P. 19. Reproduced with permission.

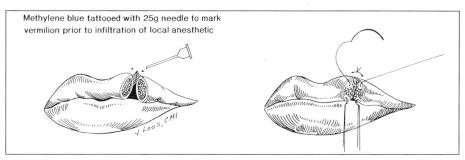

Methylene blue tattooed with 25g needle to mark vermilion prior to infiltration of local anesthetic

Fig. 33-4. Marking the vermilion border before local infiltration aids, precise repair of lacerations of the lip.

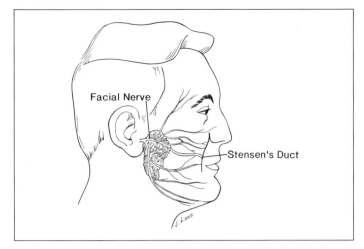

Fig. 33-5. Location of the facial nerve and Stensen's duct.

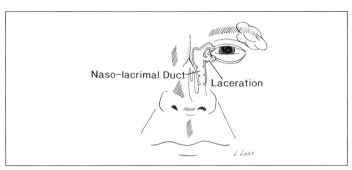

Fig. 33-6. The nasolacriminal system.

weapon and the range and path of the projectile. A complete physical examination is necessary. Low-energy entry or exit wounds should be debrided and left open to heal by contraction. Higher-energy wounds, such as a self-inflicted shotgun blast, require emergency airway control with intubation and operating room debridement and control of hemorrhage.

A key in assessment in the treatment of facial injuries is to determine whether or not a significant amount of tissue is missing. The vast majority of wounds can be closed primarily. The geometry of the laceration and reapproximation of normal landmarks, such as the eyebrow, vermilion border, or ciliary margin, will guide accurate reconstruction (Fig. 33-4). Rearrangement of local tissue with Z-plasties and local flaps is virtually never indicated for treatment of the acute injury. If major tissue loss is identified, a plastic surgery referral is indicated. If amputation of a major portion of the lip, scalp, or ear has occurred, microvascular replantation may be possible. The part is cleaned of gross debris, wrapped in gauze moistened with saline, and placed in a plastic bag on ice (*not dry ice*). Referral to a replantation center is indicated.

There are several important structures that may be injured, which should be recognized and treated appropriately. Facial nerve lacerations may be seen following sharply penetrating injuries from the level of the stylomastoid foramen to the lateral brow. These injuries are associated with palsy of the muscles of facial expression. In most cases, delayed primary microsurgical repair should be performed.

Laceration of Stensen's duct may occur following a deep penetrating injury to the cheek. Because Stensen's duct lies along the same plane as the facial nerve, concomitant facial nerve injuries are frequently present (Fig. 33-5). Proper treatment involves operative examination and microsurgical cannulation of Stensen's duct. Repair of the duct over a silicone stent is preferred. If untreated, Stensen's duct injuries can result in cutaneous salivary fistulas and prolonged swelling of the cheek.

Injury of the lacrimal duct occurs after laceration of the upper or lower lid margin medial to the lacrimal punctum. The lacrimal duct runs just below the lid margin at this level and is quite susceptible to injury if there is a vertical laceration through the lid margin at this level. If a lacrimal duct injury is suspected, specialty consultation is indicated (Fig. 33-6). Operative repair involves cannulation of the nasal lacrimal duct with Silastic tubing and microsurgical repair of the duct with repair of the lid laceration. The Silastic stent is usually left in place for 6 or more months.

Management of Facial Fractures

The treatment of facial fractures has evolved dramatically over the past 20 years. Small plates and screws are available to hold the fractures in reduction and prevent collapse. Choice of incisions for exposure and repair of facial fractures include coronal, lateral eyebrow, subciliary, intraoral buccal sulcus, and submandibular. Occasionally, adequate exposure can be obtained through an existing facial laceration. These incisions provide access to the facial skeleton, usually with quite acceptable scar camouflage. The surgical goal is anatomic reduction of the fracture fragments and restoration of preinjury dental occlusion.

After complete evaluation, facial fractures can almost always be approached in an elective setting after swelling has subsided. Exposure to the fracture is obtained through the appropriate choice of incision. Subperiosteal dissection of the fracture is performed. Fractures are reduced anatomically and held securely in place with intraosseous wires or small plates and screws. It is not uncommon to have severe comminution of critical bone segments. Acute bone grafting is recommended in these cases to replace these severely comminuted segments. Typical donor sites for acute bone grafting include split calvarium, iliac crest, and rib.

Fractures of the nose are diagnosed by history and physical examination. After complete evaluation, treatment is often successful by closed reduction and splinting. Late revisions are occasionally necessary in more severe injuries and may require cartilage or bone grafting. Revisions are usually delayed for at least 6 months from the time of injury to allow tissue to heal.

The second most common facial skeletal injury is the zygomaticomaxillary complex fracture. Displaced fractures require treatment to restore facial symmetry and to prevent enophthalmos. Occasionally orbital floor reconstruction is necessary because of severe comminution. The orbital floor can be reconstructed with an alloplastic implant or bone graft.

A blowout fracture is an isolated fracture of the orbital floor that is produced by blunt trauma to the globe. It can result in entrapment of orbital contents within the fracture site. Entrapment presents with diplopia on upward gaze. Computed tomographic scans with coronal cuts are helpful in determining optimal management of these fractures. If the orbital floor defect measures greater than 2 cm² in an adult, orbital floor reconstruction is recommended. Minimally displaced or nondisplaced fractures can be managed by observation.

Fractures of the mandible are often adequately treated by the application of maxillomandibular fixation with arch bars. Open reduction and internal fixation through intraoral or external skin incisions may reduce morbidity by minimizing time in maxillomandibular fixation. In the special case of bilateral subcondylar fractures, at least one side should be opened and fixed to restore posterior facial height. Fractures of the edentulous mandible may be especially challenging because of poor bone stock. Treatment should be individualized depending on the special needs of the patient.

Maxillary fractures require special attention to restoration of occlusal relationships (Fig. 33-7). The patient is usually placed in temporary occlusion with the use of arch bars. Fractures are then exposed through a gingivobuccal incision. Plate fixation is applied to the upper maxilla after reduction has been obtained. The patient is then usually allowed out of maxillomandibular fixation at the end of the procedure.

Displaced fractures of the upper third of the face are treated to prevent deformity

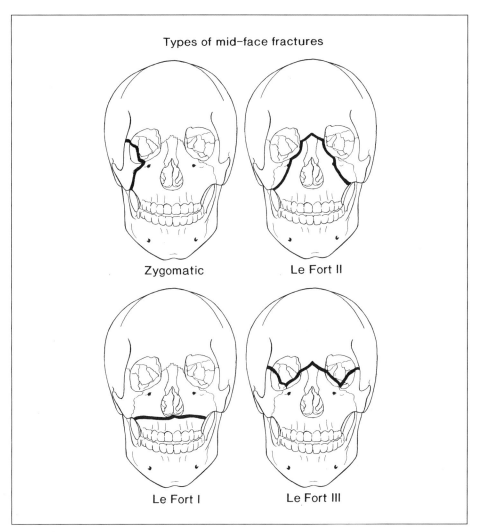

Types of mid-face fractures

Zygomatic   Le Fort II

Le Fort I   Le Fort III

Fig. 33-7. Maxillary fractures.

of the frontal area and the late complications of pyomucocele of the frontal sinus as well as the telecanthus. If the posterior table is intact and the anterior table is displaced, an assessment must be made of the nasofrontal duct. If the duct is open, simple reduction and microplate fixation of the anterior table of the frontal sinus are performed. If the duct is seriously injured, the frontal sinus is obliterated. Exposure is usually obtained either through an associated laceration or a coronal incision. The mucosa of the frontal sinus is completely removed by dissection with the aid of a high-speed bur. The nasal frontal duct is obliterated with muscle, bone, or fat grafting. Small plates are used to hold the fracture fragments of the anterior table in alignment. Bone grafting is often necessary to restore continuity of the anterior table for these patients.

Postoperative Wound Management

A few basic principles of early wound management will help minimize patient discomfort and aid healing. The patient should avoid strenuous physical exertion and preferably rest with the head elevated for the first 48 hours after the injury. Cold compresses will alleviate discomfort and help minimize swelling. Patients are allowed to wash over the sutures with soap and water within 24 hours after repair. Hydrogen peroxide may aid in keeping the suture line free of crusts. A very small amount of antibiotic ointment, that is, bacitracin, is applied to the suture line for the first 48 hours. Sutures are removed 4 to 7 days after the injury. Forty-eight hours after suture removal, the patient is encouraged to gently massage the wound with a skin moisturizer that contains a sunblock with an SPF of 15 or greater. Protection from sun exposure will help minimize pigmentation changes and massage may help desensitize the scar as healing occurs.

Surgical scar revision is not recommended until the wound has matured. A mature wound is characterized by resolution of local induration and return of pliability of the local tissues. Scar revision may be of most benefit to those patients in whom primary healing of the wound was compromised. The primary repair may have been compromised by a local wound infection or the presence of multiple other life-threatening injuries that prevented meticulous management of the facial injury. Occasionally, scar band contractures will occur around the eye, nose, or mouth. These contractures are usually readily improved by late revision. Scar revision does not result in scar removal. The scar is generally made larger by revision. For this reason, it must be undertaken conservatively. In our practice, dermabrasion has no role in the early management of facial scars, that is, less than 6 months after the injury.

Conclusion

Successful outcome after facial injury requires attention to basic surgical principles. Many common facial injuries can be appropriately managed by the trauma surgeon by following the recommendations in this chapter. More complex injuries require a cooperative multispecialty effort to optimize outcome.

Suggested Reading

Hiyama D, Appleby T, Daneker G, et al. *The Mont Reid Surgical Handbook* (2nd ed). Chicago: Mosby–Year Book, 1990.

Manson P. Facial Injuries. In J McCarthy (ed), *Plastic Surgery*. Vol 2, Part 1. Philadelphia: Saunders, 1990.

Schultz R. *Facial Injuries* (2nd ed). Chicago: Year Book, 1977.

Wolfe SA, Baker S. In J Goin (ed), *Facial Fractures*. New York: Thieme, 1993.

EDITOR'S COMMENT

Doctors Neale and Kitzmiller have provided a very straightforward and practical chapter on the treatment of facial injuries. It is important to remember that the most lasting effects of a traumatic incident may be distortion and unsatisfactory cosmesis of a facial laceration. The principles enumerated here are quite helpful, including general handling of tissues, thorough irrigation and debridement of all debris, and the use of normal guidelines such as vermilion, which can be marked with methylene blue with a No. 25 needle, so that even after the injection of local anesthetic these guidelines can be used for an appropriate approximation.

The most important message from this chapter is the appropriate evaluation of the patient. The injuries that are more severe than is initially apparent, such as a ruptured globe, lacerated Stensen's duct, lacerated lacrimal duct, laceration of the facial nerve, and complicated bony fractures, including orbital fractures, are probably beyond the expertise of most general surgeons, even in a trauma situation. Similarly, in reimplantation of tissues that may lend themselves to reimplantation with microvascular techniques, the trauma surgeon's role is to preserve the tissue on ice, irrigate it, wrap it in saline or antibiotic solution, and make certain that the patient gets to the appropriate center for microvascular reimplantation. With the current regionalization of trauma, that should not be difficult.

The overall surgical literature suggests that irrigation with antibiotic solution may be more appropriate than irrigation with saline. Since irrigation in general decreases polymorphonuclear leukocyte function, one might as well get some benefits from antibiotic irrigation. My preferred irrigating solution is kanamycin sulfate (Kantrex). In patients in whom one does not want to use Kantrex because of possible slight absorption or the dread of neuromuscular blockade (in the myasthenic, for example), cephalothin (Keflin) is an appropriate solution.

J.E.F.

34

Diagnostic and Therapeutic Approach in Penetrating Neck Trauma: Controversy of Management Techniques

John A. Weigelt

Symptomatic Patient

Controversy regarding the management of patients with penetrating wounds to the neck continues, but it must be remembered that these discussions do not apply to the symptomatic patient. Immediate neck exploration is indicated for patients with continued hemorrhage, large or expanding hematoma, or airway compromise. Operative or invasive treatment is also used for most patients who demonstrate any signs or symptoms of aerodigestive tract or vascular injury. The true management discussion centers on the asymptomatic patient.

Asymptomatic Patient

Many patients with penetrating neck wounds do not sustain injury to any organ requiring surgical repair (Table 34-1). These patients would not be expected to have signs or symptoms of injury, so it should not be surprising that many asymptomatic patients with penetrating wounds to the neck are successfully managed nonoperatively. If the presence of signs or symptoms of injury was 100 percent sensitive and specific, the controversy over managing a patient with a neck injury would disappear. However, physical examination is not 100 percent correct and the debate continues.

Table 34-1. Injured Structures from Penetrating Wounds to the Neck

SYSTEM INJURED	PATIENTS	(%)
Arterial	516	(12.3)
Venous	769	(18.3)
Digestive	354	(8.4)
Respiratory	331	(7.8)

Source: Adapted from JA Asensio, et al. Management of Penetrating Neck Injuries: The Controversy Surrounding Zone II Injuries In JA Asensio and JA Weigelt (eds.), *The Surgical Clinics of North America Contemporary Problems in Trauma Surgery.* 71:2, 1991; and LD Noyes, NE McSwain, IP Markowitz. Panendoscopy with arteriography versus mandatory exploration of penetrating wounds of the neck. *Ann Surg* 204:21, 1986.

Advocates of simple observation emphasize that a delayed diagnosis of injury does not increase mortality. However, simple observation can miss esophageal injury, which is associated with increased morbidity and mortality. Advocates of arteriography and esophagography emphasize that these tests decrease the number of negative neck explorations and the morbidity of a delayed diagnosis. However, these invasive studies increase the cost of management and have their own complication rates. Mandatory exploration is associated with at least a 50 percent negative exploration rate and associated surgical morbidity. Mandatory exploration can be appropriate when resources are limited and a low morbidity can be documented.

In summary, the debate remains unanswered.

The lack of answers might be related to our collation of the data. All penetrating wounds to the neck are considered equal in current reviews. The presence of urgent indications for operative therapy are infrequently culled from the total series. Symptomatic patients should not be grouped with asymptomatic patients. Additionally, the location of the injury in the neck should be recognized since many suggest that management of these wounds differ by location. One report suggests that for zone II injuries (Fig. 34-1), operative therapy is less costly than selective evaluation. The number of explorations in asymptomatic patients that are precipitated by diagnostic tests is also being scrutinized. Recently, the use of arteriography in the asymptomatic patient with a zone II injury has been questioned based on its low yield, incidence of complications, and potential for false-positive findings.

It might be time to rethink the issues of this controversy. A better data set with careful assessment of physical signs and symptoms would be helpful. Information needs to be stratified by location of injury and presence of symptoms. Since the debate is really about asymptomatic patients, symptomatic patients should be excluded. Collating these data points might allow us to better define management principles that provide high-quality care at a reasonable cost.

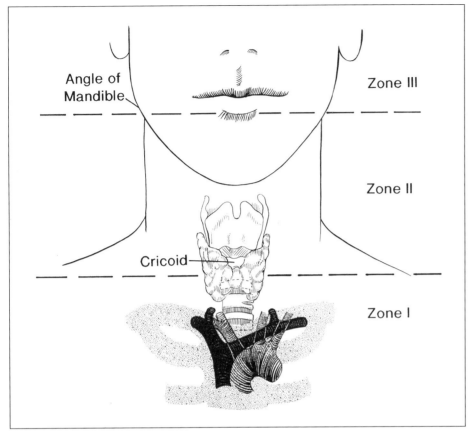

Angle of Mandible

Zone III

Zone II

Cricoid

Zone I

Fig. 34-1. Neck wounds are classified by anatomic landmarks into three zones.

Diagnosis

The physical examination of a patient with a penetrating neck wound is the first important step in any diagnostic evaluation. The presence of signs or symptoms of injury to any structure in the neck alters the subsequent evaluation. The other important aspect of managing a patient with a penetrating neck wound is the wound's anatomic location. The neck is divided into three zones (see Fig. 34-1), which helps identify the anatomy at risk for injury and helps to determine diagnostic and management approaches. Zone I extends inferiorly from 1 cm above the sternal manubrium, zone II is between zone I and the angle of the mandible, and zone III is from the angle of the mandible to the base of the skull.

Aerodigestive

Larynx
Laryngeal injuries from penetrating wounds are usually apparent on physical examination. Signs of airway injury include subcutaneous emphysema, midline swelling, laryngeal instability, or tenderness on palpation. Symptoms include hoarseness, hemoptysis, and dysphonia. Obvious signs of airway injury require no diagnostic work-up before operative exploration. Patients with equivocal findings on physical examination can require indirect or direct laryngoscopy. Examination of the larynx and trachea under anesthesia is sometimes the safest and quickest method of recognizing an upper airway injury. Management of laryngeal injuries is best done by a team approach. The general or trauma surgeon and otolaryngologist provide the core of this team. Tracheal injuries can require a team of the general or trauma surgeon and thoracic surgeon. A simple repair is all that is needed in many instances, but more complex injuries present options that are best confronted with multiple specialists. This chapter will not specifically address the management of laryngeal or tracheal injuries.

Esophagus
Signs of esophageal injury include cervical emphysema, hematoma of the neck, and blood in the oropharynx. Symptoms of injury include dysphagia, odynophagia, and hoarseness. Plain films of the neck and chest demonstrate the presence of missiles, retropharyngeal air or hematoma, and pneumomediastinum. Signs and symptoms suggestive of esophageal injury are present in the majority of gunshot wounds and in approximately one-half of stab wounds to the esophagus. Unfortunately, one-fourth of patients with no esophageal injury also have positive findings.

The two diagnostic methods helpful in identifying esophageal injuries in patients with minimal or no signs or symptoms of injury are esophagography and esophagoscopy. Esophagography requires a cooperative patient since dilute barium must be swallowed during fluoroscopy. Barium provides better roentgenographic resolution of perforations and is less toxic to the lungs if aspirated than water-soluble contrast material. False-negative rates of 0 to 40 percent have been reported with the use of esophagography in detecting perforation.

Rigid esophagoscopy is used to detect esophageal injuries in zones II and III and is more sensitive than flexible esophagoscopy. This examination requires general anesthesia and can be performed in the cooperative or uncooperative patient. When performing rigid esophagoscopy, the presence of any mucosal abnormality is presumptive evidence of an injury and mandates exploration. False-negative rates up to 40 percent have also been reported with this diagnostic modality. The combination of rigid esophagoscopy and cine esophagography is particularly sensitive in detecting esophageal injuries. Although the requirement for a general anesthetic is a drawback, patients with signs or symptoms of airway injury can also be examined with rigid laryngoscopy at the same time. Although the pharynx can be examined without general anesthesia, the examination under anesthesia is facilitated and excludes zone I injuries.

Vascular

The diagnosis of an arterial injury after penetrating trauma is most commonly made by the presence of arterial bleeding.

Bleeding can be external (visualized), contained (expanding hematoma), or internal (arteriovenous fistula). Occlusion with a pulse deficit is also possible. An injury can also be present with few or no signs of arterial injury. As previously noted, recent evidence suggests that the prevalence of asymptomatic arterial injuries in zone II of the neck is less than 1 percent.

Arteriography is the gold standard for the diagnosis of arterial injuries. Its use in zone II penetrating wounds is questionable because of the reliability of physical examination, low yield of positive findings without signs or symptoms, and the relative ease of surgical exploration. In contrast, its use in penetrating wounds of zones I and III is more common. Duplex scanning of the carotids offers another method to evaluate these patients. Availability of appropriate ultrasound machines and trained personnel limits the application of this noninvasive test in many circumstances.

Vertebral artery injuries are most commonly discovered by arteriography in patients with penetrating wounds. However, approximately 10 percent of patients with vertebral artery injuries are in hemorrhagic shock when admitted. These patients require urgent operative therapy. A knowledge of surgical anatomy is necessary to allow rapid control of a bleeding vertebral artery. As experience has grown with arteriographic embolization techniques, angiographic treatment of these injuries is also suggested since ligation is the recommended treatment.

Specific diagnostic efforts to define venous injuries are not usually used. Venous injuries are often found at the time of surgical exploration. Most likely, more are present than actually reported, but when present as isolated injuries, no specific treatment is necessary. Therefore, an aggressive diagnostic approach is inappropriate.

Indications for Exploration

Immediate neck exploration is indicated for patients with a penetrating neck wound associated with ongoing hemorrhage, large or expanding hematoma, or airway compromise. Symptomatic pa-

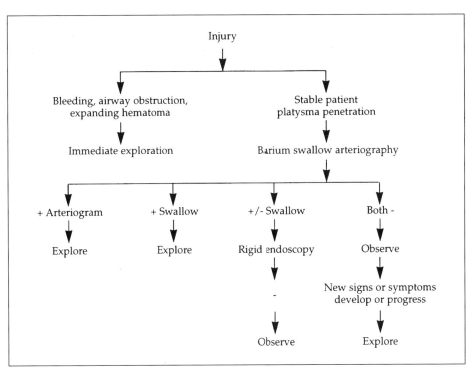

Fig. 34-2. Penetrating neck trauma treatment algorithm for selective management.

tients with injuries confined to zone II of the neck are also candidates for immediate operation. Patients with zone I or III penetrating wounds who are symptomatic but have no instability of cardiopulmonary or neurologic parameters might require diagnostic arteriography to plan a surgical approach or develop a nonoperative course of management. This nonoperative management can include embolization of nonvital but injured vessels.

Asymptomatic patients who are managed expectantly without diagnostic studies require operative therapy if symptoms or signs of injury develop. If these patients undergo a diagnostic work-up that reveals injury to the aerodigestive or arterial system, operative exploration is suggested (Fig. 34-2).

Surgical Techniques
General Exposure Principles

A standard anterior sternocleidomastoid incision provides excellent exposure when a unilateral neck exploration is planned. This incision can extend from the clavicular head to the mastoid process. It can also

be used to enter the upper mediastinum by extending the incision inferiorly as a median sternotomy. Curving the inferior aspect of this incision across the midline at the thoracic inlet can help provide exposure into the other side of the neck. A contralateral anterior incision is another method to gain exposure to both sides of the neck for a transcervical penetrating wound.

However, when a bilateral exploration is needed, a generous collar incision is often preferable. This incision is placed two fingerbreadths or 3 to 4 cm above the clavicular heads and can extend upward to the level of the mandibular angle. A large skin flap is developed superiorly providing adequate exposure to structures high in the neck (Fig. 34-3).

The sternocleidomastoid is retracted laterally to expose the carotid sheath. The omohyoid muscle passes laterally deep to the sternocleidomastoid inserting on the scapula and can be retracted or divided as necessary. Mobilization of the carotid sheath can require division of the facial vein and the ansa cervicalis loop. Division of the interior thyroid artery and middle thyroid veins is also possible to help fully mobilize the thyroid. It is important to

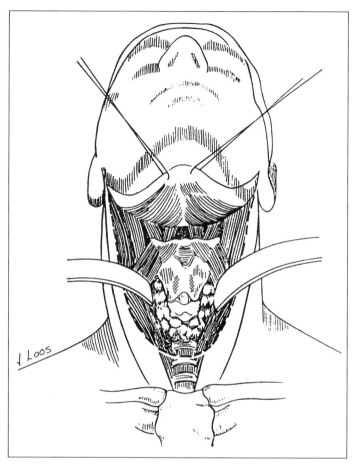

Fig. 34-3. A large skin flap is developed superiorly providing adequate exposure to structures in the midline. This approach is helpful when bilateral neck exploration is necessary.

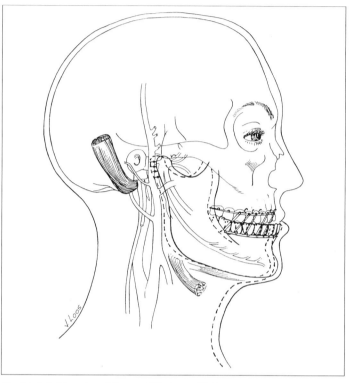

Fig. 34-4. Subluxation of the mandible is possible but requires preoperative placement of a dental appliance.

avoid injury to the recurrent laryngeal nerves. These nerves are usually located in the groove between the esophagus and trachea but can be in other locations as well, especially on the right side. Care must be taken to avoid injury to these nerves when circumferential mobilization of the esophagus is necessary.

Carotid Exposure and Repair

Exposure of the carotid artery begins in the base of the neck to avoid the suspected area of injury. When thoracic inlet injuries (carotid, innominate, and vertebral arteries) are suspected, a median sternotomy is helpful in obtaining proximal control of the arterial tree. The jugular vein and sternocleidomastoid muscles are retracted laterally. The common carotid artery is identified and a vascular tape placed around

the vessel. Dissection is adequate to safely apply a vascular clamp on the artery when inflow occlusion is necessary. Dissection is kept close to the artery to avoid injury to the vagus and hypoglossal nerves.

Distal control requires careful dissection of the internal and external carotid arteries above the carotid bifurcation. These arteries are gently encircled with vascular tapes. Again, dissection should be complete enough to allow placement of vascular clamps.

Exposure above the bifurcation requires further dissection along the anterior border of the sternocleidomastoid muscle. The trigeminal nerve must be protected as it passes near and deep to the angle of the mandible. The branches of the glossopharyngeal and vagus nerves must also be preserved. The digastric muscle belly can be transected to expose the carotid more

cephalad. Subluxation of the mandible is also possible but requires preoperative placement of a dental appliance (Fig. 34-4).

Ideally, distal and proximal control of the injured carotid is obtained before the injury is exposed, which allows vascular clamps to control blood loss (Fig. 34-5). If this step is not possible, digital pressure is often adequate to control hemorrhage while proximal and distal control are obtained. Simple lacerations can be repaired with either a running or an interrupted suture technique. A small monofilament suture is used and care is taken to coapt the intima, which should prevent the repair from becoming a source of microemboli or clotting.

Injuries causing tissue loss require resection and primary anastomosis whenever possible. Spatulation of the ends is helpful

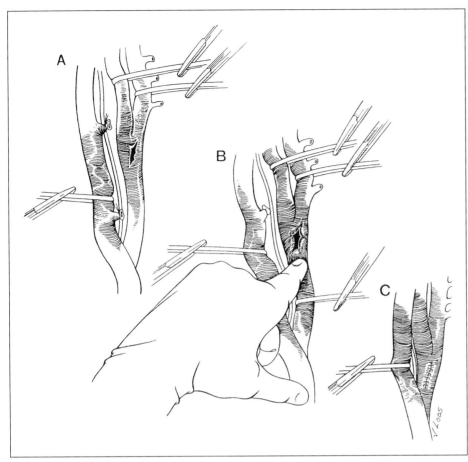

Fig. 34-5. Distal and proximal control of the injured carotid before exposure of the injury allows control of blood loss. Double looping of vascular loops can provide this control without clamps.

in avoiding stenosis at the anastomotic site. Either continuous or interrupted sutures are used. Resection and end-to-end anastomosis is particularly appropriate for common carotid artery injuries.

Internal carotid artery injuries can be repaired with a primary anastomosis but often mandate the use of an interposition graft. The external carotid artery is occasionally an adequate substitute for the internal carotid artery. When this procedure is performed, the internal carotid artery origin is carefully oversewn at the bulb. An interposition graft with a piece of reversed saphenous vein or nonreversed after valvulotomy can be used (Fig. 34-6). Size match is usually not a problem for repair of internal carotid injuries but can be a problem with common carotid injuries. The proximal saphenous vein should always be used whenever possible to lessen this problem. If the size discrepancy is too great, a polytetrafluoroethylene (PTFE)

graft is helpful in repairing these common carotid defects.

The use of temporary shunts while repairing the internal carotid artery remains controversial. They do not have a role in the management of common carotid artery injuries. If back flow from an internal carotid injury is poor and time to repair will be excessive, an indwelling shunt can help. A shunt can also be used when an interposition graft is being placed (Fig. 34-6).

Vertebral Artery Exposure and Repair

For vertebral artery exposure and repair, the anterior skin incision is used and proximal control is easy to obtain in the thoracic inlet. These vessels are usually branches of the subclavian and found lateral and in a slightly deeper plane than the common carotid. When the vertebral artery is the goal of surgical exposure, it is

helpful to turn the patient's head farther away from the side of incision, compared with the head position when exposing the carotid artery. Proximal control is obtained with a vascular loop (Fig. 34-7).

The vertebral artery enters the cervical bony canal at C6. The sternocleidomastoid muscle is retracted laterally while the internal jugular vein is retracted medially. The incision is carried deeply to expose the retrovisceral space and the prevertebral muscles. The carotid sheath, trachea, and esophagus are mobilized en masse medially to accomplish this exposure. The longus colli is identified and mobilized medial to lateral to expose the anterior surface of the vertebral body (Fig. 34-8). The anterior tubercle is a fixation point for this muscle and is the landmark for this lateral mobilization of the longus colli. A groove on the front of each transverse process, which is now palpable, is bounded laterally by the anterior tubercle and the attached longus colli muscle. The bone covering this canal can be removed using a rongeur forceps (Fig. 34-8B,C). Care must be taken to only remove the roof of the canal, leaving the anterior tubercle undisturbed. Disruption of the anterior tubercle could damage the anterior rami of the corresponding cervical nerve. The nerve lies behind the artery in the bony canal as does a venous component. A small right-angle clamp is helpful in gently dissecting the artery free from the nerve and venous attachments. Once encircled, the artery is usually simply ligated above and below the site of injury.

Ligation of the vertebral artery is also possible between C1 and C2 without the need for unroofing the bony canal. The incision is carried under the ear over the mastoid prominence (Fig. 34-9A). The sternocleidomastoid is released from its mastoid attachment. The tip of the transverse process of the atlas is a deep landmark. The spinal accessory nerve is an inferior landmark. An incision is made in the prevertebral fascia above the spinal accessory nerve from the tip of the transverse process of the atlas (Fig. 34-9B). This maneuver should expose the levator scapulae muscle, which is divided. This step can be done over an instrument allowing the muscle fibers to be splayed out as they are cut. This step exposes the vertebral artery between C1 and C2, and it can be ligated. The second cervical nerve is found crossing the vertebral

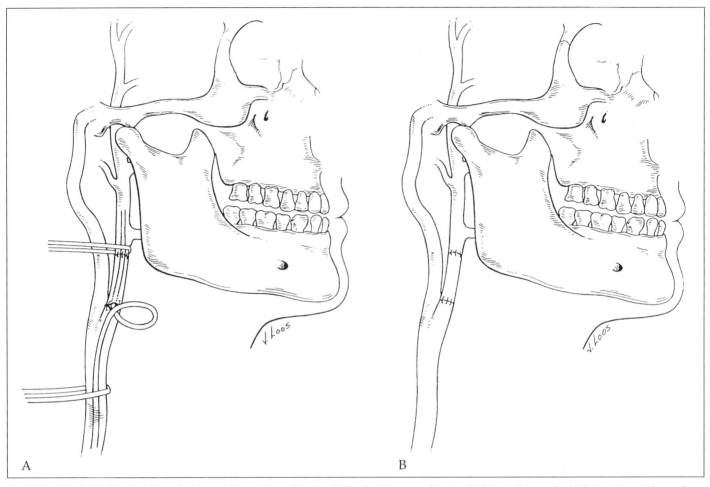

Fig. 34-6. A. A plastic shunt can be used when an interposition graft is placed. The shunt is removed just as the last stitches are placed. B. An interposition graft with a piece of reversed saphenous vein or nonreversed after vulvotomy is used to bridge large defects.

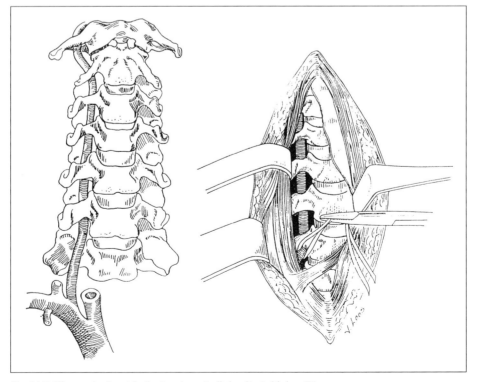

Fig. 34-7. The proximal vertebral artery is controlled or ligated below C6.

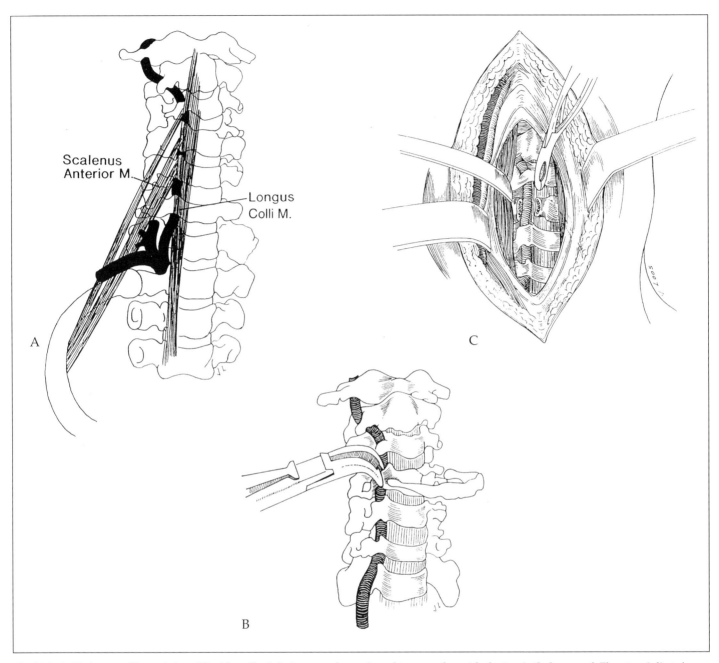

Fig. 34-8. A. The longus colli muscle is mobilized laterally. B,C. A rongeur forceps is used to expose the vertebral artery in the bony canal. The artery is ligated above and below the injury.

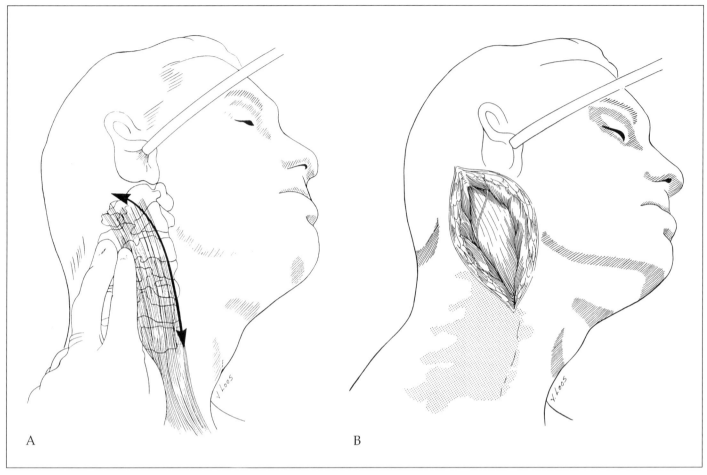

Fig. 34-9. Ligation of the vertebral artery between C1 and C2. A. The incision is carried under the ear over the mastoid prominence. B. An incision is made in the prevertebral fascia above the spinal accessory nerve from the tip of the transverse process of the atlas.

artery and should be avoided by gentle retraction. The key to this dissection is keeping the transverse process of the atlas identified throughout the dissection.

Drains are not routinely used after vascular repairs in the neck. Perioperative antibiotics are given before skin incision and for one dose after surgery. A first-generation cephalosporin is commonly used. Careful examination of cranial nerve function should be routine in the postoperative period.

Venous Repair

Venous injuries are usually managed by ligation or simple suture repair. Unless there is concomitant complete interruption of both jugular veins, it is unusual for the surgeon to attempt more extensive reconstructions.

Esophageal Exposure and Repair

The carotid sheath is usually retracted laterally when exploring the esophagus (Fig. 34-10). The tract of the penetrating object is helpful in identifying injured structures during the neck exploration. The only indication of an esophageal injury might be the missile tract and minimal blood staining of the esophageal tissues. Moving the nasogastric tube into the cervical esophagus and occluding the distal esophagus while instilling air can help identify an injury. This maneuver is best done when the wound is filled with saline. Placement of methylene blue in the nasogastric tube is another method to identify these injuries.

All injuries are debrided of devitalized tissue and bleeding controlled. Most injuries are closed in one or two layers. An inner

row of through-and-through absorbable sutures are placed. These sutures can be interrupted or continuous. Absorbable suture is used for the second row of Lembert sutures, which may be interrupted or continuous. Some larger wounds require mobilization of the esophagus to allow primary repair. It is rare to be unable to repair these wounds, but if no repair is felt possible then a lateral or end cervical esophagostomy can be performed. Complex injuries that also involve the trachea or carotid vessels can benefit from the placement of one of the strap muscles (omohyoid, sternohyoid, or sternothyroid) between the esophageal repair and the repair of the associated injury (Fig. 34-11).

A nasogastric tube is passed into the stomach before the wound is closed. All esophageal repairs are drained with a soft, silastic closed suction drain. This

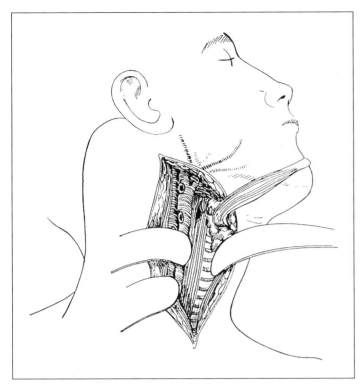

Fig. 34-10. *The carotid sheath is mobilized laterally exposing a hole in the cervical esophagus.*

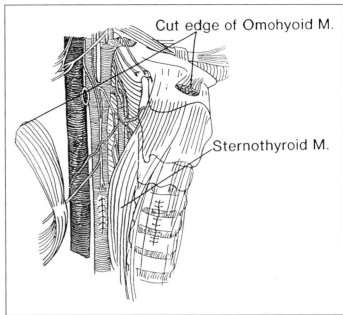

Fig. 34-11. *Complex injuries that also involve the trachea or carotid vessels can benefit from the placement of one of the strap muscles between the esophageal repair and the repair of the associated injury.*

drain is brought out behind the sternocleidomastoid muscle through a separate incision. Oral alimentation is avoided for 7 days. A barium swallow is obtained on day 7 to assess the patency of the repair, since 50 percent of esophageal leaks are asymptomatic.

Suggested Reading

Apffelstaedt JP, Muller R. Results of mandatory exploration for penetrating neck trauma. *World J Surg* 18:917, 1994.

Asensio JA, Valenziano CP, Falcone RE, et al. Management of Penetrating Neck Injuries: The Controversy Surrounding Zone II Injuries. In The Surgical Clinics of North America Contemporary Problems in JA Asensio, JA Weigelt (eds.), Trauma Surgery. 71, 1991.

Beitsch P, Weigelt JA, Flynn E, Easley S. Physical examination and arteriography in patients with penetrating zone II neck wounds. *Arch Surg* 129:577, 1994.

Carducci B, Lowe RA, Dalsey W. Penetrating neck trauma: Consensus and controversies. *Ann Emerg Med* 15:208, 1986.

Fry RE, Fry WJ. Extracranial carotid artery injuries. *Surgery* 88:581, 1980.

Henry AK. Extensile to the Vertebral Artery. In AK Henry (ed.), *Extensile Exposure*, 2nd ed. Edinburgh: Churchill-Livingstone, 1973.

Meier DE, Brink BE, Fry WJ. Vertebral artery trauma. *Arch Surg* 116:236, 1981.

Noyes LD, McSwain NE, Markowitz IP. Penendoscopy with arteriography versus mandatory exploration of penetrating wounds of the neck. *Ann Surg* 204:21, 1986.

Reid JDS, Weigelt JA. Forty-three cases of vertebral artery trauma. *J Trauma* 28:1007, 1988.

Schaefer SD. The treatment of acute external laryngeal injuries. *Arch Otolaryngol Head Neck Surg* 117:35, 1991.

Schaefer SD, Anderson RO, Carder HM. Management of the upper airway in the injured patient. In MH Meyers (ed.), *The Multiply Injured Patient with Complex Fractures*. Philadelphia: Lea & Febiger, 1984.

Thal ER. EE Moore, KL Mattox, DV Feliciano (eds.), *Injury to the Neck in Trauma*, 2nd ed. Norwalk, Appleton & Lange, 1991.

Weigelt JA, Thal ER, Synder III WH, et al. Diagnosis of penetrating cervical esophageal injuries. *Am J Surg* 154:619, 1987.

Winter RP, Weigelt JA. Cervical esophageal trauma. *Arch Surg* 125:849, 1990.

EDITOR'S COMMENT

Dr. Weigelt has presented an orderly approach to penetrating neck injuries, a problem that general surgeons are seeing more commonly. The repairs are well described. Since most of these injuries occur in young, otherwise healthy individuals, the use of shunting, for example, in repair of the internal carotid, might not be necessary because back-bleeding should be excellent provided there are no associated intracranial injuries. The lower incidence of back-bleeding is probably more of a problem of hemodynamic instability than of the intracranial vascular connections.

The controversy surrounding management continues to rage in this area. Velmahos and coworkers (*Can J Surg* 37:487, 1994) reviewed their experience at the Baragawanath Hospital of the University of Witwatersrand in Johannesburg, South Africa. Because of limited resources, they have had to adopt a policy of selective management in a number of penetrating neck injuries. Surprisingly, the results indicate that while there was a 3 percent incidence of unnecessary exploration, 4.2 percent of the mandatory exploration group died. In the group that was selectively managed, there was a 9.1 percent incidence of missed injuries, and only 2.8 percent of the patients died as a result of delayed diagnosis. Particularly damaging was the missed diagnosis of an esophageal injury, which all authorities agree should be avoided if at all possible. They present a useful decision-tree approach to vascular injuries of the neck.

The use of a selective or mandatory approach depends on many things, namely the location of the institution, its resources, the population served, and the frequency of neck lacerations as well as the expertise developed by the staff. It is likely that as penetrating neck injuries become more violent, not every zone I injury will get angiography and not every zone II injury will be explored. As Dr. Weigelt correctly points out, it may be simpler and less expensive to do a neck exploration than all the diagnostic procedures necessary to rule out an injury in zone II.

J.E.F.

FOUR

ENDOCRINE SURGERY

35

Surgical Anatomy of the Thyroid, Parathyroid, and Adrenal Glands

Clive S. Grant

Success in the surgical management of a patient can be conveniently divided into three phases: pre-, intra-, and postoperative. Vitally important is the preoperative decision-making and planning; an expertly performed operation for the wrong reason is still a bad operation. However, if the preoperative process is correctly conceived, at least in an elective procedure, a perfectly executed operation guarantees a smooth postoperative course in a high percentage of patients. The foundation for this operative success is a thorough knowledge of *surgical* anatomy. Anatomy to anatomists or pathologists is different from surgical anatomy. Because surgeons operate through limited incisions and must preserve function wherever possible, as well as control or prevent bleeding, the "anatomist's anatomy" must be applied from the surgeon's perspective. An attempt has been made to amalgamate the two "forms" of anatomy in the following sections to give a broad perspective (the anatomist's view) as well as present it through the eyes of the surgeon.

The surgical anatomy of the thyroid and parathyroid glands is so closely interrelated that much of what is important to one proves equally important to the other. Because of this overlap, the overall anatomic relationships of the region will be covered under the thyroid section, and specific differences or additions as they relate specifically to parathyroid disease will be noted under that section.

Thyroid
Embryology

From a median endodermic diverticulum on the ventral wall of the pharyngeal gut, in approximately the fourth week of embryologic development, the thyroid descends from the posterior tongue (foramen cecum) in front of the pharynx as a bilobed diverticulum. It initially remains attached to the pharynx by a hollow tube, the thyroglossal duct, which attaches to the foramen cecum. At the end of the second month, the thyroid has reached its final position in front of the trachea, and the thyroglossal duct tissue, which has become solid, usually breaks up and disappears. Distal persistence of the solid duct is represented by the pyramidal lobe of the thyroid. If parts of the ductal epithelium persist, the secretion of the epithelium expands the remnant tube, which is closed at both ends, into a cystic mass filled with colloid-like material—a thyroglossal duct cyst. It rarely has an external connection either to the skin or the tongue unless it has been infected and drained or previously operated on. Cysts can develop anywhere along the course of the thyroglossal duct but are most typically found overlying the hyoid bone in the midline just above the thyroid cartilage. Adjacent to the primary persistent thyroglossal duct remnants, other smaller duct and mucus-secreting gland remnants are often found.

To prevent cyst recurrence, the duct and remnants can be encompassed in a core of tissue that should be excised from the cyst through the mylohyoid muscle to the base of the tongue, the site of the foramen cecum (Fig. 35-1). In addition, because the hyoid bone fuses in the midline in close proximity to the thyroglossal duct, the duct can pass either anterior or posterior, or even course through the bone. The central portion of the hyoid bone should, therefore, be excised as part of the operation for a thyroglossal duct cyst. Ectopic normal thyroid tissue or papillary thyroid carcinoma can develop in a thyroglossal duct cyst or anywhere along the tract of the thyroglossal duct. Lingual thyroid represents a total failure of thyroid descent where the entire thyroid is located at the foramen cecum of the tongue, under the mucosa.

Contributing perhaps less than 1 percent of the eventual thyroid mass, yet critically important in considering thyroid malignancy, are the lateral thyroid anlagen. Originating from the fourth pharyngeal pouches, corresponding to the ultimobranchial bodies, they are responsible for production of calcitonin from the parafollicular, or C, cells. They fuse with the posterior and medial aspect of each thyroid lobe. Medullary thyroid carcinomas evolve from these small parts of the thyroid.

Surgical Anatomy

An overall view of the anatomy relevant to thyroid and parathyroid operations is shown in Fig. 35-2. For optimal surgical exposure, the patient is positioned with a small pillow placed between the scapulae, and the neck is hyperextended, bringing

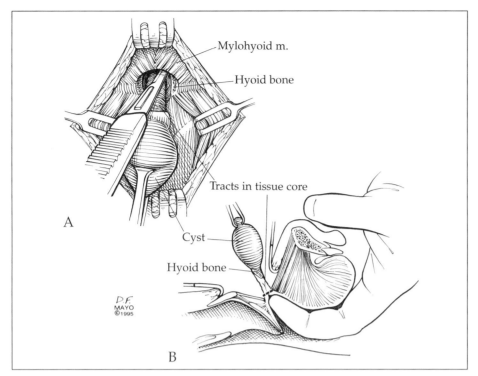

Fig. 35-1. A. A thyroglossal duct cyst is excised from its usual location just above the thyroid cartilage, in the midline, overlying, or just inferior to the hyoid bone. The central portion of the hyoid bone is excised with the specimen, as is a core of muscle tissue encompassing duct tracts leading to the former foramen cecum at the base of the posterior tongue. B. Lateral view showing the surgeon's finger through the patient's mouth to assist excision of the tract at its origin.

the thyroid gland far anteriorly. The skin incision follows Langer's lines transversely, optimally in a skin crease.

Dissection of Muscles

Beneath the skin and subcutaneous tissue is the thin platysma muscle, under which is a relatively avascular plane. In this plane, the superior and inferior flaps can be raised with minimal blood loss (Fig. 35-3). Once the flaps have been developed, the strap muscles are exposed—the sternohyoid and sternothyroid muscles. The more anterior sternohyoid muscles lie close together, but the midline can be identified between them as a thin line of fat and avascular fascia. Dissection along this line to separate these muscles is facilitated by lifting the muscles anteriorly so as to avoid the inferior thyroid veins, which course just deep, running longitudinally over the trachea. Often bordering the midline along these muscles are the anterior jugular veins. These veins can be avoided but can be ligated as the need arises.

As the sternohyoid muscle is elevated, the underlying sternothyroid muscles are ex-

posed. The fascia between these two muscles can be dissected for improved exposure. With the sternohyoid muscles retracted, as the sternothyroid muscle is dissected from the underlying thyroid lobes, care is taken to avoid the widely interconnecting venous network in the thyroid capsule. This caution is of particular importance in a larger goiter, because the strap muscles can be thinned and splayed out across the bulging thyroid lobes, and the large veins are in jeopardy. The insertion of the sternothyrohyoid muscle into the thyroid cartilage can obscure the superior pole of the thyroid gland and can be partially transected for better exposure. Both the sternohyoid and sternothyrohyoid muscles (as well as the omohyoid muscle) are innervated by the ansa cervicalis, derived from the hypoglossal nerve and C1 through C3. These muscles can be partially or completely removed as necessary for cancer operations without any significant disability. The cricothyroid muscles run obliquely from the cricoid cartilage to the thyroid cartilage and are innervated by the external branch of the superior laryngeal nerve. This muscle and nerve should be carefully preserved, be-

cause they serve the important function of fine tuning the voice.

Vascular Anatomy

The principal arterial blood supply of the thyroid gland comes from the paired superior and inferior thyroid arteries, and to a much lesser degree, the thyroidea ima (see Fig. 35-2). Even when all these arteries are ligated, remnants of thyroid often survive from other small branches derived from laryngeal and tracheoesophageal arteries. The superior thyroid artery is the first branch of the external carotid artery and courses inferiorly to reach the superior pole of the thyroid gland. It often branches at this point, with the main branch running over the anterior surface of the superior pole of the thyroid, and the other smaller branches entering more posteriorly. The inferior thyroid artery usually arises from the thyrocervical trunk, runs superiorly behind the carotid artery, then arches medially to the thyroid gland, coursing either perpendicular to or in a recurrent path to the thyroid gland. The thyroidea ima artery is encountered in less than 10 percent of patients and is almost never a relevant vessel except to ligate.

Dissection of Thyroid Lobe

Once the strap muscles have been dissected laterally, the thyroid gland is elevated anteriorly and medially, opening an areolar plane overlying the carotid artery, and traversed by one or more small middle thyroid veins (Fig. 35-4). These veins are ligated and transected, and the space anterior to the carotid from the thyroid cartilage inferiorly to the base of the neck can be dissected safety. This step exposes the transversely directed inferior thyroid artery and the obliquely coursing recurrent laryngeal nerve, a branch of the vagus nerve, which, on the right, wraps around the subclavian artery and passes behind the carotid artery to ascend in the tracheoesophageal groove (Fig. 35-5). On the left, the recurrent laryngeal nerve crosses the arch of the aorta, loops under it adjacent and lateral to the ligamentum arteriosum, and ascends in the tracheoesophageal groove. Adjacent and mostly anterior to the recurrent laryngeal nerve are the tracheoesophageal lymph nodes, which are a common site of metastasis in papillary and medullary thyroid carcinoma. Removal of these nodes requires care to protect the recurrent laryngeal nerve and should preserve not only the inferior parathyroid

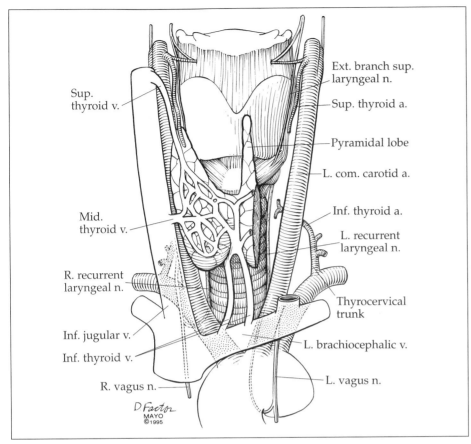

Fig. 35-2. *Overall anatomic relationships of the thyroid and surrounding structures. Note the course of the inferior thyroid artery, behind and perpendicular to the carotid artery. The superior thyroid artery and external branch of the superior laryngeal nerve run in close approximation.*

gland but also its blood supply (which usually crosses anterior to the recurrent laryngeal nerve). Damage to the recurrent laryngeal nerve on one side causes vocal cord paralysis and hoarseness, and prevents complete closure of the vocal cords to protect the trachea. This incomplete closure results in choking, especially when the patient drinks fluids. Bilateral nerve injury jeopardizes the airway and usually requires at least a temporary tracheostomy. When the right subclavian artery anomalously originates directly from the aortic arch as its fourth branch, it passes behind the trachea and esophagus. The right recurrent nerve, therefore, does not recur around this artery, and takes a direct course from the vagus nerve to the larynx. In this instance, even though it emerges posterior to the carotid artery, its perpendicular course mimics the usual course of the inferior thyroid artery and must be distinguished from it.

The inferior thyroid artery is usually the principal blood supply to both the superior and inferior parathyroid glands. These feeding vessels are small and fragile, often traveling in a course parallel if not slightly anterior to the parathyroid glands before reaching the vascular hila (Fig. 35-6). As the inferior thyroid artery intersects with the recurrent laryngeal nerve, it usually

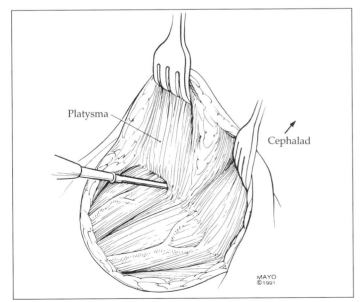

Fig. 35-3. *Following the incision, a larger superior and much smaller inferior flap are raised in the subplatysmal plane, protecting the anterior jugular veins. (From CS Grant, JA van Heerden. Technical Aspects of Thyroidectomy. In JH Donohue, JA van Heerden, JRT Monson (eds.), Atlas of Surgical Oncology. Cambridge: Blackwell, 1995. Reproduced with permission.)*

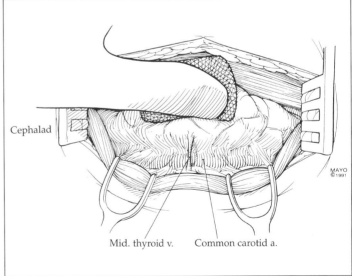

Fig. 35-4. *With traction laterally on the strap muscles that have been separated in the midline, but not transected, and countertraction on the thyroid medially, the middle thyroid vein is exposed. It runs anterior to the carotid artery and should be transected. (From CS Grant, JA van Heerden. Technical Aspects of Thyroidectomy. In JH Donohue, JA van Heerden, JRT Monson (eds.), Atlas of Surgical Oncology. Cambridge: Blackwell, 1995. Reproduced with permission.)*

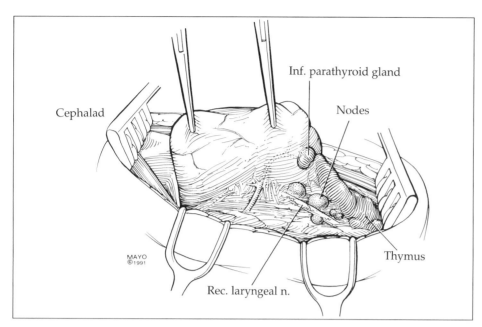

Fig. 35-5. *The right thyroid lobe is retracted anteriorly and medially, and the recurrent laryngeal nerve (RLN) is exposed, coursing obliquely in the tracheoesophageal groove, and surrounded by lymph nodes. The thymus lies anterior to the nerve and nodes, and can contain or point to the inferior parathyroid gland. The superior parathyroid gland is not yet adequately exposed. The intersection of the inferior thyroid artery and RLN is marked by branches of the artery, one crossing the nerve serving the inferior parathyroid gland. (From CS Grant, JA van Heerden. Technical Aspects of Thyroidectomy. In JH Donohue, JA van Heerden, JRT Monson (eds.),* Atlas of Surgical Oncology. *Cambridge: Blackwell, 1995. Reproduced with permission.)*

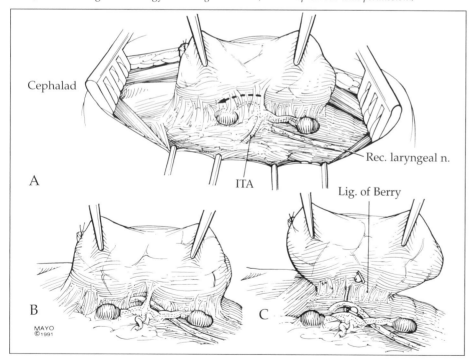

Fig. 35-6. *A. The small vessels feeding the parathyroid glands often run at least parallel if not slightly anterior to the glands. B. These vessels can usually be preserved by gently dissecting them and the parathyroid glands from the surface of the thyroid gland. C. Two significant branches of the inferior thyroid artery are routinely present, one traveling anterior and the other posterior to the RLN. The coalescence of the dense posterior thyroid capsule constitutes Berry's ligament, through which the posterior arterial branch courses. (From CS Grant, JA van Heerden. Technical Aspects of Thyroidectomy. In JH Donohue, JA van Heerden, JRT Monson (eds.),* Atlas of Surgical Oncology. *Cambridge: Blackwell, 1995. Reproduced with permission.)*

branches, typically with one branch anterior and another posterior to the recurrent laryngeal nerve. The inferior thyroid *veins* run vertically, anterior to the trachea, and are easily identified and controlled during the course of thyroidectomy. Accompanying these veins are the pretracheal lymph nodes, both infra- and supraisthmic (Delphian), which often contain metastatic thyroid cancer.

The superior thyroid artery (and vein), which is sacrificed during thyroidectomy, must be separated from the external branch of the superior laryngeal nerve. Placing inferior and lateral traction on the superior pole of the thyroid gland usually distracts the artery away from the nerve, and the artery can be cleanly isolated and individually ligated (Fig. 35-7).

Once the vascular branches to the thyroid lobe have been transected and the nodes cleared, the posterior capsule of the thyroid is all that remains before the lobe is completely removed. To reemphasize, a small vessel regularly courses in this dense posterior capsule (Berry's ligament), and the recurrent laryngeal nerve is also commonly tethered anteriorly. Gentle dissection will expose the vessel for ligation and push the recurrent laryngeal nerve down out of danger before the ligament is transected.

In addition to the pretracheal and tracheoesophageal lymph nodes already mentioned, thyroid cancer often metastasizes to lateral nodes as well (Fig. 35-8). The routes of spread roughly follow the venous drainage. Cancers of the upper lobe, in addition to the primary drainage to the supraisthmic nodes can involve the midjugular nodes both anterior and lateral to the internal jugular vein, and occasionally extend superiorly along the vein to the base of the skull. Cancers of the mid and lower thyroid lobes drain initially into the pretracheal and tracheoesophageal nodes, then to the mid and lower jugular nodes and anterior mediastinal nodes.

Parathyroid
Embryology

The parathyroid glands develop from branchial pouches III and IV. The superior parathyroid glands develop from pouch IV, travel a shorter distance than the inferior glands, and are typically located along the posterior border of the thyroid gland,

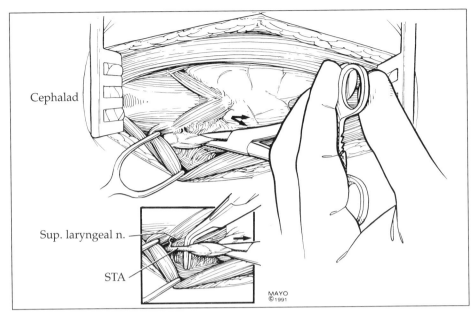

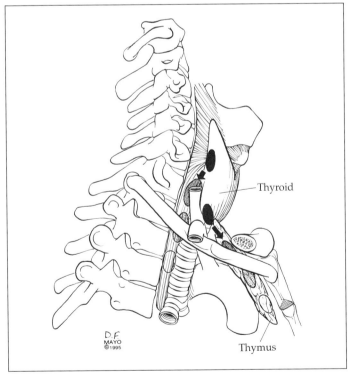

at or approximately 1 cm superior to the entrance of the inferior thyroid artery (Fig. 35-6A). Because of this location, when the superior glands descend further, they almost always remain posterior, in the tracheoesophageal groove or retroesophageal space (Fig. 35-9). Even when located quite low in the posterior superior mediastinum, they can still be retrieved through a collar incision.

In conjunction with the thymus, the inferior parathyroid glands develop from pouch III, and then descend to the posterior aspects of the lower pole of the thyroid gland. This long descent gives rise to a much more variable position for the inferior parathyroid than the superior gland. The location of the inferior gland can range from being high, anterior to the carotid artery (so-called undescended parathymus), to the anterior mediastinum within the thymus, necessitating sternotomy for retrieval (Fig. 35-9). Inferior glands associated with the thyroid gland usually re-

Fig. 35-7. With traction inferiorly and laterally on the thyroid lobe, the superior thyroid artery can be displaced from its closely associated external branch of the superior laryngeal nerve. The artery is thereby transected individually, and the nerve is preserved (insert). (From CS Grant, JA van Heerden. Technical Aspects of Thyroidectomy. In JH Donohue, JA van Heerden, JRT Monson (eds.), Atlas of Surgical Oncology. *Cambridge: Blackwell, 1995. Reproduced with permission.)*

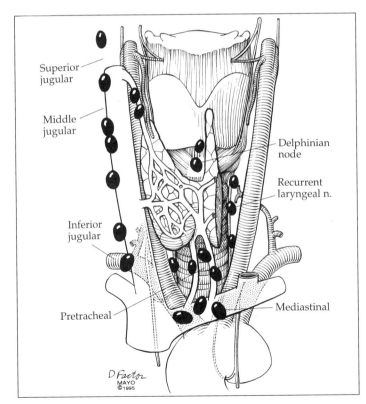

Fig. 35-8. The lymphatic drainage of the thyroid is generally divided into the central and lateral compartments. The central compartment nodes include the pretracheal and tracheoesophageal nodes. The lateral compartment nodes comprise the jugular nodes, which are found mostly lateral to the vein from the base of the neck to the base of the skull. A few nodes lie medial to the vein just above the level of the superior thyroid pole.

Fig. 35-9. Due to their embryologic origins, the parathyroid glands, particularly when enlarged, follow different but often predictable courses. The superior glands descend posteriorly in the contiguous tracheoesophageal groove or retroesophageal space, or into the posterior superior mediastinum. The inferior glands are less predictable but are usually found anteriorly in association with the thymus gland, either in the neck or in the anterior superior mediastinum.

35. Surgical Anatomy of the Thyroid, Parathyroid, and Adrenal Glands **479**

main ventral to the recurrent laryngeal nerve, whereas the superior glands are found dorsal to the nerve. The usual home for the inferior glands is on the posterolateral surface of the thyroid gland, just above, at, or within the attached remnant of the cervical thymus, the so-called thyrothymic ligament (Fig. 35-6). Rarely, this combined descent of parathyroid and thymus can be trapped within the carotid sheath, which might become relevant and evident only when the parathyroid gland is enlarged and hyperfunctioning. Moreover, because of the relationship between thymus and the developing heart, these aberrant parathyroid glands can be located adjacent to the origin of the great vessels from the aorta.

In very rare instances, the parathyroid glands can be found to be completely intrathyroidal. More commonly, they can be located on the surface of the thyroid gland, under the capsule but in clefts of the thyroid parenchyma. This location can seem intrathyroidal particularly during reoperative parathyroid surgery when the thyroid capsule is thickened with scar.

Surgical Anatomy

Virtually everyone has at least four parathyroid glands, but at least 13 percent of the population has supernumerary glands. However, only one-half of these supernumerary glands are proper glands; the others are tiny, rudimentary bits of parathyroid tissue, usually located very near another normal gland. Supernumerary glands become important surgically in four situations: 1) hyperparathyroidism caused by multiple endocrine neoplasia (MEN)—especially type I, and familial hyperparathyroidism, when all glands are abnormal; 2) secondary hyperparathyroidism, most typically resulting from chronic renal failure when all glands are stimulated to enlarge and hyperfunction; 3) sporadic cases when the four usual glands are normal, and only the supernumerary gland is abnormally enlarged and responsible for hyperfunction; and 4) when the supernumerary gland is enlarged in addition to another normal gland, representing a double adenoma situation.

Dissection of Parathyroid Glands

There are three important goals in parathyroid surgery: 1) recognition of normal parathyroid glands as well as removal of the abnormal glands, 2) safely searching in *predictable* locations for missing parathyroid glands, and 3) preserving parathyroid glands during thyroidectomy or removal of other abnormal parathyroid glands.

The dissection for parathyroid glands proceeds similarly to mobilization of a thyroid lobe, as described above. In contrast, when hyperparathyroidism is the indication for operation, the arterial supply of the thyroid is usually preserved. Once the thyroid gland has been elevated (Fig. 35-5), the inferior parathyroid gland is usually sought first. It usually resides either on the posterolateral surface of the lower pole of the thyroid gland or at the tip of the cervical thymus or thyrothymic ligament. In fact, this ligament can be used to point to the gland or conceal it within its variably atrophic and fat-replaced thymic substance. Similar to the superior gland, the inferior gland is often located in a lobule of fat, from which it can be distinguished by its reddish yellow or yellowish brown color. Normal glands are very soft, pliable, virtually nonpalpable, and can present in differing shapes depending on whether the fascial layer that flattens it against the thyroid has been teased away to yield a more globular shape. When a tiny biopsy has been taken from the *nonhilar* portion of the gland, the entire parenchymal surface will bleed from pinpoint capillaries (in contrast to fat with a single bleeding vessel). Thyroid nodules and normal or diseased lymph nodes are more firm, not soft and pliable like normal parathyroid glands, and the thymus can usually be distinguished by its pale, off-white color. When attempting to locate an inferior parathyroid adenoma, if it is not in the usual locations, it almost universally migrates along an anterior path, following the course of or located within the cervical or mediastinal thymus. The sequence to search for inferior glands not in the usual locations proceeds as follows: 1) the cervical and mediastinal thymus are drawn into the wound and searched or excised for pathologic review; 2) dissection is carried anterior to the carotid artery at least to its bifurcation to search for an undescended parathymus as described above; 3) the carotid sheath is opened, particularly if the cervical thymus is seen to deviate toward it; and 4) the lower pole of the thyroid is excised to exclude an intrathyroidal location.

The superior parathyroid glands are in a more constant location but somewhat more difficult to expose than the inferior glands. They are usually found within a globule of fat located along the posterior border of the thyroid gland, within 2 to 3 cm superior to where the inferior thyroid artery enters the thyroid gland (Fig. 35-6). Gentle dissection to strip thin fascial layers overlying the gland causes it to pop out directly, or the surrounding fat can be manipulated to expose the parathyroid gland. Initially, to identify probable locations for this gland, gentle prodding with an instrument causes the fat and contained parathyroid gland to float within the fascial envelope. They often directly overlie the recurrent laryngeal nerve, although they are separated by a delicate fascial space. When a superior gland is not in the usual position, it tends to migrate posteriorly, behind the inferior thyroid artery, drawing its blood supply with it and descending in the potential space called the tracheoesophageal groove, which is almost the same as the retroesophageal or prevertebral space. Because the recurrent laryngeal nerve is closely applied to the trachea and is located anterior to this dissection plane, the retroesophageal space can be entered and widely dissected from the level of the larynx superiorly almost to as low as the tracheal bifurcation inferiorly. The only critical structure that crosses this plane is the inferior thyroid artery, which can be protected as it enters the thyroid gland or transected. Occasionally, exposure of the superior gland can be facilitated by mobilizing the superior pole of the thyroid gland by transecting the superior thyroid artery. Very rarely is a superior gland located within the thyroid gland. Both superior and inferior glands are remarkably symmetric in their locations. Even in ectopic locations, with the exception of an inferior gland located low in the cervicomediastinal thymus, symmetry is often preserved.

Although the principal arterial blood supply to both the superior and inferior parathyroid glands originates from the inferior thyroid arteries, other anastomotic vessels certainly provide a supplementary supply in most patients. However, when a total thyroidectomy has been performed, these supplementary sources are often interrupted. As a general rule during a thyroidectomy, the inferior thyroid artery should be transected *distal* to the branches that supply the parathyroid glands. When an inferior gland is located within the substance of the thymus, it usually derives a satisfactory blood supply from thymic vessels.

Adrenal

Embryology

The adrenal glands can be separated into two distinct areas both histologically and physiologically—the *cortex* and the *medulla*. The cortex develops from mesodermic celomic epithelium of the posterior abdominal wall, at the cranial end of the mesonephros. The medulla develops from the neural crest in conjunction with the sympathetic ganglia. This group of neural cells migrates along the adrenal vein to invade the cortex and becomes the completed adrenal gland. Other small masses of these cells, which stain brown with chromic acid (thus the name chromaffin or pheochrome cells), can persist throughout life along the sympathetic chain as paraganglia. The most common location of a tumor (or paraganglioma) is at the origin of the inferior mesenteric artery on either side of the aorta, near Zuckerkandl's organs. Accessory adrenal tissue can be found occasionally in the connective tissue adjacent to the main gland but can also occur near a gonad, either ovary or testis.

Surgical Anatomy

Because the adrenal glands are situated deeply in the retroperitoneum, and because primary diseases that require adrenalectomy are rare, surgeons tend to be less familiar with the anatomic relationships of these glands (Fig. 35-10). Additionally, adrenal tumors can distort these relationships. On both sides, they cap the kidneys and derive arterial blood supply from the aorta, inferior phrenic, and renal arteries.

On the *right*, the upper part of the gland lies partially behind the inferior vena cava, against the bare area of the liver (to which it can seem somewhat adherent), and on the diaphragm. The principal venous drainage is through the adrenal vein, which is short, wide, and exits the gland just below its apex to enter the inferior vena cava on its posterior surface and is the only vein to enter the inferior vena cava posteriorly along its retrohepatic course.

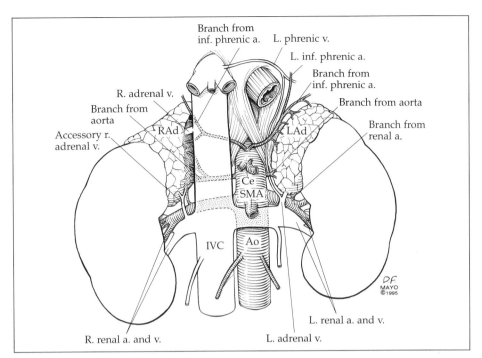

Fig. 35-10. Overall anatomic relationships of the adrenal glands. Note the origins of the three main arteries: the inferior phrenic, aortic, and renal branches. Note also the single draining veins (except a small accessory right adrenal vein), the right-located superior and medial, and the left-found inferior and medial.

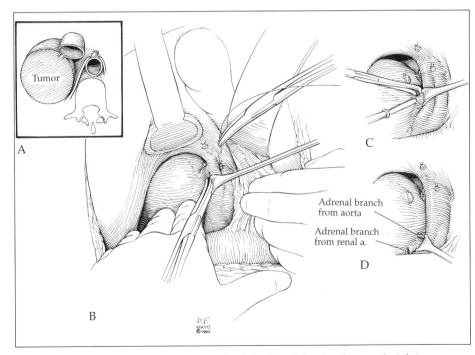

Fig. 35-11. A. Cross-sectional view of the anatomic relationships of the adrenal tumor, the inferior vena cava (IVC), and the right adrenal vein. B. With the liver elevated and the IVC retracted medially, the short, fat right adrenal vein is exposed, coursing from the adrenal tumor to the posterior surface of the IVC. C. The vein has been clipped or ligated and transected, and the minimally vascular areolar tissues between the tumor and the IVC below the level of the vein is dissected. D. Along the medial inferior aspect of the tumor, the aortic and renal arterial branches that need to be controlled are found. (From CS Grant, JA van Heerden. Technical Aspects of Adrenalectomy. In JH Donohue, JA van Heerden, JRT Monson (eds.), Atlas of Surgical Oncology. Cambridge: Blackwell, 1995. Reproduced with permission.)

The *left* adrenal gland lies on the diaphragm and is covered on its anterior surface by peritoneum superiorly and by the nonperitoneally covered pancreas on its lower portion. The adrenal *vein* exists near the lower border of the gland, often to join with the inferior phrenic vein to empty into the renal vein.

Anatomy Important to Different Surgical Approaches

Anterior (Transabdominal)

Right. After the abdominal incision is made, the posterior edge of the liver

should be dissected from the posterior peritoneum, which allows the liver to be lifted anteriorly and superiorly. This maneuver is also facilitated by transecting one or two small branches from the anterior surface of the inferior vena cava coursing to the caudate lobe of the liver. Neither the hepatic flexure of the colon nor the du-

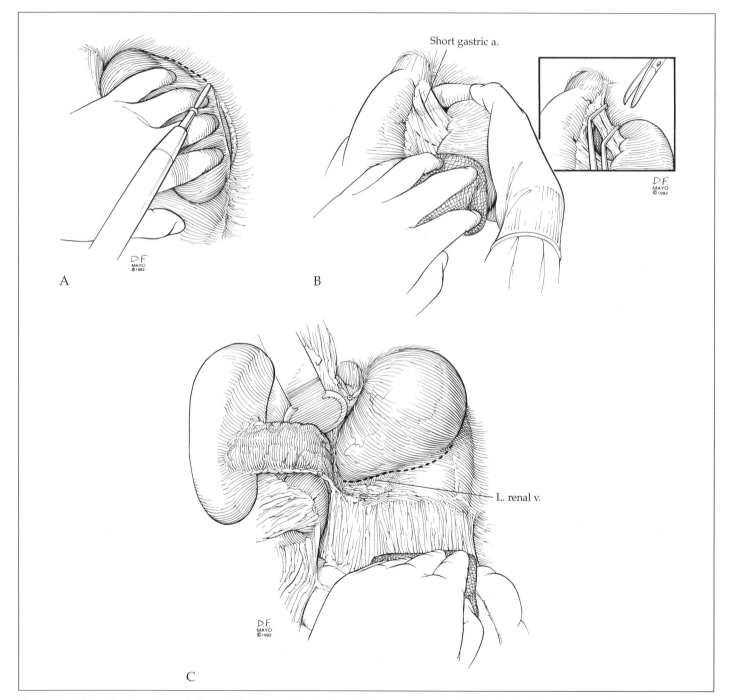

A

B

Short gastric a.

C

L. renal v.

Fig. 35-12. A. Retracting the spleen medially and inferiorly, the lateral peritoneal attachments are incised. B. The short gastric vessels are individually transected. C. With omentum dissected from the left transverse colon, the spleen and pancreas mobilized from their bed, and the short gastric vessels transected, these organs can be retracted into the patient's right upper quadrant, exposing a large adrenal tumor. (From CS Grant, JA van Heerden. Technical Aspects of Adrenalectomy. In JH Donohue, JA van Heerden, JRT Monson (eds.), Atlas of Surgical Oncology. Cambridge: Blackwell, 1995. Reproduced with permission.)

odenum usually needs to be mobilized. The arterial branch from the inferior phrenic artery is often located at the extreme superomedial aspect of the gland, higher than the adrenal vein, and requires careful control. Once this artery and the adrenal vein have been transected and the posterior peritoneal layer that covers the superior aspect of the adrenal gland has been incised, the gland can be retracted laterally as the inferior vena cava is retracted medially, separating the plane between the two (Fig. 35-11). Control of the vessels from the aorta and renal vessels completes the dissection. With reasonable frequency, at least one small but significant accessory adrenal vein drains from the inferior aspect of the gland (especially important when large tumors are present that enlarge these veins) into the right renal vein. This situation is easily controlled when recognized. Care must be taken on this side as well as on the left to avoid ligating a small polar branch of the renal artery.

Left. Access to the left adrenal gland can be gained by dissecting the omentum from the colon, elevating the stomach, and dissecting the avascular plane under the pancreas to elevate it off the adrenal gland. The spleen does not need to be mobilized in this approach, but this exposure is adequate only for small to moderate tumors. For larger tumors, including adrenal cancers, the splenic flexure of the colon can be dissected and the spleen and pancreas mobilized from their bed (including ligation of short gastric vessels) to the patient's right side (Fig. 35-12). This step exposes the adrenal gland or tumor and eventually the most critical area of dissection on the left side, inferomedially. The adrenal vein and the arterial branches from the aorta and renal artery course in this space (Fig. 35-13).

Posterior

Right. Once the incision has been made, the sacrospinalis has been retracted medially, the twelfth rib has been resected, and the pleura reflected superiorly, exposure is greatly facilitated by transecting the free edge of the diaphragm medially to the spine (Fig. 35-14). Because the adrenal gland is located against the bare area of the liver superiorly, exposure of the liver delineates the superior extent of the dissection. Nevertheless, the adrenal vein can still seem very high in its entry to the posterior aspect of the inferior vena cava and requires careful and gentle traction for safe control (Fig. 35-15).

Left. Following initial exposure similar to the right, the upper border of the dissection on the left should proceed to, and is bounded by, the diaphragm. As the perirenal fat and soft tissue are retracted down and dissection exposes the diaphragm superomedially, the vertically coursing inferior phrenic vein can often be recognized and indicates that the adrenal gland is close by, located slightly laterally (Fig. 35-16).

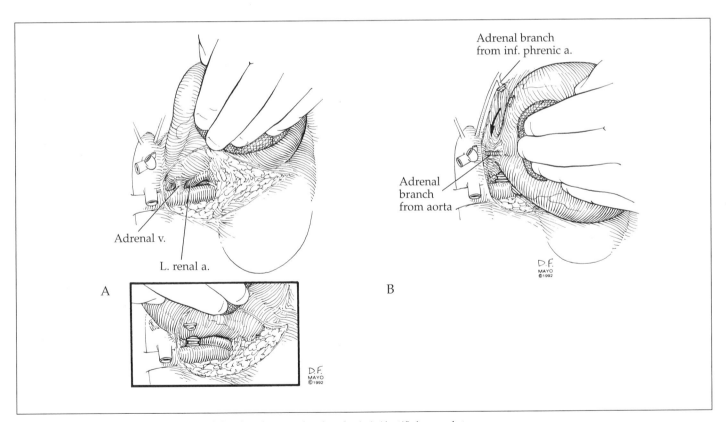

Adrenal branch from inf. phrenic a.

Adrenal branch from aorta

Adrenal v.

L. renal a.

A

B

Fig. 35-13. A. Along the inferomedial aspect of the adrenal tumor, the adrenal vein is identified, somewhat shorter than usual in the situation depicted. Care must be taken not to injure renal arterial branches coursing close by the vein as it is transected. B. The adrenal branches from the inferior phrenic and aorta can be seen in their typical locations. (From CS Grant, JA van Heerden. Technical Aspects of Adrenalectomy. In JH Donohue, JA van Heerden, JRT Monson (eds.), Atlas of Surgical Oncology. Cambridge: Blackwell, 1995. Reproduced with permission.)

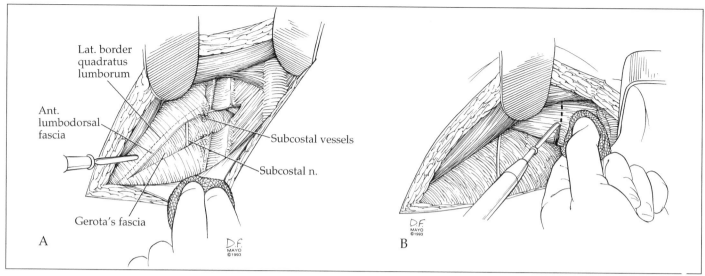

Fig. 35-14. A. From a posterior approach to the right adrenal gland, the incision has been made, the sacrospinalis muscle is retracted medially, the twelfth rib removed, and the subcostal vessels have been transected, sparing the subcostal nerve. B. The pleura has been retracted superiorly (above the gauze) and the diaphragm is divided to the midline. (From CS Grant, JA van Heerden. Technical Aspects of Adrenalectomy. In JH Donohue, JA van Heerden, JRT Monson (eds.), Atlas of Surgical Oncology. Cambridge: Blackwell, 1995. Reproduced with permission.)

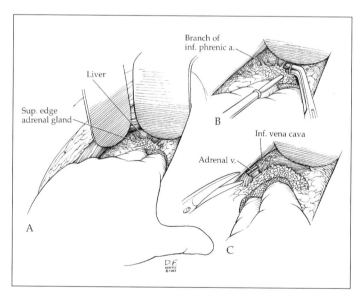

Fig. 35-15. A. The superior border of the dissection on the right is the liver. The tiny arterial branches can be seen radiating out from the adrenal gland like the spokes of a wheel. B. The tiny arterial branches can be clipped or cauterized, but the branch from the inferior phrenic artery usually requires clips or ligation. C. Exposure of the right adrenal vein is facilitated by this approach by its posterior location. (From CS Grant, JA van Heerden. Technical Aspects of Adrenalectomy. In JH Donohue, JA van Heerden, JRT Monson (eds.), Atlas of Surgical Oncology. Cambridge: Blackwell, 1995. Reproduced with permission.)

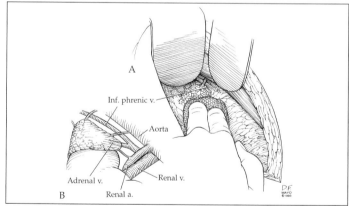

Fig. 35-16. A. The superior extent of the posterior approach on the left is the diaphragm. Medially, a clue that the adrenal is close is the vertically coursing inferior phrenic vein. Similar small and larger arteries are found on the left and the right. B. The venous drainage on the left into the renal vein causes the adrenal gland to course well down into the renal hilum. Transecting the vein and the aortic and renal arterial branches allows considerable freedom to remove the gland. (From CS Grant, JA van Heerden. Technical Aspects of Adrenalectomy. In JH Donohue, JA van Heerden, JRT Monson (eds.), Atlas of Surgical Oncology. Cambridge: Blackwell, 1995. Reproduced with permission.)

Suggested Reading

Åkerström G. Anatomy and Strategy of Parathyroid Operation. In G Åkerström, J Rastad, C Juhlin (eds.), *Current Controversy in Parathyroid Operation and Reoperation.* Auston: R.G. Landes, 1995.

Åkerström G, Malmaeus J, Bergstršm R. Surgical anatomy of human parathyroid glands. *Surgery* 95:14, 1984.

Grant CS, van Heerden JA. Technical Aspects of Adrenalectomy. In JH Donohue, JA van Heerden, JRT Monson (eds.), *Atlas of Surgical Oncology.* Cambridge: Blackwell, 1995.

Grant CS, van Heerden JA. Technical Aspects of Thyroidectomy. In JH Donohue, JA van Heerden, JRT Monson (eds.), *Atlas of Surgical Oncology.* Cambridge: Blackwell, 1995.

Grant CS, van Heerden JA, Charboneau JW, et al. Clinical management of persistent and/or recurrent primary hyperparathyroidism. *World J Surg* 10:555, 1986.

Grant JCB. *Grant's Atlas of Anatomy*, 5th ed. Baltimore: Williams & Wilkins, 1962.

Gray H. *Gray's Anatomy*, 28th ed. Philadelphia: Lea & Febiger, 1966.

Gray SW, Skandalakis JE. *Embryology for Surgeons.* Philadelphia: Saunders, 1972.

Lennquist S, Cahlin S, Smeds S. The superior laryngeal nerve in thyroid surgery. *Surgery* 102:999, 1988.

Russell CF, Grant CS, van Heerden JA. Hyperfunctioning supernumerary parathyroid glands: An occasional cause of hyperparathyroidism. *Mayo Clin Proc* 57:121, 1982.

Thompson NW, Eckhauser FE, Harness JK. The anatomy of primary hyperparathyroidism. *Surgery* 92:814, 1982.

EDITOR'S COMMENT

Special attention to the anatomy of the three endocrine glands discussed in depth in this chapter and a firm conceptual visualization of the anatomic relationships is critical to success in even simple operations on the thyroid and parathyroid glands, but are really essential in all three areas. Obviously, successful removal of a diseased gland, or glands, in the neck is considerably diminished by a serious technical complication, especially damage to the recurrent laryngeal nerve (now known as the recurrent nerve in anatomic circles) or devascularization or removal of parathyroids, rendering a patient permanently aparathyroid.

Knowledgeable surgeons seldom remove any but the most superficial portion of the thyroid, for example, the isthmus, without visualizing the ipsilateral recurrent nerve. It is neither necessary nor desirable to strip the nerve of soft tissues through its entire length, unless there is a large posterior nodule on the ipsilateral lobe of the thyroid that might be adherent to the nerve. Under those circumstances, the nerve should be gently tracked up to and slightly beyond the area of thyroid pathology. The parathyroids, especially the superior gland, are usually adjacent to the nerve, making identification of the nerve of utmost importance when resecting parathyroids.

The undescended thyroid, located at the base of the tongue in the area of the foramen cecum, is a rare condition. However, when these lesions exist at the base of the tongue, they can occasionally bleed because of ulceration of the overlying mucous membrane, or, of course, carcinoma may develop in the ectopic tissues. Although older texts describe lingual thyroid at the base of the tongue existing concurrently with thyroid in the normal position, the symptomatic lesions in the undescended position are ordinarily the only thyroid present. Thyroid scanning immediately answers the question of whether there is thyroid tissue at the base of the tongue when an unusual lesion is encountered. It can also determine the presence, extent, or absence of thyroid in the conventional cervical position. Excision of lingual thyroid is not required, even when discovered on a thyroid scan done for other purposes unless symptoms develop, such as bleeding or dysphagia, or when there is a mass that the patient often perceives.

Many surgeons have abandoned the practice of visualizing the vocal cords before operations on the thyroid and parathyroid glands and rely primarily on the anesthesiologist to detect immobility of the cords at the time of intubation (or checking the mobility of both cords at extubation). The use of a fiberoptic laryngoscope to view the cords in the office or clinic involves a capital outlay that is, however, justified if the volume of thyroid surgery is substantial in any given practice. However, in the vast majority of patients, the cords can be readily seen with a head mirror, light source, and several dental mirrors. The preparation for laryngoscopy is complete if one has a small aerosol container of local anesthetic to temporarily anesthetize the mucous membranes of the posterior tongue and pharynx and is willing to expend 5 minutes to view the cords before taking the patient to the operating room. With cancer of the thyroid, this step is an important one, since preoperative knowledge yields prognostic importance concerning the invasiveness of the tumor, and enables the physician to alert the patient to the existence of a nonfunctional cord. Although it has always been assumed that a unilateral paralysis of a vocal cord, or even a partial paralysis, results in a change in the quality and strength of the voice, it does not always, especially when the lesion has developed gradually.

Thyroidectomy and parathyroid exploration are not particularly difficult operations in most circumstances, but the safe and successful excision of lesions of either gland requires an understanding of and familiarity with the anatomic interrelationships of the various structures that are located in this small but critically important area.

R.J.B.

36

Fine-Needle Aspiration of the Thyroid: Thyroid Lobectomy and Subtotal Thyroidectomy

Jerry M. Shuck   Gregory M. Fedele

Indications

Operations on the thyroid gland are satisfying for many reasons. The first is that a significant medical problem can be diagnosed and treated quickly with prompt recovery of the patient. Complications are uncommon and patients generally are home within 24 hours. Second, the operations have clear-cut indications and are technically challenging, precise, and aesthetic exercises. As surgeons gain experience with thyroid surgery, these delicate dissections become even safer and more artistic. Unfortunately, there are many pitfalls during the course of a thyroidectomy with potential devastating long-term consequences such as permanent hypoparathyroidism or recurrent nerve injury. Such problems, however, occur very rarely in practiced hands.

There are many reasons to operate on the thyroid gland. The first, although important, is currently uncommon; that is, the operation for hyperthyroidism. Most toxic patients with thyroid disease are first treated with drugs and eventually with radioactive iodine. This protocol is particularly true in the more common diffuse thyrotoxicosis. However, there are some patients for whom an operation is the preferred alternative. Even though women can safely continue pregnancies with thyroid-suppressing drugs, thyroidectomy during the second trimester is well tolerated and definitive. Hyperthyroid crisis during delivery is obviated. The fetus is spared I-131 and prolonged exposure to drugs. Some patients simply prefer the immediate results of surgery, have a fear of

radiation, or are concerned with childbearing issues in the future. Recurrent hyperthyroidism after I-131 therapy is another indication for thyroidectomy. Patients with multinodular toxic goiters can achieve excellent results with an operation, particularly when there is a single nodule causing thyrotoxicosis (Plummer's syndrome) requiring only a lobectomy for cure. Treatment with I-131 for "hot" nodules requires a dose that will ablate the normal intervening thyroid tissue. This consideration can favor a surgical approach.

Another significant reason for thyroid operation is the cosmetic effect. Nodules, particularly in the isthmus, need not be very large to be visible. The patient sees the nodule daily in the mirror, knows it is there, and tires of answering questions about it or having it continually evaluated. Obviously, large goiters can be unsightly and are well suited to safe extirpation. Thyroid cysts can be aspirated, but when they recur, the patient again has a visible lesion that requires treatment. Our policy is to aspirate twice and recommend surgery if the cyst again recurs.

Symptoms of compression caused by enlarged thyroid glands compromising the trachea or esophagus are indications for thyroidectomy, particularly with intrathoracic extensions (substernal goiter). Occasionally, such compression occurs quite rapidly (these large goiters can hemorrhage), and emergency relief of respiratory obstruction can be necessary. If there are any symptoms caused by compression and particularly if there is a substernal extension of the goiter, an operation should be

recommended. Sternotomy is rarely required. Interpretation of roentgenograms or CT scans is important. The goiter should be looked at with respect to the position of the heads of the clavicles. Often a large mediastinal mass can be seen on a chest x-ray, but it might not extend much below the heads of the clavicle. With extension of the neck during the operation, the substernal thyroid is brought into the neck. Most are easily delivered.

The most common reason for an operation on the thyroid is to exclude cancer, or treat if present, particularly when a thyroid nodule is found in a patient with a past history of irradiation. All undiagnosed cold nodules must be evaluated, especially if solitary. In the next section we will discuss needle aspiration, but equivocal results in high-risk patients (history of irradiation, men, older age group), sheets of follicular cells, or overt cancer trigger immediate exploration and surgical treatment of such lesions.

Fine-Needle Aspiration of the Thyroid

During the past 15 years, fine-needle aspiration of thyroid nodules with cytologic examination of the material has become the standard of care. The principal indication is a solitary palpable nodule. Even if the patient has not had thyroid-function testing or scans, the first visit to the surgeon's office should include fine-needle aspiration. Obviously, a cold nodule on a thyroid scan should be followed up with needle aspiration. For routine nodules, ultrasound and CT scans are not recommended. An ultrasound can show whether the lesion is cystic or solid, and if the lesion is cystic, it will be aspirated and might disappear. If the lesion is solid, it will be aspirated and cytologic examination is performed. Therefore, since all nodules should be aspirated, there is no real indication for the ultrasound. The cost-benefit ratio of CT scans for routine situations obviates their use.

The technique of needle aspiration is shown in (Fig. 36-1). The patient lies supine on the examining table with a pillow beneath the shoulder so that the neck is hyperextended. The head and neck are positioned so that the nodule becomes most prominent. A moment should be taken to ensure that the index finger and thumb of the left hand can fix the nodule prior to proceeding with the aspiration. We use a 10-cc syringe, but the needle size tends to vary. Occasionally, an 18-gauge needle

gets a very good sample of tissues, although the standard 22-gauge needle is less traumatic, particularly in patients who are taking aspirin or have any history of bleeding. The size of the needle has not been a critical issue for us. An alcohol swab is all that is used before inserting the needle into the lesion. The senior author of this chapter does not use local anesthesia since it takes more time and causes more pain than a simple needle stick. The needle is inserted quickly into the nodule and a significant suction is placed on the syringe, which is passed back and forth 4 or 5 times through the nodule. The needle is withdrawn, pressure is placed on the needle site, and the patient is allowed to sit up. Saccamono solution is aspirated into the syringe and the material (often blood-tinged) is spread onto two clean glass slides. The slides are sprayed with fixative solution and sent for cytologic examination. Depending on the logistics and set up of the clinic, these examinations can be

done immediately. If a significant volume of bloody fluid or colloid is withdrawn, the lesion might actually disappear. If it does, cytology is performed, and the patient is seen again in 2 to 3 weeks to determine if the cyst has recurred. As mentioned above, a third appearance of the cyst carries with it some risk for malignancy and exploration and removal of the thyroid lobe is recommended.

The interpretation of cytologic examination requires cooperation between the surgeon and the surgical pathologist. At our institution, we are fortunate to have highly experienced and knowledgeable cytologists to help us. Benign lesions are the majority of what is seen in our clinic. A colloid nodule showing some red cells, colloid, and hemosiderin-laden macrophages indicates a benign condition. Such patients do not require operation, unless there is compression or cosmetic indications. When lymphocytes and follicular cells are found, Hashimoto's disease might be indicated. Solid lymphocytes in patients who have long-standing goiter with sudden growth might denote lymphoma; a definitive diagnosis requires biopsy. The most common malignant lesion of the thyroid is papillary carcinoma and this can readily be diagnosed by cytologic examination after needle aspiration. Abnormal nuclei with prominent nucleoli and nuclear grooves are reliable for the diagnosis of papillary carcinoma of the thyroid. Occasionally, psammoma bodies are seen. Sometimes a larger biopsy or core biopsy (rarely done in the office) gives enough architecture to show the papillary formation. Sheets of follicular cells pose a significant problem. In this situation, the pathologist can only diagnose a "follicular lesion" and cannot determine whether it is malignant or benign. Follicular cancer is usually diagnosed on permanent section after a definitive procedure. Malignancy is characterized by vascular invasion or capsular invasion. Needle aspiration is technically unable to make that differentiation. Occasionally, a specimen can be deemed inadequate with not enough cellularity for diagnosis. In this circumstance, the clinical judgment, history of irradiation, and even a trial of thyroid suppression can help dictate whether a surgical procedure is necessary. Aspiration can be repeated later. We perform needle aspirations on more than 95 percent of patients presenting with thyroid nodules.

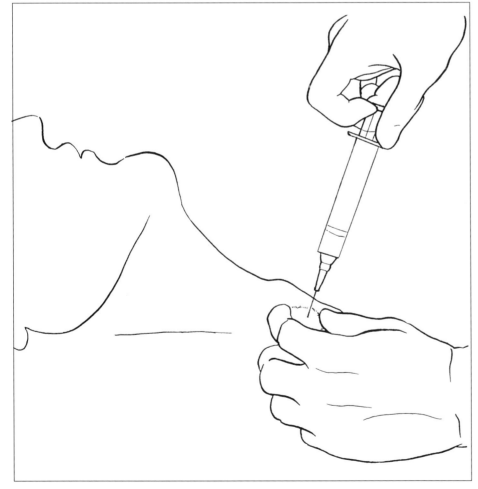

Fig. 36-1. A thyroid nodule stabilized with the left hand and aspirated.

Total Thyroid Lobectomy

Our most common operation on the thyroid is a total thyroid lobectomy and isthmusectomy. This procedure (procedure 1) is the definitive "biopsy" for thyroid nodules once indications for surgery have been met using history, physical examination, and fine-needle aspiration. In addition, the majority of patients with substernal goiters require total lobectomy and isthmusectomy. It is interesting that the majority of such substernal thyroid masses occur on the left side and deviate the trachea to the right. The opposite lobe is palpated to ensure that there are no abnormalities present. Total lobectomy is definitive for all benign lesions including cysts. Total thyroid lobectomy is the operation of choice for the single (at least 3–4 cm) toxic nodule confined to one lobe.

Small well-differentiated carcinomas can be treated adequately using total thyroid lobectomy and isthmusectomy. If there are no lymph nodes or history of irradiation, small encapsulated papillary carcinomas are adequately treated this way followed by TSH suppression by thyroid administration. The literature defines small as less than 3 to 4 cm. Patients under age 45 are low-risk individuals and certainly can be treated by lobectomy, especially for small lesions. The same approach applies to small encapsulated follicular carcinomas; these cancers have an excellent prognosis. In general, however, a total thyroidectomy is recommended for larger cancers, cancers associated with a history of irradiation, and any cancer for which I-131 might be used for scanning or adjunctive therapy. The literature is voluminous concerning the appropriate surgical management of lesions under 3 cm. We are inclined to do a complete total thyroidectomy for most patients with follicular cancers, unless the lesions are quite small and extremely well encapsulated. This chapter is not the appropriate place for the discussion of the considerable data recommending limited or extensive surgical operations. The experienced thyroid surgeon, however, is more inclined to perform a total thyroidectomy and remove the central lymph nodes since surgical risks of such an operation are extremely low.

As mentioned, the technique of total thyroid lobectomy and isthmusectomy (procedure 1) is both challenging and satisfying. Attention toward meticulous hemostasis, gentle dissection, and fine silk ligatures on small vessels are used. If these principles are followed, the anatomy can be demonstrated and important structures protected. It is unnecessary to use drains or even consider the typing and cross-matching of blood for replacement. I no longer send the patient back to the room with a tracheostomy set. Not having to open a thyroidectomy incision on the floor for 30 years has influenced the decision to avoid frightening the patients and their families with such equipment.

All patients are anesthetized and maintained with endotracheal intubation. In addition, we recommended that an esophageal probe be used, not only to monitor pulse rate but also to assist the surgeon in identifying the esophagus. To find the tracheoesophageal groove, the surgeon feels the trachea anteriorly and the tube in the esophagus posteriorly. We suggest that the endotracheal tube be taped into position on the face so that there is no material to secure the tube, such as ties or tape, below the mandible. Once the endotracheal tube and the esophageal monitor are secured, the patient is positioned. The head and chin are midline in the extended position. The neck should not be hyperextended forcibly or suspended, as risk of neck injury is real. A rolled-up sheet is placed under the shoulders and a head rest ("donut") is placed under the occiput to help hold the position. Occasionally, a piece of tape can be brought across the forehead and secured to the table but is usually not necessary. Now that the chin is midline and the neck well extended, the patient should be placed in a semi-sitting position with the knees and waist flexed so that the head and chest are elevated approximately 20 to 30 degrees. The arms are placed at the side with the elbows well padded to prevent nerve injury. At this point, the patient is ready to be prepped.

The neck is washed with a povidone-iodine solution from the angle of the mandible to the level of the fourth ribs anteriorly. Before placing the drapes, a sterile wadded-up towel is placed at both sides of the neck so that the drapes will not fall down toward the mattress. If there is any concern about a substernal extension of the goiter, the entire anterior chest beyond the xiphoid is prepared; an additional drape is placed over the chest during the cervical portion of the operation. The towels are held in position using skin staples, which keep the drapes from moving or falling away from the side of the neck during the operation. A standard laparotomy sheet finally defines the operative field.

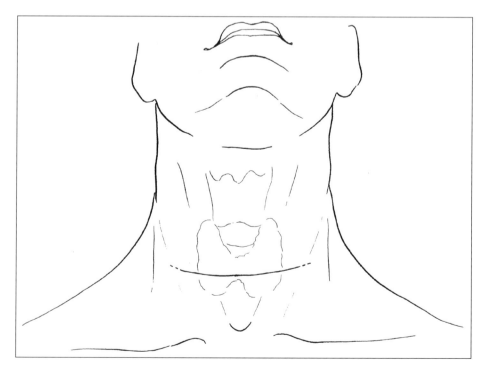

Fig. 36-2. Hand-drawn proposed incision at the base of the neck.

The proposed line of incision is marked with a pencil (Fig. 36-2). We do not use a taut suture to mark the skin. We follow skin lines, which are the primary guide for placement of the collar incision. Generally, the incision is approximately 2 cm above the heads of the clavicle. It is slightly curved and conforms to other skin folds if possible. If the incision is made too low, then the upper skin flap can become edematous because of compromised venous drainage. Once the proposed line of incision is drawn and measured for symmetry, the incision is developed through the subcutaneous fat and platysma, the latter being absent in the central portion of the neck. While developing this first incision, pressure is applied to the wound edge to compress the small skin bleeders. Persistent small bleeding vessels are caught with mosquito clamps and coagulated. The coagulation unit does not touch the tissue directly.

The skin and platysma are raised as a single flap beginning superiorly. Three Allis clamps are placed on the platysma, one each laterally and one in the midline (Fig. 36-3). Traction is applied vertically while the surgeon's left hand uses countertraction on the tissue. We use a knife with a No. 15 blade for this part of the dissection. There is an avascular plane just behind the platysma, anterior to the superficial jugular venous system. The flap is raised superiorly until the V of the thyroid cartilage is at the upper margin of the dissection. The three Allis clamps are then replaced for the lower flap in similar manner, and the dissection is carried in this same plane down to the manubrium and clavicular heads. Care must be taken to avoid going too deeply on this inferior flap since the sternocleidomastoid muscle can be raised. However, if one stays superficial, the sternocleidomastoid muscle is easily identified and its insertion is seen on the clavicular heads. At this point, two clean laparotomy tapes are placed within the skin wound margin and held in position with a sharp thyroid self-retaining retractor. Allis clamps approximate the angles of the two tapes to exclude skin in the region.

The midline strap muscles are separated with a knife (Fig. 36-4). The division between the sternohyoid muscles is identified. This line is incised superiorly and inferiorly with careful hemostasis. This superficial strap muscle is mobilized using sharp and blunt dissection on both sides so that the thyroid gland with the investing sternothyroid muscle is clearly visible. This maneuver allows palpation of the contralateral thyroid lobe, which need not be totally mobilized. If it is necessary to return to complete the thyroidectomy at a later time, the contralateral lobe is more easily dissected if the muscle is not fully raised at the first operation. Once again, using both sharp and gentle finger dissection, the sternothyroid muscle is elevated from the thyroid gland, which is then brought into view. On the side of the lesion, a small Richardson retractor holds the strap muscles laterally. It is rare for us to cut the strap muscles. This maneuver is reserved for very large goiters in which exposure is difficult. For most patients, the strap muscles can be retracted laterally and widely during the thyroid lobectomy.

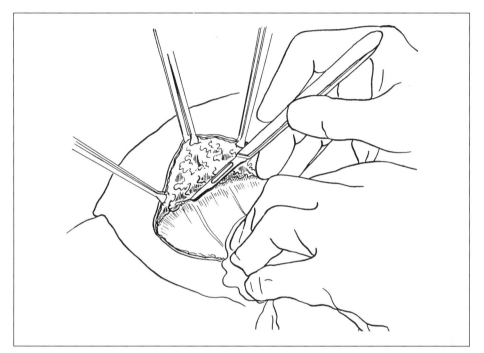

Fig. 36-3. Raising the upper flap of the platysma and skin. Countertraction with left hand is the key to clean dissection with a knife.

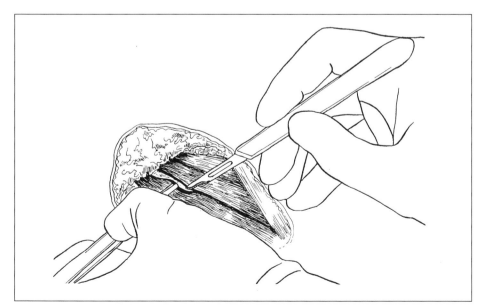

Fig. 36-4. The midline is developed between the strap muscles (sternohyoid muscle shown here).

Once the strap muscles have been reflected laterally, the surgeon gently goes around the lateral and inferior margins of the gland with an index finger to gently mobilize the lobe into the wound (Fig. 36-5). The thyroid gland is teased from lateral to medial. During the conduct of this mobilization, gentleness is necessary since the middle thyroid vein can be stretched and avulsed. When the middle thyroid vein is identified, it is immediately ligated and divided. We prefer to place ligatures around vessels and then divide the vessels between the ligatures. Most of the ligatures used for the procedure are 4–0 silk. We use 3–0 silk for larger vessels and occasionally 2–0 silk to suture or ligate superior pole vessels.

This gland mobilization is often the key to defining whether this procedure will be easy or not. When the lobe with its tumor come up easily, medial traction is placed on this lobe. Before approaching the branches of the inferior thyroid artery or even mobilizing the gland to expose the parathyroids, the superior pole is isolated. An appendiceal retractor is used in the upper corner of the incision. The areolar tissues are pushed away from this upper pole with a Küttner dissector (''peanut'' dissector). The index finger and thumb of the surgeon can often pinch the soft tissue around the upper pole and a right-angle clamp can then loop around this tissue. This clamp should be placed immediately contiguous to the thyroid tissue. If extraneous tissues are brought under this clamp, it is possible to injure the superior laryngeal nerve. If a long pedicle of the superior pole can be demonstrated, these vessels can be divided in continuity after ligating with 2–0 silk (Fig. 36-6). This maneuver is done only if there is at least a 5- or 6-mm cuff of tissue beyond the proximal ligature. Once this suture is cut, the superior thyroid vessels retract out of the wound. Occasionally, the tissue is divided between clamps and is suture-ligated with either 2–0 or 3–0 silk. Once again, this step is the last good view of the upper pole vessels. At this point, the upper pole is dissected downward from lateral to medial until Berry's ligament is encountered. Here, the recurrent laryngeal nerve is closest to the thyroid gland just before the nerve enters the larynx. Now we direct our attention more inferiorly and return to Berry's ligament later.

The thyroid lobe is retracted from lateral to medial until we identify fatty tissue near the branching of the inferior thyroid artery. We do not ligate the inferior thyroid artery or its major branches but take the finest of the capsular branches between mosquito clamps and ligate them (Fig. 36-7). Using gentle teasing and the occasional peanut dissector, these divided branches of the inferior thyroid artery allow the parathyroid gland to fall away from the thyroid and remain in the tracheal esophageal groove. This part of the operation is tedious and exacting. It does, however, allow the preservation of the inferior parathyroid gland along with its blood supply from the inferior thyroid artery. This gland is always surrounded by fat and falls back

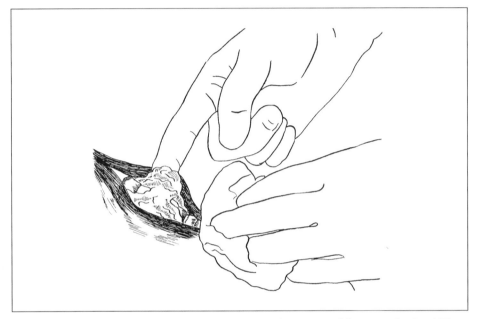

Fig. 36-5. Gentle, blunt mobilization of the nodule by an index finger. Be careful not to avulse the middle thyroid vein.

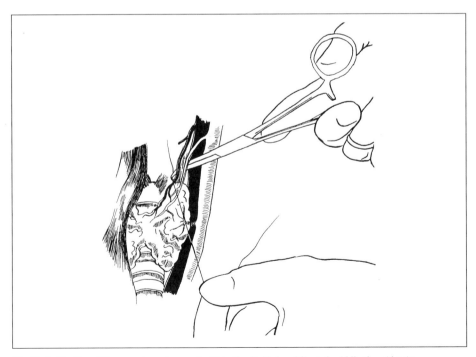

Fig. 36-6. Ligation of the superior pole vessels. Note the divided and ligated middle thyroid vein.

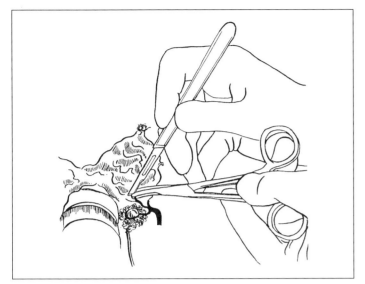

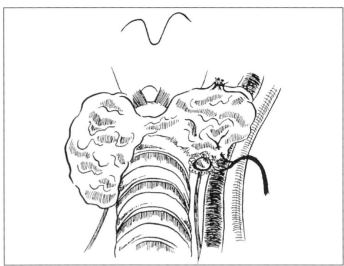

Fig. 36-7. *Careful division of the small distal branches of the inferior thyroid artery. The parathyroid gland is allowed to fall back into neck with intact vascular pedicle.*

Fig. 36-8. *Note the positions of the recurrent laryngeal nerves. The left courses vertically in the tracheoesophageal groove; the right comes into the field at a 30-degree angle.*

into position easily. At this point, the recurrent laryngeal nerve on the right side can be identified, either behind or between the major branches of the inferior thyroid artery. The right recurrent laryngeal nerve comes in at an angle of approximately 30 degrees to the tracheoesophageal groove (Fig. 36-8). The left nerve courses almost vertical in the tracheoesophageal groove. Once the nerve is identified, it is traced up to its entry into the cricothyroid muscle. Now Berry's ligament can be divided a little at a time, teasing the tissue with mosquito clamp tips. This step allows further mobilization of the thyroid gland medially.

The superior parathyroid gland, seen in fat, is usually in direct contact with the capsule of the thyroid gland. The parathyroid gland is teased away by making a plane between the parathyroid gland and the thyroid gland. Using the same techniques as above, the parathyroid gland is allowed to fall back into position. If the parathyroid gland appears to have lost its blood supply or is injured in any way, it should be removed and autotransplanted. This is done by mincing the parathyroid gland with a knife but not going all the way through the capsule. This step causes the tissue to fan out, yet be held together. The gland is placed into a pocket developed by spreading a hemostat in the substance of the sternocleidomastoid muscle. A figure-of-eight 3–0 silk stitch is used to repair the fascia overlying the muscle

and secure the autotransplant. It is unnecessary to transplant into the forearm since this is not a patient with parathyroid disease. However, the site of transplant can be marked with a silver clip. Since there can be three other functioning parathyroid glands, one never really knows how soon this transplanted parathyroid is functional.

Now that the parathyroid glands and recurrent laryngeal nerve are in view and protected, the operator easily teases the thyroid gland from lateral to medial off the trachea until directly beneath the isthmus. This dissection is performed quickly since there is very little blood supply in this region. The isthmus is mobilized all the way to the opposite lobe. The isthmus is divided to include tissue from the medial thyroid lobe on the opposite side. This maneuver is done between clamps, dividing the tissue with a knife (Fig. 36-9). Figure-of-eight sutures are used to oversew the cut edge of the thyroid gland (Fig. 36-10). The specimen is marked with various lengths of suture on the upper pole, lower pole, tumor, and isthmus so that the pathologist understands the tissue submitted and its spatial orientation.

While a frozen section is done, hemostasis is carefully achieved, ligating all small vessels and coagulating tiny ones that are clamped with mosquito tip clamps. The pathologist might diagnose a "follicular lesion". The needle aspiration cytology is

as accurate as the frozen section for follicular lesions. Unless the frozen section went directly through a point of vascular or capsular invasion, it is not possible to determine whether the lesion is benign or malignant without permanent multiple sections. At this point, the operation is terminated and the closure done.

If a lesion is demonstrated to be a carcinoma or there are indications for total thyroidectomy, the opposite lobe is removed in an identical fashion as the side with the lesion. All four parathyroid glands should be preserved and both recurrent laryngeal nerves identified and protected. During total thyroidectomies, we do not divide the isthmus but submit the specimen in toto. If it is necessary to go back and perform a completion thyroidectomy because the diagnosis of either medullary carcinoma or follicular carcinoma is made at permanent section, it is best to do the completion within 5 days of the original operation or wait at least 6 weeks. The intervening period is a difficult time to reexplore the thyroid gland, because the healing process is quite vascular and anatomy is distorted.

Closure is performed after total hemostasis. Drains are not routinely used. Occasionally, a suction catheter can be brought out through a separate stab wound if a large cavity has been created from a substernal thyroid extension. Even then, we rarely use drains. After irrigation, interrupted 3–0 silk sutures are used to bring

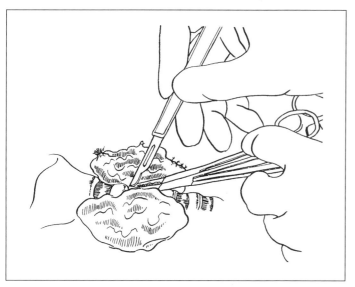

Fig. 36-9. *Isthmus divided between clamps on the medial edge of contralateral lobe.*

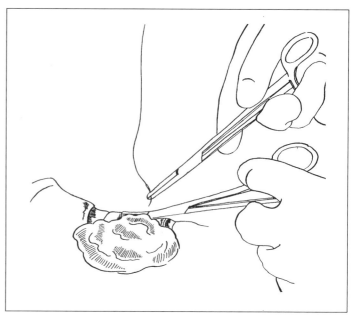

Fig. 36-10. *Isthmus tissue is suture-ligated. We suggest a figure-of-eight stitch.*

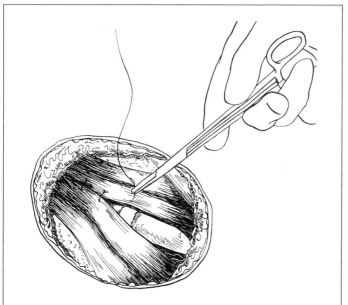

Fig. 36-11. *Closure of midline strap muscles with interrupted 3–0 silk sutures.*

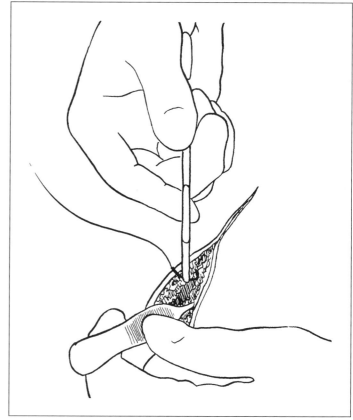

Fig. 36-12. *The platysma is closed with interrupted 4–0 silk sutures, burying the knots.*

the fascia of the sternohyoid muscles together (Fig. 36-11). The sternothyroid muscle is not repaired. Even if the muscle has been divided for a large goiter, only the sternohyoid muscle is repaired. The platysma is closed with interrupted buried 4–0 silk stitches (Fig. 36-12). All sutures are cut on the knot, since the less foreign material, the better. The skin is approximated using a running 3–0 polypropylene subcutaneous pullout stitch, which is brought out lateral to the incision on both sides. These long ends are taped into position with Steri-strips. Steri-strips are also applied to the incision. The pullout suture is removed immediately before discharge. Steri-strips on the skin edge are then in place and need not be disturbed. A small dressing is used. We do not use the large circumferential cervical dressings.

After the patient has awakened and nausea has resolved, the patient can have a clear liquid diet and progress to a regular diet almost immediately. The patient should be up and around the same night. A serum calcium level is drawn only after a total thyroidectomy. In the asymptomatic patient, it is unnecessary to measure the calcium after the lobe and isthmus are removed. As mentioned earlier, we do not keep a tracheostomy tray in the room. Narcotics are rarely required after the first 24 hours. Oral acetophentadine with codeine is sent home with the patient. The patient's voice should be normal. If there is any question about injury to the recurrent laryngeal nerves or if such nerves were not identified, the vocal cords are examined at the time of extubation. In patients with malignancies, we do use thyroxine immediately and during our long-term follow-up. With benign disease, we also recommend thyroxine to prevent hypertrophy of the residual lobe and perhaps to obviate the formation of new benign nodules. At home, the patient can shower and merely blot the Steri-strips dry. Patients are instructed not to drive or ride a bicycle for 10 to 14 days. Certain types of exercises can be resumed as tolerated.

Subtotal Thyroidectomy

We rarely perform subtotal thyroidectomies. Even in patients with diffuse toxic goiters, a total thyroidectomy is performed. This procedure allows visualiza-

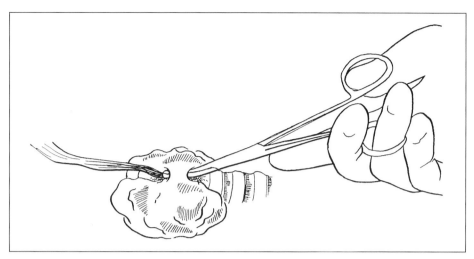

Fig. 36-13. A clamp under the isthmus pulls an umbilical tape through as a guide for the subtotal dissection.

tion and protection of nerves and parathyroid glands. Since it is difficult to determine how much of this abnormal thyroid tissue should remain in place, we prefer to remove all of it. We do use subtotal thyroidectomy for very large bilateral goiters but generally do a total lobectomy on one side. Occasionally, for reoperative thyroidectomies with a great deal of scarring, we might prefer to stay out of the tracheoesophageal groove and come directly across the thyroid gland if the lesion is anterior enough to do so with ease. We do not do subtotal thyroidectomies for cancers. We prefer total thyroidectomy or lobectomy and isthmusectomy according to indications previously described.

If we are doing a subtotal thyroidectomy, we first do the total lobectomy as described. If the operation is a subtotal thyroidectomy on both sides, we recommend first tunneling a right-angle clamp behind the isthmus (in front of the trachea) and using an umbilical tape for traction or as a guide (Fig. 36-13). The dissection, which proceeds directly through the thyroid tissue, begins just anterior to the small branches of the inferior thyroid artery. By this time, we have taken down the superior pole vessels. Clamps are placed directly across the thyroid tissue well anterior to the tracheoesophageal groove where the nerves and parathyroid glands reside. We go in a straight line toward the anterior trachea where the umbilical tape has marked the end point (Fig. 36-14). This tissue is suture-ligated with interrupted figure-of-eight 3–0 stitches and careful hemostasis is achieved. Subtotal or intracap-

sular dissections are much bloodier than total thyroidectomies. In this situation, too, we do not drain the wound.

Follow-Up Care

As described earlier, the patient usually goes home the day following the operation when the pullout suture is removed. At the first office visit (in 7–10 days), if there is any fluid collection, it can be removed by simple aspiration with an 18- or 20-gauge needle. In some large goiters, this has been necessary. It is rare to aspirate a seroma more than once. Steri-strips are removed on the first office visit and patients can return to work and resume most of their activities. We discourage weight lifting and strenuous physical activity in which a Valsalva maneuver might increase the venous pressure and cause some late bleeding. We generally see patients with benign diseases 6 months later and return them to their primary care physician at that time. During our final visit, we check TSH, T3, and T4 levels to be sure that the thyroxine dose is correct. If the patient is receiving thyroxine after an operation for malignant lesions, we prefer the TSH level to be well below the lower limits of normal. These patients are seen by the surgeon every 6 months for 5 years and once a year after that. We prefer to keep our own follow-up records of all patients on whom we have operated for malignant disease.

The use of adjunctive I-131 deserves mention. Since iodine preferentially goes to normal tissue, we should have already

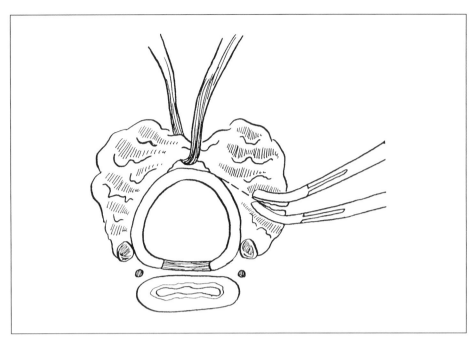

Fig. 36-14. Cross-section showing relative positions of nerves, parathyroid glands, and division of the thyroid tissue between clamps. A series of paired clamps is applied.

done a total thyroidectomy if I-131 therapy has been planned. This procedure decreases the amount of radioactive material necessary to ablate the residual tissue. We allow the patient to stop the thyroxine for approximately 4 to 6 weeks before the scan. The TSH level is checked and should be at least twice normal before a scan is performed. We often do this evaluation in association with our endocrinologist colleagues, but comprehensive care of patients with thyroidectomy remains the responsibility of the thyroid surgeon.

Suggested Reading

Alfonso A, Christondias G, Amaruddinn Q, et al. Tracheal or esophageal compression due to benign thyroid disease. *Am J Surg* 142:350, 1981.

Allo MD, Thompson NW. Rationale for the operative management of substernal goiters. *Surgery* 94:969, 1983.

Clark OH, Weber CA. Endocrine surgery. *Surg Clin North Am* 67:1967.

Croom RD, Thomas Jr CG, Reddick RL, Tawil MT. Autonomously functioning thyroid nodules in childhood and adolescence. *Surgery* 102:1101, 1987.

DeMicco C, Vasko V, Garcia S, et al. Fine-needle aspiration of thyroid follicular neoplasm: diagnostic use of thyroid peroxidase immunochemistry with monoclonal antibody 47. *Surgery* 116:1031, 1994.

Foster RS Jr. Thyroid Gland. In JH Davis, WR Drucker, RS Foster Jr, et al (eds.), *Clinical Surgery*, Vol. 2. St. Louis: Mosby, 1987.

LoGerfo P, Chabot J, Gazetas P. The intraoperative incidence of detectable bilateral and multicentric disease in papillary carcinoma of the thyroid. *Surgery* 108:958, 1990.

Shaha A, Alfonso A, Jaffe B. Acute airway distress due to thyroid pathology. *Surgery* 102:1068, 1987.

Shaha AR, DiMaio T, Webber C, Jaffe BM. Intraoperative decision-making during thyroid surgery based on the results of preoperative needle biopsy and frozen section. *Surgery* 108:964, 1990.

Tyler DS, Winchester J, Caraway NP, et al. Indeterminate fine-needle aspiration biopsy of the thyroid; identification of subgroups at high risk for invasive carcinoma. *Surgery* 116:1054, 1994.

EDITOR'S COMMENT

The authors have described a classic approach to the single most frequent indication for thyroid lobectomy—a single cold nodule in the thyroid. Occasionally, these masses can be found in the isthmus of the gland, although often those lesions prove to be large Delphian nodes overlying or contiguous to the isthmus of the gland. When isthmic nodules are encountered, it has been our practice to limit the resection to the isthmus with a wedge of normal thyroid lobe on both sides and to obtain a frozen section to ascertain whether the lesion is benign or malignant. With follicular lesions, this decision can be difficult, as the authors have emphasized, but a grossly well-encapsulated and simple appearing nodule should be dealt with in that manner.

The authors raise the issue of using CT for substernal goiter. Its purpose seldom justifies the cost, and a simple chest x-ray will reveal the lesion. Only if no goiter is palpable in the neck would CT scanning be done, particularly to rule out other causes of anterior superior mediastinal masses. The basic operative principle is that even large substernal goiters can almost invariably be removed through the cervical incision, since the blood supply to the substernal thyroid arises from the thyroid vessels in the neck. These lesions are best mobilized by putting one's fingers into the superior mediastinum and gently freeing the soft tissue connections at both sides of the thyroid. At that point, a finger on each side of the substernal component can be used to gently deliver it from the thoracic inlet. These lesions were more commonly seen when multinodular goiters were encountered more frequently, and thyroid surgeons often had two sterile teaspoons on the instrument table and delivered these glands like obstetric forceps delivered a fetal head. On only two or three occasions have I had to break up the thyroid mass to deliver it from under the superior border of the sternum. I do not advocate that maneuver, since many of the ones in older patients have enlarged because they harbor a low-grade malignancy.

The authors have also emphasized the need to use caution in aspirating or even biopsying thyroids in patients who take aspirin or a number of other drugs that affect the platelet or the clotting mechanism, including essentially all of the nonsteroidal anti-inflammatory drugs, and, of course, coumadin, dipyridamole, and pentifylline. A complete history should be obtained from the patient, as is the case when one is going to undertake a significant operative procedure, in terms of obtaining a history of previous bleeding or transfusions, drug use, and so forth.

The technique of the operation has been extremely well outlined by the authors. In women, we tend to use a lower incision, placing it just at the superior edge of the clavicular head, agreeing fully with the authors that the low incision does tend to predispose to venous edema of the flap.

However, that edema always subsides in 2 weeks or less and poses no permanent change in the appearance of the incision of the superior flap. Similarly, we seldom use drains in these patients, and, if one is used, it is always a closed suction drain that is removed in 24 hours to minimize scarring from the drain exit site. The use of absorbable suture material in the neck should be discouraged; some patients have exuberant reaction to the absorbable sutures and

are far better served by the generous use of fine silk ties and sutures, exactly as described.

Thyroid surgery in the hands of an experienced and competent surgeon is a fine example of the effective application of delicate techniques and applied anatomy in achieving minimal tissue trauma and optimal results.

R.J.B.

37

Total Thyroidectomy, Lymph Node Dissection for Cancer

Samuel A. Wells, Jr.

Carcinoma of the thyroid gland affects 15,000 persons in the United States each year. Sixty percent of thyroid cancers are of the papillary type, 20 percent are follicular carcinomas, and the remainder is almost equally divided between medullary carcinoma and anaplastic carcinomas. The range of biologic aggressiveness of the thyroid cancers is extreme and not matched in any other solid organ. For example, papillary carcinomas are generally slow growing and infrequently take the life of the host, whereas patients with giant cell anaplastic carcinomas rarely live for more than 3 years after the tumor is diagnosed. Thyroidectomy is the treatment of choice for all patients with a thyroid carcinoma except for patients with anaplastic cancers where chemotherapy and x-ray therapy are the treatments of choice.

There has been controversy regarding the extent of thyroidectomy required for a thyroid carcinoma. It is generally accepted that patients with follicular carcinoma or medullary carcinoma should be treated by total thyroidectomy. However, the management of patients with papillary carcinoma is less clear and there are generally two schools of thought. Clinicians who favor aggressive treatment for papillary carcinoma argue that in the majority of patients, microscopic disease is present in both thyroid lobes whether or not there is bilateral macroscopic disease. They further state that the disease is aggressive in certain patients, especially patients with large primary tumors that at the time of operation are found to have invaded adjacent tissues such as the trachea, strap muscles, and neurovascular structures. Conserva-

tive clinicians argue that even though the disease is bilateral microscopically, the likelihood that the patient will develop clinical evidence of papillary thyroid carcinoma following a unilateral resection of the involved thyroid lobe is only 5 percent. Also, the recurrent disease could be managed by completion thyroidectomy should it occur. Furthermore, the large majority of papillary thyroid carcinomas grow slowly and few patients die of the disease. They also cite the complications of recurrent laryngeal nerve injury and hypoparathyroidism, which are more frequent following total thyroidectomy. In addition, these complications are more common in the hands of an inexperienced thyroid surgeon.

Unfortunately, there has never been a prospective controlled trial with any of the thyroid malignancies in which patients have been staged preoperatively, randomized to either conservative (lobectomy or subtotal thyroidectomy) or aggressive (total thyroidectomy) resection, and then followed postoperatively for sufficient time to evaluate the outcomes of the various operative procedures. The data that are available suggest that the incidences of both recurrent carcinoma and death are less frequent in patients subjected to an aggressive operative procedure combined with postoperative radioiodine ablation of residual thyroid tissue and thyroid suppression.

Papillary thyroid carcinoma and medullary thyroid carcinomas metastasize first to regional lymph nodes. It is important to perform a modified neck dissection in pa-

tients with these primary thyroid malignancies when there is evidence of lymph node involvement or when the primary tumor is greater than 2 cm in diameter and occult lymph node disease is likely to be present. It is rarely necessary to perform a radical neck dissection in patients with thyroid malignancies, even though the procedure was used commonly in the past.

The two main complications associated with total thyroidectomy are damage to the recurrent laryngeal nerves and hypoparathyroidism. One must be exceedingly careful to identify both recurrent nerves and to protect them from injury during the operation. Furthermore, it is important that care be taken not to injure the external branches of the superior laryngeal nerves. It can be difficult to perform a total thyroidectomy and preserve the blood supply to the parathyroid glands. Often, at the end of a total thyroidectomy it is difficult to determine by gross observation whether the parathyroid glands are viable. We have adopted a liberal policy of performing a total parathyroidectomy and autografting the resected parathyroid glands to the sternocleidomastoid muscle if there is any question of their viability.

Total thyroidectomy, with or without lymph node dissection, has a place in the management of patients with thyroid carcinoma. The operation is generally well tolerated and can be performed with minimal disfigurement. The successful management of patients with a thyroid carcinoma depends in part on the biology of the malignancy; the clinical stage of the disease; and the philosophy, skill, and experience of the surgeon. When managing patients with thyroid carcinoma, it is important to remember that above all one should do no harm.

Preoperative Preparation

Patients should be examined carefully regarding a history of exposure to ionizing radiation to the neck. Such patients have a substantially increased risk of developing thyroid carcinoma. Furthermore, since the entire gland was almost certainly exposed to the radiation, a total thyroidectomy should be performed. The presence of familial thyroid malignancy is highly suggestive of either multiple endocrine neoplasia (MEN) type 2A, MEN-2B, or familial medullary thyroid carcinoma (FMTC). The diagnosis of a medullary thyroid carcinoma can be specifically confirmed either by detecting elevated plasma calcitonin levels or by direct DNA testing for mutations in the RET protooncogene in patients with familial disease.

It is important to ask patients if there has been a change in their voice, or if they have developed dysphagia or dyspnea. Such symptoms often indicate the presence of malignant disease. If patients have developed hoarseness, one should suspect tumor involvement of the recurrent laryngeal nerve and the vocal cords should be examined preoperatively. Dysphagia is usually caused by a large thyroid mass displacing the esophagus. A history of a rapidly enlarging thyroid mass suggests the presence of an anaplastic carcinoma.

On physical examination, it is important to determine if the mass is tender and if the nodularity is confined to one thyroid lobe. The neck should be examined for the presence of firm or enlarged lymph nodes. The preferred diagnostic procedure, for either the thyroid mass or an enlarged lymph node, is fine-needle aspiration with cytologic examination of the aspirated material. Depending on the results of the cytology, additional tests such as thyroid ultrasound and radionuclide imaging can be obtained. The patient should have a chest x-ray.

The plans for the operation should be explained to the patient. In most situations, the diagnosis is uncertain preoperatively and definitive treatment will depend on intraoperative frozen section. It must be explained that the pathologist might not be able to establish a diagnosis of malignancy on the basis of intraoperative histologic examination. Final diagnosis must await the results of the permanent section examination. When the permanent section diagnosis shows malignancy, it is usually necessary to perform a completion thyroidectomy a few days after the initial thyroid lobectomy. The patient should also understand the risk of damage to the recurrent laryngeal nerves, the external branch of the superior laryngeal nerves, and the parathyroid glands.

Positioning of the Patient

The patient should be placed in the supine position with the arms tucked close to the side. A rolled towel or half sheet is placed vertically between the scapulae and beneath the vertebral column so that the shoulders can fall away from the operative field thus exposing the neck and upper chest (Fig. 37-1A). Care should be taken that all of the tubes and lines used by the anesthesiologists are secured superiorly so that they do not drop onto the operative field. An ether screen should be placed before draping the operative field. The skin of the neck and upper chest is prepared with sterile solution, and then sterile towels are used to drape the immediate operative field. After draping with sheets, the

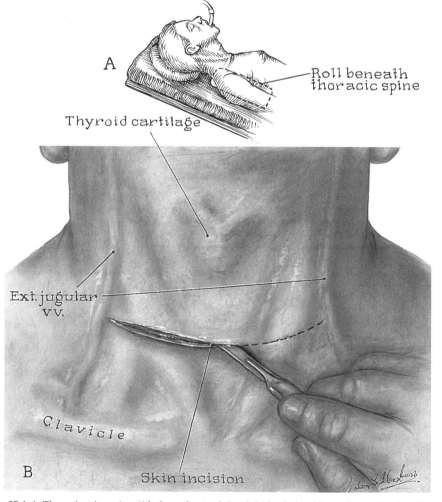

Fig. 37-1.A. The patient is supine with the neck extended and the head placed in a soft circular ring. There is a rolled half sheet (dotted outline) between the scapulae. The patient is intubated, asleep, and in the reverse Trendelenburg position. B. The skin incision is made two finger breadths above the sternal notch. If possible, the incision is placed in a skin crease.

patient is placed in the reverse Trendelen-burg position and the operation is begun.

The Operation

Skin Incision and Exposure of the Thyroid Gland and the Lateral Neck

It is important that the surgeon maintain a dry surgical field throughout the operation. Many of the vital structures encountered during total thyroidectomy are very small and can be difficult to identify even under ideal conditions. Blood staining of tissues will unnecessarily complicate the operation.

A skin incision is made about two finger breadths above the sternal notch (Fig. 37-1B). The incision should be placed in a skin crease, if possible. The incision ordinarily extends laterally to the jugular veins; however, depending on the size of the thyroid mass and the presence of enlarged lymph nodes in the neck lateral to the thyroid gland, it might be necessary to extend the incision. Once the skin incision has been deepened through the platysma (Fig. 37-2), the electrocautery is used to develop superior and inferior flaps. (For the remainder of the procedure, the electrocautery, rather than the knife, is used to develop tissue planes.) The superior flap extends to the level of the thyroid cartilage (Fig. 37-3), while the inferior flap extends to the sternal notch. Once the flaps are developed, a Mahorner self-retaining retractor is placed (Fig. 37-4). The strap muscles are then separated in the midline for the full extent of the operative field. There is seldom the need to divide the strap muscles since they can be easily retracted laterally for adequate exposure. At this point, the neck is thoroughly examined for enlarged lymph nodes. The side of the neck where the thyroid mass is located should be explored first. The strap muscles are retracted laterally, and the thyroid lobe is exposed. In the described situation, a tumor is found to be occupying the inferior pole of the left thyroid lobe (Fig. 37-5). If the thyroid mass is invading a strap muscle or is tightly adherent to muscle, a portion of the muscle should be excised to ensure that an adequate margin of tissue is obtained as the mass is resected. If the thyroid mass is small, it can be excised with a

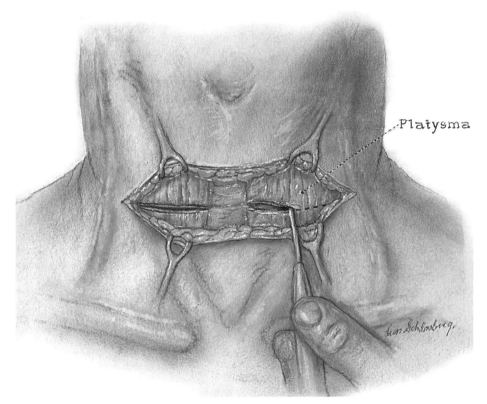

Fig. 37-2. The platysma muscle is divided with the electrocautery. The midportion of the platysma is thin. (In the figure, the lateral portions of the muscle are thicker than normal.)

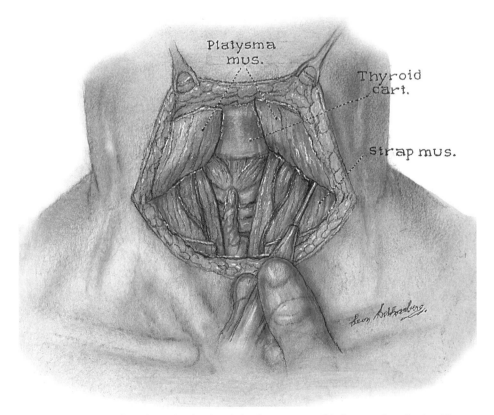

Fig. 37-3. The superior flap is being developed with the electrocautery. This flap extends to the thyroid cartilage, while the lower flap extends to the sternal notch.

rim of normal thyroid tissue and sent for immediate frozen section examination. Usually, however, the mass is large and cannot be excised without removing the entire lobe. Certainly, if the surgeon suspects thyroid malignancy, the entire lobe should be resected. Every effort should be taken to maintain the integrity of the thyroid mass. If it is ruptured, tumor cells will spill into the wound.

Mobilization of the Thyroid Lobe Containing the Nodule

For adequate exposure, it is necessary to elevate the thyroid lobe and retract it medially. This maneuver can be done either by providing gentle traction with a small cotton pledget grasped in a Kelly clamp (Küttner dissector) or by grasping the normal thyroid parenchyma adjacent to the thyroid mass with a Babcock clamp. As the lobe is elevated, the adjacent strap muscles and the associated adventitial tissues are swept away from the thyroid lobe and retracted laterally. Small blood vessels encountered are ligated and divided.

At this point, the recurrent laryngeal nerve should be identified. The normal anatomic location of the right and left recurrent laryngeal nerves are shown in the posterior and anterior views in Fig. 37-6. Also, shown in cross-sectional view is the relationship of the superior parathyroid gland and the left recurrent laryngeal nerve to the left thyroid lobe, the carotid sheath, the inferior thyroid vessels, the esophagus, and the trachea. The nerve normally ascends from the thoracic inlet parallel to the trachea until it angles to enter the larynx. However, with traction and medial rota-

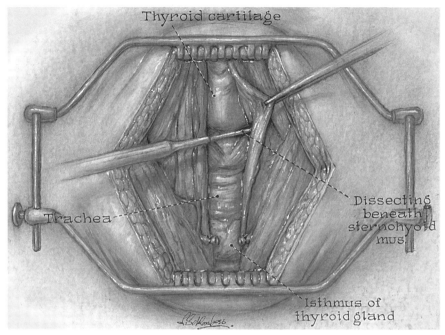

Fig. 37-4. With the Mahorner retractor in place, the medial portion of the sternohyoid muscle is elevated from the left thyroid lobe. To better show the anatomic structures, the Mahorner retractor is not shown in the subsequent figures.

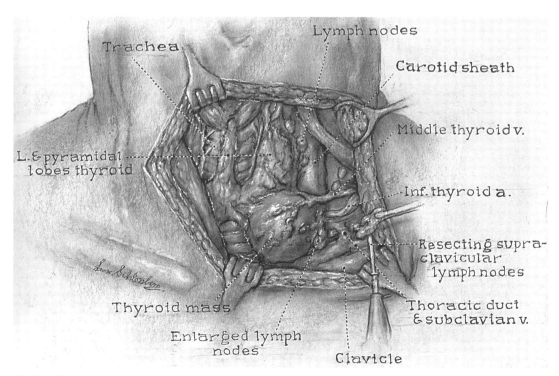

Fig. 37-5. The mass in the inferior portion of the left thyroid pole is shown. Large lymph nodes are evident adjacent to the thyroid mass and in the lateral neck.

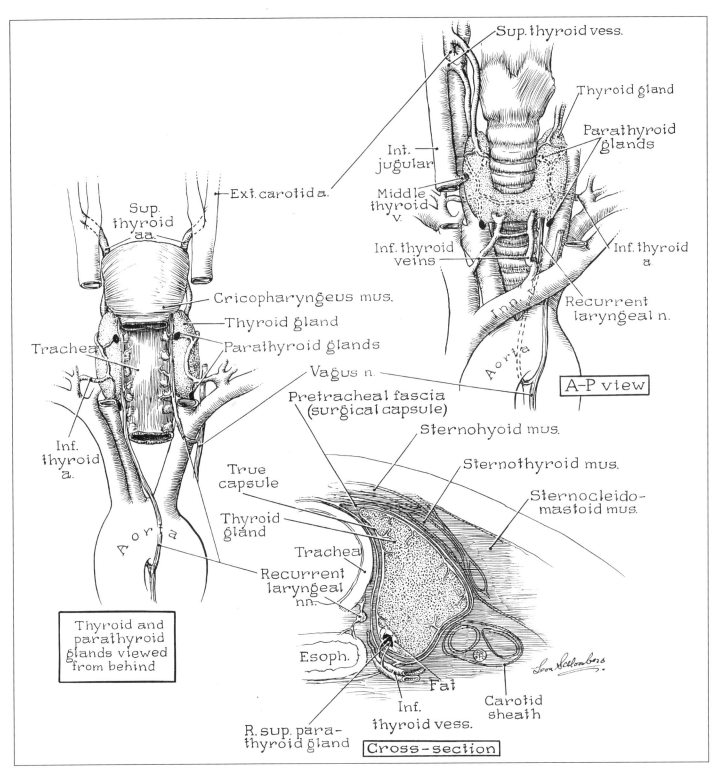

Fig. 37-6. Anterior and posterior views of the neck showing the normal anatomy of the right and left recurrent laryngeal nerves. Also, notice the location of the superior and inferior parathyroid glands. The cross-sectional view of the thyroid lobe shows the relationship of the left thyroid lobe to the carotid sheath, recurrent laryngeal nerve, superior parathyroid gland, esophagus, and trachea.

tion of the thyroid lobe, the nerve is pulled anteriorly in an oblique course from below upward. Under these circumstances, the nerve can usually be palpated against the trachea as a thin stringlike structure. On gross inspection, the nerve has a characteristic neurovasorum, which is easily recognized. It is critically important to identify this nerve and then trace it from its point of exit from the thorax to its entry into the larynx. Uncommonly, the nerve might divide low in the neck and unless detected one or more of its branches can be injured. This anatomic variant should be expected if the main trunk of the recurrent nerve is small. Usually, the nerve branches within 2 cm of its entry into the larynx. The laryngeal nerve might not be in the normal anatomic position. An anomalous recurrent laryngeal nerve most commonly arises as a direct laryngeal nerve and does not loop around the subclavian artery on the right or the aortic arch on the left. Instead, the nerve comes off of the vagus at a 90-degree angle. This anomaly is much more common on the right, and it results from an anomalous origin of the right subclavian artery from the descending thoracic aorta. This anomaly is uncommon, occurring in 1 percent of patients. If a direct laryngeal nerve is not identified, it is likely to be injured since the unwary surgeon commonly mistakes it for an inferior thyroid artery and divides it.

It is also important to identify the parathyroid glands as one prepares to resect the lobe containing the thyroid mass. The first step in finding the lower parathyroid gland is to identify the extension of the thymus gland into the neck. This structure, commonly called the "thyrothymic ligament," extends from the thorax and in most instances actually attaches to or is closely adherent to the lower pole of the thyroid gland (Fig. 37-7). The lower parathyroid gland is most often located within or immediately adjacent to this structure. The upper parathyroid gland is located on the posterior surface of the midportion of the thyroid lobe. It is usually surrounded by a lobule of fat close to the point where the inferior thyroid artery enters the thyroid parenchyma.

As a first step in resecting the thyroid lobe, the inferior thyroid artery and vein are doubly clamped, divided, and ligated. The vessels are immediately below the lower pole, and they can usually be taken together (Fig. 37-8). Attention is then di-

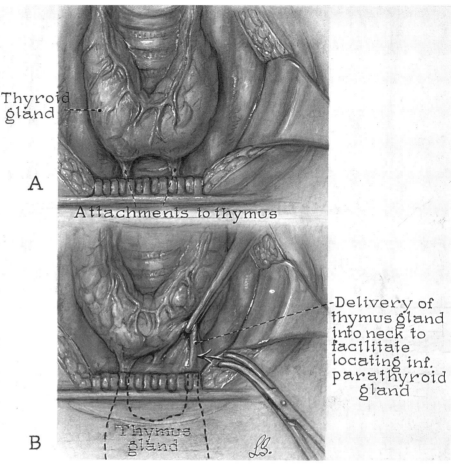

Fig. 37-7. The relationship of the thymus gland to the inferior thyroid poles of a normal gland are shown. The bilateral superior extensions of the thymus from the chest adhere to the inferior poles of the thyroid gland. The inferior parathyroid glands are almost always found within or closely adhered to this thyrothymic ligament.

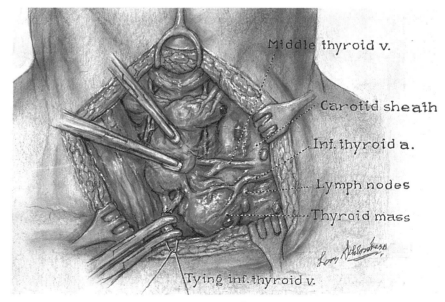

Fig. 37-8. The inferior thyroid vein is being ligated. Notice the position of the middle thyroid vein and the inferior thyroid artery.

rected to the superior pole vessels. This part of the procedure requires the adequate retraction of the strap muscles lateral to and above the upper pole of the thyroid lobe. Great care must be taken not to injure the external branch of the superior laryngeal nerve as these vessels are taken (Fig. 37-9). Because it is not always possible to visualize this nerve, the superior thyroid artery and vein should be separately ligated and divided. At this point, the pyramidal lobe extending superiorly from the thyroid gland can be dissected from surrounding tissues so that it can be removed with the thyroid lobe (Fig. 37-10). Once done, the adventitia around the upper pole is brushed away and the thyroid lobe can be further retracted medially, allowing adequate dissection and exposure of the recurrent laryngeal nerve as it nears the site of entry into the larynx. A filmy fibrous band (the ligament of Berry) covers the nerve at this point. One must exercise great care when dividing this structure to unroof the nerve (Fig. 37-11). At this point, the thyroid gland is free from its inferior and superior vascular attachments and not bound to the trachea at the point where the recurrent nerve enters the larynx. The gland is then dissected from the trachea with either a knife or electrocautery. The thyroid lobe can then be divided at the isthmus and either sent for frozen section examination, or if indicated, the surgeon can begin the dissection of the contralateral lobe.

The resected thyroid lobe is sent for frozen section examination. If the lesion is malignant a completion thyroidectomy should be performed in a manner similar to that described for the left lobectomy. If the frozen section shows that the resected tumor is benign, the opposite thyroid lobe is left intact.

During the course of the total thyroidectomy, it might be impossible to preserve the blood supply to one or more of the parathyroid glands. It is difficult to perform a total thyroidectomy and bilateral lymph node dissection for carcinoma and leave intact the blood supply to the parathyroid glands. During the course of a total thyroidectomy, every effort should be made to identify the parathyroid glands, and if their blood supply cannot be preserved, they should be resected and placed in iced saline. These glands are very hearty and will remain viable in this state for sev-

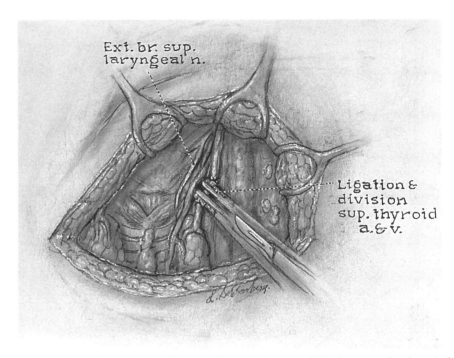

Fig. 37-9. Ligation of the superior thyroid artery. The vein is shown parallel to the artery. Also shown is the external branch of the superior laryngeal nerve. This structure is frequently not seen when the superior thyroid artery and vein are being ligated and divided.

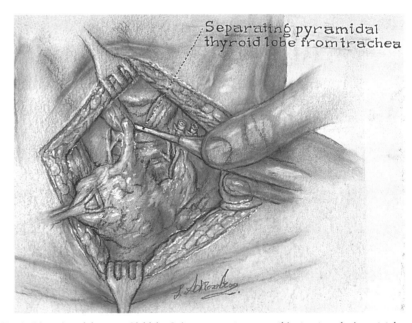

Fig. 37-10. Dissection of the pyramidal lobe. It is necessary to remove this structure during a total thyroidectomy. If left in the neck, it will frequently be evident on a radionuclide scan as residual thyroid tissue.

eral hours. If at the completion of the thyroidectomy, it has been necessary to remove all four glands, one or more of them should be autografted into a muscle bed, most often the sternocleidomastoid. This procedure will be described subsequently.

Modified Neck Dissection

In patients with a follicular carcinoma, the tumor rarely metastasizes to regional lymph nodes. Instead, the malignancy most often spreads through the blood-

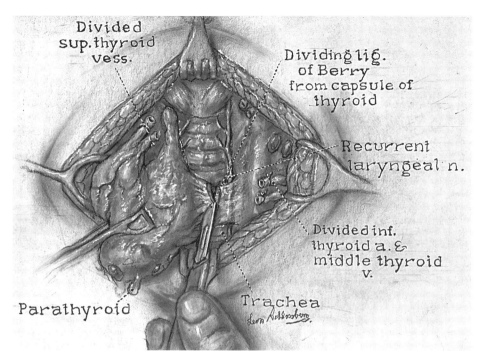

Fig. 37-11. Division of the ligament of Berry. (For the purposes of illustration, this structure is shown thicker than normal.) Notice the position of the recurrent laryngeal nerve. The inferior parathyroid gland will be removed and placed in iced saline.

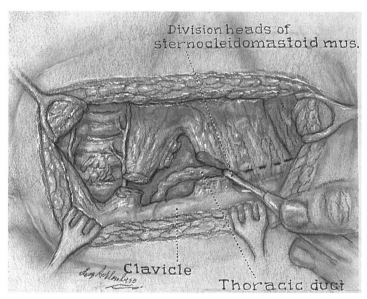

Fig. 37-12. Division of the sternal and clavicular heads of the sternocleidomastoid muscle.

stream to the lung and the bones. Therefore, it is unnecessary to perform a lymph node dissection in patients with a follicular carcinoma unless the nodes are enlarged and metastases are suspected. In patients with either papillary or medullary thyroid carcinoma, lymph node metastases are common, especially when the primary tumor is larger than 2 cm.

Metastases from these tumors are likely to remain confined to the neck region for long periods of time, and thus resection of the lymph nodes at the time of thyroidectomy for carcinoma might be curative. In our experience with medullary thyroid carcinoma, we have reoperated on patients with recurrent or persistent disease (as indicated by an elevated plasma calcitonin

level postoperatively) following total thyroidectomy. In some of these patients, the repeat neck exploration was performed several years after the primary operation. Approximately 30 percent of these patients can be cured by repeat neck exploration, as evidenced by normal plasma calcitonin levels following calcium and pentagastrin stimulation postoperatively. Our experience involves over 50 patients and has taught us three things: 1) metastases from medullary (and presumably papillary) thyroid carcinomas usually remain confined to the regional lymph node bed for a long period of time, 2) it is important to perform an adequate lymph node dissection at the time of total thyroidectomy in patients with primary tumors that are larger than 2 cm in diameter, and 3) repeat neck exploration with an extensive resection of regional lymph nodes is curative in a substantial number of patients.

The route of lymph node spread to a large degree depends on the location of the carcinoma within the thyroid lobe. For lesions located in the lateral or central portion of the lobe, the most common route of a metastasis is to the lymph nodes immediately adjacent to the thyroid gland. These nodes are situated close to the posterior surface and the inferior pole of the thyroid lobe. Some of these nodes follow the course of the recurrent laryngeal nerve and the inferior thyroid artery and vein. For carcinomas in the medial portion of the thyroid lobe or the isthmus, the most common route of spread is upward to the Delphian node and the lymphatic tissues along the pyramidal extension. If the malignancy is in the superior portion of the lobe, the tumor can spread to lymph nodes along the superior thyroid artery extending to its origin from the carotid artery. The metastases in these lymph nodes might be very small and not evident on gross examination. Some of these nodes might be unknowingly removed at the time of the total thyroidectomy. It is extremely uncommon for these thyroid carcinomas to metastasize to the lateral neck nodes without first spreading to the nodes immediately adjacent to the thyroid lobe.

During the total thyroidectomy, the lymph nodes adjacent to the lobe should be routinely removed. This removal requires additional tedious dissection along the recurrent laryngeal nerves, the inferior and superior thyroid arteries and veins, and the pyramidal lobe. On careful pathologic examination, one can expect to identify 10 to 20 lymph nodes in the resected tissue.

When the surgeon decides to perform a modified neck dissection, either because there is obvious lymph node involvement or because the primary tumor is large and microscopic nodes are suspected, it can be necessary to extend the incision laterally and superiorly. Other than extension of the incision, there is no disfigurement associated with the procedure. Specifically, it is unnecessary to sacrifice the sternocleidomastoid muscle, the internal jugular vein, or the eleventh nerve. As one extends the superior flap, care must be taken not to damage the mandibular marginal branch of the facial nerve, which can usually be identified as it crosses over the external maxillary artery and the anterior facial vein. This nerve innervates the lower lip and produces an unsightly droop if injured. The inferior flap is extended to expose the upper border of the clavicle.

At the beginning of this portion of the operation, the tendinous and muscular insertions of the sternocleidomastoid muscle into the sternum and the clavicle are divided (Fig. 37-12), and the muscle is reflected superiorly. Beginning at the superior-most extension of the field near the angle of the mandible, the lymph nodes and associated adventitia are swept inferiorly. The tissue can be removed with a combination of blunt and sharp dissection. During this portion of the procedure, it is necessary to divide the omohyoid muscle. With this exposure it is possible to remove all of the soft tissue anterior and adjacent to the carotid artery, the internal jugular vein, and the vagus nerve (Fig. 37-13). Additionally, lymph nodes and soft tissue in the anterior and the posterior triangles are removed. At the inferior portion of the field, the horn of the thymus gland, which protrudes into the neck, and the associated fatty tissue in and near the thoracic inlet are resected with care taken to preserve the recurrent laryngeal nerve and the blood supply to the inferior parathyroid gland if it has been left intact. It is unnecessary to divide the sternum and expose the mediastinum since the body of the thymus gland and associated soft tissues and lymph nodes are not removed. At the end of the dissection, the space between the vascular bundle in the lateral neck and the esophagus and trachea will be evident. In addition, the muscles bordering the ante-

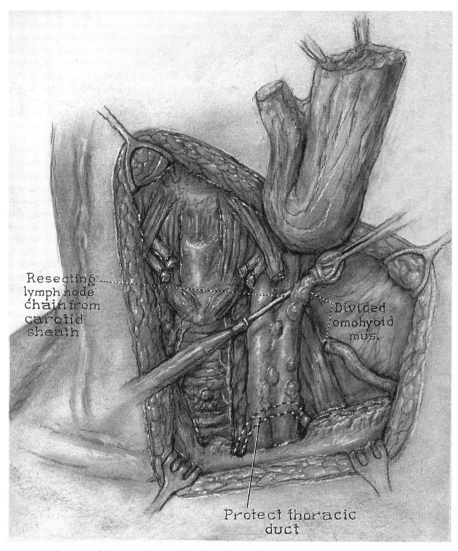

Fig. 37-13. *The sternocleidomastoid muscle has been dissected from its sternal and clavicular attachments and reflected superiorly. The lymph nodes are being dissected from the vascular sheath. The dotted line represents the course of the thoracic duct.*

rior and posterior triangles will be exposed.

In the course of removing the tissues low in the neck, care must be taken not to damage the thoracic duct on the left and the right lymphatic duct. Dissection on the left side is more problematic. The thoracic duct arises out of the thorax and extends above the left clavicle before inserting into the internal jugular vein at its junction with the subclavian vein. The duct has a very thin wall, is flat, and is not easily seen even by the experienced surgeon. Injury to this structure is usually evidenced by the presence of clear or whitish chyle in the operative field. If injury occurs, the duct should be identified and ligated or there

will be prolonged drainage of lymphatic fluid under the skin flaps in the postoperative period.

At the end of the procedure, the neck is thoroughly cleansed with large amounts of saline, and the wound is carefully checked to ensure that there are no bleeding points left uncontrolled. A suction drain is left in the lateral neck, and the sternocleidomastoid muscle is sutured to its sternal and clavicular origins. The strap muscles are then approximated in the midline.

If parathyroid glands are to be implanted, they are grafted at this point. The parathyroid glands are cleansed of all fat and then sliced into 1×3–mm pieces. These pieces are implanted into muscle pockets either in the sternocleidomastoid muscle or one of the strap muscles (Fig. 37-14). Three or four slivers of parathyroid tissue can be grafted into a single pocket, and the pocket is closed with a silk suture (Fig. 37-15). Immediately postoperatively it will be necessary to maintain patients on oral calcium and vitamin D tablets until the parathyroid grafts have developed a blood supply and begun to function. This takes approximately 6 to 8 weeks.

The neck is again cleansed with large amounts of sterile saline and after it is assured that there is no bleeding, the strap muscles are approximated with silk sutures (Fig. 37-16). The platysma is closed with interrupted sutures of an absorbable suture and then a subcuticular closure is done. The patient is sent to the recovery room with a sterile bandage in place. The postoperative period is characterized by a rapid convalescence. The patient can usually eat a regular diet on the first postoperative day and can be discharged on the second or third postoperative day. The most frequent complications that occur in the postoperative period are related to bleeding or hypoparathyroidism. It is important to make the house staff and the nursing staff aware of the possibility of postoperative bleeding. This bleeding usually results from the loosening of a vascular ligature or bleeding from an unsecured vessel that was temporarily clotted during the procedure but opened during coughing or straining postoperatively. This complication is characterized by the rapid accumulation of blood beneath the skin flaps. This situation is a surgical emergency and necessitates immediate return to the operating room with opening of the wound and control of the bleeding site. In some instances, the patient is in extremis and the neck incision must be opened at the bedside to prevent asphyxiation.

Patients should also be observed for signs and symptoms of hypoparathyroidism. The patient will rarely be symptomatic on the first postoperative day but thereafter might complain of tingling around the mouth and in the toes and fingers. Cramping of the muscles can occur, and carpal pedal spasms can develop. In examining patients in the postoperative period the surgeon should try to elicit a Chvostek sign (characterized by twitching of the facial muscles at the angle of the mouth when one taps on the zygomatic arch). Pa-

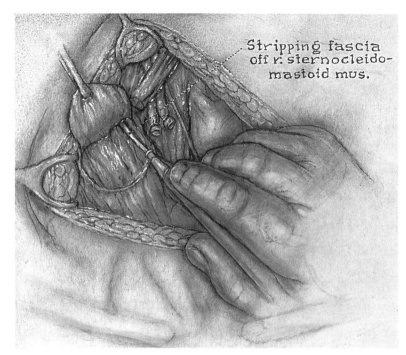

Fig. 37-14. The fascia of the right sternocleidomastoid muscle is being removed at the site of the muscle where the parathyroid tissue will be grafted.

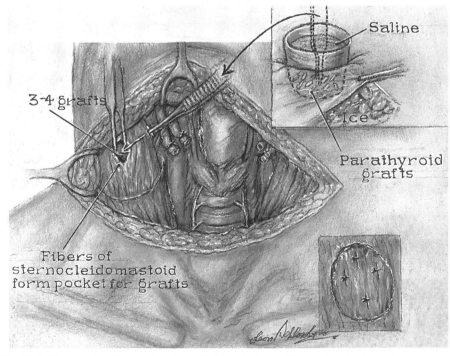

Fig. 37-15. The parathyroid glands have been sliced into 1×3–mm slivers and are implanted into the muscle. Since the parathyroid tissue is normal, three or four pieces can be grafted into a single pocket. If there was a likelihood that the parathyroid tissue would be hyperfunctional it would be grafted (as single slivers to a pocket) in the forearm. After the tissue is grafted, the pocket is closed with a black silk suture.

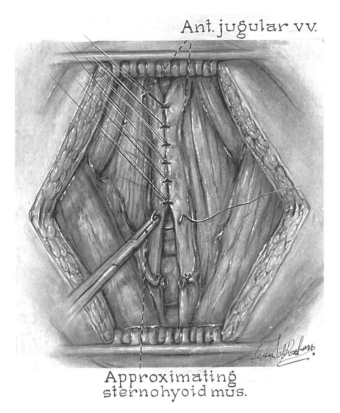

Ant. jugular vv.

Approximating
sternohyoid mus.

Fig. 37-16. The strap muscles are approximated in the midline before the platysma and the subcuticular layers are closed.

tients with a low blood calcium should be treated with calcium and vitamin D. If the blood calcium is below 7 mg per dl, and the patient is very symptomatic it can be necessary to administer the calcium intravenously.

Suggested Reading

Block MA, Horn RC, Brush BE. The place of total thyroidectomy in surgery for thyroid carcinoma. *Arch Surg* 81:236, 1960.

Favus MJ, Schneider AB, Stachura ME, et al. Thyroid malignancy occurring as a late consequence of head and neck irradiation: Evaluation of 1056 patients. *N Engl J Med* 294:1019, 1976.

Mazzaferri EL, Young RL. Papillary thyroid carcinoma: A ten-year follow-up report of the impact of therapy in 576 patients. *Am J Med* 70:511,

Schneider AB, Favus MJ, Stachura ME, et al. Incidence, prevalence and characteristics of radiation-induced thyroid tumors. *Am J Med* 64:243, 1978.

Thompson NW, Nishiyama RH, Harness JK. Thyroid carcinoma: Current controversies. *Curr Prob Surg* 25:1, 1978.

Tollefsen HR, DeCosse JJ. Papillary carcinoma of the thyroid. Recurrence in the thyroid gland after initial surgical treatment. *Am J Surg* 106:728, 1963.

Wells SA Jr, Baylin SB, Linehan WM, et al. Provocative agents and the diagnosis of medullary carcinoma of the thyroid gland. *Ann Surg* 188:139, 1978.

Wells SA Jr, Chi DD, Toshima K, et al. Predictive DNA testing and prophylactic thyroidectomy in patients at risk for multiple endocrine neoplasia type 2A. *Ann Surg* 220:237, 1994.

EDITOR'S COMMENT

Doctor Wells, an international authority in the treatment of thyroid cancer, has presented a concise description of his technique for total thyroidectomy. Any variations from an expert surgeon's technique in as standard an operation as total thyroidectomy should be a product of experience and the anatomy and pathology present in a given patient. All incisions will not necessarily be placed at precisely the same level in the neck. For example, the patient with a shorter, muscular neck would require an incision placed relatively close to the superior border of the medial end of the clavicle, whereas a longer, more slender neck would require a higher incision, generally at two finger breadths above the clavicular head.

The author has emphasized the importance of careful evaluation of the thyroid preoperatively and of discussion with the patient as to therapeutic options in the operating room, depending on frozen section findings. Of considerable importance is the point that even a very experienced surgical pathologist can have a great deal of difficulty distinguishing follicular adenoma from follicular carcinoma, unless the frozen section fortuitously includes a section with capsular invasion. The other clinical finding that is difficult to rely on is angioinvasion. Benign follicular tumors can show angioinvasion alone in a single vascular channel, and the lesion can still have a benign course. Since lymph node dissection (modified radical neck dissection) is rarely necessary for follicular carcinomas, our approach has been to do a bilateral total thyroidectomy for any patient in whom a follicular nodule is identified on frozen section, unless it is very small (<2 cm in diameter) and a total lobectomy and isthmusectomy might suffice. However, if there is any chance that the lesion can be follicular cancer, we prefer a bilateral total thyroidectomy to avoid having to reoperate to do a completion thyroidectomy. If the lesion proves to be malignant, the patient is subjected to another anesthetic, substantial emotional distress, and, if an undue delay is encountered, a somewhat difficult reentry into an operative field after several weeks.

The author doesn't cut the strap muscles routinely for total thyroidectomy, and it might not be necessary for most patients, especially patients who do not have heavy cervical musculature and in whom the thyroid lobes are normal in size or only slightly enlarged. However, in muscular individuals, we find that it is easier and contributes no undue morbidity to cut the strap muscles at the level of the cricoid cartilage, or higher. It is not desirable to cut these muscles at lower levels, since the hypoglossal nerve loops to the inferior area of the neck and then enters the strap muscles to innervate from below upward. Normally, these muscles are reapproximated at the end of the procedure to help restore the contour of the neck and to depress the hyoid bone and stabilize it during swallowing. The sternothyroid muscle holds the larynx down slightly during deglutition, aiding in complete closure of the epiglottis.

This operation is all about identifying and avoiding the recurrent laryngeal nerves, the superior laryngeal nerves (often not seen), and the parathyroid glands. The author accurately describes the palpation of the recurrent laryngeal nerve against the trachea, feeling it as a "thin, stringlike structure." The more experienced the thyroid surgeon, the better that individual is in palpating the recurrent nerve. In our experience, the nerve is palpable approximately two-thirds of the time, just as described. However, with large glands, especially if the nerve is adherent to the posterior capsule of the thyroid as is common in patients who have had thyroiditis in the past, it can be very difficult to palpate the recurrent nerve in its usual position. The author emphasizes a second important anatomic feature, which is the branching of the nerve within 2 cm of entry into the larynx. This branching can occur just before entry into the cricothyroid muscle, but occasionally occurs more proximal than that, even in the mid-portion of the neck behind the thyroid and just superior to or at the inferior thyroid artery. If the nerve appears very small, it is wise to look for a second branch, the most expeditious way being to follow the course of the nerve toward the mediastinum, separating soft tissue until one encounters a larger trunk. The second branch might appear at the Y. This anomaly is not common but can cause significant difficulty if unrecognized.

It is interesting to consider whether one should use cautery in performing thyroidectomy after the skin and platysma flaps are raised. Cautery is very helpful; I prefer sharp (scalpel) dissection for the midline separation from the thyroid cartilage to the sternal notch and for separation of the strap muscles from the pretracheal fascial investment of the thyroid lobes. Further dissection is almost invariably done with a moderately blunt hemostat or Mixter clamp, reserving the use of cautery for dissection of the gland after the recurrent nerve and parathyroids have been identified and are separated from the thyroid capsule. Bipolar cautery is a suitable instrument because it accurately contains the current between the tips of the cautery and prevents heat injury to the nerve or parathyroid blood supply. Doctor Wells' description of his technique for modified radical neck dissection is as complete a discussion as I have seen recently; it includes cutting the sternocleidomastoid muscle and reflecting it superiorly to clear the field of any impediment to the dissection. Obviously, the muscle is repaired at the end of the procedure, ordinarily with permanent (silk or synthetic) sutures, using care to include the tendinous portion of the muscle at the level of the sternum and the clavicle. However, many thyroid surgeons prefer to leave the muscle intact and retract it laterally to expose the field appropriately. Although I have rarely cut this muscle, I am persuaded by Dr. Wells' vast experience with various thyroid cancers that the performance of that step might afford not only superior exposure in the central portion of the neck but also especially in the upper reaches of the field of dissection, where the muscle does tend to cover the posterior cervical chain of nodes.

A rare, but memorable and truly frightening experience is major postoperative bleeding in the neck. Although we no longer routinely place such patients in the intensive care unit postoperatively, if there is serious concern about the possibility of postoperative bleeding and anything short of total confidence in the floor nursing staff, it can be worthwhile to do so for at least 18 hours postoperatively in order to allow immediate detection of respiratory distress, massive swelling of the neck, or both. As in most other operations, we seldom drain thyroidectomy wounds. Nevertheless, when in doubt, insert a closed suction drain, either the round or the flat (Hemovac or Jackson–Pratt).

The only death that I have ever had in a patient with thyroid surgery did not result from hemorrhage, but was in a patient who had a huge, long-standing colloid goiter. That patient was on a surgical floor, developed acute respiratory distress during the night, was seen by a house officer who started oxygen by face mask, but the patient expired 4 hours later. This event occurred years ago, before routine monitoring of oxygen saturation, at a minimum, in patients with large goiters that are resected. That patient died of tracheomalacia, a result of the pressure softening of the tracheal cartilages, caused by the impingement on the tracheal lumen by the large goiter. That patient's life would have been saved had an endotracheal tube been inserted, or an emergency tracheostomy been done. Many surgeons still order a tracheotomy set at the bedside for thyroidectomy patients, despite the fact that any complication that results from thyroidectomy, other than hemorrhage, is better treated by the immediate insertion of an endotracheal tube.

If the neck is massively swollen from hemorrhage, opening the incision, including the sutures used to reapproximate the strap muscles in the midline, will allow immediate decompression of the neck, and the patient's critical respiratory distress will be alleviated. Obviously, there is then the opportunity to revisit the operating room where the bleeding is stopped and the neck is loosely closed again.

R.J.B.

38

Parathyroidectomy for Primary Hyperparathyroidism (Adenoma and Carcinoma)

Jon A. van Heerden   Stephen L. Smith

The parathyroid glands were initially described by Sir Richard Owen in 1849. The "patient" was a Great Indian Rhinoceros (rhinoceros unicornis) undergoing an autopsy at the London Zoological Gardens. By 1909, serum calcium determinations had become a reality and the association between serum calcium levels and the parathyroid glands was established. Felix Mandl performed the first successful parathyroidectomy in 1925 in Vienna, Austria, and Oliver Cope performed the first parathyroid resection in the United States at the Massachusetts General Hospital the following year.

Primary hyperparathyroidism is a rare endocrine disorder caused by excessive secretion of parathyroid hormone by one or more of the parathyroid glands. Although the exact incidence of primary hyperparathyroidism is unknown, ranges from 28:100,000 in the United States to more than 200:100,000 in Scandinavia have been reported. With the extremely common use of automated biochemical screening, hyperparathyroidism is now recognized to be the most common cause of hypercalcemia in unselected, nonhospitalized patients and the most common cause of hypercalcemia in hospitalized patients.

Pathophysiology

Primary hyperparathyroidism is caused by excessive secretion of parathyroid hormone. Parathyroid hormone is a single-chain polypeptide consisting of 84 amino acids. The principal actions of parathyroid hormone include: 1) an increase in serum calcium and decrease in serum phosphorus levels, 2) an increase in bone osteoclast and osteoblast activity, 3) an increase in gastrointestinal absorption of calcium, 4) an increase in renal bicarbonate excretion, and 5) an increase in renal hydroxylation of 25-hydroxyvitamin D_3. The level of serum calcium in humans is under a sensitive feedback control mechanism. Hypercalcemia reduces parathyroid hormone secretion and the formation of 1,25-dihydroxyvitamin D_3 in normal individuals. Thus, a concomitant elevation of serum calcium concentration and parathyroid hormone level strongly suggests the diagnosis of primary hyperparathyroidism. We use the immunochemiluminescent technique for measurement of the entire intact parathyroid hormone molecule. This technique has essentially replaced the previous measurement of the end C and N terminals of the molecule. This whole molecule assay is highly specific, and approximately 90 percent of the patients with primary hyperparathyroidism have parathyroid hormone levels above the expected norms. The remaining 10 percent have inappropriately high parathyroid hormone levels based on their elevated calcium level, despite an absolute elevation in their parathyroid hormone assay. This concept of inappropriate parathyroid hormone secretion has important diagnostic implications and is a circumstance that can lead to a delay in diagnosis.

Diagnostic Workup

A minority of patients with primary hyperparathyroidism present with complaints specific enough to be considered symptomatic. Clinically, renal lithiasis (30%) and osteoporotic bone disease (15%) are the most common manifestations associated with complicated primary hyperparathyroidism. The diagnosis of primary hyperparathyroidism hinges on the demonstration of hypercalcemia with overproduction of parathyroid hormone and the exclusion of other possible causes of hypercalcemia.

The following is a suggested outline for an expeditious and cost-effective diagnostic work-up of hyperparathyroidism: 1) establish an elevated serum calcium level (if borderline, two or three determinations might be required), 2) rule out hypercalcemia related to medication (thiazides or lithium in particular) by taking a careful drug history, 3) order a chest x-ray to rule out other causes of hypercalcemia (bony metastases, pulmonary sarcoidosis, small cell lung carcinoma), 4) order an excretory urogram to rule out renal cell carcinoma and nephrolithiasis (the presence of hypercalcemia and nephrolithiasis is highly suggestive of hyperparathyroidism), 5) order serum protein electrophoresis to rule out multiple myeloma, 6) order a 24-hour urinary calcium determination to rule out benign familial hypocalciuric hypercalcemia (BFHH), 7) evaluate multiple endocri-

Table 38-1. Diagnostic Workup for Primary Hyperparathyroidism

1. Take a careful history (medications, symptoms, other endocrinopathies [patient and family], prior head or neck radiation therapy).
2. Establish elevated calcium (two or three determinations).
3. Order a chest x-ray (bony metastases, sarcoidosis, pulmonary tumors).
4. Order an excretory urogram (nephrolithiasis, renal tumors).
5. Order a serum protein electrophoresis (multiple myeloma).
6. Order a 24-hour urinary calcium (BFHH [hypocalciuria] or hypercalciuria).
7. Rule out MEN (usually MEN-I).
8. Check the parathyroid hormone level (absolute or relative elevation).

nopathy histories in the patient and the family to rule out multiple endocrine neoplasia (MEN) syndromes, and 8) check the parathyroid hormone level (this should be elevated or inappropriately elevated [in the physiologic situation, hypercalcemia renders parathyroid hormone levels undetectable] (Table 38-1).

Indications for Operation

It is our current philosophy that the diagnosis of primary hyperparathyroidism is, in fact, an indication for operative therapy unless undue risk factors that can prohibit general anesthesia are present. There are several reasons for this seemingly dogmatic position:

1. There is currently no effective long-term medical therapy for primary hyperparathyroidism.
2. Truly "asymptomatic" primary hyperparathyroidism probably does not exist. A minority of patients present with the well-recognized complications of renal lithiasis and bone disease. However, there is evidence that even mild hypercalcemia can influence mentation, mood, and muscle strength profoundly in a significant percentage of patients, particularly in the elderly population.
3. Operative intervention by an experienced endocrine surgeon results in a cure rate of over 99 percent with minimal morbidity and mortality.

Operative Goals

There are several operative goals:

1. To achieve a normocalcemic state.
2. To avoid injury to the laryngeal nerves (recurrent and superior).
3. To produce a cosmetically acceptable (to the patient) incision.
4. To engender minimal postoperative morbidity and negligible mortality.

Embryology, Anatomy, and Pathology

A thorough understanding of the embryology of the parathyroid glands is crucial for surgeons involved in the treatment of primary hyperparathyroidism. The inferior parathyroid glands arise from the third branchial pouch in conjunction with the thymus. They can be found anywhere from the base of the skull to the anterior mediastinum and are invariably associated with, or embedded within, thymic tissue when found in undescended or hyperdescended sites. The superior parathyroid glands arise from the fourth branchial pouch in conjunction with the thyroid gland. Normal superior glands descend minimally and remain closely associated with the posterior aspect of the superior pole of each thyroid lobe. Enlarged superior parathyroid glands tend to descend in the tracheoesophageal groove and can be found inferior to the inferior parathyroid glands. Occasionally, the superior parathyroid glands hyperdescend in a posterior plane to the aorticopulmonary window in the posterior mediastinum. The superior parathyroid glands tend to be in a more posterior plane than the inferior parathyroid glands.

The normal parathyroid gland measures $5 \times 3 \times 2$ mm and weighs between 50 and 60 mg. The majority of the blood supply for both the superior and inferior parathyroid glands comes from branches of the inferior thyroid artery. Histologic differentiation between a normal parathyroid gland and a hyperplastic gland and a parathyroid adenoma can be extremely difficult, particularly if the pathologist has to rely on small biopsies only. Therefore, the differentiation between normal and abnormal parathyroid glands essentially remains the surgeon's responsibility based

on the operative findings and is aided by intraoperative dialogue with an experienced endocrine pathologist.

The pathology encountered in patients with primary hyperparathyroidism in most reported series is 1) single adenoma (88%), 2) multiple adenomas (3%), 3) multiglandular hyperplasia (8%), and 4) parathyroid carcinoma (<1%).

In approximately 3 percent of patients, primary hyperparathyroidism is a manifestation of MEN. Thus, every patient with primary hyperparathyroidism should have a careful family history taken to search for a history of other endocrinopathies. In patients with MEN (usually MEN-I), 75 to 85 percent have multiglandular hyperplasia. In the MEN setting, the incidence of five parathyroid glands is quite high (10%); therefore, routine transcervical thymectomy is recommended even when all four glands are verified in the neck. Our surgical strategy in these patients is that of subtotal parathyroidectomy without parathyroid transplantation, leaving 50 to 80 mg of clearly viable parathyroid tissue in the neck. Hyperparathyroidism is common in patients with MEN-I (90%) and uncommon in patients with MEN-II (<5%).

Operative Therapy
Preoperative Localization

There is good evidence to support the philosophy that the patient undergoing first-time cervical exploration for primary hyperparathyroidism does not require any preoperative localization studies; this finding has been confirmed by a number of prospective, randomized studies. An experienced endocrine surgeon continues to be the most accurate and cost-effective locator of parathyroid abnormalities. Current indications for preoperative localization do exist and include: 1) the patient undergoing *reoperative* cervical exploration, 2) the patient with an acute hypercalcemic crisis, and 3) a poor-risk patient with biochemically proven hyperparathyroidism. The localizing modality of choice today is small-part (7.5 mHz) real-time ultrasound, which has an accuracy rate of 75 to 80 percent.

Patient Preparation

The patient undergoing cervical exploration for primary hyperparathyroidism should always have a secure biochemical diagnosis of hyperparathyroidism; the surgeon should never operate to make the diagnosis. Additional information required preoperatively includes evaluation to ensure the safety of general anesthesia (operative risk) and vocal cord assessment in selected patients. A thorough discussion regarding the procedure and its potential complications is carried out with the patient preoperatively.

The patient should be in the supine position on the operating room table. After general anesthesia is delivered, the patient's arms (with attention to the pressure points) are tucked to the patient's side, the neck is comfortably extended, and the head stabilized with two sandbags or a foam donut. Routine skin preparation is carried out, and draping is conducted (Fig. 38-1) using a thyroid drape. The table is placed in the reverse Trendelenburg position at a comfortable height for the operating surgeon, and lights are positioned optimally. A magnetic pad is placed on the patient's chest, which is helpful particularly with the patient in the head-up position and aids in preventing instrument slippage.

Incision

To ensure a symmetric and cosmetic incision, it is important to make sure that the patient's chin, suprasternal notch, and center of the thyroid cartilage are aligned. A collar incision is made approximately 1 ½ to 2 finger breadths above the suprasternal notch. If a skin crease should be present either slightly higher or lower than this point, it should be used. A suture can be used as a marker to ensure symmetry of this incision. The length of the incision varies with individual preference but usually need not be more than 6 cm in length. The incision is carried down to the platysma muscle. This muscle is approximately 2-mm thick in most cases and can be divided in a relatively bloodless manner with electrocautery. An avascular plane exists immediately deep to this muscle and can be readily developed. Once this plane has been identified, a superior flap is created with a combination of electrocautery and blunt or sharp dissection (Fig. 38-2). The superior extent of this dissection is to the level of the thyroid cartilage. An inferior subplatysmal flap is then created and does not need to extend more than 2 cm inferior to the incision. If bleeding ensues during

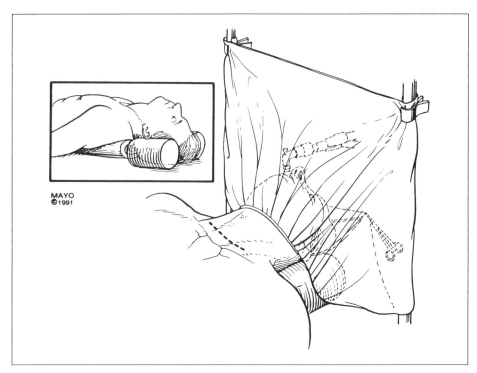

Fig. 38-1. Position of patient on operating room table with drape. (From CS Grant, JA van Heerden. Technical Aspects of Thyroidectomy. In JH Donohue, JA van Heerden, JRT Monson (eds.), Atlas of Surgical Oncology. Cambridge: Blackwell, 1995. Reproduced with permission from the Mayo Foundation.)

this phase of the procedure, the dissection is either too superficial or too deep. If dissection is too deep, injury to the external jugular and anterior jugular veins can occur.

Once the superior and inferior subplatysmal flaps are created, a self-retaining retractor is placed. The midline is usually readily identified, and the avascular fascial plane is divided using electrocautery. This dissection is carried down until the thyroid isthmus is identified (Fig. 38-3). Occasionally, small veins will be identified crossing the midline; these should be individually isolated, ligated, and divided. Once the thyroid isthmus has been identified, the side to be explored first is exposed. Medial traction is then exerted on the thyroid lobe to be exposed manually using a 4×4 sponge. The strap muscles are elevated and retracted laterally using two goiter retractors, and the avascular plane between the posterior aspect of the strap muscles and anterior aspect of the thyroid lobe is developed (Fig. 38-4). Once the edge of the thyroid lobe is reached, two Kocher clamps can be placed to facilitate anterior elevation and medial rotation of that thyroid lobe. This maneuver brings the middle thyroid vein into view, and the

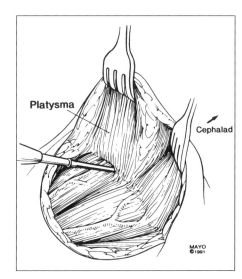

Fig. 38-2. Creating subplatysmal flaps. (From CS Grant, JA van Heerden. Technical Aspects of Thyroidectomy. In JH Donohue, JA van Heerden, JRT Monson (eds.), Atlas of Surgical Oncology. Cambridge: Blackwell, 1995. Reproduced with permission from the Mayo Foundation.)

carotid sheath is visualized posteriorly. The middle thyroid vein should be isolated, ligated, and divided. The importance of maintaining a bloodless field cannot be overemphasized. Blood staining of

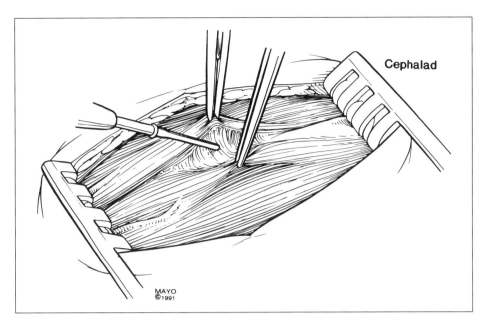

Fig. 38-3. *Dividing strap muscles in midline. (From CS Grant, JA van Heerden. Technical Aspects of Thyroidectomy. In JH Donohue, JA van Heerden, JRT Monson (eds.),* Atlas of Surgical Oncology. *Cambridge: Blackwell, 1995. Reproduced with permission from the Mayo Foundation.)*

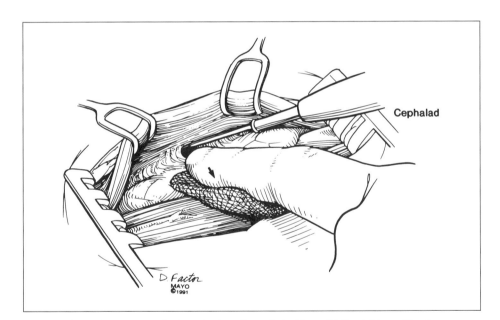

Fig. 38-4. *Separating strap muscles from the thyroid anteriorly. (From CS Grant, JA van Heerden. Technical Aspects of Thyroidectomy. In JH Donohue, JA van Heerden, JRT Monson (eds.),* Atlas of Surgical Oncology. *Cambridge: Blackwell, 1995. Reproduced with permission from the Mayo Foundation.)*

the tissues lateral to the thyroid lobe can make identification of the parathyroid glands (small normal glands, in particular) much more difficult. The operating surgeon should be traditionally positioned on the ipsilateral side of the exploration. Dissection of the tissues lateral to the thyroid lobe is greatly facilitated by medial pressure and elevated of that lobe by the sur-

geon's nondominant thumb (Fig. 38-5). Using this medial pressure on the thyroid and continued lateral traction on the strap muscles with the goiter retractors, the tissues posterior to the thyroid are now carefully inspected before any further dissection (Fig. 38-6). Obviously, surgical experience is crucial and allows the surgeon to notice any abnormalities in the

normal appearance of the tissues in this area. After careful inspection and before dissection, gentle palpation of the tissues should be undertaken. If inspection and palpation fail to reveal any areas suspicious for parathyroid pathology, then careful, meticulous, bloodless dissection is performed. A thorough understanding of the embryology and anatomic relationships and variations is crucial. Dissection can be accomplished using fine vascular forceps.

Attempts should be made in all patients to identify all four parathyroid glands. The majority of glands are oval or kidney-shaped, but can be elongated, bilobed, or flattened. The color of the normal parathyroid gland is slightly darker than the color of the adjacent fat and has been described as looking like the tongue of a jaundiced hummingbird. Adenomatous glands accurately resemble a mini-kidney, both in configuration and color. Hyperplastic glands are more yellow than the typical reddish kidney color of an adenoma. We do not recommend routine biopsy of obviously normal parathyroid glands. After an adenoma is identified, it is gently teased from the surrounding fibrofatty tissues. Care is taken to delineate the adenoma's relationship to the recurrent laryngeal nerve and preserve this structure uninjured throughout the dissection. After complete mobilization, the adenoma's vascular pedicle is ligated or clipped. We recommend routine contralateral exploration despite suggestions that unilateral, ultrasound-guided cervical exploration can be acceptable. This philosophy is based on the following: 1) multiple adenomas occur in approximately 3 percent of patients, 2) contralateral cervical exploration can be performed quickly and safely, and 3) preoperative ultrasound is truly positive in only approximately 75 to 80 percent of patients and cannot visualize any glands in the midline (tracheoesophageal groove) or behind bony structures.

Once the location of parathyroid glands has been accomplished on one side of the neck, attention should be directed to the same anatomic position when exploring the contralateral side, since mirror imaging of the parathyroid glands is a very constant finding in parathyroid surgery (symmetric parathyroid descent). Once an adenoma has been excised, the aim of contralateral exploration is to rule out a second adenoma (occurring in <2% of pa-

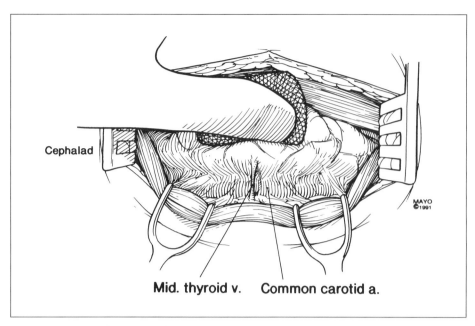

Fig. 38-5. *Retracting the strap muscle laterally and thyroid medially with left thumb. (From CS Grant, JA van Heerden. Technical Aspects of Thyroidectomy. In JH Donohue, JA van Heerden, JRT Monson (eds.), Atlas of Surgical Oncology. Cambridge: Blackwell, 1995. Reproduced with permission from the Mayo Foundation.)*

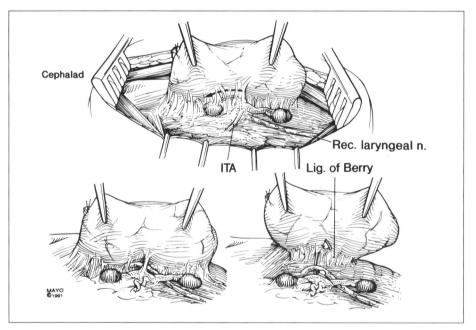

Fig. 38-6. *Normal lateral view of anatomy after taking the middle thyroid vein. (From CS Grant, JA van Heerden. Technical Aspects of Thyroidectomy. In JH Donohue, JA van Heerden, JRT Monson (eds.), Atlas of Surgical Oncology. Cambridge: Blackwell, 1995. Reproduced with permission from the Mayo Foundation.)*

tients) and not necessarily to find normal parathyroid glands. This exploration should be done expeditiously. If, on exploration, a superior parathyroid gland cannot be identified, the tracheoesophageal groove should be explored digitally by entering it in the space immediately superior to the inferior thyroid artery. This superior gland, descending in the tracheoesophageal groove, can easily be palpated between the surgeon's thumb and forefinger by gentle palpation (Fig. 38-7). It is often *inferior* to the inferior parathyroid gland, although in a more posterior plane. The inferior parathyroid gland is, in most instances, closely related to the inferior pole of the thyroid gland where it can be in the thyrothymic tongue of fatty tissue or beneath the thyroid capsule. This latter position can erroneously be interpreted as an intrathyroid parathyroid gland by the inexperienced surgeon. Access to parathyroid pathology is virtually always attainable with this approach. Transcervical thymectomy, when required in search of a hyperdescended inferior parathyroid or supernumerary gland, is almost always possible through a cervical incision by using gentle traction and blunt mobilization. It is important to stress that the search for ectopic parathyroid glands is guided by a thorough knowledge of the embryology. Ectopic parathyroid glands can "hide" in several locations (Fig. 38-8).

Treatment for parathyroid hyperplasia, as opposed to adenoma, is by excision of all but 80 to 100 mg of clearly viable, well-vascularized parathyroid tissue, which, in most cases, requires 3.5 gland resection. The gland selected to be partially resected should be dealt with first after visualization of all parathyroid glands. The gland chosen is often the smallest gland—clear viability is mandatory before proceeding with further resection of parathyroid tissue. An alternative to this course of therapy has been proposed by colleagues in Sweden who have advocated total parathyroidectomy with immediate forearm implantation of 60 to 70 mg of parathyroid tissue.

In the rare event when there is concern regarding completeness of operative therapy for primary hyperparathyroidism, a new tool is available. Intraoperative monitoring of parathyroid hormone is available through the use of a reliable 15-minute immunochemiluminescent assay. Preliminary study has shown encouraging results, and we believe that intraoperative parathyroid hormone "rapid" assay will become useful and popular in assisting surgeons and in dealing with both parathyroid and thyroid disease in the future, particularly in reoperative parathyroid surgery.

After completion of cervical exploration with parathyroidectomy as indicated, the

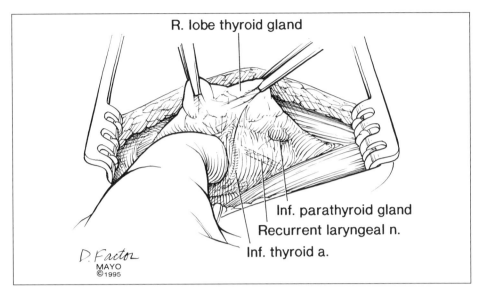

Fig. 38-7. *Digital exploration of the tracheoesophageal groove.*

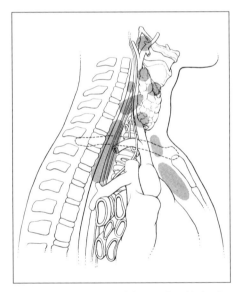

Fig. 38-8. *"Hiding places" for parathyroid glands.*

incision is closed. The deep cervical fascia should be reapproximated in the midline with a minimum number of sutures, avoiding incorporation of any of the adjacent strap muscles. If the procedure is not performed in this manner, the patient might experience a sticking sensation postoperatively when swallowing. The closure can be accomplished with absorbable sutures and should not be watertight, allowing any deep-seated hematomas to decompress into the superficial subcutaneous tissues where respiratory compromise would be less likely. There is no need for cervical drainage in the majority of parathyroid explorations. The platysma muscle

is reapproximated next with a minimal amount of absorbable sutures. Skin closure can be performed with absorbable subcuticular running suture, which need not be removed. A small occlusive dressing is applied and removed the morning after surgery, at which time the patient may bathe.

Parathyroid Reexploration

Reexploration for either persistent or recurrent hypercalcemia following initial cervical exploration for primary hyperparathyroidism should be rare. A recent review of our experience showed that in patients requiring reexploration, 75 percent required cervical exploration only, 19 percent required cervical and mediastinal exploration, and 6 percent required mediastinal exploration only with cure of hypercalcemia achieved in 90 percent of patients (±9% less than in primary exploration). The vast majority of reoperative surgery for primary hyperparathyroidism revealed single gland disease. There was not mortality among the 224 patients reviewed undergoing cervical reexploration. Hypoparathyroidism was evident in 15 percent and permanent recurrent laryngeal nerve paralysis occurred in 3.5 percent of patients.

If reexploration can be scheduled within 7 days of the initial operation, the inflammatory response will not preclude a safe operation. However, in patients who underwent cervical exploration more than 7 days before presentation, a period of 3 to 6 months should elapse before consideration of reexploration, if the clinical situation allows, to allow safe dissection and reduce the operative morbidity. Cervical exploration, as previously described, affords the advantage of a familiar approach. However, if there is significant scarring and if the scarring is severe, a lateral approach might be considered, dissecting between the strap muscles and the sternocleidmastoid muscle and resecting the omohyoid muscle if necessary. This approach often allows easy access to the posterior aspect of the thyroid and tracheoesophageal groove, which facilitates the approach to the superior parathyroid glands. To expose the area of the inferior glands and thymus using this method, the strap muscles must either be dissected or transected. In contrast to the primary situation, preoperative localization is of prime importance. The most useful localizing modalities in our practice are small-part ultrasound (for cervical disease) and sestamibi radionuclide scanning (for mediastinal disease). Computed tomography, MRI, and venous sampling are used, although rarely. Our experience with venous sampling techniques for detection of parathyroid disease has led us to essentially abandon this invasive procedure over the past 15 years.

It should be noted that true intrathyroidal parathyroid glands are extremely rare. It is far more common to find a parathyroid gland located beneath the "pseudocapsule" of scarring that envelops the thyroid gland after the initial operation. Prior resection of the thyroid gland at the time of the initial operation increases the risk of reoperation by removing the "protection" of the recurrent laryngeal nerve and carotid sheath structures by the thyroid lobe. The search for the unidentified inferior parathyroid gland can require resection of the thymus. Gentle but firm traction on the cervical thymus plus finger dissection along the thymus into the mediastinum retrieves a considerable portion of the gland; rarely the tip of the thymus extends into the carotid sheath concealing an ectopic parathyroid gland. Additionally, the "undescended parathymus" may be identified and can contain the associated inferior parathyroid gland. The inferior gland is thus *superior* to the superior parathyroid gland. This inferior gland is identified by dissecting anterior to the carotid artery to the level of its bifurcation and using bimanual palpation. Mediastinal exploration, as discussed, is seldom required (<2%). Once assured that the missing parathyroid gland is not in the neck, the surgeon can choose to proceed with mediastinal exploration using either a partial or full-length median sternotomy. If the gland can be identified, it is excised. If not, complete removal of the mediastinal thymus is carried out with careful pathologic sectioning. Resection should proceed to the great vessels arising from the aortic arch, which is the second most common location for mediastinal glands. Rarely middle mediastinal glands are located behind the aortic arch, between it and the pulmonary artery anterior to the trachea (aorticopulmonary window).

There are other surgical approaches to mediastinal parathyroid adenomas: thoracoscopy or limited anterior thoracotomy by resection of the costochondral junction (Chamberlin procedure). We and others have had limited experience with these evolving approaches, but thus far these alternatives seem most promising.

Parathyroid Carcinoma

Parathyroid carcinoma is excessively rare, occurring in approximately 1 percent of patients with hyperparathyroidism and has several distinguishing features. The most important of these features, which separate it from benign hyperparathyroidism, include:

1. Marked hypercalcemia. The mean serum calcium in this group of patients is usually approximately 14.5 mg per dL. Any patient with a serum calcium greater than 15.0 mg per dL should be suspected of having parathyroid carcinoma until disproved.
2. Marked elevations of parathyroid hormone levels. In our experience, the parathyroid hormone level is usually elevated tenfold above the upper limit of normal; levels that are seldom seen in patients with either adenoma or hyperplasia.
3. A high percentage of nephrolithiasis (56% of patients) and severe bone disease (91% of patients).

4. Palpable neck mass. In contrast to primary hyperparathyroidism secondary to adenoma or hyperplasia where a neck mass is palpable in less than 1 percent of patients, 50 percent of patients with parathyroid carcinoma might have a palpable cervical mass.
5. Invasive features. Parathyroid carcinoma appears "stuck" to surrounding tissues and is grayish white and firm, which is significantly different from the characteristics of benign hyperparathyroidism (adenoma or hyperplasia).
6. Recurrence of hypercalcemia soon after surgical treatment of hyperparathyroidism should raise the suspicion of malignancy and possible regional or distant metastasis.
7. Histologic criteria suggestive of malignancy. In contrast to benign disease, microscopic sectioning of parathyroid carcinoma reveals capsular and vascular invasion, cellular mitosis, thick fibrous bands separating lobules of the tumor, and trabecular growth pattern.

Treatment of patients with parathyroid carcinoma requires en bloc resection of the malignancy with the overlying musculature and adjacent thyroid gland. Lymph node metastases are present in 30 percent of patients, and, therefore, a prophylactic modified neck dissection is indicated in all patients. Locally recurrent disease as well as seemingly localized distant disease (lung and bone) are best treated surgically. Both radiation therapy and chemotherapy have been of minimal benefit. Three-year survival for patients with parathyroid carcinoma is 85 percent, with a 5-year survival of 60 percent in our most recent review. Sixty percent of these patients required more than one operation for recurrent disease.

Surgical Results in the Treatment of Primary Hyperparathyroidism

In our most recent 2-year review (1983–1984) of our experience, all four parathyroid glands were visualized in 44 percent of patients. Single adenomas were encountered in 88 percent of the patients, multiple adenomata in 3 percent and hyperplasia in 8 percent overall. Permanent hypocalcemia occurred in 0.3 percent and permanent recurrent laryngeal nerve palsy in 0.8 per-

cent of patients. One of 379 consecutive patients died in the immediately postoperative period from an acute myocardial infarction for an overall operative mortality of 0.3 percent. Initial operation cured 98.6 percent of these patients. Of the five patients not initially cured, three were reoperated on within days of the initial operation and cured for an overall cure rate of 99.5 percent.

Parathyroid "Pearls"

We believe it is essential for the endocrine surgeon to remember the following:

1. A patient can have primary hyperparathyroidism despite a "normal" parathyroid hormone level. "Normal" is inappropriately high if the calcium level is elevated.
2. The diagnosis of primary hyperparathyroidism is an indication for operative therapy.
3. An experienced endocrine surgeon is the best and only necessary localizing tool for a patient undergoing first-time cervical exploration for primary hyperparathyroidism.
4. Knowing parathyroid embryology is the key to surgical success.
5. Maintain a bloodless operative field.
6. After gaining adequate lateral exposure, first look for abnormalities, then palpate for abnormalities, and finally begin meticulous dissection.
7. Attempt to identify all four glands, but do not spend excessive (?wasted) time once an adenoma has been identified and removed.
8. Primary hyperparathyroidism can be diagnosed with a very high degree of accuracy, and once recognized, can be treated by the experienced endocrine surgeon with an extremely high rate of cure and very low morbidity and mortality.

Suggested Reading

Carlson GL, Farndon JR, Clayton B, Rose PG. Thallium isotope schintigraphy and ultrasonography: Comparative studies of localization techniques in primary hyperparathyroidism. *Br J Surg* 77:327, 1990.

Clark OH (ed). *Endocrine Surgery of the Thyroid and Parathyroid Gland*. St. Louis, MO: Mosby, 1985.

Grant CS, et al. Clinical management of persistent and/or recurrent primary hyperparathyroidism. *World J Surg* 10:555, 1986.

Grant CS, Weaver A. Treatment of primary parathyroid hyperplasia: Representative experience at Mayo Clinic. *Acta Chir Aust* 26(Suppl.):112, 1994.

Heath H III, Hodgson SF, Kennedy MA. Primary hyperparathyroidism: Incidence, morbidity, and potential economic impact in the community. *N Engl J Med* 302:189, 1980.

Herrera M, Grant CS, van Heerden JA, Fitzpatrick LA. Parathyroid autotransplantation. *Arch Surg* 172:825, 1992.

Kao PC, van Heerden JA, Taylor RL. Intraoperative monitoring of parathyroid procedures by a 15-minute parathyroid hormone immunochemiluminometric assay. *Mayo Clin Proc* 69:432, 1994.

Malmaeus J, et al. Parathyroid surgery in the multiple endocrine neoplasia type 1 syndrome: Choice of surgical procedure. *World J Surg* 10:668, 1986.

O'Riordain DS, et al. Surgical management of primary hyperparathyroidism in multiple endocrine neoplasia types 1 and 2. *Surgery* 114:1031, 1993.

Prinz RA, et al. Thoracoscopic excision of enlarged mediastinal parathyroid glands. *Surgery* 116:999, 1994.

Thompson GB, et al. Parathyroid imaging with technetium-99m-sestamibi: An initial institutional experience. *Surgery* 116:966, 1994.

van Heerden JA, Grant CS. Surgical treatment or primary hyperparathyroidism: An institutional perspective. *World J Surg* 15:688, 1991.

Wynne AG, van Heerden J, Carney JA, Fitzpatrick LA. Parathyroid carcinoma: Clinical and pathologic features in 43 patients. *Medicine* 71:197, 1992.

EDITOR'S COMMENT

The incidence with which primary hyperparathyroidism is encountered is in part a function of the frequency with which routine serum calciums are measured. Although frequently when patients are questioned closely about feelings of lethargy, lack of energy, or episodes of weakness they may give a positive history, these symptoms are often not investigated in the usual primary care practice. The absolute incidence has been reported to be as high as 1:700 or as low as 1:3500 by these authors, so a busy surgeon with an interest in endocrine surgery should encounter several patients annually. This chapter has a wealth of valuable information, but should be coupled with Chapter 35, Dr. Grant's introductory chapter on anatomy of the parathyroid glands, in which he describes a very important topic: embryology of the parathyroid glands. When these glands are in the typical position, operative exposure is not demanding, and appropriate definitive treatment is a straightforward matter. However, one of the most frustrating experiences that any surgeon can have is to explore the neck in a patient with chemically demonstrated hyperparathyroidism, only to find one, or often two, glands that are not readily discernible and extending the search in the usual places without finding one or two of the glands. Knowledge of the embryology is essential to direct the surgeon to appropriate places to look for these missing glands.

Competent surgeons should cure primary hyperparathyroidism in at least 95 percent of instances at the first operation. Whether high-resolution real-time ultrasound should be used preoperatively has been addressed by the authors, but many surgeons are more comfortable with performance of the test. Obviously, both ultrasound and sestamibi scanning should be used when the operation has failed to uncover the lesion and reoperation will undoubtedly be required. Arteriography has become obsolete for work-up with the reoperative management of persistent hypercalcemia, although venography continues to be used in some centers coupled with parathormone assay at appropriate levels. Interestingly, there are several roentgenographic reports of ablation of a functioning mediastinal adenoma by injection of a bolus of angiographic dye when the lesion has been definitely identified, destroying the ectopic mediastinal adenoma. This situation obviously would spare the patient a median sternotomy and mediastinal exploration, and if the lesion can be definitely identified, would perhaps be worth that approach, especially in elderly patients.

Intraoperative ultrasound in the reoperative setting is an attractive alternative to mechanical exploration alone; this ultrasound is done with a 5- or 7.5-mHz probe and can be quite specific for intrathyroidal parathyroid adenoma if such a lesion truly exists. This test has great appeal, but does require an individual with considerable experience in ultrasound, which few surgeons have at this point. A radiologist with a special interest in ultrasound, assuming a willingness to come to the operating room, would be a very helpful consultant, and the test might disclose the site of the ectopic lesion.

The clinical causes of hypercalcemia that have nothing to do with hyperparathyroidism should be considered in all patients before exploration. These causes include:

Chlorothiazide therapy

Metastatic malignant disease

Oat cell carcinoma of the lung

Sarcoidosis

Hypernephroma

Multiple myeloma

Paraneoplastic syndrome

Benign familial hypocalciuric hypercalcemia

Metastatic malignant disease to bone, most importantly carcinoma of the breast, lung, and occasionally of the prostate, should always be ruled out.

R.J.B.

39

Parathyroidectomy for Hyperplasia and Secondary Hyperparathyroidism

Jeffrey A. Norton

Primary Hyperparathyroidism

Primary hyperparathyroidism is a primary abnormality of the parathyroid gland(s) associated with excessive parathyroid hormone secretion, elevated serum and urinary levels of calcium, and decreased bony levels of calcium.

Primary hyperparathyroidism is diagnosed by elevated serum levels of calcium and concomitant elevated serum levels of parathyroid hormone. The current widespread availability of excellent immunologic assays for measurement of intact parathyroid hormone has greatly simplified the diagnosis of primary hyperparathyroidism. If the patient has elevated serum levels of calcium and intact parathyroid hormone, the diagnosis of primary hyperparathyroidism can be quickly ascertained. Twenty-four–hour urinary calcium excretion can be measured in select individuals to exclude familial hypocalciuric hypercalcemia.

For a great majority of patients with primary hyperparathyroidism, a parathyroid adenoma is the cause of the primary hyperparathyroidism (85%). Most experts now believe that approximately 1 to 3 percent of patients have multiple adenomas, and these can be treated by simply removing the two abnormal parathyroid glands. Except for the minority of patients with parathyroid carcinoma, 1 percent or less of patients with primary hyperparathyroid-

ism, the remainder (13–15%), parathyroid hyperplasia is the cause of the primary hyperparathyroidism.

Parathyroid hyperplasia can occur as a sporadic disease, usually in elderly females, associated with marked enlargement of all the parathyroid glands. Parathyroid hyperplasia can also occur as a familial disease, usually in younger individuals with one of two multiple endocrine neoplasias (MEN types IIA and I). The genetic defect in patients with MEN IIA has been recognized recently as missense mutations in the RET proto-oncogene, which is in the pericentrimeric region of chromosome 10. The exact genetic abnormality in patients with MEN I has not been clearly determined. However, recent studies have carefully mapped the genetic defect to the long arm of chromosome 11. The differentiation of type of parathyroid hyperplasia from the sporadic type to the familial type is important for the surgeon. The familial form has a high probability of recurrent disease (30–80% in some series) and needs a more aggressive operative procedure than the sporadic form of parathyroid hyperplasia. A 3½ gland parathyroidectomy is recommended for individuals with the sporadic form of parathyroid hyperplasia, whereas total parathyroidectomy, thymectomy, and parathyroid transplantation to the forearm is recommended for individuals with the familial form.

Another familial form of parathyroid disease that must be excluded is familial hypocalciuric hypercalcemia (FHH). Individ-

uals with FHH have elevated serum levels of calcium and parathyroid hormone but no symptoms related to primary hyperparathyroidism. These individuals have marked hypocalciuria. The 24-hour urinary calcium excretion is less than 3 mEq per 24 hours. The genetic defect in patients with FHH has been mapped to the long arm of chromosome 3. It appears to be related to the cellular calcium "set point" for parathyroid hormone secretion. FHH is an important diagnosis to exclude, because parathyroid surgery is not indicated for these individuals.

Clear indications for surgery in patients with primary hyperparathyroidism include significant hypercalcemia (serum levels of calcium greater than 12 mg/dl); nephrolithiasis; and parathyroid bone disease as documented by decreased bone density on bone densitometry studies, abnormal bone pathology on skeletal x-rays, or elevated serum levels of bony alkaline phosphatase. Many patients with primary hyperparathyroidism are "asymptomatic." Often these individuals have subtle symptoms of primary hyperparathyroidism that include fatigue, memory loss, difficulties in concentration, poor work performance, bone pain, peptic ulcer disease and pancreatitis, and other mild symptoms that are not uncommon in daily living. Furthermore, primary hyperparathyroidism has been shown to progress if left untreated. Therefore, unless individuals have significant medical contraindications that limit their life expectancy, parathyroid surgery is recommended for most patients with clear documentation of primary hyperparathyroidism.

Secondary Hyperparathyroidism

In secondary hyperparathyroidism, there is an increase in parathyroid hormone secretion in response to low plasma concentrations of ionized calcium. This increase occurs because of renal disease and malabsorption of oral calcium intake. This increase in parathyroid hormone secretion results in secondary chief cell hyperplasia. When secondary hyperparathyroidism occurs as a sequela of renal disease, the serum phosphorus level is usually elevated. Factors that play a role in the development of renal osteodystrophy are 1) phosphate retention, secondary to a decrease in the number of nephrons, 2) failure of the kidneys to hydroxylate 25-hydroxyvitamin D to the biologically active metabolite 1,25-dihydroxyvitamin D with resultant decreased intestinal absorption of calcium, 3) resistance of the bone to the action of parathyroid hormone, and 4) increased concentrations of serum calcitonin. These factors initiate the development of severe bone disease, which can be very debilitating. Most patients with secondary hyperparathyroidism can be treated medically by maintaining relatively normal serum concentrations of calcium and phosphorus during dialysis and treatment with vitamin D_3 decrease the incidence of bone disease.

Occasionally, a patient with secondary hyperparathyroidism develops relatively autonomous parathyroid function, which is then called tertiary hyperparathyroidism. Tertiary hyperparathyroidism is diagnosed by elevated serum levels of calcium and intact parathyroid hormone in patients with renal failure. The indications for parathyroid surgery in individuals with either secondary or tertiary hyperparathyroidism include: 1) persistent hypercalcemia (serum calcium levels >11.5 mg/dl), 2) intractable and severe pruritus that fails to respond to dialysis or other medical treatments, 3) evidence of progressive extraskeletal calcification, 4) severe skeletal pain, fractures, and bony deformities, and 5) the syndrome of calciphylaxis. When the patient does not have significant hypercalcemia, hyperphospha-

temia that is refractory to management, or progressive calciphylaxis, a therapeutic trial with intravenous or oral calcitriol can be indicated before parathyroidectomy. Hypercalcemia can occur in patients with aluminum-related bone disease, and aluminum toxicity must be excluded before parathyroid surgery.

In patients with secondary or tertiary hyperparathyroidism secondary to renal failure, total parathyroidectomy with autotransplantation is recommended. The procedure includes removal of each of four parathyroid glands and transplantation of twenty 2×1–mm slices of parathyroid tissue into the nondominant forearm. Some parathyroid tissue should also be cryopreserved in case the transplanted tissue does not function. These patients usually respond with dramatic relief of symptoms including decreased bone pain, decreased pruritus, and decreased pain associated with calciphylaxis.

Operative Procedures

Subtotal Parathyroidectomy (3½ Gland Parathyroidectomy)

Subtotal (3½ gland) parathyroidectomy is recommended for individuals with sporadic primary hyperparathyroidism who are found at neck exploration to have multiple gland disease without any family history of MEN-I or II-A. The patient is placed in the semi-sitting position with the neck extended (Fig. 39-1). The incision is made as a transverse cervical incision 1 to 2 finger breadths above the sternal notch (Fig. 39-2). The skin is incised with the knife. The remainder of the procedure is done with the cautery. The skin, subcutaneous tissue, and platysma muscle are divided. Flaps are raised just deep to the platysma muscle to the level of the thyroid cartilage with the cautery (Fig. 39-3). Similar flaps are raised inferiorly to the level of the sternal notch. A large self-retaining retractor, called the Mahorner retractor, is used to secure exposure by elevating the flaps and holding them out of the way. The flaps are carefully protected by placement of moist laparotomy tape to protect the edges. In previously unoperated individuals, the strap muscles are opened in the midline down to the level of the thyroid gland with the cautery (Fig. 39-4). Each thyroid lobe is

exposed and elevated medially by dissecting away the adherent strap muscles and lifting it with a Babcock clamp (Fig. 39-5, center). Most of the dissection can be done bluntly with a pusher or by using a fine-tipped clamp and asking the assistant to cauterize the selected tissue between the tips. Care should be used to avoid arcing of the current from the cautery to the instrument performing the dissection. Minor veins to the thyroid gland including the middle thyroid vein are ligated and divided in continuity with 3–0 silk suture.

A peanut dissector is used to identify the inferior thyroid artery and the recurrent laryngeal nerve. These structures should not be divided or injured, but the surgeon must clearly identify them in order to locate the parathyroid glands. The inferior thyroid artery generally exists superficially and at a right angle to the recurrent laryngeal nerve, although in some patients the recurrent laryngeal nerve can be superficial to the inferior thyroid artery. The recurrent laryngeal nerve is always in the tracheoesophageal groove. The esophagus can be readily identified if the anesthesiologist passes an esophageal stethoscope before the procedure. The left recurrent laryngeal nerve runs a more medial course in the tracheoesophageal groove and is seldom injured. The right recurrent laryngeal nerve can be nonrecurrent or runs a more oblique course in the tracheoesophageal groove, so it is injured more often. It is important to realize that both parathyroid glands have a uniform relationship to these structures. The upper parathyroid gland is always superior to the inferior thyroid artery and posterolateral to the recurrent laryngeal nerve. The lower parathyroid gland is inferior to the inferior thyroid artery and anteromedial to the recurrent laryngeal nerve. The lower parathyroid gland can commonly be within thymus tissue. Individuals with parathyroid hyperplasia can have supernumerary (>4 glands) fragments of parathyroid tissue that become hyperplastic. These supernumerary fragments are almost always located within the cervical thymus. Therefore, cervical thymectomy (removing thymus tissue to the level of the innominate vein) is recommended as part of the operative procedure for all individuals with parathyroid hyperplasia.

In patients with sporadic hyperplasia, it is necessary to carefully identify each of the

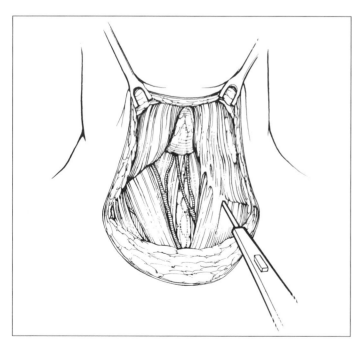

Fig. 39-1 Positioning of the patient for parathyroid surgery. The patient is placed in the semi-sitting position with the neck extended. A roll is placed longitudinally between the scapulae.

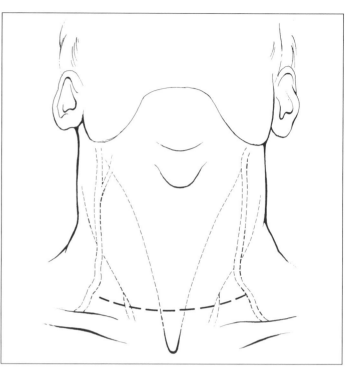

Fig. 39-2. Skin incision for parathyroid exploration. A skin incision is made 1 to 2 finger breadths superior to the sternal notch. The incision is made as far laterally as the external jugular vein on each side.

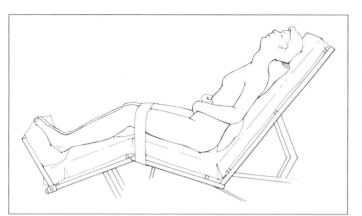

Fig. 39-3. Superior flap. The skin, subcutaneous tissue, and platysma muscle have been incised and retracted with skin hooks. The superior flap is raised just deep to the platysma with the cautery. The superior flap is raised to the level of the thyroid notch.

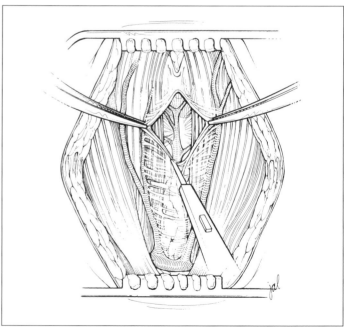

Fig. 39-4. Strap muscles are opened in midline. After insertion of the Mahorner retractor to hold the superior and inferior flaps, the strap muscles are opened in the midline to the depth of the thyroid gland with the cautery.

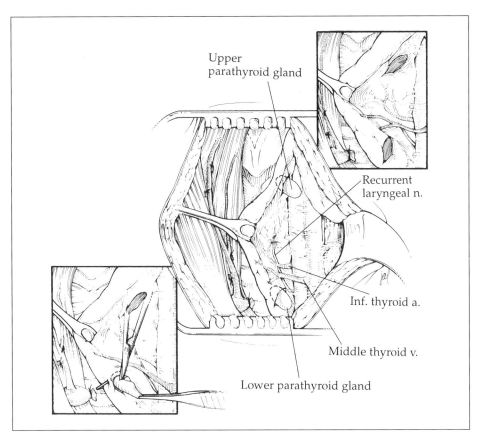

Upper
parathyroid gland

Recurrent
laryngeal n.

Inf. thyroid a.

Middle thyroid v.

Lower parathyroid gland

Fig. 39-5. Parathyroid resections for individuals with hyperplasia
Center. The left lobe of the thyroid is elevated by a Babcock clamp. The left recurrent laryngeal nerve is seen within the tracheoesophageal groove. The left inferior thyroid artery is seen superficial to the recurrent laryngeal nerve and running at right angles to it. The enlarged inferior parathyroid gland is identified inferior to the inferior thyroid artery and anteromedial to the recurrent laryngeal nerve. The enlarged superior parathyroid gland is identified superior to the inferior thyroid artery and posterolateral to the recurrent laryngeal nerve.
Lower left. In patients with sporadic hyperplasia 3½ gland resection is recommended. The superior gland has been removed and the inferior gland is being subtotally resected. The location of the remainder of the inferior gland is marked by a hemoclip placed on the thyroid.
Upper right. In patients with familial primary hyperparathyroidism or secondary or tertiary hyperparathyroidism, resection of all four enlarged parathyroid glands is recommended. The space where two left-sided glands were located is shown following excision.

four enlarged parathyroid glands. It is important to decide which gland is the most normal in appearance (most normal in size and color). Normal parathyroid glands are usually 3×2×4 mm in size, thin, and tan to light brown. Abnormal parathyroid glands are usually enlarged (>1 cm), thick, and reddish brown. Hyperplasia can be asymmetric in that some glands will appear to be more normal, that is closer to a normal size, color, and thickness. When the most normal appearing gland is identified, the three more abnormal appearing glands are removed and sent for frozen section. Frozen section is used to determine if parathyroid tissue has been ex-

cised. It might also be able to suggest whether the gland is hyperplastic based on the ratio of parathyroid cells to fat. However, cellularity determined by frozen section is not as useful as the surgeon's judgment based on size and color such that the frozen section diagnosis is used to identify the type of tissue. The fat that envelopes the most normal appearing gland is dissected free, and the blood supply is clearly identified. The surgeon should try to remove approximately three-fourths of this parathyroid gland leaving only approximately 30 to 50 mg of parathyroid tissue (Fig. 39-5, lower left). An effort to keep the blood supply intact is done by removing

the parathyroid tissue contralateral to the vessels. After subtotal resection, parathyroid gland location is identified with a surgical hemoclip. The hemoclip should be placed on the thyroid gland pointing toward the parathyroid tissue. A cervical thymectomy is also performed to remove any supernumerary fragments of parathyroid tissue that can be present.

Subtotal parathyroidectomy works very well in patients with sporadic hyperplasia. If 3½ glands are removed as described, patients have a very low incidence of persistent and recurrent primary hyperparathyroidism. If only two or three glands are identified, a patient can have persistent disease or later develop recurrent primary hyperparathyroidism. It is important that the operating surgeon can reliably identify four glands at exploration. Parathyroid glands can have some variability in location. In general, if the inferior thyroid artery and the recurrent laryngeal nerve are identified, the parathyroid glands will usually be found.

Total Parathyroidectomy and Transplantation

Total parathyroidectomy and immediate forearm transplantation is indicated for individuals with familial MEN-I or MEN-IIA primary hyperparathyroidism and individuals who have secondary or tertiary hyperparathyroidism. The goal of the operation is to remove all parathyroid tissue from the neck and transplant the normal gland equivalent into the musculature of the nondominant forearm. Parathyroid tissue should also be saved by cryopreservation in case the parathyroid graft does not function. The operation is done the same way as the previous operation except that during this operation, no parathyroid tissue is left in the neck (Fig. 39-5, upper right). A cervical thymectomy is also indicated (Fig. 39-6).

The most normal appearing gland is used for the graft. Patients with the familial form of the disease or renal failure have the highest probability of developing recurrent hyperparathyroidism. Placing the graft in the forearm allows easy access to the tissue, which can be partially excised if recurrent disease develops. The most normal appearing parathyroid gland is kept in iced saline solution on the operating table. The gland is diced and sliced

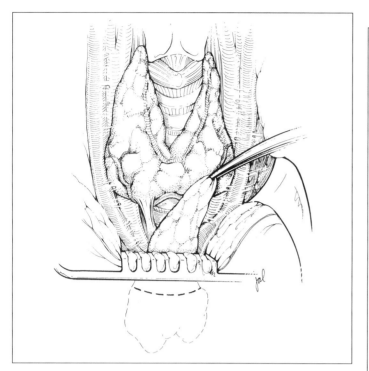

Fig. 39-6. Cervical thymectomy. The left superior horn of the thymus has been mobilized and is being removed down to the level of the innominate vein. The right superior horn of the thymus will also need to be mobilized and removed with the specimen because frequently supernumerary fragments of parathyroid tissue are present within the thymus.

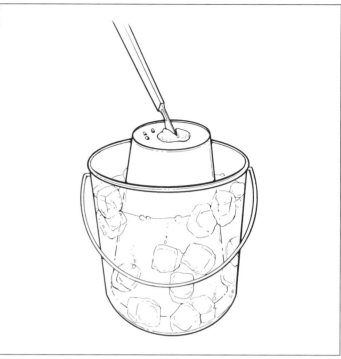

Fig. 39-7. Preparing parathyroid tissue for grafting. The removed parathyroid gland is kept in iced saline solution. It is sliced into approximately twenty 2×1 mm fragments, which are suitable for grafting. The tissue should be kept cold at all times.

into 2×1 mm fragments (Fig. 39-7). Most of the 2×1 mm fragments are sent to the laboratory for cryopreservation. Twenty are immediately grafted into the nondominant forearm (Fig. 39-8).

Cryopreservation is performed in a programmed freezer that will freeze the tissue 1°C per minute until it reaches a temperature of −40°C, then the tissue is transferred to a liquid nitrogen freezer. For cryopreservation, the tissue is mixed with 85 percent 1640 RPMI tissue culture media, 5 percent dimethyl sulfoxide (DMSO), and the remainder autologous serum. After complete closure of the neck incision, the nondominant forearm is extended and placed with the palm up, such that the volar aspect of the forearm is exposed. A small 1 to 2 cm longitudinal incision is made over the fleshy forearm muscles on the thumb side of the forearm. This incision is made distal to the antecubital fossa such that the veins in the antecubital fossa can be used to measure parathyroid hormone to document subsequent graft function. The muscles are exposed using a self-retaining retractor. Twenty 1×2 mm

fragments of parathyroid tissue are placed into the muscle. Each fragment is marked with a 4–0 silk suture. The grafts are placed in rows of five to facilitate subsequent partial resection in case recurrent hyperparathyroidism develops.

Fresh hyperplastic parathyroid tissue will have a high probability (95–100%) of graft function. Tissue is kept cryopreserved in case the immediate graft does not completely ameliorate the hypoparathyroidism. The advantage of this procedure is in the treatment of recurrent disease. If recurrent disease occurs, it can be documented by measuring parathyroid hormone levels in the antecubital fossa (as compared to the opposite antecubital fossa) to determine if the source of the parathyroid hormone is the grafted tissue. If the graft is hyperfunctioning, then resection of part of the graft can be performed in a subsequent procedure under local anesthesia. In addition, if the graft is hypofunctioning, cryopreserved tissue can be taken from the freezer and inserted into the same area under local anesthesia to supplement graft function.

Reoperations for Parathyroid Hyperplasia

Reoperations for parathyroid hyperplasia are fairly common. Patients who have primary hyperparathyroidism secondary to hyperplasia commonly have inadequate initial surgical procedures because the operating surgeon fails to identify four abnormal glands. Persistent disease can develop in these individuals, which means that the postoperative serum level of calcium is still elevated despite parathyroid surgery. Recurrent disease can also develop in patients, which means that the serum level of calcium normalized for a period of 6 months but subsequently became elevated, suggesting recurrent growth of hyperplastic parathyroid tissue. Therefore, reoperations are common in individuals with hyperplasia.

The documentation of primary hyperparathyroidism is as described initially. The indications for reoperative surgery include the presence of significant symptoms such as marked elevation of serum calcium levels (>12 mg/dl), significant bone disease as documented by bone densitometry, or nephrocalcinosis and nephrolithiasis. Because the incidence of recurrent laryngeal nerve injury is greater in reoperations (5% versus initial operations <1%), and the probability of unsuccessful surgery is greater (approximately 5–10% versus 2%), the individual patient should not undergo reoperation unless he or she has symptomatic hyperparathyroidism.

Operative records from the initial operation are reviewed in an attempt to determine the existence and location of clearly hyperplastic parathyroid glands that were previously removed. The pathology slides should also be reviewed to determine the size of the abnormal glands previously removed. If one or two abnormal glands were removed previously, reoperation should not be terminated until a total of four hyperplastic glands are removed, combining the first and second operation.

It is not unusual to find some confusion and poor documentation of the full extent of surgery at the original operation. Before the reoperation, imaging studies are used in an attempt to localize remaining abnormal parathyroid glands. Imaging studies include sestamibi scan, ultrasound, and CT. In most individuals with hyperplasia (85%), a combination of these studies will identify one abnormal parathyroid gland, but they will seldom identify more than one abnormal gland. The surgeon must carefully reexplore the neck with a plan to remove a total of four abnormal parathy-roid glands when the results of both the initial and reoperation are added together. Intraoperative determination of urinary levels of cAMP or parathyroid hormone can be helpful as a functional assay to determine when all abnormal parathyroid tissue has been removed.

The operation is performed by positioning the patient as before. The neck incision is reopened. Flaps are raised as before. The same retractor is used. However, the subsequent approach is not through the midline but along the medial border of the sternocleidomastoid (SCM) muscle (Fig. 39-9). Each side of the neck is explored using a separate lateral approach along the medial border of the ipsilateral SCM muscle. This step avoids dissection through the

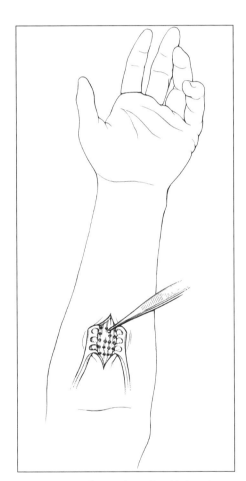

Fig. 39-8. Engraftment of parathyroid tissue into the musculature of the nondominant forearm. Twenty 2×1 mm fragments of parathyroid tissue are placed into the volar muscle distal to the antecubital fossa. Each graft is marked with a 4–0 silk suture. The grafts are placed in uniform rows to facilitate reexcision, if necessary.

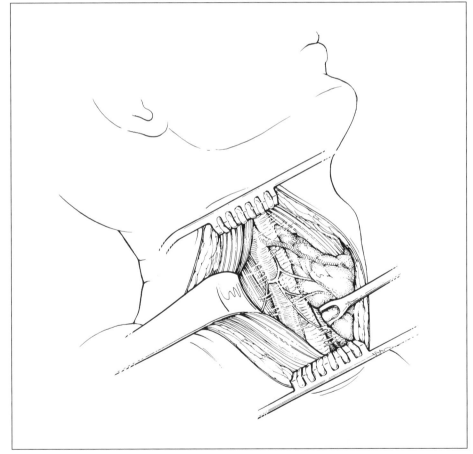

Fig. 39-9. Reoperation for parathyroid hyperplasia. In this reoperation, the patient has been positioned, the skin incised, and the superior and inferior flaps have been raised as shown in Figs. 39-1 through 39-3. However, instead of opening the strap muscles in the midline as is shown in Figure 39-4, the right side of the neck is explored separately by opening along the medial border of the ipsilateral SCM. After dissecting along the SCM, the omohyoid muscle is exposed and is divided to expose the right internal jugular vein and common carotid artery. The dissection proceeds along the medial border of the vessels to expose the tissues posterior to the thyroid and along the esophagus, which commonly contain the hyperplastic parathyroid glands.

dense scar tissue in the midline and allows a direct posterior approach to the parathyroid glands. The medial border of the SCM is identified, then the jugular vein and the common carotid arteries are identified and retracted laterally. The omohyoid muscle is divided. The inferior thyroid artery and recurrent laryngeal nerve can then be easily identified. Intraoperative ultrasound can be used to help identify the parathyroid glands. Abnormal parathyroid glands appear sonolucent. Ultrasound allows identification of the enlarged hyperplastic parathyroid glands quickly with minimal dissection. The reoperative procedure is focused based on the prior operative records, preoperative imaging studies, and findings of intraoperative ultrasound. Most frequently, in the reoperative setting for hyperplasia, both sides of the neck will need to be reexplored. The procedure is not terminated until four abnormal parathyroid glands have been removed considering the total of the first and second operation. For example, if two glands were removed at the initial operation, then two glands must be removed at the reoperation. Abnormal hyperplastic parathyroid tissue is not reimplanted during the reoperation. Often it is confusing to determine the amount of parathyroid tissue that has been removed. Because all the parathyroid tissue is hyperplastic, it is not desirable to reimplant it unless one is certain that all the abnormal tissue has been removed from the neck. Therefore, one should cryopreserve all abnormal tissue that is removed during the reoperation and wait to see if the patient is permanently hypoparathyroid (vitamin D and calcium are required to maintain a normal serum level of calcium) before grafting the cryopreserved tissue into the nondominant forearm. It usually takes approximately 6 months to determine if calcium replacement therapy can be discontinued. The engraftment of cryopreserved tissue is done exactly as the description of the grafting procedure at the time of surgery except the tissue is thawed and then taken to the operating room.

Postoperative Management

Postoperatively, individuals with sporadic primary hyperparathyroidism who undergo 3½ gland parathyroidectomy might need a significant amount of calcium replacement. However, they usually do not need as much replacement as individuals who have had a four gland parathyroidectomy and transplant. Individuals who have had a four gland parathyroidectomy and transplant are clearly hypoparathyroid. These individuals need approximately 1 to 2 g of oral calcium carbonate a day, with 1 to 2 μg of calcitriol. Patients with hyperparathyroidism and renal failure have severe bone disease and need a large amount of postoperative calcium and calcitriol replacement. Following surgery, serum levels of calcium and phosphorus should be monitored every 12 to 24 hours. By 24 to 36 hours after surgery, marked hypocalcemia with serum calcium levels less than 7 mg per dl can occur. If this occurs, an infusion containing calcium gluconate should be initiated. Enough ampules of calcium gluconate (calcium content approximately 110 mg/10 ml ampule) should be added to an intravenous infusion to provide 100 mg of calcium ion per hour, and the infusion should be continued for 8 to 12 hours or longer if the serum calcium level does not rise above 8 mg per dl. During this infusion, the serum calcium levels should be measured every 6 to 12 hours. Oral calcium carbonate instituted in doses of 2 to 3 g of calcium per day and oral calcitriol in doses of 1 to 2 μg per day or higher should be added if the hypocalcemia persists. Most patients require intravenous calcium for only approximately 2 to 3 days, and then the oral calcium and calcitriol will maintain serum levels of calcium. After approximately 1 to 2 months, an attempt should be made to decrease the oral calcium and calcitriol. The dose of oral calcium and calcitriol is decreased by 50 percent and then the calcitriol dose is reduced by 50 percent at 2-week intervals. After 6 to 8 weeks, most patients (90%) with a parathyroid graft will be able to have oral calcium and calcitriol replacement completely stopped. However, occasional individuals (<5%) might not be able to be completely weaned off these medications and are candidates for repeat engraftment with cryopreserved tissue. In individuals who have had reoperations for parathyroid hyperplasia and need the same dose of oral calcium and calcitriol for 3 to 6 months following surgery, then autologous cryopreserved parathyroid tissue is removed from the freezer and grafted into the nondominant forearm.

Outcome of Operations for Hyperplasia

In general, using the methods described here, the outcome of individuals with either sporadic or familial parathyroid hyperplasia is excellent. In addition, the outcome for reoperations is excellent, having a greater than 95% success rate with minimal recurrent disease. The key to these operations is meticulously identifying all the parathyroid glands and leaving either a small portion of a gland with a good blood supply or keeping the tissue on ice and functional before grafting it into the nondominant forearm. In patients with hyperplasia, if four glands are identified and removed and a small portion of one is either left intact or grafted, the outcome is excellent.

Suggested Reading

Clark OH. Secondary Hyperparathyroidism. In OH Clark (ed.), *Endocrine Surgery of the Thyroid and Parathyroid Glands*. St. Louis: Mosby, 1985.

Clark OH, Way LW, Hunt TK. Recurrent hyperparathyroidism. *Ann Surg* 184:391, 1976.

Norton JA. Reoperative parathyroid surgery: indication, intraoperative decision-making and results. *Prog Surg* 18:133, 1986.

Norton JA, Brennan MF, Saxe AW, et al. Intraoperative urinary cyclic adenosine monophosphate as a guide to successful reoperative parathyroidectomy. *Ann Surg* 200:389, 1984.

Norton JA, Cornelius MJ, Doppman JL, et al. Effect of parathyroidectomy in patients with hyperparathyroidism, Zollinger–Ellison syndrome, and multiple endocrine neoplasia type 1: a prospective study. *Surgery* 102:958, 1987.

Thompson NW. Surgical Considerations in the MEN I Syndrome. In IDA Johnston, NW Thompson (eds.), *Endocrine Surgery. Butterworths International Medical Reviews*. London: Butterworths, 1983.

Thompson NW, Vinik AI. The Technique of Initial Parathyroid Exploration and Reoperative Parathyroidectomy. In NW Thompson, AI Vinik (ed.), *Endocrine Surgery Update*. New York: Grune & Stratton, 1983.

Wells SA Jr, Ellis GJ, Gunnells JC, et al. Parathyroid autotransplantation in primary parathyroid hyperplasia. *N Engl J Med* 295:57, 1976.

Wells SA Jr, Leight GF, Ross A. Primary hyperparathyroidism. *Curr Probl Surg* 17:398, 1980.

Wells SA Jr, Ross RJ, Dale JK, Gray RS. Transplantation of the parathyroid glands. *Surg Clin North Am* 59:167, 1979.

Wells SA Jr, Farndon JR, Dale JK, et al. Long-term evaluation of patients with primary parathyroid hyperplasia managed by total parathyroidectomy and heterotopic autotransplantation. *Ann Surg* 192:451, 1980.

EDITOR'S COMMENT

The two chapters by Drs. van Heerden, Smith, and Norton have summarized in depth current thinking about parathyroidectomy for both adenoma and hyperplasia. Multiple endocrine neoplasia syndromes involving the parathyroid glands (MEN-I and MEN-IIA) are infrequent occurrences in clinical practice but have a very high incidence of parathyroid hyperfunction. Whenever a patient with medullary cancer of the thyroid is encountered, the hyperparathyroidism should have been detected preoperatively. At the very least, serum calcium levels should always be obtained with patients with surgical thyroid disease, both to rule out hyperparathyroidism as in MEN syndrome and as a baseline in the unlikely event that the patients were to become hypocalcemic in the postoperative period.

Doctor Norton notes the occurrence of peptic ulcer disease or pancreatitis with patients with parathyroid hyperplasia, a concept which has waxed and waned in acceptance over the past three decades. Many endocrine surgeons believe that these two clinical entities do not have an increased incidence in parathyroid adenoma but can occasionally be seen with hyperplasia. Although uncommon, it is necessary to screen patients with peptic ulcer or pancreatitis for hypercalcemia. If a patient is encountered with acute pancreatitis and the calcium is normal, the finding might be misleading, since that patient without severe acute pancreatitis would have an elevated serum calcium, and the normal level reflects the calcium lowering that is commonly encountered in severe pancreatitis. Obviously, repeat calcium levels when the patient has recovered from acute pancreatitis are always in order.

Most endocrine surgeons are now in agreement that it is wise to visualize all parathyroids when exploring for hyperparathyroidism, that enlargement of two or more glands usually represents hyperplasia as the underlying cause of primary hyperparathyroidism (only 1–3% of adenomas are multiple), and that even a normal size gland can represent a hyperplastic parathyroid. An area of disagreement is whether the normal gland should be biopsied, opposite the hilus (blood supply), looking for hypercellularity with little or no fat interspersed among the parathyroid cells that is characteristic of adenoma or hyperplasia.

The use of cautery, on or about the thyroid and parathyroids, is reasonable if one uses the bipolar instrument. Many surgeons have some concern about using a monopolar cautery in this area, because of the inherent risk of thermal damage to the recurrent nerve even if that structure is 1 cm from the end of the cautery tip. The bipolar instrument for hemostasis alone has proved to be safer with much less risk of adjacent structure injury, unless that structure is included between the jaws of the end of the instrument.

The operation for recurrent hyperparathyroidism is a formidable undertaking and one which the occasional surgeon probably should not attempt. The lateral approach espoused by the author is the current method of choice for finding the recurrent nerve and the parathyroids that remain, but it, like the anterior incision, can uncover a good deal of scar tissue and a pair of binocular loupes can be most helpful in dissecting in the previously operated on area. Doctor Norton's experience with intraoperative ultrasound is substantial, some done in conjunction with Dr. Bernard Sigel, one of the authors of Chapter 14, Intraoperative Ultrasound, but the experience required to interpret the ultrasound under these trying circumstances is not readily available in every institution. As in most other reoperative surgery, the best solution is to complete the task at the first procedure and not have to embark on the second.

R.J.B.

Transsternal, Transcervical, and Thoracoscopic Thymectomy for Benign and Malignant Disease

Michael S. Nussbaum

The thymus gland is one of the more common structures in the anterior mediastinum that requires surgical extirpation. Most commonly, the indications for thymectomy are either for thymic neoplasm or in the treatment of the autoimmune disorder, myasthenia gravis. Thymus removal should be a safe, straightforward procedure. The key elements in successful and complete thymectomy depend on a comprehensive knowledge of the physiology of thymic disease and the anatomic and embryologic characteristics of thymic development.

Embryology and Anatomy

The thymus is a lymphoepithelial organ that is embryologically derived primarily from the third pair of pharyngeal pouches. In the fifth week of embryonic life, the paired thymic primordia appear as buds on the ventral aspects of the third pharyngeal pouches (Fig. 40-1). It is believed that the ventral portion of the fourth pharyngeal pouch also gives rise to a small amount of thymus that might disappear soon after its formation. The entire third pouch separates from the pharynx during the seventh week and through a complex series of migrations, these anlagen migrate in a caudal and medial direction. These hollow primordia rapidly become solid epithelial bars, and, during the eighth week, the caudad ends of the paired components of the thymus fuse together to form what is generally a four-lobed gland

that attaches to the anterior pericardium. This attachment enhances the descent of the thymus into the thorax while the cephalic extremes of the organ become attenuated and generally disappear. However, migration can be incomplete and remnants might appear anywhere along the excursion of the primordia. In addition to being embedded within the thyroid gland or associated with the parathyroid glands (see below), aberrant thymic rests can occur independently, along the entire path of thymic descent, in as many as 20 percent of humans. The lower lobe capsule tends to be less distinct, and thymic corpuscles, as well as abundant lymphocytes, trail off into the surrounding mediastinal fat and nodal tissue. The thymus gland itself can

occupy a cervical position reaching occasionally as far cephalad as the hyoid bone. The caudad extremes of the gland can extend as far downward as the xiphoid process.

The thyroid, parathyroid, and thymus share a common origin from the primordial pharynx and its pouches. The inferior parathyroid glands are derived from the dorsal wings of the third pair of pharyngeal pouches. As the thymus migrates downward to its definitive position in the anterior mediastinum, the inferior parathyroid glands are pulled down and left behind at the level of the lower poles of the thyroid. The superior parathyroid glands and the ultimobranchial bodies, the

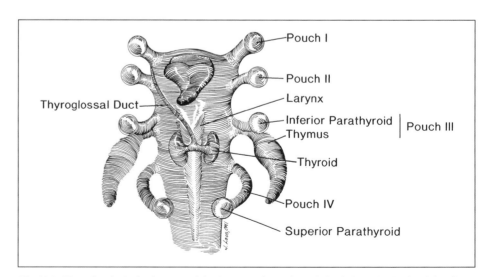

Fig. 40-1. The embryologic development of the thymus and parathyroid glands from the third and fourth pharyngeal pouches.

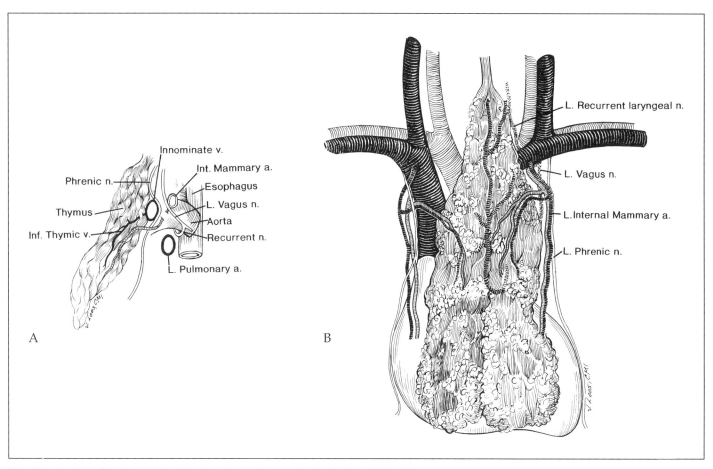

Fig. 40-2. Anatomy of the thymus gland. A. Lateral view, showing the relationship with the left brachiocephalic vein, the inferior aspect of the thyroid gland, and the phrenic and recurrent laryngeal nerves. B. Anterior view, showing the relationship with the pericardium and great vessels. The major arterial supply originates from the internal thoracic arteries, and the major venous drainage empties posteriorly into the left brachiocephalic vein.

source of parafollicular (calcitonin) cells, develop from the fourth pair of pharyngeal pouches, which can also contribute to the development of the thymus. The parathyroid glands are also "parathymic" glands. In autopsy studies, as many as 20 percent of inferior parathyroid glands invade the thymic capsule in the neck or mediastinum. Although intrathymic parathyroid is well established, there have also been isolated reports of intrathymic thyroid. Ectopic thyroid is usually found along the normal route of its descent from the base of the tongue to the thyroglossal duct. However, rests of thyroid tissue can be found throughout the mediastinum, including the thymus and can be mistaken as thymic tumors.

At the completion of its development, the thymus is separated from the sternum by a thin film of loose connective tissue lying anterior to the pericardium and great vessels and is in especially close contact with the left brachiocephalic (innominate) vein (Fig. 40-2). The gland can extend laterally to the phrenic nerves and is partially covered on either side by the pleural reflections. The arterial supply to the thymus is derived from three sources: the internal thoracic (mammary), inferior thyroid, and pericardiophrenic arteries. However, the principal blood supply is from the internal thoracic arteries. The veins from both lobes ascend between the lobes posteriorly and usually drain into the left brachiocephalic vein or, rarely, directly in the superior vena cava. The numerous veins that leave the lobes generally converge, forming one or two major trunks, although the number of trunks is quite variable (usually between one and five trunks). The inferior thyroid

and thyroid ima veins can receive minor tributaries from the cervical portion of the gland. At birth, the thymus weighs 10 to 35 g and continues to grow in size until puberty, when it achieves a maximum weight of 20 to 50 g. It then undergoes progressive atrophy to little more than 5 to 15 g in the elderly, with the thymic parenchyma being replaced by fibrofatty tissue.

Physiology and Pathophysiology

The thymus gland is a central lymphoid organ that performs the important immunologic function of transforming null lymphocytes into thymic or T-lymphocytes, which are responsible for cellular immunity. The maturation of T-lymphocytes appears to be promoted by one or more thymic-derived factors, such as the peptide thymosin. The thymus gland is involved in a variety of immunologic, hematologic, endocrine, infectious, and neoplastic diseases. The thymus can display morphologic changes that can be categorized as anomalies associated with abnormal development, immune deficiencies, hyperplasia, and neoplasia. Symptoms related to thymic disease are categorized as the ones arising directly from the thymic lesion either by compression or invasion; symptoms associated with a previously described clinical syndrome (i. e., myasthenia gravis, red cell aplasia, or hypogammaglobulinemia); or nonspecific systemic symptoms such as anorexia and fatigue. Developmental anomalies can involve the location of the thymus or its development. Failure of the thymus to descend into the anterior mediastinum might account for cervical thymic tissue, which can be mistaken for neoplasm, lymphadenopathy, or an enlarged parathyroid. This aberrant tissue can cause compressive symptoms such as respiratory stridor or dysphagia. In general, symptoms are more common and specific in patients with malignancy, whereas patients with thymic cysts and germ cell tumors have symptoms less frequently.

Thymic Neoplasms

Thymoma is one of the most common solid neoplasms of the mediastinum, accounting for 20 to 25 percent of all mediastinal tumors. They are usually found in the anterosuperior mediastinum but on rare occasions (<10%), thymic tumors can also be encountered in other areas within the thorax and the neck. Adults between the age of 45 and 50 years old are most frequently affected. The clinical presentation of thymoma is extremely varied. In up to 50 percent of instances, these neoplasms are entirely asymptomatic, discovered incidentally on chest x-ray or at autopsy. Approximately 30 percent of patients present with local symptoms related to pressure or direct invasion such as cough, dyspnea, dysphagia, hoarseness, Horner's syndrome, or signs of superior vena caval compression. In anywhere from 20 to 70 percent of patients, thymoma is associated with systemic disorders that are primarily of autoimmune origin. When present, these concomitant diseases worsen the prognosis. These associated disorders include (in order of frequency): myasthenia gravis, cytopenia, nonthymic cancer, hypogammaglobulinemia, polymyositis, systemic lupus erythematosus, and others. Whenever a patient has an autoimmune disease the possibility of a thymoma must be considered, and in some cases removal of the thymic tumor induces a cure or remission of the immunologic disorder. There is no clear-cut relationship between the histologic pattern of the thymoma and the appearance or nature of the associated disease. The prognosis is directly related to aggressiveness of the tumor as well as the presence and nature of an associated systemic disease.

In terms of classification and determination of malignancy, no mediastinal tumor is subject to more disagreement among pathologists than thymic tumors. There are no clear histologic differences between benign and malignant neoplasms. The most significant determinant of survival is invasiveness. The malignant potential of thymoma is determined by its gross invasive character. Benign thymomas are well-encapsulated lesions that are easily dissected away from contiguous structures. Malignant tumors invade lymphatics, blood vessels, and adjacent structures within the anterior mediastinum and chest and can defy complete excision. Between 7 and 35 percent of thymic tumors are malignant. Malignant thymomas usually cause death by progressive local involvement of the surrounding tissue within the thorax. A concomitant systemic disease has a strong adverse effect on survival. Distant metastases to the lungs, liver, bone, or other sites are rare.

Previously, all primary tumors of the thymus were referred to as thymomas. However, the thymus is composed of two basic cells types, lymphocytes and epithelial cells. The term *thymoma* should be restricted to neoplasms of thymic epithelial cell origin. All thymomas have, as their neoplastic component, a greater or lesser component of thymic epithelial cells in a variable amount of lymphocytic infiltrate. Clinically, patients with predominantly lymphocytic cell–type thymoma have a much better survival rate than patients with mixed or predominantly epithelial cell type. Lymphomas derived from the lymphocytes can also arise in the thymus, and such neoplasms are called thymic lymphomas.

Conventionally, thymic carcinoma has been included in the category of malignant thymoma. However, since the concept of thymic squamous cell carcinoma was first advocated, thymic carcinoma has increasingly become included in a group different from that of thymoma. Squamous cell carcinoma of the thymus has been clearly differentiated microscopically and histologically as a thymic epithelial tumor consisting of clearly atypical cells with a strong tendency for invasion and does not involve immature T-lymphocytes. Thymoma originates from epithelial cells in the periphery of the thymic cortical area, whereas thymic carcinoma originates from thymic medullary cells. Thymoma can often be cured since it is associated with less possibility of extrathoracic distant metastases, and it grows slowly even when invasive. In contrast, thymic carcinoma is associated with a higher incidence of distant metastases, and the outcome is generally poor when compared with thymoma. Well-differentiated thymic carcinomas have the highest association with myasthenia gravis among all thymic epithelial tumors. These carcinomas might develop from preexisting cortical thymomas, which could initiate the paraneoplastic myasthenia gravis before the carcinomatous transition. However, the well-differentiated thymic carcinoma might provide the minimal but most effective prerequisite for an intratumorous pathogenesis of myasthenia gravis. Squamous cell carcinoma of the thymus is highly sensitive to radiation therapy. Since the efficacy of chemotherapy has not been established, it has been considered reasonable to resect as extensively as possible and follow with adjuvant radiation therapy.

An anterior mediastinal mass can develop following therapy for cancer. Recurrence or metastasis of the malignant disease must be ruled out first. The differential diagnosis of a mediastinal mass recurring after the successful treatment of a malignant lesion by chemotherapy or radiation therapy would also include thymoma, thymic hyperplasia, and benign thymic cyst. Recent studies to evaluate the frequency of thymic changes after chemotherapy indicate that the problem is more common than previously thought. Thymic hyperplasia has been reported after chemotherapy in children and adolescents as a rebound phenomenon and might actually be a good prognostic sign, indicating restoration of the host's immunity. These patients often respond to a 7-day course of high-dose steroids (prednisone 60 mg/m^2/day), and, if the mediastinal changes regress, the patient should be followed by serial chest roentgenography. If the mass remains unchanged or enlarges, then open biopsy or excision of the mass should be performed. The development of a benign cystic lesion in the thymus after radiation therapy for Hodgkin's disease has also been reported. The cyst usually occurs after successful radiation-therapy to a thymus previously involved with lymphoma, and most patients can be followed without additional lymphoma therapy or biopsy.

Thymic follicular hyperplasia is defined by the presence of lymphoid follicles with large germinal centers within the thymus. The gland may be normal in weight but usually is slightly enlarged. The germinal centers are located principally in the medulla, resulting in compression and atrophy of the cortex. Thymic hyperplasia is classically associated with myasthenia gravis but it also has been found in association with other autoimmune disorders such as Grave's disease, Addison's disease, systemic lupus erythematosus, scleroderma, and rheumatoid arthritis as well as in a variety of liver diseases less clearly immunologic in origin. In children, certain severe stresses such as starvation, serious infection, high fever, or thermal burn may cause involution of the thymus. At recovery the thymus will sometimes grow to be larger than its former size. In adults, on the other hand, thymic hyperplasia of benign etiology is rare.

Myasthenia Gravis

Myasthenia gravis was first described clinically in 1672 by the physiologist Thomas Willis. However, only over the last two decades has the pathophysiology of this disorder become better elucidated. It is truly one of the best understood of the autoimmune diseases. The prevalence of myasthenia gravis has been estimated at 43 to 64 per million population. It affects all ages and both sexes with peaks in the second and fifth decades. Younger females and older males are the most commonly affected. The natural history of the disease is one of insidious onset of generalized weakness. Often these patients present initially with external ocular symptoms, such as ptosis and diplopia, so that the diagnosis is made by ophthalmologists in a sig-

nificant number of patients. Spontaneous remissions do occur, and there appears to be an association with other autoimmune diseases. Approximately 75 percent of patients with this muscular disorder have thymic abnormalities. Approximately 85 percent of these abnormalities constitute follicular hyperplasia, and the remainder are thymomas. Between 8 and 13 percent of patients with myasthenia gravis have an associated thymoma. However, the incidence of myasthenia gravis in patients with thyomoma varies between 10 and 40 percent. Since small tumors might not be detected preoperatively and, until recently, only selected patients with myasthenia gravis were referred for thymectomy, the association of thymomas with myasthenia gravis might be more common than currently estimated.

Myasthenia gravis is caused by a loss of immunologic tolerance leading to an antibody-mediated attack on the nicotinic acetylcholine receptors of the muscle endplate. The factors that are responsible for initiating this autoimmune disorder are not well understood. However, the attack on the receptors appears to involve both T-cell–mediated and humoral components of the immune system, causing the destruction of the receptor and thus interfering with neuromuscular transmission. The involvement of the B-lymphocyte is evident by several findings in myasthenia gravis. Approximately 80 to 90 percent of myasthenia patients have serum antibodies to the acetylcholine receptor (AChR). B-lymphocytes, which secrete anti-AChR-IgG, have been found in both circulating blood as well as intrathymic germinal centers. This antibody interacts with the target antigen, the acetylcholine receptor. In addition, the pathogenic effect of this antibody is evident as myasthenia gravis is induced by transfer of IgG from patients with myasthenia to mice. Treatment aimed at decreasing the circulating antibody levels, using either immunosuppression or plasmapheresis, will result in clinical improvement in the majority of affected individuals.

The role of cell-mediated immunity and the thymus in the pathogenesis of myasthenia gravis is not well understood, but several facts are known. The number of AChR-reactive T-cells are increased in cell culture when compared to cells from normal controls and patients with other neurologic diseases. These reactive T-cells

may represent a cell population with suppressor effects because there is a reduction of interleukin-2 and interferon-gamma production by T-lymphocytes in myasthenia gravis. These defects in T-cell function are most pronounced in nonthymectomized patients and are partially reversed with thymectomy. In addition to lymphocytes and epithelial cells, the thymus gland contains myoid cells that bear an AChR-like receptor. In myasthenia gravis an alteration in these myoid cells or the adjacent lymphocytes may lead to a loss of immunologic tolerance and the development of an autoimmune response that may activate intrathymic T- and B-lymphocytes against the AChR. Activated B-lymphocytes have been demonstrated in the thymus and a thymic T-suppressor cell population might also be triggered by the acetylcholine receptors on thymic myoid cells, leading to the described impairment of circulating T-lymphocyte cytokine production.

Thymectomy has long been an accepted treatment for this disorder and is the treatment that offers the best chance of complete remission. In 1939, Blalock brought the potential value of thymectomy in myasthenia to the forefront when he excised a benign thymic cyst in a 19-year-old female with myasthenia and demonstrated dramatic clinical improvement. Since that time, thymectomy has played an important role in the treatment of this disease. Thymectomy removes the source of autosensitization and depletes the specific T-suppressor cell population, normalizing T-cell function. B-cells and suppressor T-cells primed before thymectomy would theoretically remain in circulation, thus accounting for incomplete recovery in many thymectomized patients as well as the relatively prolonged period (up to 2 years) between operation and remission in many patients.

Thymectomy should be considered early in the treatment of all patients affected with myasthenia gravis. Although the exact role of the thymus in myasthenia gravis has not been thoroughly elicited, the embryology and recent immunologic discoveries reinforce the need to resect all thymic tissue via a mediastinal clearing approach. In children, it is preferable to delay this procedure until puberty, if possible, because of the role that the thymus plays in the maturation of the immune system. In patients with thymomas, the clinical course is influenced favorably by the smaller size of the tumors. Since approximately 50 percent of thymic tumors less than 5 cm in longest diameter are not diagnosed preoperatively, early surgical intervention is essential in this subgroup of patients. Using an aggressive approach of early thymectomy, one can expect to achieve either drug-free remission or significant palliation in the majority (>90%) of patients.

Thymectomy

The majority of thymic abnormalities are treated by surgical extirpation. However, the surgical approach to thymectomy has been a matter of considerable controversy. Thymectomy must be complete in order to achieve lasting remission or improvement of malignant thymomas or autoimmune disorders such as myasthenia gravis. In the early experience with the transsternal approach, there was a relatively high mortality, primarily caused by inadequate respiratory and perioperative support. Thus, transcervical thymectomy was long advocated despite the abundant documentation of residual thymic tissue following this approach. More recently, with improved perioperative support and increased experience with median sternotomy, this procedure has become a relatively innocuous approach to the anterior mediastinum and affords far greater opportunity for adequate exposure of the mediastinal structures, allowing complete removal of the gland. Proponents of the transcervical route argue that improved techniques in the exposure and visualization of the anterior mediastinum via a cervical incision allow complete excision under direct vision with equivalent results. The advantage of this less invasive approach in terms of morbidity, length of hospital stay, and acceptance of the procedure early in the disease are obvious. However, this method is clearly more difficult to learn and requires considerably more experience than the sternotomy approach. The recent advances in videoscopic technology have led to the use of thoracoscopic visualization of the anterior mediastinum in conjunction with a transcervical incision. This method will possibly provide a minimally invasive technique that might not compromise the exposure and extent of the dissection.

Preoperative Evaluation and Preparation

Regardless of the method of thymectomy chosen, preoperative evaluation of the thymus and accurate localization of the mediastinal lesion are very important. When a mass is discovered in the anterior mediastinum (usually on routine chest roentgenogram) or in a patient with myasthenia gravis, the initial work-up should include a careful history and physical examination; the neck and particularly the thyroid gland requires careful palpation. A complete blood count, serum electrolytes, thyroid function tests, acetylcholine-receptor antibody assay, immunoglobulin assay, bone marrow biopsy, and cervical lymph node biopsy may be indicated. Routine chest roentgenography can demonstrate a mass or reveal obliteration or displacement of mediastinal structures. Ultrasound can be used to differentiate between solid and cystic masses. Computed tomography of the chest is far superior to the other methods in evaluating suspected mediastinal tumors. Computed tomography defines the anatomic location, nature, and extent of mediastinal tumors, identifies pulmonary metastases, and evaluates the status of mediastinal lymph nodes. However, CT cannot always determine invasiveness. Magnetic resonance imaging (MRI) can provide additional views of the thymus as well as more detail concerning invasion and its relationship to adjacent structures.

Removal of the thymus is never an emergency, and preoperative preparation of the patient should be complete before the operation. This step is especially important when performing thymectomy for myasthenia gravis. The myasthenic's strength and respiratory status should be optimized with the use of pyridostigmine and immunosuppressive agents when indicated. Preoperative plasmapheresis can be beneficial in severe myasthenia and in instances in which the patient's pulmonary function is markedly diminished by the disease (vital capacity <2 L).

Unless patients require preoperative parenteral steroids, hemodynamic stabilization, or plasmapheresis, they can be admitted to the hospital on the day of surgery. In general, anticholinesterase agents (pyridostigmine) should be discontinued 8 hours before surgery. Discontinuing these medications any earlier, especially in patients with severe myasthenia, can result in a myasthenic crisis, whereas continuing the medications, particularly in patients with mild symptoms, can result in a postoperative cholinergic crisis. In severe cases, an additional intramuscular injection of a small dose of pyridostigmine can be administered just before the operation. If the patient is on steroids, perioperative parenteral steroid coverage is provided, beginning with 100 mg of hydrocortisone 1 hour before surgery and continuing every 8 hours for the first 24 hours, then every 12 hours, then resuming the preoperative oral dosage. Perioperative antibiotics (usually a first-generation cephalosporin) are administered until the mediastinal tubes are removed. Neuromuscular relaxant agents are avoided if possible because of their adverse effects on myasthenic patients. Aminoglycoside antibiotics and ether are also contraindicated because they increase the neuromuscular block.

Transsternal Thymectomy

The patient is positioned on the operating table in the supine position. A transverse shoulder roll is placed behind the patient and the neck is extended with the occiput of the head resting on a "donut" pillow. Following induction of anesthesia, a Foley catheter and arterial line should be placed. The operation is carried out via a median sternotomy. The incision can be a midline incision from the sternal notch to below the xiphoid process. Since many of these patients are young women, a more cosmetic incision might be preferable, such as a Y-shaped skin incision that follows the upper contours of the breasts and converges on a point in the midline approximately 10 cm below the sternal notch and continues down the midline to the tip of the xiphoid (Fig. 40-3). A cephalad skin/subcutaneous flap is carefully developed so that cosmesis of the upper chest area is maintained. The superior limit of the subcutaneous dissection is the sternal notch. Electrocautery is used to divide the fascia overlying the sternum. The cleidocleido ligament, which is attached to the posterior surface of manubrium at the sternal notch, is divided vertically and the sternum is separated from the upper mediastinal structures by blunt finger dissection.

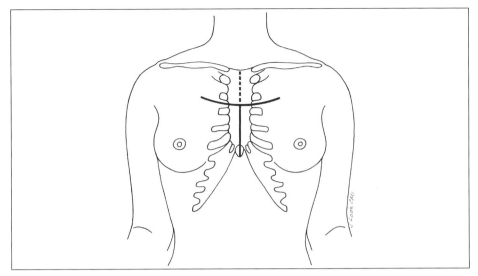

Fig. 40-3. The Y-shaped skin incision, with a cephalad skin/subcutaneous flap, allows access to the entire sternum for midline sternotomy while maintaining cosmesis (especially in females) of the upper chest area.

Inferiorly, the avascular anterior mediastinal space is entered with finger dissection just below the xiphoid and developed as far cephalad as possible. The sternum is divided longitudinally with a sternal saw.

In adults, obese individuals, and patients on long-term steroids, it is often not possible to distinguish thymus from mediastinal fat until the specimen is removed and examined microscopically. Gross and microscopic thymus is found outside the confines of the classic cervical mediastinal lobes in the neck in approximately 30 percent of specimens and in the mediastinum in approximately 98 percent of studies. Therefore, wide exposure and meticulous dissection is needed to remove all of the potential thymic tissue completely and safely. An en bloc dissection from diaphragm to thyroid gland and from phrenic nerve to phrenic nerve is undertaken by means of a combination of cautery and sharp dissection of the mediastinal pleura and pericardium. All thymus, suspected thymus, and mediastinal fat including both mediastinal pleural sheets are removed.

The mediastinal dissection begins at the diaphragm. The mediastinal fat, including the anterior pericardiophrenic fat pad, is elevated bilaterally and continued superiorly with the lower lobes of the thymus. The mediastinal pleura is incised anteriorly and once the lower lobes are mobilized bilaterally, the phrenic nerves should

be clearly identified. The lymph nodes and fat that course along the nerves are separated from the phrenic nerves on either side anteriorly as part of the en bloc specimen. The thymus is elevated off the pericardium using upward traction and electrocautery. The main arterial supply to the thymus is derived from the internal thoracic arteries, which enter the gland laterally at the level of the isthmus that joins the two lobes. Once identified, the arteries and accompanying veins should be isolated and divided in continuity between ligatures. These lateral vessels tend to tether the gland in position, and their division allows the en bloc specimen to be rotated upward, exposing the undersurface of the gland (Fig. 40-4). This method is the safest approach to the brachiocephalic vein and the venous drainage of the thymus. The brachiocephalic vein should be exposed and the thymic veins isolated and divided in continuity between ligatures. The thymus can then be elevated from the brachiocephalic vein and dissection is continued laterally anterior to the phrenic nerves until the entire specimen is tethered only by the cephalic horns of the thymus in the vicinity of the thyroid and inferior parathyroid glands. An attempt should be made to identify and spare the inferior parathyroids and their blood supply, but this step is not always possible. The cephalad extent of the thymus should be carefully isolated, and the branches of the inferior thyroid vessels entering the

two horns should be clamped at the point where they enter the superior thymic lobes, divided, and ligated.

It is important to include in the en bloc dissection the fatty thymic tissue lying in the sulcus between the superior vena cava and the aorta and the tissue in the region of the aortopulmonary window deep under the brachiocephalic vein. During this part of the dissection, it is essential to identify and avoid the left phrenic and vagus (recurrent laryngeal) nerves, which are especially at risk here. Injury to either of these nerves would be catastrophic, particularly in a patient with myasthenia gravis. The wide mediastinal exposure obtained by opening both pleural spaces not only ensures complete thymus removal but also helps safeguard the phrenic and vagus nerves.

Malignant thymic tumors are notorious for local extension and lack of distant metastases as well as a deceptively benign appearance on microscopic examination. Gross evidence of invasiveness is the most important prognostic sign. When a thymoma is present, the same extensive removal of thymic tissue is performed en bloc with the thymoma. The initial exploration includes palpation and visualization of each hemidiaphragm for possible tumor implants. If the pericardium, lungs, brachiocephalic vein, or sternal periosteum are adherent to the tumor, they are removed en bloc since there can be tumor invasion. Unless a phrenic nerve is nonfunctional from tumor invasion, it should be preserved if at all possible. Postoperative radiation therapy can be used as adjuvant therapy and to control residual unresected tumor.

After the thymectomy and anterior mediastinal dissection is completed, two angled chest tubes are placed through separate incisions in the superior epigastrium and positioned along the diaphragms in both pleural cavities. The sternum is reapproximated using No. 5 stainless steel wires, and the fascia and skin incisions are closed.

Previously, the mortality and considerable morbidity associated with transsternal thymectomy in myasthenia gravis were primarily caused by respiratory complications. Improvements in the surgical technique, anesthesia, respiratory care, and the use of plasmapheresis in severe cases of myasthenia gravis have markedly

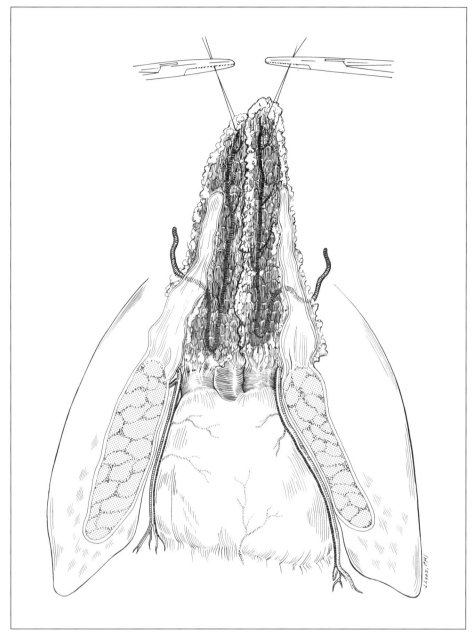

Fig. 40-4. The thymus, along with the adherent mediastinal pleura, is elevated from the pericardium and separated from the phrenic nerves bilaterally. Division of the branches from the internal thoracic vessels allows the en bloc specimen to be rotated upward, exposing the undersurface of the gland and the draining veins.

sternal and cervical incisions. Their rationale for this extensive exposure was to clear all potential thymic rests of tissue from the mediastinum and neck. This decision was based on the hypothesis that it is not always possible to perform complete thymectomy with only a mediastinal approach since islands of aberrant thymic tissue can be located anywhere in the retrothyroid space, as far proximal as the level of the hyoid bone. The results from this group (46% remission and 96% improved) were similar to our series. Therefore, the additional morbidity of a cervical incision might not be warranted if one performs an extended transsternal dissection as described above. Drug-free remission in our current series was achieved only in patients classified as Osserman's I or II, although patients with more advanced stages of the disease have responded to surgery with overall improvement in their symptoms and drug requirements. This finding confirms the findings of other investigators that early thymectomy, before progression of symptoms, influences the progression of this disease and should routinely be offered to patients early in the course of their disease.

Transcervical Thymectomy

The transcervical approach to the anterior mediastinum is the preferred exposure for nonthymic abnormalities such as retrosternal thyroid and mediastinal parathyroid adenomas. This method has also been advocated by some as an appropriate approach for thymectomy in certain clinical situations. Proponents of transcervical thymectomy claim superior cosmetic results and lower morbidity. They believe that, in selected patients, the clinical results are the same as with transsternal thymectomy. The advantage of the transcervical approach appears to be related to the selection of patients. The approach is applied most commonly in the treatment of myasthenia gravis with thymic hyperplasia. Patients with myasthenia gravis might choose transcervical removal of the thymus earlier in the course of their disease because of the perceived cosmetic benefits and lesser morbidity. Since duration of the disease before thymectomy has an adverse effect on the effectiveness of surgery, the tendency toward earlier intervention can have a positive effect on the long-term outcome. When a thymoma is diagnosed or suspected preoperatively, the transsternal

reduced the mortality and morbidity of the procedure. Thymectomy is now recognized as a standard procedure in combination with medical management for myasthenia gravis. In a recent series of 48 patients with myasthenia gravis managed with a transsternal mediastinal clearing–extended thymectomy at the University of Cincinnati, we reported a drug-free remission in 42 percent of patients and improvement in 94 percent. These results are sim-

ilar to the ones reported in other recent studies of transsternal thymectomy for myasthenia. In particular, Maggi and colleagues reported on a large series of 662 patients operated on over a 15-year period and demonstrated a remission rate of 38 percent and an improvement in 87 percent in 500 patients without thymoma. In 95 patients, Jaretzki and colleagues used a ''maximal'' approach to thymectomy, which involved exposure via both trans-

approach is generally preferable because it allows complete exposure and removal of the tumor and the entire gland. When an occult tumor is removed by this approach, the tumors are generally smaller and less likely to have invaded adjacent structures. In a series of 2097 patients with myasthenia gravis treated at the Mt. Sinai Medical Center (New York), thymomas were present in 239 (11%). Patients with occult thymomas treated with the transcervical approach had a clinical course superior to patients with tumors diagnosed before surgery and treated with the transsternal approach. Occult thymomas were accessible through the transcervical approach, with some operations necessitating a complementary median sternotomy.

Before proceeding with a transcervical thymectomy, preoperative evaluation and preparation are the same as for transsternal thymectomy. If a thymoma is diagnosed or suspected, then the transcervical approach should not be used. The patient is positioned on the operating table, prepared, and draped exactly as described for a median sternotomy, since conversion to a transsternal approach might be required if an unanticipated tumor is encountered or if the surgeon, for any reason, is not satisfied with the transcervical exposure. A transverse curvilinear incision is made between the sternocleidomastoid muscles with the midpoint of the collar incision approximately 2 cm above the sternal notch. After dividing the platysma muscle, skin flaps are developed in the avascular subplatysmal plane using electrocautery dissection. The upper skin flap is dissected to the level of the thyroid cartilage, and the lower skin flap is dissected to the sternal notch. The strap muscles are separated in the midline. The upper poles of the thymus gland are found lying immediately below the strap muscles and superficial to the inferior thyroid vessels. The en bloc dissection is begun cephalad to the brachiocephalic vein, posterior to the strap muscles, medial to the recurrent nerves, anterior to the trachea, and is terminated at the level of the thyroid isthmus. The thyroid lobes are mobilized, and thymic tissue is searched for behind and superior to the thyroid gland. It is important to identify and preserve both superior parathyroid glands since one or both inferior parathyroid glands can lie within the superior poles of the thymus gland or within accessory cervical thymic tissue and might be

included in the en bloc resection. When it is difficult to distinguish thymic tissue from a parathyroid gland, a biopsy for frozen section examination should be routinely performed.

The left superior thymic pole is isolated, dissected to its most superior point, and the branches from the inferior thyroid vessels are isolated and divided. The right upper pole is similarly mobilized. The two upper poles usually come together in the midline just above the sternal notch and anterior to the brachiocephalic vein. Once the upper poles have been fully mobilized, the cleidocleido ligament is divided vertically, and a finger is passed into the mediastinum anterior to the thymus gland for palpation and for blunt dissection of the anterior surface of the gland from the surrounding tissue. A special, narrow, right-angle retractor is passed behind the sternal notch and attached to a self-retaining apparatus for upward traction of the sternum. With the use of a headlight or a lighted suction device, the anterior mediastinum can now be well visualized with the surgeon seated on a stool at the head of the table. The superior thymic poles are then retracted forward, and the posterior portion of the gland is dissected free down to the brachiocephalic vein. The veins draining from the thymus gland into the brachiocephalic vein are identified, isolated, ligated, and divided under direct vision.

Once the thymic veins have been divided, dissection can be carried along the poste-

rior surface of the thymus gland, anterior to the brachiocephalic vein. Sharp dissection is used to separate the gland from the pericardium over the anterior surface of the ascending aorta. The remainder of the dissection is carried out using a combination of traction, sharp dissection, and electrocautery as described for the transsternal operation, beginning with the right lower pole, followed by the posterior surface of the gland, and, finally, by the left lower pole (Fig. 40-5.) If the thymus is adherent to the pleura, a portion of the pleura should be taken en bloc with the thymus gland. Care should be taken to avoid injury to the phrenic nerves. Once the thymus gland and anterior mediastinal fat are removed, the mediastinum is carefully inspected to ensure that hemostasis is satisfactory and thymectomy is complete. A chest tube is not usually required; instead a red rubber catheter is placed into the mediastinum and brought out through the incision during closure of the wound. This catheter is withdrawn after closure of the platysmal layer. The strap muscles are reapproximated in the midline with 2–0 absorbable sutures, the platysma is closed with interrupted 3–0 absorbable sutures, and the skin incision is approximated with running 4–0 subcuticular sutures.

Complete removal of the thymus via a cervical incision has been regarded by many authors as unfeasible, and studies of surgical anatomy support this view. Surgeons who use the transsternal approach claim it allows complete removal of the thymus

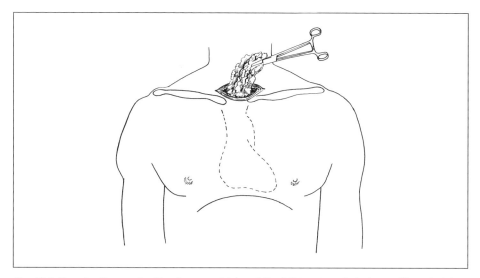

Fig. 40-5. Once the thymus gland has been completely mobilized, it is extracted via the curvilinear incision in the neck.

and believe that the transcervical approach leads to a high incidence of incomplete thymectomy. The excellent surgical anatomic studies by Jaretzki and colleagues confirm the extreme difficulty or even impossibility of performing complete thymectomy by transcervical approach alone. The incidence of failure of transcervical thymectomy has been reported to be as high as 27 percent in some series. The occasional mediastinal thymoma that develops following transcervical thymectomy, the discovery of thymoma at cervical operations with possible spreading of the tumor by incomplete resection, and the finding of two distinct thymomas of different cell type in separate mediastinal lobes are additional reasons for not favoring the transcervical approach. There is no longer much difference in morbidity and mortality between the transsternal and transcervical procedures. The cosmetic benefit of the cervical incision is offset by the lower rates of remission reported in most series involving myasthenia gravis. There are surgeons who advocate performing the transcervical procedure first with the more extensive procedure reserved for the patients whose conditions fail to improve after the initial procedure. However, such a policy might commit up to one-third of patients to persistent symptoms and repeat operations.

Thoracoscopic-Assisted Thymectomy

The debate continues between surgeons who advocate the less invasive transcervical thymectomy and surgeons who adhere to the more extensive transsternal approach. Acceptable clinical results have been reported by surgeons who are expert at their particular approach. A compromise between the more extensive exposure afforded by the sternal splitting incision and the presumed lesser morbidity of the cervical approach is video-assisted minimally invasive access to the anterior mediastinum. Thoracoscopy is useful in the diagnosis and treatment of certain anterior mediastinal disorders. Recent reports of thoracoscopic-assisted thymectomy have been limited to situations in which the extent of the resection is ensured, such as diagnostic procedures requiring adequate biopsy, and to the management of new onset myasthenia gravis in small series of patients with relatively normal thymus glands.

Several techniques for thoracoscopic-assisted thymectomy have been described. Currently, the best approach to ensure a safe and complete resection involves a combined transcervical and thoracoscopic exposure. The patient is intubated with a double lumen endotracheal tube and positioned supine on the operating table. The thymus gland is initially exposed and mobilized via a neck incision as previously described. Once the superior poles are mobilized and the veins draining into the left brachiocephalic vein are divided, the gland is dissected away from the brachiocephalic vein posteriorly and the manubrium anteriorly, is tucked down into the mediastinum, and the neck is closed.

The patient is then positioned at a 45-degree left anterolateral decubitus position, and the anterior mediastinum is approached via the left chest. Split-lung ventilation is begun, allowing the left lung to collapse. Three ports are placed in a triangular orientation at the level of the isthmus of the thymus gland, which is usually in the vicinity of the fourth or fifth interspace (Fig. 40-6). The camera port is placed laterally in the fifth intercostal space midway between the anterior axillary and the midclavicular lines. Using an angled (30° or 45°) thoracoscope, the mediastinal anatomy is assessed with the heart and pericardium providing excellent anatomic orientation. The two working ports are then placed under direct vision. The medial port is placed in the fourth or fifth interspace approximately 2 to 3 cm lateral to the sternum. The other port is placed lateral and superior to the camera port in the fourth or fifth interspace, depending on the location of the thymus. The left lobe of the thymus is mobilized by applying traction inferiorly from the lateral port and dissecting with scissors or cautery via the medial port. The lobe is elevated off the pericardium and pleura until the branches from the left internal thoracic vessels are

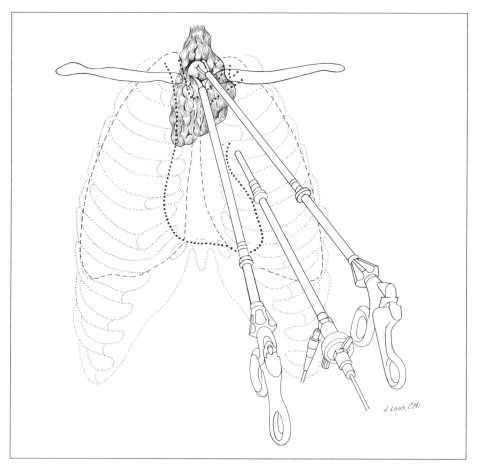

Fig. 40-6. Three thoracoscopic ports are placed at the level of the fourth or fifth interspace in a triangular orientation. The exact location of the two working ports depends on the size of the heart, the shape of the chest cavity, the position of the thymus, and any abnormalities (neoplasms) of the thymus.

identified, controlled with clips, and divided. Dissection is continued anterior to the phrenic nerve, until the previously mobilized superior pole is reached. The right lobe of the thymus is then grasped from the lateral port, pulled upward and to the left, and is dissected off the pericardium, pleura, and internal thoracic vessels in a similar manner as done on the left. When the thymus is completely mobilized, the gland can be placed in a specimen retrieval bag and removed through one of the chest incisions. One or two chest tubes are placed through the medial or lateral working port(s) and the other incision(s) are closed.

The thoracoscopic procedure is generally more time consuming and requires additional technical expertise as compared with the "open" procedures. Careful patient selection is required. The patient must be able to tolerate single lung ventilation for a prolonged period of time. At present, the technique cannot be advocated for invasive thymomas because of the risk of leaving residual tumor behind. This evolving technique holds much promise as a less invasive approach to the thymus and is particularly appealing in patients with early myasthenia gravis. However, the efficacy of this approach compared with the other two "open" methods of thymectomy has not been established and will require confirmation through larger clinical trials with adequate follow up.

Postoperative Management

Patients are usually extubated in the operating room or within 30 minutes after the conclusion of the operation. They are usually kept in the recovery room or intensive care unit overnight. Parenteral analgesia is administered as small intravenous doses of morphine or self-administered in the form of patient-controlled analgesia. Continuous infusions and large boluses of narcotic should be avoided and parenteral ketorolac can be used adjunctively for breakthrough pain. On the morning after the operation, a clear liquid diet is begun and advanced as tolerated. Patients are transferred out of the special care unit unless they require continued intensive monitoring or respiratory support. The mediastinal or chest tubes are removed when there is no air leak or significant output and the lungs are fully expanded on chest x-ray. These tubes can

usually be removed by the second postoperative day. Antibiotics are discontinued, and oral narcotic analgesics are started once the chest tubes are removed. The patients are discharged when they are taking a regular diet well. Patients with myasthenia gravis are discharged when their symptoms are adequately controlled with oral medication. Most patients are able to return to normal activity and work within 2 to 3 weeks for transsternal and within 1 to 2 weeks following transcervical and thoracoscopic thymectomy.

Postoperatively, the greatest threat to the patient's life in myasthenia gravis is weakness and fatigability of the respiratory and oral or pharyngeal musculature. Anticholinesterase medication is generally not given in the immediate postoperative period because many patients have an increased sensitivity to these drugs, poor relief of their weakness, or a decreased need for these medications. Additionally, drug toxicity can be confused with symptoms of myasthenic crisis. A postoperative myasthenic crisis is rare, but when it occurs the patient is unable to maintain an open airway free of secretions or an adequate ventilatory exchange because of failing muscle function. If the patient develops respiratory difficulties or signs of an exacerbation of myasthenic symptoms, a trial dose of edrophonium chloride should be given. If this medication results in prompt improvement in the patient's strength, small doses of a long-acting anticholinesterase drug such as pyridostigmine (approximately one-thirtieth of the oral dose) should be cautiously administered by intramuscular or very slow intravenous injection until a salutary effect is achieved. The patient should be monitored for signs of overmedication. Stress doses of intravenous hydrocortisone or ACTH (80–100 international units) should be administered in conjunction with the cholinesterase inhibitor. If such medical therapy does not result in rapid improvement, plasmapheresis should be instituted and continued daily for 3 days, then every other day until the symptoms are controlled by oral medication.

Tapering of medications in patients with myasthenia gravis begins at various times after operation, depending on the judgment of the neurologist caring for the patient. In most patients, tapering can be started in the early postoperative period. However, some patients require more

gradual attempts at weaning. This situation is particularly true for patients on large preoperative doses of steroids and patients who had long-standing symptoms before the operation. Such individuals can require anywhere from weeks to months after the operation to begin a substantial tapering in dosage. Patients who do not achieve drug-free remission by 2 years after thymectomy are unlikely to do so subsequently.

Suggested Reading

Blalock A, Mason MF, Morgan HJ, et al. Myasthenia gravis and tumors of the thymic region: Report of a case in which the tumor was removed. *Ann Surg* 110:544, 1939.

Cooper JD, Al-Jilaihawa AN, Pearson FG, et al. An improved technique to facilitate transcervical thymectomy for myasthenia gravis. *Ann Thorac Surg* 45:242, 1988.

Drachman DB. Myasthenia gravis. *N Engl J Med* 330:1797, 1994.

Fukai I, Funato Y, Mizuno T, et al. Distribution of thymic tissue in the mediastinal adipose tissue. *J Thorac Cardiovasc Surg* 101:1099, 1991.

Henze A. Biberfeld P, Christensson B, et al. Failing transcervical thymectomy in myasthenia gravis, an evaluation of transsternal re-exploration. *Scand J Thor Cardiovasc Surg* 18:235, 1984.

Jaretzki A III, Penn AS, Younger DS, et al. "Maximal" thymectomy for myasthenia gravis. *J Thorac Cardiovasc Surg* 95:747, 1988.

Kaiser LR: Video-assisted thoracic surgery: Current state of the art. *Ann Surg* 220:720, 1994.

Kirchner T, Schalke B, Buchwald J, et al. Well-differentiated thymic carcinoma: An organotypical low-grade carcinoma with relationship to cortical thymoma. *Am J Surg Pathol* 16:1153, 1992.

Kirchner T, Tzartos S. Hoppe F, et al. Pathogenesis of myasthenia gravis: Acetylcholine receptor-related antigenic determinants in tumor-free thymuses and thynmic epithelial tumors. *Am J Pathol* 130:268, 1988.

Large SR, Shneerson JM, Stovin PG, et al. Surgical pathology of the thymus: 20 years' experience. *Thorax* 41:51, 1986.

Maggi G, Casadio C, Cavallo A, et al. Thymectomy in myasthenia gravis: results of 662 cases operated upon in 15 years. *Eur J Cardiothorac Surg* 3:504, 1989.

Nussbaum MS, Rosenthal GJ, Samaha FJ, et al. Management of myasthenia gravis by extended thymectomy with anterior mediastinal dissection. *Surgery* 112:681, 1992.

Papatestas AE, Pozner J. Genkins G, et al. Prognosis in occult thymomas in myasthenia gravis following transcervical thymectomy. *Arch Surg* 122:1352, 1987.

Shimizu J, Hayashi Y, Morita K, et al. Primary thymic carcinoma: A clinicopathological and immunohistochemical study. *J Surg Oncol* 56:159, 1994.

Sugarbaker DJ. Thoracoscopy in the management of anterior mediastinal masses. *Ann Thorac Surg* 56:653, 1993.

EDITOR'S COMMENT

This chapter on thymectomy for benign tumor, myasthenia gravis, and total thymectomy for malignant thymoma does not deal with other lesions that occur in the superior or anteroinferior mediastinum. The most common lesion in the superior mediastinum is unquestionably substernal goiter, although parathyroid adenoma, bronchogenic cysts, teratoma, aneurysms, lymph nodes from lymphoma or other hematodyscrasias and lipomas are also found in this location. With the exception of substernal goiter, most are best approached through the median sternotomy, including mediastinal thymic lesions and even aortic arch branch trauma. With trauma to the superior mediastinum, it is often necessary to extend a median sternotomy into the third or fourth interspace on the appropriate side, with section of the mid-portion of the clavicle and the first four ribs, in order to turn an anatomic trap door for optimal exposure of the proximal carotid or subclavian vessels.

The thymus commonly, unlike the thyroid, lies in both the neck and mediastinum. The approach to the thymus through the neck, in which excision is sometimes used in a search for a missing parathyroid, illustrates well the difficulties with complete thymic excision through the cervical approach. In myasthenia gravis, in which complete excision of the thymus is important, the combined cervical and mediastinal approach has the advantages that the author has outlined. Thymic carcinoma is a relatively rare lesion, although it, too, can be associated with myasthenia gravis. Under no circumstances should a lesion that is suspected of being malignant be dealt with through the cervical approach, since the transsternal exposure is far superior and the lateral and sometimes convoluted extremities of the tumor can best be excised with the broadest possible exposure. As emphasized, clinical invasiveness is as important in the evaluation of a thymic tumor as is the microscopic appearance, specifically with regard to benign versus malignant varieties, since the common phenomenon seen in endocrine tumors, namely that the invasive characteristics and the histologic characteristics are not necessarily correlated, applies to the thymus as it does to other endocrine organs.

The specific approach to pre- and postoperative management of the patient with myasthenia gravis is of critical importance and has been well outlined by Dr. Nussbaum. Postoperative complications, specifically respiratory, are less common than formerly, but the cooperation between an experienced neurologist and the operating surgeon is of utmost importance to guarantee a functional airway and to maximize the pharamcologic agents and their efficacy. Myasthenic patients, like thyrotoxic patients, have a relatively narrow margin of safety, and close monitoring in the immediately postoperative period is essential to success.

R.J.B.

41

Adrenalectomy

Jon A. van Heerden   Richard T. Schlinkert

Anatomy

The adrenal glands lie within the retroperitoneum immediately superior to the kidneys. The left adrenal is bordered by the aorta medially, the left kidney and left renal vein inferiorly, and the diaphragm superiorly and laterally. The tail of the pancreas is anterior to the left adrenal. The right adrenal is bordered by the inferior vena cava medially, the right kidney inferiorly, and the diaphragm superiorly and laterally. The liver lies anterior to the right adrenal. The adrenal glands derive their blood supply from branches of the renal and inferior phrenic arteries and branches directly from the aorta. Along the surface of the adrenal, these branches make up a delicate arcade. The left adrenal venous drainage is via the left adrenal vein, which arises from the inferomedial aspect of the left adrenal and empties into the left renal vein. The right adrenal drains through the right adrenal vein, which is short and arises from the posteromedial aspect of the adrenal gland, to empty directly into the posterior lateral aspect of the inferior vena cava.

The adrenal glands are composed of two major layers: the cortex and the medulla. The cortex is subdivided into three layers: the zona glomerulosa, zona fasciculata, and zona reticularis. These layers produce aldosterone, cortisone, and sex hormones, respectively. The medulla produces epinephrine, norepinephrine, and dopamine.

Pheochromocytoma

Pheochromocytomas arise from the adrenal medulla (Table 41-1). Approximately 10 percent of tumors can also arise in extra-adrenal locations (paraganglioma). Symptoms are produced by excessive secretion of catecholamines and include spells of hypertension, which can be associated with palpitations, headache, abdominal pain, pallor, and sweating. Less commonly, a patient might present with chronic, sustained hypertension.

Diagnosis and Localization

The measurement of 24-hour urinary metanephrines provides an excellent

Table 41-1. Diagnostic Aspects, Preoperative Preparation, and Neurons Employed for the Most Common Adrenal Tumors

Pathology	Diagnosis	Preoperative Preparation	Incision
Pheochromocytoma	24-hour urinary metanephrines; fractionated urinary catecholamines	Alpha blockade; $\pm$ beta blockade; fluids	Anterior; posterior; laparoscopy
Aldosteronoma	Serum potassium; plasma resin activity; aldosterone level	Replace total body potassium	Posterior; laparoscopy
Cushing's (solitary adrenal adenoma)	Screen A.M. and P.M. cortisol; urinary free cortisol; overnight DMST* Confirm low-dose DMST Identify source high-dose DMST, ACTH level	Steroid preparation	Posterior (<5 cm); abdominal (>5 cm); laparoscopy
Carcinoma	Test Function 24-hour urinary metanephrines; cortisol A.M., P.M.; 24-hour urinary cortisol		Abdominal; thoracoabdominal
Incidentaloma	Low-dose DMST		Posterior or laparoscopic if >4 cm; no surgery if <4 cm

DMST = dexamethasone suppression test.

screening test for pheochromocytoma and will be abnormally high in the majority (approximately 98%) of patients. Measurement of fractionated urinary catecholamines (epinephrine, norepinephrine, and dopamine) is highly accurate. It is important to be familiar with medications or drugs (i.e., intravenous contrast) that can occasionally interfere with these assays.

CT of the abdomen will localize the majority of pheochromocytomas. Met-iodo-benzyl-guanidine (MIBG) scanning will provide confirmation that the visualized tumor is functioning and can aid in the localization of extra-adrenal or metastatic tumors. MRI studies will show a characteristic white tumor on the T2-weighted images but are seldom used in our practice.

Preoperative Preparation

The sudden release of catecholamines from the tumor intraoperatively can lead to severe hypertension or arrhythmias with disastrous consequences. In addition, patients with pheochromocytomas experience persistent contraction of the intravascular space because of catecholamine excess. Following removal of the tumor, sudden vasodilation can produce fatal hypotension. For these reasons, excellent preoperative preparation is essential. Initial treatment is alpha blockade (phenoxybenzamine) for 5 to 7 days to control hypertension and dilate the intravascular space. Following alpha blockade, if the patient remains tachycardic, beta blockade (e.g., propranolol) is instituted for 2 to 4 days before the operation. It is a catastrophic error to administer beta blockade first, because this agent leads to unopposed vasoconstriction and can cause acute right heart failure.

Operative Approach

Patients with pheochromocytoma can have wide swings of blood pressure intraoperatively, even if adequate preoperative preparation has been given. Therefore, all patients should be monitored with an arterial line. Central venous or pulmonary arterial catheters should be used in patients with significant cardiac disease. Hypertension is controlled with nitroprusside, and hypotension with fluid administration and dopamine. In addition, lidocaine can be used to control cardiac arrhythmias, although this complication is rare. The mild hypotension that often oc-

curs following removal of the tumor is best managed with volume expansion–reserving vasopressors for refractory hypotension.

We prefer an abdominal approach for most patients with pheochromocytoma because of the tumor's potential for malignancy (10%), multicentricity (10%), and extra-adrenal location (10%). This approach can be accomplished through a midline or subcostal incision. In select patients with small tumors (< 5 cm), which have been localized by both CT and MIBG scans, a posterior or flank incision can be appropriate. Alternatively, laparoscopy can be used.

During dissection, it is imperative that the tumor not be disturbed excessively. The surgical strategy is to dissect "the patient away from the tumor." The adrenal vein should be identified and ligated as early in the operation as possible to prevent excessive release of catecholamines. Frequently, the surgeon encounters more than one adrenal vein, making it relatively unsafe to manipulate the tumor until the gland has been extensively devascularized.

Postoperative Course

Patients who have been adequately blocked preoperatively should have a smooth postoperative course. It is not uncommon for patients to display mild hypotension (systolic blood pressure in the 90s), which invariably responds to fluid administration.

Aldosteronoma

Primary hyperaldosteronism can be caused by adrenal hyperplasia, a solitary aldosterone-secreting adenoma, and rarely an adrenocortical carcinoma. The adenomas are generally approximately 1 cm in size and are a golden-yellow. The presence of hypertension with hypokalemia in the absence of a loop diuretic should raise the clinical suspicion of primary hyperaldosteronism.

Diagnosis and Localization

Measurement of plasma renin level is an excellent screening test. An elevated plasma renin level virtually excludes the diagnosis of primary hyperaldosteronism. Further evaluation, however, depends on measurement of urinary aldosterone levels. Elevated aldosterone levels in the set-

ting of suppressed renin levels confirm the diagnosis of primary hyperaldosteronism. The differentiation between an aldosteronoma and bilateral adrenal hyperplasia is then made based on postural studies. In difficult instances in which this differentiation cannot be made, adrenal venous sampling can be of considerable help. CT scans will localize most lesions, and NP-59 scanning can be of benefit in select situations.

Preoperative Preparation

Aldactone (spironolactone) controls hypokalemia in patients with primary hyperaldosteronism. However, the long-term side effects of this medication, as well as the frequent need for multiple antihypertensive medications, make an operation the preferred option for patients with an aldosteronoma. Patients with bilateral adrenal hyperplasia are best managed medically. Before the operation, the patient's serum potassium levels should be returned to normal, and attempts should be made to replenish the patient's total body potassium store adequately.

Operative Approach

The small size and benign nature of aldosteronomas allow for removal using either a posterior or laparoscopic approach. Indeed, these tumors are ideal to approach early in the surgeon's experience with the evolving technique of laparoscopic adrenalectomy.

Postoperative Course

Patients can be discharged within 24 hours of laparoscopic adrenalectomy or within 4 to 5 days after an open adrenalectomy. Biochemical disturbances are few, and the patient's serum potassium level should return to normal rapidly. Hypertension might resolve. However, there can still be a need for antihypertensive medications, although the number and dosages are usually reduced.

Cushing's Syndrome

Cushing's syndrome represents the physical manifestations of the endogenous overproduction or excessive exogenous intake of glucocorticoids. It is characterized by typical features, including a moon facies, truncal obesity, abdominal and thigh stria, hirsutism, muscle weakness, acne, and the presence of a "buffalo hump." Mild hypertension is common. Cushing's disease represents the overproduction of glucocorticoids secondary to a pituitary adenoma, and this is beyond the scope of this chapter.

Diagnosis and Localization

Screening tests for Cushing's include A.M. and P.M. cortisol levels (showing elevation or lack of diurnal variation), urinary free cortisol levels, and an overnight dexamethasone suppression test evaluating the adrenocorticotropic hormone (ACTH) axis. A low-dose dexamethasone suppression test is then used to confirm the diagnosis of Cushing's syndrome. A high-dose dexamethasone suppression test identifies pituitary Cushing's. ACTH levels differentiate ectopic production of ACTH (markedly elevated levels) from a primary adrenal source (low levels of ACTH). Localization of adrenal tumors is accomplished with a CT scan, and radionucleotide scanning with NP-59 can be beneficial in select situations.

Preoperative Preparation

Patients with Cushing's syndrome might be unable to respond to a stressful situation with an appropriate response of glucocorticoid secretion. Therefore, it is reasonable to give patients a steroid preparation preoperatively (i.e., 40 mg Solumedrol intravenously). Electrolyte disturbances, if present, require correction preoperatively. Careful attention to the details of physically handling a patient is essential, because these patients' skin is invariably thin and easily injured. Heavy adhesive tape is to be avoided on the operative incision.

Operative Approach

Small- to moderate-sized tumors and bilateral hyperplasia not amenable to hypophysectomy are managed through a posterior approach. Laparoscopy can also be considered. Large carcinomas presenting with Cushing's syndrome should be approached transabdominally or through a thoracoabdominal incision.

Postoperative Course

Patients should be continued on a steroid taper until normal adrenal function returns. If a bilateral adrenalectomy has been performed, replacement of both glu-

cocorticoid and mineralocorticoid will be required.

Adrenocortical Carcinoma

Cancers of the adrenal gland can be either functioning or nonfunctioning, and often these tumors secrete more than one hormone. The rapid onset of symptoms related to overproduction of adrenocortical hormones should be a tipoff to the diagnosis. Conversely, tumors can be nonfunctioning and present with pain or a mass.

Preoperative considerations are similar to the ones for other functioning adrenal tumors. Curative resection can be feasible for localized disease. Palliative resections can prove beneficial in select patients with functioning tumors to decrease symptoms of hormonal excess. Most adrenocortical carcinomas are large (mean diameter approximately 12.0 cm) at the time of diagnosis, suggesting an advanced stage of the disease. This situation is reflected in the almost universal poor long-term prognosis of these patients.

Incidentaloma

Many patients harbor unsuspected adrenal tumors that are found incidentally dur-

ing a CT scan performed for nonadrenal reasons. Tumors less than 4 cm that have been shown to be nonfunctional can be safely observed with repeat CT scans at 6 and 12 months. Tumors greater than 4 cm should probably be removed, because the incidence of cancer rises as tumor size increases.

Technique

The adrenal gland can be approached through a variety of incisions (Fig. 41-1), and the appropriate choice of a procedure is based on the size, biologic behavior, and biochemical profile of the adrenal tumor. In general, small tumors measuring less than 5 cm in size can be approached through a posterior or flank incision. Larger tumors need to be approached transabdominally with a thoracoabdominal incision (rarely) reserved for the largest tumors. Pheochromocytomas, although small tumors, are often approached transabdominally to allow exploration of the abdominal cavity, as well as the opposite adrenal gland, and to minimize tumor manipulation. With the high quality of CT scans and the functional MIBG studies, a posterior approach can be used for select patients with pheochromocytomas. The role of laparoscopic surgery is not clearly defined. However, this

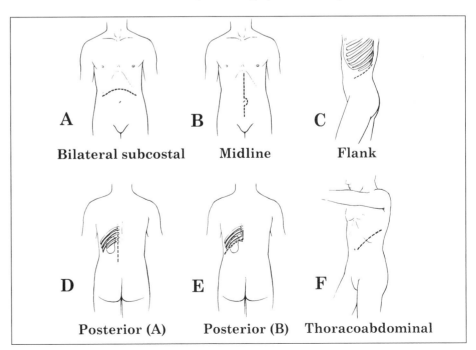

| A | B | C |
| Bilateral subcostal | Midline | Flank |

| D | E | F |
| Posterior (A) | Posterior (B) | Thoracoabdominal |

Fig. 41-1. Potential incisions for adrenalectomy.

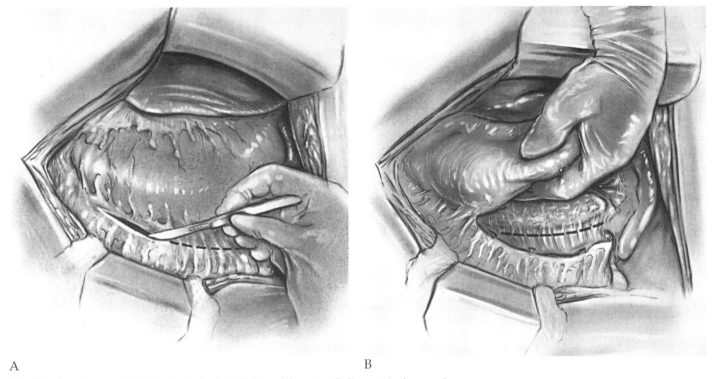

A   B

Fig. 41-2. Anterior approach to left adrenal gland. A. Division of the gastrocolic ligament in the avascular plane. B. Division of the peritoneum inferior to the pancreas.

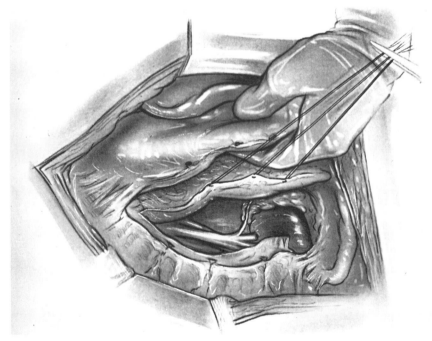

Fig. 41-3. Anterior left adrenalectomy. The pancreas is reflected superiorly to expose the left adrenal.

procedure does appear to be a reasonable approach for small benign tumors of the adrenal gland or for benign hyperplasia of the adrenal glands in patients with Cushing's disease following failed transsphenoidal hypophysectomy.

Abdominal Incisions

The abdomen can be explored through either a bilateral subcostal or a midline incision. The left adrenal gland is exposed by reflecting the splenic flexure of the colon inferiorly and dividing the attachments of the omentum to the transverse mesocolon (Fig. 41-2A). This step allows entry into the lesser sac and exposure of the inferior border of the pancreas. The peritoneum in this region is opened (Fig. 41-2B), as is Gerota's fascia, and the pancreas and superior aspect of Gerota's fascia are retracted anterosuperiorly. The kidney is retracted inferiorly to allow exposure of the left adrenal gland (Fig. 41-3). The left adrenal vein exits the adrenal on its inferomedial aspect and should be ligated initially when resecting a pheochromocytoma. The gland is then dissected from surrounding tissue. In general, if dissection is carried along the surface of the adrenal, only small vessels will be encountered, which can be controlled using electrocautery or, in some instances, clips or ligatures. The anterior and posterior surfaces of the adrenal are essentially avascular. Dissection of the upper pole of the adrenal can be facilitated by leaving the attachments between the adrenal and superior pole of the kidney intact and retracting the kidney inferiorly. This maneuver allows the adrenal gland to be pulled inferiorly. For larger tumors of the left adrenal gland, it might be necessary to mobilize the spleen and tail of the pancreas (Fig. 41-4). After mobilization of the splenic flexure, as described previously, the lienophrenic ligament is divided, and the avascular plane posterior to the spleen and pancreas is developed. This step allows exposure of the anterior surface of the adrenal gland, which is then dissected from surrounding tissue, as described above.

Exposure of the right adrenal gland is obtained by reflecting the hepatic flexure of the colon inferiorly. The duodenum is kocherized (Fig. 41-5A) to expose the vena cava, and the inferolateral peritoneal attachments of the liver are divided. Traction is placed inferiorly on the kidney to allow visualization of the adrenal gland. On the right side, the adrenal vein is short and drains from the posteromedial aspect of the adrenal directly into the vena cava (Fig. 41-5B). Again, this vein should be ligated and divided early in the dissection of a pheochromocytoma.

During abdominal procedures for pheochromocytoma, the periaortic region must be carefully explored to rule out accessory tumors. This step has become less important with the excellence of current preoperative roentgenographic localizing modalities.

Posterior Approach

For the posterior approach, the patient is placed prone on two chest rolls. The hips are supported on a pillow and the legs are bent at the knees. The lower rib cage should be located in the area of the kidney rest or the break in the operating table to allow increased exposure, if necessary. An incision is made along the course of the twelfth rib with a superior extension medially, or alternatively a vertical incision can be performed (Fig. 41-1D, E). The twelfth rib is exposed and the periosteum

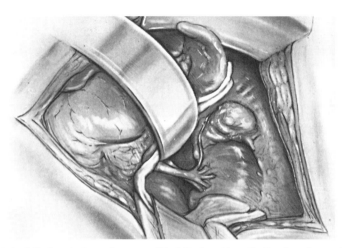

Fig. 41-4. Anterior left adrenalectomy. Exposure of the left adrenal by reflecting the spleen and tail of the pancreas medially.

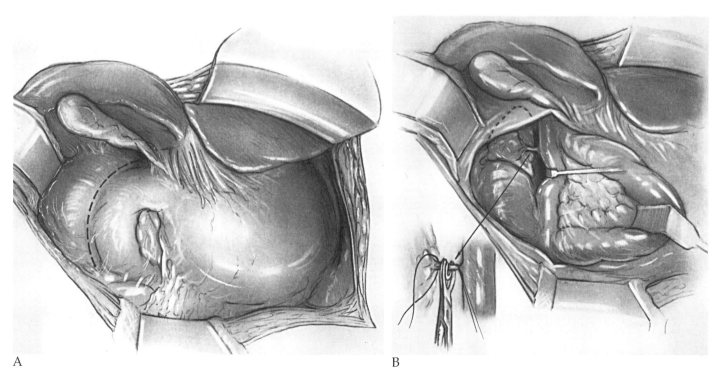

A   B

Fig. 41-5. Anterior right adrenalectomy. A. The duodenum is kocherized. B. The adrenal is exposed with the short right adrenal vein.

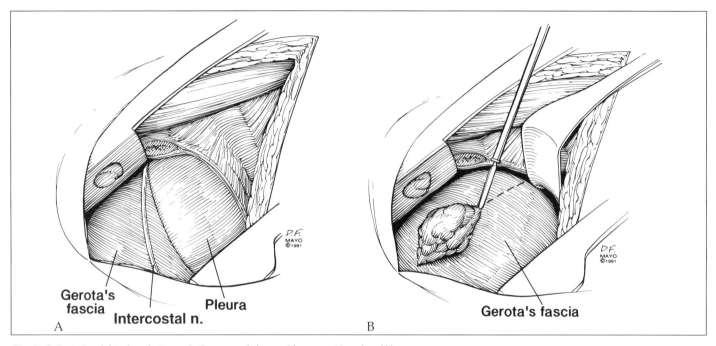

Fig. 41-6. Posterior right adrenalectomy. A. Exposure of pleura with preservation of twelfth nerve.
B. Division of Gerota's fascia.

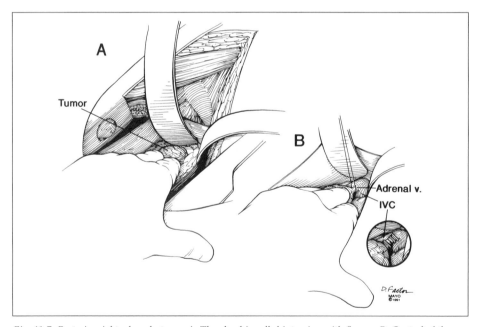

Fig. 41-7. Posterior right adrenalectomy. A. The gland is pulled into view with fingers. B. Control of the
right adrenal vein.

hands and sweeping the tissues inferiorly using gauze sponges, dissection is carried in the direction of the diaphragmatic hiatus and the adrenal exposed (Fig. 41-7). Again, dissection is carried along the surface of the adrenal and the gland removed. Closure is performed in layers using absorbable sutures, with particular attention to preservation of the neurovascular bundles. It is not uncommon to create a small hole in the pleura during dissection, and this hole can be dealt with at the conclusion of the procedure by closing the incision over a small catheter placed in the pleural space. Following closure of the muscles and subcutaneous tissues, the catheter is placed under a water seal and the lungs inflated. When the air leak stops, the catheter is removed. There is no need for chest tube placement on these occasions.

In select instances in which a slightly larger tumor needs to be excised, a flank incision can be used. The patient is placed in a lateral decubitus position, and an incision made along the twelfth rib. Dissection is carried out in a similar manner to the posterior approach; however, the incision is somewhat larger. The direction of this incision, as well as the larger size, allows the surgeon to place both hands into the incision for adequate mobilization.

elevated. It is imperative that the intercostal nerves be preserved during this resection. The rib is dissected as far medially as possible, and the rib excised preserving the periosteum. The paraspinous muscles are left intact. The lower portion of the diaphragm with the pleura along its superior surface is now exposed (Fig. 41-6A). The pleura is dissected free from the diaphragm and reflected superiorly. The diaphragm can then be incised and Gerota's fascia exposed. Gerota's fascia is opened and the fatty tissues in this region reflected inferiorly (Fig. 41-6B). By alternating

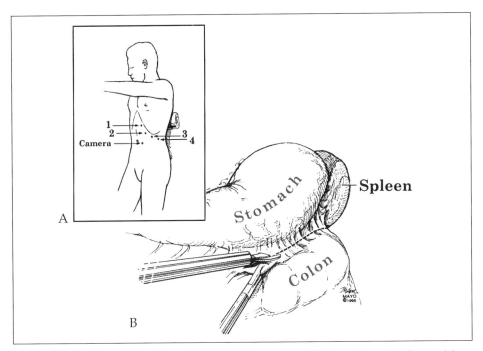

Fig. 41-8. Laparoscopic left adrenalectomy. A. Port placement. B. Mobilization of the splenic flexure of the colon.

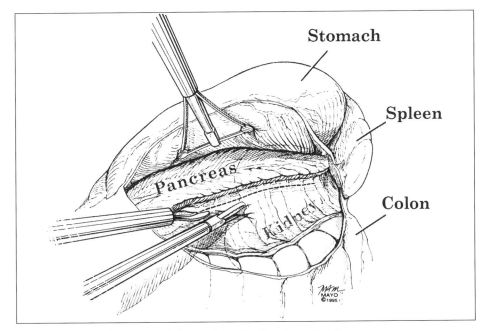

Fig. 41-9. Laparoscopic exposure of left adrenal. Mobilization of the tail of the pancreas.

Thoracoabdominal

The patient is placed in a supine position with a roll under the thorax to be incised. An incision is made along the tenth rib and extended onto the abdominal cavity. The incision is deepened through the subcutaneous tissues and muscular layers, and a portion of the costal cartilage is excised. This step prevents the edges of the costal margins from rubbing against each other after closure, which can lead to significant patient discomfort. On entering the chest through the ninth or tenth interspace, the lung is reflected superiorly and the diaphragm exposed. The diaphragm is di-

vided peripherally in a circumferential manner. On the left side, the spleen and tail of the pancreas are reflected anteriorly. On the right side, the triangular ligament of the right lobe of the liver is divided, and the liver is reflected medially. This incision is generally reserved for large adrenocortical carcinomas. Tissue surrounding an adrenal carcinoma should be removed in continuity with the gland. If the tumor is invading adjacent structures, they can be removed with the specimen.

Laparoscopic Adrenalectomy

The indications for laparoscopic adrenalectomy are, as yet, not fully delineated. Certainly, the technique is feasible and early results are encouraging for the removal of small adrenal tumors. The safety of this procedure has to date not been documented in a large number of patients. Despite these shortcomings, patients can frequently be discharged within 24 hours of laparoscopic surgery, and further cautious testing is warranted. Because of the relative infrequency with which this procedure has been performed, the ideal techniques have yet to be determined.

The left adrenal gland can be approached with the patient in the lateral position with a roll under the left rib cage (Fig. 41-8A). Carbon dioxide is insufflated through a needle inserted through the umbilicus and four trocars are placed around the left costal margin. A fifth trocar is placed to the left side of the umbilicus and is used for the camera location. Dissection is carried out as described for a transabdominal left adrenalectomy. The splenic flexure of the colon is mobilized inferiorly (Fig. 41-8B), and the omentum is removed from the transverse colon for a short distance. The peritoneum along the inferior surface of the pancreas and Gerota's fascia are opened, and they are retracted anteriorly and superiorly with a fan-type retractor inserted through the highest subcostal port (Fig. 41-9). A fan retractor is placed through the most lateral port to provide inferior traction on the kidney. The two medial subcostal ports are used by the surgeon for dissection. The adrenal gland and the left adrenal vein come into view, and the adrenal vein can be divided between clips or ligatures (Fig. 41-10). The gland is then mobilized from surrounding tissues using electrocautery and clips for hemo-

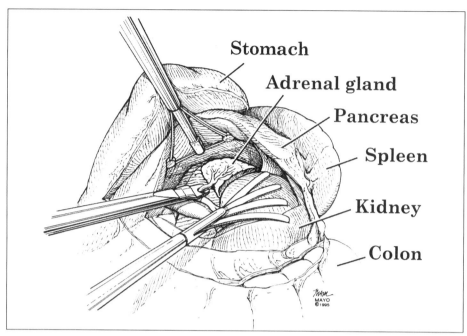

Fig. 41-10. Laparoscopic left adrenalectomy. Division of the left adrenal vein. Note the inferior traction on the left kidney.

Suggested Reading

Gagner M, Lacroix A, Prinz RA, et al. Early experience with laparoscopic approach for adrenalectomy. *Surgery* 114:1120, 1993.

Gajraj H, Young AE. Adrenal incidentaloma. *Br J Surg* 80:422, 1993.

Herrera MF, Grant CS, van Heerden J, et al. Incidentally discovered adrenal tumors: An institutional perspective. *Surgery* 110:1014, 1991.

Kaye TB, Crapo L. The Cushing syndrome: An update on diagnostic tests. *Anns Intern Med* 112:434, 1990.

Ross NS, Aron DC. Hormonal evaluation of the patient with an incidentally discovered adrenal mass. *N Engl J Med* 323:1401, 1990.

Sheps SG, Jiang N-S, Klee GG, et al. Recent developments in the diagnosis and treatment of pheochromocytoma. *Mayo Clin Proc* 65:88, 1990.

Stein PP, Black HR. A simplified diagnostic approach to pheochromocytoma: A review of the literature and report of one institution's experience. *Medicine* 70:46, 1990.

van Heerden J. Bilateral Anterior Adrenalectomy. In RA Malt (ed.), *Surgical Techniques Illustrated*. Boston: Little, Brown, 1978. Pp 43–50.

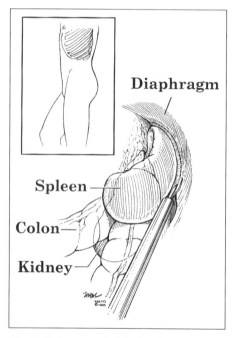

Fig. 41-11. Laparoscopic left adrenalectomy. Exposure of the left adrenal by dividing lienophrenic and lienorenal ligaments with the patient in the right lateral decubitus position.

stasis. Once the gland is completely freed, it is placed in a small plastic bag, and the open end of the bag is delivered through one of the incisions. The incision might need to be enlarged slightly to allow removal of the adrenal gland. The left upper quadrant is irrigated to reduce the incidence of left shoulder pain postoperatively, and trocars are removed under direct vision. The incisions are closed in layers using absorbable sutures. Alternatively, the patient can be placed in the right lateral decubitus position. From this approach, the splenic flexure is mobilized (Fig. 41-11), and the lienophrenic ligament is divided. The spleen and tail of the pancreas are reflected anteriorly to expose the adrenal gland.

For a right-sided laparoscopic adrenalectomy, the patient is placed in the left lateral decubitus position. Trocars are placed, and the triangular ligament of the right lobe of the liver is mobilized. This step allows the liver to drop out of the way medially with the effect of gravity. The adrenal vein and vena cava can then be exposed and the adrenal removed as described previously. Again, irrigation of the right upper quadrant is performed. Trocars are removed under direct vision and the incisions closed in layers using absorbable sutures.

Because of the theoretical possibility of significant hemorrhage during laparoscopic adrenalectomy, instrumentation to perform a laparotomy must be available and open at the time of laparoscopic surgery.

EDITOR'S COMMENT

As an international authority on surgery of the endocrines, Dr. van Heerden's very important contribution summarizes the required work-up and preparation of patients for surgery for adrenal disease. He and Dr. Schlinkert emphasize the importance of understanding the anatomy, particularly the blood supply, of these small but vital organs. The reader is referred to Chapter 35, by Dr. Grant, detailing the anatomy of the adrenal glands. The average general surgeon seldom encounters patients with indications for adrenalectomy, unilateral or bilateral, but surgeons with a special interest in surgical endocrine disease operate on patients with pheochromocytoma, particularly, often enough to have an abiding interest in the technical considerations.

Pheochromocytomas can produce both epinephrine and norepinephrine, as well as dopamine. There can be a predominance of one hormone over the others. Most of these lesions produce an excess of norepinephrine, but most require both alpha-adrenergic blockade as well as beta blockade. Oral phenoxybenzamine is almost invariably the initial drug used, although beta blockade with propranolol can be required for persistent tachycardia for several days before the operation, or occasionally during and for several days postoperatively. It is important to have these patients appropriately monitored or in the intensive care unit in the immediately preoperative and postoperative periods, for at least 24 hours, because the patients are prone to sudden, precipitous hypotension or even arrhythmias and heart failure. The use of exogenous catechol to maintain blood pressure can always be minimized or avoided entirely with fluid loading. It is wise to monitor patients preoperatively, and our preference is to use a pulmonary artery catheter with wedge pressure monitoring to assess most effectively intravascular volume and then to fluid load the patient based on the comprehensive data accumulation that this device allows. Obviously, a monitoring unit or monitored step down bed is necessary in both the preoperative and postoperative periods.

Aldosterone-producing tumors or bilateral adrenal hyperplasia with high aldosterone levels are rare indications for adrenalectomy. Patients with these conditions are characterized as having weakness, hypertension, and hypokalemia. Conn's syndrome, as this lesion was known, is characteristic of hyperaldosteronism, since aldosterone causes reabsorption of sodium and water from the renal tubule and inhibits reabsorption of potassium from the tubule. The lesions are almost invariably benign, and the adrenal size is usually unremarkable, making these lesions simpler to deal with surgically than Cushing's syndrome. The authors have summarized the common findings in Cushing's syndrome. In addition, there is hyperglycemia, usually interpreted as diabetes, a function of the profound wasting of protein caused by the action of cortisol, converting protein to carbohydrate. With the exception of adrenal carcinoma, the surgical challenge is greatest among the various surgical diseases of the adrenal because of the truncal obesity, which is frequently formidable. Therefore, many experienced endocrine surgeons prefer to approach patients with Cushing's syndrome through the posterolateral or posterior approach. Although there is a large amount of fat necessitating a somewhat longer incision, once the adrenal gland is approached, the dissection is far less difficult than when retracting other viscera and coping with a heavy omentum and other large fat deposits.

Most adrenocortical carcinomas are nonfunctioning and rapidly growing. When functional, the symptoms are rapid in onset and of short duration, since the tumors grow at an extremely rapid rate. Surgical cure of symptomatic adrenocortical carcinoma is not common, but palliative resections should always be attempted. When pain is the presenting complaint, it is not uncommon for these patients, regardless of surgical attack, to be dead of rampant disease in a matter of months.

The adrenal gland is a frequent site of metastases from other primary cancers, most commonly from the lung or breast. These metastases are often bilateral and represent absolute evidence for far advanced metastatic disease, which is difficult to treat with radiation or chemotherapy. When an adrenal lesion is discovered, metastases should be suspected. Bilateral adrenal enlargements can be subjected to fine-needle aspiration cytology to identify malignant cells and prevent a needless adrenalectomy.

Adrenal surgery has arrived at the new era, as has much of abdominal surgery, with the advent of laparoscopic surgical techniques that allow removal of all but very large glands. As instrumentation improves almost daily, appropriate instruments to simplify and make this approach more practical will be forthcoming. Nevertheless, despite the longer operative time required to excise the adrenal, as is the case with other organs, the prospect of being able to discharge a relatively pain-free patient with unilateral, or even bilateral, adrenalectomy in 48 hours is a very exciting prospect.

R.J.B.

42

Surgical Approach to Pancreatic Islet Cell Tumors

Thomas F. Wood   Edward Passaro, Jr.

Pancreatic islet cell tumors are rare lesions that cause clinical syndromes related to the endocrine hormones that they secrete. These tumors include gastrinomas, insulinomas, glucagonomas, vasoactive intestinal polypeptideoma (VIPomas), somatostatinomas, pancreatic polypeptideomas (PPomas), and nonfunctional (nonsecretory) islet cell tumors. Of these tumors gastrinomas and insulinomas are by far the most common, and together make up the large majority of pancreatic endocrine cell tumors. Therefore, we will present in depth surgical strategies for gastrinomas and insulinomas while emphasizing important considerations for the less common pancreatic endocrine tumors.

Pathophysiology

The clinical syndromes caused by pancreatic endocrine tumors are dependent on the cell type and the resultant hormone excess (Table 42-1). The origin of the pancreatic islets is uncertain. One theory is that they arise from pluripotent periductal cells throughout the pancreas. If tumors were to arise from these cells, their expected distribution in the pancreas would be equal. However, pancreatic endocrine tumors can be clustered into two groups depending upon which side of the superior mesenteric artery (SMA) they are found. Gastrinomas, somatostatinomas, and PPomas are found on the right side of the SMA in 75 percent of cases while insulinomas and glucagonomas are found to the left of the SMA in a similar proportion. This observation implies that these tumors may orig-

inate from differentially distributed precursors.

Gastrinoma

The syndrome of acid hypersecretion, peptic ulcers, and pancreatic islet cell tumor was first described in 1955 by Zollinger and Ellison. The Zollinger-Ellison syndrome (ZES) results from hypergastrinemia that is often refractory to conventional medical therapy. Ulcers seen in ZES can be multiple and located from the gastrum to the proximal jejunum. Diarrhea can result from the acid hypersecretion.

Diagnosis

The diagnosis of gastrinoma is based on an elevated basal gastrin level (>200 pg/ml), basal acid secretion (>10 meq/hr), and a paradoxical rise in gastrin after stimulation by intravenous infusion of secretin (elevation of 200 pg/ml or twofold increase of gastrin). Once the diagnosis of gastrinoma is confirmed, it must be determined whether the gastrinoma is sporadic versus part of the inherited multiple endocrine neoplasia type I (MEN-I) syndrome. Twenty-five percent of patients with gastrinoma will have the associated multiglandular (pancreatic endocrine, pituitary,

Table 42-1. Synopsis of Pancreatic Islet Cell Tumor Syndromes.

Tumor/Syndrome	Cell Type	Symptoms	Diagnostic Studies
Gastrinoma (Zollinger-Ellison)	G	Acid hypersecretion, diarrhea, ulcers	Secretin stimulation, basal acid output, endoscopy
Insulinoma	Beta	Hypoglycemia, mental status changes, adrenergic symptoms	Insulin/glucose ratio, C peptide, 72-hr fast
Somatostatinoma	Delta	Diabetes, gallstones, steatorrhea, hypochlorhydria, weight loss	Somatostatin
Glucagonoma	Alpha	Diabetes, weight loss, rash	Glucose tolerance, arginine test
VIPoma (WDHA, Verner-Morrison)	Delta$_1$	Watery diarrhea, hypokalemia, achlorhydria	VIP
Pancreatic polypeptideoma	F (PP)	Diarrhea, abdominal pain, weight loss; often asymptomatic	PP level
Nonsecretory tumor	?	Mass effect or found serendipitously	Negative RIA for known hormones

WDHA = watery diarrhea, hypokalemia, achlorhydria; RIA = radioimmunoassay.

and parathyroid tumors) involvement of MEN-I. Family history may reveal peptic ulcer disease or symptoms of hyperparathyroidism. Ionized serum calcium and parathyroid hormone levels are checked to rule out parathyroid hyperplasia, while prolactin levels are useful to determine pituitary involvement.

Localization

Preoperative localization of gastrinomas is a topic of controversy. Computed tomographic scan of the abdomen is commonly the first localization study performed. Quite often (75%), however, no tumor is found by CT. The utility of CT and MRI scanning is to exclude liver metastases. Although some authorities advocate portovenous sampling with or without secretin stimulation, we have not found it to be especially helpful (Table 42-2).

Table 42-2. Pancreatic Islet Cell Localizing Modalities and Sensitivities

Modality	Localization Sensitivity (%)
Ultrasound	25–50
CT scan	25–60
PVS–gastrinoma	50–65
PVS–insulinoma	60–80
Angiography	
Insulinoma	60–80
Secretin	>80
Octreotide scan	>80

PVS = portovenous sampling.

A new localization test we use that appears helpful is the octreotide uptake scan. Radiolabeled octreotide, a somatostatin analog, is injected intravenously and gamma ray scans are taken 24 to 48 hours later. Gastrinomas, more than other pancreatic endocrine tumors, have high concentrations of somatostain receptors on their cells' surface. Areas with increased uptake (i.e., high concentration of somatostatin receptors) appear "hot" on the scan (Fig. 42-1). Frequently, gastrinomas not seen on CT scan will be shown on octreotide scan. Several series have reported that gastrinomas can be localized by the octreotide scan in 80 to 100 percent of cases. In patients with MEN-I and recurrent elevation of serum gastrin, we believe that it is important to image not only the abdomen but also the neck since we have treated patients with recurrent parathyroid disease manifested as a "hot" spot in the neck.

Indications for Operation

Surgical resection represents the only chance for cure in patients with pancreatic endocrine tumors. In gastrinoma, patients can be cured after excision of a pancreatic tumor (or tumors) in lymph nodes. As many as 80 percent of patients with sporadic gastrinomas can be clinically cured with operation. Exploration for resection of tumor is appropriate except in cases of extensive metastatic disease to the liver.

Although the reported cure rate for ZES in MEN-I is only in the range of 10 percent, we recommend operation on these pa-

tients to decrease the risk of ulcer diathesis–related complications. Surgical correction of hyperparathyroidism, if present, should precede attempts at gastrinoma resection. Serum gastrin levels may decrease or normalize, or both, after parathyroidectomy in patients with the MEN-I syndrome. These patients have multiple pancreatic tumors and it is difficult to determine which of these are functional and responsible for the disease. Therefore, the octreotide scan may be important to show the surgeon which tumors are gastrinomas.

Preoperative Considerations

In patients with gastrinomas, preoperative antacid therapy with either H$_2$ blockers or omeprazole is given. Patients with active ulcers should be given at least 6 weeks of medical therapy to allow ulcers to begin healing before operation.

Operative Technique

We prefer an upper midline incision although a bilateral subcostal incision can be used. If hepatic lesions are present, frozen sections are taken. If positive for metastatic tumor, these can be resected if they are few and small and if it is technically feasible. If multiple large metastases are present, the decision must be made as to whether to perform palliative total gastrectomy. In general, we perform total gastrectomy in patients whose disease has been refractory to medical therapy; otherwise, these pa-

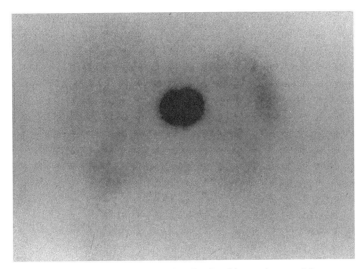

Fig. 42-1. Octreotide scan demonstrating the signal from a 1-cm gastrinoma on the surface of the head of the pancreas. This tumor was missed by CT scan but was easily found at exploration.

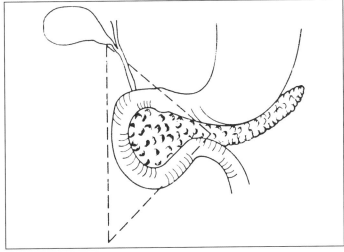

Fig. 42-2. The gastrinoma triangle. (From BE Stabile, DJ Morrow, E Passaro. The gastrinoma triangle: Operative implications. Am J Surg 147:25–31, 1984. With permission.)

tients' symptoms are controlled with either H₂ blockers or omeprazole. In selected patients, referral for orthotopic liver transplantation can be considered, as death is most often secondary to liver failure from extensive intrahepatic tumor growth, but not widespread tumor growth. Because of the general slow progression of gastrinomas, patients can have a chance at increased survival with removal of the liver and tumor burden.

If no hepatic lesions are present, the remainder of the abdomen is explored, with concentration on the most common locations of gastrinomas. Eighty-five percent of gastrinomas occur in the "gastrinoma triangle," an anatomic area bounded by the junction of the cystic and common bile ducts superiorly, the junction of the second and third portions of the duodenum inferiorly, and the junction of the neck and body of the pancreas medially (Fig. 42-2). Our experience has also shown that 85 percent of sporadic gastrinomas are located to the right of the superior mesenteric artery, which is distinct from insulinomas and glucagonomas, which occur most frequently on the left side of these vessels. It should also be kept in mind that a large number of gastrinomas (40%) are located in extrapancreatic locations while insulinomas are almost exclusively intrapancreatic. In females, palpation of the pelvic organs is performed to rule out rare ectopic locations of tumors such as ovarian gastrinomas, particularly in the right ovary. With careful exploration, more than 80 percent of gastrinomas can be found and excised at operation even if no tumor is localized preoperatively. This is accomplished by careful search and removal of not only obvious tumor(s), but all lymph nodes found in the region.

With these caveats in mind, a diligent search for the gastrinoma is undertaken. The lesser sac is sharply opened by incision of the avascular plane between the colon and omentum. With this exposure of the pancreas, a wide Kocher's maneuver is performed with scissors or electrocautery to completely mobilize the head of the pancreas. Any masses that are discovered by direct vision or palpation are excised and submitted for frozen section. Most gastrinomas (80–90%) are found around or on the surface of the pancreas and only rarely within the pancreas. Therefore, most of these tumors easily "shell out" and simple enucleation using electrocau-

tery is performed. If the tumor is large, located in the head of the pancreas, and enucleation not possible, then a formal resection (pancreaticoduodenectomy) is performed. Any lymph nodes found in the triangle, as well as any other enlarged or suspicious nodes outside the area, are excised. Once all masses in the triangle have been excised, further exploration of the omentum, porta hepatis, splenic hilum, celiac axis, and root of the mesentery is performed for either obvious tumor or lymph nodes. Confirmation of tumor within a lymph node ("nodal" gastrinoma) is easily performed by frozen section.

Intraoperative duodenoscopy with transillumination is then performed to look for duodenal wall gastrinomas. The jejunum at the ligament of Treitz is gently occluded temporarily so that the duodenum can be distended. The endoscope is guided through the duodenum with the assistance of the surgeon. The operating theater lights are turned off and the duodenum is systematically transilluminated circumferentially from the ligament of Treitz to the pylorus as the endoscope is withdrawn. Duodenal tumors as small as 2 to 3 mm in diameter can be found by this method. Duodenal tumors can be simply wedge excised in a longitudinal direction. Full-thickness excision need not be performed unless the tumor extends to the mucosal layer. The wedge defect then can be repaired anatomically in one or two layers. In general, we do not perform routine formal duodenotomies to look for tumors. If, after excision, there is concern about pancreatic or duodenal leakage, a soft Silastic closed suction drain is placed.

With a thorough exploration, gastrinomas can be found at operation in greater than 80 percent of patients who carry that diagnosis. In those patients in whom primary gastrinomas cannot be found, we do not perform blind or "prophylactic" distal or subtotal pancreatectomy or pancreaticoduodenectomy. With current pharmacologic agents (H₂ blockers and omeprazole), the hypersecretion of acid in these patients can usually be controlled. Total gastrectomy is reserved for the patient in whom medical management has failed, either after unsuccessful tumor extirpation, or in the patient with extensive unresectable tumor burden. Total gastrectomy is a well-tolerated procedure after which patients can still enjoy a good quality of life.

Postoperative Considerations

Fasting and secretin stimulation gastrin levels are checked one month postoperatively. If these are normal, they should be rechecked in 6 to 12 months to assess for tumor recurrence.

If full abdominal exploration fails to localize the gastrinoma or if postoperative gastrin levels remain elevated, then medical therapy is continued. Because of the general slow progression of this disease, patients can be maintained on medical therapy for extended periods. The usefulness of repeating localization studies or exploration must be weighed by the surgeon on a case-by-case basis. The patient's best chance of cure is a thorough exploration with complete tumor resection.

Insulinoma

Insulinoma is the second most common pancreatic islet cell tumor. The majority of patients with insulinoma present with neuropsychiatric symptoms related to hypoglycemia. Symptoms include altered mental status, blurred vision, and adrenergic symptoms of sweating, palpitation, nervousness, and weakness related to insulin excess. Whipple's triad consists of mental status changes related to fasting, serum glucose level less than 50 mg/dl, and prompt relief of symptoms with glucose ingestion.

Insulinomas are usually small (< 1.5 cm diameter), solitary, benign, and intrapancreatic. Three-fourths of insulinomas are located left of the SMA. Insulinoma is part of the MEN-I syndrome in only about 5 percent of patients. Extrapancreatic insulinomas are exceedingly rare.

Diagnosis

The presence of an insulinoma is confirmed by a fasting insulin-glucose ratio of greater than 0.3 (μU per ml/mg% glucose) in conjunction with elevated C-peptide levels. Provocation tests are rarely needed for this diagnosis.

Localization

Insulinomas are most frequently embedded within the pancreatic parenchyma. However, since insulinomas are commonly small in size, CT scans are often uninformative. Arteriography and porto-venous sampling may be helpful. Recent reports have shown that intraoperative ultrasound (IOUS), along with manual palpation at operation, can localize greater than 90 percent of tumors. In fact, some authorities recommend reserving arteriography and portovenous sampling for reoperative cases.

Indications for Operation

Almost all (75–95%) patients with insulinomas can be cured by tumor excision. Because the symptoms of the insulinoma syndrome are life threatening, we recommend an aggressive operative approach in these patients.

Preoperative Considerations

Preoperative and intraoperative glucose control are crucial and insertion of an arterial catheter facilitates easy, serial glucose monitoring during operation.

Operative Technique

As with gastrinoma, either an upper midline or bilateral subcostal incision can be performed. After thorough exploration of the abdomen, the lesser sac is opened to expose the pancreas. A wide Kocher's maneuver is then performed. If the tumor is not evident, the body and tail of the pancreas can be mobilized by careful incision of its inferior peritoneal attachments. Unlike gastrinomas, 75 percent of insulinomas lie to the left of the superior mesenteric artery. The entire pancreas is palpated bimanually. If the tumor is still not localized, then IOUS can be used with attention given to the relationship of the tumor to the pancreatic duct.

Once the tumor has been found, simple enucleation with electrocautery is performed. Insulinomas, like gastrinomas, often are encapsulated and a plane of dissection can be developed directly adjacent to the tumor. Care is taken not to injure the pancreatic duct if it is in proximity to the tumor. Pancreatic resection is considered if the tumor is large in size or has infiltrating characteristics.

Postoperative Considerations

With tumor excision, the insulin and glucose levels should become normal. If no insulinoma is found at operation, or the patient remains hypoglycemic, arteriography and portovenous sampling should be considered if they were not done preoperatively.

Approaches to the Less Common Pancreatic Islet Cell Tumors

Glucagonomas

Glucagonomas are often large and bulky, and may be unresectable at operation. Their borders tend to be indistinct. These tumors always occur in the pancreas, but are often metastatic to the lymph nodes, liver, adrenals, and bone. They have a poor prognosis, but debulking by means of pancreatic resection is indicated for control of symptoms.

Somatostatinomas

Somatostatinomas are also often large and found to be metastatic at operation. They frequently occur in the head of the pancreas and may encroach on the duodenum; therefore, they often require pancreaticoduodenectomy. The prognosis of patients with somatostatinomas is also poor.

VIPomas

Patients with VIPomas usually present with a secretory diarrhea that does not abate when the patient fasts. Preoperative correction of fluid and electrolyte imbalance is imperative. These tumors are usually large, single, and located in the tail of the pancreas, and therefore distal pancreatectomy is the most often performed operation. VIPomas are metastatic in approximately one-half of patients. In cases of unresectable disease, octreotide is effective in controlling the diarrhea.

Pancreatic Polypeptideomas

Polypeptideomas cause minimal or nonspecific symptoms. These tumors are often small, multiple, and extrapancreatic. They are managed in a manner similar to that for gastrinomas. Both serum pancreatic polypeptide levels and immunohistologic staining help establish the diagnosis.

Nonsecretory (Nonfunctional) Tumors

Because nonsecretory tumors have no recognized hormonal excess syndrome, they are usually found incidentally or when they cause obstructive symptoms. With improved imaging techniques, more of these tumors are being found. While these tumors stain for enolase and chromogranin A, markers for pancreatic endocrine tumors, no secretory products for these tumors have been reported to date.

Nonsecretory tumors are often large when found. They are most often located in the head of the pancreas. Therefore, a pancreaticoduodenectomy is often required to prevent pain, gastrointestinal bleeding, and obstructive jaundice.

Summary

Successful excision represents a chance for cure in patients with pancreatic islet cell tumors. Gastrinomas and insulinomas, the most common pancreatic endocrine tumors, are usually small and may be difficult to localize preoperatively or even at operation. All pancreatic endocrine tumors other than gastrinomas and insulinomas tend to be large, obvious, and frequently metastatic or unresectable at the time of operation. Cure in these cases is infrequent.

For a localization study to be considered truly helpful to the surgeon, it must localize tumors not found by the surgeon at operation; as many as 20 percent of patients with gastrinomas and insulinomas may have tumors not localized at operation. To date, no localization study is helpful in these cases, although the octreotide scan may show promise for gastrinomas. At operation, the best approach to the most common tumor, gastrinoma, is thorough exploration of the gastrinoma triangle with complete excision of all obvious tumors and lymph nodes.

Suggested Reading

Howard TJ, Zinner MJ, Stabile BE, Passaro E. Gastrinomas excision for cure: A prospective analysis. *Ann Surg* 211:9, 1990.

Howard TJ, Stabile BE, Zinner MJ, et al. Anatomic distribution of pancreatic endocrine tumors. *Am J Surg* 159:258, 1990.

Meko JB, Norton JA. Endocrine tumors of the pancreas. *Curr Opinion Gen Surg* 186, 1994.

Norton JA. Neuroendocrine tumors of the pancreas and duodenum. *Curr Probl Surg* February 1994.

Norton JA, Doppman JL, Jensen RT. Curative resection in Zollinger-Ellison syndrome: Results of a 10-year prospective study. *Ann Surg* 215:8, 1992.

Sawicki MP, Howard TJ, Dalton M, et al. The dichotomous distribution of gastrinomas. *Arch Surg* 125:1584, 1990.

Shepard JJ, Challis DR, Davies PF, et al. Multiple endocrine neoplasm, type I: Gastrinomas, pancreatic neoplasms, microcarcinoids, the Zollinger-Ellison syndrome, lymph nodes, and hepatic metastases. *Arch Surg* 128:1133, 1993.

Stabile BE, Morrow DJ, Passaro E. The gastrinoma triangle: Operative implications. *Am J Surg* 147:25, 1984.

Thompson NW, Pasieka J, Fukuuchi A. Duodenal gastrinomas, duodenotomy, and duodenal exploration in the surgical management of Zollinger-Ellison syndrome. *World J Surg* 17:455, 1993.

Van Eyck CHF, Bruining HA, Reubi JC, et al. Use of isotope labelled somatosatin analogs for visualization of islet cell tumors. *World J Surg* 17:444, 1993.

Wise SR, Johnson J, Sparks J, et al. Gastrinoma: The predictive value of preoperative localization. *Surgery* 106:1087, 1989.

Zeiger MA, Shawker TH, Norton JA. Use of intraoperative ultrasonography to localize islet cell tumors. *World J Surg* 17:448, 1993.

EDITOR'S COMMENT

Neuroendocrine or islet tumors of the pancreas have now been well catalogued, and the symptoms have been outlined by the author. The clinical syndromes of gastrinoma and insulinoma, the two most commonly encountered lesions in this group, can often be ameliorated or cured by excision of the lesion or lesions elaborating the involved peptides, but the ultimate result is dependent on the localization of the tumor, its successful extirpation, and whether or not metastases have already occurred. The classic teaching is that at least 60 percent of gastrinomas have metastasized when first encountered, and that almost 10 percent of insulinomas have likewise spread. Interestingly, although 90 percent of the islets are in the distal 70 percent of the pancreas (to the left of the superior mesenteric vessels), insulin-producing tumors are distributed uniformly throughout the pancreas, and, in fact, gastrinoma is commoner in the "gastrinoma triangle" than it is in the distal portion of the gland.

The use of total gastrectomy for patients with gastrinoma that cannot be completely removed is a more controversial issue. Doctors Zollinger and Ellison were firm on this issue, as are Drs. Passaro and Wood, in the event that the gastrinoma cannot be completely removed, but most surgeons now would consider a vagotomy (parietal cell or truncal) in conjunction with intensive and lifelong medical management, including omeprazole and antacid therapy, rather than proceed directly to total gastrectomy.

The other pancreatic islet cell tumor subsets (glucagonoma, somatostatinoma, etc.) are seldom encountered, even in major endocrine surgical centers, but the incidence of metastatic cancer is extremely high. Among the more interesting of these tumors is the nonsecretory (nonfunctional) lesions, which are often malignant and can occur in the head or body of the pancreas. Unlike adenocarcinomas of the pancreas, these lesions are less likely to involve the superior mesenteric and portal vessels, and total excision of large malignant lesions is frequently possible. It is important to debulk metastatic disease, even to the point of excising numerous small metastases on the surface of the liver, lymph nodal metastatic disease where it occurs, and omental spread. The responsiveness of these lesions to radiotherapy or chemotherapy, or both, is not predictable, but the chemotherapeutic regimens, which usually embody streptozocin and other agents, have had variable response in these lesions.

R.J.B.

FIVE

BREAST, CHEST, AND MEDIASTINUM

I

The Breast

43

Anatomy of the Breast

Kirby I. Bland   Michael P. Vezeridis

The mammary glands are modified sweat glands. They are a unique feature of mammals. Embryologically paired mammary glands develop along the milk lines that extend between the limb buds from the primordial axilla distally to the inguinal region. The number of paired glands varies widely among the various mammalian species, but in the human and in most primates, normally only one pair of glands develops in the pectoral region, one gland on each side. In about 1 percent of the female population, supernumerary breasts (polymastia) or nipples (polythelia) may develop, usually along the milk lines. While there is normally little additional development of the mammary gland during postnatal life in the male, in the female extensive growth and development are evident. This postnatal development of the female mammary gland is related to age and is regulated by hormones that influence reproductive function. The greatest development of the breast is attained by the age of 20 years and atrophy begins at the age of 40 years. During pregnancy and lactation striking changes occur in both the amount (volume) of glandular tissue and the functional activity of the breast. Structural changes also occur during the menstrual cycles that result from variations in ovarian hormone levels. During menopause, with the changes occurring in the hormonal environment, the mammary gland undergoes involution and is replaced by fat and connective tissue.

Gross Anatomy of the Breast

The breast is located within the superficial fascia of the anterior chest wall. It consists of 15 to 20 lobes of tubuloalveolar glandular tissue and fibrous connective tissue that supports its lobes and the adipose tissue that resides in parenchyma between the lobes. Subcutaneous connective tissue typically does not form a distinctive capsule around breast components, but, rather, surrounds the gland and extends as septa between the lobes and lobules, providing support to the glandular elements. The deep layer of the superficial fascia that lies on the posterior surface of the breast fuses with the deep (pectoral) fascia of the chest wall. A distinct space, the retromammary bursa, can be identified anatomically on the posterior aspect of the breast and resides between the deep layer of the superficial fascia and the deep investing fascia of the pectoralis major and the contiguous muscles of the thoracic wall (Fig. 43-1). The retromammary bursa contributes to the mobility of the breast on the chest wall. Fibrous thickenings of supportive connective tissue interdigitate between the parenchymal tissue of the breast and extend from the deep layer of the superficial fascia to attach to the dermis of the skin. These suspensory structures, known as Cooper's ligaments, insert perpendicular to the delicate superficial fascial layers of the dermis, permitting remarkable mobility of the breast while providing structural support and breast contour.

The mature female breast extends from the level of the second or third rib inferiorly to the inframammary fold that is located at the level of the sixth or seventh rib. Laterally the breast extends from the lateral border of the sternum to the anterior or midaxillary line. Breast tissue extends commonly into the anterior axillary fold as the axillary tail of Spence. The upper half of the breast, particularly the upper outer quadrant, contains more glandular tissue than the remainder of the breast. The posterior or deep surface of the breast rests on portions of the fasciae of the pectoralis major, serratus anterior, and external oblique muscles and also resides on upper portions of the anterior rectus sheath.

Anatomy of the Axilla

The axilla is a pyramidal compartment located between the upper extremity and the thoracic wall; this structure has four boundaries inclusive of a base and an apex (Fig. 43-2). The curved base is comprised of the axillary fascia. The apex of the axilla is not a roof but, rather, an aperture that extends into the posterior triangle of the neck via the cervicoaxillary canal. Most structures that course between the neck

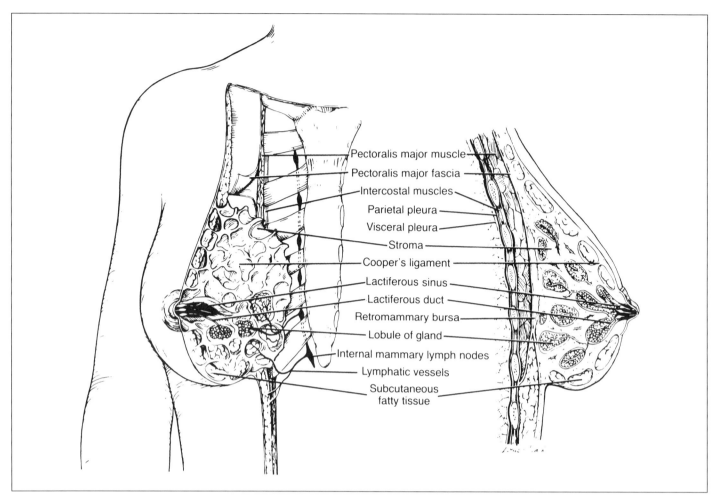

Fig. 43-1. *A tangential view of the breast on the chest wall and a cross-sectional (sagittal) view of the breast and associated chest wall. The breast lies in the superficial fascia just deep to the dermis. It is attached to the skin by the suspensory ligaments of Cooper and is separated from the investing fascia of the pectoralis major muscle by the retromammary bursa. Cooper's ligaments form fibrosepta in the stroma that provide support for the breast parenchyma. Fifteen to 20 lactiferous ducts extend from lobules composed of glandular epithelium to openings located on the nipple. A dilation of the duct, the lactiferous sinus, is present near the opening of the duct in the subareolar tissue. Subcutaneous fat and adipose tissue distributed around the lobules of the gland give the breast its smooth contour and, in the nonlactating breast, account for most of its mass. Lymphatic vessels pass through the stroma surrounding the lobules of the gland and convey lymph to collecting ducts. Lymphatic channels ending in the internal mammary (or parasternal) lymph nodes are shown. The pectoralis major muscle lies adjacent to the ribs and intercostal muscles. The parietal pleura, attached to the endothoracic fascia, and the visceral pleura, covering the surface of the lung, are shown. (From LJ Romrell, KI Bland. Anatomy of the Breast, Axilla, Chest Wall, and Related Metastatic Sites. In KI Bland, EM Copeland III (eds),* The Breast: Comprehensive Management of Benign and Malignant Diseases. *Philadelphia: Saunders, 1991. Reproduced with permission.)*

and the upper extremity pass through the cervicoaxillary canal, which is bounded anteriorly by the clavicle, medially by the first rib, and posteriorly by the scapula. The anterior wall of the axilla includes the pectoralis major and minor muscles and their associated fasciae. The posterior wall is composed primarily of the subscapularis muscle, located on the anterior surface of the scapula, and to a lesser extent by the teres major and latissimus dorsi muscles. The lateral wall is the bicipital groove, a thin strip of the arm between the insertion of the muscles of the anterior and posterior compartments. The medial wall is composed of the serratus anterior muscle.

The fascia of the pectoralis major and minor muscles are evident in two distinct planes. The superficial layer, called the pectoral fascia, invests the pectoralis major muscle, while the deep layer, called the clavipectoral or costocoracoid fascia, extends from the clavicle to the axillary fascia in the floor of the axilla and encloses the subclavius and the pectoralis minor muscle (Fig. 43-3).

The upper portion of the clavipectoral fascia, the costocoracoid membrane, is pierced by the cephalic vein, the lateral pectoral nerve, and branches of the thoracoacromial trunk. The medial pectoral nerve does not pierce the costocoracoid membrane, but enters the deep surface of the pectoralis minor and passes through the anterior investing layer of the pectoralis minor to innervate the pectoralis ma-

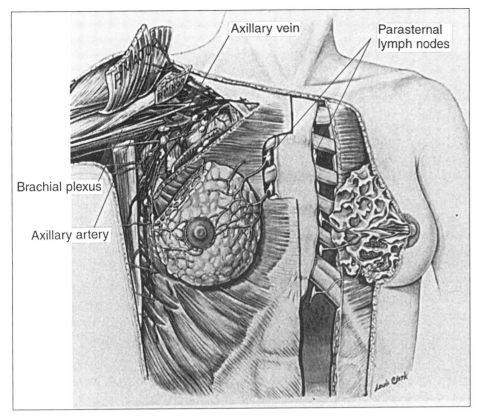

Fig. 43-2. *The anterior chest illustrating the structure of the chest wall, breast, and axilla. See text for details of the structure of the axilla and a description of its contents. On the right side, the pectoralis major has been cut lateral to the breast and reflected laterally to its insertion into the crest of the greater tubercle of the humerus. This exposes the underlying pectoralis minor and the other muscles forming the walls of the axilla. The contents of the axilla, including the axillary artery and vein, components of the brachial plexus, and axillary lymph node groups and lymphatic channels, are exposed. On the left side, the organ is cut to expose the structure of the breast in sagittal view. The lactiferous ducts and sinuses can be seen. Lymphatic channels passing to parasternal lymph nodes are also shown. (From LJ Romrell, KI Bland. Anatomy of the Breast, Axilla, Chest Wall, and Related Metastatic Sites. In KI Bland, EM Copeland III (eds),* The Breast: Comprehensive Management of Benign and Malignant Diseases. *Philadelphia: Saunders, 1991. Reproduced with permission.)*

jor muscle. The lower portion of the clavipectoral fascia, located below the pectoralis minor, is sometimes referred to as the suspensory ligament of the axilla or the coracoaxillary fascia. Halsted's ligament represents a dense condensation of the clavipectoral fascia that extends from the medial aspect of the clavicle, attaches to the first rib, and invests the subclavian artery and vein as each traverses the first rib.

The axilla contains the great vessels and nerves of the upper extremity, which, together with the other axillary contents, are surrounded by loose connective tissue. These vessels and nerves are anatomically contiguous and are enclosed within an investing layer of fascia, the axillary sheath.

The axillary artery can be divided into three parts within the axilla:

1. The first portion, located medial to the pectoralis minor muscle, gives rise to one branch, the supreme thoracic, that supplies the upper thoracic wall inclusive of the first and second intercostal spaces.
2. The second portion of this artery, located immediately posterior to the pectoralis minor, gives rise to two branches, the thoracoacromial trunk and the lateral thoracic artery. Pectoral branches of the thoracoacromial and lateral thoracic arteries supply the pectoralis major and minor muscles. Identification of these vessels during surgical dissection of the

axilla is imperative to safely conduct the procedure. The lateral thoracic artery gives origin to the lateral mammary branches.
3. The third portion of this vessel, located lateral to the pectoralis minor muscle, gives rise to three branches. These include the anterior and posterior humeral circumflex arteries that supply the upper arm, and the subscapular artery, which is the largest branch within the axilla. After a short course, the subscapular artery gives origin to its terminal branches, the subscapular circumflex and the thoracodorsal arteries. The thoracodorsal artery crosses the subscapularis muscle, providing branches to it and to the serratus anterior and latissimus dorsi muscles.

The tributaries of the axillary vein follow the course of the branches of the axillary artery, usually in the form of venae comitantes, paired veins that follow an artery. The cephalic vein passes in the groove between the deltoid and pectoralis major muscles and thereafter enters the axillary vein after piercing the clavipectoral fascia.

The axillary artery is associated with various portions of the brachial plexus throughout its course in the axilla. The cords of the brachial plexus are named according to their relationship with the axillary artery—medial, lateral, and posterior—rather than their anatomic position in the axilla or on the chest wall.

Three nerves of particular interest to surgeons are located in the axilla. The long thoracic nerve, located on the medial wall of the axilla, arises in the neck from the fifth, sixth, and seventh cervical roots and enters the axilla via the cervicoaxillary canal. This medially placed nerve lies on the lateralmost surface of the serratus anterior muscle and is invested by the serratus fascia such that it might be accidentally divided together with resection of the fascia during surgical dissection (sampling) of lymphatics of the axilla. The long thoracic nerve, while diminutive in size, courses a long distance to supply the serratus anterior muscle; injury or division of this nerve will result in the "winged scapula." The thoracodorsal nerve takes origin from the posterior cord of the brachial plexus and innervates the laterally placed latissimus dorsi muscle. Injury or division is inconsequential to shoulder function; however, preservation of this nerve is essential to transfer survival and motor function of the myocutaneous flap utilized for reconstructive purposes. The intercostobrachial nerve is formed by the merging of the lateral cutaneous branch of the second intercostal nerve with the medial cutaneous nerve of the arm; this nerve provides sensory innervation of skin of the axilla and the upper medial aspect of the arm. A second intercostobrachial nerve may sometimes form an anterior branch of the third lateral cutaneous nerve.

Blood Supply of the Breast

The breast receives its blood supply from perforating branches of the internal mammary artery, lateral branches of the posterior intercostal arteries, and several branches of the axillary artery. The latter vessels include the highest thoracic, lateral thoracic, and pectoral branches of the thoracoacromial artery (Figs. 43-4, 43-5). Branches from the second, third, and fourth anterior perforating arteries pass to the breast as medial mammary arteries.

The lateral thoracic artery gives origin to branches to the serratus anterior muscle, both pectoralis muscles, and the subscap-

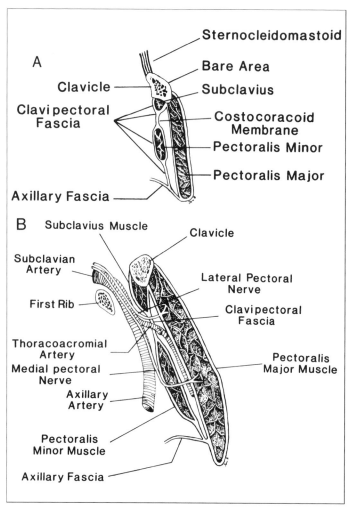

Fig. 43-3. Sagittal sections of the chest wall in the axillary region. A. The anterior wall of the axilla. The clavicle and three muscles inferior to it are shown. B. Section through the chest wall illustrating the relationship of the axillary artery and medial and lateral pectoral nerves to the clavipectoral fascia. The clavipectoral fascia is a strong sheet of connective tissue that is attached superiorly to the clavicle and envelops the subclavius and pectoralis minor muscles. The fascia extends from the lower border of the pectoralis minor to become continuous with the axillary fascia in the floor of the axilla. (From LJ Romrell, KI Bland, Anatomy of the Breast, Axilla, Chest Wall, and Related Metastatic Sites. In KI Bland, EM Copeland III (eds), The Breast: Comprehensive Management of Benign and Malignant Diseases. Philadelphia: Saunders, 1991. Reproduced with permission.)

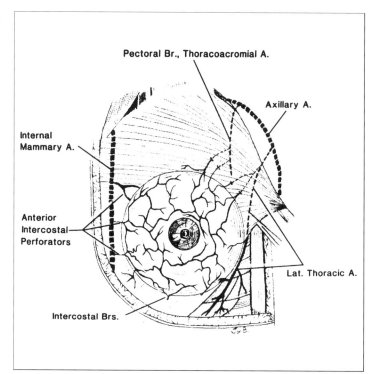

Fig. 43-4. Arterial distribution of blood to the breast, axilla, and chest wall. The breast receives its blood supply via three major arterial routes: 1) medially from anterior perforating intercostal branches arising from the internal thoracic artery, 2) laterally from either pectoral branch of the thoracoacromial trunk or branches of the lateral thoracic artery (the thoracoacromial trunk and the lateral thoracic arteries are branches of the axillary artery), and 3) from lateral cutaneous branches of the intercostal arteries that are associated with the overlying breast. The arteries indicated with a dashed line lie deep to the muscles of the thoracic wall and axilla. Many of the arteries must pass through these muscles before reaching the breast. (From LJ Romrell, KI Bland. Anatomy of the Breast, Axilla, Chest Wall, and Related Metastatic Sites. In KI Bland, EM Copeland III (eds), The Breast: Comprehensive Management of Benign and Malignant Diseases. Philadelphia: Saunders, 1991. Reproduced with permission.)

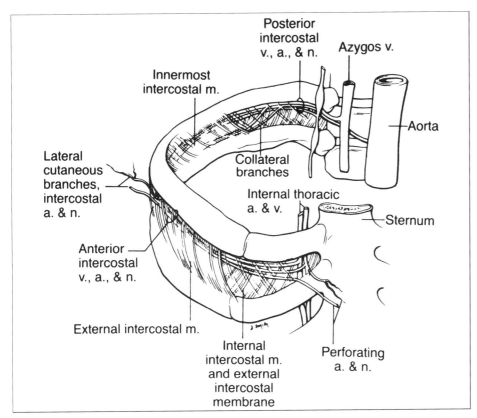

Fig. 43-5. A segment of the body wall illustrating the relationship of structures to the ribs. Two ribs are shown as they extend from the vertebrae to attach to the sternum. The orientation of the muscle and connective tissue fibers is shown. The external intercostal muscle extends downward and forward. The muscle layer extends forward from the rib tubercle to the costochondral junction, where the muscle is replaced by the aponeurosis, called the external intercostal membrane. The internal intercostal muscle fibers with the oposite orientation can be seen through this layer. The innermost intercostal muscle fibers are present along the lateral half of the intercostal space. The intercostal nerve and vessels pass through the intercostal space in the plane between the internal and innermost (or intima of the internal) intercostal muscle layers. Anterior intercostal arteries arise from the internal thoracic artery; anterior intercostal veins join the internal thoracic vein. Posterior intercostal arteries arise from the aorta; posterior intercostal veins join the azygos system on the right and the hemiazygos system on the left. Lymphatics follow the path of the blood vessels. Anteriorly, lymphatics pass to parasternal (or internal mammary) nodes that are located along the internal mammary vessels; posteriorly, they pass to intercostal nodes located in the intercostal space near the vertebral bodies. (From LJ Romrell, KI Bland. Anatomy of the Breast, Axilla, Chest Wall, and Related Metastatic Sites. In KI Bland, EM Copeland III (eds), The Breast: Comprehensive Management of Benign and Malignant Diseases. *Philadelphia: Saunders, 1991. Reproduced with permission.)*

ularis muscle, and also supplies the axillary lymph nodes. The posterior intercostal arteries give rise to mammary branches in the second, third, and fourth intercostal spaces.

Although the thoracodorsal branch of the subscapular artery does not contribute to the blood supply of the breast, this vessel is intimately associated with the central and scapular lymph node groups of the axilla. This fact should be taken into consideration during axillary node dissection, as

bleeding that is difficult to control can result when branches of this vessel are severed.

Major venous drainage of the breast is directed toward the axilla with the veins basically following the path of the arterial distribution. The superficial breast veins have extensive anastomoses that may be evident through the overlying skin. Around the nipple, these superficial veins form an anastomotic circle, the circulus venosus. Veins from this circle and from

deeper aspects of the gland drain blood to the periphery of the breast and thereafter into vessels that terminate in the internal mammary, axillary, and internal jugular veins.

The three principal groups of veins essential to venous drainage of the breast and the thoracic wall include 1) perforating branches of the internal mammary vein, 2) tributaries of the axillary vein, and 3) perforating branches of posterior intercostal veins. The posterior intercostal veins lie in direct continuity with the vertebral plexus of veins (Batson's plexus) that surround the vertebrae and extend from the base of the skull to the sacrum. This plexus may provide an important pathway for hematogenous dissemination of breast cancer that explains metastases to the skull, vertebrae, pelvic bones, and central nervous system in the absence of pulmonary metastases.

Innervation of the Breast

The sensory innervation of the breast is primarily supplied by the lateral and anterior cutaneous branches of the second through the sixth intercostal nerves (Fig. 43-5). These sensory nerves of the breast originate principally from the fourth, fifth, and sixth intercostal nerves, although the second and third intercostal nerves may provide cutaneous branches to the superior aspect of the breast. Nerves arising from the cervical plexus, specifically the anterior or medial branches of the supraclavicular nerve, supply a limited region of the skin of the upper portion of the breast. Collectively, these nerves convey sympathetic fibers for innervation to the breast and the overlying skin.

The lateral branches of the intercostal nerves exit the intercostal space via the attachment sites of the slips of the serratus anterior muscle. These nerves divide into anterior and posterior branches as they exit the muscle. Anterior branches of the intercostals supply the anterolateral thoracic wall. The third through the sixth branches, known as the lateral mammary branches, supply the majority of the surface of the breast. The intercostal brachial, a large nerve, takes origin from the lateral branch of the second intercostal nerve. The intercostal brachial nerve courses through the fascia of the floor of the axilla to commonly join the medial cutaneous nerve of the arm. This nerve is of little functional significance; with injury to the intercostal brachial nerve during axillary dissection, the only consequence for the patient will be modest loss of cutaneous sensation in the upper medial aspect of the arm. No motor loss will be evident following injury or division of the intercostal brachial nerve.

The anterior branches of the intercostal nerves exit the intercostal space near the lateral border of the sternum to allow arborization of branches medially and laterally over the thoracic wall. The branches that course laterally innervate the medial aspect of the breast and are sometimes called medial mammary branches.

Lymphatic Drainage of the Breast

The main route of lymphatic drainage of the breast is through the axillary lymph node groups (Fig. 43-6). There have been considerable variations in the names given to the lymph node groups because the boundaries of nodal groups in the axilla are not well demarcated. These variations are particularly evident in level I nodal groups. Anatomists usually describe four groups of axillary lymph nodes, while surgeons typically identify six groups at three anatomic levels. The most commonly used terms to describe the axillary nodes are the following.

1. The *axillary vein group*, usually identified by anatomists as the *lateral group*, consists of four to six lymph nodes that lie medial or posterior to the axillary vein. These nodes receive the majority of lymphatic contents from the upper extremity with the exception of lymph that drains into the deltopectoral lymph nodes, a group also referred to as the infraclavicular nodes (Fig. 43-7).
2. The *external mammary group*, usually identified by anatomists as the *anterior or pectoral group*, consists of four or five lymph nodes positioned along the lower border of the pectoralis minor muscle contiguous in association with the lateral thoracic vessels. These nodes receive the principal volume of lymph drainage from the breast. From these

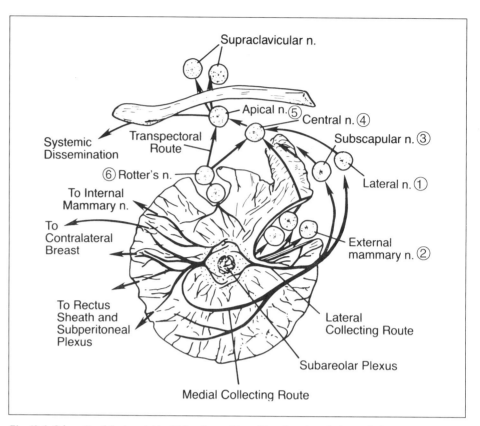

Fig. 43-6. Schematic of the breast identifying the position of lymph nodes relative to the breast and illustrating routes of lymphatic drainage. The clavicle is indicated as a reference point. See the text and Figs. 43-8 and 43-9 to identify the group or level to which the lymph nodes belong. Level I lymph nodes include the external mammary (or anterior) axillary vein (or lateral) and scapular (or posterior) groups; level II, the central group; and level III, the subclavicular (or apical). The arrows indicate the routes of lymphatic drainage (see text). (From LJ Romrell, KI Bland. Anatomy of the Breast, Axilla, Chest Wall, and Related Metastatic Sites. In KI Bland, EM Copeland III (eds), The Breast: Comprehensive Management of Benign and Malignant Diseases. Philadelphia: Saunders, 1991. Reproduced with permission.)

nodes, lymph drains primarily into the *central lymph nodes*. However, lymph may pass directly from the external mammary nodes to the subclavicular lymph nodes.
3. The *scapular group*, usually identified by anatomists as the *posterior or subscapular group*, consists of six or seven lymph nodes positioned near the posterior wall of the axilla in juxtaposition to the lateral border of the scapula and contiguous with the subscapular vessels. These nodes receive lymph primarily from the lower aspects of the neck, the posterior skin and subcutaneous tissues of the trunk (as low as the iliac crest), and posterior portions of the shoulder region. Lymph from the scapular nodes drains into the central and subclavicular nodes.
4. The *central group*, considered to be cen-

trally positioned by both anatomists and surgeons, consists of three or four large lymph nodes that are embedded in the fat of the axilla, usually behind the pectoralis minor muscle. These nodes receive lymph from the preceding nodal groups (axillary, external mammary, and scapular nodal sites) and may also receive afferent lymphatic vessels directly from the breast. Lymph from the central group drains directly to the subclavicular (apical, level III) nodes. This group is often placed superficially beneath the skin and the fascia of the midaxilla and it is centrally located between the posterior and anterior axillary folds. This nodal group is often palpable, because of its superficial position, thus allowing clinical assessment of metastatic disease.

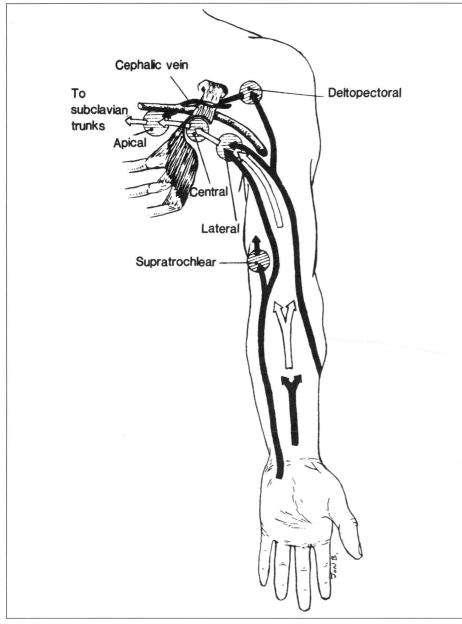

Fig. 43-7. Schematic illustrating the route of lymphatic drainage in the upper extremity. The relationship of this drainage to the major axillary lymph node groups is indicated by the arrows. All the lymph vessels of the upper extremity drain directly or indirectly through outlying lymph node groups into the axillary lymph nodes. The outlying lymph nodes are few in number and are organized into three groups: 1) supratrochlear lymph nodes (one or two, located above the medial epicondyle of the humerus adjacent to the basilic vein), 2) deltopectoral lymph nodes (one or two, located beside the cephalic vein where it lies between the pectoralis major and deltoid muscle just below the clavicle), and 3) variable, small, isolated lymph nodes (few and variable in number; may be located in the cubital fossa or along the medial side of the brachial vessels). Note that the deltopectoral lymph node group drains directly into the subclavicular, or apical, lymph nodes of the axillary group. (From LJ Romrell, KI Bland. Anatomy of the Breast, Axilla, Chest Wall, and Related Metastatic Sites. In KI Bland, EM Copeland III (eds), The Breast: Comprehensive Management of Benign and Malignant Diseases. Philadelphia: Saunders, 1991. Reproduced with permission.)

5. The *subclavicular group*, identified by anatomists as the *apical group*, consists of 6 to 12 lymph nodes that are located partially posterior to and partially above the upper border of the pectoralis minor muscle. This nodal group extends into the apex of the axilla along the medial aspect of the axillary vein. These nodes receive lymph from all the other axillary lymph node groups. The efferent lymphatic vessels from the subclavicular lymph nodes unite to form the subclavian trunk. The course of the subclavian trunk is highly variable anatomically. It may join and directly enter the internal jugular vein or the subclavian vein, or their junction. On the right side of the trunk, the right lymphatic duct may enter this structure, while on the left side confluence with the thoracic duct is common. Efferent vessels from the subclavicular lymph nodes may also pass to the deep cervical lymph nodes.

6. The *interpectoral or Rotter's group*, usually identified by surgeons but not by anatomists, consists of one to four small lymph nodes located between the pectoralis major and minor muscles and is contiguous with pectoral branches of the thoracoacromial vessels. Lymph from these nodes enters the central and subclavicular nodes.

The axillary lymph node groups are also divided according to their lateral and medial relationships with the pectoralis minor muscle into three distinct levels and are identified as levels I through III (Figs. 43-8 and 43-9). *Level I nodes* are located *lateral to* or *below* the lower border of the pectoralis minor; this level includes the external mammary, axillary vein, and scapular lymph node groups. *Level II nodes* are located *deep to* or *behind* the pectoralis minor and include the central lymph node group and possibly some of the subclavicular lymph node group. *Level III nodes* are located superomedial to the upper margin of the pectoralis minor and include the subclavicular (apical) lymph node group.

The British surgeon W. Sampson Handley is credited with the recognition of metastatic spread of breast carcinoma to the internal mammary nodes as a primary route of lymphatic dissemination. Extensive clinical and anatomic research confirmed that central and medial breast lymphatics pass

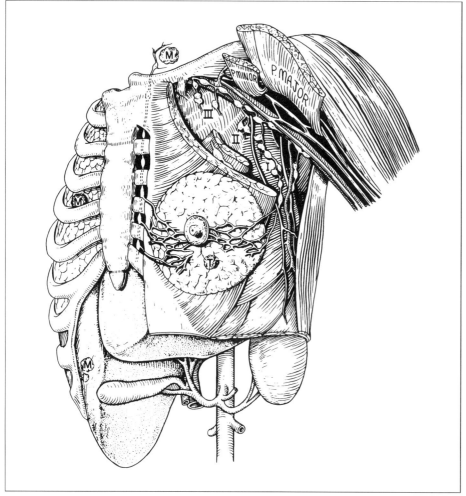

Fig. 43-8. Lymphatic drainage of the breast. The pectoralis major and minor muscles, which contribute to the anterior wall of the axilla, have been cut and reflected. This exposes the medial and posterior walls of the axilla as well as the basic contents of the axilla. The lymph node groups of the axilla and the internal mammary nodes are depicted. Also shown is the location of the long thoracic nerve on the surface of the serratus anterior muscle (on the medial wall of the axilla). The scapular lymph node group is closely associated with the thoracodorsal nerve and vessels. (From LJ Romrell, KI Bland. Anatomy of the Breast, Axilla, Chest Wall, and Related Metastatic Sites. In KI Bland, EM Copeland III (eds), The Breast: Comprehensive Management of Benign and Malignant Diseases. Philadelphia: Saunders, 1991. Reproduced with permission.)

medially and parallel the course of major blood vessels to perforate the pectoralis major muscle and terminate in the internal mammary nodal chain.

The internal mammary nodal group is located in the retrosternal interspaces between the costal cartilages approximately 2 to 3 cm within the sternal margin (see Fig. 43-8). This nodal group traverses and parallels the internal mammary vasculature and is invested by endothoracic fascia. The internal mammary lymphatic trunks terminate in the subclavicular nodal groups (see Figs. 43-6 and 43-9). The right internal mammary nodal group enters the right lymphatic duct while the left enters the main thoracic duct (Fig. 43-10).

Three interconnecting groups of lymphatic vessels drain the breast:

1. A primary set of vessels originates as channels within the gland in the interlobular spaces and along the lactiferous ducts.

2. The vessels draining the glandular tissue and the overlying skin of the central part of the gland pass into the subareolar plexus, an interconnecting network of vessels located beneath the areola.

3. A plexus on the deep surface of the breast communicates with minute vessels in the deep fascia underlying the breast. Along the medial border of the breast, lymphatic vessels within the substance of the gland anastomose with vessels passing to parasternal nodes.

More than 75 percent of the lymph from the breast flows directly to the axillary lymph nodes, while the majority of residual lymph passes to parasternal nodes. This anatomic fact provides support for the rationale for lymph node dissection (sampling) of the axilla to determine the histologic status of these nodes and, hence, accurate clinical and pathologic staging. Although some authorities have suggested that the parasternal nodes receive lymph primarily from the medial part of the breast, others report that *both* the axillary and the parasternal lymph node groups receive lymph from all quadrants of the breast, with no specific tendency for any quadrant to drain medially or laterally. The skin of the breast drains via the superficial lymphatic vessels to the axillary lymph nodes. The anterolateral chest and the upper abdominal wall cephalad to the umbilicus show a striking directional flow of lymph toward the axilla. Lymphatic vessels near the lateral margin of the sternum pass through intercostal spaces to the parasternal lymph nodes that are associated with the internal thoracic vessels. In the upper pectoral region, small numbers of lymphatic vessels pass over the clavicle to inferior deep cervical lymph nodes.

The lymphatic vessels of the deeper structures of the thoracic wall drain primarily into three groups of lymph nodes: *the parasternal, intercostal, and diaphragmatic lymphatics*. The parasternal or internal thoracic lymph nodes are a group of smaller lymphatics positioned about 1 cm lateral to the sternal border in the intercostal spaces along the internal mammary vessels. These nodes reside in the areolar tissue just under the endothoracic fascia bordering the space between the adjacent costal cartilages.

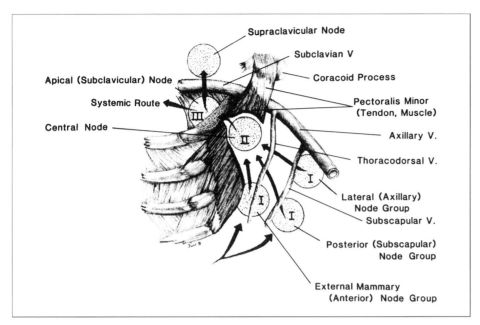

Fig. 43-9. Schematic illustrating the major lymph node groups associated with the lymphatic drainage of the breast. The Roman numerals indicate three levels or groups of lymph nodes that are defined by their location relative to the pectoralis minor. Level I includes lymph nodes located lateral to the pectoralis minor; level II, lymph nodes located deep to the muscle; and level III, lymph nodes located medial to the muscle. The arrows indicate the general direction of lymph flow. The axillary vein and its major tributaries associated with the pectoralis minor are included. (From LJ Romrell, KI Bland. Anatomy of the Breast, Axilla, Chest Wall, and Related Metastatic Sites. In KI Bland, EM Copeland III (eds), The Breast: Comprehensive Management of Benign and Malignant Diseases. *Philadelphia: Saunders, 1991. Reproduced with permission.)*

The intercostal lymph nodes represent a small group located in the posterior portion of the thoracic cavity within the intercostal spaces near the head of the ribs. One or more nodes are found in each intercostal space with relationship to the intercostal vessels. These nodes receive deep lymphatics from the posterolateral thoracic wall, including lymphatic channels from the breast. The upper efferent lymphatics from the intercostal lymph nodes on the right side terminate in the right lymphatic duct, while the efferent lymphatics from the corresponding nodes on the left side terminate in the thoracic duct.

The diaphragmatic lymph nodes consist of three sets of small lymph nodes located on the thoracic surface of the diaphragm. The anterior group includes two or three small lymph nodes, also known as prepericardial nodes, that are located behind the sternum at the base of the xiphoid process. Efferent lymphatics from the anterior diaphragmatic nodes pass to the parasternal nodes. The lateral set of diaphragmatic lymph nodes is comprised of two or three small nodes on each side of the diaphragm adjacent to the pericardial sac where the phrenic nerves enter the diaphragm. They lie near the vena cava on the right side and near the esophageal hiatus on the left. The posterior set of diaphragmatic nodes consists of a few lymph nodes located next to the crura of the diaphragm. These nodes receive lymph from the posterior aspect of the diaphragm and convey it to posterior mediastinal and lateral aortic nodes.

Microscopic Anatomy of the Breast

The adult mammary gland is made of 15 to 20 irregular lobes of branched tubuloalveolar glands. These lobes, separated by fibrous bands of connective tissue, radiate from the mammary papilla or nipple and are further subdivided into multiple lobules. The fibrous bands that support the parenchyma and connect with the dermis are termed the suspensory ligaments of Cooper. The tubuloalveolar glands lie in the subcutaneous tissues. Each lobe of the primary gland ends in a lactiferous duct, 2 to 4 mm in diameter, that empties into the subareolar ampulla via a constricted orifice onto the nipple (see Fig. 43-1). Beneath the areola on each duct is a dilated portion, the lactiferous sinus. The lactiferous ducts are lined near their openings with stratified squamous epithelium. The epithelial lining of the duct has evidence of gradual transition to two layers of cuboidal cells in the lactiferous sinus to become a single layer of columnar or cuboidal cells throughout the remainder of the duct system.

The morphology of the secretory portion of the mammary gland varies greatly with age and also during pregnancy and lactation. The glandular component is sparse in the inactive gland and consists predominantly of duct elements. The inactive breast undergoes slight cyclical changes throughout the menstrual cycle. During pregnancy, the mammary glands undergo dramatic proliferation via cellular hypertrophy, lactation, and development. These events are accompanied by relative decreases in the volume of connective and adipose tissue. With pregnancy, the epidermis of the nipple and areola becomes deeply pigmented and somewhat corrugated. It is covered by keratinized, stratified squamous epithelium. The areola contains sebaceous glands, sweat glands, and accessory areolar glands of Montgomery, which are intermediate between true mammary glands and sweat glands in their structure. The accessory areolar glands produce small elevations on the surface of the areola. The sebaceous and sweat glands are located along the margin of the areola. The tip of the nipple contains numerous free sensory nerve endings and Meissner's corpuscles in the dermal papillae, while the areola contains fewer of these structures. Neuronal plexuses are also present around hair follicles in the skin peripheral to the areola; pacinian (pressure) corpuscles are present in the dermis and in the glandular tissue. The rich sensory innervation of the breast is of great functional significance in lactation.

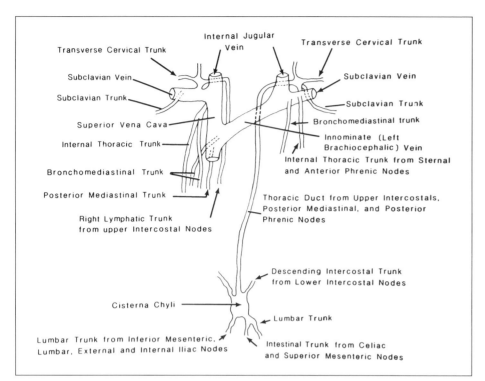

Fig. 43-10. *Schematic of the major lymphatic vessels of the thorax and the root of the neck. The thoracic duct begins at the cisterna chyli, a dilated sac that receives drainage from the lower extremities and the abdominal and pelvic cavities via the lumbar and intestinal trunks. Lymph enters the systemic circulation via channels that join the great veins of the neck and superior mediastinum. The lymphatic vessels demonstrate considerable variation as to their number and pattern of branching. A typical pattern is illustrated here. Most of the major trunks, including the thoracic and right lymphatic ducts, end at or near the confluence of the internal jugular with the subclavian. (From LJ Romrell, KI Bland. Anatomy of the Breast, Axilla, Chest Wall, and Related Metastatic Sites. In KI Bland, EM Copeland III (eds),* The Breast: Comprehensive Management of Benign and Malignant Diseases. *Philadelphia: Saunders, 1991. Reproduced with permission.)*

Suggested Reading

Anson BJ, McVay CB. Thoracic walls: Breast or mammary region. In BJ Anson, CB McVay, *Surgical Anatomy*. Philadelphia: Saunders, 1971. Pp 330–369.

Batson OV. The function of the vertebral veins and their role in the spread of metastases. *Ann Surg* 112:138, 1940.

Bland KI, Copeland EM III. Breast. In SI Schwartz (ed), *Principles of Surgery* (6th ed). New York: McGraw-Hill, 1994. Pp 531–594.

Copeland EM III, Bland KI. The Breast. In DCJ Sabiston (ed), *Essentials of Surgery*. Philadelphia: Saunders, 1987. Pp 288–326.

Cunningham L. The anatomy of the arteries and veins of the breast. *J Surg Oncol*. 9:71, 1977.

Gray H. The Lymphatic System. In CD Clemente (ed). *Anatomy of the Human Body* (30th American ed). Philadelphia: Lea & Febiger, 1985. p 866.

Haagensen CD. Anatomy of the Mammary Glands. In CD Haagensen (ed.), *Diseases of the Breast* (2nd ed). Philadelphia: Saunders, 1971. Pp 1–28.

Henriques C. The veins of the vertebral column and their role in the spread of cancer. *Ann R Coll Surg Engl* 31:1, 1962.

Romrell LJ, Bland KI. Anatomy of the Breast, Axilla, Chest wall and Related Metastatic Sites.

In KI Bland, EM Copeland III (eds), *The Breast: Comprehensive Management of Benign and Malignant Diseases*. Philadelphia: Saunders, 1991. Pp 17–35.

Sakki S. Angiography of the female breast. *Ann Clin Res*. 6:1, 1974.

Sykes PA. The nerve supply of the human nipple. *J Anat (Lond)* 105:201, 1969.

Turner-Warwick R. The lymphatics of the breast. *Br J Surg* 46:574, 1959.

EDITOR'S COMMENT

The authors have presented a comprehensive and extremely important exposition of the gross, microscopic, and topographic anatomy of the female breast, with appropriate emphasis on the blood supply and the lymphatic drainage. The frequency with which breast operations are done is increasing rapidly, as routine mammography and discovery of small, nonpalpable lesions become commonplace. Halsted's radical mastectomy has all but disappeared from the surgical scene, and is now performed only for those lesions that grossly invade the pectoralis major muscle. Modified radical mastectomy, or lumpectomy with axillary sampling, is described in subsequent chapters and is now the mainstay of the management of breast cancer at any stage.

A solid understanding of the vital structures in the breast, adjacent soft tissue, and, perhaps most important, the axilla is the basis for modern surgical management of breast lesions, specifically infiltrating cancer of the breast. The key steps for identifying vital nerves and major blood vessels are outlined subsequently, but locating those structures and protecting them from surgical injury are dependent on the information that has been presented.

R.J.B.

44

Diagnostic Approaches to Breast Masses

Susan M. Love   Kelly K. Hunt

It is estimated that 182,000 women in the United States were diagnosed with breast cancer in 1995. The majority of breast cancers are self-detected and present as palpable, usually painless, lumps in the breast. The advent of screening mammography has introduced a new diagnostic challenge to physicians: nonpalpable breast masses. Although the incidence of breast cancer is rising, physicians are presented with many breast masses that will not prove to be malignant disease. Approximately 560,000 open breast biopsies are performed each year in the United States, with over 80 percent revealing benign disease on final pathology. While diagnostic accuracy is paramount in the evaluation of a woman with a breast mass, unnecessary surgical procedures should be avoided. As newer diagnostic approaches have become available, it is possible to approach the diagnosis of breast masses in a systematic and less invasive fashion.

Diagnostic Approaches

A complete history and physical examination should always be performed when a woman presents with a palpable breast mass or mammographic abnormality. Risk factors for breast cancer should be gleaned from the history while keeping in mind that 80 percent of patients with a diagnosis of breast cancer have no identifiable risk factors. Physical examination includes inspection of the breasts in both the sitting position and with the patient's arms raised upward. The breast should be palpated with the patient in the supine and upright positions with the arms raised. The cervical, supraclavicular, and axillary nodal ba-

sins should also be examined with the patient in the upright position.

Once the surgeon identifies a dominant lump in the breast, a diagnostic evaluation is warranted. Figure 44-1 illustrates an algorithm for the diagnostic approach to a dominant lump. It is helpful to separate suspicious from nonsuspicious masses. If the patient has a mass that is suspicious for carcinoma, she should proceed to diagnostic mammography. The mammogram is performed with a marker placed over the palpable lesion so that the radiologist can correlate the palpable mass with any radiographic abnormalities in the breast. With the results of mammography available, ultrasound can be used to distinguish a solid from a cystic lesion. Ultrasound can be especially helpful in the patient who has a suspicious mass on examination but no visible abnormality on mammogram.

The next step is to obtain a tissue diagnosis. In most situations, this is best performed with a needle biopsy. Fine-needle aspiration biopsy (FNA) and core needle

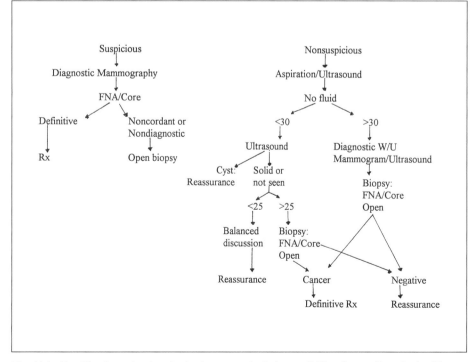

Fig. 44-1. Algorithm for evaluation of a dominant mass in the breast. FNA = fine-needle aspiration biopsy; W/U = workup; Rx = treatment. (From SM Love. Revlon/UCLA Breast Center Practice Guidelines. Unpublished.)

biopsy both have advantages and disadvantages in the diagnosis of breast disease. An FNA is easily performed with minimal discomfort to the patient and offers a rapid cytologic diagnosis. The major drawback is the number of cases with insufficient material for diagnosis. With a skilled aspirator and an experienced cytopathologist, over 95 percent of aspirates should be of sufficient quality for diagnosis. A diagnosis of malignancy by FNA allows the physician and patient to plan definitive treatment. There is a reported false-positive rate of up to 1.6 percent and therefore it is important that the physical examination, mammogram, and FNA are all in concordance.

Core needle biopsies are easier for the pathologist to read since they provide a piece of tissue rather than merely cells. They are, however, more difficult for the surgeon to perform and for the patient to undergo. Core biopsies provide a histologic diagnosis whereas FNA provides a cytologic diagnosis. This can be important in distinguishing invasive from noninvasive breast cancer. Core biopsy may be most appropriate in patients with large breast masses who are candidates for preoperative chemotherapy and need histologic confirmation before initiation of treatment.

Whether a suspicious mass is biopsied with an FNA or a core biopsy, it is important that the tissue diagnosis matches the clinical and mammographic impressions. If this is not the case or when the needle biopsy is nondiagnostic, the surgeon should proceed to open biopsy. Another indication for open biopsy is a diagnosis of atypia. When atypical cells are seen, it is important to remove additional tissue to make sure that ductal carcinoma in situ (DCIS) or invasive cancer is not adjacent to the area that has been sampled with the needle biopsy.

When a woman presents with a lump in the breast that is not suspicious for malignancy, the approach is different. If the mass is cystic in character, needle aspiration can be performed in the office or under ultrasound guidance. If the mass resolves completely, no further evaluation is needed. In patients who are over 50 years of age or who have recurrent cysts after repeated needle aspiration, pneumocystography is indicated. This mammographic study can identify an intracystic lesion, which would be an indication for open biopsy. Bloody cyst fluid, which may be indicative of an intracystic carcinoma, is another reason to perform a pneumocystogram.

If the initial impression on physical examination is consistent with a cyst, needle aspiration in the office may be both diagnostic and therapeutic. If the mass resolves completely on both physician examination and patient self-examination, a costly diagnostic workup can be avoided. Cyst fluid does not need to be sent for cytology if it has the typical greenish or yellowish appearance, and the patient can be reassured. Bloody fluid should be evaluated further with a pneumocystogram or open biopsy.

When aspiration of a lump in the breast does not reveal any fluid, the patient needs further evaluation before biopsy. Needle biopsies can lead to hematomas in the breast that can make further evaluation or open biopsy difficult. Women over the age of 35 should have a diagnostic workup including mammogram and ultrasound before FNA. The surgeon can then proceed with biopsy based on the clinical and mammographic impressions. Using FNA to distinguish pseudolumps from dominant ones requires a close working effort between the surgeon and the cytologist. If the area in question is not truly a dominant abnormality then needle biopsy is best performed with either mammographic or ultrasound guidance. This approach will prevent sampling errors, which can mislead the practitioner. Again, the rule of concordance should be followed; the clinical, mammographic, and histologic impressions must conform.

When a woman under 35 years old has a nonsuspicious mass in the breast that does not reveal fluid on aspiration, an ultrasound should be obtained. If a simple cyst is seen on the sonogram, the patient can be reassured and returned for routine follow-up study. If a solid mass is imaged or no abnormality is seen, the workup will vary depending on age. Women under age 25 are unlikely to have a malignancy and the decision to perform a needle biopsy or open biopsy should be preceded by a balanced discussion. Women over the age of 25 should have a tissue diagnosis either by FNA or core or open biopsy. If the biopsy is benign and the clinical impression is in agreement, then the patient can be reassured. If the biopsy reveals cancer, definitive treatment can be discussed.

Patients will frequently present with a nondominant but palpable lump in the breast. These masses are often described as thickenings or nodularity of the breast. An

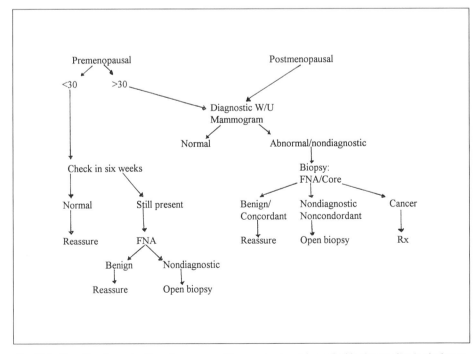

Fig. 44-2. Algorithm for evaluation of a woman with a nondominant but palpable abnormality in the breast: lumps, thickenings, nodularity. FNA = fine-needle aspiration biopsy; W/U = workup; Rx = treatment. (From SM Love. Revlon/UCLA Breast Center Practice Guidelines. Unpublished.)

algorithm for this patient population can be developed based on the menopausal status (Fig. 44-2). Premenopausal women under the age of 30 should be re-examined in 6 weeks. If no palpable abnormality is present at that time, the patient can be reassured that the lesion was hormonal. If the abnormality is still present, an FNA can be performed. With a diagnosis of benign ductal epithelium, the patient can be reassured; however, if the FNA is nondiagnostic, she should be considered for an open biopsy.

Women who are over the age of 30 and have an indistinct thickening or nodular area in the breast should have a diagnostic evaluation including mammography and ultrasound. A normal diagnostic workup can offer the patient and physician reassurance. Mammography and ultrasound will not image up to 15 percent of breast cancers and therefore it is important that a palpable area or suspicious lesion be biopsied. An abnormal or nondiagnostic study should always be evaluated with a needle biopsy.

Screening mammography can reduce the mortality of breast cancer by 30 percent in women over the age of 50. This is possible because mammography can identify nonpalpable breast cancers that are localized and more amenable to cure. The widespread use of screening mammograms also identifies a large number of breast masses that are not malignant. The interpretation of mammograms by the radiologist without communication between the surgeon and the radiologist can lead to unnecessary biopsies. Figure 44-3 illustrates the appropriate workup and use of different biopsy techniques dependent on the mammographic characteristics of the mass.

When mammography identifies a well-circumscribed mass that is interpreted as benign by the radiologist, no biopsy is needed. Ultrasound can be used to further characterize the mass. Examples of benign tumors identified using these techniques include lipomas, galactoceles, fat necrosis, fibroadenomas, and intramammary or low axillary lymph nodes. Ultrasound can distinguish a cyst from a solid lesion when a rounded mass is seen on mammography. Simple cysts do not require intervention but complex cysts should be evaluated with a pneumocystogram.

Additional mammographic views are indicated when a "density" is seen on rou-

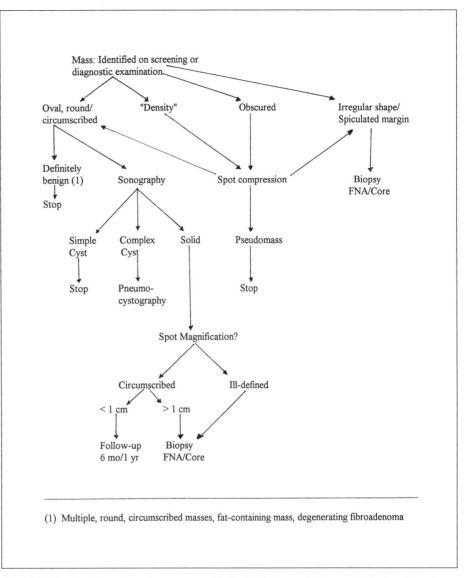

(1) Multiple, round, circumscribed masses, fat-containing mass, degenerating fibroadenoma

Fig. 44-3. Algorithm for workup of a mammographically detected, nonpalpable mass in the breast based on the mammographic characteristics of the lesion. FNA = fine-needle aspiration biopsy. (From SM Love. Revlon/UCLA Breast Center Practice Guidelines. Unpublished.)

tine mammography or when breast tissue is obscured or distorted. A pseudomass will no longer be seen when the area is pressed out on spot compression views. If an irregularly shaped or spiculated mass is identified on compression, a stereotactic FNA or core biopsy should be done. Spot magnification views can better assess the margins of a mammographic mass and may identify calcifications not seen on a routine study. A well-circumscribed mass that is less than 1 cm in size can be followed with repeat mammography in 6 months to 1 year. A mass with ill-defined borders or a circumscribed mass greater than 1 cm in size should be biopsied.

The limitations of stereotactic FNA are the same as those of FNA for palpable masses: inadequate material or difficulty in cytologic diagnosis. Stereotactic core biopsy obviates most of these problems by obtaining more tissue and being easier for most pathologists to read. The core biopsy has the additional advantage of yielding enough tissue to allow the determination of invasive or in situ disease. A diagnosis of cancer on core biopsy can lead to definitive therapy. The stereotactic core biopsy may also be useful in patients who have masses that are read by the radiologist as possibly but not definitely benign. These patients have traditionally undergone frequent mammographic follow-up study or open surgical biopsy. If a benign histologic diagnosis is obtained with the aid of stereotactic core biopsy, these patients can undergo routine mammographic screening on an annual basis and avoid open biopsy. Benign-appearing masses that would not normally be biopsied should not be referred for stereotactic biopsy.

Techniques
Fine-Needle Aspiration Biopsy

The area in question should be fixed between the fingers of the nondominant hand (Fig. 44-4). A small wheal of lidocaine is raised intradermally with a 25-gauge needle. A 22-gauge needle attached to a 10-ml syringe is held in the dominant hand and the needle is passed into the area while suction is held. This is repeated in several different directions, with care taken not to release the vacuum. The suction is then released and the needle is withdrawn. A holder for the syringe can be used to do the aspiration but this can be awkward for the aspirator and intimidating to the patient. The needle and syringe should be given immediately to the pathologist or evacuated onto a glass slide.

The slide can then be fixed as with a Papanicolaou (Pap) smear. The procedure should be repeated two to three times to ensure that adequate tissue has been obtained. On-the-spot evaluation by the cytopathologist makes this technique more successful because the aspiration can be repeated if sufficient tissue was not obtained from the initial aspirations. Adequate tissue must be obtained for a reliable cytologic diagnosis with FNA. Some series report inadequate tissue in up to 30 percent of FNA biopsies. This technique can be easily mastered and performed by both surgeons and pathologists.

Core Needle Biopsy

A core needle biopsy can be done on palpable masses with a Tru-cut needle or on nonpalpable masses with ultrasound guidance or use of a stereotactic mammography unit. In the case of a palpable breast mass, the lesion is fixed by the surgeon's nondominant hand and local anesthesia is injected into the skin. A small nick is made in the skin with a scalpel to facilitate passage of the Tru-cut needle. The needle is passed into the lesion and the outer sheath then slides over the needle, slicing out a core of tissue. The number of cores needed for a definitive diagnosis is not known. For stereotactic biopsies it is recommended that five cores be obtained. It is important

that mammography be performed on all the specimens when biopsy is done for calcifications.

Excisional Breast Biopsy

An open biopsy or excisional breast biopsy is performed when needle biopsies are nondiagnostic or when a small lesion needs to be removed. If the lesion is thought to be benign, the tumor can be removed with only a small rim of normal tissue. If there is a strong suspicion of malignancy, excision can be performed with a 1-cm margin. This decreases the need for re-excision if, indeed, the final histology reveals a malignant tumor. Planning the location and size of the incision is probably the most critical part of the procedure. The incision should be placed directly over the lesion along the natural resting skin tension lines (Fig. 44-5). These are different from Langer's lines, which encircle the breast. The natural skin tension lines are best seen in the breast in the upright position. The proper incision can be marked out with the patient in a sitting position before starting the procedure. Circumareolar incisions should only be used when the lesion is adjacent to or under the nipple. Tunneling out to the periphery of the breast from a circumareolar incision should be avoided since it is associated with more complications and jeopardizes

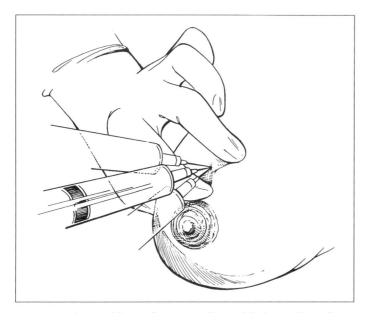

Fig. 44-4. Technique of fine-needle aspiration biopsy of the breast. The needle is passed in and out of the lesion several times while suction is maintained with the syringe. Samples should be fixed immediately to allow for the best possible material for cytologic diagnosis.

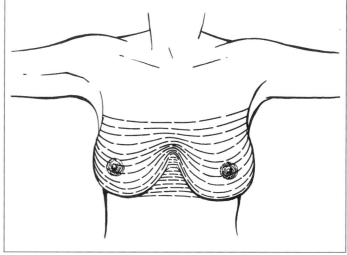

Fig. 44-5. The natural resting skin tension lines of the breast. Placement of a biopsy incision is best done along these natural lines of the breast. The incision can be marked with the patient in the sitting position before starting the procedure. (From S Love. Benign and Malignant Breast Disease. In WP Ritchie, G Steele, RH Dean (eds) General Surgery. Philadelphia: Lippincott, 1994. Reproduced with permission.)

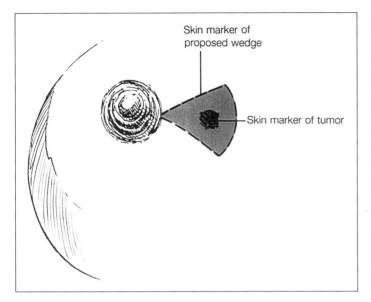

Skin marker of
proposed wedge

Skin marker of tumor

Fig. 44-6. Placement of biopsy incision directly over the palpable abnormality in the breast with the area of proposed excision marked out on the breast. This planned excision and placement of incision is critical in management of the patient who proves to have malignancy on open biopsy. (From S Love. Benign and Malignant Breast Disease. In WP Ritchie, G Steele, RH Dean (eds) General Surgery. Philadelphia: Lippincott, 1994. Reproduced with permission.)

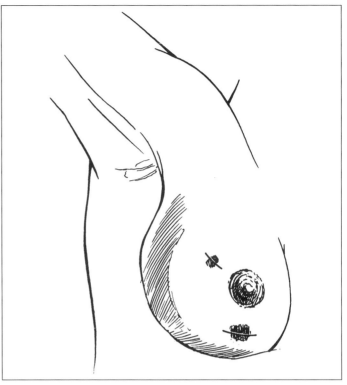

Fig. 44-7. Placement of skin incisions in different areas of the breast directly overlying the palpable lump. Circumareolar incisions should only be used for lesions directly under or adjacent to the nipple-areolar complex. (From S Love. Benign and Malignant Breast Disease. In WP Ritchie, G Steele, RH Dean (eds) General Surgery. Philadelphia: Lippincott, 1994. Reproduced with permission.)

the patient's chances for breast conservation surgery if a malignancy is found.

Most excisional biopsies can be performed with local anesthesia with or without the use of intravenous sedation. The breast is prepped and draped and the area of proposed excision is marked out on the skin (Fig. 44-6). The incision is marked out directly over the lesion (Fig. 44-7). Local anesthetic is then used to infiltrate the skin and deeper tissues. This should be done slowly and with a small (27 gauge) needle to minimize the discomfort experienced by the patient. The incision is made sharply and carried down through the subcutaneous tissue. Excision of the lesion should also be done with a knife or Metzenbaum scissors since electrocautery can obscure the margins and interfere with hormone receptor assays. The tumor should be removed with a rim of normal tissue and marked for orientation for the pathologist with a short stitch superior and a long stitch lateral. The specimen should be de-

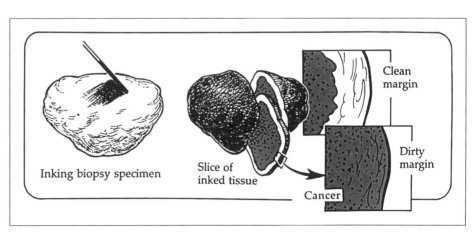

Inking biopsy specimen

Slice of inked tissue

Cancer

Clean margin

Dirty margin

Fig. 44-8. The biopsy specimen is marked with sutures to orient the specimen for the pathologist. Placing a short stitch in the superior position and a long stitch in the lateral position is easy for the physician and pathologist. The specimen is inked by the pathologist to allow for proper margin assessment. (From SM Love. Dr. Susan Love's Breast Book. Reading, MA: Addison-Wesley, 1990. Reproduced with permission.)

livered fresh to the pathologist, who then inks the perimeter of the tumor with India ink before the lesion is cut to allow for proper assessment of margins (Fig. 44-8).

Once the specimen is removed, hemostasis is obtained with the electrocautery. This is an important part of the procedure since hematomas are painful and can delay re-excision or other necessary procedures postoperatively. The breast tissue is not re-approximated with suture material. The subcutaneous tissue is closed with inter-rupted absorbable suture and the skin is closed with an absorbable stitch in a sub-cuticular fashion. Frozen section diagnosis at the time of excisional biopsy is rarely indicated since in general it would not al-ter the immediate management of the pa-tient. Examination of resection margins with frozen section is difficult to do since this is too time consuming and inaccurate to warrant the effort.

Mammographic Localization Biopsy

When a stereotactic core or FNA cannot be done or if there is any question about a mammographic abnormality, a diagnostic wire localization biopsy is indicated. The hook wire technique with a Homer, Sa-dowski, or Kopans wire is easiest for both the mammographer and the surgeon. It is important that the the wire is within 0.5 cm of the lesion. Any further distance re-quires excision of excessive amounts of tis-sue and increases the risk of a missed le-sion. Injection of methylene blue by the radiologist through the needle before the wire is passed serves as an additional marker of the area of concern. The proce-dure can usually be done with a local an-esthetic, as described previously for pal-pable lesions.

Once the localization has been completed, the surgeon can plan the operative ap-proach. It is important to place the incision as close to the lesion as possible. This al-lows for future re-excision or radiation therapy if the lesion is malignant. Since only 20 percent of these biopsies reveal cancer, the amount of tissue excised at the initial procedure should be minimized. Gently palpating the breast and watching the direction of movement of the wire will help to estimate where the lesion will be. Once this is marked, the area of the inci-

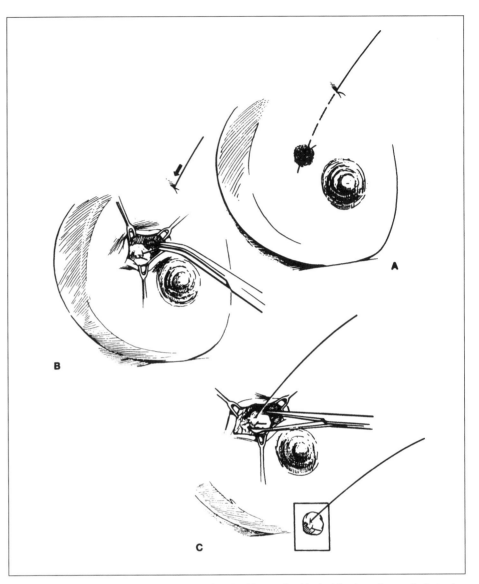

Fig. 44-9. Technique of mammographic wire localization biopsy. The skin incision is made over the lesion by palpating the end of the wire in the breast. The incision is made and sharp dissection carried out in the area of the hook of the wire. Once the area is dissected away from the deep tissues, the mammography wire is pulled through the incision. The specimen is sent for radiography with the wire in place. (From S Love. Benign and Malignant Breast Disease. In WP Ritchie, G Steele, RH Dean (eds), General Surgery. Philadelphia: Lippincott, 1994. Reproduced with permission.)

sion can then be injected with local anes-thetic. The incision is made and then dis-section is carried sharply down to the wire (Fig. 44-9). The wire can then be passed into the incision and the tissue to be ex-cised is grasped with an Allis clamp. The lesion is removed and marked with su-tures for orientation (short superior and long lateral). The specimen is then taken to radiology for a specimen radiograph. The incision can be closed while one waits to

hear from the radiologist. If there is any question, the wound is reopened and the blue dye is used to help locate the area that needs to be removed. The patient should have a postbiopsy mammogram taken 6 to 8 weeks after operation to confirm that the lesion in question was removed and to document any residual abnormality or cal-cifications. The specimen should be inked for margin assessment as in the excisional biopsy for a palpable mass.

Conclusion

The options for treatment of primary breast cancer have significantly changed over the past decade. Patients should participate in decisions regarding definitive treatment after a firm diagnosis has been established. The approach one uses to obtain a diagnosis should be based on an understanding of both benign and malignant breast diseases. A thorough evaluation of each patient is important when considering the potential diagnoses, overall cost, and trauma to the patient.

Suggested Reading

Donegan WL. Evaluation of a palpable breast mass. N Engl J Med 327:937, 1992.

Kinne DW, Kopans DB. Physical Examination and Mammography in the Diagnosis of Breast Disease. In JR Harris, S Hellman, IC Henderson, DW Kinne (eds), Breast Diseases (2nd ed). Philadelphia: Lippincott, 1991. Chap 5, p 81.

Layfield LJ, Chrischilles EA, Cohen MB, Bottles K. The palpable breast nodule. A cost effectiveness analysis of alternate diagnostic approaches. Cancer 72:1642, 1993.

Parker SH, Lovin JD, Jobe WE, et al. Nonpalpable breast lesions: Stereotactic automated large-core biopsies. *Radiology* 180:403, 1991.

EDITOR'S COMMENT

The vast majority of breast masses in the United States are treated by surgeons who, unlike the authors, have some interest in breast disease but do not devote their full time and effort to it. Therefore, having the benefit of the vast experience and focused approach to breast disease in general and breast masses in particular, as exemplified by Drs. Love and Hunt, affords the surgeon the advantages of this experience when dealing with breast masses. Doctor Love documents that over 500,000 open breast biopsies are performed in the United States each year, and that the rate of malignancy that is found varies substantially from institution to institution and even from surgeon to surgeon. The authors report a 20 percent rate of malignancy in all biopsy specimens, probably higher than in many institutions. There is always concern that a higher rate of malignancy may indicate that some lesions that truly do harbor cancer are missed in favor of doing fewer open breast biopsies. Obviously, a balance must be struck, and the authors have presented three practical algorithms for the proper approach to these lesions.

Pneumocystography is not described in this chapter, but is occasionally performed in patients with cysts of the breast, which are aspirated under ultrasound control, at the end of which a minimal amount of air is injected. The patient is then subjected to immediate mammography, which affords a good contrast medium to evaluate the breast cyst wall. This is usually used when the mass reforms promptly after aspiration, or when the aspirate is bloody.

A significant issue that the authors do not address is definitive therapy based on fine-needle aspiration alone, important primarily in larger lesions, which are then subject to modified radical mastectomy. Even though one has extreme confidence in the cytopathologist who interprets the fine-needle aspirate, it is still essential that a diagnosis be arrived at either by a core tissue biopsy or by open incisional biopsy. As with any cytopathologic diagnostic procedure, a small but finite number of misdiagnoses are made, and the sacrifice of a breast that on final pathology turns out to have benign disease is something that must be assiduously avoided.

Doctor Love's approach to the skin incision, of great importance to the patient, is somewhat different from the conventional teaching; she chooses not to use Langer's lines above the nipple and a radial incision below the nipple, which is the conventional teaching, popularized by the National Surgical Adjuvant Breast Project (NSABP) group in the late 1980s, but rather uses largely transverse or occasionally oblique incisions in all locations in the breast. Because of this and a number of other different opinions among various experts in the field, this chapter and the two following will, on occasion, seem somewhat discordant in advice about breast incisions. All points of view are being presented to show that there is no absolute uniformity of opinion as to how an incision should be made. Nevertheless, all of these techniques have the primary goal of a workable approach to diagnosis of the mass, a good cosmetic result, and, most importantly, an adequate margin of normal tissue around the lesion that proves to be cancer.

R.J.B.

45

Segmental Mastectomy and Axillary Dissection

Monica Morrow

For many years, total mastectomy was believed to be the only appropriate surgical procedure for the treatment of breast carcinoma. The Halstedian view of tumor biology, in which breast cancer was thought to spread in an orderly fashion from the site of the primary tumor to the axillary lymph nodes, and then via the lymphatics to distant sites, mandated an operation that would remove the primary tumor with a large margin of normal tissue and widely extirpate the draining lymphatics. Over time, it became apparent that distant metastases develop in many women with breast cancer in spite of radical surgical procedures, prompting a re-examination of our understanding of breast cancer biology. The demonstration that moderate doses of radiation successfully eradicate microscopic deposits of breast cancer, coupled with the increasingly frequent detection of smaller cancers by mammography and an increasing emphasis on the use of systemic adjuvant therapy, opened the door for the use of breast-conserving surgery in the treatment of breast cancer.

A major concern with the removal of less than the entire breast for cancer treatment is the multifocality and the multicentricity of breast cancer. However, in contrast to mastectomy, the goal of which is to remove all of the breast tissue that is potentially tumor bearing, the goal of breast-conserving surgery is to remove all of the gross tumor and to depend on postoperative irradiation to eradicate microscopic residual tumor deposits. This principle has now been tested in six modern, prospective randomized trials comparing some form of breast-conserving surgery and irradiation

to mastectomy for the management of invasive cancer. No survival advantage for mastectomy was demonstrated in any of these studies, and breast-conserving surgery should be regarded as an equal alternative to mastectomy for properly selected patients.

Patient Selection

Appropriate patient selection is critical to the success of breast-conserving surgery, and is an attempt to balance an acceptably low rate of local recurrence in the breast with a good cosmetic outcome. Standard guidelines for the use of breast-conserving surgery have been developed by a multidisciplinary group of surgeons, radiation oncologists, pathologists, and radiologists. Absolute contraindications to the procedure include the following: 1) Multiple gross primary tumors in separate quadrants of the breast: In this circumstance, the likelihood of the presence of a large amount of tumor in the residual breast tissue is great, and local failure rates are high. 2) Diffuse indeterminate or suspicious microcalcifications on mammography: This mammographic picture raises the possibility of extensive carcinoma, and even when some of the calcifications are surgically proved to be benign, makes follow-up difficult. It is important to note that diffuse benign-appearing calcifications are not a contraindication to breast-conserving surgery. 3) First and second trimester of pregnancy: It is not possible to safely deliver therapeutic doses of radiation at any time during pregnancy. It is unknown whether segmental mastectomy in the

third trimester, with a delay in radiation therapy until after delivery, is safe. I favor the use of mastectomy for breast cancer diagnosed during pregnancy unless the diagnosis is made late in the third trimester. 4) History of prior irradiation to the breast field: Therapeutic irradiation cannot be readministered without excessive damage to normal tissues. This contraindication is most commonly encountered in the management of the breast cancer patient with a history of treatment for Hodgkin's lymphoma with mantle irradiation. Women who received such treatment during childhood or adolescence have a markedly increased risk of breast cancer development and are not usually candidates for breast-conserving therapy.

In addition to these absolute contraindications, there are several relative contraindications to breast-conserving surgery. The most important of these is a large tumor-breast ratio. The purpose of breast-conserving surgery is to maintain a breast that is cosmetically acceptable to the patient. The impact of tumor size on cosmetic outcome will vary with the quadrant of the breast in which the tumor is located and the depth of the tumor. There is no absolute tumor size for which breast-conserving surgery is contraindicated. Many women prefer to retain their own sensate breast, even with some degree of cosmetic deformity, rather than to have a "perfect," but insensate, breast reconstruction. Another relative contraindication is the presence of active collagen vascular disease, primarily scleroderma and systemic lupus erythematosus. This contraindication is based on anecdotal reports of severe fibrosis and soft-tissue necrosis after irradiation in these patients. In the past, the need to sacrifice the nipple-areolar complex as part of a segmental mastectomy was considered to be a contraindication to the procedure. While it is true that this worsens the cosmetic result, there is no evidence that tumor location impacts on local recurrence rates, and this probably should not be considered a contraindication.

The previously discussed contraindications to breast-conserving surgery apply to women with ductal carcinoma in situ (DCIS) and clinical stages I and II breast cancer. In my experience with 456 unselected patients, only 25 percent had medical contraindications to breast-conserving surgery. The frequency of contraindications varied with stage, and breast conservation was possible in 90 percent of patients with stage I disease. Nationally, fewer than 50 percent of patients with early-stage breast cancer are treated with breast-conserving surgery, suggesting some degree of misunderstanding of the selection criteria for the procedure. It is important to remember that tumor features that are associated with poor prognosis, such as large size, palpable adenopathy, and high histologic grade, are not contraindications to breast-conserving surgery. Similarly, breast-conserving surgery is appropriate for all types of invasive carcinomas, providing that negative margins can be obtained. Excision of infiltrating lobular carcinoma is often more difficult than excision of infiltrating ductal carcinoma due to the tendency of many lobular carcinomas to be ill defined and to grow in a discontinuous pattern. However, if negative margins are obtained, local recur-

Table 45-1. Selection Criteria
for Breast-Conserving Surgery

Patient desire for procedure

Single primary tumor

Able to excise to negative margins

Tumor-breast ratio that allows a cosmetic
result that is acceptable to the patient

Able to deliver postoperative radiotherapy
  No history of prior irradiation to breast field
  No active collagen vascular disease
  Not pregnant

Able to follow patient
  Mammogram without diffuse indeterminate
    microcalcifications
  Reliable

rence rates for infiltrating lobular cancers are no greater than those seen with infiltrating ductal carcinoma. Selection criteria for breast-conserving surgery are summarized in Table 45-1.

While it is clear that survival after breast-conserving surgery is equal to survival after mastectomy for invasive carcinoma, more controversy exists regarding the use of the procedure for DCIS. Mastectomy for the treatment of DCIS has a failure rate of 1 percent or less with long-term follow-up study. When breast-conserving surgery is used in DCIS, breast recurrence rates of 10 to 15 percent at 10 years are seen. Half of these recurrences are invasive carcinomas, raising the possibility of a small but real (2–3% at 10 years) increase in breast cancer mortality when compared to treatment with mastectomy. This does not mean that breast-conserving surgery for DCIS is contraindicated, but rather that particular attention must be paid to patient selection and follow-up.

Preoperative Evaluation

High-quality bilateral mammography, before surgical biopsy, is essential in assessing a patient's suitability for breast-conserving surgery. The site of the palpable tumor should be marked with a radiopaque marker, and magnification views of the primary tumor site should be obtained to assess the extent of any calcifications associated with the primary tumor. Other abnormalities detected in the ipsilateral breast should be evaluated with spot compression and magnification views to assess their significance, and the contralateral breast should be closely scrutinized. About 2 percent of patients will be found to have a clinically occult contralateral breast cancer. However, the major benefit of this detailed mammographic approach is to determine the extent of the breast excision needed to achieve negative margins, and to exclude patients with extensive multifocal or multicentric disease from attempts at breast-sparing surgery. Using such an approach, I have found that only 3 percent of patients selected for breast-sparing surgery were unable to successfully undergo the procedure. When microcalcifications are the presenting sign of cancer, a mammogram with magnification views of the tumor site should be obtained

after the segmental mastectomy before one concludes that the procedure is complete, even if the histologic margins are negative.

Extensive evaluations for metastatic disease in the asymptomatic patient are unwarranted. Bone scans should be reserved for patients with palpable adenopathy, an elevated alkaline phosphatase level, or symptoms of bone pain. Imaging studies of the liver and brain are only indicated if symptoms are present. Obviously, metastatic workups for women with DCIS are unnecessary, since this disease, by definition, does not metastasize.

Technique of Segmental Mastectomy

A number of imprecisely defined terms, including segmental mastectomy, lumpectomy, partial mastectomy, wide local excision, and tylectomy, are used to describe the removal of a breast cancer and a variable amount of normal breast tissue. The extent of the surgical resection is determined by the clinical and mammographic extent of the cancer. The procedure described is for a combined segmental mastectomy and axillary dissection.

The patient is positioned with the arm at 90 degrees to the body on an armboard. A small folded sheet is placed under the shoulder to elevate the axilla. The entire arm is prepped and draped in a stockinet in case manipulation of the arm is necessary during the axillary dissection (Fig. 45-1). Antibiotics are given if a surgical biopsy has been performed to establish the diagnosis of carcinoma. The anesthesiologist should be asked to avoid long-acting muscle relaxants to allow reliable identification of the motor nerves of the axilla.

The segmental mastectomy incision should be placed in a skin line and be large enough to allow the specimen to be removed as a single piece of tissue (Fig. 45-1). In the upper half of the breast, incisions should be curvilinear, while radial incisions are used for tumors at the 3 o'clock and 6 o'clock positions. Circumareolar incisions give the best cosmetic result, but should be reserved for lesions in the peri-areolar area since they rarely give adequate exposure for lesions in the periphery of the breast. Incision placement for lesions in the inferior half of the breast is more difficult to generalize. Whether a radial incision or a curvilinear incision is utilized will vary with both the breast shape and the tumor size. I have found that, in general, radial incisions maintain the position of the nipple better than curvilinear approaches, and give the best cosmetic result. Excision of the skin overlying the tumor is neither necessary nor desirable unless the tumor is extremely superficial, and may alter the position of the nipple.

An important step in segmental mastectomy is the preservation of the subcutaneous fat overlying the tumor. Preservation of this layer will result in the maintenance of a normal breast contour, even when large amounts of breast tissue are removed. Tumors within the substance of the breast are approached by incising the breast tissue overlying the tumor to a point approximately one centimeter above the tumor (Fig. 45-2). The tissue superficial to the tumor is retracted with double-pronged skin hooks, and thick flaps are raised with a knife (Fig. 45-3). I attempt to excise a margin of one centimeter of grossly normal breast tissue around the tumor site, recognizing that the actual margin of tissue removed will vary. After the flaps are raised, the skin hooks are replaced with Richardson retractors of an appropriate size (Fig. 45-4). The surgeon controls the tumor with the nondominant hand and the tumor is sharply excised. The use of Allis clamps or other similar devices to grasp the tumor and surrounding breast tissue should be avoided, since this technique makes it extremely difficult to determine if the tumor is being excised with an adequate margin of normal tissue. Removal of the pectoral fascia is unnecessary, and should be reserved for those tumors adherent to or in close proximity to this structure. When the segmental mastectomy specimen is removed it is carefully inspected for evidence of tumor extending to the margins. Frozen sections of margins are only done for clinically suspicious areas since it is impossible for the pathologist to adequately sample all of the margin surfaces with random frozen sections.

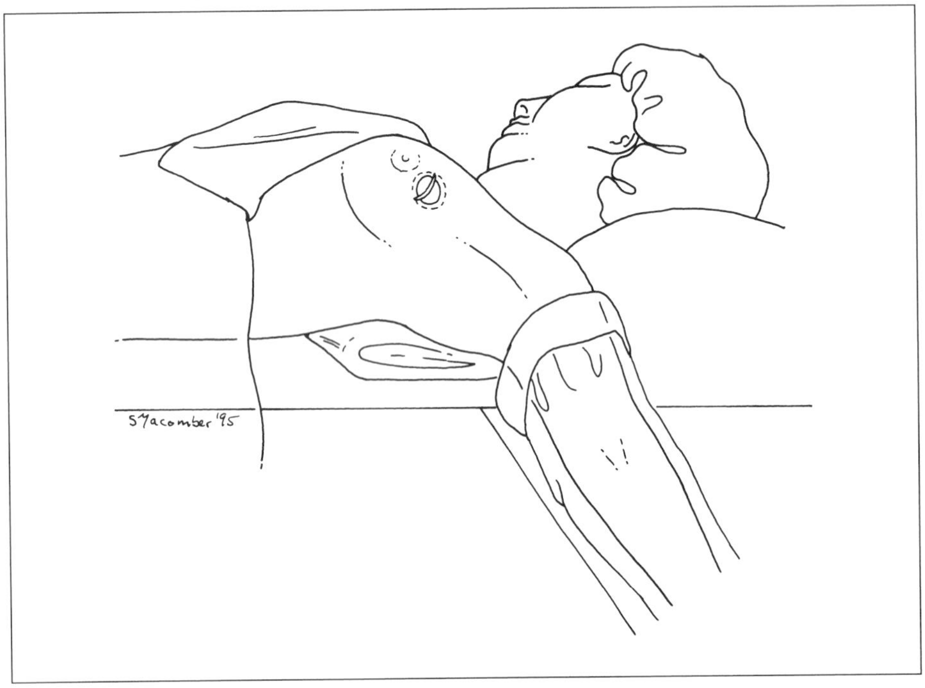

Fig. 45-1. Patient position for combined segmental mastectomy and axillary dissection. The extent of the tumor is shown with the solid line and the extent of the planned segmental mastectomy with the dotted line.

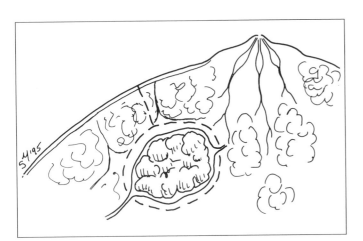

Fig. 45-2. Breast tissue superficial to the tumor is incised (dotted line) to a point approximately one centimeter above the lesion before the segmental mastectomy is begun.

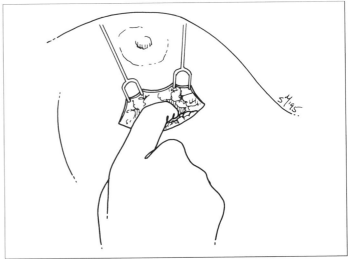

Fig. 45-3. Thick skin flaps are raised to allow access to the tumor while the tumor is retracted with the nondominant hand.

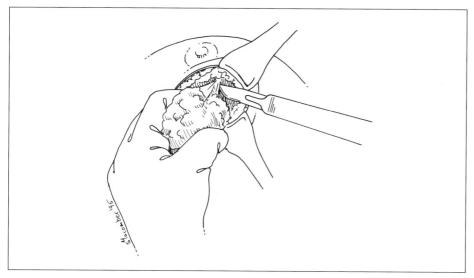

Fig. 45-4. *The tumor is elevated into the incision and sharply excised.*

After the specimen is delivered, meticulous hemostasis is obtained with the cautery. Re-approximation of the lumpectomy cavity should be avoided, since this will usually distort the contour of the breast. This distortion may not be evident with the patient supine with her arms relaxed on the operating table. Drains are not employed since the dead space in the breast will fill in with seroma, helping to maintain the breast contour. The use of metallic clips to outline the margins of the lumpectomy cavity is useful for radiation treatment planning. The incision is closed with an interrupted layer of 3-0 Vicryl, which is placed in the deep dermis to take the tension off the skin closure. A running 4-0 nylon subcuticular pull-out suture is used to re-approximate the skin. A single Steri-Strip is placed over the length of the incision and a light dressing is used. Large pressure bandages are not employed.

Specimen Management

Proper management of the segmental mastectomy specimen is essential to the success of the procedure. The specimen should be removed as a single piece of tissue; otherwise margins cannot be assessed. Two marking sutures are placed to orient the pathologist: a short suture in the superior margin and a long suture in the lateral margin. The specimen is sent fresh to pathology for determination of the estrogen and progesterone receptor status.

The surface of the specimen is painted with ink to allow an assessment of the proximity of the tumor to the margin. The pathology report should include a statement regarding the presence or absence of tumor at the margins of resection, which margins are involved, and the extent (gross, extensive microscopic, or single microscopic focus) of involvement of the margins.

Indications for Re-Excision

Re-excision is indicated when the margins of the initial excision (whether it is a biopsy or an attempted segmental mastectomy) contain gross or extensive amounts of microscopic tumor, or when the margin status is unknown. The need for re-excisions for small amounts of microscopic disease at the margin is unclear, and must be decided on a case-by-case basis.

Attempts to perform re-excision by removing the entire previous biopsy site as a single piece of tissue usually result in the sacrifice of excessive amounts of breast tissue and a poor cosmetic result. I prefer to sample each wall of the biopsy cavity as a separate specimen, or, if the site of the positive margin is known, to confine the re-excision to that area. The previous incision is re-opened and any fluid in the biopsy cavity is evacuated. The cavity is carefully palpated for evidence of gross tumor. The

cavity walls are then excised using a knife. The pieces that are excised should include most of the surface of the old biopsy cavity and be approximately 1 cm in thickness. The new margin surface of each specimen is marked with a suture, since what is important is not whether tumor is present in the re-excision specimen, but whether tumor is present at the final margin. Each specimen is separately labeled and sent for permanent section. Frozen sections are only used if an area of concern is palpated. Hemostasis is obtained and the cavity is closed in the same fashion as described for a primary segmental mastectomy.

Technique of Axillary Dissection

The boundaries of the axillary triangle are the axillary vein superiorly, the serratus anterior medially, and the latissimus dorsi laterally. Within this space, the axillary contents are divided into three levels, with the level 1 nodes found lateral and inferior to the pectoralis minor, the level 2 nodes below the axillary vein and behind the pectoralis minor, and the level 3 nodes medial to the pectoralis minor against the chest wall. Removal of the level 1 and 2 nodes provides accurate staging information since isolated nodal metastases in level 3 ("skip metastases") are seen in fewer than 1 percent of patients. If gross nodal metastases are evident at the time of operation, all three levels of nodal tissue should be removed to maintain local control. In the clinically node-negative patient, level dissection is appropriate.

The axillary incision is placed in a skin crease at the inferior margin of the hair-bearing portion of the axilla (Fig. 45-5). The incision extends from just below the free edge of the pectoral muscle anteriorly to the latissimus dorsi posteriorly, and should not cross either of these structures. If the axillary space is wide, a transverse incision in this space will provide adequate exposure. When the axilla is narrow, the ends of the incision should be curved superiorly, parallel to the muscles, resulting in a U-shaped incision.

The dissection is begun by raising flaps superiorly to the estimated level of the axillary vein, medially to expose the free edge of the pectoralis major, laterally to expose

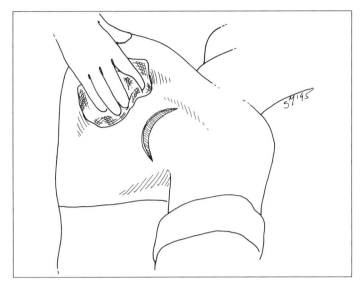

Fig. 45-5. The incision for axillary dissection is placed in one of the inferior axillary skin creases. It should not cross the plane of the pectoralis major or the latissimus dorsi.

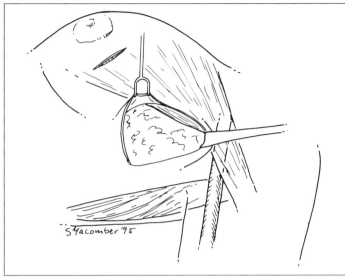

Fig. 45-6. Extent of the axillary flaps: superiorly to the axillary vein, medially to the edge of the pectoralis major, laterally to the latissimus dorsi. The inferior flap has not been raised yet.

the edge of the latissimus dorsi, and inferiorly to the junction of the axillary tissue and the tail of the breast (Fig. 45-6). Failure to raise the inferior flap will result in the lowest axillary nodes being left in place, with the potential for inaccurate staging and inadequate local control. The flaps can be raised using the knife or the cautery. The purpose of this part of the operation is to obtain exposure, and the subcutaneous fat should be left on the flaps.

After the flaps have been raised, the clavipectoral fascia is incised along the length of the pectoralis major, and the pectoralis major and minor are freed from the surrounding fat and a Richardson retractor placed beneath them. The medial pectoral neurovascular bundle will usually be encountered during this dissection and should be preserved. The axillary vein is then identified by following the latissimus cranially until its tendon is identified (Fig. 45-7). At the point where the latissimus turns tendinous it is crossed by the axillary vein. The dissection is done sharply, and accomplishes both the identification of the axillary vein and mobilization of the lateral border of the specimen. The only important structure that is encountered during this approach is the intercostobrachial nerve, which is usually found one-half to two-thirds of the way to the vein. In the clinically node-negative axilla, the intercostobrachial nerve should be identified and preserved to avoid the numbness of

the upper inner arm associated with its transection. Continued division of the fat and axillary fascia superior to the intercostobrachial nerve will result in identification of the axillary vein.

Once the vein is identified, it is cleared of overlying fat in a lateral to medial direction. If dissection is confined to the anterior surface of the vein, no major vessels will be encountered. It is important to avoid both "stripping" the axillary vein of all its overlying fat and dissection above the level of the axillary vein, both of which increase the risk of lymphedema postoperatively. The purpose of clearing the fat off the axillary vein is to allow visualization of the vein so that its branches can be dissected. In a level 3 dissection, the clearance of the vein extends to the chest wall. If level 2 dissection is being done, the fat is divided to a point behind the pectoralis minor.

When exposure of the vein is completed, dissection of the venous branches is carried out from lateral to medial (Fig. 45-8). Dissecting approximately 5 mm below the vein will avoid the problem of a side hole in the vein if a branch is accidentally transected. At this point a large collateral lymphatic that runs parallel to the vein is often encountered, and this structure should be preserved if possible. The fatty tissue of the axilla is manually retracted inferiorly and sharply dissected in a systematic fash-

ion from lateral to medial. No effort is made to identify neurovascular structures at this point. As branches of the axillary vein are encountered, they are clamped with right-angle clamps, divided, and tied with 3-0 silk ties.

The thoracodorsal neurovascular bundle is usually identified as the first deep branch of the axillary vein that is encountered laterally. The thoracodorsal nerve is found medial to the thoracodorsal vein. After the nerve is identified, the thoracodorsal bundle is dissected free from the anterior axillary fat. The thoracodorsal vein usually has a number of small anterior branches that must be ligated to avoid annoying bleeding. After the identification of the thoracodorsal bundle, any remaining superficial branches of the axillary vein medial to the thoracodorsal bundle are ligated. The long thoracic nerve is readily identified at this point by inserting two fingers into the space between the axillary fat and the chest wall immediately below the axillary vein (Fig. 45-9) and gently spreading along the chest wall. The axillary tissue is retracted laterally, and the long thoracic nerve is usually visible lying against the chest wall. If the nerve is not seen against the chest wall it has been pulled laterally with the specimen. The nerve is dissected free from the specimen by sharp dissection on its anterior and lateral surface. Dissection between the long thoracic nerve and

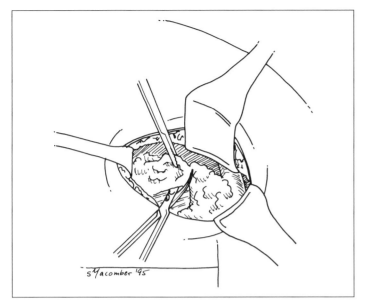

Fig. 45-7. Dissection along the latissimus dorsi to expose the axillary vein. The vein is exposed in the illustration for clarity, but would be encased in fat at this point.

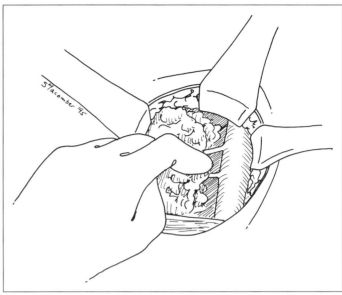

Fig. 45-8. Exposure of branches of the axillary vein.

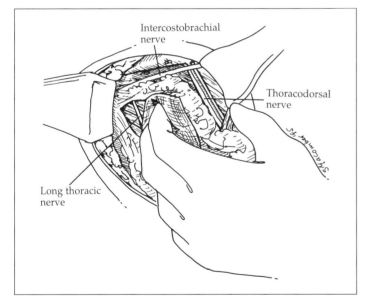

Fig. 45-9. Exposure of the long thoracic nerve by retracting the axillary contents laterally.

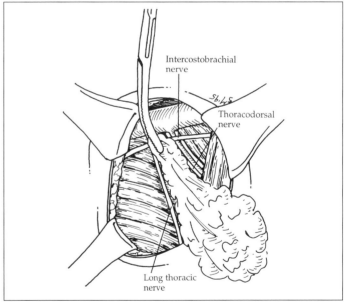

Fig. 45-10. The axillary tissue between the long thoracic nerve and the thoracodorsal nerve is lifted anteriorly in preparation for encircling it with a right-angle clamp.

the chest wall should be avoided. The safest way to dissect the nerve is by keeping it under direct vision and sharply dissecting immediately on top of it, and the nerve should be followed inferiorly until it is seen to penetrate the serratus anterior.

Once both the long thoracic nerve and the thoracodorsal nerve have been identified, the axillary fat remaining between the two nerves can be encircled with a right-angle clamp and divided (Fig. 45-10). At this point, if the intercostobrachial nerve is to be preserved, it must be dissected free from the axillary specimen. The maneuver to expose the long thoracic nerve will usually expose the medial end of the intercostobrachial nerve. The axillary tissue over-

lying the remainder of the nerve is sharply divided until the nerve is free for its entire length. The nerve is then gently retracted upward while the dissection of the upper portion of the axilla is completed. After dealing with the intercostobrachial nerve, the tissue between the long thoracic and thoracodorsal nerves is bluntly swept down with a sponge, using a posterior and inferior sweeping motion (Fig. 45-11). The dissection of the thoracodorsal neurovascular bundle is then completed inferiorly, until the nerve and accompanying vessels are seen to enter the latissimus on its deep medial surface. The inferior axillary contents are then freed from the chest wall and the tail of the breast using the cautery. Large veins crossing the axilla are usually encountered at this point and are clamped and tied. Care must be taken before freeing the inferior attachments of the specimen that the long thoracic nerve has been identified and dissected free down to the point where it penetrates the serratus anterior since immediately before entering the serratus, the nerve hooks laterally into the axillary specimen and may be inadvertently transected at this point if it has not been completely dissected.

After the specimen is removed the wound is irrigated with warm saline and hemostasis is obtained. A single No. 10 flat suction drain is shortened and placed through a stab wound inferior to the incision (Fig. 45-12). Care should be taken to avoid placing the drain exit site too far anteriorly, where it will be visible, or too far posteriorly, where it will not be accessible for the patient to strip. The axillary incision is closed with a deep dermal layer of interrupted 3-0 Vicryl sutures and the skin is closed with a 4-0 Vicryl running subcuticular stitch. A light fluff dressing is placed until the following morning.

Postoperative Care

Patients are instructed in drain care and discharged after an observation period of 23 hours or less. Drain output is recorded on a 24-hour basis, and the drain is removed when the 24-hour output is less than 40 ml for 2 consecutive days. Patients are not maintained on antibiotics during the time that their drains are in place. Arm exercises are begun on the day after operation and continued until a normal range of motion is achieved. Radiation is begun 2 weeks postoperatively unless the axillary drain is still in place. Patients have a new baseline posttreatment mammogram of the treated breast approximately 2 months after the completion of radiation, and mammograms of the treated breast are obtained at 6-month intervals until the changes from surgery and radiation stabilize (usually about 2 years); then annual mammography is resumed. With this technique of segmental mastectomy and axillary dissection, 89 percent of patients have assessed their cosmetic outcome as excellent or good and the incidence of severe lymphedema (>4-cm discrepancy in arm circumference) is less than 1 percent.

Suggested Reading

Fisher B, Costantino J, Redmond C, et al. Lumpectomy compared with lumpectomy and radiation therapy for the treatment of intraductal breast cancer. *N Engl J Med* 328:1581, 1993.

Gluck BS, Dershaw DD, Liberman L, Deutch BM. Microcalcifications on postoperative mammograms as an indicator of adequacy of tumor excision. *Radiology* 188:469, 1993.

Gwin JL, Eisenberg BL, Hoffman JP, et al. Incidence of gross and microscopic carcinoma in specimens from patients with breast cancer after re-excision lumpectomy. *Ann Surg* 218:729, 1993.

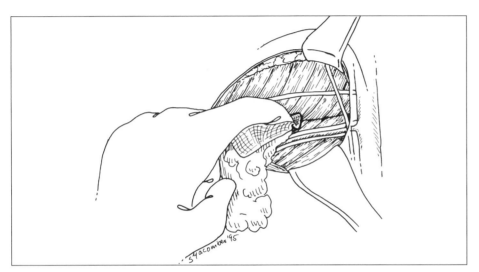

Fig. 45-11. *The axillary tissue between the long thoracic nerve and the thoracodorsal nerve is bluntly swept down with a sponge.*

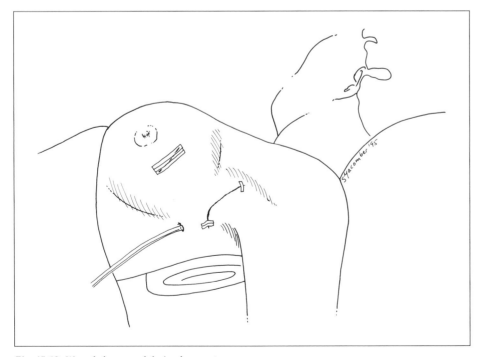

Fig. 45-12. *Wound closure and drain placement.*

Harris JR, Morrow M. Local Management of Invasive Breast Cancer. In *Diseases of the Breast*. JR Harris, ME Lippman, M Morrow, S Hellman, Philadelphia: Lippincott-Raven, 1996. Pp. 487–547.

Kearney T, Morrow M. Effect of reexcision on the success of breast conserving surgery. *Ann Surg Oncol* 2:303, 1995.

Margolese R, Poisson R, Shibata H, et al. The technique of segmental mastectomy (lumpectomy) and axillary dissection: A syllabus from the National Surgical Adjuvant Breast Project Workshops. *Surgery* 102:828, 1987.

Morrow M, Schmidt R, Hassett C. Patient selection for breast conservation: Identification of multifocality with magnification mammography. *Surgery* 118:621, 1995.

Rose MA, Olivotto I, Cady B, et al. Conservative surgery and radiation therapy for early breast cancer. Long term cosmetic results. *Arch Surg* 124:153, 1989.

Veronesi U, Volterrani F, Luini A, et al. Quadrantectomy versus lumpectomy for small size breast cancer. *Eur J Cancer* 26:671, 1990.

Winchester DP, Cox JD. Standards for breast-conservation treatment. *CA* 42:134, 1992.

EDITOR'S COMMENT

Doctor Morrow, in her usual scholarly and highly precise fashion, has written a classic description of the indications for and technique of segmental mastectomy with axillary dissection. She has covered essentially all of the important technical features of this operation, which to most surgeons seems very simple, but to the accomplished breast surgeon is a demanding and more complex operation. The major goals are to preserve the function and appearance of the breast but at the same time to eliminate, with a high degree of certainty, all gross and, it is hoped, microscopic tumor.

Doctor Morrow, in the new approach to excisions for breast cancer, believes that there is no absolute tumor size for which conservation is contraindicated. More traditional surgeons who learned a decade ago that T1 and smaller T2 lesions are appropriately treated by this procedure will need to rethink what may be too conservative a position. If 4- and 5-cm tumors can be excised and allow a satisfactory cosmetic result to be obtained, there is no logical, perhaps even rational, reason for not doing so. Unfortunately, a favorite truism is that "being logical doesn't make it correct." However, as the boundaries of the procedure are delineated and as appropriate amounts of data are collected, with careful follow-up, the answers should become available in the not too distant future. The simplest judgment parameter is the presence or absence of recurrent cancer in the ipsilateral breast; the more difficult issue, and one that may be a nonissue, is the incidence of recurrent disease elsewhere. The familiar "biologic predeterminism" principle of 30 years ago was probably one of the most reliable biologic observations of that era of the behavior of breast cancer; the work of numerous clinical investigators in breast cancer has, of course, changed our outlook. As the author points out, however, some surgeons still believe that breast conservation is not necessary or in the best interest of the patient, an archaic view.

This form of treatment does, however, require that the patient be reliable and understand the importance of the postoperative radiation therapy management, with or without chemotherapy, and be willing to cooperate fully in obtaining the best possible adjunctive treatment. It is also important that the radiation therapist, in concert with the surgeon, have the opportunity to fully inform the patient about the implications of and complications of radiotherapy, so that the patient has full information available to participate actively in the decision-making process.

Many patients with early breast cancer and no symptoms are investigated beyond what is really necessary; the best example is the use of bone scans in asymptomatic patients, although the author appropriately emphasizes that significant palpable axillary nodes or an elevated alkaline phosphatase suggest that the tumor may be advanced, and both bone scans and CT scanning may be necessary. The finding of an abnormality of the liver on CT scan is always a source of considerable concern and occasionally some consternation, since it then becomes incumbent on the surgeon and consultants to determine whether the lesion in the liver is metastatic and of breast origin or whether it is an unrelated benign lesion. Without the elevated alkaline phosphatase, CT scan is not used in my practice in the asymptomatic patient.

The use of metal clips to outline the cavity has been emphasized by the author. These are primarily of use if the lesion is not directly below the skin incision, although outlining the cavity certainly cannot be faulted, both for directing radiotherapists in terms of radiation ports and also in helping the surgeon in the unlikely but finite possibility that a re-excision becomes necessary, since exposure of the clips will assure the surgeon that the cavity has been exposed in its entirety.

The concise and highly specific description of the exposure of the axilla and its contents and the technique of axillary resection warrants no further comment except to compliment the author on a fine essay for this purpose.

R.J.B.

46

Management of Minimally Invasive and Noninvasive (In Situ) Carcinoma of the Breast

Cheryl A. Ewing   Richard B. Arenas

Breast cancer is the most commonly diagnosed cancer in American women, accounting for approximately 18 percent of malignant diagnoses in the female population. It is estimated that during 1995, 182,000 women were diagnosed with breast cancer, and 46,000 will eventually die from breast cancer. The incidence of breast cancer in the United States has increased 2 percent per year since 1973. However, since 1982, breast cancers have been diagnosed at earlier stages.

The overall diagnosis of in situ breast cancer has nearly quadrupled over the past decade, increasing from 1.4 percent of all breast biopsy specimens before 1975 to 9.6 percent after 1987. Over the last two decades, the diagnosis of stage I breast cancer has increased from 26 to 37 percent.

In order to appreciate the indications for breast conservation surgery for early cancer, an understanding of the pathophysiology of in situ breast carcinoma and its subsequent transformation into invasive cancer is required. Similar to carcinoma of the colon or bladder, breast cancer is a progression from atypical hyperplasia within the ducts or lobules to formation of in situ disease and subsequent invasion beyond the basement membrane.

The incidence of noninvasive cancer of the breast has increased dramatically since 1987 based solely on the improvement of early detection. Before the development and routine practice of screening mammography, noninvasive cancer included 1 to 3 percent of all breast cancers. Now as many as 30 to 45 percent of breast cancers may be in situ. This trend toward the di-

agnosis of breast cancer at an early stage has helped to bring about the current treatment modalities of breast conservation.

Ductal Carcinoma In Situ

Ductal carcinoma in situ (DCIS) describes cancer limited to the extralobular terminal ductal segments of the breast. Similar to invasive ductal carcinoma, the majority of noninvasive cancers are ductal in nature. Rarely palpable, DCIS accounts for about one-third of all mammographically detected cancers. DCIS pathologically consists of an array of histologic subtypes (solid, micropapillary, cribriform, and comedo). The accurate grading of DCIS can predict the associated presence of microinvasion; comedocarcinoma as determined by the presence of necrosis within the ducts tends to be clinically more malignant.

Indications for Surgery

Breast conservation surgery for DCIS requires minimizing the chance of local recurrence and the eradication of any potentially coexisting invasive component. Axillary nodal metastases from DCIS are rare and in cases of extensive intraductal cancer, any nodal involvement is probably the result of occult invasion. Total mastectomy for DCIS therefore rarely requires a formal axillary node dissection; the need for node dissection should be re-evaluated in cases in which invasion is later determined or suspected.

Excision alone for DCIS results in a local recurrence rate of about 30 percent; however, a significant majority of local failures will present with invasive disease. Such recurrences occur after a latent interval of 5 to 10 years. With the addition of radiotherapy, local recurrence is substantially decreased (Table 46-1) but never reaches the local failure rate for total mastectomy (1–3%). The discrepancy between the re-

Table 46-1. Incidence of Recurrence After Wide Excision and Radiation Therapy (DCIS)

Authors*	No. of Pts	Median Follow-up (mo)	No. of Recurrences (%)	
Fisher et al	399	43	28	(7%)
Bornstein et al	38	81	8	(21%)
Kurtz et al	43	61	3	(7%)
McCormick et al	54	36	10	(18%)
Recht et al	40	44	4	(10%)
Silverstein et al	103	63	10	(10%)
Solin et al	172	84	6	(3%)

*See Suggested Reading List.

sults of breast conservation and mastectomy diminishes when comparing overall survival; cancer-related mortality after breast conservation for DCIS should be close to zero.

The indications for local excision in the treatment of noninvasive breast cancer require that all the disease be excised with negative margins. Acceptable cosmesis will be determined by the relative size of the lesion to the entire breast. Ductal carcinoma generally follows a segmental distribution, but in some instances, DCIS is extensive or multifocal in nature. Such cases of multifocal or extensive intraductal cancer would contraindicate breast conservation surgery. Axillary node dissection is generally not required for intraductal cancer unless invasive cancer is determined after excision or in cases of extensive disease when microinvasion is suspected.

Lobular Carcinoma In Situ

Lobular carcinoma in situ (LCIS) is generally diagnosed as an incidental finding on routine biopsy. Although clinically and mammographically silent, it is increasing in incidence, probably reflective of the increase in the number of breast biopsies performed. The significance of LCIS as a marker for cancer is based upon the high incidence of bilaterality compounded by the associated risk to develop cancer of ductal origin in either breast. Since the significance of LCIS is based upon the relative risk of developing cancer away from its origin, wide excision with free margins is not required. Therapy is directed to the surveillance and early detection of cancer unless prophylactic mastectomy is contemplated after sufficient patient counseling.

Method of Evaluation and Diagnosis of Breast Cancer

Stage I and stage II breast cancers are considered early-stage breast cancer, and account for 75 percent of newly diagnosed breast cancer. In comparison to the long-term survival for patients diagnosed with breast cancer in the last 50 years, the future long-term survival rates are expected to improve due to increased early diagnosis

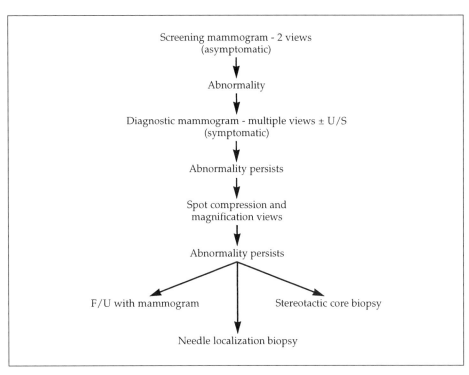

Fig. 46-1. Algorithm for mammography. U/S = ultrasound; F/U = followup.

and the use of adjuvant chemotherapy, particularly in node-negative patients.

It has been clearly demonstrated in six prospective randomized trials, evaluating some 4077 women, that breast conservation (partial mastectomy, axillary node dissection, and radiation therapy) is an acceptable alternative treatment for breast cancer to the modified radical mastectomy, if the patient is an appropriate candidate. With breast cancer early detection, surgeons interested in breast disease should know all approaches for diagnosis and treatment for in situ and early-stage breast cancers (see Chapter 44). Before any invasive procedures are performed, a diagnostic mammogram is obtained to evaluate a potential breast cancer and possible treatment with breast conservation, if a breast malignancy is diagnosed. If the mammogram is obtained after the invasive procedure, a breast hematoma may confuse the issue.

For women under the age of 30 with clinically benign breast lesions, we do not routinely obtain a mammogram or ultrasound examination. A diagnostic aspiration cytology or core biopsy for vague indefinite lesions and excisional biopsy for palpable breast masses are recommended. With clinically suspicious lesions, we use the

same algorithm as for women over the age of 30. We use a similar algorithm for nonpalpable mammographic lesions (Fig. 46-1).

Selection for Breast Conservation

Following the diagnosis of minimal breast cancer, defined as intraductal carcinoma or invasive cancer less than 5 mm in size, and early-stage breast cancer (stages I and II), each patient should be evaluated as a possible candidate for breast conservation. The National Cancer Institute recently published their 10-year results comparing total mastectomy to partial mastectomy (lumpectomy) and radiation therapy. The disease-free survival (Fig. 46-2) and overall survival (Fig. 46-3) are very similar. The risk for recurrent disease is slightly higher in the breast conservation group (5–10% per year compared to 1% per year for the total mastectomy group at 10 years).

It is important for the surgeon to understand the principles of breast conservation, that is, interpretation of mammograms, methods of diagnosis, which patients are candidates for conservation, technical considerations for performing a lumpectomy for palpable and nonpalpable lesions, ra-

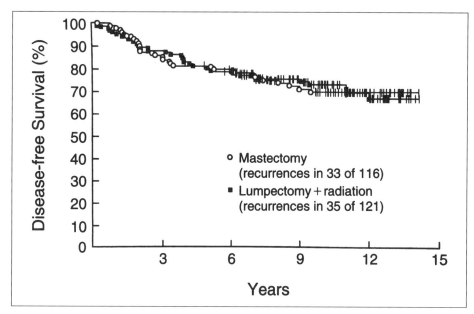

Fig. 46-2. *Disease-free survival. (Modified from JA Jacobson, DN Danforth, and KH Cowan. Ten year results of a comparison of conservation with mastectomy in the treatment of Stage I and Stage II breast cancer.* NEJM 332:907, 1995.

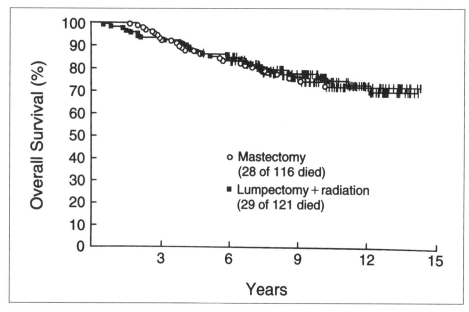

Fig. 46-3. *Overall survival. (Modified from JA Jacobson, DN Danforth, and KH Cowan. Ten year results of a comparison of conservation with mastectomy in the treatment of State I and Stage II breast cancer.* NEJM 332:907, 1995.

diation therapy, risks and treatment for local failure, and long-term follow-up study.

For any patient who is an appropriate candidate for breast conservation, we provide a lengthy and detailed discussion with the patient and family, often with the radiation oncologist in attendance, concerning the risks and benefits of breast conservation, in order that the patient can make an informed decision. The surgeon's particular

biases for breast conservation or mastectomy should not cloud the discussion.

When given the choice of breast conservation or mastectomy for the treatment of breast cancer, 75 percent of our patients chose breast conservation. Patients with early breast cancer, not considered candidates for breast conservation, are treated with skin-sparing mastectomy if an immediate reconstruction is desired by the

Table 46-2. Patients Not Considered Candidates for Breast Conservation

Previous history of breast irradiation

First and second trimester of pregnancy

Tumor size relative to breast size (results in unacceptable cosmesis) or tumor size greater than 4 cm

Women with 2 or more malignancies in the same breast (multicentric breast cancer)

Disseminated suspicious microcalcifications on mammogram

Extensive multifocal intraductal carcinoma in situ

Negative tumor margin cannot be achieved surgically without loss of cosmesis

Table 46-3. Patients with No Contraindication to Breast Conservation

Contralateral breast cancer
Clinically positive axillary lymph nodes that are not fixed
Tumor histology (invasive lobular carcinoma, poorly differentiated carcinomas, lymphatic or venous invasion)
Tumor location in breast
Tumor fixation to pectoralis major
Age > 65 yr

patient. The patient's history, physical examination, mammogram, and breast pathology (Tables 46-2 and 46-3) will determine if breast conservation should be offered.

The diagnosis of breast cancer can usually be determined preoperatively in palpable breast masses with aspiration cytology using a 21-gauge needle and syringe or Tru-cut core biopsy. We favor aspiration cytology, as it is quick, painless, and usually atraumatic, and the diagnosis can be obtained immediately from the cytopathologist. A preoperative diagnosis of breast cancer can facilitate definitive therapy with lumpectomy (with or without axillary node dissection) or mastectomy with appropriate frozen section as a one-stage procedure.

Technical Considerations for Lumpectomy

If an open breast biopsy is necessary, either as an excisional breast biopsy or needle localization breast biopsy, the procedure

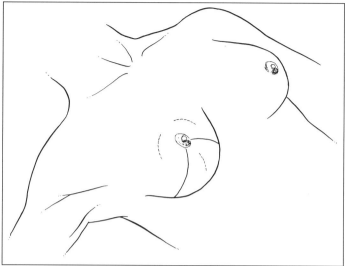

Fig. 46-4. Cosmetically pleasing incision lines for lumpectomy.

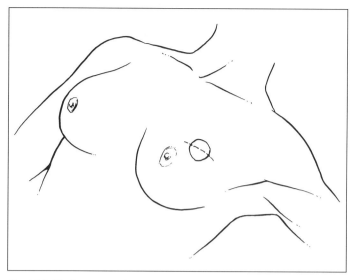

Fig. 46-5. The lumpectomy incision is placed over the breast mass.

should be performed as a lumpectomy to avoid the need for re-excision of the biopsy cavity for residual carcinoma. The surgeon should pay great attention to all technical details when performing breast lumpectomies. This will assure an adequate lumpectomy with complete tumor excision without tumor extending to the margins, avoid the need for re-excision, and optimize the cosmetic outcome.

To obtain optimal cosmetic results, the lumpectomy incision is placed in a curvilinear fashion following Langer's lines of tension of the skin, with the exception of the lower inner quadrant of the breast (approximately between 7 o'clock and 4 o'clock). We favor a radial incision to prevent shortening the distance between the areolar margin and inframammary fold (Fig. 46-4). Excision of the skin is not necessary unless the tumor directly invades the skin or if the tumor is very superficial (just below the skin), and excision of the skin is necessary to achieve an adequate tumor-free anterior margin.

The skin incision is always placed directly over the breast mass (Fig. 46-5). Tunneling from the areolar margin is to be avoided, as this can result in tumor seeding the tunnel, an excessive amount of normal breast tissue excised with increased risk of breast deformity, increased risk of postoperative hematoma, and increased difficulty for the radiation oncologist to accurately direct the radiation boost.

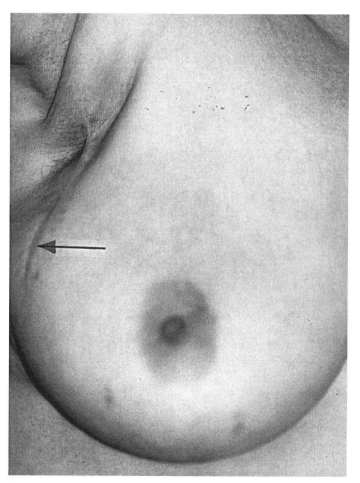

Fig. 46-6. Unacceptable scarring results from a continuous incision for a tumor in the upper outer quadrant and an axillary node dissection.

For breast tumors located in the upper outer quadrant and if an axillary node dissection is planned, a separate incision at the base of the axillary hairline, for the axillary node dissection, will result in better cosmetic outcome. A radial incision extending from the upper outer quadrant into the axilla to perform the lumpectomy and axillary node dissection is to be condemned, as this will result in unacceptable breast deformity (Fig. 46-6). The lumpectomy and axillary node dissection can be performed through one curvilinear incision at the base of the axillary hairline only for carcinomas located high in the axillary tail of Spence, without significant scarring of the breast.

The incision for the lumpectomy is kept as small as possible, usually between 2 and 3 cm in length. The incision is deepened into the breast tissue to a depth of approximately 1.0 to 1.5 cm from the tumor. This will maintain breast tissue under the incision to prevent depression of the incision after closure and to minimize the amount of normal tissue excised. For needle localization, the surgeon uses the needle localization radiograph to estimate how deep the incision is to be carried into the breast tissue before doing a lumpectomy around the localization needle to remove the non-palpable breast lesion.

The lumpectomy is performed with great care and attention to detail. To facilitate retraction in a very small incision, we use double-pronged skin hooks, Senn retractors, and long narrow retractors such as Army/Navy retractors, Richardson appendiceal retractors, and S-shaped retractors. The retractors used are based on the depth of the lumpectomy in the breast (Fig. 46-7). The operative field is kept dry to inspect the breast tissue for any abnormalities. We recommend electrocautery in the cut mode, which does not cause histologic artifact or interfere with hormonal receptor studies. The breast tissue is carefully palpated to feel for suspicious nodules distant from the primary carcinoma and to assure the surgeon that an adequate margin of normal breast tissue surrounds the tumor, to avoid cutting through the tumor. The breast tumor is removed, with an ellipse of normal tissue around it, as one specimen. The lumpectomy specimen should never be removed in fragments as this will prevent determination of the

pathologic tumor size and eliminate evaluation for tumor-free margins.

Before the lumpectomy specimen is excised from the breast, sutures are placed in the specimen to orient the pathologist for margins (Fig. 46-8). We place a short stitch at the superior margin and a long stitch at the lateral margin. The lumpectomy specimen is then excised from the breast. If there is tumor invasion into the pectoralis major muscle, a wedge of muscle is excised as part of the lumpectomy specimen. Before the lumpectomy specimen is taken to the pathology department, each margin is carefully palpated to assess how close the

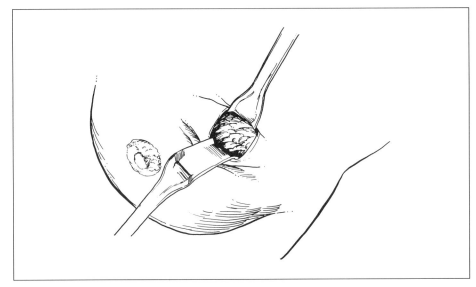

Fig. 46-7. The retractors used to expose the specimen are based on the depth of the tumor in the breast.

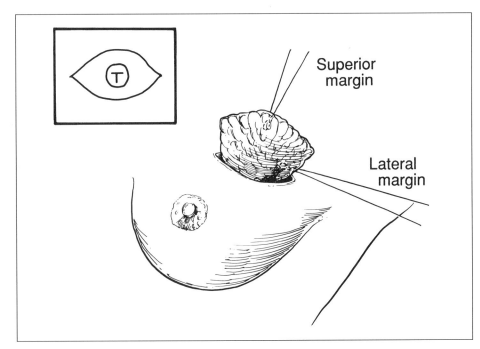

Fig. 46-8. Sutures are placed in the specimen to orient the pathologist—a short suture at the superior margin and a long suture at the lateral margin.

tumor is to the margin. If the tumor is close to the margin, a re-excision of that margin is performed, with a single stitch to mark the new margin on the re-excision specimen. Frozen section examination of the lumpectomy specimen and re-excision specimen is rarely done, unless the preoperative fine-needle aspiration is nondiagnostic and an axillary node dissection is planned for breast conservation. Frozen section examination is not necessary for very small needle localization specimens. All needle localization specimens should be radiographed to assure that the mammographic lesion is excised.

For proper handling of the specimen in the pathology department, the surgeon should speak directly to the pathologist for correct margin orientation and to express any concern about multifocal cancers or residual tumor at the lumpectomy site if re-excision is not possible. The lumpectomy specimen and any re-excised margins are covered with India ink to mark the margins and are sectioned with proper margin orientation. Hormonal receptor analysis, flow cytometry, and other prognostic tumor markers are obtained.

Before the skin closure, complete hemostasis is necessary in the lumpectomy cavity, as drains are never used. If muscle is exposed at the base of the lumpectomy cavity, we cover it with breast tissue located at the bottom of the lumpectomy cavity, using 3-0 Vicryl suture with interrupted stitches. This will prevent the skin incision from adhering to the muscle with healing, particularly in women with small breasts and lesions located in the upper inner quadrant. We usually leave a small hemoclip at the base of the lumpectomy cavity, to aid targeting for the breast irradiation boost. The lumpectomy cavity is never sutured closed as this will only lead to increased fibrosis and breast deformity. The skin incision is closed in two layers, with absorbable sutures (Fig. 46-9). The dermis is re-approximated with buried 3-0 Vicryl interrupted stitches. The skin is closed with a 4-0 Vicryl suture as a running subcuticular stitch (Fig. 46-9).

In stage I or stage II breast carcinomas that involve the nipple-areolar complex, the nipple-areolar complex is completely excised as a transverse ellipse. The incisions are deepened into the breast tissue and a lumpectomy is performed as described previously.

Skin-Sparing Mastectomy

If a breast carcinoma is diagnosed in any patient not considered a candidate for breast conservation for reasons of contraindication to breast conservation or personal preference, and when the plan is a mastectomy with immediate reconstruction, the diagnosis should be obtained with fine-needle aspiration (with definitive cytology for carcinoma for a palpable breast mass) or with stereotactic core biopsy for nonpalpable, suspicious mammographic lesions. This will facilitate optimal cosmesis of the skin-sparing mastectomy by obviating the need to excise the skin of a previous open biopsy incision.

The skin-sparing mastectomy is done through a circular incision around the nipple-areolar complex (Fig. 46-10). If an axillary node dissection is necessary, or for large breasts, a teardrop incision is made with the V end pointed toward the axilla (Fig. 46-11) The skin flaps are raised from the breast in the subcutaneous plane using electrocautery in a circular spiral around the breast, until all the surgical boundaries of the breast are identified (Fig. 46-12). The superior flap is raised to the clavicles and the fascia of the pectoralis major muscle is incised. The medial flap is raised to the lateral sternal border. The inferior flap is raised to the insertion of the pectoralis major on the fascia of the rectus abdominis and sixth rib, and laterally to the latissimus dorsi. The skin flaps can easily be elevated from the breast with skin hooks or Adair clamps on the skin for traction and a laparotomy pad over the breast for countertraction. The breast is excised in a subfascial plane started at the most superior aspect of the previously incised pectoralis fascia. The breast is excised in the subfascial plane of the pectoralis major muscle

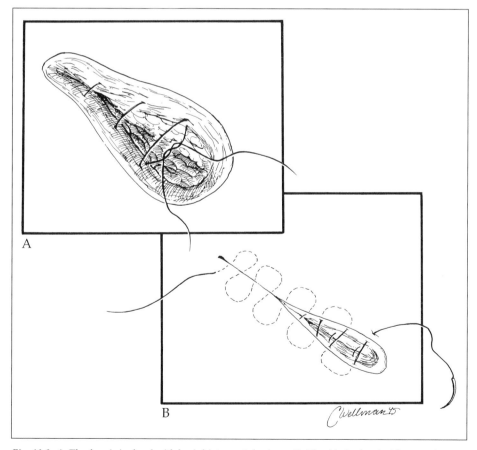

Fig. 46-9. A. The dermis is closed with buried interrupted sutures. B. The skin is closed with a running subcuticular suture.

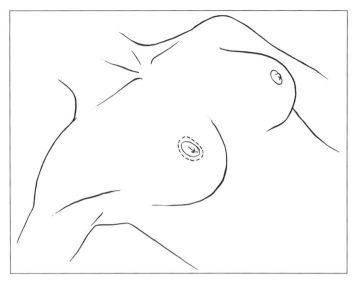

Fig. 46-10. *A circular incision around the nipple-areolar complex is used for a skin-sparing mastectomy.*

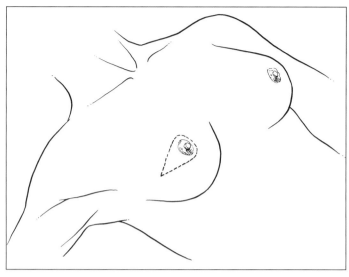

Fig. 46-11. *A teardrop incision is used for a skin-sparing mastectomy if the breasts are large or an axillary node dissection is necessary.*

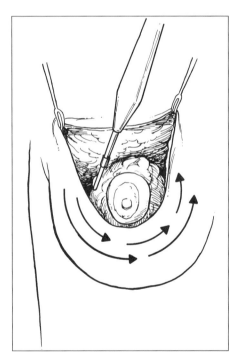

Fig. 46-12. *The skin flaps are raised in a skin-sparing mastectomy.*

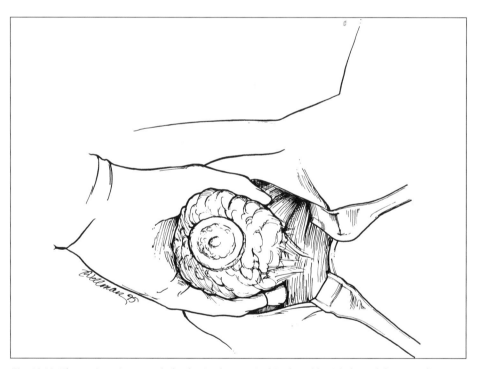

Fig. 46-13. *The specimen is removed after having been excised in the subfascial plane of the pectoralis muscle.*

from lateral to medial, then medial to lateral, following the striae of pectoralis major muscle fibers. We have found this dissection to be simple and it will avoid cutting into muscle, which can lead to unnecessary blood loss. Near the sternal border care must be observed to avoid transecting the perforating arteries and veins

from the internal mammary vessels. The breast is delivered through the incision attached to the serratus anterior laterally (Fig. 46-13). The level I and II axillary node dissection is done at this time with care to avoid injury to the thoracodorsal vessels if a free TRAM (*t*ransfer of *r*ectus *a*bdominis *m*yocutaneous) flap is planned. The cos-

metic appearance of a skin-sparing mastectomy with reconstruction is far superior to that of the standard modified mastectomy. The natural contour of the breast is maintained, particularly the inframammary fold. The only incision line on the reconstructed breast is at the reconstructed nipple-areolar complex (Fig. 46-14).

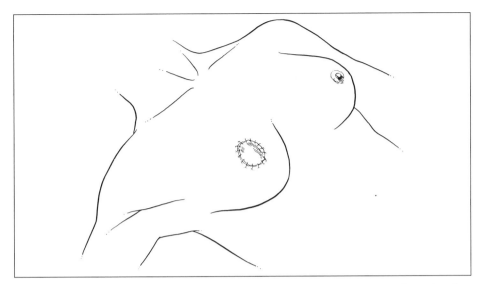

Fig. 46-14. The final appearance of the skin-sparing mastectomy with reconstruction is excellent. The only incision line is at the nipple-areolar complex.

Silverstein MJ, Cohlan BF, Gierson DH, et al. Duct carcinoma in situ: 227 cases without microinvasion. *Eur J Cancer* 28:630, 1992.

Smith RA. Epidemiology of Breast Cancer. In AG Hans, MJ Yaffee, (eds). *Syllabus: A Categorical Course in Physics. Technical Aspects of Breast Imaging.* Oakbrook, IL: RSNA, 1993.

Solin LJ, Yeh I-T, Kurtz J, et al. Ductal carcinoma in situ (intraductal carcinoma) of the breast treated with conservation surgery and definitive irradiation. *Cancer* 71:2532, 1993.

Veronesi U, Banfi A, Del Vecchio M, et al. Comparison of Halsted mastectomy with quadrantectomy, axillary dissection and radiotherapy in early breast cancer: Long-term results. *Eur J Cancer Clin Oncol* 22:1085 1986.

EDITOR'S COMMENT

Doctors Ewing and Arenas, both of whom devote most of their surgical activities to breast disease, have presented what proves to be an important discussion of a lesion that is far more commonly recognized today than was previously the case. Routine mammography and investigation of abnormal mammograms are now so much a part of daily surgical life that the discovery of ductal carcinoma in situ, especially, is quite commonplace. Patients with one or several groups of microcalcifications have at least a 30 to 40 percent chance of having ductal carcinoma in situ, and this chapter outlines very well the best therapeutic approach to these lesions.

There are, as would be expected, several areas where differences of opinion almost inevitably will arise. For example, the authors advocate breast conservation for invasive ductal cancers of the breast up to 4 cm in size (stage II). The data support conservatism versus breast sacrifice for lesions of 2.5 to 3.0 cm; the newer approach to larger lesions still should be evaluated with considerable caution. In Table 46-3, the authors urge breast conservation in patients with lymphatic or venous invasion, with tumor fixation to the pectoralis major, and in patients who have been treated for contralateral breast cancer, among other considerations. Certainly these are debatable issues, and the only one about which I have serious concern is the patient with lymphatic or venous invasion, although I am sure that the authors' rationale is that patients who already have lymphatic or venous spread are not better served by

Suggested Reading

Bader J, Lippman M, Swain S, et al. Preliminary report of NCI early breast cancer (BC) study: A prospective randomization comparison of lumpectomy (L) to radiation (XRT) to mastectomy (M) for stage I and II BC. *Int J Radiat Oncol Biol Phys* 13 (Suppl 1):160, 1987.

Bartelink H, Van Dongen JA. Randomized clinical trial to assess the value of breast conserving therapy (BCT) in stage I and stage II breast cancer (abstract). In *Proceedings of the 5th European Conference on Clinical Oncology*, 1989.

Blichert-Toft M, Brinker H, Anderson JA, et al. A Danish randomized trial comparing breast preserving therapy with mastectomy in mammary carcinoma: Preliminary results. *ACTA Oncol* 27:671, 1988.

Bornstein BA, Recht A, Connelly JL, et al. Results of treating ductal carcinoma in situ of the breast with breast-conservation surgery and radiation therapy. *Cancer* 67:7, 1991.

Cancer Statistics 1995. *Ca Cancer J Clin* 45:8, 1995.

Fisher B, Constantino J, Redmond C, et al. Lumpectomy compared with lumpectomy and radiation therapy for the treatment of intraductal breast cancer. *N Engl J Med* 328:1581, 1993.

Fisher B, Redmond C, Poisson R, et al. Eight year result of randomized clinical trial comparing total mastectomy and lumpectomy with or without irradiation in the treatment of breast cancer. *N Engl J Med* 320: 822, 1989.

Frykberg ER, Bland KJ, Management of in situ and minimally invasive breast carcinoma. *World J Surg* 18: 45, 1994.

Jacobson JA, Danforth DN, Cowan KH. Ten-year results of a comparison of conservation with mastectomy in the treatment of stage I and stage II breast cancer. *N Engl J Med* 332:907, 1995.

Kurtz JM, Jacquemier J, Torhorst J, et al. Conservation therapy for breast cancers other than infiltrating ductal carcinomas. *Cancer* 63:1630, 1989.

McCormick B, Rosen PP, Kinne D, et al. Duct carcinoma-in-situ of the breast: Does conservation surgery and radiotherapy provide acceptable local control? (abstract). *Int J Radiat Oncol Biol Phys.* 19 (Suppl):132, 1990.

Recht A, Connelly JL, Schnitt S, et al. The effect of young age on tumor recurrence in the treated breast after conservation surgery and radiotherapy. *Int J Radiat Oncol Biol Phys* 14:3, 1988.

Recht A, Danoff BS, Solin LJ, et al. Intra ductal carcinoma of the breast: Results of treatment with excisional biopsy and irradiation. *J Clin Oncol* 3:1339, 1985.

Ries LG, Hankey BF, Miller BA, et al. *Cancer Statistics Review 1973–88.* NIH Publication No. 91-2789. Bethesda, MD: National Cancer Intstitute, 1991.

Sarrazin D, Lê MG, Arrigada, et al. Ten year result of a randomized trial comparing a conservative treatment to mastectomy in early breast cancer. *Radiat Oncol* 14:177, 1989.

Schnitt S, Connelly JL, Recht A, et al. Breast relapse following primary radiation for early breast cancer. II. Detection, pathologic features, and prognostic significance. *Int J Radiat Oncol Biol Phys* 11:1277, 1985.

eradication of the breast and the axillary contents, since surgical treatment is most likely palliative and not curative. Despite minor differences of opinion, it appears that the authors are on the right track, and that modified radical mastectomy will become less commonly used in the future.

A very interesting surgical approach to subtotal mastectomy is the one performed through a circumareolar incision and in which the breast is, in essence, "cored out" through a relatively small incision. I have not personally performed the procedure through this incision, although I have used a somewhat extended "teardrop"-shaped incision in women with small breasts and have found that to be totally satisfactory. The entire concept is contrary to the classic Haagensen principles that breast tissue extends almost to the dermis, that thinner flaps are better than thicker flaps, and that one should reach to the subclavicular fascia at the level of the subclavius muscle, as advocated by Drs. Bland and Vezeridis, to assure excision of all breast tissue possible. As in other controversial areas in breast cancer management, a great deal of data will need to be accumulated to show that chest wall recurrence with this particular type of excision is no greater than chest wall recurrence in patients subjected to modified radical mastectomy through the wider incisions.

R.J.B.

47

Modified Radical Mastectomy with Early or Delayed Breast Reconstruction

Kirby I. Bland   Michael P. Vezeridis

The term *modified radical mastectomy* includes a total mastectomy and removal of the axillary lymphatics with preservation of the pectoralis major muscle, a technique that enhances cosmesis of the chest wall when compared to the Halsted radical mastectomy. As early as 1912, JB Murphy acknowledged that he had abandoned the Halsted radical mastectomy and did not resect either pectoral muscle. Murphy's practice of pectoral muscle preservation was based on the original report by Bryant of London, who found only one case of recurrent breast carcinoma in the pectoral muscles of patients followed during a clinical experience of 40 years. However, modified radical mastectomy was not established as appropriate therapy for T1 and T2 breast lesions unfixed to the pectoralis major muscle until the widely regarded contribution of DH Patey.

The value of modified radical mastectomy in the management of breast cancer was established by retrospective and prospective studies. Five retrospective studies analyzed the 5- and 10-year local and regional recurrence rates for chest wall, scar, operative field, and axilla (Table 47-1). De Larue and associates reported no recurrence at any site in 43 patients with stage I disease at 5-year follow-up. Leis found no recurrence in any site for stage 0; 5 percent scar, chest wall, and operative field recurrence for stage I; and 13.8 percent for stage II disease. In 1936, David Patey of London began the routine application of modification of the Halsted mastectomy with preservation of the pectoralis major muscle. The Patey modified radical mastectomy approach resected level I, II, and

III nodes with sacrifice of only the pectoralis minor muscle. Leis subsequently observed the very low axillary recurrence rate of 0.8 percent when using the Patey mastectomy technique for stage I and II lesions. Handley also observed low axillary recurrence rates, of 1.8 percent for Columbia Clinical Classification stage A and 0.1 percent for stage B lesions. Recurrence of the chest wall, scar, or operative field for Columbia Classifications A, B, and C was 10.0, 22.6, and 63.6 percent, respectively. Madden and associates extolled the virtues of the Auchincloss technique and stressed the necessity to dissect completely the low (level I/II) axillary contents. The

local recurrence rate reported in these series was 10 percent, while no recurrences were observed in the axilla. Baker and associates compared the results of modified radical to radical mastectomy in the treatment of operable breast cancer and found no statistically significant differences in 5-year survival. Furthermore, when they compared the results of the two surgical procedures, they confirmed no statistically significant differences in the incidence of local or regional recurrence. In contrast, patients with stage III disease treated with modified radical mastectomy had a statistically significant ($P = 0.002$) higher incidence of chest wall and axillary recurrence

Table 47-1. Local and Regional Recurrence Rates Following Modified Radical Mastectomy

Author and Year	Clinic or Study Group	Number of Pts	Disease Stage[a]	Chest Wall, Scar, or Operative Field	Axilla
				Site (%)	
DeLarue et al, 1969	Toronto General[b] (Canada)	43	I	0	0
		32	II	12.5	—
		25	III	15.0	—
Madden et al, 1972	NYC[c]	94	I–III	10	0
Handley, 1976	UK[c]	77	A[d]	10.0	1.8
		58	B	22.6	0.1
		8	C	63.6	9.1
Baker et al, 1979	Johns Hopkins[b]	91	I	13.2	1.1
		22	II	9.1	4.5
		31	III	22.6	22.6
Leis, 1980	NY Medical College[c]	116	0	0	0
		397	I	5.0	0.08
		333	II	13.8	0.08

[a]Staging is tumor, node, metastasis (TNM) unless otherwise noted.
[b]5-year recurrence rates.
[c]10-year recurrence rates.
[d]Columbia Clinical Classification.

compared to patients treated with radical mastectomy alone. These authors concluded that modified radical mastectomy is the treatment of choice for patients with stage I and II breast cancer. Thereafter, Nemoto and Dao observed that modified radical mastectomy using the Patey technique can recover as many axillary lymph nodes as the radical mastectomy. All these observations support the conclusion that removal of the pectoralis major muscle is not essential for local and regional control in stage I and II cancer of the breast.

The value of the modified radical mastectomy for the treatment of carcinoma of the breast was also established by prospective trials. In the Manchester trial, Turner and coworkers prospectively randomized and treated T1 and T2 (N0 or N1) breast cancers with either Halsted radical or modified radical mastectomy. At a median follow-up period of 5 years, no statistically significant differences in disease-free or overall survival were observed between the two surgical treatment groups. In addition, the 5-year local/regional recurrence rates for the chest wall, axilla, and skin were equivalent in the two treatment groups for patients with clinical and pathologic stage I and stage II disease. Further, there was a trend that favored the modified radical mastectomy technique (21% local recurrence rate for modified radical vs 25% for radical mastectomy). Thus, the Manchester trial supports the comparability of modified radical and radical mastectomy with regard to recurrence, local-regional control, and overall and disease-free survival.

Another prospective randomized trial (1975–1978) was conducted at the University of Alabama by Maddox and associates. Patients with histologically positive metastatic axillary lymph nodes were randomized to receive adjuvant chemotherapy. At a median follow-up period of 5.5 years, no statistically significant difference in disease-free survival was found between the two operative groups. However, a trend toward improvement in the 5-year survival rate was present for the radical mastectomy and this trend became more evident when analysis was completed at 10 years. At 10-year follow-up, Maddox and associates confirmed that the local recurrence rate for the modified radical mastectomy technique was twice that of the radical mastectomy technique ($P = 0.04$).

This increase in recurrence was evident with subset analysis of the more advanced stage lesions and it was greatest for stage III disease. The results of this study indicate that although the overall survival was similar for patients treated with the two techniques, patients with more advanced disease had better ultimate survival when treated with radical mastectomy.

Fisher and other investigators at 34 American and Canadian institutions participated in protocol B-04 of the National Surgical Adjuvant Breast Project (NSABP), a prospectively randomized trial comparing alternative local and regional treatments of breast cancer, all of which employed breast removal. The results of this study, reported by Fisher and coworkers in 1985, confirmed that the modified radical mastectomy is equivalent to radical mastectomy in overall and disease-free survival.

Surgical Technique

The patient is positioned on the operating table in the supine position for induction of general endotracheal anesthesia. A rolled sheet provides modest elevation of the ipsilateral hemithorax and shoulder such that there is no limitation of range of motion of the arm and shoulder with abduction and adduction. The positioning of the patient at the margin of the operating table is important to allow the surgeon and the assistant ample access without undue retraction on the pectoralis muscle groups or the brachial plexus (Fig. 47-1). With positioning, the surgeon should be cognizant of potential subluxation on abduction of the shoulder. This complication is best prevented by padding the armboard to avoid stretch of the brachial plexus and denervation of major muscle groups of the shoulder and arm. The surgeon must confirm adequate mobility of the ipsilateral arm for adduction and extension during operation.

The ipsilateral breast, neck, shoulder, and hemithorax are prepped with povidone-iodine to the table margin and well beyond the midline (Fig. 47-2). In addition, the axilla, arm, and hand are fully prepped within the operative field. Towels are secured with clips or stainless steel staples to the skin within the operative field, which includes the shoulder, lower neck, sternum, and upper abdominal musculature.

Alternative methods exist for including the arm and hand in the operative field. Our preference is to isolate the hand and forearm with an occlusive Stockinette

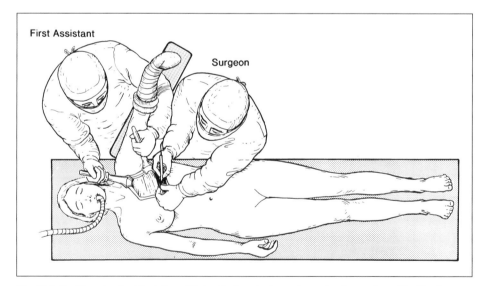

Fig. 47-1. Position of patient for left modified radical mastectomy at margin of operating table. The first assistant is cephalad to the armboard and shoulder of the patient to allow access to the axillary contents without undue traction on major muscle groups. Depicted is the preferential isolation of the hand and forearm with an occlusive Stockinette cotton dressing secured distal to the elbow. This technique allows free mobility of the elbow, arm, and shoulder to avoid undue stretch of the brachial plexus with muscle retraction. (From KI Bland, EM Copeland III (eds), The Breast: Comprehensive Management of Benign and Malignant Diseases. *Philadelphia: Saunders, 1991. Reproduced with permission.)*

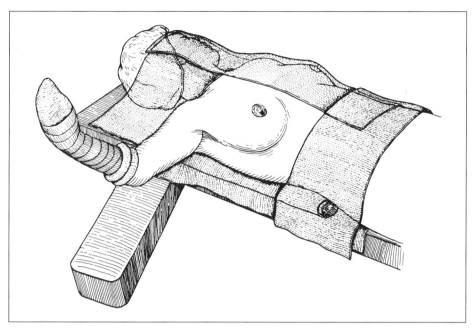

Fig. 47-2. Typical position for draping patient for operations of cancer of the right breast. The ipsilateral hemithorax is positioned at the margin of the operating table with a sheet roll that provides slight elevation to the ipsilateral shoulder and hemithorax. This position potentially prevents subluxation and abduction of the shoulder with stretch of the brachial plexus. Draping of the periphery of the breast is inclusive of the supraclavicular fossa and the entire shoulder to allow adequate mobility for adduction of the shoulder and arm across the chest wall. The elbow should be easily flexed and extended without undue tension. (From KI Bland, EM Copeland III (eds), The Breast: Comprehensive Management of Benign and Malignant Diseases. *Philadelphia: Saunders, 1991. Reproduced with permission.)*

(DeRoyal Industries, Powell, TN) cotton dressing that is further secured with Kling or Kerlix cotton roll (Johnson & Johnson, New Brunswick, NJ) distal to the elbow. Free mobility of the elbow, arm, and shoulder must be ensured with isolation of the forearm and hand.

We position the first assistant over the shoulder of the ipsilateral breast, cranial to the armboard, so that appropriate muscle retraction at the time of the axillary dissection can be accomplished with free mobility of the shoulder to allow extension, abduction, and adduction without undue stretch of neuromuscular structures of the axilla.

The incision should incorporate the previous biopsy scar. We prefer incisions that are slightly oblique from the transverse line and extend cephalad toward the axilla. The design of a cosmetic scar should not compromise in any way the successful extirpation of the primary tumor. Incisions appropriate for primary tumors of various locations in the breast are shown in Fig. 47-3A through 47-3G. Regardless of the skin

incision utilized, the limits of the modified radical mastectomy are defined laterally by the anterior margin of the latissimus dorsi muscle, medially by the midline of the sternum, superiorly by the subclavius muscle, and inferiorly by the caudal extension of the breast 3 to 4 cm inferior to the inframammary fold (Fig. 47-4).

The design of the skin flaps is planned with relation to the quadrant of the primary tumor so that adequate margins can be obtained. Primary closure should be possible in the majority of cases. Incisions and skin flaps should be developed perpendicular to the subcutaneous plane. Retraction hooks and clamps or towel clips are then placed on the skin edges for appropriate elevation under tension to enhance visualization of anatomic tissue planes. Flaps are retracted with constant tension on the periphery of the elevated margin at right angles to the chest wall to expose the superficial and deep layers of the superficial fascia.

The thickness of the flaps varies with patient habitus and proportional lean body

mass. Ideally, the flap thickness should be 7 to 8 mm including skin and tela subcutanea. The interface for flap elevation is developed deep to the cutaneous and subcutaneous vasculature and superficial to parenchymal vessels. The surgeon must be aware of the necessity for flap elevation with consistent thickness to avoid creation of devascularized subcutaneous tissues that contribute to wound seroma, skin necrosis, or flap retraction.

We prefer to elevate the cephalad skin flap with constant thickness to the level of the subclavius muscle. Dissection proceeds from lateral to medial with the use of the cold scalpel or the electrocautery. The pectoralis major fascia is dissected from the pectoralis musculature in a plane parallel with the course of the muscle bundle from the origin of ribs 2 to 6 to its insertion on the humerus (Fig. 47-5). The surgeon places inferior traction on the breast and fascia perpendicular to the clavicle and this traction is maintained constantly with elevation of the fascia from the muscle.

Multiple perforator vessels from the lateral thoracic or anterior intercostal arteries are invariably encountered during this part of the dissection. These vessels are end arteries that supply the pectoralis major and minor muscles, and they should be identified, clamped, and ligated with 2-0 or 3-0 nonabsorbable sutures.

The breast and skin, including the elevated pectoralis fascia from the lateral humeral extension to the medial costochondral junction, are elevated en bloc to approximately the fifth or sixth rib, leaving intact the most inferior portion of the breast. If access to the central and lower aspect of the breast is not possible because of the location of the lesion, the inferior flap should be elevated using the same technique described for the superior flap. The lateral flap is elevated to the anterior margin of the latissimus dorsi (Fig. 47-6). The loose areolar tissue of the lateral axillary space is elevated with identification of the later-almost extent of the axillary vein in its course anterior and caudal to the brachial plexus and axillary artery. Dissection above the axillary vein is inadvisable because of fear of damage to the brachial plexus and the infrequent observation of nodal tissue cephalad to the vein.

The axillary vein should be dissected sharply with cold scalpel following divi-

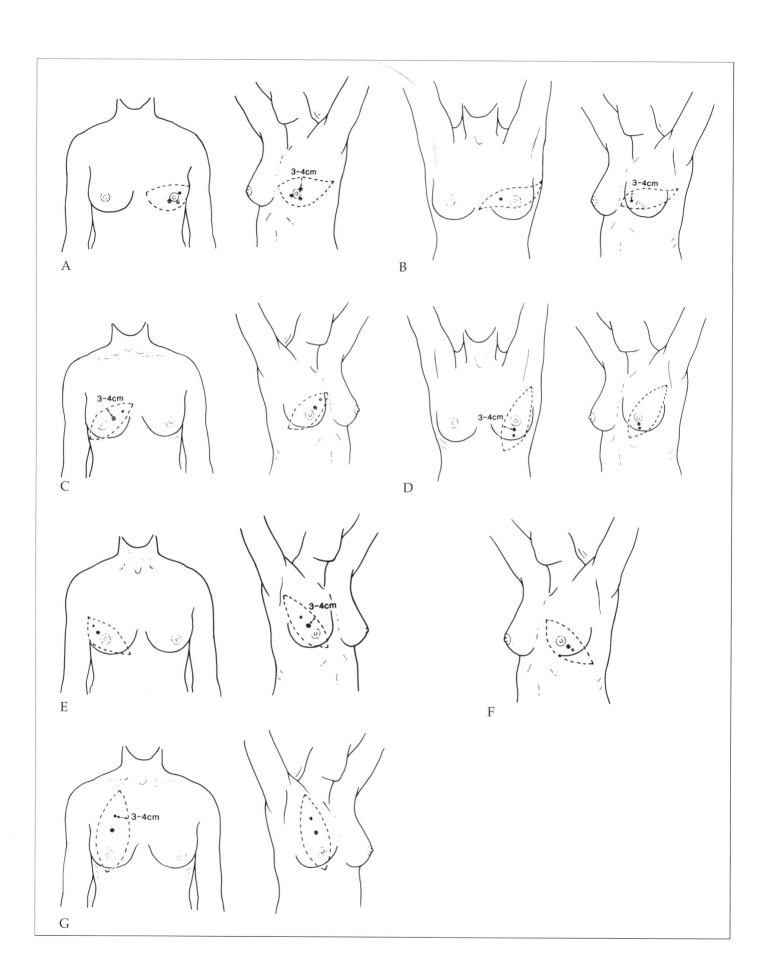

A

B

C

D

E

F

G

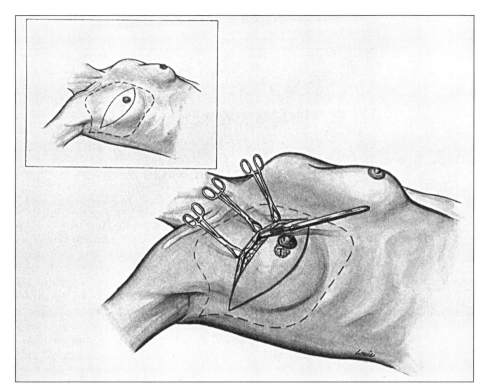

Fig. 47-4. Inset. Limits of the modified radical mastectomy are delineated superiorly by the subclavius muscle, laterally by the anterior margin of the latissimus dorsi muscle, medially by the midline of the sternum, and inferiorly by the caudal extension of the breast approximately 3 to 4 cm inferior to the inframammary fold. Skin flaps for the modified radical technique are planned with relation to the quadrant in which the primary neoplasm is located. Adequate margins are ensured by developing skin edges 3 to 5 cm from the tumor margin. Incisions are planned so that they are developed perpendicular to the subcutaneous plane and are inclusive of skin and parenchymal tissue 3 to 5 cm around the neoplasm. Flap thickness is dependent on patient habitus and proportional lean body mass. Flaps should be 7 to 8 mm in thickness inclusive of the skin and tela subcutanea. Flap tension should be perpendicular to the chest wall with flap elevation deep to the cutaneous vasculature, which is accentuated by flap retraction. (From KI Bland, EM Copeland III (eds), The Breast: Comprehensive Management of Benign and Malignant Diseases. Philadelphia: Saunders, 1991. Reproduced with permission.)

sion of the investing deep layer of the superficial fascia of the axillary space. The use of electrocautery for this dissection can cause thermal damage to the surface of the anterior or inferior vein wall. The electrocautery can also cause electrical stimulation of the brachial plexus or its motor branches to the muscles of the arm and the shoulder.

As the surgeon proceeds medially to complete dissection of the lateralmost margin of the pectoralis major, abduction of the shoulder and extension of the arm with finger dissection of the lateral and inferior margin of the pectoralis major allow visualization of the insertion of the pectoralis minor on the coracoid process of the scapula. The tendinous portion of the pectoralis minor is divided near its insertion on the coracoid process (Fig. 47-7).

The surgeon must be aware of the anatomic location of the lateral neurovascular bundle in which the medial pectoral nerve (laterally placed with origin from the medial cord) courses to innervate the pectoralis major and minor muscles. This nerve should be preserved, if possible, to prevent atrophy of the lateral head of the pectoralis major—a significant cosmetic and functional defect. However, if the entire nerve trunk penetrates the pectoralis minor, sacrifice may be necessary. It may also be necessary to sacrifice penetrating branches of the medial pectoral nerve with elevation and medial retraction of the pectoralis minor to its origin on ribs 2 through 5.

◀ Fig. 47-3. A. Design of the classic Stewart elliptical incision for central and subareolar primary lesions of the breast. The medial extent of the incision ends at the margin of the sternum. The lateral extent of the skin incision should overlie the anterior margin of the latissimus dorsi. The design of the skin incision should incorporate the primary neoplasm en bloc with margins that are 3 to 4 cm from the cranial and caudal edges of the tumor. B. Design of the obliquely placed modified Stewart incision for cancer of the inner quadrant of the breast. The medial extent of the incision often must incorporate skin to the midsternum to allow a 3- to 4-cm margin in all directions from the edge of the tumor. Lateral extent of the incision ends at the anterior margin of the latissimus. C. Design of the classic Orr oblique incision for carcinoma of the upper outer quadrants of the breast. The skin incision is placed 3 to 4 cm from the margin of the tumor in an oblique plane that is directed cephalad toward the ipsilateral axilla. This incision is a variant of the original Greenough, Kocher, and Rodman techniques for flap development. D. Variation of the Orr incision for lower inner and vertically placed (6 o'clock) lesions of the breast. The design of the skin incision is identical to that of Fig. 47-5, with attention directed to margins of 3 to 4 cm. E. Design of skin flaps for upper inner quadrant primary tumors of the breast. The cephalad margin of the flap must be designed to allow access for dissection of the axilla. With flap margins 3 to 4 cm from the tumor, variation in the medial extent of the incision is expectant and may extend beyond the edge of the sternum. On occasion, the modified Stewart incision can incorporate the tumor en bloc, provided that the cancer is not too high on the breast and craniad from the nipple-areolar complex. All incision designs must be inclusive of the nipple-areola when total mastectomy is planned with primary therapy. F. Incisions for cancer of the lower outer quadrants of the breast. The surgeon should design incisions that achieve margins of 3 to 4 cm from the tumor with cephalad margins that allow access for dissection of the axilla. The medial extent is the margin of the sternum. Laterally, the inferior extent of the incision is the latissimus. G. Depiction of skin flaps for lesions of the breast that are high lying, infraclavicular, or fixed to the pectoralis major muscle. Fixation to the muscle necessitates Halsted radical mastectomy with skin margins of a minimal 3 cm. Skin grafting is necessary when large margins of skin are resected for T3 and T4 cancers. Primary closure for T1 and some T2 tumors is often possible. (From KI Bland, EM Copeland III (eds), The Breast: Comprehensive Management of Benign and Malignant Diseases. Philadelphia: Saunders, 1991. Reproduced with permission.)

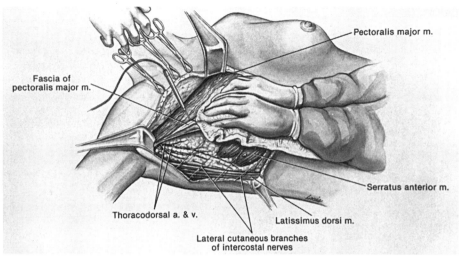

Fig. 47-5. *Elevation of the superior flap to the level of the subclavius muscle at the superiormost extent of breast parenchyma. Skin flap thickness is constant at 7 to 8 mm from lateral to medial. Thereafter, dissection of the pectoralis major fascia from the pectoralis musculature can be completed with cold scalpel or electrocautery. Dissection commences lateral to medial in a plane that parallels the muscle bundles of the pectoralis major muscle from the origin of ribs 2 to 6 to the insertion on the humerus. Countertraction in a caudal direction allows tension on the fascia to facilitate its removal from the pectoralis major. Perforator vessels from the lateral thoracic or anterior intercostal arteries are encountered as end arteries that supply the pectoralis major and minor muscles. Thereafter, the inferior flap is elevated medially in similar fashion to the midline, inferiorly to the aponeurosis of the rectus abdominis tendon, and laterally to the anterior margin of the latissimus. The inferiormost portion of the breast is left intact following clearing of the supralateral margin of the pectoralis major. This maneuver ensures an en bloc resection of the axillary contents with the breast, leaving the axillary tail of Spence intact. (From KI Bland, EM Copeland III (eds).* The Breast: Comprehensive Management of Benign and Malignant Diseases. *Philadelphia: Saunders, 1991. Reproduced with permission.)*

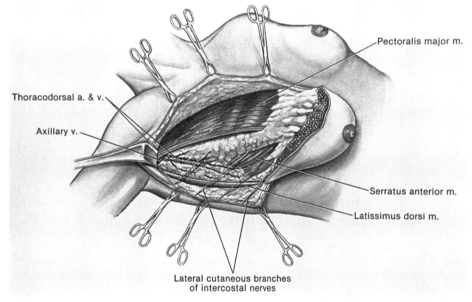

Fig. 47-6. *The completed superior and inferior flap with breast parenchyma intact with the axillary tail of Spence and the axillary contents. The pectoralis major is completely cleared of its fascia en bloc with the breast parenchyma. At this juncture, the pectoralis minor has not been exposed to allow access to the axilla (level II and III nodes). The latissimus dorsi muscle has been dissected on its anterior surface to delineate the lateral boundary of dissection. Illustrated in this view is the cutaneous innervation of skin of the lateral chest, axilla, and medial arm by intercostobrachial sensory nerves. These nerves are commonly divided in the course of dissection of the axilla and lateral skin flap following identification of the latissimus dorsi. (From KI Bland, EM Copeland III (eds).* The Breast: Comprehensive Management of Benign and Malignant Diseases. *Philadelphia: Saunders, 1991. Reproduced with permission.)*

With the use of this maneuver, the interpectoral nodes (Rotter's nodes) are included en bloc with the operative specimen. Furthermore, resection of the pectoralis minor allows full visualization of the extent of the axillary vein in its course beneath the pectoralis minor and its entry into the chest wall at its confluence with the subclavian vein beneath the costoclavicular ligament (Halsted's ligament). With resection of the pectoralis minor muscle, complete exposure of level II and III nodes is possible.

Dissection should continue from lateral to medial with complete visualization of the anterior and ventral surfaces of the axillary vein. The investing fascia of the axillary vein is dissected with elevation of the deep layer of the superficial fascia and division with cold scalpel following exposure. Ligation and division of all venous tributaries are then performed. With identification and retraction of the superomedial aspect of the pectoralis major, the lateral pectoral (anterior thoracic) nerve with origin from the lateral cord is exposed with the medial neurovascular bundle. This structure should also be protected to preserve innervation to the medial heads of the pectoralis major (Fig. 47-8).

Dissection commences medially on the anterior/ventral surface of the axillary vein to the costoclavicular ligament, which represents the condensation of the clavipectoral fascia. The loose areolar tissue at the juncture of the axillary vein with the anterior margin of the latissimus dorsi muscle is swept inferomedially to include the lateral (axillary) nodal group (level I nodes).

The surgeon should preserve the thoracodorsal artery and vein, which are located deep in the axillary space and are fully invested with loose areolar tissue and nodes of the lateral and subscapular groups. The surgeon should also be aware of the origin of the thoracodorsal nerve from the posterior cord medial to the thoracodorsal artery and vein. This nerve has a variable inferolateral course en route to its innervation of the latissimus dorsi muscle and must be visualized and protected throughout its course, particularly if subsequent breast reconstruction with the use of myocutaneous flaps that incorporate the latissimus dorsi muscle is planned.

The lateral axillary nodal group is retracted inferomedially and anterior to the

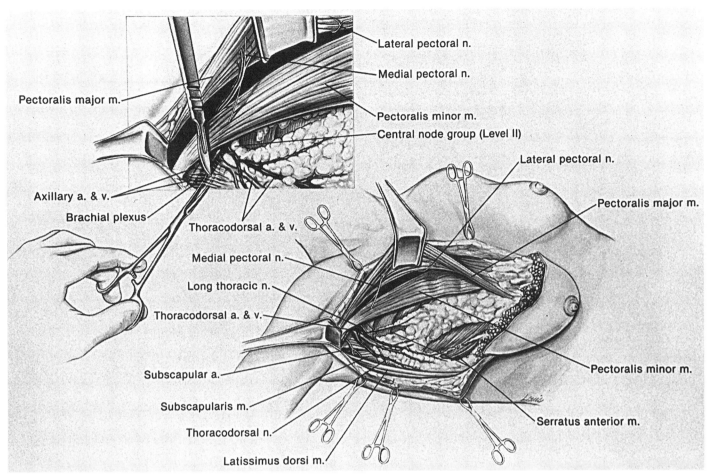

Fig. 47-7. Inset. Juncture of the latissimus (unexposed) with the ventral surface of the axillary vein. Sharp division with scalpel to incise the investing fascia of the axillary space. Following isolation of the tendinous portion of the pectoralis minor muscle with finger dissection, the insertion of this tendon on the coracoid process of the scapula can be readily identified. The surgeon must be cognizant of the anatomic location of the lateral neurovascular bundle and the laterally placed medial pectoral nerve, which takes origin from the medial cord. Every attempt should be made to preserve the medial pectoral nerve, as sacrifice of the main trunk may allow atrophy of the lateral head of the pectoralis major. Further, the lateral pectoral nerve, which takes origin from the lateral cord and is medially placed, should also be preserved. (From KI Bland, EM Copeland III (eds). The Breast: Comprehensive Management of Benign and Malignant Diseases. *Philadelphia: Saunders, 1991. Reproduced with permission.)*

thoracodorsal neurovascular bundle and dissected en bloc with the subscapular group of nodes (level I), which are medially located between the thoracodorsal nerve and the lateral chest wall. Dissection of the posterior contents of the axillary space and division of multiple tributaries from the thoracoacromial artery and vein allow free access to exposure of the posterior boundary of the axilla with visualization of the heads of the teres major muscle laterally and the subscapularis muscle medially.

Dissection then commences medially with extirpation of the central nodal groups (level II) and, on occasion, the apical/subclavicular (level III) nodes when grossly evident. The superomedialmost aspect of the dissection at the level of the costocla-

vicular ligament represents the point of termination of the dissection. This nodal group should be identified with a metallic marker or suture to give the pathologist the opportunity to examine for extension of nodal disease, which may have therapeutic and prognostic significance.

It is important that the surgeon continue this dissection en bloc to avoid the separation of nodal groups and disruption of lymphatic vessels in the axilla. Inferomedial retraction of levels II and III nodes en bloc with the specimen, which is inclusive of the external mammary group (level I), is conducted in a cephalad to caudad direction in parallel with the thoracodorsal neurovascular bundle. This dissection maneuver incorporates nodal groups en bloc and avoids neural injury while providing

direct access to and exposure of venous tributaries posterior to the axillary vein.

With medial dissection, the surgeon encounters the chest wall deep in the medial axillary space and is able to identify the long thoracic nerve (respiratory nerve of Bell) applied in the deep investing (serratus) fascia of the medial axillary space. This nerve is constant in its location, anterior to the subscapularis muscle, and it is closely applied to the investing fascial compartment of the chest wall. The surgeon should make every effort to preserve the long thoracic nerve. Damage to the long thoracic nerve will cause permanent disability, with shoulder apraxia and the "winged scapula" deformity secondary to denervation of the serratus anterior muscle.

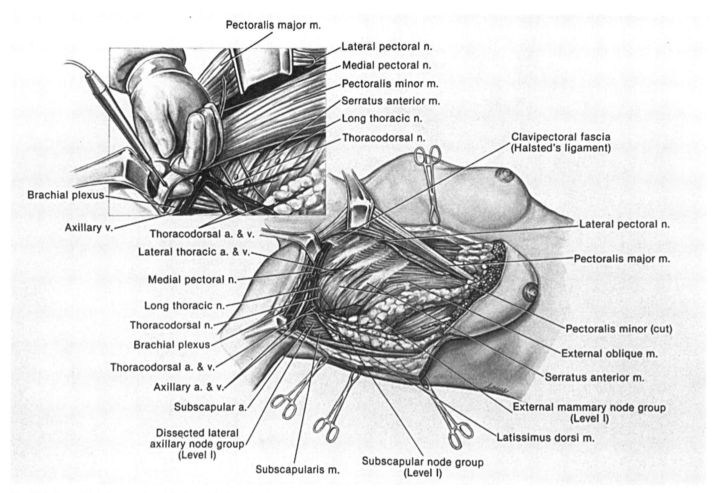

Fig. 47-8. Inset. Digital protection of the brachial plexus for division of the insertion of the pectoralis minor muscle on the coracoid process. All loose areolar and lymphatic tissues are swept en bloc with the axillary contents to ensure resection of the interpectoral (Rotter's) nodes. Dissection commences lateral to medial with complete visualization of the anterior and ventral aspects of the axillary vein. Dissection craniad to the axillary vein is inadvisable, for fear of damage to the brachial plexus and the infrequent observation of gross nodal tissue cephalic to the vein. Investing fascial dissection of the vein is best completed with the cold scalpel following exposure, ligation, and division of all venous tributaries on the anterior and ventral surfaces. Caudal to the vein, loose areolar tissue at the junction of the vein with the anterior margin of latissimus is swept inferomedially inclusive of the lateral (axillary) nodal group (level I). Care is taken to preserve the neurovascular thoracodorsal artery, vein, and nerve in the deep axillary space. The thoracodorsal nerve is traced to its innervation of the latissimus dorsi muscle laterally. Lateral axillary nodal groups are retracted inferomedially and anterior to this bundle for dissection en bloc with the subscapular (level I) nodal group. Preferentially dissection commences superomedially before completion of dissection of the external mammary (level I) nodal group. Superomedial dissection over the axillary vein allows extirpation of the central nodal group (level II) and apical (subclavicular) level III group. The superomedialmost extent of the dissection is the clavipectoral fascia (Halsted's ligament). This level of dissection with the Patey technique allows the surgeon to mark, with metallic clip or suture, the superiormost extent of dissection. All loose areolar tissue just inferior to the apical nodal group is swept off the chest wall, leaving the fascia of the serratus anterior intact. With dissection parallel to the long thoracic nerve (respiratory nerve of Bell), the deep investing serratus fascia is incised. This nerve is closely applied to the investing fascial compartment of the chest wall and must be dissected in its entirety, cephalic to caudal to ensure innervation of the serratus anterior and avoidance of the ''winged scapula'' disability. (From KI Bland, EM Copeland III (eds). The Breast: Comprehensive Management of Benign and Malignant Diseases. Philadelphia: Saunders, 1991. Reproduced with permission.)

The long thoracic nerve is dissected throughout its course to the serratus anterior muscle (see Figs. 47-7 and 47-8). The axillary contents anterior and medial to the nerve are swept inferomedially with the specimen. The surgeon should ensure that innervations of the long thoracic and thoracodorsal nerves are visualized before division of the inferiormost extent of the axillary contents. Incompletely divided or-

igins of the pectoralis minor muscle from ribs 2 through 5 are resected with the electrocautery, and the remaining portions of the muscle are swept en bloc with the axillary contents to include Rotter's interpectoral and retropectoral nodal groups.

Thereafter, the dissection commences in a caudal direction so that the entire breast and fascia are cleared medially and infe-

riorly from the aponeurosis of the rectus abdominis muscle (Fig. 47-8). The specimen is sent immediately to the pathology department for examination, sectioning, and procurement of hormone receptors, if the latter was not done at the time of the initial biopsy. Hormone receptor analyses are thermo- and ischemia-labile within the ambient temperature of the operating room environment, and, therefore, it is essential that tissue is forwarded promptly after removal to the laboratory.

The operating field is carefully inspected and bleeding points are identified, clamped, and ligated individually with nonabsorbable 2-0 and 3-0 sutures. Before closure, the margins of the wound are carefully examined for devascularization caused by the trauma of flap retraction or by dissection of thin, poorly vascularized skin. Incision sites that are obviously devascularized are debrided parallel with the original skin incision so that satisfactory closure without tension is possible. When equivocal areas of devascularized tissue are present, systemic intravenous injection of 4 to 5 ml fluorescein will allow the surgeon to visualize viable skin margins with a Wood's ultraviolet lamp.

It is advisable that the surgeon, assistants, and scrub nurse reglove and optionally regown. In addition, new instruments are used for wound closure to avoid the potential for implantation of exfoliated tumor cells in the wound. Before closure, the operating field is copiously irrigated with sterile water or saline, which augments the evacuation of residual tissue, blood clots, and serum. The wound is again inspected for the presence of bleeding sites, and if none are found, closed suction (No. 18–20 French) or soft, flat Silastic catheters are placed through separate stab incisions that enter the inferior flap at approximately the anterior axillary line (Fig. 47-9).

The laterally placed Silastic catheter is positioned in the axillary space approximately 2 cm inferior to the axillary vein on the ventral surface of the latissimus dorsi muscle to provide drainage of the axilla. A longer, second catheter placed through the medial stab incision is positioned in the superomedial aspect of the defect to provide continual evacuation of serum and blood that may accumulate within the large surface area of the dissected pectoralis major muscle. Both catheters are secured on the skin with a 2-0 nonabsorbable suture. We prefer not to secure the catheters to the pectoral muscles or to the latissimus dorsi muscle for fear of creating bleeding at the time of their removal.

The wound is closed in two layers with 2-0 or 3-0 absorbable synthetic sutures placed in the subcutaneous tissues. Undue tension on the margins may necessitate extensive undermining of these tissues to re-

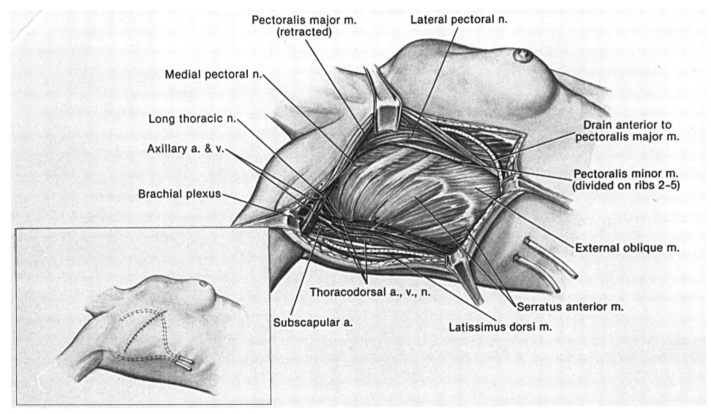

Fig. 47-9. The completed Patey axillary dissection variant of the modified radical technique. The dissection is inclusive of the pectoralis minor muscle from origin to insertion on ribs 2 to 5. Both medial and lateral pectoral nerves are preserved to ensure innervation of the lateral and medial heads, respectively, of the pectoralis major. With completion of the procedure, remaining portions of this muscle are swept en bloc with the axillary contents to be inclusive of Rotter's interpectoral and the retropectoral groups. Inset. Following copious irrigation with distilled water and saline, closed suction Silastic catheters (18–20 French) are positioned via stab incisions placed in the inferior flap at the anterior axillary line. The lateral catheter is placed approximately 2 cm inferior to the axillary vein. The superior, longer catheter placed via the medial stab wound is positioned in the superomedial aspect of the defect anterior to the pectoralis major muscle beneath the skin flap. The wound is closed in two layers with 2-0 absorbable synthetic sutures placed in subcutaneous planes. Undue tension on margins of the flap must be avoided; this may necessitate undermining of tissues to reduce mechanical forces. The skin is optionally closed with subcuticular 4-0 synthetic absorbable sutures or stainless steel staples. Following completion of wound closure, both catheters are irrigated copiously with saline to ensure patency and are connected and maintained on low to moderate continuous suction provided by reservoir portable vacuum bottles. Light, bulky dressings of gauze are placed over the dissection site and taped securely in place with occlusive dressings. The surgeon may elect to place the ipsilateral arm in a sling to provide immobilization. (From KI Bland, EM Copeland III (eds). The Breast: Comprehensive Management of Benign and Malignant Diseases. *Philadelphia: Saunders, 1991. Reproduced with permission.)*

duce mechanical forces and maximize adherence to the underlying pectoralis major muscle.

The skin is optionally closed with subcuticular 4-0 synthetic absorbable sutures or stainless steel staples. Wounds closed with subcuticular sutures should have Steri-Strips applied to the skin perpendicular to the incision to enhance wound repair. Both catheters are copiously irrigated with saline to ensure patency and they are connected and maintained on continuous low to moderate suction by large-reservoir portable vacuum bottles. Light bulky (noncompressive) dressings of cotton are applied to the dissection site and are taped securely in place. Optionally, the ipsilateral arm can be immobilized in an arm sling.

The dressings should remain intact on the wound until the second or third postoperative day, unless the surgeon is concerned about the viability of the dissected flaps. The drains should remain in the site of dissection until the drainage becomes predominantly serous and decreases to 20 to 25 ml during a 24-hour interval. Shoulder and arm exercises are initiated on the day after the removal of the drainage catheters.

Postmastectomy Breast Reconstruction

The significant advancements in breast reconstruction techniques that have occurred in recent years have resulted in the wide acceptance of breast reconstruction following mastectomy among physicians who treat breast cancer. This acceptance by physicians and the increasing awareness of the availability and success of this option among patients with breast cancer have resulted in a substantial increase in the number of postmastectomy breast reconstructions performed in the last 5 years.

The timing of breast reconstruction in relation to the mastectomy requires careful consideration by the surgeon of the tumor biology and stage of disease; complete understanding by the patient of reconstruction implications is essential for exercise of this option. Delayed reconstruction has been the traditional approach for most clinics in North America. A contemporary trend has been that of simultaneous (immediate) reconstruction for favorable (stage 0, I, II) disease.

The rationale for delayed reconstruction is based on important considerations. Observation for a relatively long period of time following mastectomy provides some assurance that the neoplasm is controlled. Delay in breast reconstruction provides adequate time for completion of adjuvant treatment when indicated. In addition, delayed reconstruction allows time for the mastectomy scar to undergo repair and maturation, and gives the patient the opportunity to live with the deformity of the mastectomy and, thus, to better appreciate the cosmetic and functional benefits of the reconstruction.

Several studies confirm that immediate reconstruction provides significant psychological benefits such as positive body image and decreases postmastectomy stress. In fact, support for the belief that a woman should live with the mastectomy deformity to better appreciate the reconstruction was negated by Wellisch and associates. Additionally, it has been shown that immediate reconstruction does not portend a negative impact on patient outcome. Immediate breast reconstruction has gained increasing popularity in the last few years, particularly for women with noninvasive or minimally invasive breast cancers. Delayed reconstruction can be performed at any time after the mastectomy although traditionally a waiting period of 6 to 9 months is recommended.

Immediate reconstruction is a team effort that requires proper coordination and communication between the team members, which include the general surgeon, the plastic surgeon, and, if needed, the radiation and medical oncologists. It is essential that the general surgeon has familiarity with the technical and psychological aspects of immediate breast reconstruction. The patient must be well informed about the procedure, its complications, and its limitations.

Careful patient selection is of great importance to the success of immediate postmastectomy breast reconstruction. Oncologic and psychological considerations are essential to patient selection. Women with ductal carcinoma in situ who are not candidates for local excision are highly suitable for immediate reconstruction. Women with early invasive breast cancer (stages I/II) are also proper candidates for

immediate reconstruction and should be so counseled in this regard. This group includes patients with tumors of 2 cm in size or less with no clinical evidence of axillary nodal involvement. Women with larger tumors and clinically negative axillary lymph nodes may be proper candidates if the surgeon is technically satisfied with the resection margins. Formerly, the necessity of postoperative radiation to the chest wall was considered a contraindication to immediate reconstruction. While this consideration is essential to the decision of whether to reconstruct, the increasing experience with postreconstruction methods suggests that therapeutic radiotherapy can be completed with excellent local-regional control results. When adjuvant treatment is indicated, immediate reconstruction should not initiate compromise or delay.

Assessment of the patient's psychological status is of great importance. The patient's motivation should be examined and her strong desire for breast reconstruction should be established. The reconstructive goals and potential for achievement of the desirable aesthetic result should be thoroughly discussed and clearly understood by the patient before she gives informed consent. The patient should also realize that a number of subsequent procedures may be necessary before the final reconstructive goal is achieved.

The surgical options for breast reconstruction are depicted in Table 47-2. These options include a wide spectrum of procedures that range from a simple implant placement to the transfer of free flaps using microvascular anastomotic techniques. The technique that is selected should conform to the needs and requirements of the individual patient. The management of the skin and fascia by the surgeon who performs the mastectomy should be meticulous and atraumatic, as technique affects the outcome of immediate reconstruction. The skin flaps should not be developed into the dermis in order to avoid ischemic necrosis of the flaps; variation in technique

Table 47-2. Surgical Options for Breast Reconstruction After Mastectomy

Placement of implant (subpectoral)

Placement of tissue expander (subpectoral)

Myocutaneous flap (latissimus dorsi, TRAM)

Free flap (TRAM, gluteal, gracilis, tensor fascia lata)

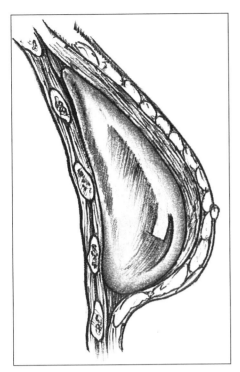

Fig. 47-10. Reconstruction with implant placement. Cross section showing the implant placed beneath the musculofascial flap.

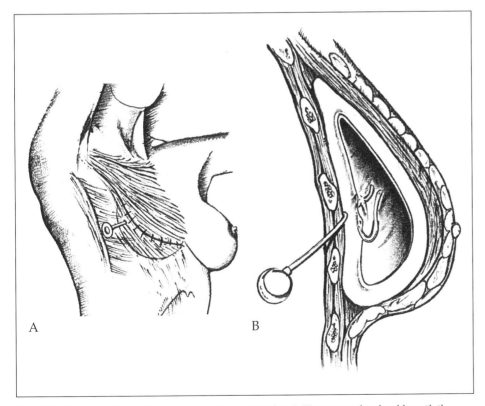

A   B

Fig. 47-11. Reconstruction with placement of a tissue expander. A. Tissue expander placed beneath the musculofascial flap. B. Cross section of tissue expander.

increases the complication rate. Careful examination of the flaps under the Wood's lamp with the use of fluorescein to determine viability is advisable. Tissues with questionable viability should be excised. The surgeon who performs the mastectomy should also preserve as much skin as possible without compromise of basic oncologic principles (e.g., removal of the tumor with adequate skin and parenchymal margins). Careful dissection with preservation of the subdermal vascular plexus is essential to the viability of the skin. When implant placement is chosen as the appropriate option, muscular and neural preservation is an important consideration. Further, efforts should be made to preserve the pectoral nerves and the skin branches of the internal mammary perforators.

The simplest technique of immediate reconstruction is the placement of an implant under the available tissues (muscle, skin). The ideal candidates for this technique include 1) patients with early breast cancer who require minimal skin excision, 2) patients with a nipple-areolar complex of small diameter, and 3) patients with small- to moderate-sized breasts without ptosis. Satisfactory results are obtained with placement of an implant beneath the pectoralis major muscle. After completion of the mastectomy, following the principles of skin and fascia preservation outlined earlier in this chapter, a musculofascial incision is performed at the lower level of the inframammary crease, and a musculofascial flap, including the pectoralis major, serratus anterior, external oblique, and rectus abdominis muscles, is elevated. An implant of appropriate size, matching the size of the opposite breast, is selected and placed on the chest wall beneath the musculofascial flap. The flap is then sutured to the lower skin flap with absorbable sutures placed approximately 3 cm above the inframammary crease (Fig. 47-10). Scar encapsulation, known as capsular contracture, is a common complication of implant placement and may require reoperation.

The placement of a tissue expander is an appropriate and desirable option when an implant of adequate size cannot be placed at the initial operation. A tissue expander is a saline-filled balloon with a valve that allows periodic inflation of the implant. The tissue expander is eventually replaced with a polyurethane-covered implant when inflation to the desirable size has been achieved. The expander can be used with immediate or delayed reconstruction. It is positioned using the same technique as for placement of an implant, described earlier in this chapter (Fig. 47-11). Tissue expansion should begin during the second to third postoperative week and before wound contracture; expansion should be delayed if a seroma is present, to avoid contamination caused by the percutaneous injections of the expander. The use of a tissue expander with an integrated port avoids a separate valve and connective tubing with the associated problems of malpositioning and kinking. The complication rate with the use of tissue expanders is higher than that observed with simple implantation. Complications include infection, capsular contracture, implant exposure, extrusion, and deflation.

Reconstruction with autogenous tissue transfer avoids the use of foreign materials, and this is the only material that can successfully mimic/conform to the shape, form, and consistency of the contralateral breast. Recent technical refinements have significantly decreased the probability of flap loss. Autogenous tissue transfer requires fewer operations than the usage of implantation techniques, since the size, shape, and conformity of the neobreast are achieved during the initial procedure, in the majority of cases.

When the standard latissimus dorsi myocutaneous flap is used, an implant is usually necessary due to the lack of sufficient bulk for the creation of an adequate breast mound. The use of the ''J'' latissimus dorsi reconstruction obviates the need for an implant. The J design incorporates a long horizontal ellipse of skin with a vertical extension into redundant fatty tissue of the posterior axillary fold. This technique is very appropriate for immediate reconstruction because of the favorable donor site and the predictable healing, and also because it does not add an excessive amount of time for completion of the mastectomy procedure.

The transverse rectus abdominis myocutaneous (TRAM) flap has been widely used in breast reconstruction. Smoking and obesity are relative contraindications for this procedure because the former can lead to flap necrosis, while the latter may predispose to the formation of an abdominal wall hernia. The major advantage of the TRAM flap is that it provides maximal

symmetry relative to the contralateral breast. However, the creation of this flap is a major operation that often necessitates blood transfusions and prolongation of operative time. Candidates for this procedure should be carefully selected.

The TRAM flap uses the rectus abdominis muscles to transfer redundant skin and fat of the lower abdomen to the site of the resected breast. The blood supply to this flap is based on the superior epigastric vessels. The flap is rotated on its vascular pedicle and passed upward to the area of reconstruction through a subcutaneous tunnel (Fig. 47-12). Thereafter, the flap is tailored with conformity to the mastectomy wound and sutured to the pectoralis major muscle. The abdominal wall defect created by the harvesting of the flap is then closed in layers.

The major drawbacks of the TRAM flap are the length of the procedure and the requirement of longer hospitalization and convalescence periods. The most significant complications of this procedure are loss of the flap and loss of abdominal wall competency. The former is usually the result of twisting or excessive tension on the vascular pedicle and can be largely prevented with the use of proper operative

technique. Abdominal wall hernia is a rather uncommon occurrence and is clearly preventable with proper closure of the abdominal wall defect. Abdominal wall competency is not compromised in most patients. The great majority of patients are able to resume their usual work and sports activities following recovery from this operation. Less serious complications associated with this procedure are infection, fluid collection, and skin wound separation.

Recent innovations in microvascular techniques have made free tissue transfers reasonable alternatives for breast reconstruction. Several donor sites for free flaps can be utilized, and include 1) the free TRAM flap, 2) the superior and the inferior gluteal flap, and 3) the transverse lateral thigh flap. The selection of the free flap should be based on the reconstructive needs of the individual patient. Excessive operating time is a major criticism of the free tissue transfers. Although the vascular anastomosis can be completed in less than 1 hour, the overall operative time is significant due to the complex and tedious flap dissection. An advantage of the free flap technique is that breast reconstruction can usually be accomplished in one stage.

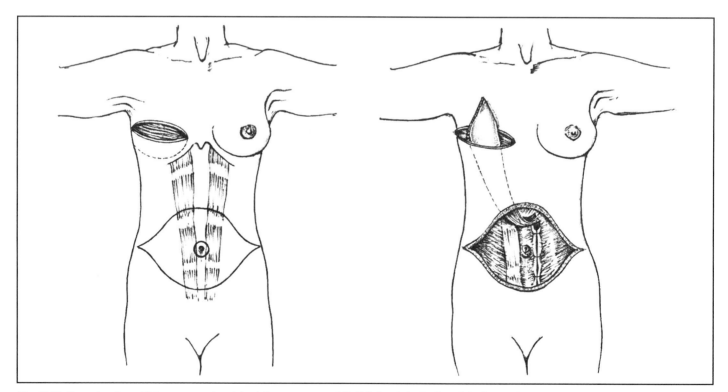

Fig. 47-12. Reconstruction with transverse rectus abdominis myocutaneous (TRAM) flap. Left. Outline of the flap. Right. After harvesting, the flap is passed to the mastectomy through a subcutaneous channel.

Immediate and delayed breast reconstruction following mastectomy have been used with increasing frequency during the last decade. Technical advances in the area of breast reconstruction have increased significantly the array of available options. These options improve the potential for successful reconstruction but also make the selection of the most appropriate option for the individual patient a greater challenge. Breast reconstruction following mastectomy requires a team effort that includes the patient. Clearly, the final decision to undergo a breast reconstruction should be made by a fully informed patient. Further, proper communication among these team members is of paramount importance. Comprehensive evaluation of the patient's oncologic, psychological, and general health status is essential to a successful outcome.

Suggested Reading

Baker R, Montague A, Childs J. A comparison of modified radical mastectomy to radical mastectomy in the treatment of operable breast cancer. *Ann Surg* 189:553, 1979.

Bostwick JI III. *Plastic and Reconstructive Breast Surgery*. St. Louis: Quality Medical Publishing, 1990.

DeLarue N, Anderson W, Starr J. Modified radical mastectomy in the individualized treatment of breast carcimoma. *Surg Gynecol Obstet* 129:79, 1969.

Ellis L, Wittliff J, Bryant M, et al. Lability of steroid hormone receptors following devascularization of breast tumors. *Arch Surg* 124:39, 1989.

Fisher B, Redmond C, Fisher E, et al. Ten-year results of a randomized clinical trial comparing radical mastectomy and total mastectomy with or without radiation. *N Engl J Med* 312:674, 1985.

Frykberg ER, Bland KI. Evolution of Surgical Principles for the Management of Breast Cancer. In KI Bland, EM Copeland III (eds), *The Breast: Comprehensive Management of Benign and Malignant Diseases*. Philadelphia: Saunders, 1991, Pp. 539–568.

Handley R. The conservative radical mastectomy of Patey: 10 year results in 425 patients' breasts. *Dis Breast* 2:16, 1976.

Johnson C, Van Heerden J, Donohue J, et al. Oncological aspects of immediate breast reconstruction following mastectomy for malignancy. *Arch Surg* 124:819, 1989.

Madden J, Kandalaft S, and Bourque R. Modified radical mastectomy. *Ann Surg* 175:624, 1972.

Maddox W, Carpenter JJ, Laws H, et al. A randomized prospective trial of radical (Halsted) mastectomy versus modified radical mastectomy in 311 breast cancer patients. *Ann Surg* 198:207, 1983.

Margarrey C. Aspects of the psychological management of breast cancer. *Med J Aust* 148:239, 1988.

McCraw JB, Gamer AR, Horton CE. Breast Reconstruction Following Mastectomy. In KI Bland, EM Copeland III (eds), *The Breast: Comprehensive Management of Benign and Malignant Diseases*. Philadelphia: Saunders, 1991, Pp 656–693.

Murphy J. Carcinoma of the breast. *Surg Clin* 1: 779, 1912.

Noone R, Frazier T, Hayward C, Skiles M. Patient acceptance of immediate reconstruction following mastectomy. *Plas Reconstr Surg.* 69:632, 1982.

Patey D. A review of 146 cases of carcinoma of the breast operated on between 1930 and 1943. *Br J Cancer* 21:260, 1967.

Patey D, Dyson W. The prognosis of carcinoma of the breast in relation to the type of operation performed. *Br J Cancer* 2:7, 1948.

Schaim W, Wellisch D, Pasmau R, Landsverk J. The sooner the better: A study of psychological factors in women undergoing immediate versus delayed breast reconstruction. *Am J Psychiatry* 142:40, 1985.

Turner L, Swindell R, Bell W, et al. Radical versus modified radical mastectomy for breast cancer. *Ann R Coll Surg Engl* 63:239, 1981.

Wellisch D, Schain W, Noone R, Little JI. Psychosocial correlates of immediate versus delayed reconstruction of the breast. *Plast Reconstr Surg* 76:713, 1985.

EDITOR'S COMMENT

The authors have produced a classic chapter on various considerations, especially technical, in modified radical mastectomy for infiltrating breast cancer. Even for surgeons with a very wide experience with this operation, a review of the technical information provided in this chapter, with superior illustrations, is worthwhile. There has been a significant increase in the numbers of patients who are subjected to local excision, axillary dissection, and radiation therapy in the past 5 to 8 years. Five years ago in a discussion of the subject of modified radical mastectomy in the second edition of this text, I made the point that "three-quarters of all patients with breast cancer still require or are treated by modified radical mastectomy." Today, in most centers, those data have been reversed, as more and more patients are now encountered whose cancer is very small or with mammographic findings only, and as knowledgeable surgeons who operate on the breast recognize that local excision plus radiation therapy has enormous advantages with minimal, if any, increase in risk of recurrence in properly selected patients.

A sizable proportion of our patients still require modified radical mastectomy, including the following:

Patients with tumors 2.5 to 3.0 cm in diameter or larger

Patients with central lesions that necessitate resection of the nipple and areola to encompass the tumor

Patients with multicentric collections of true microcalcifications in the affected breast, one or more of which is malignant on biopsy

Pregnant patients with carcinoma of the breast

Intractable patients who refuse to accept radiation therapy

Patients with very large breasts in whom radiation therapy is ineffective

Patients who cannot be relied upon to have good follow-up and to pursue appropriate adjunctive courses of management

Patients with ductal spread of tumor with substantial invasive intraductal lesion seen on excisional biopsy

Patients with two synchronous tumors in the breast or recurrence of a cancer in a previously treated and irradiated breast

Formerly, when patients were informed of the presence of breast cancer, a substantial number elected mastectomy in the belief that this afforded the best chance of cure. With appropriate public education, many more women are now opting for local excision, and axillary dissection plus radiation therapy. The net result has been an appropriate decrease in the frequency with which modified radical mastectomy is performed.

The authors comment on the lability of hormone receptors, pointing out the importance of prompt processing of the tumor specimen with immediate freezing of tissue for hormone receptor determination later. In most instances, the tumor will have been removed, or at least generously sampled, before the performance of the mastectomy, making this a somewhat less important concern than was previously the case. Even if Tru-cut needle biopsy of a larger tumor is performed, enough tissue is obtained to enable estrogen and progesterone receptors, S-phase protein, ploidy, and other tumor markers to be determined on those specimens. Nevertheless, the point is still an important one when frozen section biopsy and mastectomy are done at the same time. Related to marker lability is the concern about the use of cautery in performing breast biopsy. Cautery is a local form of intense heat that can be expected to have an effect on the levels of hormone receptors that are measured in the biopsy specimen. Although the data are not conclusive, it would still seem wise to excise the lesion first, and then to achieve hemostasis with cautery when the specimen is on its way to the surgical pathologist.

The authors have produced a superior description of the technique of this operation, and any difference of opinion is simply a matter of habit and learned practice; for example, I usually start the breast removal on the medial side of the field, and dissect from medial to lateral; this has an advantage in that the weight of the breast, especially a large breast, tends to expose the plane of dissection below the anterior pectoralis major fascia and allows that plane to be pursued without an assistant having to retract the breast. The authors, on the other hand, prefer the superior to inferior dissection of the breast, leaving the breast attached at the inferior margin of the field of resection, which has the advantage of stabilizing the breast and keeping it a bit out of the surgeon's way, so that it does not interfere with the axillary dissection. Either technique appears to be a matter of personal preference of the surgeon, but the width and length of the field of excision should be the same, this being largely a square field of excision, as is illustrated in this chapter.

An item of lessening disagreement at this time is the question of immediate reconstruction of the breast following modified radical mastectomy, which means that simultaneous mastectomy and performance of some form of reconstruction are done, as opposed to a delay of 6 to 9 months before reconstruction is carried out. There are forceful proponents of both courses, but the approach of the surgeon has a great deal to do with the decision of the patient. It is interesting that many patients who talk enthusiastically about reconstruction of the breast in the preoperative period who are not subjected to simultaneous reconstruction will, after several months, decline any further surgical treatment, despite its being available and suggested.

Especially in older women, modified radical mastectomy can be accompanied by significant morbidity if the individual allows the shoulder to become frozen. Like Drs. Bland and Vezeridis, I always emphasize to patients that at the end of 7 to 10 days, when the wound is healed and the drains have been removed, it is very important for them to commence shoulder exercises. Patients who are recalcitrant or intolerant of discomfort, or who simply have a physical infirmity, should be seen by the physical therapy department on a daily basis. In more cooperative patients, I like to demonstrate two significant exercises. The first is a circumduction exercise in which the patient flexes at the waist to 90 degrees, has the affected arm hanging down toward the floor, and begins to swing the arm in a circle with an ever-increasing radius, so that ultimately, after several days, the complete abduction and adduction of the arm can be achieved by this simple maneuver. A second exercise is one in which the patient stands with the trunk at a right angle to a wall, places the hand on the wall as high as is comfortable, and then begins to inch the hand up by "climbing" the wall with the fingers; as the shoulder is abducted higher, the patient moves closer to the wall, and ultimately the patient stands with the lateral trunk against the wall and the arm fully abducted. These exercises generally take from 7 to 14 days to achieve a full range of motion of the shoulder, but both circumduction and abduction exercises are the key to restoring full functional mobility to the shoulder.

Management of early breast cancer is now being sharply focused upon, as mammography is unearthing substantial numbers of women with early and noninvasive breast cancers. For those women whose tumors are discovered at a later stage, however, this operation still offers the best chance of appropriate excision and the highest probability of preventing local recurrence.

R.J.B.

II

The Chest and Mediastinum

48

Applied Anatomy of the Chest Wall and Mediastinum

Jemi Olak

A thorough knowledge of chest wall anatomy enables the surgeon to select optimal sites and patient positioning for a variety of thoracic surgical procedures from thoracentesis to thoracotomy. Knowledge of mediastinal anatomy is likewise important to the extent that mediastinal masses are more likely to occur in one compartment than another and their diagnostic evaluation can be focused on the appropriate compartment based on patient history, physical examination, and the chest radiograph.

This chapter approaches the anatomy of the chest wall and mediastinum from a practical perspective as it pertains to the diagnosis, workup, and treatment of thoracic diseases. The anatomy of the diaphragm is covered in Chap. 52 and the anatomy of the esophagus in Chap. 58.

Chest Wall

Thoracentesis

One of the most commonly performed procedures for which an understanding of chest wall anatomy is necessary is thoracentesis. The rate of complications, such as bleeding, pneumothorax, or failure of the procedure to accomplish its objective, will increase if such knowledge is lacking.

When thoracentesis is performed to diagnose or treat a free-flowing pleural effusion, the patient is usually sitting with the legs hanging over the side of the bed. He or she is asked to lean forward and to rest the arms on a table adjusted to the height of the patient's elbows. This position moves the scapulae anterolaterally, thereby exposing most of the patient's back. It is important to adjust the height of the bed as well as the height of the table over which the patient leans in order that both the patient and the physician can be comfortable. It is advisable to consider placing the patient on oxygen via nasal cannula for the duration of the procedure. These maneuvers help to optimize the chance of a successful outcome.

When the patient is unable to assume a sitting position, a lateral approach may be appropriate. If this approach is selected, the patient is propped up with a rolled towel placed lengthwise beneath the back with the upper arm resting over the ear to open up the intercostal spaces. Likewise, when the pleural effusion is loculated, as evidenced by failure of the fluid to layer out on decubitus chest radiographs or chest CT scan, alternative areas are chosen to perform the thoracentesis and may warrant a change in patient positioning. Successful evacuation of loculated fluid may be aided by the use of fluoroscopy, ultrasound or, less commonly, computed tomographic scan to localize the collection. When localization of the effusion is needed, however, it is important to be certain that it be done with the patient in the same position as he/she will be in for the thoracentesis to keep the surface landmarks constant.

Thoracentesis is performed after review of old and new chest radiographs. The fluid level is percussed and the ribs in the region are palpated to identify the intercostal space through which the needle will be placed. In general, the posterior aspect of the seventh intercostal space is an appropriate site for thoracentesis. This site is localized by palpating the tip of the scapula with the patient sitting upright. The parietal pleural reflection in this region is at the level of the tenth thoracic vertebra Fig. 48-1).

The patient is prepped and draped, and a local anesthetic (e.g., 1% lidocaine) is used to raise a wheal in the epidermis (Fig. 48-2A). The most important aspect of the procedure from the patient's point of view is that it should be painless. Pain is avoided by anesthetizing the periosteum over the eighth rib as well as the parietal pleura in the seventh intercostal space. This is done by infiltrating the subcutaneous tissues and then guiding the needle over the superior margin of the eighth rib, remaining perpendicular to the rib (Fig. 48-2B). Damage to the intercostal neurovascular bundle of the eighth rib, which lies in the intercostal groove of that rib, can be avoided by maintaining a perpendicular orientation (Fig. 48-2C). At the level of the rib, infiltration of the tissue is alternated with aspiration with the syringe to ascertain when the pleural space has been reached. Once fluid has been aspirated, confirming that the needle has reached the pleural space, the needle is slowly withdrawn while a further 2 to 3 ml of local anesthetic is injected. If this is done correctly, the parietal pleura will be well anesthetized. If fluid cannot be aspirated from the pleural space, it is advisable to attempt to anesthetize and aspirate one intercostal space lower. It is not recommended, how-

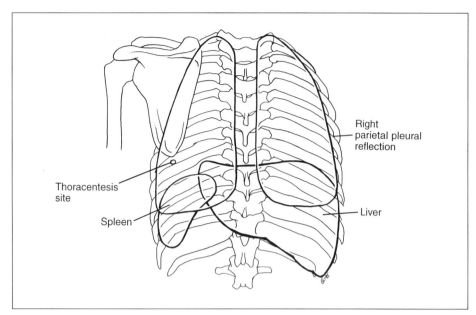

Fig. 48-1. Posterior view of the thorax demonstrating the posterior reflection of the right and left parietal pleura and outlining the space occupied by the liver and spleen. The site for a left seventh intercostal space thoracentesis is marked.

ever, that one go any lower than the eighth intercostal space because of the risk of lacerating the liver on the right or the spleen on the left. The spleen lies adjacent to the bed of ribs 9 to 11 and an enlarged spleen or liver will elevate the respective hemidiaphragm (see Fig. 48-1).

The thoracentesis catheter is inserted into the pleural space next. The catheter should be kept perpendicular to the chest wall to avoid inadvertent injury to the intercostal neurovascular bundle of the seventh rib (Fig. 48-2D). Fluid is removed into a 60-ml syringe and then injected into a sterile bag or bottle connected to the catheter with a stopcock.

A chest radiograph should be obtained subsequent to any attempt at thoracentesis to check for the presence of either a pneumothorax or residual fluid collection.

Conditions that might alter the approach to thoracentesis, outlined previously, include any condition that causes elevation of the hemidiaphragm (phrenic nerve paralysis, previous lung resection, concurrent volume loss, ascites, or morbid obesity). It is helpful to review the chest radiograph with the radiologist to understand the likely position of the hemidiaphragm. Bilateral thoracentesis is discouraged because of the risk of bilateral complications.

Chest Tube Insertion

The two most common locations to place chest tubes are the second intercostal space anteriorly and the fifth intercostal space in the anterior axillary line (Fig. 48-3). An anterior chest tube is usually placed to treat a pneumothorax or a loculated apical fluid collection. The lateral site is appropriate for the treatment of pneumothorax, hydrothorax (from blood or pus), and hydropneumothorax.

Understanding the anatomic landmarks will minimize misadventures with this commonly performed procedure. Before insertion of a chest tube, the chest radiograph should be reviewed with a radiologist to verify the side and optimal site for insertion. It is also advisable to review a chest radiograph that predates the current illness to gain a better understanding of the position of the diaphragm and the size of the cardiopericardial silhouette at baseline. In patients who have had prior lung resection, the ipsilateral diaphragm ascends and the mediastinum shifts to the side of the surgery. This may mandate placement of the chest tube one interspace higher. The complication rate associated with insertion of chest tubes using the method described below is 1 percent.

The recommended site for the insertion of most chest tubes is the fifth intercostal space in the anterior axillary line (Fig. 48-3A). The following surface landmarks will enable accurate localization of this position. The anterior axillary line is created by the lateral border of the pectoralis major muscle. In the male, the nipple overlies the fourth intercostal space. By tracing a line from the nipple to the anterior axillary line and then palpating one intercostal space lower the site is localized. In the female, the inframammary fold intersects the anterior axillary line over the fifth intercostal space. In this region, the parietal pleural reflection is at the level of the eighth thoracic vertebra and the risk of injuring the liver, spleen, or diaphragm is very low.

The second intercostal space anteriorly is an appropriate site for insertion of chest tubes to treat pneumothoraces or apical fluid collections although cosmetically it is considerably less attractive (Fig. 48-3B). In an emergency situation, however, access to the pleural space can be accomplished quickly, as there is less musculature and adipose tissue in this area and the patient remains in the supine position. The following surface landmarks will help to localize the second intercostal space. The angle of Louis, which represents the joint between the manubrium and the sternum, is the point at which the second costal cartilage meets the sternum. By palpating the second costal cartilage at this level and moving caudad into the next interspace approximately 3 cm from the sternal margin, the tube thoracostomy site is localized (Fig. 48-4). The internal mammary arteries and veins run beneath the parietal pleura approximately 1 cm on either side of the sternal margin.

After selecting the site for chest tube insertion and verifying the patient's coagulation status, informed consent is obtained. Generally, a No. 20 to 24 French chest tube is adequate to treat a pneumothorax while a 28 to 40 French chest tube is used to treat pleural effusions, blood, and pus. In all trauma cases, a 28 to 32 French chest tube should be used because of the frequent coexistence of hemothorax with pneumothorax.

The patient is positioned toward one edge of the bed with the affected side elevated by placing a rolled towel lengthwise under the spine. The arm is placed over the patient's ear to help spread the intercostal spaces. The bed is elevated to an appro-

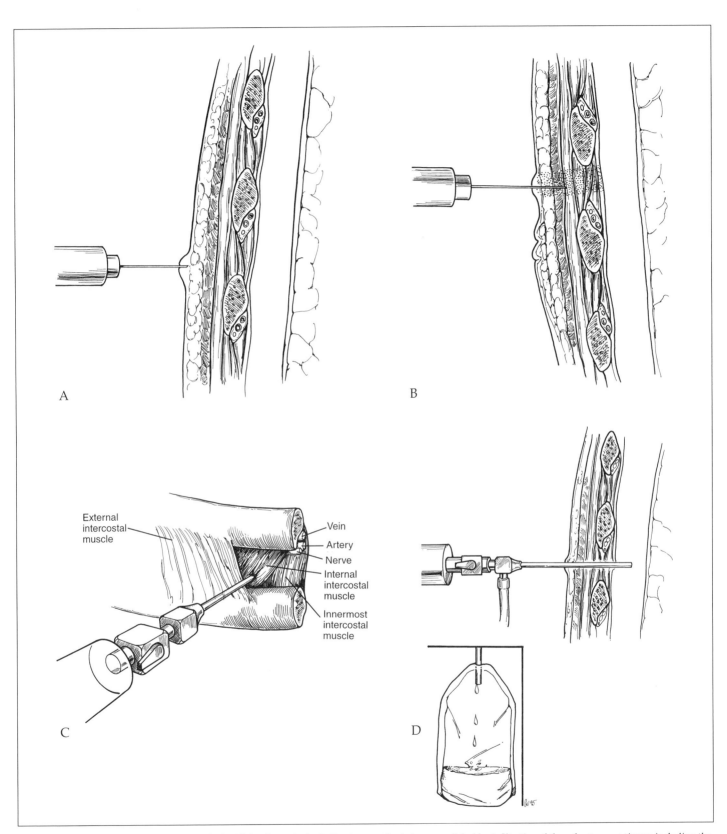

Fig. 48-2. Thoracentesis. A. Raising a skin wheal with local anesthetic. B. Further anesthesia is accomplished by infiltration of the subcutaneous tissues including the parietal pleura. C. Maintenance of a perpendicular orientation to the needle will avoid injury to the intercostal neurovascular bundle, which sits in the intercostal groove of the rib above. D. Insertion of the thoracentesis catheter and aspiration of pleural fluid first into a syringe and then into a sterile container using a three-way stopcock.

Labels in figure C:
External intercostal muscle
Vein
Artery
Nerve
Internal intercostal muscle
Innermost intercostal muscle

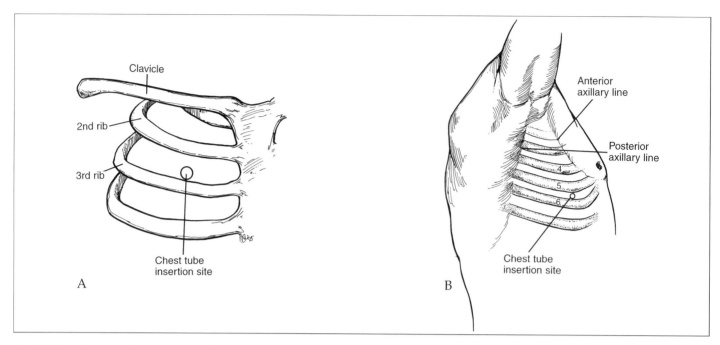

Fig. 48-3. Chest tube insertion sites: A. Second intercostal space at the junction of the medial one-third and lateral two-thirds of the clavicle. B. Fifth intercostal space in the anterior axillary line.

priate height so that the physician is not bending over the patient. Oxygen is delivered via nasal cannula. In selected cases, an anxiolytic or a narcotic drug, or both, may be administered parenterally; however, for most patients, the use of local anesthetic (e.g., 1% lidocaine [Xylocaine]) as described in the section on thoracentesis is sufficient. It is helpful to have a nurse present to reassure the patient and to help maintain the patient's arm position.

After prepping and draping the patient's chest, local anesthetic (e.g., 1% Xylocaine) is used as shown in Fig. 48-2A and B. Verification that the correct interspace has been chosen is obtained by aspirating air or fluid at this point. It is not advisable to proceed with chest tube insertion at this site if the aspiration is not successful. A one-centimeter incision is made in the skin over the sixth intercostal space. In most elective circumstances it is desirable to tunnel the chest tube over one rib. The reason for doing so is that when the chest tube is removed the parietal pleural entry site will be covered immediately by subcutaneous tissue, thereby decreasing the likelihood that air will be sucked into the pleural space. In situations in which the chest

tube was placed to remove fluid, tunneling will limit the amount of leakage at the skin site after the tube is removed.

The skin is retracted superiorly in order to create a subcutaneous tunnel and a hemostat is used to spread the muscles horizontally and vertically until the parietal pleura is reached (Fig. 48-4A). The parietal pleura is then punctured with the closed tip of a blunt hemostat and the hole enlarged by spreading the hemostat as it is withdrawn. The chest tube is mounted on a hemostat and advanced through the incision (Fig. 48-4B). Once the tip of the hemostat is in the pleural space and turned so that it is oriented posteriorly, the chest tube is advanced into the pleural space and directed posteriorly and toward the apex of the chest (Fig. 48-4C). Failure to do so will result in the chest tube resting in the major fissure, and may not completely address the problem for which it was inserted (Fig. 48-4D). This is because the major fissures follow the course of the sixth rib from the root of the spine of the scapula posteriorly to the sixth costochondral junction anteriorly. The chest tube is then fixed to the skin with a heavy silk tie. A pull-out stitch can be placed if desired. The chest

tube should be connected to a drainage system and appropriate fluctuation of the underwater seal column verified (Fig. 48-4E). Finally, an occlusive dressing of gauze and adhesive tape is applied to the chest tube to prevent air from being sucked into the chest or fluid from draining around the chest tube. Vaseline-impregnated gauze can be placed around the chest tube to improve the seal.

An upright portable chest radiograph is obtained to verify that the chest tube is properly positioned in the pleural space and the last side hole within the space, and that the hemothorax or pneumothorax is being appropriately treated.

Acute hemothoraces should be evacuated in their entirety as soon as possible. It is generally recommended that other pleural effusions be evacuated more slowly (for example, 1500 ml acutely, then 500 ml hourly) to minimize the risk of re-expansion pulmonary edema. Incentive spirometry and chest physical therapy will help re-expand atelectatic lung.

While some chest tubes are manufactured with internal trocars, the use of a trocar to guide chest tube insertion as opposed to

Fig. 48-4. Chest tube insertion. A. Spreading the subcutaneous tissues and intercostal muscles using a hemostat. B. A chest tube mounted on a hemostat or Kelly ▶ clamp is advanced into the pleural space. C. The chest tube is directed posteroapically by rotating the hemostat 180 degrees counterclockwise. D. The chest tube is advanced toward the apex of the pleural space. E. Final position of the chest tube.

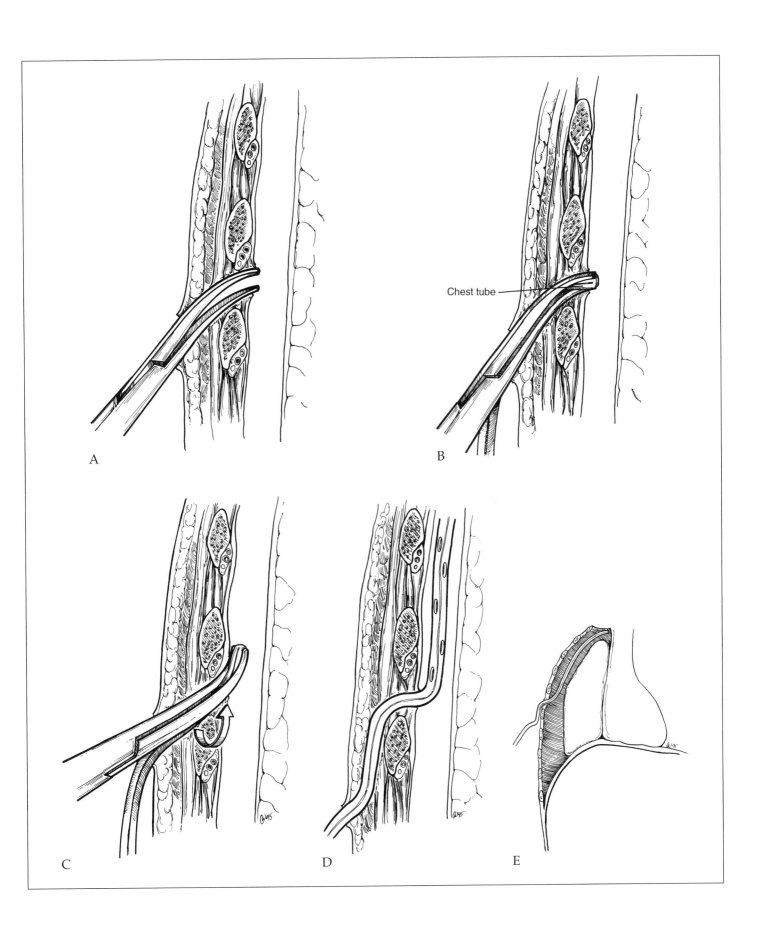

Chest tube

A

B

C

D

E

the method outlined previously should be discouraged for all but the most experienced surgical personnel. It is much more difficult to control entry of a trocar chest tube into the pleural space, and the trocar's sharp tip can easily lacerate the underlying lung or a cardiac chamber, or penetrate a high-lying diaphragm.

Anatomy of the Mediastinum

Boundaries

The mediastinum is bounded superiorly by the thoracic inlet, inferiorly by the diaphragm, and laterally by the mediastinal pleura. Classically, the mediastinum was divided into superior, anterior, middle, and posterior compartments. Practically, however, the separation of the mediastinum into three compartments—anterosuperior, middle, and posterior—is more practical. Dividing the mediastinum into these compartments helps to direct the investigation and treatment of mediastinal masses since most masses have a predilection for a particular compartment.

The boundaries of the mediastinal compartments illustrated in Fig. 48-5 were first proposed by Shields in 1972. Each compartment extends from the thoracic inlet to the diaphragm and is bounded laterally by the adjacent mediastinal parietal pleura.

The anterosuperior compartment is bounded anteriorly by the inner table of the sternum and posteriorly by the pericardium and the reflection of the pericardium onto the great vessels. The anterosuperior compartment is also known as the prevascular compartment. The middle mediastinum, also known as the visceral compartment, is bounded anteriorly by the pericardium and its reflection onto the great vessels. Its posterior limit is the prevertebral fascia. The posterior mediastinum is a bilateral compartment also known as the paravertebral sulcus. The posterior mediastinum projects on either side of the vertebral column and adjacent proximal portions of the ribs.

Contents

The anterosuperior mediastinum normally contains the thymus gland, lymph nodes and lymphatic vessels, connective tissue, and adipose tissue. Displaced or ectopic parathyroid glands and ectopic thyroid tissue also may be found in this location.

The middle mediastinum contains the pericardium, heart, great vessels, trachea, proximal portion of the bronchial tree, and esophagus. In addition, the vagus and phrenic nerves, thoracic duct, and lymph nodes reside in this compartment.

The posterior mediastinum contains the proximal portion of the intercostal nerves, the thoracic spinal ganglia, and the sympathetic chains, as well as connective tissue and lymphatics.

A list of tumors commonly found in each compartment is provided in Table 48-1.

Anterior Compartment

Thymus
The thymus arises as ventral primordia from the third and possibly the fourth pharyngeal pouches during the latter part of the sixth week of gestation. By the eighth week, the thymic primordia have enlarged and moved toward the midline caudal to the thyroid and meet but do not fuse in this location. Further caudal migration into the anterosuperior mediastinum represents the final step in its development.

The thymus can weigh as much as 15 g in the newborn. It reaches a maximum of 30 to 40 g at puberty, and then involutes in the adult to weigh between 5 and 25 g.

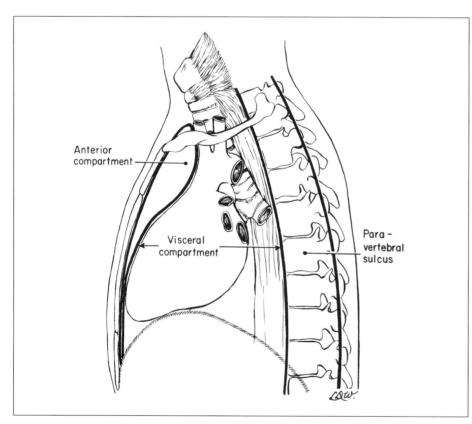

Fig. 48-5. *Anatomic subdivisions of the mediastinum as proposed by Shields. (From TW Shields (ed). Mediastinal Surgery [1st ed]. Philadelphia: Lea & Febriger, 1991. P 4. With permission.)*

Table 48-1. Classification of Mediastinal Tumors and Masses by Location

Anterior	Middle	Posterior
Thymoma	Foregut cyst, duplication	Neurilemmoma
Lymphoma	Lymphoma	Neurofibroma
Germ cell tumor	Pleuropericardial cyst	Malignant schwannoma
Other mesenchymal tumor	Granulomatous disease	Ganglioneuroma
Thymic cyst	Mesenchymal cyst	Neuroblastoma
Endocrine tumor	Mesenchymal tumor	

Mediastinal Lymph Nodes

Lymph nodes in the anterior compartment are found in either the internal mammary or the prevascular regions. The internal mammary chain drains the anterior chest wall, upper anterior abdominal wall, anterior diaphragm, and medial aspect of the breast. The prevascular chain lies anterior and lateral to the thymus and anterior to the great vessels. Lung cancers in the left lung, particularly those in the left upper lobe, metastasize to this lymph node region. Biopsy of lymph nodes in this region requires a parasternal incision through the second intercostal space or by left thoracoscopy.

Mediastinal Thyroid and Parathyroid Glands

The four parathyroid glands, derived from the third and fourth pharyngeal pouches, are found in the neck in 99 percent of patients. Ectopic glands usually originate from the third pharyngeal pouch and migrate in close association with or embedded within the thymus and as such are more often found in the mediastinum. Six percent of 527 patients in one autopsy study were found to have supernumerary glands and approximately two-thirds of these were located in the mediastinum.

When thyroid tissue is found in the mediastinum, it most often represents mediastinal extension of a goitrous gland in the neck as opposed to true ectopic tissue. Intrathoracic thyroid goiters project into the anterosuperior mediastinal compartment on the chest radiograph. Most patients with goiter are over 50 years of age, and women are affected approximately three times more often than men. The glands are located in the prevascular (anterosuperior) compartment in 75 percent and in the middle (visceral) compartment in 25 percent of cases. Glands in the visceral compartment often displace the carotid vessels and recurrent laryngeal nerves anteriorly. Glands that project behind the vasculature occur more often in patients who have undergone previous thyroid surgery in whom the tissue planes have been violated. When true ectopic thyroid tissue is identified on an iodine-131 scan, a normal-sized cervical gland will usually also be demonstrated. Ectopic thyroid always has an anomalous blood supply from locoregional vessels.

Middle Compartment

Mediastinal Lymph Nodes

Lymph nodes in the middle compartment are often of clinical importance, as they may be involved in a variety of pathologic processes, both benign and malignant. When lung cancers metastasize to mediastinal lymph nodes, the nodes in this compartment are involved most often. A mediastinal lymph node map has been developed for use in staging lung cancer Fig. 48-6. Strictly speaking, the prevascular lymph nodes (level 6) lie in the anterosuperior mediastinal compartment while all other groups lie in the middle compartment. Lymph flows from the right hilum to both right tracheobronchial angle and subcarinal lymph node stations and then upward to right lower paratracheal and right upper paratracheal lymph node stations. On the left, lymph flows from the hilum to either aorticopulmonary window and prevascular lymph node stations and then to left tracheobronchial angle and subcarinal lymph nodes or directly to

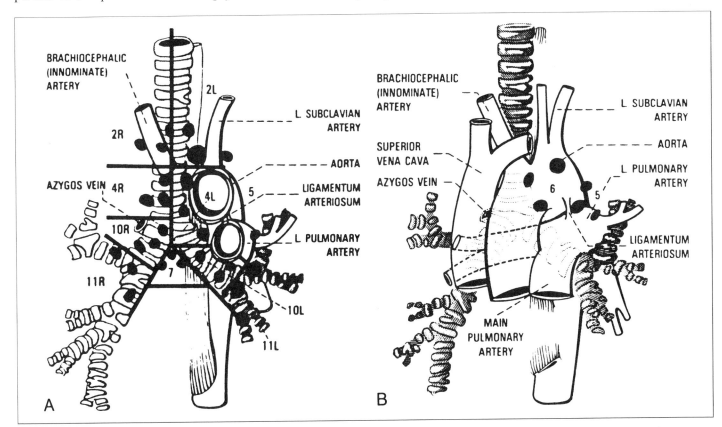

Fig. 48-6. Mediastinal lymph node map developed by the American Thoracic Society. (From the American Thoracic Society. Clinical staging of primary lung cancer. Am Rev Respir Dis 127:659, 1983. With permission.)

these latter two nodal groups. It ascends to paratracheal lymph stations on either side of the trachea. The lymphatic drainage of the left lower lobe of the lung is such that lymphatic spread of cancer to right-sided nodal stations occurs in up to 25 percent of patients. Left upper lobe tumors and tumors in the right lung metastasize less often to contralateral lymph node stations.

Foregut Structures

The trachea extends from the lower border of the cricoid cartilage in the neck to the level of the angle of Louis, which corresponds to the level of the fourth intervertebral disk. At this point, it bifurcates into right and left main stem bronchi. The left main stem bronchus is longer and follows a more horizontal course than the right main stem bronchus. Upon leaving the mediastinum the left main stem bronchus bifurcates into left upper and left lower lobe bronchi while the right main stem bronchus gives off the right upper lobe bronchus and continues on as the bronchus intermedius upon leaving the mediastinum.

The anatomy of the esophagus is discussed in Chap. 58.

Thoracic Duct

The thoracic duct is renowned for its anatomic variability. Duplications, left-sided ducts, and bilateral termination of the duct account for much of this variability. The pattern described below is found in approximately 65 percent of humans and is illustrated in Fig. 48-7.

The thoracic duct originates at the cisterna chyli and ascends into the thorax through the aortic hiatus to the right of the aorta at the level of the twelfth thoracic vertebra. It proceeds upward on the anterior surface of the vertebral column behind the esophagus and between the aorta and azygos vein. It crosses the midline behind the aorta at the level of the fifth or sixth thoracic vertebra and proceeds toward the left side of the neck close to the left side of the esophagus and the mediastinal pleural reflection. It then arches 2 to 3 cm above the clavicle and swings laterally anterior to the

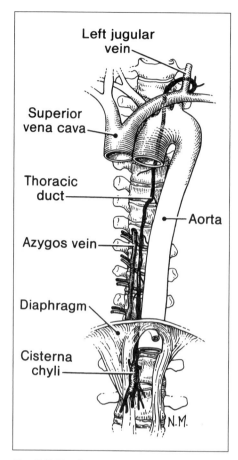

Fig. 48-7. Usual anatomic route of the thoracic duct. (From JI Miller. Anatomy of the thoracic duct. In TW Shields (ed), Mediastinal Surgery [1st ed]. Philadelphia: Lea & Febiger, 1991. P 24. With permission.)

left subclavian artery and thyrocervical trunk. It passes behind the carotid sheath and empties into the subclavian-jugular venous junction. It is important to understand the course of the thoracic duct, particularly when operating on the esophagus, since inadvertent injury might result in a postoperative chylothorax and cause significant morbidity.

Neural Structures

Vagus Nerves. The right vagus enters the thorax within the carotid sheath and crosses anterior to the first part of the right subclavian artery, where it gives off its recurrent laryngeal branch. The recurrent

branch loops beneath and behind the right subclavian artery and ascends in the tracheoesophageal groove to the larynx. The vagus continues caudally on the right side of the trachea, passing behind the right hilum. It forms a plexus of nerve fibers on the posterior surface of the esophagus and reconstitutes into a single posterior vagal trunk in the region of the lower third of the esophagus. It passes into the abdomen through the esophageal hiatus in the diaphragm, which is located at the level of the tenth thoracic vertebra.

The left vagus nerve enters the thorax between the left common carotid and left subclavian arteries. It descends over the aortic arch, passing between the aorta and left main pulmonary artery, where it gives off the left recurrent laryngeal nerve. The recurrent nerve sweeps beneath the ligamentum arteriosum and behind the aortic arch and then ascends in the tracheoesophageal groove toward the larynx. The left vagus passes behind the left hilum and forms a plexus of nerve fibers on the anterior surface of the esophagus. It reconstitutes into a single trunk before passing into the abdomen through the esophageal hiatus in the diaphragm. The thoracic courses of both vagus and phrenic nerves are illustrated in Fig. 48-8.

Phrenic Nerves. The right phrenic nerve enters the thorax between the right subclavian artery and vein. It crosses the origin of the right internal mammary artery in this region before descending on the anterior surface of the superior vena cava. It passes in front of the hilum of the right lung onto the lateral surface of the pericardium. It divides into at least two terminal branches above the right hemidiaphragm, which it innervates.

The left phrenic nerve enters the thorax behind the thoracic duct between the left common carotid and left subclavian arteries. It moves ventrally as it descends, and lies medial to the left vagus nerve as it crosses over the aortic arch. It crosses in front of the hilum of the left lung and then onto the pericardium. It also terminates in at least two branches above the left hemidiaphragm, which it innervates.

Fig. 48-8. A. Right side of the mediastinum demonstrating the course of the right phrenic and vagus nerves as well as the right sympathetic chain. B. Left side of ▶ the mediastinum demonstrating the course of the left phrenic and vagus nerves and the left sympathetic chain. (From RA Snell. Clinical Anatomy for Medical Students [1st ed]. Boston: Little, Brown, 1973. Pp 93, 94. With permission.)

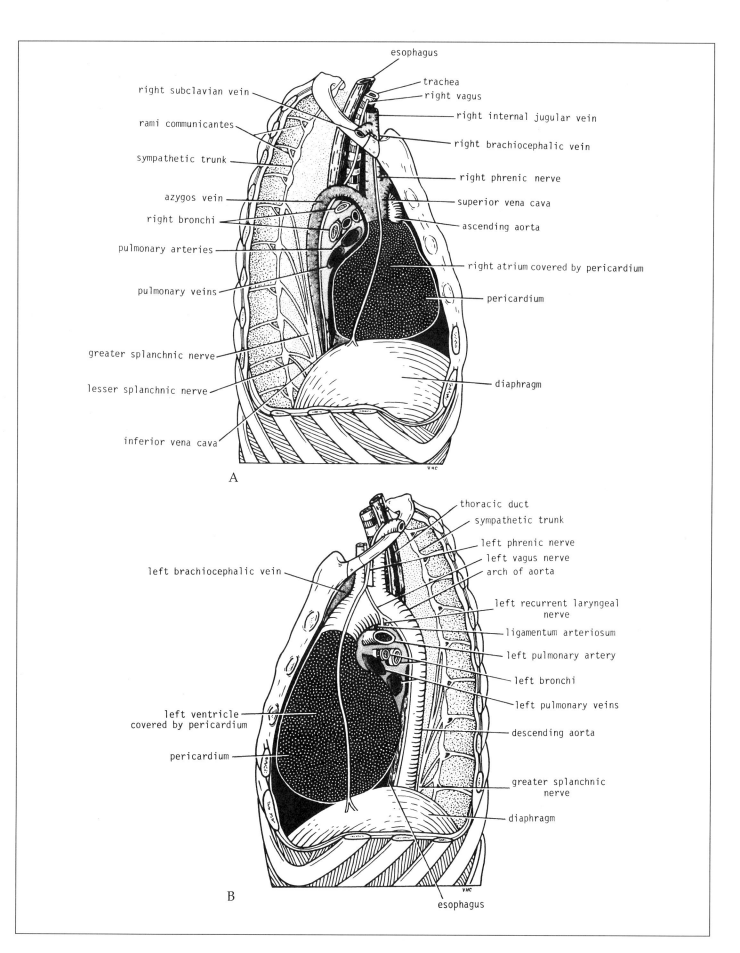

esophagus

trachea
right vagus
right internal jugular vein
right brachiocephalic vein
right phrenic nerve
superior vena cava
ascending aorta
right atrium covered by pericardium
pericardium

right subclavian vein
rami communicantes
sympathetic trunk
azygos vein
right bronchi
pulmonary arteries
pulmonary veins
greater splanchnic nerve
lesser splanchnic nerve
inferior vena cava
diaphragm

A

thoracic duct
sympathetic trunk
left phrenic nerve
left vagus nerve
arch of aorta
left recurrent laryngeal
nerve
ligamentum arteriosum
left pulmonary artery
left bronchi
left pulmonary veins
descending aorta
greater splanchnic
nerve
diaphragm

left brachiocephalic vein
left ventricle
covered by pericardium
pericardium

B

esophagus

Posterior Compartment

Neural Structures

Sympathetic Chain. The right and left sympathetic trunks lie ventral to the heads of ribs 1 through 10 immediately beneath the parietal pleura. At this level they move ventrally to lie on the eleventh and twelfth thoracic vertebral bodies. The chains are made up of a variable number of ganglia connected by the sympathetic trunk. The first thoracic ganglion, for example, is often fused with the inferior cervical ganglion and named the stellate ganglion (Fig. 48-8). Removal of the lower one-half to two-thirds of this ganglion has been shown to relieve palmar hyperhidrosis, reflex sympathetic dystrophy, and Raynaud's disease in selected individuals.

Intercostal Nerves. These paired structures emerge from intervertebral foramina below their corresponding vertebrae. They divide into four branches: an anterior and a posterior primary division; a ramus communicans, which is connected to the sympathetic chain; and a ramus meningeus, which returns to the spinal cord. The anterior primary divisions become the intercostal nerves and run in the intercostal grooves of each rib with the corresponding intercostal artery and vein (see Fig. 48-2A). The smaller posterior primary divisions leave the thoracic cavity and branch to supply the soft tissues of the back.

Neurogenic tumors are found most often in this mediastinal compartment and commonly originate from either the intercostal nerves or the sympathetic trunk.

Suggested Reading

Ravitch MM, Steichen FM (eds). *Atlas of General Thoracic Surgery* (1st ed). Philadelphia: Saunders, 1988.

Shields TW (ed). *Mediastinal Surgery* (1st ed). Philadelphia: Lea & Febiger, 1991.

Snell RS. *Clinical Anatomy for Medical Students* (1st ed). Boston: Little, Brown, 1973.

Waldhausen JA, Orringer MB (eds). *Complications in Cardiothoracic Surgery* (1st ed). St. Louis: Mosby–Year Book, 1991.

EDITOR'S COMMENT

Doctor Olak's chapter provides a considerable amount of information, ranging from the simple procedures on the chest wall and pleural space of thoracentesis and tube thoracostomy insertion to the anatomic relationships in the mediastinum, with special emphasis on a number of anatomic structures that bear directly on surgery of the lung and mediastinum.

The author's description of chest tube insertion is one that is commonly employed in elective tube thoracostomy. Trauma surgeons, who are apt to encounter blood and air under pressure, make a skin incision under local anesthesia, insert a hemostat into the muscle, and spread it, but follow that with the gloved finger to open the pleura and be certain that the lung is free and that the pleural space is not adhered to the point of insertion. Inserting the finger is followed by the rush of air or blood, or both; the lung can be felt at the tip of the finger, and the chest tube is inserted precisely as described by Dr. Olak with the assurance that the lung or diaphragm is safe and will not be injured by the firm tube or the hemostat.

Ectopic mediastinal thyroid, except for very tiny fragments that have descended with the thymus, is most unusual in the mediastinum. Much commoner and frequently encountered in clinical practice is the substernal extension of a thyroid goiter or neoplasm. In fact, in older patients, in whom this lesion is usually seen, the development of symptoms from a substernal goiter often heralds the development of carcinoma in the thyroid in that portion of the lobe or lobes that has enlarged and extended into the superior mediastinum. For that reason, considerable care should be exercised when bluntly dissecting and delivering the thyroid into the cervical incision from its mediastinal location. It is most important that the capsule is not ruptured. The seeding of thyroid cancer in the superior mediastinum would have serious implications, and is to be strictly avoided. In actuality, once the soft tissue adjacent to the thyroid is gently dissected away, delivery of the mass is difficult. Under the very unusual circumstance of a thyroid that is densely adherent and cannot be delivered as previously described, there is a valid indication for a median sternotomy, to avoid any possibility of rupture or of damage to the innominate vein or other structures to which a thyroid cancer may be adherent.

The thoracic duct is rarely operated on, but when it presents surgical problems because of acute trauma, persistent chylothorax, or persistent chylous ascites, knowledge of the anatomy is most important. Chyle flows, in the fasting state, at approximately 60 ml per hour. Further, enteral alimentation with a solution with high fat content can markedly increase that volume for short periods after feedings. Malnutrition often occurs with major loss of chyle into the chest, primarily because of the loss of protein and fat in the lymph. Obviously, a thoracostomy tube to keep the pleural space open and relatively dry is essential in management. Repair of protein malnutrition may require total parenteral nutrition and cessation of oral feedings to diminish lymph flow.

Surgical trauma to the thoracic duct can occur after any mediastinal operation or esophagectomy, or in the abdomen following retroperitoneal resection for tumor or abdominal aortic operations. It is somewhat surprising that it is not encountered more commonly in transhiatal esophagectomy performed without thoracotomy.

Regardless of the location of a thoracic duct injury, ligation of the duct proximal and distal to the defect is the preferred treatment if the more conservative measures do not effect closure. Without exception, collateral flow through various accessory lymphatic channels is quite sufficient to allow normal lymph transport into the venous circuit, and distal lymph collections, once the primary injury to the thoracic duct is isolated by proximal and distal ligation, are almost unknown. Unfortunately, management of chylothorax or chylous ascites by relying on intravenous hyperalimentation has not proved to be as successful as was once thought. One can certainly diminish the flow of lymph by intravenous hyperalimentation, but permanent sealing of the defect, unless it is quite small, will generally not occur, and surgical ligation will be required.

R.J.B.

49

Surgical Approach to the Chest Wall and Mediastinum: Incisions, Excisions, and Repair of Defects

Mark K. Ferguson

The pleural cavities and mediastinum are notoriously difficult regions to access. The bony thorax serves as a framework for muscles of respiration, as an anchor for the shoulder girdle, and as protection for vital organs of the thorax. This bony structure, and compartmentalization of organs within the thorax, prevent simple access to all intrathoracic contents through a single incision. In addition, adequate ventilation is dependent on the existence of a semirigid thoracic cage in which volume and pressure changes can be controlled. Thoracotomies and chest wall excisions are planned to minimize disruption of chest wall integrity as much as possible.

Incisions

Lateral and Posterolateral Thoracotomies

The lateral thoracotomy is the most common incision used to access intrapleural structures, including the lungs, esophagus, chest wall, and mediastinum. It replaces the posterolateral thoracotomy in this regard, which is used in selected circumstances for improved access to the mediastinum and superior sulcus. Many intrathoracic operations are facilitated by the use of single lung ventilation, which is achieved with use of a double lumen endotracheal tube or a bronchial blocker. The patient is placed in a true lateral position with the ipsilateral arm extended anteriorly and suspended on a sling fixed to the operating table, taking care not to put traction on the brachial plexus. This position rotates the scapula anterosuperiorly, exposing the auscultatory triangle and paraspinous muscles so that if necessary, the incision can be extended into a posterolateral thoracotomy.

The incision is placed 1 to 2 cm below the tip of the scapula, extending from the angle of the ribs posteriorly to the anterior edge of the latissimus dorsi muscle anteriorly, parallel to the intercostal spaces (Fig. 49-1). The body of the latissimus dorsi muscle is divided in the bed of the incision.

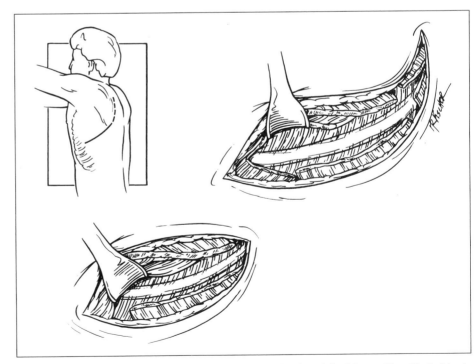

Fig. 49-1. A lateral thoracotomy is performed with the patient in a lateral decubitus position. The incision is oriented parallel to the direction of the ribs (inset). The latissimus dorsi muscle is divided, and the serratus anterior muscle is either divided or is retracted anteriorly (left). A posterolateral thoracotomy incision extends medial to the scapula in a curvilinear manner, and the trapezius and rhomboid major muscles are divided (right).

The fascial layer overlying the auscultatory triangle is incised, and a finger is inserted under the posterior edge of the serratus anterior muscle to elevate it. A retractor is placed under the tip of the scapula to lift it off the chest wall, and the proper interspace for the incision is identified. Counting rib interspaces is performed by reaching under the scapula and identifying the second rib, which is usually the highest rib that is palpated easily. Alternatively, opening the subscapular space is avoided by counting from below, starting with the twelfth rib. Access to the upper thorax (upper lobe, trachea, and upper esophagus) is best gained through the fourth or fifth interspace. The fifth or sixth interspace gives optimum exposure to the hilum, lower lobes, and lower esophagus; and the seventh interspace provides the best access to the diaphragm and esophageal hiatus.

The intercostal incision is made on the superior surface of the rib at the lower margin of the interspace, which helps to avoid injury to the intercostal neurovascular bundle. The superficial intercostal muscles are oriented from posterosuperior to anteroinferior in the interspace. Beginning the incision posteriorly and extending it anteriorly helps to keep the blade on the superior margin of the lower rib by making use of the orientation of these muscles.

The pleura is entered bluntly to avoid injury to the underlying lung and is divided the length of the intercostal incision. A small rib spreader is placed, and the intercostal incision is extended from inside the chest to permit further displacement of the ribs. In older patients, rib fractures are common and are minimized by excising a 1-cm segment of the lower rib to permit greater distraction of the rib. This step is performed medially, deep to the paraspinous muscles, which prevents the cut edge of the rib from putting pressure on the overlying skin.

In some patients, exposure is difficult because of adhesions of the lung to the chest wall that are caused by inflammatory disease or previous thoracotomy. Improved exposure is achieved by resecting the rib at the lower margin of the interspace in a subperiosteal manner, entering the pleural space through the bed of the resected rib.

Short incisions are completed by retracting the serratus anterior muscle anteriorly without dividing it. Longer incisions require division of this muscle, which is performed at the inferior margin of the incision to preserve the neural supply that originates superiorly from the long thoracic nerve.

To perform a posterolateral thoracotomy, the standard lateral thoracotomy incision is continued in a curvilinear manner medial to the scapula. This incision can be extended as high as the second rib if necessary. The trapezius and rhomboid major muscles are incised to provide access to the chest wall, and the intercostal incision is extended posteromedially to the transverse process of the vertebra.

Once the intrathoracic portion of the operation is completed, chest drainage is instituted. The position and number of chest tubes that are used depend on the type and amount of drainage that is expected. If little fluid accumulation and no air leak from the lung are anticipated, a single tube placed laterally through a separate intercostal incision to the apex of the hemithorax is sufficient. Usually two drainage tubes are used, particularly after a standard lung resection. One is placed laterally and the other posteriorly, and both are positioned at the apex of the hemithorax. In some situations, such as following decortication for an empyema, a third drain is placed inferiorly across the hemidiaphragm. All tubes are connected to underwater seal and suction as the chest is closed.

The ribs on either side of the incision are reapproximated using a heavy absorbable suture. Two or three figure-of-eight stitches are placed, encircling both ribs but excluding the neurovascular bundle of the inferior rib, to restore the normal width of the interspace. The intercostal muscle is closed with a running suture if there is sufficient soft tissue available. The divided muscles of the shoulder girdle are reapproximated using a running suture. Retracting the shoulder inferiorly helps to take tension off the muscular closure. A simple cuticular closure is performed.

Muscle-Sparing Thoracotomy

The muscle-sparing thoracotomy is used by many surgeons as the incision of choice for most pulmonary operations. The advantages of this approach are decreased operative time, improved cosmesis, decreased initial postoperative pain, and improved early postoperative shoulder girdle function. However, the exposure is not as good as the exposure provided by traditional lateral or posterolateral thoracotomies, and use of this incision can be difficult for surgeons with limited experience operating in the thorax.

Two approaches to this incision are used. The first is similar to the anterior portion of a standard lateral thoracotomy and provides the ability to convert a muscle-sparing thoracotomy to a standard lateral or posterolateral thoracotomy when necessary. The patient is placed in a full lateral decubitus position, and the ipsilateral arm is positioned on a sling or is fixed overhead. An incision is performed 1 to 2 cm below the tip of the scapula, extending from the posterior edge of the serratus anterior muscle to the anterior margin of the latissimus dorsi muscle (Fig. 49-2). Flaps are raised superficial to the fascia, extending 5 to 8 cm superiorly and inferiorly at the center of the incision. The edge of the latissimus dorsi muscle is freed to the limits of the flaps, and the muscle is retracted from the chest wall and dissected bluntly from the underlying serratus anterior muscle. The posterior edge of the serratus anterior muscle is freed and is dissected from the chest wall and retracted anteriorly, exposing the ribs. Identifying the appropriate interspace is best accomplished by counting ribs from below. After opening the interspace, a small rib spreader is used to retract the ribs, which permits the interspace to be opened further from inside the chest. A second rib spreader is placed at right angles to the first to retract the latissimus dorsi and serratus anterior muscles.

The second muscle-sparing incision requires less traction on the serratus anterior and latissimus dorsi muscles, but, because it is placed higher on the chest wall than the incision described above, it is less able to be extended into a formal lateral or posterolateral thoracotomy in case the scope of the operation changes unexpectedly. The patient is placed in a lateral or semilateral position, and the ipsilateral arm is suspended overhead. The skin incision is made in the direction of the ribs from just posterior to the anterior edge of the latissimus dorsi muscle to several centimeters anterior to the anterior axillary line (Fig.

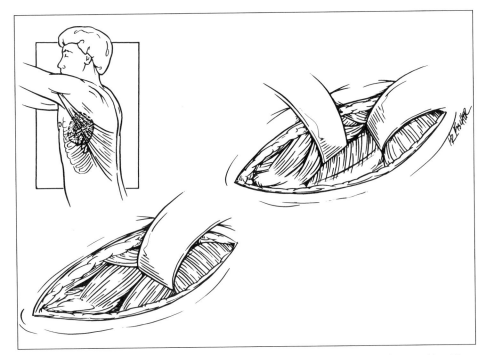

Fig. 49-2. A muscle-sparing thoracotomy is performed with the patient in a lateral decubitus position. The extent of dissection of the subcutaneous flaps is indicated by shading (inset). The latissimus dorsi muscle is mobilized and retracted posteriorly, exposing the edge of the serratus anterior muscle (left). The serratus anterior muscle is mobilized and retracted off the chest wall (right).

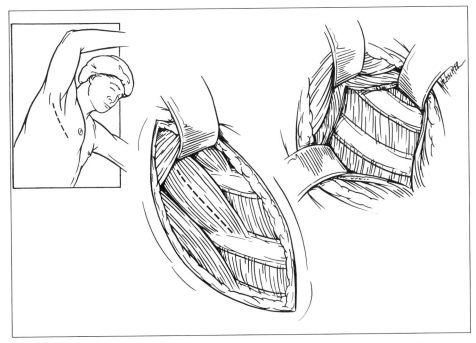

Fig. 49-3. A second type of muscle-sparing thoracotomy is performed with the patient in a lateral or semilateral position. The incision is angled vertically (inset). After retracting the latissimus dorsi muscle (left), the fibers of the serratus anterior muscle overlying the interspace to be opened are separated (right).

49-3). Small flaps are dissected posteriorly, and the belly of the latissimus dorsi muscle is retracted posteriorly. The appropriate interspace is identified, and the serratus anterior muscle is divided along the direction of its fibers over this interspace. After opening the interspace, rib spreaders are placed at right angles to each other as described previously.

The ease of closure of a muscle-sparing thoracotomy is one of its main attractions. After placing appropriate pleural drains, the ribs are reapproximated. The muscles are allowed to retract back into place, and if fibers of the serratus anterior muscle were separated, they are approximated. The skin and subcutaneous tissues are closed in one or two layers. It is unnecessary to place drains under the skin flaps unless very large flaps were created, which would increase the risk of seroma formation.

Anterior Thoracotomy

The anterior thoracotomy is used for performing small open lung biopsies for diffuse pulmonary disease, for standard thoracic operations on patients in whom simultaneous access to the abdomen is necessary, and for selected operations on the lower and middle lobes. Access to the posterior and apical thorax is often limited.

The patient is placed in a semirecumbent position, and the ipsilateral arm is suspended overhead. For small biopsies through a very limited thoracotomy, a 6- to 8-cm incision is made in the inframammary crease, ending laterally at the anterior axillary line. The pectoralis and intercostal muscles are divided and the fifth or sixth interspace is entered. For performing small lung biopsies it is often unnecessary to insert a rib spreader. Once the procedure is complete and a chest drain is placed, the pectoralis fibers are approximated and the superficial tissues are closed in one or two layers using a continuous suture technique.

A formal anterior thoracotomy incision extends from just lateral to the sternal border to the anterior or middle axillary line, following the course of the inframammary crease (Fig. 49-4). A suprafascial flap is raised superiorly to the level of the fifth interspace, and the pectoralis and intercostal muscles are divided, permitting entry

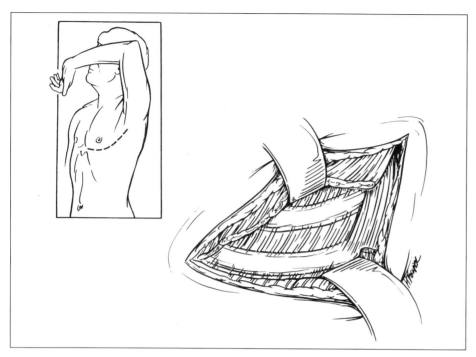

Fig. 49-4. *An anterior thoracotomy is performed with the patient in a semirecumbent position (inset). The incision follows the inframammary crease, and the pectoralis major muscle is divided.*

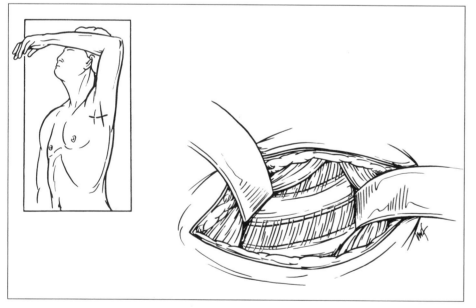

Fig. 49-5. *An axillary thoracotomy is performed with the patient in a lateral or semilateral position (inset). The incision is placed over the third rib, and the pectoralis major and latissimus dorsi muscles are retracted.*

Axillary Thoracotomy

A true axillary thoracotomy is used for diseases involving the apices of the lungs and pleural spaces, such as bullous disease with spontaneous pneumothorax. Access to the remainder of the hemithorax is quite limited. The patient is placed in a lateral or semilateral position with the ipsilateral arm suspended toward the ceiling. A 6- to 8-cm incision is made just below the axillary hairline, and dissection is carried down between the latissimus dorsi and pectoralis major muscles, taking care to preserve the long thoracic nerve (Fig. 49-5). The pleura is entered in the third intercostal space or through the bed of the resected third rib. Following the conclusion of the procedure and placement of a chest drain, the superficial tissues are closed in one or two layers using a continuous suture technique.

Transverse Sternothoracotomy (Clamshell Incision)

This approach recently has been repopularized for use in double lung transplantation, in bilateral pulmonary operations, and for operations on anterior mediastinal tumors or extensive lung cancers involving the mediastinum. The transverse incision causes less injury to the intercostal nerves than does a standard thoracotomy and is cosmetically superior to a median sternotomy. Exposure of the phrenic nerves, vagi, and recurrent laryngeal nerves is superior to the exposure provided by a median sternotomy. The disadvantages of the transverse sternothoracotomy are that the most superior aspect of the mediastinum at the thoracic inlet is sometimes difficult to reach and the closure sometimes is not as stable as lateral thoracotomy and sternotomy closures.

The patient is positioned supine with the arms abducted on arm boards or flexed at the elbow and anchored to an overhead frame. The incision is made in a curvilinear manner from the anterior axillary line on each side, following the inframammary crease across the sternum (Fig. 49-6). The pectoralis major muscles are incised, the pleural spaces are entered, and the internal mammary vessels are divided. The sternum is transected with a saw, and rib spreaders are placed bilaterally. The pleu-

into the pleural space. Because the anterior portions of the ribs have an exaggerated curve, angling the rib spreader superiorly off the chest wall displaces the superior rib above the inferior rib ("clamshell" fashion), providing good access to the pleural space. If additional exposure is required,

the cartilage of the superior rib is divided at its medial end, which necessitates division of the internal mammary vessels. Once the procedure is completed and a chest drain is placed, the ribs are reapproximated, and the muscles and skin are closed in layers in a standard manner.

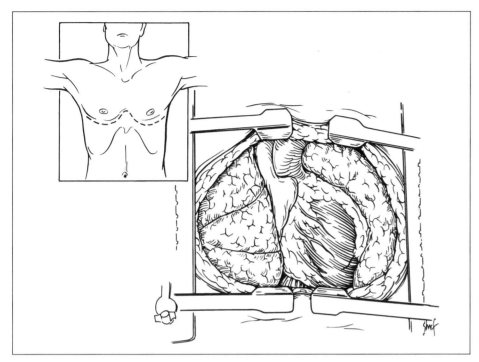

Fig. 49-6. *A transverse sternothoracotomy is performed with the patient supine (inset). The incision follows the inframammary crease. The fourth or fifth interspace is opened, and the sternum is divided.*

ral reflections along the anterior mediastinum are divided to expose the mediastinal structures. Following the conclusion of the intrathoracic portion of the procedure and placement of bilateral chest drains, the sternum is approximated using two or three sternal wires. Placement of Kirschner wires or Steinmann pins across the sternotomy can help prevent sternal override that sometimes occurs following this approach. The pectoralis muscles and skin are closed in a standard manner.

Sternotomy and Its Variations

In addition to being the standard surgical approach for most open heart procedures, sternotomy incisions provide excellent exposure for surgery of the anterosuperior mediastinum and, in selected patients, the lung. The advantages of these incisions are decreased postoperative pain, lack of interference with the muscles of the shoulder girdle, and simultaneous access to both pleural spaces. Disadvantages include the inability to expose the posterior aspects of the lungs, relatively poor visualization of the phrenic and vagus nerves, and potential contamination of the sternotomy during operations on infected structures.

A standard sternotomy is performed with the patient in a supine position and with the arms positioned at the sides. A pad or roll is placed along the thoracic spine to elevate the sternum. It is often convenient to place the grounding pad for monopolar electrocautery units on the patient's back as well. The incision is performed from the sternal notch to the xiphoid process (Fig. 49-7). Shorter incisions that still permit complete division of the sternum can be used for operations limited to the anterior mediastinum. The incision is carried along the decussation of the pectoralis major, which is a useful guide to the midline of the sternum. The interclavicular ligament at the sternal notch is divided with electrocautery. If bleeding from the innominate vein occurs, it is controlled with pressure until the sternum is divided. The periosteum is scored in the midline of the sternum, which then is divided from superior to inferior using a sternal saw. The edges of the sternum are elevated, and bleeding from the anterior and posterior tables is controlled with electrocautery. A sternal retractor is placed, and the edges of the sternum are gradually spread apart. Placing the retractor below the level of the manubrial-sternal junction helps to avoid stretch injury to the brachial plexus and fracture of the first rib.

At the conclusion of the operation, a mediastinal drain is placed through the fascia and is positioned with its tip inferior to the innominate vein. Additional pleural drains are placed if the pleural spaces have been entered and either air leak from pulmonary parenchyma or fluid accumulation is anticipated. The sternal edges are then approximated using sternal wires that pass through the bone in larger individuals or around the sternum (excluding the internal thoracic vessels) in smaller patients. Alternative closure techniques include the use of plates anchored in the sternum or bands that encircle it. The fascia and skin are closed in separate layers.

Modifications of the standard sternotomy are tailored to specific problems. Limited exposure of the superior mediastinum using a partial sternotomy often is sufficient for tracheal resection, thyroidectomy, parathyroidectomy, thymectomy for benign disease, and exposure of the upper esophagus. The skin incision extends only to the midsternum, and the sternal division is performed to the level of the third or fourth costal cartilage (Fig. 49-8). Exposure of the mediastinum is provided by alternately raising one side of the sternum or the other by angling the ipsilateral blade of the sternal retractor toward the ceiling before spreading the retractor. For operations on the superior vena cava or innominate artery and its branches, a "trap door" incision is often useful. This incision is performed by creating a partial sternotomy and extending each end of the incision laterally to the patient's right. The superior extension of the incision is carried immediately superior to the clavicle and reaches to its middle third, necessitating division of the insertions of the strap muscles on the manubrium and clavicle. In some instances, it is helpful to resect the medial half of the clavicle. The inferior extension is brought through the fourth interspace for a distance of approximately 10 cm, dividing the internal thoracic vessels and the intercostal muscles. A standard sternal retractor placed at an angle then elevates the trap door above the level of the sternum.

Postoperative Care

Most thoracotomy incisions are accompanied by postoperative pain and impairment of the function of muscles of respiration, which cause acute decreases in forced vital capacity (FVC), forced expi-

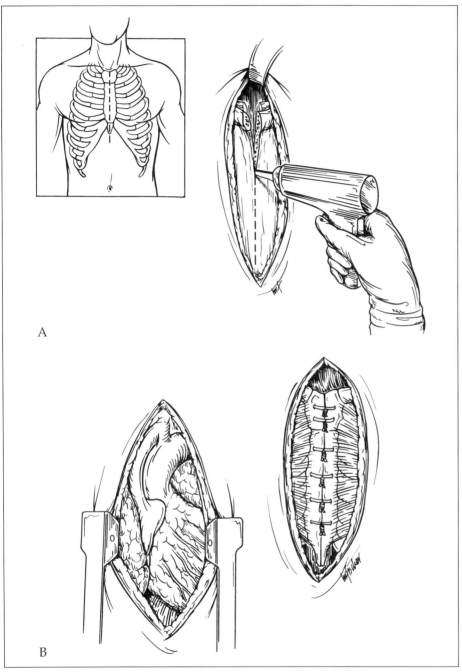

The duration of chest drainage is based on the operation and the patient's postoperative course. If the lung is completely expanded, chest tubes are typically removed when drainage is minimal (<200 ml over 24 hr) and there is no evidence of air leak from the lung for a period of 24 hours. Drains are left in for longer periods following an operation for empyema, when there is incomplete lung expansion, or following operations on the esophagus when anastomotic leakage is thought to be a risk.

Chest Wall Excision

Chest wall resection is performed for primary chest wall malignancies, for some primary lung cancers that directly invade the chest wall, for breast cancer with chest wall invasion, occasionally for an isolated metastasis to a rib, and for trauma or infections of the chest wall. This discussion will focus on management of primary chest wall tumors and sternal infections.

Approximately one-half of all chest wall tumors are malignant, and approximately one-half of all malignant chest wall tumors are primary chest wall cancers. It is often impossible to determine the true nature of a chest wall mass unless permanent histologic sections can be reviewed. This necessity makes decisions about appropriate therapy for chest wall masses difficult because many chest wall tumors, such as Ewing's sarcoma, multiple myeloma, lymphoma, and most metastases, are not appropriately treated by resection. However, the most important determinant of survival for most primary chest wall malignancies is the completeness of the resection. Indiscriminate incision into a malignant tumor should be avoided because it requires any subsequent resection to be approached as if the tumor had invaded the skin.

If clinical signs indicate that a chest wall mass is likely manageable by nonsurgical means, a small incisional biopsy or a percutaneous needle core biopsy or aspiration is appropriate. Under most other circumstances, wide excision is performed for masses measuring less than approximately 4 cm in diameter, which will leave a defect that is easily closed and is unlikely to require major reconstruction. Larger masses are best approached by initial incisional biopsy, reserving major resection for tumors

Fig. 49-7. A sternotomy is performed with the patient in a supine position. A. After separating the pectoralis muscles at the decussation of their fibers and dividing the interclavicular ligament, the sternum is opened with a saw. B. The mediastinum is exposed. Sternal closure is accomplished with heavy wires.

ratory volume in 1 second (FEV_1), and negative inspiratory force (NIF). The impaired respiratory function often leads to the development of retained secretions, atelectasis, and pneumonia. Pain control is best managed with use of continuous thoracic epidural infusions of a combination of narcotic and local anesthetic or with use of commercially available patient-controlled analgesia (PCA) pumps. The routine use of chest percussion, inhaled expectorants and bronchodilators, and an incentive spirometer helps prevent retention of secretions and atelectasis. Early ambulation also helps prevent pulmonary and other cardiovascular complications.

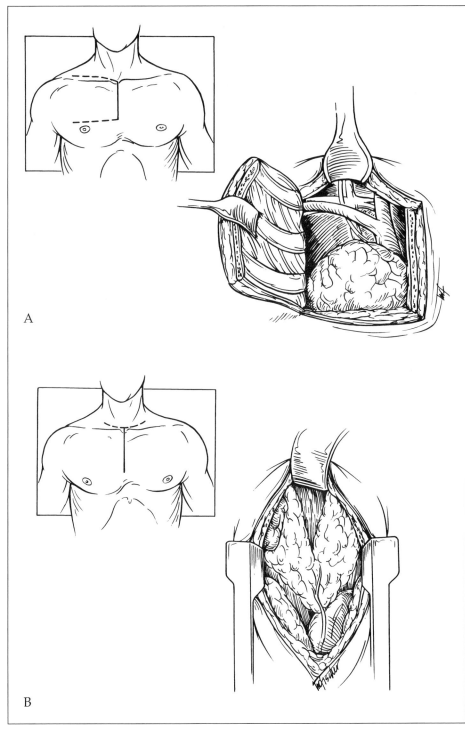

A

B

Fig. 49-8. Limited sternotomy incisions. A. These incisions are used for improved exposure of the great vessels and their branches ("trap door" incision). B. Partial sternotomy incisions are used for limited exposure of the superior mediastinum (when combined with a collar incision).

sues are removed en bloc so that a generous plane of normal tissue surrounds the resected specimen.

Rib Resection

Malignant chest wall tumors most commonly arise in the ribs and are approached with relative ease. The area to be resected is carefully mapped out before making a skin incision, and potential reconstructive tissues are protected in advance. If skin is to be removed, a circumferential incision is made, and dissection is carried through the chest wall musculature to the level of the ribs. Segments of ribs are resected so that one normal rib above and below the affected ribs is taken en bloc. This step is performed with electrocautery, dividing the intercostal muscles on the margins of the ribs and in the interspaces at the lateral limits of the resection. The lateral extent of rib resection includes margins at least 5 cm from any gross abnormalities in the affected ribs (Fig. 49-9). The intercostal vessels are controlled, and an angled rib cutter is used to divide the ribs. If lung tissue is adherent to the underlying pleural surface, it is also is resected en bloc by dividing the lung with a linear cutting stapler.

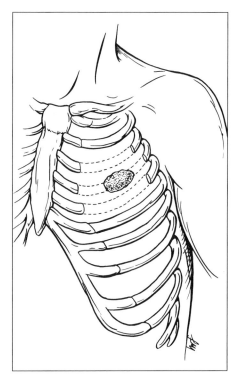

Fig. 49-9. Resection of a malignant chest wall tumor encompasses the affected ribs, an adjacent normal rib on each side, and all involved soft tissues.

that are histologically demonstrated to require it.

Techniques of chest wall resection for malignancy require that we observe several general principles. Margins of resection are generous, because local recurrence is a frequent problem, even for some so-called low-grade malignancies. Incisions are planned to permit subsequent reconstruction without violating the principles of en bloc resection. Adjacent bony and soft tis-

Resection of tumors of the ribs that are adjacent to the costovertebral junction sometimes necessitates disarticulation of the rib or, on occasion, formal lateral vertebral osteotomy. Disarticulation is accomplished by dividing the transverse process of the vertebral body with an osteotome and incising the costotransverse ligament with electrocautery. The osteotome or a periosteal elevator is inserted medial to the rib head, and the rib head is disarticulated from the articular process with a levering action (Fig. 49-10). The affected nerve root is put on a mild stretch as the articular head is retracted laterally and is ligated to prevent leakage of cerebrospinal fluid. If a lateral osteotomy is also necessary, the osteotome is then used, taking care not to violate the neural foramen in the process.

Resection of Tumors Arising in the Sternum

The sternum is a common location for primary malignant chest wall tumors. Because the sternum provides stability to the chest wall, its complete removal should be avoided unless preserving a part of the sternum compromises the cancer operation. Tumors often will exclusively involve either the manubrium or the sternum proper, allowing preservation of the unaffected component (Fig. 49-11). It is usually necessary to excise skin en bloc with the sternum because the margin between skin and bone is shallow. Once the skin is incised, dissection is carried down to the costal cartilages adjoining the affected portion of the region to be resected, which are divided along with the adjoining intercostal muscles. The internal thoracic vessels are divided at the superior and inferior extent of the resection, and the mobilized bone is elevated to evaluate any potential posterior adhesions to mediastinal tissues. It is sometimes necessary to perform an en bloc resection of the thymus or pericardium.

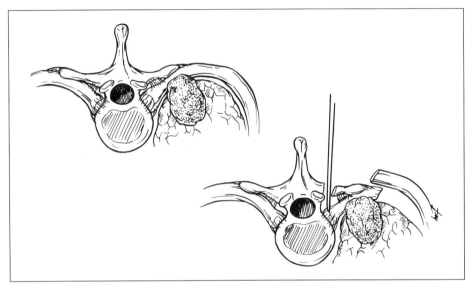

Fig. 49-10. Resection of a malignant chest wall tumor in proximity to a vertebral body requires transection of the transverse process and disarticulation of the rib.

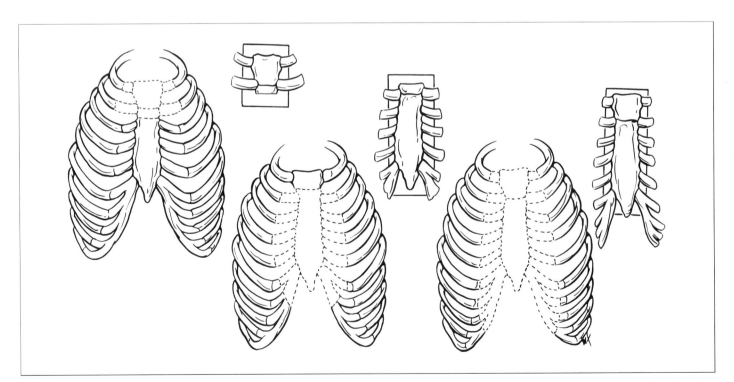

Fig. 49-11. Operations for malignant tumors affecting the sternum can consist of limited resection of the manubrium (left), the sternum proper (center), or the entire breast plate (right).

If the resection is limited to the manubrium or sternum proper, the sternomanubrial junction is incised, and the specimen is removed. Reconstruction usually is unnecessary under these circumstances because the remaining bone provides sufficient stabilization to the chest wall. If the entire sternum is removed, the need for reconstruction is determined by the degree of paradoxical motion with breathing and the need to protect the heart and great vessels from trauma. Resections in some patients are accompanied by severe paradoxical motion with respiration, often leading to ineffective ventilation, particularly in patients with underlying impaired lung function. In contrast, patients who have had mediastinal irradiation or mediastinitis often have sufficient fixation of the mediastinum that little ventilatory compromise is evident. Younger patients who wish to pursue active endeavors might require reconstruction to protect the heart and great vessels.

Resection for Sternal Infections

Sternal wound infection is an infrequent but disastrous consequence of sternotomy. Resection usually is necessary to avoid systemic sepsis and infection of any underlying prosthetic materials. Once the patient is stabilized and the purulence has been evacuated from the wound, the sternum is dissected from the overlying pectoralis muscle. The manubrium is freed from the heads of the clavicles, the strap muscles to the manubrium are divided, and the costosternal junctions are separated. After removing the sternum, the anterior perichondrial surfaces are sectioned, and each costal cartilage that was attached to an affected portion of the sternum is resected to its junction with bony rib. The blood supply to this cartilage typically is insufficient to permit healing in the face of a severe infection. Reconstruction is performed at the same time or is staged, depending on the condition of the patient and the degree of contamination.

Chest Wall Reconstruction

Chest wall reconstruction is necessary most often for defects following resection of tumors but is sometimes needed after resections for sternal osteomyelitis and for traumatic injuries. The objectives of chest wall reconstruction are to preserve or restore ventilatory efficiency; to improve cosmesis, usually through tissue flap rotation or transfer; and to limit loss of function in the region from which tissues for reconstruction are obtained.

If the chest wall defect is of such a size that neither respiratory paradox nor protection of underlying viscera is a concern, simple closure of adjacent muscle and skin, without reconstruction of the bony chest wall, is all that is required. For example, the resection of one to three ribs anteriorly does not cause significant paradoxical respiratory motion, whereas resection of four ribs can often be done posteriorly without reconstruction because the scapula provides additional protection against paradoxical motion. Bony reconstruction is necessary for most larger defects, when paradoxical motion is problematic, or when underlying viscera require protection.

Options for bony reconstruction include the use of autologous material, including ribs, other bone grafts, and fascia lata, and prosthetic materials such as polypropylene mesh or a patch of expanded polytetrafluoroethylene (PTFE). The objective of bony reconstruction is to restore rigidity to the chest wall, which is accomplished by fastening the reconstructive material to the remaining thoracic cage under tension (Fig. 49-12). Nonabsorbable sutures of appropriate strength are passed through or around the ribs or sternum at the edges of the defect, which sometimes requires a bone awl or drill to pass the suture material through the bone. The material is cut to size, and all the sutures from one edge of the defect are passed through it before any is tied down. After tying these sutures, the material is stretched tightly before placing the remaining sutures through it to ensure that it will be placed under adequate tension.

Bone grafts, either free or pedicled, are used when protection of underlying viscera is of paramount importance. Free grafts supply a framework for bone ingrowth but must be adequately stabilized for months to prevent the development of a pseudarthrosis. Pedicled grafts also require stabilization, but healing occurs much more rapidly using this type of reconstruction. Fixation is performed with

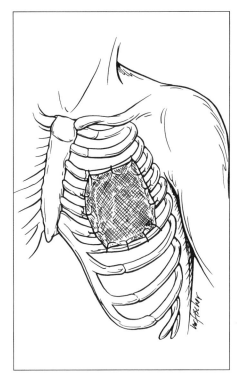

Fig. 49-12. Defects of the bony chest wall often require reconstruction with prosthetic material sutured under tension to the edges of the remaining bones.

Kirschner wires, screw-plates, or wiring of the bones together.

Additional soft tissue is often necessary to complete the reconstruction of large chest wall defects. A variety of muscle flaps have been described for this purpose, many of which can also be prepared as musculocutaneous flaps if additional skin coverage is necessary (see the Special Comment at the end of this chapter). These flaps are characterized by the presence of a single dominant vascular pedicle that permits transposition of the flap over a large arc of rotation. Many can also be used as free flaps, requiring microvascular anastomoses to donor vessels in the vicinity of the defect. The advantages of transposing autologous tissues into chest wall defects include the ability to obtain primary closure with rapid healing, control of residual infection, elimination of dead space, and added protection for underlying viscera.

The most versatile flap is the latissimus dorsi muscle, which is based on the thoracodorsal artery and is innervated by the thoracodorsal nerve. It is prepared as either a muscle flap or a myocutaneous flap and is capable of being transposed as far as the midline of the sternum anteriorly and to the contralateral side posteriorly. Unfortunately, many patients who require chest wall reconstruction have had a lateral or posterolateral thoracotomy, resulting in transection of this muscle. An alternative flap based laterally is the serratus anterior muscle, which is based on branches of the thoracodorsal artery and innervated by the long thoracic nerve. Because this muscle is relatively small, it does not provide much bulk, and it is poorly adapted for use as a myocutaneous unit.

Anterior defects are often reconstructed with pectoralis major flaps, which also can be mobilized as myocutaneous units if desired (see the Special Comment at the end of this chapter). These flaps are based on the thoracoacromial artery and are innervated by the anterior thoracic nerve. They are particularly useful in the reconstruction of defects remaining after sternal resection. An alternative flap for anterior chest wall reconstruction is the rectus abdominis muscle flap, which can also be raised as a myocutaneous unit. It is based on the superior epigastric artery and is innervated by branches of the lower thoracic nerve. This flap is not of value in many patients who have undergone sternal resection because the internal thoracic vessels, which supply the superior epigastric vessels, usually have been transected.

An alternative flap for use in soft-tissue reconstruction is the greater omentum, which is based on the right gastroepiploic artery. The omentum provides soft-tissue bulk and forms a good base for skin grafts. Although versatile in promoting healing and in overcoming bacterial contamination, its use is avoided if its mobilization exposes the patient to intra-abdominal infection.

Suggested Reading

Allen MS, Mathisen DJ, Grillo HC, et al. Bronchogenic carcinoma with chest wall invasion. *Ann Thorac Surg* 51:948, 1991.

Bains MS, Ginsberg RJ, Jones WG II, et al. The clamshell incision: An improved approach to bilateral pulmonary and mediastinal tumor. *Ann Thorac Surg* 58:30, 1994.

Burt M, Fulton M, Wessner-Dunlap S, et al. Primary bony and cartilaginous sarcomas of chest wall: Results of therapy. *Ann Thorac Surg* 54:226, 1992.

DeMeester TR, Albertucci M, Dawson PJ, et al. Management of tumor adherent to the vertebral column. *J Thorac Cardiovasc Surg* 97:373, 1989.

Fry WA, Kehoe TJ, McGee JP. Axillary thoracotomy. *Am Surg* 56:460, 1990.

Gordon MS, Hajdu SI, Bains MS, et al. Soft tissue sarcomas of the chest wall. *J Thorac Cardiovasc Surg* 101:843, 1991.

Kohman LJ, Auchincloss JH, Gilbert R, et al. Functional results of muscle flap closure for sternal infection. *Ann Thorac Surg* 52:102, 1991.

Lemmer JH Jr, Gomez MN, Symreng T, et al. Limited lateral thoracotomy. *Arch Surg* 125:873, 1990.

Lubenow TR, Faber LP, McCarthy RJ, et al. Post-thoracotomy pain management using continuous epidural analgesia in 1,324 patients. *Ann Thorac Surg* 58:924, 1994.

Mansour KA, Anderson TM, Hester TR. Sternal resection and reconstruction. *Ann Thorac Surg* 55:838, 1993.

Mathisen DJ, Grillo HC, Vlahakes GJ, et al. The omentum in the management of complicated cardiothoracic problems. *J Thorac Cardiovasc Surg* 95:677, 1988.

Mitchell RL. The lateral limited thoracotomy incision: Standard for pulmonary operations. *J Thorac Cardiovasc Surg* 99:590, 1990.

Morgan RF, Edgerton MT, Wanebo HJ, et al. Reconstruction of full thickness chest wall defects. *Ann Surg* 207:707, 1988.

Pairolero PC, Arnold PG, Harris JB. Long-term results of pectoralis major muscle transposition for infected sternotomy wounds. *Ann Surg* 213:583, 1991.

Ratto GB, Piacenza G, Frola C, et al. Chest wall involvement by lung cancer: Computed tomographic detection and results of operation. *Ann Thorac Surg* 51:182, 1991.

EDITOR'S COMMENT

The most widely used thoracotomy incision for operations on the lung and posterior mediastinum has been and continues to be the posterolateral thoracotomy. This incision affords the greatest versatility, the best opportunity for extension, and the widest exposure, not only to the lung and posterior mediastinum but also to the great vessels at the thoracic inlet. However, when a very rapid approach to the heart or aorta is required, with trauma to either structure, for example, or when a rapid thoracotomy to minimize blood loss by abdominal cross-clamping is needed, an anterolateral incision can be invaluable. This incision bleeds very little, there are only intercostal muscles and the serratus anterior to traverse, and an incision can be made even by a moderately talented surgeon or surgical resident in 1 or 2 minutes. This incision is an intercostal one, under these circumstances, and it is often necessary, even with a rib spreader inserted, to cut a costochondral junction above, or perhaps both above and below, so that a hand can be inserted into the chest to control bleeding or to guide the placement of a vascular instrument. The most basic thoracotomy tray suffices, cautery is unnecessary, and with a modicum of care, the internal thoracic artery will not be transected.

The median sternotomy is used in the operating room, not only for cardiac and ascending aortic trauma but also for excellent exposure of the injured liver and vena cava, as well as injury to the aorta just distal to the aortic hiatus. Obviously, under most of these circumstances, the sternotomy will be the superior extension of the midline or right subcostal incision, most often for penetrating trauma, rather than blunt injury.

A major problem with thoracotomy incisions is the postoperative discomfort, which is generally worse than the discomfort of the abdominal incision. However, this pain can be minimized by placing catheters adjacent to the intercostal nerves at a level posterior to the incision for local anesthetic injection with immediate postoperative pain relief. Alternatively, repeated needle nerve blocks can be done with longer acting local anesthetic agents. However, many patients continue to experience significant pain, even after months have passed since the operation was performed. Accordingly, some thoracic surgeons intentionally section the intercostal nerves at one interspace above and one below the intercostal incision, and, of course, include the nerve supplying the interspace that has been opened. This section does not appear to have a significant effect on respiratory function and is a reasonable step to take for a smoother postoperative course.

Removal of a portion of the chest wall for tumor is an uncommon operation, except for carcinomas of the lung or mesotheliomas of the pleura that have invaded the parietal tissues, or occasionally for patients with recurrent breast cancer in the chest wall. In centers doing trauma, an important indication is for debridement and closure of the often very substantial defects that occur with high-velocity gunshot wounds or with major blast injuries, the most common in civilian practice being shotgun wounds at close range. Military injuries or injuries in areas with military-like operations can result in chest wall defects from exploded land mines or from planned explosions. Shotgun blasts usually cause underlying lung damage, the destruction of ribs, and loss of a substantial amount of soft tissue. Debridement of the lung, control of air leak, and appropriate debridement of the chest wall defect are always required. Blood loss is substantial, but after appropriate debridement and closure of lung substance, the chest wall defect remains.

The simplest option for closure is the formation of a chest wall strut, using horizontal and vertical lattices of permanent suture material attached to the intact ribs superiorly and inferiorly, and to the ends of the debrided injured ribs horizontally. This bridge must then be covered with soft tissue, obtaining something closely approximating an airtight seal, if possible. A better alternative is to use a musculocutaneous flap to close the defect. However, patients who have been subjected to major chest trauma of this nature are seldom candidates for another 3 to 4 hours of operation for such a closure, although there is considerably less difficulty from that approach in the long run, provided the patient's general condition permits the formation of a formal flap. A newer mesh prosthetic device is Vicryl mesh, which can be sewn to the edges of the defect and covered with soft tissue. This mesh has the advantage of being an absorbable structure that becomes incorporated into the flap or soft tissue covering it but provides sufficient tension to maintain the respiratory integrity of the thoracic cage for a considerable length of time. When any prosthetic is used, either absorbable or permanent, one should always fold the edge of the mesh over to create a 1- to 1.5-cm cuff, so that sutures can be placed through a double thickness of the prosthetic patch, resulting in greater holding power and much less tendency for the sutures to tear through the edge of the patch.

It is important that the mesh be put in under some tension; otherwise a large defect will result in paradoxical movement of the chest wall, analogous to a substantial flail segment following a crush injury of the chest. Under any circumstances, prolonged suction drainage of the pleural space is required, although the former principle that endotracheal intubation with ventilator support for 5 to 7 days or more is required is no longer an operative principle. In general, once the patient has achieved respiratory stability, as evidenced by adequate pulmonary function studies, oxygen saturation, and a low A-a gradient, extubation can be accomplished, and the chest wall will promptly heal.

R.J.B.

SPECIAL COMMENT

Chest Wall Reconstruction with Flaps

Chest wall defects result mainly from ablative procedures for tumors, radiation damage, infection, and trauma. These defects can be superficial, including only the soft tissue of the chest wall, or they can extend to the bony-cartilaginous framework and even beyond into the thoracic cavities and the mediastinum.

Superficial defects can be easily managed with skin grafts or local flaps, but full-thickness defects are much more difficult to manage and require the coordinated efforts of the plastic surgeon and the cardiothoracic surgeon in order to achieve the best possible functional and aesthetic long-term results while reducing the rate of complications.

The reconstructive techniques for chest wall defects have changed substantially and improved in the past 15 years, primarily because of a better understanding of tissue vascularity; experience with axial flaps; and the extensive use of muscle, musculocutaneous flaps, or the greater omentum alone or in combination for the successful obliteration of residual cavities and coverage of a variety of large thoracic defects. The availability of these large flaps provides well-vascularized tissue for coverage of chest wall defects, thus enabling the surgeon to undertake wide excision of malignant tumors with clear margins or to

perform aggressive debridement of all devitalized soft tissues, cartilage, and bone. Such a debridement is a prerequisite for successful long-term management of defects caused by infection or radiation necrosis.

There are several advantages to using autogenous tissue for the reconstruction of chest wall defects. Healthy, well-vascularized flaps with considerable bulk are transposed from areas distant from the zone of injury, infection, or radiation to obliterate all potential dead space in the thoracic cavity or the mediastinum and provide immediate coverage of a chest wall defect. The muscles, through their excellent blood supply, promote healing and eliminate any residual local infection. With their bulk, the muscle flaps help protect the underlying heart, great vessels, and lungs and stabilize the chest wall, improving respiratory function and eliminating paradoxical movement during breathing.

The choice of flap to be used for the reconstruction varies, depending primarily on the size, extent, and location of the defect, as well as tissue availability and the surgeon's preference. However, the basic reconstructive principles are standardized and widely accepted. The surgeon should firmly adhere to these principles to achieve a successful outcome and minimize the possibility of complications or recurrent infections. These principles include control of infection with systemic antibiotics; appropriate local wound care; extensive debridement of all devitalized soft tissues, cartilage, and bone; obliteration of residual cavities with muscle flaps or omentum, or both; and early definitive coverage of the tissue defect with well-vascularized tissues.

Structural defects of the osteocartilaginous framework of the chest need to be addressed simultaneously in some instances. There is no consensus regarding the necessity for reconstruction of bony defects and reestablishment of skeletal continuity. The decision for bony reconstruction depends on the location and size of the defect and the patient's respiratory reserve. Bone grafting is strongly discouraged in the presence of infection. Thus, bony defects of the manubrium following en bloc resection of malignant tumors can be immediately stabilized with autogenous bone grafting material, such as ribs or synthetic mesh, before soft-tissue reconstruction with muscle flaps, whereas midline defects following sternal debridement for an infected median sternotomy are covered only with muscle flaps and will remain stable because of the fibrosis and scarring of the tissues. Lateral thoracic defects following resection of more than two consecutive ribs are better stabilized with synthetic mesh, a patch, or methylmethacrylate to provide support and prevent paradoxical movement.

Most muscles of the chest wall have a single dominant vascular pedicle and can be transposed to cover a variety of extrathoracic and intrathoracic defects. The latissimus dorsi muscle based on the thoracodorsal vascular pedicle and the pectoralis major muscle based on the thoracoacromial pedicle are the muscles most commonly used because of their size, location, and arc of rotation. The rectus abdominis muscle based on its superior epigastric pedicle is a primary alternative flap. If a large musculocutaneous unit is needed for the reconstruction, a transverse rectus abdominis musculocutaneous (TRAM) design can be used. The greater omentum based on the right or left gastroepiploic artery can be mobilized from the greater curvature of the stomach and the transverse colon and delivered as a flap from the abdominal cavity to obliterate the mediastinal or thoracic cavity or to cover a chest wall defect. The rich lymphatic plexus of the omentum is ideal for the management of local infection, and its soft and pliable texture allows obliteration of small spaces in the mediastinum. However, use of omentum has been limited since the introduction and extensive use of muscle flaps because of the lesser bulk and structural stability that the omentum provides, the risk of spreading infection into the peritoneal cavity, and the additional morbidity associated with a laparotomy. The serratus anterior, the pectoralis minor, and the external olique muscles are also used independently but primarily in combination with the larger muscles of the chest wall and abdomen when additional bulk is required (Fig. 49-13).

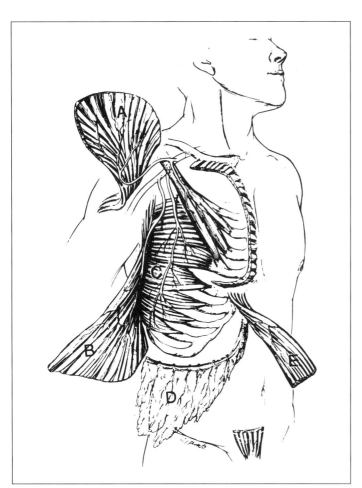

Fig. 49-13. Flaps available for the reconstruction of chest wall defects and obliteration of intrathoracic cavities. A. The pectoralis major muscle flap based on the thoracoacromial artery. B. The latissimus dorsi muscle flap based on the thoracodorsal artery. C. The serratus anterior muscle flap based primarily on branches of the thoracodorsal artery. D. The omentum flap based on the right or left gastroepiploic artery. E. The rectus abdominis muscle flap based on the superior epigastric artery.

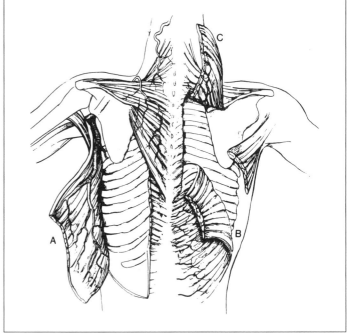

Fig. 49-14. Flaps available for the reconstruction of defects in the posterior chest wall. A. The latissimus dorsi muscle flap based on the thoracodorsal artery. B. The latissimus dorsi muscle flap based on intercostal and lumbar arteries. C. The trapezius muscle flap based on the descending branch of the transverse cervical artery.

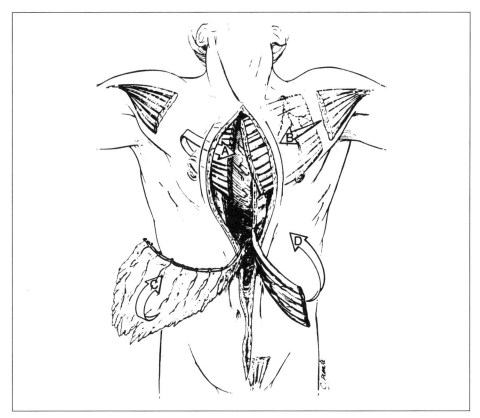

Fig. 49-15. *Flaps available for the reconstruction of infected median sternotomy wounds. A. The turnover pectoralis major muscle flap based on perforators of the internal thoracic artery. B. The pectoralis major flap based on the thoracoacromial artery. C. The omentum flap based on the right gastroepiploic artery. D. The rectus abdominis muscle flap based on the superior epigastric artery.*

Defects of the posterior chest wall can be reconstructed with muscles of the back. Midline defects are better managed with a lower trapezius muscle flap based on the descending branch of the transverse cervical artery, whereas lower back defects are better managed with a latissimus dorsi muscle flap based on its segmental blood supply from perforating branches of the intercostal and lumbar arteries (Fig. 49-14).

An interdisciplinary approach with a combined preoperative evaluation of the patient by the cardiothoracic and plastic surgical teams is necessary to establish a careful plan and decrease the margin of error or complications. Before embarking on a major reconstructive procedure, the surgeon should carefully evaluate the patient for previous scars on the chest wall or abdomen that might have divided the muscles or injured their vascular pedicles. A detailed discussion with the cardiothoracic surgeon will provide information about

the estimated size of the defect, about whether the internal thoracic artery has been used as a bypass conduit, or if the artery was injured or ligated during previous debridements. However, the final decision and flap selection can be made only intraoperatively, after the resection or debridement has been completed and the size of the defect can be properly evaluated. Thus, the reconstructive surgeon should plan for several options and be prepared to use a second or third reconstructive option as required.

Chest Wall Resection

Resection of primary or secondary malignant tumors arising from the soft tissues, bone, or even the lung and excision of radionecrotic areas result in large partial or full-thickness defects of the chest wall. The bony defect can be reconstructed with syn-

thetic mesh, or a PTFE (Goretex) patch. Immediate, soft-tissue coverage with appropriate muscle or musculocutaneous flaps should follow. The latissimus dorsi muscle or musculocutaneous unit is the flap of choice for the reconstruction of large anterior or lateral chest wall defects. The rectus abdominis and the pectoralis major muscles can also be used. The omentum represents an excellent alternative for superficial defects in this area. It can even be transposed directly over a synthetic mesh or patch, and covered with a split-thickness skin graft to provide immediate coverage of the synthetic material and closure of the defect.

Intrathoracic Cavities

Large postpneumonectomy residual intrathoracic cavities with empyema or persistent bronchopleural fistulas are extremely difficult to manage. Several techniques have been described, including drainage, filling the cavity with sclerosing antibiotic solution, and partial thoracoplasty. Obliteration of the thoracic cavity with intrathoracic transposition of extrathoracic muscles has proved to be a reasonable alternative technique. After evacuation of all purulent collections and debridement of all devitalized tissues, the entire residual intrathoracic space is filled with one or several extrathoracic muscles, thus achieving obliteration of the dead space with well-vascularized healthy tissues. Additionally, a muscle flap can be wrapped around the bronchial stump, thus promoting healing and preventing recurrence of a bronchial leak and fistula formation.

Infected and Dehisced Median Sternotomy

An infected and dehisced median sternotomy is a devastating complication of cardiac operations, which greatly increases the morbidity and mortality among already debilitated patients. The method of choice to treat the infection and dehiscence includes immediate drainage of all purulent collections, debridement of devitalized tissues, and rewiring of the sternum over suction-irrigation catheters. However, a number of patients do not respond to this treatment and require a more aggressive approach with radical debridement and immediate reconstruction with muscle flaps or omentum. Extensive debridement of all devitalized sternum, costal cartilages, ribs, and soft tissues before the reconstruction is of paramount importance and is considered the key to a successful long-term reconstruction without recurrence of infection.

A variety of flaps have been described for the soft-tissue coverage of median sternotomy wounds (Fig. 49-15). Several flaps can be combined when necessary to provide complete obliteration of the dead space and coverage of the chest wall defect.

The pectoralis major muscle, because of its location on the chest wall, its bulk, and its arc of rotation, is currently the primary muscle used to obliterate the mediastinal defect and provide coverage. In some instances, one muscle is sufficient, but in most patients the use of both pectoralis major muscles is necessary. The muscle is mobilized from its attachments to the chest wall and can be based superiorly on its thoracoacromial vascular pedicle or medially on perforators of the internal thoracic artery and vein. This last flap design cannot be performed when the internal mammary artery has been used for a bypass conduit or has been ligated during debridement. The use of the rectus abdominis muscle based on the superior epigastric pedicle represents a prime alternative technique. This flap can be used as a muscle or as a musculocutaneous unit to cover the defect completely, or in combination with the pectoralis major muscle flap when this muscle cannot obliterate the inferior portion of the sternotomy wound. If these reconstructive options are not available, then the greater omentum can be used to obliterate the mediastinal cavity. The latissimus dorsi muscle flap represents the last resource for reconstruction when other options are unavailable. As soon as the mediastinum has been obliterated, the overlying skin can be mobilized with wide undermining to achieve primary closure. When necessary, a split-thickness skin graft can be applied directly over the muscle flap or the omentum for immediate definitive coverage.

Mimis Cohen
Sai S. Ramasastry

Suggested Reading

Cohen M. Reconstruction of Chest Wall. In M. Cohen (ed.), *Mastery of Surgery: Plastic and Reconstructive Surgery*. Boston: Little, Brown, 1994.

Mathes SS, Nahai F (eds.). *Clinical Applications for Muscle and Musculocutaneous Flaps*. St. Louis: Mosby, 1982.

McGraw JB, Arnold PG (eds.). *McGraw and Arnold's Atlas of Muscle and Musculocutaneous Flaps*. Norfolk: Hampton, 1986.

Meland NB, Arnold PG. Intrathoracic Transposition of Soft Tissue. In M Cohen (ed.), *Mastery of Surgery: Plastic and Reconstructive Surgery*. Boston: Little, Brown, 1994.

Seyfer A, Graeber G, Wind G. *Atlas of Chest Wall Reconstruction*. Rockville: Aspen, 1986.

50

Thoracic Trauma Management for the General Surgeon

L. D. Britt   Sidney Trogdon

Approximately 20 percent of trauma deaths are caused by chest injuries that usually occur as a result of cardiac and aortic ruptures. The majority of thoracic trauma patients, fortunately, do not require operative intervention but can be managed successfully with supportive measures, such as pain management (systemic or nerve blocks) or tube thoracostomy. The initial treatment of the chest trauma patient is the same as for any other injured person; the primary survey (i. e., airway, breathing, circulation, disability, and exposure to environmental control) is always the mainstay of management.

There are important anatomic considerations that must be taken into account in the management of thoracic trauma, such as lower chest wall blunt trauma with associated intra-abdominal solid organ injuries. In addition to abdominal injuries, trauma to the thorax can also be associated with neck and spinal column injuries. Also, lower chest (i. e., thoracoabdominal) penetrating injuries (Fig. 50-1) can actually traverse the abdominal cavity through the diaphragm. Penetrating injuries in the thoracoabdominal region (from nipple to costal margin) need to be aggressively assessed for the possibility of diaphragmatic injuries and intra-abdominal penetration. Unfortunately, there is no noninvasive diagnostic modality that can conclusively rule out a diaphragmatic injury. Although plain chest roentgenography, CT scan, and diagnostic peritoneal lavage (DPL) have all been advocated, their sensitivity in detecting diaphragmatic rents is clearly less than acceptable. Currently, the most appropriate methods to determine diaphrag-

matic penetration are laparoscopy (or thoracoscopy) or mandatory celiotomy. In fact, the best indication to date for the use of laparoscopy in the trauma setting is with penetrating thoracoabdominal injuries to rule out diaphragmatic penetration with possible associated intra-abdominal injuries. Although a learning curve does exist, this invasive modality should ultimately replace the need for mandatory celiotomy in the patient who has sustained a thoracoabdominal penetrating injury without any overt sign or clinical findings suggestive of an intra-abdominal injury.

Another important anatomic consideration is the possibility of a transmediastinal penetrating wound. Even if the patient remains hemodynamically stable and requires only tube thoracostomies, the surgeon must rule out injury to the mediastinal organs. The density of the mediastinum with many vital structures makes it imperative that detection of occult injuries be discovered expeditiously. Therefore, the following diagnostic paradigm is recommended for transmediastinal penetrating injuries:

Diagnostic Paradigm for
Transmediastinal Injuries

Transmediastinal Gunshot Wounds in the
    Hemodynamically Stable Patient
    Bilateral tube thoracostomies
        ↓
Operating Suite
    Subxiphoid pericardial window (vs
        transesophageal echocardiogram)
        (definite)
    Bronchoscopy (definite)
    Esophagoscopy (definite)

Laparoscopy (vs laparotomy)
        ↓
Radiology Suite
    Angiography (definite)
    Esophagogram (controversial)
        ↓
Monitor

Specific Indications for Thoracotomy

Often, the surgeon does not have the luxury of using a diagnostic modality, not even plain roentgenography, to assist in determining the need for urgent operative intervention. Interestingly enough, of the generally accepted acutely life-threatening conditions (Table 50-1), only two necessitate emergency thoracotomy: massive hemothorax and cardiac tamponade. It is essential for a general surgeon managing the trauma patient to know the indications for an emergency thoracotomy. The specific indications for the so-called ED (emergency department) thoracotomy will be specifically addressed subsequently. However, in the acute setting, an operating room or emergency room thoracotomy is indicated for the following:

Cardiac arrest (acute deterioration associated with *penetrating* chest injuries)

Documented cardiac tamponade (pericardiocentesis vs pericardial window vs echocardiography)

Proven specific thoracic injuries (esophageal injury, tracheal or bronchial disruption, great vessel injury)

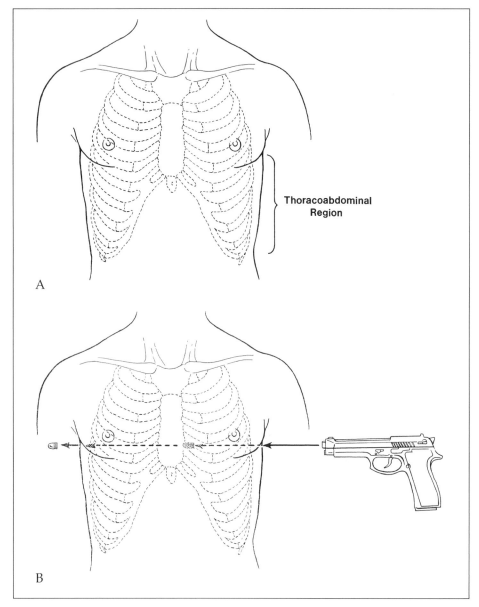

Fig. 50-1. Thoracoabdominal regional injury. A. The thoracoabdominal region includes that zone between the nipple and costal margin. B. Because the diaphragm does elevate to the level of the nipples, diaphragmatic injuries and intra-abdominal penetration can occur.

Table 50-1. Chest Trauma: Acute Life-Threatening Pathophysiologic Changes

Airway obstruction
Tension pneumothorax
Open pneumothorax
Massive hemothorax
Flail chest
Cardiac tamponade

Table 50-2. Chest Roentgenographic Signs Suggestive of Traumatic Aortic Disruption

Widened mediastinum
Obliteration of the aortic knob
Pleural cap
Obliteration of the pulmonary-aortic window
Depression of the left mainstem bronchus
Elevation and shift (rightward) of the right mainstem bronchus
Tracheal deviation (rightward)
Fractures of the first and second ribs

In addition, fortunately, there are some rare occasions in which a thoracotomy will be required, for example, a cardiac or pulmonary vasculature gunshot wound resulting in bullet embolus or thoracic penetration and subsequent contamination with industrial oils or products (e. g., coal tar). With respect to massive hemothorax, the often quoted figure of 1500 to 2000 ml of blood initially removed from the pleural space as an indicator for an urgent thoracotomy is not absolute. In fact, more often it is the hourly amount of chest tube output of blood (2000/hr) that mandates thoracotomy.

Diagnostic Modalities Used in Thoracic Trauma

There is no substitute for a thorough physical examination of a patient presenting with thoracic trauma. Clinical findings frequently dictate the optimal management approach. However, there are numerous diagnostic modalities that can be used in the thoracic trauma setting, including plain roentgenography, endoscopy (esophagoscopy and tracheoscopy or bronchoscopy), contrast studies, arteriography, CT scan, MRI, ultrasound, transesophageal echocardiography, pericardiocentesis, pericardial window, and thoracoscopy. Although many of these modalities have been advocated in the overall management paradigm, there is still ongoing debate. For example, traumatic aortic disruption is one of the most common causes of sudden death following motor vehicle accidents. Of the survivors (10–20%) who arrive at a hospital (because of a tamponade effect of the residual aortic or periaortic tissue), a significant percentage of the patients die each day if the diagnosis is not made and definitive management accomplished. Because of the subtleties of this injury, a high index of suspicion is imperative.

Plain chest roentgenography is often the initial screening study. Roentgenographic findings suggestive of traumatic aortic disruption are noted in Table 50-2. Although arch angiography is still the gold standard in making the definitive diagnosis of this injury, other diagnostic modalities are being advocated in the work-up of this life-threatening injury. Transesophageal echocardiography (TEE) has recently been proposed as an adjunct and probable replacement for arch angiography in detecting traumatic aortic injuries. A possible drawback to this modality is that associated great vessel injuries can be missed because of inadequate visualization. Dynamic CT scan has been used to provide another ancillary screening modality to lessen the number of negative arch angiograms. The appropriate caveat is the fact that this modality is a screening device, at best, and it requires an experienced radiologist or trauma surgeon to interpret the findings.

Another controversy has been the role of pericardiocentesis in the acute trauma setting. When a surgeon is involved in the management of the trauma patient, there is no role for a pericardiocentesis in the acute trauma setting. A pericardial window, performed in the operating room, is a much better option and certainly of less risk to the patient than the relatively blind insertion of a needle into the mediastinum. If the patient is hemodynamically stable and the personnel and equipment are available, TEE has a role. Obviously, if the patient is significantly hemodynamically labile or in full cardiac arrest, an emergency thoracotomy is the procedure of choice.

Operative Exposure and Techniques

Selecting the best incision for optimal exposure is important. For the general surgeon, there are just a few incisions to consider. Each has a distinct advantage, depending on the specific injury. Thoracotomy (usually a left anterolateral incision) in the emergency department or trauma bay setting is discussed in a subsequent section of this chapter. In the operating room, the median sternotomy (Fig. 50-2) is often the incision selected, especially when a cardiac injury is suspected after performing a positive subxiphoid pericardiotomy ("window") (Fig. 50-3). Although other incisions might provide better access to certain areas of the heart, pulmonary hilum, and peripheral pulmonary vasculature, the median sternotomy enables the patient to be in the supine position, which allows concomitant access to the abdomen, if necessary. This incision, along with possible extensions into the neck when appropriate, provides ade-

quate exposure for some of the thoracic great vessel injuries. A "trap door" incision (Fig. 50-2D) is one in which a partial median sternotomy is performed along with supraclavicular and fourth intercostal space extensions. For the trauma surgeon, this incision is the best one for expeditious exposure of injuries in the thoracic outlet. In respect to the other options in a more elective setting, a left posterolateral thoracotomy (Fig. 50-2C) allows access to the left posterior heart, the distal esophagus, and descending aorta. Exposing the proximal esophagus and tracheal injuries will usually require a right posterolateral thoracotomy.

Although not always possible, choosing the correct incision avoids critical delays in the definitive management of the often lethal injuries.

The Role of Emergency Department Thoracotomy

The indications for an emergency department thoracotomy are much more specific than a decade ago. These indications include the following:

1. Pericardial penetrating trauma and acute deterioration in the emergency center,
2. Penetrating thoracic trauma with documented prehospital cardiac arrest less than 4 to 5 minutes before arrival at a trauma center,
3. Suspected systemic air embolism in a previously stable patient with penetrating chest injury, and
4. Selected cases of penetrating abdominal trauma in which cardiac arrest occurs in the trauma bay.

There are surgeons who have advocated broader indications for an emergency department thoracotomy; however, the survival rates have been dismal to nil. In this era of containing costs and protecting health care providers from unnecessary blood exposure and inadvertent injury, the need to keep the indications for emergency department thoracotomy appropriately few is imperative. Table 50-3 highlights the procedure set-up and necessary intrathoracic maneuvers.

Adjunctive Modalities in the Management of Thoracic Trauma

Video thoracoscopy offers another diagnostic and therapeutic modality in the management of blunt and penetrating chest trauma. Its specific indications are still being evaluated and its final place in the skills of the trauma surgeon is evolving. Useful settings demonstrated so far include evaluation of acute blunt or penetrating trauma and their sequelae, such as a clotted hemothorax and empyema. Thoracoscopy offers a means of visualization of the pleural space in one hemithorax and somewhat less sensitivity in evaluating the mediastinal structures. Disadvantages of the technique include the necessity for the patient to be hemodynamically stable, ability to tolerate the lateral decubitus position and one lung anesthesia, and the obvious inability to easily evaluate the opposite hemithorax or abdominal cavity.

Thoracoscopy for the acutely injured patient has been used to evaluate and treat the source of ongoing blood loss from the chest in patients with blunt or penetrating trauma. Such continuing bleeding is often caused by chest wall vessel lacerations that can be readily controlled using endoscopic techniques. High-volume air leaks from pulmonary parenchymal injuries can also be controlled with stapling devices or laser coagulation. This procedure must, of course, be preceded by airway endoscopy to rule out a major tracheobronchial injury. Thoracoscopy can also be used in an extremely selective manner for the evaluation of diaphragmatic injury, although currently it is more practical to assess possible diaphragmatic injury with laparoscopy. Determining a diaphragmatic rent is particularly important in the patient with penetrating thoracoabdominal injury, which would necessitate intra-abdominal exploration if a diaphragmatic rent were detected on laparoscopy. Thoracoscopy might be appropriate in a patient who has a blunt rupture of the diaphragm and is otherwise stable without evidence of other intra-abdominal injury. The repair of a diaphragmatic defect is readily accomplished using minimally invasive techniques.

The sequelae of chest trauma can include a clotted hemothorax, empyema, and chy-

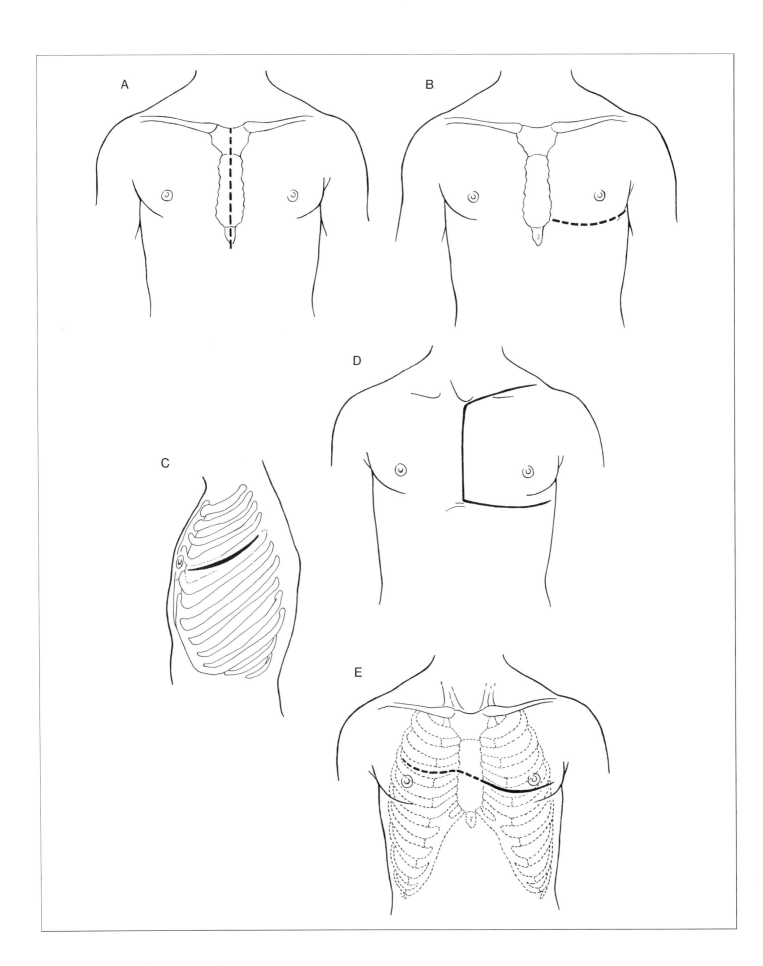

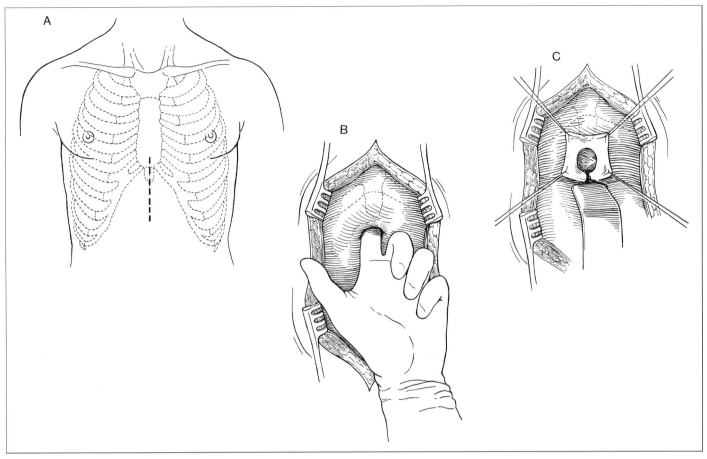

Fig. 50-3. Subxiphoid pericardial window. A. Subxiphoid pericardial window; the incision is made through the skin or subcutaneous tissue and the linea alba is divided. The xiphoid can either be retracted or excised to access the pericardium. B,C. With blunt and sharp dissection, the pericardium is exposed and incised in order to determine if there is blood in the pericardial sac.

lothorax. Clotted hemothorax is a common sequela of delayed or inadequate drainage of traumatic hemothorax. It usually responds to additional tube thoracostomy drainage, and successful treatment with intrapleural thrombolytic agents has also been reported. Thoracoscopy is evolving as a possible method of treatment for a clotted hemothorax of significant size that does not respond to these initial management techniques. It should probably be used early in the course of treatment, within 1 week, to prevent further sequelae of infection and trapped lung. Drainage of an infected hemothorax or empyema, especially loculated empyema, is another possible application of thoracoscopy. Once the empyema has entered the subacute phase, after 2 weeks, the lung is frequently

covered with an inflammatory peel. Decortication of the trapped lung can be attempted thoracoscopically at this point. Once the peel has matured and become fibrous, decortication is much more difficult and usually requires open operation. Persistent chylothorax after chest trauma can also be approached with a thoracoscopically guided talc pleurodesis with or without obliteration of the injured thoracic duct.

Several important points must be emphasized regarding the technique of thoracoscopy for diagnosis and treatment of chest trauma. The patient must be able to tolerate one lung ventilation and the lateral decubitus position. Thoracoscopy in the supine position is reported, but visualization

of the thorax is much more difficult. A double lumen left endobronchial tube (Carlen's tube) is placed by anesthesia, which is essential to provide adequate visualization of the hemithorax. Intermittent periods of ventilation of the injured side can be used to detect and evaluate air leaks. Oxygen flow, with or without continuous positive alveolar pressure (CPAP), into the nonventilated side can aid in maintaining oxygenation. The most common cause of hypoxemia during one lung anesthesia is migration of the endobronchial tube distally to occlude the left upper lobe bronchial orifice. Deflation of the balloon with slight withdrawal of the tube quickly alleviates this problem. Appropriate incision sites for access to the entire hemithorax are essential. The principle

◄ Fig. 50-2. Incisions for thoracic trauma. A. Median sternotomy incision. B. Anterolateral incision. C. Posterolateral thoracotomy incision. D. A ''trap door'' incision (partial median sternotomy with supraclavicular and fourth intercostal extensions). E. Anterolateral thoracotomy with transsternal extension into the right chest.

Table 50-3. Emergency Department Thoracotomy Setup and Maneuvers

SETUP

Emergency department/trauma bay/operating room

Thoracotomy tray
  Finocchietto
  Skin knife
  Heavy scissors
  Lebsche knife, electric sternal saw, Gigli saw
  Tissue forceps
  Hemostats
  Dissecting scissors
  Vascular clamps (2)
  3-0 and 4-0 polypropylene suture
  30-ml Foley catheter

MANUEVERS

  Open pericardium
  Release tamponade
  Control cardiac wound (if applicable)
  Cardiac massage
  Defibrillation (if applicable)
  Aortic cross-clamping
  Hilum cross-clamping (if applicable)

generally followed is that of triangulation, with one incision for the camera and two working incisions. Generally the camera is placed first under direct vision through the seventh or eighth intercostal space in the midaxillary line. Additional incisions are made two or three ribs higher in the anterior and posterior axillary lines. These incisions provide sites for the camera and instruments, which can be interchanged as necessary to best approach the injury as it is identified. The telescope that is best for diagnostic and therapeutic purposes is usually the 30- or 45-degree angled instrument, which enables visualization of all the lateral chest wall as well as the recesses of the pleural space.

Gas insufflation for maintenance of pneumothorax is unnecessary and is contraindicated in the presence of a pulmonary parenchymal injury because of the risk of gas embolism. Conventional instruments are often easily used through the small thoracoscopy incisions. A long, flexible tonsil sucker is a very useful instrument for breaking up loculated clot or infection effusion. An electrocautery extension can be used for dividing pleural adhesions. The most useful specialized instruments include endoscopic clip appliers and stapling devices. Special 45-mm endoscopic staplers are particularly useful for resecting and closing larger segments of lung.

The Nd:YAG laser as well as argon beam coagulator have also been used to seal pulmonary air leaks and control oozing. Although not widely accepted, the role of thoracoscopy should continue to be objectively assessed in the evaluation and therapy of selected aspects of thoracic trauma. Currently, it is best used for evaluation and therapy of persistent chest bleeding in the stable patient and treatment of loculated hemothorax and its infectious complications.

Being able to initiate supportive measures in the overall management of thoracic trauma is as important as the definitive operative procedure. Autologous transfusion (autotransfusion) has proved to be a safe and efficient method of maintaining the oxygen-carrying capacity in a patient who is undergoing significant blood loss. In the trauma setting, this transfusion is usually achieved by salvaging a patient's own blood in either the pre- or postoperative period or intraoperatively. With the increased awareness of the many risks of homologous transfusion (e. g., malaria, hepatitis, and AIDS), the concept of autologous transfusion is widely accepted. Currently, there are several autotransfusion devices on the market, including Haemonetics Cell Saver (Braintree, MA) and Sorenson (Salt Lake City, UT).

With standard approaches to overall trauma management continually being challenged and revised, there is no doubt that more avenues will be explored in our attempt to establish the optimal treatment protocols for thoracic trauma.

Suggested Reading

Chen JC, Wilson SE. Diaphragmatic injuries. *Am Surg* 57:810, 1991.

Feliciano DV, Cruse PA, Mattox KL, et al. Delayed diagnosis of injuries of the diaphragm after penetrating wounds. *J Trauma* 28:1135, 1988.

Ivatury RR, Simon RJ, Weksler B, et al. Laparoscopy in the evaluation of the intrathoracic abdomen after penetrating injury. *J Trauma* 33:101, 1992.

Mariadason JG, Parsa MH, Ayuyao A, Freeman HP. Management of stab wounds to the thoracoabdominal region. *Ann Surg* 207:335, 1988.

Merlotti GJ, Dillon BC, Lange DA, et al. Peritoneal lavage in penetrating thoracoabdominal trauma. *J Trauma* 28:17, 1988.

Meyers BF, McCabe CJ. Traumatic diaphragmatic hernia. Occult marker of serious injury. *Ann Surg* 218:783, 1993.

Pagliarello G, Carter J. Traumatic injury to the diaphragm: Timely diagnosis and treatment. *J Trauma* 33:194, 1992.

Pate JW. Chest wall injuries. *Surg Clin North Am* 69:59, 1989.

Sharma OP. Traumatic diaphragmatic rupture: Not an uncommon entity—personal experience with collective review of the 1980s. *J Trauma* 29:678, 1989.

Sparks H, Falcone R. The ruptured diaphragm revisited. *Pan Am J Trauma* 3:76, 1992.

EDITOR'S COMMENT

As is appropriate for thoracic trauma management, the authors have chosen to focus their primary attention on the diagnosis of the thoracic injury, rather than on the precise technique of treatment, at least in most applications. Unilateral chest wall injury without an abdominal component is not often a surgical problem, at least in patients who are alive on arrival at the hospital. Obviously, the most lethal penetrating wounds are those of the heart, great vessels, and pulmonary hilus, in which massive blood loss occurs and optimal surgical management is sometimes unsuccessful. Of great interest are the transmediastinal penetrating wound, which has several important diagnostic as well as therapeutic implications and blunt injuries to the heart and aortic arch. The former is frequently surgically treated, and the latter is among the most interesting of all nonpenetrating wounds, since the results of surgery in patients who arrive alive in the emergency department are excellent. Myocardial contusion is one of the more common reasons for admitting patients with vehicular trauma. It is diagnosed far less often than it actually occurs, but has important diagnostic potential because severe contusions behave very much like acute anteroseptal infarcts, requiring similar work-up and management.

The authors have proposed extreme solutions to the question of the presence of diaphragmatic injury with thoracic gunshot wounds below the nipple (fourth intercostal space), including laparotomy in one proposed protocol. There are several simpler options, including a chest x-ray of the patient in the upright position, followed by DPL, followed by a repeated upright posteroanterior chest x-ray. If a pleural effusion, even minimal, appears between the first and second films, it is diagnostic of a hole in the diaphragm through which the peritoneal fluid infused in the peritoneal lavage has entered the chest. A more direct approach, and one that is possible under local anesthesia, is to view the anterior aspect of the right hemidiaphragm and most of the left hemidiaphragm with a laparoscope. There is a substantial difference of opinion among various trauma surgeons concerning the value of diagnostic laparoscopy, but the diaphragm is one of the easier organs to visualize, and therefore such laparoscopic evaluation is relatively straightforward. However, it has the obvious disadvantage of allowing a significant pneumothorax to occur if there is a hole in the diaphragm. The gas will promptly fill the ipsilateral pleural space and can conceivably cause a critical tension pneumothorax. Therefore, in the case of unilateral chest injury, it is imperative to place a large thoracostomy tube before the laparoscopy in order to provide a vent in case there is a diaphragmatic rent and to prevent tension pneumothorax. Thoracoscopy, as has been indicated, is a very good way to observe the diaphragm but does require bronchial intubation and a general anesthetic. Another disadvantage is that a hole in the diaphragm is often accompanied by intra-abdominal injury. Therefore, at least a CT scan of the abdomen should be performed before thoracoscopy, if the patient is stable, in order to rule out significant intra-abdominal or retroperitoneal injury. Coupled with DPL, abdominal injury can be considered to be trivial if both modalities (DPL and CT) yield no definitive diagnostic information, although the elusive diaphragmatic wound can still be missed unless one directly views the diaphragm.

One of the concerns in performing a subxiphoid pericardial window is that it is a fine test for ruling out cardiac injury; it is very good at ruling in cardiac injury, if there is a sudden rush of blood from the pericardium, causing the surgeon's blood pressure to rise dramatically and the patient's blood pressure often to fall or disappear equally dramatically. There is still a place for diagnostic pericardiocentesis and very definitely a place for transesophageal echocardiogram (TEE) in a patient with a penetrating wound of the thorax in the central portion in which a cardiac injury is a likely possibility. If pericardiocentesis is negative, a subxiphoid pericardial window should still be performed, but the chance of being greeted by a life-threatening (occasionally life-ending) bleed is less likely.

The working rule for thoracotomy or thoracoscopy for hemothorax is not necessarily the amount of blood that one initially retrieves, as the authors indicate, but a bleed that continues for 2 hours or more at 500 ml per hour. To look for 2000 ml per hour is to wait too long, and even 1000 ml per hour is a massive bleed in anyone's lexicon. Most significant pulmonary wounds bleed initially at between 200 and 500 ml per hour and often stop; therefore, the figure cited is the operative one. However, wounds of the pulmonary hilus or the intercostal bundle, with intercostal artery transection or partial transection, are the ones that will bleed in a major way and need to be dealt with directly. Many pulmonary hilar wounds, if a survivor can be brought to the operating room and opened, will require pneumonectomy. The intercostal bleeders are ideally handled with thoracoscopy, but the time and effort required to prepare the patient for that procedure are probably not appropriate for patients with major hemorrhage from the pleural space, which can be handled with a rapid incision into the chest wall through one of several incisions.

An interesting debate that the authors did not address is whether esophagoscopy is an effective diagnostic procedure to uncover or rule out penetrating esophageal injury, as compared with an esophagogram. In gunshot wounds, it is not uncommon for the bullet to traverse the muscularis of the esophagus, usually posteriorly, which might not show initial extravasation on esophagogram, but can result in enough contact burn injury to allow leakage to develop over the next 24 to 48 hours. Such a wound viewed through the esophagoscope should show a bluish purple discoloration of the esophageal mucosa, which is highly important information for the trauma surgeon, since it strongly suggests the need for exploration and repair. If 24 hours or more have elapsed, esophagogram is undoubtedly as reliable as the esophagoscopy, and either modality can be used.

R.J.B.

51

Pulmonary Resection

David J. Sugarbaker   Malcolm M. DeCamp, Jr.   Michael J. Liptay

History and Epidemiology

The evolution of thoracic surgery parallels developments in endotracheal anesthesia and selective lung ventilation. These techniques allow for safe operations on an open thoracic cavity. Pulmonary surgery has evolved from the simple management of pleural infection in the early 1900s, through parenchymal resection for the consequences of tuberculosis in the mid 1900s, to the extirpation of lung cancer, which is now its current focus.

In the last 50 years, there has been an epidemic rise in the number of reported cases of lung cancer in the United States. Over 174,000 new cases were reported in 1994. In that same year, 152,000 patients died of lung cancer. Twenty percent of these patients had small-cell (oat cell) carcinoma, a disease rarely treatable with resection alone. The majority, 80 percent of patients with lung cancer, present with non–small–cell lung cancer (NSCLC). NSCLC can be subdivided into three subtypes: adenocarcinoma (accounting for 50% of all NSCLC), squamous cell carcinoma (35%), and large cell–undifferentiated carcinoma (15%).

The first successful resection for lung cancer, a pneumonectomy, was performed by Evarts Graham in St. Louis in 1933. Over the next six decades, the introduction of lesser parenchymal resections for lung cancer met with skepticism and accusations of compromising the curative intent of the operation. Today the accepted standard resection for a localized NSCLC is the removal of the involved lobe of the lung along with its draining peribronchial and hilar lymph nodes.

Surgery remains the cornerstone for curative therapy for NSCLC. Between 20 and 30 percent of all patients with new lung cancers will have disease that is amenable to surgical treatment. The balance of patients present with locally unresectable disease or distant metastases. Neoadjuvant strategies involving chemotherapy or thoracic radiation, or both, can render some of these patients subsequently resectable. In patients thought to have resectable lesions without mediastinal nodal involvement, surgery remains the best curative modality.

Staging Non–Small Cell Lung Cancer

Before recommending resection to a patient with lung cancer, a thorough examination of the extent of disease is necessary. In 1986, the International Staging System for lung cancer was developed for four distinct stages of the disease (Table 51-1) that were validated with survival data. The TNM system was developed to enable classification of tumor extension (T1–4), nodal involvement (N0–3), and distant metastatic spread (M0–1). Surgical therapy is generally offered as monotherapy or in combination with chemotherapy and radiation for stages I through IIIA.

Noninvasive Roentgenographic Staging

A standard posteroanterior and lateral chest x-ray can reveal discrete mass lesions or the consequences of endobronchial tumors (atelectasis and postobstructive pneumonia). Hilar and mediastinal adenopathy along with pleural effusion might also be noted. In almost all cases of suspected lung cancer, a CT scan is obtained to include examination of the liver and adrenal glands along with mediastinal lymph node stations. The exclusion of metastatic disease in the liver and adrenal glands (present in up to 20% of patients at diagnosis) and ipsilateral or contralateral, synchronous, pulmonary parenchymal lesions dictates whether surgical treatment will be of any value. Head CT scans and bone scans are often part of the metastatic evaluation to rule out central nervous system (CNS) and bone involvement. The four most common sites of NSCLC metastases (stage IV disease) are the brain, bone, liver, and adrenal glands. If these sites are excluded, the disease is confined to the chest (stages I–IIIB). The presence of pleural effusion, unresectable T4 tumors or contralateral nodal involvement can be suggested by chest CT scan.

Surgical Staging

With the growing interest in a multimodality approach to NSCLC, accurate pretreatment pathologic staging has become paramount. Noninvasive roentgenographic staging can reliably determine the absence of distant metastatic spread. Involvement of the mediastinal lymph nodes is suggested by the finding of nodes that are greater than 1.5 cm in cross-sectional diameter. The accuracy of CT scanning in definitively identifying tumor-bearing nodes is 60 to 70 percent. Because of the high false-positive rate with chest CT scanning, we do not consider a patient inoperable without performing a cervical mediastinoscopy to sample mediastinal lymph nodes bilaterally for histologic examination. The presence of only ipsilateral tumor-bearing lymph nodes renders a patient's disease stage IIIA. There are many

Table 51-1. International Staging System of Lung Cancer

T:TUMOR STATUS

T1   3.0 cm or less without invasion of visceral pleura of proximal to lobar bronchus

T2   > 3.0 cm or any size with associated atelectasis or obstructive pneumonitis, may invade visceral pleura, proximal extent must be > 2 cm from carina

T3   Any size with direct extension into chest wall, diaphragm, mediastinal pleura without involvement of great vessels or vital mediastinal structures, cannot involve carina

T4   Any size with invasion of heart or mediastinal vital structures or carina, malignant pleural effusion

N:NODAL INVOLVEMENT

N0   None

N1   Peribronchial or ipsilateral hilar lymph nodes

N2   Ipsilateral mediastinal lymph nodes including subcarinal

N3   Contralateral mediastinal or hilar lymph nodes, ipsilateral or contralateral scalene or supra-clavicular lymph nodes

M:DISTANT METASTASES

M0   None

M1   Distant metastases present

STAGE:

Occult	TX	N0	M0
0	TIS	Carcinoma	In situ
I	T1	N0	M0
	T2	N0	M0
II	T1	N1	M0
	T2	N1	M0
IIIA	T3	N0	M0
	T3	N1	M0
	T1-3	N2	M0
IIIB	Any T	N3	M0
	T4	Any N	M0
IV	Any T	Any N	M1

Source: Adapted from CF Mountain. A new international staging system for lung cancer. *Chest* 89 (Suppl):225S, 1986; and TW Shields. *General Thoracic Surgery* (3rd ed.). Philadelphia: Lea & Febiger, 1989. Pp 911–913.

ongoing protocols using a multimodality approach including induction chemotherapy, radiation therapy, or concomitant chemoradiation to downstage such patients, thereby enhancing resectability and survival.

Bronchoscopy

Before thoracotomy for lung cancer resection, the surgeon performs a bronchoscopy using a flexible, fiber-optic bronchoscope to evaluate for any anatomic abnormalities, endobronchial tumor extent, and previously undetected lesions.

Mediastinoscopy

The intrathoracic lymph nodes are divided into anatomic stations (Fig. 51-1). Mediastinoscopy is used to diagnose N2 or N3 nodal involvement. The patient is positioned supine with the neck fully extended. A small transverse incision is made a finger breadth above the sternal notch, and the tissue planes are dissected between the strap muscles down to the pretracheal fascia. This plane is entered,

and finger dissection is used to develop a plane along the anterior surface of the trachea posterior to the innominate artery down to the aortic arch (Fig. 51-2). The mediastinoscope is inserted, and the paratracheal nodes at stations 2 and 4 are sampled bilaterally. On the left (level 4), care is taken to identify and preserve the left recurrent laryngeal nerve as it courses medially to reach the tracheoesophageal groove. Further dissection along each mainstem bronchus allows the surgeon to sample the tracheobronchial angle nodes bilaterally (level 10). The subcarinal nodes (level 7) are visualized next and biopsied.

The information gained from these nodal biopsies allows for accurate pathologic staging of the extent of disease before the decision for definitive resection. In instances in which the disease has spread to the contralateral mediastinal lymph nodes or to the supraclavicular nodes on either side (stage IIIB), curative resection is not possible, and surgery is offered only in a multimodality protocol setting.

The presence of nodal spread to the ipsilateral mediastinal stations confirms the diagnosis of stage IIIA disease, and surgery is offered only after preoperative therapy, usually involving a platinum-based regimen of chemotherapy with or without radiation therapy. Mediastinoscopy is more than 90 percent accurate in staging the mediastinum in NSCLC, whereas CT scanning misses 15 to 20 percent of mediastinal nodal metastases.

Anterior Mediastinoscopy

For tumors originating in the left upper lobe, the first stations of mediastinal lymph nodes most frequently involved with tumor are the periaortic and aortopulmonary (AP) window nodes (levels 5 and 6) (Fig. 51-1). These nodes are difficult to access through a standard cervical approach. In this setting, we prefer to use a limited anterior mediastinotomy (Chamberlain procedure) through the left parasternal second interspace (Fig. 51-3). An extrapleural dissection is continued down onto the aortic arch and AP window. The internal mammary vessels are identified and swept medially and rarely need to be ligated. Level 5 and level 6 lymph nodes (see Fig. 51-1, inset) are sampled, and care is taken to avoid the use of electrocautery near the recurrent laryngeal nerve, which arises from the left vagus nerve and travels under the aortic arch medially to the ligamentum arteriosum.

Preoperative Evaluation

Estimate of Pulmonary Reserve

The extent of surgery necessary for complete resection is often uncertain before the operation. Therefore, most patients should be able to tolerate a pneumonectomy if anatomic resection of their tumor is considered. The most important factor in determining patients' ability to undergo pulmonary resection is their preoperative status. The majority of patients are either current or former smokers; coexistent emphysema or obstructive pulmonary insufficiency are frequent companions to the primary malignancy. For these reasons, a careful preoperative assessment of pulmonary reserve and cardiac function is mandatory. Cessation of smoking at least 2 weeks before resection aids in the peri-

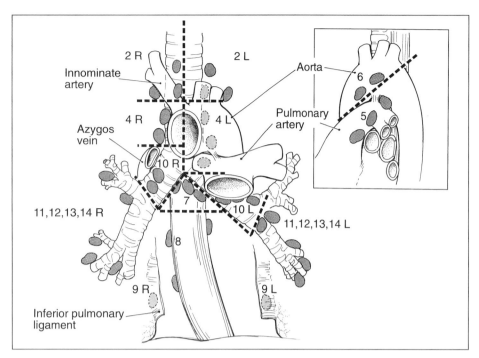

Fig. 51-1. *Intrathoracic lymph node map depicting mediastinal and hilar nodal stations. N1 nodal stations include levels 11, 12, 13, and 14. Stations 2 through 10 indicate N2 or N3 disease, depending on the side of the primary lesion.*

operative control of secretions and the avoidance of pneumonitis.

Postoperative pulmonary function is calculated by the use of preoperative pulmonary function tests measuring forced expiratory volume in one second (FEV_1). An equation to estimate the postoperative FEV_1 is:

$$\text{Predicted postoperative } FEV_1 = \text{Preoperative } FEV_1 - (\text{preoperative } FEV_1 \times \% \text{ lung to be removed})$$

In general, a predicted postoperative FEV_1 greater than 800 cc per second is desirable. There are several exceptions to this rule, including obstructing or central lesions and coexistent pleural disease. Quantitative ventilation/perfusion scanning and cardiopulmonary exercise testing can help clarify uncertain situations.

Pneumonectomy

Indications

In patients whose tumor is centrally located, adherent to hilar structures, or

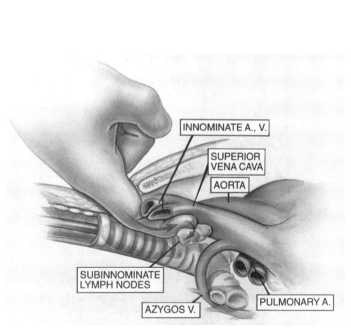

Fig. 51-2. *Incision for cervical mediastinoscopy. The mediastinoscope is inserted after digital dissection in the pretracheal space. Frequently palpable nodes and their relationship to the major vascular structures are shown. (From DJ Sugarbaker, and GM Strauss. Advances in surgical staging and therapy of non-small-cell lung cancer. Semin Oncol 20:163, 1993. Reprinted with permission.)*

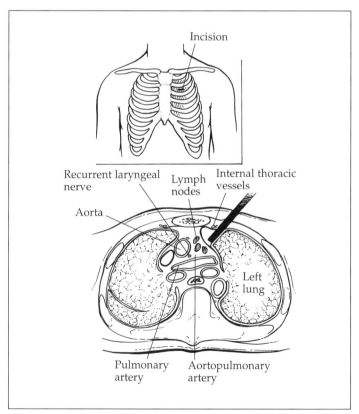

Fig. 51-3. *Anterior mediastinoscopy (Chamberlain procedure) (inset) incision. (Figure) Cross-sectional anatomic view of extrapleural plane of dissection with mediastinoscope to access aortopulmonary lymph nodes.*

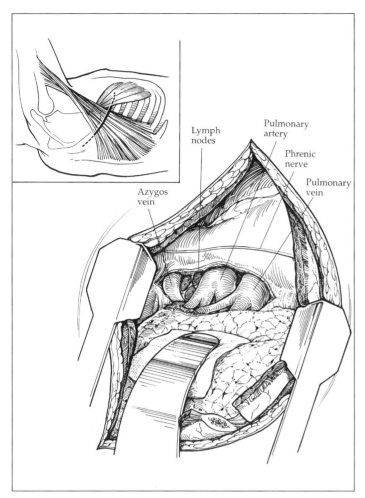

Fig. 51-4. Exposure for pulmonary resection. (Inset) Standard posterolateral incision. Solid line depicts complete division of latissimus dorsi. Hash marked line indicates options for extension to provide additional exposure. (Figure) View of right anterior hilar structures.

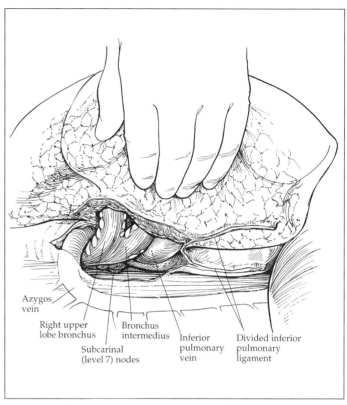

Fig. 51-5. Posterior right hilar view after division of the mediastinal pleura and inferior pulmonary ligament.

crossing the fissure (left-sided lesions), a pneumonectomy is necessary for a curative resection. Reported operative mortality varies but is generally 4 to 8 percent.

After general anesthesia is induced, a flexible bronchoscopy is performed to evaluate the patient for synchronous endobronchial lesions and anatomic anomalies. For endobronchial primary lesions, at least a 2-cm margin of grossly uninvolved mainstem bronchus is desired to ensure a curative resection.

Preparation

For left-sided lesions, a bronchial blocker or right-sided double-lumen endotracheal tube is positioned to aid in left lung deflation; for right-sided tumors the standard left-sided double-lumen endotracheal tube

is preferred. The patient is then placed in the lateral decubitus position, and the chest is prepped and draped.

Right Pneumonectomy

A standard posterolateral thoracotomy incision is made and the latissimus dorsi muscle is completely divided (Fig. 51-4, inset). The border between the serratus muscle and latissimus is freed. The ribs are counted by placing the hand beneath the scapula and counting down posteriorly. The sixth rib is marked, and the intercostal muscle is divided along the superior border of this rib. The pleural space is entered through the fifth interspace, and care is taken not to damage the underlying lung. A small segment of posterior rib can be isolated subperiosteally and divided with

a rib cutter ("shingling") to aid in exposure and avoid unintentional rib fracture with retraction.

After insertion of the chest retractor, the surgeon systematically evaluates the lung and mediastinum to document the extent of disease. A histologic diagnosis of NSCLC is made by biopsy if tissue has not been obtained preoperatively. Pleural metastases or adherence to the spine or unresectable mediastinal structures (T4 lesions) should be ruled out.

After documenting localized lung cancer, the resectability of the tumor is evaluated. This step requires a circumferential evaluation of the hilar structures with a goal of ligation and division of major vessels and the bronchus with clear margins. The pulmonary artery, veins, and bronchus must be inspected before proceeding with any ligation of these structures and committing the patient to resection.

The lung is gently retracted posteroinferiorly to access the hilar structures (main pulmonary artery, right mainstem bronchus, superior pulmonary vein, and azygos vein (Fig. 51-4). The azygos vein can

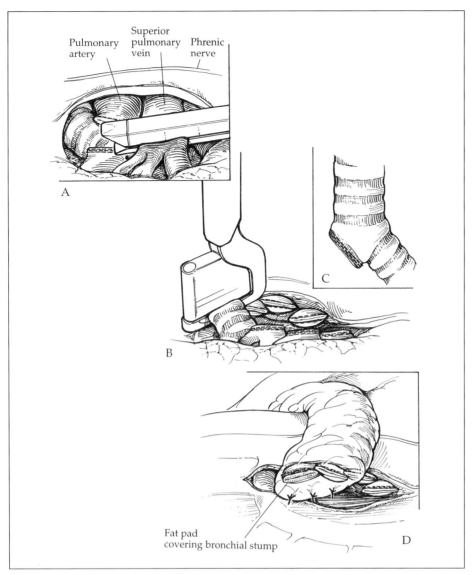

Fig. 51-6. Right pneumonectomy. A. The right main pulmonary artery has been divided, and the stapler is across the superior pulmonary vein. B. The right pulmonary vessels have been divided, and the heavy wire 30-mm stapler is placed across the proximal right mainstem bronchus. C. Right pneumonectomy stump. D. Mobilized pericardial fat pad used to cover the pneumonectomy stump.

rior pulmonary veins are evaluated for resectability. The last question to be answered is whether a lesser resection such as a lobectomy or sleeve lobectomy can be performed. If not, then attention is directed toward division of the hilar structures. The order of division of the vascular structures or bronchus is not critical and usually proceeds along the lines of the ease of dissection. Our preferred technique involves division of the right main pulmonary artery first.

After sharply dividing the adventitial sheath of the main pulmonary artery, most of the isolation of the vessel can be carried out with gentle, blunt dissection. Occasionally, the truncus anterior branch of the pulmonary artery can be divided separately to provide more room for division of the right main pulmonary artery. If there is sufficient length to accommodate the surgeon's finger, we prefer to use an endovascular stapler to divide the artery (Fig. 51-6). Other surgeons prefer to ligate the artery with nonabsorbable sutures and suture ligate the proximal end.

After division of the artery is complete, the superior pulmonary veins are isolated by dissecting anteriorly in the groove of pericardial reflection between the superior and inferior pulmonary veins. These veins can be similarly divided with separate applications of the stapler (Fig. 51-6A).

The lung is now tethered only by the bronchus. Reflecting the lung anteriorly affords access to the membranous side of the mainstem bronchus. The bronchus can be divided with suture closure or stapler. We staple the bronchus with a heavy wire 30-mm stapler (Fig. 51-6B). The stump should be left as short as possible, flush with the carina to avoid the dependent pooling of secretions and the higher likelihood of breakdown incumbent with a longer stump (Fig. 51-6C). The chest is then irrigated, and the stump is tested for air leakage with 20 to 30 cm H_2O of static positive pressure ventilation.

We routinely cover any pneumonectomy stump with vascularized tissue. A pericardial fat pad based on the superior thymic vessels can easily be mobilized to cover the stump in most instances (Fig. 51-6D). The flap is anchored to the airway with absorbable suture. Other local flap coverage options include an intercostal muscle flap, parietal pleura, or pericardium.

usually be spared in the dissection but can be divided with impunity. The adventitial sheath of the proximal pulmonary artery is dissected superomedially near the origin of the right upper lobe bronchial takeoff. Level 10 lymph nodes should be swept up onto the specimen side revealing the right mainstem bronchus in the space beneath the azygos vein. The vagal afferents to the bronchus are divided, and visible bronchial arteries are ligated.

The lung is then retracted anteriorly exposing the right mainstem bronchus and subcarinal space (Fig. 51-5). Level 7 subcarinal lymph nodes are removed, and a finger is passed behind the bronchus to ensure resectability. With the lung retracted superiorly, the inferior pulmonary ligament is divided to the edge of the inferior pulmonary vein, and the level 9 lymph nodes are swept up with the specimen (Fig. 51-5).

The lung is then retracted posteroinferiorly, and the hilar pleura is opened posterior to the phrenic nerve. The main pulmonary artery and superior and infe-

The empty pleural space is examined for hemostasis, and the wound is closed without the use of chest tube drainage. A catheter and syringe are used to evacuate 1000 to 1200 cc of air from the hemithorax after the patient is placed supine to aid in repositioning the mediastinum to the midline.

Left Pneumonectomy

The left pneumonectomy differs from one on the right side mainly because of the anatomy near the aortic arch (Fig. 51-7). The level 5 AP window lymph nodes and the level 6 nodes over the anterior aortic arch are dissected and removed during the initial exploration. The recurrent laryngeal nerve branches off the vagus and courses anteriorly then inferiorly to the aortic arch. This structure should be protected except in instances of direct tumor involvement.

All hilar structures are inspected and confirmation of tumor resectability is made before ligating or dividing these structures. The vessels are divided in a manner similar to the procedure described for the right side. The left mainstem bronchus is significantly longer than the right, and attaining the desired short stump can be more challenging. Tissue coverage of the stump remains important, and the pedicled pericardial fat pad is used when available.

Occasionally, in an otherwise resectable situation, the tumor involves the proximal hilum where a safe margin cannot be obtained on the vessels. In this setting, the pericardium can be opened away from the tumor and an intrapericardial plane established for safe ligation of the pulmonary veins or main pulmonary artery of the involved side. Small pericardial defects need not be covered or closed, whereas larger defects require patch closure, usually using a surgical membrane, to prevent cardiac herniation into the empty thorax. Such approaches do not increase operative mortality, although the incidence of postoperative supraventricular arrhythmias approaches 30 percent.

Lobar Resections

A lobectomy is considered the standard oncologic resection for most NSCLC. It involves removal of the involved anatomic lobe of lung parenchyma as well as the N1 hilar, interlobar, and segmental lymph nodes draining the area. An intimate understanding of the anatomy of the main pulmonary artery and its branches is necessary for the safe performance of a lobectomy (Fig. 51-8). The pulmonary artery is a delicate, thin-walled vessel requiring meticulous dissection to avoid injury.

Right Upper Lobectomy

After positioning the patient in the left lateral decubitus position, the right chest is typically entered through a serratus-sparing, limited posterolateral thoracotomy through the fifth interspace (see Fig. 51-4, inset). We routinely shingle the fifth rib posteriorly, removing a 2- to 3-cm portion, to allow for atraumatic exposure during spreading of the ribs. After insertion of the

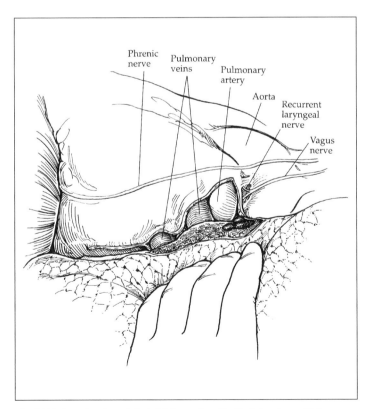

Fig. 51-7. Anterior view of the left hilar and mediastinal structures. Note relationship of the recurrent laryngeal nerve to the left main pulmonary artery and aorta.

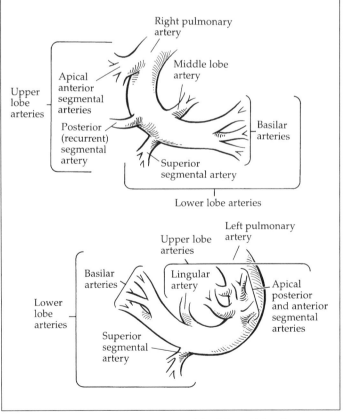

Fig. 51-8. Right upper lobectomy. Anatomy of the right and left pulmonary arteries.

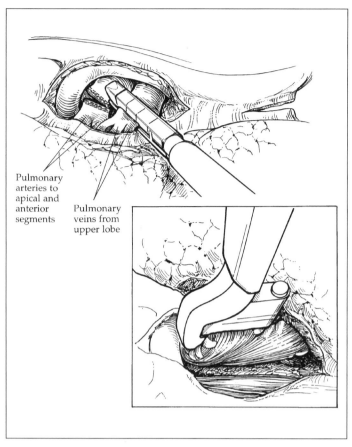

Fig. 51-9. (Figure) The truncus anterior pulmonary artery has been divided, and the veins draining the right upper lobe are next divided with a vascular stapler. (Inset) Posterior approach to division of right upper lobe bronchus.

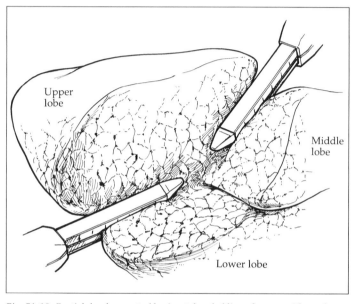

Fig. 51-10. Partial development of horizontal and oblique fissures with staplers.

chest retractor, the lung and pleural cavity are inspected for any evidence of local metastases such as pleural seeding or effusion.

Next, the inferior pulmonary ligament is divided to allow for mobility of the remaining lung in filling the apex of the pleural cavity. The oblique and horizontal fissures are examined to assess the need for further dissection. The sequence in dissection and ligation is again based on the anatomic setting and convenience. The dissection proceeds initially at the anterior hilum. The phrenic nerve is seen coursing over the superior vena cava. The mediastinal pleura is divided posterior to the nerve at its junction with the visceral pleura of the lung anteriorly. This dissection plane is carried superiorly and posteriorly after gently elevating the upper lobe anteriorly. Blunt dissection reveals the right mainstem bronchus and the upper lobe origin with the bronchus intermedius coursing distally.

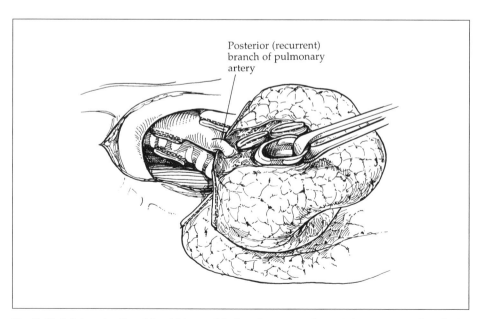

Fig. 51-11. Inferior retraction of the right upper lobe bronchus exposes the posterior or recurrent branch of the pulmonary artery.

Within the anterior hilum, the pulmonary artery is dissected as it exits the mediastinum inferior to the azygos vein. The truncus anterior branch giving off the arteries to the apical and anterior segments of the upper lobe is isolated and ligated first using either a vascular stapler or suture ligatures (Fig. 51-9).

Attention is next directed toward the superior pulmonary vein, which includes the venous drainage of the upper and middle lobe. The veins draining the upper lobe are identified and ligated with a vascular stapler (Fig. 51-9); care is taken to spare the venous drainage of the middle lobe lying inferiorly. If necessary, at this point the oblique and horizontal fissures are partially developed with a stapler (Fig. 51-10). We next divide the right upper lobe bronchus by developing a plane posteriorly between the bronchus intermedius and upper lobe bronchus. With the truncus anterior branch of the pulmonary artery already divided, pulmonary arterial injury is avoided. We prefer to use a 30-mm stapler, but suture closure of the bronchus is acceptable (Fig. 51-9, inset). The divided distal bronchus is then grasped with an Allis clamp and retracted inferiorly exposing the recurrent, posterior, or ascending pulmonary artery branch to the posterior segment of the upper lobe, which is suture ligated and divided (Fig. 51-11).

The specimen is now attached only by its remaining fissures and parenchyma, which are divided with a stapler to provide an airtight resection (Fig. 51-12). After removal of the specimen, the bronchial staple line is tested under water for integrity. We do not routinely cover nondependent stumps. Two chest tubes are inserted through separate stab incisions for drainage. The wound is closed after irrigation of the chest and confirmation of hemostasis.

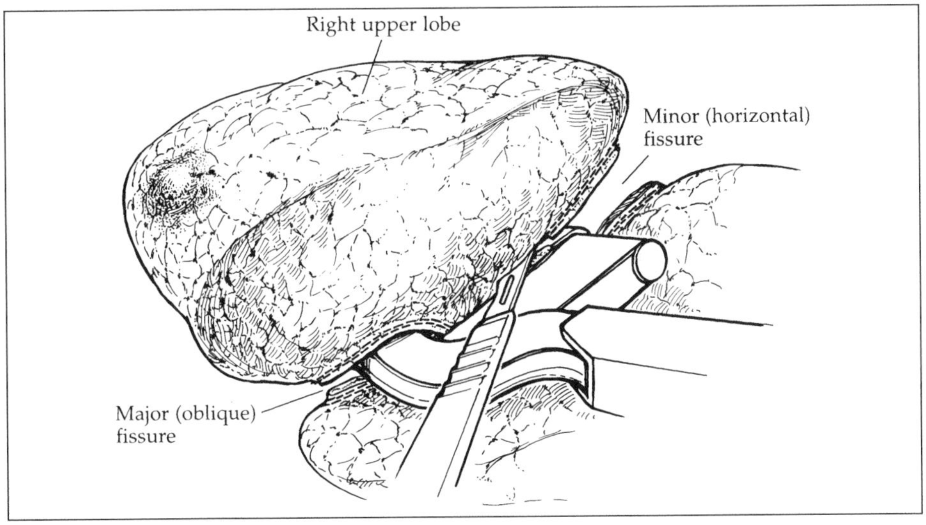

Right Middle Lobectomy

The right middle lobe is less commonly involved as the primary site of tumor. More

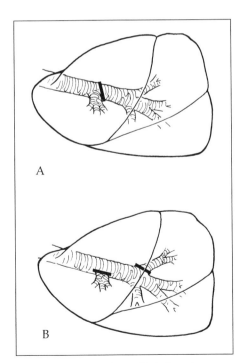

Fig. 51-12. Division of remaining right upper lobe fissural attachments.

Fig. 51-13. Bilobectomies. A. Right bronchus intermedius division site for a right middle and lower lobe bilobectomy. B. Separate right upper lobe and middle lobe bronchial division sites for bilobectomy of the right upper and middle lobes.

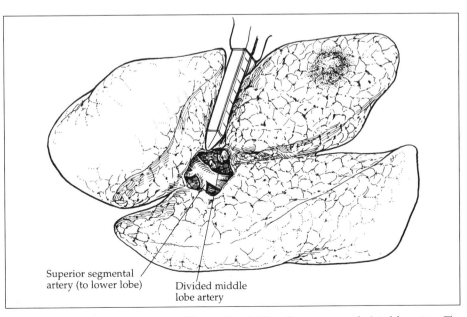

Fig. 51-14. Dissection at the intersection of horizontal and oblique fissures exposes the interlobar artery. The middle lobe branch (divided) is just opposite the artery to the superior segment of the lower lobe.

often, it is removed along with the upper or lower lobe as a bilobectomy specimen for tumors that cross fissures. In the case of the right middle and lower bilobectomy, the bronchus intermedius can be divided just distal to the upper lobe bronchus take off (Fig. 51-13A). In the setting of the right upper and middle bilobectomy, the bronchi are divided separately (Fig. 51-13B).

To perform an isolated right middle lobectomy, an anterolateral thoracotomy is preferable. The dissection begins in the oblique fissure at its intersection with the horizontal fissure. The visceral pleura is opened, and the interlobar pulmonary artery is identified. With gentle traction anteriorly on the middle lobe, the one or two middle lobe arteries are identified and ligated (Fig. 51-14). If necessary, the horizontal fissure is completed with a stapler.

After division of the arteries, the hilum is approached anteriorly, reflecting the lung posteroinferiorly. The anterior mediastinal pleura is incised, revealing the middle lobe vein, which empties into the lower portion of the superior pulmonary vein (Fig. 51-15). The vein is isolated and divided, leaving the middle lobe tethered by its bronchus. The middle lobe bronchus is easily identified and divided (Fig. 51-15, inset). The stump is stapled or sutured closed with interrupted sutures and is not usually reinforced with tissue coverage because the stump is well covered by the parenchyma of the remaining lobes. Problems with bronchial healing after middle lobectomy are rare. The inferior pulmonary ligament is divided to allow the remaining lung mobility to fill the pleural space.

Right Lower Lobectomy

As is the case in most lobectomies, the completeness of the fissures determines the ease of initial exposure. Typically for a right lower lobectomy, the first step after gaining entry into the chest involves retracting the upper and middle lobes anteriorly and the lower lobe posteroinferiorly, spreading open the oblique fissure.

Dissection of the visceral pleura reveals the interlobar pulmonary artery. Identification of the middle lobe artery anteromedially aids in the detection of the superior segmental artery posteriorly and

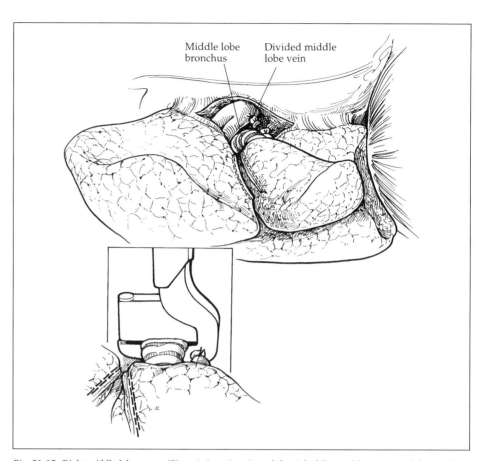

Fig. 51-15. Right middle lobectomy. (Figure) Anterior view of the right hilum with exposure of the middle lobe vein (already divided) and bronchus. (Inset) Division of the bronchus with a stapler.

opposite the middle lobe artery (Fig. 51-16). After dividing the superior segmental artery, the basilar arteries are isolated and ligated.

The inferior pulmonary vein is approached posteriorly, and the inferior pulmonary ligament is divided to the lower border of the vein, sweeping any level 9 lymph nodes up with the specimen. Division of the mediastinal pleura posteriorly allows for clearance of the inferior pulmonary vein away from the lower border of the bronchus and the superior pulmonary vein. After freeing the inferior pulmonary vein anteriorly, a clamp is passed to aid in the stapling of the vein with a vascular stapler. Before division, anomalous middle lobe venous drainage into the inferior pulmonary vein should be ruled out.

If the oblique fissure is incomplete, a stapler is applied to separate the middle lobe

from the specimen. The lower lobe is now attached by only its bronchi. Most often it is safer to divide the superior segmental bronchus separately from the ongoing bronchus to the basal segments (Fig. 51-16, inset). After division of these bronchi with the 30-mm stapler, we cover the dependent stumps of the lower lobe bronchi with vascularized tissue. A pericardial fat pad, intercostal muscle, parietal pleura, or pericardium can be used as described earlier for pneumonectomy stumps.

Left Upper Lobectomy

The chest is entered through a fourth or fifth interspace thoracotomy. The hilum is approached anteriorly by gentle lateral and inferior retraction of the left lung. The mediastinal pleura is incised over the pulmonary artery as it courses beneath the aortic arch. The phrenic nerve anteromedially and the vagus nerve with its recur-

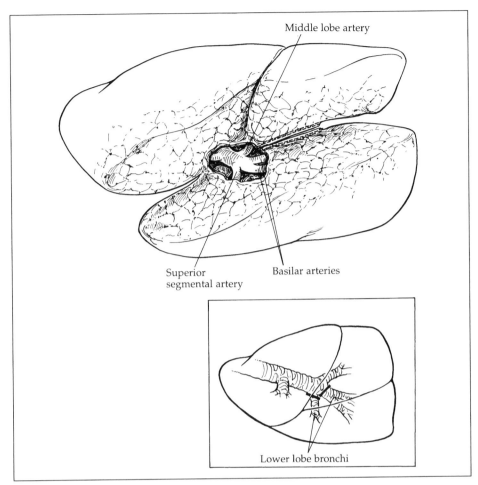

Fig. 51-16. Right lower lobectomy. (Figure) Interlobar arterial dissection exposing lower lobar arteries. (Inset) Sites of sequential division of lower lobe superior segmental and basilar bronchi.

rent laryngeal branch coursing below the aortic arch form the boundaries of the pleural dissection (see Fig. 51-7).

Working from the top of the fissure posteriorly with the upper lobe retracted superomedially and lateral reflection of the lower lobe, the interlobar left pulmonary artery is exposed (Fig. 51-17A). The most common anatomic variability encountered is the number of segmental pulmonary arterial branches to the upper lobe. Most commonly four branches (apicoposterior, anterior, superior lingular, and inferior lingular), one to each of the segments, are present. However, between three and seven branches can be present, and careful dissection is required. The segmental arteries are identified and ligated. After arterial ligation is complete, attention is shifted to circumferential isolation of the

upper lobe bronchus, which is carefully freed from the posterior surface of the superior pulmonary vein. The stapling device is used to divide the bronchus, and the superior vein is then exposed for similar ligation with a vascular stapling device.

Left Lower Lobectomy

The dissection for left lower lobectomy begins posteriorly in the fissure with opening of the pleura and sheath over the main left pulmonary artery. Reflection of the lower lobe posteriorly allows visualization of the artery to the superior segment of the lower lobe, which is isolated and ligated (see Fig. 51-17A). Next, the basilar arterial branches are isolated and divided distal to the lingular artery (see Fig. 51-17A). The inferior extent of the fissure can then be

completed by applying a stapler (Fig. 51-17B). The lower lobe is reflected anteriorly and the inferior pulmonary ligament divided to the lower border of the inferior pulmonary vein. The posterior mediastinal pleural attachments to the inferior vein and the plane between the vein and the membranous bronchus are developed. The inferior pulmonary vein is freed circumferentially and then divided with a vascular stapler. The lower lobe is now attached only by its bronchus, which in most cases can be divided with a single stapler fired across both the basal bronchi and superior segmental bronchus without compromising the left upper lobe bronchial orifice. We cover the stump with locally derived vascularized tissue.

Conclusions and General Considerations

Safe pulmonary resection requires careful dissection under ideal conditions of exposure. Contralateral single lung ventilation and care in obtaining proximal control of the pulmonary artery before performing difficult dissections are mandatory. The use of epidural anesthesia both intraoperatively and postoperatively allows for the majority of patients to be extubated immediately following the procedure and to begin pulmonary rehabilitation promptly in the early postoperative period. Supraventricular arrhythmias are common within the first 5 days (especially after pneumonectomy, occurring in up to 30% of patients). Cardiac monitoring of these patients postoperatively allows for timely intervention for these most often benign arrhythmias. Ninety percent of patients achieve sinus rhythm with correction of electrolyte abnormalities, supplemental oxygen, and the judicious use of digoxin or calcium channel blockers. The use of routine beta blockade is discouraged, because of the frequent association of reactive airway disease in these patients. Vigilant postoperative monitoring of pulmonary function with liberal use of bedside bronchoscopy for pulmonary toilet can avoid the debilitating complication of postoperative pneumonia and respiratory failure.

The authors wish to thank Mary Sullivan Visciano for editorial assistance and Marcia Williams for illustrations.

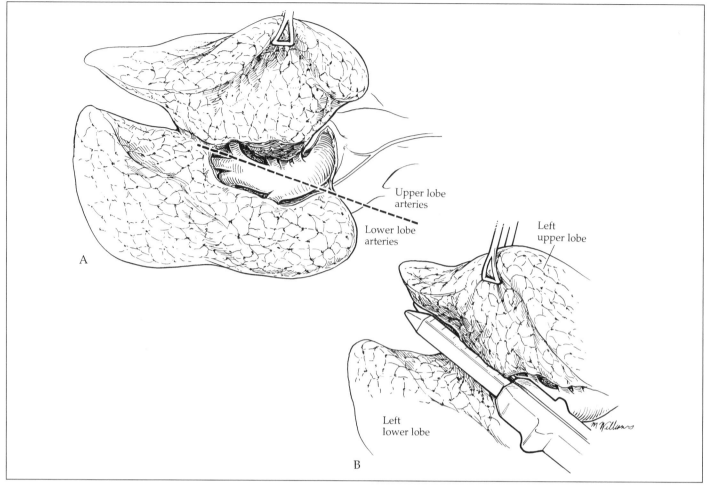

Fig. 51-17. Exposure of the left interlobar pulmonary artery. A. Segmental arteries above the dotted line are divided for left upper lobectomy. Those below are ligated for lower lobectomies. B. The incomplete portion of the fissure anteroinferiorly is completed with a stapler.

Suggested Reading

Carlens E. Mediastinoscopy: a method for inspection and tissue biopsy in the superior mediastinum. *Dis Chest* 36:343, 1959.

Fell SC, Kirby TJ. Technical Aspects of Lobectomy. In TW Shields (ed.), *General Thoracic Surgery*, 4th ed. Malvern, PA: Williams & Wilkins, 1994.

Ginsberg RJ, Hill LD, Eagan RT, et al. Modern thirty-day operative mortality for surgical resections in lung cancer. *J Thorac Cardiovasc Surg* 86:654, 1983.

Goldstraw P. Pneumonectomy and Its Modifications. In TW Shields (ed.), *General Thoracic Surgery*, 4th ed. Malvern, PA: Williams & Wilkins, 1994.

Hood RM. *Techniques in General Thoracic Surgery*, 2nd ed. Malvern, PA: Lea & Febiger, 1993.

Mountain CF. A new international staging system for lung cancer. *Chest* 89 (Suppl):225S, 1986.

Naruke T, Tomoyuki G, Tsuchiya R, et al. Prognosis and survival in resected lung carcinoma based on the new international staging system. *J Thorac Cardiovasc Surg* 96:440, 1988.

Ravitch MM, Steichen FM. *Atlas of General Thoracic Surgery*, Philadelphia: Saunders, 1988.

Sugarbaker DJ, Strauss GM. Advances in surgical staging and therapy of non-small-cell lung cancer. *Semin Oncol* 20:163, 1993.

EDITOR'S COMMENT

The authors have presented an elegant exposition of the indications for and techniques in surgical management of cancer of the lung. As the authors have stated, this disease has become one of epidemic proportions in the past several decades, with an especially alarming rise in frequency in women. It has become the leading cause of cancer deaths in individuals irrespective of gender. Unfortunately, symptoms are not necessarily predictable, and many smokers with chronic coughs do not seek medical help or chest x-ray when they experience the earlier symptoms but wait until the disease process has become function-limiting.

With far more sophisticated pulmonary function testing and evaluation than was formerly available, fewer patients are now subjected to resections that result in extreme pulmonary dysfunction in the postoperative period. Three decades ago, every house officer had vivid memories of patients whose lung cancer was apparently cured by pneumonectomy or bilobectomy, only to have the patient become progressively worse in the postoperative period as hypercarbia and respiratory acidosis gradually destroyed the quality and length of life remaining to such individuals. In fact, some thoracic surgeons were noted to be very "brave" in doing major resections in patients who were not able to climb two flights of stairs without stopping. House officers who had been through such experiences walked patients up two hospital flights at a modest pace, and the patient who was unable to walk up the second flight without stopping was, predictably, likely to succumb to pulmonary insufficiency if major resection was undertaken the next day in order to "cure the cancer." Modern technology has eliminated such scenarios, with pulmonary function laboratories providing data predicting the physiologic results of a particular resection with a 95 percent accuracy. Postoperative infection in the remaining lobe or lung has become substantially less common, with a predictable drop in mortality and morbidity.

An advance of great merit has been the advent of stapling techniques for the pulmonary vasculature and the bronchial stump. In the gastrointestinal tract, there is no evidence that hand-sewn closures or anastomoses are superior to stapled anastomoses; they are equal. However, in the chest, including both lung and esophagus, the generous application of staples has undoubtedly saved lives, since a catastrophic technical misadventure can result from the attempt to hand sew the stump of the pulmonary artery, a very fragile and delicate structure. A tear in that artery can and does result in torrential hemorrhage that often requires intrapericardial control. As long as there is room for the instrument, the vascular staples are far more efficient and much faster at dealing with a vessel that is often encased in inflammatory reaction because of endobronchial inflammatory disease on which the cancer is superimposed.

R.J.B.

SIX

THE DIAPHRAGM

52

Surgical Anatomy of the Diaphragm

Lee J. Skandalakis   Gene L. Colborn   John E. Skandalakis

The diaphragm alone is responsible for the ease of inhalation and exhalation. However, when exhalation becomes difficult, then intercostal muscles, pectoral muscles, shoulder and neck muscles participate as well.
MOSES MAIMONIDES

Embryogenesis

The mammalian diaphragm is a composite organ formed from four embryonic sources: transverse septum, mediastinum, pleuroperitoneal membranes, and muscles of the body wall.

Transverse Septum

The growing head fold of the embryo brings a wall of mesoderm to a position cranial to the open midgut and caudal to the heart during the third embryonic week (Fig. 52-1). This mesoderm forms the ventral component of the future diaphragm, which is the largest part.

The cranial surface of the septum also contributes to the connective tissue of the pericardium, whereas from the caudal surface comes the connective tissue of the capsule and stroma of the liver.

Mediastinum

The mediastinum is the thick dorsal mesentery of the foregut, containing the future esophagus and the inferior vena cava (Fig. 52-2A). It is continuous anteriorly with the transverse septum and posteriorly with the axial mesoderm. By posterior and caudal extension, it splits to form the diaphragmatic crura.

Pleuroperitoneal Membranes

The pleuroperitoneal membranes close the right and left communication between the pleural and peritoneal cavities at about the eighth embryonic week. Originally they form a large part of the developing diaphragm (see Fig. 52-2A), but relative growth of other elements reduces their contribution to a small area (Fig. 52-2B).

Muscles of the Body Wall

Myotomes of the seventh to twelfth segments contribute the lateral component of the diaphragm by caudal excavation of the thoracic wall to form the costodiaphragmatic recesses. This process produces the final domed shape of the diaphragm.

Phrenic nerve fibers are present in the diaphragm by the seventh week, and muscle fibers can be found a week later. Before birth, there is a preponderance of white, fast-twitch, low-oxidative fibers. An increase in red, slow-twitch, high-oxidative fibers takes place until, by the eighth postnatal month, about 55 percent of the fibers are of the red, slow-twitch type. These fibers are less easily fatigued than are white fibers.

It is not certain whether all muscle fibers originate from the thoracic wall and migrate centrally or originate in the transverse septum and migrate peripherally. With the data currently available, it is not possible to delineate on the adult diaphragm the exact boundaries of the four embryonic components.

Descent of the Diaphragm

In the third week, the transverse septum lies at the level of C3, and the developing diaphragm descends to its final position at the level of L1 by the eighth week (Fig. 52-3). The phrenic nerve, which originates from the third to fifth cervical levels, is carried caudad with the descending diaphragm.

Diaphragmatic Anomalies
Duplication and Accessory Diaphragms

In rare instances, the hemithorax is divided into two spaces by an accessory sheet, which can be fibrous, muscular, or both. The anomaly is usually on the right and equally distributed between the sexes. Hart and his colleagues were able to collect 27 reports since the first report by Haeberlin in 1945. Typically the membrane originates in the pericardial reflection; its attachment ranges from the seventh rib to the apex of the pleura. Hypoplastic lung tissue is usually present in the lower cavity. A hiatus in the membrane permits the passage of pulmonary vessels and bronchi. Anomalous pulmonary venous drainage into the inferior cava is frequently associated. Accessory diaphragm was reported in 1993 by Bruce and colleagues and Doi and colleagues; both instances were associated with pulmonary problems. Differing from accessory diaphragm is an apparent duplication of the transverse septum, the ventral component of the diaphragm, as reported by Krzyzaniak and Gray. Both this defect and accessory dia-

Fig. 52-1. Formation of the transverse septum. A. The heart and pericardium form anterior to the head of the embryo in the third week. B. Rapid growth of the head rotates the heart and the mesoderm, which will become the transverse septum, in the direction indicated by the arrows the fourth week.

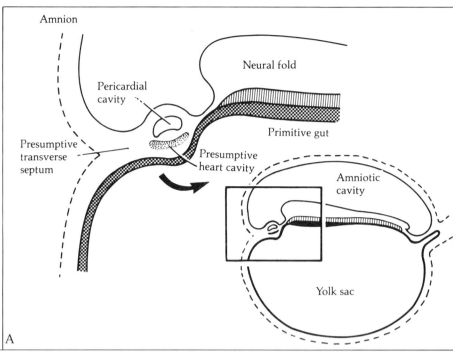

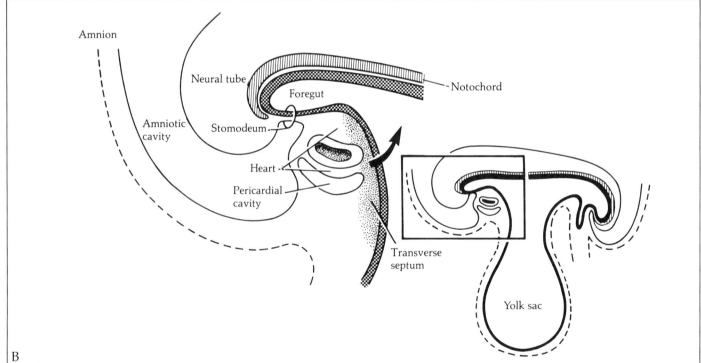

phragm are amenable to surgical correction if no other severe defects are present.

Anatomy of Congenital and Acquired Diaphragmatic Hernias

During the first 2 months of fetal life, there is no pressure on the developing dia-phragm from above or below. Above, the lungs are not inflated; below, the growth of the gut is taking place extra-abdominally, into the umbilical cord. The first mechanical pressure on the diaphragm comes during the tenth week when the intestines return from the umbilical cord to the abdomen. By that time, all of the diaphragmatic components are normally in place and have sufficient strength to contain the abdominal viscera, which might not be the case if the normal developmental timetable is disturbed.

A number of areas of the diaphragm can give way under pressure from the abdominal viscera. Most diaphragmatic hernias start in these small areas of weakness and

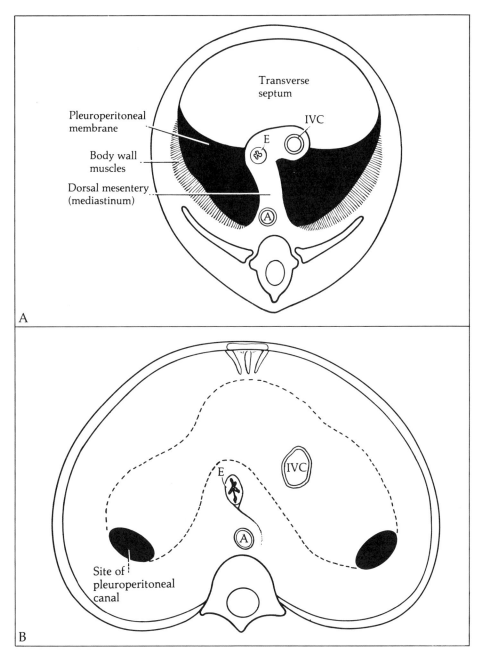

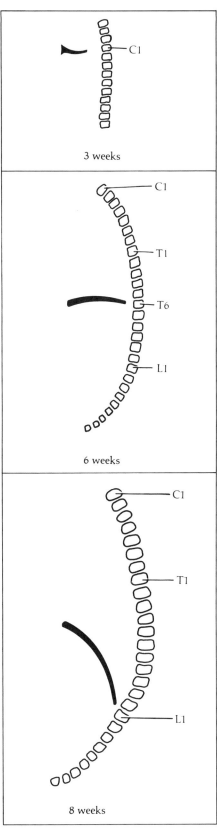

Fig. 52-2. Comparison of embryonic and adult diaphragms. A. The four embryonic components of the diaphragm. B. The adult diaphragm. The sites of the closed pleuroperitoneal canals occupy a relatively small area in the adult diaphragm. E, esophagus; IVC, inferior vena cava; A, aorta.

Fig. 52-3. The descent of the diaphragm during development. The phrenic nerve arises from the third to the fifth cervical segments and follows the diaphragm down to its final position.

enlarge with age. The specific hernias are described below and summarized in Table 52-1.

It has been reported that the abnormal development of the diaphragmatic anlage and the production of congenital diaphragmatic hernia in embryo were noted at the age of 13 to 14 days. A defect at the dorsal part of the diaphragm will permit an early hepatic entrance, but intrathoracic position of the gut will be seen in very late stages approximately on the twenty-first or twenty-second day. There is disagreement with the theory that the pleuroperitoneal canals fail to close at the end of the embryonic period.

Hiatal Hernia

Ascent of the stomach into the thorax through the esophageal hiatus of the diaphragm is a common and poorly under-

Table 52-1. Characteristics of Diaphragmatic Hernias

Hernia	Anatomy	Sac and Herniated Organs	Remarks

Hernia through the foramen of Morgagni (retrosternal hernia, parasternal hernia, anterior diaphragmatic hernia)	Congenital potential hernia through muscular hiatus on either side of the xiphoid process
	Usually on the right; bilateral hernias are known. Actual herniation usually the result of postnatal trauma
		Sac present at first. Can rupture later, leaving no trace
		Contents
		  Infants: liver
		  Adults: omentum
		    Can be followed by colon and stomach later
			Rare in infants and children

Hernia through the foramen of Bochdalek (posterolateral hernia of the diaphragm)	Congenital hernia through the lumbocostal trigone Can expand to include almost whole hemidiaphragm. More common on left	Sac present in 10–15% Contents: small intestine usual; stomach, colon, spleen, frequent. Pancreas and liver rare. Liver only in right-sided hernia	Heart and mediastinum shifted to contralateral side Ipsilateral lung collapsed but usually not hypoplastic Secondary malrotation is common Craniorachischisis, tracheoesophageal fistula, and heart defects are common
Traumatic hernia	Acquired hernia Tear, usually from esophageal hiatus across dome to left costal attachment of diaphragm	No sac Herniated organs: none at first. Spleen, splenic flexure of colon, stomach, left lobe of liver later	
Peritoneopericardial hernia (defect of the central tendon, defect of the transverse septum)	Congenital hernia through central tendon and pericardium	Sac rarely present Contents: stomach, colon	Has been seen in newborns and adults. Perhaps traumatic in adults Rare
Eventration of the diaphragm	Congenital hernia Diaphragm is thin with sparsely distributed, but normal, muscle fibers Either or both sides can be affected Phrenic nerve appears normal Acquired: paralysis of normal muscle resulting from phrenic nerve injury	"Sac" is formed by the attenuated diaphragm Contents: normal abdominal organs under elevated dome of hemidiaphragm No sac	Heart and mediastinum shifted to contralateral side. Ipsilateral lung collapsed, but normal. Malrotation and inversion of abdominal viscera are common As above, without malrotation and inversion

Hiatal hernia
  Sliding hiatal hernia
  Fixed hiatal hernia
	Congenital potential hernia. The enlarged esophageal hiatus of the diaphragm permits the cardia of the stomach to enter the mediastinum above the diaphragm. The phrenoesophageal ligament is attenuated and stretched. The gastroesophageal junction can be freely movable or fixed in the thorax	Sac lies anterior and lateral to the herniated stomach
		Contents: cardiac stomach
			A large hiatus (admitting three fingers) can be a predisposing factor; actual herniation usually occurs in late adult life
			Has been seen in newborn infants

Paraesophageal hernia	Congenital potential hernia. The cardia is in the normal position. The fundus has herniated through the hiatus, into the thorax	Sac lies anterior to the esophagus and posterior to the pericardium Contents: fundus of stomach. Body of stomach, transverse colon, omentum, and spleen can enter the sac later	An esophageal hiatus larger than normal can be the predisposing factor Actual herniation occurs in late adult life
Short esophagus	Congenital hernia The cardia of the stomach is fixed in the mediastinum	No sac	This lesion is rare. It appears to be the result of failure of the embryonic esophagus to elongate sufficiently to bring the gastroesophageal junction into the abdomen

stood lesion. It has been found in stillborn infants, but its congenital origin is not well established.

The two requirements for a sliding hiatal hernia appear to be an enlarged hiatus and a weakened phrenoesophageal ligament.

Because both conditions are exacerbated by the hernia, the opening is further dilated and the ligament further stretched. When actual herniation occurs, there is an empty hernial sac of peritoneum on the left side of the stomach. On the right, the small bare area of the stomach has no peritoneal covering (Fig. 52-4A).

Congenital short esophagus can simulate hiatal hernia. It is present in children, although it might be asymptomatic. The phrenoesophageal ligament is normal, there is no hernial sac, and the left gastric artery is not displaced upward. The condition is often familial, and it is more common in males. It is sometimes associated with pyloric stenosis, malrotation, and Marfan syndrome. We believe that although it is rare, short esophagus is a true congenital malformation.

Nyhus believes that short esophagus is not congenital and the shortening is caused by secondary factors in an esophagus of normal length. He stated that infants with chalasia develop peptic esophagitis and then shortening of the esophagus.

Congenital short esophagus has long been the subject of debate. Three conditions must be considered.

1. Grossly normal esophagus. The lower portion of the esophagus is lined with gastric mucosa (Barrett's esophagus) (Barrett 1950). This condition can also be described as heterotopic gastric mucosa. Far from being a benign anomaly, as Gray and colleagues believe, it can be a precursor of adenocarcinoma, as Starnes and coworkers and Saubien and colleagues suggest. As Skinner and colleagues and Sanfey and colleagues report, this metaplasia is often associated with gastroesophageal reflux.
2. Irreducible partially supradiaphragmatic true stomach. The stomach has herniated into the thorax through an en-

larged diaphragmatic esophageal hiatus and become fixed. This condition is true fixed hiatal hernia.
3. Partially supradiaphragmatic true stomach existing from birth and not reducible. This condition is true congenital short esophagus and is very rare.

Barrett believed that congenital short esophagus could be recognized by the absence of a hernial sac. Branches of the left gastric artery do not pass upward through the hiatus. According to Gray and Skandalakis, only a small percentage of hiatal hernias belong to this group. Gozzetti and colleagues stated that acquired short esophagus is the result of gastroesophageal reflux of gastric and biliopancreatic fluids.

If the gastroesophageal junction remains in its normal position, the fundus of the stomach can herniate through an enlarged hiatus anterior to the esophagus producing a paraesophageal hiatal hernia (Fig. 52-4B). There is a peritoneal sac anterior to the esophagus containing stomach and, in extreme instances, transverse colon and

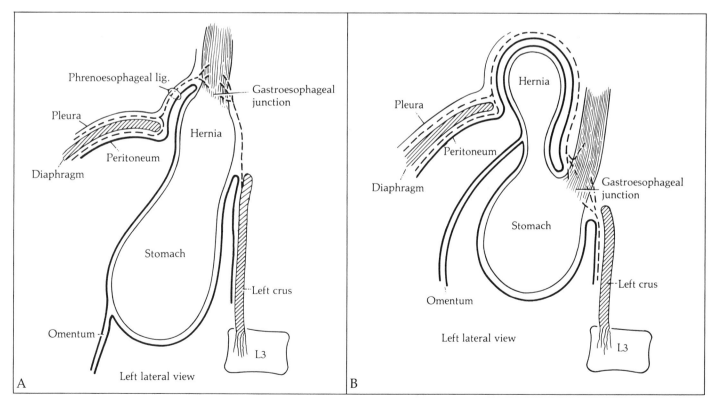

Fig. 52-4. Hiatal hernias. A. Sliding hiatal hernia seen from the left. The gastroesophageal junction is in the thorax. B. Paraesophageal hernia seen from the left. The gastroesophageal junction is in its normal location; the fundus has herniated into the thorax through the hiatus anterior to the esophagus.

omentum. Obstruction of the distal esophagus or the stomach is the usual result.

Posterolateral (Bochdalek) Defects

The defect begins at the vertebrocostal trigone, above and lateral to the left lateral arcuate ligament (Fig. 52-5). At the time of intestinal return to the abdomen, this trigone is membranous, with few muscle fibers; even at maturity it is variable in size and degree of muscular development. Spreading of the muscle fibers permits a defect, the foramen of Bochdalek, to form and spread upward and forward on the dome of the diaphragm to include the site of the embryonic pleuroperitoneal canal.

The defect can be as small as 1 cm in diameter or it might involve almost the entire hemidiaphragm. It is much more common on the left. During an operation, usually no hernial sac is found. The small intestine, stomach, colon, or spleen can be present in the thorax at birth. The lung on the affected side is usually hypoplastic (Fig. 52-6).

Bilateral defects have been reported.

Parasternal (Morgagni) Defects

Between attachments of the diaphragm to the xiphoid process and to the seventh costal cartilage, there is a small gap in the musculature on either side of the xiphoid process (foramina of Morgagni). Herniation at these sites represent only approximately 3 percent of surgically treated hernias of the diaphragm. The gaps are filled with fat, and the superior epigastric arteries and veins pass through them (see Figs. 52-5 and 52-12).

Herniation through these muscular gaps is almost always the result of postnatal trauma. The hernia is more often on the right, and the herniated organs are usually the omentum, colon, and, eventually, stomach. A sac can be present, or it might have ruptured and disappeared. There might be a predisposition to herniation in persons with large foramina or in individuals with more fat between muscle fibers, but this pattern has not been demonstrated. Harrison and colleagues have performed intrauterine repair of congenital hernias, and increased experience has resulted in success in seven infants. Al-

though Nyhus expresses some concern about the procedure (*Mastery of Surgery* [2nd ed]. P 409), he nevertheless feels it offers "truly amazing therapeutic vistas." We call this procedure the triumph of pediatric surgery.

Omental herniation through the foramen of Morgagni has been reported. Laparoscopic procedure has been used to repair this defect.

A very rare case of diaphragmatic hernia in identical twins has been reported. This instance suggests the possibility that diaphragmatic hernia is an inheritable defect.

Eventration of the Diaphragm

Congenital eventration describes the abnormal elevation of one leaf of the diaphragm. The entire leaf bulges upward in contrast to the localized defect of a foramen of Bochdalek hernia (Fig. 52-7). The left side is affected more often than the right, and males are affected more often than females. The phrenic nerve appears normal, but the eventrated leaf can consist of a fascial layer with few or no muscle fibers between the pleura and peritoneum. The failure is of muscularization rather than fusion of embryonic components. Intestinal malrotation is often associated. The lung is usually partially collapsed but not hypoplastic; the mediastinum is shifted to the contralateral side, which further reduces ventilation.

By contrast, acquired eventration is the result of phrenic nerve injury with normal musculature. The acquired lesion can be temporary; the congenital lesion is permanent unless repaired.

Eventration can be unilateral or bilateral and can rupture in later life. Eventration and acute gastric volvulus have been seen in pediatric patients.

Peritoneopericardial Hernia

Peritoneopericardial hernia is a rare hernia that is embryologically inexplicable. It has been reported in newborn infants and in adults. A hernial sac, or a trace of one, has been found in a few instances. Because the defect is in the central tendon and the overlying pericardium, it originates in that part of the diaphragm formed by the transverse septum.

Liver herniation into the pericardium through the central tendon has been reported. Investigators have found that

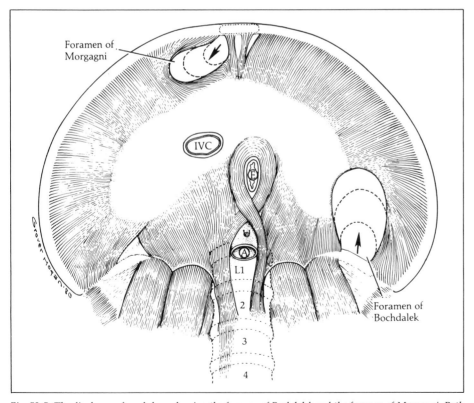

Fig. 52-5. The diaphragm from below, showing the foramen of Bochdalek and the foramen of Morgagni. Both are weak areas of potential herniation. Arrows indicate the direction of enlargement after herniation has begun.

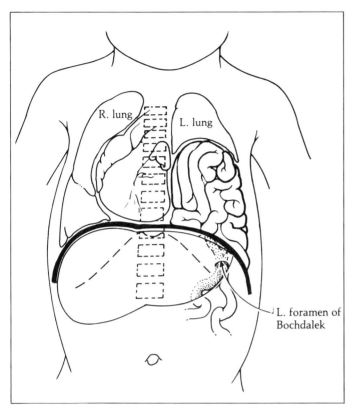

Fig. 52-6. Herniation of intestines through the foramen of Bochdalek compressing the left lung. The mediastinum is shifted to the right, reducing the volume of the right lung also.

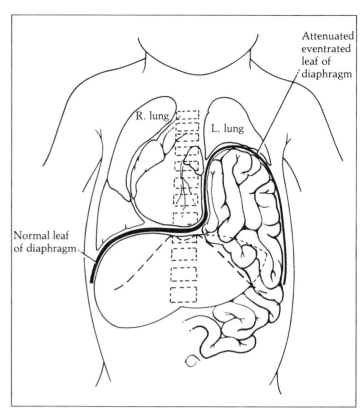

Fig. 52-7. Eventration of the (left) diaphragm. The herniated abdominal organs remain beneath the attenuated but intact leaf of the diaphragm. Both lungs are compressed and the mediastinum is shifted to the right. Compare with Fig. 52-6.

symptoms of diaphragmatic hernia might not appear until viscera incarcerate in it years after a causal injury.

Other Anomalies Associated with Diaphragmatic Defects

Diaphragmatic anomalies can be associated with other congenital anomalies such as Cantrell's pentology, tracheal agenesis, genetic syndromes with omphalocele, gastroschisis, intestinal atresias and stenoses, and obstructive uropathies.

Anatomy of the Diaphragm

It is not within the scope of this chapter to present the physiology of the diaphragm, but the following information is pertinent. Roentgenographic findings support the hypothesis that the cardiac mass is responsible for the caudad displacement of the related hemidiaphragm; this finding is contrary to the classic teaching that it is the liver that lifts the corresponding hemidiaphragm.

The function of the diaphragm, which is composed of skeletal voluntary muscle, is as automatic as the function of the heart, with the difference that the cardiac myocytes function as a syncytium. It has been suggested that the diaphragm is second in importance only to the heart in maintaining life.

The Pediatric Diaphragm

The following observations have been made from anatomic and ultrasonographic studies of the diaphragm in newborn infants:

1. The diaphragm inserts only on the anterior costodiaphragmatic rib cage border.
2. From anterolaterally to posteriorly, the diaphragmatic insertion has increasingly greater distance from the rib cage.
3. The dorsal diaphragm ends its free course at the eleventh rib and continues caudally, ending between the twelfth rib and the crista iliaca. The diaphragm in the newborn acts as a bellows moving

mainly in the posterior part, whereas in the adult it acts as a piston (Fig. 52-8). The diaphragm of the newborn, which has a flat curve because of its large angle of insertion on the rib cage and small area of apposition, has only one physiologic destiny—"to suck in the rib cage rather than air." It is this rib cage action that reduces the area of apposition and results in an increase in chest volume.

Origins and Insertions of the Diaphragmatic Musculature

The diaphragm is composed of a central tendinous area from which muscle fibers radiate in all directions toward their peripheral attachments (Fig. 52-9).

Sternal Portion (Anterior). Paired slips of muscle originate from the xiphoid process and the aponeurosis of the transversus abdominis muscle. Small triangular spaces (foramina of Morgagni) separate those slips from the costal fibers and from each other (see Figs. 52-5 and 52-9).

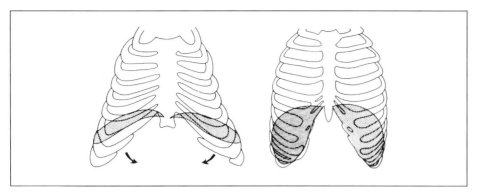

Fig. 52-8. Developmental changes of the rib cage and the anterior and lateral diaphragmatic insertions from birth (left) to adulthood (right). The stippled surface represents the anterior projection of the diaphragm. (From H Devlieger, H Daniels, G Marchal, et al. The diaphragm of the newborn infant: anatomical and ultrasonographic studies. J Dev Physiol 16:321, 1991. Reproduced with permission.)

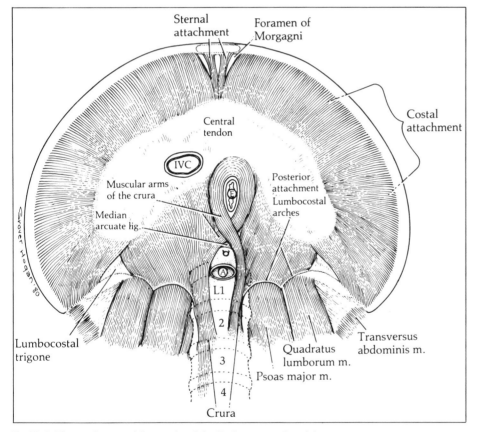

Fig. 52-9. The attachments of the muscles of the diaphragm seen from below.

The Crura.

The crura arise from the anterior surface of L1 to L4 on the right, and L1 to L2 or L3 on the left, as well as from the intervertebral disks and the anterior longitudinal ligament. The crural fibers pass superiorly and anteriorly, forming the muscular arms that surround the openings for the aorta and the esophagus; they insert on the central tendon. At their origin on the vertebrae, the crura are tendinous, becoming increasingly muscular as they ascend into the diaphragm proper (Fig. 52-10). In our studies of cadavers, we found the crura to be tendinous, posteriorly and medially, from their vertebral origins to the level of the tenth thoracic vertebra, in 90 percent of cadavers. Sutures to approximate the crura should always be placed through the tendinous portions.

The pattern of the crural arms at the esophageal hiatus is variable. In one-half or more of persons, both right and left arms arise from the right crus (Fig. 52-11A). In another one-third or more, the left arm arises from the right crus, and the right arm arises from both crura (Fig. 52-11B). The remaining persons present a variety of uncommon patterns. Hiatal hernia is not associated with any specific hiatal pattern.

The Arcuate Ligaments.

The lateral arcuate ligaments (lumbocostal arches) compose the thickened fascia of the upper surface of the quadratus lumborum muscles, which attach to the twelfth ribs laterally and to the transverse processes of L1 medially. The medial arcuate ligaments (medial arches) compose the similarly thickened fascia of the psoas muscles, which attach to the transverse processes of L1 laterally and to the body of L1 or L2 medially. The medial arcuate ligaments are separated from each other by the crura and the median arcuate ligament to be described later. From these two pairs of arcuate ligaments on either side arise the muscle fibers of the posterior portion of the diaphragm (see Fig. 52-9).

The Central Tendon

All the musculature described so far inserts on the fibrous central tendon of the diaphragm. The thickened portion anterior to the esophageal hiatus and to the left of the caval aperture is sometimes called the *cruciform* (transverse) *ligament*. Fibers on the superior surface of the central tendon blend with those of the fibrous peri-

Costal Portion (Anterolateral).

Muscle fibers arise from the cartilages of the seventh and eighth ribs, the cartilage and bony portions of the ninth rib, and the distal bony portions of the tenth to twelfth ribs. Anteriorly these origins are related to the origins of the transversus abdominis; on the twelfth rib they are related to the attachment of the thoracolumbar fascia.

Lumbar Portion (Posterior).

Posteriorly the diaphragmatic muscle arises from the crura and the medial and lateral arcuate ligaments (lumbocostal arches).

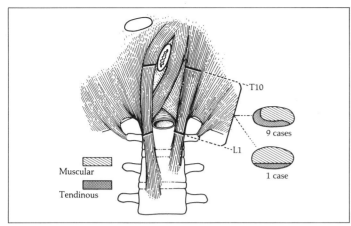

Fig. 52-10. The crura consist of both tendinous and muscular tissue; only the tendinous portion holds sutures. In 9 out of 10 persons, the medial edge of the crura is tendinous. (From SW Gray, JS Rowe Jr, and JE Skandalakis. Surgical anatomy of the gastroesophageal junction. Am Surg 45:575, 1979. Reproduced with permission.)

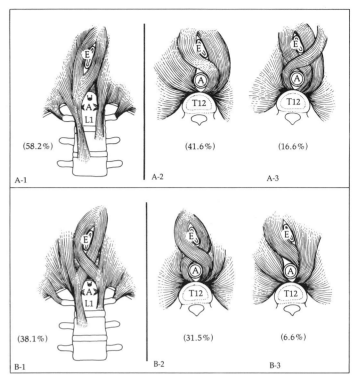

Fig. 52-11. The most common patterns of the diaphragmatic crura. A-1 and B-1 seen from below. A-2, A-3 and B-2, B-3 seen from above. (Data from V A Pataro et al. Anatomic aspects of the esophageal hiatus: distribution of the crura in its formation. J Int Coll Surg 35:154, 1961.)

cardium. Patches of muscle are often present among the fibers of the central tendon.

The Openings of the Diaphragm

The Hiatus of the Inferior Vena Cava.
The hiatus of the inferior vena cava lies in the right lobe of the central tendon approximately 1 inch to the right of the midline and at the level of T8. The margins of the hiatus are fixed to the vena cava, which is accompanied by branches of the right phrenic nerve (Fig. 52-12).

The collagen fiber bundles forming the right margin of the caval hiatus cross inferiorly to the bundles forming the medial and posterior margins to form a fibrous limb that can be traced to the edge of the central tendon. The tendinous fibers forming the medial margin of the hiatus are attached to the muscle fibers of the right crus. This arrangement is often omitted in textbook illustrations of the caval hiatus. Whether this arrangement of fibers constricts or enlarges the caval hiatus during inspiration has been a source of controversy for many years. Constriction of the

vena cava during inspiration is known to occur in diving mammals such as the seal. In these animals, a muscular sphincter takes the place of the fibrous bundles found in the human diaphragm. No parallel can be drawn between seal and human.

The Esophageal Hiatus.
The elliptical esophageal hiatus is in the muscular portion of the diaphragm an inch or less to the left of the midline at the level of T10 (Figs. 52-13 and 52-14). The anterior and lateral margins of the hiatus are formed by the muscular arms of the diaphragmatic crura, and the posterior margin is formed by the median arcuate ligament (see Fig. 52-9). The anterior and posterior vagal trunks and the esophageal arteries and veins from the left gastric vessels pass through the hiatus with the esophagus. In this region, the portal circulation (left gastric vein) communicates with the systemic circulation (esophageal branches of the azygos veins).

The esophageal hiatus is of great surgical importance and is considered in more detail later.

In a study of 50 human diaphragms there were five variations in the formation of the esophageal hiatus. In 62 percent, the hiatus was formed by both crura, with the right constituting most of the border and the left sharing only in the formation of the posterior border. In 10 percent, the hiatus was formed by the medial parts of both crura equally. In 10 percent, the hiatus was formed by the right crus only. In 2 percent, the left crus exclusively formed the hiatus. In 16 percent, both crura were located posteriorly and the hiatus was bounded from the median arcuate ligament by a V-shaped band.

Hiatal hernia can be defined as the protrusion of a portion of the stomach into the thoracic mediastinum through the esophageal hiatus of the diaphragm. A hernial sac is present. Akerlund was one of the first to classify hernia in this area, and he might have been first to use the term "hiatal hernia." He recognized three types of hernia that occur: sliding, paraesophageal, and congenital short esophagus. Today we recognize an additional type: combined sliding and paraesophageal. The anatomy

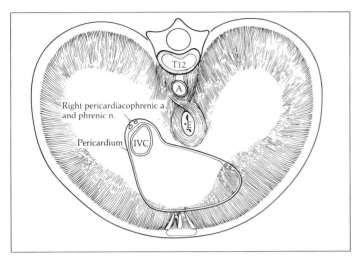

Fig. 52-12. *The diaphragm viewed from above. The area in contact with the pericardium is indicated. The pericardial fibrous tissue is continuous with that of the diaphragm.*

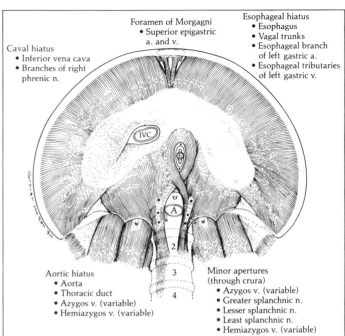

Esophageal hiatus
• Esophagus
• Vagal trunks
• Esophageal branch of left gastric a.
• Esophageal tributaries of left gastric v.

Foramen of Morgagni
• Superior epigastric a. and v.

Caval hiatus
• Inferior vena cava
• Branches of right phrenic n.

Aortic hiatus
• Aorta
• Thoracic duct
• Azygos v. (variable)
• Hemiazygos v. (variable)

Minor apertures (through crura)
• Azygos v. (variable)
• Greater splanchnic n.
• Lesser splanchnic n.
• Least splanchnic n.
• Hemiazygos v. (variable)

Fig. 52-13. *The apertures of the diaphragm seen from below and the structures transversing them.*

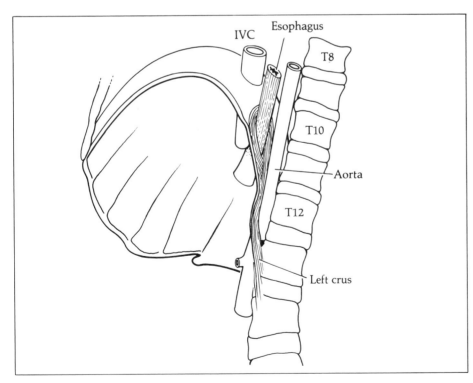

Fig. 52-14. *The diaphragmatic openings for the inferior vena cava (IVC), the esophagus, and the aorta as seen from the left.*

of the normal esophageal hiatus is shown in Fig. 52-15A.

Sliding Hiatal Hernia. The esophagus moves freely through the hiatus with the gastroesophageal junction being in the thorax or in the normal position at different times. It is usually found in the normal position at autopsy. Sliding hernias (Fig. 52-15B) constitute 90 percent of all hiatal hernias. Although these hernias do slide back and forth through the hiatus, they are called sliding hernias because the stomach composes part of the wall of the hernial sac. Thus, they are analogous with sliding inguinal hernias.

A sliding hernia can become secondarily fixed in the thorax by adhesion. In such instances, the esophagus appears to be too short to reach the diaphragm because of contraction of the longitudinal muscle coat. This type is uncommon.

Paraesophageal Hiatal Hernia. In this type of hernia (Fig. 52-15C), the gastro-esophageal junction remains in its normal location. The gastric fundus and greater curvature bulge through the hiatus anterior to the esophagus. Volvulus of the herniated stomach is a major complication.

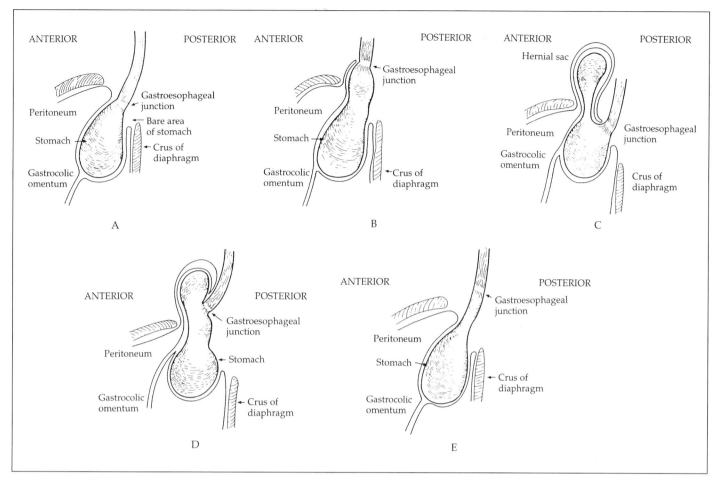

Fig. 52-15. The esophageal hiatus in sagittal section with the (A) normal anatomy and the various abnormalities described in the text, (B) sliding hiatal hernia, (C) paraesophageal hiatal hernia, (D) combined sliding and paraesophageal, (E) congenital short esophagus. (From SW Gray, LJ Skandalakis, and JE Skandalakis. Classification of Hernias Through the Oesophageal Hiatus. In GG Jamieson (ed.), Surgery of the Oesophagus. Edinburgh: Churchill Livingstone, 1988. Reproduced with permission.)

Combined Sliding and Paraesophageal. The gastroesophageal junction is displaced upward as in a sliding hernia, and the fundus and greater curvature are herniated as in a paraesophageal hernia. Paraesophageal hernias usually are of the combined type (Fig. 52-15D).

Congenital Short Esophagus. This type (Fig. 52-15E) has been discussed under the heading Hiatal Hernia.

Abdominal Esophagus. Anatomically, the last 0.5–4 cm of the esophagus lies below the diaphragm, forming the abdominal esophagus. With decrease in the length of the abdominal esophagus, the pressure necessary for competence of the sphincter rises exponentially. Normal lower esophageal sphincter pressure values vary from 14.5 to 34 mmHg. Ninety percent of pa-

tients with lower esophageal sphincter pressure below 5 mmHg experience reflux, regardless of the length of the abdominal esophagus. Similarly, reflux occurs in 90 percent if the length of the abdominal esophagus is less than 1 cm. Thus, sphincteric incompetence is the result of a low sphincter pressure, a short abdominal esophagus, or both.

If the abdominal esophagus were the only factor governing reflux, all patients with hiatal hernia would have esophagitis. This situation is not the case. If the hernial sac, carried up into the mediastinum, can transmit intra-abdominal pressure to the distal esophagus it can support the sphincter. It seems clear that the abdominal esophagus plays a role in the prevention of reflux; precisely what that role is remains to be determined.

The Phrenoesophageal Ligament (Membrane). A strong, flexible, airtight seal is necessary at the esophageal hiatus of the diaphragm. The seal is provided by the pleura above and the peritoneum below; strength and flexibility are provided by the phrenoesophageal ligament.

The major component of the ligament is collagenous, elastic fibers that arise as a continuation of the endoabdominal (transversalis) fascia beneath the diaphragm. One leaf of this fascia passes upward through the hiatus forming a truncated cone that inserts in the adventitia and intermuscular connective tissue of the esophagus 1 or 2 cm above the diaphragm. A second leaf of the fascia turns downward and inserts into the adventitia of the abdominal esophagus and the stomach. A weaker and less constant component can

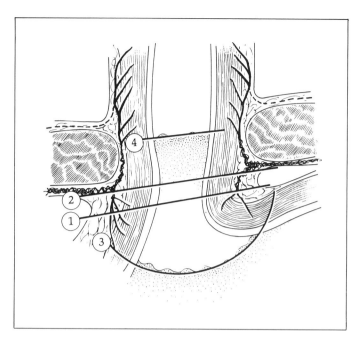

Fig. 52-16. Structures at the gastroesophageal junction and the diaphragmatic hiatus. (From Anatomical Complications in General Surgery, by John E. Skandalakis, Stephen W. Gray, Joseph S. Rowe, Jr., published by McGraw-Hill, New York, 1983. Reproduced with permission.)

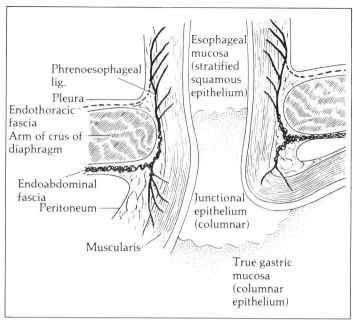

Fig. 52-17. The gastroesophageal junction from the point of view of (1) the anatomist, (2) the surgeon, (3) the radiologist, and (4) the endoscopist. (From Anatomical Complications in General Surgery, by John E. Skandalakis, Stephen W. Gray, Joseph S. Rowe, Jr., published by McGraw-Hill, New York, 1983. Reproduced with permission.)

arise from the endothoracic fascia, passing upward to join the fibers of the endoabdominal fascia. The relations of these components of the phrenoesophageal ligament are shown in Fig. 52-16.

The upper leaf of the phrenoesophageal ligament inserts into the esophagus an average of 3.35 cm above the squamocolumnar epithelial junction. In 227 patients with esophagitis, as noted by Bombeck and colleagues, the insertion was only about 0.5 cm above the epithelial junction.

The development of the phrenoesophageal membrane has been studied by Botros and his group. They agree with Carey and Hollinshead that loose connective tissue with collagenous and elastic fibers arises from both surfaces of the diaphragm and attaches to the esophagus. Between these fascial components, a layer of crural striated muscle is found in the 10-week-old fetus. With age, the muscle fibers undergo gradual regression and replacement with collagen fibers. Muscle fibers in the adult phrenoesophageal membrane should be considered vestigial.

Botros and colleagues found that the superior component, from the superior diaphragmatic fascia, appears first and forms about two-thirds of the total thickness at 16 weeks of embryonic age. By 20 weeks of age, the superior and inferior diaphragmatic fasciae contribute equally to the membrane. The first result in postnatal life is the fusion of the inner, compact layers from the upper and lower surface of the diaphragmatic fascia before reaching the esophagus and their fanning out to end in the esophageal adventitia. We agree with Botros and associates' conclusion that further development of the membrane occurs after birth.

Descriptions of the phrenoesophageal ligament vary because the tissue changes with age. In the fetus, the esophagus and diaphragm are tightly joined at the hiatus by connective tissue. With the onset of respiratory movements and swallowing in postnatal life, the two structures become less firmly attached, and the space between them fills with loose connective tissue and fat.

The development of the phrenoesophageal ligament can be summarized as follows (per investigations by Androvlakis and colleagues):

1. In newborn infants, the phrenoesophageal ligament is present.

2. In adults, the ligament is attenuated and subperitoneal fat accumulates at the hiatus.

3. In adults with hiatal hernias, the ligament for all practical purposes does not exist.

The Gastroesophageal Junction. The external gastroesophageal junction can be described as the point at which the esophageal tube becomes the gastric pouch. From 0.5 to 2.5 cm of the tube lies in the abdomen. The external junction lies at the level of T11 or T12.

Internally, the junction is marked by an irregular boundary between stratified squamous esophageal epithelium and columnar gastric epithelium. This boundary can lie as far as 1 cm above the external junction. A biopsy specimen of esophageal mucosa should be taken at least 2 cm above the external junction.

The columnar epithelium below the internal junction contains mucus-secreting glands, the cardiac glands of the histologists, without the chief and parietal cells that characterize the true gastric glands of the body of the stomach. The term *junctional epithelium* has been proposed by Hayward.

The external and internal junctions do not coincide; in addition, the loose submucosal connective tissue permits considerable movement between the mucosa and the muscularis externa, changing the relation between them as the stomach fills with food. Figure 52-17 shows the gastroesophageal junction from several points of view.

The Lower Esophageal Sphincter. A sphincter at the distal end of the esophagus normally permits swallowing but not reflux. No specialized muscular ring guards this opening, such as is found in the pylorus, although several investigators have reported a thickening of the circular muscle in most individuals.

A number of mechanisms for closing the distal esophagus have been suggested: the angle (of His), at which the esophagus enters the stomach; the pinchcock action of the diaphragm; a plug of redundant mucosa (mucosal rosette); the sling of oblique fibers of the gastric musculature; and factors relating to wall tension of the stomach as a force contributing to sphincter opening. Regardless of the mechanism, the average resting pressure of the lower esophageal sphincter is 35 mm Hg. This mechanism permits one to stand on one's head without losing one's lunch. Incompetence of this closing mechanism with esophageal reflex might or might not be associated with sliding hiatal hernia.

The Aortic Opening. The oblique course of the aorta takes it behind the diaphragm rather than through it (see Fig. 52-14). At the level of T12, the anterior border of the opening is the median arcuate ligament; laterally the diaphragmatic crura form its margins. The thoracic duct and sometimes the azygos vein accompany the aorta.

Other Openings in the Diaphragm. Anteriorly the superior epigastric vessels pass through the parasternal spaces (foramina of Morgagni). In the dome of the diaphragm, the phrenic nerves pierce the upper surface to become distributed over the lower surface between the muscle and the peritoneum.

The azygos vein can pass behind the diaphragm with the aorta, to the right of the right crus, or it can pierce the right crus. Also passing through the crura are the greater, lesser, and least splanchnic nerves (see Fig. 52-13).

The Median Arcuate Ligament. The esophageal hiatus is separated from the aortic hiatus by fusion of the arms of the left and right crura. If the tendinous portions of the crura are fused, the median arcuate ligament is present as a fibrous arch passing over the aorta, connecting the right and left crura. If the fusion is muscular only, the ligament is ill defined or absent.

The median arcuate ligament passes in front of the aorta at the level of L1 just above the origin of the celiac trunk (see Figs. 52-6 and 52-9). The celiac ganglia lie just below and lateral to the celiac trunk. The ligament and the origin of the celiac artery become slightly lower with increasing age. In 16 percent of patients, a low median arcuate ligament covers the celiac artery and can compress it. At angiography, such compression can simulate atherosclerotic plaques. Adequate collateral circulation exists, since such patients usually do not have symptoms. The median arcuate ligament has been implicated in abdominal angina in instances in which substantial, tense, fibromuscular tissue at the hiatus exerted a constrictive effect on the celiac trunk or the aorta.

If there is no true ligament, and the muscular arms of the crura are thinned by posterior extension of the esophageal hiatus, the aortic and esophageal openings can become practically confluent, although there is always some connective tissue between them.

In approximately one-half of the cadavers with hiatal hernia that we examined, the ligament was sufficiently well developed to use in surgical repair of the esophageal hiatus. In the remainder, there was enough preaortic fascia lateral to the celiac trunk to perform a posterior fixation of the gastroesophageal junction. The celiac ganglion, just below the arcuate ligament, must be avoided.

Diaphragmatic/Pleural/Mediastinal Relations

Over much of the anterosuperior surface of the diaphragm, the fibrous tissue of the central tendon is continuous with the fibrous pericardium (see Fig. 52-12).

In addition to the pericardium, the mediastinum on the right contains the inferior vena cava, the right phrenic nerve, the right pulmonary ligament, the esophagus with the right vagal trunk, the azygos vein, the vertebral bodies, and the right sympathetic trunk (Fig. 52-18).

In the left mediastinum (Fig. 52-19) are the pericardium, the left phrenic nerve, the esophagus, the left vagal trunk, the descending aorta, the vertebral bodies, and the left sympathetic trunk. The triangle (of Truesdale) formed by the pericardium, the aorta, and the diaphragm contains the left pulmonary ligament and the distal esoph-

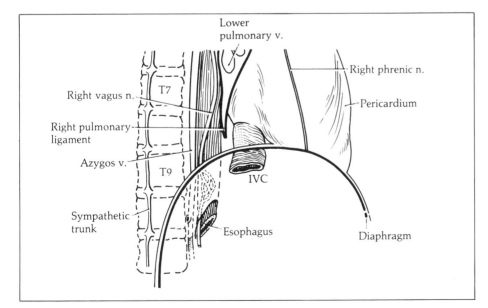

Fig. 52-18. Structures in the inferior portion of the right mediastinum.

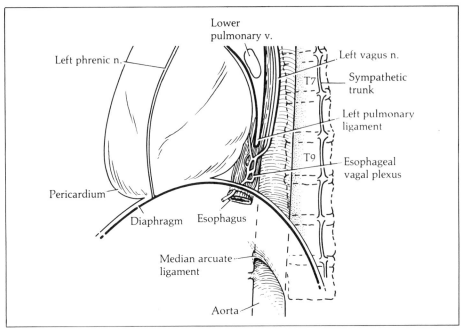

Fig. 52-19. Structures in the inferior portion of the left mediastinum.

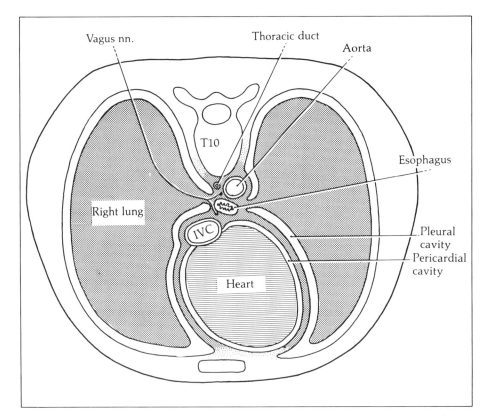

Fig. 52-20. Cross section through the thorax at the level of T10 showing the relation of the pleura to the distal esophagus. (From SW Gray, JS Rowe Jr, and JE Skandalakis. Surgical anatomy of the gastroesophageal junction. Am Surg 45:575, 1979. Reproduced with permission.)

agus. In sliding hiatal hernia, the stomach is in this triangle.

The remainder of the superior surface of the diaphragm is covered with parietal pleura. The approximation of the right and left pleurae between the esophagus and the aorta forms the so-called mesoesophagus. The right pleura is in contact with the lower third of the esophagus almost down to the esophageal hiatus (Fig. 52-20). This situation creates the risk of accidental entrance into the pleural cavity during abdominal operations on the esophageal hiatus. In spite of this proximity of the right pleura, the surgeon, working on the right side of the operation table, is more likely to produce a pneumothorax or hemopneumothorax on the left.

The diaphragmatic pleura is part of the parietal pleura and covers all parts of the diaphragm except the part of the central tendon that is in contact with the pericardium. It is heavily fixed to the diaphragm through the phrenopleural fascia of the endothoracic fascia in such a way that separation from the diaphragm is practically impossible. This situation is in contrast to the costal pleura, which can be stripped away along with the endothoracic fascia.

The costodiaphragmatic recess is located at the reflection of the parietal pleura from the ribs to the diaphragm. The phrenomediastinal recess is between the mediastinum and the diaphragm.

The blood supply of the diaphragmatic pleura springs from the internal thoracic artery, thoracic aorta, and abdominal aorta or celiac artery. At the inferior surface of the diaphragm, these arteries form internal and external branches that anastomose with the vascular plexus of the costal pleura.

The inferior phrenic veins drain into the inferior vena cava and the superior phrenic (pericardiophrenic) veins, which run parallel with the internal thoracic artery to terminate in the right and left internal thoracic veins.

Table 52-2 summarizes the lymphatic drainage of pleural structures.

Peritoneal Reflections of the Inferior Surface of the Diaphragm and the Gastroesophageal Junction

The primitive dorsal and ventral mesenteries of the abdomen form a number of ligaments related to the diaphragm and the gastroesophageal junction (Fig. 52-21).

Falciform, Coronary, and Triangular Ligaments. The falciform ligament, a remnant of the primitive ventral mesentery, arises from the anterior abdominal wall and extends to the anterior surface of the liver and the diaphragm. In its free edge runs the round ligament, the obliterated left umbilical vein.

The leaves of the falciform ligament separate over the liver to form the anterior and posterior layers of the coronary ligament. Enclosing the bare area on the right, these leaves unite laterally to form the right triangular ligament. On the left, the leaves are in apposition to each other, forming the left triangular ligament. One approach to the gastroesophageal junction is to section the left triangular and left portion of the posterior layer of the coronary ligament.

In operating, one must be careful in mobilization of the liver, especially the left lobe, not to injure the left hepatic vein or the inferior vena cava.

Hepatogastric (Gastrohepatic) Ligament. The abdominal esophagus lies between the two layers of the hepatogastric ligament. This area is the superior part of the lesser omentum, derived from the primitive ventral mesentery. The inferior portion is the hepatoduodenal ligament. The hepatogastric ligament extends from the porta hepatis to the lesser curvature of the stomach and the abdominal esophagus. The ligament contains the left gastric artery and vein, the hepatic division of the left vagus nerve, and lymph nodes. It can also contain both vagal trunks, branches of the right gastric artery and vein, and the

Table 52-2. Lymph Nodes Draining Pleural Structures in the Human

Groups of Lymph Nodes	Pleural Structures Drained
Sternal	Parietal pleura: anterior thoracic wall Diaphragmatic pleura: anterior portion
Intercostal	Parietal pleura
Middle mediastinal	Diaphragmatic pleura: middle portion Visceral pleura
Anterior mediastinal	Diaphragmatic pleura: anterior portion Mediastinal pleura
Posterior mediastinal	Diaphragmatic pleura: posterior portion Visceral pleura: lower lobes

Source: From JF Bernaudin, J Fleury. Anatomy of the Blood and Lymphatic Circulation of the Pleural Serosa. In J Chretien, J Bignon, A Hirsch (eds.), *The Pleura in Health and Disease.* New York: Marcel Dekker, 1985. Reproduced with permission.

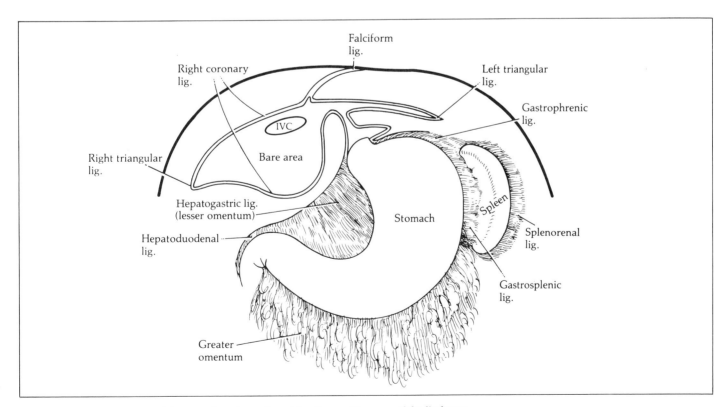

Fig. 52-21. Peritoneal reflections of the stomach, gastroesophageal junction, and bare area of the diaphragm. (From Anatomical Complications in General Surgery, *by John E. Skandalakis, Stephen W. Gray, Joseph S. Rowe, Jr., published by McGraw-Hill, New York, 1983. Reproduced with permission.)*

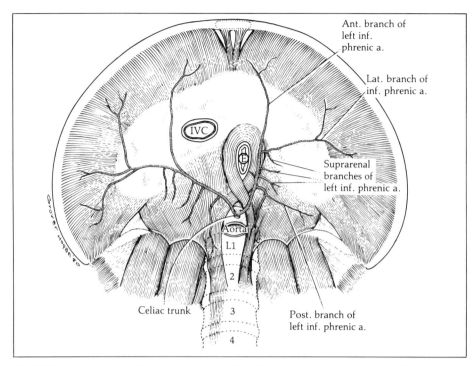

Fig. 52-22. *Arterial supply of the diaphragm from below. The inferior phrenic arteries can arise from the celiac trunk or directly from the aorta.*

left hepatic artery if it arises from the left gastric artery (26%).

Gastrosplenic (Gastrolienal) Ligament.

On the right, the hepatogastric ligament divides to enclose the abdominal esophagus; its leaves rejoin on the left to form the gastrosplenic ligament, which is part of the primitive dorsal mesentery. The hepatogastric ligament separates the lesser sac from the rest of the peritoneal cavity. The hepatogastric ligament is formed by the anterior leaf; the posterior leaf does not reach the gastroesophageal junction. Thus, a small bare area is left on the posterior wall of the stomach that lies over the left crus of the diaphragm and is easily separated from it by the surgeon's finger.

The upper portion of the gastrosplenic ligament contains the short gastric vessels and the pancreaticosplenic lymph nodes; the lower portion contains the left gastroepiploic vessels, lymph nodes, and the terminal branches of the splenic artery.

Gastrophrenic Ligament.

The gastrophrenic ligament, the superior portion of the dorsal mesentery, arises from the greater curvature of the fundus and extends upward to the diaphragm. The up-

per part is transparent and avascular, continuous with the posterior layer of the coronary ligament on the left. The lower part is continuous with the gastrosplenic ligament and contains some short gastric vessels and lymph nodes.

The upper, avascular area can be perforated by the surgeon's finger in order to insert a Penrose drain around the cardia. The surgeon can thus apply gentle traction on the esophagus, a useful maneuver in vagotomy.

Vascularization of the Diaphragm

Arteries. The arterial supply to the superior surface of the diaphragm consists of two branches from the internal thoracic arteries—the pericardiophrenic and musculophrenic arteries—and two branches from the thoracic aorta—the superior phrenic arteries. All these branches are small.

The major blood supply to the diaphragm is to the inferior surface and comes from the inferior phrenic arteries, which arise from the aorta or the celiac axis just below the median arcuate ligament of the diaphragm. In a small percentage of individuals, the right inferior phrenic artery arises

from the right renal artery. The inferior phrenic arteries also supply branches to the suprarenal glands (Fig. 52-22).

Left Inferior Phrenic Artery and Left Gastric Artery. The abdominal esophagus and the proximal stomach are supplied by esophageal branches of the left gastric artery. These branches usually, but not always, anastomose above the diaphragm with esophageal arteries from the aorta (Fig. 52-23A). In some persons, the lower esophagus also receives twigs from the left inferior phrenic artery (Fig. 52-23B). In still others, branches of the inferior phrenic artery supply the lower esophagus, whereas branches of the left gastric artery are confined to the cardia and fundus of the stomach (Fig. 52-23C). The margin of the hiatus is always supplied by a branch of the left inferior phrenic artery.

Aberrant Left Hepatic Artery. An aberrant left hepatic artery arising from the left gastric artery lies in the hepatogastric ligament in approximately 26 percent of persons. One must consider the possibility of such an artery before dividing the ligament to reach the gastroesophageal junction.

A study of the diaphragmatic circulation in dogs found the following:

1. Anastomosis between the phrenic arteries and internal thoracic arteries forms an arterial circle around the medial leaflet of the tendinous diaphragm.
2. From the circle described above, vascular branches travel toward the periphery of the diaphragm and anastomose with branches of the intercostal arteries forming costophrenic arcades along the costal diaphragm.
3. Anastomosis of the intercostal arteries to one another within the muscular diaphragm forms another arterial ring at the area of origin of the diaphragm from the ribs.

Veins. On the superior surface, small tributaries form the pericardiophrenic and musculophrenic veins, which run with the corresponding arteries and empty into the internal thoracic veins. Posteriorly there is some local drainage into the azygos and hemiazygos veins.

On the inferior surface, the right inferior phrenic vein runs with the artery and

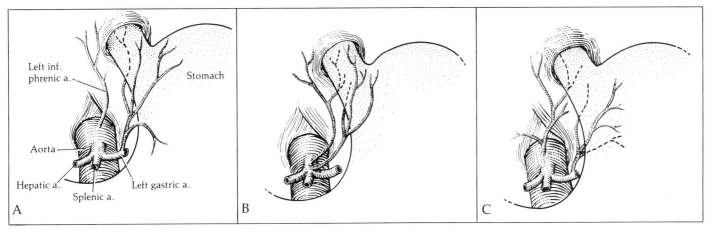

Fig. 52-23. *Variations in the blood supply to the distal esophagus and the esophageal hiatus. A. The inferior phrenic artery supplies the margin of the hiatus. An esophageal branch of the left gastric artery supplies the esophagus and anastomoses with thoracic esophageal arteries. This pattern is the most frequent one. B. The esophagus is supplied by esophageal branches of the left gastric and the inferior phrenic arteries without cranial anastomoses. C. The esophagus is supplied entirely by a branch of the inferior phrenic artery, which anastomoses with thoracic esophageal arteries. This pattern is rare. (From* Anatomical Complications in General Surgery, *by John E. Skandalakis, Stephen W. Gray, Joseph S. Rowe, Jr., published by McGraw-Hill, New York, 1983. Reproduced with permission.)*

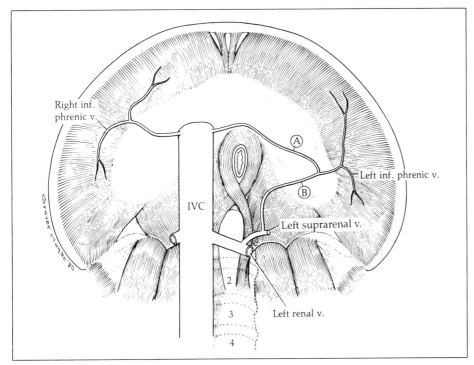

Fig. 52-24. *Venous drainage of the diaphragm from below. The left inferior phrenic vein may enter the inferior vena cava (A), the left suprarenal vein (B), or both.*

empties into the inferior vena cava. The left inferior phrenic vein enters the inferior vena cava, but it usually has a posterior branch that descends posteriorly to enter the left suprarenal vein (Fig. 52-24).

Left Inferior Phrenic Vein. The left inferior phrenic vein can drain into the left suprarenal vein or the inferior vena cava, or both. The branch draining into the vena cava passes in front of the esophagus closely enough to be injured.

Left Gastric (Coronary) Vein. The left gastric vein passes upward along the lesser curvature to a point 2 to 3 cm from the esophageal hiatus, where it receives one to three esophageal tributaries. From this point, it turns downward and obliquely to the right to join the portal vein or backward to enter the splenic vein.

In our own dissections of 22 cadavers, we found the left gastric vein entering the portal vein in 16 and entering the splenic vein in six instances. It is important to remember that the severed distal tributaries of the left gastric vein bleed from anastomoses with esophageal and hemiazygos veins in the thorax.

Other Vessels. The celiac trunk, the aorta, and the inferior vena cava are all close enough to the esophageal hiatus to be at risk during operations on the hiatus.

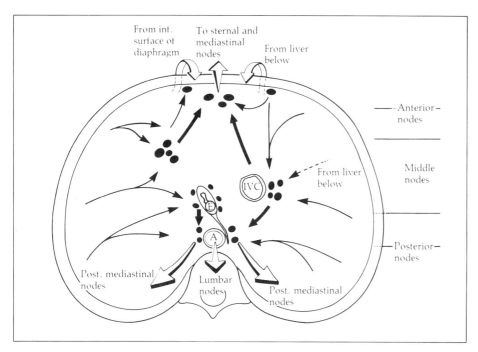

Fig. 52-25. Lymphatic drainage of the diaphragm seen from above. The diaphragm receives lymph from the liver below and sends it to ascending sternal, anterior, and posterior mediastinal nodes.

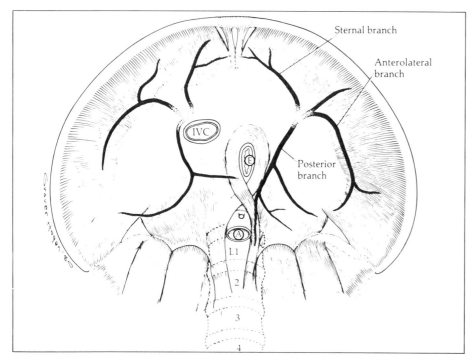

Fig. 52-26. The major branches of the phrenic nerves from below. Each phrenic nerve divides just before entering the diaphragm from above.

All the diaphragmatic lymph nodes lie on the superior surface of the diaphragm. These nodes can be divided into anterior, middle, and posterior groups (Fig. 52-25). They receive drainage from the upper surface of the liver, the gastroesophageal junction, and the abdominal surface of the diaphragm.

Efferent lymph vessels from these nodes drain upward to parasternal and mediastinal nodes anteriorly, and to posterior mediastinal and brachiocephalic nodes posteriorly.

Both thoracic and abdominal serosal surfaces of the diaphragm are active in the removal of fluid and cells from the pleural and peritoneal cavities. Pores between mesothelial cells from 4 to 12 μm in diameter open directly into the lymphatic vessels of the diaphragm. First seen in 1863 by von Recklinghausen, their existence has been confirmed by electron microscopy.

Thoracic Duct. The cisterna chyli, when present, lies on the bodies of L1 and L2 between the right crus of the diaphragm and the aorta. Division of the thoracic duct or other large lymph vessels in this area can result in chylous ascites. Ligation of the thoracic duct produces no ill effects.

Nerve Supply to the Diaphragm

The right phrenic nerve enters the diaphragm through the central tendon just lateral to the opening for the inferior vena cava. Occasionally, it passes through that opening with the vena cava. The left phrenic nerve pierces the superior surface of the muscular portion of the diaphragm just lateral to the left border of the heart.

Both nerves divide or trifurcate at or just above the diaphragm, and the branches travel together into the musculature. Small sensory branches are given off to the pleura and to the peritoneum over the central part of the diaphragm. The larger motor branches separate within the diaphragm into three or four major nerve trunks: sternal, anterolateral, posterolateral, and crural; the last two usually have a common trunk. These nerve trunks travel partly within the diaphragmatic musculature and partly on the inferior surface covered only by the peritoneum. The sternal branches of the two sides can anastomose behind the sternum (Fig. 52-26).

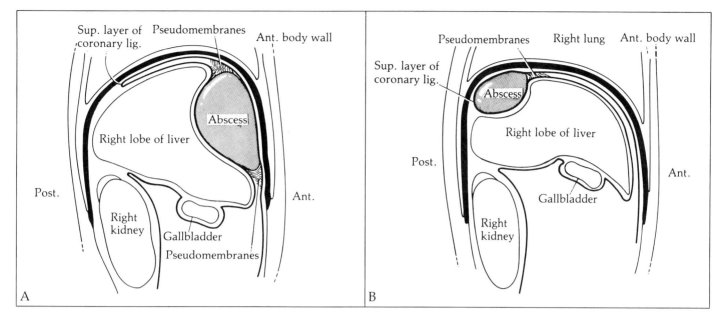

Fig. 52-27. *Right parasagittal sections. A. Fluid accumulation in the anterior portion of the right subphrenic space. B. Fluid accumulation in the posterior portion of the right subphrenic space. The fluid-filled spaces are usually walled off by pseudomembranes. The diaphragm is abnormally elevated over the region of fluid accumulation. (From* Anatomical Complications in General Surgery, *by John E. Skandalakis, Stephen W. Gray, Joseph S. Rowe, Jr., published by McGraw-Hill, New York, 1983. Reproduced with permission.)*

The peripheral portions of the pleura and peritoneum have an independent sensory innervation that arises from the seventh to the twelfth intercostal nerves.

In addition to the phrenic and intercostal nerves, fibers to the inferior surfaces of the right posterior portion of the diaphragm arise from the celiac ganglion, often forming a phrenic ganglion before their distribution. A connection has been claimed between these fibers and a posterior branch of the right phrenic nerve.

Vagal Trunks. Among 100 cadavers dissected by our group, the anterior and posterior vagal trunks passed through the hiatus with the esophagus in 88. In three others, the esophageal plexus was present at the hiatus and the trunks lay entirely within the abdomen. In another nine, the trunks had divided above the hiatus and their major divisions passed through the hiatus.

Celiac Ganglia. The celiac ganglia are closely adherent to the celiac artery at its origin from the aorta, and closely related to the crura of the diaphragm bilaterally. Sutures to approximate the crura must be placed above the ganglia and behind the celiac division of the posterior vagal trunk.

Subphrenic Spaces

A portion of the inferior surface of the diaphragm is attached directly to the liver without a serosal covering. This area is the bare area of the diaphragm (or liver). The margins of the bare area are peritoneal reflections that form the falciform, coronary, and triangular ligaments of the liver (see Fig. 52-21).

Outside the bare area, the serous (peritoneal) surfaces of the diaphragm and the liver are in apposition with a potential space between. This potential space is divided by the falciform ligament into right and left subphrenic (suprahepatic) compartments (see Fig. 52-21). These spaces can become the sites of peritoneal fluid collection and subphrenic abscesses.

The right and left compartments are defined as follows. The right subphrenic space is bounded above by the inferior surface of the right leaf of the diaphragm and below by the anterosuperior leaf of the diaphragm, the anterosuperior surface of the right lobe of the liver, and the medial segment of the left lobe. It is bounded medially by the falciform ligament and posteriorly by the right anterior coronary and right triangular ligaments. Anteriorly and inferiorly the space opens into the greater peritoneal cavity.

The left subphrenic space is bounded above by the inferior surface of the left leaf of the diaphragm and below by the superior surface of the lateral segment of the left lobe of the liver, and the fundus of the stomach. It is bounded medially by the falciform ligament and posteriorly by the left anterior coronary and left triangular ligaments. Anteriorly and laterally the space communicates with the infrahepatic space and the greater peritoneal cavity. On the left, the anterior and posterior leaves of the coronary ligament are in apposition.

In the absence of disease there is no distinction between anterior and posterior portions of the right space, but fluid may collect or an abscess may form anteriorly between the liver and diaphragm just beneath the sternum (right anterior subphrenic abscess) (Fig. 52-27A), or one may form at the reflection of the anterior leaf of the coronary ligament between the liver

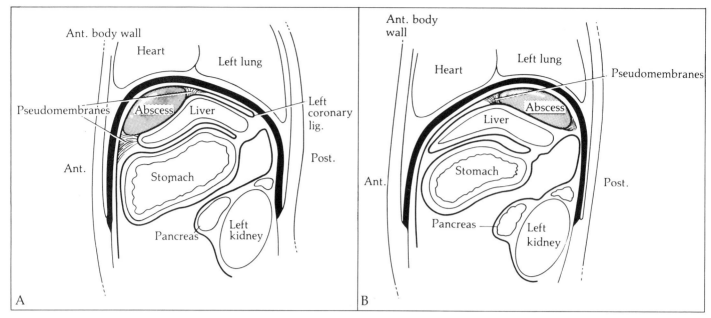

Fig. 52-28. Left parasagittal sections. A. Fluid accumulation in the anterior portion of the left subphrenic space. B. Fluid accumulation in the posterior portion of the left subphrenic space. Pseudomembranes limit the space occupied by fluid accumulations. (From Anatomical Complications in General Surgery, *by John E. Skandalakis, Stephen W. Gray, Joseph S. Rowe, Jr., published by McGraw-Hill, New York, 1983. Reproduced with permission.)*

and the diaphragm (right posterior subphrenic abscess) (Fig. 52-27B). Thus the single normal space can become compartmentalized by pseudomembranes into the anterior or posterior abscess sites of the clinician.

On the left, the subphrenic space can be similarly compartmentalized by pseudomembranes between the liver and diaphragm or abdominal wall (Fig. 52-28). If the collection of fluid is large, it can spread from the left subphrenic space into the communicating subhepatic space, where the stomach and spleen as well as the liver participate in walling off the infection. The diaphragm is usually elevated over the space occupied by the fluid collection.

The surgical approach to fluid collections in the subphrenic spaces is chosen after localization and determination of size and degree of extension of the abscess. Changes in the anatomy caused by the formation of pyogenic membranes and pressure of the abscess must be evaluated. Close cooperation between the surgeon and radiologist is necessary.

There are no anatomic complications using the anterior approach from beneath the costal margin. The posterior approach requires an incision at the level of the spinous process of L1 to avoid entering the pleura (Fig. 52-20 and Table 52-3).

Table 52-3. Approximate Rib Levels of Liver, Lung, and Pleura

Aspect	Upper Extent of Liver	Lower Extent of Lung	Lower Extent of Pleura
Anterior Lateral border of sternum	5th rib	6th rib	8th rib
Lateral Midaxillary line	6th rib	8th rib	10th rib
Posterior Level of vertebral spines	7th rib	10th rib	12th rib

Source: From RD Lockhart, GF Hamilton, FW Fyfe. *Anatomy of the Human Body*. Philadelphia: Lippincott, 1959. Reproduced with permission.

Suggested Reading

Akerlund A, Ohnell A, Key E. Hernia diaphragmatica hiatus oesophagi vom anatomischen und rontgenologischen gesichtspunkt. *Acta Radiol* 6:3, 1926.

Androulakis JA, Skandalakis JE, Gray SW. Contributions to the pathological anatomy of hiatal hernia. *J Med Assoc Ga* 55:295, 1966.

Barrett NR. Hiatus hernia: a review of some controversial points. *Brit J Surg* 42:231, 1954.

Bombeck CT, Dillard DW, Nyhus LM. Muscular anatomy of the gastroesophageal junction and role of phrenoesophageal ligament. *Ann Surg* 164:643, 1966.

Botros KG, El-Ayat AA, El-Naggar MM, State FA. The development of the human phreno-oesophageal membrane. *Acta Anat* 115:23, 1983.

Botros KG, Bondok AA, Gabr OM, et al. Anatomical variations in the formation of the human oesophageal hiatus. *Anat Anz* 171:193, 1990.

Carey JM, Hollinshead WH. Anatomic study of esophageal hiatus. *SGO* 100:196, 1955.

Comtois A, Gorczyca W, Grassino A. Anatomy of diaphragmatic circulation. *J Appl Physiol* 62:238, 1987.

DeMeester TR, Wernly JA, Bryant GH, et al. Clinical and in-vitro determinants of gastroesophageal competence: a study of the principles of antireflux surgery. *Am J Surg* 137:39, 1979.

Devlieger H, Daniels H, Marchal G, et al. The diaphragm of the newborn infant: anatomical and ultrasonographic studies. *J Dev Physiol* 16(6):321, 1991.

Ehren H, Frenckner B, Palmer K. Diaphragmatic hernia in infancy and childhood—20 years' experience. *Eur J Pediatr Surg* 2:327, 1992.

Fadhli HA. Congenital diaphragmatic obstruction of the aorta and the celiac artery. *J Thorac Cardiovasc Surg* 55:431, 1968.

Gahagan R. The function of the musculature of the esophagus and stomach in the esophagogastric sphincter mechanism. *Surg Gynecol Obstet* 114:293, 1962.

Gozzetti G, Pilotti V, Spangaro M, et al. Pathophysiology and natural history of acquired short esophagus. *Surgery* 102:507, 1987.

Gray SW, Skandalakis JE. *Embryology for Surgeons*. Philadelphia: Saunders, 1972.

Gray SW, Skandalakis LJ, Skandalakis JE. Classification of Hernias Through the Oesophageal Hiatus. In GG Jamieson (ed.), *Surgery of the Oesophagus*. Edinburgh: Churchill Livingstone, 1988.

Gray SW, Rowe JS Jr, Skandalakis JE. Surgical anatomy of the gastroesophageal junction. *Am Surg* 45:575, 1979.

Harris GJ, Soper RT, Kimura KK. Foramen of Morgagni hernia in identical twins: is this an inheritable defect? *J Pediatr Surg* 28:177, 1993.

Harrison MR, Langer JC, Adzick NS, et al. Correction of congenital diaphragmatic hernia in utero, V. Initial clinical experience. *J Pediatr Surg* 25:47, 1990.

Hart JC, Cohen IC, Ballantine TVN, Varrano LF. Accessory diaphragm in an infant. *J Pediatr Surg* 16:947, 1981.

Hidayet MA, Wahid HA, Wilson AS. Investigations on the innervation of the human diaphragm. *Anat Rec* 179:507, 1974.

Kaplan LJ, Bellows CF, Whitman GJR, Barnes AU. Coexistent diaphragmatic herniation and eventration: embryologic rationale for therapeutic intervention. *Clin Anat* 7:143, 1994.

Kleinman PK, Raptopoulos V. The anterior diaphragmatic attachments: an anatomic and radiologic study with clinical correlates. *Radiology* 155:289, 1985.

Kluth D, Tenbrinck R, von Ekesparre M, et al. The natural history of congenital diaphragmatic hernia and pulmonary hypoplasia in the embryo. *J Pediatr Surg* 28:456, 1993.

Krzyzaniak R, Gray SW. Accessory septum transversum: The first case report. *Am Surg* 52:278, 1986.

Leak LV. Gross and ultrastructural morphologic features of the diaphragm. *Am Rev Respir Dis* 119:3, 1979.

Libshitz I, Holbert JM. Anterior diaphragmatic lymph nodes. *Lymphology* 21:99, 1988.

Linder HH, Kemprud E. A clinicoanatomical study of the arcuate ligament of the diaphragm. *Arch Surg* 103:600, 1971.

Mishalany HG, Nakada K, Woolley MM. Congenital diaphragmatic hernias, eleven years' experience. *Arch Surg* 114:1118, 1979.

Mitchell TE, Ridley PD, Forrester-Wood CP. Spontaneous rupture of a congenital diaphragmatic eventration. *Eur J Cardiothorac Surg* 8:281, 1994.

Nyhus LM, Baker RJ. *Mastery of Surgery* (2nd ed.). Boston: Little, Brown, 1992. P 395.

O'Sullivan GC, DeMeester TR. The interaction between distal esophageal sphincter pressure and length of the abdominal esophagus as determinants of gastroesophageal competence. *Am J Surg* 143:40, 1982.

Payne WS, Ellis FH Jr. Esophagus and Diaphragmatic Hernias. In SI Schwartz (ed.), *Principles of Surgery*. New York: McGraw-Hill, 1984.

Pearl RK. *Gastrointestinal Endoscopy for Surgeons*. Boston: Little, Brown, 1984.

Pearson AA, Sauter RW, Oler RC. Relationship of the diaphragm to the inferior vena cava in human embryos and fetuses. *Thorax* 26:348, 1971.

Pettersson GB, Bombeck CT, Nyhus LM. The lower esophageal sphincter: Mechanisms of opening and closure. *Surgery* 88:307, 1980.

Pettersson GB, Bombeck CT, Nyhus LM. Influence of hiatal hernia on lower esophageal sphincter function. *Ann Surg* 193:215, 1981.

Reddy V, Sharma S, Cobanoglu A. What dictates the position of the diaphragm—the heart or the liver? A review of sixty-five cases. *J Thorac Cardiovasc Surg* 108:687, 1994.

Sabiston DC, Spencer FC (eds.). *Surgery of the Chest*. Philadelphia: Saunders, 1990.

Sanfey H, Hamilton SR, Smith RL, et al. Carcinoma arising in Barrett's esophagus. *Surg Gynecol Obstet* 161:570, 1985.

Saubier EC, Gouillat C, Samaniego C, et al. Adenocarcinoma in columnar-lined Barrett's esophagus. Analysis of 13 esophagectomies. *Am J Surg* 150:365, 1985.

Schmid C, Prokop M, Scheumann GF, et al. [Morgagni's Hernia: diagnosis and therapy] [German]. *Dtsch Med Wochenschr* 117:1057, 1992.

Sharp JT. Respiratory muscle: a review of old and newer concepts. *Lung* 157:185, 1980.

Skinner DB, Belsey RHR, Hendrix TR, et al. *Gastroesophageal Reflux and Hiatal Hernia*. Boston: Little, Brown, 1972.

Skinner DB, Walther RC, Riddell RH, et al. Barrett's esophagus: comparison of benign and malignant cases. *Ann Surg* 198:554, 1983.

Starnes VA, Adkins RB, Ballinger JF, et al. Barrett's esophagus. A surgical entity. *Arch Surg* 119:563, 1984.

Trutmann M, Sasse D. The lymphatics of the liver. *Anat Embryol* 190:201, 1994.

Walther B, DeMeester TR, LaFontaine E, et al. Effects of paraesophageal hernia on sphincter function and its implications on surgical therapy. *Am J Surg* 147:111, 1984.

Walker WF, Attwood HD. The inferior vena caval opening in the diaphragm. *Br J Surg* 48:86, 1960.

Wastell C, Nyhus LM, Donahue PE. *Surgery of the Esophagus; Stomach and Small Intestine*, 5th ed. Boston: Little, Brown, 1995.

West JB (ed.). *Best and Taylor's Physiological Basis of Medical Practice* (11th ed.). Baltimore: Williams & Wilkins, 1985. P 646.

Whalen JP. *Radiology of the Abdomen: Anatomic Basis*. Philadelphia: Lea & Febiger, 1976.

Wolf BS. Sliding hiatal hernia: The need for redefinition. *AJR* 177:231, 1973.

Zamir O, Eyal F, Lernau OZ, Nissan S. Bilateral congenital posterolateral diaphragmatic hernia. *Am J Perinatol*. 3:56, 1986.

EDITOR'S COMMENT

The debate concerning the fine points of the lower esophageal sphincter and its relationship to esophageal reflux continues. It is of interest that the computer age is making an impact in this area. We are now able to build three-dimensional computer-generated models of our patients' entire sphincter complex (Bombeck CT, Vaz O, DeSalva J, et al. *Ann Surg* 206:465, 1987). When this technology is applied to the detailed anatomic information presented herein, we can devise improved operative methods to cure our patients.

Since the authors comment on chalasia in children, I found the observation by Perdikis and Hinder (In LM Nyhus and RE Condon [eds.], *Hernia* [4th ed.]. Philadelphia: Lippincott, 1995. Pp 546–547) that the incidence of paraesophageal hiatal hernia was common following a Nissen fundoplication for treatment of chalasia. This finding was especially common if a crural repair had not been performed.

Please note the inconsistency of the median arcuate ligament as presented by the authors. This anatomic structure is extremely important in the proper completion of the Hill repair for the treatment of reflux peptic esophagitis. The identification of this strong fascial band and its use to secure the Hill gastropexy posteriorly is key to the successful completion of this operation. The fact that only one-half of the cadavers examined by the authors had a ligament sufficiently well developed to be used in a surgical repair causes some concern about the merit of the entire procedure.

L.M.N.

53

Congenital Diaphragmatic Hernia

Jayant Radhakrishnan

The term *congenital diaphragmatic hernia (CDH)* is generally used for the posterolateral diaphragmatic hernia of Bochdalek. In this chapter, management of the posterolateral hernia of Bochdalek, eventration of the diaphragm, and the anterior retrosternal hernia of Morgagni are described.

History

In 1848, Bochdalek described the posterolateral diaphragmatic foramen and herniation through it so accurately that CDH is called the Bochdalek hernia even though Riverius was the first to describe a congenital diaphragmatic hernia in 1679. In 1946, Dr. Robert Gross first successfully repaired a CDH in a neonate under 24 hours of age. In 1761, Morgagni reviewed cases of congenital diaphragmatic hernia and he credited Stehelinus with observing pulmonary hypoplasia in a fetus with diaphragmatic hernia. In this same manuscript he also described a patient with a substernal diaphragmatic hernia (hernia of Morgagni).

Embryology of the Diaphragm

The adult diaphragm develops from two paired and two unpaired components. The pleuroperitoneal membranes and contributions from the dorsal esophageal mesenteries are paired whereas the unpaired components are the septum transversum and contributions from the body wall as the lungs and pleural cavities burrow and excavate into the mesoderm of the lateral body wall. During the fourth week of ges-

tation the septum transversum develops as a membranous infolding in the mesenchyme between the pericardium and coelomic cavity. After forming at the cervical level, it migrates to the thoracic area, where it fuses with the pleuroperitoneal membranes and the ventral esophageal mesenchyme to separate the chest from the abdominal cavity. In the adult it forms the central tendon of the diaphragm. Dorsal to the septum, on either side of the mediastinum, are the pleural canals, which connect the pericardial and peritoneal cavities. The lung buds develop within the mediastinum and bulge into the pleural canals, which later form the pleural cavities. The pleuroperitoneal membranes form as a result of progressive narrowing of the communication between the developing pleural cavities and the pericardium. This process of narrowing leaves a very small aperture to be covered by membrane, its closure being completed by the eighth week.

Following closure of the pleuroperitoneal canal, the pleural cavities enlarge as the lungs develop. Caudally, the pleural cavities burrow into the body wall, which then contributes the costal component of the diaphragm during the third month. Dorsally, this expansion transfers thoracic muscles to the diaphragm, forming the crura, while anteriorly and laterally the innermost layer of thoracic muscles is stripped from the thoracic wall and added to the diaphragm. The triangular space at which the dorsal and lateral muscle groups join is the lumbocostal trigone, which, if unfused when intestinal loops return to the abdominal cavity, forms the site of herniation through the foramen of Bochdalek. The associated pulmonary hypoplasia is believed to be due to pressure from abdominal vis-

cera in the thorax. The above theory is generally accepted as the cause of CDH; however, another school of thought is that the primary problem is failure of development of the lung buds, which do not fill the developing pleural space. The pleural space then does not contribute to normal closure of the pleuroperitoneal canal.

Eventration of the diaphragm is believed to occur because of failure of muscular tissue to spread over the entire area of the diaphragm following normal fusion of the embryonic components.

Hernias through the foramen of Morgagni may be the result of failure of fusion of the septum transversum with the sternum and anterior chest wall, or they may be due to failure of muscular tissue to develop in the retrosternal portion of the diaphragm.

Congenital Posterolateral Diaphragmatic Hernia of Bochdalek

Incidence

The estimated incidence of CDH is 1 : 4000 to 5000 live births, with the incidence rising as high as 1 : 2000 if all stillbirths are included. Associated anomalies, especially of the central nervous system, are very common in stillborn infants with CDH.

Anatomy

Usually a 1- to 2-cm defect is present in the posterolateral part of the diaphragm, but it can vary significantly in size and the entire hemidiaphragm may be absent. The size of the diaphragmatic defect does not correlate with the mass of herniated organs. The defect occurs on the left side in 80 to 85 percent of patients. Very occasionally, it is bilateral. In fewer than 10 percent of cases, a hernia sac is seen. Intestinal malrotation and malfixation are always present. In left-sided CDH herniated viscera consist of stomach, small intestine, colon, spleen, and the left lobe of the liver. Rarely, the left kidney, adrenal gland, and pancreas are displaced into the chest. In right-sided defects, the liver usually herniates along with the small bowel and occasionally the colon.

There is significant hypoplasia of both lungs, with the weight of the ipsilateral lung being as low as 31 percent and that of the contralateral lung being 60 percent that of control subjects. Along with reduction in the size of bronchi, bronchial branching is reduced and the surface area of alveolae is decreased. In addition, the total size of the pulmonary vascular bed is decreased. There are fewer vessels per unit of lung. Pulmonary vascular resistance is elevated due to increase in the thickness of

arteriolar smooth muscle with muscular growth extending down to the capillary level.

Herniated viscera compound the problem by forming a space-occupying lesion in the hemithorax that displaces the mediastinum to the contralateral side, thus kinking the venae cavae and compressing the contralateral lung (Figs. 53-1 and 53-2).

Pathophysiology

Infants with CDH have to deal with two distinct pathophysiologic entities: pulmonary hypoplasia, which results in inadequate gas exchange, and pulmonary hypertension, which disrupts pulmonary blood flow. Of these two elements pulmonary hypertension seems to be the more dangerous problem. The highly reactive pulmonary vessels are sensitive to acidosis, hypoxia, and hypercarbia. Resultant pulmonary hypertension produces persistence of fetal circulation with shunting of blood through the patent ductus arteriosus and the foramen ovale. The shunt further aggravates acidosis, hypoxia, and

hypercarbia, thus perpetuating a vicious cycle. This pulmonary hypertension may also be due to lack of production or early depletion of pulmonary vasodilators such as prostaglandins and nitric oxide.

Barotrauma caused by ventilation and a transpulmonary pressure gradient (airway pressure minus intrapleural pressure) seem to play a role in the deterioration in these patients. Surfactant deficiency also is noted in infants with CDH.

Clinical Findings

Congenital diaphragmatic hernia is often diagnosed antenatally when ultrasonography is carried out for evaluation of polyhydramnios. Sometimes it is an incidental discovery on a routine antenatal ultrasound. Ultrasonography will demonstrate a mediastinal shift and loops of intestine, stomach, or liver in the thoracic cavity. Herniation of the stomach is indicative of a serious lesion. In most patients not diagnosed antenatally, respiratory distress, tachypnea, and cyanosis develop at birth. On examination, breath sounds are absent

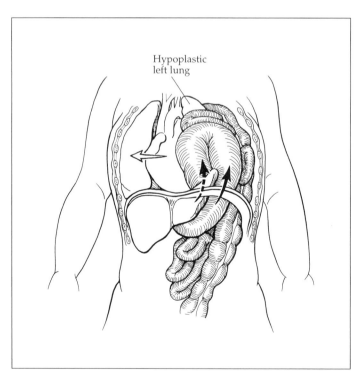

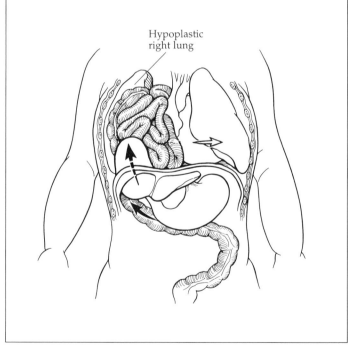

Fig. 53-1. Left-sided CDH with the stomach (dark arrow) and left lobe of the liver (interrupted arrow) in the left hemithorax along with small and large bowel. The mediastinum is displaced to the right (light arrow). The hypoplastic left lung is visualized at the apex of the left hemithorax.

Fig. 53-2. Right-sided CDH with herniated intestines (dark arrow) and right lobe of the liver (interrupted arrow) causing mediastinal displacement (light arrow). The hypoplastic right lung is at the apex of the right hemithorax. Note that the stomach is stretched across the midabdomen.

on the ipsilateral side and the heart is displaced toward the contralateral hemithorax. In addition, the abdomen is scaphoid. A few patients do not develop symptoms until after 24 hours of life and occasionally not until a few months or years. Patients in whom symptoms are delayed more than 24 hours have well-developed lungs, and they do very well after surgery. It is essential to identify associated anomalies, particularly chromosomal abnormalities (trisomy 13), central nervous system malformations (myelomeningocele), and cardiovascular anomalies (ventricular septal defect).

Diagnosis

Plain anteroposterior radiographs of the chest and abdomen are generally sufficient to make the diagnosis of CDH. Typically, the ipsilateral hemithorax has a "soap-bubble" appearance with contralateral displacement of the mediastinum. In addition, there is a paucity of intestinal gas in the abdomen. On occasion the nasogastric tube may be seen entering the chest. If liver constitutes the major part of herniated viscera, one may find a solid shadow in the hemithorax, and a normal amount of intestinal gas may be present in the abdomen. In such cases cystadenomatoid malformation of the lung and intralobar pulmonary sequestration have to be differentiated from CDH, and an upper GI examination may be required.

Management

Preoperative Care

If diagnosis of CDH is made antenatally, the infant should be delivered at a tertiary care center. In cases in which the diagnosis is suspected at birth due to respiratory distress, immediate nasogastric or orogastric intubation with a No. 10 French sump (Replogle) tube should be carried out to decompress the stomach, thus avoiding further displacement of the mediastinum, which would compound the hypoventilation and also reduce venous return to the heart. Immediate endotracheal intubation is also indicated since ventilation by mask increases gastrointestinal distention. Manual ventilation with low peak pressures (20–25 cm H_2O) and high ventilatory rates (80–100 breaths/minute) should be used. Acidosis, hypercarbia, and hypoxia should

be corrected and the patient placed on an FIO_2 of 1.0. A chest radiograph should be obtained after initiation of resuscitation. The patient should then be placed on conventional ventilation. One tries to attain a

PaO_2 of greater than 100 mm Hg, a $PaCO_2$ of less than 40 mm Hg, and a pH of greater than 7.5. If conventional ventilation is not successful, high-frequency ventilation (800–1800 breaths/minute) may be of

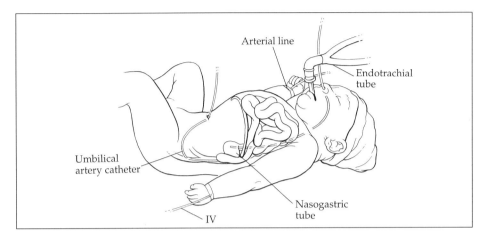

Fig. 53-3. Preoperative management of these babies consists of ventilation via an endotracheal tube, nasogastric tube for gastric decompression, umbilical and right radial arterial lines for post- and preductal blood gas determinations, and an intravenous line on the dorsum of the left hand. Note the scaphoid abdomen.

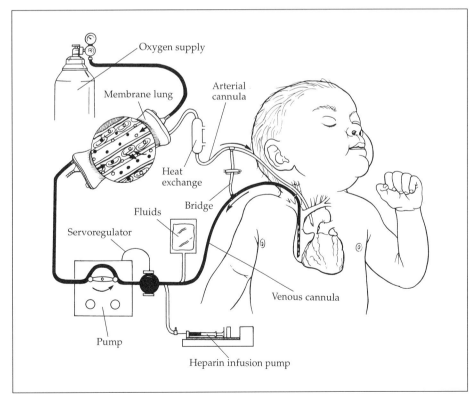

Fig. 53-4. The ECMO circuit. Blood is drawn from the superior vena cava (arrow). It passes through a pump and membrane oxygenator and is returned to the aorta after being warmed (arrow).

value. In addition, the baby should be kept warm, well sedated, and paralyzed. Paralysis not only improves mechanical ventilation but possibly also directly reduces pulmonary artery hypertension. Vasodilators (tolazoline) are also of value along with an infusion of inotropic agents (dopamine or dobutamine) to maintain the blood pressure.

By careful monitoring of postductal (umbilical artery) and preductal (right radial artery) blood gases, one determines the degree of shunting. A pulse oximeter or transcutaneous oxygen monitor placed on the right upper extremity and a lower extremity can also be used to detect shunting (Fig. 53-3). During resuscitation careful and repeated radiographic examinations ensure that a contralateral pneumothorax does not occur.

Metabolic disturbances such as hypoglycemia and hypocalcemia should be avoided, and sodium bicarbonate or trisaminomethane (THAM) can be administered to correct acidosis. It must be remembered that adequate ventilation is essential to blow off carbon dioxide when using sodium bicarbonate to correct acidosis. Antibiotics should be administered since surgical correction will definitely be indicated. Although all infants with CDH require operative repair, immediate surgical reduction may, in fact, impair pulmonary function by elevating the contralateral diaphragm and reducing contralateral lung compliance. If the child's condition can be stabilized with respiratory management for 24 to 48 hours, a better result is obtained with semi-elective hernia repair. If the child's condition cannot be stabilized by conventional and ultra–high-frequency ventilation, he or she should be placed on extracorporeal membrane oxygenation (ECMO) (Fig. 53-4) to give the hyperreactive pulmonary vascular bed a chance to stabilize over a 7- to 10-day period. ECMO also permits the lung to recover from the trauma of initial resuscitative efforts. Veno-arterial ECMO is the method of choice. Numerous indices have been utilized to identify candidates for ECMO. In general, the use of ECMO is indicated if the patient is on an FIO_2 of 1.0, PaO_2s are less than 50 mm Hg, and $PaCO_2$s are greater than 50 mm Hg. Cardiac dysfunction that does not respond to dopamine and epinephrine is also an indication for ECMO.

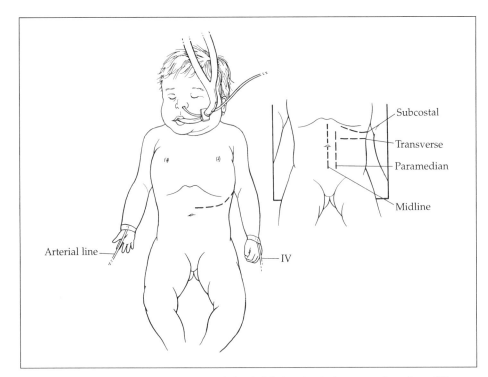

Fig. 53-5. Preferred abdominal incision. The medial end of the incision is about 1 cm above the umbilicus, and it is curved toward the costal margin at its lateral extent. Inset. Demonstrates other incisions that can be used.

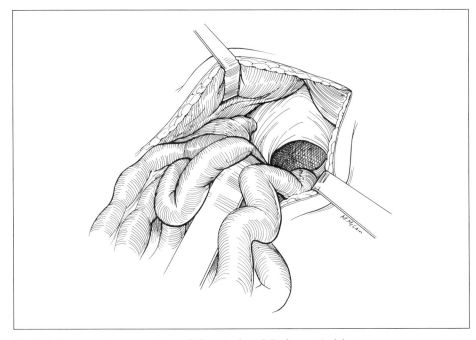

Fig. 53-6. Diagrammatic representation of left posterolateral diaphragmatic defect.

Once the child's condition is stabilized on ECMO for 24 hours, he or she should be weaned off and the CDH repaired another 24 to 48 hours later. CDH can be repaired on ECMO but the incidence of complications is increased. If the child cannot be weaned from ECMO after 2 to 3 weeks, the chances of survival are poor. Such children may be repaired on ECMO but the family should understand that ECMO support will be withdrawn if no significant improvement is seen within 4 to 5 days after the repair.

As was previously mentioned, the prognosis of babies with CDH is dependent on the degree of pulmonary hypoplasia and pulmonary hypertension that is present. It is difficult to predict whether a degree of pulmonary hypoplasia is incompatible with survival before institution of ECMO; however, evaluation of functional residual capacity of the lungs may be a valid predictor of survival early during the course of ECMO.

Operation

The operating room should be prewarmed, heat lamps placed at the operating table, and the infant's head and extremities wrapped to prevent development of hypothermia during the procedure. High-frequency ventilation at low pressures should be continued during the surgical procedure. CDH is repaired transabdominally since viscera are more easily reduced by this approach and the defect is better visualized for repair. In addition, this permits placement of the malrotated intestines appropriately in the abdomen to avoid a possible midgut volvulus, and, on those rare occasions when Ladd's bands have to be lysed, an abdominal approach is essential. Finally, either stretching of the abdominal wall or creation of a ventral hernia is usually required to prevent excessive pressure on the diaphragm by the viscera.

We prefer a transverse abdominal incision about 1 cm above the umbilicus in the midline with a gentle upward curve at its lateral extent to bring it to the costal margin in the midaxillary line (Fig. 53-5). This incision gives a better exposure to the posterolateral aspect of the defect than does a straight transverse incision. Other possible incisions are demonstrated in the inset of Fig. 53-5. After the abdominal cavity is entered, the herniated viscera first are reduced. Occasionally, intrathoracic negative pressure makes it difficult to reduce the viscera. In such cases, instead of pulling on the viscera, one should pass a red rubber catheter through the defect adjacent to the viscera or elevate the anterior lip of the defect with a retractor. Both maneuvers permit air to enter the thoracic cavity and correct the negative pressure. Once the viscera are reduced, the size of the defect is visualized and a careful search is made in the left hemithorax for a hernial sac. The sac must be resected if found. The hypoplastic lung is also visualized and a gross estimate of its size and degree of differentiation into lobes can be made. This hypoplastic lung must not be distended

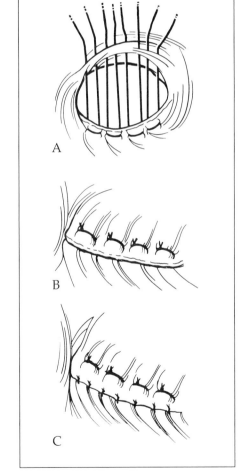

Fig. 53-8. *A. Horizontal mattress sutures are placed in the two edges of the diaphragm. B. The sutures are tied after all of them have been placed. C. A second layer of simple sutures is placed in the edge of the diaphragm.*

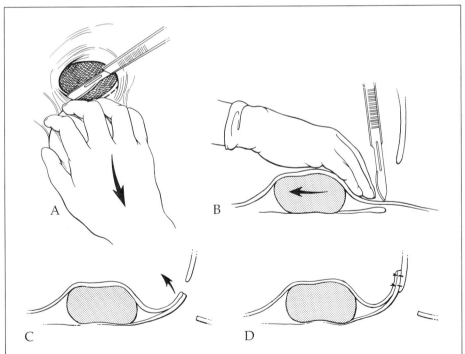

Fig. 53-7. *A. Posterior edge of the diaphragm being released by incising the posterior peritoneum over it. The kidney is manually displaced inferiorly (**arrow**). B. Longitudinal section demonstrating inferior displacement of kidney and incision in the peritoneum. C. Posterior edge of diaphragm is mobilized. D. Anterior and posterior edges of the defect are sutured.*

forcefully by the anesthesiologist or it will develop a leak. Before repair of the defect, a No. 10 French chest tube is placed in the left hemithorax and secured to the chest wall. It is connected to a three-way stopcock and a syringe. Smaller defects in the diaphragm are repaired by directly suturing the anterior and posterior margins (Fig. 53-6). However, the small, rolled-up posterior edge of diaphragm is not easily visualized, as it is covered by posterior peritoneum superior to the kidney. To release the posterior edge of diaphragm, the kidney is displaced downward and the peritoneum over the rim of the diaphragm is incised (Fig. 53-7A and B).). Once dissected the free edge of the posterior diaphragm is displaced anteriorly (Fig. 53-7C) and it is sutured to the anterior margin of the defect (Fig. 53-7D). We place a layer of horizontal mattress sutures of 4-0 nonabsorbable material (Ethibond) approximately 2 to 3 mm from the edge of the defect and 2 to 3 mm apart (Fig. 53-8A). The sutures are tied only after all of them have been placed (Fig. 53-8B). A second layer of simple, interrupted sutures is then placed in the free margin of the repaired diaphragm (Fig. 53-8C).

After the defect is repaired, the abdominal cavity is explored and the intestines are replaced in such a fashion as to prevent a midgut volvulus. Although malrotation and malfixation of the small bowel are always present, lysis of Ladd's bands or a formal Ladd's procedure is not always required. If a Ladd's procedure is required, we do not remove the appendix in children with CDH. The abdominal wall is then stretched circumferentially to obtain a tension-free closure. If it appears that stretching alone is not adequate, a ventral hernia is created using a prosthetic patch on the fascia. The overlying skin is undermined and closed. Very rarely, a silo may be required if tension is too great to even permit skin closure.

Before the patient is transferred off the operating table, an anteroposterior chest radiograph is obtained and the mediastinum is stabilized in the midline by instilling or withdrawing air from the left hemithorax with a syringe attached to the three-way stopcock on the chest tube. After the mediastinum is stabilized, the stopcock is closed and the child is transferred back to the neonatal intensive care unit with all the previously placed monitors in position (Fig. 53-9).

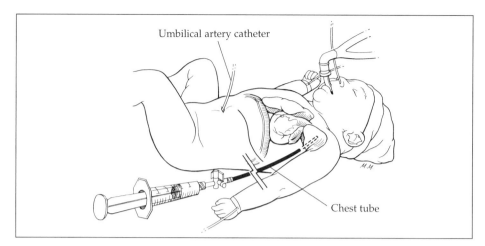

Fig. 53-9. Postoperative appearance. The previously placed monitors are in place. The left chest tube is connected to a three-way stopcock and a syringe to instill or evacuate air as required to maintain the mediastinum in the midline.

Postoperative Care

A chest radiograph is again obtained on admission to the neonatal intensive care unit to confirm the position of the mediastinum and also to identify any contralateral pneumothorax. Chest radiographs are repeated at 6- to 8-hour intervals for the first 48 hours.

Preoperatively instituted medical management is continued and the child is carefully monitored. The baby must be weaned off respiratory support very slowly since significant pulmonary vasoconstriction and pulmonary hypertension can develop with small decreases in FIO_2. The child must continue to be sedated and paralyzed during this time. If hypoxia, pulmonary hypertension, or a right-to-left shunt redevelops and is refractory to conventional therapy, ECMO should be instituted.

Prognosis

Infants whose symptoms develop after 24 hours of life have a survival rate close to 100 percent. On the other hand, if symptoms develop within 24 hours of birth, the survival rate has remained around 50 percent for the past two decades. With the use of ECMO, 60 to 80 percent survival can be expected in high-risk babies. Infants who survive the neonatal period usually have normal growth and development, and their long-term outcome is good although respiratory problems are common in the first few years of life and there is some morbidity. Patients who require ECMO af-

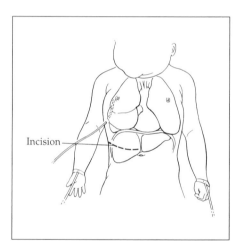

Fig. 53-10. The incision for a right-sided CDH. A right chest tube is left after the repair and is connected to a three-way stopcock and syringe.

ter repair of CDH or are repaired while on ECMO unfortunately appear to have significant long-term pulmonary dysfunction.

Future Considerations
Antenatal Repair of CDH

This technique is physiologically sound and has been carried out at the University of California at San Francisco; however, the results so far are poor. This approach requires extensive experience in fetal surgery, it is very expensive, and availability is limited.

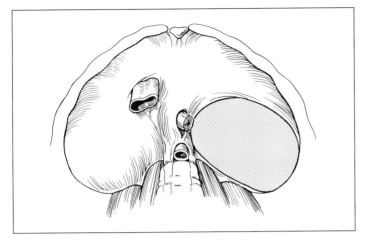

Fig. 53-11. *Large defect involving the left hemidiaphragm.*

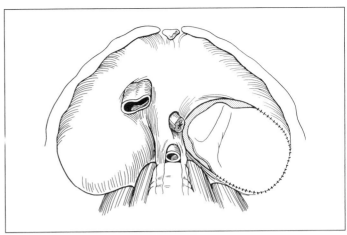

Fig. 53-12. *Goretex patch being sutured into the defect.*

Lung Transplantation

This is based on the concept of using a downsized adult lobe of lung in patients with CDH who have undergone repair but cannot be weaned off ECMO because of the presence of bilateral pulmonary hypoplasia. Of two infants treated in this fashion, one is a long-term survivor.

Right-Sided Congenital Diaphragmatic Hernia

Right-sided lesions occur in 10 to 15 percent of all patients with CDH. Presentation of right-sided CDH is often delayed since the liver plugs the opening. Once herniation occurs small bowel and occasionally large bowel are found in the right chest. In these infants the right lung is more hypoplastic. The stomach does not enter the thoracic cavity (see Fig. 53-2) and on an anteroposterior radiograph it is often seen as a midabdominal, transversely placed, "banana-shaped" air shadow. Preoperative evaluation, monitoring, and management are the same as for a left-sided CDH. The typical posterolateral defect is exposed transabdominally by making an incision that is the mirror image of that described for a left-sided CDH (Fig. 53-10). Upon entering the abdominal cavity the intestines are first reduced. Next, the right lobe of the liver is gently displaced medially and anteriorly, with reduction being completed by passing a hand along its lat-

eral aspect up to the dome, which is then displaced downward. The repair is carried out in the same fashion as described for a left-sided CDH after leaving a chest tube in the right hemithorax (Fig. 53-10).

Postoperative management of a right-sided CDH is also similar to that of a left-sided CDH.

Absent Diaphragm

On occasion, upon reduction of CDH, one finds a near-complete or total absence of the hemidiaphragm. This cannot be predicted preoperatively since neither the severity of symptoms nor the amount of herniated viscera noted on a radiograph correlates with the size of the diaphragmatic defect. In such patients primary closure of the diaphragm is not feasible. If the low transverse abdominal incision described in Fig. 53-5 is made, one may be able to turn the cut edge of the transversus abdominis muscle inward to suture it to the posterior rim of the diaphragm or to the ribs posteriorly. If a high transverse incision or a subcostal incision is used, the length of muscle is insufficient to permit such a repair. If the muscle flap is of inadequate size, a prosthetic patch is sutured into the defect (Figs. 53-11 and 53-12). We prefer to use Goretex (polytetrafluoroethylene). We have not noted the higher incidence of disruption and recurrence of hernia reported in the literature. We have

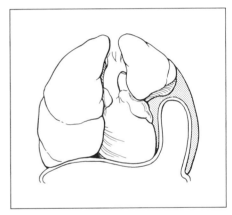

Fig. 53-13. *Eventration of the left hemidiaphragm with a hypoplastic left lung.*

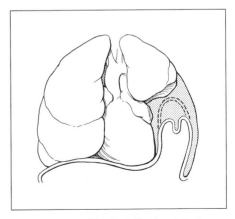

Fig. 53-14. *Transabdominal plication of diaphragm. The dome of the diaphragm is being inverted.*

seen seepage of abdominal fluids and blood into the left hemithorax through the suture line, and in these patients the chest tube is used to evacuate fluid to maintain the mediastinum in the midline. These babies invariably require the creation of a ventral hernia.

Eventration of the Diaphragm

Eventration of the diaphragm may be congenital, due to defective muscular development of the diaphragm resulting in a membranous diaphragm, or it may be acquired because of damage to the phrenic nerve. It may involve either the entire hemidiaphragm or a part of it. Congenital eventrations usually occur on the left side. In left-sided lesions partial or complete inversion of the stomach along with malro-

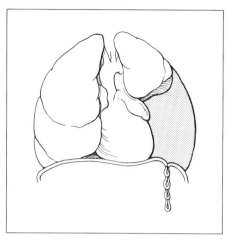

Fig. 53-15. Completed transabdominal plication.

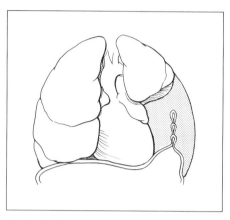

Fig. 53-16. Technique of transthoracic plication of diaphragm.

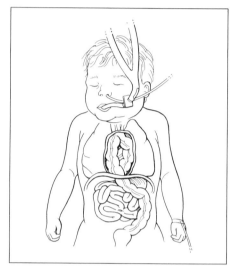

Fig. 53-17. Hernia of Morgagni. The sac is usually occupied by colon.

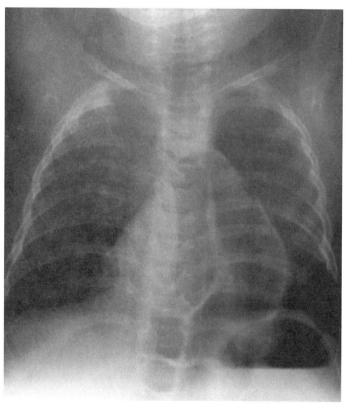

Fig. 53-18. Posteroanterior chest radiograph of Morgagni hernia with colon in the pericardial sac.

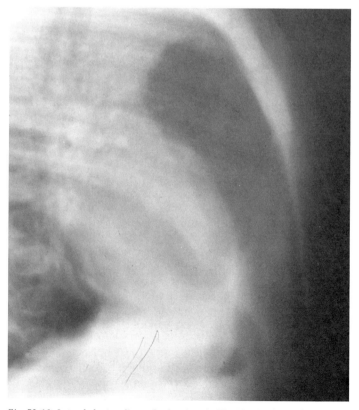

Fig. 53-19. Lateral chest radiograph of patient in Fig. 53-18. The air-filled colon is visible anterior to the cardiac shadow.

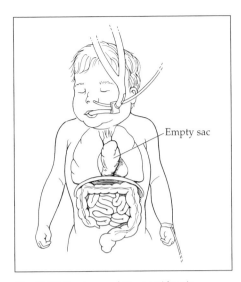

Fig. 53-20. Empty sac of Morgagni hernia.

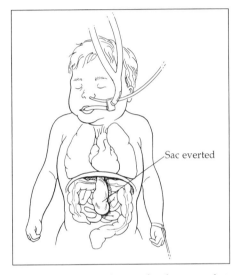

Fig. 53-21. Hernia sac is everted and amputated at its neck.

tation of the small bowel is often present. Hypoplasia of the ipsilateral lung does occur but to a lesser degree than with CDH.

Clinical Findings

Patients with congenital eventration are often asymptomatic whereas those with acquired eventration develop significant symptoms due to respiratory inadequacy or displacement of the mediastinum. The stomach may also undergo a volvulus.

Diagnosis

On occasion eventration is difficult to differentiate from CDH. Fluoroscopy usually demonstrates an intact elevated hemidiaphragm that does not move with respiratory activity in congenital cases, whereas paradoxical movement is seen in patients with phrenic nerve paralysis. On ultrasonography the intact diaphragm is visualized above the abdominal viscera.

Treatment

Surgical treatment is only required for respiratory, cardiac, or gastrointestinal symptoms. Replacement of the diaphragm into its normal position should stabilize the mediastinum and restore pulmonary functions, and it should replace abdominal organs into their normal positions. Occasionally, in a very young infant with an extremely high hemidiaphragm that severely compresses the ipsilateral lung, repair may be of value in permitting adequate lung growth.

The leaf of diaphragm can be excised, overlapped, or plicated. In congenital cases, since the phrenic nerve is intact and functional, we believe that the safest approach is plication using horizontal mattress sutures of 4-0 Ethibond. This can be carried out transabdominally (Figs. 53-13 through 53-15) or transthoracically (Fig. 53-16). There may be some theoretical benefit in plicating the left side transabdominally since the stomach and other viscera can then be placed in their normal positions under direct vision. On the right side a transthoracic approach may be worthwhile since one would not have to displace the liver to approach the dome of the diaphragm.

Retrosternal Hernia of Morgagni

Anatomy

The foramina of Morgagni are small triangular areas on either side of the inferior end of the sternum at the anterior aspect of the diaphragm. They are bound by muscle fibers from the xiphoid process medially and from the costal cartilages laterally. These small gaps, also known as the spaces of Larrey or parasternal spaces, permit the passage of the superior epigastric vessels. Morgagni hernias usually occur on the right side but they can be bilateral. A hernia sac is always formed and the superior epigastric artery is located lateral to it. Transverse colon and omentum are

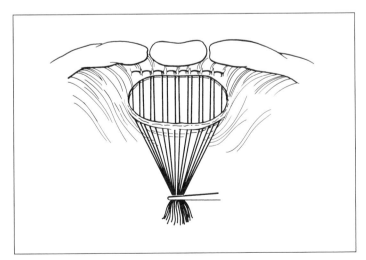

Fig. 53-22. Horizontal mattress sutures are placed between the posterior margin of the defect and the anterior rectus sheath and sternum.

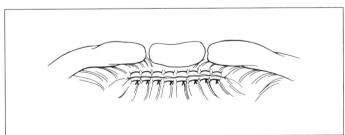

Fig. 53-23. The sutures are tied after they have all been placed.

the most common contents of these hernias (Fig. 53-17).

Clinical Findings

Since patients are often asymptomatic, clinical findings may be discovered incidentally on a chest radiograph (Figs. 53-18 and 53-19). If the hernia is difficult to differentiate from an anterior mediastinal mass, an upper GI series is helpful.

Treatment

Due to the potential of Morgagni hernia for incarceration, surgical repair is indicated. An upper abdominal transverse incision gives adequate exposure. After reduction of the viscera, the empty sac is grasped through the defect (Fig. 53-20), everted (Fig. 53-21), and excised at its neck. The defect is repaired by placing horizonal mattress sutures of nonabsorbable material of appropriate size between the lip of diaphragm at the posterior edge of the defect and the undersurface of the sternum and posterior rectus sheath (Fig. 53-22). The sutures are tied after they have all been placed (Fig. 53-23).

Suggested Reading

Adzick NS, Harrison MR, Glick PL, et al. Diaphragmatic hernia in the fetus: Prenatal diagnosis and outcome in 94 cases. *J Pediatr Surg* 20:357, 1985.

Bohn D, Tamura M, Perrin D, et al. Ventilatory predictors of pulmonary hypoplasia in congenital diaphragmatic hernia, confirmed by morphologic assessment. *J Pediatr* 111:423, 1987.

Bos AP, Tibboel D, Koot VCM, et al. Persistent pulmonary hypertension in high-risk congenital diaphragmatic hernia patients: Incidence and vasodilator therapy. *J Pediatr Surg* 28:1463, 1993.

Burge DM, Atwell JD, Freeman NV. Could the stomach site help predict outcome in babies with left sided congenital diaphragmatic hernia diagnosed antenatally? *J Pediatr Surg* 24:567, 1989.

Glick PL, Leach CL, Besner GE, et al. Pathophysiology of congenital diaphragmtic hernia III. Exogenous surfactant therapy for the high risk neonate with CDH. *J Pediatr Surg* 27:866, 1992.

Harrison MR, Adzick NS, Flake AW, et al. Correction of congenital diaphragmatic hernia in utero: VI. Hard-earned lessons. *J Pediatr Surg* 28:1411, 1993.

Kinsella JP, Neish SR, Ivy DD, et al. Clinical responses to prolonged treatment of persistent pulmonary hypertension of the newborn with low doses of inhaled nitric oxide. *J Pediatr* 123:103, 1993.

Langer JC, Filler RM, Bohn DJ, et al. Timing of surgery for congenital diaphragmatic hernia: Is emergency operation necessary? *J Pediatr Surg* 23:731, 1988.

Lotze A, Knight GR, Anderson KD, et al. Surfactant (Beractant) therapy for infants with congenital diaphragmatic hernia on ECMO: Evidence of persistent surfactant deficiency. *J Pediatr Surg* 29:407, 1994.

Lund DP, Mitchell J, Kharasch V, et al. Congenital diaphragmatic hernia: The hidden morbidity. *J Pediatr Surg* 29:258, 1994.

Nakayama DK, Motoyama EK, Tagge EM. Effect of preoperative stabilization on respiratory system compliance and outcome in newborn infants with congenital diaphragmatic hernia. *J Pediatr* 118:793, 1991.

Nio M, Haase G, Kennaugh J, et al. A prospective randomized trial of delayed versus immediate repair of congenital diaphragmatic hernia. *J Pediatr Surg* 29:618, 1994.

Norden MA, Butt W, McDougall P. Predictors of survival in infants with congenital diaphragmatic hernia. *J Pediatr Surg* 29:1442, 1994.

Sakai H, Tamura M, Hosokawa Y, et al. Effect of surgical repair on respiratory mechanics in congenital diaphragmatic hernia. *J Pediatr* 111:432, 1987.

Shah N, Jacob T, Exler R, et al. Inhaled nitric oxide in congenital diaphragmatic hernia. *J Pediatr Surg* 29:1010, 1994.

Shochat SJ. Pulmonary vascular pathology in congenital diaphragmatic hernias. *Pediatr Surg Int* 2:331, 1987.

Skandalakis JE, Gray SW, Ricketts RR. Diaphragm. In JE Skandalakis, SW Gray (eds), *Embryology for Surgeons* (2nd ed). Baltimore: Williams & Wilkins, 1994. Chap. 15, Pp 491–539.

Tracy TF Jr, Bailey PV, Sadiq F, et al. Predictive capabilities of preoperative and postoperative pulmonary function tests in delayed repair of congenital diaphragmatic hernia. *J Pediatr Surg* 29:265, 1994.

Vazquez WD, Cheu HW. Hemorrhagic complications and repair of congenital diaphragmatic hernias: Does timing of the repair make a difference? Data from the Extracorporeal Life Support Organization. *J Pediatr Surg* 29:1002, 1994.

West KW, Bengston K, Rescorla FJ, et al. Delayed surgical repair and ECMO improves survival in congenital diaphragmatic hernia. *Ann Surg* 216:454, 1992.

Wilson JM, Bower LK, Lund DP. Evolution of the technique of congenital diaphragmatic hernia repair on ECMO. *J Pediatr Surg* 29:1109, 1994.

EDITOR'S COMMENT

Congenital diaphragmatic hernia continues to present the surgeon with multiple challenges. Unfortunately, to date the in utero correction of the defect has not been as successful as initially hoped. The team at the Fetal Treatment Center, University of California at San Francisco, has resolved many of the intraoperative technical problems, resulting in a few successful repairs (Harrison MR et al. *J Pediatr Surg* 28:1411, 1993).

This same group has analyzed the cost of medical care (hospital bills and professional fees) for all 35 infants who underwent postnatal CDH repair at their institution between January 1990 and December 1993. The cost averaged $137,000 per patient, and use of the extracorporeal membrane oxygenator dramatically increased the cost. The cost per survivor was $98,000 in the non-ECMO group and $365,000 in the ECMO group. The estimated cost of CDH per year in the United States is more than $230 million (Metkus AP et al. *J Pediatr Surg* 30:226, 1995). Recognizing that the survivors from this initial hospitalization frequently are plagued with respiratory problems, thus increasing the short-term—and possibly long-term—morbidity, costs can escalate to astronomical levels.

The continuing search for answers to these difficult problems is applauded.

L.M.N.

54

Eventration of the Diaphragm

Frederick C. Ryckman   Daniel von Allmen

Eventration of the diaphragm is a patho-logic condition in which the diaphragm is immobile and elevated, and does not par-ticipate in respiratory activity. The condi-tion can be congenital, due to incomplete muscularization of the diaphragm, or ac-quired secondary to phrenic nerve paral-ysis. Its incidence in adults is estimated at 1 in 10,000 to 1 in 13,000, as judged by ra-diographic screening studies using chest radiography.

Congenital eventration of the diaphragm is, by definition, present at birth. It is associated with a failure of normal muscularization of the fused pleuroperitoneal membrane that forms the diaphragm. Whether this arises secondary to a defective distribution of the phrenic nerve fibers, or is secondary to abnormal muscularization of the prim-itive diaphragm, is not proven. The most acceptable theory suggests failure of mi-gration of the myoblasts along the phrenic nerve branches as the primary etiology. Eventration can involve the entire dia-phragm or only a portion of the hemidia-phragm, or it may be bilateral in rare cases. The phrenic nerve and the site of attach-ment of the diaphragmatic margins are normal. The muscle fibers in the dia-phragm are sparsely distributed and me-chanically nonfunctional but not atrophic. As a result, the diaphragm is lax, thin, and elongated, rising as a smooth arched mem-brane into the involved hemithorax.

Congenital eventration differs from a con-genital diaphragmatic hernia (CDH) in that the diaphragm is intact and no com-munication exists between the thoracic and the abdominal cavity. The distinction between a congenital diaphragmatic her-nia with a hernia sac and a partial even-tration of the diaphragm is often less clear.

Both conditions can have an intact rim of normal diaphragmatic muscle around the peripheral diaphragmatic margins. How-ever, the diaphragmatic defect in CDH is at the fusion plane of the embryonic tis-sues, in the posterolateral diaphragmatic sulcus, whereas the defect in congenital eventration is more often at the apex of the dome of the diaphragm. In the extreme case in which eventration involves the whole diaphragm, with only the fused pleuroperitoneal membrane remaining, eventration is indistinguishable from a large diaphragmatic hernia with an intact sac. As the pulmonary developmental con-sequences of these anomalies are similar, further distinction between these defects is rarely of any benefit to the patient. Both defects cause a significant decrease in the intrathoracic volume in the involved hemi-thorax, and can lead to pulmonary hypo-plasia of varying degrees.

Acquired or paralytic eventration of the dia-phragm can result from a wide variety of causes. These include 1) birth trauma, 2) infection (poliomyelitis, fetal rubella, cy-tomegalovirus), 3) local inflammation of the phrenic nerve from a primary pulmo-nary or pleural source, 4) malignant tumor invasion involving the phrenic nerve, 5) congenital absence of the anterior horn cells (Werdnig-Hoffmann disease), 6) tri-somy 13–15 or 18, and 7) operative injury during mediastinal, cervical, or cardiac procedures. In children, birth trauma is by far the most common cause of acquired paralytic eventration. This is often related to a difficult vaginal delivery, with shoul-der dystocia or breech birth, leading to a stretch injury to the C3–C5 nerve roots, af-fecting the origin of the phrenic nerve, and the brachial plexua (Erb-Duchenne or Klumpke's palsy). Fractures of the hu-

merus or clavicle are often seen in associ-ation with these neural injuries and should be sought. A wide spectrum of injury se-verity is possible. When the nerve roots are avulsed, no improvement can be expected. Lesser degrees of injury or edema are po-tentially recoverable with time.

The diaphragm in patients with acquired phrenic nerve paralysis is initially normal with appropriate muscle development and position. With time, muscle atrophy de-velops, and the diaphragm becomes atten-uated and rises into the hemithorax. This is accompanied by progressive respiratory or gastrointestinal symptoms, or both. Again, symptoms are more severe in in-fants and young children.

Clinical Presentation

Most adult patients with diaphragmatic eventrations are asymptomatic, and re-quire no specific surgical therapy. When present, symptoms arise as a result of in-adequate ventilation or displacement of the abdominal viscera within the eventra-tion. Respiratory distress, cyanosis, tachy-pnea, tachycardia, and atelectasis with or without pneumonia predominate. Signifi-cant respiratory symptoms are most com-mon in infants and children secondary to the greater mobility of the mediastinum and their reliance upon diaphragmatic rather than intercostal muscles for respi-ration. On inspiration, the involved hemi-diaphragm rises, causing mediastinal shift to the opposite side. This impairs the ven-tilation of the involved hemithorax, com-presses the contralateral lung, and places torsion on the great vessels and heart. The degree of paradoxical diaphragmatic motion is slightly greater but not restricted to patients with acquired eventrations.

In infants, the respiratory symptoms increase during feedings or with abdominal distention. In addition, patients with asymptomatic eventrations can develop significant respiratory distress when mild respiratory infections occur. Symptoms associated with displacement of the abdominal viscera include abdominal pain, dysphagia, belching, heartburn, and epigastric pain in older patients. Infants with congenital eventration can also have a variety of other anomalies, including malrotation of the intestine, megacolon, hypospadias, situs inversus, congenital heart disease, Ehlers-Danlos syndrome, cleft palate, tracheomalacia, and bony abnormalities. The presence of these associated anomalies is a strong argument for a congenital etiology in these infants.

Infants and children with diaphragmatic eventration are also predisposed to acute gastric volvulus. Although this condition is rare, it requires prompt recognition and operative treatment. Organoaxial volvulus is more common than mesenteroaxial volvulus. However, both have been described. Eventration may predispose the patient to gastric volvulus by elongation of the gastrophrenic and gastrosplenic ligaments, allowing free rotational mobility of the stomach. This diagnostic possibility, heralded by unexplained vomiting, requires urgent investigation in infants with a known eventration.

Diagnosis

Dullness of the involved hemithorax, poor diaphragmatic excursion, and findings that suggest pneumonitis are the hallmarks on physical examination. Although the diagnosis can be suggested by physical examination, in most cases, eventration is first recognized during the radiographic investigation of respiratory distress. Chest radiographs demonstrate the characteristic elevation of the involved hemidiaphragm (Fig. 54-1). Demonstration of paralysis or paradoxical motion of the diaphragm requires chest fluoroscopy or ultrasonography. Radionuclide ventilation-perfusion scans often show a 50 to 75 percent decrease in ventilation on the involved side; however, this quantification of the ventilation defect is not always closely correlated with the severity of symptoms. Radiographic differentiation between CDH with a sac and eventration is difficult, if not impossible, in extensive cases.

The characteristic physical findings and radiographs depicting eventration are not present in patients undergoing mechanical ventilation at the time of examination. Positive-pressure ventilation reverses the diaphragmatic displacement, and pulmonary ventilation appears normal. Chest radiographs with the patient breathing spontaneously are necessary to identify the characteristic radiographic findings, and should be undertaken in all patients who fail ventilator discontinuation. In addition, eventration must be considered in infants with unexplained respiratory distress who require urgent intubation before baseline chest radiography can be obtained.

Indications for Operation

The indications for operation include 1) progressive respiratory distress, atelectasis, and/or pneumonia; 2) eventration as-

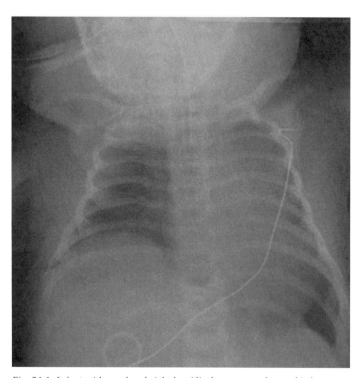

Fig. 54-1. Infant with paralyzed right hemidiaphragm secondary to birth trauma.

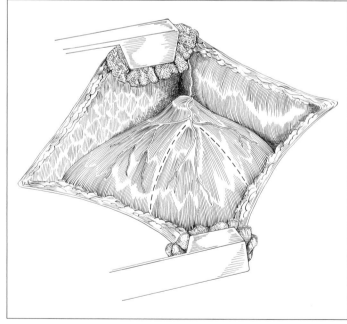

Fig. 54-2. Phrenic nerve descending over the central dome of the diaphragm. Right posterolateral thoracotomy. Dotted line indicates site of diaphragmatic plication.

sociated with birth injury in infants who do not improve during observation; and 3) patients with known phrenic nerve injury during thoracic or mediastinal operation. Infants with progressive respiratory symptoms due to congenital eventration should undergo surgery without delay, as their mediastinal anatomy limits their tolerance of this defect. Infants with birth trauma, where the potential for phrenic nerve recovery exists, present a greater dilemma. Although a waiting period of 2 weeks to allow recovery is recommended by some authors, the great improvement seen following surgical correction, and the excellent tolerance of the operative procedure, have driven many pediatric surgeons to proceed with correction at the time of diagnosis if mechanical ventilation is required. Failure to improve during conservative observation, or deterioration of respiratory status, merits immediate operative intervention.

A relative indication for operation in the infant with congenital eventration is the presence of significant elevation of the hemidiaphragm, compromising the growth of the ipsilateral lung. The eventrated diaphragm and displaced abdominal viscera represent a space-occupying lesion within the chest that restricts lung growth in a manner similar to that of CDH. Normal lung growth occurs following operative correction. This consideration should be entertained when selecting treatment options for infants with severe congenital eventration.

Operative Correction

The goals of surgical therapy should be 1) to restore the diaphragm to a normal location within the involved hemithorax, 2) to restore normal capacity to the hemithorax to allow lung growth in infants and children, 3) to restore normal visceral location in the abdomen, and 4) to stabilize the mediastinum by eliminating paradoxical motion of the diaphragm. These goals have been achieved by two different surgical procedures, one using plication and the other resection of the redundant hemidiaphragm. Either procedure should effectively eliminate the passive redundant diaphragmatic tissue, and establish in its place a rigid diaphragmatic structure. Although the potential for recovery of

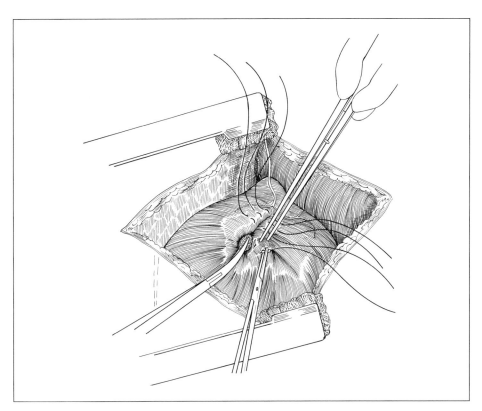

Fig. 54-3. Multiple interrupted imbricating sutures are placed between the phrenic nerve branches at the site of the diaphragmatic plication.

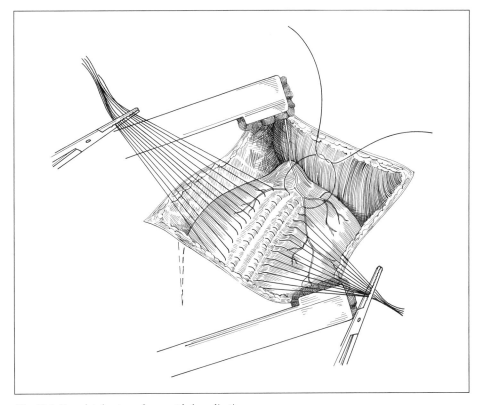

Fig. 54-4. Completed suture placement before plication.

phrenic nerve function may exist in cases of neural paralysis, the recovery of normal neuromuscular function cannot be predicted or anticipated.

The operative approach uses a posterolateral thoracotomy in most cases. All right-sided eventrations are best approached through the chest. Left-sided lesions can be approached via a thoracotomy or laparotomy. Our preference is to proceed with thoracotomy due to the better exposure of the phrenic nerve branches. Bilateral eventrations, although rare, are best approached through a laparotomy incision. Patients who present with gastric volvulus and eventration should undergo laparotomy for gastric fixation and diaphragmatic plication.

Our preference is for diaphragmatic plication, rather then resection. The procedure is performed through a standard posterolateral thoracotomy incision, using the seventh to eighth intercostal space. The initial examination of the diaphragmatic tissue should concentrate on the identification of the phrenic nerve branches (Fig. 54-2). Their preservation should be planned even though their potential for recovery is often limited.

The desired outcome of surgical intervention should be the construction of a rigid, flat hemidiaphragm that does not participate in or detract from ventilatory movement. This can be achieved by placing two rows of sutures to imbricate the redundant hemidiaphragm. The initial row of plication sutures is placed along the posterolateral one-third of the diaphragm, beginning at the central portion of the diaphragm and proceeding toward the periphery. The sutures are placed parallel to the branches of the phrenic nerve. Each suture placed should pick up several centimeters of tissue in two to three equally spaced bites. During this imbrication maneuver, the diaphragmatic tissue should be elevated to lift it off the liver in the case of a right-sided eventration, or stomach/spleen in left-sided defects (Fig. 54-3). The entire row of interrupted sutures is placed; then all are tied to imbricate the diaphragm (Fig. 54-4). The suture material selected should be permanent; we prefer 2-0 braided nylon, or monofilament nylon. A second row of sutures is then placed from the center of the diaphragm along the anterior one-third of the diaphragm. Following plication of the diaphragm, the tissue

should be taut, not redundant. If this is not achieved following the placement of these two suture lines, the tissue along the suture lines can be plicated again over itself to continue the imbrication of the redundant hemidiaphragm until proper correction is achieved (Fig. 54-5).

A thoracostomy tube is placed for pleural drainage, and can usually be removed after 24 to 48 hours. We provide antibiotic coverage until thoracostomy tube removal is accomplished. The patient can often be weaned from mechanical ventilatory support immediately after operation.

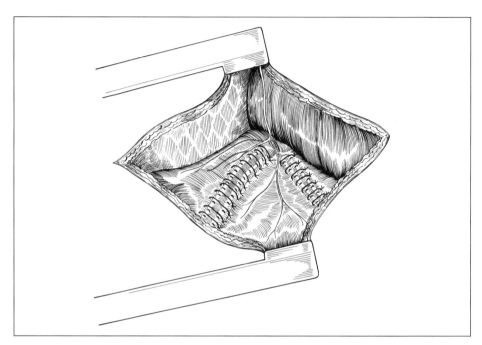

Fig. 54-5. Completed diaphragmatic plication removing the redundacy within the hemidiaphragm.

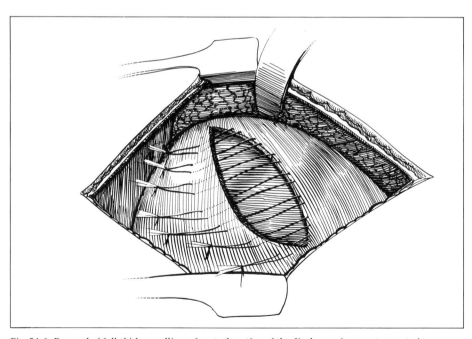

Fig. 54-6. Removal of full-thickness ellipse of central portion of the diaphragm in an anteroposterior direction. (From AJ Ross III and HC Bishop. Congenital and Acquired Enervation of the Diaphram. In LM Nyhus, and RJ Baker [eds]. Mastery of Surgery *[2nd ed]. Boston: Little, Brown, 1992.)*

An alternative procedure involves resection of the redundant portion of the eventrated diaphragm. A full-thickness ellipse of the central portion of the diaphragm is removed, and the remaining portions are imbricated to achieve a two-layer closure. The diaphragm resected should not include the major branches of the phrenic nerve, and care must be exercised to avoid abdominal visceral injury when the resection margins are established. The first row of sutures is placed, and then tied, to imbricate the diaphragm margins. The second row of sutures that secures the imbrication should not transgress the diaphragm to avoid abdominal organ injury (Fig. 54-6). This procedure also reconstructs a flat, noncompliant diaphragm.

Extubation is expected following recovery from the anesthetic administered. Recurrence is uncommon, and recovery of motion within the involved hemidiaphragm is rarely a problem.

Suggested Reading

Anderson KD. Congenital Diaphragmatic Hernia. In KJ Welch, JG Randolph, MM Ravitch, et al (eds), *Pediatric Surgery* (4th ed). Vol 1. Chicago: Year Book, 1986.

deLorimier AA. Diaphragmatic Hernia. In KW Ashcraft, TM Holder (eds), *Pediatric Surgery* (2nd ed). Philadelphia, Saunders, 1993.

The Diaphragm. In JE Skandalakis, SW Gray (eds), *Embryology for Surgeons* (2nd ed). Baltimore: Williams & Wilkins, 1994.

McIntyre RC Jr, Bensard DD, Karrer FM, et al. The pediatric diaphragm in acute gastric volvulus. *J Am Coll Surg* 178:234, 1994.

Pomerantz M. The Diaphragm. In DC Sabiston Jr, FC Spencer (eds), *Gibbon's Surgery of the Chest* (4th ed). Vol II. Philadelphia: Saunders, 1983.

Reynolds M. Diaphragmatic Anomalies. In JG Raffensperger (ed), *Swenson's Pediatric Surgery* (5th ed). Norwalk, CT: Appleton & Lange, 1990.

Ross AJ, Bishop HC. Congenital and Acquired Eventration of the Diaphragm. In LM Nyhus, RJ Baker (ed), *Mastery of Surgery* (2nd ed). Vol II. Boston: Little, Brown, 1992.

EDITOR'S COMMENT

The presentation on eventration of the diaphragm in newborn infants and young children is found in the preceding chapter. We are reminded that unilateral elevation of the diaphragm (eventration) in adults is a clinically distinct syndrome. Surgical intervention frequently is required in infants but is rarely necessary in adults. This clinical difference is related almost entirely to the effects of eventration on pulmonary function. When an infant sustains diaphragmatic paresis, compromise of lung function is sudden and leads to disastrous sequelae if not corrected immediately. The onset in adults is usually insidious and more tolerable. Surgical repair may not be indicated, but when it is necessary, incision, excision, plication, and insertion of prosthetic material are techniques available to the surgeon.

It is unusual to find good follow-up data after operative treatment. Kizilcan and associates (*J Pediatr Surg* 28:42, 1993) made an assessment of the long-term functions of plicated diaphragms 1.5 to 11 years postoperatively. This was achieved by fluoroscopic, ultrasonographic, and spirometric studies in 12 patients. The absence of paradoxical motion with normal localization of the diaphragms in all patients, and satisfactory motions of diaphragms in nine patients, were documented by fluoroscopy. Measurements of diaphragmatic thicknesses showed that plicated diaphragms of all patients maintained their growths in proportion to the contralateral sides. Additionally, normal values of pulmonary function tests in five of six patients of suitable age for spirometry were obtained. All the clinical studies demonstrated that diaphragmatic plication did not interfere with further development of diaphragms, and late functional results of the plication were acceptable.

L.M.N.

55

Traumatic Rupture of the Diaphragm

Erwin R. Thal   David A. Provost

Sennertus was the first to report the post-mortem finding of a strangulated stomach associated with a diaphragmatic hernia in 1541. Three hundred years later, in 1853, Bowditch recognized the injury before death and is given credit for describing some of the classic clinical findings, such as mediastinal shift, dullness to percussion, and bowel sounds auscultated in the chest.

Diaphragmatic rupture resulting from blunt or penetrating trauma is a relatively common occurrence in the injured patient. While the true incidence is unknown, autopsy series of patients with blunt trauma who died before arrival at a hospital suggest that approximately 5 percent have a ruptured diaphragm. The injury is found more frequently in patients who sustain penetrating trauma, and in some subsets, such as anterior wounds below the nipple, the occurrence may be as high as 30 percent.

Anatomy

The diaphragm is a large structure consisting primarily of muscle and fascia that divides the two major torso cavities. The word *diaphragm* is of Greek derivation: "dia," meaning in between, and "phragma," meaning fence. The peripheral muscle fibers of the diaphragm insert into a central tendon, the superior surface of which is partially fused with the fibrous portion of the pericardium. The central tendon consists of a left, median, and right lobe. The lateral aspects of the muscle attach to the lateral chest wall while the posterior portion inserts on the periosteal surfaces of the first three lumbar vertebrae.

Anteriorly, it attaches to the sternum (Fig. 55-1).

The motor supply comes from the phrenic nerve, as does the sensory innervation to the central tendon, parietal pleura, and peritoneum. The nerve inserts into each leaflet near the junction of the pericardium and the central tendon. It then splays out laterally over the dome. Care must be taken to avoid the large branches when repairing traumatic injuries (Fig. 55-2). The sensory supply to the peripheral part of the diaphragm comes from the lower five intercostal nerves.

The blood supply arises inferiorly from direct branches off the aorta. Additional

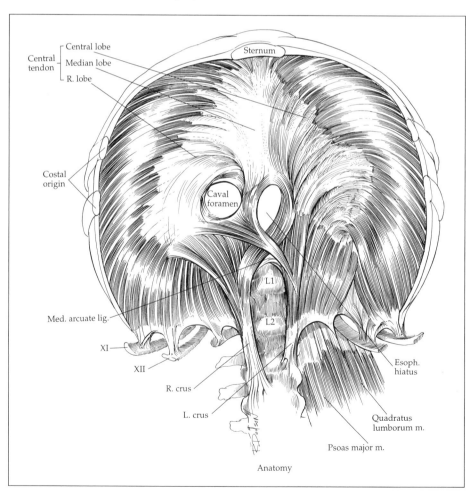

Fig. 55-1. Anatomy of the diaphragm; view from below.

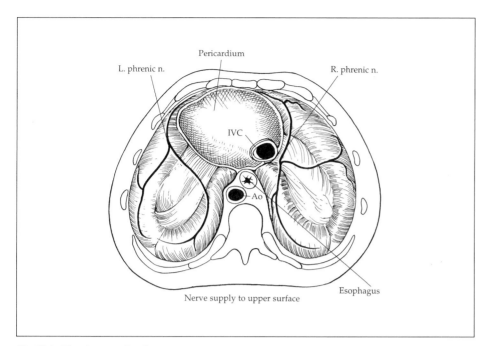

Fig. 55-2. Phrenic nerve distribution.

blood supply comes peripherally from the intercostal vessels and vessels traveling with the phrenic nerve.

During the normal respiratory cycle diaphragmatic excursion is significant. The right diaphragm on deep expiration may rise as high as the fourth intercostal space anteriorly, which is slightly higher than its left-sided counterpart. Both sides ascend to the seventh or eighth intercostal space posteriorly. These landmarks serve as guidelines to potential diaphragmatic injury when associated with penetrating trauma.

Mechanism of Injury

Although diaphragmatic injuries occur with both blunt and penetrating trauma, the latter is far more prevalent. The relative risk of injury associated with knife wounds is dependent upon variables that are frequently unknown. These include the size and length of the offending weapon, the position of the diaphragm in the respiratory cycle, and the effect of concurrent diseases. The large surface area of the diaphragm leaves it susceptible to injury with gunshot and shotgun wounds. These may be more difficult to assess because of the unpredictable trajectory often taken by missiles. Missiles may enter the chest, perforate the diaphragm, injure intra-abdom-

inal organs, and somehow end up back in the chest cavity. Awareness of these erratic pathways will alert the astute physician to the possibility of diaphragmatic injury in patients who on first assessment seem to have their injuries limited to the chest. Seemingly innocuous external wounds may be deceptive and despite their minuscule size may traverse the diaphragm.

Penetrating injuries often leave a small rent in the diaphragm. The combination of intra-abdominal pressure, which may be as high as 150 mm Hg; negative intrathoracic pressure; and the constant motion of the diaphragm may prevent spontaneous healing of the injury. On the contrary it is not unusual for these small injuries to increase in size with time to the point where they allow herniation and subsequent strangulation of intra-abdominal viscera.

Blunt trauma may cause a burst type of injury to the diaphragm when associated with a sudden increase in intra-abdominal pressure. This is commonly seen in patients wearing lap-type seat belts who are suddenly compressed with rapid deceleration-type collisions. Victims of lateral impact collisions may be more likely to sustain a ruptured diaphragm than those subjected to frontal collisions. Deformation of the chest wall, which creates a shearing force on the diaphragm; crush injuries; and other types of trauma that cause an increase in pressure in the ab-

dominal cavity are all forces that are capable of producing a disruption. The injury usually extends in a posterolateral fashion from the central tendon and is more common on the left. The same mechanism occurs on the right; however, it is thought that some of the force may be dissipated by the liver, which in turn may afford some protection to the right hemidiaphragm. The defect in the diaphragm tends to be larger when associated with blunt trauma. The diaphragm may be avulsed from its lateral attachments to the chest wall and less frequently may involve its pericardial surface. Fragments of rib fractures can also cause penetration of the diaphragm.

It is often reported that diaphragmatic injuries occur more frequently on the left side. In patients who sustain stab wounds, this is attributed to the fact that most assailants are right handed. The preponderance of left-sided wounds associated with blunt trauma is explained on the basis of the left posterior leaf being the weaker portion of the diaphragm. Recent reports seem to describe a more equal distribution of these injuries, which is certainly the case with penetrating injuries and many blunt injuries as well.

Pathophysiology

Minor injuries may be difficult to detect and, hence, a high index of suspicion must be ever present. On the other hand patients who sustain acute injury may manifest several pathophysiologic changes that facilitate the diagnosis but also place them at considerable risk.

Hemodynamic instability may occur secondary to acute blood loss. This usually occurs as a result of associated injuries and is rarely attributed to the diaphragm. Blood from the abdominal cavity can translocate into the chest and cause ventilatory compromise. Massive blood loss may accumulate in the ipsilateral pleural space and on rare occasion can result in a shift of the mediastinum, with resultant decrease in ventilation both on the involved and uninvolved side. One must guard against blindly attributing blood in the pleural cavity to a primary hemothorax when in reality it may be coming from the abdomen via the rent in the diaphragm. Visceral organs may be displaced into the chest through large defects more commonly seen with blunt trauma. On rare occasions these organs compromise left ventricular function simulating cardiac tamponade.

Respiratory function can be significantly reduced when the positive intra-abdominal pressure equilibrates with the negative intrathoracic pressure, causing collapse of the ipsilateral lung. The mechanical effect of herniated abdominal viscera may cause the mediastinum to shift to the contralateral side, with resultant compromise of ventilatory function and possible decrease in venous return, diminished cardiac output, and hypotension.

Blood supply may become compromised if an organ is trapped in a small defect. Signs and symptoms of nonviable tissue may ensue as the patient becomes toxic. If a hollow organ ruptures in the chest cavity a severe pleural reaction may occur and if colonic contents are extravasated the patient may become septic.

Diagnosis

The high incidence of associated intra-abdominal injuries results in early diagnosis and surgical exploration in many patients. In those without indications for surgical intervention, the recognition of this injury becomes much more difficult. Although history and physical examination are the hallmark of clinical diagnosis, their accuracy is disappointing in detecting diaphragmatic injury. With visceral herniation one may detect decreased breath sounds, the presence of bowel sounds on auscultation, or dullness and on occasion tympany to percussion. More commonly these injuries produce no abnormal physical signs. Aronoff and coauthors reported normal physical findings in 55 percent of blunt injuries and 44 percent of penetrating injuries. Moore and colleagues reported that 30 percent of patients with stab wounds and 20 percent of patients who sustained gunshot wounds to the lower chest and abdomen had negative clinical findings despite significant injuries found at operation. This difficulty in recognizing diaphragmatic injuries can be explained by the infrequency of herniation with both penetrating and blunt trauma as well as the protection provided by the large right lobe of the liver.

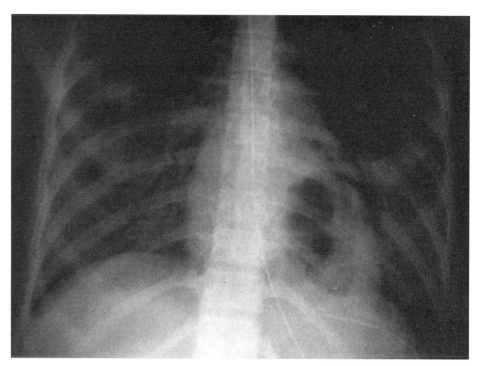

Fig. 55-3. Chest roentgenogram demonstrating herniation of the colon into the left thoracic cavity.

Routine chest roentgenograms are limited in their ability to identify a diaphragmatic defect unless abdominal visceral herniation has occurred (Fig. 55-3). Gelman and associates, in a retrospective review of 50 patients with surgically proven diaphragmatic injuries due to blunt trauma, noted that the chest radiograph was diagnostic in only 46 percent of left-sided injuries. Another 18 percent were suspicious enough to warrant additional studies. The chest x-ray was diagnostic of the injury in one of seven patients (14 percent) with right-sided injuries. Although some authors found abnormal x-rays in almost all patients, the majority of series now report that at least one-third of the chest films obtained in these patients are normal.

Nonspecific findings suggestive of this injury are a hemothorax, basal subsegmental atelectasis, elevation of the injured hemidiaphragm, or irregularity in the diaphragmatic contour. The seemingly elevated hemidiaphragm may represent the arcuate contour of a partially herniated gastric fundus or a portion of the liver. On the contrary, elevation of the hemidiaphragm caused by phrenic nerve damage or eventration may permit the abdominal viscera to occupy a position high in the thorax, thus mimicking herniation. This confusion may be resolved by instilling contrast material in either the stomach or colon. A contrast study may demonstrate constriction of the viscera as it passes through the defect in the diaphragm. With the routine use of nasogastric tubes in trauma patients, one may occasionally see the tube in the chest on the routine chest film.

Serial x-rays may be of some value. Because of the pressure differential between the chest and abdominal cavity, the visceral organ may be sucked into the chest and become apparent at a later time. It is also possible that the defect will expand with time, allowing herniation to occur, hence delaying the diagnosis.

Pneumoperitoneum may be seen on a preoperative chest x-ray. If a hollow viscus injury is not found at celiotomy, one should be suspicious of a diaphragmatic injury. Pneumoperitoneum has been used in the past as a diagnostic test; however, it is unreliable and has essentially been discarded. The omentum or herniated viscus often plugs the defect rendering the study useless.

Diagnostic peritoneal lavage has been a poor predictor of diaphragmatic injury. The defect in the diaphragm rarely produces significant bleeding and unless there is hemorrhage from associated injuries the lavage is likely to be negative. Most series report a 20 to 25 percent incidence of false-negative lavages. On occasion useful information is gained, by lavage, if the patient has a chest tube inserted before the study. If a large clear effluent is noted consistent with the infusion of fluid into the peritoneal cavity, one can surmise that a defect is present in the diaphragm.

In spite of the frequent use of computed tomography, its ability to demonstrate diaphragmatic injuries has been disappointing. Gelman and associates reported the study as being diagnostic in only one of seven patients with proven injury in whom it was performed. These authors noted that an MRI identified the injury in the two patients in whom it was utilized. There has not been enough experience with this study to determine its efficacy at this time.

With the current interest in laparoscopy varying reports are beginning to appear in the literature. Many are favorable; however, there is no question that some of these injuries are missed. The accuracy is dependent upon the laparoscopic technique that is used and the location of the injury. Possible insufflation of the chest cavity with its potential pulmonary complications was an early concern, but at present has not been a major problem. Ivatury and his coauthors reported finding eight clinically unsuspected diaphragmatic injuries in a series of 40 patients who sustained penetrating trauma to the lower chest. They concluded that laparoscopy is an excellent modality for the evaluation of the intrathoracic abdomen and the diaphragm. Rossi and colleagues reported missing three of eight diaphragmatic injuries in their laparoscopic study. Other series have noted missed injury rates of 20 to 25 percent.

The newest and perhaps most accurate study in the evaluation of diaphragmatic injuries is video-assisted thoracoscopy. Ochsner and associates were the first to report an experience with this modality. They evaluated thoracoscopy in 14 patients, the last 9 of whom had videothoracoscopy, which was believed to be easier and faster to perform. Their findings were confirmed by either laparoscopy or laparotomy and they correctly identified an injury in nine patients and no injury in five. They found the procedure to be safe, ac-

curate, and less invasive than laparotomy. Fry and his coauthors evaluated 24 consecutive patients with chest trauma, 22 of whom sustained penetrating injuries and 2 who had blunt trauma. Diaphragmatic laceration was suspected in 10, 2 because of an abnormal chest x-ray and 8 because of proximity. Videothoracoscopy confirmed five injuries, four of which were repaired with thoracoscopic techniques. These authors concluded that videothoracoscopy is an accurate, safe, and minimally invasive method for the assessment of diaphragmatic injuries. Spann and colleagues reported their experience with video-assisted thoracoscopic surgery in 22 patients who sustained either blunt or penetrating injuries to the lower chest or upper abdomen and who were suspected of having a diaphragmatic injury. Each of these patients underwent a celiotomy after thoracoscopy. Only two of eight patients suspected of having the injury based on physical examination and chest radiography had it confirmed at operation. Six of the 22 patients had an injury and all 6 were seen at thoracoscopy. No injuries were missed, leading the authors to conclude that video-assisted thoracoscopy is a safe, expeditious, and accurate method of evaluating the diaphragm in injured patients and is comparable in diagnostic accuracy to exploratory celiotomy.

Injury to the diaphragm is rare in the pediatric population. Brandt and coauthors reported only 13 children with the injury in an 18-year period, noting that 9 of the children had associated injuries as well. They suggest that, as a result of the increased compliance of the thoracic cage in children, rupture of the diaphragm can occur without external evidence of injury and hence should be considered in any child who suffers blunt or penetrating thoracoabdominal trauma.

Feliciano and associates caution that diaphragmatic injuries can be missed in patients with penetrating trauma even when they are taken to the operating room. During a 9-year period they identified 16 patients who had a delay in diagnosis that ranged from 16 hours to 14 years. Three patients had the injury missed at operation. Three patients had x-rays that did not identify the injury, two patients had a false-negative lavage, and one patient in the acute group did not have a chest film taken. They recommend careful review of

early and late follow-up chest x-rays as the easiest mechanism to avoid significant delays in diagnosis.

Finally, a small group of authors believe that the best diagnostic study is a celiotomy without extensive preoperative studies. Stylianos and King reported their experience with 41 consecutive patients with stab wounds to the left lower anterior chest. The first 21 patients were operated on only after demonstrating peritoneal signs or continued blood loss. Ten of the 21 patients required celiotomy, with 2 having an isolated diaphragmatic injury. Two of the 11 patients not explored returned within 18 months with an incarcerated hernia. The next 20 patients in their series were studied prospectively and all had a routine celiotomy. Ten patients (50 percent) were found to have isolated diaphragm injuries and seven had a negative exploration. These authors suggested that the true incidence of occult diaphragm injuries may be underestimated and concluded that in the absence of a reliable, noninvasive test to diagnose penetration of the diaphragm, celiotomy should be considered in light of the risks of late strangulation.

Madden and his coauthors reported, in their review of 95 patients with stab wounds to the lower chest and abdomen who underwent routine exploration, that 18 had a diaphragmatic injury, and in 5 it was the only injury found. They reported that a delayed recognition of an incarcerated diaphragmatic hernia had an associated mortality of 36 percent. They concluded that exploratory laparotomy is necessary until a reliable nonoperative method is established that can exclude injuries to the diaphragm.

Treatment

Patients with diaphragmatic hernia are resuscitated in the usual fashion. A nasogastric tube is routinely inserted as part of the initial assessment; however, resistance may be encountered if there is distortion of the esophagogastric junction. Placement of the tube in the distal esophagus will often evacuate air from the stomach; however, forceful attempts to pass the tube should be avoided. If there has been visceral herniation with resultant respiratory compromise, it may be necessary to intubate the patient. Caution must be exercised if there is an associated pneumothorax or hemothorax as chest tube insertion may cause further injury to the herniated abdominal viscus.

Acute injuries are best approached through an abdominal incision. This affords the advantage of being able to assess and treat any associated abdominal injury. Most chest injuries can be managed non-operatively, thus eliminating the need for two operations. Thoracotomy is reserved for chronic hernias, where adhesions between the herniated organs and the lung are difficult to take down from an abdominal approach and associated injuries are not a concern.

The patient is placed on the operating table in the supine position. Pneumatic compression stockings are used for prophylaxis of thromboembolism if permitted by the patient's condition. A wide surgical prep extending from the proximal thighs to the neck is performed. The chest should always be included in the surgical field in case urgent anterolateral thoracotomy or tube thoracostomy is required. The patient is draped before induction of anesthesia, which will allow rapid access to the abdomen should rapid deterioration occur.

The abdomen is entered through a midline incision from the xiphoid process to just below the umbilicus. If present, intraperitoneal blood and clot are rapidly evacuated, and packs are placed to control ongoing hemorrhage. The abdomen is explored in a systematic and thorough fashion. Blood loss is controlled and gross soilage is limited by closing any hollow organ perforation. The diaphragm is carefully evaluated by both visual inspection and manual palpation.

Herniated viscera are reduced from the thoracic cavity by gentle traction. When resistance is met, careful passage of a small nasogastric tube alongside the herniated organs into the chest will often release a vacuum, facilitating reduction (Fig. 55-4). Extending the phrenotomy a short distance allows reduction when other maneuvers are unsuccessful. Lateral extension for central ruptures and anterior phrenotomy for medial and parahiatal defects avoid the phrenic nerve branches, minimizing postoperative diaphragmatic dysfunction (Fig. 55-5).

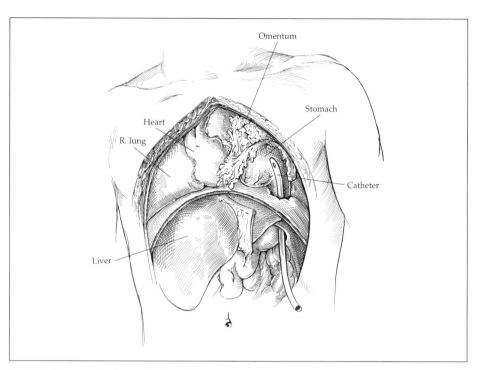

Fig. 55-4. Nasogastric tube passed through the injured diaphragm into the chest to release a vacuum, facilitating reduction of herniated viscera.

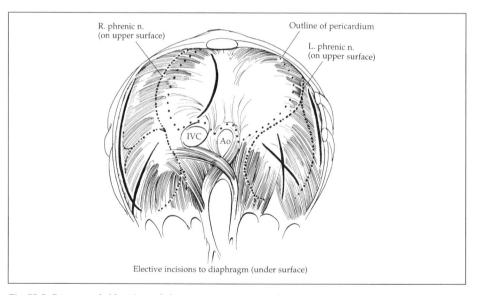

Fig. 55-5. Recommended locations of phrenotomy extension to allow reduction and avoid phrenic nerve injury.

The pleural space is thoroughly irrigated with warm saline to remove retained blood and clot. Several liters are required in the presence of a perforated viscus. The diaphragmatic defect is closed using interrupted figure-of-eight or horizontal mattress sutures of 2-0 polypropylene (Fig. 55-6). The tail of the previously placed suture is used as a handle to provide expo- sure, permitting careful suture placement during repair of the posterior portion of the defect (Fig. 55-7). Teflon pledgets are occasionally used when the diaphragm is attenuated or the closure is tenuous. Some authors recommend a two-layer closure for defects greater than 2 cm. The inner layer is an interlocking horizontal mattress that everts the edges of the diaphragm.

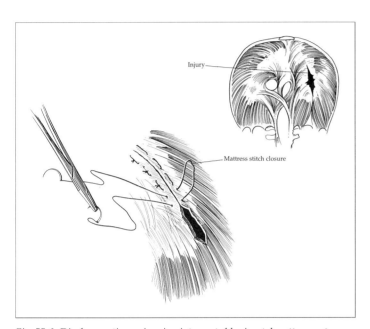

Fig. 55-6. *Diaphragmatic repair using interrupted horizontal mattress sutures.*

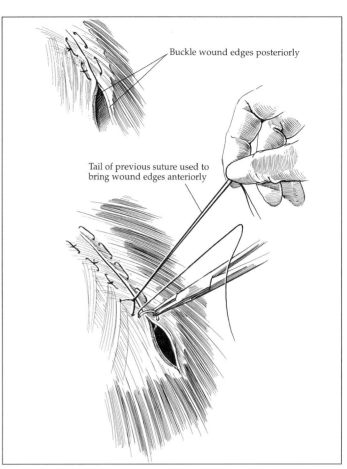

Fig. 55-7. *The tail of the previously placed suture used as a handle to improve exposure for repair of the posterior portion of the defect.*

This is reinforced with a running 3-0 polypropylene or similar type of nonabsorbable suture.

When tube thoracostomy has not been performed preoperatively and no underlying lung injury is present, residual air and fluid can be aspirated from the pleural space, thereby eliminating the need for a postoperative chest tube. A No. 24 French red rubber catheter is placed through the final mattress suture into the chest (Fig. 55-8). Air and fluid are then withdrawn under suction. With the lungs held in full inspiration, the catheter is extracted while the final mattress suture is tied.

The diaphragm is occasionally avulsed from the rib cage following blunt injuries. Closure of the defect is accomplished using interrupted mattress sutures placed through the diaphragm and around the appropriate rib (Fig. 55-9). It is often necessary to reattach the diaphragm one or

two ribs higher than its insertion to permit closure without tension. Synthetic material such as Marlex mesh is rarely needed, but may be indicated in occasional patients with large defects. The mesh is sutured to the free edges of the defect using interrupted sutures of 2-0 polypropylene (Fig. 55-10).

A postoperative chest x-ray is obtained and tube thoracostomy may be necessary if a residual pneumothorax is large. Diaphragmatic dysfunction varies, and ventilator support may be required in the immediate postoperative period. This is rarely needed for isolated injuries but may be necessary for significant chest injuries or other associated injuries. Postoperative atelectasis is common and respiratory complications can be minimized by aggressive pulmonary support. Recurrence of diaphragmatic hernias repaired in the acute postinjury period is rare.

Chronic Herniation

A small defect in the diaphragm may not produce symptoms and therefore may not be recognized at the time of injury. On occasion visceral herniation may occur early, but the patient will remain asymptomatic for varying periods of time. Symptoms may be vague and range from nonspecific pleuritic or chest pain to frank sepsis resulting from free perforation into the thoracic cavity. The diagnostic workup is similar to that for patients who present with acute injury.

Patients who are operated on more than a week or two after the acute injury are best approached through the thoracic route. The lack of a peritoneal hernia sac allows the bowel to adhere to the lung, thus making reduction through a celiotomy difficult. Solid organs may also become adherent to the lung, thus requiring tedious and

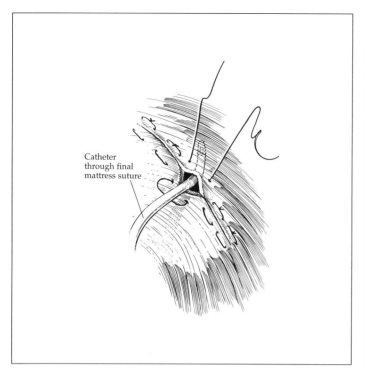

Fig. 55-8. Aspiration of residual pneumothorax with a No. 24 French red rubber catheter. The catheter is extracted as the final suture is tied.

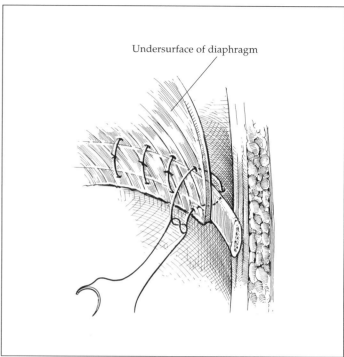

Fig. 55-9. Re-attachment of diaphragm avulsed from costal origin with interrupted mattress sutures placed around the rib.

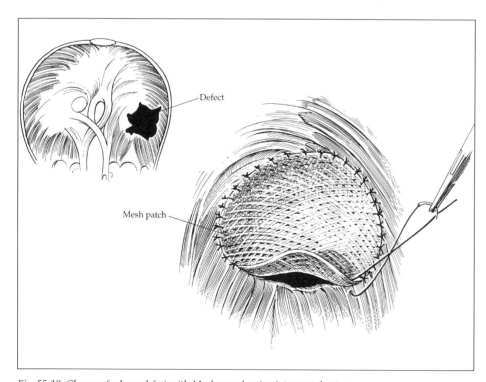

Fig. 55-10. Closure of a large defect with Marlex mesh using interrupted sutures.

meticulous dissection. Once reduction is accomplished the diaphragm is repaired using the same techniques as described for patients with an acute injury. Delayed recognition, especially when associated with incarceration or strangulation, is associated with significant mortality.

Suggested Reading

Aronoff RJ, Reynolds J, Thal ER. Evaluation of diaphragmatic injuries. *Am J Surg* 144:671, 1982.

Brandt ML, Luks FI, Spigland NA, et al. Diaphragmatic injury in children. *J Trauma* 32:298, 1992.

Brown GL, Richardson JD. Traumatic diaphragmatic hernia: A continuing challenge. *Ann Thorac Surg* 39:170, 1985.

Feliciano DV, Cruse PA, Mattox KL, et al. Delayed diagnosis of injuries to the diaphragm after penetrating wounds. *J Trauma* 28:1135, 1988.

Gelman R, Mirvis SE, Gens D. Diaphragmatic rupture due to blunt trauma: Sensitivity of plain chest radiographs. *AJR* 156:51, 1991.

Ivatury RR, Simon RJ, Weksler B, et al. Laparoscopy in the evaluation of the intrathoracic abdomen after penetrating injury. *J Trauma* 33:101, 1992.

Kearney PA, Rouhana SW, Burney RE. Blunt rupture of the diaphragm: Mechanism, diagnosis, and treatment. *Ann Emerg Med* 18:1326, 1989.

Madden MR, Paull DE, Finkelstein JL, et al. Occult diaphragmatic injury from stab wounds to the lower chest and abdomen. *J Trauma* 29:292, 1989.

Moore JB, Moore EE, Thompson JS. Abdominal injuries associated with penetrating trauma in the lower chest. *Am J Surg* 140:724, 1980.

Ochsner MG, Rozycki GS, Lucente F, et al. Prospective evaluation of thoracostomy for diagnosing injury in thoracoabdominal trauma: A preliminary report. *J Trauma* 34:704, 1993.

Root HD. Injury to the Diaphragm. In EE Moore, KL Mattox, DV Feliciano (eds), *Trauma*, (2nd ed.), Norwalk, CT: Appleton & Lange, 1991.

Rossi P, Mullins D, Thal E. Role of laparoscopy in the evaluation of abdominal trauma. *Am J Surg* 166:707, 1993.

Smith RS, Fry WR, Tsoi EK, et al. Preliminary report on videothoracoscopy in the evaluation and treatment of thoracic injury. *Am J Surg* 166:690, 1993.

Spann JC, Nwariaku FE, Wait MA. Evaluation of video-assisted thoracoscopic surgery in the diagnosis of diaphragmatic injuries. *Am J Surg* 170:628, 1995.

Stylianos S, King TC. Occult diaphragm injuries at celiotomy for left chest stab wounds. *Am Surg* 58:364, 1992.

EDITOR'S COMMENT

We have been pleased by the ability to view a chest roentgenogram in an adult patient and, on seeing the air fluid levels in the right or left chest, announce to the gathered throng, "Aha, this patient has a diaphragmatic hernia, probably traumatic in origin!" Further discussion ensues, outlining how to confirm this evidence of diagnostic acumen. The list of diagnostic methods presented by Fildes (in Nyhus, and Condon [eds], *Hernia* (4th ed). Philadelphia: Lippincott, 1995) is formidable, but at the same time helpful. His long list includes: history and physical examination, chest roentgenogram, diagnostic peritoneal lavage, computed tomography, contrast studies of the stomach and colon, magnetic resonance imaging, laparoscopy or thoracoscopy, fluoroscopy, pneumoperitoneum, sonography, liver-spleen radionuclide scan, intraperitoneal contrast, and laparotomy. Classically, acute traumatic diaphragmatic hernias are repaired through the abdomen, whereas thoracotomy is the preferred approach for chronic hernias repaired one month or more after injury. The major differences between the two forms of diaphragmatic rupture are 1) acute hernias from either blunt or penetrating trauma may be accompanied by other intra-abdominal injuries, requiring celiotomy for evaluation and definitive treatment, and 2) chronic hernias are occasionally encountered in which the herniated viscus (or viscera) is densely adherent to the lung or parietal pleura, making good visibility through extensive exposure mandatory. With a significant amount of pleural reaction seen on the chest roentgenogram, thoracotomy is especially useful, because the original injury is highly likely to have caused dense adherence between the lung and the viscus. If a chronic traumatic diaphragmatic hernia is approached through the abdomen and reduction of the herniated viscus, usually colon, is not easily accomplished by dissecting the diaphragmatic defect, excessive traction of the viscus must be avoided in order to prevent tearing and contamination of the pleural space with intestinal content. Rather than face this dilemma, our authors recommend that the patient be positioned appropriately on the operating table and the chest wall prepared so that it is easy to open, if necessary, for proper reduction of the chest contents and repair of the hernia defect. It should be remembered, that, in this setting, a combined thoracoabdominal incision is the worst choice, as the diaphragm will almost certainly end up with two defects, and denervation of the diaphragm or a recurrent hernia is a likely sequela.

L.M.N.

56

Surgical Management
of Paraesophageal Herniation

Rodney J. Landreneau

Paraesophageal herniation is an uncommon disorder of the gastroesophageal hiatus characterized by the potential for life-threatening complications resulting from mechanical obstruction and vascular compromise of the stomach. This scenario of paraesophageal hernias contrasts with the more common sliding esophageal hiatal hernia, which is principally defined by its frequent association with symptomatic gastroesophageal reflux.

The sliding esophageal hiatal hernia is anatomically characterized by a laxity in the phrenoesophageal ligament, which usually anchors the gastroesophageal junction to its normal intra-abdominal location and maintains the relationship of the distal esophagus to the gastric cardia and fundus. A variable cephalad migration of the gastroesophageal junction through the hiatus into the posterior mediastinum is characteristic (Fig. 56-1). These abnormalities in the phrenoesophageal ligamentous attachments of the gastroesophageal junction also increase the risk for impaired function of the lower esophageal sphincter. This in part explains the common association of pathologic gastroesophageal reflux with sliding (*type I*) hiatal hernias.

In distinction, primary paraesophageal (*type II*) hiatal hernias are associated with preservation of the normal posterior phrenoesophageal ligamentous anchorage of the gastroesophageal junction within the abdomen. These true hernias are defined by a large peritoneal lined opening in the esophageal hiatus anterior to a normally positioned gastroesophageal junction (Fig. 56-2).

The combination of sliding and paraesophageal hernia components (*type III hiatal hernia*) is also commonly encountered. Patients with this combined hernia process will often have symptoms related to pathologic gastroesophageal reflux and to mechanical obstruction of the stomach within the paraesophageal component of the hernia.

In the vast majority of circumstances, the body of the gastric fundus is the lead point of the paraesophageal herniation; however, other intra-abdominal viscera may also herniate (*type IV hiatal hernia*) into the mediastinum anterior to the stationary gastroesophageal junction (Fig. 56-3). Air within the obstructed stomach or other herniated hollow viscera results in the

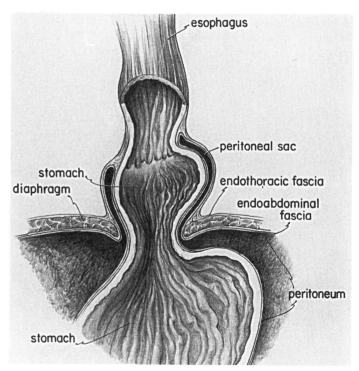

Fig. 56-1. *Illustration of the anatomic characteristics of the "sliding" hiatal hernia. The phrenoesophageal ligament is attenuated, resulting in cephalic migration of the gastroesophageal junction into the chest. This is commonly associated with functional disturbance in the integrity of the lower esophageal sphincter and pathologic gastroesophageal reflux.*

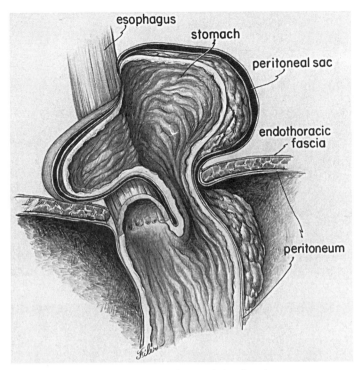

Fig. 56-2. Illustration of the anatomic characteristics of a primary paraesophageal hiatal hernia demonstrating preservation of the posterior phrenoesophageal ligament attachments and a true peritoneal lined herniation of the gastric fundus through an anterior expansion of the esophageal hiatal opening.

esophagus
stomach
peritoneal sac
endothoracic fascia
peritoneum

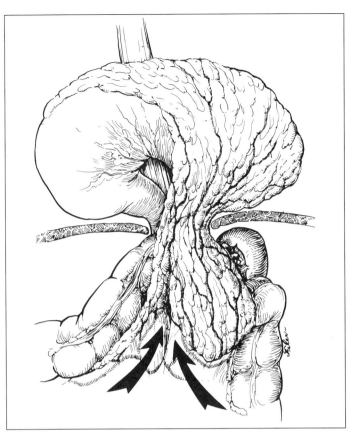

Fig. 56-3. Illustration of large paraesophageal hernia with stomach and omentum migrating into the intrathoracic hernia sac.

characteristic roentgenographic findings of an air fluid level within a retrocardiac mass (Fig. 56-4).

Clinical Presentation

As with other true hernias of the abdominal cavity, paraesophageal hernias are primarily distinguished by symptoms related to intermittent mechanical obstruction of the herniated gastric fundus. Typically, patients with paraesophageal hernia are older than patients identified with sliding hiatal hernias. On careful questioning paraesophageal hernia patients will usually admit to having a long history of upper aerodigestive complaints that can be attributed to their hiatal hernias. This has led some investigators to believe that paraesophageal hernias are simply a more advanced stage of the commoner sliding hiatal hernia. The physiologic case against this is that only a minority of patients with primary paraesophageal hernias admit to having classic gastroesophageal reflux symptoms and anatomically the gastro-

esophageal junction usually remains in its normal intra-abdominal position. Indeed, the primary complaints of patients with paraesophageal hernia are intermittent substernal chest pain, cough, and aspiration events related to distention and obstruction of the esophagus and intrathoracic stomach. The patient may also present with occult or frank gastrointestinal bleeding from the intrathoracic stomach related to "acid stasis" ulceration or chronic mucosal venous engorgement. The gastroesophageal reflux symptoms of regurgitation and heartburn are usually minor complaints unless the patient also has impairment in the integrity of the lower esophageal sphincter mechanism. This latter circumstance is usually associated with the anatomic, physiologic, and roentgenographic findings found with the minority of patients who have "truly" mixed (type III) sliding and paraesophageal herniation (Fig. 56-5).

The most devastating complications of paraesophageal hernias are gastric incarceration and vascular strangulation, which

can be associated with a mortality approaching 50 percent. Surgical treatment is generally indicated to avoid these catastrophes related to gastric obstruction or volvulus.

We believe in individualizing the operative approach utilized for paraesophageal hernia repair to the patient's pathophysiologic condition rather than attempting to apply a single repair for all patients with this heterogeneous clinical problem. Accordingly, we advocate selective application of primary repair alone or the alternative of repair with fundoplication in the management of paraesophageal herniation. This chapter describes our surgical approach to the broad clinical spectrum of paraesophageal herniation.

Diagnostic Workup

The primary diagnostic approach to paraesophageal herniation is the barium esophagogram and upper GI series. Endoscopic assessment is also an important

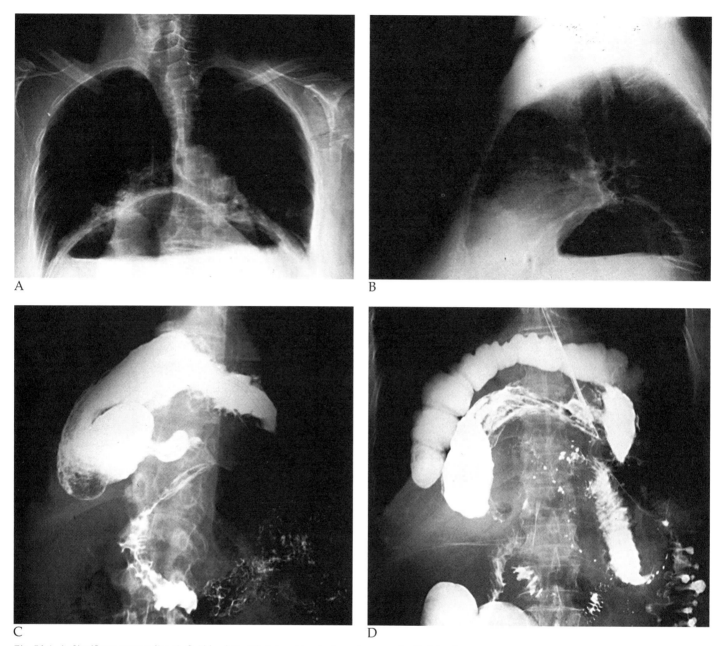

A

B

C

D

Fig. 56-4. A. Significant retrocardiac air fluid level identified at routine chest roentgenography. B. Lateral chest roentgenogram demonstrating large air fluid level within the intrathoracic stomach in the characteristic retrocardiac position. C. Barium upper GI series demonstrating total intrathoracic stomach (type II hiatal hernia). D. Large paraesophageal hernia (type IV) characterized by herniation of the entire stomach and colon into the chest.

preoperative evaluation. Because insufflation during the endoscopic procedure can precipitate acute gastric incarceration requiring urgent surgery, we usually defer this intervention until the time of the proposed elective surgical procedure. If significant esophagitis is identified at the endoscopic examination, fundoplication should be included in the management of the good-risk paraesophageal hernia patient with a clinical history consistent with symptomatic gastroesophageal reflux.

Because of technical difficulty in passing the manometric catheters into the stomach for the assessment of lower esophageal sphincter function, esophageal manometry is not routinely performed in the elective evaluation of patients with primary paraesophageal hernias who do not have reflux symptoms. The diagnostic importance of esophageal manometric studies in this clinical setting of primary paraesophageal herniation is therefore limited to determining the integrity of esophageal body function. A relatively normal lower esophageal sphincter pressure is usually noted among patients with paraesophageal hernia, which contrasts with the low mean sphincter pressure noted among patients

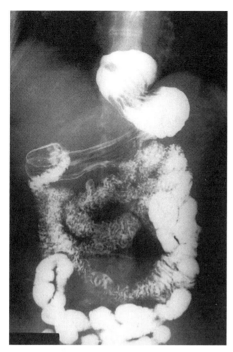

Fig. 56-5. Barium esophagram demonstrating mixed sliding and paraesophageal hernia (type III).

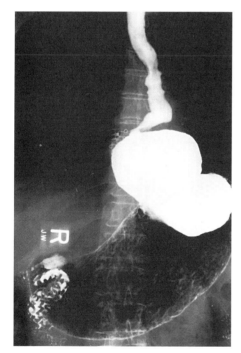

Fig. 56-6. Esophageal "shortening" associated with mixed sliding and paraesophageal hernia.

with sliding hiatal hernias and pathologic reflux esophagitis. Even among paraesophageal hernia patients with visible esophagitis, the most consistent manometric abnormality identified is a reduction in the overall length of the lower esophageal

sphincter. At the present time, our primary use of esophageal manometric testing is to determine the adequacy of esophageal body peristalsis before adding fundoplication to the elective repair of mixed sliding and paraesophageal hernias.

Prolonged intraesophageal pH testing is also of limited benefit in the evaluation of patients with primary paraesophageal hernia, as the primary cause of increased esophageal acid exposure is impaired emptying of gastric acid from the herniated intrathoracic gastric fundus. Reduction of the herniated stomach to its normal intra-abdominal position during the course of the repair of the paraesophageal hernia usually results in normal gastric emptying and resolution of the abnormal esophageal acid exposure. This consideration has dissuaded us from relying on prolonged esophageal pH studies in the preoperative assessment of the integrity of the lower esophageal sphincter for most paraesophageal hernia patients.

Preoperative Decision Making Regarding the Operative Approach

For the most part, the operative approach to paraesophageal herniation is determined by the clinical urgency of the situation, and the age and functional status of the patient. The preoperative determination of associated pathologic gastroesophageal reflux will also affect the operative strategy. We will usually include a fundoplication with the paraesophageal hernia repair if significant esophagitis is identified in a patient with a consistent clinical history for gastroesophageal reflux. If esophageal mucosal injury is absent and the gastroesophageal junction is in its normal intra-abdominal location, we rely upon anatomic repair of the paraesophageal hernia defect and reduction of the stomach to its normal intra-abdominal position.

Under most circumstances, an abdominal approach is used to accomplish the paraesophageal hernia repair; however, thoracotomy is chosen for the management of "primary" paraesophageal hernias when significant esophageal shortening is identified by preoperative barium contrast studies and endoscopy examination (Fig. 56-6). We also favor the transthoracic ap-

proach to manage the patient with symptomatic paraesophageal herniation that occurs after a previous antireflux surgical procedure.

Transabdominal Repair of Paraesophageal Herniation

Anatomic Repair

After induction of general anesthesia, esophagoscopy is routinely performed to identify the presence of significant esophagitis and the degree of anatomic shortening of the esophagus. We usually defer this endoscopic evaluation until the time of operation because of the potential risk of inducing gastric incarceration within the paraesophageal hernia when insufflation maneuvers are utilized during the examination. We attempt to examine the stomach and duodenum at this endoscopic procedure; however, it is often impossible to negotiate the endoscope through the gastroesophageal junction when the entire stomach is herniated into the chest. The finding of significant esophagitis in the patient with significant reflux symptoms will usually lead us to include fundoplication with the paraesophageal hernia repair.

Following the endoscopic examination, the patient is surgically prepared in the supine position. The abdomen is opened through an upper midline abdominal incision extending from the xiphoid process to the umbilicus. Attention is directed to the esophageal hiatus and the left upper quadrant after a general exploration of the abdominal cavity is performed. The fundus of the stomach is usually found to have migrated within the enlarged esophageal hiatal opening. When the paraesophageal herniation is large, it is also common to have the omentum and even the transverse colon within the hernia (see Figs. 56-3 and 56-4).

The technical aspects of anatomic repair of paraesophageal hernias are straightforward. The primary management principles are reduction of the herniated abdominal viscera, hernia sac excision, and crural repair. We begin by grasping the gastric fundus with an atraumatic Babcock clamp at the hiatal opening and gently reducing the stomach back into the abdomen. Remarkably, significant adhesions are rarely present between the stomach and the her-

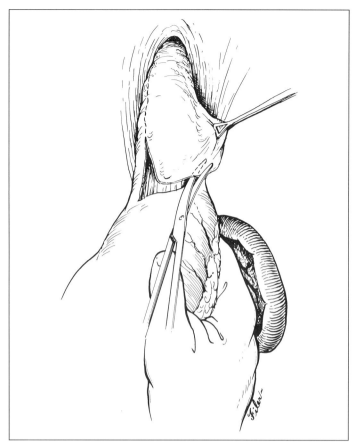

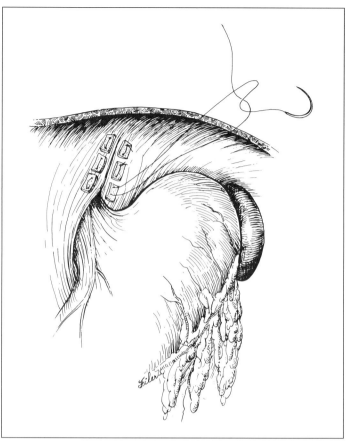

Fig. 56-7. Manual retraction of the gastric cardia hernia sac can result in clear definition of the extent of the hernia sac.

Fig. 56-8. Illustration of the usual extent of peritoneal-lined hernia sac resection, which results in exposure of the anterior aspect of the gastroesophageal junction and the crural margins.

nia sac. Serial applications of these clamps will usually be necessary to reduce the entire gastric fundus through the hiatus opening. After the stomach has been reduced into the abdomen, the surgeon grasps the greater curvature side of the gastric cardia with his or her hand to apply traction on the hernia sac (Fig. 56-7). The peritoneum is then elevated and incised at the greater curvature side of the gastroesophageal junction to begin the hernia sac excision. This excision progresses along the greater curvature and over the left crus in a counterclockwise fashion to encompass the entire hiatal arch (Fig. 56-8). The excision of the hernia sac over the distal esophagus is carried toward the lesser curvature of the stomach. In doing so, care is taken to avoid injury to the anterior vagal nerve trunk, which can be easily injured during the final aspects of this dissection.

After the paraesophageal hernia sac is excised, inspection of the gastroesophageal junction will usually reveal a normal relationship with the esophageal hiatus

opening. This is because the posterior phrenoesophageal membranous attachments to the gastroesophageal junction are anatomically and functionally preserved in patients with pure paraesophageal hernias. These posterior phrenoesophageal attachments are left intact. Division of these structures will increase the likelihood of lower esophageal sphincter incompetence and the iatrogenic development of postoperative pathologic gastroesophageal reflux in patients without this preoperative problem, necessitating the need for an otherwise unnecessary fundoplication.

After excision of the hernia sac, crural approximation is performed anterior to the esophagus as described originally by Collis. The crural arch at the hiatus is usually quite wide and the muscular tissues are often weak. This "anterior" crural repair is performed to avoid disruption of the posterior phrenoesophageal ligamentous attachments and to prevent excessive suture line tension along the crural approximation (Fig. 56-9). We routinely use heavy

nonabsorbable sutures buttressed with felt pledgets to reinforce the crural repair and to prevent any "tearing through" of the stitches as the crural margins are approximated.

After the crural approximation has been accomplished, division of the upper short gastric vessels is also performed to interrupt the elongated mesenteric connection between the stomach and the spleen. We believe the risk for postoperative recurrent paraesophageal herniation is increased when the fundus is allowed to torque about its elongated short gastric mesentery. Pexy of the gastric fundus to the undersurface of the left leaf of the diaphragm is also performed to reduce the likelihood of postoperative recurrent paraesophageal herniation (Fig. 56-10). Alternatively, a gastrostomy can be used to pex the fundus of the stomach. The use of a pexing gastrostomy also avoids the need for postoperative nasogastric tube drainage (Fig. 56-11). It is important to perform this gastrostomy relatively high upon the greater

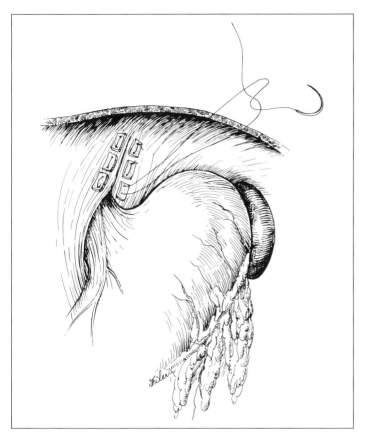

Fig. 56-9. *Anterior crural repair of "collis." Teflon-felt reinforcement of the crural sutures are routinely performed.*

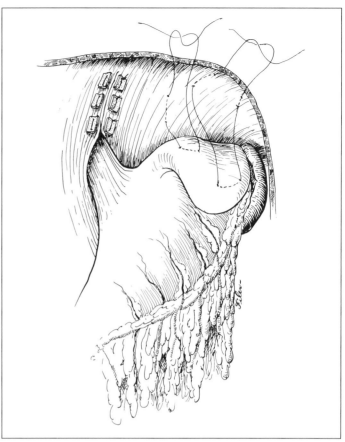

Fig. 56-10. *Depiction of a fundic pexy to the undersurface of the left-leaf of the diaphragm.*

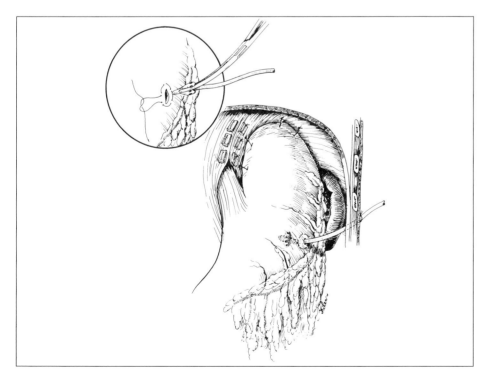

Fig. 56-11. *Pexing gastrostomy established in a high-fundic position, which is frequently employed with anatomic paraesophageal hernia repair.*

curvature to fix the fundus in a position that will avoid postoperative recurrence of the paraesophageal herniation. Performance of the gastrostomy in a low fundic or antral position will not adequately control the greater curvature of the fundus.

Laparoscopic Approach

Familiarity with the technical nuances of endosurgical instrumentation and the general conduct of laparoscopic surgical approaches is a vital prerequisite before laparoscopic repair of paraesophageal hernias is attempted. Likewise, the surgeon should be experienced with the "open surgical" approaches to repair of paraesophageal hernias, as the technical standards of "open surgical" management must be maintained to avoid suboptimal results. The surgeon must also be prepared to convert to an open surgical approach when the operative conditions preclude a safe or effective surgical repair of the paraesophageal hernia.

Laparoscopic techniques can be readily applied in the management of paraesophageal herniation. The trocar access utilized to conduct the laparoscopic intervention is illustrated in Fig. 56-12. Five sites of trocar access are routinely employed. Unless the patient has had a previous abdominal surgical intervention, a "Veress needle puncture" approach is used to gain access to the abdominal cavity for coelomic insufflation. A supraumbilical site for this needle entry is chosen.

After abdominal insufflation is achieved with the Veress needle approach, the initial trocar access used for the laparoscopic camera unit is established. We choose a left paramedian location 3 to 5 cm above the umbilicus for this access, as this gives the greatest direct visibility of the esophageal hiatal anatomy. After making an appropriately sized skin incision to accommodate an 11-mm sealed endosurgical trocar, two towel clips are positioned laterally to provide upward traction on the abdominal wall during the introduction of the trocar through the rectus sheath and into the abdominal cavity.

When the possibility of intraperitoneal adhesions exists, an open approach to the initial trocar cannulation is performed to visually confirm the freedom of adhesions at the site of the initial trocar access. This same left paramedian site would be used when the "open" cutdown method for initial trocar access is used. A careful laparoscopic exploration of the peritoneal cavity follows. Subsequent trocar access is then achieved under direct laparoscopic visibility using the same towel clip countertraction technique described.

The second 11-mm trocar access achieved is in the right upper quadrant 3 cm below the costal margin. It is best to keep this trocar access site in a far lateral position to prevent crowding of subsequent instrumentation. This right upper quadrant site is primarily utilized to introduce an expandable retracting instrument beneath the left lobe of the liver to expose the esophageal hiatus. The hiatal exposure is facilitated by leaving the triangular ligamentous attachments of the liver intact. A third trocar access site is established in the left upper quadrant for the "right-handed" endoscopic instrument access used to accomplish the hiatal dissection. A fourth trocar access is placed approximately 4 to 5 cm below the first left upper quadrant site. This site is primarily used for retraction of the gastric fundus during

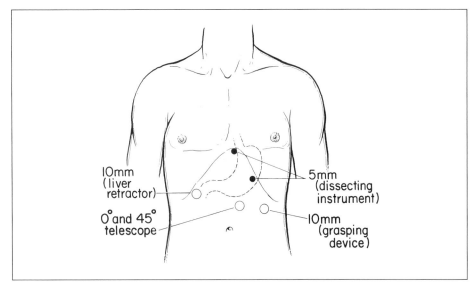

Fig. 56-12. The usual sites of trocar access used to accomplish laparoscopic repair of paraesophageal hernias.

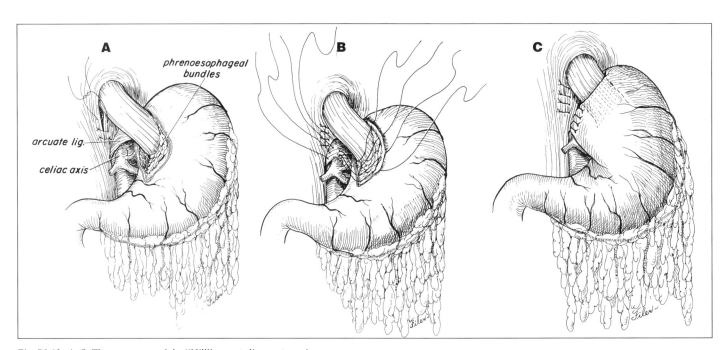

Fig. 56-13. A–C. The appearance of the "Hill" arcuate ligament repair.

the hiatal dissection. A final trocar access is achieved in the midline subxiphoid position to introduce the "left-handed" endoscopic dissecting instrumentation. The basic operative technique for the hiatal dissection is the same as that utilized for "open" anatomic repair of paraesophageal hernias. Endoscopic suturing is accomplished using coaxially oriented endoscopic needle holders and extracorporeal knot-tying techniques.

Concomitant Antireflux Procedures

To reiterate, we selectively utilize fundoplication as a specific antireflux procedure in the management of patients with paraesophageal hernia. The decision to include fundoplication with the repair is based upon the endoscopic findings of esophagitis, a redo operative status, or the intraoperative evidence of a significant sliding hiatal hernia and esophageal shortening.

In general, patients with primary paraesophageal hernia who are elderly or physiologically impaired, and those without evidence of clinical esophagitis, are not considered for fundoplication. In these circumstances, the "anatomic repair of Collis" is the primary antireflux mechanism relied upon. When equivocal clinical findings of significant gastroesophageal reflux are identified, we utilize the "Hill" arcuate ligament repair to anchor the gastroesophageal junction within the abdomen and restore an effective antireflux barrier (Fig. 56-13A–C).

When a fundoplication procedure is necessary, dissection about the esophageal hiatus is completed with division of the posterior phrenoesophageal ligamentous attachments along the entire circumference of the distal esophagus and the lesser curvature of the stomach. The fundoplication procedure chosen is dictated by determination of the severity of the reflux process and the integrity of the esophageal peristaltic pump. This is determined by preoperative esophageal barium studies and standard esophageal manometric testing of esophageal body function.

When the adequacy of esophageal peristalsis is in question, we rely upon a partial fundoplication to avoid potential postoperative dysphagia related to too competent a wrap following total fundoplication. The "D'or" anterior partial fundoplication is usually chosen for patients approached through the abdomen. The "Toupet" posterior partial fundoplication procedure is avoided because of the inherent difficulties in providing adequate posterior diaphragmatic crural support for the mobilized fundus resulting from the anatomic distortion in the esophageal hiatus. The "Belsey" partial fundoplication is chosen when thoracotomy is used to approach the para-

esophageal hernia patient with impaired esophageal peristalsis. When esophageal peristalsis is normal, a standard "floppy" Nissen fundoplication (2–3 cm in length) about a No. 50 to 60 French intraesophageal bougie is utilized (Fig. 56-14A–D). The extensive pexy of the gastric fundus to the diaphragm utilized with anatomic repair alone is not necessary when a total fundoplication is created. We do include a

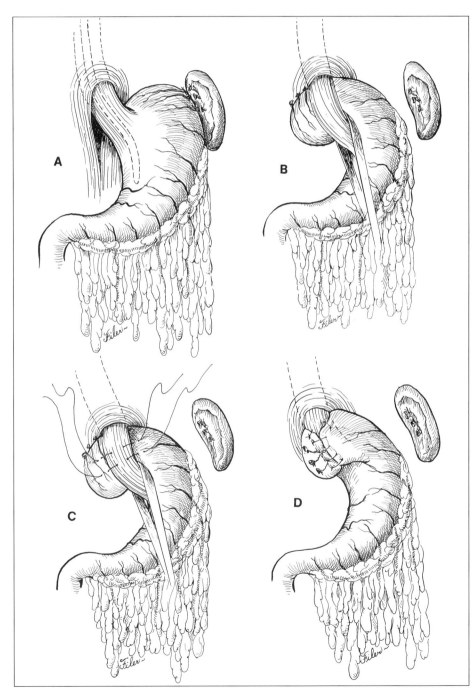

Fig. 56-14. A–D. Serial steps to accomplishing transabdominal Nissen fundoplication.

few pexing stitches at the completion of the repair between the fundus and the crural margins to secure the redundant aspect of the fundus. Pexing gastrostomy is only utilized with fundoplication in the management of the patient with pulmonary functional impairment whose postoperative respiratory hygiene will be potentially compromised by the discomfort associated with an indwelling nasogastric tube.

Whether or not fundoplication is included with the paraesophageal hernia repair, a postoperative barium esophagogram is performed once the postoperative ileus has resolved. This study can usually be accomplished 3 to 5 days after open surgical approaches. An earlier recovery can often be seen after laparoscopic repair. The patient is also allowed clear liquid oral intake shortly after operation. The diet is advanced to a six small feedings, mechanical soft regimen that spares the introduction of gas-forming foods and beverages.

Management of Incarcerated Paraesophageal Herniation

Gastric incarceration most commonly occurs in patients with large paraesophageal hernias associated with chronic intrathoracic displacement of the entire stomach. Before the incarcerating event, the individual's chief complaint is chronic substernal pain related to intermittent distention/obstruction of the intrathoracic stomach. Incarceration of the stomach within the paraesophageal hernia defect results when the distended fundus of an intrathoracic stomach slips back into the abdomen. This results in the development of two closed loop obstructions of the stomach: one within the intrathoracic antrum and the other within the gastric fundus that has slipped back into the abdomen through the hiatal opening. The distal esophagus and the proximal duodenum are also obstructed by the incarcerated mass bound at the diaphragmatic hiatus (Fig. 56-15). In spite of the acute upper abdominal distress, the patient is unable to vomit, although retching attempts are commonly observed. Chest roentgenography will usually demonstrate a characteristic distended, retrocardiac air-filled mass representing the intrathoracic gastric antrum. A similarly distended gastric fundus will be noted beneath the diaphragm on chest film

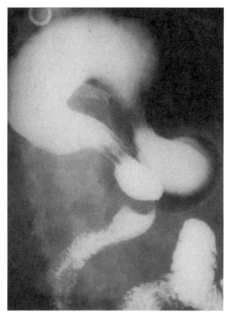

Fig. 56-15. Barium radiograph demonstrating prolapse of the previously intrathoracic gastric fundus back into the abdomen, resulting in gastric volvulus and closed loop obstruction of the fundus and antrum of the stomach.

or on flat plate roentgenographic examination of the abdomen. The primary therapeutic maneuver for this emergency situation is passage of a nasogastric tube to decompress the distended gastric fundus. Immediate relief of the patient's symptoms can be seen if the nasogastric tube can be successfully passed into the fundus of the stomach. The patient can then be prepared for semielective paraesophageal hernia repair since relief of the gastric volvulus has been accomplished.

An emergency situation exists when nasogastric decompression of the stomach cannot be accomplished. Mesenteric vascular compromise of the obstructed antrum and fundus is imminent. We approach these patients through an upper midline laparotomy; however, the left chest is always surgically prepared for thoracotomy should this approach be necessary to facilitate reduction of the stomach or resection of a devitalized gastric segment. On entry into the abdomen, the ischemic and distended fundus is immediately visualized in the upper abdomen. The surgeon should attempt to gently reduce the gastric antrum into the abdomen through the hiatal opening. Decompressive gastrotomy to reduce the intragastric tension may allow for successful reduc-

tion. If the reduction of the antrum is not possible after decompression of the fundus, we incise the anterior rim of the diaphragm at the hiatal margin to gain a larger opening for hernia reduction. If the antrum remains incarcerated, thoracotomy will be necessary to accomplish decompression of this distended gastric segment before it can be reduced into the abdomen.

After reduction of the stomach has been accomplished, the general principles of paraesophageal hernia management outlined for anatomic repair are used. In this clinical circumstance, we are less likely to include a fundoplication to the paraesophageal hernia repair. Creation of a fundoplication with the edematous gastric fundus about similarly distorted distal esophageal tissue is prone to result in suboptimal operative results. This, taken together with the fact that fewer than one-third of patients with paraesophageal hernia have a history of classic gastroesophageal reflux symptoms, leads us to avoid fundoplication in this urgent clinical setting unless definitive evidence of pathologic gastroesophageal reflux exists.

When gastric necrosis has occurred, resection of the devitalized segment must be performed. We usually rely upon stapled transection of the esophagus at the gastroesophageal junction and resection of the segment of devitalized stomach. Distal gastrostomy and jejunostomy are performed. A colonic interposition is utilized to restore gastrointestinal continuity at a later date once the patient has recovered from this primary surgical intervention.

Thoracic Management of Paraesophageal Hernias

As was previously mentioned, our primary indication for the thoracotomy approach to paraesophageal hernia repair is the situation in which significant "shortening" of the esophagus is noted roentgenographically and endoscopically (see Figs. 56-5 and 56-6). Thoracotomy is also preferred when approaching symptomatic paraesophageal hernias that develop after a previous antireflux surgical procedure. In this latter circumstance, thoracotomy can provide the best exposure of the hernia process. The thoracotomy approach also allows for improved mobilization of the esophagus so that tension-free positioning of the gastroesophageal junction is accomplished within the abdomen at the completion of the hernia repair.

Although selective lung ventilation is not necessary to accomplish the thoracotomy approach to paraesophageal herniation, we find it helpful in improving our overall operative exposure. Of course this method of intraoperative ventilation requires that the anesthesia team and the surgeon be familiar with the nuances and technical details of proper double-lumen endotracheal tube positioning and management. Once successful induction of anesthesia and ventilation has been accomplished, the patient is positioned in the right lateral decubitus position and the chest is surgically prepared and draped for thoracotomy. A left seventh interspace lateral thoracotomy is routinely employed (Fig. 56-16). The latissimus dorsi muscle is divided as low as possible and the serratus anterior muscle is mobilized without division by incising this muscle's attachments from the underlying ribs and intercostal tissues. The seventh rib can be excised within its periosteal bed when wider exposure is necessary. Once into the chest, the paraesophageal hernia mass will be seen in its lateral and retrocardiac position.

We begin by dividing the inferior pulmonary ligament to the level of the inferior pulmonary vein. We then identify the distal esophagus by incising the posterior parietal pleura behind the pulmonary vein. Careful dissection in the posterior mediastinal space anterior to the thoracic aorta will bring the surgeon into the proper plane to identify the distal esophagus. This identification is important to establish the primary relationship of the distal esophagus to the herniated stomach (Fig. 56-17). A one-inch Penrose drain is positioned around the esophagus above the paraesophageal hernia mass. The next important maneuver is to incise the true hernia sac of the paraesophageal hernia and identify the normal orientation of the stomach to the distal esophagus (Fig. 56-18). The redundancy of the hernia sac about the intrathoracic stomach can sometimes make this identification difficult. After clearly determining the margins of the hiatal opening, we routinely excise the paraesophageal hernia sac and prepare the gastric fundus for fundoplication. Care must be taken to avoid injury to the vagal nerve trunks and gastroesophageal junction during the course of this dissection. A formal antireflux procedure is required when a transthoracic approach to paraesophageal hernia repair is chosen, as the phrenoesophageal membranous attachments anchoring the gastroesophageal junction are necessarily divided during the course of the intrathoracic dissection of the paraesophageal hernia sac. The upper three short gastric vessels are divided to accomplish a tension mobilization of gastric fundus about the distal esophagus for fundoplication (Fig. 56-19). The intrathoracic esophagus is then to the level of the aortic arch so that the fundoplication can be positioned beneath the diaphragm without tension. Heavy nonabsorbable sutures are then placed in the posterior margins of the diaphragmatic crura to restore a normal aperture of the esophageal hiatus after completion of the repair. These sutures are reinforced with Teflon felt pledgets in most circumstances, as is the practice for crural approximation during the transabdominal approach to paraesophageal hernia repair. A No. 50 to 56 French intraesophageal bougie should be positioned within the esophagus to avoid postoperative dysphagia related to excessive closure of the hiatal opening.

After placement of the crural sutures, we perform a total fundoplication of 2 to 3 cm in length about the distal esophagus. To accomplish a loose, floppy repair, the fundoplication should be performed over the same intraesophageal bougie that will be used later during the crural approximation. Additionally, an adequate portion of the fundus must be mobilized around the distal esophagus to avoid torquing, distortion, and tension about the fundoplication. A Babcock clamp is positioned on the leading edge of the fundus once it is seen behind the right side of the esophagus. The fundus is advanced around the esophagus by placing traction on this leading edge of

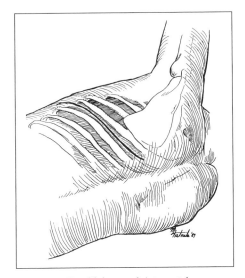

Fig. 56-16. Usual left seventh intercostal space thoracotomy incision used for selected cases of paraesophageal hernia repair.

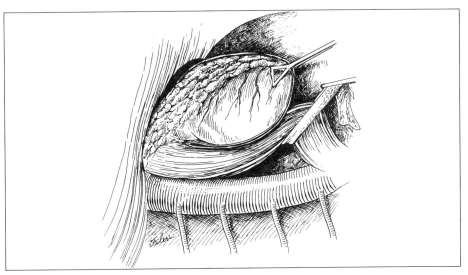

Fig. 56-17. Illustration of the usual pathologic relationship of the herniated stomach and the esophagus seen with paraesophageal herniation.

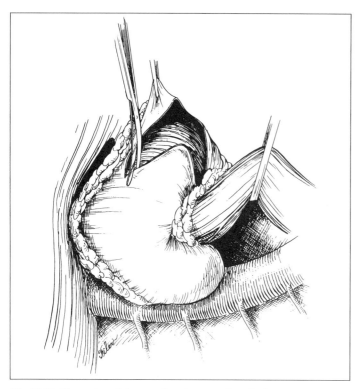

Fig. 56-18. *Illustration of the transthoracic approach to the dissection of the paraesophageal hernia sac.*

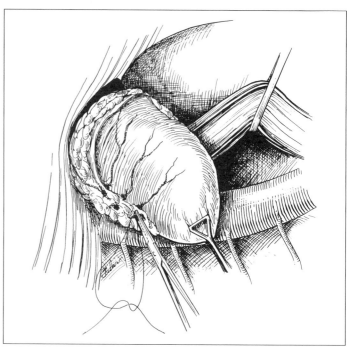

Fig. 56-19. *Illustration of division of the short gastric vessels during the mobilization of gastric fundus and resection of the paraesophageal hernia sac.*

the fundus with the Babcock clamp and with concomitant advancement of the fundus behind the esophagus with the surgeon's hand. Before placement of the fundoplication sutures, the surgeon should approximate the proposed areas of the fundus to be used for the fundoplication about the distal esophagus with opposing Babcock clamps. The intraesophageal bougie should be left in place during this maneuver to ensure that the fundoplication is created without excessive tightness or tension. Three to four heavy interrupted sutures are then placed between the opposed areas of the fundus to accomplish a total fundoplication of 2 to 3 cm in length (Fig. 56-20A, B). The lowest of these plicating sutures is also placed through the muscular wall of the distal esophagus at the gastroesophageal junction to prevent "slippage" of the fundoplication. As is the case in transabdominal repairs, care is taken to avoid injury or encroachment of the vagal nerve trunks during this mobilization and fundoplication stitch placement.

In some instances, the gastroesophageal junction will be impossible to reduce beneath the diaphragm despite extensive intrathoracic mobilization of the esophagus to the level of the aortic arch. In these

cases, a "Collis" gastroplasty (esophageal lengthening procedure) should be used to restore enough esophageal length to position the fundoplication beneath the diaphragm without undo tension (Fig. 56-21).

The previously placed crural sutures are then approximated after the fundoplication has been positioned beneath the diaphragm. To avoid problems of excessive closure or inadequate repair of the hiatus, the esophageal hiatal opening should be reduced to a diameter that allows for passage of the surgeon's index finger along the esophagus with the bougie still in place.

After completion of the repair, a single No. 28 French chest tube is placed in a posterior and medial intrapleural location. The lung is re-expanded and the chest is closed. The chest tube is initially placed on underwater seal drainage with 20 cm of additional negative pressure. This chest tube is removed on the second or third postoperative day once pleural drainage has reduced to less than 150 ml per day. Postoperative roentgenographic assessment of the repair and dietary management are similar to those following transabdominal approaches.

Conclusions

Elective repair of these "true" hernias of the esophageal hiatus is usually recommended, regardless of the severity of symptoms, to avoid the life-threatening complications of obstruction, perforation, bleeding, and gastric strangulation. This elective surgical management approach to paraesophageal herniation is supported by us for all but the seriously unfit patient.

Although we recognize that symptomatic reflux may be seen in 10 to 15 percent of patients with primary paraesophageal hernias (*type II*) following anatomic repair, we do not favor universal application of fundoplication in their management. Our approach is affected by our belief that the risk of significant postfundoplication problems outweighs the possible benefits of obtaining total control of reflux symptoms in this characteristically elderly group of patients. If mild to moderate postoperative reflux symptoms develop in these patients, present-day antisecretory and prokinetic medical therapies will almost always control the patient's symptoms. It is also important to realize that the routine addition of

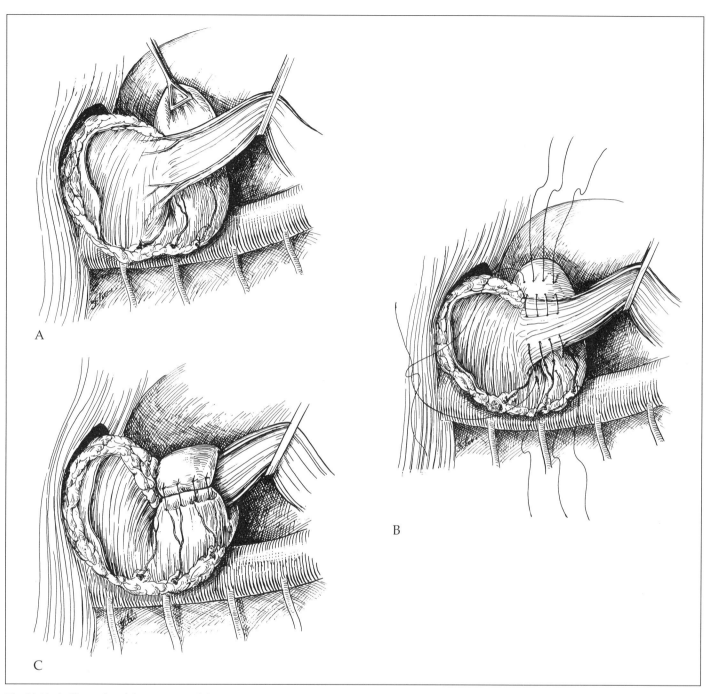

Fig. 56-20. A. Illustration of the posterior mobilization of the gastric fundus and its positioning about the distal esophagus in preparation for performing fundoplication. B. Placement of fundoplication sutures. C. Completed fundoplication illustrated before its reduction beneath the diaphragmatic crura.

fundoplication to the paraesophageal hernia repair does not reliably protect against postoperative reflux symptoms. Actually the occurrence of significant postoperative reflux symptoms has been found to be similar whether anatomic repair alone or repair with routine fundoplication is applied

for patients with primary paraesophageal herniation *(type II hiatal hernias)*. However, the use of fundoplication does appear to be valid when managing patients with pathologic gastroesophageal reflux associated with a "mixed" *(type III)* sliding and paraesophageal hernia.

One should tailor repair of paraesophageal hernias to each patient's pathophysiologic condition rather than applying one universal surgical treatment policy. Accordingly, a good clinical result can be expected in over 90 percent of patients with paraesophageal hernia when appropriate

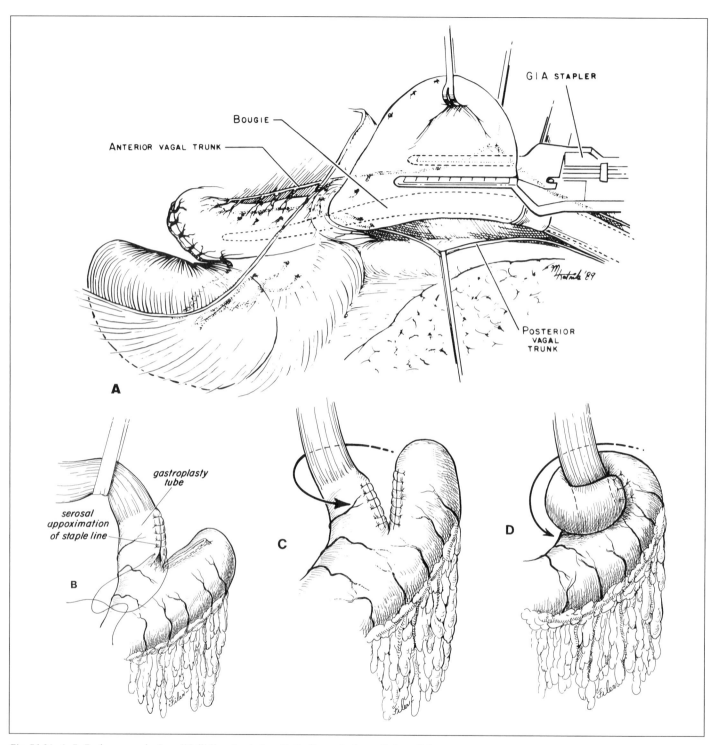

Fig. 56-21. A, B. Performance of a 5-cm ''Collis'' gastroplasty with the linear stapler applied parallel to an intraesophageal bougie. C–D. Completion of ''Collis'' elongation of neoesophagus.

surgical management principles are followed. The surgeon addressing such complex problems of the esophageal hiatus should utilize a flexible repair approach adapted to the individual needs of the patient rather than narrowly following preconceived doctrines. Likewise, it is important that the esophageal surgeon approaching paraesophageal hernia repair be well versed in the various options available for the management of these challenging cases.

Suggested Reading

Collis JL. Surgical control of reflux in hiatus hernia. *Am J Surg* 115:465, 1968.

Deitel M. Chronic or recurring organoaxial rotation of the stomach. *Can J Surg* 10:195, 1973.

Ellis FH, Crozier RE, Shea JA. Paraesophageal hiatus hernia. *Arch Surg* 121:416, 1986.

Harriss DR, Graham TR, Galea M, Salama FD. Paraoesophageal hiatal hernias. When to operate. *J Roy Coll Surg Edinburgh* 37:97, 1992.

Hill LD. Incarcerated paraesophageal hernia: A surgical emergency. *Am J Surg* 126:286, 1973.

Landreneau RJ. Surgical management of gastroesophageal reflux disease. *Postgrad Med* 85:117, 1989.

Landreneau RJ, Hazelrigg SR, Johnson JA, et al. The giant paraesophageal hernia: A particularly morbid condition of the esophageal hiatus. *Missouri Med* 87:884, 1990.

Landreneau RJ, Marshall JM, Hazelrigg SR, et al. The clinical spectrum of paraesophageal herniation. *Dig Dis Sci* 37:537, 1992.

Landreneau RJ, Marshall JM, Johnson JA, et al. A new balanced operation for complex gastroesophageal reflux disease. *Ann Thorac Surg* 52:325, 1991.

Mercer CD, Velasco N, Hill LD. Paraesophageal Hernia. In L Hill, R Kozarek, R McCallum, CD Mercer (eds), *The Esophagus: Medical and Surgical Management*. Philadelphia: Saunders, 1988. Pp 148–156.

Ozdemir IA, Burke WA, Ikins PM. Paraesophageal hernia: A life-threatening disease. *Ann Thorac Surg* 16:547, 1973.

Pearson FG, Cooper JD, Ilves R, et al. Massive hiatal hernia with incarceration: A report of 53 cases. *Ann Thorac Surg* 35:45, 1983.

Skinner DB, Belsey RHR, Russell PS. Surgical management of esophageal reflux and hiatus hernia: Long term results with 1030 patients. *J Thorac Cardiovasc Surg* 53:33, 1967.

Treacy PJ, Jamieson GG. An approach to the management of para-oesophageal hiatus hernias. *Aust NZ J Surg* 57:813, 1987.

Walther B, DeMeester TR, Lafontaine E, et al. Effect of paraesophageal hernia on sphincter function and its implication on surgical therapy. *Am J Surg* 147:111, 1984.

Weinstein EC, Kohn BS. Paraesophageal hiatus hernia in the aged. *J Am Geriat Soc* 24:37, 1976.

Wichterman K, Geha AS, Cahow CE, Baue AE. Giant paraesophageal hiatus hernia with intrathoracic stomach and colon: The case for early repair. *Surgery* 86:498, 1979.

Williamson WA, Ellis FH, Streitz JM, Shahian DM. Paraesophageal hiatal hernia: Is an antireflux procedure necessary? *Ann Thorac Surg* 56:447, 1993.

EDITOR'S COMMENT

Paraesophageal hiatal hernia is a unique problem seen infrequently by the solo practitioner of surgery. It is only in the large surgical clinics that enough experience is gained with the treatment of this disorder to allow a comprehensive review.

I am in general agreement with the presentation. In our clinic, we do not perform a Nissen fundoplication routinely after repair of this type of hiatal hernia.

If there is preoperative endoscopic evidence of reflux peptic esophagitis or if manometric studies confirm a defective lower esophageal sphincter, we always have added the floppy Nissen fundoplication to the anatomic repair. I reviewed this matter in an invited commentary (*World J Surg* 12:422, 1988) and at that time concluded: "Because so few patients with paraesophageal hernias have serious gastroesophageal reflux, I err on the side of no antireflux procedure unless I have full knowledge of the presence of reflux peptic esophagitis in a given patient." I plan to hold to this therapeutic posture. Although I favor the transabdominal approach to repair, there can be no argument against the transthoracic approach presented so well by our authors.

Since I have chosen the Nissen fundoplication as the method of choice when an antireflux procedure is indicated, I comment on a frequent complication that follows this fine operation, namely, the gas-bloat syndrome. The valve produced is simply too effective. Eructation and vomiting are made difficult or impossible, leading to an accumulation of ingested air with distention of the fundic portion of the stomach. This in turn results in a sensation of early satiety, bloating, or "gas" in the left upper quadrant, which is often painful and which may be accompanied by weight loss secondary to voluntary restriction of food intake. There is also excessive borborygmi and flatulence, which may render these patients social outcasts. The "floppy" Nissen of Donahue and Bombeck (*Rev Surg* 34:223, 1977) in large measure prevents this common complication and is still effective in preventing gastroesophageal reflux.

Csendes and colleagues (in C Wastell, et al, *Surgery of the Esophagus, Stomach and Small Intestine* (5th ed). Boston: Little, Brown, 1995) remind us that paraesophageal hernia can occur as a late complication when an extensive periesophageal dissection with mobilization of the gastric fundus is performed in the initial treatment of esophageal achalasia.

L.M.N.

57

Gastroesophageal Reflux in Infants and Children

Brad W. Warner

Gastroesophageal reflux is an important surgical disorder in the pediatric population since it is fairly common, the consequences may be life threatening, and its persistence during growth can result in permanent developmental morbidity. Several factors have contributed to an enhanced appreciation of this clinical entity and include recognition of the importance of enteral feeding and its preference over the parenteral route. Further, survival for smaller preterm infants and patients with severe neurologic deficits has improved. Finally, methods for the detection of significant reflux have become fairly sensitive.

Clinical Presentation

The signs and symptoms of gastroesophageal reflux in infants and children range from being quite subtle to very obvious. A high index of suspicion is therefore important in children at high risk. Reflux is very common in preterm infants, patients with psychomotor mental retardation, and patients with developmental anomalies of the esophagus. For this reason, a reflux workup should be considered in neurologically impaired children who are referred for feeding tube placement. One of the most visible signs of reflux is persistent vomiting, which usually occurs shortly after meals and consists of undigested food. Bilious emesis in a child mandates urgent investigation to exclude midgut volvulus/malrotation (with an upper gastrointestinal series) and should not be attributed to simple reflux. The vomiting may be so se-

vere as to cause failure to thrive and diminished growth due to inadequate caloric intake.

Acid injury of the esophageal mucosa may be painful. In young infants and children, this meal-associated pain can result in food aversion and failure to thrive. Sandifer syndrome (facial asymmetry and spasmodic torticollis associated with gastroesophageal reflux) occurs when the child twists his or her head in an attempt to straighten the esophagus and promote clearance of the acid. Additional symptoms of reflux include gagging or retching. Continued acid injury to the esophagus will result in the same spectrum of findings, such as ulcer, chronic blood loss, and stricture formation, as in adult patients.

Reflux may contribute acid injury to the respiratory tract, both at the level of the larynx and the lungs. Laryngeal edema can result in stridor. Acute acid contact with the larynx can induce laryngospasm, and this has been considered by some to be an important component of the sudden infant death syndrome. Similarly, episodes of apnea and bradycardia may be related to reflux and should be considered in preterm infants in whom other causes have been excluded. Recurrent pneumonias that are otherwise unexplained as well as episodes of bronchospasm should raise the suspicion for aspiration due to reflux.

Growth failure may occur due to several mechanisms. Persistent vomiting with inadequate caloric intake is probably the most common cause. Other mechanisms include aversion to food intake, as the pain of reflux is aggravated by eating. Less

common causes of failure to thrive include protein loss from the denuded esophageal mucosa as well as the chronic illness associated with repeated episodes of aspiration pneumonia.

Preoperative Evaluation

A thorough preoperative evaluation of children for antireflux surgery should generally consist of an upper gastrointestinal series, a pH probe, esophagoscopy, and a radionuclide gastric emptying study. Although reflux can be detected by any of these tests, each test is important for different reasons. Not every test needs to be done, however, as clinical reflux may be obvious and its documentation by multiple different methods is unnecessary and cost ineffective.

Upper Gastrointestinal Series

The barium upper gastrointestinal series (UGI) is probably the best initial test to evaluate the infant or child suspected of having gastroesophageal reflux. The UGI is not done for the purpose of making the diagnosis of reflux since it is not the most sensitive method. Further, reflux that is demonstrated during a UGI study cannot be assumed to be pathologic. For example, it is not uncommon for normal infants to spit up after feeding. When this normal event is observed during a UGI study, the diagnosis of gastroesophageal reflux is made. This information is not useful in deciding which children are candidates for antireflux surgery.

The value of the UGI study is to evaluate the esophagogastroduodenal anatomy as well as to exclude other potential anatomic causes of reflux. Esophageal strictures are best evaluated by this test. Motility of the esophagus can be evaluated and possibly reveal aspiration from an oral motor swallowing disorder, unrelated to gastroesophageal reflux. Important causes of reflux that a UGI study may be useful in documenting include congenital microgastria, gastric volvulus, antral web, pyloric stenosis, duodenal stenosis or atresia, or other causes of gastric outlet obstruction.

Esophageal pH Monitoring

This is presently the most sensitive and specific test for the diagnosis of gastroesophageal reflux. A nasoesophageal catheter is inserted and continuous pH readings are recorded during a 12- or 24-hour period from the lower and midesophagus. The value of this test is that pathologic reflux can be separated from reflux that is physiologic. This is done by computing a score for each patient based upon such factors as the total time the lower esophageal pH is less than 4, the duration of time the esophageal pH stays less than 4 after a reflux episode (suggesting the effectiveness of esophageal clearance), and the number of episodes of reflux during the period of time studied. A pH of the lower esophagus of less than 4 for greater than 4 percent of the time is considered abnormal. Additionally, episodes of reflux can be temporally correlated with such activities as facial grimacing, irritability, bronchospastic episodes, or coughing.

Esophagoscopy

Endoscopy of the lower esophagus may reveal the presence of Barrett's esophagitis. Long-term endoscopic surveillance is crucial in these patients. Erythema, mucosal friability, and frank ulcer formation all gauge the severity of the reflux. Serial endoscopic examinations during a course of medical management of the reflux may be important to document response to therapy. Severe, erosive esophagitis may increase the risk of esophageal perforation during the performance of an antireflux procedure and, thus, endoscopy is important in the early preoperative period.

Radionuclide Gastric Emptying Study

The value of this test in the preoperative evaluation of the child with gastroesophageal reflux is uncertain. For the detection of reflux, it is too sensitive and cannot distinguish between pathologic and physiologic reflux. If gastric emptying is delayed, a trial of medical therapy to improve gastric emptying may alleviate the reflux. Some pediatric surgeons advocate the performance of a pyloroplasty at the time of the antireflux operation in neurologically impaired patients who have been shown to have delayed gastric emptying. While this is theoretically attractive, pyloroplasty has not been shown to improve the results of the antireflux procedure and may introduce further morbidity such as alkaline reflux or the dumping syndrome.

Esophageal Manometry

Mean lower esophageal sphincter (LES) pressures are lower in children than in adults and do not reliably correlate with reflux. Further, the recent realization that mean resting pressure is less important in determining the presence of pathologic reflux than is inappropriate relaxation of the LES has made manometry less valuable in the evaluation of children with reflux.

Medical Management

Medical management of gastroesophageal reflux is effective in the majority of cases. Positioning of the child in an upright position, thickened foods, and more frequent and smaller volume feedings are all important in the initial management. Medications to augment gastric emptying (metoclopramide) may be useful in patients in whom gastric emptying has been shown to be delayed. Acid-reducing medications serve primarily to reduce the acid injury to the lower esophagus.

The primary indications for antireflux surgery in the pediatric population include persistent symptoms or significant endoscopic evidence of esophageal acid injury despite a trial of maximal medical management. Generally, a period of 6 to 8 weeks should be allowed for the alleviation of symptoms. Absolute surgical indications include an episode of near-miss sudden infant death syndrome and esoph-

ageal stricture. Attempts at medical management of reflux for these latter two conditions are not recommended.

Failure to thrive is an important indication and the response to surgical intervention can be dramatic. Aspiration pneumonia is another important indication since a cornerstone of the medical management of reflux includes the administration of acid-reducing medications. Alkalinization of the stomach may worsen the aspiration pneumonia by allowing for bacterial overgrowth.

Another critical indication for antireflux surgery includes the neurologically impaired patient who needs a gastrostomy tube for feeding and in whom reflux has been documented. There appears to be a high incidence of reflux in these patients and a preoperative workup is therefore prudent. The exception to this rule would be if the patient is already tolerating nasogastric feeding without clinical evidence for reflux.

Surgical Technique

Multiple operative procedures have been designed to correct gastroesophageal reflux in the pediatric population and include the Thal fundoplication, the Hill repair, and the anterior gastropexy. The Nissen fundoplication is probably the most frequently performed procedure and the gold standard by which other procedures are compared. This is my own preferred technique. Preoperative parenteral antibiotics should be administered and a first-generation cephalosporin should suffice. Consideration should be given to flexible esophagoscopy after induction of general endotracheal anesthesia. This may be useful in identifying patients who require more aggressive medical therapy for esophagitis before embarking on operative therapy since the presence of severe, edematous esophagitis may make manipulation around the esophagus more hazardous. Indications for endoscopy include a long period of time since the previous examination, patients who have not previously been evaluated, or patients with known esophageal stricture.

In infants and young children with a broad costal margin, a left upper quadrant transverse incision is used. If the costal margin is narrow, access to the esophageal hiatus is best achieved via a midline incision. On entering the peritoneal cavity, the falciform ligament is divided between ties, and the membranous component of the ligament that attaches the anterior aspect of the liver to the body wall is taken down using electrocautery to the level of the inferior vena cava posteriorly (Fig. 57-1). The liver in neonates and young children is very fragile and care must be excercised when it is handled. This maneuver allows for greater mobility of the liver during exposure of the hiatus and helps to prevent liver injury during retraction. Next, a handheld body wall retractor is placed in the left upper quadrant to expose the left triangular ligament of the liver. Exposure is facilitated by placing a dry lap pad on the anterior aspect of the left lobe and applying downward traction. A right-angled hemostat is inserted below the ligament to present it to the electrocautery and minimize the potential of injury to the underlying anterior gastric wall (Fig. 57-2). This ligament is dissected medially to the level of the inferior vena cava. With the liver freed from attachment to the diaphragm and anterior abdominal wall, a self-retaining Thompson retractor is placed. Richardson retractors are placed in the upper midline body wall, as well as one on either side. The left lobe of the liver is then folded over inferiorly and retracted medially using a curved malleable retractor and a moist lap pad between the liver and retractor. The esophagogastric junction is now exposed (Fig. 57-3).

A Babcock clamp is placed on the greater curvature of the stomach and used to pull the stomach outward from the abdominal cavity. This allows for exposure of the short gastric vessels. These are divided in continuity between ties to enter the lesser sac and separate the greater curvature from the spleen (Fig. 57-4). Care must be taken not to injure the spleen during division of these vessels. This is most critical near the top of the spleen as the attachments to the stomach in this area are very short. Moving the Babcock clamp more superiorly along the greater curvature and retracting the stomach more cephalad as the dissection proceeds allow for better exposure of this critical area. Once the stomach is completely separated from the spleen, the spleen should fall away posteriorly. There may be an additional few small vessels going toward the greater cur-

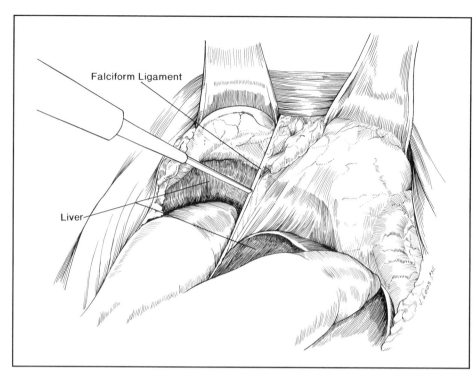

Fig. 57-1. On entering the abdominal cavity, the membranous portion of the falciform ligament is divided with electrocautery from its attachment to the anterior abdominal wall and anterior aspect of the diaphragm. This is carried posteriorly to the inferior vena cava and will help to minimize the potential of iatrogenic injury to the liver during retraction.

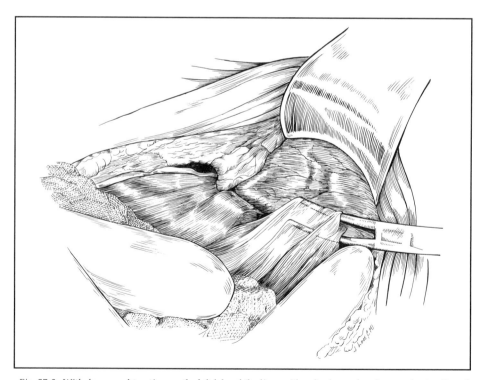

Fig. 57-2. With downward traction on the left lobe of the liver with a dry lap pad and upward retraction of the body wall, the left triangular ligament is divided to the level of the inferior vena cava. Insertion of a right-angled hemostat behind the ligament and in front of the stomach will help prevent the possibility of electrocautery injury to both the anterior stomach and diaphragm.

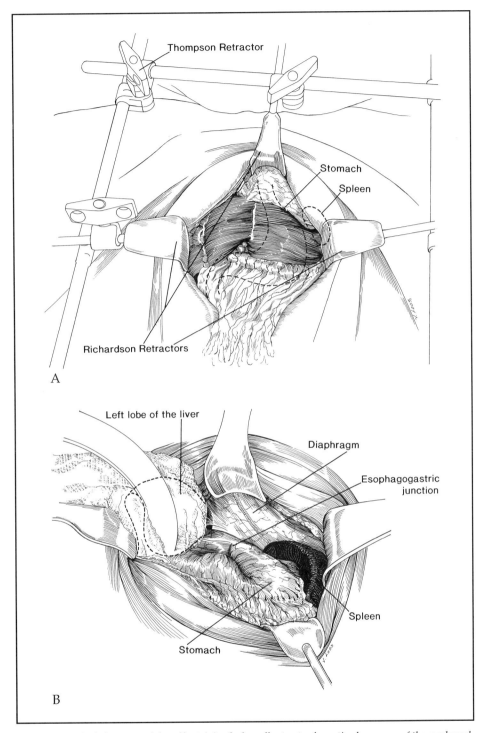

Labels in figure A: Thompson Retractor, Stomach, Spleen, Richardson Retractors, A

Labels in figure B: Left lobe of the liver, Diaphragm, Esophagogastric junction, Spleen, Stomach, B

Fig. 57-3. A. Final placement of the self-retaining body wall retractor for optimal exposure of the esophageal hiatus. B. The left lobe of the liver has been folded over and a moist lap pad has been placed between it and the malleable retractor to guard against the possibility of retractor injury.

vature area from the top of the pancreas that will require division.

With the spleen completely separated, a plane is entered between the esophagus and the peritoneum overlying the esophagogastric junction as well as the phrenoesophageal ligament. This tissue plane is most easily entered from the left side of the esophagus near the last short gastric vessel (Fig. 57-5). A right-angled clamp is inserted between the esophagus and the peritoneum and electrocautery is utilized to divide the tissue surrounding the esophagus. On the anterior esophagus, care must be taken to identify and preserve the anterior vagus nerve. As the dissection is carried from the anterior esophagus to the right, the cephalad portion of the gastrohepatic ligament is divided, thus exposing the right of the esophagus and crus of the diaphragm. In this area, several veins as well as hepatic branches of the vagus may be encountered and must be divided between ties. One potential structure in this area, important to identify and preserve, is a replaced left hepatic artery. This arises from the left gastric artery and is seen in roughly 15 percent of patients. More caudal dissection of the peritoneum of the lesser sac will reveal the left gastric artery. If the distance between the left gastric artery and the inferior aspect of the esophageal hiatus is so short that it does not allow for the fundic wrap, the artery may be divided. This is not necessary in the majority of cases. After division of the gastrohepatic ligament, exposure of the right crus and right side of the esophagus is facilitated by repositioning the malleable retractor deeper into the abdomen to include the caudate lobe of the liver. The posterior vagus nerve is identified on the posterior aspect of the esophagus and the esophagus is encircled to include both vagi using a vessel loop. Three to 4 cm of the lower esophagus is mobilized bluntly into the abdomen using either finger or Kittner dissection (Fig. 57-6).

After full mobilization of sufficient length of intra-abdominal esophagus has been completed, a bougie is passed by the anesthesiologist through the mouth and into the lower esophagus. The size of bougie to be used should be the largest size that the esophagus will comfortably accept. In very small infants, this may be in the range of No. 18 to 24 French. Once the bougie has been passed, a vein retractor is used to re-

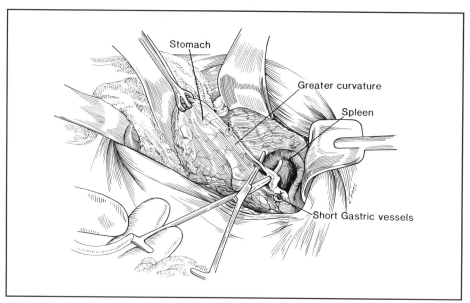

Fig. 57-4. *The spleen is separated from its attachment to the stomach by division of short gastric vessels between ties from a point midway along the greater curvature of the stomach upward to the gastroesophageal junction. This is facilitated by placement of a Babcock clamp on the greater curvature and pulling the stomach anterior and more cephalad as the dissection proceeds upward. The attachment of the upper portion of the spleen to the greater curvature is short and the possibility of a capsular tear of the spleen is greatest in this area.*

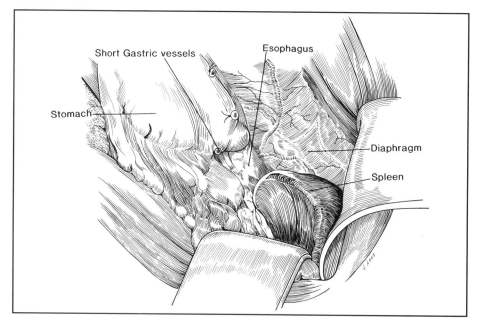

Fig. 57-5. *The plane between the esophagus and peritoneum and phrenoesophageal ligament is most easily entered on the patient's left side of the esophagus after the highest short gastric vessel has been divided. A right-angled instrument is inserted here to facilitate dissection circumferentially around the esophagus. Care should be taken to identify and preserve the anterior and posterior vagus nerves.*

tract the esophagus to the patient's left and the crura and esophageal hiatus are visualized. The crura are then reapproximated up to the esophagus using interrupted, braided, nonabsorbable nylon or silk suture material (Fig. 57-7). It is important to take deep bites of tissue and to avoid strangulation of the tissue by tying the knots too tightly. The aorta can be palpated deep to the esophageal hiatus, and this should be avoided during placement of these sutures.

After the crura have been reapproximated, the lower end of the bougie is pulled back into the thoracic esophagus. This maneuver facilitates wrapping the fundus. With downward traction on the vessel loop around the gastroesophageal junction, the upper portion of the greater curvature of the fundus is passed posterior and to the right side of the esophagus. The lower portion of the bougie is then passed back into the lower esophagus and stomach. The wrap is then created by placing nonabsorbable, braided sutures through the edge of the greater curvature (as marked by the sutures around the previously divided short gastric vessels), the lower esophagus (with care not to injure the anterior vagus nerve), and the fundus of the stomach on the left side of the esophagus. Two to three sutures are placed over a distance of 1 to 2 cm and are tied down. A second layer of Lembert's sutures is then placed to reinforce the previous suture line (Fig. 57-8). At this point, the bougie may be removed. Two final sutures are then placed to finish the fundoplication. The first is placed anteriorly through the upper portion of both sides of the wrap (Fig. 57-9) and the phrenoesophageal ligament to fix the wrap to the diaphragm. The second suture is placed through the upper portion of the wrap posteriorly and then into the most cephalad portion of the crural repair. This suture is important in preventing posterior herniation of the wrap into the mediastinum. The fundoplication is now complete (Fig. 57-10).

Because of the possibility of the gas-bloat syndrome as well as the need for gastric drainage in the postoperative period, a Malecot gastrostomy tube is placed in all patients. An inversion appendectomy is also recommended since it adds little additional time or morbidity. This is perhaps more important in neurologically impaired children in whom the potential de-

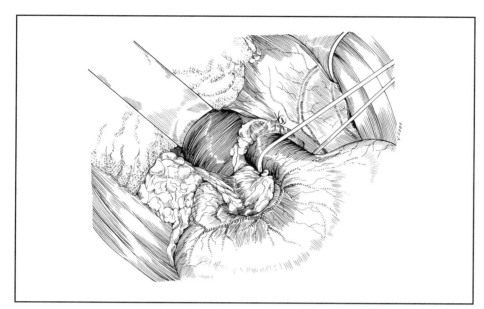

Fig. 57-6. The esophagus has been detached circumferentially from its peritoneal and ligamentous attachments to the diaphragm and crura, and a vessel loop has been placed around the esophagus to include both anterior and posterior vagus nerves. Three to 4 cm of esophagus is mobilized into the abdomen using blunt dissection. This becomes easy once the appropriate plane has been entered within the loose areolar tissue around the esophageal wall. Note the left gastric artery and its relationship to the inferior aspect of the esophageal hiatus. Rarely, this vessel may need to be divided to allow room for the fundic wrap.

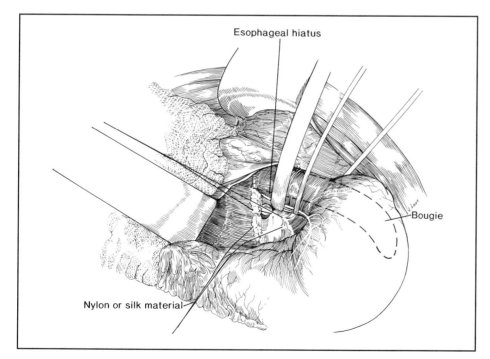

Fig. 57-7. With an appropriate-sized bougie inserted into the esophagus, the crura are reapproximated using interrupted, braided, nonabsorbable suture. Exposure for placement of the sutures is facilitated using a vein retractor to pull the esophagus toward the patient's left.

velopment of appendicitis may be difficult to recognize.

Postoperative Care

In the postoperative period, the gastrostomy tube is left to gravity drainage until the return of bowel function is confirmed by the passage of flatus or stool, or both. When this occurs, or if this has not happened by the fifth postoperative day, the end of the gastrostomy tube is elevated above the level of the stomach and attached to rubber tubing, which is then attached to a large graduated cylinder. This will promote gastric emptying of liquid secretions, at the same time allowing for egress of air. If this is tolerated over a 24 hour period as dictated by the absence of high gastric residuals (greater than 10–15 ml/kg when checked every 4 hours) or abdominal discomfort, clear liquids are begun. In neurologically normal patients, the gastrostomy may then be clamped and should be opened to vent air at any sign of abdominal pain, distention, or discomfort. In neurologically abnormal patients in whom the gastrostomy is the only source of feeding, gas or fluid buildup in the stomach may be difficult to detect. In these patients the gastrostomy should remain elevated and open throughout the 4- to 5-day period whereby the feedings are advanced up to full calories. At this point, the gastrostomy may be clamped between feedings. Gastric residuals should be checked before each feeding to prevent overdistention of the stomach and potential breakdown of the wrap.

Results

The most important determinant in outcome for antireflux procedures in children is the neurologic status of the patient. Normal children with gastroesophageal reflux can be expected to have excellent results over 90 percent of the time. In neurologically impaired patients, excellent or good long-term outcome can be expected in only 65 to 75 percent. This difference is due primarily to the difficulty in determining when the stomach is full and the ability to vent the gastrostomy effectively. Further, prolonged or frequent intermittent elevations in mean intra-abdominal pressure due to such factors as seizures, rhythmic

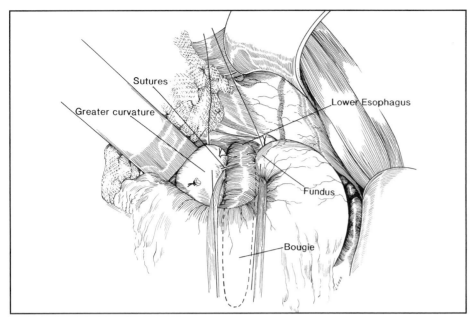

Fig. 57-8. *The vessel loop around the esophagus is now placed on downward traction and the upper portion of the fundus has been passed posteriorly behind the esophagus to rest on the right side. With the appropriate-sized bougie within the esophagus, interrupted, nonabsorbable, braided sutures are then placed through the fundic wrap on the right, the anterior esophageal wall (with care to avoid the anterior vagus nerve), and the fundus on the left side of the esophagus over a distance of 1 to 2 cm. After these sutures are tied down, a second layer of Lembert's sutures is placed through the wrap on either side to reinforce the previously placed sutures.*

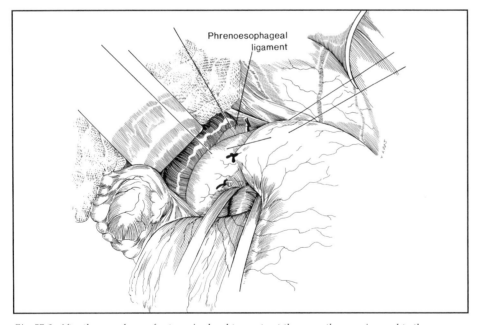

Fig. 57-9. *After the second row of sutures is placed to construct the wrap, the wrap is pexed to the diaphragm by a suture placed through the upper portion of the wrap on the right, through the phrenoesophageal ligament anteriorly, and next through the other side of the wrap, and then is tied down. One final suture is placed posterior to the upper portion of the wrap and the crura to prevent herniation of the wrap into the mediastinum.*

body movements, or hypertonia characteristic of patients with neurologic impairment all contribute to placing stress on and encouraging breakdown of the fundic wrap. Finally, whatever central nervous system factors are present that contribute to the high frequency of gastroesophageal reflux in this patient population probably also contribute toward breakdown of the wrap in the long-term postoperative period. When the fundoplication procedure needs to be redone (as is the case in up to 20% of neurologically impaired patients) as a result of either recurrent reflux or the development of a paraesophageal hernia, the greater risk of iatrogenic vagal nerve injury should be appreciated. In these cases, the pylorus should be ablated by either a pyloroplasty or pyloromyotomy. In some instances, gastroesophageal reflux may recur after one or two reoperations. Consideration may be given at this point to transpyloric feeding via a tube placed through the gastrostomy into the proximal jejunum, placement of a surgical jejunostomy for feeding while leaving the gastrostomy to gravity drainage, or, in extreme cases, total esophageal disconnection from the stomach with a Roux-en-Y esophagojejunostomy. Because of the less than optimal results in the population of neurologically impaired children, the perfect procedure has yet to be designed. The surgical management of gastroesophageal reflux in infants and children therefore commands continued refinement, modification, and critical evaluation.

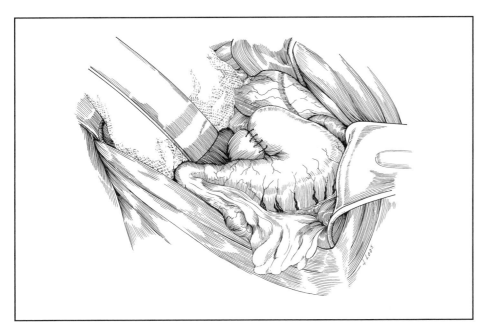

Fig. 57-10. The completed fundoplication. A gastrostomy is routinely placed and in neurologically impaired patients, an incidental appendectomy is strongly urged.

Suggested Reading

DeCou JM, Shorter NA, Karl SR. Feeding Roux-en-Y jejunostomy in the management of severely neurologically impaired children. *Pediatr Surg* 28:1276, 1993.

Hebra A, Hoffman MA. Gastroesophageal reflux in children. *Pediatr Clin North Am* 40:1233, 1993.

Jolley SG. Current surgical considerations in gastroesophageal reflux disease in infancy and childhood. *Surg Clin North Am* 72:1365, 1992.

Martinez DA, Ginn-Pease ME, Caniano DA. Recognition of recurrent gastroesophageal reflux following antireflux surgery in the neurologically disabled child: High index of suspicion and definitive evaluation. *J Pediatr Surg* 27:983, 1992.

Maxson RT, Harp S, Jackson RJ, et al. Delayed gastric emptying in neurologically impaired children with gastroesophageal reflux: The role of pyloroplasty. *J Pediatr Surg.* 29:726, 1994.

Orenstein SR. Controversies in pediatric gastroesophageal reflux. *J Pediatr Gastroenterol Nutrition* 14:338, 1992.

Othersen HB Jr, Ocampo RJ, Parker EF, et al. Barrett's esophagus in children. Diagnosis and management. *Ann Surg.* 217:676, 1993.

Pearl RH, Robie DK, Ein SH, et al. Complications of gastroesophageal antireflux surgery in neurologically impaired versus neurologically normal children. *J Pediatr Surg.* 25:1169, 1990.

Smith CD, Othersen HB Jr, Gogan NJ, Walker JD. Nissen fundoplication in children with profound neurologic disability. High risks and unmet goals. *Ann Surg.* 215:654, 1992.

Taylor LA, Weiner T, Lacey SR, Azizkhan RG. Chronic lung disease is the leading risk factor correlating with the failure (wrap disruption) of antireflux procedures in children. *J Pediatr Surg.* 29:161, 1994.

Veereman-Wauters G, Bochner A, Van Caillie-Bertrand M. Gastroesophageal reflux in infants with a history of near-miss sudden infant death. *J Pediatr Gastroenter Nutrition* 12:319, 1991.

Wheatley MJ, Wesley JR, Tkach DM, Coran AG. Long-term follow-up of brain-damaged children requiring feeding gastrostomy: Should an antireflux procedure always be performed? *J Pediatr Surg.* 26:301, 1991.

EDITOR'S COMMENT

I am always surprised at the large number of children who seem to require surgical intervention for gastroesophageal reflux. When did I last treat an adult for peptic reflux esophagitis who gave a history of classic symptoms from early childhood? I have never seen such a patient. Commonly, adult complaints begin during or after the fifth decade of life, and they are frequently associated with increasing girth, or obesity. Are the etiologic factors in any way similar in the two age groups? The entire problem is complex; there are certain similarities and some differences, but similar therapy, whether medical or surgical, seems to give the same overall, generally good results.

To underscore the admonition to operate sparingly, Tunell and colleagues found significant late complications following use of the Nissen fundoplication in children (*Am Surg* 197:560, 1983). Because of subsequent paraesophageal hiatal hernia, small-intestinal obstruction, and wrap malalignment, they recommend the following steps for avoidance of complications in children: 1) Nissen fundoplication in children should be accompanied by an accurate multisuture crural repair and by suture fixation of the fundal wrap to the crura and to the abdominal surface of the diaphragm, 2) appropriate alignment of the fundal wrap and of the crural repair is best accomplished with a large indwelling esophageal bougie of sufficient size to efface and blanch the esophageal musculature, and 3) appropriate care in avoiding small-intestinal obstruction mandates meticulous avoidance of trauma to the liver capsule and small-intestinal serosa.

The reference to Barrett's esophagitis is noted. This mucosal change to abnormal cells with a propensity for malignant transformation actively is under study in the adult esophagus. During Digestive Disease Week (May 1995) several scientific posters were presented that suggested electrocoagulation of the altered mucosa would allow healing with normal squamous cell mucosa. If this finding is confirmed, a major breakthrough in our approach to the treatment of Barrett's esophagus has been found.

I agree that alkaline reflux through a malfunctioning pylorus must always be considered in patients with gastroesophageal reflux disease. Tovar and colleagues (*J Pediatr Surg* 28:1386, 1993) rightfully stress the need to exclude alkaline reflux as the succus entericus of cause: It is not always acid reflux.

L.M.N.

SEVEN
THE GASTROINTESTINAL TRACT

I

The Esophagus

58

Anatomy of the Esophagus

Mario Albertucci   Francis D. Ferdinand

The esophagus passes through three body areas: the neck, the thorax and the abdomen; the safe and effective performance of most surgical procedures can be attained in these areas. To be considered are only those anatomic features most relevant to surgical procedures. The anatomic boundaries utilized consist of the area posterior to the trachea and pericardium, anterior to the thoracic spine, and between the reflections of the right and left parietal pleura. Specifically, we concentrate on the esophagus, including its vasculature, innervation, lymphatic drainage, and passage through the hiatus and gastroesophageal (GE) junction.

Embryology

The esophagus develops from the initially uniform primitive foregut comprised of two germ layers: endoderm and mesoderm. It is thought that the tracheal bud (later the trachea and lungs) and the esophagus separate as a result of proliferating ridges. The esophagus then elongates, the distal portion more so than the mid and proximal portions. Derived from the mesoderm, skeletal striated muscle forms in the pharynx, larynx, and upper esophagus, and smooth muscle forms in the middle to distal esophagus. The former is derived from caudal branchial arches and is innervated by branchiomotor branches of the vagus, while the latter is derived from visceral splanchnopleural mesoderm and is innervated by sympathetics. The lumen of the esophagus forms through a process of endodermally derived mucosal proliferation, vacuole formation, and subsequent dissolution.

The developing arterial vasculature of the foregut is derived from the branchial arch arteries, which form the thyroid and bronchial arteries, and the celiac, which will give rise to the left gastric, hepatic, and splenic arteries. This developmental pattern of arterial supply causes branchial arch–derived arterial blood to flow caudad while celiac axis–derived arterial blood flows cephalad. The venous and lymphatic vasculature develop concomitantly; however, their flow pattern is reversed, that is, with flow from above the tracheal bifurcation coming cephalad and below the tracheal bifurcation coursing caudad. In summary, arterial blood flows toward the tracheal bifurcation while venous blood flows away from it.

Surgical Implications

From this very brief description of the embryologic development, we can begin to understand the origins of some common congenital abnormalities seen by the surgeon. Failure of the full development of the esophagus leads to esophageal atresia, either partial or complete. The intimate relationship of the developing trachea and esophagus explains the association of tracheoesophageal fistula with esophageal atresia. Failure of complete muscular development may lead to, or predispose to, later diverticular formation. Incomplete recanalization or vacuole resolution is the probable etiologic process in the formation of esophageal duplications, webs, or rings.

Topography

The esophagus starts at the termination of the pharynx and ends at the cardia of the stomach. Thus, the esophagus starts in the neck, passes through the thorax, and ends in the abdominal cavity. The total length in the adult is approximately 25 cm. This course, through three body areas or cavities, and the relations to other structures have great relevance to any diagnostic or therapeutic maneuvers. For the purposes of this discussion, we reference all measurements or distances in centimeters from the incisors (Fig. 58-1). This corresponds to those measurements made at endoscopy and gives a common reference for accurate diagnosis and implementation of treatment. All distances are generally within ±1 cm between male and female adults. With swallowing or tilting of the head, there is a 1 to 2 cm movement of the esophagus, cephalad in the former and cephalad or caudad in the latter.

The origin of the esophagus at the termination of the pharynx corresponds to a distance of 15 cm from the incisors. This is also at the level of the sixth cervical vertebra (C6), just above the thoracic inlet. This is the narrowest portion of the entire GI tract and corresponds to the first of three indentations seen on barium esophagogram and at endoscopy. Radiologically (barium study or CT scan), this area appears flattened because of compression by surrounding structures. At the level of the cricopharyngeal muscle, the internal diameter is approximately 1.5 cm. This is the area of the upper esophageal sphincter (UES), formed by three broad flat muscles of the pharynx: the superior, middle, and inferior constrictors. Each passes obliquely and inserts posteriorly into a median raphe. The cricopharyngeal muscle arises from the cricoid cartilage and passes transversely in a continuous fashion. An inherent weakness between

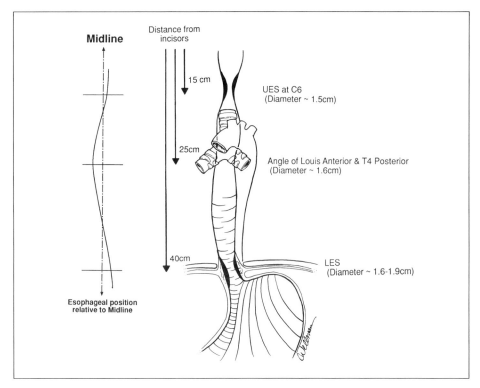

Fig. 58-1. Topography of the esophagus. UES = upper esophageal sphincter; LES = lower esophageal sphincter.

these oblique and transverse-oriented muscle fibers, in addition to distal dysmotility, provides a rather consistent location for pharyngoesophageal or Zenker's diverticulum. This area is the most common site of iatrogenic perforation of the esophagus. Great care must be exercised during rigid esophagoscopy to allow for proper positioning and gentle manipulation to avoid perforation of the posterior wall of the esophagus against the cervical spine. Elderly patients with decreased mobility of the cervical spine and cervical vertebral osteophytes are at an increased risk.

The esophagus is in the midline posterior to the trachea and just to the left at the level of the thoracic inlet. Anteriorly, it is separated from the membranous wall of the trachea by loose fibrous tissue. Posteriorly, it is separated from the prevertebral fascia by alar fascia. This retroesophageal space continues from the base of the skull to the mediastinum and may be a route for infections extending into the mediastinum. The recurrent laryngeal nerves lie in the tracheoesophageal groove with the left side being closer to the esophagus and the right lying more lateral in the neck. Ex-

posure of the cervical esophagus is easier via a left neck incision by dissecting in a plane between the sternocleidomastoid and carotid sheath, gently retracting laterally with the trachea and strap muscles positioned medially.

As the esophagus enters the thorax, it will assume a more rounded configuration on barium esophagogram or CT scan due to the relative negative intrathoracic pressure. Its position is just to the left of the midline at the thoracic inlet and gradually courses to the right in its midportion (Fig. 58-1). As in the neck, from the thoracic inlet to the tracheal bifurcation, the esophagus is bounded anteriorly by the membranous or posterior wall of the trachea, and posteriorly by the prevertebral fascia. The second indentation seen on barium esophagogram or at endoscopy occurs on the anterior aspect and left side of the esophagus at a distance of approximately 25 cm. The internal diameter at this location is usually 1.6 cm. This indentation is caused by the left main stem bronchus and the aortic arch. The corresponding surface landmarks are the angle of Lewis or sternomanubrial junction anteriorly and the fourth thoracic vertebra posteriorly. The

esophagus continues its slightly right-of-midline course until its distal one-third, where it gently curves to the left. This distal portion of the esophagus is bounded anteriorly by the subcarinal lymph nodes and then the pericardium until it enters the esophageal hiatus. Most lesions located in the proximal to midintrathoracic esophagus are best approached via a right thoracotomy because of its slightly right-of-midline position and the left-sided aortic arch.

The distal one-third of the intrathoracic esophagus is, again, on the left side. In addition, it leaves its close association in contour and location to the thoracic spine and passes anteriorly to traverse the diaphragmatic hiatus. This anterior and leftward deflection of the esophagus starting at T8 puts it at risk, and this is the second most common site of iatrogenic perforation. This area of the esophagus is only covered by parietal pleura due to the aorta continuing posteriorly to enter the abdominal cavity beneath the median arcuate ligament. Spontaneous perforation of the esophagus (Boerhaave syndrome) occurs at this location, on the left and posterior aspect of the distal intrathoracic esophagus. Just distal to the esophageal hiatus, the esophagus passes into the abdominal cavity for a distance of approximately 2 cm before ending at its insertion into the cardia of the stomach. This 2-cm segment of esophagus corresponds to the third indentation and occurs at a distance of 40 cm. Its internal diameter is 1.6 to 1.9 cm and radiologically appears flattened because of the relative positive intra-abdominal pressure. This area corresponds to the lower esophageal sphincter (LES) or, more precisely, the distal esophageal high-pressure zone (HPZ).

Most pathology of the distal esophagus, such as distal or GE junction adenocarcinomas, spontaneous perforations, and parahiatal hernias are best approached via a left thoracotomy. Entering through the seventh interspace usually gives optimal exposure.

At 1 to 2 cm proximal to the esophageal hiatus in the diaphragm, the phrenoesophageal membrane inserts into the esophageal intramuscular fibrous tissues (Figs. 58-1 and 58-2). This membrane is a continuation of the transversalis fascia of the abdomen and is composed of fibrous and elastic tissues. It extends from the sub-

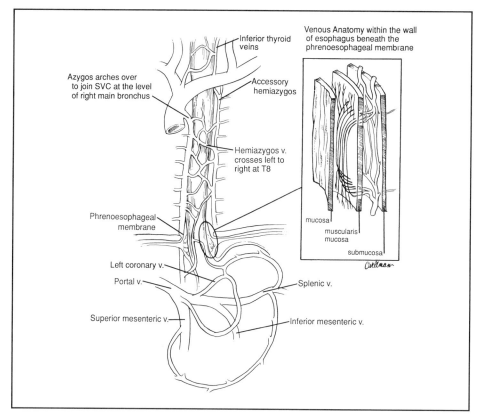

Azygos arches over
to join SVC at the level
of right main bronchus

Inferior thyroid
veins

Accessory
hemiazygos

Venous Anatomy within the wall
of esophagus beneath the
phrenoesophageal membrane

Hemiazygos v.
crosses left to
right at T8

Phrenoesophageal
membrane

mucosa

muscularis
mucosa

submucosa

Left coronary v.

Portal v.

Splenic v.

Superior mesenteric v.

Inferior mesenteric v.

Cuellman

Fig. 58-2. Venous drainage of the esophagus. SVC = superior vena cava.
Inset. Venous drainage within the wall of the distal esophagus (Adapted from CAF deCarvalho. Sin l' angio-
architecture veineuse de la zore de transition aesophagogastrique et son interpretation fonctionelle. Acta
Anatomica 64:125, 1966.)

diaphragmatic fascia into an ascending and descending leaf. The ascending leaf passes up through the diaphragmatic hiatus, extending circumferentially from the margins of the hiatus to the esophagus. This membrane, in addition to tethering the esophagus, also separates mediastinal from retroperitoneal structures. The descending leaf, which is thinner and shorter, inserts on and becomes continuous with the visceral peritoneum of the stomach. Beneath this membrane overlying the GE junction lies the gastric fat pad. The phrenoesophageal membrane must be accurately identified for any surgical procedures involving the distal esophagus or GE junction.

Gross Structure

The esophagus has no true serosa. Its close association with surrounding structures, however, gives a serosa-like relationship: the close apposition to the membranous wall of the trachea, and the continuation

of its outer muscle fibers blend with the right and left parietal pleura surfaces and the pericardium. While this serosa-like relationship cannot be considered a layer to be incorporated within sutures during an anastomosis, it has great importance when considering spread of tumor to adjacent tissues, performing dissections to obtain clear margins, and avoiding entering the pericardial or contralateral pleural spaces.

Because they have different embryologic origins, the muscles that comprise the esophagus are of two types. The cephaladmost one-third, or 6 to 10 cm, contains striated muscle. Then, there is a gradual transition of striated to smooth muscle. The two muscular layers of the esophagus, outer longitudinal and inner circular, also have different transitions from striated to smooth muscle. The inner circular muscle layer has its transition to smooth muscle more proximally than the outer or longitudinal muscle layer. At about 25 cm, greater than 50 percent of the muscle fibers are smooth.

The orientation of the longitudinal and circular muscle fibers is also not uniform. The longitudinal fibers take a gradual 90-degree leftward turn throughout the length of the esophagus. In addition, the longitudinal fibers have a more abundant deposition on the lateral aspects of the esophagus in the proximal one-third, and a more uniform deposition below this level. The circular muscle layer is thicker than the outer layer. This inner layer takes a spiral course throughout its length, keeping a more elliptical rather than horizontal orientation. These patterns give a sinusoidal peristalsis.

The importance of these aspects of muscular type and orientation bears on disorders of esophageal motility. Motility disorders of the proximal esophagus involving striated muscle are usually secondary to central nervous system lesions, such as a brainstem cerebrovascular accident. Motility disorders intrinsic to the esophagus involve smooth muscle and can have a corkscrew pattern seen on barium esophagogram. Surgical myotomies need only be performed upon the distal esophagus below the aortic arch.

The esophageal submucosa can be separated from the muscle layers without much difficulty, greatly facilitating surgical myotomy. The submucosa is well developed and contains a rich network of arteries, veins, lymphatics, nerves, and parasympathetic ganglion cells, and abundant areolar tissue. The submucosa also contains mucus-secreting glands, which are more heavily concentrated in the proximal and distal ends of the esophagus. There is surprising mobility of the submucosa and its overlying muscularis mucosa and mucosa relative to the outer circular and longitudinal muscle layers. Thus, tumor spread, estimating margins for resection, identifying accurate levels for measurements of lesions, and performing an anastomosis, which requires mucosa-to-mucosa apposition, all require that these subtleties of the submucosa be kept in mind. In fact, after transection of the esophagus, the mucosa, muscularis, and submucosa may all retract up to 1 to 2 cm within the outer, circular, and longitudinal muscle layers. It is imperative that the surgeon gently grasp this mucosal layer while placing sutures for an anastomosis to ensure mucosa-to-mucosa apposition. Similarly, placement of stay sutures in the esophagus before transection must be deep enough to include the submucosa as well as the circular and longitudinal muscles.

The muscularis mucosa is a thin layer of smooth-muscle fibers oriented longitudinally, of the type that is typically found throughout the bowel. The mucosa is comprised of squamous endothelium except where it ends abruptly in the distal 1 to 2 cm of the esophagus. This is called the Z line or squamocolumnar junction and forms a jagged line that is easily visualized at endoscopy. Abnormally proximal extension (greater than 3 cm above the GE junction) of the columnar gastric mucosa occurs in Barrett's esophagus. The distal mucosa at the GE junction is slightly heaped up, forming a rosette that may have a secondary role in preventing gastroesophageal reflux.

Vasculature

Arterial Supply

The arterial blood supply to the esophagus is much maligned. Although the distribution of arterial in-flow is segmental based on the embryologic development (see the section on embryology), there exist extensive intramural arterial collaterals. Virtually the entire esophagus can be adequately perfused via the cervical vessels. In fact, it would be a rare situation in which postoperative anastomotic complications are a result of "poor blood supply" to the esophagus. Such complications are usually produced by tension on the anastomosis due to insufficient mobilization, poor postoperative decompression, failure to clearly identify a retracted mucosa to ensure mucosa-to-mucosa apposition, and poor surgical or suture technique.

The cervical esophagus is perfused mainly by the inferior thyroid arteries (Fig. 58-3), either directly or via collaterals from the thyroid gland and small branches from the common carotid and subclavian arteries. Bronchial arteries arising from the distal aortic arch supply the intrathoracic esophagus in its proximal portion. In most patients, there is usually one bronchial artery from the right side and one to two on the left. Additionally, two esophageal branches usually arise directly from the aorta at the level of the sixth and eighth thoracic vertebrae. The most distal intra-

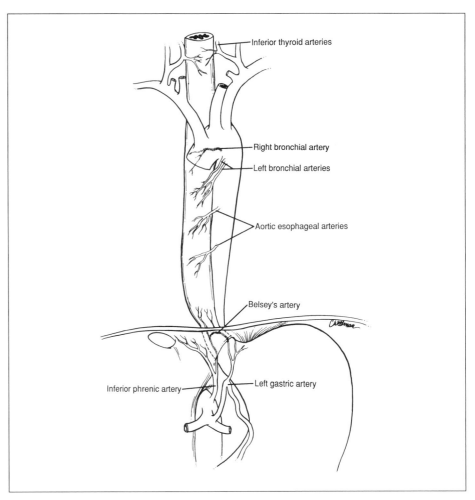

Fig. 58-3. Arterial supply of the esophagus.

thoracic esophagus and the intra-abdominal portion receive arterial blood supply from ascending branches of the left gastric and the inferior phrenic arteries. This vessel passes superiorly beneath the phreno-esophageal membrane. There is often a communicating vessel between the inferior phrenic and left gastric systems, usually referred to as Belsey's artery. Great care must be exercised in mobilizing the distal esophagus beneath the phreno-esophageal membrane during distal resections or fundoplications to avoid inadvertently injuring these vessels without adequate control. This is especially important with left thoracotomy approaches as these vessels may retract into the abdominal cavity causing difficult-to-control hemorrhage.

As these segmental arteries enter the esophagus, their caliber is usually quite small. After penetrating the muscular

wall, they assume a T-type configuration within the submucosa and between the circular and longitudinal muscle fiber layers to form an extensive intramural anastomosing network. This configuration of small-caliber vessels penetrating from outside to inside the esophagus and the extensive intramural arterial network allow for blunt mobilization of the esophagus during a transhiatal esophagectomy. As was previously noted, the entire esophagus may be mobilized with its blood supply based on cervical or inferior thyroid-derived vessels. An exception exists when a prior partial or complete thyroidectomy or any cervical procedure has compromised the inferior thyroid vessels.

Venous Drainage

Similar to the arterial system, the venous system has an extensive intramural venous plexus in the submucosa. These veins drain out through the circular and longitudinal muscle layers to a series of veins on the outer surface of the esophagus. Venous drainage then continues via vessels that parallel the arteries in a more or less segmental fashion.

In the cervical portion of the esophagus, drainage is via the inferior thyroid vein to the brachiocephalic veins (see Fig. 58-2). The intrathoracic esophagus drains principally via the azygos system, and to a lesser extent, the intercostal and accessory hemiazygos veins. On the right side, the azygos vein originates in the abdomen, either directly from the inferior vena cava or the right lumbar vein. It lies posterolateral to the esophagus, and to the right of the thoracic duct, until it arches over to drain into the superior vena cava (SVC) above the right main stem bronchus. In addition to helping to define the boundaries of the lymph node stations No. 4 (lower paratracheal) and No. 10 (hilar), the azygos vein is a useful landmark for defining the level of the esophagus relating to the main stem bronchus and aortic arch. The azygos is also useful during esophagectomy and reconstruction with colonic interposition or gastric pull-up in that one can pass the new conduit beneath the azygos as it arches over to insert into the SVC. This forms a natural tether to keep the colon or stomach in line and to help avoid redundancy. It also helps to prevent postoperative distention provided a functioning nasogastric (NG) tube is in place. While this ancillary use of the azygos arch can be useful in cases in which its sacrifice is not required for an appropriate ''cancer'' procedure, there also exists a potentially serious risk if there is unrecognized tumor extension into the azygos. Thus, during closed or transhiatal esophageal resections for tumor, one must be cognizant of the fact that continuing attempts to free up a ''stuck'' esophagus by blunt mobilization in the region of the azygos vein can lead to uncontrollable hemorrhage due to tearing of the azygos vein.

The hemiazygos vein arises on the left either directly from the left renal vein or the left lumbar vein. It lies along the left anterior aspect of the thoracic vertebral bodies. At the level of the eighth thoracic vertebra, the hemiazygos vein crosses over posterior to the esophagus to connect with the azygos vein on the right side.

In the distal esophagus, beneath the phrenoesophageal membrane, there exists a vast venous plexus that passes from the submucosa to directly under the mucosa (see Fig. 58-2, inset). This then continues on to the outer surface of the cardia of the stomach and, ultimately, the coronary vein. This plexus, then, can serve as one of the five collateral pathways connecting the caval or systemic with the portal venous systems. With sustained portal hypertension, this vast plexus with only scant supporting tissues undergoes marked distention and, ultimately, variceal formation. This area beneath the phrenoesophageal membrane is the most common location for variceal rupture and potentially fatal hemorrhage. It is highly unusual for esophageal varices to extend above the level of the azygos/SVC junction.

Lymphatic Drainage

An extensive network of lymphatics is contained within the wall of the esophagus, similar to that seen with the vasculature. Interconnections between the mucosal and submucosal networks essentially create one large system. This mucosal/submucosal network drains via lymph channels to the adventitia and periesophageal lymph nodes (Fig. 58-4). The periesophageal lymph nodes form groups that are the basis for the numbered system of

mediastinal nodes and the N classification of the TNM staging system.

Based on the embryologic development, lymphatic drainage, like venous drainage, flows away from the tracheal bifurcation. Thus, lymphatic drainage proximal to 25 cm (the level of the tracheal bifurcation/aortic arch) would be to the tracheobronchial, paratracheal, cervical, internal jugular, and superclavicular nodes. Distal to 25 cm, drainage would be to the subcarinal, posterior mediastinal, diaphragmatic, celiac, and left gastric nodes (Fig. 58-5).

This general schema is approximate at best when considering nodal involvement in esophageal carcinoma. The rich mucosal and submucosal networks allow tumor to extend intramurally. In addition, there is shared lymphatic drainage of the trachea and esophagus, thus making en bloc esophagectomy impossible for lesions above the tracheal bifurcation.

Extensive mapping of lymph nodes for patients with esophageal cancer demonstrates areas of lymph nodes most likely to be involved, but there is much overlap for tumors at different levels within the esophagus. Perhaps the most important consideration is that peri- and paraesophageal lymph nodes be sampled and specifically labeled at surgical resections, so that proper staging can be performed. This is especially true for nodes below the diaphragm.

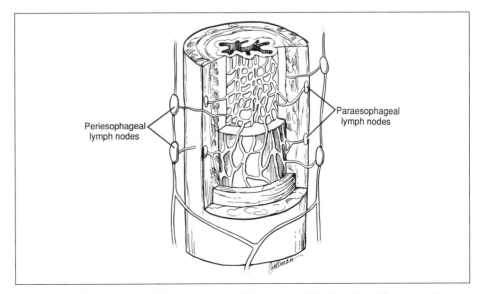

Fig. 58-4. Lymphatic drainage of the esophagus. Detailed anatomy within the wall and the surrounding tissues.

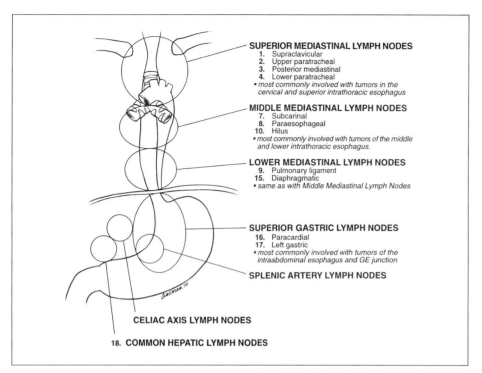

SUPERIOR MEDIASTINAL LYMPH NODES
1. Supraclavicular
2. Upper paratracheal
3. Posterior mediastinal
4. Lower paratracheal
• *most commonly involved with tumors in the cervical and superior intrathoracic esophagus*

MIDDLE MEDIASTINAL LYMPH NODES
7. Subcarinal
8. Paraesophageal
10. Hilus
• *most commonly involved with tumors of the middle and lower intrathoracic esophagus.*

LOWER MEDIASTINAL LYMPH NODES
9. Pulmonary ligament
15. Diaphragmatic
• *same as with Middle Mediastinal Lymph Nodes*

SUPERIOR GASTRIC LYMPH NODES
16. Paracardial
17. Left gastric
• *most commonly involved with tumors of the intraabdominal esophagus and GE junction*

SPLENIC ARTERY LYMPH NODES

CELIAC AXIS LYMPH NODES

18. **COMMON HEPATIC LYMPH NODES**

Fig. 58-5. Lymph node groups in relation to the esophagus. Boldface numbers correspond to the lymph node stations utilized by the American Joint Committee on Cancer Staging. (Adapted from H Akiyama, et al. Principles of surgical treatment for carcinoma of the esophagus: Analysis of lymph node involvement. Ann Surg *194:438, 1981.)*

Suggested Reading

Akiyama H, et al. Principles of surgical treatment for carcinoma of the esophagus: Analysis of lymph node involvement. *Ann Surg* 194:438, 1981.

Butler H. The views of the aesophagus. *Thorac* 6: 276, 1951.

deCarvalho CAF. Sin l' angio-architecture veineuse de la zore de transition aesophagogastrique et son interpretation fonctionelle. *Acta Anatomica* 64:125, 1966.

Hermann JD, Minngasia JJ. The blood supply of the aesophagus in relation to aesophageal surgery. *Aust NZ J Surg* 35:195, 1966.

Hollinshead WH. *Anatomy for Surgeons* Vol 2 (2nd ed). New York: Harper Row, 1971. Pp 168-219.

Shields TW. *General Thoracic Surgery*, (4th ed). Philadelphia: Williams & Wilkins, 1994. Pp 1335-1377, 1529-1540.

Skinner DR, Belsey RHR. *Management of Esophageal Disease*. Philadelphia: Saunders, 1988. Pp 9–17.

Tisi GM, et al. Clinical staging of primary lung cancer. *Am Rev Respir Dis* 127:659, 1981.

EDITOR'S COMMENT

The authors have presented a practical orientation to the anatomy of the esophagus in the mediastinum. In the cervical and proximal thoracic portion of the esophagus, it is essentially a striated muscle-lined hollow viscus that is really a tube within a tube. The mucosa and submucosa form a single fused tube, and the space between the submucosa and the muscularis has enough loose areolar tissue so that tumor cells can traverse the space between the inner layer and the outer muscular tube, perhaps being transported in part by active peristalsis, especially in the upper third. The muscular coat has been extensively described by the authors, who have emphasized the absence of a serosal layer; this makes the esophagus a most treacherous hollow viscus to anastomose, since apposition of serosa to serosa across the anastomosis is not possible in the absence of esophageal serosa. Furthermore, the somewhat discontinuous character of the inner mucosa-submucosa and outer muscularis makes the anastomosis to another viscus less secure than it would be if this was a single fused layer, as is the case in the rest of the gastrointestinal tract.

Experimental studies have shown that injection of a marker such as carbon black submucosally at the very distal end of the esophagus in experimental animals will result in a short period of time that those particles are retrievable from the upper end of the esophagus, primarily by transport through the lymphatics of the deep submucosa and those in the space between the submucosa and the muscularis layers. These observations are interpreted to translate into the principle that tumors of the esophagus are very apt to spread throughout the submucosa-muscularis interface, and that it is common to have tumors of the lower or midesophagus with tumor cells microscopically apparent at both the proximal and distal end of the esophagus. For this reason, a truly curative operation for primary esophageal cancer usually requires total esophagectomy, with only enough cervical esophagus remaining to provide a convenient anastomotic site.

It is apparent that an understanding of both the external anatomy and the functional internal anatomy of the esophagus is crucial to operation design and successful procedures for improving esophageal function or excising esophageal tumors, both benign and malignant. This is discussed in subsequent chapters.

R.J.B.

59

Transthoracic Antireflux Procedures

Tom R. DeMeester   Jeffrey A. Hagen

A great advance in the surgical treatment of hiatal hernia occurred when it was recognized that the symptoms associated with hernia were actually caused by gastroesophageal reflux (GER). This view directed surgeons toward improving the function of the cardia rather than simply reducing the hernia and closing the crura. The Allison transthoracic repair represented the first effort in this direction and emphasized the need to place the gastroesophageal junction in its normal intra-abdominal position to improve its function. Recognition of a high incidence of symptomatic and anatomic recurrences after the Allison repair led to the development of procedures designed to more effectively place and anchor the lower esophagus in the intra-abdominal position. One of these procedures, the Belsey Mark IV antireflux repair, is a partial fundoplication done only through a thoracic incision, whereas the other procedure, the Nissen fundoplication, is done through either a thoracic or an abdominal incision. Although the Nissen procedure consists of constructing a 360-degree gastric fundoplication of the distal esophagus, the techniques of accomplishing this through an abdominal or thoracic approach are somewhat different.

The recognition that the esophagus shortens and loses its propulsive force as a consequence of long-standing severe mucosal damage led to the development of the Collis gastroplasty, a procedure designed to lengthen the esophagus in order to reduce tension on a repair by tubing, over a No. 45 French bougie, 4 to 5 cm of the lesser curve of the stomach. This procedure is best performed by the thoracic approach to allow maximal mobilization of the esophagus

and the construction of a Belsey partial fundoplication over the gastroplasty tube.

Medical treatment of gastroesophageal reflux is directed toward changing the pH of the reflux material and decreasing the incidence and duration of reflux episodes by postural and dietetic therapy. Changing the pH reduces the symptoms of heartburn but has minimal effect on regurgitation. Avoiding certain positions reduces the number of reflux episodes, and assuming the upright position improves esophageal clearance. Eating a bland diet with low fat content neutralizes gastric acidity during and after a meal and improves gastric emptying. Both lessen postprandial heartburn and regurgitation. Despite these efforts, however, the cardia remains incompetent. Thus, the monitoring of medical therapy is necessary since patients may continue to regurgitate and have persistent mucosal damage without the symptom of heartburn, and chronic cough may develop as the result of repetitive occult aspiration or dysphagia emerging from progressive mucosal injury. In contrast, antireflux operations can provide immediate correction of an incompetent cardia after one short surgical procedure. Long-term studies indicate that this correction stops symptoms of heartburn and regurgitation, heals esophagitis, prevents progression of the disease, and lasts well over 9 years (Fig. 59-1).

The pain associated with an operation and the somewhat prolonged recuperative time, especially following transthoracic procedures, has created some reluctance to consider surgical therapy. The recent addition of laparoscopic procedures to the armamentarium of the surgeon has de-

creased the significance of this issue. Surgical therapy becomes more attractive when one considers the restraints of medical therapy on the patient's lifestyle, and the expense associated with a lifetime of medication and repetitive endoscopic procedures to monitor the health of the mucosa.

The primary goal of an antireflux operation is to make the cardia competent by improving its function. To accomplish this, it is paramount that the surgeon understand the physiology of the foregut and how its function can be improved by a surgical procedure. An antireflux operation is different from the simple extirpation of a diseased organ, in which function is of no concern because the organ is destroyed with its removal. Rather, an antireflux operation is designed to improve the function of an organ that will be left in the patient with the expectation of complete and permanent relief of all symptoms and complications of gastroesophageal reflux while allowing the patient to swallow normally. After an antireflux operation, a patient should not need further medical, postural, or dietetic therapy. As antireflux operations achieve these goals more dependably, safely, and with less morbidity, requests for this operation will increase.

Indications for Surgical Therapy

Patients with persistent or recurrent symptoms and/or complications of GER disease such as esophagitis or stricture, despite an 8- to 12-week course of intensive acid suppression therapy, are potential candidates

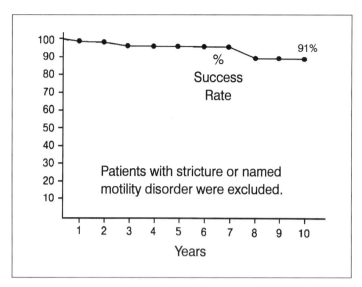

Fig. 59-1. *Actuarial success of a primary Nissen fundoplication to relieve reflux symptoms in 100 patients. Patients with stricture and severe motility disorders were excluded.*

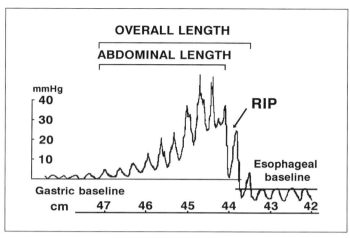

Fig. 59-2. *Normal manometric tracing obtained by pulling the transducer through the gastroesophageal junction from the stomach into the esophagus. Note the positive deflections with inspiration in the intra-abdominal portion and the negative deflections in the intrathoracic portion.*

for an antireflux operation. This is particularly so if they have a long life expectancy or are unwilling to become dependent on continuous pharmacologic therapy. Antireflux surgery is an appropriate therapeutic option, especially when the reason for the increased esophageal acid exposure is a mechanically defective lower esophageal sphincter (LES), as defined by low resting pressure (<6 mm Hg), short overall length (<2 cm), or short intra-abdominal length (<1 cm) on standard manometry (Fig. 59-2). If a mechanical defect of the cardia is not present on esophageal manometry, gastric causes of reflux, such as delayed emptying, should be evaluated before one proceeds with an operation. Chronic aspiration that persists, or emerges, during medical therapy is an indication for surgical therapy. Twenty-four–hour esophageal pH monitoring has proved to be helpful in objectively relating the symptoms of aspiration, that is, coughing, choking, and shortness of breath, with a reflux episode.

Patients who are drug dependent for the control of their symptoms should have the option of surgical therapy. Medical therapy may prove to be too confining or expensive on a long-term basis. It is not necessary that these patients have esophagitis before surgical therapy is considered, but abnormal reflux must be shown on 24-hour esophageal pH monitoring when they are off medication. Again, if a me-

chanical defect of the cardia is not present, gastric causes of reflux should be evaluated, particularly in patients who reflux only during the day when they are eating.

Patients who are to undergo an operation for another upper abdominal disease, such as chronic cholelithiasis or peptic ulceration, and who have *objectively proved symptomatic gastroesophageal reflux* should have a concomitant antireflux procedure if a mechanically defective cardia is present.

Children with *severe esophagitis, recurrent pneumonia, or failure to thrive* should be considered for surgical therapy if gastroesophageal reflux is documented. Esophagitis is rapidly progressive in this age group, and peptic stricture can develop in a matter of weeks, even while the child is undergoing an acceptable form of medical therapy. Once the diagnosis of grade III esophagitis has been confirmed in children, the need for a surgical antireflux procedure becomes urgent if further complications are to be avoided. Failure to thrive, anemia, and aspiration pneumonia in infants may be the only evidence that reflux is present. Once gastroesophageal reflux is objectively established by 24-hour esophageal pH monitoring, surgical correction should be performed.

The presence of *gastroesophageal reflux in association with scleroderma or a severe motility disorder* should merit careful evaluation

before one proceeds with surgical therapy, as the results in such patients are disappointing. Reflux in the presence of a severe motility disorder progresses rapidly to esophagitis with stricture formation and is frequently associated with pulmonary aspiration. Esophagectomy and esophageal replacement with stomach or colon may be the only solution for such patients.

The presence of a Barrett's columnar-lined esophagus is usually associated with reflux complicated by ulceration and stenosis at the squamocolumnar interface. An antireflux procedure should be done to control the reflux in these patients since they almost always have a mechanically defective cardia. These patients are at risk for adenocarcinoma of the esophagus and should have biannual endoscopic evaluations after repair. It is uncertain, but highly likely, that the risk of developing carcinoma is reduced following the elimination of reflux by a surgical procedure. Before one proceeds with surgery, extensive biopsies should be taken of the metaplastic epithelium to exclude severe dysplasia or intramucosal carcinoma. If found, these patients should have an esophagectomy.

The presence of a mechanically defective cardia in association with delayed gastric emptying after vagotomy or partial gastric resection can result in the reflux of gastric and pancreatobiliary secretions into the esophagus. This problem can cause severe esophagitis and pulmonary aspiration. Therapeutic measures that selectively control either the acid or alkaline reflux components alone usually fail; hence, bile-diverting procedures are of little benefit. These patients should have an antireflux operation and a bile-diverting procedure if symptomatic alkaline gastritis is present. If gastric emptying is severely impaired, a partial or total fundoplication with a near-total gastrectomy and Roux-en-Y gastrojejunostomy should be done.

Biomechanics of an Antireflux Repair

Four principles are important to the reconstruction of the antireflux mechanism and should be understood by all surgeons who attempt to perform such procedures. First, the technique should permanently restore 1.5 to 2.0 cm of abdominal esophagus and ensure its response to changes in intra-abdominal pressure. The degree of competence provided by a segment of intra-abdominal esophagus, in the absence of intrinsic muscle tone, is a direct function of its length (Figs. 59-2 and 59-3). As the intra-abdominal pressure increases, the length of abdominal esophagus necessary for competence decreases (Fig. 59-4). The presence of intrinsic muscle tone augments the effectiveness of the intra-abdominal esophagus as an antireflux barrier; the shorter the abdominal length, the greater is the muscle tone required to maintain competence (Fig. 59-5). The permanent restoration of 1.5 to 2.0 cm of the abdominal esophagus in a patient with normal sphincter tone maintains the competence of the cardia over a wide range of intra-abdominal pressures and ensures reflux control during fluctuations of abdominal pressure even though these pressure changes tend to force the cardia up into the hiatus and reduce the length of abdominal esophagus. Mobilization of the lower esophagus so that an adequate segment can be placed below the diaphragm is fundamental to any antireflux operation.

The construction of a conduit that ensures the transmission of intra-abdominal pressure changes around the abdominal esophagus is an important aspect in achieving this goal. The fundoplication in the Nissen and Belsey repairs serves this

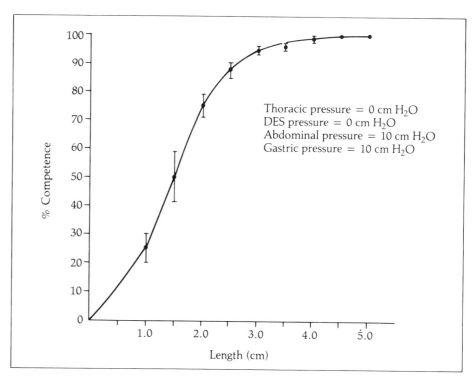

Fig. 59-3. The relation of length of the abdominal esophagus, in the absence of intrinsic sphincter tone, to competence of the cardia. DES = distal esophageal sphincter.

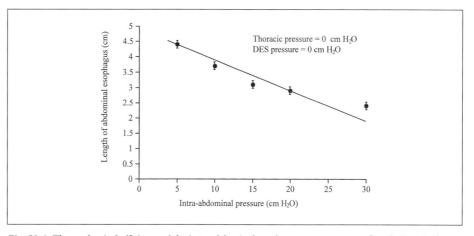

Fig. 59-4. The mechanical efficiency of the intra-abdominal esophagus to counteract reflux during challenges of increased intra-abdominal pressure. DES = distal esophageal sphincter.

purpose. In the absence of a conduit, the development of postoperative periesophageal adhesions can prevent the transmission of changes in intra-abdominal pressures to the abdominal esophagus and allows posturally induced pressure changes in the abdominal cavity to act unequally on the stomach and abdominal esophagus, resulting in reflux.

The second principle is to use a technique that permanently augments the resting distal esophageal sphincter pressure equal to or greater than three times the resting gastric pressure or about 15 mm Hg and maintains an overall sphincter length of at least 2 cm. It has been shown that up to 60 percent of reflux episodes, rather than related to changes in intra-abdominal pres-

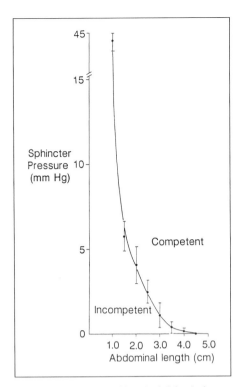

Fig. 59-5. *The relation of length of abdominal esophagus and distal esophageal sphincter pressure (DESP) to achieve competency against intra-abdominal pressure changes.*

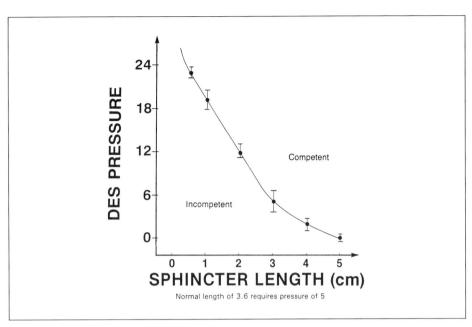

Fig. 59-6. *The relation of overall lower esophageal sphincter length and sphincter pressure to achieve competency against intragastric pressure changes.*

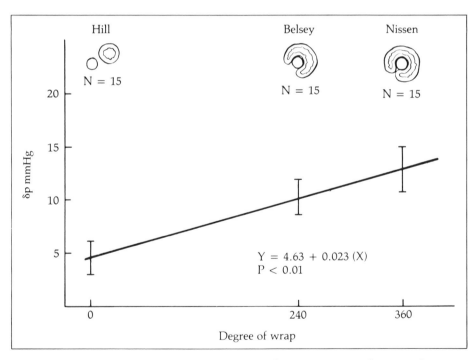

Fig. 59-7. *The relation between the increase in postoperative sphincter pressure over the preoperative pressure (δp) and the degree of fundoplication.*

sure, are related to independent increases in intragastric pressure, which overcome the esophageal sphincter tone or cause gastric dilations and shortening of the overall sphincter length resulting in reflux. In gastric dilation, the overall length of the sphincter decreases as the neck of a balloon shortens during inflation, and a greater sphincter pressure is required for competence (Fig 59-6). The resting esophageal sphincter pressures can be surgically augmented over the preoperative pressure values. This increase is a function of the degree of fundoplication around the distal esophagus (Fig. 59-7). The final pressure values achieved are thought to be caused by the transfer of gastric muscle tone around the distal esophagus. This restores normal length-tension characteristics and improves the myogenic function of the cardia.

The third principle is to use only the fundus of the stomach to construct the fundoplication and avoid damage to the vagus nerves. To facilitate normal swallowing, the distal esophageal sphinc-ter must relax after the operation. On deglutition, a vagally mediated relaxation of the distal esophagus and fundus of the stomach occurs. This relaxation lasts for approximately 10 seconds and is followed by rapid recovery to its former tonicity. To ensure relaxation of the reconstructed cardia, only the fundus of the stomach should be used in constructing a fundoplication since it is known to relax with the distal

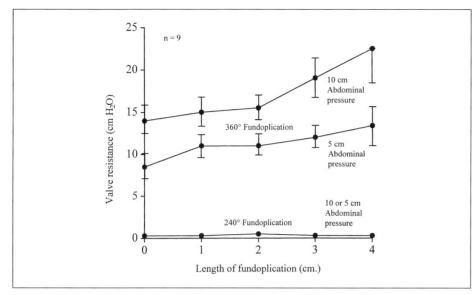

Fig. 59-8. The amount of pressure the esophageal body must generate to overcome the resistance of a 360-degree or 240-degree fundoplication of various lengths, in the absence of intrinsic tone, at different levels of abdominal pressure.

esophageal sphincter. It is paramount that the innervation of the cardia be protected, since vagal damage results in failure of relaxation of the gastric fundus and achalasia-like symptoms.

The fourth principle is to use a technique that matches the resistance of the reconstructed valve to the propulsive power of the esophagus. The choice between a 360-degree or partial 240-degree wrap is influenced by the strength of the peristaltic contractions in the body of the esophagus. Normal wave progression and strong contractions do well with a Nissen 360-degree fundoplication. When the peristaltic wave progression is lost or its prevalence reduced below 50 percent, or esophageal contractions are below 20 mm Hg, the Belsey two-thirds fundoplication is preferred. Inappropriate matching of the body of the esophagus to the resistance of the reconstructed valve results in a delay in the passage of food through the cardia and symptoms of dysphagia. The Nissen 360-degree fundoplication provides excellent control of reflux but adds considerable resistance to the cardia even in the relaxed state. This resistance is directly related to the length of the fundoplication, and for this reason it should rarely exceed 1.5 to 2.0 cm (Fig. 59-8). Whenever there is a question as to the strength of esophageal peristalsis, a Belsey 240-degree fundoplication should

be done. This fundoplication has no measurable resistance to esophageal emptying.

Indications for the Thoracic Approach

The thoracic approach to an antireflux procedure should be used in the following situations:

1. A patient who has had a previous antireflux repair.
2. A patient with esophageal contraction amplitude below 20 mm Hg in the distal one-third of the esophagus. These patients do not have sufficient propulsive force to cope with the outflow resistance of a full fundoplication and require a partial fundoplication to avoid dysphagia from developing after operation. Since a partial fundoplication does not withstand tension, the esophagus must be fully mobilized by a thoracic approach in order to construct a tension-free repair.
3. A patient with shortening of the esophagus. Again, the thoracic approach is preferred for maximum mobilization of the esophagus to place the repair, without tension, in the abdomen or, if necessary, a gastroplasty can be added to lengthen the esophagus.

4. A patient with a sliding hernia that measures greater than 4 cm between the crura and the gastroesophageal junction on endoscopy or does not reduce below the diaphragm on an upright barium swallow. These signs suggest esophageal shortening.
5. A patient with associated pulmonary disease that requires a biopsy or removal.
6. A patient who needs a concomitant esophageal myotomy for achalasia or diffuse spasm.
7. A patient who is obese.

Choice of Surgical Procedure

The operations performed for gastroesophageal reflux by the transthoracic route include the Belsey Mark IV, the Nissen, and the Collis gastroplasty. The operation chosen depends on the effectiveness of esophageal wave progression contraction amplitude and the presence of esophageal shortening. Figure 59-9 depicts the algorithm utilized in selecting the appropriate antireflux procedure. In patients with preserved esophageal body function and length, a Nissen fundoplication can be performed. A Belsey Mark IV procedure causes less outflow resistance and is utilized wherever the esophageal body function is diminished. When the esophageal length is shortened, a Collis gastroplasty with a partial fundoplication is utilized. When the patient is obese, we prefer the transthoracic approach for ease of exposure. Table 59-1 shows the outcome of this approach in 85 consecutive patients who were followed after operation for a median of 4 years, with 40 patients followed beyond 5 years.

Surgical Technique
Belsey Mark IV Partial Fundoplication

The Belsey partial fundoplication was originally introduced by Ronald Belsey of Great Britain in 1967. The steps in the Belsey or the transthoracic Nissen operation are the same, differing only in the completeness of the gastric fundoplication and the length of tension-free intra-abdominal

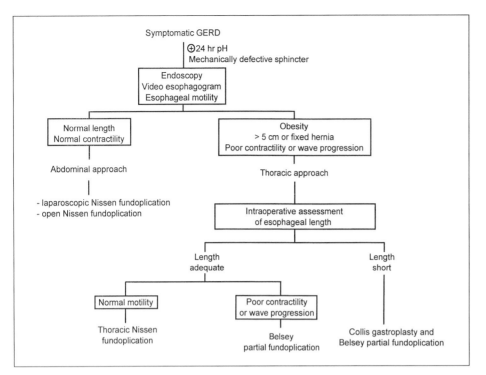

Fig. 59-9. Algorithm of decisions in selecting the appropriate antireflux procedure based on clinical and manometric evaluation. GERD = gastroesophageal reflux disease.

Table 59-1. Improvement of the Primary Symptom Responsible for Surgery After the Various Tailored Antireflux Procedures

Procedure	No. of Pts	No. of Pts Cured	No. of Pts Failed	% Cured
Abdominal Nissen	49	44	5	90
Thoracic Nissen	20	19	1	95
Belsey	6	4	2	67
Collis Belsey	10	8	2	80
Total	85	75	10	89

esophagus necessary to do the repair. The former requires a minimum of 4 cm and the latter 1.5 cm. Consequently, the clinical success of a Belsey repair deteriorates progressively from 90 percent in patients with no esophageal shortening to 50 percent in those with significant shortening.

The hiatus is approached through a left posterolateral thoracotomy in the sixth intercostal space, that is, over the upper border of the seventh rib. For patients who are undergoing a second procedure because of a previous failed antireflux repair, we prefer to use the seventh intercostal space over the upper border of the eighth rib to obtain better exposure of the abdomen through a peripheral diaphragmatic incision. The incision in the diaphragm is made circumferentially 2 to 3 cm from the chest wall for a distance of 10 to 15 cm. A sufficient fringe of diaphragm must be left along the chest wall to allow for easy closure of the incision. If further abdominal exposure is necessary, the thoracic incision can be extended across the costal margin and diagonally down to the abdominal midline, dividing the fibers of the left rectus muscle. The operation is made easier if a double-lumen endobronchial tube is used for anesthesia and the left lung is selectively deflated.

The esophagus is mobilized from the diaphragm to underneath the aortic arch. Care is taken not to injure the vagus nerves. Branches of the vagal plexus going to the left and right lung must be divided to obtain sufficient esophageal length to construct, without tension, a partial fun-

doplication over 4 cm of abdominal esophagus. Two vessels arise from the proximal descending thoracic aorta and pass over the esophagus to the left main stem bronchus. They are the left superior and inferior bronchial arteries. Ligation of these arteries is necessary to fully mobilize the esophagus underneath the aortic arch. In addition to these arteries, two to three direct esophageal branches come off the distal descending thoracic aorta and go directly to the distal esophagus. These are also ligated and divided without concern about ischemic necrosis of the esophagus. There is sufficient blood supply through the intrinsic arterial plexus of the esophagus fed by the inferior thyroid artery in the neck and by branches from the right bronchial artery in the thorax to maintain its integrity. This degree of mobilization is necessary to place the reconstructed cardia into the abdomen without undue tension. Failure of adequate mobilization is one of the major causes for subsequent breakdown of a repair and return of symptoms.

Freeing the cardia from the diaphragmatic hiatus is the most difficult portion of the procedure but can be completed through the hiatus. It is unnecessary to make an incision through the central tendon of the diaphragm or to enlarge the hiatus by an incision through the crura. The dissection is started by gaining access to the abdominal cavity through the phrenoesophageal membrane. It can be difficult at times to find the correct tissue plane once the membrane has been divided due to the protrusion of the properitoneal fat. Persistence and dissection underneath the retracted left crus, away from the gastric vessels, eventually yield entry into the free peritoneal space. Entering the abdominal cavity is easier when a hiatal hernia is present than when it is not.

The proper stance of the surgeon at the operating table aids in freeing the hiatus. With the patient in the left posterior thoracotomy position, the surgeon should stand adjacent to the patient's back, facing the head of the table. The left index and middle fingers are placed through the diaphragmatic hiatus into the abdominal cavity with the palm facing the patient's feet. The surgeon's line of vision is down and backward under his or her left axilla. With judicious use of the left thumb, index, and middle fingers, the surgeon is able to spread the hiatal tissues and divide them with a scissors controlled by the right hand. In this position, the left hand is also used to retract the esophagus and protect the vagal trunks. Although it sounds somewhat awkward, this stance greatly facilitates the most difficult part of the operation.

All the attachments between the cardia and diaphragmatic hiatus are divided. The short gastric vessels are divided and ligated to allow good mobilization of the fundus. When free, the fundus and part of the body of the stomach are withdrawn up through the hiatus into the chest (Fig. 59-10).

The vascular fat pad, which lies on the anterolateral surface of the cardia, is excised back to the vagi on each side. The fundus of the stomach must adhere firmly to the lower esophagus; this fat pad, if not removed, interferes with the healing between these two structures.

The completely mobilized esophagus, encircled with a Penrose drain, is retracted forward to the anterior border of the hiatus to give exposure for closure of the hiatus posteriorly. The right and left crura of the diaphragmatic hiatus are identified and approximated with interrupted 0 silk sutures, taking generous bites of muscle. Usually there is a decussation of muscle fibers from the right crus anteriorly around the aorta, but occasionally the aorta lies free within the enlarged hiatus. In either situation, the first crural suture is placed close to the aorta. Traction on this first posterior crural stitch elevates the right crus toward the surgeon and facilitates the placement of subsequent crural sutures. Occasionally it is necessary to mobilize the pericardium off the diaphragm to give better exposure of the fascia and muscle making up the right crus. The subsequent crural sutures should incorporate the fascia from the periphery of the central tendon that blends in with the muscle fibers making up the right crus.

On the left side, the sutures are passed through the muscle fibers on the left crus and the firmly adherent overlying pleura. Approximately six sutures, placed 1 cm apart, are necessary to approximate the crura and to adequately reduce the size of the hiatus. All six sutures are placed at this time since it is easier to remove those not needed than to add additional sutures after completion of the repair. To insert the last of the six sutures, it is often necessary to push the esophagus posteriorly against the previously placed sutures. The sixth suture is then placed into the right crus anterior to the esophagus, passed posteriorly to the esophagus, and then through the left crus. The crural sutures are not tied until reconstruction of the cardia is completed (Fig. 59-11).

The construction of the gastric fundoplication is the keystone of the antireflux repair in that its proper function is responsible for fulfilling the four principles necessary to re-establish the competence of the cardia. In the Belsey Mark IV operation, the fundus of the stomach is plicated around the anterior two-thirds of the lower 4 cm of esophagus. The partial fundoplication is held in place by two rows of three horizontal mattress sutures placed equidistantly between the seromuscular layers of the stomach and the muscular layers of the esophagus. Number 000 silk sutures are used, and each suture obtains a firm grip of the esophageal muscle fibers by passing down to, but not through, the muscularis mucosae. The first row of sutures is placed 1.5 cm above the cardia and is tied only tightly enough to obtain tissue apposition without disrupting the muscle fibers of the esophagus. It is important to remember that the hiatus is approached surgically from the left lateral position. To construct the fundoplication over the anterolateral two-thirds of the esophagus, it is necessary that the far right suture be placed in the right lateral wall of the esophagus. This is out of the surgeon's view and requires rotation of the esophagus before placement of the suture. A common mistake is placing this suture too far anteriorly, resulting in an anterolateral fundoplication displaced to the left (Fig. 59-12).

A second row of 00 sutures is placed 2.0 cm above the first row, using the position of the previously placed first row of sutures as a guide (Fig. 59-13). Once again the second row of sutures is tied carefully so as to give tissue apposition without strangulation. The tails of these sutures are not cut but are separately rethreaded on a large thin Ferguson needle and passed 0.5 cm apart from each other through the diaphragm from the abdominal to the thoracic surface, 1.0 to 1.5 cm from the edge of the hiatus. The diaphragmatic sutures are placed at the 4, 8, and 12 o'clock posi-

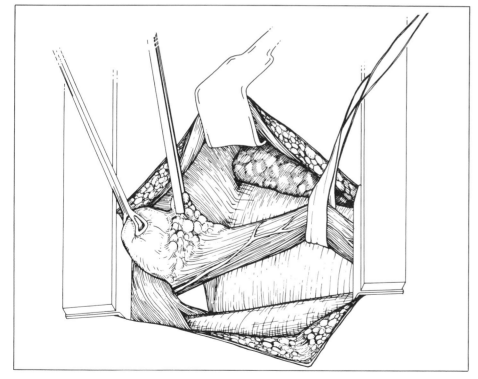

Fig. 59-10. A transthoracic mobilization of the esophagus and stomach through a left posterolateral thoracotomy showing the esophagus and cardia from the diaphragmatic hiatus and mediastinal tissue. The fundus of the stomach is drawn through the hiatus into the chest with a Babcock clamp. The forceps is on the vascular fat pad at the cardioesophageal junction.

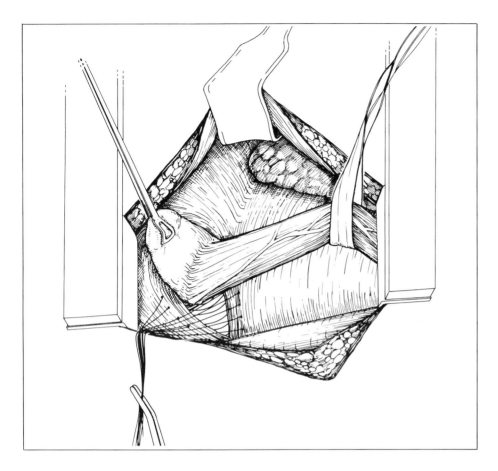

Fig. 59-11. A transthoracic exposure showing the vascular fat pad removed and anterior retraction of the esophagus with placement of the crural sutures for closure of the hiatus posteriorly.

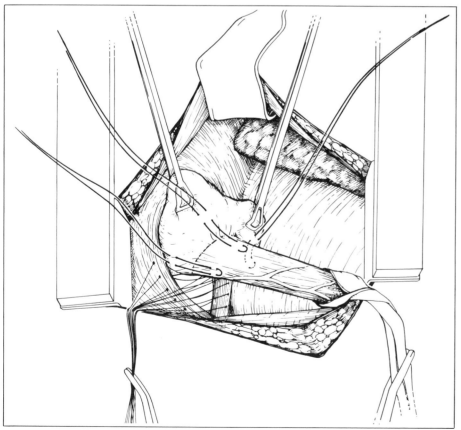

Fig. 59-12. Construction of a Belsey 240-degree partial fundoplication showing placement of the first row of sutures 1.5 to 2 cm above the gastroesophageal junction. Particular attention must be given to placement of the right lateral suture.

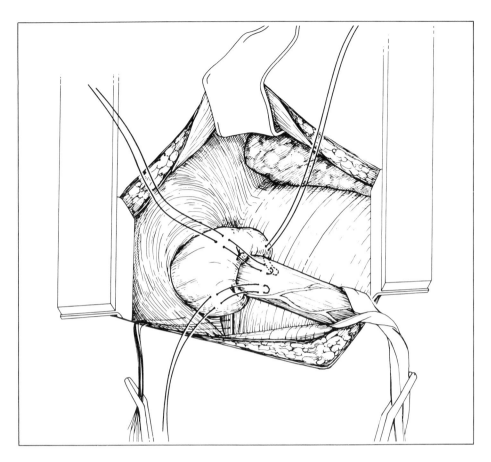

Fig. 59-13. Continued construction of the Belsey 240-degree partial fundoplication showing placement of the second row of sutures 2.0 cm above the previously tied sutures of the first row.

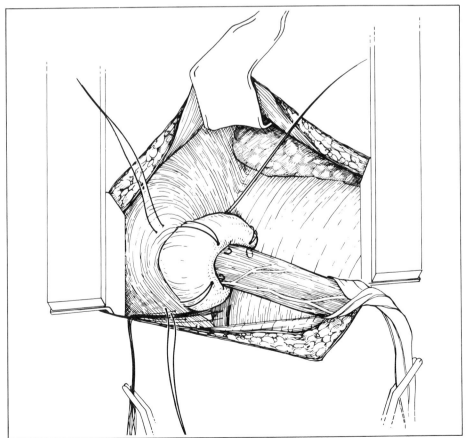

Fig. 59-14. Continued construction of the Belsey 240-degree partial fundoplication showing placement of the tails of the previously tied second row of sutures through the diaphragm, 0.5 cm apart and 1.0 to 1.5 cm from the edge of the hiatus. Note the placement of the sutures at the 4, 8, and 12 o'clock positions on an imaginary clock face oriented with the 6 o'clock position posterior in the hiatus between the right and left crura just anterior to the aorta.

tions on a clock face, oriented with the 6 o'clock position on the posterior margin of the hiatus between the right and left crura just anterior to the aorta (Fig. 59-14). It is important to properly place the right lateral, or 4 o'clock, suture to avoid the common error of putting this suture too far anteriorly, in the 1 or 2 o'clock position, and constructing an anterolateral fundoplication displaced to the left. These sutures must be carefully placed to avoid injury to the abdominal structures. A spoon retractor has become a popular aid in placing these sutures without snagging abdominal mesentery or omentum. The needle is guided along the inner surface of a spoon held firmly against the undersurface of the diaphragm before it is passed through the diaphragm.

The reconstructed cardia is massaged through the hiatus and into the abdomen. It is not dragged down into the abdomen by pulling on the diaphragmatic sutures but rather is placed into the abdomen by compressing the fundic ball with the hand and manually maneuvering it through the hiatus. Resistance to placing the repair into

the abdomen can result from the shoelace obstruction of the previously placed crural sutures. Opening the crural sutures, as loosening the laces of a shoe, relieves the obstruction and helps in placing the reconstructed cardia into the abdomen. Once in the abdomen, the cardia should remain there without tension on the holding sutures. A gentle up-and-down motion on the diaphragm should not allow the cardia to emerge back through the esophageal hiatus. If the repair remains in the abdomen unaided, the previously placed crural sutures are tied. The holding sutures are then tied, approximating the knot against the previously tied knot so as to avoid any redundancy in the suture between the repair and the diaphragm (Fig. 59-15). An additional safety factor of the double knot technique is that if one of the tails of the holding sutures breaks while it is being tied, it is not necessary to take the repair down, pull the stomach back up into the chest, and insert a new suture. Simple anchoring of the single remaining tail to the diaphragm is sufficient to hold the cardia in position. The technique also prevents tying the sutures too tight and causing ne-

crosis of the incorporated esophageal and gastric tissue.

If the fundoplication tends to ride up through the hiatus, tension on the repair is too great. It is usually caused by inadequate mobilization of the esophagus. If, after further attempts at mobilization, the tendency still exists, a Collis gastroplasty may be necessary.

Transthoracic Collis Gastroplasty

The concept of a gastroplasty was initially introduced by Collis of Great Britain in 1957 as an antireflux procedure. It was modified in 1987 by Pearson to include a Belsey-type fundoplication over the Collis gastroplasty. The Collis-Belsey procedure is performed in patients with gastroesophageal reflux disease complicated by esophageal fibrosis and shortening. As a result of the severe alterations in esophageal body structure and function, many of these patients present with dysphagia in addition to heartburn and regurgitation.

The gastroplasty lengthens the esophagus by tubing the lesser curve of the stomach to create a ''neo-esophagus,'' allowing tension-free construction of a Belsey Mark IV or Nissen fundoplication over the tube, and reducing the risk of subsequent breakdown or displacement of the fundoplication into the chest. We prefer to combine the Belsey partial fundoplication rather than the Nissen full fundoplication with a gastroplasty because of the likelihood of poor contraction amplitude of the esophageal body when it has been shortened from long-standing reflux disease. The gastroplasty component of the procedure, in addition to adding esophageal length, provides relatively uninflamed tissue to which the stomach can be sewn in performing the Belsey partial fundoplication. The improved competency of the cardia provided by the partial fundoplication results in the healing of reflux-induced esophageal inflammation and ulceration, softening of strictures and tissue fibrosis, and some restoration of esophageal compliance. The loss in contraction amplitude is usually not reversible.

Surgical staplers have made the construction of the gastroplasty tube simple and reliable and prevent spillage of gastric contents into the chest or abdomen. The relative ease with which a gastroplasty

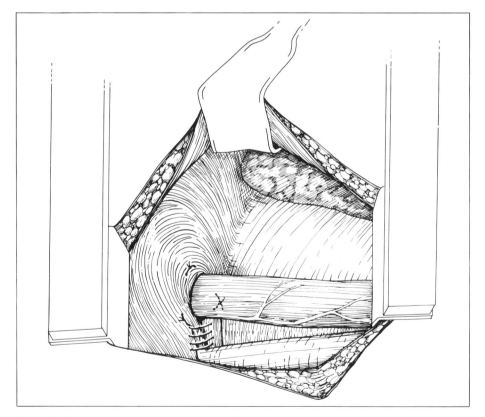

Fig. 59-15. The completed Belsey 240-degree partial fundoplication showing the right and left crura approximated by tying the previously placed sutures. The position of the tied holding sutures is also shown.

and partial fundoplication can be performed has made the procedure particularly suited for patients with the sequelae of advanced disease and has reduced the need for esophageal resection and replacement.

The esophageal and gastric mobilizations are performed in a manner identical to that described previously for the Belsey Mark IV repair. The Collis gastroplasty tube is created along the lesser curvature of the stomach, in continuity with the distal esophagus and for a length of 4 to 5 cm, over a No. 48 French Maloney bougie (Fig. 59-16). The tube can be readily constructed using a single fire of the GIA stapler. To aid in achieving a uniform diameter along the length of the gastric tube, traction is exerted on the greater curvature before the jaws of the stapler are closed (Fig. 59-17). The resultant staple lines, both on the tube and the remaining fundus, are oversewn with a running absorbable suture (Fig. 59-18). A Belsey fundoplication is performed, as described previously, over and around the gastroplasty tube (Figs. 59-19 through 59-21). This sutured reinforcement is essential to prevent subsequent leakage or fistulization from the staple lines. Caution must be exercised in constructing gastroplasty tubes in patients with previous or concomitant gastric surgery, such as highly selective vagotomy, that interrupted blood supply to the lesser curvature. This can cause devascularization of the tubularized portion of stomach with subsequent ischemic necrosis.

Transthoracic Nissen Fundoplication

The Nissen fundoplication was initially described in the German literature by Rudolph Nissen in 1956 and subsequently in the English literature in 1961. A modification of the originally described procedure was made in 1986 to reduce the incidence of side effects associated with the original repair. This consisted of constructing the fundoplication over a No. 60 French bougie, reducing the length of the fundoplication to 1.5 to 2.0 cm, and holding the fundoplication in place with a single U stitch of permanent suture material reinforced with Teflon (polytetrafluoroethylene [PTFE]) pledgets. When completed, the approximated lips of the fundoplication lie over the anterior right lateral surface of the lower esophagus.

In patients who complained of recurrent heartburn and regurgitation, traces of a previous fundoplication were completely absent, due to disruption of the fundic sutures. This suggested the need for stronger sutures placed in a more durable manner. Other patients had marked dysphagia and inability to belch, even though an endoscope could be passed easily into the stomach. In these patients, the fundoplication was either too tight or too long. From these clinical observations, along with observations made from a model on the biomechanics of the cardia, it became evident that the fundoplication should be at least No. 60 French in diameter, only 1.5 to 2.0 cm long, and held in place with permanent reinforced sutures. The technique that emerged used one permanent 00 polypropylene suture placed in a U-shaped pattern over two 1.5 × 0.5 cm PTFE pledgets

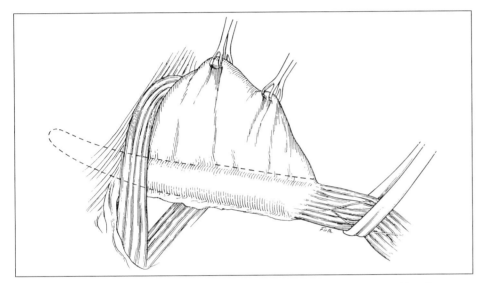

Fig. 59-16. Preparation for forming a Collis gastroplasty. A No. 48 French bougie is passed into the stomach. The dotted line indicates the proposed site of division of the gastric wall for construction of the gastric tube in continuity with the esophagus.

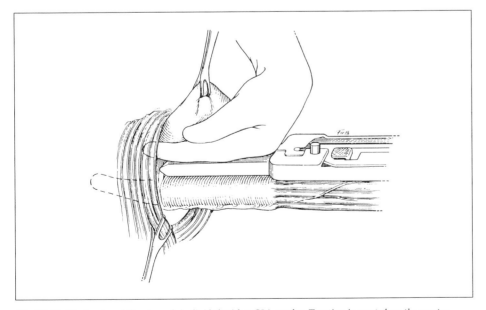

Fig. 59-17. The fundus of the stomach is divided with a GIA stapler. Traction is exerted on the greater curvature side of the fundus before the jaws of the stapler are closed. This ensures that the gastric tube closely approximates the diameter of the indwelling No. 48 French bougie throughout its length.

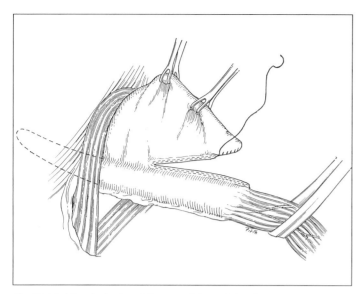

Fig. 59-18. *After the fundus of the stomach is stapled and cut, a 5-cm gastric tube is formed along the proximal portion of the lesser curvature. This effectively lengthens the esophagus by approximately 4 to 5 cm. The exposed staple line is inverted by a running suture to avoid fistulization.*

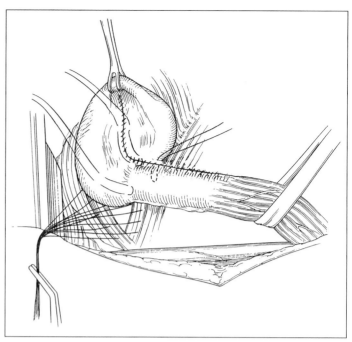

Fig. 59-19. *Construction of a Belsey 240-degree partial fundoplication around the gastroplasty tube. The first row of sutures is placed 1.5 cm above the end of the gastroplasty tube. Particular attention must be given to place the right lateral suture far to the right in order to avoid constructing a partial fundoplication that covers only the left anterior lateral portion of the gastroplasty tube.*

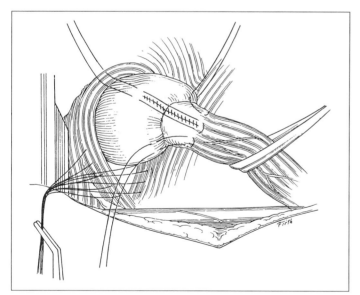

Fig. 59-20. *Continued construction of the Belsey 240-degree partial fundoplication over the gastroplasty tube. A second row of sutures has already been placed 1.5 cm above the first row of sutures. A third row of sutures is placed 1.0 to 1.5 cm above the previously tied sutures of the second row.*

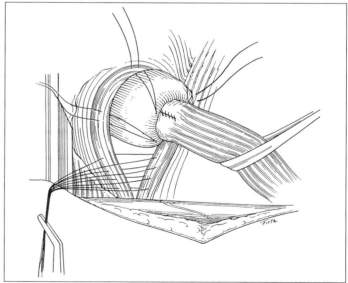

Fig. 59-21. *Continued construction of the Belsey 240-degree partial fundoplication showing placement of the tails of a third row of sutures through the diaphragm, 0.5 cm apart and 1.0 cm from the edge of the hiatus. Note the placement of the sutures at the 4, 8, and 12 o'clock positions on an imaginary clock face oriented with the 6 o'clock position posterior in the hiatus between the right and left crura just anterior to the aorta.*

for reinforcement. It is important that the PTFE pledgets are cut to exact size to keep the fundoplication a standard length and give reproducible results. Standardization of the diameter of the fundoplication was achieved by loosely constructing it over a No. 60 French bougie.

To perform the transthoracic Nissen procedure, the esophagus and cardia are mobilized, and the fundus of the stomach is brought up through the hiatus as described for the Belsey operation. When completely mobilized, the fundus of the stomach is placed in its normal left lateral relationship to the esophagus and then plicated around the distal esophagus by pulling with Babcock clamps, with the posterior fundic wall posterior and the anterior fundic wall anterior to the esophagus (Fig. 59-22). A No. 60 French bougie is then passed by the anesthesiologist into the stomach for accurate sizing of the fundoplication. The lips of the fundoplication are secured in an anterior–right lateral position with a U stitch, using a double-arm 00 polypropylene suture and a 1.5 × 0.5 cm PTFE pledget on the outside of the right and left lips. A portion of the anterior–right lateral esophageal wall down to, but not through, the muscularis mucosa, is incorporated into the stitch. The two limbs of the U suture are separated by 1 cm and placed 1 cm above the gastroesophageal junction identified by the site of insertion of the phrenoesophageal membrane. This sandwiches the esophageal wall between the two lips of the fundoplication and maintains it in the proper position (Fig. 59-23).

The polypropylene suture slides through the tissue without sawing and allows a test sizing of the fundoplication without producing damage to the tissue of the esophagus or stomach. When the edges of the fundoplication are drawn together, the diameter of the wrap should be large enough to accept the insertion of the surgeon's index fingertip between the stomach and the esophagus containing the No. 60 French dilator (Fig. 59-24). If the surgeon's fingertip cannot fit, the fundoplication is too tight and the U stitch must be placed more laterally and inferior in the stomach, enlarging the internal diameter of the fundoplication. If the surgeon's fingertip inserts too easily, the fundoplication is too floppy and the U stitch must be placed more medially and superior in the stom-

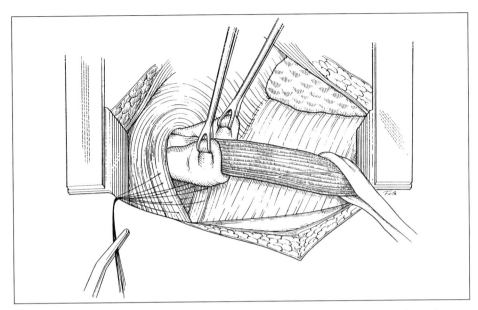

Fig. 59-22. Construction of a Nissen 360-degree full fundoplication showing the posterior and anterior fundic wall brought up through the hiatus and plicated around the lower esophagus.

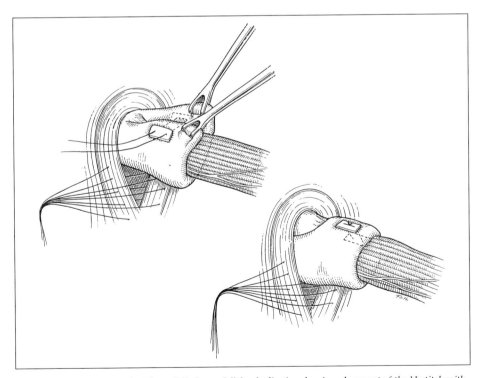

Fig. 59-23. Construction of a Nissen 360-degree full fundoplication showing placement of the U stitch with the PTFE pledgets. A No. 60 French bougie is passed into the stomach to allow accurate sizing of the fundoplication. The fundoplication is placed 1 cm above the gastroesophageal junction on the right anterior-lateral wall of the esophagus.

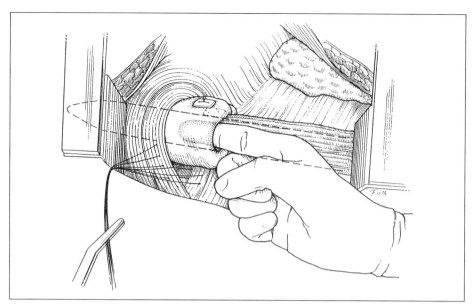

Fig. 59-24. Continued construction of a Nissen 360-degree full fundoplication. The size of the diameter of the fundoplication is tested by insertion of the tip of the surgeon's index finger between the fundoplication and the esophagus containing the No. 60 French dilator. The stomach and esophagus are in their normal position with the U stitch located on the right anterior-lateral wall of the esophagus.

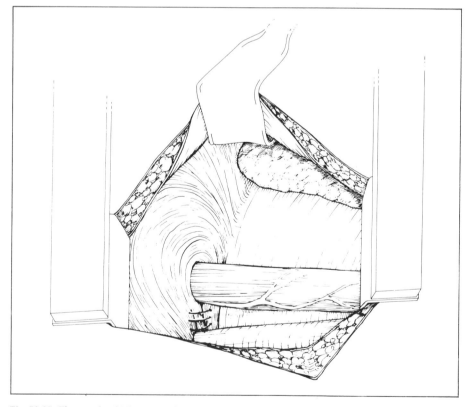

Fig. 59-25. The completed Nissen 360-degree full fundoplication. The repair is in the abdomen, and the right and left crura have been approximated by tying the previously placed sutures.

ach, reducing the internal diameter of the fundoplication. When the fundoplication is of proper size, the bougie is removed and the limbs of the U stitch are tied securely. Since only one suture is used to secure the fundoplication, it is important that this suture be of permanent material and that PTFE pledgets be used to reinforce its purchase on the tissues.

When complete, the fundoplication is massaged into the abdomen in a manner similar to that described for the Belsey Mark IV operation. No sutures are used in the Nissen procedure to hold the repair in the abdomen; the fundoplication serves as the anchoring device. Again, as with the Belsey Mark IV operation, the fundus should not ride out of the hiatus when the repair is placed in the abdomen. If it does, the reconstruction is under too much tension and the problem is managed similarly to the Belsey procedure, that is, performing a Collis gastroplasty.

Once the repair is in the abdominal position, the crural sutures are tied, starting posteriorly at the aortic hiatus and progressing anteriorly until the size of the hiatal opening allows easy insertion of the surgeon's index finger adjacent to the empty esophagus. Any unused sutures are removed (Fig. 59-25). It is much better to leave the hiatus too loose than too tight. In the Belsey repair, the closure of the crura provides a posterior buttress against which the intra-abdominal segment of the esophagus is compressed, whereas in the Nissen procedure, the crural closure helps anchor the repair in the abdomen by preventing the fundoplication from riding up through the hiatus into the chest. The Nissen repair should not be left in the chest since it essentially converts a sliding hernia into a paraesophageal hernia with all its potential hazards.

In both repairs, it is important that the vagi be protected and not injured and that only the fundus of the stomach be used in constructing the fundoplication. This precaution ensures the relaxation of the fundoplication in concert with the distal esophageal sphincter at the time of deglutition. At the completion of the procedure, a nasogastric tube should pass without guidance from the surgeon directly into the stomach to ensure that there has been no angulation of the distal esophagus. A chest tube for drainage of the pleural cavity is placed and the chest incision is closed.

Nasogastric suction is used to avoid over-distention of the stomach during the immediate postoperative period. Gastric distention can cause a breakdown of the repair, particularly with the Belsey partial fundoplication. This is less likely to occur with the Nissen full fundoplication and even less so if pledgets are used. A barium swallow is performed on the seventh postoperative day to check the repair and demonstrate free passage of barium into the stomach. A slight dysphagia may initially be experienced by the patient when oral intake of solid food is resumed, but it disappears as the traumatic edema subsides. Occasionally, dysphagia persists for a longer period, and is usually caused by the presence of an intramural gastric hematoma at the site of the repair. When present, it generally is absorbed within 4 to 6 weeks, and the dysphagia subsides. From the time the patient recovers from anesthesia, there is relief from heartburn and regurgitation. Before discharge the patient should be counseled that until the habit of air swallowing is broken, he or she may experience increased flatus. Early satiety is usual until the patient gains confidence and ingests a meal with fewer swallows and, as a consequence, takes in less air with the food.

Postoperatively, we have evaluated our patients with esophageal manometry and 24-hour esophageal pH monitoring and a questionnaire about their esophageal symptoms and eating habits. Comparison of the results of these studies with results of similar studies obtained from healthy volunteers has helped to evaluate objectively what has been accomplished by the surgical repair. Consequently, the described technique represents a refinement of the method initially published by the originators of the operation and gives excellent results. The surgeon must keep in mind that the operation is designed to improve function of the cardia, and simple alterations in technique can have a profound effect on its postoperative function. No change in technique should be made unless its effects on function are known.

Suggested Reading

Collis JL. An operation for hiatus hernia with short esophagus. *J Thorac Cardiovasc Surg* 34:768, 1957.

DeMeester TR, Bonavina L, Albertucci M. Nissen fundoplication for gastroesophageal reflux disease: Evaluation of primary repair in 100 consecutive patients. *Ann Surg* 204:9, 1986.

DeMeester TR, Wernly JA, Bryant GH, et al. Clinical and in vitro determinants of gastroesophageal competence: A study of the principles of antireflux surgery. *Am J Surg* 137:39, 1979.

Kauer WKH, Peters JH, DeMeester TR, et al. A tailored approach to antireflux surgery. *J Thorac Cardiovasc Surg*, 110:141, 1995.

Nissen R. Eine einfache operation zur beeinflussung der refluxesophagitis. *Schweiz Med Wochenschr* 86:590, 1956.

Nissen R. Gastropexy and "fundoplication" in surgical treatment of hiatus hernia. *Am J Dig Dis* 6:954, 1961.

Pearson FG, Cooper JD, Patterson GA, et al. Gastroplasty and fundoplication for complex reflux problems. *Ann Surg* 206:473, 1987.

Saloma FD, Lamont G. Long-term results of the Belsey Mark IV antireflux operation in relation to the severity of esophagitis. *J Thorac Cardiovasc Surg* 100:517, 1990.

Skinner DB, Belsey RHR. Surgical management of esophageal reflux with hiatus hernia: Long-term results with 1,030 cases. *J Thorac Cardiovasc Surg* 53:33, 1967.

Zaninotto G, DeMeester TR, Schwizer W, et al. The lower esophageal sphincter in health and disease. *Am J Surg* 155:104, 1988.

EDITOR'S COMMENT

The authors, recognized experts in the field of gastroesophageal reflux disease (GERD), have presented a number of concepts that are not commonly recognized by the occasional surgeon who deals with this disease relatively infrequently. It has been well established that 24-hour esophageal pH monitoring is critical in deciding whether the symptoms of aspiration are due to reflux episodes, but it is not well recognized that surgery is indicated in patients with abnormal reflux who are off medication even if no gross morphologic evidence of severe esophagitis is seen on endoscopy. Likewise, it is most important that failure of adequate gastric emptying for any reason should be considered carefully as a cause of reflux in patients who reflux primarily during the day or in the immediate postprandial period, but do not reflux at night. These patients may have a satisfactory cardia from a functional stand-point, and will not benefit from an antireflux procedure, but, instead, may actually be made worse by such an operation when the real need is to improve gastric emptying.

The authors have emphasized the need to restore a minimum of 1.5 to 2.0 cm of the abdominal esophagus in patients with a cardia that is herniated into the chest. Previously, it was not uncommon to see a Nissen fundoplication herniate into the chest some months after the repair was done. Although these patients tended to remain asymptomatic in some instances, recent experience has shown that reflux can occur into the esophagus with an intrathoracic wrap, and it should always be a goal to maintain at least a minimum amount of esophagus in the abdomen. The wrap should always be located within the abdomen.

The authors have documented the significant difference in the Nissen gastric wrap, which encompasses 360 degrees of the circumference of the esophagus, as opposed to a wrap done with the Belsey Mark IV, which results in a wrap of only 240 degrees. The complete wrap is most frequently performed on patients operated on through the transabdominal approach, unless the patient is identified as having inadequate esophageal motility, in which case a partial wrap is done either through the transthoracic or transabdominal approach. The abdominal incomplete wrap (270 degrees) was popular two decades ago, but is seldom used now. Rather, a logical and highly effective modification known as the "floppy Nissen" fundoplication has essentially replaced it (see Chap. 63).

Doctors DeMeester and Hagen have advocated a Nissen wrap held in place by a single polypropylene suture, a U stitch buttressed with nonabsorbable pledgets. General surgeons who perform this wrap ordinarily use three or even four sutures, but it is extremely important to ensure that the wrap is loose and gently approximating, rather than tight. One should be able to insert the finger between the wrap and the esophagogastric junction, assuring that the wrap is performed over a No. 50 French dilator that accompanies a nasogastric tube. Seeing patients who have had a successful antireflux procedure done by the Nissen procedure but in whom the gas-bloat syndrome has developed is a frustrating experience since many of these individuals would have preferred to have continued with reflux on medical management rather than to have had this syndrome develop. Characteristically, the inability to relieve intragastric gaseous pressure by eructation is a most uncomfortable sensation and the inability to vomit is a source of extreme discomfort, and perhaps even danger. We agree that an intra-abdominal antireflux procedure that does not succeed and requires revision is an excellent indication for the transthoracic approach. On the contrary, if a transthoracic approach fails, it may be considerably easier to redo the antireflux operation through the abdomen.

R.J.B.

60

Nissen–Rossetti Antireflux Fundoplication (Open Procedure)

Mario E. Rossetti   Dorothea Liebermann-Meffert

Development, Concept, and Rationale

In 1946, Rudolf Nissen (1896–1981) was faced with the necessity of operating on a huge, bleeding paraesophageal hernia. The diaphragmatic crura had chronically incarcerated the stomach, and the food passage was completely obstructed. The 69-year-old patient was in extremely poor general health but had a clear indication for surgical treatment. Nissen was at this time Head of Surgery in the Jewish Hospital at Brooklyn, New York. He did not succeed in persuading the patient, who actually was the well-known and experienced New York radiologist, Bucky, to undergo a thoracotomy, which was the common approach in this situation but of great risk in those days. Nissen mobilized and reduced the stomach into the abdomen from below the diaphragm through a less demanding laparotomy. He then sutured the stomach to the anterior abdominal wall using a strip of aponeurosis of the rectus abdominis muscle. The patient recovered without complications or a recurrence and cared for his own patients for several years. The operation, which Nissen called a *gastropexy* to repair a hiatal hernia, became the principal procedure for abdominal correction of hiatal hernia. In 1952, Nissen became chairman of the Surgical Department at the University Hospital in Basel, Switzerland. There, he and his colleagues used this technique not only for paraesophageal and mixed hernias but also for sliding hernias with gastroesophageal reflux. One of us (M. R.), coworker of Nissen, had become intensely involved in this topic.

The aim of the fundoplication was to plicate parts of the anterior and posterior walls of the gastric fundus around the lesser curvature without opening either esophagus or stomach and to construct a one-way valve for fluid and solid food. The method required the complete separation of the posterior wall of the fundus and incision of the lesser omentum with dissection of the vagal branches. This procedure remained our routine technique for approximately 10 years. In this initial phase, fundoplication acted as a mildly functioning one-way valve able to compensate for an increasing pressure or volume within the stomach, as shown in simple animal experiments and on cadavers.

The operation, called a *Nissen fundoplication*, became widely used, and, despite our warnings, the fundoplication was often made too narrow and too long. Consequently, postfundoplication syndromes developed, such as postoperative dysphagia, inability to belch and vomit, and persistent gas bloat caused by permanent stricture.

However, in the long term, the results proved to be unsatisfactory; gastropexy alone prevented the sliding element but not the lower esophageal sphincter (LES) incontinence. A former observation delineated the concept of fundoplication as a potential reflux barrier.

In 1937, Nissen was faced with an insecure esophagogastric anastomosis after transpleural resection for an ulcer of the cardia, which had penetrated into the pericardium. He decided to dunk the remaining end of the esophagus into the stomach, similar to a feeding rubber tube described by Witzel for gastrostomy, and plicated the gastric wall over it (Fig. 60-1). The patient was lost to follow-up; but 15 years later, Nissen learned that the patient was well; despite a resected cardia he never did develop clinical symptoms of reflux. So, when shortly later in 1955 a patient, suffering from severe reflux esophagitis but without obvious hiatal hernia, was admitted to his hospital in Basel, Nissen decided to plicate the fundus around the cardia of this patient, which in fact, was the first "fundoplication."

In 1965, we modified the initial fundoplication by using the anterior wall of the fundus alone to build up a complete 360-degree fundic wrap. Careful anatomic studies confirmed the concept and function of the modified technique, which not only follows the principle of a one-way valve but also becomes a true substitute for the insufficient LES. The specific reactivity of this musculature was first shown by Siewert and was later confirmed by others in animal experiments. Since the first procedure, we have performed more than 2000 fundoplications.

Indications for an Antireflux Operation

A sliding hernia per se does not necessitate an operation. A fundoplication, however,

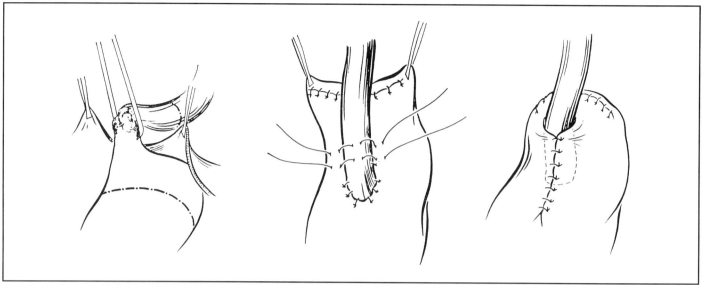

Fig. 60-1. *Transthoracic resection of the cardia. The esophagogastric anastomosis (so-called continent anastomosis) is wrapped into the wall of the stomach, which protects the suture and constitutes a barrier against postoperative reflux. The idea of the later fundoplication was born. (From Nissen R. Die Transpleurale resektion der Kardia. Dtsch. Z. Clin. 249:311, 1937.)*

is indicated in any instance of established symptomatic reflux disease and its clinical manifestations. These manifestations are as follows:

1. Severe persistent or progressive esophagitis with intolerance to medical treatment or failure of 2 to 3 months of intensive medical treatment.
2. Juvenile esophagitis of long duration without spontaneous remission or improvement by conservative treatment.
3. Massive functional reflux without esophagitis but with a risk of pulmonary complications, tracheobronchial aspiration, asthma, and chronic persistent severe laryngitis.
4. Barrett's esophagus with or without actual complications. In our experience, an antireflux operation best prevents stricture, ulceration, and malignant growth.
5. Peptic stricture caused by endobrachyesophagus or secondary brachyesophagus with or without functional or Barrett's ulceration.
6. Mixed and paraesophageal hernia, complemented by a gastropexy.
7. Recurrent reflux or complications after surgical therapy.

Patients with severe insufficiency of the cardia (antireflux mechanism) should be operated on fairly quickly because of the high risk of rapid stricture development.

Surgical Diagnostic Evaluation

In addition to a general examination to ensure fitness for an operation, detailed assessment of the clinical findings is necessary with evaluation of the history of reflux symptoms and potential associated disorders. It is essential to review results of endoscopy, biopsy of all suspicious areas, and conventional x-ray contrast study in order to recognize the space related and dynamic function of the gastroesophageal junction, as well as 24-hour pH monitoring. Especially in instances of functional disturbances, manometry provides the essential criterion for the indication for fundoplication. The more recent diagnostic imaging (CT) is mainly used to exclude concomitant disease, advanced organic stage, recurrence, findings suspicious for malignancies, assessment of operability, and approach.

Special Instruments

Long surgical instruments and right-angled retractors are useful, particularly when the patient is obese.

Good exposure is essential. The application of a rib cage retractor in combination with an abdominal wall retractor mounted on the operating table lifts the costal arch and enlarges the working space. We use the Rochard autostatic retractor, which has two blade widths. A narrow blade is used for thin patients with an acute costal angle, and a wide blade is used for obese patients with a wide costal angle. Excessive pressure on soft tissues can lead to postoperative pain and impaired breathing. The retractor should, therefore, be removed as soon as possible.

Gastric Tubes

A nasogastric tube is a wise precaution and makes the postoperative period more comfortable. We also insert a large-bore gastric tube of at least 10- to 12-mm diameter, which corresponds to a No. 46 to No. 50 French Maloney esophageal dilator. Inserting the tube helps identify and free the subdiaphragmatic esophagus. The tube also avoids dangerous compromise of the esophageal lumen because of a too-tight fundoplication. Our anesthetist inserts this tube alongside the nasogastric tube and leaves both in place until the end of the operation. Frequently, the tube can be positioned only at a laparotomy by palpating and stretching the esophagus and stomach.

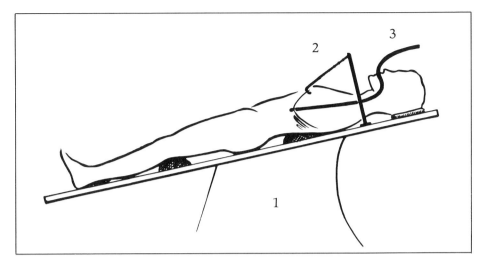

Fig. 60-2. Positioning for reflux operations. 1. Anti-Trendelenburg adjustment. 2. Autostatic rib retractor. 3. Gastric tube.

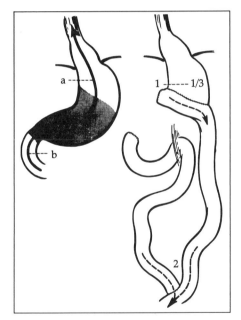

Fig. 60-3. Distal gastric resection and isoperistaltic long Roux-en-Y loop for biliopancreatic alcaline diversion to treat complicated brachyesophagus, ulcerostenotic complications in the thoracic esophagus, and recurrence owing to severe panmural fibrosis. Arrows show flow direction of intestial content.

Positioning the Patient

For the *transabdominal approach*, the patient is placed on the operating table in a supine position. The upper part of the body must be slightly raised (Fig. 60-2). The table is tilted approximately 20 degrees toward the right.

In the *thoracoabdominal approach*, a procedure only exceptionally necessary in our experience, the patient is positioned with the left side raised 45 degrees so that a midline laparotomy can be supplemented by a left anterolateral thoracotomy in case the pathologic findings make one necessary.

Surgical Approach

The transthoracic approach is rarely used in our department. Its only advantage is that it provides direct vision of the lower and middle esophagus, easier mobilization of the middle esophagus, and more appropriate treatment of unexpected panmural esophagitis. We have used the transthoracic approach for fundoplication for secondary brachyesophagus and for certain lesions that cannot be approached safely through the abdomen.

Dissection by the transabdominal approach can be difficult in the presence of panmural esophagitis; marked periesophageal inflammation; an extremely scarred or shortened esophagus; adhesions from previous repairs; a large, incarcerated sliding hiatal hernia; or penetrating ulceration. In these situations, we prefer a conventional distal gastric resection with a long Roux-en-Y gastrojejunostomy (Fig. 60-3). This procedure has technical and biologic advantages. First, healthy tissue is used. Second, the resection of the stomach with biliopancreatic diversion prevents

peptic and alkaline damage to the esophagus.

Surgical Technique
Access to the Cardia

The upper midline incision is most satisfactory. The incision can deviate to avoid the xiphisternum and to extend around the umbilicus. A simple epigastric incision should be used only for slender patients with a small costal angle. A bilateral subcostal incision can be used for obese patients with a wide costal angle. The less favorable the anatomic conditions, the greater the assistance required by the surgeon. Obesity and barrel chest with emphysema are unfavorable conditions.

The Original Nissen Plication

The original method of fundoplication consisted of uniting the posterior and anterior walls of the stomach in front of the esophagus with sutures, including the wall of the esophagus in one or two stitches to prevent the cardia from slipping back in eversion, or the so-called telescope effect. The exposure of the posterior wall necessitated opening the omental bursa by a partial separation of the cranial part of the gastrohepatic ligament (Figs. 60-4 and 60-5). As a result, the vagal branch to the liver and several branches to the pyloric region were unavoidably severed. Furthermore, the triangular connective tissue binding the cardia to the retroperitoneum was deliberately partly severed to improve the mobilization of the back wall at the expense of the stabilization afforded by this tissue. This procedure is justified only in special situations such as a combined operation after a proximal selective vagotomy or in certain recurrences of reflux. The disadvantages of the original method of fundoplication as a primary procedure were potential injury to the vagus nerve, detachment of the posterior wall of the stomach from the vagus, and potential eversion of the wrap despite the suture through the wall of the esophagus. According to the present knowledge of the arrangement of the musculature of the stomach, the original method of fundoplication was effective only because it acted as a valve rather than forming a real substitute for the sphincter.

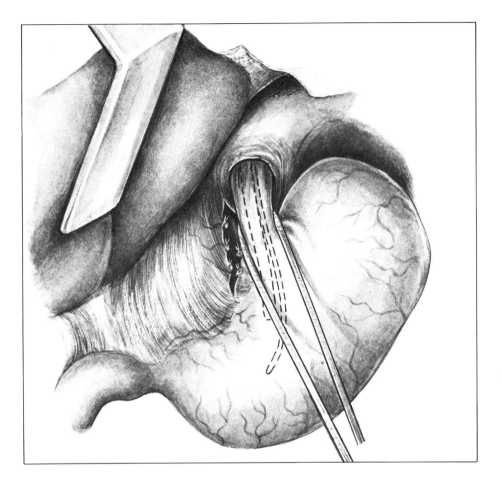

Fig. 60-4. Opening of the omental bursa by division of the upper part of the gastrohepatic ligament severs a part of vagal branches to the liver. (From R Nissen, M Rossetti, and JR Siewert. Fundoplicatio und Gastropexie bei Refluxkrankheit und Hiatushernien. *Stuttgart: Thieme, 1981. Reprinted with permission.*)

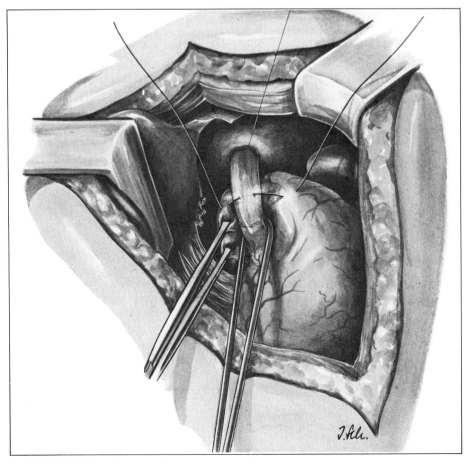

Fig. 60-5. The original fundoplication uniting the posterior and the anterior fundic wall. (From R Nissen, M Rossetti, and JR Siewert. Fundoplicatio und Gastropexie bei Refluxkrankheit und Hiatushernien. *Stuttgart: Thieme, 1981. Reproduced with permission.*)

The Nissen–Rossetti Modified Fundoplication: The So-Called Anterior Wall Technique

Principle

A complete 360-degree cuff or wrap is made by folding the anterior wall of the gastric fundus around the terminal esophagus. This maneuver forms form not only an antireflux valve but also an actual substitute for the insufficient sphincter. Our anatomic studies (Fig. 60-6) and the pharmacomanometric studies by Siewert on animals have supported the rationale for this technique.

Procedure

After careful exploration of the abdomen, the configuration of the hiatus and sliding element is judged by palpation along the lesser curvature of the stomach into the esophageal hiatus. The left lobe of the liver is displaced to the right and ventrally with a rectangular retractor to expose the fundus and the cardia. Depending on the patient's anatomy, one can mobilize the left lobe of the liver by transecting the triangular ligament and displacing the lobe medially to gain access to the esophagogastric junction. We usually find this maneuver unnecessary except when the liver is enlarged or the lobe extends extremely far to the left.

The stomach is retracted downward and the exact position of the nasogastric tube is assessed. The peritoneum is incised from its upper end through the entire gastrophrenic ligament without interrupting the short gastric vessels and toward the right as far as the hepatic–gastro ligament extends. The lower 4 to 6 cm of the esophagus must be freed above the esophagogastric junction (Figs. 60-7 and 60-8).

During mobilization of the lower end of the esophagus, great care is exercised to protect and preserve all the branches of the vagus nerves. The anterior branches have many anatomic variants abut the esophagus and are visible below the phrenoesophageal membrane. They are included in the fundoplication. The posterior vagus nerve is usually not near the esophagus and remains outside the fundoplication. If, however, it is attached by a thick layer of connective tissue, we include the posterior vagus nerve in the fundic wrap (Fig. 60-9).

The phrenoesophageal membrane can be recognized by its well-defined lower edge and slightly yellow color, even in the presence of severe periesophagitis. This membrane is removed gently from the distal esophagus by a soft sponge. The longitudinal muscle of the esophagus is gradually and atraumatically freed from its surroundings over a length of about 6 cm by finger dissection. This step is the most dangerous of the operation, especially if the esophageal wall is inflamed, edematous, or friable. The risk of perforation is greater on the posterior wall, where a transmural lesion is most easily overlooked. With the large tube inserted, one can run a finger along the esophagus to determine whether the wall is intact. As long as the incision is in the correct layer, there is no risk of hemorrhage because the ligaments contain only very small vessels. However, the surgeon must watch for the esophageal branch of the left gastric artery with its numerous accompanying veins. If the branch is damaged, it can bleed or cause intraligamentous hematomas. The esophageal artery runs anteromedially, or, rarely, posteromedially, up along the esophagus. It is possible, but not necessary, to spare it during exposure of the esophagus. The left inferior phrenic artery runs dorsally to the cardia and fundus with one or more branches directly from the aorta or celiac trunk. It can be, but is not often, damaged

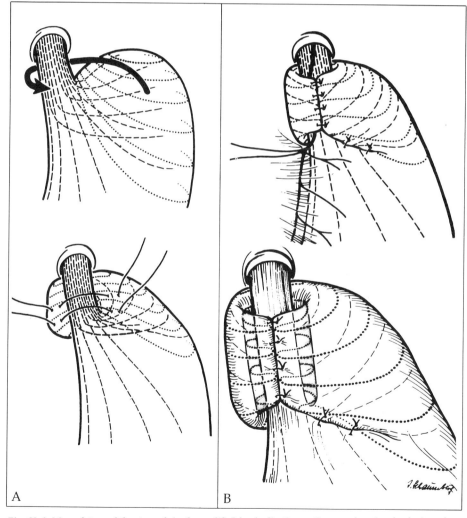

A   B

Fig. 60-6. Musculature of the stomach in the modified fundoplication, acting as a functional substitute for the lower esophageal sphincter rather than forming a rigid valve. The dotted lines indicate the lines of muscular force; these are initially vertical (A) but are transverse in the completed repair (B). (From R Nissen, M Rossetti, and JR Siewert. Fundoplicatio und Gastropexie bei Refluxkrankheit und Hiatushernien. *Stuttgart: Thieme, 1981. Reproduced with permission.)*

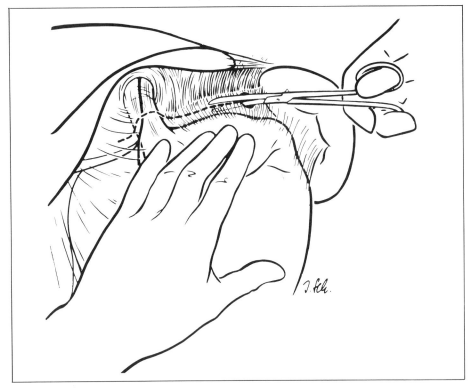

Fig. 60-7. Mobilization of the gastric fundus. The gastrophrenic ligament is cut. (From R Nissen, M Rossetti, and JR Siewert. Fundoplicatio und Gastropexie bei Refluxkrankheit und Hiatushernien. *Stuttgart: Thieme, 1981. Reproduced with permission.)*

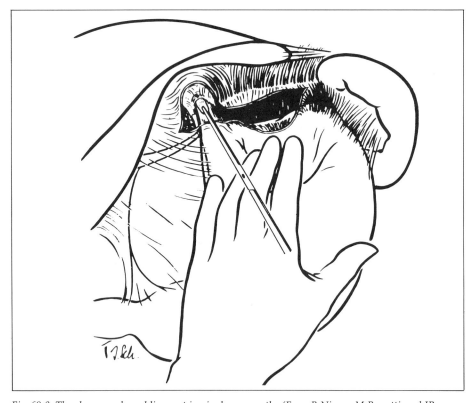

Fig. 60-8. The phrenoesophageal ligament is wiped away gently. (From R Nissen, M Rossetti, and JR Siewert. Fundoplicatio und Gastropexie bei Refluxkrankheit und Hiatushernien. *Stuttgart: Thieme, 1981. Reproduced with permission.)*

during mobilization of the anterior surface of the fundus.

Fine Penrose drains or atraumatic rubber bands are passed behind the esophagus with the aid of a curved clamp. If necessary, as it is in approximately 5 percent of fundoplications, the upper short gastric vessels can be divided, and the posterior portion of the upper portion of the stomach might have to be freed. The exposure is now complete and the fundoplication is anatomically ready.

Plication of the Fundus

The anterior wall of the fundus is passed behind the esophagus with one or two fingers of the right hand until it appears in the medial gap. The flap is held in this position with two long atraumatic clamps, either Babcock or Allis (see Fig. 60-9). A second fold is formed from the more distal part of the anterior fundic wall and held with a clamp so that the flaps can be wrapped around the esophagus without pulling or stretching the distal section of the esophagus. The fundus should comfortably form a cuff around the lower part of the esophagus. Four or five interrupted, deeply placed seromuscular sutures of nonabsorbable 000 material are placed to hold the cuff loosely in position; the esophageal wall is not included (Fig. 60-10). To obtain adequate hold, the sutures are passed through both muscle layers down to but never through the submucosa. Gently tying these sutures achieves tissue apposition without tissue strangulation. It is advisable to tie each stitch immediately; otherwise, subserous hematomas at the point of puncture might appear at the site of the sutures.

The fundoplication should be approximately 4 cm long. It is very important that the flaps be loosely wrapped around the esophagus. With the bougie in place, the surgeon should be able to insert a large, so-called crocodile clamp (Fig. 60-11) or two fingers easily between the esophagus and the wrap around the cardia (Fig. 60-12). If these steps are taken, a constriction is almost impossible or unlikely. We place two or more sutures in the bottom edge of the gastric wall and the fundic wrap to stabilize the fundoplication (Fig. 60-13). This step prevents the cardia from telescoping within the wrap. As an alternative, Siewert includes in the most distal suture the connective tissue covering the junction of the terminal esophagus and the stomach.

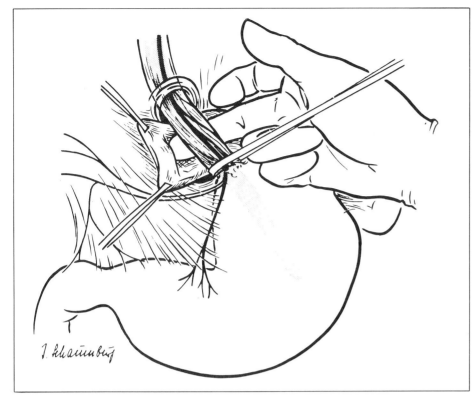

Fig. 60-9. Passing the anterior fundic fold around the esophagus. (From R Nissen, M Rossetti, and JR Siewert. Fundoplicatio und Gastropexie bei Refluxkrankheit und Hiatushernien. Stuttgart: Thieme, 1981. Reproduced with permission.)

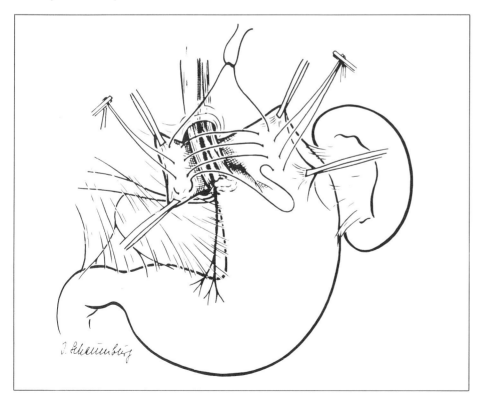

Fig. 60-10. Bringing the two folds together with four seromuscular stitches of nonabsorbable 000 suture material. (From R Nissen, M Rossetti, and JR Siewert. Fundoplicatio und Gastropexie bei Refluxkrankheit und Hiatushernien. Stuttgart: Thieme, 1981. Reproduced with permission.)

Additional sutures, as have been recommended by some surgeons to constrict the hiatus or to attach the fundoplication to the diaphragm, are not part of the technique of repair.

Postoperative Care

After the fundoplication, we remove the large gastric tube. The nasogastric tube is left in place for at least 12 to 24 hours. We drain the region of the cardia for approximately 2 days with a fine Penrose drain and the subcutis with a suction drain. Oral feeding is started from the second day and gradually increased. Thereafter, postoperative treatment is the same as for any abdominal operation.

The Nissen–Rossetti Technique for Mixed and Paraesophageal Hernias

A factor predisposing to this form of hiatal hernia is a wide "hiatus communis" with the aorta posteriorly. Paraesophageal hernias and mixed forms are often combined. They initially can present without symptoms. Progressive migration of the stomach into the chest, however, will increase the sliding and rolling element and finally lead to twisting of the esophagogastric junction, gastric volvulus, and incarceration. The predominantly mixed form is frequently associated with reflux and brachyesophagus (primary or postoperative after simple gastropexy). The event is signified by the onset of dysphagia, postprandial distress, severe heartburn, vomiting, and chronic or acute blood loss. Of our 298 surgical cases, one-third presented with anemia, 10 percent of them combined with an ulceration at the constriction ring; in the second third, the food passage was largely impaired, and the last third was asymptomatic. In all these situations, immediate surgical intervention is mandatory.

Our surgical strategy for the repair of the paraesophageal and mixed hiatal hernias is a combination of various surgical steps:

1. Decompression of the herniated stomach using a nasogastric tube
2. Careful reduction of the stomach, preferably through the abdominal approach leaving the hernial sac in place
3. Narrowing of the wide hiatus with 2 to 4 nonabsorbable sutures from the lateral or anterior aspect.

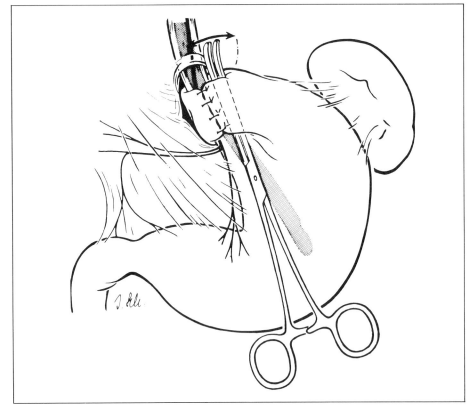

Fig. 60-11. The loosely wrapped fundoplication is checked with an instrument, the so-called crocodile clamp. (From R Nissen, M Rossetti, and JR Siewert. Fundoplicatio und Gastropexie bei Refluxkrankheit und Hiatushernien. *Stuttgart: Thieme, 1981. Reproduced with permission.)*

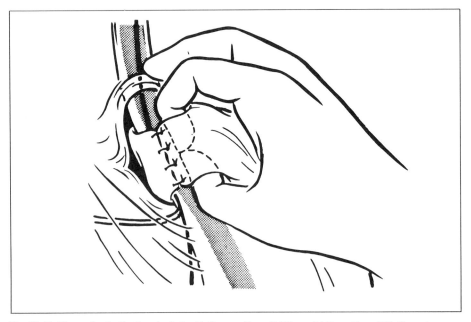

Fig. 60-12. Floppy fundoplication checked with fingers. (From R Nissen, M Rossetti, and JR Siewert. Fundoplicatio und Gastropexie bei Refluxkrankheit und Hiatushernien. *Stuttgart: Thieme, 1981. Reproduced with permission.)*

4. Fundoplication completed with a two-fold gastropexy, one to the diaphragm and another to the anterior abdominal wall (Fig. 60-14)

Complications and Sequelae

Intraoperative Complications

Intraoperative complications are rare. The spleen is subject to unintentional injury during transabdominal fundoplication.

Capsular avulsion or small tears causing persistent hilar bleeding occurred in 3 percent of our patients and is reported in the literature to occur in approximately 7 percent of patients. Most lesions that occurred in our patients were unimportant and easy to repair either with tamponade, or with carefully placed sutures. The advantages of saving the spleen are great, both in young and adult patients. Preservation of the organ also lessens operative risk. Subphrenic abscesses almost never were reported in our series. Another possible complication is injury to the vagal trunks, which can occur in the presence of marked inflammation of the cardioesophageal junction or after a previous operation. The sequelae are rarely of clinical relevance.

The most serious complication, accidental perforation of a severely inflamed esophagus, can cause a great deal of difficulty. This disaster occurs either during difficult mobilization of the cardia or during the attempt to pass an instrument around the esophagus. An unrecognized perforation of the esophagus is a life-threatening complication. Thorough evaluation of the situation, particularly of the posterior aspect of the esophagus, before encircling the distal esophagus with any instrument is therefore mandatory. Simple closure of a perforated esophagus is usually doomed to failure. When the esophagus perforated in our patients, we closed the defect very loosely with 4–0 absorbable synthetic sutures and covered the suture line with the fundoplication. We encountered no further complications in these patients.

Transient Functional Digestive Disturbances

Frequently, a patient has an overfull feeling in the stomach or even some postprandial discomfort in the first postoperative

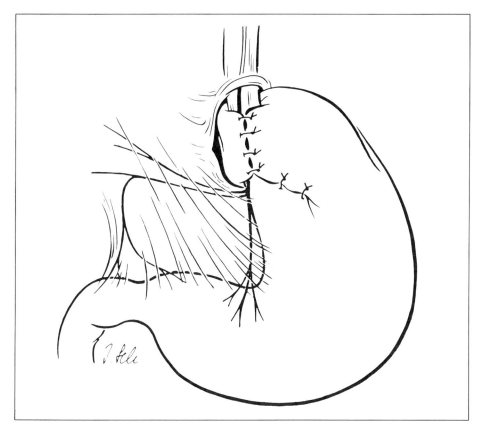

Fig. 60-13. Two sutures stabilize the bottom edge of the fundic sleeve to avoid the telescope phenomenon. (From R Nissen, M Rossetti, and JR Siewert. Fundoplicatio und Gastropexie bei Refluxkrankheit und Hiatushernien. *Stuttgart: Thieme, 1981. Reproduced with permission.)*

days. This discomfort can be consistent with edema formation at the cardia and a slight transient gas-bloat syndrome. Eating small amounts frequently and possibly taking prokinetic drugs usually help to overcome these functional disturbances.

Aerophagia is common in the early postoperative period. Many patients become accustomed to swallowing air during the course of reflux disease to overcome the painful foreign-body sensation in their esophagus that results from esophagitis. Along with repeated swallowing, aerophagic patients have greater problems postoperatively. Patients should be taught to control the tendency to try to swallow their discomfort away. Drinking water is helpful. Since we perform a loose fundoplication, the problem of aerophagia is diminished. The loose fundic wrap allows easy belching, or eructation, the physiologic reflux of air.

Postfundoplication Syndromes

Dysphagia was the most common complaint we encountered in one-third of our patients during early trials of the fundoplication. The onset typically occurred on the tenth postoperative day, and the dysphagia disappeared by the end of 3 weeks. It was found to be the result of local edema

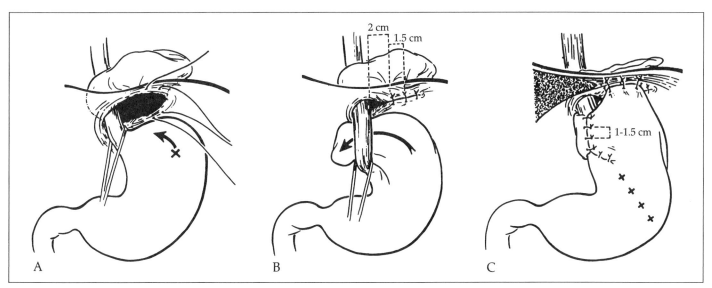

Fig. 60-14. Technique to correct mixed and paraesophageal hiatal hernias. A. The stomach is retracted through the "hiatus communis" and the plication is prepared. B. The hiatal gap is narrowed and a fundoplication is performed. C. Completion with double gastropexy: one to the diaphragm and a second to the anterior abdominal wall (crosses). (From R Nissen, M Rossetti, and JR Siewert. Fundoplicatio und Gastropexie bei Refluxkrankheit und Hiatushernien. *Stuttgart: Thieme, 1981. Reproduced with permission.)*

and was usually caused by a too-tight wrap. The looser plication and the use of a larger gastric tube have proved to be of great help in preventing postoperative dysphagia. The late onset of dysphagia can be attributed to excessive scar formation within the terminal esophagus or to migration of the collarlike wrap that constricts the fundus and gastroesophageal junction. Incomplete vagotomy and drainage procedures can allow ulcers to recur. Total vagotomy can result in diarrhea and other postvagotomy problems.

Ill-advised complementary procedures, such as inadequate vagotomy and drainage procedures, can lead to digestive disturbances.

The measure of success is the continued amelioration of a patient's symptoms. In our and others' experience, failure to correct gastroesophageal reflux was mainly the result of disregard for the technique and the correct indications.

Vagotomy as an Additional Procedure

Some authors believe that the addition of a vagotomy facilitates the fundoplication and, therefore, advocate the operation. However, vagotomy, whether selective or truncal, in normal fundoplication is virtually never required. Adding a highly selective vagotomy (HSV) does not significantly change the function of the esophagogastric sphincter, and reduction of secretion is not the solution. The reason that adding vagotomy has not become more popular is the high incidence of disabling postoperative symptoms, such as dumping, postoperative diarrhea, or nausea.

Combined fundoplication and vagotomy is indicated when gastroesophageal reflux disease is accompanied by a duodenal ulcer. However, only 8 percent of our patients with clinical manifestations of reflux disease had a duodenal ulcer. If a pentagastrin test indicates considerable hyperacidity, and if the reflux disease is in the organic stage (as in grade IV reflux esophagitis, transitional ulcer, Barrett's ulcer, and stenotic esophageal ulcer), we recommend the antireflux operation in combination with ulcer-treating procedures.

The combined fundoplication and vagotomy has, in addition to biologic consequences, certain procedural consequences, which must be well understood if both parts of the operation are to be a success.

The vagotomy can be performed in different ways.

Highly Selective Proximal Vagotomy and Fundoplication

Selective proximal vagotomy and fundoplication is illustrated in Figs. 60-15 through 60-17. The necessity for exposing the distal esophagus and the lesser curvature as far as the angulus alters the type of fundoplication. It is no longer possible to form a flap of the anterior fundic wall without impairing the vagal branches. Thus, in accordance with the original Nissen technique, we plicate and connect the anterior and posterior walls of the medial fundus of the stomach. Once again, the sleeve formed must be loose and cover a reasonable section of the esophagus. Approximately four seromuscular stitches of

nonabsorbable 000 suture material are used. The lowest suture should include the wall of the lesser curvature in order to prevent erosion. Caudad to the fundoplication, the lesser curvature is covered by fine gastric seromuscular sutures as far as the angulus. This step protects the gastric wall, prevents adhesions to the surrounding tissues, and avoids vagal nerve regeneration.

Truncal Vagotomy and Selective Gastric Vagotomy

Truncal vagotomy and selective gastric vagotomy should be combined with a pyloroplasty because the simultaneous denervation of the antropyloric region leads to gastric stasis. A proximal highly selective vagotomy leaves the pyloric region unaffected. Advantages of a truncal vagotomy are speed and ease of performance. The drawbacks are the consequences of hepatic pancreatic and intestinal denervation, primarily the tendency toward diarrhea. Proximal highly selective vagotomy re-

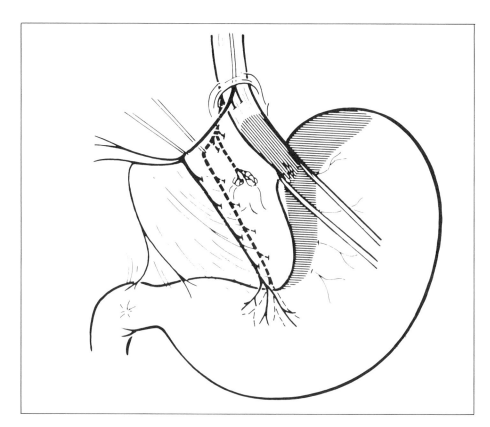

Fig. 60-15. Diagram illustrating proximal selective vagotomy. (From R Nissen, M Rossetti, and JR Siewert. Fundoplicatio und Gastropexie bei Refluxkrankheit und Hiatushernien. *Stuttgart: Thieme, 1981. Reproduced with permission.*)

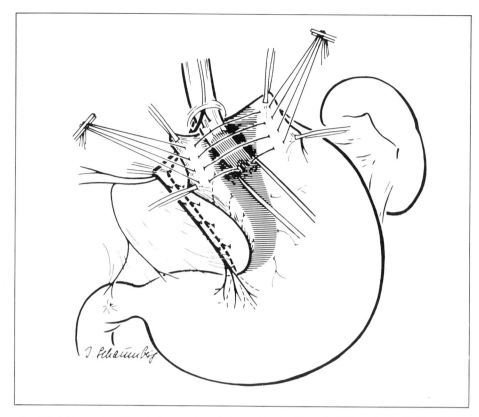

Fig. 60-16. Proximal highly selective vagotomy to be combined with original Nissen fundoplication. (From R Nissen, M Rossetti, and JR Siewert. Fundoplicatio und Gastropexie bei Refluxkrankheit und Hiatushernien. *Stuttgart: Thieme, 1981. Reproduced with permission.)*

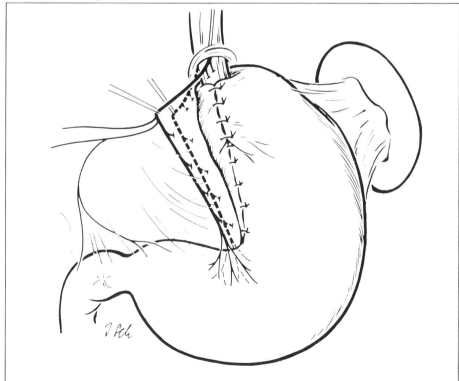

Fig. 60-17. Proximal highly selective vagotomy with fundoplication completed. (From R Nissen, M Rossetti, and JR Siewert. Fundoplicatio und Gastropexie bei Refluxkrankheit und Hiatushernien. *Stuttgart: Thieme, 1981. Reproduced with permission.)*

quires time and care. Because it affects secretion and not the function of the stomach, most surgeons prefer proximal highly selective vagotomy. Unfortunately, the inflammatory changes at the gastroesophageal junction, a result of reflux disease, can complicate or make this form of vagotomy impossible. Truncal vagotomy often is the only possible procedure to combine with fundoplication, although the periesophageal scar formation can make it difficult to isolate the vagal trunks.

Dissection of the main vagal branches after exposure of the cardia makes it easy to mobilize the terminal esophagus and perform the fundoplication by the anterior wall technique. One should search for and isolate the nerves carefully, keeping in mind the danger of perforating the inflamed esophagus. We hold the nerve with a curved clamp, fulgurate it by coagulation, and sever it. The distal esophagus is then mobile, and the fundoplication is facilitated. The fundoplication is always supplemented by a pyloroplasty or an antrectomy (Fig. 60-18).

Surgical Treatment of Peptic Stenoses

Notes and Preparation

Most peptic esophageal stenoses develop along with an endobrachyesophagus, or short esophagus, usually at the boundary between the healthy epithelium and the metaplastic epithelium. We distinguish between two types, short annular stenosis and elongated stenosis (Fig. 60-19). The second type can involve the major part of the thoracic esophagus and strongly resemble cicatrization by acid or base. A long history of reflux complaints is characteristic of elongated stenosis. It culminates in severe dysphagia that has changed from intermittent to increasingly frequent episodes. In approximately one-third of instances, however, dysphagia is reported to occur without preceding subjective reflux symptoms. Serious dysphagia is often a compelling indication for surgical intervention. A simple bougienage often brings temporary relief, and, if frequently repeated in combination with extensive antacid therapy, it can give acceptable long-term results. The tendency toward recurrence is high.

The surgical strategy is based on a thorough diagnosis. A roentgenographic ex-

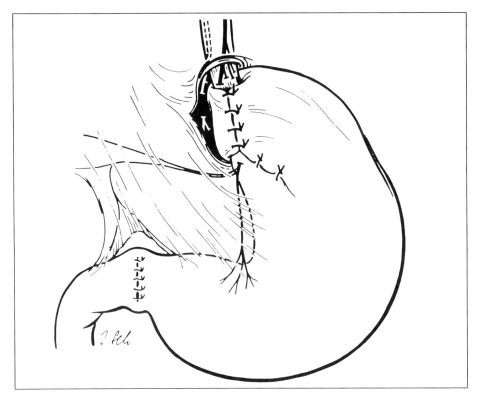

Fig. 60-18. Truncal vagotomy and fundoplication with anterior extramucosal partial pylorectomy. (From R Nissen, M Rossetti, and JR Siewert. Fundoplicatio und Gastropexie bei Refluxkrankheit und Hiatushernien. *Stuttgart: Thieme, 1981. Reproduced with permission.)*

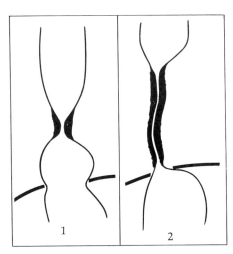

Fig. 60-19. Stenotic reflux disease. 1. Short annular stenosis. 2. Elongated stenosis of the lower esophagus.

amination shows the morphology and dynamics of the whole functional system of the esophagus, stomach, and duodenum, the localization and extent of stenosis, and the remaining mobility of a sliding element of the cardia. Endoscopy reveals the level of the ulcerostenotic process, struc-tures above and at the start of the stenosis, the distensibility of the stenotic segment, and the histology by means of multiple bi-opsies. One should keep precise records of the extent and level of the biopsies. An ex-perienced pathologist can help determine the stage of the disease and whether or not malignant degeneration has occurred. It should be noted that adenocarcinomas are found in 10 percent of instances in this crit-ical part of the esophagus, occasionally as carcinomas-in-situ. Dysplasia can pose considerable problems in the histologic interpretation, for the therapeutic con-sequences and the choice of pure obser-vation, medical treatment, functional conservative surgery, and esophagectomy. Possible or confirmed malignant disease necessitates a radical change in treatment.

Approach

Most stenoses are located in the thoracic esophagus, often high up and accessible only through a thoracotomy. The transtho-racic approach is indicated when there is doubt about the benignity of the lesion and if resection of the esophageal stenosis ne-cessitates an intestinal bypass. The high in-cidence of adenocarcinoma associated with reflux disease seems to justify such a radical approach. In respect to all other in-dications, experience has demonstrated that these radical methods are subject to considerable mortality and morbidity and are often of questionable benefit to the pa-tient. For these reasons we prefer to use methods that do not involve reconstruc-tion. The abdominal approach has the ad-vantage that it is less traumatic, especially for elderly patients, and allows better ex-amination of the upper stomach.

Surgical Technique

The intraoperative examination is a most important extension of the roentgeno-graphic and endoscopic findings. In en-dobrachyesophagus, the area of the junc-tion is often found to be anatomically well preserved; the convexity of the fundus is easily seen and can be used for the fun-doplication; and the vessels and the vagus nerves are also in good condition. In con-trast, advanced inflammatory changes with cicatrization and mediastinal funnel formation are found in secondary brachy-esophagus. Here, the exposure is difficult and traumatic; danger of esophageal per-foration exists.

Intraoperative Dilation

It is a great advantage if the anesthetist is able to push a fine stomach tube through the stenosis. If this cannot be achieved de-spite manually straightening the cardia, it is advisable to introduce the tube from the abdomen. By means of a miniature gas-trostomy, a thin tube is pushed through the cardia retrograde under digital control until the tube appears in the patient's mouth. This retrograde dilation is often re-quired. The diameter of the inserted tube is increased in small steps until the tube is about as thick as a finger. This maneuver is achieved by sewing a slightly larger tube to the end of the first tube and pulling through from the opening in the stomach toward the mouth. In this way, progres-sively larger tubes can be introduced with-out using excessive force to pass them through the stenosis. The last tube is left in position and acts as a dilator until the end of the operation (Fig. 60-20).

Antireflux Operation

Fundoplication is normally possible with-out any additional technical problems. In

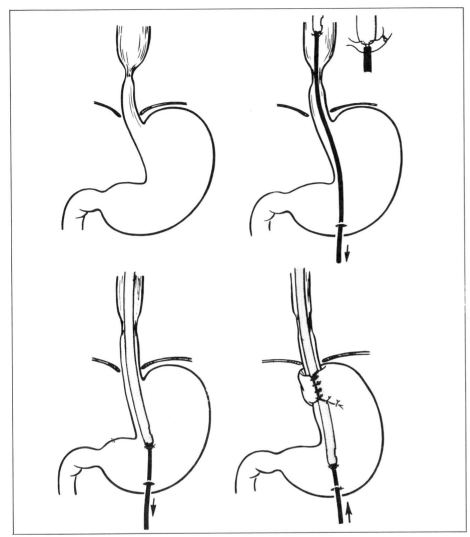

Fig. 60-20. Techniques of operative dilation and fundoplication for stenotic reflux disease either orthograde (↓) or retrograde (↑) via a minigastrostomy. (From R Nissen, M Rossetti, and JR Siewert. Fundoplicatio und Gastropexie bei Refluxkrankheit und Hiatushernien. *Stuttgart: Thieme, 1981. Reproduced with permission.)*

the presence of a secondary brachyesophagus with periesophageal fibrosis, however, fundoplication is difficult and requires special competence in this type of procedure. If the plication of the anterior wall is difficult because of tissue contraction and insufficient mobility of the fundus, the original Nissen technique is used. The omental bursa is separated. A fold is formed out of the anterior wall, and a second fold is formed from the posterior wall. Both folds are fixed loosely in front of the cardia by the usual row of sutures.

In this situation, the transthoracic fundoplication can be advantageous. To perform this procedure, the greater curvature of the stomach is mobilized after separation of the gastrosplenic ligament, if this proves necessary. After a thoracotomy is made through the seventh intercostal space, the hiatal diaphragm is stretched or split over a short distance, the fundus is pulled up, and the sleeve is formed and fixed in position.

Roux-en-Y Anastomosis and Gastric Resection

We have treated several esophageal stenoses successfully with two-thirds gastric resection and a long isoperistaltic Roux-en-Y loop. The biliopancreatic diversion and the acid reduction proved to be especially helpful in instances of severe trans-

mural fibrosis. Preoperative or intraoperative dilation of the stenosis was performed regularly in anticipation of fundoplication.

Review and Conclusion

Fundoplication has celebrated its fortieth anniversary. Clinical experience, experimental research, a tremendous literature, and innumerable symposia worldwide verify its efficiency as an antireflux procedure in the sense of true functional sphincter replacement. The modification of a short, tension-free floppy fundoplication has reduced the undesirable side effects (postfundoplication syndrome) provided the indication and the technique were correct.

Our results and those of other surgeons after careful follow-up can be summarized as follows: 90 percent of patients are free of reflux symptoms and satisfied in the short and medium term, and 80 percent are at 10 to 20 years after the operation.

Development of a broad and effective pharmacology, which includes the wide range of antacids, acid-inhibitors, cytoprotective agents, prokinetic drugs, and H_2-receptor blockers, most applied as long-term medication over years, has drastically decreased the number of operations from 1970 to 1990 to a minimum. This fact has reduced surgical experience and rendered practical training of residents difficult. Therefore, many centers treat only advanced and complicated pathology; these situations demand innovative technical variants instead of standard operations.

More recently, the minimal invasive surgery seems to open a new era for fundoplication, if the indication is correct and the technical principles are observed.

Suggested Reading

Bombeck CT. Gastroesophageal Reflux. In LM Nyhus, RE Condon (eds.), *Hernia*, 3rd ed. Philadelphia: Lippincott, 1989.

Donahue PE, Larson GM, Stewardson, RH, Bombeck CT. Floppy Nissen fundoplication. *Rev Surg* 34:223, 1977.

Ireland AC, Holloway RH, Toculi J, Dent J. Mechanisms underlying the antireflux action of fundoplication. *Gut* 34:303, 1993.

Jamieson G. (ed.). *Surgery of the Oesophagus*. Edinburgh: Churchill-Livingstone, 1988.

Liebermann-Meffert D. Architecture of the musculature at the gastroesophageal junction and in the fundus. *Chir Gastroenterol* 9:425, 1975.

Liebermann-Meffert D, Allgöwer M, Schmid P, Blum AL. Muscular equivalent of the lower esophageal sphincter. *Gastroenterology* 76:31, 1979.

Liebermann-Meffert D, Heberer M, Allgöwer M. The Muscular Counterpart of the Lower Esophageal Sphincter. In TM DeMeester, DB Skinner (eds.), *Esophageal Disorders: Pathophysiology and Therapy*. New York: Raven, 1985.

Luostarinen M, Isolauri J, Laitinen J, et al. Fate of Nissen fundoplication after 20 years. A clinical, endoscopic and functional analysis. *Gut* 34:1015, 1993.

Nissen R. Die transpleurale Resektion der Kardia. *Dtsch Z Chir* 249:311, 1937.

Nissen R. Eine einfache Operation zur beinflussung der Refluxesophagitis. *Schweiz Med Wochenschr* 86:590, 1956.

Nissen R, Rossetti M, Siewert JR. *Fundoplicatio und Gastropexie bei Refluxkrankheit und Hiatushernien*, 2nd ed. Stuttgart: Thieme, 1981.

Rossetti M. *Die Refluxkrankheit des Oesophagus*. Stuttgart: Hippokrates, 1966.

Rossetti M. Thirty years of Nissen procedure: Development of fundoplication. In JR Siewert AH Hölscher (eds.), *Diseases of the Esophagus*. Berlin: Springer Verlag, 1987.

Rossetti M, Allgöwer M. Fundoplication for treatment of hiatal hernia. *Progr Surg* 12:1, 1973.

Samelson SL, Bombeck CT, Nyhus LM. Lower Esophageal Sphincter Competence: Anatomic-Physiologic Correlation. In TR DeMeester, DB Skinner (eds.), *Esophageal Disorders: Pathophysiology and Therapy*. New York: Raven, 1985.

Savary M, Miller G. Der Oesophagus. Lehrbuch und endoscopischer Atlas. Solothurn, Gassmann 1977.

Skinner DB, Klementschitsch P, Little AG, et al. Assessment of Failed Antireflux Repairs. In TR DeMeester DB Skinner (eds.), *Esophageal Disorders: Pathophysiology and Therapy*. New York: Raven, 1985.

EDITOR'S COMMENT

The authors, having worked with Dr. Nissen, have outlined the important indications for this operation. An internist or gastroenterologist will frequently tolerate the failure of medical treatment for months or even years, until patients become totally discouraged and insist on surgical treatment. Surgery has become a more attractive consideration with the advent of laparoscopic fundoplication, which will be described in Chap. 62. The incidence of pulmonary complications in patients with major reflux but without esophagitis is considerable and has become the most common indication for this operation in children, especially in children who have mental handicaps.

Open to question is whether an antireflux procedure prevents the progression of established Barrett's esophagus to frank malignancy. Healing of the Barrett's esophagus is unlikely, and patients must be monitored with endoscopy at 6-month intervals for the rest of their life, even after a procedure that has effectively prevented reflux. However, it appears that progression or worsening of the Barrett's esophagus is lessened or even prevented with an effective antireflux procedure.

As technology of laparoscopic procedures progresses, the performance of an open antireflux procedure as described in this chapter will soon be limited to patients who have had significant upper abdominal surgery, including gastric operations, previous antireflux procedures, or other operative interventions that render the left upper quadrant difficult to approach with a laparoscope. This procedure can be a challenging open operative one, especially in obese patients, despite the straightforward concept of fundoplication. The required retraction is best provided with one of the newer mechanical retractors (we prefer the Omni) that has the option of fitting several retracting blades to the two arms. The Upper Hand can be fitted with two or three blades, but it is limited to retraction in the cephalad direction and is not as useful overall as is the Omni. Both instruments have the disadvantage of allowing excessive traction to be placed on the costal margin with the possibility of significant trauma to the rib cage and excessive postoperative pain. All mechanical retractors should be repositioned periodically (at 20- to 30-minute intervals) in order to prevent excessive and prolonged pressure on one portion of the rib cage, which occasionally causes costochondral fracture.

In a significant number of patients, there is dense and severe adherence of the distal 5 to 8 cm of esophagus to the phrenoesophageal ligament, the hiatus, the distal mediastinal structures including the vagus nerves, and other surrounding structures, making the dissection difficult and hazardous. This adherence can frequently be predicted by the severe esophagitis demonstrated during preoperative esophagogastroscopy. The major catastrophic complication of this operation is severe damage to or perforation of the terminal esophagus during this tedious dissection. This complication can be the result of a previously unrecognized perforation of the posterior or posterolateral esophageal wall that sealed spontaneously against the periaortic fascia or phrenoesophageal ligament. The authors' solution to this problem is to abandon the fundoplication, perform a distal gastrectomy (of at least two-thirds of the stomach), and perform a long Roux-en-Y gastrojejunostomy. This sensible alternative has considerable merit, but there are two concerns: The Roux-en-Y procedure has occasionally resulted in a gastric pouch that empties poorly, and gastroparesis can occur perhaps because of the loss of duodenal motilin control of gastric emptying. These complications have led us away from the Roux-en-Y procedure. These problems have occurred in 20 percent of instances in which we have used Roux-en-Y gastrojejunostomy. Usually, careful dissection of the esophagus with a tube in the esophagus that is smaller than the large Maloney dilator, avoiding encircling the esophagus with a metal right-angled instrument, and good visibility while retracting the esophagus gently with a sponge and index finger allow mobilization of the esophagus without breaching the esophageal wall or damaging the vagus nerves. Nevertheless, Professor Rossetti's idea has considerable merit for an occasional patient in whom persistent dissection by a surgeon not totally comfortable in the area should be avoided. Diverting bile and pancreatic juice away from the gastroesophageal junction plays a major role in decreasing esophagitis, but the Roux limb must be 60 cm or longer to achieve total diversion.

The concept of draining the area of the cardia is one that is logical enough, but if the esophagus has been perforated during the mobilization of that viscus, or if there is even minimal concern about the integrity of the gastric wall at or near the placement of the fundoplication sutures, drainage would probably be best used as an early indicator of the presence of a luminal leak, although the development of a controlled fistula might not occur. Subcutaneous drainage has not been used in most instances in the United States for some years; it is perceived to be a "two-way street" through which it is as likely that bacteria would invade a wound as it is that a wound hematoma or collection of fluid would be drained out, preventing infection.

An unresolved issue is the possibility of migration of the wrap into the mediastinum. Professor Rossetti underscores the questionable value of tacking the wrap to the esophagus but does use an inferior tacking to the gastric corpus with interrupted permanent sutures from the wrap to the gastric wall to minimize the possibility that the wrap will migrate. Furthermore, in the combined paraesophageal and sliding esophageal hiatal hernias, the wrap is fixed to the diaphragm after the markedly enlarged hiatus is closed. Whether the migration of the wrap into the chest is sufficient reason to assume that the operation has failed has not been established. It is logical, although not necessarily true, that the ultimate fate of a displaced wrap will be a function not of its position in the chest or abdomen, but of its integrity as an antireflux mechanism. In general, the wrap should remain intra-abdominal, if at all possible.

R.J.B.

61

Modified Hill
Repair for Gastroesophageal Reflux

Attila Csendes Juhasz   Italo Braghetto Miranda
Patricio Burdiles Pinto   Juan Carlos Diaz Jeraldo

There are five main factors responsible for the pathogenesis of chronic gastroesophageal reflux with reflux esophagitis: 1) incompetence of lower esophageal sphincter or mechanically defective cardia, 2) volume and composition of the refluxed material, 3) delayed gastric emptying, 4) impaired esophageal clearance, and 5) resistance of esophageal mucosa. Ideally, surgical procedures should correct these factors. However, the primary surgical techniques are directed only toward the restoration of an incompetent lower esophageal sphincter. We have developed a surgical technique based on the original work of Hill, which accomplishes some of the factors mentioned above.

Posterior gastropexy was introduced by Hill in 1967 in order to create a lower and permanent intra-abdominal segment of the esophagus by anchoring the anterior and posterior phrenoesophageal fascial bundles to the median arcuate ligament. This operation was modified by Larrain, who added calibration of the cardia because several surgical observations indicated that the distal portion of the esophagus and esophagogastric junction was dilated in patients with reflux esophagitis. This calibration or decrease of the diameter of the muscular esophagogastric junction to normal or less than normal diameter was achieved by invaginating a finger into the stomach and the distal end of the esophagus. This surgical step was sporadically accepted. In 1985, Skinner defined three essential steps that must be achieved for a proper antireflux operation: 1) ensure there is a long intra-abdominal segment of the esophagus, 2) increase the resting pressure to normal values of the lower esophageal sphincter, and 3) calibrate the cardia by application of the law of Laplace.

We have introduced some modifications to Hill's original technique to make a more objective and reproducible operation and to accomplish a more physiologic approach to surgical treatment of reflux esophagitis. Any surgeon performing antireflux procedures must be aware of the several abnormalities that can be found in a patient with gastroesophageal reflux disease (GERD). These surgeons must also know how an operation can resolve the clinical symptoms and laboratory abnormalities and improve quality of life.

Principles of Antireflux Surgery

The main steps for performing an antireflux procedure are:

1. Highly selective vagotomy
2. Closure of the right crus of the diaphragm
3. Calibration of the cardia using a No. 30 French bougie as a guide for calibration
4. Posterior gastropexy with two stitches to the median arcuate ligament
5. Anterior fundogastropexy to avoid a late anterior iatrogenic paraesophageal hernia

Highly Selective Vagotomy

This step is a new and important one for a more physiologic approach to surgical treatment of patients with reflux esopha-

gitis. The principal reasons to perform it are:

1. It provides excellent visualization and recognition of the lower esophagus and esophagogastric junction. Any surgeon who has performed highly selective vagotomy (HSV) for duodenal ulcer will understand this point. Patients with chronic reflux esophagitis and hiatal hernia have increased fatty tissue surrounding the esophagogastric junction, which makes identification of this segment difficult. In addition, in patients with severe esophagitis and Barrett's esophagus, transmural inflammation can alter the external surface of the esophageal wall so that it resembles gastric serosa, which is why it is easy to confuse the dilated distal esophagus with a hiatal hernia. Without thorough dissection, stitches can easily grasp fatty tissue; this loosening of the stitches might cause a late recurrence. After performing several hundred HSV procedures for duodenal ulcer, it is clear that the surgical exposure of the esophagogastric junction is excellent, setting the stage for a very precise antireflux operation combined with the physiologic advantages of the vagotomy.
2. In many procedures reported by several authors, it is necessary to divide the lesser omentum and the hepatic branch of the anterior vagal trunk in order to obtain an adequate exposure of the esophagogastric junction. This step might not be important in some populations, but it is in countries with a high prevalence of gallstone disease such as

Chile. A prospective study that we conducted demonstrated that gallstones developed in 42 percent of patients after 5 years of observation, compared with 8 percent in controls during the same period (p <0.001). Therefore we believe it is very important to preserve the hepatic branch.

3. During any of the procedures used in patients with reflux esophagitis, vagal trunks and Latarjet's branches are not clearly visualized. Therefore, they can be injured or, perhaps more frequently, entrapped in the sutures for calibration or fundoplication. This partial or complete vagotomy can be responsible for several symptoms at the late postoperative period such as diarrhea, delayed gastric emptying, development of gastric ulcer, and so forth. With our procedure, we can and should completely avoid any vagal damage.

4. Gastric acid secretion has an essential role in the pathogenesis of reflux esophagitis; 20 percent of patients with GERD have shown hypersecretion at basal and stimulated studies. This figure rises up to 48 percent when GERD patients with normal manometric lower esophageal sphincter (LES) pressures are studied. Medical treatment with H_2 blockers or proton-pump inhibitors tends to decrease dramatically both acid secretion and volume and therefore, acid reflux to the esophagus. HSV has a similar permanent effect as a "surgical acid secretion blocker," although the reduction is only 60 percent of peak acid output and never produces anacidity.

5. Delayed gastric emptying is observed in 30 to 50 percent of patients with reflux esophagitis. As a collateral beneficial effect of HSV, there is an increase of gastric emptying of fluids after surgery.

6. In patients undergoing a fundoplication, the addition of HSV has a favorable effect by increasing intragastric pressure through a loss of the capacity for accommodation after distention and loss of receptive relaxation. The wrap around the distal esophagus created by the Nissen procedure produces an increased intragastric pressure that improves competence of the LES.

The majority of surgeons have difficulty accepting the performance of HSV for two principal reasons: 1) unfamiliarity with the procedure, believing that it is very difficult to perform and is a time-consuming op-

eration. Actually, it can be very easy to perform and it takes an experienced operator less than 30 minutes. 2) HSV promotes changes at the LES by the extensive dissection and denervation of the distal esophagus. However, several studies in our patients demonstrated clearly that HSV did not alter the characteristics of the LES because resting pressure is not changed, gastroesophageal reflux does not increase after HSV, length and location of the LES are not changed, the response of the sphincter to cholinergic stimulation is not changed; and sphincter relaxation, increase of pressure after step-by-step increase of intragastric pressure, and amplitude of distal waves are not changed.

Calibration of the Cardia

This step is essential for antireflux surgery and was developed to decrease the dilated diameter of the distal esophagus and cardia in patients with reflux esophagitis. This point was an old surgical truism, but had never been measured objectively. Therefore, we performed a prospective study measuring the external circumference of the perimeter of the esophagogastric junction in 20 patients with duodenal ulcer without reflux and in 40 patients with reflux esophagitis. In the control group, the mean perimeter was 6 cm (which corresponds to a diameter of 2 cm) and in reflux esophagitis patients the circumference measured almost 10 cm, which correlates with the severity of reflux esophagitis and the enlargement of the circumference of the cardia, measuring as much as 14 to 15 cm in patients with Barrett's esophagus. These clinical studies were confirmed by DeMeester in experimental studies, demonstrating that the competence of the sphincter depends on

its length and the diameter of the cardia. With a diameter of the cardia of 1 cm (which is obtained in our patients with the No. 30 French bougie), a sphincter length of 2 cm can achieve 100 percent competence, whereas a cardia of 3-cm diameter needs a sphincter 5 cm long for proper competence.

Surgical Technique

Patients are placed in a supine position with the chest elevated relative to the feet (Grassi's position) (Fig. 61-1). A midline supraumbilical incision is made. A sternal retractor is always used. HSV is performed mainly with electrocautery, beginning the procedure at the crow's foot at the antrum, cutting the proximal branch. Dissection continues proximally by dividing the insertion of the anterior leaf of the lesser omentum at the lesser curvature and later dividing the posterior leaf of the lesser or hepatic–gastro omentum. The arterial branches are ligated. The dissection continues to the angle of His and 6 to 7 cm of the distal esophagus. This step leads to displacement of the vagal trunks and Latarjet's nerves along with the lesser omentum to the right of the patient. The lesser curvature is reperitonealized by interrupted stitches, and HSV is then complete (Fig. 61-2).

Closure of the Hiatus

This step is mandatory when true hiatal hernia exists. Otherwise, this point is not an important step in antireflux surgery. However, to avoid a postoperative hiatal hernia caused by surgical dissection of the phrenoesophageal membrane, the hiatus is closed with two sutures posterior to the esophagus (Fig. 61-3).

A Hurst or Maloney No. 30 French bougie is always used to avoid a too tight or too

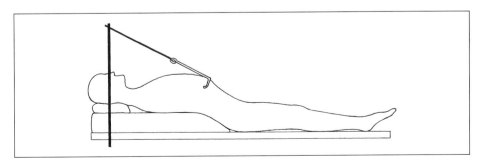

Fig. 61-1. Position of the patient for antireflux surgery.

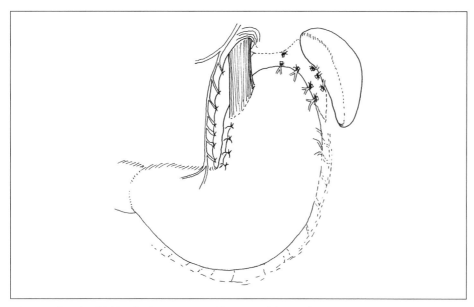

Fig. 61-2. Complete highly selective vagotomy with section of the vessels.

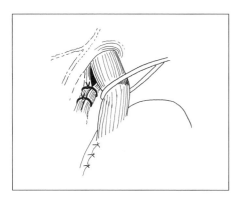

Fig. 61-3. Closure of the hiatus.

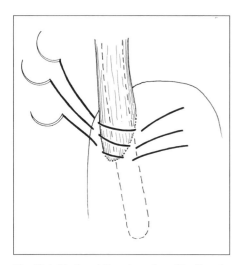

Fig. 61-4. Placing of the sutures for calibration of the cardia, with the bougie inside the lumen.

loose calibration of the cardia. Nonabsorbable silk sutures are used. This stitch is placed on the anterior surface of the stomach 2 cm distal to the cardia; therefore, it is perpendicular to it. The suture is placed at the anatomic border of the cardia, without including the esophagus. It should not include gastric mucosa or submucosa in order to avoid perforation or an ulcer. This suture includes the esophagogastric muscular junction and the same portion of the sling fibers. The stomach is then rotated easily to the left position to expose the posterior gastric wall. The suture is placed at the same level as the calibrating suture of the anterior wall (Fig. 61-4). Therefore, it enters at the posterior esophagogastric junction and emerges 2 cm distally on the posterior surface of the stomach. This suture is called the "mirror" suture. Three or four similar sutures are then placed extending to the left toward the angle of His. The sutures are tied, and the final calibration is then evaluated by moving the No. 30 French bougie back and forth into the stomach. A muscular ring created by the sutures should be palpated at the cardia. The bougie must pass easily but the cardia should be felt to close completely when it is withdrawn into the esophagus. Calibration of the cardia is completed, and the dilated distal esophagus and esophagogastric junction is decreased to a 1-cm diameter, restoring the resting LES pressure to a normal value (Fig. 61-5).

Posterior Gastropexy

This step was created by Hill and was designed to obtain a long intra-abdominal segment of the esophagus. However, we believe that it is unnecessary to dissect the median arcuate ligament as Hill did. Instead, we pick up this ligament together with the crus of the diaphragm just above the celiac trunk. This surgical step is performed with two stitches of the calibration of the cardia, which have been tied previously (Fig. 61-6). Usually we use the midpoint sutures of the calibration, because using the more distal or more proximal sutures can produce an undesirable angulation of the abdominal esophagus. By using a large special Babcock clamp, which firmly grasps the distal crus, preaortic fascia, and median arcuate ligament, the two stitches are passed through this fibromuscular tissue by lifting the clamp upward. The sutures must be passed easily without damaging the aorta.

Anterior Fundophrenopexy

In a previous study we noted that some patients developed an anterior paraesophageal hernia 3 to 5 years after surgery caused by the mobilization of the fundus of the stomach, which is left loose in order to proceed with the surgical repair. The hiatus has been dissected by the performance of HSV. The permanent positive intra-abdominal pressure exerts pressure on the loose fundus, which slowly migrates to the posterior mediastinum just in front of the esophagus. To avoid this complication, two nonabsorbable stitches are placed on the anterior surface of the gastric fundus and attached to the diaphragm (Fig. 61-7). The calibration is checked again, and the bougie is removed. A soft nasogastric tube is passed into the stomach for 24 hours. No abdominal drainage is used. Oral feeding starts the second day after surgery, and patients are discharged 4 to 5 days after surgery.

Results

It is very important to stress that we use this procedure only in patients with gastroesophageal reflux or erosive esophagi-

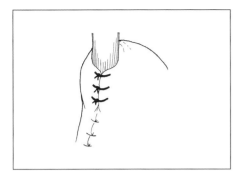

Fig. 61-5. Completion of the calibration of the cardia.

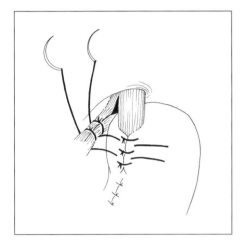

Fig. 61-6. Stitches for posterior gastropexy.

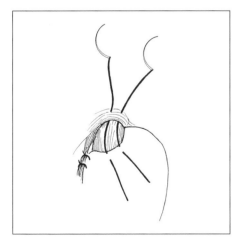

Fig. 61-7. Stitches for fundophrenopexy.

tis that has not responded to comprehensive long-standing medical treatment. Do *not* use this procedure in patients with Barrett's esophagus, because late recurrence rates are very high. In patients with severe reflux esophagitis and Barrett's esopha-gus, some type of bile diversion procedure is used.

In the last 13 years, we have used this surgical technique in 325 patients with uncomplicated reflux esophagitis. There has been no operative mortality, and postoperative complications have occurred in only 5 percent. Patients are investigated each 6 months the first year and each year thereafter. Complete clinical, roentgenographic, endoscopic, manometric, and 24-hour pH studies are performed to ensure that the procedure has achieved the goals of successful antireflux surgery: 1) to obtain a permanent relief of reflux symptoms, 2) to avoid the appearance of complications of severe reflux esophagitis, and 3) to restore the ability to vomit, to eat, and to eructate normally. These goals can be achieved if the surgical procedure produces an increase in LES pressure, an increase in sphincter length, an increase in abdominal length of the esophagus, and a decrease in the size of the dilated esophagogastric junction or cardia. Our recent results have shown a permanent control of reflux in 85 percent of the patients and failure in 15 percent.

Suggested Reading

Barlow AP, DeMeester TR, Ball CS. The significance of the gastric secretory state in gastroesophageal reflux disease. *Arch Surg* 124:937, 1989.

Bonavina L, Evander A, DeMeester TR. Length of the distal esophageal sphincter and competence of the cardia. *Ann Surg* 151:25, 1986.

Csendes A. Highly Selective Vagotomy Posterior Gastropexy and Calibration of the Cardia for Reflux Esophagitis. In JR Siewert, AM Holscher (eds.), *Disease of the Esophagus*. Springer Verlag, 1272, 1987.

Csendes A. Modified Posterior Cardiogastropexy for Surgical Treatment of Gastroesophageal Reflux with the Adding of Highly Selective Vagotomy and Bougie Calibration. In RB Belsey, A Moraldi (eds.), *Medical and Surgical Problems of the Esophagus*. London and New York: Academic, 91, 1981.

Csendes A, Braghetto I, Korn O, Cortes C. Late subjective and objective evaluation of antireflux surgery in patients with reflux esophagitis: Analysis of 215 patients. *Surgery* 105:374, 1989.

Csendes A, Braghetto I, Velasco N. A Comparison of Three Surgical Techniques for the Treatment of Reflux Esophagitis: A Prospective Study. In TR DeMeester, DB Skinner (eds.), *Esophageal Disorders: Pathophysiology and Therapy*. Raven, New York: 177, 1985.

Csendes A, Oster M, Brandsborg O, et al. Effect of vagotomy on human gastroesophageal sphincter pressure in the resting state and following increases in intra-abdominal pressure. *Surgery* 85:419, 1979.

Csendes A, Oster M, Moller IJ, et al. Effect of extrinsic denervation of the lower end of the esophagus on resting and cholinergic stimulated gastroesophageal sphincter pressure in man. *Surg Gynecol Obstet* 148:375, 1979.

Csendes A, Oster M, Moller IJ, et al. Gastroesophageal reflux in duodenal ulcer patients before and after vagotomy. *Ann Surg* 188:804, 1978.

Dodds WJ, Hogan WI, Kelin JI. Pathogenesis of reflux esophagitis. *Gastroenterology* 81:376, 1981.

Hill LD. An effective operation for hiatal hernia. An eight-year appraisal. *Ann Surg* 166:681, 1967.

Larrain A. Technical consideration in posterior gastropexy. *Surg Gynecol Obstet* 122:299, 1971.

Oster M, Csendes A, Furch-Jensen P, et al. PCV and modified Hill procedure as surgical treatment for reflux esophagitis: results in 108 patients. *World J Surg* 6:412, 1982.

Skinner DB. Pathophysiology of gastroesophageal reflux. *Ann Surg* 202:546, 1985.

EDITOR'S COMMENT

The conventional Hill operation has been used by some surgeons for almost thirty years. The operation is relatively straightforward, does not require a great deal of dissection, and involves only two steps: closing the esophageal hiatus and tacking the phrenoesophageal bundles of soft tissue to the arcuate ligament overlying the aorta just above the celiac axis. Professor Csendes's modification involves the performance of a highly selective (parietal cell) vagotomy, a procedure that I like but that some surgeons in the United States do not perform. This procedure can be technically difficult in obese patients or patients who have had a prior operation on the stomach.

The concept of "calibration of the cardia" seems very familiar, although the term describing the maneuver can be different; the stitches that tighten the cardia around the terminal esophagus would appear to have the same effect (not the same procedure) as the initial Nissen procedure. In actuality, tightening the cardia should be a useful modification of the standard Hill repair in the hands of most surgeons, because Dr. Hill's reported results of 95 percent good-to-excellent responses to his procedure have not been equaled by most surgeons, regardless of the surgical technique used. These authors present 85 percent good results, even with the additional step of the calibration of the cardia, or modified fundoplication, which they have added to the procedure.

Like these authors, in my relatively small experience with the Hill repair, it is often very difficult to isolate a strong median arcuate ligament, especially in elderly, obese patients, and the authors' practice of picking up the soft tissue that represents the preaortic fascia and sewing it with the repair of the crus is an attractive modification. Whether is it preferable to perform that step, rather than another type of antireflux procedure such as a floppy Nissen fundoplication, remains to be seen.

I have some concerns about using a No. 30 French dilator as the measure of the degree of tightness of the repair around the terminal esophagus. Most other authors in the past decade have advocated a looser repair as being better and use a No. 50 French dilator, coupled with the concept that one should be able to insert one's finger or a cervical dilator between the repair and the wall of the esophagus and lesser curvature of the stomach. Results that the author reports suggest that his technique does not result in the gas-bloat syndrome or inability to vomit. Whether there is actually some loosening of those sutures later, which presumably is what happens, or whether the importance of a looser wrap repair is overestimated is probably no longer open to question.

Conceptually, results of careful study of operations to prevent gastroesophageal reflux indicate that reflux is not absolutely prevented, but continues, albeit at a considerably abated level. Episodes of reflux continue, but they require a substantially greater increase in intra-abdominal pressure or straining. They last a shorter period of time, and there is more rapid esophageal emptying than before the operation. Esophagitis symptomatically improves, although it seldom disappears completely if microscopic study of biopsy specimens is carried out. Most important, patients feel symptomatically improved. One can, however, overdo a good thing, and the consequences of a too tight repair are sometimes worse than the consequences of no repair.

R.J.B.

62

Laparoscopic Nissen Fundoplication

Nathaniel J. Soper   Daniel B. Jones

Nissen fundoplication is a highly effective treatment for gastroesophageal reflux disease (GERD). Originally described by the Swiss Rudolf Nissen in 1955, the 360-degree gastric wrap performed through an upper abdominal incision has resulted in a greater than 90 percent long-term control of reflux symptoms. The fundoplication is accomplished by circumferentially dissecting the distal esophagus, mobilizing the gastric fundus, and encircling the esophagus with the fundus to create a high-pressure zone. Increasing the resting tone of the sphincter mechanism improves its response to elevated intragastric pressure yet allows "normal" swallowing, belching, and vomiting. Randomized trials comparing transabdominal open Nissen fundoplication with medical therapy in patients with complicated GERD proved surgical therapy to be more effective. Despite these findings, many patients and physicians opted instead for lifelong medication and significant lifestyle limitations until 1991 when Bernard Dallemagne in Belgium performed the first laparoscopic Nissen fundoplication. Although the actual gastric fundoplication follows the same surgical principles as the open operation, the laparoscopic approach appears to reduce postoperative pain and shorten the hospital stay and recovery period. Short-term functional outcome is similar to the outcome of the open operation.

GERD is a common disorder; an estimated 61 million Americans complain of heartburn and indigestion. In one survey of the U. S. population, approximately 15 percent experienced reflux on a monthly basis, 14 percent weekly, and 7 percent daily. GERD usually presents as heartburn and regur-

gitation and can progress to dysphagia. A relatively small subset of patients with esophageal reflux do not have heartburn but present with atypical symptoms such as postprandial fullness, belching, odynophagia, anginalike chest pain, nocturnal aspiration, chronic cough, wheezing, and hoarseness. Eating, drinking, and simply bending over can aggravate reflux and associated symptoms.

Gastroesophageal reflux is usually attributed to an incompetent lower esophageal sphincter (LES) mechanism. However, other diseases that impair esophageal clearing or gastric emptying such as achalasia, esophageal spasm, esophageal carcinoma, and pyloric stenosis can initially present with symptoms similar to the symptoms of GERD. Reflux symptoms can be confused with symptomatic cholelithiasis, peptic ulcer disease, or coronary artery disease. Before operative therapy, a thorough evaluation is essential since antireflux operations are designed solely to correct a mechanically defective gastroesophageal sphincter.

Roentgenographic imaging, endoscopy, pH monitoring, and esophageal manometry are performed as part of a complete work-up. The latter three tests should be performed in virtually all patients before an antireflux operation. A barium swallow can demonstrate ulceration, stricture, and hiatal hernia, but it is most useful to exclude a foreshortened esophagus. Endoscopy with biopsy determines the extent and severity of esophagitis and excludes Barrett's metaplasia or malignancy, and 24-hour esophageal pH monitoring objectively records the frequency and duration of gastroesophageal reflux. Manometry characterizes the location and tone of the

LES and rules out primary motility disorders of the proximal esophagus, which would contraindicate a Nissen antireflux operation.

Medical therapy is aimed at decreasing gastric acidity and reducing esophageal exposure to gastric contents. Antacids neutralize corrosive gastric juices, and H_2 blockers and omeprazole inhibit acidic secretion. Metoclopramide and newer prokinetic agents, such as cisapride, enhance gastric emptying and augment LES tone, thereby decreasing intragastric pressure and improving esophageal clearance. Virtually all our patients receive a short-term (2 month) trial of intensive medical therapy before considering an antireflux operation.

Lifestyle modifications are recommended to all patients receiving medical treatment for GERD. Patients with reflux are counseled to lose weight if they are obese and are discouraged from eating within 2 hours of bedtime. Since reflux is often aggravated while the patient is asleep, the head of the bed is elevated to promote nocturnal gravity-dependent clearance of the esophagus. Patients are advised to avoid foods and other substances known to diminish LES tone, especially fats, chocolate, alcohol, and tobacco. Commonly prescribed medications such as theophylline, calcium channel blockers, nitrates, and tricyclic antidepressants also promote reflux. Unfortunately, significant lifestyle modifications are usually ignored, symptoms usually persist, and many patients are ultimately referred for surgical relief of gastroesophageal symptoms.

Complications of GERD can develop if reflux is not adequately controlled. Ulceration, stricture, and bleeding are commonplace, but malignancy occurs rarely. By the time patients seek medical attention for reflux, 10 percent already have esophageal strictures and 5 to 20 percent have Barrett's esophagus. Although many patients initially respond well to medical therapy, withdrawal of antisecretory drugs is associated with a high recurrence. Furthermore, omeprazole induces human hepatic cytochrome P450 and can be carcinogenic if used in high doses for prolonged duration, although this finding has not been documented clinically in patients followed for 5 years. The laparoscopic antireflux operations have become an appealing alternative to chronic medical therapy.

Indications for Surgical Therapy

Surgical therapy improves the LES barrier and is recommended for patients with proven gastroesophageal reflux whose symptoms are unresponsive to a trial of medical therapy or who develop complications. The most common indications for operation for documented gastroesophageal reflux are:

1. Symptomatic GERD refractory to medical therapy
2. Esophageal ulcers
3. Stricture
4. Aspiration
5. Barrett's esophagus
6. Inability or unwillingness to remain on life-long acid suppression therapy
7. Children with severe esophagitis, recurrent pneumonia, or failure to thrive

Preoperative work-up including endoscopy, pH testing, and manometry is necessary to rule out other etiologies for symptoms that are not correctable with a fundoplication, or primary esophageal motility disorders that would be worsened by a traditional 360-degree wrap. Ideal patients for the Nissen fundoplication have an incompetent LES with normal proximal esophageal peristaltic contraction amplitude, esophagitis documented by endoscopic biopsy, and 24-hour esophageal pH monitoring demonstrating frequent reflux events.

Absolute contraindications to a laparoscopic Nissen fundoplication include patients who cannot tolerate general anesthesia or have an uncorrectable coagulopathy. Chronic reflux can cause stricturing and shortening of the esophagus and prevent the creation of a tension-free intra-abdominal gastric wrap causing wrap disruption or intrathoracic displacement. The propulsive force of the esophagus must also be sufficient to propel food across a reconstructed valve. If peristalsis is diminished, a partial wrap might be preferable. Obesity is a relative contraindication to laparoscopy, because these patients can require longer ports to traverse the abdominal wall and extra ports to retract omentum or elevate the liver. Obviously, patients with documented symptomatic gastroesophageal reflux who undergo laparotomy for some other reason should have a concomitant antireflux operation rather than accept chronic medical therapy or a later laparoscopic procedure. A history of upper abdominal surgery (especially prior fundoplication, vagotomy, or gastrectomy) is a relative contraindication to laparoscopic antireflux surgery. Scarring and adhesion formation distort anatomy and render the dissection more difficult.

Principles for Reconstruction of the Cardia

The laparoscopic Nissen fundoplication performed by an experienced surgeon is deceptively simple, and surgeons performing antireflux procedures should be familiar with principles for reconstructing the cardia (see Chap. 59) as well as be skilled in minimally invasive surgical techniques. Principles for reconstruction of the cardia are:

1. The length of the intra-abdominal esophagus determines the degree of competence in the absence of intrinsic muscle tone. The Nissen procedure permanently restores 1.5 to 2.0 cm of abdominal esophagus, which will respond to intra-abdominal pressure changes.
2. The resting distal esophageal sphincter pressure must be three times the resting intragastric pressure to overcome gastric distention.
3. The fundus of the stomach must be used in the wrap, and the vagus nerves must be protected. These structures are necessary to allow receptive relaxation, whereby the distal esophageal sphincter and fundus relax during deglutition, allowing normal swallowing.
4. The propulsive power of the esophagus should overcome the resistance of the reconstructed valve. For a Nissen fundoplication, the patient should have normal or near-normal esophageal peristalsis.

Whether the short gastric vessels need to be divided during a laparoscopic Nissen fundoplication is controversial and was not performed originally by Nissen. We believe the short gastrics should be divided to allow full fundic mobilization, to diminish tension on the wrap, and to ensure that the fundus, rather than the gastric body (which does not exhibit receptive relaxation), is used for the wrap.

Laparoscopic Nissen fundoplication is considered an advanced laparoscopic procedure because of its delicate dissection, suturing, and knot-tying. Several knot-tying devices have recently been manufactured to facilitate intra- and extracorporeal knot-tying; however, we feel that the surgeon performing laparoscopic procedures should be comfortable suturing before embarking on antireflux procedures. We recommend practicing with an endoscopic pelvic-trainer, in the animal laboratory, and during other laparoscopic procedures (ligation of the cystic artery during cholecystectomy and closure of the peritoneum during herniorrhaphy). Before attempting this procedure alone, the operation should be performed with the supervision of a proctor. Once skilled in both intra- and extracorporeal suturing techniques, the surgeon can choose either. We prefer extracorporeal knot-tying for the laparoscopic Nissen procedure because the gastric wall is strong and successive knots can be thrown quickly with a knot-pusher. With this technique, the surgeon must be careful not to pull up forcibly on the suture and inadvertently tear the esophagus. Laparoscopic expertise is critical to perform the operation with a low morbidity and mortality.

Preoperative Preparation

During the preoperative office visit, the expectations and risks of a laparoscopic Nissen fundoplication are discussed with the patient. Patients are counseled that if at any point a laparoscopic operation cannot be continued safely, the operation will be converted to an open approach. Gastric or esophageal perforation, injury to the vagal nerve or spleen, pneumomediastinum, dysphagia, and bloating are potential complications. The crural repair can also slip over time or break down and require re-operation.

Healthy patients are admitted the day of surgery after an overnight fast. In the operating room, the patient is placed in a modified lithotomy position on a ''bean bag'' cushion (Fig. 62-1). After induction of general anesthesia, the stomach is decompressed with an orogastric tube and the bladder emptied with a urinary catheter. The arms are tucked and protected at the sides. Inflatable compression stockings are worn on the lower extremities for deep venous thrombosis prophylaxis. The legs are abducted and supported on cushioned spreader bars. The bean bag is aspirated while ''cupping'' the patient's body wall and perineum; this step prevents subsequent slippage during extremes of tilt of the operating table. The abdomen is prepped and draped sterilely.

The operating room personnel and equipment are arranged with the surgeon between the patient's legs, the assistant surgeon on the patient's right, and the camera-holder to the left. Other surgeons prefer to work from the patient's side for the entire procedure or prefer to place the first assistant on the patient's left side. Video monitors placed at either side of the

head of the table are viewed easily by all members of the operating team. Irrigation, suction, and electrocautery connections come off the head of the table on the patient's left side. Special instruments include an endoscopic Babcock grasper, cautery scissors, curved dissectors, clip applier, atraumatic liver retractor, and 5-mm needle-holders. A mechanical self-retractor for the liver can also be used if readily available in the operating room. We occasionally use the Leonard Arm (Leonard Medical, Inc., Huntingdon Valley, PA) to stabilize the liver retractor if the assistant is relatively inexperienced with operating laparoscopically with two hands. We recently had a favorable experience using a device that coagulates blood vessels by ultrasonic vibration of apposable jaws (UltraCision, Inc., Smithfield, RI) to divide the gastrosplenic ligament.

Surgical Technique

Access to the abdominal cavity is achieved by either a closed or open technique. Before incision and trocar placement, bupivacaine 0.5% is injected at the port sites to augment postoperative pain control. With a closed technique, a 2-mm skin incision is made at the umbilicus, and a Veress needle is inserted blindly away from the aortic bifurcation and into the abdominal cavity. Two pops should be heard as the needle penetrates the fascial layers, and before in-

sufflation the needle's position should be confirmed with a drop test. Alternatively, with an open technique, the initial port is inserted similar to the way it is for peritoneal lavage cutdown. Fascial sutures secure an airtight seal around the Hasson (wedge-shaped) port. Open insertion is particularly helpful in patients with adhesions and distorted anatomy from previous abdominal surgery.

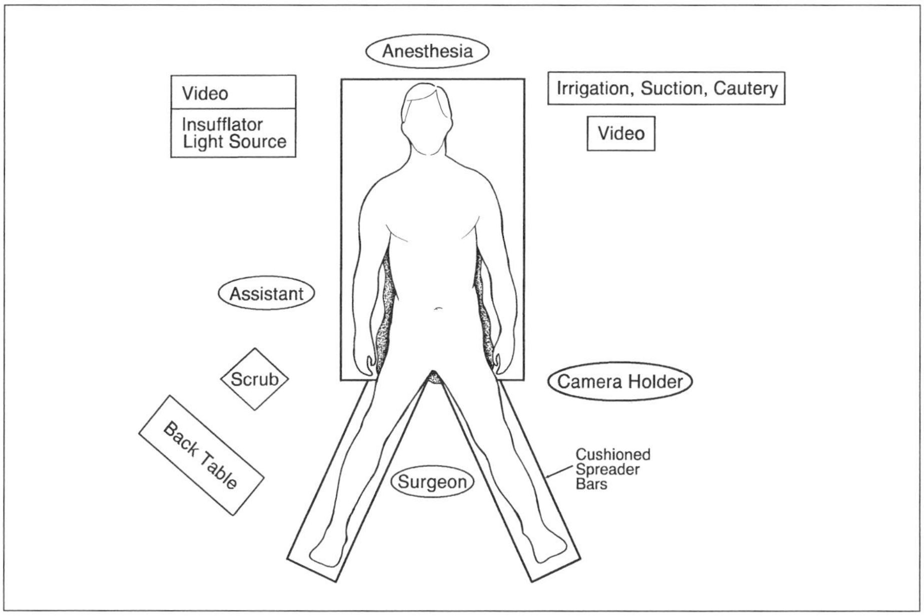

A carbon dioxide pneumoperitoneum expands the abdominal cavity and creates a working space. The abdominal cavity is insufflated with carbon dioxide to a pressure of 12 mm Hg. After establishing the pneumoperitoneum, the anterior abdominal wall is manually lifted, and a 10- to 12-mm port is placed in the left midrectus muscle superior to the umbilicus approximately 13 to 15 cm below the xiphoid process. The entire abdomen is explored with an angled laparoscope (usually 30-degree oblique) beginning at the area deep to the insertion site. Adhesiolysis might be necessary if the patient has had previous surgery. After thorough inspection of the pelvis, right upper quadrant, and left upper quadrant, four additional 10-mm ports are placed under direct vision of the videolaparoscope. Ports are typically placed in the following locations to optimize visualization and tissue manipulation, and to facilitate suturing (Fig. 62-2A): right subcostal, 15 cm from the xiphoid process; a point midway between the first two ports in the right midrectus region; in the left subcostal region 8 to 10 cm from the xiphoid; and in the right paramedian location at the same horizontal level as the left subcostal trocar (usually 5 cm inferior to the xiphoid). This port arrangement allows access to the hiatus and permits comfortable suturing. The gastroesophageal junction is usually deep to the xiphoid, and from a point 15 cm distant, only one-half of the laparoscopic instrument must be introduced to reach the hiatus. This distance establishes the fulcrum at the midpoint of the instrument and maximizes its range of motion during tissue manipulation. With the laparoscope directed between the suturing hands, the surgeon operates straight ahead, avoids the problem of video ''mirror images'' caused by working with the back toward the camera, and maximizes visual cues allowing accurate perception of three-dimensional relationships. Using 10-mm diameter sheaths for all ports allows the surgeon to easily introduce the

Fig. 62-1. Operating room layout. Patient is supine with legs abducted on a cushioned spreader bar.

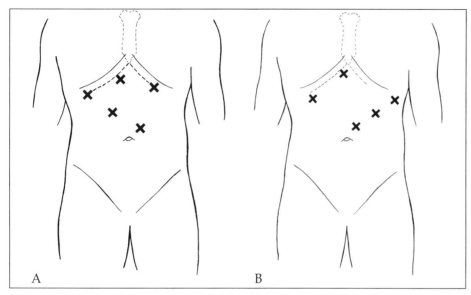

Fig. 62-2. Cannula placement. A. Standard placement if the surgeon sutures from between the patient's legs. B. Alternate port placement if the surgeon prefers to work from the patient's side.

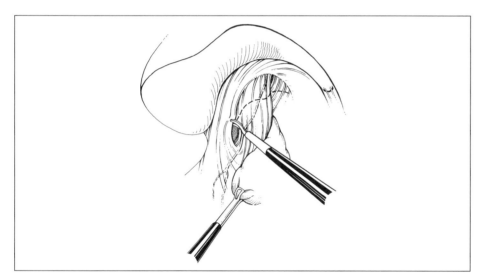

Fig. 62-3. Retraction of the liver exposes the esophageal hiatus while the phrenoesophageal ligament is divided.

laparoscope from any port for different viewing angles.

Alternatively, ports can be arranged for the surgeon to operate from the patient's side (Fig. 62-2B): a 10-mm port in the midline, midway between the xiphisternum and umbilicus; a subcostal 5-mm port in the right midclavicular line; a 5-mm port in the right epigastrium; a 10-mm port in the left subcostal anterior axillary line; and a 10-mm port in the left midclavicular line. All ports should be at least 8 cm apart to avoid "sword-fighting" of instruments, and two ports should be in the upper ab-

domen within 15 cm of the hiatus from which to suture.

Trocar insertion and insufflation can potentially cause life-threatening complications of hemorrhage and air embolism, which if suspected, require prompt action by the surgeon. Brisk return of blood can occur if the trocar mistakenly enters the aorta or spleen. A laparotomy tray should be immediately available if emergent laparotomy is necessary. Just as with other penetrating trauma, the trocar should not be removed before gaining proximal and distal control. Air embolism on the other

hand presents with a noticeable drop in end tidal carbon dioxide, hypotension, and "mill-wheel" heart murmur. If suspected, the pneumoperitoneum should be deflated and the patient positioned head down in the left lateral decubitus position. Attempts should be made to aspirate air after inserting a central line. These complications are extremely uncommon and should be avoided by applying careful laparoscopic technique.

Once access is safely achieved, exposure of the esophageal hiatus is facilitated by gravity and maintained by an assistant. Positioning the patient in the reverse Trendelenburg (Fowler) position lets gravity displace the bowel and stomach from the diaphragm. A skilled camera-holder and an angled laparoscope are important. The assistant uses a retractor introduced through the right subcostal port to elevate the left lobe of the liver and a Babcock forceps through the right midrectus port to pull the stomach and epiphrenic fat pad inferiorly and to the left (Fig. 62-3). The left triangular ligament is not divided but is left to help suspend the liver anteriorly. Next, both crura and the anterior vagus nerve are identified after opening the phrenoesophageal ligament. If a hiatal hernia is present, it is reduced fully into the abdominal cavity with gentle traction after cutting all adhesions to the hernial sac. The right crus is retracted laterally, while the right side of the esophagus is carefully dissected to visualize the aorto-esophageal groove and posterior vagus nerve (Fig. 62-4). On the other side of the esophagus, the left crus is similarly dissected from the esophagus and fundus to its point of origin from the right crural leaflet. A "window" is created between the crura and posterior esophageal wall. It is important never to grasp the esophagus with the jaws of the laparoscopic instruments, which risks perforation, a potentially life-threatening complication. Violation of the pleura can accidentally occur during dissection, but the resulting pneumothorax usually resolves without intervention as long as the patient is ventilated with positive pressure.

The fundus is then fully mobilized by dividing the proximal gastrosplenic ligament. Beginning at a point on the greater curve 8 to 10 cm distal to the esophageal junction, the short gastric vessels are placed on traction, a window is created into the lesser sac, and the anterior peri-

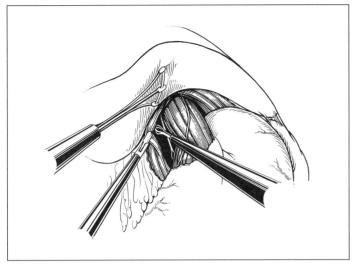

Fig. 62-4. With the right crus retracted laterally, the anterior and posterior vagus nerves are clearly visible. (From DB Jones and NJ Soper. Laparoscopic Nissen fundoplication. Surgical Rounds 17:573, 1994. Reproduced with permission.)

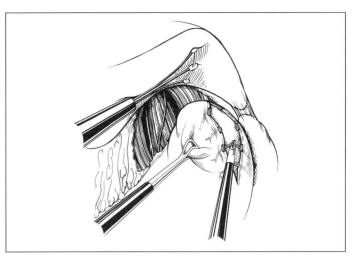

Fig. 62-5. The short gastric vessels are clipped and divided from inferiorly to superiorly until the fundus is completely mobilized. (From DB Jones and NJ Soper. Laparoscopic Nissen fundoplication. Surgical Rounds 17:573, 1994. Reproduced with permission.)

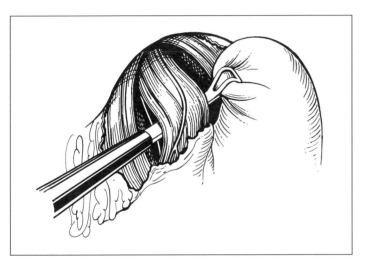

Fig. 62-6. A Babcock clamp is passed through the postesophageal "window" to grasp the lateral wall of the gastric fundus. (From DB Jones and NJ Soper. Laparoscopic Nissen fundoplication. Surgical Rounds 17:573, 1994. Reproduced with permission.)

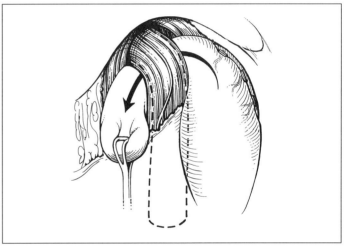

Fig. 62-7. The fundus is wrapped posterior to the esophagus and anterior to the crura and posterior branch of the vagus nerve. The 360-degree fundoplication is calibrated over a 60 French esophageal dilator. A tension-free wrap will not recoil back around the esophagus when the Babcock releases the fundus. (From DB Jones and NJ Soper. Laparoscopic Nissen fundoplication. Surgical Rounds 17:573, 1994. Reproduced with permission.)

toneum is scored proximally. The short gastric vessels are then serially divided. This step can be done by clipping and dividing them (Fig. 62-5) or by serial application of the LCS ultrasonic coagulator (UltraCision, Inc., Smithfield, RI). To complete mobilization of the proximal stomach, all posterior retroperitoneal adhesions to the fundus are divided sharply.

After fundic mobilization, a Babcock clamp is passed right to left in front of both crura and the posterior vagus nerve, and behind the esophagus (Fig. 62-6).The Babcock grasps the fundus near the insertion of the short gastric vessels and pulls the fundus left to right around the esophagus (Fig. 62-7).When the surgeon lets go of the fundus it should lie in place; if it springs

back around the esophagus, the wrap is too tight. Next, the esophagus is serially dilated before leaving a 60 French Maloney bougie. The bougie calibrates the wrap and prevents excessive narrowing of the esophagus during the actual fundoplication. Dilation must be performed cautiously if the patient has esophageal strictures or severe inflammation, and the

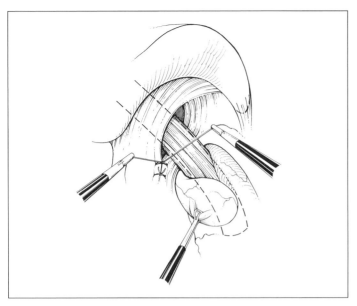

Fig. 62-8. The crura are approximated beginning posteriorly and inferiorly. Closure is usually performed posterior to the esophagus.

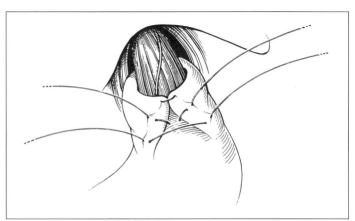

Fig. 62-9. The fundoplication is secured with two or three 0-nonabsorbable sutures. Sutures should include bites of seromuscular left fundus, superficial anterior esophageal wall, and seromuscular right fundus. (From DB Jones and NJ Soper. Laparoscopic Nissen fundoplication. Surgical Rounds 17:573, 1994. Reproduced with permission.)

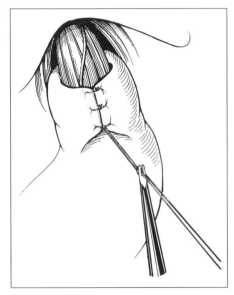

Fig. 62-10. After the knot is formed extracorporeally, it is advanced with a knot-pusher apparatus to secure the wrap and complete the laparoscopic Nissen fundoplication. (From DB Jones and NJ Soper. Laparoscopic Nissen fundoplication. Surgical Rounds 17:573, 1994. Reproduced with permission.)

dilator should never be forced. Instead, the surgeon should watch the bougie pass smoothly through the gastroesophageal junction as a bulge on the video monitor. If the bougie appears hung up at the gastroesophageal junction, the surgeon can sometimes improve the angulation by re-

tracting the stomach anteriorly or caudally.

If the esophageal hiatus is enlarged by hiatal hernia or dissection, the hiatus should be closed with several 0-Ethibond sutures. Reapproximation of the right and left crura to restore the esophageal hiatus is usually performed posterior to the esophagus (Fig. 62-8), although anterior closure can be appropriate.

With the dilator in the esophagus, a "short, floppy" Nissen fundoplication is performed using three interrupted 0-Ethibond sutures (silk suture can degrade and lose tensile strength after 2 years). Seromuscular bites of fundus to the left of the esophagus, the anterior esophageal wall away from the anterior vagus nerve, and the fundus to the right are all incorporated in the 360-degree fundoplication (Fig. 62-9). The esophageal wall should be incorporated in at least one of the sutures to prevent slippage of the wrap around the body of the stomach or into the thoracic cavity. We use extracorporeal knotting techniques, tying square knots and pushing them into position (Fig. 62-10),whereas other surgeons prefer intracorporeal suturing. Regardless of the method used, the surgeon should take generous tissue bites and oppose the gastric wall without strangulation of the tissues. Ideally, the wrap should be only 1.5 to 2 cm in length, be-

cause longer wraps are associated with a higher incidence of postoperative dysphagia. After three sutures secure the fundoplication, one additional suture tacks the wrap to the right crus to further prevent thoracic migration and diminish rotational stress. The esophageal dilator is withdrawn by the anesthesiologist. At this point, the laparoscopic Nissen fundoplication is complete.

The abdominal cavity is thoroughly irrigated with saline and aspirated dry. The suture line is inspected at the end of the operation to ensure that there is no leak or hemorrhage. The gastroesophageal angle can be checked by passing a nasogastric tube smoothly through the hiatus. Similarly, a 10-mm Babcock should slide easily under a loose wrap. If the gastroesophageal junction is steeply angled by the hiatal closure or the wrap seems too tight, removing a stitch or two might partially release the hiatus or fundoplication, respectively. The pneumoperitoneum is evacuated, and the ports are removed under direct vision as a last check to ensure no bleeding from the trocar sites. Incision sites are irrigated with saline and infiltrated with the remaining 0.5% bupivacaine (maximal dose of 2.5 mg/kg). The fascia of each incision is closed using an absorbable No. 1-Vicryl suture, and the skin is closed using running subcuticular 4–0 absorbable sutures. Steri-strips (3M, St.

Paul, MN) are applied, and before leaving the operating room the urinary catheter and gastric tube are removed while the patient is still anesthetized. Pneumatic compression stockings are left in place until the patient is awake and ambulating. Injectable or oral narcotics are administered as needed for pain control. Postoperatively, all antireflux and antacid medications (e. g., antacids, H$_2$ blockers, omeprazole, and metoclopramide) can be discontinued. Clear liquids are permitted on the morning following surgery. The diet is rapidly advanced to mechanical soft as tolerated and the soft diet is maintained for 2 weeks while esophageal edema resolves. The patient is followed serially as an outpatient, and postoperative manometry is routinely performed at approximately 3 months; however, many asymptomatic patients are difficult to persuade to undergo additional uncomfortable and costly studies.

Preliminary reports with short-term follow-up after the laparoscopic Nissen fundoplication have been encouraging. As with other "minimally invasive" operations, we find that our patients have less postoperative pain, shorter hospitalization, and faster recovery after a laparoscopic Nissen rather than they would with an open approach. At Barnes Hospital–Washington University Medical Center, more than 150 patients underwent the laparoscopic antireflux operation from May 1992 to December 1995. In our series, symptomatic reflux has completely resolved in more than 95 percent of our patients. Two patients were converted to open Nissen fundoplication because of extensive adhesions; one patient had a diaphragmatic hernia repair during childhood, and the other patient had extensive gastrosplenic adhesions. Five patients complained of transient early postoperative dysphagia and underwent esophageal dilation; further evaluation revealed no evidence of stricture, motility disorder, esophagitis, or sphincter dysfunction, and dysphagia resolved by 3 months. Two additional patients required laparoscopic reoperation. In one patient, the fundoplication migrated into the chest because of inadequate crural closure, and in the other patient the wrap was disrupted after a high-impact train accident.

Operative time ranges from 1.5 to 5.5 hours, with a median of 2.0 hours. With additional experience and new instrumentation, the duration of operation should approach the time typically required for a standard open Nissen. Following the open Nissen fundoplication at our hospital, patients were discharged on average 10 to 12 days postoperatively. Following a laparoscopic Nissen fundoplication, patients are usually discharged within 24 to 72 hours and return to work or full activity within 12 days of surgery. Early hospital discharge and discontinuation of expensive medication represent substantial savings in health care dollars, and rapid return to employment should markedly decrease indirect costs.

The laparoscopic Nissen fundoplication has proved to be highly effective treatment of GERD in several large series with short follow-up. Since the laparoscopic fundoplication follows well-established principles of antireflux surgery, patients should enjoy the same effective long-term control of GERD as they would with open Nissen fundoplication. In addition, by avoiding a major laparotomy incision, patients experience less pain, shorter hospitalization, faster recovery to full activity, and improved cosmesis with the laparoscopic operation compared with its open counterpart. For these reasons, patients who previously endured significant lifestyle restrictions and chronic medication are now more likely to consider operative therapy of GERD. Multi-institutional studies with long-term follow-up are needed to assess the durability of the repair before the laparoscopic Nissen procedure is deemed the "gold standard" surgical treatment of GERD.

The authors gratefully acknowledge the Washington University Institute for Minimally Invasive Surgery as funded by an educational grant from Ethicon-Endosurgery, Inc.

Suggested Reading

Dallemagne B, Weents JM, Jehaes C, et al. Laparoscopic Nissen fundoplication: Preliminary report. *Surg Lap Endosc* 1:138, 1991.

DeMeester TR, Bonavina L, Albertucci M. Nissen fundoplication for gastroesophageal reflux disease—evaluation of primary repair in 100 consecutive patients. *Ann Surg* 204:9, 1986.

Howard PJ, Heading RC. Epidemiology of gastroesophageal reflux disease. *World J Surg* 16:288, 1992.

Hinder RA, Filipi CJ, Wetscher G, et al. Laparoscopic Nissen fundoplication is an effective treatment for gastroesophageal reflux disease. *Ann Surg* 220:472, 1994.

Jamieson GG, Watson DI, Britten-Jones R, et al. Laparoscopic Nissen fundoplication. *Ann Surg* 220:137, 1994.

Jones DB, Soper NJ. Laparoscopic Nissen fundoplication. *Surg. Rounds* 17:573, 1994.

Nissen R. Eine einfache operation zur beeinflussung der refluxoesophagitis. *Schewiz Med Wochenschr* 86:590-592, 1956.

Skinner DB. Pathophysiology of gastroesophageal reflux. *Ann Surg* 202:546, 1985

Spechler SJ and the Department of Veterans Affairs Gastroesophageal Reflux Disease Study Group. Comparison of medical and surgical therapy for complicated gastroesophageal reflux disease in veterans. *New Engl J Med* 326:786, 1992.

Stein HJ, DeMeester TR, Hinder RA. Outpatient and physiologic testing and surgical management of foregut motility disorders. *Curr Probl Surg* 31:415, 1992.

EDITOR'S COMMENT

Doctor Soper is an acknowledged expert in the field of laparoscopic surgery. He and Dr. Jones have presented as concise and clear a description of this very interesting operation as I have encountered. Doctor Soper's laparoscopic skills have made him one of the most widely sought-after teachers of laparoscopic surgery, and his role as a leader at Washington University in the Institute for Minimally Invasive Surgery is well known.

The preoperative considerations in performing this operation have been fully displayed, and it is impossible to disagree with any. As for surgical technique, the use of the Veress needle to establish the pneumoperitoneum is completely safe in Dr. Soper's hands, but for less experienced operators (the vast majority of general surgeons who perform laparoscopic surgery), the Hasson 10-mm port inserted through an open fascial incision is most attractive. Truly serious and even life-threatening complications occur far more commonly with the blind introduction of the Veress needle and the trocar than with the open insertion in which one sees omentum or intestine. In addition, it is unnecessary to use a sharp trocar at all for the initial port and camera placement. Ninety percent of laparoscopic procedures in the United

States are initiated with the Hasson open technique.

It is very interesting that the authors place the initial 10-mm port in the left midrectus muscle. Most of us have either used the midline or have taken care to place a large port lateral to the rectus muscle, with the concern that traversing the rectus muscle with a trocar can damage the deep superior epigastric vessels or cause bleeding from the muscle itself. This obviously is not the experience of the authors, and Dr. Soper's placement of the port for insertion of the laparoscope has obvious advantages, if one is operating in the left upper quadrant.

The authors have properly identified the difficulties that can occur with the use of silk sutures to perform the fundoplication or the closure of the right crus of the diaphragm to restore the esophageal hiatus. It was somewhat disconcerting to learn years ago that silk is not permanent, and its use in hernia repair or in repair of any defect of the abdominal wall or parietes is not indicated. There are many good, almost inert and readily available synthetic sutures that are permanent; silk should not be used for any type of surgery, including laparoscopic surgery, when the longevity of the repair can depend on the integrity of the sutures. Intestinal anastomoses are not included in this sweeping generalization, since serosa-to-serosa apposition and healing are complete long before silk begins to deteriorate.

It is very interesting that Dr. Soper uses one or two stitches through the esophageal wall, as well as the two sides of the gastric wall, to anchor the fundoplication. Several authors in this Esophageal Surgery section have cautioned against using esophageal stitches in open fundoplication and have preferred to anchor the wrap using the gastric wall alone. There is no question that there is a mechanical advantage with the esophageal incorporation in the closure, since the gastric wall is quite loose and might not always anchor the wrap. In open Nissen fundoplication, I have done it both ways and have not been dissatisfied with or concerned about the esophageal suturing technique for anchoring the wrap. Doctor Soper's expertise with the laparoscope enables him to accurately gauge the depth of the suture in the esophageal wall, despite the fact that he is viewing this three-dimensional field on a two-dimensional monitor. For surgeons commencing this operation laparoscopically, it would be wise to consider the consequences of too deep a suture in the esophagus, and either obtain extensive experience in the animal laboratory with sewing to the esophagus before attempting it in the human, or using another variation of wrap immobilization including a stitch through the right crus of the diaphragm or perhaps even one or two stitches through the phrenoesophageal ligament to anchor the superior portion of the wrap.

R.J.B.

63

Nissen Fundoplication: Reflux Control in Disease States

Philip E. Donahue

Reflux of gastric contents into the esophagus occurs in many circumstances; in patients of all ages; and is categorized as physiologic, pathologic, congenital, neuropathic, primary, secondary, or idiopathic. When possible, detailed barium studies as well as motility studies should be obtained on all patients preoperatively to characterize the anatomy and physiologic function of each particular individual. With these studies, one can assess the depth of esophageal ulcers (when present), recognize anatomic relationships of the diaphragm and stomach precisely, and identify any gastric or duodenal pathology or malformations that might predispose to reflux.

Whether reflux is accompanied by inflammation or irritation of the esophageal mucosa depends on cofactors in the pathogenesis of erosive esophagitis, which include the composition of the refluxate, the exposure time for susceptible mucosa, and the innate resistance of the target tissue. Each of these variables can be independently assessed. For example, refluxate can be evaluated by considering the concentration of acid or bile salts present. Some patients with severe reflux symptoms, especially atypical symptoms such as asthma, choking, dysphagia, or chest pain, might not have endoscopically visible evidence of reflux disease and can still be candidates for elective operation.

Etiology of Reflux

Allison, the father of modern antireflux surgery, was one of the first to realize that a mechanism at the lower end of the esophagus prevented increases in gastric or intra-abdominal pressure, or both, from propelling gastric contents toward the oropharynx; he proposed that a sling mechanism of the esophageal hiatal musculature is a central part of reflux control. He thought that the angulation of the distal esophagus caused by the esophageal hiatus was analogous to the angulation of the rectum caused by the puborectalis muscle. The Allison repair for hiatal hernia was based on reconstituting this angle (angle of His) but was ineffective in the control of reflux.

As for sliding hiatal hernia, it is now generally agreed that it has little to do with the causation of reflux. A hernia can be demonstrated in many individuals who are over 50 years of age, with an incidence approaching its occurrence in the population of patients with reflux esophagitis, most of whom do not have the disease. The size of the hernia, however, is related to the severity of the reflux. Actually, one-third of patients with a hiatal hernia will *not* have evidence of gastroesophageal reflux disease (GERD).

The single most important factor accounting for the competence of the gastroesophageal junction is the lower esophageal sphincter (LES). There was uncertainty about the importance of the LES, partly because of the absence of an obvious anatomic sphincter in the distal esophagus. However, the LES and cardia have been shown to be a two-component arrangement of clasplike bands of muscle above and a slinglike muscle below. The clasps are clustered on the lesser curve of the esophagus, extending for several centimeters above and below the true gastroesophageal junction; the sling is a condensation of the oblique muscle layer of the stomach located on the greater curvature of the stomach, at the angle of His. More recently, investigators have provided convincing data relating to the function of the sling muscles. The sling muscle contraction can contribute to the well-known asymmetry of the LES, which has higher pressures in the left and posterior aspects of the sphincter; these higher pressures correspond to the area of the sling fibers.

Pathophysiology of Reflux Esophagitis

The general requirement for reflux esophagitis is the presence of reflux. However, since we now know that normal patients have acidic pH levels in the distal esophagus up to 4.0 percent of the time, the patient with severe esophagitis is expected to have considerably more reflux. This difference is indeed what we have observed in the clinical evaluation of reflux complications; patients with free reflux and with the worst complications of reflux (i. e., ulcer, stricture, Barrett's esophagus) all had reflux times that were considerably longer than in controls.

Refluxate

Normal acid-peptic gastric contents produce mild esophagitis if left in contact with the esophagus for sufficient periods of time. However, the most pronounced and severe degrees of esophagitis are associated with reflux of a mixture of gastric and duodenal contents. The bile salts from the duodenum, a known barrier breaker and surface-tension lowering agent, exacerbate the inflammatory process. Control of acid secretion leads to marked improvement in symptoms, without necessarily improving the degree of inflammation observed in the target organ. The amount of acid present in the esophagus is the critical issue in patients with reflux, not the total amount of acid secreted in various circumstances; patients whose refluxate is at a pH of 0 to 2 can have severe esophagitis when the total time of abnormal reflux is within normal limits. Reflux changes can be quite severe even in patients who have *no* endogenous acid secretion. For example, if intestinal continuity is re-established with an Omega loop or Braun anastomosis after total gastrectomy, some patients will develop frank esophagitis because of the noxious effects of jejunal content on the esophageal mucosa. After total gastrectomy, the surgeon should always divert bile and jejunal contents away from the esophagus. The general principle of diversion of duodenal content from the esophagus is an important one and is used in the treatment of refractory esophagitis from a variety of causes.

Abnormal Antireflux Mechanism

Although we refer to the patient with severe reflux as an individual with a ''failed'' LES, it might be more appropriate to consider pathologic GERD as a failure of gastric and esophageal components of the reflux barrier. However, until we have a better means to evaluate the gastric component, surgeons should consider reflux primarily a function of LES dysfunction.

Pathology of Reflux Esophagitis

The pathologic changes encountered with GERD are subtle. Microscopic changes range from simple increases in the length of the squamous epithelial papillae with or without neutrophil infiltration in the milder degrees of esophagitis to extrusive mucosal destruction with acute inflammatory cell infiltration into the muscularis,

with varying degrees of circumferential fibrosis. Recently, a variation of inflammation in the esophageal wall has been reported in a group of patients without frank inflammation, for whom the evidence for reflux was based on pH testing and the biopsy findings consisted of an eosinophilic infiltrate in the submucosa of the esophagus. The implication of this finding is that all symptomatic patients should undergo biopsies, and patients with symptoms such as dysphagia referable to the esophagus should be completely evaluated.

Fibrosis can extend through the wall of the esophagus and involve contiguous structures. All stages of acute and chronic ulceration can be present between these extremes. In the aftermath of ulceration, there is a tendency for fibrous scar formation. Depending on the depth of the original inflammatory process, a stricture might be noted at the locus of the most severely affected esophagus. It is worth noting that many esophageal strictures are rather superficial in location, involving only the mucosa and submucosa of the esophagus; the relative obstruction produced by a stricture of this type is aggravated by the edema that accompanies the healing process. The superficial stricture is easily dilated and is reversible early in the course of treatment by any means that will correct its underlying cause. Superficial strictures often require one or several dilations in the course of treatment.

The second type of stricture is a true fibrous scar of the distal esophagus. The submucosal and at least part of the muscular layers of the esophagus are replaced by fibrous tissue. Dilation of this type of stricture is extremely difficult, and the stricture promptly recurs.

The Columnar-Lined Esophagus

The columnar-lined esophagus, first described by Barrett in 1954, is an end-stage mucosal response to chronic gastroesophageal reflux. Most investigators now believe that it is acquired, resulting from metaplasia of lower esophageal epithelium in response to severe chronic esophagitis. It is most often described as the columnar-lined lower esophagus and is frequently associated with a stricture at the upper extent of the metaplastic process. Chronic peptic ulceration is not infrequent in the abnormal epithelium, and adeno-

carcinoma is thought to occur in up to 10 percent of the Barrett's epithelium population over many years.

Indications for Surgical Treatment

There are several indications for surgical intervention (Table 63-1):

1. Severe objective evidence of GERD unresponsive to treatment. The presence of inflammatory esophagitis, with or without ulcer, stricture, and bleeding, is the most obvious indication for operation. Interestingly, the availability of H_2 blockers and proton-pump inhibitors (e. g., omeprazole) has changed the natural history of reflux conditions; severe ulcers and strictures are not seen as commonly now as previously. However, some patients are intolerant of reflux symptoms after years of medical treatment, and they request definitive surgical intervention.
2. Severe atypical symptoms of GERD *without* inflammatory changes in the esophagus. The patient with adult-onset asthma, aspiration symptoms, or atypical chest pain might not have inflammatory changes in the esophageal epithelium and might still be an appropriate candidate for surgical treatment. In such instances, there is a particular need for documentation of reflux to identify the source of the symptoms and to use as a reference point for measuring the efficacy of the treatment; 24-hour pH testing is the most important element of this documentation.
3. Chronic bleeding in long-term anticoagulation patients.

Table 63-1. Indications for Surgical Treatment of GERD

1. Severe objective findings of GERD unresponsive to medical treatment; young patient with typical disease who recognizes risks of life-long medical treatment (i. e., risk of Barrett's epithelium, and so forth)
2. Severe atypical symptoms of GERD unresponsive to medical treatment
   a. Pulmonary asthma
   b. Frequent nocturnal choking
3. Severe chronic bleeding in patients requiring long-term anticoagulation
4. Severe typical symptoms of GERD that resist medical treatment

4. Severe typical symptoms of GERD, resistant to medical treatment, without inflammatory complications of GERD.

The last group of patients is an extremely small fraction of the surgical treatment cohort. However, when a patient has severe problems with regurgitation, pain, heartburn, or other reflux symptoms, it is reasonable to undertake surgical correction if the treatment is suited to the patient's need.

Surgical Treatment of Gastroesophageal Reflux

The Nissen fundoplication is the most effective mechanical barrier against reflux. The Nissen operation was originally proposed as a treatment for hiatal hernia and was thought to be effective because it resulted in reduction of the hernia. However, it soon became apparent that a hernia reduction was not essential for reflux prevention. We (Bombeck and Daeselare) later proposed a modification of the Nissen operation, the *"floppy"* Nissen, whose essence was that it was loose enough to allow physiologic reflux while preventing pathologic reflux. In the follow-up of patients with a floppy Nissen, it became evident that the goals of the modification had been realized; reflux was prevented *without* a marked increase in postoperative LES pressures and with few postoperative symptoms.

The Floppy Nissen Fundoplication

The operation is identical whether performed laparoscopically or via laparotomy. Since the laparoscopic approach is proving extremely useful, this approach to fundoplication will be briefly illustrated (see Chap. 62).

Insertion of Ports for Laparoscopic Surgery

I use the Hasson technique for all cases. This approach facilitates safe entry to the peritoneal cavity and has proved its merit. Four working ports are placed in addition to the camera (Hasson) site (Fig. 63-1). The use of 10-mm ports in all locations allows flexibility in the use of dissectors or other necessary instruments. The camera site

port is extremely important for perihiatal dissection; the ordinary position is approximately 10 cm above the umbilicus, although in the very obese patient, it might be advisable to insert the Hasson cannula even higher, mid way between xiphoid and umbilicus.

General Setup of the Operative Field

The first retractor placed elevates the left lobe of the liver. The size and consistency of the left lobe are of importance to exposure of the proximal stomach and the esophageal hiatus, since a fatty liver or a liver with a fragile capsule can bleed or tear when retracted; therefore, caution and gentle retraction are essential. The best approach is the use of a mechanical retractor holder, since these devices hold the instruments immobile.

Adhesions to the spleen are of particular interest and should be divided cautiously if present, just as in open surgical procedures. Then, the proximal stomach is grasped with a Babcock clamp and retracted inferiorly and to the left.

The reverse Trendelenburg position is used, and occasionally if necessary, a left or right tilt is used to assist in the exposure of the lateral aspect of the stomach.

Mobilization of the Fundus of the Stomach

The initial maneuver is separation of the short gastric vessels from the proximal portion of the stomach. Although division of the short gastric vessels can be tedious and difficult, it has become apparent that the short gastric vessels can be safely divided, provided that hemostasis is meticulous and the surgeon is patient. Several technical factors have facilitated this exposure, including the use of 30- or 45-degree angled telescopes, which are invaluable and essential for the safe dissection of the distal esophagus and proximal stomach. While performing dissection of the proximal greater curve, it is useful to have the telescope inserted at the level of the left midclavicular line.

The division of the short gastric vessels is the first maneuver and is readily accomplished with the assistance of metallic clips, bipolar coagulator, or harmonic scalpel. A mobile fundus is the key to a tension-free fundoplication.

Exposure of the Distal Esophagus

Identification of the pillars of the esophageal hiatus, and identification of the posterior vagus nerve are most important. When the proximal stomach is completely separated from its peritoneal attachments, the left pillar of the esophageal hiatus is clearly seen. The surgeon directs dissection upward toward the anterior border of the esophageal hiatus. By continuing dissection along the rim of the hiatus, the right crus becomes apparent. With a combination of blunt and sharp dissection, often with the assistance of a laparoscopic "peanut" dissector, the posterior vagus nerve trunk is seen coursing from above left toward the inferior right lower part of the visual field (Fig. 63-2). Subsequently, the wall of the esophagus is seen, and the process of clearing a window behind the esophagus is continued. The remaining part of prefundoplication dissection is the creation of a retroesophageal window and closure of the diaphragm.

Closure of the Esophageal Hiatus

The posterior vagus nerve can be clearly seen, and following identification of both crura of the diaphragm, the surgeon plans

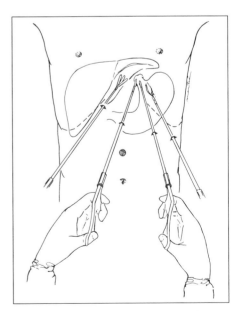

Fig. 63-1. Five ports are used for laparoscopic fundoplication. The camera will be inserted in the midline, approximately one-third the distance from the umbilicus toward the xiphoid. The left midclavicular port is used to retract the stomach and the right midclavicular port to retract the liver.

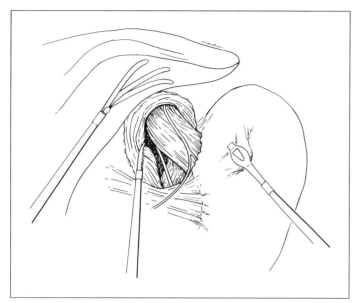

Fig. 63-2. At the completion of mobilization of the short gastric vessels and the esophageal hiatus, the vagus nerves are clearly seen. The window behind should be at least 4 cm long to allow the fundic wrap to lie without tension posterior to the esophagus.

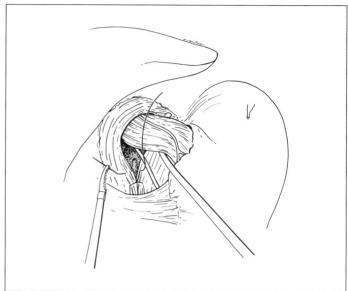

Fig. 63-3. Suture closure of the widened esophageal hiatus is an important part of the closure. The surgeon ensures that the esophagus is not tightly constricted. Because there are no tubes in the esophagus at this point, one must make an allowance for the dimensions of the esophagus when distended by the bougie.

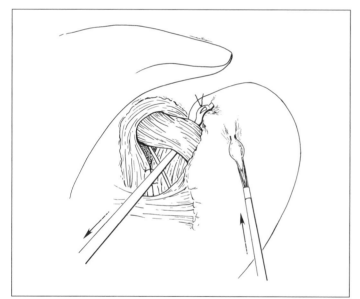

Fig. 63-4. The mobilized fundus is passed behind the esophagus, and it is important that the fundus lies behind the esophagus without being held tightly by clamps. When the clamps are released, the fundus should remain in situ, and not "snap back" to the anatomic position. Before tying the sutures, a large bougie (50–60 Fr) is placed within the lumen of the esophagus to assist in the calibration of a floppy wrap.

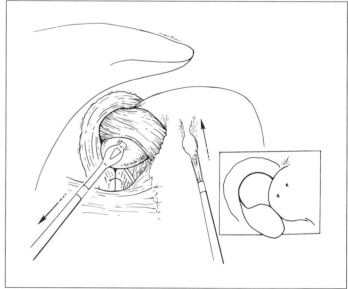

Fig. 63-5. The anterior wall of the stomach is advanced cephalad and the fundus is passed behind the esophagus, anterior to the posterior vagus nerve. The site of the fundoplication suture on the anterior gastric wall is noted (inset).

suture closure of the widened esophageal hiatus (Fig. 63-3). It is necessary to close the esophageal hiatus, even when no hiatal hernia was present preoperatively, because there is inevitable damage to phrenoesophageal support structures in the course of mobilizing the esophagogastric junction. As a result, there is a definite risk of postoperative transhiatal migration of the fundoplication and proximal stomach. Patients with an "acquired" paraesophageal hernia are liable to the same complications of incarceration, bloating, and perforation as are patients with a primary paraesophageal hernia.

The esophageal hiatus is closed with permanent suture material, and one or two

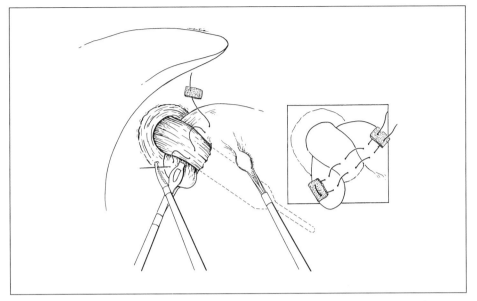

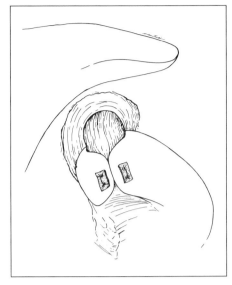

Fig. 63-7. Completed fundoplication.

Fig. 63-6. A No. 50 French bougie has been passed into the stomach beside the nasogastric tube. The mattressed fundoplication suture is placed, encompassing the muscularis only of the esophagus, buttressed by Teflon pledgets.

sutures of 2–0 or 0 material are used. The major question, "How tight should the hiatus opening be?" is one that is not easily answered. As in the open cases, the hiatus is not closed tightly around the esophagus; leave approximately 1.0 cm of space between the esophagus and the hiatus.

Fundoplication (Figs. 63-4 through 63-7)

The fundus is passed behind the esophagus using one of several approaches. One useful maneuver is to elevate the esophagogastric junction (with a Penrose drain or retractor) and ensure that the posterior window is adequate. A suture can be placed on the upper aspect of the anterior gastric wall (see Fig. 63-3); that suture can be passed behind the esophagus on a curved clamp and the stomach subsequently pulled behind the esophagus: *It is essential that at this time, no tubes are in the esophagus.*

Next, a large (50–60 Fr) bougie is advanced into the stomach by the anesthesiologist. With the esophagus distended, the fundoplication sutures can be placed; the surgeon assesses the mobility of the gastric wall and tries to ensure that the wrap will be as loose as possible. This step is the essence of the "floppy Nissen" fundoplication. Sutures incorporate the anterior gastric wall, an adventitial muscular "bite" of the esophagus, and the posterior shoulder

of the fundoplication. Permanent suture material is used, and Teflon pledgets can be used to minimize the chance of suture disruption. A total of two sutures are used.

Postoperative complaints after fundoplication are identical to the ones encountered after the open operation. The most frequent complaints are dysphagia, gasbloat (if a floppy wrap is not done), and early satiety. The incidence of dysphagia appears to be greater than the incidence observed after open procedures, possibly related to the fact that the gastropancreatic fold is not divided during laparoscopic operations. It seems that the division of the short gastric vessels allows the gastric fundus to be placed under less tension, another important feature in avoiding postoperative dysphagia.

Original Nissen Procedure (Figs. 63-8 and 63-9)

As mentioned previously, dissections of the cardia and esophageal hiatus are performed. Narrowing of the esophageal hiatus is performed before the insertion of bougies. In the classic Nissen fundoplication, the short gastric vessels are divided and the gastropancreatic attachments of the posterior cardia are divided to allow the use of both anterior and posterior gastric walls in the construction of the wrap. If this approach is used, at least 6 cm of the

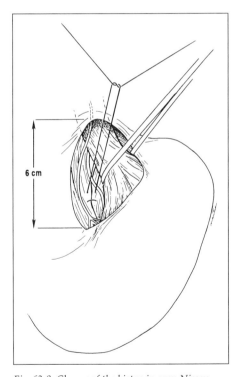

Fig. 63-8. Closure of the hiatus in open Nissen fundoplication. The fundus is mobilized as in Figures 63-2 and 63-3. It is usually necessary to dissect a wider space for the open Nissen procedure, since the crura cannot be dissected and seen clearly without division of the gastropancreatic fold. At least two, and often three, sutures are placed; the sutures are nylon or other permanent suture material (not silk), and can be used with or without Teflon pledgets.

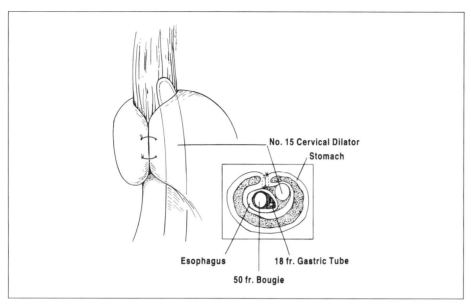

Fig. 63-9. *Nissen fundoplication. Two sutures are placed at the gastroesophageal junction, and a series of four to six "collar" stitches are placed between the apex of the wrap and the esophageal wall. Nylon suture material is preferred.*

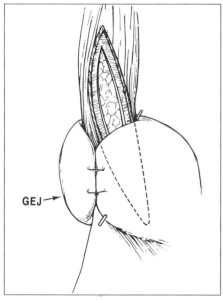

Fig. 63-10. *The fundoplication is performed in a floppy manner after mobilization of the fundus; a large (50-60 Fr) bougie is placed within the esophagus before suture placement. Two or three sutures are required for a 1- to 1.5-cm length of fundoplication. Each suture includes the anterior gastric wall, the right lateral wall of the esophagus (at the right margin of the esophagocardiomyotomy), and the posterior shoulder of the wrap. Note the hemoclips, which facilitate roentgenographic localization of the fundoplication. GEJ, gastroesophageal junction.*

gastric fundus must be freed from splenic attachments to allow the anterior and posterior gastric walls to be plicated in front of the esophagus. The length of the fundoplication (formerly 3–4 cm) has been shortened to 1 to 1.5 cm, the length used over a period of years with good results.

Nissen–Rossetti Procedure

In the Rossetti modification of the Nissen fundoplication, the wrap is performed with the anterior wall of the stomach only. The advantage of using the Rossetti approach is the avoidance of division of the posterior (gastropancreatic) and lateral (short gastric) attachments of the stomach. Some surgeons who perform the Nissen–Rossetti operation laparoscopically have found that postoperative dysphagia is a common complaint; however, there are many enthusiastic reports that attest to the absence of postoperative complaints in the majority of patients.

Fundoplication in Patients with Achalasia of the Esophagus

Effective surgical treatment for achalasia of the esophagus facilitates swallowing by

division of muscles that fail to relax normally during swallowing. If esophagocardiomyotomy is performed, a complementary antireflux procedure is mandatory to prevent postoperative gastroesophageal reflux, specifically with floppy Nissen fundoplication (Fig. 63-10). This approach is an effective treatment for achalasia; there is no clinical evidence of obstruction of the esophagus, and manometric data in postoperative patients do not suggest that the sphincter is obstructive in any way.

Esophagocardiomyotomy with Fundoplication

The division of the hypertrophied lower esophageal segment is done in the usual way, and the preparation of the fundus is performed as for Nissen fundoplication (above). The plication is performed with a dilator in place, requires only two sutures for completion, and does not constrict the distal esophagus (Fig. 63-10). Alternative methods of fundoplication, such as the 270-degree Toupet fundoplication, are of great interest to laparoscopic surgeons. The use of this anti-reflux procedure avoids much of the post–Nissen dysphagia, which was previously thought "inevitable."

Among surgeons who treat achalasia, the primary differences in approach relate to the length of the myotomy, and the need for the type of antireflux procedure that should be performed. The reported incidence of postoperative reflux is variable. Although some individuals are apparently unaffected, others find reflux a more common problem. Most would agree that the potential for reflux is great if the myotomy includes the gastric oblique sling fibers. Our manometric data suggest that esophagocardiomyotomy followed by fundoplication is not obstructive.

Suggested Reading

Barrett NR. Hiatus hernia: a review of some controversial points. *Br J Surg* 42:231, 1954.

Behar J, Sheahan DC. Histologic abnormalities in reflux esophagitis. *Arch Path* 99:387, 1975.

Bjerkeset T, Edna T-H, Fjosne U. Long-term results after a Floppy Nissen/Rossetti fundoplication for gastroesophageal reflux disease. *Scan J Gastroenterol* 27:707, 1991.

Bombeck CT, Vaz O, DeSalvo J, et al. Computerized axial manometry of the esophagus; a new method for the assessment of antireflux operations. *Ann Surg* 206:465, 1987.

Bremner RM, Crookes PF, DeMeester TR, et al. Concentration of refluxed acid and esophageal mucosal injury. *Am J Surg* 164:522, 1992.

Csendes A, Maluenda F, Braghetto I, et al. Location of the lower esophageal sphincter and the squamous columnar mucosal junction in 109 healthy controls and 778 patients with different degrees of endoscopic oesophagitis. *Gut* 34:21, 1993.

Donahue PE, Bombeck CT. The modified Nissen fundoplication: reflux prevention without gasbloat. *Chir Gastroenterol* 11:15, 1977.

Hinder RA, Filipi CJ, Wetscher G, et al. Laparoscopic Nissen fundoplication is an effective treatment for gastroesophageal reflux disease. *Ann Sug* 220:137, 1994.

Janssen IMC, Gouma DJ, Klementschitsch P, et al. Prospective randomized comparison after cardiopexy and Nissen fundoplication in the surgical therapy of gastro-oesophageal reflux disease. *Br J Surg* 80:875, 1993.

Liebermann-Meffert D, Allgower M, Schmid P, Blum AL. Muscular equivalent of the lower esophageal sphincter. *Gastroenterology* 76:31, 1979.

Stein HJ, De Meester TR, Naspetti R, et al. Three-dimensional imaging of the lower esophageal sphincter in gastroesophageal reflux disease. *Ann Surg* 214:374, 1991.

EDITOR'S COMMENT

Although it might seem redundant, it is often useful to present two authors' viewpoints on the same disease process and even on the same operation. Doctor Soper has described the laparoscopic approach to the Nissen fundoplication, whereas Dr. Donahue has presented a description of the same procedure with greater emphasis on the loose nature of the wrap. The reader about to embark on this very important laparoscopic approach can cull complementary information on the approach to symptomatic gastroesophageal reflux with both authors' modifications. Doctor Donahue's career has been devoted to the study of the LES and the reflux conditions that follow failure of sphincter function; his approach is a function of years of study of this challenging condition.

Doctor Donahue has reflected on the pathophysiology of gastroesophageal reflux and of reflux esophagitis, both of which are of critical importance in performing the operation, since correction of the underlying reflux is essential to correction of the deleterious effects of persistent esophagitis. In the past decade, it has become routine to measure 24-hour pH levels in the distal esophagus on an ambulatory basis, and from this type of information has come the principle that a minimal amount (4% or less) of acid reflux occurs in the distal esophagus of many patients for very short periods of time, without any pathologic change. Normal patients often experience some mild substernal burning, especially after eating a very full meal and assuming the supine position. With patients with significant esophagitis, however, the reflux not only occurs more often but it also takes considerably longer for the distal esophagus to empty than in patients with a normal esophagus. The author emphasizes the importance of the bile salts from the duodenum refluxing into the esophagus; it is important to remember that 50 percent of the contents of the proximal (first and second portions) duodenum refluxes into the antrum of the stomach under normal circumstances. With significant reflux disease, this duodenal content proceeds as far proximal as the esophagus and is probably even more damaging to the esophageal mucosa than the acid from the corpus of the stomach. Therefore, a number of authors have advocated an alternative to the Nissen operation when the pathology encountered at operation makes Nissen fundoplication or other antireflux procedures difficult. The simplest alternative is the Roux-en-Y reconstruction following subtotal gastrectomy, as has been commented on in previous chapters. Reducing gastric acid by removing the antrum and distal corpus deals with the acid issue, and the construction of a long Roux limb (at least 60 cm measured) should effectively eliminate bile salt entry into the esophagus.

Although it is desirable to preserve carefully the vagus nerves during this operation, it is not always possible to do so. When the procedure is performed by a laparotomy, the vagus nerves are preserved with less difficulty. However, when the laparoscopic approach is used, it is even more important to protect the vagi, since laparoscopic performance of a pyloromyotomy is possible but is more difficult than is the procedure done open. There is some difference of opinion about whether the pyloromyotomy (or pyloroplasty) is necessary. Many thoracic surgeons would not be concerned about transecting the esophagus and the vagus nerves and not doing the pyloroplasty when the stomach is used to replace the esophagus. However, others, perhaps because of an occasional unpleasant experience, always perform some pyloric sphincter ablation procedure. My inclination is to protect the vagus nerves, if possible; if not, a drainage procedure should be performed, often a Heineke-Mikulicz pyloroplasty.

R.J.B.

64

Achalasia, Diffuse Esophageal Spasm, and High-Amplitude Peristaltic Contractions

Alex G. Little

Esophageal motility disorders vary in their presentation. Typically, the clinical picture of each esophageal motility disorder is predominantly either dysphagia or chest pain. Achalasia, diffuse esophageal spasm, and high-amplitude peristaltic contractions represent paradigms of these dichotomous clinical pictures. These disorders are discussed individually; however, because the surgical considerations tend to be similar, the technical operative aspects are presented together in the final section of the chapter.

Achalasia

Achalasia is a motility disorder with the principal characteristics of a tonically contracted lower esophageal sphincter (LES) and absence of esophageal body peristalsis. These motor defects combine to result in a functional distal esophageal obstruction with no assistance for emptying provided by the esophageal body. Not surprisingly, all patients with achalasia have a history of dysphagia. The patient has to accumulate a column of food in the esophagus such that the hydrostatic pressure at the bottom can overcome the nonrelaxing sphincter and push some food into the stomach. Over time, the esophagus steadily distends and finally can reach such an enormous size that the patient no longer feels a sensation of dysphagia; each new food bolus simply drops into a now large reservoir organ. In this advanced disease setting, patients begin to regurgitate and frequently present with evidence of pulmonary soilage including episodes of aspiration pneumonia. The roentgenograms

in Fig. 64-1 illustrate these early and late stages.

The etiology of achalasia is unknown. Pathologic examination of the achalasia esophagus reveals hypertrophy of the two muscle layers, an absence of myenteric neural ganglia, and hypertrophy of nerve fibers. The hypersensitivity response that can be elicited with cholinergic drugs is consistent with a denervation sensitivity phenomenon. This picture suggests that this disorder is an acquired one in which

esophageal innervation is disrupted or lost. In addition, nitric oxide synthetase (NOS) levels in the LES muscle are considerably lower than normal. Whether this diminished availability of the potent smooth-muscle relaxant, NO, is a primary or a secondary phenomenon is unclear.

The diagnosis of achalasia is suggested by history and barium x-ray findings but can be unequivocally established only by esophageal manometry. Diagnostic findings are shown in Fig. 64-2 and include a

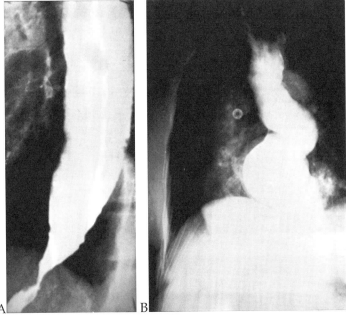

Fig. 64-1. Barium contrast x-rays illustrating features of achalasia. A. The typical features of achalasia are shown: moderate dilation and a smooth distal tapering. B. The features of long-standing achalasia are illustrated: the massively dilated esophagus has assumed a sigmoid configuration.

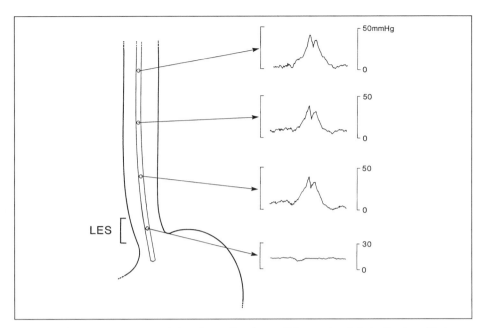

Fig. 64-2. This manometry tracing depicts the motility abnormalities seen in achalasia. Esophageal body contractions are not peristaltic; they are simultaneous rather than sequential. The LES does not relax completely down to gastric baseline pressure with swallowing.

Table 64-1. Treatment of Achalasia: Results of Pneumatic Dilation

Report Authors	Year	Improved (%)	Mortality (%)	Postoperative GERD (%)
Vantrappen and Hellemans	1980	77	0.2	Not mentioned
Fellows, et al.	1983	58	0	27
Robertson, et al.	1988	48	0	26
Sauer, et al.	1989	50	1.5	30
Barnett, et al.	1990	78	0	7

GERD = Gastroesophageal reflux disease.

failure of LES relaxation, which either does not occur or is incomplete and sporadic. The other diagnostic finding is that all esophageal body contractions are simultaneous so that no functional peristalsis occurs. Other findings that are inconsistently present include a high-resting pressure in the LES and low pressure esophageal body contractions.

Treatment

Treatment of achalasia is limited to correction of the LES dysfunction. Options include forceful pneumatic dilation, open surgical myotomy, and minimally invasive laparoscopic or thoracoscopic myotomy.

The track record of pneumatic dilatation is well established and reveals a success rate of approximately 75 percent with up to two pneumatic dilation sessions. The dilator is passed across the gastroesophageal junction under endoscopic or fluoroscopic control. As the bag is rapidly inflated, the balloon indentation caused by the lower sphincter is effaced. The patient typically experiences mild-to-moderate epigastric pain, and when the bag is deflated and removed after 60 seconds of inflation there is usually blood staining, suggesting that there has been forceful disruption.

In addition to achieving a reasonably good success rate, pneumatic dilatation is accomplished with surprisingly few complications. The perforation rate in large series is consistently under 5 percent. Long-term follow-up shows that symptomatic gastroesophageal reflux through the dilated LES occurs in up to one-third of patients, but the majority are able to eat satisfactorily and are happy with their outcome. Table 64-1 provides results from representative reports in the literature.

Historically, surgical myotomy has been performed through either a laparotomy or, more commonly, a thoracotomy and has been generally reserved for patients whom balloon dilation fails to help. My preference has been the thoracic approach, which allows a generous myotomy to be performed under direct vision following mobilization of the gastroesophageal junction from the hiatus. This last maneuver ensures ideal exposure of and access to the distal esophagus and the gastroesophageal junction so that the surgeon can be confident that the muscular fibers that constitute the LES have been completely divided and the myotomy extended onto the stomach itself. Complete disruption of the LES is essential because the primary indication for intervention is dysphagia, and the surgeon should be certain that this symptom is relieved. The dissection of the hiatus necessitates the addition of an antireflux procedure to prevent iatrogenic reflux. This step is accomplished with a modified Belsey fundoplication, which involves reapproximating the hiatus posteriorly and performing a 270-degree partial fundoplication using a total of four instead of the usual six sutures. The hypertrophied esophageal muscle permits reassuringly generous bites of muscle to be taken with each suture. Several large series document that this operation can be performed with mortality ranging from 0 to 5 percent and minimal morbidity. Long-term follow-up shows significant improvement of symptoms in approximately 90 percent of patients treated in this manner. Although most reports have documented a low incidence of postoperative reflux, recent series have documented a somewhat disturbing incidence of the late development of clinically important reflux. This series suggests, at least, the need for continuing follow-up of these patients following surgery.

There are new minimally invasive surgical approaches for this motility disorder. Either thoracoscopically or laparoscopically the esophagus can be mobilized and a myotomy performed. An endoscope placed in the distal esophagus is manipulated both to provide countertraction on the esophagus and to confirm that a sufficient myotomy has been accomplished. As with the open procedure, there is some controversy regarding the role of an antireflux procedure. If an antireflux procedure is added, it should not incorporate a 360-degree fun-

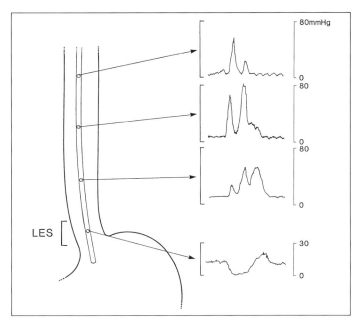

Fig. 64-3. This manometry tracing shows the motility abnormalities seen in DES. Most contractions are simultaneous and, as shown here, frequently are repetitive. Some contraction waves are peristaltic, and the LES is usually normal. These characteristics distinguish this disorder from achalasia.

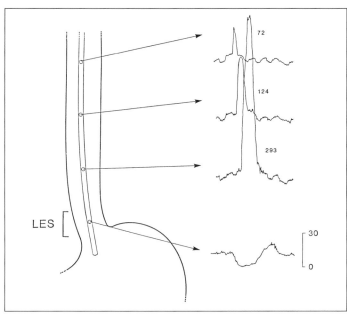

Fig. 64-4. This manometry tracing shows the typical motility features of HAPC. Esophageal body contraction amplitudes are exceedingly high, occasionally exceeding 300 mm Hg. Peristalsis is present, and the LES is normal.

doplication, which will cause obstruction. A better choice is a partial gastric wrap such as is developed by the Belsey and Toupet procedures.

Early results show that, following completion of a learning curve, both thoracoscopic and laparoscopic myotomies can be performed with appropriately low mortality and morbidity. It must be emphasized that long-term results are not available, and therefore, the role of this approach is undefined. It is possible that it will be successful enough to compete with pneumatic dilation as the initial treatment. Alternatively, it might replace the open procedures but have similar indications or, finally, it might simply be another surgical alternative.

Diffuse Esophageal Spasm and High-Amplitude Peristaltic Contractions

Diffuse esophageal spasm (DES) is a motility disorder characterized by an abnormal pattern of contractions, and high-am-

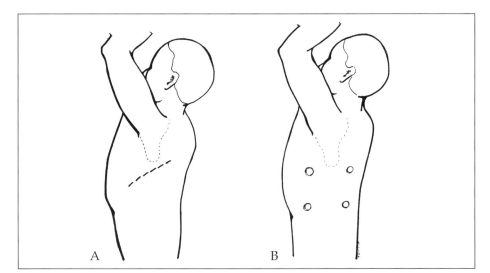

Fig. 64-5. A. The standard left thoracotomy approach to esophagomyotomy. A lateral thoracotomy extending from the midaxillary line to the angle of the ribs provides sufficient exposure. I prefer to enter the pleural cavity in the seventh intercostal space with resection of a short portion of the eighth rib beneath the paraspinous muscles to prevent unplanned mid-rib fractures. B. Port placement for thoracoscopic myotomy. Important principles include maximizing the distance between ports to avoid "fencing" of instruments and operating in the direction the camera is facing. An endoscope is placed in the esophagus and used to manipulate the esophagus and visualize the gastroesophageal junction.

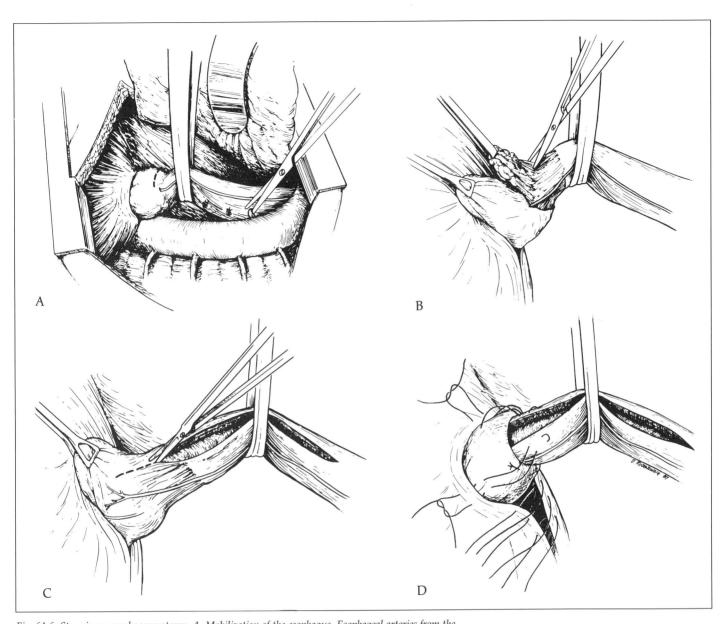

Fig. 64-6. Steps in an esophagomyotomy. A. Mobilization of the esophagus. Esophageal arteries from the aorta require ligation and division so that the esophagus can be mobilized to the aortic arch. The vagus nerves are protected. The dotted line depicts the incision to be made in the phrenoesophageal membrane so that the cardia can be completely mobilized. B. The fat pad from the cardia, including the phrenoesophageal membrane remnant, is being excised to provide complete exposure of this region for accurate performance of the myotomy. The fat pad is excised from vagus nerve to vagus nerve. C. The myotomy is being performed. Proximally the myotomy is carried to the level of the aortic arch unless the esophagus is grossly enlarged. Distally, as shown by the dotted line, the myotomy is carried unequivocally onto the stomach to ensure complete division of the fibers of the LES. The edges of the muscle are freed from the mucosa for a distance sufficient to prevent rehealing. D. The modified Belsey Mark IV fundoplication is being completed. Because the muscle of the esophagus is hypertrophied, secure bites of the esophagus can be achieved. The sutures have been placed in the hiatus, and after reduction of the cardia into the abdomen, they will be sequentially tied until the hiatal aperture is approximately the size of an index finger.

plitude peristaltic contractions (HAPC) is a separate disorder characterized by an abnormal magnitude of contractions. With DES, there are frequent simultaneous contractions in the esophageal body. Although there is some argument over the frequency with which simultaneous contractions must occur for the diagnosis, some normal peristalsis must be present to distinguish this disorder from achalasia in which there is no peristalsis. Patients with elevated contraction pressure are diagnosed as having HAPC, sometimes called a nutcracker esophagus, and are distinct from patients with DES. The LES in both patient groups is usually normal. The manometric characteristics of DES and HAPC are illustrated in Figs. 64-3 and 64-4.

The clinical pictures of both DES and HAPC are predominated by chest pain. This pain is usually perceived as squeezing but can also be described as crushing or burning. The pain is usually not related to eating, and it is common for patients to undergo evaluation for a cardiac etiology before the correct identification of the esophageal disorder. As with all esophageal motor disorders, the essential diagnostic test is esophageal manometry.

Treatment

The majority of patients with DES or HAPC do not require specific treatment, which is not surprising in light of the inability to elucidate a direct relationship between the abnormal contractions and the chest pain. Coexistence is not the same as cause and effect. The gastroenterology community has documented that reassurance of disease benignancy and psychological support are the therapeutic mainstays and are sufficient for most patients.

Surgical intervention is appropriate for only a minority of patients and only after medical or supportive management has failed. Relief of dysphagia can be expected, but the impact of a long esophagomyotomy on the chest pain is less predictable. Although the LES is usually normal, when I operate on these patients I routinely extend the myotomy across it. This step requires a Belsey antireflux procedure, but it ensures completeness of the myotomy, which seems more appropriate than risking an inadequate operation.

Historically, this operative approach has been performed via a thoracotomy; however, there is documentation that the thoracoscopic alternative is feasible. As with other types of minimally invasive surgery, both the short- and long-term results must be documented to determine the role of this surgical option.

Surgical Technique

Access for an esophagomyotomy is gained through the left chest. Figure 64-5 depicts the options of a lateral thoracotomy for an open approach and the appropriate port placements for a thorascopic procedure.

Figure 64-6 illustrates the steps in performance of an esophagomyotomy. After the chest is entered, the first step, whether open or thoracoscopic, is to divide the inferior pulmonary ligament and either retract the lung or pack it out of the way with a lap pad. Dissection within the opening of the mediastinal pleura developed by dividing the pulmonary ligament leads to the enlarged esophagus.

With the chest open, the surgeon can encircle the esophagus with blunt finger dissection and pass a Penrose drain for traction. The esophagus is mobilized from the hiatus to the aortic arch. The gastroesophageal junction is dissected free of its attachments at the hiatus and fully released. The fat usually present anteriorly at the gastroesophageal junction is removed. With this exposure, an esophagomyotomy from the aortic arch across and on to the stomach is performed. Relief of dysphagia is the operative goal, and division of all fibers of the LES is essential to achieve this outcome. This technique optimizes the achievement of the operative goal but necessitates the addition of an antireflux procedure to avoid postoperative, iatrogenic reflux.

As shown in Fig. 64-6D, the antireflux procedure of choice is a modified Belsey fundoplication. Sutures are placed in the posterior limbs of the esophageal hiatus. A 270-degree gastric wrap is constructed with two rows of horizontal mattress sutures with the second row incorporating the diaphragm. Only two sutures are placed in each row, one on each side of the myotomy. The crural sutures are tied after the fundoplication sutures.

Most surgeons performing thoracoscopic myotomy are not adding an antireflux procedure. The key is to be sure that the myotomy crosses the musculature of the LES but does not otherwise disturb the hiatus. The myotomy can be discerned through an esophageal endoscope, and this control ensures that the myotomy reaches the stomach. This procedure is similar to the one depicted in Fig. 64-6 but without such extensive mobilization of the esophagus or dissection of the hiatus. When the myotomy is performed laparoscopically, an anterior fundoplication of the Dor type is frequently added and consists of suturing the anterior gastric wall over the myotomized lower esophagus.

Suggested Reading

Ancona E, Peracchia A, Zaninotto G, et al. Heller laparoscopic cardiomyotomy with antireflux anterior fundoplication (DOR) in the treatment of esophageal achalasia. *Surg Endosc* 7P:459, 1993.

Barnett JL, Eisenman R, Nostrant TT, Elta GH. Witzel pneumatic dilation for achalasia: safety and long-term efficacy. *Gastrointest Endosc* 36:482, 1990.

Chakkapahak S, Chakkapahak K, Ferguson MK, Little AG. Disorders of esophageal motility. *Surg Gynecol Obstet* 172:325, 1991.

Dalton GB, Castell DO, Huwson EG, Wu WC, et al. Diffuse esophageal spasm. *Dig Dis Sci* 36:1025, 1991.

Ellis FH, Watkins E, Gibb SP, Heatley GJ. Ten to twenty-year clinical results after short esophagomyotomy without an antireflux procedure for esophageal achalasia. *Eur J Cardiothorac Surg* 6:86, 1992.

Ferguson MK, Little AG. Angina-like chest pain associated with high amplitude peristaltic contractions of the esophagus. *Surgery* 104:713, 1988.

Little AG, Soriano A, Ferguson MK, Wynans CS, et al. Surgical treatment of achalasia: results with esophagomyotomy and Belsey repair. *Ann Thorac Surg* 45:489, 1988.

Orr WC, Robinson MG. Hypertensive peristalsis in the pathogenesis of chest pain: further exploration of the "nutcracker" esophagus. *Am J Gastroenterol* 77:607, 1982.

Pellegrini C, Wetter LA, Patti M, Leichter R, et al. Thoracoscopic esophagomyotomy: initial experience with a new approach to the treatment of achalasia. *Ann Surg* 216:291, 1992.

EDITOR'S COMMENT

Achalasia of the esophagus is a disease that is successfully treated surgically both through the chest and through the abdomen. Surgeons who operate in the left upper quadrant of the abdomen far more frequently than in the chest are most able to deal with achalasia through the abdomen, since the 5- to 8-cm esophagomyotomy can usually be performed without difficulty through the left upper quadrant subcostal incision, and a Nissen fundoplication can be added to the procedure without undue extra difficulty or operative time. After opening the phrenoesophageal ligament, the vagus nerves are protected, and the distal 6 to 8 cm of esophagus is carefully exposed.

The myotomy can be performed over a 50 French dilator, and the myotomy, not dissimilar from the pyloromyotomy for pyloric stenosis in the infant, should extend to the submucosa with no circular muscle fibers left intact. In addition, the myotomy should extend down onto the stomach, for at least 2 to 3 cm, to be sure that none of the LES fibers is left intact. Great care should be exercised when the gastric wall is reached, since it is more difficult to separate the gastric musculature from the submucosa without perforating it than is the case with the esophagus, where there is a clear plane between the submucosa and the circular muscle.

If a tiny perforation occurs in the mucosa or submucosa of the stomach, it will be simple to repair that with one or two fine absorbable sutures. That defect will be covered with the Nissen fundoplication, which is always performed now to protect the esophagus from reflux. A floppy Nissen as popularized by Donahue and colleagues is the preferred antireflux procedure of choice, whether performed for restoration of an antireflux mechanism in patients with achalasia or for pure reflux.

As Dr. Little notes, in treating achalasia, it seems to make little difference whether the myotomy that is done is short on the esophagus or extends to the arch of the aorta. However, treatment of diffuse esophageal spasm and high-amplitude peristaltic contractions (nutcracker esophagus) must include a very long esophagomyotomy, often extending to the thoracic inlet. Bleeding is minimal, and many surgeons prefer not to use cautery on the muscularis of the esophagus, for fear of causing thermal injury to the submucosa and mucosa, perhaps resulting in delayed perforation in the postoperative period. However, the thoracoscopic approach to esophagomyotomy requires cautery, and there appears to be no particular difficulty when minimally invasive surgery is undertaken. Enthusiasts for thoracoscopic operations on the esophagus are convinced that the operations are not only safe but will also ultimately be considerably shorter than the conventional ones, since there is no long posterolateral thoracotomy incision to open or close. The enormous advantage of minimal postoperative pain with the thoracoscopic approach makes this option an attractive one, and it is quite obvious that many esophageal and pulmonary operations will be accomplished with the thoracoscope in both the near future and the long term.

In patients with dysphagia, one cannot overemphasize the importance of endoscopic examination of the esophagus before any operation for achalasia or other myoneural motility disorders. A small but finite percentage of these patients have a carcinoma as the actual cause of the dysphagia, and the myotomy simply delays the appropriate treatment for the tumor, resulting in a tragedy. The endoscopist always enters the stomach and the duodenum to rule out other or associated causes of dysphagia but most importantly to rule out neoplasm.

R.J.B.

65

Esophagectomy Without Thoracotomy (Transhiatal Esophagectomy) and Gastric or Colonic Replacement of the Esophagus

Hiroshi Akiyama

Principal Techniques of Esophagectomy Without Thoracotomy

The technique of esophagectomy without thoracotomy had been forgotten for many years since its discovery in the late nineteenth and early twentieth centuries. Later, the technique was proved by many authors to be a useful method. It is still considered useful in light of recent developments in thoracoscopic esophagectomy. Although there is some overlap in terminology, this chapter details techniques of esophagectomy without thoracotomy. Mechanical systems and instruments developed for video-assisted surgery can also be used in the mediastinal phase of esophagectomy without thoracotomy.

Esophagectomy without thoracotomy is not a surgical procedure specifically indicated for the treatment of a particular esophageal lesion. Instead, it is a useful technique that surgeons should use as necessary when indicated. If serious abnormal bleeding arises during blunt extraction of the esophagus, it should be discontinued immediately and the mediastinum packed so that the resection can be completed under direct vision via thoracotomy. However, this occurrence should be rare.

The indications for performing esophagectomy without thoracotomy are important to know. Carcinoma of the hypopharynx and cervical esophagus with or without concomitant mucosal cancers of the tho-racic esophagus, wide or multicentric intraepithelial or lamina propria muscularis cancers of the esophagus, and benign esophageal lesions are the common indications. In many of these patients, the vagi can be preserved. It is also indicated for some of the palliative resections of malignant lesions of the lower esophagus and cardia. In attempted curative resection of advanced cancer, vagal preservation is not possible. Thoracoscopic esophagectomy is valuable in the management of esophageal lesions. However, when its aim is only a simple esophagectomy and when cervical and abdominal incisions are already made, conventional esophagectomy without thoracotomy seems superior because of its simplicity and rapidity.

There are several techniques for esophagectomy without thoracotomy. Blunt dissection (blunt finger dissection) and eversion stripping are the two basic principles (Fig. 65-1). The other techniques are modifications or combinations of these principles. Selection of the procedure in terms of

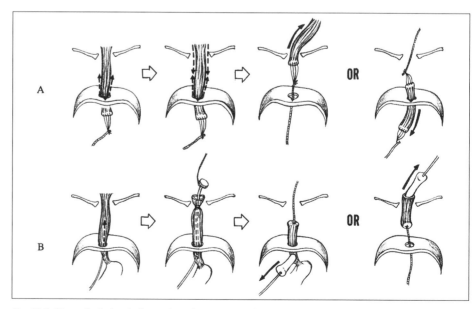

Fig. 65-1. Two principal techniques of esophagectomy without thoracotomy. A. Blunt finger dissection. B. Eversion stripping.

the nature and location of the esophageal lesion must be carefully considered before application of the technique. Although this technique violates one of the most fundamental principles of surgery, that the surgical procedure should be done under direct vision, it can be safely performed using the following techniques.

Blunt Finger Dissection

The skin incision is from the xiphoid process to just above the umbilicus. Longer incisions extending below the umbilicus are unnecessary. After dividing the left triangular ligament, the lateral segment of the left lobe of the liver is retracted to the right as necessary. In order to have a wide opening of the esophageal hiatus, an incision is made in the anterior portion of the crus of the diaphragm and along the midline through the central tendon of the diaphragm (Fig. 65-2A). The central tendon is dissected away from the pericardial sac. When necessary, the heart is gently elevated using a flat malleable intestinal retractor behind the freed pericardial sac. The right and left mediastinal pleurae are pushed laterally so that the esophageal hiatus is widely opened and good exposure

of the lower mediastinum is obtained. The lower half of the esophagus is exposed in the enlarged esophageal hiatus and can easily be dissected under direct vision (Fig. 65-2B). Only the small segment of the middle thoracic esophagus, not within the reach of direct vision, is blindly and bluntly dissected. Although the dissection can be performed bluntly with fingers, the use of various instruments designed for thoracoscopic or laparoscopic surgery is recommended as necessary.

The esophagus is transected a few centimeters above the cardioesophageal junction. Blunt finger dissection of the thoracic esophagus is performed by maintaining downward traction of the esophagus (Fig. 65-3A). One of the most important procedures is the handling of the vagus nerves. The bilateral vagi running along the esophagus are hooked with the index finger (Fig. 65-3B) and dissected inferiorly until they can be reached via the esophageal hiatus. The vagal nerve trunks are preferably preserved (see Preservation of the Vagus Nerves). However, for instances in which the vagi cannot be preserved because of tumor or for clinical reasons, the nerves are divided with scissors. The ceph-

alad dissection of the esophagus is further continued via the esophageal hiatus to the level of the tracheal bifurcation. It is essential to free the esophagus from the surrounding tissue along its adventitia.

The upper portion of the thoracic esophagus is dissected from the thoracic inlet down toward the tracheal bifurcation using blunt finger dissection. There are no difficulties in this dissection. However, care should be taken not to traumatize the membranous portion of the trachea and the recurrent laryngeal nerves, particularly on the left side. Upward traction of the cervical esophagus is maintained while blunt finger dissection along the adventitia of the esophagus is used. Once the dissection is completed, the surgeon can feel that the entire esophagus has become mobile. The esophagus can then be extracted via the neck. Alternatively, after transection at the cervical level, the esophagus can also be extracted caudally via the hiatus. However, upward extraction of the esophagus is preferable, because anatomically the nerve fibers are more easily detached from the esophagus in this direction (Fig. 65-1A). When the posterior mediastinal tunnel is used as the route for esophageal

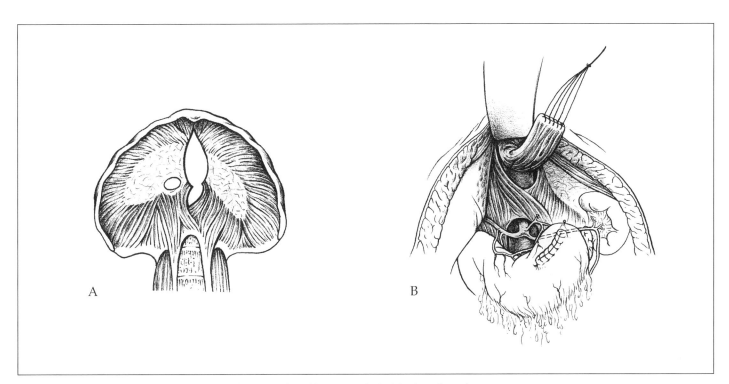

Fig. 65-2. Techniques for obtaining a wide surgical field of esophageal hiatus. A. The incision is made on the midline of the central tendon of the diaphragm. B. With this procedure, a much wider space in the lower mediastinum between the esophagus and aorta is available for direct vision and manual maneuver.

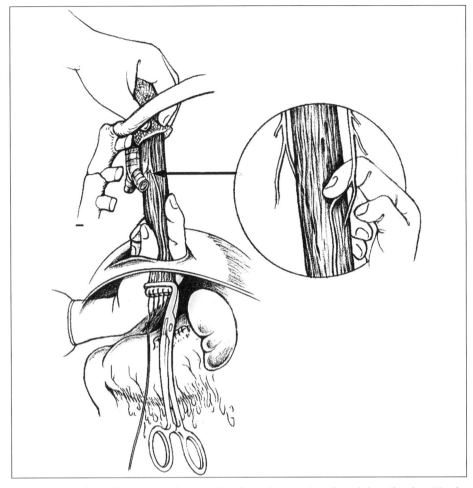

reconstruction, a tape is tied to the end of the esophagus before extraction. This tape is later used to guide and bring up the stomach or colon as the esophageal substitute.

Eversion Stripping

Among various surgical techniques, eversion or invagination stripping is a technically simple method of extracting the thoracic esophagus. For this procedure, a vein stripper is useful (Fig. 65-4A). A small perforation is made on the anterior wall of the abdominal portion of the esophagus or on the anterior wall of the cardia of the stomach. The wire of the vein stripper is inserted via the perforation into the lumen of the thoracic esophagus. The wire is then advanced upward until it can be palpated through the wall of the cervical esophagus. The cervical esophagus is then perforated by the tip of wire and an obturator, or bead, is attached for subsequent stripping. The end of the wire is secured in place by a heavy tie just distal to the perforation. The cervical portion of the esophagus is then transected just above the perforation. Both cut ends are disinfected.

Before stripping the esophagus, the abdominal cavity should be thoroughly prepared to isolate the field with a sterile towel. The stripper is gently pulled downward. The entire length of the thoracic esophagus is thus extracted, being invag-

Fig. 65-3. Blunt finger dissection technique. A. Blunt finger dissection is performed along the adventitia of the esophagus. B. Esophageal branches of the vagus nerve (here, left vagus) are hooked with the index finger and are dissected downward until they are seen via the enlarged esophageal hiatus.

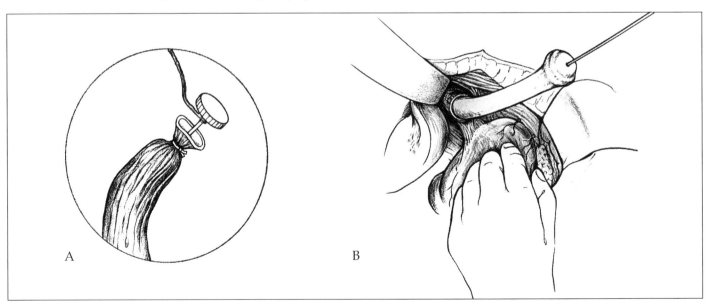

Fig. 65-4. Eversion stripping. A. Appropriate size of tubes or guides of any materials can be used. However, a vein stripper is useful. After insertion of a wire intraluminally, a head, or obturator, is placed on the tip of wire. A tape is attached to the wire for passage of an abdominal organ for esophageal replacement. B. The esophagus is being extracted by invagination and the mucosal surface everted.

inated with its mucosal surface everted. It should be extracted smoothly by gentle, steady traction and without much bleeding (Fig. 65-4B).

Modified Techniques of Esophagectomy Without Thoracotomy

Turnover Stripping

Blunt dissection is performed using a narrow flat retractor in the prevertebral space throughout the posterior mediastinum (arrow in (Fig. 65-5). A guide is introduced into the space thus created and is connected to the distal divided end of the esophagus in the neck. By drawing down the guide, turnover stripping of the esophagus is completed. Upward stripping is also possible in the same manner.

Preservation of the Vagus Nerves

Although correct management of the vagus nerve is a key aspect of esophagectomy without thoracotomy, vagal preservation has only recently been described. In esophagectomy without thoracotomy, the vagi are too often transected without any particular attention being paid to the consequences. Weight loss, intermittent diarrhea or steatorrhea, the dumping syndrome, and postvagotomy biliary disease are characteristic features of the postvagotomy syndrome. It has been suggested that postvagotomy diarrhea is related to division of the celiac and hepatic fibers of the vagus nerves, and that the incidence of diarrhea following truncal vagotomy can be reduced from 25 percent to only 2 percent by selective vagotomy when the celiac

and hepatic branches are preserved. Therefore, preservation of these branches is worthwhile, even when total preservation is not possible. By using the techniques herewith described, the vagus can be preserved and development of the postvagotomy syndrome avoided.

The techniques of vagal preservation differ depending on 1) the method of esophagectomy, 2) whether the whole vagus or only the celiac and hepatic branches are preserved, 3) the primary esophageal disease, and 4) the mode of esophageal reconstruction. After giving off the right and left recurrent laryngeal nerves and pulmonary branches, both vagus nerves enter the esophagus. From this point, the vagal trunks and the vagal plexus run down to the cardia embedded in the esophageal wall. The method of vagal preservation used is determined by anatomic relationship and the angle between the esophagus and the nerves.

Vagal Preservation in Blunt Dissection Esophagectomy

In the conventional method of blunt dissection using the fingers, the esophageal branch of the vagus nerve is hooked with the index finger at the level where it enters the esophagus. Vagal preservation can be achieved by continuing further dissection of the nerves down to the cardia (Fig. 65-3B). This preservation can also be achieved by initially freeing the vagi at the level of the esophageal hiatus and dissecting the nerves upward (Fig. 65-6).

Vagal Preservation in Eversion Stripping

Vagal Preservation in Downward Eversion Stripping. From the anatomic point

of view, no particular preparation is needed before downward eversion stripping, unless the vagi are carelessly cut when the abdominal esophagus is transected (Fig. 65-7A).

Vagal Preservation in Upward Eversion Stripping. With upward eversion stripping of the esophagus, the main vagal trunks are pulled downward for countertraction, so that the vagi are separated from the esophagus. Some small esophageal branches are torn off when stripping is completed (Fig. 65-7B). There is no damage to the recurrent laryngeal nerves and the pulmonary branches because they diverge from the main vagal trunks at some distance from the esophagus.

Type of Vagal Preservation

Partial Vagal Preservation. When the stomach is used as an esophageal substitute, the gastric branches must be sacrificed and the nerves of Laterjet divided. In order to preserve the celiac and hepatic branches, the gastric branches are severed close to the gastric wall. When the blood supply to the upper lesser curvature and cardia becomes insufficient as a result, partial gastrectomy can be necessary (Fig. 65-8A).

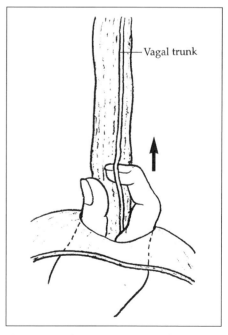

Fig. 65-6. Vagal preservation in blunt finger dissection technique.

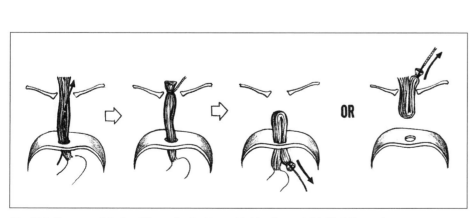

Fig. 65-5. Turnover stripping. The mediastinal tunnel is bluntly created behind the esophagus.

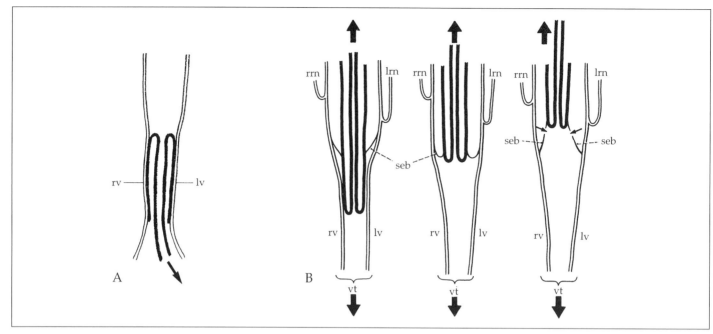

Fig. 65-7. Vagal preservation in eversion stripping technique. A. Downward eversion stripping. No particular attempts are needed. B. Upward eversion stripping. The main vagal trunks are pulled downward for countertraction. Small esophageal branches are automatically torn (arrows). (rrn, lrn = right, left recurrent nerves; rv, lv = right, left vagal trunks; seb = small esophageal branches; vt = vagal trunk.)

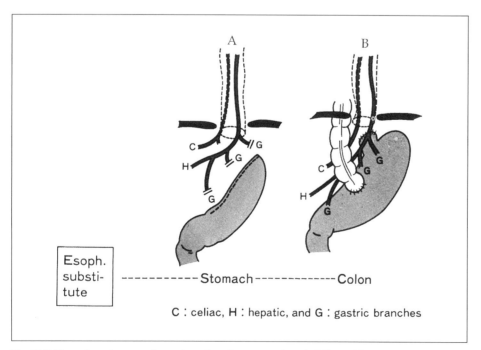

Fig. 65-8. Type of vagal preservation and esophageal reconstruction. A. Celiac and hepatic branches are preserved. B. Total vagal preservation. (C = celiac branches; H = hepatic branches; G = gastric branches.)

Total Vagal Preservation. This type includes preservation of the celiac, hepatic, and gastric branches of the vagus. For total vagal preservation, the vagal trunks are separated from the esophagus, and the abdominal portion of the esophagus is transected with the vagal trunks intact. Thus, the whole stomach is preserved in situ (Fig. 65-8B). Esophageal reconstruction is then performed with the colon.

Transoral Esophagectomy

The principal techniques for transoral esophagectomy are shown in Fig. 65-9. An orogastric tube is inserted. This tube is securely fixed to the abdominal esophagus by a heavy suture. The esophagus is then transected below the level of ligation. The cervical esophagus is identified via a small neck incision (Fig. 65-9A). In the abdomen, by holding the vagus nerves downward as a countertraction, the tube inserted via the mouth is pulled outward. The thoracic esophagus is then transorally stripped out, being invaginated with the mucosal surface facing outside. One of the cut ends of

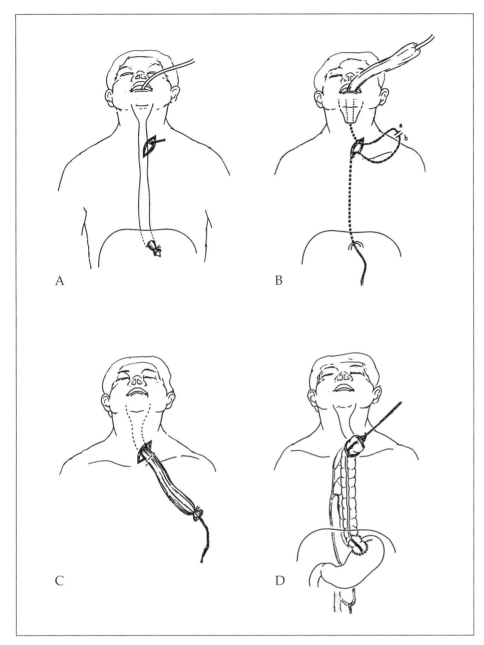

Mucosal Stripping of the Esophagus

This operation has a limited but special indication as described below. A tape is placed around the cervical esophagus. A transverse incision is made in the adventitio-muscular layer of the esophagus so that the mucosal column is separated from the remaining esophageal wall. The incision is placed only on the anterior wall of the cervical esophagus, which facilitates identification and creation of the mucosal column (Fig. 65-10).

A guide is inserted into the lumen of the abdominal esophagus and is pushed upward. The mucosal column in the neck is fixed around the end of the guide. The remaining posterior wall of the cervical esophagus is then divided above the point of fixation. As the guide is being pulled down, only the mucosal layer is stripped out (Fig. 65-10B, C).

In our series, mucosal stripping of the esophagus was used for an intractable old empyema caused by delayed diagnosis and inappropriate treatment for a spontaneous rupture of the esophagus. This technique is a suitable, safe, and lifesaving technique for such a very poor risk patient. The advantages of mucosal stripping of the esophagus are that a smaller dead space is left minimizing the risk of contamination from the empyema, and bleeding will not occur. Use of this technique for malignancies is not appropriate.

Techniques of Esophageal Reconstruction Using the Stomach or Colon After Esophagectomy Without Thoracotomy

Use of the Stomach

The greater curvature of the stomach is freed preserving the right gastroepiploic arteries and veins. The short gastric arteries and veins are all divided and ligated. The left gastric artery and vein are severed at their roots in order to preserve the entire length of the marginal vascular arcade along the lesser curvature. Thus, the whole stomach receives its blood supply from the

Fig. 65-9. Transoral esophagectomy techniques. A. A guide is inserted via the mouth and fixed to the abdominal esophagus. The cervical esophagus is palpated until extraction is completed up to this point (arrow). B. Transorally stripped out esophagus. By pulling the end of the tape (a), the esophagus is re-extracted via the neck (see C). C. Re-extracted esophagus. The esophagus is then transected (arrow). D. By pulling tape "b" in B, the colon (or stomach) is elevated as an esophageal substitute. The vascular pedicle of the colon is placed behind the stomach.

the tape (a in Fig. 65-9A) is used to extract the transorally stripped esophagus outside the neck (Fig. 65-9B). The everted esophagus is returned to normal condition with the adventitia outside. The stripped out esophagus is then resected at any level according to the primary lesion (Fig. 65-9C).

The other cut end of the tape (b in Fig. 65-9B) is used to bring an esophageal substitute up to the neck (Fig. 65-9D). The advantages of this operation are minimal tissue dissection, minimal chance of contamination, and preservation of the vagus nerves.

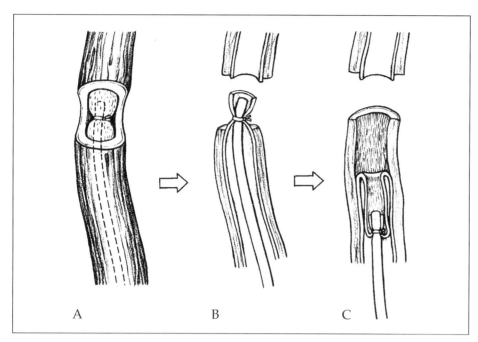

Fig. 65-10. *Mucosal stripping of the esophagus. A. In order to make it easier to dissect the entire circumferential mucosal column in the neck, only the anterior wall of the muscle layer is incised before the esophagus is entirely severed. A guide is tightly fixed to the mucosal column. B. The esophagus is transected. C. The mucosal column is extracted.*

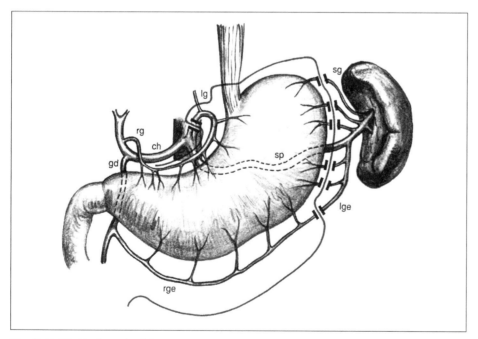

Fig. 65-11. *The blood supply of the entire stomach as an esophageal substitute. (rge, lge = right, left gastroepiploic artery; rg, lg = right, left gastric artery; sp = splenic artery; sg = short gastric artery; ch = common hepatic artery; gd = gastroduodenal artery.) (From H Akiyama.* Surgery for Cancer of the Esophagus. *Baltimore: Williams & Wilkins, 1990. Reprinted with permission.)*

right gastric and gastroepiploic arteries (Fig. 65-11). The abdominal esophagus is transected, and both ends are closed.

Before transposition of the stomach via the mediastinum, accurate selection of the "highest point of the stomach" is of the utmost importance (Fig. 65-12). The stomach is gently stretched and the highest point at the fundus is identified and chosen for the site of anastomosis in the neck. After esophagectomy without thoracotomy, the posterior mediastinum is usually chosen as the route of transposition (Fig. 65-13). When the operation is for malignancy of the thoracic esophagus, division of the left gastric artery at its origin and resection of the left gastric area of the lesser curvature is mandatory.

In the majority of reconstructions using the stomach, pyloroplasty is unnecessary. In functional postoperative pyloric dysfunction, balloon dilatation of the pylorus is effective.

Use of the Colon

In esophageal reconstruction after esophagectomy without thoracotomy, use of the colon is particularly advantageous when it is used in conjunction with preservation of the vagus nerves and the stomach in situ. When indicated and possible, this method of esophageal reconstruction (Fig. 65-8B) probably represents the ideal in terms of full capacity of a food reservoir with satisfactory function.

The effective design and use of the colon are achieved in an isoperistaltic manner. Entire mobilization of the colon is essential for the appropriate selection of vessels as a vascular pedicle. The selection is usually made from the right colon toward the left. The occlusion test is made in the order of the ileocolic, right colic, and middle colic arteries and veins. The middle colic and left colic vessels are frequently and conventionally used as the nutrient vessels for the use of the right and transverse or left colon substitute, respectively (Fig. 65-14). In transposition of the colon, the vascular pedicle lies behind the stomach (Fig. 65-9D).

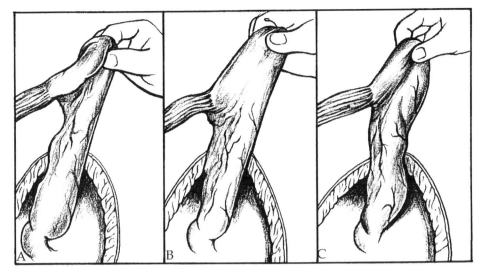

Fig. 65-12. Selection of the highest point of the stomach. A. Too close to the cardia. B. Appropriate. C. Too far from the cardia.

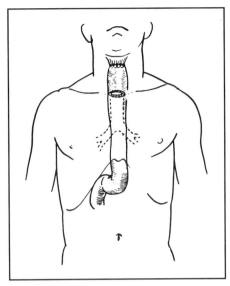

Fig. 65-13. Transposition of the stomach to the neck. After esophagectomy without thoracotomy, the posterior mediastinum is the common route for esophageal reconstruction (pharyngogastrostomy is shown here).

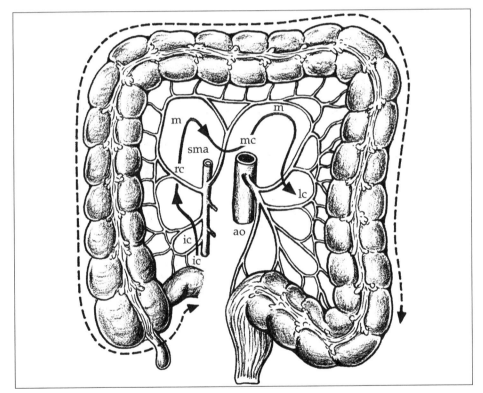

Fig. 65-14. Selection of the nutritional vessel for isoperistaltic colonic transposition. The order of checking the result of vascular clamping is shown by the arrow (in the order of 1, 2, 3). Entire freeing of the colon (dotted line) is important for this selection. (ao = aorta; lc = left colic artery; sma = superior mesenteric artery; mc = middle colic artery; rc = right colic artery; ic = ileocolic artery; m = marginal artery.)

Suggested Reading

Akiyama H. *Surgery for Cancer of the Esophagus.* Baltimore: Williams & Wilkins, 1990.

Akiyama H, Hiyama M, Miyazono H. Total esophageal reconstruction after extraction of the esophagus. *Ann Surg* 182:547, 1975.

Akiyama H, Miyazono M, Tsurumaru M, Hashimoto C. Use of the stomach as an esophageal substitute. *Ann Surg* 188:606, 1978.

Akiyama H, Sato Y, Takahashi F. Immediate pharyngogastrostomy following total esophagectomy by blunt dissection. *Jpn J Surg* 1:225, 1971.

Akiyama H, Tsurumaru M, Kawamura T, Ono Y. Esophageal stripping with preservation of the vagus nerve. *Int Surg* 67: 125, 1982.

Akiyama H, Tsurumaru M, Kawamura T, Ono Y. Principles of surgical treatment for carcinoma of the esophagus. *Ann Surg* 194:438, 1981.

Akiyama H, Tsurumaru M, Ono Y, et al. Esophagectomy without thoracotomy with vagal preservation. *J Amer Coll Surg* 178:83, 1994.

Akiyama H, Tsurumaru M, Ono Y, et al. Mucosal stripping of the esophagus. *Dis Esoph* 6:27, 1993.

Akiyama H, Tsurumaru M, Ono Y, et al. Transoral esophagectomy. *Surg Gynecol Obstet* 173:399, 1991.

Dorothea MI, Liebermann-Meffert D, Luescher URS, et al. Esophagectomy without thoracotomy: Is there a risk of intramediastinal bleeding? A study on blood supply of the esophagus. *Ann Surg* 206:184, 1987.

LeQuesne LP, Ranger D. Pharyngolaryngectomy with immediate pharyngogastric anastomosis. *Br J Surg* 53:105, 1966.

Liebermann-Meffert D, Siewert JR. Arterial anatomy of the esophagus. A review of the literature with brief comments on clinical aspects. *Gullet* 2:3, 1992.

Ong GB. Carcinoma of the Hypopharynx and Cervical Oesophagus. In R. Smith (ed.), *Progress in Clinical Surgery.* London: J & A Churchill, 1969.

Orringer MB, Orringer JS. Esophagectomy without thoracotomy: A dangerous operation? *J Thorac Cardiovasc Surg* 85:72, 1983.

Pinotti HW, Zilberstein B, Pollara W, Raia A. Esophagectomy without thoracotomy. *Surg Gynecol Obstet* 152:345, 1981.

Saidi F. Endoesophageal pull through. A technique for the treatment of cancers of the cardia and lower esophagus. *Ann Surg* 207:446, 1988.

EDITOR'S COMMENT

Professor Akiyama has provided a concise and valuable description of the technique of esophagectomy without thoracotomy. However, he modified the concept somewhat when he discussed the mediastinal dissection of the esophagus with the thoracoscope. In fact, this relatively new instrumentation has provided a substantial safety factor in two respects: 1) in direct visualization of the tumor and separation of the tumor from the posterior wall of the trachea or bronchus and 2) in avoiding or promptly dealing with bleeding that, although uncommon, can occur in the middle third of the mediastinum, particularly behind the arch of the aorta or at the level of the azygos vein.

Although the text describes transecting the esophagus a few centimeters above the cardioesophageal junction, Fig. 65-2B illustrates what most surgeons do for squamous cell cancer (i. e., transect the terminal esophagus with a small cuff of stomach in order to eliminate the possibility of submucosal spread of tumor inferiorly and recurrence at that site). Further, it is easier to pass the stomach into the neck through the posterior mediastinum if the esophageal stump does not remain, but there is a smooth, usually stapled, closure of the lesser curvature of the gastroesophageal junction. In fact, some esophageal surgeons purposely resect much of the lesser curve of the stomach with a stapler to decrease the bulk of stomach to be brought to the neck and to facilitate passage of the gastric tube through the thoracic inlet.

A very important advance in esophagectomy is the management of the vagus nerves where they become intramuscular in the central portion of the thoracic esophagus. Professor Akiyama has shown conclusively that esophagectomy does not infer automatic vagotomy, and the technique that he originally described of preserving the vagus nerves would appear to have great promise. Not having performed this maneuver to preserve the vagi, I am unable to comment on its effectiveness, but fully accept that the author's modification should add considerably to the quality of life and the function of the gastric reservoir as well as the hepatobiliary branch function which is described as being preserved. This aspect of the operation would definitely be enhanced by doing the procedure with the thoracoscope, under direct vision, rather than using digital dissection through the mediastinum where actually seeing the structures must be quite difficult.

Two techniques herein described, transoral esophagectomy and mucosal stripping of the esophagus are very interesting and undoubtedly useful modifications of the technique with, however, very specific and limited indications. Mucosal stripping of the esophagus in patients with Barrett's esophagus for significant esophagitis would, I would think, be extremely difficult, and perhaps not possible, as the inflammatory process is often transmural and would lead to shredding or incomplete removal of the esophageal mucosa and submucosa. Whether this procedure would have any use in patients with diffuse esophageal spasm when thoracotomy cannot be performed is more problematic.

Overall, the indications for the three-stage operation (the Ivor Lewis procedure), performed simultaneously, of cervical exploration, usually on the left, right thoracotomy to remove the esophagus, and midline abdominal laparotomy to assess operability and to free the stomach or colon, has in most centers been largely supplanted by transhiatal total esophagectomy, or esophagectomy without thoracotomy. There is no question about the advantages of transhiatal esophagectomy in patients with poor pulmonary function, serious myocardial disease, or other serious systemic entities that formerly were considered contraindications to esophagectomy. Overall, the complication rates are probably not dissimilar, but the morbidity is substantially less with this procedure than with the transthoracic esophagectomy. Numerous studies have demonstrated that the difference in survival rates for esophageal cancer are not statistically significant in both the operative procedures (Hankins JR, et al. *Ann Thorac Surg* 47:700, 1989), and blood loss appears to be approximately the same. Because of the possibility of cardiac arrhythmias during the manipulation in the mediastinum, as well as the finite, possibility of significant bleeding, most surgeons and anesthesiologists perform this procedure with the use of central cardiac hemodynamic monitoring, specifically with a pulmonary artery catheter. Since the surgical approach to the neck, or even to the mediastinum, may be necessary, a subclavian catheter can be placed prior to or at the induction of anesthesia, and these catheters prove their worth many times over both during the operation and in the postoperative period. Mixed venous oxygen saturation can, likewise, be used for this purpose, but the advantages of the pulmonary artery catheter, and the obtaining of wedge pressure data, makes this device most useful.

A particularly important use of thoracoscopy, in addition to assisting in the dissection of the central portion of the esophagus where the tumor is frequently located, is the staging of the tumor; with smaller tumors, which are less likely to be bulky and have probably not invaded the full thickness of the esophageal wall, it is possible to sample nodes if not actually dissect the mediastinum, particularly in the area of the tumor for staging. However, under any circumstances, the patient will undoubtedly be subjected to radiation therapy and chemotherapy in the postoperative period, or, with some of the newer protocols, in the preoperative period. Although cure rates for squamous cell cancer of the esophagus are improving slightly, these are still highly unfavorable tumors, in general, and the expeditious removal as with this technique is an attractive option in terms of lesser patient discomfort and perhaps lesser morbidity overall.

R.J.B.

66

The Esophageal Anastomosis in Excision of the Esophagus

John Wong   Manson Fok

Surgery for carcinoma of the esophagus carries one of the highest morbidity and mortality risks associated with any elective operation. The three most common causes of hospital deaths are respiratory failure, advancing malignancy, and surgical sepsis. The principal cause of the latter is anastomotic leakage. The absence of a sturdy serosal layer in the esophagus and the apparent precarious blood supply of the substitute organ are often blamed as factors predisposing to anastomotic breakdown. However, careful preparation of the organs for anastomosis, meticulous attention to technical details, and ensuring that the union is tension-free result in a low occurrence of anastomotic leakage. The surgeon's technique is probably more important than whether the method of anastomosis is one- or two-layered, interrupted or continuous hand suturing, or circular stapling.

In our practice, all hand-sewn anastomoses are performed in a standard manner regardless of the level of anastomosis or type of substitute used. The circular stapler (EEA, U. S. Surgical Corporation, Norwalk, CT, or ILS, Ethicon, Inc., Somerville, N.J.) can be used for anastomosis in the chest or abdomen, but it is awkward to use in the neck because of limited bowel length and confined space. A detailed description of how the esophagus and the substitute organs are prepared for anastomosis is described in Chap. 85. For illustration, esophageal anastomoses made by circular stapling and by hand in the right thoracic apex are described below.

Preparation of the Esophagus

For the common middle third esophageal cancer, the patient is placed in a left lateral position and a right posterolateral thoracotomy is performed through the fifth intercostal space. The entire esophagus including the tumor is mobilized together with the paraesophageal, paratracheal, parabronchial, and subcarinal lymph nodes; and the thoracic duct; and the mediastinum is bared. The esophagus is freed proximally to the triangular apex of the right thoracic cavity bordered by the membranous trachea in front, vertebra behind, and the subclavian artery cranially.

Before the esophagus is divided, the nasogastric tube is withdrawn to a position just proximal to the intended line of division, with suction being applied to the tube for gastric decompression and for removal of secretions within the esophageal lumen. With the esophagus slightly stretched, a medium Satinsky clamp is placed across the freed esophagus approximately 2 cm distal to the thoracic apex. An adequate in situ proximal margin of at least 6 cm from the tumor is ascertained before the esophagus is divided flush with the Satinsky clamp by electrocautery.

The distal esophagus bearing the tumor remains attached to the intra-abdominal stomach. The previously mobilized stomach is then gently delivered into the thoracic cavity via the diaphragmatic hiatus and its proper orientation confirmed. The esophagus with the tumor is then removed

after the stomach has been stapled by a 90-mm linear stapler applied across from the angle of His to the middle of the gastric lesser curve. The stomach should be lying in the esophageal bed and brought up without tension for anastomosis with the esophagus (Fig. 66-1).

The Stapled Anastomosis

When the Satinsky clamp on the proximal divided esophagus is released, the esophagus retracts upward. Its wall is gently picked up with serrated forceps, and six 3–0 silk stay sutures are placed at equal distances from each other, incorporating all layers of the esophagus and at depth of 1 cm from the divided margin. These stay sutures are slid from adventitia toward the lumen and outward to expose the mucosa for the anastomosis.

An EEA sizer is then inserted into the esophagus to gauge the size of stapler to be used. The stay sutures are gently pulled outward to facilitate insertion. The size of circular stapler used is determined by the following criteria: if the small (25 mm) sizer cannot be admitted, a 25-mm stapler is used. If the small sizer can be admitted comfortably but the medium (28 mm) sizer cannot, a 28-mm stapler is used. If the medium sizer can be admitted but the large (31 mm) sizer cannot, a 29-mm stapler is used. If the large sizer can be inserted either sparingly or comfortably, a 31-mm stapler or a 33-mm stapler is chosen, respectively. We select the largest size stapler

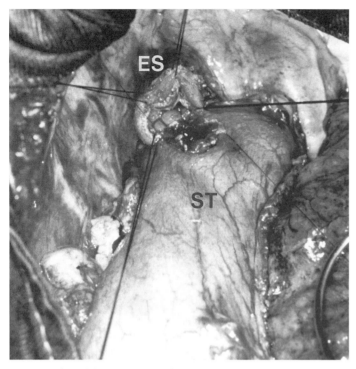

Fig. 66-1. The mobilized stomach, with its arcade (blood supply) based on the right gastroepiploic and right gastric vessels, is delivered into the right thoracic cavity via the diaphragmatic hiatus. For a hand-sewn anastomosis, a clear area near the apex of the fundus is chosen as the site of anastomosis. (ES = esophagus; ST = stomach.)

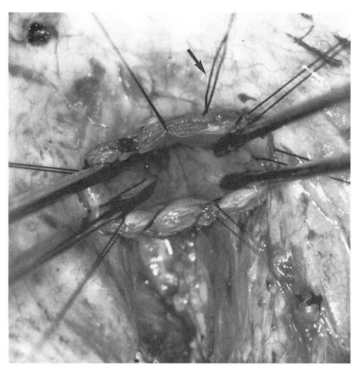

Fig. 66-2. The stapled anastomosis (Figs. 66-2 through 66-6). The esophagus is divided at the thoracic apex, six 3–0 silk stay sutures are placed at equal distances apart to keep the esophageal lumen open. For stapling, a continuous pursestring suture using 0-Prolene (polypropylene) is first made around the margin of the esophagus (arrow).

that can be inserted safely into the esophagus because of the increased incidence of anastomotic stricture associated with the smaller size staplers.

Following the selection of stapler size, a pursestring is placed around the proximal esophagus using a 0-Prolene (polypropylene) suture. We choose a strong monofilament suture for its sliding property and strength. The pursestring suture is placed from adventitia to mucosa starting at the middle of the anterior lip of the esophagus 5 mm from the edge. It is then brought out (mucosa to adventitia), and the subsequent suturing follows this direction over the edge of the esophagus to complete the circle, ending with both ends of the pursestring on the outside. The stay sutures are kept tight during the placement of the pursestring to ensure each bite takes in an adequate tissue depth and is of full thickness but without catching other adjacent tissues. After the placement of the pursestring, the esophageal lumen is irrigated with normal saline and dilated again with the chosen sizer in preparation for the anastomosis (Fig. 66-2).

For the insertion of the stapler shaft into the stomach, a 2-cm anterior gastrotomy is made in its mid-body with electrocautery. Held apart by three Babcock forceps, the gastrotomy is dilated with the chosen sizer. The stapling instrument (without the anvil) is inserted into the stomach toward the gastric fundus. The center rod of the stapler shaft is advanced through a clear area on the back of the fundus near the apex, away from blood vessels and the linear staple line. Once the center rod has perforated the gastric wall, the anvil nut is securely fitted and the center rod is advanced maximally to allow easy maneuverability of the anvil without traction on the stomach. No pursestring is necessary on the gastric side.

With the stay sutures held tightly apart, the anvil is inserted into the esophageal lumen (Fig. 66-3). To facilitate insertion, the anvil is first tilted under the anterior lip of the esophageal wall, then followed by the posterior lip. The alternate pulling of the anterior stay sutures and the posterior stay sutures will maneuver the esophageal circumference around the anvil more easily

and minimizes the risk of splitting the esophagus. Occasionally, when there is limited space between the trachea and the vertebra, the anvil can be more easily inserted inside the posterior lip of the esophagus before the anterior lip. After the placement of the entire anvil into the esophageal lumen, the pursestring is tightened by sliding the monofilament suture back and forth to close the edge of the esophagus around the center rod. The suture is securely fastened with a triple throw of surgeon's knot (Fig. 66-4). The stay sutures should be relaxed when the pursestring is being tied and can be removed after the knot is secured.

Before closure of the anvil onto the stapler shaft, the anvil with the proximal esophagus is pulled downward and outward to avoid incorporating the membranous trachea. The sheen of the metallic part of the anvil can sometimes be seen through the esophageal muscle. The wall of the stomach is also examined to ensure a smooth gastric surface on stapling. The anvil is then apposed to the shaft and fired. The stapler is disengaged and removed by first

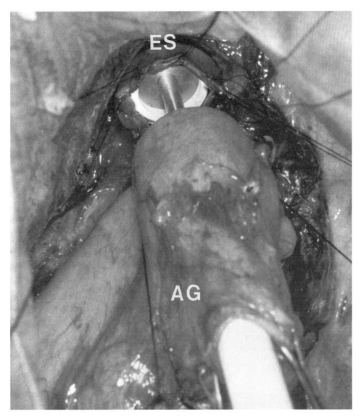

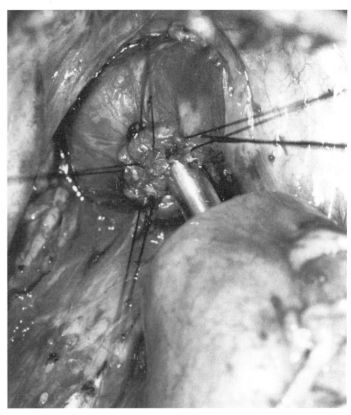

Fig. 66-3. After the stapling instrument without the anvil is introduced into the stomach via an anterior gastrotomy, the center rod is advanced through a clear area at the back of the gastric fundus near the apex. With the anvil securely fitted onto the center rod, it is placed into the esophagus. (ES = esophagus; AG = anterior gastrotomy.)

Fig. 66-4. Appearance of the esophagus after tying the pursestring around the anvil of the stapler. The whole device and the esophagus are gently pulled downward and outward away from the back of the trachea and the mediastinum to avoid accidental inclusion of these structures. The stay sutures are cut and removed at this point.

tilting the posterior part of the anvil through the anastomosis ring. Doughnuts from the esophagus and stomach are recovered from within the shaft and examined for completeness (Fig. 66-5). The integrity of the anastomosis is inspected externally (Fig. 66-6). and internally by placing two small retractors into the stomach. The anterior gastrotomy is closed with a continuous layer of 4–0 Maxon suture (polyglyconate, Davis & Geck) after advancement of the nasogastric tube into the stomach.

It is unnecessary to tag the stomach to the thoracic wall to avoid gastric rotation or to avoid tension on the anastomosis. Hemostasis in the mediastinum is secured and the thoracotomy closed with drainage.

The Hand-Sewn Anastomosis

For the hand-sewn anastomosis, the steps in the preparation of the proximal esoph-

agus and the substitute are the same as described for the stapled anastomosis. Usually only four 3–0 silk stay sutures are placed on the proximal esophagus. For a grossly dilated esophagus, more stay sutures are needed.

Whatever is used as the esophageal substitute, the technique for the anastomosis is the same. When the whole stomach is used, a small gastrotomy is first made at a clear area on the back of the fundus close to the apex, or at the apex itself, for the anastomosis.

A mosquito forceps is used to pick up the gastric wall at the center of the selected anastomotic site, and a ring of seromuscular wall of 2-cm diameter is cut with cautery. The exposed mucosa is then grasped with another pair of mosquito forceps, stretched and divided flush with the previous cut on the serosa. This step allows a greater ring of mucosa to be removed, which prevents excessive mucosal eversion. When the distal stomach is used, the

anastomotic site is the tip of the stomach tube and a defect is made by a similar technique, incorporating the uppermost part of the linear staple line.

The preparation of the colon and the jejunum is described in Chap. 85. An end-to-end anastomosis is our preferred configuration. A 1-cm cuff of bowel free of vascular and omental appendages is required for the anastomosis. The bowel is cut in two steps (as described above) with proportionally more mucosa removed than the seromuscular layer to avoid mucosal eversion. A soft bowel clamp or Satinsky clamp is placed a few centimeters from the margins and the opened end of the bowel is cleansed with aqueous chlorhexidine solution. Care is taken to ensure proper orientation of the bowel and its mesentery.

When a jejunal loop or an ileocolic loop is delivered into the neck for anastomosis, the upper end of the loop usually angulates to the right toward the mesentery and

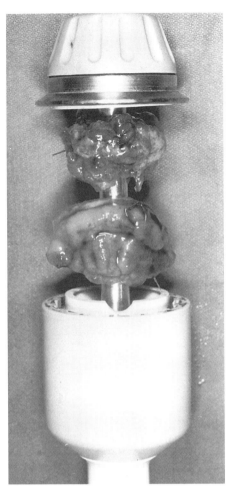

Fig. 66-5. *After firing and disengagement of the stapler from the anastomosis, two complete rings of tissues are recovered from within the stapling instrument, one from the esophagus and one from the stomach.*

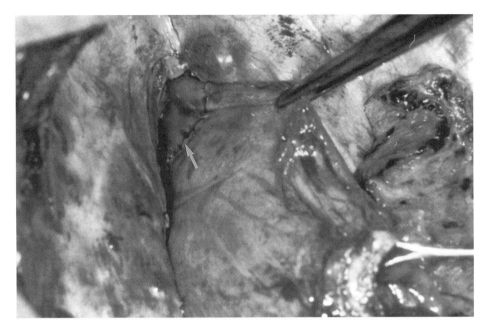

Fig. 66-6. *The integrity of the stapled anastomosis is inspected externally. The staple line is clearly visible (arrow). Often, the anastomosis might have retracted out of sight toward the neck and has to be pulled downward to be seen.*

is often redundant. A short length of jejunum has to be resected to straighten the loop for an end-to-end anastomosis.

The hand-sewn anastomosis is performed with a single layer of continuous monofilament absorbable sutures, such as 4–0 Maxon (polyglyconate) (Figs. 66-7 through 66-11. This method of anastomosis requires two single-armed sutures to be securely tied at the ends. The knot is used to anchor the two parts for anastomosis. The first step is to pass one needle from the inside of the substitute to the outside and from the outside of the esophagus into its lumen, beginning on the left border with the surgeon standing on the right side. By pulling the suture on the esophageal side,

the knot brings the substitute to the esophagus. This suture is then continued in an over-and-over manner to complete the posterior wall anastomosis. Full thickness bites of the substitute of at least 5 mm and full thickness bites of the esophageal wall at 5-mm depth and 5 mm apart are incorporated in the suture (Fig. 66-7). When the posterior wall is completed, the suture is continued around the corner in a similar manner to approximately one-third the way across the anterior wall. At the right lateral angle, the suture takes the full thickness of the esophagus with a minimum of mucosa, and on the substitute only the seromuscular layer is incorporated, thus inverting the mucosa on both sides (Fig. 66-8). When this step is completed, the suture is brought from the lumen to the outside of the substitute.

With the distal stomach used as the substitute, the uppermost portion of the linear staple closure is included in the anastomosis. This T junction can be inverted by taking slightly deeper bites of the seromuscular wall only on both sides of the staple line (Fig. 66-9).

The rest of the anterior wall anastomosis is begun on the left side with the other needle, which is first brought to the outside through the esophageal wall. The anterior wall is then completed by taking only the seromuscular wall of the substitute but a full thickness of the esophagus with minimal mucosa. Once again, big bites are picked up by the needle. Before the anterior layer is finished, a radiopaque nasogastric tube is advanced through the anastomosis into the substitute by the anesthetist. Alternatively, a sterile tube is introduced into the substitute by the surgeon, and the proximal end of the tube is passed upward into the pharynx and brought out through the nose by the anesthetist. At the end of the anastomosis, the two sutures should be on opposite sides and can be simply tied. After tying, a metal clip is placed near the knot to mark the anastomosis, which helps its identification when a contrast study is performed (Figs. 66-10 and 66-11).

Throughout the anastomosis, the esophagus and the substitute are only lightly apposed.

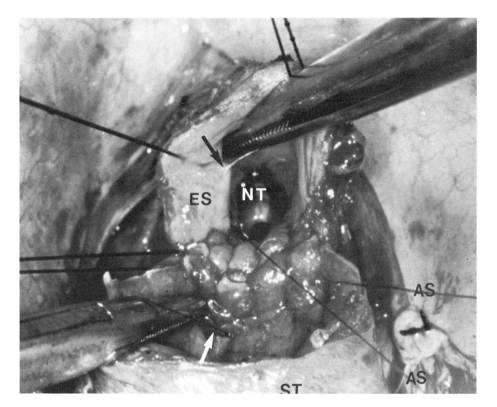

Fig. 66-7. The hand-sewn esophageal anastomosis (Figs. 66-7 through 66-11). The thoracic esophagus at the apex of the right pleural cavity is being anastomosed to a stomach tube, the resection line of which has been stapled. The anastomosis is made using a continuous single-layer technique with two single-armed monofilament absorbable sutures tied at the ends. The posterior wall is being completed. The needle is seen passing from inside the stomach tube to the inside of the esophagus (arrow). Large bites are taken on both sides. The esophagus is held open by stay sutures. (ES = esophagus; ST = stomach tube; AS = anastomotic sutures; NT = nasogastric tube.)

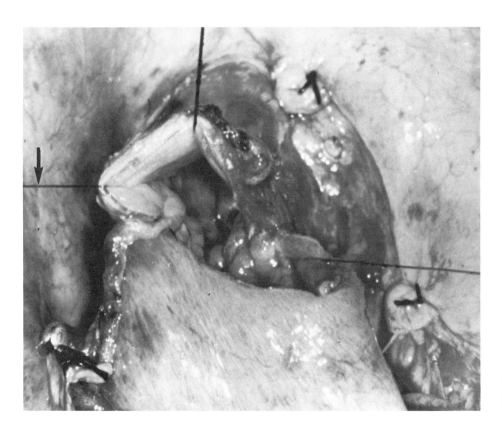

Fig. 66-8. The suture (arrow) has emerged from the lumen of the esophagus after the posterior wall has been completed.

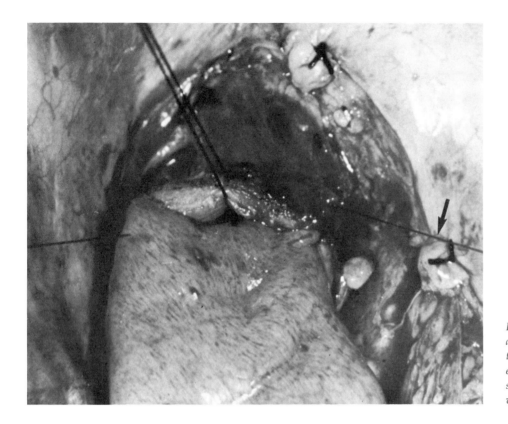

Fig. 66-9. *After completion of the posterior wall and approximately one-third of the anterior wall, the suture is brought from the lumen of the esophagus (see Fig. 66-7) to the outside of the stomach tube. Anterior wall anastomosis is begun with the other needle (arrow).*

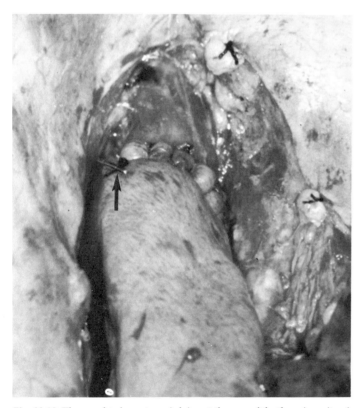

Fig. 66-10. *The completed anastomosis lying at the apex of the thoracic cavity. A metal clip (arrow) is placed near the knot to mark the site of the anastomosis for identification in a chest x-ray and subsequent contrast study.*

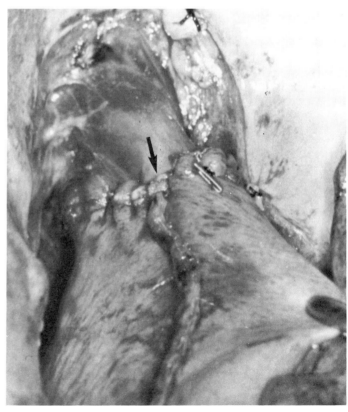

Fig. 66-11. *The posterior wall of the anastomosis and the T junction between the line of gastric resection and the esophagus are shown (arrow).*

The Abdominal Anastomoses

Distal anastomoses in the abdomen are necessary only when the colon or jejunum is used. The duodenum is usually selected as the site of anastomosis. When the colon is used, the distal end of the loop is anastomosed directly to the duodenum.

For a jejunal loop, a Roux-en-Y configuration is an alternative. If the duodenum is selected for distal anastomosis, the site on the jejunum is marked by a pair of Babcock forceps. To allow the distal end of the jejunal loop to return to the infracolic compartment, a segment of approximately 15 to 20 cm of jejunum has to be resected distal to the duodenojejunal anastomosis. A third and final anastomosis establishes intestinal continuity. All intra-abdominal anastomoses are performed by the one-layer continuous method. The mesenteric defects are closed. A final inspection for bleeding points is made before abdominal closure.

Postoperative Care

Avoid Hypoxia

Hypoxia and hypotension predispose to anastomotic and nonanastomotic breakdown because of decreased oxygenation of the tissues. Patients with increased pulmonary risk should be ventilated postoperatively, and all patients should have adequate analgesia such as epidural morphine infusion or patient-controlled analgesia.

Meticulous attention is paid to ensure that the airway is free of sputum and secretions leading to atelectasis and bronchopneumonia. In addition to vigorous chest physiotherapy and the use of incentive spirometry, patients with weak cough effort require frequent bronchoscopy with the flexible fiberoptic bronchoscope under local anesthesia. A liberal policy should be adopted in performing tracheotomy to facilitate sputum clearance if the patient requires more than three episodes of bronchoscopic suction in 24 hours, exhibits weak cough effort, has a vocal cord paralysis, has already suffered from episodes of hypoxia, or shows the development of arrhythmia.

Avoid Fluid Overload

Circulatory overload predisposes to hypoxia, pulmonary edema, and heart failure. Since most of our patients are elderly, chronic smokers with restrictive lung function, it is best to maintain patients on strict fluid balance in the early days after surgery. Inotropic agent support can adequately maintain the blood pressure and renal perfusion in place of more fluids. Diuretics are given periodically, if necessary. After the operation, the serum albumin can fall leading to interstitial edema in the lungs and at the anastomosis. These patients should be given serum albumin to optimize plasma oncotic pressure.

Early Ambulation

Stable patients should be out of bed within 24 hours after the operation to facilitate full lung expansion. Bed-bound patients are more likely to develop sputum retention, atelectasis, bronchopneumonia, and deep vein thrombosis.

Early Detection and Management of Leakage

When the anastomosis is in the chest, anastomotic leakage is suspected if there is excessive output from the chest drain, which may be turbid in color or bile stained. Large volume output of clear fluid can indicate chylothorax. Confirmation of a leak is done by giving the patient methylene blue dye orally and observing this dye appearing in the chest drainage. The location and magnitude of the leak can be visualized by a noniodine-containing water-soluble contrast study under fluoroscopic screening. The extent of the dehiscence and the viability of the esophagus and the substitute can be determined by a carefully performed flexible endoscopic examination.

For a cervical anastomosis, leakage is suspected when there is inflammation and pain around the neck wound, and the release of turbid infected discharge when the skin stitches are removed and the wound laid open.

The presentation of anastomotic leakage can vary from as early as 5 days up to 3 weeks after the operation. A predisposing perioperative event such as prolonged hypoxia, hypotension from postoperative bleeding, or sepsis might be evident. Leakage that occurs within the first 3 days after the surgical procedure is primarily nonanastomotic in nature and is the result of pinpoint, partial, or complete necrosis of the substitute, or results from a nonanastomotic staple line. Re-exploration is mandatory for these nonanastomotic leakages, with direct repair if the involved area is small, or the taking down of the substitute and performing a cervical esophagostomy with a feeding jejunostomy. Reconstruction is subsequently performed.

The treatment of anastomotic leakage should be individualized according to its location and magnitude, and the presence or absence of systemic sepsis. Occasionally, a small leak even in the chest can be treated conservatively with broad-spectrum antibiotics, adequate drainage, and total parenteral nutrition. Larger leaks require early re-exploration with decortication and more comprehensive drainage. Direct repair of the perforation is seldom possible or effective. For major leakage, the anastomosis is taken down and stomas established.

Results

Since adopting the techniques we described, the leakage rate fell from 18 percent between 1964 and 1982 to just under 4 percent between 1982 and 1993. It is currently 2 percent.

The leakage rate is lowest when using the whole stomach (2.7%), which is our preferred substitution and was used in 92 percent of reconstructions. The leakage rates of the other substitutes are: jejunum (4%), distal stomach (6%), and colon (13%). The leakage rate for the hand-sewn anastomosis was 3 percent in 361 esophageal anastomoses after resection and was 4 percent in 298 stapled anastomoses. The hospital mortality of an anastomotic leak remained high at 46 percent, although in many instances the anastomotic leak might have healed. Cervical and intrathoracic anastomoses had similar incidences of leakage (3.5%), and the incidence of fatal leaks were 37 percent and 27 percent, respectively. By contrast, the risk of developing a leak and the risk of dying from an abdominal esophageal anastomosis were comparatively higher at 10 percent and 60 percent, respectively.

The incidence of fibrotic stricture of the anastomosis was significantly higher with the circular stapler and was dependent on the stapler size. The relative risks of developing fibrotic strictures with a small-size (25 mm), medium-size (28 mm and 29 mm) and large-size (31 mm and 33 mm) stapler at 1 year were 46 percent, 26 percent, and 15 percent, respectively. For the hand-sewn anastomosis, the incidence of fibrotic stricture was 14 percent.

Therefore, we have found the anastomosis constructed by the hand-sewn method using 4–0 Maxon (polyglyconate) to be satisfactory and superior to the stapled anastomosis with respect to leakage and the development of stricture. The proper use of the anastomotic technique and selection of the anastomotic site and substitute, together with the avoidance of factors that predispose to anastomotic leakage should further reduce the occurrence of this potentially lethal and largely avoidable complication. A near-zero leakage rate should be achievable.

Suggested Reading

Chasseray VM, Kiroff GK, Buard JL, et al. Cervical or thoracic anastomosis for esophagectomy for carcinoma. *Surg Gynecol Obstet* 169:55, 1989.

Dewar L, Gelfand G, Finley R, et al. Factors affecting cervical anastomotic leak and stricture formation following esophagogastrectomy and gastric tube interposition. *Am J Surg* 163:484, 1992.

Fok M, Ah-Chong AK, Cheng SWK, Wong J. Comparison of a single layer continuous hand-sewn method and circular stapler in 580 oesophageal anastomoses. *Br J Surg* 78:342, 1991.

Fok M, Law SYK, Wong J. Operable esophageal carcinoma: current results from Hong Kong. *Progress World J Surg* 18:355, 1994.

Fok M, Wong J. Cancer of the oesophagus and gastric cardia. Standard oesophagectomy and anastomotic technique. *Ann Chirurg Gynaecol* 84:179, 1995.

Hermreck AS, Crawford DG. The esophageal anastomotic leak. *Am J Surg* 132:794, 1976.

Hopkins RA, Alexander JC, Postlethwait RW. Stapled esophagogastric anastomosis. *Am J Surg* 147:283, 1984.

Lam TCF, Fok M, Cheng SWK, Wong J. Anastomotic leakage following oesophageal reconstruction using whole stomach or distal stomach. *Gullet* 1:114, 1991.

Lam TCF, Fok M, Cheng SWK, Wong J. Anastomotic complications after esophagectomy for cancer: a comparison of neck and chest anastomosis. *J Thor Cardiovasc Surg.* 104:395, 1992.

Lorentz T, Fok M, Wong J. Anastomotic leakage after resection and bypass for esophageal cancer: lessons learned from the past. *World J Surg* 13:472, 1989.

Wong J, Cheung HC, Lui R, et al. Esophagogastric anastomosis performed with a stapler: the occurrence of leakage and stricture. *Surgery* 101:408, 1987.

Wong J. Stapled esophagogastric anastomosis in the apex of the right chest after subtotal esophagectomy for carcinoma. *Surg Gynecol Obstet* 164:568, 1987.

EDITOR'S COMMENT

Professor Wong and his colleagues have had a remarkably extensive experience with treatment of esophageal cancer, probably unparalleled anywhere in the world. They have had an enormous number of patients, the results have been superior, and they are ideally qualified to provide a time- and experience-based description of the best methods of dealing with the esophagogastric or esophagocolic anastomosis. Unlike other authors in this chapter, they have used operative photographs to illustrate the operative principles, with considerable success. Although there is nothing dramatically new in their technique, meticulous attention to detail and establishment of important principles are always very useful to the reader if applied as described.

As is being more frequently shown in other parts of the gastrointestinal tract, their best results with fewer complications have occurred with a single-layer hand-sewn anastomosis. The authors advocate the use of absorbable polyglycolate (Maxon), using a relatively small 4–0 suture material with very carefully placed bites. They report that this method results

in fewer leaks, fewer strictures and overall is the best technique available for restoring continuity of the upper esophagus to the interposition. They appropriately emphasize the need to take relatively deeper bites than usual, with the conclusion that incorporating more tissue into the knots (not tied so tightly that they cause ischemic changes at the anastomosis) leads to the best chance of achieving a watertight secure anastomosis.

Another noteworthy modification of theirs is that they do not tack the stomach to adjacent fascia to hold it in place. The conventional wisdom in this part of the operation has been to take secure seromuscular bites of the posterior gastric wall or colon and tack the viscus with interrupted sutures to the prevertebral fascia. We have always thought that this step was worthwhile to prevent undue tension on the suture line, but it does have the disadvantage of a potential for kinking of the stomach or even of the anastomosis when the patient sits, stands erect, or swallows.

The authors describe dividing the esophagus "at least 6 cm away from the tumor," which raises several questions. First, is this distance far enough from the tumor to ensure that there will not be submucosal spread in the residual esophagus? Second, with an intrathoracic anastomosis, is the cuff sometimes too long, requiring re-excision of the proximal esophagus and the potential for transecting through tumor? Presumably, the authors always subject a portion of the proximal end of the esophageal site of transection to frozen section and rule out any possibility of tumor at the new anastomosis. If no tumor is seen, it does not rule out skip areas in this portion of the esophageal resection, but seeing tumor at the frozen section site makes a significantly higher resection than might be used otherwise mandatory.

The authors differ with numerous published reports in which the esophagogastric anastomosis is always at some distance from the stapled closure of the lesser curvature of the stomach. Figure 66-11 shows the suture line abutting on the lesser curvature closure, making a Y-anastomosis. Although this step can be a bit awkward for the occasional surgeon, with sufficient care the anastomosis should be as secure as ones that are done at some distance from the lesser curvature closure. However, if the most superior portion of the stomach is away from that lesser curvature closure and lies closer to the esophagus, it would seem logical to do the anastomosis at the higher point.

The care and attention to detail that the authors give to this most critical part of the operation for removal of esophageal or esophagogastric cancer are a measure of the way in which they perform their surgery and are indicators of the reason for their outstanding success with this demanding procedure.

R.J.B.

67

Jejunal Interposition in Esophageal Replacement

J. Rüdiger Siewert   Arnulf H. Hölscher

After partial or total resection, the esophagus can be replaced by stomach, colon, or small intestine. In this chapter, the use of jejunal interposition in esophageal replacement is discussed. Actually, substitution by small intestine is only occasionally used since anatomic factors in forming a sufficiently long small-intestinal segment are often unfavorable. Jejunal interposition is used only in the following circumstances: substitution of the entire esophagus after total or subtotal resection (hypopharyngojejunostomy or esophagojejunostomy); substitution for the cervical esophagus, or to complete partial esophageal substitution, for example, with a short colonic segment; and substitution for the distal esophagus with or without simultaneous total gastrectomy.

Replacement of the Entire Esophagus

Surgical Technique

Jejunal interposition using the method of Yudin is technically simple because only one anastomosis is performed in the abdomen. The vessels can be examined with a source of cold light, which is held behind the stretched mesentery; the intestine is not mobilized for this purpose. It is recommended that the vessels and the intestine temporarily be clamped on the planned cutting lines. Large amounts of fat in the mesentery are more of a hindrance to jejunal preparation than to preparation of the colon. Long segments of mobilized small intestine cannot be relied on. The length of the mesentery, which is much

shorter than the corresponding length of intestine, is the decisive factor.

Vascular distribution is of great importance. It cannot be determined which of the many possible variations is present until the abdomen has been opened. Preoperative angiography of the superior mesenteric artery as a rule provides little clarification as to vascular distribution. It is better to illuminate the stretched mesentery with a cold light source at the operating table in order to identify the blood supply.

Two extreme situations are possible (Fig. 67-1A). In a favorable situation, the superior mesenteric artery divides into a few main branches. These are joined together by sturdy marginal arcades near the intestine ("bunch-type" vessel structure). In unfavorable situations, the superior mesenteric artery splits into many small separate branches. The anastomoses between the individual jejunal arteries are numerous but weak ("ladder-type" vessel structure). Between these two extremes are numerous variations. It is frequently observed that the marginal arcade on the intestine is completely interrupted somewhere between two jejunal arteries or joined only by a very thin vessel.

The aforementioned ladder-type vessel structure provides unsatisfactory blood supply for jejunal interposition. It is better not to carry out a jejunal interposition in this situation.

The length of available jejunum depends on the length of the vascular trunk and, thus, on the mesentery. This vascular trunk

can be lengthened operatively only insofar as the mesenteric root can be prepared from the aorta in the retroperitoneum. In principle, the small intestine would always be long enough if it could be stretched; however, the mesentery does not permit stretching of this kind. Occasionally, lengthening the small-intestinal segment may be attempted after dissection of the vascular trunk by radial incisions of the mesentery. As a rule, only a few centimeters are gained by such measures.

The various methods of jejunal interposition differ according to their anastomoses with the intestinal tract in the abdomen. Roux used an isolated loop of small intestine and anastomosed the distal end with the front wall of the stomach, while the continuity of the small intestine was achieved by side-to-side enteroanastomosis. Herzen transected the jejunum and pulled it up toward the pharynx in a Y shape, achieving intestinal continuity in the abdomen by end-to-side enteroanastomosis. He also added an end-to-side gastrojejunostomy to this technique so that the stomach was not completely bypassed.

Yudin simplified this method even more by leaving out the gastroenterostomy. We recommend the procedure described by Yudin.

Jejunal Interposition According to Yudin

The abdomen is opened by a midline epigastric incision or by an upper left paramedian incision. The upper jejunum is pulled forward and the vascular distribution is critically examined. The fourth or

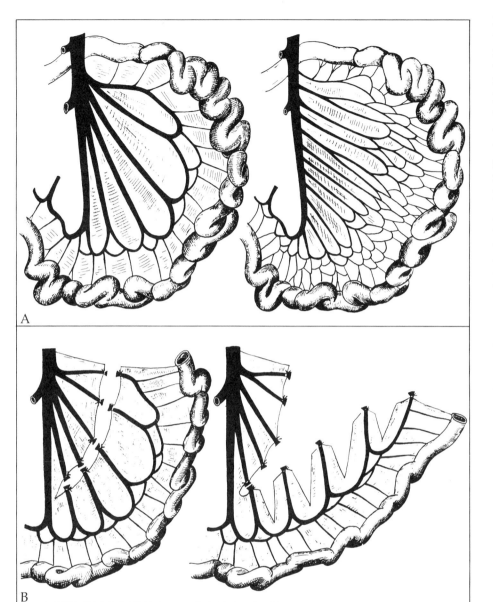

Fig. 67-1. A. Vascular distribution of the small intestine. Two extreme situations are possible. The superior mesenteric artery splits into a few main branches ("bunch-type") (left); the superior mesenteric artery splits into many small separate branches ("ladder-type") (right). B. Lengthening of the small-intestinal segment by parallel incisions of the mesentery.

lon. The mobilized small intestine is pulled up behind the colon through an opening in the mesocolon. Finally, the thin part of the lesser omentum (gastrohepatic ligament) is cut, and the small intestine is pulled through this opening into the upper abdomen behind the stomach.

We routinely use the former esophageal bed in the posterior mediastinum as the route for reconstruction (Fig. 67-3). This route is the shortest, which is important for jejunal interposition.

An alternative route is to use a retrosternal tunnel. The disadvantage of this method is that postoperative development of intestinal necrosis with its serious complications is handled only with great difficulty. The technical procedure is as follows. The xiphoid process can, but need not, be resected. The loose tissue layer behind the sternum is carefully separated from the back of the sternum from below and above simultaneously with a finger and sponge, thus forming a tunnel. The surgeon should be working directly on the back surface of the sternum, observing the large vessels, which are gently retracted posteriorly. The pleural layers are likewise carefully pushed down laterally on both sides. If a pneumothorax occurs, which almost always can be avoided, it can be decompressed with a chest tube for 48 hours.

The small intestine must then be pushed up from the abdomen toward the neck with the finger and a swab through the preformed tunnel. The long suture ends may be used only to guide the intestine through the tunnel, or the delicate mesenteric vessels will be damaged. The anastomosis in the neck can be done at the same operation, or the jejunum can be exteriorized and the anastomosis done as a second stage.

We select the interpleural passage for the jejunum only after distal esophageal resection with an intrathoracic anastomosis.

Abdominal Anastomosis

The intestinal passage is reconstructed in the abdomen by an end-to-side jejunostomy (Roux en Y). The small intestine that has been pulled up is secured by several interrupted sutures in the mesocolic slit (Fig. 67-4). The mesenteric vessels of the interposed intestine must be meticulously observed during these maneuvers. The jejunal interposition can be condemned to

fifth jejunal artery should not be automatically selected as the vascular trunk, but the existing anatomic configuration should be evaluated and the largest artery chosen as the trunk. A fat small-intestinal mesentery causes difficulties. The vascular distribution can best be judged with transillumination of the mesentery. The loop chosen for the interposition is dissected from the distal toward the proximal end at a safe distance from the marginal arcade (Fig. 67-1B). It is advisable first to free the vessels to be severed and then to close

them off temporarily with vascular bulldog clamps (Fig. 67-2). If compressing the proximal end of the intestine with a soft clamp leads to vascular impairment (cyanosis, heavy bleeding in the mesentery), interposition is not carried out, and another method is chosen. Otherwise, the jejunum is cut with the stapler (TA55) as far proximally as possible, and the proximal jejunal end is oversewn with interrupted sutures, leaving long suture ends. Next, the gastrocolic omentum is opened between the stomach and the transverse co-

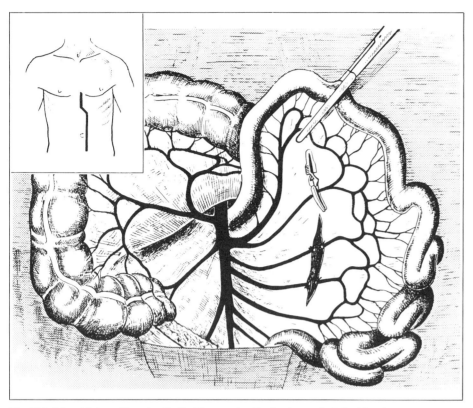

Fig. 67-2. Jejunal interposition after Yudin. The vascular distribution can be judged best by temporary occlusion with bulldog clamps; the intestine is clamped with a soft clamp at the proximal end.

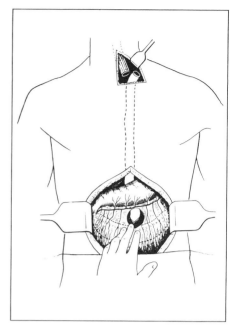

Fig. 67-3. The mobilized small intestine is pulled up into retrocolic and retrogastric positions through an opening in the mesocolon. The jejunal interposition is then pushed up toward the neck from the abdomen through the posterior mediastinum.

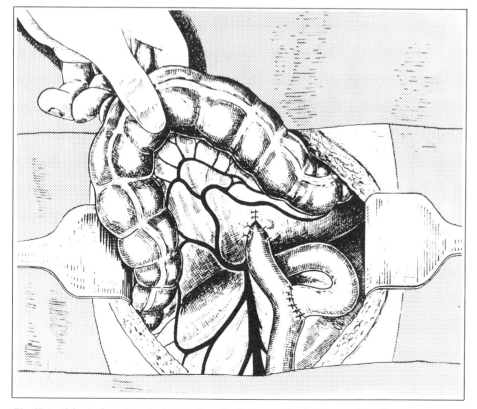

Fig. 67-4. Abdominal anastomosis. Intestinal continuity is reconstructed by an end-to-side jejunojejunostomy (Roux en Y).

failure by even moderate traction on the fragile jejunal veins.

Cervical Anastomosis

The anastomosis between the hypopharynx or cervical esophagus and the small intestine should, whenever possible, be carried out simultaneously with the jejunal interposition (Fig. 67-5A). The anastomosis poses no problems when the two lumens are the same size. It is carried out with a single row, all-layer, interrupted suture technique. For 5 to 7 days after the operation, decompression of the interpositioned small-intestinal loop should be accomplished by a transnasal suction silicone tube.

If the interposed jejunum seems to have a limited blood supply at its superior end, the anastomosis can be performed later. In this situation, the small intestine is not opened, and the sutures that have been left long are brought through the skin and knotted. This prevents retraction of the small intestine into the mediastinal tunnel. The cervical esophagus can then be sewn into the upper end of the wound as a salivary fistula, and the operation is completed.

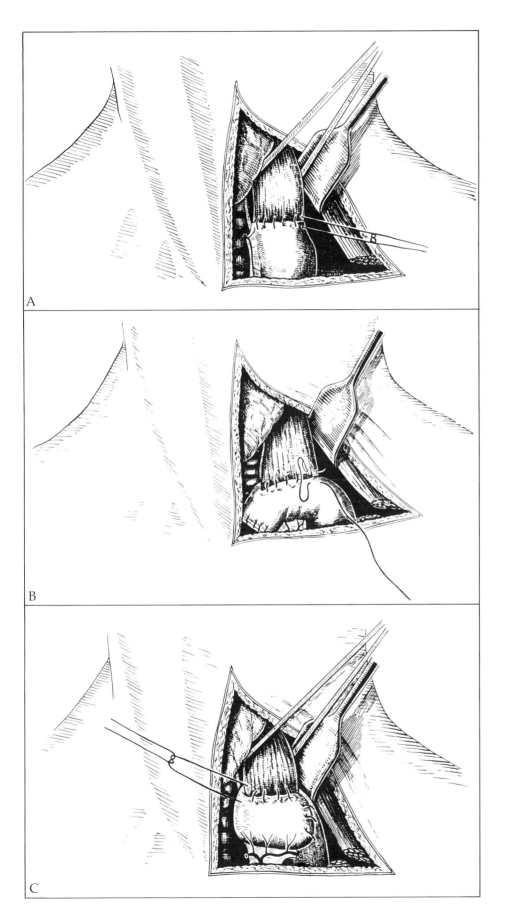

Fig. 67-5. A. The cervical anastomosis is performed as an end-to-end anastomosis. B. The anastomosis can also be performed end to side. C. If a long movable end is present, it can be folded over and used for covering the front wall of the anastomosis.

67. Jejunal Interposition in Esophageal Replacement   **805**

The second operation should be done between the fifth and the seventh day. At this time the vitality of the jejunum can be judged with certainty. It has not become densely adherent and can easily be prepared. If postponed for too long, the preparation becomes much more difficult.

The surgical wound is reopened, and the jejunum is freed from all adhesions so that it can be folded over forward. The cervical muscles are then cut horizontally on the left-hand side, and the cervical esophagus is freed and encircled with a soft rubber drain. The incision of the sternal part of the sternocleidomastoid muscle broadens the operative field and renders easier access to the cervical esophagus. The anastomosis can now be performed according to the aforementioned principles.

Frequently, the jejunal loop appears bent because of the tension on the mesentery, and the uppermost point of the jejunal loop lies opposite the mesentery. In these instances the cervical anastomosis can also be performed end to side (Fig. 67-5B).

If a long jejunal end is present, it can be folded over and used for covering the front wall of the anastomosis (Fig. 67-5C). After the anastomosis has been completed, the mediastinum is drained superiorly with a Silastic drain. The drain is removed between the fifth and seventh day. If the patient has an uneventful postoperative recovery, the tube in the small-intestinal interposition can be removed after the fifth day.

Suture line leaks are not infrequent, and salivary fistulas in the neck usually close spontaneously. Necrosis of the small intestine, on the other hand, is a serious complication that endangers the patient's life.

Results

The fatality rate of jejunal interposition in esophageal replacement is given as between 15 and 25 percent. The fact that jejunal interposition is performed only infrequently is certainly responsible for the relatively high fatality rate. Complications without fatality are observed in about 50 percent of instances. Only 25 percent proceed without complications.

Esophagojejunostomy Using Stapler Technique

The CEEA stapler is ideally suited to complete an end-to-side esophagojejunos-

tomy; the instrument carries the jejunum to the esophageal stump.

A circular border stitch pursestring suture is performed at the edge of the opening of the esophagus. Alternatively, a pursestring clamp can be used before the esophagus is cut in order to place this suture mechanically. After the anvil from the CEEA stapler is disconnected, it is introduced into the esophagus and the pursestring suture is tied. The stapler instrument is then

introduced through the open cut end of the jejunum abutting the antimesenteric border of the jejunal wall about 10 cm from the open introduction site of the stapler. The sharp tip of the central rod is driven out and perforated through the jejunal wall. After removal of the sharp tip, the stapler is connected to the anvil in the esophagus and the stapler is closed and fired (Fig. 67-6). By this activation of the instrument, a circular, inverting end-to-side esophagojejunostomy is made. The

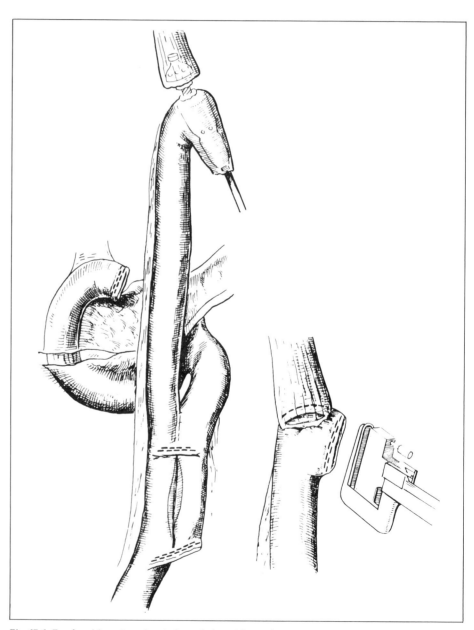

Fig. 67-6. Esophagojejunostomy by stapler technique. The stapler instrument is introduced through the open cut end of jejunum, and a circular, inverting end-to-side esophagojejunostomy is made. After removal of the EEA, the jejunum is closed (vertical) to its long axis with a TA55 instrument.

instrument is withdrawn by opening the gap between the anvil and the cartridge and then turning the instrument obliquely (Fig. 67-6).

After removal of the CEEA stapler, the excised circular tissue doughnuts of esophagus and jejunum are examined for completeness. The anastomosis can be controlled by digital palpation from inside with a finger introduced via the open end of the jejunum. The jejunum is then closed perpendicular to its long axis with the TA55 instrument, flush with the lateral aspect of the esophagus. The excess jejunum is excised and the stapler line is oversewn with seromuscular stitches. The Roux en Y end-to-side anastomosis of the two jejunal loops is performed at least 40 cm below the esophagojejunostomy by stapling technique (Fig. 67-6).

Replacement of the Cervical Esophagus

Seidenberg and Hurwitt, in 1959, reported a technique of revascularizing isolated jejunal segments to replace the cervical esophagus in dogs. The mesenteric vessel was anastomosed to the superior thyroid artery, and the anterior facial vein was anastomosed to the mesenteric vein by a ringed cuff. Roberts and Douglass replaced the cervical esophagus and hypopharynx successfully with a revascularized free jejunal graft.

The largest series of patients with free visceral grafts, with blood supply brought in by local collateral or vessel anastomosis, was reported by Nakayama and associates in 1964. They reported 21 autografts of intestine using a vascular anastomosis stapling device. A segment of ileum was used in only one patient; the sigmoid colon was used in the other 20 patients.

Green and Som published their experience of free grafting and revascularization of intestine for replacement of the cervical esophagus and oral pharynx in the dog. They used revascularized segments of small intestine and accomplished the vascular anastomosis with the aid of a Zeiss operating microscope. Green and Som were able to demonstrate patency of vessels as small as 1 to 2 mm in diameter using 9–0 monofilament nylon.

Free Ileum or Jejunal Interposition

A midline incision is made in the abdomen, and a gastrostomy is performed. The ileocolic vessels are carefully dissected near their junction with the superior mesenteric artery and vein. The vessels are proximally ligated and are then cut cleanly across at a slight angle to increase the diameter. A segment of terminal ileum approximately 25 cm long is isolated by dividing between clamps (Fig. 67-7). If necessary, a portion of cecum can be left attached to the ileum. The vessels are immediately irrigated with a cold serum albumin solution to which heparin has been added to remove all the blood from the vessels of the severed intestinal segment. Gastrointestinal continuity in the abdomen is restored by single-layer anastomosis between the terminal ileum and ascending colon after the cervical vascular anastomoses are finished, and the abdomen is closed in layers.

The intestinal segment is placed in the neck (Fig. 67-8). Vascular continuity is restored between the ileocolic artery and the left external carotid artery in an end-to-side manner using interrupted 6–0 sutures. The ileocolic vein is anastomosed end to side to the internal jugular vein on the left side. It is necessary to use magnifying loupes for these anastomoses. Immediately after removal of the vascular clamp, there must be good blood flow with visible pulsation in the mesenteric arteries and bleeding from the cut edges of the terminal ileum. The cecum is then removed if it was taken with the ileum. The ends of the terminal ileum are closed with running 3–0 or 4–0 polyglycolic acid sutures and an outer layer of interrupted permanent sutures. Anastomosis is then accomplished end to side in an isoperistaltic manner between the pharynx and the ileum above, and the cervical esophagus and the terminal ileum below, using one layer of interrupted 4–0 polyglycolic acid sutures (Fig. 67-8). Silastic drains

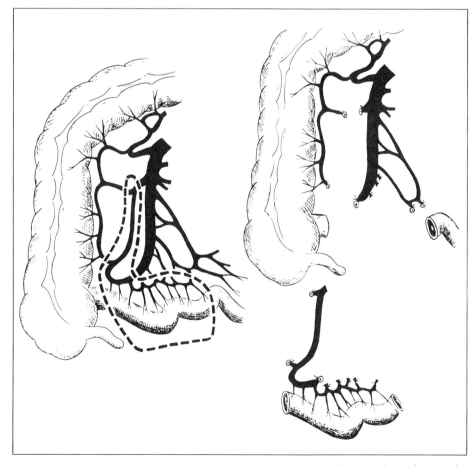

Fig. 67-7. Method of obtaining ileal autograft. The ileocolic vessels are carefully dissected near their junction with the superior mesenteric artery and vein, and a segment of terminal ileum is divided between clamps.

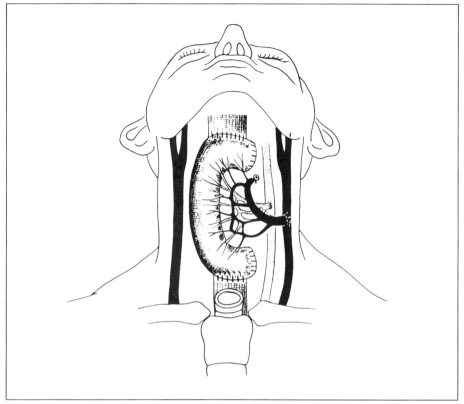

Fig. 67-8. Pharyngeal reconstruction with free ileal graft. Arterial anastomosis is performed between the ileocolic artery and the left carotid artery in an end-to-side manner. The ileocolic vein is anastomosed end to side to the internal jugular vein. The intestinal anastomosis is accomplished end to side or end to end in an isoperistaltic manner between the pharynx and the terminal ileum and the oral part of the esophagus and the ileum below.

are placed in the left lateral side of the neck.

It is also possible to select a segment of the proximal small intestine. The segment should be supplied by a vascular arcade, arising from a single artery and vein that correspond in size to the recipient vessels in the neck. A pedicle can usually be found without dissection into the root of the mesentery. At appropriate points, the intestine is cleaned and divided between clamps (Fig. 67-9). The mesentery is then divided, careful attention being given to preserving the vessels chosen as the vascular pedicle. Without separating the vessels from the surrounding fat, a suitable site for division is selected. The isolated segment is cooled during the period of anoxia.

At this point, the recipient vessels in the neck have been prepared for anastomosis, and adequate flow in the artery has been demonstrated. The intestine and mesentery are divided and the lumen is irrigated. Until now, blood has been perfusing the loop through the vascular pedicle of the autograft. The vascular pedicle is divided between clamps, and the isolated segment is brought to the neck.

The intestinal segment is situated isoperistaltically and is secured in the wound to prevent movement. Under the operating microscope, the graft artery and vein are dissected from the surrounding fatty tissue for a distance of 1.5 cm. The portion of vessel crushed in the clamp is discarded. The anastomoses are carried out using a standard operating microscope with 4 to 25 magnification, Acland approximator clamps, and interrupted sutures of 9–0 monofilament nylon on a flat-bodied microvascular needle. Both anastomoses are completed before the vascular clamps are released.

Before circulation is re-established in the autograft, the cooling process is reversed by circulating water at body temperature through the perfusion tube in the lumen. The venous clamps are released before the arterial clamps to avoid venous congestion. The anoxic period varies from 40 to 60 minutes. To ensure satisfactory circulation, as demonstrated by rapid and sustained return of normal color, bleeding from the cut ends, and peristalsis, the graft is observed for 10 to 15 minutes before being sutured into place.

Replacement of the Distal Esophagus Combined with Total Gastrectomy

The main indication for replacement of the distal esophagus by small intestine is when gastrectomy is necessary at the same time, as in carcinoma of the cardia, or when operations on the stomach, such as partial gastrectomy, have previously been performed.

The proximal and distal visceral anastomoses in the neck are performed in one layer (Fig. 67-10).

The terminal ileum supplied by the ileocolic vessels appears to be the most suitable segment for transplantation because of the constancy and size of the vessels. However, depending on the vascular architecture, jejunal segments may also be as appropriate for this procedure as the terminal ileum. The terminal ileum or the jejunum is preferable to the colon because the small intestine more closely approximates the diameter of the cervical esophagus and pharynx, and it has a thicker wall and better blood supply.

Merendino Operation

The replacement of the distal esophagus only after distal esophagectomy without combined total gastrectomy—so-called Merendino operation—is rarely performed. It is indicated in all benign stenoses of the distal esophagus that do not respond to bougienage. Pathogenesis of such a stenosis would be scar stenosis (e.g., after caustic burn or peptic stenosis). The operation comprises a resection of the distal esophagus and an interposition be-

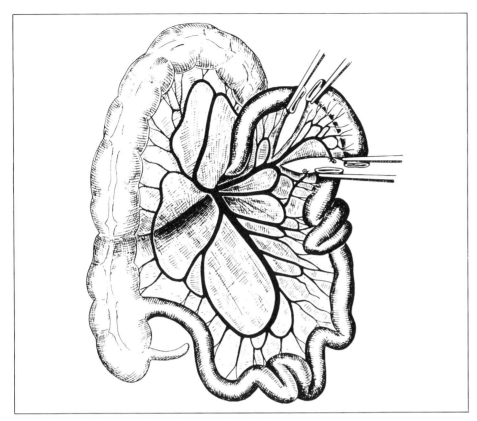

Fig. 67-9. Preparation of a jejunal segment. The segment should be supplied by a vascular arcade arising from a single artery and vein. A pedicle can usually be found without dissection into the root of the mesentery.

tween esophageal remnant and stomach. This operation is performed by an abdominotranshiatal approach using a wide incision of the diaphragm from in front of the esophageal hiatus and exposure of the lower mediastinum by insertion of two long hook retractors. Thus, the distal esophagus can easily be resected after placement of a staple line on the subcardial stomach. A pursestring suture is placed at the margin of the esophageal remnant either manually or by pursestring clamp. The anvil of the stapler instrument (size 25 or 28) is inserted in the esophageal lumen and the pursestring suture is tied.

A 25-cm segment of the upper jejunum is dissected by taking care to preserve the vascular pedicle. This preparation is most easily performed using transillumination of the small-bowel mesentery. After transection of the small bowel the continuity of the gut is restored by end-to-end anastomosis. The jejunal segment with its vascular pedicle is carefully advanced by a

retrocolic and retrogastric route into the lower mediastinum. The jejunal segment must be isoperistaltic. Now the stapler is inserted via the oral end of the jejunal loop and the sharp tip of the center rod is perforated at the antimesenteric side of the jejunum. After closing and firing of the stapler, the instrument is removed and the circular tissue doughnuts are examined for completeness. The remaining blind oral part of the jejunum is shortened and closed by a linear stapler line. The length of the jejunum is adjusted to the distance to the stomach and eventually the aborad end of the jejunum is shortened. Finally, the jejunogastrostomy is performed on the anterior surface of the stomach with [extramucosal] manual suture technique and a gastric tube is inserted through the esophageal remnant and the jejunal interposition into the stomach. Usually the vagal nerves can be preserved during resection of the distal esophagus. If this is not possible or they have been damaged, dilatation of the pylorus with a long clamp via

the gastrostomy is recommended before the jejunogastrostomy is completed.

The most simple form of jejunal interposition is the Roux en Y loop. Preparation of the loop of small intestine is the same as that described for jejunal interposition according to Yudin (see p. 802). The loops can be correspondingly shorter. For this reason, substitution of the distal esophagus by small intestine is almost always possible. In instances of simultaneous gastrectomy, the end-to-side implantation (Roux en Y) of the afferent loop is the best and easiest method. The same is also true for the gastric remnant, which is often not worth keeping intact.

The esophagojejunal anastomosis usually proceeds end to side with interrupted all-layer sutures. The most secure structure of the esophagus is the mucosa, which must, therefore, be pulled into the suture. The anastomosis lies in the thorax and must be especially secure (small intestine and esophagus edges well vascularized, tension-free anastomosis). Today a stapler anastomosis is usually favored for the intrathoracic esophagojejunostomy because it is an easy and very safe procedure. (For technique see pp. 806–807.)

Great anastomotic security can also be achieved by the principle of jejunoplication. Moreover, 8 to 10 cm of small intestine is necessary in addition to the usual length. A further advantage of this anastomosing technique is the favorable influence on or prevention of intestinoesophageal reflux.

Jejunoplication

The jejunal loop is prepared as described for Yudin jejunal interposition (see p. 802). It must be about 10 cm longer than necessary. The anastomosis is placed correspondingly about 10 cm distally to the upper, blind, closed end of the small intestine (Fig. 67-10). The anastomosis is done as a modified end-to-side connection. For this purpose, the esophagus is implanted on the antimesenteric side of the small intestine. An oblique angle of about 45 degrees is cut on the implantation surface. Interrupted single-layer, full-thickness, permanent sutures are used. The envelopment of the anastomosis is relatively easy to achieve by the oblique implantation. The loop of small intestine at the back of the esophagus is placed around the esophagus

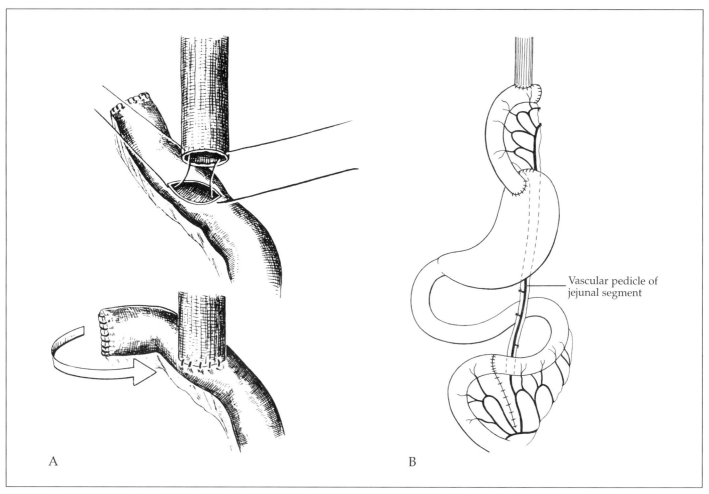

Fig. 67-10. A. The anastomosis between the distal esophagus and the jejunum is placed about 10 cm distal to the upper, blind, closed end of the small intestine. An oblique angle of about 45 degrees is prepared on the implantation surface. After the anastomosis is finished, the loop of the small intestine at the back of the esophagus is placed around the anastomosis and then sewn onto the front wall with the distal part of the small intestine. B. Final position of the jejunum after replacement of the distal esophagus by jejunal interposition and esophagojejunostomy + jejunogastrostomy (Merendino operation).

and then is sewn onto the front wall with the distal part of the small intestine (jejunoplication).

Occasionally, anatomically favorable situations allow the partial replacement of the distal esophagus with a jejunal pouch and a jejunoplication. This is successful only when the mesentery is especially long and mobile. The surgical technique is as follows.

Subsequent to total gastrectomy, distal esophageal resection, and closure of the duodenum, intestinal continuity is restored using the first jejunal loop, which is prepared in a Roux en Y manner and is passed retrocolically into the upper abdomen. A side-to-side enteroanastomosis about 15 cm long between ascending and descending limbs of the loop is done approximately 8 cm below the crest of the loop (Fig. 67-11A). The blind end of the ascending loop is closed using a stapler. The arc of the loop should admit about three fingers. In the area superior to the ventral suture of the anastomosis, an opening about 3 to 4 cm long should remain; it corresponds with the size of the lumen of the esophagus. The esophageal stump is then sewn into this aperture, utilizing a full-thickness, all-layer, interrupted suture (Fig 67-11B). After completion of the esophagojejunostomy, the lateral segments of the jejunal loop are pulled forward around the front wall of the esophagus and sewn together with seromuscular interrupted sutures. The establishment of a tensionless cuff can be guaranteed only if the crescent of the jejunal loop is constructed in the manner described. The cuff tends to embrace the distal esophagus, especially the anastomosis. Finally, the jejunal loop is fixed to the edges of the opening of the mesocolon. This procedure can also be performed in the thorax if the jejunal loop is prepared as described earlier (see p. 808). The esophagojejunoplication today is mostly performed using stapler technique.

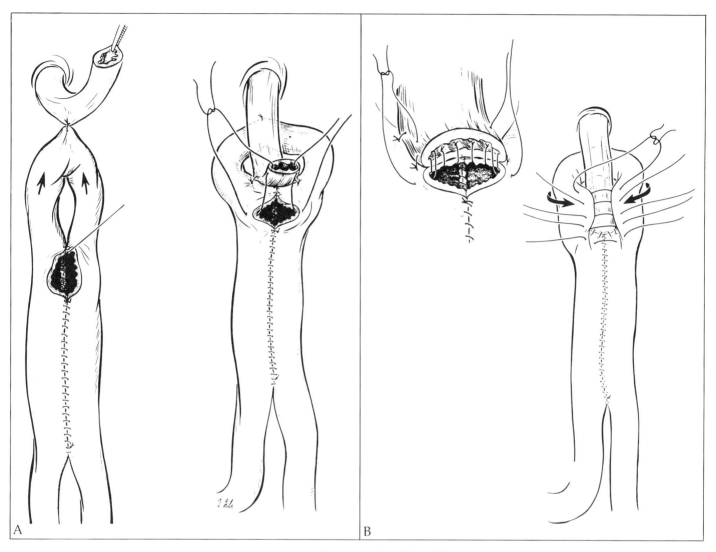

Fig. 67-11. A. A side-to-side enteroanastomosis about 15 cm long is established approximately 8 cm below the crest of the loop. The esophageal stump is then sewn into the opening of the ventral suture. The blind arc of the loop is brought behind the esophagus. B. After completion of the esophagojejunostomy, the lateral segments of the jejunal crescent are pulled forward around the front wall of the esophagus and fastened together with seromuscular interrupted sutures.

Suggested Reading

Behl PR, Holden MP, Brown AH. Three years' experience with esophageal stapling device. *Ann Surg* 198:134, 1983.

Ellis FH Jr. Treatment of carcinoma of the esophagus and cardia. *Mayo Clin Proc* 64:945, 1989.

Flynn MB, Acland RD. Free intestinal autografts for reconstruction following pharyngolaryngoesophagectomy. *Surg Gynecol Obstet* 149:858, 1979.

Green GE, Som ML. Free grafting and revascularization of intestine: I. Replacement of the cervical esophagus. *Surgery* 60:1012, 1966.

Iascone C, DeMeester TR, Little AG, et al. Barrett's esophagus: Functional assessment, proposed pathogenesis, and surgical therapy. *Arch Surg* 118:543, 1983.

Kasai M, Nishihira T. Reconstruction using pedicled jejunal segments after resection for carcinoma of the cervical esophagus. *Surg Gynecol Obstet* 163:145, 1986.

Nakayama K, Yamamoto K, Tmaiya T, et al. Experience with free autografts of the bowel with a new venous anastomosis apparatus. *Surgery* 55:796, 1964.

Ngan SYK, Wong J. Lengths of different routes for esophageal replacement. *J Thorac Cardiovasc Surg* 91:790, 1986.

Omara K, Misaki T, Watanabe Y, et al. Reconstruction with free jejunal autograft after pharyngolaryngoesophagectomy. *Ann Thorac Surg* 57:112, 1994.

Parker EF, Ballenger JF, Shull KC. Esophageal resection and replacement for carcinoma. *Ann Surg* 187:629, 1978.

Seidenberg B, Hurwitt ES. Immediate reconstruction of the cervical esophagus by a revascularized isolated jejunal segment. *Surg Forum* 9:413, 1958.

Siewert JR, Hölscher AH (eds). *Diseases of the Esophagus: Pathology, Diagnosis, Conservative and Surgical Treatment.* Berlin: Springer-Verlag, 1988.

Siewert JR, Hölscher AH. Eingriffe am Oesophagus. In JR Siewert (ed), *Breitner Chirurgische Operationslehre*. Bd IV: *Chirurgie des Abdomens II. Oesophagus, Magen und Duodenum*. Baltimore: Urban and Schwarzenberg, 1989.

Siewert JR, Peiper HJ. Clinical results of esophago-jejunoplication: A special reconstructive procedure after total gastrectomy. *Surg Gastroenterol* 1:55, 1982.

Yudin SS. The surgical construction of 80 cases of artificial esophagus. *Surg Gynecol Obstet* 78:561, 1944.

EDITOR'S COMMENT

The use of jejunum to replace the distal esophagus, most often performed in patients who have had their stomach resected for tumor or another disease process, is not necessarily a straightforward operation, and one that is quite difficult or not possible when the patient has a very fat thickened mesentery or with substantial inflammation in the jejunum from intrinsic small-intestinal disease (Crohn's disease, lipodystrophy, etc.). When most or all of the esophagus is to be replaced, the stomach is the first choice and a segment of colon is second, since the blood supply of these two organs is more reliable, and it is far easier to mobilize the viscus to be used for bypass and bring it to the neck or even the hypopharynx. Nevertheless, two procedures that utilize the jejunum are available. The first is the Yudin procedure, in which the mobilized jejunum is passed through a substernal tunnel or through the bed of the resected esophagus. In general, it is helpful to resect the xiphoid, and if the bypass is to reach the cervical esophagus in the neck or even the hypopharynx, it is often advantageous to resect the medial end of the clavicle and a portion of the left side of the sternum at its superior margin, enlarging the thoracic inlet and putting less pressure on the transposed esophageal substitute. Either colon or jejunum should be passed behind the antrum of the stomach, since this will put less traction on the mesentery of either viscus, and help to secure and protect the blood supply to the transposed viscus. The second procedure is a free jejunal graft, with microvascular anastomoses.

The authors describe a reliable method to assure that the blood supply at the superior end of the jejunum (or colon) is adequate by bringing the viscus to the neck, but not performing a simultaneous anastomosis. After one week, the neck incision is reopened, the jejunum or colon is readily assessed as to adequacy of blood supply, and the anastomosis is performed with considerable confidence that the blood supply is indeed going to sustain the interposed viscus.

Under any circumstances, it is important to perform a feeding jejunostomy, in our hands by Witzel's technique, so that early enteral feeding can be started. If any complication develops at the anastomosis, it can be dealt with by conservative measures since alimentation through the feeding jejunostomy tube is preferable to intravenous hyperalimentation. We have abandoned the "fine-needle tube jejunostomy" because of a significant number of complications, primarily leak or failure of the tube to remain in appropriate position, and now prefer to use a No. 14 French rubber tube introduced through a small jejunotomy distal to the anastomosis in the abdomen with the tube fed aborally. The Witzel tunnel should be 3 to 4 cm in length, and we like to wrap the tube in omentum or fasten the jejunum to the parietal peritoneum at the site where the tube exits the abdominal wall.

The authors appropriately emphasize the difficulties with this operation, especially the fact that only one of four patients who are operated on and have this procedure performed have no complications; unfortunately, one of four patients operated on with this operation die of complications of the procedure, and at least one-half of the patients undergoing jejunal esophageal replacement have serious complications. Both the stomach and the colon replacement of the esophagus have substantially fewer complications, the procedures allow very good swallowing function, and the mortality and morbidity are substantially less than with the jejunal replacement procedure reported by Professor Siewert and Dr. Hölscher.

The usefulness of the free jejunal graft to replace the esophagus has been markedly enhanced by the substantial number of surgeons who have now been trained in microvascular surgical techniques. General surgeons, plastic surgeons, and orthopedic surgeons who have been involved with limb replantation and are familiar with microvascular techniques done with an operating microscope are ordinarily experienced in and understand the principles that allow a free jejunal graft to be placed, most commonly as a cervical esophageal substitute. Further, if this graft were to fail because of vascular occlusion, having it in the neck significantly diminishes the seriousness of the resultant ischemic necrosis of the jejunal graft, although the need to replace that graft is obviously a most unfortunate occurrence. Professor Siewert and Dr. Hölscher's experience with this procedure is among the largest reported anywhere in the world, and their candor about its shortcomings is both refreshing and educational.

R.J.B.

68

Perforation of the Esophagus

Alex G. Little

Perforations of the esophagus are caused by three mechanisms: 1) external trauma, which includes blunt and penetrating injuries; 2) barogenic rupture, also called Boerhaave syndrome; or 3) iatrogenic disruption during esophageal instrumentation, including endoscopic examination or esophageal dilation, or both. Leaks from disrupted esophageal anastomoses are a separate issue, which is not considered in this chapter. The common therapeutic theme for all esophageal perforations is that the shorter the time interval from diagnosis to treatment, the better are the chances for a successful outcome following surgical intervention.

External Esophageal Trauma

Either blunt trauma or penetrating injuries can result in damage to the esophagus. With improvements in both the efficiency of patient retrieval from the field and resuscitation techniques, more patients with extensive and multiorgan trauma are surviving their initial injury to reach the hospital and, subsequently, the operating room than in earlier times. In addition, recent years have shown a relative decrease in the frequency of esophageal trauma due to instrumentation. These two events in combination have made external injury the most common cause of esophageal trauma.

Penetrating Injuries

The esophagus can be injured in any of its three anatomic body compartments—the neck, the chest, or the abdomen. When the neck is the site of injury, the approach to

the patient is dictated in part by the location. Figure 68-1 demonstrates the anatomic zones of the neck that are used in trauma patients to guide diagnosis and therapy. Zone 1 extends from the clavicles to the cricoid cartilage. Zone 2 spans the area between the cricoid cartilage and the angle of the mandible, and zone 3 is the remaining neck above the angle of the mandible.

Injuries in zone 2 mandate automatic and immediate surgical exploration, at which time the esophagus should be visualized and inspected. Unstable patients with injuries in zone 1 or 3 also must proceed quickly to the operating room and, again, the esophagus should be explored. However, patients in clinically stable condition with injuries in either zone 1 or zone 3 typically undergo diagnostic arteriographic

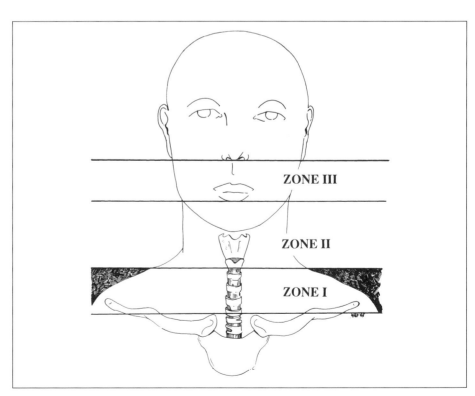

Fig. 68-1. *Anatomic neck zones used to determine the diagnostic and therapeutic approach to individual trauma patients. Injuries in zone 2 mandate surgical exploration while clinically stable patients with zone 1 or 3 injuries can be evaluated with diagnostic modalities such as radiology and endoscopy before definitive therapy is selected.*

evaluation before a decision is made regarding surgery. This also provides an opportunity to assess the esophagus. Unfortunately, contrast esophagograms have a high false-negative rate in penetrating trauma, especially for gunshot injuries, and therefore esophagoscopy is especially useful in these patients. An endoscopic examination that fails to disclose injury is sufficient to withhold surgical exploration.

When the injury is to the chest, surgery is usually performed for bleeding, for gunshot or stab injuries where the bullet or wounding instrument is known to have crossed the midline, or when the level of suspicion of cardiac or great vessel injury is high. The esophagus is able to be visualized during the exploration. When the patient has no clear indication for urgent surgical exploration but there is a clinical suspicion of esophageal injury then both esophagogram and esophagoscopy provide accurate information and are a sufficient evaluation for esophageal injury.

Injury to the abdominal esophagus is uncommon because of its short length. However, criteria for abdominal exploration are well developed and include all the standard indications for exploration of the abdomen of a trauma victim. They can be supplemented by an abnormal esophagogram or esophagoscopy when injury of the esophagus or upper stomach is suspected.

Blunt Trauma

Although uncommon, injury to the esophagus by blunt trauma is being reported with increasing frequency. Esophageal injuries in the neck are often associated with damage to other organs, such as the trachea, great vessels, and cervical spine. Blunt trauma can also cause rupture of the thoracic esophagus or the esophagogastric junction. In these instances a high index of clinical suspicion coupled with expeditious radiologic study or early surgical exploration, or both, are essential for good patient outcome.

Iatrogenic Injuries

With the almost complete disappearance of elective rigid esophagoscopy, the frequency of rupture of the esophagus during endoscopic examination has diminished considerably. Rupture still occurs during other types of esophageal manipulations,

particularly dilation of peptic strictures. However, the overall incidence of rupture during instrumentation has significantly diminished, and this is now the second most common cause of esophageal perforation in most centers.

The essential feature in the care of these patients is having a high index of suspicion of perforation following esophageal instrumentation. Most of these procedures are performed on an outpatient basis or even in the office setting. Many patients experience mild and nonspecific epigastric and chest discomfort following esophageal dilation, but the key word is "mild"—the pain should be clearly resolving by the time the patient is sent home. In addition to persistence or severity of pain, tachycardia and fever must also be taken seriously. Even though it may be an inconvenience to the patient, it is wise to obtain a contrast esophagogram before discharge from the recovery room or office if there is any significant clinical suspicion of esophageal perforation.

Barogenic Injuries (Boerhaave Syndrome)

Herman Boerhaave diagnosed postemetic esophageal rupture in his patient, Admiral von Wassenauer, in 1724. Although some instances of what is now known as Boerhaave syndrome have occurred in patients with no apparent provocation, the majority are related to vomiting or retching. Presumably, in these instances esophageal pressure is raised when both the upper, that is, the cricopharyngeus muscle, and the lower esophageal sphincter are closed. The resulting intraluminal pressure is sufficient to disrupt the esophageal wall.

The patient presentation is frequently deceptively innocuous. Depending on whether from the onset the tear is full thickness or only partial, and/or the parietal pleura remains intact and prevents leakage outside the mediastinal compartment, the extent of contamination of pleura, mediastinum, or abdomen by esophagogastric contents is quite varied. The one constant symptom is chest or epigastric pain, or both, which all patients experience. However, if other signs or symptoms have not yet developed, the initial presentation suggests a diagnosis such as peptic ulcer disease or myocardial is-

chemia. On physical examination, subcutaneous crepitus may be present and is a pathognomonic indicator of esophageal injury. A chest x-ray may show a hydropneumothorax, usually on the left side, but this may not be present depending upon the depth of the esophageal perforation. The key to diagnosis and achieving a good outcome is obtaining a contrast esophagogram early in the evaluation process.

Therapy for Esophageal Perforation

As was emphasized earlier, the key to a good patient outcome is establishing the diagnosis in an expeditious fashion and following with speedy surgical exploration. Many series have documented that morbidity and mortality, regardless of the cause of the esophageal perforation, increase rapidly with time. Although there is no longer believed to be a distinct golden period during which operative repair can be performed, it does remain true that the shorter the time interval from injury to operation, the greater is the likelihood of success.

Cervical Injuries

Most injuries to the cervical esophagus are due to external trauma. Common sense dictates that injury to the esophagus is tended to after all vascular injuries have been repaired. As shown in Fig. 68-2, the esophagus is mobilized from the back of the trachea by dissecting directly on the esophageal muscle as far distally as is possible. This allows entry into the tracheoesophageal groove without disturbing the recurrent nerve. The esophagus can more easily be separated from the trachea in the mediastinum, where it is less intimately attached than more proximally, near the pharynx. After beginning the dissection, I press the esophagus posteriorly with a Kuttner dissector while the assistant provides upward traction on the thyroid gland with a hand rather than a metal retractor, which can traumatize the recurrent nerve. After the esophagus is mobilized, all injuries can be visualized and closed in a transverse direction after debridement of necrotic material.

When a vascular injury has also been repaired, it is protective to mobilize and interpose a convenient strap muscle between

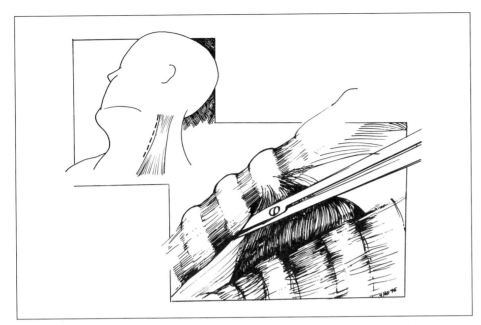

Fig. 68-2. As the inset shows, access to the cervical esophagus has been gained through a neck incision along the anterior border of the left sternocleidomastoid muscle. The esophagus is mobilized from the trachea by incising the tissue on the anterior aspect of the esophagus. If the incision and subsequent dissection are kept close to the esophagus, the recurrent nerves will be undisturbed. The esophagotracheal attachments are less intimate in the upper mediastinum than close to the pharynx and dissection is accordingly easier in this location.

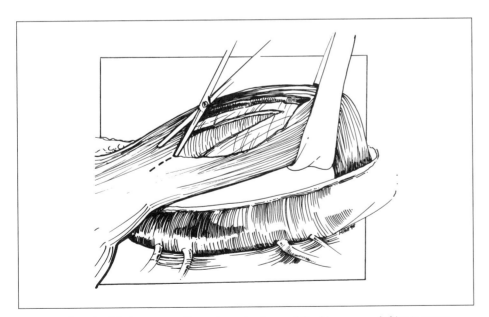

Fig. 68-3. Through a left thoracotomy, the esophagus has been mobilized in generous fashion to ensure complete visualization and exploration and to permit easy manipulation. Necrotic esophageal muscle and mediastinal tissue are debrided. The scissors are external to the mucosa and submucosa and are used to incise esophageal muscle until the proximal and distal limits of the mucosal-submucosal defect are uncovered and clearly identified. In this drawing, the proximal end of the mucosal tear has been identified and distal esophageal muscle is being incised to expose the distal mucosal tear.

the esophageal suture line and the vascular suture line to minimize the chance of development of an esophagovascular fistula. Following repair of an esophageal injury, all neck wounds should routinely be well drained with a suction-type drainage system. Even when a postoperative suture line leak is evidenced by drainage of saliva, there will be ultimate healing of all injuries if adequate and efficient drainage prevents saliva from gaining access to the rest of the neck tissues. In this setting, it is best to support the patient with parenteral nutrition. In my opinion, antibiotics are not routinely necessary and should be reserved for use when there is evidence of actual infection.

Thoracic Esophagus

Injuries to the thoracic esophagus can be caused either by external trauma, esophageal instrumentation, or barogenic rupture. Independently of the cause, the surgical therapeutic principles are constant. First, an accurate preoperative diagnosis of the location and number of injuries should have been unequivocally defined. This may not be applicable for patients with significant thoracic vascular injuries who have been taken quickly and directly from the emergency department to the operating room. When possible, however, all patients should have an esophagogram before operation to avoid the possibility of leaving an injury untreated.

During surgery, the esophagus should be fully mobilized in the area in which the injury exists. When perforation is related to external trauma or iatrogenic rupture, the extent of mediastinal and pleural contamination is usually minimal and simple irrigation is sufficient to clean these spaces. In patients with Boerhaave syndrome, contamination and mediastinal and pleural sepsis may be extensive. In this setting, not only should all foreign material be evacuated but necrotic tissue must be debrided and the mediastinal pleura should be opened widely from the esophageal hiatus to above the aortic arch so that all infected tissues are adequately drained.

The esophageal injury should be carefully inspected and nonviable muscle must be debrided. Particularly with Boerhaave syndrome–type injuries, the muscle at the injury site must be opened sufficiently so that the ends of the mucosal disruption are clearly identified beneath the overlying muscle (Fig. 68-3). Otherwise, one runs the risk that the mucosal defect, which frequently is larger than the muscular tear, will not be completely approximated during the surgical closure.

Small defects are closed transversely. The typical larger injuries have to be closed longitudinally (Fig. 68-4). I prefer to approximate the mucosa using a running suture with either 4–0 polypropylene suture material or a similar sized absorbable suture material. I then approximate the esophageal muscle separately, over the mucosal closure, using an interrupted suture technique, again with 4–0 size and a non-absorbable suture material. Continuing experience suggests that it is reasonable to attempt to close most esophageal perforations. Only those that are associated with extensive necrosis and established mediastinal sepsis should not be closed. Although the outcome is related to the time interval from diagnosis to operation, it can no longer be said that there is a time after which no esophageal perforation should be primarily repaired.

Following closure of a thoracic perforation, it is prudent to buttress the suture line for reinforcement. If the perforation is quite distal, particularly if the patient has an underlying reflux stricture that has been sufficiently dilated, a transthoracic Nissen fundoplication can be safely performed through the hiatus. There is some chance of contaminating the abdominal cavity but if the chest has been cleaned and the perforation closed, this is a small and acceptable risk. For perforations that are more proximal in the chest, as shown in Fig. 68-5, a pleural flap should be developed and sutured in place around the suture line. Although it has not been clearly demonstrated that this is a necessity, it certainly adds integrity to the closure and, given the ease of performance, I think it should be routinely utilized.

Patients with perforation that occurs during esophageal instrumentation typically have known esophageal pathology. The more common types are esophageal stricture related to chronic gastroesophageal reflux and achalasia. These patients should have definitive therapy of their underlying obstructive disease, since the risk of suture line disruption is increased by the distal obstruction. Even if primary healing occurs, the patient's underlying pathology will continue to cause symptoms and necessitate further treatment.

In patients with achalasia this means that after the perforation is closed, a distal myotomy should be carried out. A modified Belsey fundoplication should also be performed, both to prevent iatrogenic reflux and to buttress the suture line. Treatment of patients with esophageal stricture has to be individualized. When the stricture has been sufficiently dilated, then the esophageal perforation can be closed and a transthoracic antireflux procedure performed. However, when the stricture has not been sufficiently dilated, it makes little sense to attempt to salvage a nonfunctional esophagus. Accordingly, esophagectomy is reasonable in this setting. This is an ideal patient to treat using the transhiatal technique, as all patients with benign disease are best reconstructed with an esophagogastrostomy performed in the neck, which

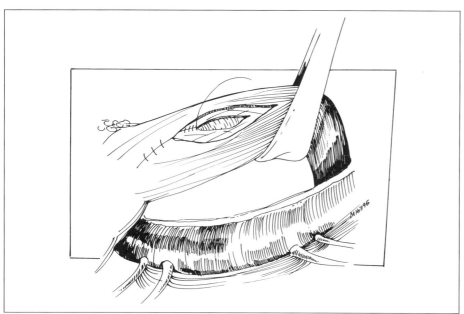

Fig. 68-4. The esophageal mucosa-submucosa is approximated with a running suture technique. The muscle is closed separately, over the submucosa, with interrupted sutures. See the text for details.

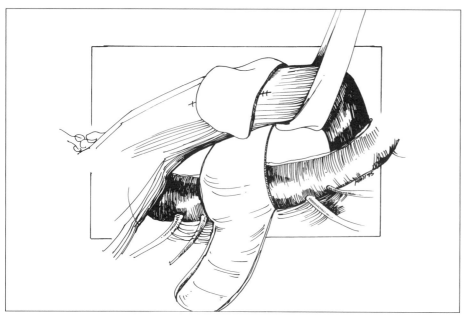

Fig. 68-5. A pleural flap is elevated from the lateral chest wall to a base near the aorta. This pleura is frequently thicker than normal because of the inflammatory process. The mobilized pleural flap is rotated to cover the suture line where it is sutured in place.

the transhiatal technique encompasses. A transthoracic esophagectomy can also be performed with reconstruction either with an intrathoracic colon interposition or by bringing the stomach up into the neck. An intrathoracic esophagogastrostomy is undesirable because of the unremitting gastroesophageal reflux that always ensues, and should only be accepted under exceptional circumstances.

Suggested Reading

Attar S, Hankins JR, Suter CM, et al. Esophageal perforation: A therapeutic challenge. *Ann Thorac Surg* 50:45, 1990.

Goldstein LA, Thompson WR. Esophageal perforations: A fifteen-year experience. *Am J Surg* 143:495, 1982.

Gouge TH, Depan HJ, Spencer FC. Experience with a grillo pleural wrap procedure in eighteen patients with perforation of the thoracic esophagus. *Ann Surg* 209:612, 1989.

Hatzitheofilou C, Strahlendorf C, Kakoyiannis S, et al. Penetrating external injuries of the oesophagus and pharynx. *Br J Surg* 80:1147, 1993.

Horwitz B, Krevsky B, Buckman RF Jr, et al. Endoscopic evaluation of penetrating esophageal injuries. *Am J Gastroenter* 88:1249, 1993.

Kirgan D, Pennathur A, Little AG. Esophageal Trauma: A Modern Perspective. In K Nabeya, T Hanaoka, Nogami (eds), *Recent Advances in Diseases of the Esophagus*. Munich: Springer, 1994. Pp 386–388.

Walker WS, Cameron EW, Walbaum PR. Diagnosis and management of spontaneous transmural rupture of the oesophagus (Boerhaave's syndrome). *Br J Surg* 72:204, 1985.

Wood J, Fabian TC, Mangiante EC. Penetrating neck injuries: Recommendations for selective management. *J Trauma* 29:602, 1989.

Yellin A, Schacter P, Lieberman Y. Spontaneous transmural rupture of esophagus—Boerhaave's syndrome. *Acta Chir Scand* 155:337, 1989.

EDITOR'S COMMENT

Perforation of the esophagus occurs from iatrogenic trauma (instrumentation with an endoscope), external trauma, penetrating or occasionally blunt perforation due to forceful emesis (Boerhaave syndrome), or perforation from foreign bodies. The most likely type of instrumental perforation, in addition to endoscopy, is that which occurs with esophageal dilatation. With endoscopy, the common site of perforation is the upper end of the esophagus, at the cricopharyngeus muscle, for example, whereas the lower esophagus, just above the esophageal hiatus, is where perforation due to dilatation occurs. Perforation from foreign bodies occasionally occurs, but more often is a consequence of attempts at removal. An impressive array of instruments is currently available to remove all types of esophageal foreign bodies, but the danger always exists in endoscopic removal that damage may be done to the esophageal wall; this is particularly true when the foreign body has been present in the esophagus for some time. Perforation from sharp, ingested foreign bodies, such as a fish bone, sewing needles, or other sharp objects, can occur, and may result in serious consequences.

Trauma to the esophagus, either blunt or penetrating, should be approached aggressively. It is important that an adequate diagnostic evaluation of the esophagus be carried out in any patient in whom even a remote possibility exists that the esophagus has perforated, and the workup can either be done by giving oral contrast or by endoscopy. If the cause of the suspected esophageal perforation has been endoscopy, it is most logical to give contrast by mouth, using meglumine diatrizoate (Gastrografin) as the agent of choice, unless there is a risk that the patient may aspirate. Gastrografin aspirated into the tracheo-bronchial tree is more dangerous than is thin barium, which is well tolerated by the mucosa of the upper respiratory tract compared to Gastrografin. If the perforation is thought to be associated with a foreign body, the foreign body should be removed by endoscopy and the esophagus can be evaluated at the same time.

Boerhaave syndrome characteristically occurs on the left posterolateral aspect of the distal esophagus, usually just above the phrenoesophageal ligament. The majority of patients with spontaneous perforations of the distal esophagus will have ingested a substantial amount of alcohol, in addition to a full meal, and these perforations are large and frequently longer than one would expect, as the author has described. The author mentions continuous absorbable suture material for repair of esophageal perforations, although the more commonly used suture material is nonabsorbable, usually interrupted. The esophagus is closed in two layers, the mucosal-submucosal inner layer and the outer muscular coat. Buttressing the repair in the mid or upper esophagus with adjacent soft tissue such as mediastinal pleura is routine, but perforations at the lower end of the esophagus can often be buttressed by the gastric wall, often as an intrathoracic fundoplication.

When the perforation is neglected, or operative treatment has been delayed, mediastinitis is often severe, and attempts at surgical closure alone will often result in secondary perforation, extensive morbidity, and high mortality. When in doubt, the safest course remains complete esophageal diversion by cervical esophagostomy, and if it is technically feasible based on the site of the perforation in the mediastinum, the esophagostomy should be brought out through the skin below the clavicle, so that a suitable stoma bag can be fitted. The distal end of the esophagus should be closed with a simple staple line, and a gastrostomy and feeding jejunostomy should be performed. If there is any question about the viability of the esophagus because of the nature of the trauma or perforation, or because mediastinitis has progressed to the point where the esophagus itself has become irreversibly damaged, it may be necessary to perform esophagectomy without reconstruction, that is, with the cervical esophagostomy, gastrostomy, and jejunostomy.

Cervical esophageal perforations, unless caused by bullet wounds, may be very difficult to find. In the event that the upper esophagus is explored, most commonly through the left cervical approach, and the perforation is not one that is readily identified, extensive drainage of the prevertebral space is the preferred treatment, coupled with gastrostomy to decompress the stomach and feeding jejunostomy. When such transcervical drainage is performed, it is important to be sure that the posterior mediastinum is adequately drained by careful dissection and insertion of a drain into the superior portion of the posterior mediastinum. If the defect is found, primary closure is indicated, but the drains are placed as a last step. Gastrostomy and jejunostomy are not indicated after satisfactory cervical esophageal repair, but total parenteral nutrition (TPN) may be used. Regardless of the site of repair, an esophagogram should always be obtained to rule out leak before one attempts to feed the patient.

R.J.B.

69

Surgical Repair of Tracheoesophageal Fistula and Esophageal Atresia

Jay L. Grosfeld   Scott A. Engum

Esophageal atresia and tracheoesophageal (TE) fistula is a common neonatal condition that remains a significant challenge to children's surgical specialists. The first description of esophageal atresia is attributed to Thomas Durston in 1670. In 1696, Thomas Gibson described the association of atresia with a distal tracheoesophageal fistula. In 1939, Dr. Thomas Lanman in Boston and Dr. Logan Leven of Minneapolis reported the successful management of babies with esophageal atresia using a staged repair that initially created a gastrostomy followed by ligation of the fistula and subsequent esophageal replacement using an antethoracic skin tube. The first successful primary repair was performed by Dr. Cameron Haight of Ann Arbor, Michigan, in 1941. Over the past 50+ years continuous refinements in clinical management have occurred associated with improved surgical technique, advances in neonatal anesthesia, development of infant ventilators, and modern sophisticated neonatal intensive care. These advances have allowed survival of even low birth weight infants, many of whom have associated anomalies that formerly decided the issue in a negative way.

Clinical Presentation

Common findings on presentation include excessive salivation due to pooling of secretions in the proximal atretic esophageal pouch, and respiratory distress and cyanosis due to aspiration. Abdominal distention may occur as a result of inspired air passing through the fistula into the stomach causing gastric dilatation (Fig. 69-1) with subsequent reflux of gastric juice upward through the fistula and into the lungs resulting in pneumonitis. Some babies have severe respiratory distress and require mechanical ventilation before their admission to specialized high-risk neonatal centers. Associated congenital anomalies are very common, occurring in 146 of 227 cases (65%) treated in our facility; con-

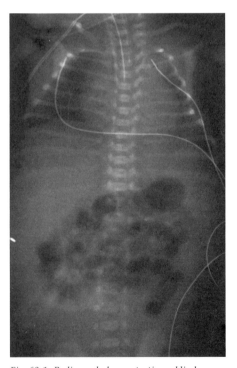

Fig. 69-1. Radiograph demonstrating a blind-ending proximal esophageal pouch with feeding tube, and the presence of gas in the gastrointestinal tract, indicating a distal tracheoesophageal fistula (type C).

genital heart defects are the most common defect, noted in 38 percent of cases. Musculoskeletal anomalies were seen in 19 percent, central nervous system abnormalities in 15 percent, renal anomalies in 15 percent, and associated abnormalities of the alimentary tract in 13 percent, including duodenal atresia, malrotation, and imperforate anus.

There are five major anatomic variants of esophageal atresia. Type A, atresia without a fistula, occurs in approximately 13 percent of cases; type B, in which a proximal atresia and fistula are present, occurs in 1 percent; and the most common variant, type C, with proximal esophageal atresia and a distal TE fistula, occurs in 78 percent of cases. We experienced five type D patients (2%), who have a double fistula, and in 6 percent of cases an H-type TE fistula may occur in the absence of esophageal atresia (type E). For the purpose of this chapter, we will describe the operative management of the most common variants, beginning with type C and also discussing types A and E.

The timing of operation must be individualized according to the specific infant's clinical condition. Although the Waterston classification system, devised in 1962 to categorize babies with esophageal atresia, was used extensively in the past, we no longer employ these guidelines but simply individualize each patient according to his or her clinical status. Immediate thoracotomy and primary repair are performed in reasonably healthy infants with early diagnosis and no associated anomalies. Smaller infants, even with minimal respiratory compromise and associated anomalies after appropriate stabilization, will undergo similar repair within 24 hours. Poor-risk infants, especially the premature with severe respiratory ailments or congestive heart failure, or both, may require some delay in therapy and are initially treated with an emergency gastrostomy (often under local anesthesia), continuous proximal atretic pouch suction, and administration of intravenous antibiotics. Definitive repair is attempted when the infant's condition stabilizes, usually in the first few days (2–5) of life.

Preoperative Preparation

Repair is carried out in the operating theater. The room temperature is adjustable and is kept at approximately 80°F to maintain thermal neutrality. The baby is placed on a warming blanket and carefully monitored with an arterial line, ECG monitor, pulse oximeter, and thermal probe. The legs are wrapped in swaddling cloth and a cap is placed on the baby's head to retain body heat. An awake intubation is performed and the endotracheal tube is positioned with the bevel facing posteriorly to occlude the fistula, if possible, to avoid gastric distention. A small, flexible fiberoptic bronchoscope is passed down the endotracheal tube to ascertain the location of the end of the tube and the fistula opening. The procedure is performed under an

overhead warmer, which also helps maintain the baby's thermal equilibrium. The patient is positioned for a right lateral thoracotomy. A folded towel or soft rubber support is placed under the left axilla to make sure that the left chest can expand appropriately. The baby's skin is prepared with an iodophor solution and alcohol and draped appropriately for a posterolateral thoracotomy. A Replogle tube is placed in the proximal esophageal pouch. If a previous gastrostomy was performed, this is opened and placed on straight drainage to avoid gastric distention during the procedure.

A short posterolateral incision is made below the level of the tip of the scapula (Fig. 69-2), and hemostasis is effected with an infant electrocoagulator. The latissimus dorsi muscle is identified and divided (Fig. 69-3), the auscultatory space of Korotkov is identified, and the scapula is retracted superiorly and the serratus anterior muscle medially. It is usually unnecessary to divide the serratus muscle, thus avoiding the risk of developing a winged scapula. The fourth intercostal space is identified and entered. The intercostal muscles are carefully divided to avoid entering the pleura. An extrapleural dissection is carried out using either a small periosteal elevator or a moistened cotton-tipped applicator. An extrapleural plane is established and an infant rib spreader is inserted to improve exposure. The intact pleura is dissected superiorly to the thoracic inlet and

posteriorly to identify the azygos vein. The intact pleura and underlying lung are dissected and retracted medially with moistened sponges under a soft malleable retractor. The dissection continues with the use of a moist peanut sponge until the azygos is fully mobilized and the mediastinal pleura over the vein is opened (Fig. 69-4). The azygos vein is divided between two 4–0 silk suture ties. This vein is often the marker for the site of the tracheoesophageal fistula as it enters the trachea. A branch of the vagus nerve usually passes over the area as well.

Following ligation and division of the vein, the TE fistula (TEF) is identified and carefully dissected free near the trachea (Fig. 69-5A). It is important to avoid dividing small vessels to the midesophagus that arise directly from the aorta. A vascular loop is placed around the TE fistula and a fine 5–0 suture of Maxon (Davis and Geck, Manati, PR) or PDS (Ethicon/Johnson & Johnson, Somerville, NJ) on a small tapered needle is placed at the end of the TE fistula on the esophageal side to avoid tracheal narrowing by the closure (Fig. 69-5B). The TEF is divided by a fine tenotomy scissors and the tracheal side is oversewn (Fig. 69-5C) with fine bites of a running or interrupted 5–0 suture. The suture line is then placed under saline and the anesthesiologist is requested to slightly hyperinflate the lungs to assure that the tracheal closure is airtight. Mediastinal pleura is used to cover the tracheal suture line to

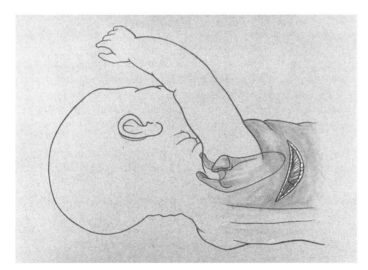

Fig. 69-2. A posterolateral incision is made just below the tip of the scapula. The latissimus dorsi muscle is divided while the serratus anterior muscle is retracted anteriorly and medially.

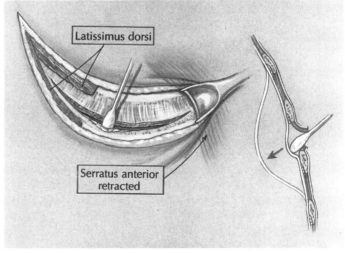

Fig. 69-3. The fourth intercostal space is identified and entered, and an extrapleural dissection is carried out using a moistened cotton-tipped applicator.

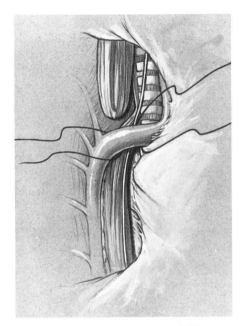

Fig. 69-4. The intact pleura is retracted. The azygos vein is isolated, divided, and retracted anteriorly with the pleura. This allows identification of the tracheoesophageal fistula.

reduce the risk of a recurrent TE fistula should an anastomotic leak occur postoperatively.

The upper atretic esophageal pouch is identified with the aid of the anesthesiologist, who pushes down on the end of the pouch with a previously placed tube. The dissection of the proximal pouch is facilitated by placing a 3–0 traction suture in the tip of the pouch (Fig. 69-6). The atretic esophagus is mobilized up to the level of thoracic inlet and into the neck to acquire adequate length to achieve primary repair by constructing an anastomosis without tension. The rich blood supply to the more hypertrophic upper pouch is derived from the inferior thyroid artery. Clearing the esophagus from the mediastinal tissues can be done by blunt dissection and a fine-tipped infant electrocoagulator. Dissection of the proximal atretic pouch from the tracheal wall can be difficult and requires meticulous attention and gentle technique to avoid injury of or entry into the trachea.

Rarely (in 2% of cases), a type D variant (double fistula) is encountered, with the second fistula located in the upper pouch. Traction sutures are placed at the 3 and 9 o'clock positions on the open distal esophagus, and by placing gentle traction in opposite directions, the proximity of the upper and lower esophageal ends is determined. Extensive distal esophageal mobilization should be avoided to reduce the risk of ischemia to the midesophagus by damaging the small arterial branches that come directly from the aorta. The major blood supply to the midesophagus in these cases comes through the TE fistula, which has already been divided. If the distal rim of the esophageal tissue is cyanotic, it should be carefully debrided. The distal esophageal opening is gently dilated with a right-angle clamp. Full-thickness lateral sutures of 4–0 Vicryl (Ethicon), PDS, or Maxon are placed in the distal esophagus. Each suture must include a healthy full-thickness bite, including mucosa as well as the smooth muscle of the esophageal wall.

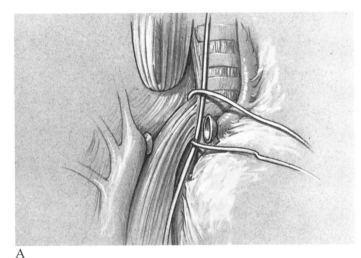

A

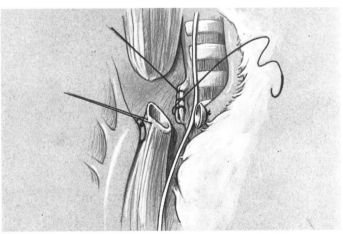

B

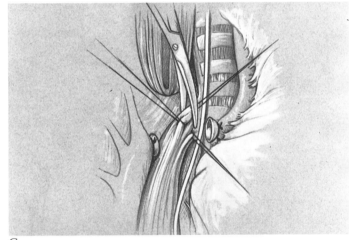

C

Fig. 69-5. A. The TE fistula site is mobilized circumferentially distal to the fistula and the area is encircled with a vessel loop. B. Traction sutures are placed, with great care taken not to encroach on the lumen of the trachea, which can result in narrowing with closure. Division of the fistula is then performed using a tenotomy scissors. C. The tracheal end is closed with either a 5–0 continuous or interrupted suture. The closure is tested with positive-pressure ventilation to rule out a leak. The tracheal suture line is covered with mediastinal pleura to reduce the risk of recurrent TE fistula should an anastomotic leak occur.

The needles should be left in place so that the esophageal wall can be sutured to the upper pouch.

The distal portion of the larger, thicker proximal atretic pouch is incised directly over the tube located in the pouch lumen to determine its dependent area. Entry can be accomplished with either a scalpel or tenotomy scissors. The size of the opening should be similar to or just slightly larger than the distal esophagus after it has been dilated. A full-thickness suture bite is placed in the midportion of the posterior wall of both ends of the esophagus with the knots tied on the outside (Fig. 69-7A). Using this suture and the previously placed corner sutures for traction, the one-layer posterior suture line is completed with a few additional interrupted sutures.

All the sutures are placed before any are tied in order to distribute the tension evenly along the suture line. An orogastric tube (No. 8–10 French size) is then passed from above by the anesthesiologist through the anastomosis into the stomach. The anterior wall of the anastomosis is completed with full-thickness, interrupted, 4–0 PDS, Maxon, or Vicryl suture (Fig. 69-7B and C), completing the single-layer repair. A No. 5 French catheter is placed in the upper esophagus and 5 to 10 ml saline is carefully instilled to test the anastomotic suture line for a leak. The traditional two-layer Haight telescopic anastomosis is no longer employed. Although some authors recommend the use of 5–0 suture material for the anastomosis, the finer suture has more of a tendency to cut through the tissues if there is any tension on the anastomosis, which cannot be avoided in a significant number of cases. The use of silk in the anastomosis is more often associated with both an increased incidence of leak and stricture formation.

In some instances, the two ends of the esophagus are too far apart (>2.0 cm) for a safe primary anastomosis. A circular myotomy (Fig. 69-8), as described by Livaditis, can lengthen the proximal end. The myotomy is performed approximately 2 cm above the blind proximal atretic end, using a Beaver blade and right-angle clamp to divide the longitudinal and circular smooth muscle. This will increase the

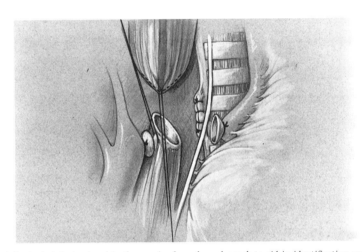

Fig. 69-6. A Replogle tube is placed in the proximal esophageal pouch to aid in identification and dissection. While the proximal esophageal pouch is mobilized, a proximal fistula should be excluded. The proximal esophagus is mobilized to the thoracic inlet within the neck. When opening the proximal esophagus, care should be taken to ensure that the opening is at the lowermost point recognized with the feeding tube tip. The distal esophagus is freed only as much as necessary to approximate the ends of the esophagus.

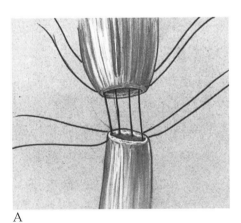

A

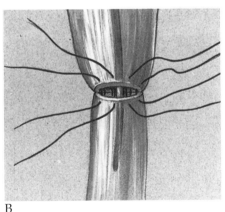

B

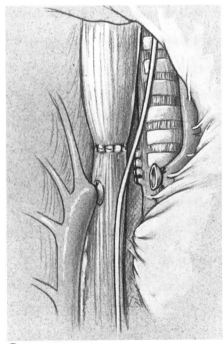

C

Fig. 69-7. A. A single-layer anastomosis is performed with full-thickness, interrupted 4–0 sutures involving mucosa and muscularis. The posterior sutures are placed with the suture knots on the outside. B. After the posterior suture line is completed, a feeding tube is advanced into the distal esophagus and stomach. The anterior sutures are inserted to complete the single-layer anastomosis. C. An extrapleural chest tube is placed adjacent to, but not on, the anastomosis.

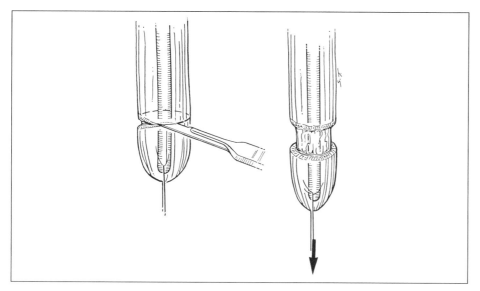

Fig. 69-8. Circular myotomy of the proximal esophageal pouch is useful to gain 1 cm of esophageal length for a tension-free anastomosis.

length of the proximal esophagus approximately 1 cm and often facilitates a primary anastomosis without tension. Occasionally, a second myotomy may be required at a more proximal level. A spiral myotomy has been described but its use is not routinely advocated.

At the conclusion of the anastomosis, the pleura should be checked for possible holes and then a No. 12 French chest tube is placed, entering the posterior mediastinal space below the incision, being careful to avoid injury to the pleura during insertion. The tip of the tube is situated superiorly, near, but not on, the anastomosis, and it is kept in place with a 4–0 Vicryl suture, fixing the tube to the chest wall should a leak occur. A 3–0 polypropylene suture affixes the tube to the skin at the exit site. The tube is then attached to an underwater seal closed drainage system. The lung is gently expanded and the chest wound is closed using 2–0 Vicryl paracostal sutures to oppose the ribs and a running 3–0 Vicryl suture to close the divided latissimus dorsi muscle. The anesthesiologist can aid in the closure by pushing down on the infant's right arm and shoulder, taking tension off the wound. The subcutaneous fascia is approximated with a continuous running 4–0 Vicryl suture and the skin edges are closed with 4–0 subcuticular suture. Steri-Strips and a dry occlusive dressing are applied using gauze and Opsite.

Postoperative Care

The infant is extubated if the respiratory effort is satisfactory and blood gas determinations are acceptable. It is not unusual to keep the endotracheal tube in place overnight and to remove it in the newborn intensive care unit after stabilization. A suction catheter, carefully marked in the operating room to limit maximum extent of tube insertion, is used by the nursing staff to avoid injury to the suture line. If the baby is intubated and the endotracheal tube comes out, reintubation should be performed only by experienced personnel with direct visualization of the vocal cords to avoid injury to the anastomosis. Tracheomalacia can occur in anywhere from 8 to 15 percent of cases and may require long-term ventilatory support. If compression of the trachea is observed by pulsatile external vascular compression on bronchoscopy, an aortic suspension procedure may relieve these symptoms. Otherwise a tracheostomy may eventually be necessary.

The orogastric tube that was placed in the stomach at the time of the procedure should be fixed and not moved. If it comes out, replacement should not be attempted. Feedings are often initiated through the orogastric tube on postoperative day 3 or 4. Gastrostomy tubes are not routinely used for healthy babies. The chest tube is left in place until postoperative day 6, when a

contrast barium swallow confirms that no anastomotic leak is present. Oral feedings may be initiated at that time. Care should be exercised during oral feedings because of the high incidence of esophageal dysmotility problems (greater than 30%) and the risk of gastroesophageal reflux, which is seen in 50 percent of cases. When observed, the patient should be placed on reflux precautions, using an incline board, antacids, H$_2$ blockers, and prokinetic agents (cisapride). If an anastomotic leak is noted, it is usually minimal and closes spontaneously. Rarely, a major anastomotic disruption may require reoperation.

Stricture at the anastomotic suture line may be related to gastroesophageal reflux with acid juice injuring the site of repair. A stricture may occur in from 16 to 30 percent of cases. Half of the patients who demonstrate gastroesophageal reflux will require an antireflux operation. Because of the poor motility experienced by many of these babies, if a 360-degree wrap (Nissen) is used this should be constructed as a short, loose floppy fundoplication. Most anastomotic strictures respond to esophageal dilatation using either a balloon dilator or more traditional dilators of the Tucker, Maloney, or Savorie type.

Esophageal Atresia Without a Fistula (Type A)

Management of neonates with long-gap type A esophageal atresia is often complex, and there is some controversy regarding the choice of operation. A number of therapeutic options are available, including esophageal replacement with stomach or colon as a gastric pull-up or reversed gastric tube and right or left colon interposition. Jejunal interposition has also been used; however, it has not been as popular a primary procedure. During the past decade, many surgeons have attempted to preserve the native esophagus and perform a delayed esophageal anastomosis. The diagnosis of type A atresia is usually achieved when an esophageal tube cannot be passed into the stomach and it is observed on chest or abdominal radiographs that no air is present in hollow viscera beneath the diaphragm (Fig. 69-9). Initial clinical management involves the use of a Replogle tube in the proximal

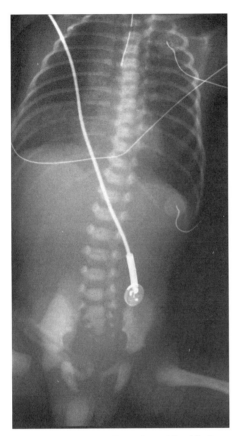

Fig. 69-9. Radiograph of an infant with a blind-ending proximal esophageal pouch containing a Replogle tube and a gasless abdomen, indicating an isolated (type A) esophageal atresia.

esophagus placed on constant suction to decompress the pouch and control secretions and placement of a gastrostomy tube for feeding purposes. The proximal atretic pouch is dilated daily with an esophageal bougie for 6 to 8 weeks (or occasionally longer) as gastrostomy feedings continue and the baby grows. Occasionally, a dilator can be placed through the gastrostomy site into the lower end of the esophagus and retrograde dilatations can be accomplished from below, as well. Reflux of bolus gastrostomy feedings may also be useful. The gap between the two ends of the esophagus can be measured by placing a radiopaque dilator in the proximal esophagus, refluxing contrast material into the lower esophagus through the gastrostomy, and obtaining a radiograph (Fig. 69-10).

When the gap is less than 2.0 cm, a thoracotomy can be attempted. Delayed anastomosis is possible in the majority of cases; however, frequently an esophageal

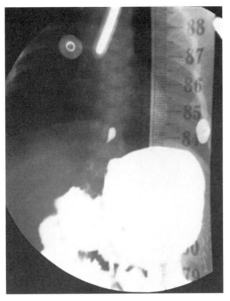

Fig. 69-10. Chest radiograph with proximal bougie and distal contrast study in a baby with type A isolated esophageal atresia illustrating the length of esophageal gap. This patient has a 2.5-cm gap.

myotomy to bridge the gap may be necessary. Staged stretching of the proximal esophagus by formation of an esophagostomy that is stretched inferiorly onto the anterior chest wall, as described by Kimura and Soper, is an alternative method of achieving additional length of the proximal esophagus. The technical aspects of the operative anastomosis are similar to those previously noted for type C cases. Despite the dilatation, an esophagomyotomy is often required. Following primary esophageal anastomosis for type A atresia, the leak rate is slightly higher than that noted after type C repair, and many of the cases develop a stricture that requires subsequent dilatation. Gastroesophageal reflux is also more common in this group of patients. An antireflux procedure (fundoplication) is required more often in these cases than in other variants of esophageal atresia.

Alternative management of type A atresia utilizes a temporary cervical esophagostomy to divert secretions and stimulate the swallowing reflux with sham feedings. Subsequent reconstruction of the esophagus can be performed either using the colon (Fig. 69-11) or stomach. A gastric tube (Fig. 69-12) is developed by maintaining the blood supply to the left gastroepiploic artery. The right gastroepiploic vessels are

then divided approximately 2 cm proximal to the pylorus and the greater omentum is divided up to the splenic hilum. The gastric tube will be fashioned along the greater curvature of the stomach. A No. 18–24 Fr tube is placed in the stomach tube and the division of the stomach along the greater curvature is accomplished using a GIA autostapler (U.S. Surgical Corporation, Norwalk, CT). A left cervical neck incision is made around the proximal esophagostomy, which is mobilized. A left thoracotomy incision is made over the sixth interspace. The tube is brought up through the hiatus into the chest behind the hilum of the lung and brought up into the neck, where an end-to-end anastomosis is performed with the esophagus. An alternative procedure is the gastric pull-up operation, as described by Spitz and others, in which the proximal stomach is pulled up through the hiatus to the neck level and an anastomosis to the esophagus is performed without a formal thoracotomy.

The upward passage of the stomach is done in a blunt manner, passing it through the posterior mediastinum. The major postoperative problems in these cases are related to the anastomosis. The incidence of leak and stricture is common and dilatations are often required. Babies frequently have food aversion for 6 to 12 months after the operation. The incidence of tracheomalacia is similar in type A babies despite the fact that they have no TE fistula.

H-Type Tracheoesophageal Fistula

Tracheoesophageal fistula without atresia (type E) often occurs at a cervical level at or above the second thoracic vertebra but can occur more distally. Diagnosis in these cases may be delayed; however, frequently they are associated with coughing or choking during a feeding, particularly with liquids. Abdominal distention may be impressive because of filling of the stomach with inspired air. Recurring episodes of pneumonia are also a common finding. Contrast studies of the esophagus and trachea using isosmolar contrast material are often successful in demonstrating

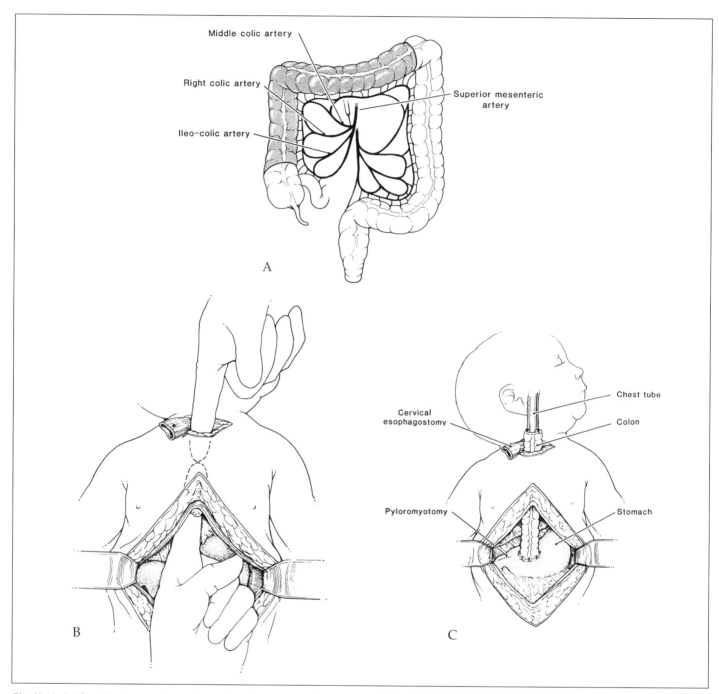

Fig. 69-11. A. The right colon may be used for esophageal replacement. The cecum (and ileocecal valve) are preserved, and the blood supply for the vascular pedicle is based on the middle colic artery. B. Blunt dissection is used to create the substernal tunnel for the colon conduit. Alternatively, the left colon can be used via the left chest (Waterston's technique). C. A concomitant gastric drainage procedure (pyloromyotomy or pyloroplasty) is an important adjunct to the colon conduit technique.

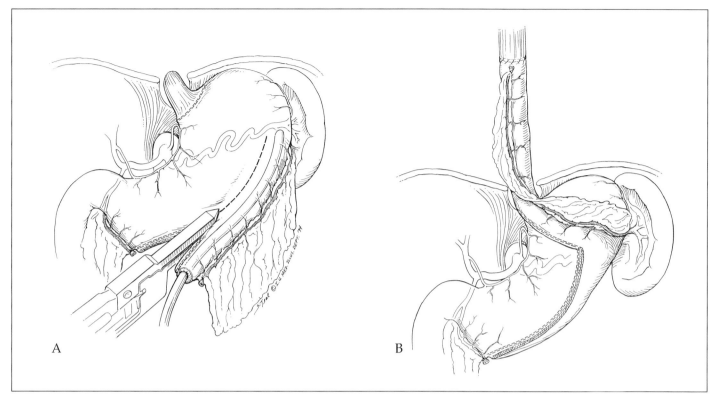

Fig. 69-12. A reversed gastric tube is fashioned along the greater curvature of the stomach, incising both anterior and posterior walls to conform to the size of a No. 18–24 French catheter.

the site of the fistula; however, we have found rigid fiberoptic bronchoscopy to be the most accurate method of detecting the site of the fistula.

Since the vast majority of fistulas occur in the neck, most cases can be approached through a right cervical incision in the lower neck, extending from the sternal notch laterally to beyond the level of the sternocleidomastoid muscle. The esophagus can be identified by palpating an oral esophageal tube placed from above. At the time of bronchoscopy, a fine Fogarty dilator catheter is placed through the fistula, and during the procedure the balloon is inflated and pulled back in the esophagus to the level of the fistula, which will help guide the dissection (Fig. 69-13). The actual shape of the fistula is more like an N, with the tract passing downward from the esophagus to the posterolateral portion of the trachea near its membranous and cartilaginous components. Once the fistula has been identified, a vascular loop is placed around the fistula and it is divided on the esophageal side to avoid narrowing of the trachea. The defect is closed with interrupted 4–0 PDS, Vicryl, or Maxon sutures on both the tracheal and esophageal

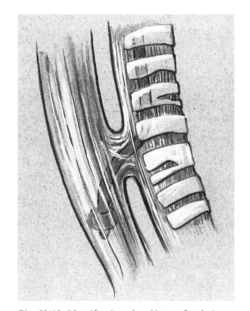

Fig. 69-13. Identification of an H-type fistula is aided by placing a Fogarty catheter through the fistula at bronchoscopy.

side. The suture lines are separated by placing mobilized strap muscle from the neck between these two areas to prevent recurrence of the fistula if an esophageal leak occurs. A small drain is left near the

TE fistula repair and brought out through a separate skin exit site lateral to the wound. The drain is maintained until an esophagogram is performed on the sixth postoperative day and shows no evidence of a leak. A right thoracotomy in the third intercostal space should be used when the fistula is located in the chest. Division of the fistula is carried out as described earlier. Success in the management of H-type TE fistula requires a high degree of suspicion, precise localization, and meticulous operation tailored to the location of the fistula.

Summary

The overall survival of infants with the several variants of esophageal atresia and TE fistula is 90 to 95 percent, with most deaths attributed to complex cardiac anomalies and chromosomal disorders that are incompatible with life. Although complications are common, these can often be prevented by careful attention to detail in the operating room and, when they occur, early recognition along with aggressive treatment of strictures, gastroesophageal reflux, and tracheomalacia.

Suggested Reading

Ashcraft KW, Holder TM. The story of esophageal atresia and tracheoesophageal fistula. *Surgery* 65:332, 1969.

Ein SH, Shandling B. Pure esophageal atresia: A 50 year review. *J Pediatr Surg* 29:1208, 1994.

Engum SA, Grosfeld JL, West KW, et al. Analysis of morbidity and mortality in 227 cases of esophageal atresia (EA) and/or tracheoesophageal fistula (TEF) over two decades. *Arch Surg* 130:502, 1995.

Haight C, Towsley HA. Congenital atresia of the esophagus with tracheoesophageal fistula: Extrapleural ligation of fistula and end-to-end anastomosis of esophageal segments. *Surg Gynecol Obstet* 76:672, 1943.

Kimura K, Soper RT. Multistaged extrathoracic esophageal elongation for long gap esophageal atresia. *J Pediatr Surg* 29:566, 1994.

Livaditis A. Esophageal atresia, a method of overbridging large segmental gaps. *Z Kinderchir* 13:298, 1973.

Louhimo I, Lindahl H. Esophageal atresia: Primary results of 500 consecutively treated patients. *J Pediatr Surg* 18:217, 1983.

Manning P, Morgan RA, Coran A, et al. Fifty years' experience with esophageal atresia and tracheoesophageal fistula. *Ann Surg* 204:446, 1986.

Randolph JG, Newman KD, Anderson KD. Current results in repair of esophageal atresia with tracheoesophageal fistula using physiologic status as a guide to therapy. *Ann Surg* 209:526, 1989.

Rescorla FJ, West KW, Scherer LR III, et al. The complex nature of type A (long-gap) esophageal atresia. *Surgery* 116:658, 1994.

Spitz L, Kiely E, Brereton RJ, Drake D. Management of esophageal atresia. *World J Surg* 17:296, 1993.

Waterston BJ, Bonham-Carter RE, Aberdeen E. Esophageal atresia with tracheoesophageal fistula: A study of survival in 218 infants. *Lancet* 1:819, 1962.

EDITOR'S COMMENT

The commonest congenital anomaly of the esophagus is proximal esophageal atresia with distal tracheoesophageal fistula, the so-called type C atresia encountered in approximately 80 percent of cases of esophageal atresia. The success rate with operation for esophageal atresia in full-term infants is in excess of 90 percent; the major complications in that group center around associated congenital defects, including several varieties of congenital heart disease, imperforate anus, and duodenal stenosis or atresia. The preoperative preparation includes careful survey of the entire gastrointestinal tract, echocardiography, and evaluation for other less commonly seen anomalies. At this time, the majority of infants are operated on very promptly, although those encountered after considerable delay in arriving at the appropriate diagnosis often have significant respiratory complications, which can usually be dealt with by performance of a gastrostomy, use of the head-up position with proximal pouch suction, and peripheral hyperalimentation. It is important to remember that the placement of the gastrostomy may complicate the creation of a reversed gastric tube later if it is necessary to interpose a portion of the gastrointestinal tract between the proximal end of the pouch, when it is quite short, and the stomach. The colon is also a satisfactory esophageal substitute under these circumstances, but placement of the gastrostomy at the lesser curvature side of the stomach should always be considered in those babies who require that procedure.

Small H-type tracheoesophageal fistulas in older babies have the most subtle presentation of this anomaly. Most of the fistulas are above the second thoracic vertebra, a few are multiple with two fistulas, and the diagnosis can be delayed for weeks or even months. The symptoms that are ordinarily encountered are coughing or choking with feeding, and greater or lesser abdominal distention, depending on the size of the fistula. Any child with frequent episodes of pneumonia should be assumed to be aspirating from a specific anomaly, and gastroesophageal reflux and H-type tracheoesophageal fistula are important considerations in evaluating such a child. Contrast studies of the esophagus, under cine control, may be quite helpful, but the most precise localization is undoubtedly made with bronchoscopy or esophagoscopy, or both, where the orifice can usually be seen. Nevertheless, if that orifice is tiny, it is possible to miss it with either rigid or flexible endoscopic examination.

As with esophageal operations in older patients, the commonest problem encountered after the immediate postoperative period is that of stricture at the anastomosis, usually due to a small anastomotic leak that has closed. The unfortunate necessity for repeated dilatations in these children is not rare, but interrupted suture lines of minimally reactive suture material (polydioxanone or polypropylene) are necessary to allow growth of the esophagus and maximize effectiveness of dilatation.

R.J.B.

II

The Stomach and Duodenum

70

Anatomic Considerations in Gastroduodenal Surgery

Charles A. Griffith†

This section on the stomach and duodenum is concerned primarily with operations for peptic ulcer and carcinoma. Accordingly, the topics in this chapter are confined to anatomic points that pertain to these operations.

The Omentum

Iatrogenic Injury to the Spleen

A variable number of peritoneal folds from the greater omentum may attach directly onto the medial or anterior surfaces of the spleen, particularly at its lower pole. Excessive traction on the omentum or stomach can be transmitted to these folds and can disrupt the splenic capsule and pulp. This accident is the most common cause of iatrogenic splenic injury and is prevented by looking for omental attachments to the spleen when the abdomen is first explored. Some attachments are flimsy and avascular; others are bulky and contain aberrant vessels. Snipping the former or ligating and transecting the latter is often expedient, for the stomach and omentum may then be retracted without injury to the spleen as the operation progresses.

Necrosis of the Greater Omentum

Omental necrosis after gastric resection is caused by devascularization of the arc of Barkow (Fig. 70-1). This sequela has occurred frequently enough for some surgeons to recommend excising the greater

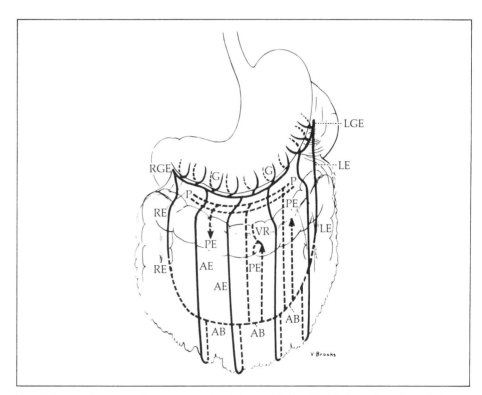

Fig. 70-1. Arterial supply to the greater omentum. The arc of Barkow (AB) in the posterior layer of the omentum is formed by the anastomosis of the right and left epiploic branches (RE and LE) from the right and left gastroepiploic arteries (RGE and LGE). The anterior epiploic arteries (AE) from RGE and LGE descend in the anterior layer of the omentum, wind around its free edge, and enter AB posteriorly. Only a few of the posterior epiploic arteries (PE) from the transverse, dorsal, or great pancreatic arteries (P) enter AB; other PE enter the transverse colon directly or anastomose with the vasa recta (VR) of the middle colic circulation. (G = gastric branches from RGE and LGE.) (From CA Griffith. Anatomy. In LM Nyhus, C Wastell [eds], Surgery of the Stomach and Duodenum [4th ed]. Boston: Little, Brown, 1986. Reproduced with permission.)

†Deceased

omentum routinely during gastrectomy or, if the omentum is retained, preserving all epiploic branches and ligating only the gastric branches of the gastroepiploic vessels when separating the omentum from the greater curve, a tedious and time-consuming task. A quicker technique, one that preserves blood flow through the arc of Barkow and maintains omental viability, entails transecting the gastrocolic ligament and ligating the anterior epiploic arteries. On the left, only the gastric branches of the left gastroepiploic artery are ligated; the left epiploic branches are preserved. On the right, the right gastroepiploic artery is ligated distal to the origin of its right epiploic branch. Even if this branch is ligated in some instances, the left and posterior epiploic branches furnish enough supply to the arc of Barkow to prevent omental necrosis.

When the greater omentum is removed in instances of carcinoma, the bloodiness of the dissection for separating the omentum from the transverse colon varies according to the sizes and numbers of the posterior epiploic branches. Similarly, the bloodiness of the dissection for mobilizing the splenic flexure of the colon varies according to the sizes and numbers of the left epiploic branches within the splenocolic ligament.

The Abdominal Vagi

The abdominal vagal system has three components: 1) the esophageal plexus from the left and right vagus nerves, 2) the two trunks from the plexus, and 3) the four truncal divisions. The anterior and posterior gastric divisions innervate the stomach; the hepatic and celiac divisions innervate all derivations of the midgut (Fig. 70-2).

Total Abdominal (Truncal) Vagotomy at the Hiatus

In reference to Dragstedt's technique of transecting all vagal fibers at or just above or below the diaphragmatic esophageal hiatus, the term *total abdominal* defines a vagotomy of the stomach plus the midgut. Continued use of the more popular term *truncal vagotomy* perpetuates the fallacy that the surgeon always cuts trunks. Recognition of the anatomic basis of the fallacy affords explanation of why incomplete vagotomy occurs and how it can be avoided.

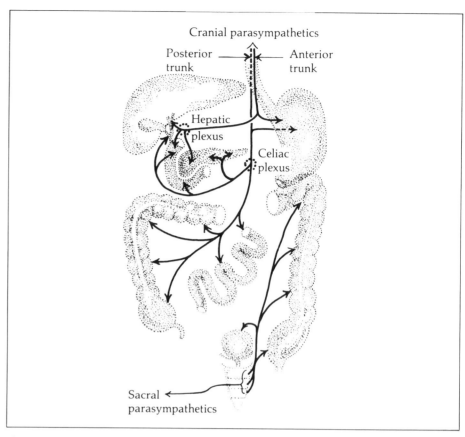

Fig. 70-2. Distribution of the abdominal vagi. The gastric, hepatic, and celiac vagal branches are preganglionic fibers. The hepatic branches pass through the hepatic plexus without synapse to innervate the biliary tract and liver. The celiac branches pass through the celiac and superior mesenteric plexuses without synapse to innervate the remainder of the midgut. (From CA Griffith. Courtesy of Surgical Clinics of North America and W. B. Saunders Company.)

Multiple Nerves
The vagal system may descend through the hiatus as the esophageal plexus or as the two trunks or the four truncal divisions (Fig. 70-3). In approximately one-fourth of dissections, the surgeon encounters variable numbers of large fibers of the esophageal plexus or small fibers of the truncal divisions. When these fibers are transected, the vagotomy is not truncal in the strict anatomic sense. Thus, the term *truncal vagotomy* perpetuates the misconception that the surgeon cuts only the two vagal trunks.

Variable Positions of the Vagi at the Hiatus
The embryologic rotation of the stomach accounts for considerable variation in the positions of the vagi at the hiatus (Fig. 70-4). Also, but not diagrammed in Fig. 70-4, some of the vagi may lie well *away* from the esophagus. For example, the anterior trunk may lie closer to the left hiatal margin, and the posterior trunk may lie closer to the aorta than to the esophagus.

Primary Cause of Inadequate Incomplete Vagotomy
A dissection confined to the hiatus does not afford enough exposure to identify the vagi as the esophageal plexus, the trunks, or the truncal divisions. Therefore, the surgeon cannot know how many nerves there are or where they are. Under these circumstances, one or more fibers lying well away from the esophagus may be excluded as the surgeon encircles the esophagus. Thus, rather than a small fiber closely applied to the esophagus being overlooked, an entire trunk or large fiber of the esophageal

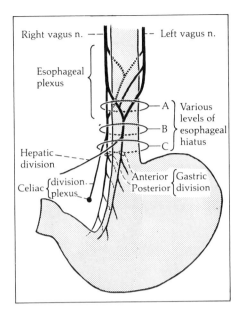

Fig. 70-3. Variations of the vagi at the hiatus. In the lower thorax, the right and left vagus nerves branch and communicate with each other to form the esophageal plexus. The branches of this plexus then unite to form two trunks—one anterior and the other posterior to the esophagus. Each trunk contains fibers from both right and left nerves. The anterior trunk divides into the anterior gastric and hepatic divisions, and the posterior trunk divides into the posterior gastric and celiac divisions. The gastric divisions continue along the lesser curve as the greater anterior and posterior gastric nerves (of Latarjet), which send off terminal branches to the stomach. The hepatic division consists of a few small, closely applied fibers that run parallel within the lesser omentum to the hepatic autonomic plexus at the porta hepatis. The celiac division, largest of the four truncal divisions, can be considered a continuation of the posterior trunk. This posterior trunk–celiac division descends within the gastropancreatic peritoneal fold to the celiac and superior mesenteric autonomic plexuses. A. Multiple fibers of the esophageal plexus at the hiatus. B. The two trunks at the hiatus. C. Multiple fibers of the four truncal divisions at the hiatus. (From CA Griffith. Anatomy. In LM Nyhus, C Wastell [eds], Surgery of the Stomach and Duodenum [3rd ed]. Boston: Little, Brown, 1977. Reproduced with permission.)

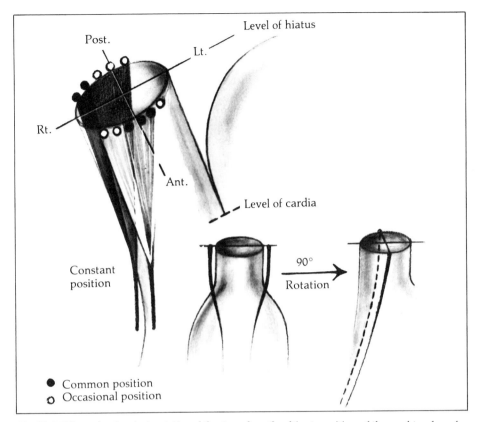

Fig. 70-4. Effects of embryologic rotation of the stomach on the ultimate positions of the vagal trunks and gastric truncal divisions in the adult. At the level of the distal esophagus and gastric cardia, the gastric truncal divisions rotate completely with the stomach so that their anterior and posterior positions are constant. At the level of the hiatus, well removed from the rotating stomach, the vagal trunks may or may not rotate completely and their positions vary accordingly. (From CA Griffith. Courtesy of Surgical Clinics of North America and W. B. Saunders Company.)

plexus may be missed by failure to bring it into the surgical field (Figs. 70-5 and 70-6).

Total Vagotomy at the Distal Esophagus

In contrast to variable numbers of fibers in variable positions at the hiatus, the area at the level of the distal esophagus provides three constant anatomic landmarks—the cardioesophageal angle of His, the hepatic vagi, and the celiac vagal division. These three landmarks delimit a surgical field within which all gastric vagal branches are included (Figs. 70-5 and 70-6). Encirclement of all gastric vagi is a sine qua non for a complete gastric vagotomy whether it be total or selective.

Selective Gastric Vagotomy

Selective gastric vagotomy entails transection of all gastric vagi with preservation of the hepatic and celiac vagi. The extent of the dissection is dictated by the occurrence of essentially two anatomic variations. Both concern the variable origins of the terminal gastric vagal branches.

Adequate Dissection of the Distal Esophagus

The most proximal of the terminal gastric vagal branches to the fundus may arise from a nerve of Latarjet or a trunk or a fiber of the esophageal plexus (Fig. 70-7). When proximal branches arise well above the gastric cardia, they descend closely applied to the esophagus in their course to the fundus. Therefore, to transect these branches, the technique of selective or total vagotomy entails an adequate dissection of the esophagus. The gastric branches in question may lie within or beneath the esophageal fascia propria but not in the esophageal muscle. Nerves in the muscle innervate the esophagus and not the stomach. Therefore, the esophageal muscle is laid bare in its circumference, but the muscle is not violated.

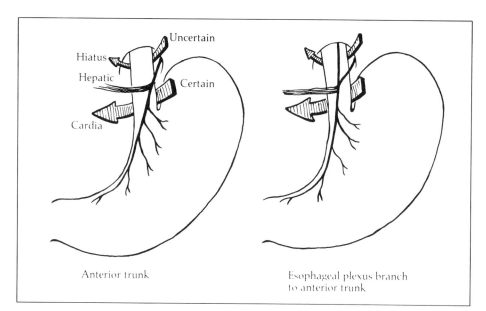

Fig. 70-5. Encirclement of the anterior vagi. At the hiatus, the anterior trunk (left), or a branch of the esophageal plexus contributing to the anterior trunk (right), may lie well to the patient's left of the esophagus. Failure to find this trunk (left) should lead to continued search for it. However, the encirclement of a branch of the esophageal plexus may dissuade further search, and the residual branch is overlooked (right). In contrast to this uncertain encirclement at the hiatus, all anterior gastric vagi are encircled with certainty at the distal esophagus. The lower arrows enter the cardioesophageal angle of His (no vagi lie to the left of this angle) and emerge through the avascular area of the lesser omentum below the hepatic vagal branches and well to the right of the gastric cardia. No gastric vagi lie to the patient's right of this area in the lesser omentum. (From CA Griffith. In R Maingot [ed], Abdominal Operations [7th ed]. New York: Appleton-Century-Crofts, 1980. Reproduced with permission.)

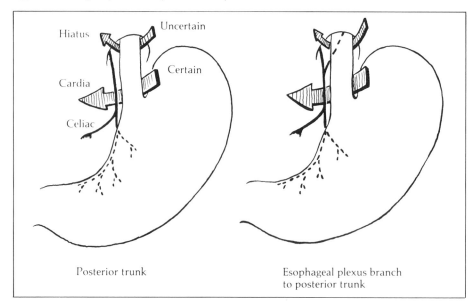

Fig. 70-6. Encirclement of the posterior vagi. At the hiatus, the posterior trunk (left), or a branch of the esophageal plexus contributing to the posterior trunk (right), may lie well posterior to the esophagus in an extremely dorsal position adjacent to the right diaphragmatic crus. In this circumstance the posterior trunk (left), or a contributing branch of the esophageal plexus (right), may be excluded from the encirclement at the hiatus. In contrast, at the distal esophagus and gastric cardia all posterior gastric vagi are encircled because the celiac vagal division may always be positively identified by palpating its course to the celiac plexus. No gastric vagi lie posterior to the celiac division. (From CA Griffith. In R Maingot [ed], Abdominal Operations [7th ed]. New York: Appleton-Century-Crofts, 1980. Reproduced with permission.)

The Descending Left Gastric Artery

The distal origins of the posterior gastric vagi are diagrammed in Fig. 70-8. To ensure transection of all posterior gastric vagal branches that may accompany the left gastric artery to the stomach, the descending branch of the left gastric artery must be ligated and transected.

Proximal Gastric (Parietal or Highly Selective) Vagotomy

As originally devised, proximal gastric vagotomy entails transection of *all* vagal branches to the parietal cell mass with preservation of the branches to the antrum. The hepatic and celiac vagi are also preserved.

Proximal gastric vagotomy is based on two findings. First, vagal innervation of the stomach is segmental: Each terminal gastric branch innervates its own segment of gastric mucosa. Thus, the intact nerves to the antral mucosa do not innervate the denervated parietal mucosa through Meissner's submucosal plexus. Second, the intact nerves to the antral mucosa after proximal gastric vagotomy do not significantly reinnervate the denervated parietal cell mucosa by the process of sprouting.

Proximal Parietal Cell Mass

The proximal extent of proximal gastric vagotomy requires an adequate dissection of the distal esophagus *identical to that described for selective gastric vagotomy*. Failure to apply this anatomic lesson learned from selective gastric vagotomy to the technique of proximal gastric vagotomy has resulted in unacceptable rates of recurrent ulcer.

Distal Parietal Cell Mass

The termination of the anterior nerve of Latarjet along the distal lesser curve is often called the "crow's foot." Some descriptions of proximal gastric vagotomy imply that the pattern and location of the crow's foot are constant, and further imply that the most distal claw of the crow's foot is always distal to the antral-parietal border. Both implications are erroneous. No gross landmarks exist to localize the mucosal border.

First, the distal extents of the nerves of Latarjet show great variation. In some bodies, the anterior nerve extends all the way

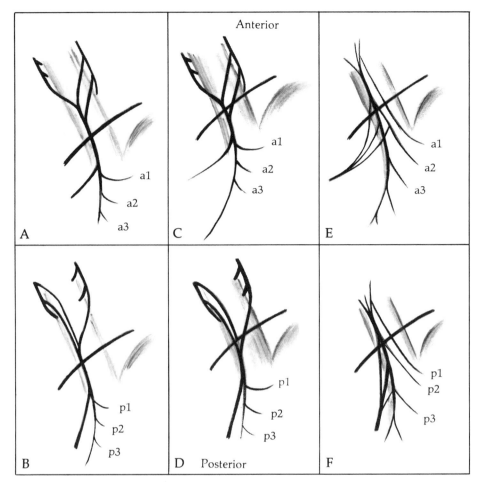

Fig. 70-7. Variable origins of proximal gastric vagi to the fundus. A and B. The two trunks at the hiatus. The most proximal anterior (a1, a2, a3) and posterior (p1, p2, p3) gastric vagal branches arise from the greater anterior and posterior gastric nerves below the origins of the hepatic and celiac branches, and also below the esophagogastric junction. C and D. The esophageal plexus at the hiatus. The patterns are similar to those of A and B. E and F. The truncal divisions at the hiatus. The gastric vagal branches (a1, a2, a3 and p1, p2, p3) may arise from the trunks or esophageal plexus well above the esophagogastric junction and even above the hiatus. In this case, p1 has been called the "criminal nerve." This nerve and other proximal nerves to the fundus may also arise independently from the trunks or esophageal plexus when the trunks (A and B) or esophageal plexus (C and D) are at the hiatus. (From CA Griffith. Courtesy of Surgical Clinics of North America and W. B. Saunders Company.)

to the pylorus and, rarely, onto the proximal duodenum. In other bodies, the nerve of Latarjet is considerably shorter and ends 8 cm or more proximal to the pylorus. In these bodies, the distal antrum and pylorus are supplied by either or both a well-defined pyloric nerve of McCrea and several fibers that descend from the hepatic vagal division within the hepatoduodenal ligament.

Second, the location of the antral-parietal mucosal border also varies considerably. Of particular importance is the occasional occurrence of the exceedingly small antrum, which I have seen by the Congo red

spray method to measure less than 3 cm from the pylorus. Thus, in patients with relatively short nerves of Latarjet plus small antra, complete vagotomy of the distal parietal cell mass is anatomically impossible by proximal gastric vagotomy. When proximal gastric vagotomy is done in these patients, significant innervation to the parietal cell mass remains, and recurrent ulcer may be a problem.

Residual Innervation of the Antrum

The antral mucosa receives vagal innervation from two sources—an *extramural*

source from the end branches of the nerves of Latarjet, and an *intramural* source from more proximal branches that descend in the submucosa beneath the distal parietal cell mass to the antrum. This intramural supply is transected by proximal gastric vagotomy, leaving intact only the extramural supply. Thus, the shorter the nerve of Latarjet, the less is the residual antral innervation and, in turn, the possibility of decreased motility with occult stasis and excessive release of gastrin from the innervated antral mucosa. This may be a factor in recurrence as a prepyloric rather than a duodenal ulcer.

Extended Parietal Vagotomy: The Gastroepiploic Nerves

Endoscopic study with Congo red after parietal vagotomy in some patients reveals variable amounts of residual innervation along the greater curve. This innervation presumably arises from the intact branches of the distal nerves of Latarjet to the antrum and pylorus, which pursue an intraduodenal course to the greater omentum, where, as the gastroepiploic nerves, they accompany the main gastroepiploic arteries and veins to the greater curve. Cutting the gastroepiploic nerve denervates the residually innervated mucosa along the greater curve and completes the vagotomy. One of our editors (Nyhus) and his associate Donahue pioneered much of this work, and applied the word "extended" to mean that transecting the gastroepiploic nerves extends the conventional dissection for parietal vagotomy.

Anatomic Types and Adequacy of Incomplete Vagotomy

Figures 70-5 and 70-6 illustrate how an incomplete vagotomy occurs because an intact trunk or a branch of the esophageal plexus is missed. This inadequate vagotomy is compared in Fig. 70-9 with another error; an incomplete vagotomy occurs because an intact terminal branch to the fundus (e.g., an intact "criminal nerve" in Fig. 70-7E and F) is missed. The large area of innervated mucosa in the inadequate vagotomy provides *inadequate* protection against ulcer, whereas the small area in the incomplete vagotomy provides *adequate* protection. In patients with incomplete va-

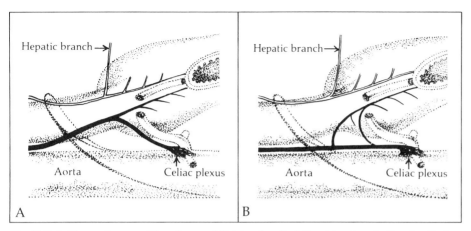

Fig. 70-8. A. The usual course of the celiac vagal division along the left gastric artery. B. Occasionally the celiac division runs adjacent to the diaphragmatic crura and aorta. Note the posterior gastric vagal branches accompanying the left gastric artery to the stomach.

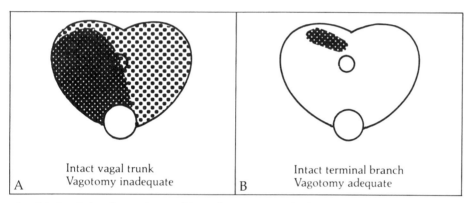

Fig. 70-9. Correlation of anatomic type of incomplete vagotomy with adequacy. A. With one intact vagal trunk, the ipsilateral wall of the stomach remains innervated and continues to secrete (dark shading). The vagal release of gastrin causes a delayed and lesser secretion from the denervated contralateral wall (light shading). Secretion remains high. The insulin response is large-early. Ulcers develop in 75 percent of Shay rats, an inadequate vagotomy. The same secretion occurs after incomplete vagotomy of an intact branch of the esophageal plexus contributing to a vagal trunk, as in Figs. 70-5 and 70-6. B. With an intact terminal branch (e.g., criminal nerve) to the fundus, only a small area of gastric mucosa remains innervated. The amount of secretion is only slightly greater than with complete vagotomy. The insulin response is small-late. No ulcers develop in Shay rats, an adequate vagotomy. After 1 year, the area of innervated mucosa does not increase in size by reinnervation owing to sprouting, and the amount of secretion remains the same. Thus, this adequate incomplete vagotomy is permanently adequate. (From GR Pritchard et al. By permission of Surgery, Gynecology and Obstetrics. Reproduced with permission.

gotomy and recurrent ulcer, completion of the vagotomy may be indicated if it is inadequate but not if it is adequate.

Hepatic and Celiac Vagotomy

The hepatic vagi can be injured during gastric resection, hiatal hernia repair, or fundoplication. The celiac vagal division can be injured during ligation of the left gastric artery (see Fig. 70-8A). These unrecognized injuries may account for unexpected postoperative sequelae. Conversely, the unknown occurrence of incomplete hepatic vagotomy (see Fig. 70-5) and incomplete celiac vagotomy (see Fig. 70-6) accounts for the absence of postvagotomy sequelae in patients with allegedly complete total vagotomy.

Mucosa and Mucosal Borders

Brunner's Glands (Billroth I or II Anastomosis)

The proximal duodenum contains a dense concentration of Brunner's glands, which secrete an alkaline mucus that resists peptic ulceration. Brunner's glands are absent from the jejunum; therefore, the proximal duodenum possesses a greater intrinsic resistance to ulcer. This difference in resistance is one of many factors in the issue of gastroduodenostomy or gastrojejunostomy.

Location of Peptic Ulcers

Oi's group showed that ulcers form adjacent to mucosal borders. Duodenal ulcers usually occur just distal to the gastroduodenal border, and gastric ulcers occur just distal to the antral-parietal border.

Prepyloric Duodenal Ulcer

The gastroduodenal mucosal border may lie distal or proximal to the pylorus. If the border is proximal to the pylorus, a prepyloric ulcer may actually be duodenal rather than gastric. (Any hypersecretion associated with this prepyloric duodenal ulcer will be overlooked if only the serum gastrin level is determined and gastric secretion is not tested.)

High and Low Gastric Ulcers

A prepyloric ulcer may also be gastric in patients with exceedingly small antra. Oi's group found that the antral-parietal border varied in location from 4 to 12 cm proximal to the pylorus on the lesser curve and from 5 to 10 cm on the greater curve. The variable location of this border is a factor in the formation of high and low gastric ulcers—the higher the border, the higher the ulcer. In addition, even higher ulcers may form in the parietal cell mass rendered nonacid by "antralization" or "intestinalization" from biliary reflux.

Arteries

The usual arterial pattern supplying the stomach and duodenum is diagrammed in Fig. 70-10. Like many similar diagrams, this figure neglects both the submucosal

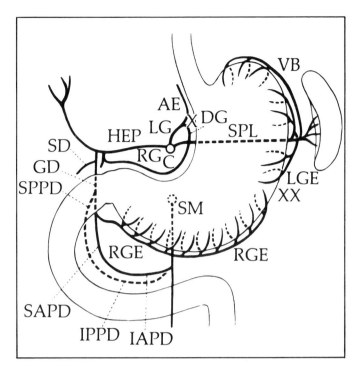

Fig. 70-10. Arterial supply to stomach and duodenum. C = celiac; HEP = hepatic; RG = right gastric; GD = gastroduodenal; SD = supraduodenal; SPPD = superior posterior pancreaticoduodenal (retroduodenal); SAPD = superior anterior pancreaticoduodenal; RGE = right gastroepiploic; IAPD = inferior anterior pancreaticoduodenal; IPPD = inferior posterior pancreaticoduodenal; LG = left gastric; AE = ascending esophageal branch; DG = descending gastric branch; SPL = splenic; VB = vasa brevia; LGE = left gastroepiploic; X = bifurcation LG; XX = anastomosis RGE and LGE; SM = superior mesenteric. (From CA Griffith. Anatomy. In LM Nyhus, C Wastell [eds], Surgery of the Stomach and Duodenum [4th ed]. Boston: Little, Brown, 1986. Reproduced with permission.)

plexus and frequent variations of the main arteries.

Submucosal Plexus

The right and left gastric arteries along the lesser curve and the right and left gastroepiploic arteries along the greater curve each send off anterior and posterior branches that penetrate the muscular walls to enter the submucosa, where they ramify and communicate with each other to form the submucosal plexus. This plexus is an important collateral circulation for it maintains viability of the partially devascularized stomach following various gastric operations. However, necrosis does occur, although rarely.

Necrosis of the Lesser Curve After Proximal Gastric Vagotomy

Factors other than iatrogenic injury to the lesser curve (e.g., gouging it with a clamp

or burning it with a cautery) merit consideration. First of all, the gastric wall is thinnest along the lesser curve because the inner oblique muscle is absent. Of more importance is the vascularity unique to the lesser curve. Angiographic study in cadavers shows that the arteries ligated during parietal vagotomy are more or less end arteries with sparse connections to the submucosal plexus. Furthermore, this part of the plexus has a weaker collateral circulation than the rest of the plexuses throughout the stomach. Also, the submucosal plexus along the lesser curve has sparse connections to the richer plexus adjacent to it. Thus, after parietal vagotomy, angiography shows a definite ischemic band of the gastric wall, 2 cm wide, coursing along the operated part of the lesser curve. Ischemic perforations occur through this avascular band, but are prevented by covering the ischemic area with the technique of imbrication.

Necrosis of Gastric Remnant

This complication is also rare, even after ligation of the left gastric artery and splenectomy. In this instance, the remnant is supplied by communications between the ascending and descending esophageal vessels, the esophageal and gastric submucosal plexuses, and the vasa brevia not ligated during splenectomy. Necrosis of this type of remnant and also of the smaller remnant after higher resection with ligation of all vasa brevia is caused by insufficient blood descending from the esophageal circulation. This sequela usually occurs in the elderly with arteriosclerotic occlusive disease.

The Hepatogastric Artery and Left Hepatic Lobar Necrosis

In about 10 percent of persons, the main left gastric artery sends off a large left hepatic artery just before bifurcating into its descending gastric and ascending esophageal branches. This aberrant left hepatic (hepatogastric) artery reaches the porta hepatis along with the hepatic vagi in the lesser omentum and may be either a part of or the entire supply to the left lobe of the liver. If the latter, its ligation during resection or its injury during selective or proximal gastric vagotomy can cause necrosis of the left hepatic lobe. When looked for routinely during the initial exploration, the presence of a hepatogastric artery can be established and precautions can be taken to protect it.

Vascular Landmarks for Resection

If the stomach is transected between points X and XX in Fig. 70-10, the resection approximates 50 percent. When vagotomy is added, a less extensive resection can be done, but as previously discussed, no landmarks exist to perform a precise antrectomy. When vagotomy is not added, more extensive resections require resections higher than point XX on the greater curve. Also, the higher the transection of the lesser curve (at or above point X), the greater is the amount of vagal denervation of the gastric remnant, particularly when the gastric vagal branches are as diagrammed in A and B but not as in E and F in Fig. 70-7.

Ligation of the Celiac Axis

A direct and rich anastomosis between the inferior and superior pancreaticoduodenal vessels provides extensive collateral circulation between the celiac and superior mesenteric arteries. This collateral circulation permits ligation of the celiac axis, which, nevertheless, is hazardous because of arterial variations, for example, the gastroduodenal artery arising from the superior mesenteric artery or the superior mesenteric artery arising from the celiac axis.

Lymphatics

Lymphatic drainage of the stomach is both intrinsic and extrinsic. The intrinsic routes are in the submucosal lymphatic plexus. The extrinsic channels follow the arteries, but lymphatic flow is the reverse of arterial flow.

Intrinsic Lymphatic Spread of Carcinoma

A carcinoma localized to a small area of mucosa may spread all over the stomach by the submucosal lymphatic plexus. This plexus has abundant anastomoses with the esophageal submucosal lymphatics. Thus, submucosal invasion of gastric carcinoma into the esophagus is common. In contrast, the duodenum has a scanty submucosal lymphatic plexus, and invasion of the duodenum is unusual.

The intrinsic spread of carcinoma plus the frequency of multicentric origins of carcinoma provide the rationale of total gastrectomy or at least extensive resections to remove all tumor. Also, a liberal resection of the distal esophagus is included for carcinoma in the proximal stomach.

Extrinsic Lymphatic Spread of Carcinoma

The extrinsic lymphatic vessels may be conceived in terms of four primary channels that correspond to the arteries—the right gastroepiploic, the right gastric, the left gastric, and the left gastroepiploic. The common collecting point is in nodes surrounding the celiac axis. En route to this common point, however, the primary channels may communicate with secondary channels of the pancreas, liver, and spleen (Fig. 70-11). These extensive lymphatic communications account for the widespread metastases that frequently occur with gastric carcinoma.

Suggested Reading

Agossou-Voyeme AK, Hureau J, Germian M. Arterial vascularization of the operated stomach. *Surg Radiol Anat* 12:247, 1990.

Donahue PE, Richter HM, Liu KJM, et al. Experimental basis and clinical application of extended highly selective vagotomy for duodenal ulcer. *Surg Gynecol Obstet* 176:39, 1993.

Grassi G, Orecchia C. A comparison of intraoperative tests of completeness of vagal section. *Surgery* 75:155, 1974.

Griffith CA. Selective gastric vagotomy. Parts I, II. *West J Surg Obstet Gynecol* 70:107, 175, 1962.

Griffith CA. A new anatomic approach to the problem of incomplete vagotomy. *Surg Clin North Am* 44:1239, 1964.

Griffith CA. Selective Gastric Vagotomy. In R Maingot (ed), *Abdominal Operations* (7th ed). New York: Appleton-Century-Crofts, 1980.

Griffith CA. Anatomy. In LM Nyhus, C Wastell (eds), *Surgery of the Stomach and Duodenum* (4th ed). Boston: Little, Brown, 1986.

Nielsen HO, Munoz JD, Kronborg O, et al. Relationship between antrum size, nerve of Latarjet. *Scand J Gastroenterol* 16:491, 1981.

Oi M, Oshida K, Sugimura S. The location of gastric ulcer. *Gastroenterology* 36:45, 1959.

Poppen B, Delin A, Sandstedt B. Parietal cell vagotomy: Localisation of the microscopical an-

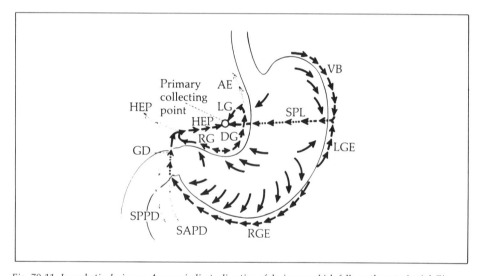

Fig. 70-11. Lymphatic drainage. Arrows indicate direction of drainage, which follows the arteries (cf. Fig. 70-10). Dotted arrows indicate immediate secondary routes of lymphatic drainage.

The right gastroepiploic route (RGE) of metastasis begins with lymph nodes in the greater omentum and proceeds to subpyloric nodes around the gastroduodenal (GD) artery. Communications with the pancreaticoduodenal lymphatics (SPPD, SAPD) account for metastasis to nodes anterior and posterior to the head of the pancreas.

The right gastric (RG) route starts with lymph nodes in the distal lesser omentum and joins the right gastroepiploic (RGE) route at the hepatic artery, where the lymphatics communicate with hepatic (HEP) lymphatics and permit metastasis to nodes in the porta hepatis. The right gastric and right gastroepiploic routes then follow the common hepatic artery to the celiac axis, which is the common collecting point for the entire stomach.

The left gastric (LG) route begins with lymph nodes in the proximal lesser omentum. On its way to the celiac axis, the left gastric route communicates with nodes around the esophagus by the ascending esophageal (AE) vessels. This communication allows metastasis upward along the esophagus.

The left gastroepiploic (LGE) route drains across the gastrosplenic ligament to pancreaticosplenic nodes in the hilus of the spleen and tail of the pancreas. These nodes also receive lymphatic vessels that accompany the vasa brevia (VB). It then follows the splenic (SPL) artery through nodes along the pancreas to the celiac axis. (From CA Griffith. Anatomy. In LM Nyhus, C Wastell [ed], Surgery of the Stomach and Duodenum [4th ed]. Boston: Little, Brown, 1986. Reproduced with permission.)

tral-fundic boundary in relation to the macro-scopical. *Acta Chir Scand* 142:251, 1976.

Pritchard GR, Griffith CA, Harkins HN A physiologic demonstration of the anatomic distribution of the vagal system to the stomach. *Surg Gynecol Obstet* 126:791, 1968.

Skandalakis JE, Gray SW, Saria RE, et al. Distribution of the vagus nerve to the stomach. *Am Surg* 46:130, 1980.

Taylor TV. Lesser curve myotomy. *Ann Surg* 191:414, 1980.

Yoshida J, Polley EH, Nyhus LM, Donahue PE. Brain stem topography of vagus nerve to the greater curvature of the stomach. *J Surg Res* 46:60, 1989.

EDITOR'S COMMENT

Charles A. Griffith (Fig. 70-12) was a superb surgical scientist. He was born in Oak Park, Illinois, where his father was a respected physician. Doctor Griffith received

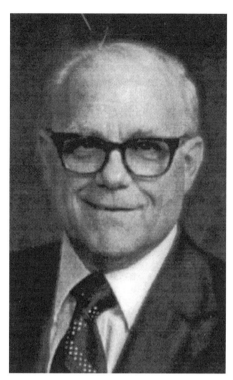

Fig. 70-12. Charles A. Griffith (1921–1994).

both his BA and MD degrees from Harvard University. Following his surgical residency, he worked with Henry N. Harkins at the University of Washington at Seattle before entering the private practice of surgery. In 1957, he and Professor Harkins published the first experimental studies that set the entire basis for the clinical change from truncal to selective vagotomy in the operative treatment of duodenal ulcer (*Gastroenterology* 32:96, 1957).

For those surgeons who love the anatomic correlations of our specialty, Griffith's anatomic study of 1959 (*Surg Clin North Am* 39:531) relating to the inguinal area and hernias, will find the exposition of 38 years ago fresh and filled with observations that have "stood the test of time."

Charles A. Griffith died on December 30, 1994. The world of anatomy-surgery has lost one of its best.

L.M.N.

71

Open Gastrostomy

Jerry M. Jesseph

Gastrostomy as a surgical technique is an old one and has been described in many forms and detail. Its usefulness has increased in proportion to the growth of abdominal visceral surgery and, thus, has grown a good deal in the last 30 years. The history of early efforts is interesting but will not be detailed here.

Direct access to the lumen of the stomach is designed to be either temporary, as in patients who will soon be able to return to normal alimentation, or permanent, for people who will need to be fed or emptied directly through the stomach. These procedures have great utility, and the basic methods will be shown for both. The specific methods described are selected because of their simplicity and wide applicability.

Temporary Gastrostomy

As an alternative to postoperative nasogastric intubation, gastrostomy has a number of advantages. It is vastly more comfortable and allows the patient greater mobility. It does not interfere with respiration or pulmonary toilet. In very old people or in patients with chronic pulmonary diseases, gastrostomy averts some potentially lethal postoperative difficulties.

Temporary tube gastrostomy is useful as a means of feeding patients who are undergoing a series of operations on the mouth and oropharynx and cannot ingest food orally for weeks or months. Since food is broken down into its constituent parts better in the stomach than in the jejunum, gas-

trostomy is preferred over jejunostomy when more than a week or two of alimentation is needed.

Caution is recommended when considering long-term feeding by gastrostomy. Patients who are being fed directly into the stomach should be alert and able to clear upper-airway secretions. There is evidence that a gastrostomy itself can predispose to gastroesophageal reflux, aspiration, and pneumonia. Therefore, an alternative technique or the addition of an antireflux procedure is suggested for comatose patients.

Of all forms of temporary gastrostomy, the method of Stamm has had the widest application. It is quickly and easily done, is safe when correctly done, and provides efficient venting of the stomach. The procedure can be performed laparoscopically with results equal to an "open" gastrostomy.

With this method, a point is chosen on the middle anterior surface of the stomach where it lies against the anterior abdominal wall without tension. In this way, the tube exits in the left hypochondriac region (Fig. 71-1). A small puncture is made through the stomach wall, and a large (No. 20 to 26 French) Malecot or dePezzar catheter is inserted an inch or two into the lumen. One or two concentric pursestring sutures of silk or other semipermanent material are used to invert the stomach wall about the tube, forming a snug seal and a serosal lining for the tube tract. (One must make certain there is no bleeding from submucosal vessels, since one of the few complications of tube gastrostomy is intragastric bleeding.) The tube is then brought out through a tightly fitting stab wound in the left upper quadrant, and the

stomach is attached firmly to the abdominal wall by several heavy sutures around the exit site of the tube to prevent retraction and leak, especially if the tube is dislodged earlier than intended. No suction device is needed for drainage; a simple gravity collection system will do.

Postoperative care is easy. It is probably a good idea to irrigate the tube once or twice each day to prevent occlusion by mucus.

The tube can be safely removed as early as 3 or 4 days after the operation, but it can be left in place much longer. Given normal or near normal nutrition, the tube will not lead to erosion or digestion of the skin, and it is well tolerated by most patients for many weeks. Removal is easy: The tube is simply pulled out. Patients are often apprehensive about the removal, imagining all sorts of pain and visceral trauma, but the experience is a minor one. Furthermore, if the tube falls out prematurely, it can quickly and easily be replaced by percutaneous techniques.

Many variations on the technique of Stamm have been described. Most of these propose special tubes. It is doubtful that any of these is of special advantage, since the effectiveness of the method depends on a relatively short tube of large internal diameter. As noted earlier, the Malecot (mushroom) catheter is probably best, in No. 20 to 26 French, depending on circumstances. The dePezzar and Foley catheters are acceptable but tend to drain less well, and the latter is more liable to accidental displacement. A number of gastrostomy "button" appliances are available, most for long-term feeding in infants and children. These have the advantage of an internal flap valve, which prevents leakage

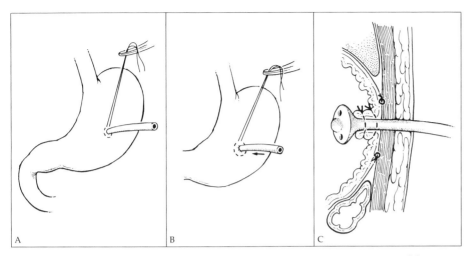

Fig. 71-1. Stamm gastrostomy. A and B. The mushroom catheter is retained within the stomach by two concentric pursestring sutures. C. The catheter is brought through a stab wound, and the anterior stomach wall is sutured to the peritoneum so that solid fusion takes place, preventing leakage into the peritoneal cavity.

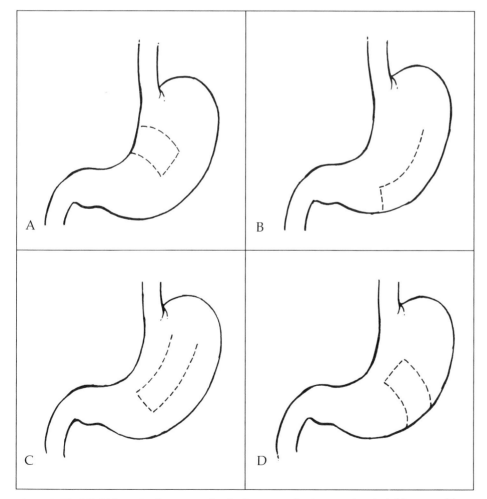

Fig. 71-2. The full-thickness flap for constructing the Janeway gastrostomy can be oriented in any position on the anterior wall of the stomach.

of gastric contents, and no external tube. They can be easily changed as the child grows and when the device wears out.

One of the older forms of temporary tube gastrostomy is that described by Witzel. In this method (not illustrated), a tunnel or inverted tract is fashioned along the anterior stomach wall, so that the tube penetrates the stomach at a distance from the point where it exits the abdominal wall. The concept of the method is to prevent leakage around the tube. In fact, this method is probably *more* liable to leakage than is the Stamm, because the tube tract is longer and requires more suturing, and the tube itself is required to bend acutely in two places.

Permanent Gastrostomy

The distinguishing anatomic feature of the permanent gastrostomy is that it comprises a tube of stomach wall that is brought to the surface so that the mucosa of the stomach forms the inner layer or lining of the tube. This layer forms a fistula to the skin surface that will not close spontaneously whether or not a tube or catheter is left in place through the tube into the stomach. The advantage of this method is obvious: Nutrition can be provided for long periods, and a tube or other mechanical device is needed only when food is actually being introduced. Between feedings, the patient needs only to keep the external stoma covered.

While there are advantages to permanent gastrostomy, all forms of this procedure require more skill and operating time than the simpler tube methods. Better exposure is needed, more of the stomach is used up in the construction of the full-thickness tube, and there are many more details that provide chances for failure or complication. Nevertheless, a permanent gastrostomy can be a blessing to the patient and those responsible for his or her care.

Fortunately, the stomach lends itself very well to the construction of full-thickness tubes. It has a rich blood supply, is large and in a sense redundant, and is tough enough in texture to be easily sewn. In Fig. 71-2 four examples of full-thickness flaps that can safely and easily be raised from the stomach are diagrammed; these flaps

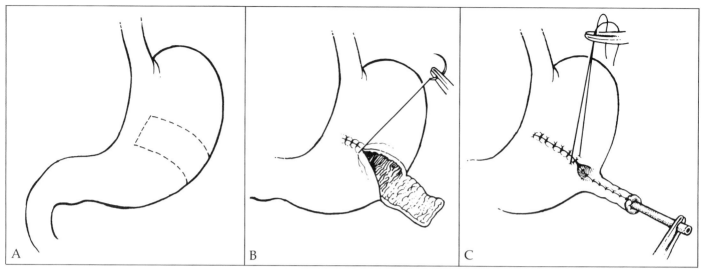

Fig. 71-3. Depage-Janeway gastrostomy. As shown, the flap of stomach wall is converted into a tube by a two-layer closure. A catheter makes formation of the tube simple. The tube is brought out through a full-thickness excised tract and its mucosa is sutured to the skin.

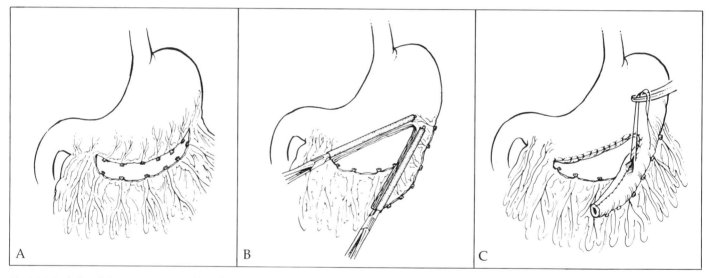

Fig. 71-4. Beck-Carrel-Jianu gastrostomy. This technique provides a long tube that can be brought through an oblique abdominal wall tunnel. A two-layer closure is used throughout.

are the basis for all the currently useful forms of permanent gastrostomy.

The simplest and probably most widely used method is that of Janeway, as shown in Fig. 71-3. A flap is formed with its base at the greater curvature, which is then converted into a tube by two-layer closure of the defect in the stomach in continuity to the distal (skin) end of the flap. The dimensions of the flap are not as critical as in certain skin flaps, but the width should be sufficient to easily accommodate a No. 18 to 20 French tube for introduction of semiliquid foodstuffs, and the length

should be sufficient to reach the skin surface without tension.

The completed gastric tube is brought to the skin surface through a stab wound made 3 to 5 cm from the primary incision. The stab wound, or tunnel, should fit the tube loosely. The full thickness of the end of the tube is everted slightly and sewed to the skin. The latter point is important to avoid stenosis. A plastic or rubber catheter should be left in place for 4 to 5 days, after which it can be inserted for feedings only.

It is unusual to have difficulty with the Janeway gastrostomy. Even though it does

not contain a valve or flap of gastric mucosa, the leakage of gastric juice is small in the absence of distal obstruction. A gauze pad is usually adequate coverage.

Beck-Carrel-Jianu Gastrostomy

The Beck-Carrel-Jianu gastrostomy is a variation on the simple flap-tube method and is shown in Fig. 71-4. This tube, which is made from the greater curvature, is the forerunner of the Gavriliu–Heimlich tube

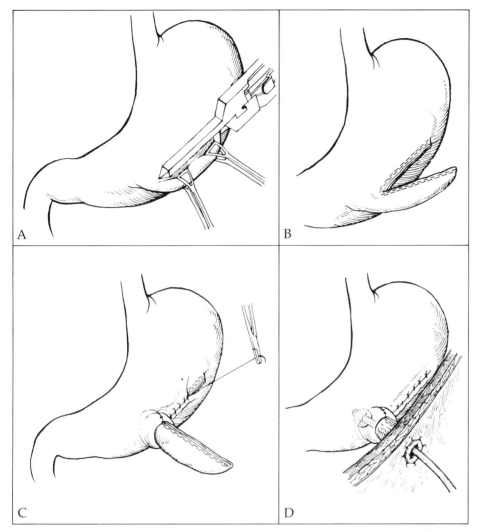

Fig. 71-5. Permanent gastrostomy using the GIA stapler. The stomach is grasped with a Babcock forceps, and the GIA stapling device is oriented along the greater curvature (A). The gastric tube is formed, and the gastric side of the stomach incision is inverted with silk sutures (B and C). The gastric tube is exteriorized, and after the abdomen is closed, the tip is amputated (D). The mucosa is approximated to the skin with absorbable suture and a catheter is inserted.

for esophageal substitution. As depicted in Fig. 71-4, the tube is isolated from the greater curvature by the use of noncrushing clamps, and the cut edges of stomach and tube are closed with two layers of suture: inner running, seromuscular interrupted. The tube is otherwise managed identically to the Janeway gastrostomy tube.

Stapling Method

A variation on construction of gastrostomy tubes comes from the stapling devices. Figure 71-5 shows the raising of a tube from the greater curvature using the GIA stapler (Autosuture Co, U.S. Surgical Corp. Stamford, CT). Here the tube is based in the distal stomach; it can also be based in the corpus or raised transversely across the stomach as with the flap methods. The staple rows can be inverted by Lembert sutures, but if the staple rows are left exposed, care must be taken to control bleeding along the staple line using electrocautery. (The staples are intentionally noncrushing, and bleeding can be of considerable volume.) The tip of the tube is amputated, and a catheter is inserted into the stomach. The remainder of the procedure and aftercare are as for the Janeway gastrostomy.

As a variation, a catheter can be inserted into the stomach through a small stab wound *before* the tube is raised. The catheter is then grasped with Babcock clamps, thus wrapping the stomach about the catheter, which serves as a mandrel and guide for the stapling operation.

Spivack-Watsuji Method

Over a span of many years, surgeons have described technical variations of permanent gastrostomy that were intended to provide an internal valve to leakproof the tube. This notion undoubtedly has merit. The simpler methods are worth knowing about and can be done by an experienced surgeon in an occasional instance.

As shown in Fig. 71-6A and B, the Spivack-Watsuji gastrostomy is a flap-tube method, with the variation that a ridge or collar of stomach wall is inverted at the base of the flap, so that when the edges are approximated, this ridge becomes a doughnut of tissue and acts as an occluding device. A catheter is easily inserted for feeding, but in principle, the mucosal doughnut is pliable enough to occlude with the action of normal intragastric pressure. There are several variations on this general technique, but none of them is fundamentally different.

Jejunal Interposition Gastrostomy

Jejunal interposition gastrostomy was described originally by Tavel and modified by Nyhus and associates (Fig. 71-7). The advantage of this method is that it is entirely leakproof as long as the interposed jejunal segment is at least 30 cm long. The method has had limited use in humans and is much more complex than necessary for the ordinary indications for gastrostomy. It is an elegant procedure, however, and is included so that it will not be forgotten.

Percutaneous Endoscopic Gastrostomy

Percutaneous endoscopic gastrostomy is the most commonly performed gastros-

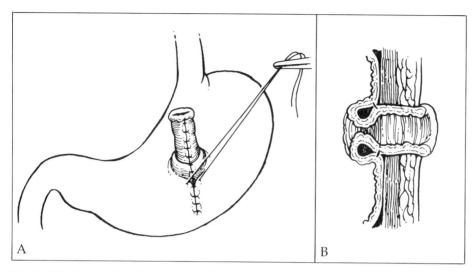

Fig. 71-6. The Spivack-Watsuji gastrostomy. This method forms a true valve at the base of the tube by inverting a roll of stomach wall (A and B). After formation of the tube, leakage is prevented by the mucosal roll within the stomach lumen. Seromuscular sutures are used to retain the tube within its tract, and the mucosal end of the tube is sutured to the skin edge. A soft rubber catheter should be kept in the tube throughout the first week.

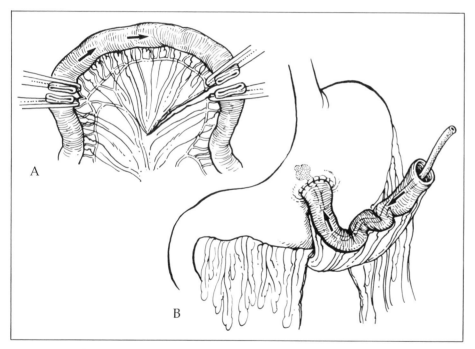

Fig. 71-7. Jejunal gastrostomy. A. The jejunal segment is prepared by division of the intestine at either end of the 30-cm segment. The venous arcade at the distal end is left intact to ensure drainage. The segment is brought through the transverse mesocolon, and the omentum is split up to the greater curvature of the stomach so that the vascular pedicle of the segment is not compromised. B. A Foley catheter is passed through the segment before the anastomoses are completed.

tomy today. Experience suggests that although this procedure can have complications, such as intraperitoneal leak, retroperitoneal perforation, hemorrhage, and peristomal leakage and infection, sur-

gical gastrostomy also has a high morbidity rate. It is widely used and now is an accepted treatment modality. Radiologists have become adept at placing percutaneous gastric feeding tubes under fluoros-

copy without the use of an endoscope. By this method the anterior gastric wall is not apposed to the anterior abdominal wall. Naturally there has been concern about the safety of this method. Radiologists expert with this technique have proved to their own satisfaction that in patients who are at poor risk for a surgical procedure, percutaneous gastrostomy is a satisfactory nonoperative method. Laparoscopic gastrostomy is an acceptable alternative for patients who cannot undergo endoscopy because of head and neck cancer or esophageal disease.

As in most other areas of surgical craft, many technical variations in gastrostomy have come and gone. The methods shown here are the durable few and should suffice for nearly every use.

Suggested Reading

Benson M, Slater G. Technique for the replacement of a feeding gastrostomy tube. *Am J Surg* 138:732, 1979.

Burtch GD, Shatney CH. Feeding gastrostomy: Assistant or assassin? *Am Surg* 51:204, 1985.

Davis JB Jr, Bowden TA, Roves DA. Percutaneous endoscopic gastrostomy: Do surgeons and gastroenterologists get the same results? *Am Surg* 56:47, 1990.

Ditesheim JA, Richards W, Sharp K. Fatal and disastrous complications following percutaneous endoscopic gastrostomy. *Am Surg* 55:92, 1989.

Ho CS, Yee ACN, McPherson R. Complications of surgical and percutaneous nonendoscopic gastrostomy: Review of 233 patients. *Gastroenterology* 95:1206, 1988.

Lee WI, Chao SH, Yu SC, et al. Laparoscopic assisted gastrostomy tube replacement. *J Laparoendoscopic Surg* 4:201, 1994.

Meguid MM, Williams LF. The use of gastrostomy to correct malnutrition. *Surg Gynecol Obstet* 149:27, 1979.

Nyhus LM, McDade WC, Condon RE, et al. Further experience with jejunal gastrostomy. *Arch Surg* 83:864, 1961.

Ochsner A. The relative merits of temporary gastrostomy and nasogastric suction of the stomach. *Am J Surg* 133:729, 1977.

Pomerantz MA, Salomon J, Dunn R. Permanent gastrostomy as a solution to some nutritional problems in the elderly. *J Am Geriatr Soc* 28:104, 1980.

Sacks BA, Glotzer DJ. Percutaneous re-establishment of feeding gastrostomies. *Surgery* 85:575, 1979.

Shellito PC, Malt RA. Tube gastrostomy: Techniques and complications. *Ann Surg* 201:180, 1985.

Torosian MH, Rombeau JL. Feeding by tube enterostomy. *Surg Gynecol Obstet* 150:918, 1980.

Wilkinson WA, Pickleman J. Feeding gastrostomy: A reappraisal. *Am Surg* 48:273, 1982.

EDITOR'S COMMENT

Since our studies of the jejunal gastrostomy (*Arch Surg* 83:864, 1961), each new presentation on this age-old subject is of interest to me. On this occasion, I write about an older gastrostomy technique that has been proved to be very effective: the Glassman aseptic tubovalvular gastrostomy.

From 1939 to 1942, Glassman and MacNealy (*Surg Gynecol Obstet* 74:843, 1942) described a mucosa-lined gastrostomy in which leakage of gastric juice is prevented by creating two areas of constriction in a cone-shaped diverticulum formed from the anterior wall of the stomach.

Those interested in the origins of atraumatic (noncrushing) intestinal clamps and forceps and the abdominal viscera retainer ("fish" in our parlance) should peruse the Glassman monograph *Gastric Surgery* (Springfield: Thomas, 1970). It is clear that many of these advances in instrumentation originated with Jacob Glassman and Raymond MacNealy.

L.M.N.

72

Percutaneous Endoscopic Gastrostomy

Jeffrey L. Ponsky

Although surgical gastrostomy has been performed safely and effectively for decades, the introduction of the percutaneous endoscopic technique of gastrostomy placement (PEG) has permitted the creation of long-term gastric access for feeding or decompression without the need for general anesthesia or laparotomy. Reports of comparisons with traditional gastrostomy suggest that the method offers equivalent results with less patient discomfort and a lower cost. Complications, although consistent with those noted with the open procedure, can be minimized by appropriate patient selection and attention to technical details. Although a number of modifications of the originally described technique have been suggested, the original "pull" method and the closely related "push" approach are the most well-accepted and widely practiced techniques.

Indications

The most common and appropriate indication for PEG is the need for long-term alimentation in patients who are unable to eat but have functional gastrointestinal tracts. Such individuals include those with progressive neurologic diseases, stroke victims, children with birth asphyxia or severe psychomotor retardation, and patients with head or facial trauma. The method has also been useful in administering unpalatable medications to children, in the administration of nighttime supplemental feedings to patients with inflammatory bowel disease, as a route for returning external biliary drainage to the gastrointestinal tract, and in providing gastric decompression in patients with carcinomatosis or radiation enteritis.

Percutaneous gastrostomy has not proved particularly useful in patients with aspiration secondary to gastroesophageal reflux, and in some cases may exacerbate the problem. The procedure should be avoided in patients with massive ascites or severe malnutrition, as tract formation is impaired and leakage can result. Multiple system organ failure or systemic sepsis should be corrected before placement of a PEG, as infectious complications are more likely to occur. Feedings may be provided by the nasoenteric route until these problems are resolved. Also, the performance of PEG in patients with very limited life expectancy is meddlesome and costly, contributing to the high in-hospital mortality reported following the procedure.

Technique

The patient is prepared by fasting overnight or withholding enteral feedings for 6 to 8 hours before the procedure. A preoperative intravenous antibiotic, usually a cephalosporin, is administered to reduce the incidence of wound infection in the abdominal wall surrounding the tube. Swabbing of the oropharynx with an antiseptic solution will help to reduce bacterial counts in the mouth and may thus help protect against wound infection.

Intravenous access is established for the administration of analgesia and sedation, and the patient is placed on the endoscopy table in the supine position. While this position is most appropriate for the performance of the gastrostomy, it predisposes to the accumulation of secretions in the patient's oropharynx and may lead to aspiration. Therefore, frequent evacuation of this material by suctioning is imperative.

Titrated sedation and analgesia are usually provided by the sequential administration of a narcotic and a benzodiazepine, while respiration, blood pressure, and oxygen saturation are monitored. The abdomen can be minimally shaved in the left upper quadrant, washed with a preparatory solution, and steriley draped.

The procedure begins with the introduction of the gastroscope into the patient's esophagus. This can be somewhat difficult with the patient in the supine position and may be facilitated by slightly turning the patient to the left for passage of the instrument. The scope is then advanced into the stomach and the room lights dimmed. A rapid but thorough inspection of the stomach and duodenum should be performed to rule out pathology or pyloric obstruction. The instrument is then pulled back into the gastric body and turned anteriorly as the assistant inspects the external aspect of the abdominal wall looking for transillumination. Transillumination of the abdominal wall by the light of the endoscope indicates close contact of the gastric and abdominal walls and the absence of intervening tissue. Should light not be apparent, finger palpation of the abdominal wall may reveal a point of light when gentle pressure is applied. Once the point of brightest transillumination is identified, continued finger pressure is applied to this site by the assistant, which should create a clear and prominent indentation of the gastric wall visible to the endoscopist. Multiple sites may be palpated until the best transillumination and gastric indentation are achieved. Extra time spent at this stage of the procedure is well worth the effort and will help reduce inadvertent puncture of adjacent organs (Fig. 72-1).

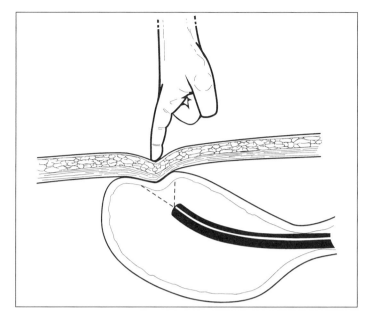

Fig. 72-1. *The site for gastric puncture should be carefully selected, using transillumination of the abdominal wall and gastric indentation with finger pressure as a guide.*

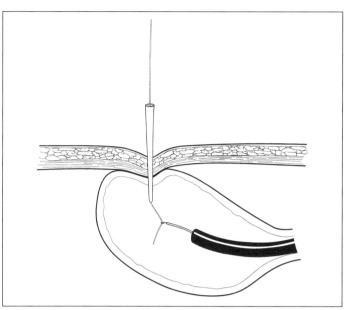

Fig. 72-2. *Once several inches of suture have entered the gastric lumen, the snare is loosened from around the cannula, repositioned on the suture, and once again tightened.*

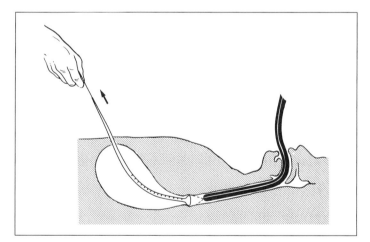

Fig. 72-3. *The suture is affixed to the end of the gastrostomy catheter, and the catheter is pulled down the esophagus, into the stomach, and out of the abdominal wall. The scope is re-introduced to follow the progress of the tube, and care is taken to avoid undue tension.*

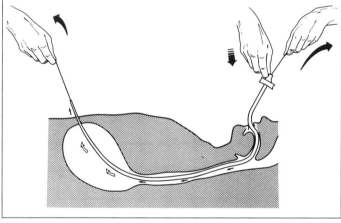

Fig. 72-4. *In the "push" method, both ends of the guidewire are held taut as the tube is pushed over the wire and out of the abdominal wall. (From JL Ponsky.* Techniques of Percutaneous Gastrostomy. *New York: Igaku-Shoin, 1988. Reproduced with permission.)*

Several milliliters of local anesthetic is infiltrated into the skin at the selected site, and an incision 1 cm in length is made through the skin and into the subcutaneous tissue. While the assistant anesthetizes the abdominal wall skin, the endoscopist uses a polypectomy snare, passed through the biopsy channel of the endoscope, to surround the area of gastric indentation. When the endoscopist is ready, the assistant passes a needle cannula with an outer plastic sheath through the skin incision and into the stomach. The open polypectomy snare in the gastric lumen will surround the cannula and is tightened around it. The inner needle is then removed and a long suture or wire is threaded through the cannula into the stomach. After several inches of the suture have entered the stomach, the snare is slightly loosened, the cannula pulled back a bit, and the snare retightened around the suture itself (Fig. 72-2). The gastroscope is then withdrawn from the patient's mouth, pulling the suture along with it.

The two most frequently used techniques for PEG are the "pull" and "push" methods. In the pull method, the gastrostomy tube is affixed to the suture exiting the patient's mouth and pulled down through the esophagus and into the stomach, its end emerging from the abdominal wall

(Fig. 72-3). In the push method, a guidewire instead of a suture is used and the tube is threaded over the wire and pushed down the esophagus and into the stomach as tension is applied to both ends of the guidewire (Fig. 72-4). In each method, when the tube emerges from the abdominal wall, it is grasped and pulled upward. The gastroscope is re-introduced to monitor the position of the head of the catheter and to assure that it comes to lie in contact with the gastric mucosa. When the latter position has been ascertained, pull is discontinued on the tube. An outer bolster is applied to the tube and moved close to the skin (Fig. 72-5). It need not apply pressure to the skin, and a distance of 1 to 2 mm from the skin is advisable. Tension is not necessary to hold the stomach in contact with the abdominal wall and, in fact, has been associated with ischemic necrosis of the intervening tissue with subsequent abdominal wall infection, tube extrusion, and occasionally separation of the stomach from the abdominal wall. The tube and crossbar can be sutured to the abdominal wall or secured with additional rubber "O rings." An occlusive dressing is to be discouraged, as it encourages skin maceration and fungal infection. Preferably, the site should be left open and cleansed with saline or peroxide twice a day. Feedings are generally begun in 12 to 18 hours.

Complications

Most of the complications associated with PEG are trivial, but some may be life threatening. Minor irritation around the tube, wound exudate, and skin irritation can be handled by close attention to cleansing and use of appropriate skin creams. When fungal infection seems likely, antifungal powders or creams are beneficial. Redness, swelling, tenderness, or fluctuance around the tube should initiate concern regarding the presence of an abdominal wall infection. When this suspicion exists, the area may be aspirated or incised, looking for pus. Antibiotics should be started, and any tension between the outer bolster and the skin relieved. When the infection seems to be spreading or the patient's condition deteriorating, one may suspect a necrotizing abdominal wall infection, and surgical debridement is carried out.

Migration of the gastrostomy tube through the abdominal wall has been reported and

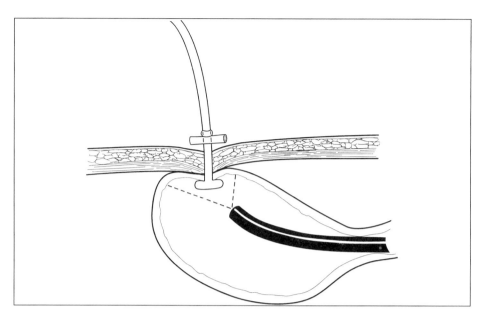

Fig. 72-5. An outer bolster is applied to prevent the tube from migrating inward. This should be placed several millimeters from the skin.

is almost always secondary to excessive traction with necrosis of the intervening abdominal wall tissue. Again, this can be prevented by avoidance of tension. If the outer bolster is placed too far from the skin, greater than several inches, the tube may migrate inward, obstructing the pylorus. Should this occur with the original or replacement gastrostomy tube, it is a simple matter to pull the catheter back and place the bolster closer to the skin.

Gastrocolic fistula has been known to occur following PEG. This can be the result of puncture of the colon at the time of the performance of the procedure, or be a result of pinching the colon between the stomach and abdominal wall. This problem may present long after placement of the gastrostomy or at the time of tube replacement. Frequently, the patient will have diarrhea. This should prompt an upper or lower gastrointestinal study using barium. When identified, these fistulas are usually easily managed by simply removing the gastrostomy catheter, and the abnormal tract closes within several days.

Separation of the stomach from the abdominal wall may occur soon after performance of the PEG. Early after performance of the procedure, the tube may be inadvertently pulled out by patient or staff. If this is recognized, treatment with nasogastric suction and intravenous antibiotics may be all that is required, with the procedure being repeated in 5 to 7 days. Should the patient show signs of deterioration or sepsis, laparotomy is indicated without delay. Separation may also be the result of tissue necrosis due to excessive tension on the tube. When signs of abdominal sepsis develop following a PEG, it is wise to stop feedings and confirm the intragastric position of the tube with a contrast study. Contrast agent is introduced through the tube and its position in the stomach assured.

Summary

Percutaneous endoscopic gastrostomy has become the method of choice for the establishment of a tube-feeding gastrostomy. Improvements in details of technique, familiarity with the prevention and management of complications, and new developments in tube design have helped improve the safety and expand the applications of the method. Attention to details of the technique and careful patient selection will assure that the best results are achieved.

Suggested Reading

Foutch GP. Complications of percutaneous endoscopic gastrostomy and jejunostomy: Recognition, prevention, and treatment. *Gastrointest Endosc Clin North Am* 2:231, 1992.

Hogan RB, DeMarco DC, Hamilton JK, et al. Percutaneous endoscopic gastrostomy: To push or pull, a prospective randomized trial. *Gastrointest Endosc* 32:253, 1986.

Mellinger JD. Percutaneous endoscopic gastrostomy: An evaluation after a decade. *Gastrointest Endosc Clin North Am* 2:187, 1992.

Ponsky JL, Gauderer MWL. Percutaneous endoscopic gastrostomy: A nonoperative technique for feeding gastrostomy. *Gastrointest Endosc* 27:9, 1981.

Russell TR, Brotman M, Forbes N. Percutaneous gastrostomy: A new simplified and cost-effective technique. *Am J Surg* 148:132, 1984.

Sacks BA, Vine HS, Palestrant AM, et al. A nonoperative technique for establishment of a gastrostomy in the dog. *Invest Radiol* 18:485, 1983.

Tellato TA, Gauderer MWL, Ponsky JL. Percutaneous endoscopic gastrostomy following previous abdominal surgery. *Ann Surg* 200:46, 1984.

Wolfsen HC, Kozarek RA. Percutaneous endoscopic gastrostomy: Ethical considerations. *Gastrointest Endosc Clin North Am* 2:259, 1992.

EDITOR'S COMMENT

Percutaneous endoscopic gastrostomy has been a successful new technique largely because of the work of Ponsky and colleagues. Pay especial attention to his clear remonstrations of when not to use PEG. Indeed, he has written (*Surg Endosc* 8:667, 1994), "Get Away from Get Away." Although one can often "get away" with something, there is frequently a price to pay. Strict adherence to established procedure may be a safer approach. The endoscopic removal of PEG tubes is expensive, invasive, and frequently unnecessary. The literature has demonstrated that most, when just cut off, will pass harmlessly through the gastrointestinal tract. It is clear, however, that this approach in some cases will lead to impaction of the catheter head in the intestinal lumen with resultant bowel obstruction. This is only one of many, many details that are so important in recognizing what may or may not keep us from the "get away" syndrome.

PEG has advantages over open gastrostomy, and is an accepted technique for children. However, a number of technical problems may be encountered during insertion. Recognized major complications include esophageal injury, colonic perforation, wound infection, gastric erosion by the gastrostomy tube, and later symptomatic gastroesophageal reflux requiring correction by fundoplication (*J Pediatr Surg* 30:671, 1995).

L.M.N.

73

Billroth I Gastrectomy

J. Rüdiger Siewert   Arnulf H. Hölscher

Billroth partial gastrectomies consist in the removal of the distal portion of the stomach. According to the type of disease (ulcer or carcinoma) and the location of the basic disease (duodenal ulcer, gastric ulcer, high-gastric ulcer), they are performed as antral, two-thirds, four-fifths, or subtotal gastrectomy. The distal partial gastrectomy is named according to the type of anastomosis between the small intestine and the gastric remnant, regardless of the extent of the gastrectomy.

The Billroth I operation is a gastroduodenostomy that can be performed both end to end and end to side. A decisive difference between this method and the Billroth II procedure is that the duodenal passage remains intact in the former method. Because of anastomotic requirements, the Billroth I operation is, as a rule, performed as an antral or a two-thirds gastrectomy. Gastroduodenostomy is difficult after extended gastrectomies. Direct anastomoses of this kind between gastric fundus and duodenum are followed by postoperative complications in a large number of patients.

Historical Note

After failed attempts at partial gastrectomy by Péan (1879) and Rydigier (1880)—both patients died after the operation—Theodor Billroth in 1881 performed the first successful partial gastrectomy, on a patient with antral carcinoma. He reconstructed the gastrointestinal passage by a superior end-to-end duodenostomy with the duodenum anastomosed to the lesser curvature side of the stomach (Fig. 73-1A). He later changed his surgical technique by effecting the anastomosis to the greater curvature (Fig. 73-1B). The reconstruction of the gastroduodenal passage in the Billroth I operation underwent numerous modifications in the time that followed: The end-to-end anastomosis was performed as a posterior or anterior gastroduodenostomy, or the duodenal end was connected to the entire circumference of the cut edge of the stomach (Fig. 73-1C–E). End-to-side gastroduodenostomy was performed by anastomosing the stomach to the side of the duodenum opposite the major duodenal papilla or entirely below the level of the papilla (Fig. 73-1F and G). Further modifications are the tube-shaped resection for ulcers high on the stomach and subsequent reanastomosis of the duodenum to the side of the greater curvature of the stomach (Fig. 73-1H), and antrectomy performed in combination with vagotomy and followed by an end-to-end anastomosis (Fig. 73-1I).

The technique most frequently used today is the Schoemaker modification of the Billroth I operation, with partial closure of the stomach remnant along the lesser curvature and an inferior gastroduodenostomy.

Arguments in Favor of Billroth I Gastrectomy

A decisive argument in favor of Billroth I anastomosis as compared with other forms of gastrectomy, such as Billroth II, is the preservation of the duodenal passage. The question arises as to whether the important functions of the duodenum are dependent on the presence or absence of the food passage.

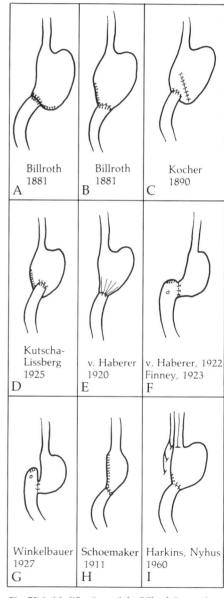

Fig. 73-1. Modifications of the Billroth I resection from the historical point of view.

Acids are neutralized in the duodenum by pancreatic and duodenal bicarbonate through neural and hormonal regulation. After distal stomach resection, this regulation is disturbed regardless of the type of anastomosis. Proportioned, regulated stomach emptying is no longer possible because the antrum and pylorus are gone.

The value of providing a duodenal passage cannot be properly assessed because the rapid and uncoordinated emptying of the stomach precludes the function of the digestive process that normally takes place in the duodenum. The value of the duodenal passage is clearer with regard to the function of the pancreas, the changes in the stomach remnant, and the function of the cardia.

Experimental and clinical investigations may indicate undisturbed pancreatic function, even after gastrectomy, but altered pancreatic function is apparent after gastrojejunostomy (Billroth II). Fat loss in the feces is considerably greater after Billroth II resection than after gastroduodenostomy. This loss may indicate insufficient digestion of food by pancreatic enzymes.

Even histologic changes of the stomach mucosa characteristic of chronic atrophic gastritis seem to be present to a lesser degree after a Billroth I resection than after gastrojejunostomy (Billroth II). The same is true for the frequency of carcinoma of the stomach remnant.

Examinations of the function of the cardia after partial gastrectomy show that the lower esophageal sphincter tends to react to a test meal after gastroduodenostomy in the same way as before the operation. After Billroth II resection, the tonicity of the lower esophageal sphincter disappears, but this functional disturbance of the cardia is rarely of clinical relevance.

Indications
Gastric Ulcer

The main indication for the Billroth I operation is gastric ulcer, which gives evidence of a high recurrence rate after vagotomy. The following arguments favor Billroth I resection: 1) The gastric ulcer is removed in toto during distal resection and can be examined histologically. 2) The point of least resistance on the antrum-corpus border of the lesser curvature is

eliminated. 3) The number of chief cells is reduced by removal of a part of the fundus. 4) The antrum as a point for the formation of gastrin is eliminated. 5) The remainder of the stomach is partly vagotomized by dissection of the lesser curvature from above the resection border.

Prepyloric Ulcer

Even prepyloric ulcers represent a good indication for Billroth I resection. Because of its secretory behavior, this ulcer type was, as far as the surgical and therapeutic consequences were concerned, previously included with the duodenal ulcers and, thus, normally represented an indication for vagotomy. However, results after 5 years of using this procedure show relatively high recurrence rates, so that it can be concluded that prepyloric ulcers would better be regarded as gastric ulcers as far as surgical treatment is concerned. Billroth I resection for prepyloric ulcers should be combined with selective gastric vagotomy.

Recurrent Ulcer in Both the Stomach and the Duodenum After Vagotomy

With recurrent ulcer in both the stomach and the duodenum after vagotomy, the Billroth I distal gastrectomy is, as a rule, a component of a combined operation. In consideration of the vagotomy performed simultaneously (selective gastric or truncal), the distal resection can be kept small (antrectomy). However, resection of the stomach after vagotomy, especially proximal gastric vagotomy, is technically difficult. If a recurrent ulcer is present in the duodenum, or if a pyloroplasty has been performed during the first operation, dissection of the duodenum can present problems, and occasionally an end-to-side anastomosis must be performed.

Early Carcinoma and Carcinoma of the Lesser Antrum

The Billroth I operation is not recommended for gastric cancer because a more radical procedure is required. Early carcinoma in the distal stomach without lymph node metastases ($T_1 N_0$) could prove an exception, and complete removal of the tumor can be achieved here with Billroth I resection.

Surgical Technique
Gastroduodenostomy with Anastomosis to the Side of the Greater Curvature of the Stomach

As a rule, the midline epigastric incision is the best approach (Fig. 73-2). Alternatively, a transverse epigastric rectus muscle-cutting incision or an upper vertical muscle-splitting incision to the right can be made.

The dissection of the stomach begins at the middle of the greater curvature by incising the gastrocolic ligament (Fig. 73-3A). Thus, the omental bursa is opened. The dissection for gastric ulcers can be done between the gastroepiploic vessels and the gastric wall. In carcinoma, a length of greater omentum corresponding to the extent of the resection of the greater curvature must be removed at the same time. When the omental bursa has been opened, the flimsy part of the gastrohepatic omentum may be pierced by the finger, and a soft rubber Penrose drain can be placed around the stomach. The dissection is then continued step by step along the greater curvature toward the duodenum. Near the pylorus, the greater curvature omentum becomes thick and divides into a front and back layer. The dissection should be continued bluntly in the loose intermediate tissue in the direction of the duodenum; the layers of tissue carrying the vessels should then be severed individually.

The preparation of the duodenum begins above or just below the second portion of the duodenum from a lateral direction, the so-called Kocher's maneuver (Fig. 73-3B). The peritoneal duplication is sharply cut along the lateral duodenal wall between the second portion of the duodenum and the beginning of the hepatoduodenal ligament. By stretching the second portion of the duodenum medially, the retroperitoneal tissue is loosened (part bluntly, part sharply) until the duodenum is mobilized. In this way a good general exposure can be achieved; this important maneuver facilitates the gastroduodenostomy. The preparation of the free first part of the duodenum is then continued.

By stretching the stomach, the dissection then proceeds along the greater curvature toward the left medial duodenal wall, then toward the back wall, and finally toward the lateral duodenal wall as far as the be-

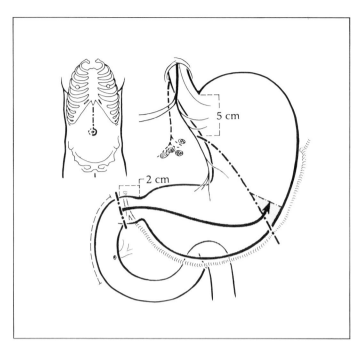

Fig. 73-2. The Billroth I resection. Midline epigastric incision and extent of the gastric resection. (From JR Siewert. Chirurgische Gastroenterologie. Berlin, Heidelberg, New York, Tokyo: Springer, 1981. Reproduced with permission.)

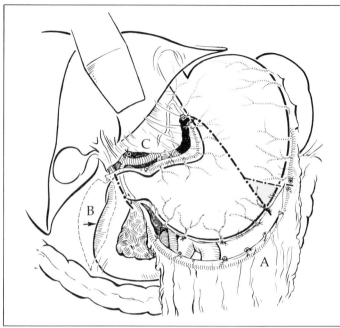

Fig. 73-3. Dissection of the stomach. A. Cutting of the gastrocolic omentum. B. Mobilization of the duodenum. C. Preparation of the lesser curvature. (From JR Siewert. Chirurgische Gastroenterologie. Berlin, Heidelberg, New York, Tokyo: Springer, 1981. Reproduced with permission.)

ginning of the hepatoduodenal ligament. In this way, 3 to 5 cm of the back wall of the duodenum can be made free, usually without technical difficulty. The transition from the free first part of the duodenum to the part fixed dorsally on the pancreas can be recognized from the course of the gastroduodenal artery. At this point, the serosa goes from the duodenum to the head of the pancreas. The surgeon must be especially careful because the artery is important for the blood supply to the duodenum.

After mobilization of the duodenum, the dissection is continued along the lesser curvature of the stomach (Fig. 73-3C). Difficulties could arise as a result of penetration of a gastric ulcer. Frequently, a penetrating gastric ulcer can be pinched off by fingers.

It is then advisable to coagulate the base of the ulcer and to oversew the hole in the stomach. The dissection must in every instance be continued far enough orally for a sufficiently large area of intact stomach wall to be prepared. According to the localization of the ulcer, the dissection of the stomach along the lesser curvature can be continued directly into the area of the cardia. The layers of the gastrohepatic omentum rest at varying intervals on the front

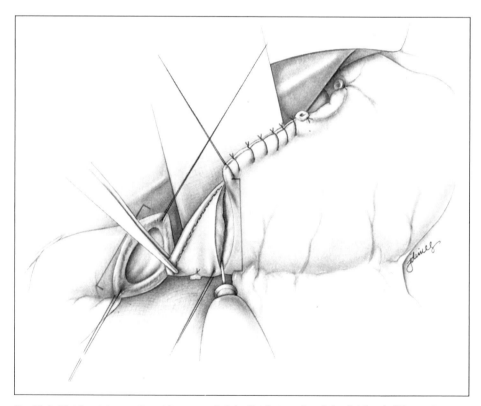

Fig. 73-4. Distal gastric resection. After removal of the distal stomach and the distal end of the greater curvature, the two cut surfaces are placed on each other. (From JR Siewert, AH Hölscher. Billroth I Operation (Gastroduodenostomie). In JR Siewert, Breitner Chirurgische Operationslehre Bd IV. Chirurgie des Abdomens II. Ösophagus, Magen, und Duodenum. Baltimore: Urban and Schwarzenberg, 1989. Reproduced with permission.)

or back wall of the stomach. These layers encircle a tissue rich in fat, within which the branches of the left gastric artery are found. The dissection proceeds by bluntly forcing the intermediate tissue apart and by individually severing the front and back layer of the gastrohepatic omentum. As long as the ascending trunk of the left gastric artery is not directly included, it remains intact during the ulcer resection.

The resection starts with the cutting of the duodenum between holding or guy sutures. The duodenum is temporarily closed with a sponge; the resection borders in the stomach are then determined.

A sewing machine (e.g., stapler technique TA90) facilitates the final step of stomach removal. The incision follows at an angle of 45 degrees to the lesser curvature (Fig. 73-3). The line can but need not be oversewn (Fig. 73-4). After removal of the distal portion of the stomach, a clamp is fitted at right angles to the greater curvature. The clamp is thus pushed far enough orally for the removal level to correspond to the duodenal lumen. The remaining aboral end is cut off after stay sutures are placed at each cut edge (Fig. 73-4). It is recommended that the so-called von Haberer submucous sutures (4–0 polyglycolic acid) be used in the front and back walls to

achieve hemostasis. The anastomosis should be performed without clamps.

The end-to-end gastroduodenostomy is done by anastomosing duodenum to the end of the greater curvature. For this purpose, the two cut surfaces are placed on each other and the two corner stitches are taken, starting at the stomach through the seromuscular layers with tangential grasping of the mucosa. At the duodenum, this stitch is done the other way around from inside to outside. The corner suture at the lesser curvature is tied, whereas the suture on the opposite side is left open (Fig. 73-5). The back wall is joined by interrupted

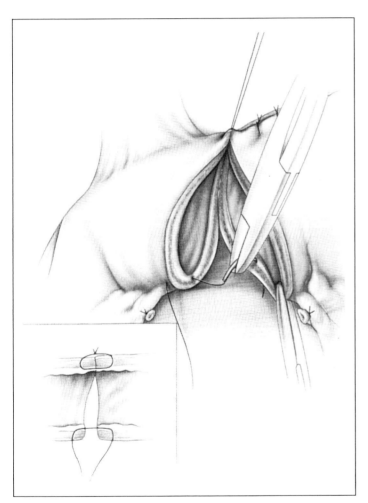

Fig. 73-5. Gastroduodenostomy with duodenum connected to the stomach on the side of the greater curvature. Corner sutures are seromuscular stitches that grasp the mucosa tangentially. The suture is tied on the lesser curvature side and left open on the opposite side. (From JR Siewert, AH Hölscher. Billroth I Operation (Gastroduodenostomie). In JR Siewert, Breitner Chirurgische Operationslehre Bd IV. Chirurgie des Abdomens II. Ösophagus, Magen, und Duodenum. Baltimore: Urban and Schwarzenberg, 1989. Reproduced with permission.)

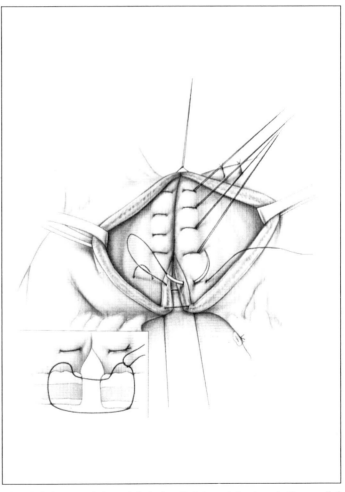

Fig. 73-6. Suture technique of the back wall. Interrupted sutures in the so-called back stitch technique, first through all layers of the stomach and duodenum and back, grasping only the mucosal edges. (From JR Siewert, AH Hölscher. Billroth I Operation (Gastroduodenostomie). In JR Siewert, Breitner Chirurgische Operationslehre Bd IV. Chirurgie des Abdomens II. Ösophagus, Magen, und Duodenum. Baltimore: Urban and Schwarzenberg, 1989. Reproduced with permission.)

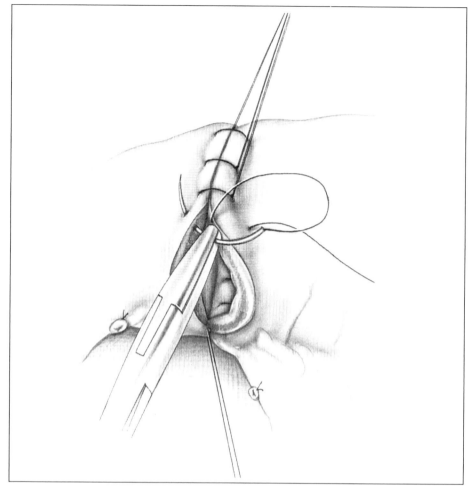

Fig. 73-7. The front wall is closed by interrupted sutures with seromuscular stitches, which grasp the mucosa tangentially. (From JR Siewert, AH Hölscher. Billroth I Operation (Gastroduodenostomie). In JR Siewert, Breitner Chirurgische Operationslehre Bd IV. Chirurgie des Abdomens II. Ösophagus, Magen, und Duodenum. Baltimore: Urban and Schwarzenberg, 1989. Reproduced with permission.)

back stitches (3–0 polyglycolic acid). These stitches start through all layers of the back wall at the cut edge of the lesser curvature from inside to outside and go through all layers of the posterior wall of the duodenum from outside to inside. The suture is led back grasping only the mucosa, first of the duodenum and then of the stomach. The knotting of these sutures leads to an exact adaptation, especially of the mucosa (Fig. 73-6). The front wall is best covered with one row of interrupted sutures through all layers with tangential stitches of the mucosa in the same technique as the corner stitches (Fig. 73-7). Special attention must be paid to the so-called Jammerecke (angle of sorrow) on the lesser curvature (Fig. 73-8). It is advisable to use a triple seromuscular suture, which includes the

duodenal wall as well as the front and back wall of the stomach. Another alternative is shown in (Fig. 73-9.)

Finally, the anastomosis is checked for openings with the finger. The position of the stomach tube is also checked to be sure it is crossing the anastomosis. The operative area is drained thoroughly by a soft silicone drain (Fig. 73-10).

Alternative Method: End-to-Side Gastroduodenostomy

In difficult duodenal ulcers, it can be impossible to preserve enough duodenal wall to be able to construct a tension-free anastomosis. In this situation, it is safer to

close the duodenum with a row of TA55 staples.

The reconstruction of the intestinal passage can proceed by end-to-side anastomosis (Fig. 73-11). For this purpose, the stomach is removed as previously described; the dissected stomach lumen is then anastomosed onto the front wall of the duodenum. Usually, an oblique incision should be made on the duodenal front wall so that the incision level starts from oral-medial and goes to aboral-lateral. The suturing technique is the same as for the end-to-end anastomosis. In technically difficult duodenal stump closures, additional covering of the stump with the back wall of the stomach can be obtained.

Anastomosis Using the Stapler Technique

The preparation of the stomach and duodenum proceeds as described previously. After the duodenum is cut, a circular border stitch pursestring suture is performed at the edge of the opening. The removable anvil of the EEA stapler (size 28 of 31) is introduced in the duodenum and the pursestring suture is tied around the center rod of the anvil (Fig. 73-12). Now the EEA stapler is introduced transpylorically into the stomach and at the posterior wall of the stomach the sharp tip of the center rod of the EEA stapler is perforated through the gastric wall. After removal of the tip, the center rod is connected with the anvil and the stapler is closed. After firing of the instrument, the stapler is removed and the excised circular tissue doughnuts of duodenum and stomach are controlled for completeness. The stomach resection is performed aborally to the anastomosis after closure of the proximal stomach with a TA90 stapler. The cut surface of the stomach can but need not be oversewn (Figs. 73-13 and 73-14).

Postoperative Complications

After Billroth I resection of the stomach, the following complications can occur: anastomotic leak in the area of the gastroduodenostomy (3–4%), bleeding (2%), passage disorders (2–5%), and postoperative pancreatitis (0.9%) (Table 73-1; Fig. 73-15).

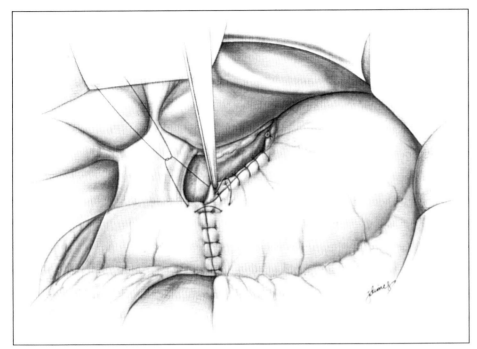

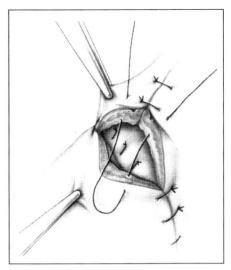

Fig. 73-8. The so-called Jammerecke is traditionally covered by a triple seromuscular suture, including the front wall of the stomach, the duodenum, and the back wall of the stomach. (From JR Siewert, AH Hölscher. Billroth I Operation (Gastroduodenostomie). In JR Siewert, Breitner Chirurgische Operationslehre Bd IV. Chirurgie des Abdomens II. Ösophagus, Magen, und Duodenum. Baltimore: Urban and Schwarzenberg, 1989. Reproduced with permission.)

Fig. 73-9. Alternative method for closing the Jammerecke in a single-row stitch technique. Seromuscular stitches are taken in the front wall of the stomach from outside to inside, including seromuscular layers of the duodenal wall from outside to inside and finally the back wall of the stomach in the same way from inside to outside. This suture does not achieve exact adaptation of all layers, but it leads to good closure of this corner by pulling the duodenal wall between the sutures at the lesser curvature. (From JR Siewert, AH Hölscher. Billroth I Operation (Gastroduodenostomie). In JR Siewert, Breitner Chirurgische Operationslehre Bd IV. Chirurgie des Abdomens II. Ösophagus, Magen, und Duodenum. Baltimore: Urban and Schwarzenberg, 1989. Reproduced with permission.)

Suture insufficiency in the area of the gastroduodenostomy can be managed well with conservative therapy, as long as the suture line does not occur in the first 3 or 4 days after the operation. It is imperative that the leak be well drained. With good drainage by a gastric tube, external drainage, and high doses of H_2 blockers or omeprazole and parenteral nutrition, it is usually possible for the anastomotic leak to heal.

Gastric emptying problems should not occur after gastroduodenostomy. If gastric stasis is a problem, it usually is the consequence of anastomotic edema or a hematoma and resolves within 10 to 14 days of good drainage to the stomach. Revisions are rarely necessary.

Intragastric or intraperitoneal bleeding is infrequent. Management depends on the extent of bleeding. Reoperation should follow if more than six units of blood per 24 hours are needed for substitution of the lost volume. For bleeding from the anastomosis or the stomach remnant, the stomach must be reopened with a horizontal incision about 3 to 5 cm above the anastomosis. The anastomosis and the stomach remnant can be surveyed easily from here and hemostasis can be obtained. Closure of the incision follows in a horizontal direction. Extraluminal bleeding sources are dealt with in the typical way. If the spleen represents the source of bleeding, hemostasis by coagulation, application of polyglactin 910 net, or, if inevitable, splenectomy should be done.

Postoperative pancreatitis is usually of the edematous variety, and the prognosis is relatively good. If it is hemorrhagic necrotizing pancreatitis, however, a high mortality must be expected. In postoperative pancreatitis of this kind, a mechanical alteration of the pancreatic duct should always be suspected.

Results and Postsurgical Diseases

A mortality of 1 to 2 percent must be expected for Billroth I resection for an uncomplicated gastric ulcer. Ulcers recur in 0 to 4 percent of patients; serious postgastrectomy problems are observed in 3 to 5 percent of patients.

Chronic Gastritis

In 80 to 90 percent of patients who have undergone partial gastrectomy, chronic gastritis of varying extent occurs in the stomach remnant 5 to 10 years after resection. The fact that the atrophic mucosal changes are slighter after Billroth I resection than after Billroth II resection has not yet been sufficiently proved.

Most patients who have undergone gastrectomy do not complain of symptoms despite extensive histologic changes. Only about 10 percent complain of symptoms requiring treatment. The cause of these

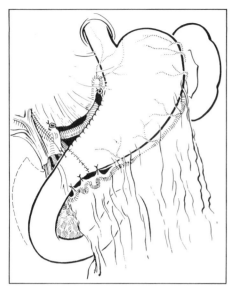

Fig. 73-10. Final aspect of the completed Billroth I gastrectomy. (From JR Siewert. Chirurgische Gastroenterologie. *Berlin, Heidelberg, New York, Tokyo: Springer, 1981. Reproduced with permission.*)

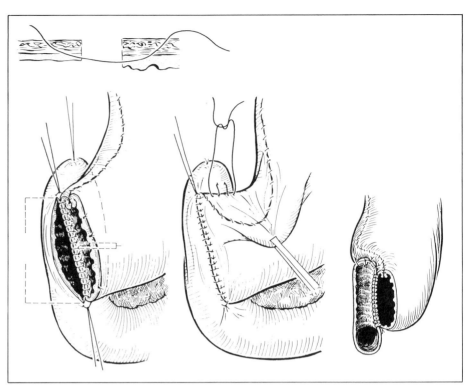

Fig. 73-11. End-to-side gastroduodenostomy. After removal of the distal stomach, the gastric lumen is anastomosed onto the front wall of the duodenum. The suturing technique is the same as described in Figs. 73-5 through 73-10. The duodenal stump is covered with the back of the gastric wall. (From JR Siewert. Chirurgische Gastroenterologie. *Berlin, Heidelberg, New York, Tokyo: Springer, 1981. Reproduced with permission.*)

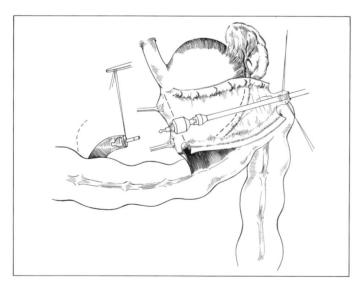

Fig. 73-12. Billroth I, stapler technique. The removable anvil of the stapler is introduced in the opening of the duodenum and the pursestring suture is tied around the center rod of the anvil. The EEA stapler is introduced transpylorically and the sharp tip of the central rod of the stapler is driven out and perforated through the back wall of the stomach. (From JR Siewert. Chirurgische Gastroenterologie. *Berlin, Heidelberg, New York, Tokyo: Springer, 1981. Reproduced with permission.*)

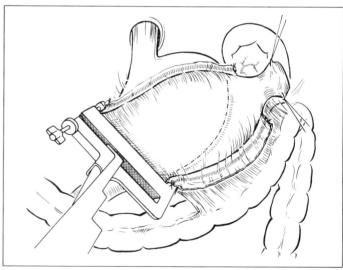

Fig. 73-13. The gastric resection is performed aborally to the anastomosis after closure of the proximal stomach with a TA90 stapler. (From JR Siewert. Chirurgische Gastroenterologie. *Berlin, Heidelberg, New York, Tokyo: Springer, 1981. Reproduced with permission.*)

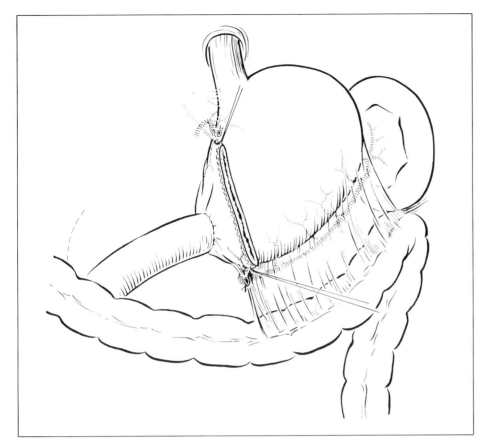

Fig. 73-14. After removal of the distal stomach, the cut surface can but need not be oversewn. (From JR Siewert. Chirurgische Gastroenterologie. Berlin, Heidelberg, New York, Tokyo: Springer, 1981. Reproduced with permission.)

Table 73-1. Early Postoperative Complications of Billroth I Gastrectomy for Gastric or Duodenal Ulcer

Author	Year	No. of Pts	Atony/ Stenosis	Suture Insufficiency/ Peritonitis	Secondary Hemorrhage	Pancreatitis
				Incidence (%)		
Horsburgh	1965	113	—	0	0	—
Semb	1973	130	3.8	0	0	—
Nielsen	1973	97	5.1	2.1	4.1	—
Duthie	1973	50	6.0	6.0	4.0	—
Madsen	1976	22	4.5	—	—	—
Winkler	1977	302	6.3	7.3	2.3	0.7
Kraft–Kinz	1977	1023	0	1.0	0	—
Hollender	1978	228	1.3	1.3	—	0.9
Hollender[a]	1978	2303	—	1.7	—	—
Baehrlehner[b]	1979	155	0	3.9	0.6	—
Baehrlehner[c]	1979	157	2.5	8.3	3.8	—

[a]Compilation from the literature.
[b]Single-row anastomosis.
[c]Double-row anastomosis.

complaints is apparently not the chronic gastritis, but the enterogastric reflux. The clinical signs and symptoms are epigastric pain, feeling of fullness, nausea, and bile vomiting. The disappearance of epigastric symptoms after bile vomiting is characteristic, as is its intensification by stimulation of the bile or pancreatic secretion. Conservative treatment includes metoclopramide, spasmolytics and maybe cholestyramine, antacids, and dietary regulations. An antiperistaltic jejunal interposition is rarely necessary.

Dumping

Dumping problems in the sense of early dumping are less frequent after Billroth I resection than after Billroth II resection. The frequency is between 7 and 29 percent of patients. The most important conservative measure of treatment is dietary (no sweet meals, small meals frequently, no liquid intake with food, moist food). All attempts with drugs, including serotonin antagonists, have until now proved disappointing, except somatostatin, which, however, is only available in the intravenous or intramuscular form but not for oral intake. The most serious dumping forms can be an indication for antiperistaltic jejunal interposition.

Gastroesophageal Reflux

Gastroesophageal reflux does not frequently occur after resection of the distal part of the stomach. A carefully taken history often reveals that gastroesophageal reflux was present before the operation; this frequently occurs among patients with ulcers. There has been no investigation into whether or not reflux after Billroth I resection is more infrequent than after other forms of stomach resection. The function of the lower esophageal sphincter after gastrojejunostomy seems to be defective. The diagnostic examination of reflux esophagitis after stomach resection requires endoscopy, 24-hour pH measurement, and an examination of the material drawn out of the esophagus for bile acids. Metoclopramide or domperidone can be useful, but antacids also are helpful because of their bile-acid absorbing qualities. Serious reflux esophagitis can be an indication for a conversion to a Roux en Y gastrojejunostomy with a long efferent loop.

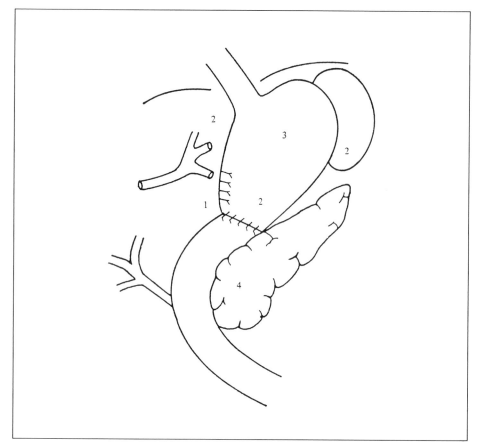

Fig. 73-15. Possible early complications of Billroth I gastrectomy. 1. Suture insufficiency in the area of the gastroduodenostomy. 2. Secondary hemorrhage from the gastroduodenostomy into the intraluminal or extraluminal space. 3. Impairment of passage because of obstruction of anastomosis. 4. Postoperative pancreatitis.

Suggested Reading

Alexander-Williams J, Hoare AM. Partial gastric resection. *Clin Gastroenterol* 8:321, 1979.

Baron JH. The Rationale of the Different Operations for Peptic Ulcer. In AG Cox, J Williams (eds), *Vagotomy on Trial*. London: Heinemann, 1973.

Blum AL, Siewert JR. *Ulcus-Therapie*. Berlin: Springer, 1982.

Domellof L, Eriksson S, Janunger KG. Late precancerous changes and carcinoma of the gastric stump after Billroth I resection. *Am J Surg* 132:26, 1976.

Duthie HL, Kwong H-K. Vagotomy or gastrectomy for gastric ulcer. *Br Med J* 4:79, 1973.

Emas S, Hammerberg C. Prospective randomized trial of selective proximal vagotomy with ulcer excision and partial gastrectomy with gastroduodenostomy in the treatment of corporal gastric ulcer. *Am J Surg* 146:631, 1983.

Fiser WP, Wellborn JC, Thompson BW, Read RC. Age and morbidity of vagotomy with antrectomy or pyloroplasty. *Am J Surg* 144:694, 1982.

Hoare AM, McLeish A, Thompson H, Alexander-Williams J. Hydrotalcite in the treatment of bile vomiting after gastric surgery. *Br J Surg* 64:849, 1977.

Hölscher AH, Bumm R, Siewert JR. Chirurgische Therapie prinzipièn bei der Rezidivprophylaxe. In P Bauerfeind, AL Blum (eds), *Ulkusalmanach*. 1 + 2. Berlin: Springer, 1990. Pp 87–113.

Koelz HR, Lepsien G, Blum AL, Siewert JR. The duodenum regulates the lower esophageal sphincter. *Gastroenterology* 75:283, 1978.

Lundquist G, Hedenstedt S. Jejunal transposition in stomach surgery: Indications and results. *Acta Chir Scand*. [Suppl] 457, 1975.

Madsen P, Kronborg O, Hansen OH, Pedersen T. Billroth I gastric resection versus truncal vagotomy and pyloroplasty in the treatment of gastric ulcer. *Acta Chir Scand* 142:151, 1976.

Schumpelick V, Werner B. Postoperative alkalische Refluxgastritis. *Dtsch Med Wochenschr* 103:220, 1978.

Siewert JR, Hölscher AH. Billroth I Gastrectomy. In LM Nyhus, C Wastell (eds), *Surgery of the Stomach and Duodenum* (4th ed). Boston: Little, Brown, 1986.

Siewert JR, Hölscher AH. Billroth I operation (gastroduodenostomie). In JR Siewert, *Breitner Chirurgische Operationslehre Bd. IV. Chirurgie des Abdomens. II. Ösophagus, Magen und Duodenum*. Baltimore: Urban and Schwarzenberg, 1989.

Siewert JR, Hölscher AH. Operative Therapie des unkomplizierten Ulcus ventriculi. In JR Siewert, F Harder, M Allgöwer, et al (eds), *Chirurgische Gastroenterologie* (2nd ed). Berlin: Springer, 1990.

Skandalakis JE, Skandalakis LJ, Colbŏrn GL, et al. The duodenum: Surgical anatomy. *Am Surg* 55:291, 1989.

EDITOR'S COMMENT

In the early 1950s, gastric resection ad modum Billroth II (subtotal gastric resection with gastrojejunal anastomosis) was the surgical approach in the treatment of either gastric or duodenal ulcer. I credit the late Henry N. Harkins of Seattle for demonstrating to the surgical world several important technical details that helped make the gastroduodenal anastomosis feasible in most patients. Today, most surgeons prefer to use the gastroduodenal anastomosis after gastric resection. This is an important change in surgical approach that should not be unnoticed.

The thrust of this presentation by our German colleagues is the use of the Billroth I gastrectomy for the treatment of benign gastric ulcer. I am in complete agreement that resection of the stomach with Billroth I anastomosis is sufficient, and that the addition of vagotomy is unnecessary; perhaps it is even meddlesome.

The authors take a very conservative approach to the problem of alkaline reflux gastritis; that is, they emphasize a nonoperative approach. Again, I agree. A patient with bona fide symptomatic alkaline reflux gastritis, following either a Billroth I or a Billroth II anastomosis, deserves to have some type of procedure to divert this alkaline chyme away from the susceptible gastric mucosa. The problem rests in selection of the appropriate patients for the operation. There is too much overlap in patient symptoms, endoscopic appearance of the gastric mucosa, and mucosal biopsy findings between those who do well and those who do not do well after such diversion. Until we have greater specificity in our diagnoses, we should err on the side of performing too few rather than too many diversion operations.

Silen and colleagues (*J Am Coll Surg* 180:648, 1995) have had excellent results with the Henley jejunal interposition (40 cm) procedure in their treatment of alkaline reflux gastritis. This approach did not have the motility problems so frequently seen after the Roux en Y reconstruction.

L.M.N.

74

Billroth II Gastrectomy

Frank James Branicki   Leslie Karl Nathanson

Duodenal Ulcer: Etiology and Management Strategies

A 1989 National Institutes of Health (NIH) consensus statement documented that bleeding was estimated to occur in 100,000 of four million patients with peptic ulceration in the United States annually. Globally, peptic ulceration reaches almost epidemic proportions in the Chinese populations of Hong Kong, the People's Republic of China, and Taiwan. Genetic influences are believed to play a part and it is not uncommon to encounter the disorder in children. Nevertheless, there is now overwhelming evidence for a role for *Helicobacter pylori* in the etiology of peptic ulcer and the intestinal type of gastric adenocarcinoma.

Therapy of duodenal ulceration has evolved in the past decade with a greater understanding of therapeutic options and more recently with the advent of minimal access surgery. At least 90 percent of duodenal ulcers have an association with *H. pylori*, which may be diagnosed by histologic examination of endoscopic mucosal biopsy or by the rapid urease test. Occasionally, culture of *H. pylori* is employed particularly in patients who have antibiotic allergies or failed previous therapies, or in countries where *H. pylori* has a high level of background antibiotic resistance. There is no justification for treatment of patients for periods longer than 14 days. Breath tests to detect urease can indicate cure of *H. pylori* 4 weeks after antibiotic therapy, at a time when serologic antibody tests will still give a positive result. Cure has been defined as failure to demon-

strate *H. pylori* by a sensitive technique 4 weeks after cessation of all antimicrobial therapy and proton pump inhibitors, the latter having been shown to interfere with diagnosis. The 1994 NIH consensus conference guidelines for duodenal ulcer include assessment of *H. pylori* status and eradication of the organism. Recurrence will develop in 10 percent of patients with duodenal ulceration, usually as a result of persistent basal acid hypersecretion or an underlying mucosal defect. Basal acid secretion is increased sixfold in patients with duodenal ulcer but returns toward normal within 6 months after *H. pylori* eradication.

The efficacy of various drug regimens for eradication of *H. pylori* has led physicians to adopt a conservative approach to referral for consideration of surgical intervention for peptic ulcer. This policy has been supported by the finding that reinfectivity rates for *H. pylori* are very low, for example, less than 1 percent in Western societies. It has now become inappropriate to recommend elective surgical intervention for complicated peptic ulcer unless there is evidence that ulceration persists in the absence of *Helicobacter* infection. Indeed, it has been documented in two reports that subsequent eradication of the organism in patients undergoing nonsurgical management of bleeding peptic ulcer was associated not only with ulcer healing but with no subsequent hemorrhage during follow-up studies.

Thus, it is now considered that the indications for elective surgical intervention in complicated ulcer disease require better definition. Surgery in patients with recurrent duodenal ulceration is warranted for 1) poor patient compliance with medical

therapy, 2) patient preference when ulcer relapse occurs frequently despite intermittent medication, and 3) definitive alternative treatment to long-term maintenance therapy in younger patients. The introduction of a variety of laparoscopic techniques, including posterior truncal vagotomy and anterior seromyotomy, highly selective vagotomy (HSV), vagotomy and antrectomy, and partial gastrectomy, now provide opportunities for treatment of duodenal ulceration without the short-term morbidity related to open upper abdominal incisions. It is essential, however, that the procedure of choice at open surgery for the majority of patients with duodenal ulcer (HSV) is also adopted as optimal laparoscopic treatment when a gastric resection is deemed unnecessary. Truncal vagotomy and antrectomy retain a place in the management of some patients with pyloric/duodenal stenosis, prepyloric ulceration, and recurrence despite previous HSV or truncal vagotomy and a drainage procedure. Billroth II gastrectomy is an alternative in some circumstances; even in the recent past, its usage has been widespread in China but it is occasionally associated with side effects of diarrhea and dumping. The role of truncal vagotomy and antrectomy or Billroth II gastrectomy is largely confined to the management of patients with primary ulceration with bleeding or perforation arising from a large ulcer, for example, 2 cm or greater in size, or recurrent ulceration following previous truncal vagotomy. Although truncal vagotomy and antrectomy are associated with a recurrence rate of less than 3 percent, on long-term follow-up studies they have the distinct disadvantage of delayed gastric emptying, which occurs in about 6 percent of patients, regardless of whether continuity has been restored with gastro-duodenal or gastrojejunal anastomosis. The combination of vagotomy, which interferes with gastric motor function, and excision of the antral pacemaker mechanism occasionally gives rise to gastric remnant stasis. This may take between 2 and 6 weeks to resolve but always does so spontaneously in our experience. Obviously, nutritional support needs to be provided during this period. Enteral fine-bore tube feeding is sometimes problematic with proximal migration of the distal tube to the stomach with gastric distention; parenteral nutrition is preferred. As truncal vagotomy and antrectomy may require protracted hospitalization in the postoperative period, there is a reluctance to undertake this procedure in the elderly, who often have concomitant illness and run the risk of atelectasis or deep vein thrombosis. Billroth II gastrectomy is therefore favored for older patients, whereas truncal vagotomy and antrectomy offer the benefits of a larger gastric remnant in the younger age group.

The first successful gastric resection was performed by Theodor Billroth on January 29, 1881, in a 43-year-old woman with gastric cancer, the gastric remnant being anastomosed to the duodenum (Billroth I). On January 15, 1885, Billroth performed the first gastrectomy (Billroth II) with closure of both the duodenal stump and the gastric remnant, continuity being restored by fashioning an anterior gastrojejunostomy. Following gastric resection for duodenal ulcer, although gastroduodenal anastomosis has perhaps the greatest physiologic appeal for restoration of continuity, it is well established that lower rates of recurrent ulceration are achieved by a two-thirds gastric resection, duodenal stump closure, and gastrojejunal anastomosis. In addition, gastroduodenostomy is often technically difficult in the presence of a scarred or fibrotic duodenum, necessitating extensive mobilization of both duodenum and remnant to ensure a tension-free anastomosis. Doubts may also be harbored as to whether the reconstructed gastroduodenal outlet will have sufficient caliber for adequate gastric emptying to take place. The Billroth II procedure can be performed with the confidence that a safe adequate stoma is always possible. Gastrojejunal reconstruction is also favored in the management of patients with gastric cancer, as it obviates potential obstructive

problems should recurrent disease arise in the vicinity of the pancreatic head. Early gastric cancer may require only a 2-cm resection margin and, depending on the site of the lesion, gastroduodenal anastomosis may be appropriate. In contrast, all advanced cancers are best dealt with by gastrojejunal reconstruction following gastric resection, which does not compromise the extent of lymphadenectomy undertaken.

An awareness of technical variations is important to the gastric surgeon, who may select which is most appropriate according to anatomic and pathologic findings. The variation promoted by Franz Hofmeister (1867–1929) with closure of much of the lesser curvature side of the cut gastric remnant proved popular, as it is said to ensure that the stoma is placed at the most dependent part of the stomach and avoids acute angulation of the jejunum at the lesser curvature, which is claimed to be a disadvantage of the Polya technique (Fig. 74-1). Nevertheless, our own practice of the Polya operation described by Jeno (Eugene) Polya (1876–1944) in which the whole of the cut end of the gastric remnant is su-

tured to the jejunum has provided satisfactory functional results in a large majority (Fig. 74-2). There appears to be little or no advantage for the crosscut technique with a transverse jejunal incision, as described by Hoerr and Turnbull (Fig. 74-3). Indeed, theoretical considerations concerning uncut Roux en Y loops suggest that a crosscut jejunum may have a greater possibility of impaired motility.

More than two dozen variations of the Billroth II procedure have been described since its introduction in 1885. These encompass variations that involve siting of the loop gastroenterostomy with regard to the gastric remnant and transverse colon and Braun enteroenterostomy or Roux en Y modifications. Anastomosis of the afferent limb of the loop to the greater (Moynihan; Fig. 74-4) or lesser (Balfour; Fig. 74-5) curvatures is an option, and much controversy has centered on whether a loop should be sited in an antecolic or retrocolic position. Tanner held the view that antecolic placement was advantageous, as it rendered revision gastric surgery much simpler should the need ever

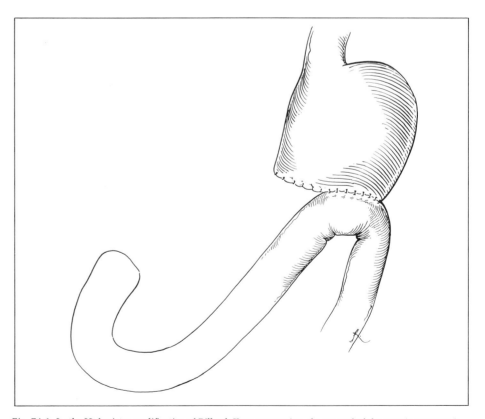

Fig. 74-1. In the Hofmeister modification of Billroth II reconstruction, the cut end of the gastric remnant is closed in two layers on the lesser curvature side, except for an opening at the greater curvature, which is used for anastomosis to the jejunum.

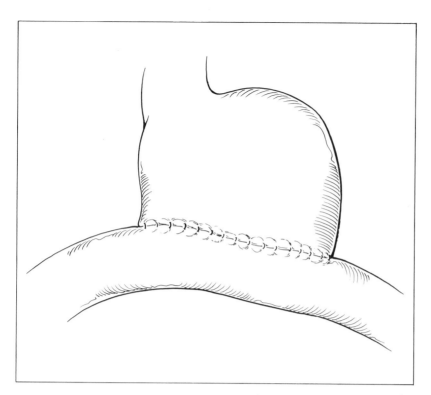

Fig. 74-2. In the Polya technique of Billroth II reconstruction, the entire cut end of the gastric remnant is used to fashion an anastomosis with the jejunum.

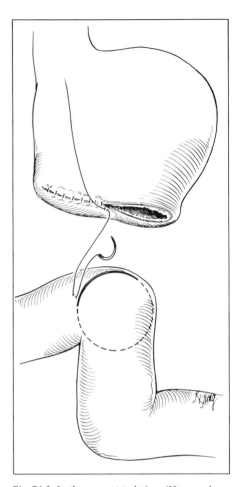

Fig. 74-3. In the crosscut technique (Hoerr and Turnbull), the incision is made transversely to correspond to the gastric stoma in the Hofmeister modification of the Billroth II.

arise and that carcinoma of the colon occurred frequently enough in England to raise concerns regarding the hazards of radical colonic resection in patients in whom a retrocolic gastrojejunostomy had been performed. These technical considerations were considered sufficient argument for advocating antecolic anastomosis, as this does not appear to compromise function. It has, however, been voiced that antecolic anastomosis is associated with a greater likelihood of colonic or small-bowel obstruction. This risk is believed to be reduced by bringing the colon with gentle traction to the right side of the anastomosis at the conclusion of the procedure. Our preference for Billroth II gastrectomy involves mobilization of the distal stomach, closure of the duodenal stump, and gastric resection followed by antecolic (Balfour) gastrojejunostomy.

Timing of Surgical Intervention

The timing of surgery in the management of complicated duodenal ulceration is cru-

cial to outcome measurements. Emergency surgical intervention for gastrointestinal bleeding is associated with a 10-fold increase in mortality compared with elective surgery. If at all possible the patient presenting with bleeding duodenal ulcer should undergo urgent therapeutic endoscopy for immediate management, followed in selected patients by elective surgical intervention when operation is deemed essential. Experience with such a policy in the management of over a thousand patients with bleeding peptic ulcer has recorded no operative mortality for elective or early operative intervention during the same admission. In the selection of management strategies for patients who present with acute hemorrhage, it is necessary to identify the "high-risk" patient with coexisting medical illness or hemodynamic instability, or both, and the "high risk" lesion. Therapeutic endoscopy for bleeding peptic ulcer is believed to be of value for active spurting/oozing hemorrhage, or when a nonbleeding visible vessel with or without sentinel clot has been visualized at endoscopy on initial presentation. Endoscopic stigmata of recent hemorrhage are more likely to be seen

in large ulcers, greater than 1 cm, in diameter, large ulcers being more frequently encountered in patients over 60 years of age. Ulcer size of greater than 1 cm is associated with an increased risk of rebleeding and mortality, with rebleeding carrying a 10-fold increase in mortality. Postoperative gastrointestinal bleeding from bleeding peptic ulcer has a mortality of 40 percent if reoperation is required. Injection sclerotherapy is considered the procedure of choice for control of postoperative hemorrhage that continues or recurs. Obvious reservations exist regarding distention of the stomach in the immediate postoperative period, but using as little insufflation as possible we have successfully managed suture line bleeding in this way. The portable nature and minimal cost of equipment required have been responsible for the increasing popularity of injection

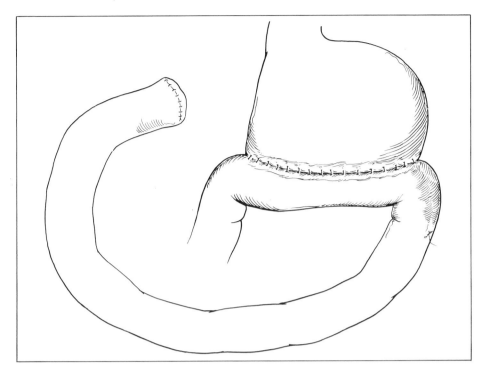

Fig. 74-4. Proximal jejunum is brought to the greater curvature end of the Polya anastomosis (Moynihan).

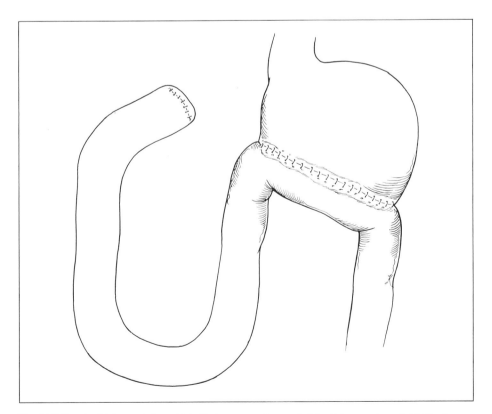

Fig. 74-5. Proximal jejunum is brought to the lesser curvature end of the Polya anastomosis (Balfour).

sclerotherapy (with alcohol, epinephrine, polidocanol, or saline) in preference to electrocoagulation, heater probe application, or laser therapy. Sclerotherapy has been shown to be equally efficacious and may be repeated if so required. Gastric wall necrosis and jaundice due to bile duct fibrosis have been reported with the use of epinephrine and polidocanol, respectively. Thus, overzealous injection treatment with excessive injections of aliquots is to be avoided.

Bleeding

When surgical intervention for gastrointestinal hemorrhage is required, adequate control of the bleeding site in an ulcer that is to remain in situ is essential. Figure-of-eight plication of a bleeding vessel may suffice but, occasionally, control may only be obtained with the aid of prior ligation of the gastroduodenal artery adjacent to its origin from the hepatic artery. Nonabsorbable sutures, for example, 2–0 linen, are preferred for transfixion of the bleeding site and suture ligation of feeding vessels required to control oozing hemorrhage from the ulcer base. If hemorrhage is such that there is hemodynamic instability at induction of anesthesia, then pyloroduodenotomy with direct suture of the bleeding point is essential before one embarks on gastric mobilization. Difficulty is sometimes encountered in securing hemorrhage in the fibrotic base of an ulcer. It is important to use a wide-nosed needle holder that has a firm grip on the needle without any free rotational movement of the needle in its holder. When bleeding from extensive ulceration proves difficult to control by direct plication following pyloroduodenotomy, it may be necessary to identify the origin of the gastroduodenal artery and ligate the vessel medially and lateral to the duodenum as it courses posteriorly on the head of the pancreas. Extensive ulceration of the medial duodenal wall may encroach on the ampulla of Vater or the accessory pancreatic duct of Santorini. Encroachment on the ampulla is usually recognized endoscopically or at open operation without too much difficulty, whereas the presence of an accessory pancreatic duct opening may easily be overlooked. Particularly when hemorrhage is brisk, it is necessary to be wary of the possible inadvertent suture ligation of the ampulla of Vater. If ulceration extends to the second part of the duodenum, the location of the ampulla must be identified by palpation or visually, once hemostasis has been achieved. The risk of rebleeding in the postoperative period is believed to be greater in patients with large peptic ulcers greater than 2 cm in size. Accordingly, we hold the view that all large ulcers that have given rise to life-threatening hemorrhage be resected if surgery is required. Penetrating ulcers of the head or body of the pancreas are generally left in situ with exclusion from the gastrointestinal tract when continuity is restored. Plication of the bleeding point in small posteromedial duodenal ulcers may be followed by exclusion of the ulcer base from access to the duodenal lumen by suture closure of the mucosa at the ulcer margins.

Perforation

Large duodenal ulcers, greater than 5 cm in size, are most commonly found in a posteromedial position in the first part of the duodenum. Anterior ulcers generally perforate into the peritoneal cavity before attaining such a size, whereas posteromedial ulceration into the pancreas may not give rise to complication unless bleeding supervenes. In the low-risk patient with a free intraperitoneal perforation from duodenal ulceration, definitive anti-ulcer surgery may have a place. Definitive intervention, some form of vagotomy or excisional surgery, is not recommended 1) if the patient has a history of coexistent medical illness, for example, diabetes; 2) the duration of intraperitoneal contamination exceeds 24 hours; or 3) hemodynamic instability is evident on first presentation, for example, systolic blood pressure less than 100 mm Hg. In such circumstances simple omental patch repair is advisable with the exception of the large ulcer defect, greater than 2 cm in diameter, for which excisional surgery is the preferred option. Omental patch repair of ulcers greater than 2 cm in size is believed to be associated with an increased risk of peripatch leakage of duodenal contents postoperatively. In addition, closure in such circumstances may give rise to obstruction in the duodenum, which may already have some degree of stenosis from chronic scarring. There is, therefore, support for excisional ulcer surgery, duodenal stump closure followed by antrectomy with truncal vagotomy, or Billroth II gastric resection and anastomosis.

Billroth II Gastrectomy

Prior usage of H_2 receptor antagonists or proton pump inhibitors may have resulted in hypochlorhydria with endogenous bacterial overgrowth and a greater likelihood of infective postoperative complications. Gastroduodenal resections are classified as "clean contaminated" in nature and prophylactic antibiotic therapy is indicated; a single cephalosporin injection an hour before operation is usually sufficient. Prior upper endoscopy will have provided in most instances, except perforation, information crucial to decision making as regards the nature of the procedure to be performed. Patients with pyloric/duodenal stenosis need to be fasted and undergo repeated gastric lavage, with nutrition being maintained intravenously for up to a week preoperatively. This helps to ensure adequate motility in the remnant stomach should resection be performed. Truncal vagotomy and pyloroplasty or gastroenterostomy may, however, be ineffective for the treatment of vomiting when there has been chronic gross distention of the stomach with resultant atony. Alternatively, the Billroth II procedure may be considered in patients over 60 years of age with pyloric/duodenal stenosis.

Our preference at open surgery is an upper midline incision that extends to the left side of the xiphisternum to provide adequate exposure of the proximal lesser curvature of the stomach. Access is greatly enhanced with the use of a self-retaining retractor (Hepco, Kansas City, KS), which comprises two vertical poles that are attached by fixators to the operating tube and a central horizontal bar that is then used to bridge the poles. A variety of self-retaining Hepco retractors for xiphisternum, costal margin, and liver are available to facilitate excellent abdominal exposure without the need for manual retraction of wound or liver. Any adhesions to the lower pole of the spleen are divided before gastric mobilization.

Duodenal Transection and Closure

At open operation, the duodenum, stomach, gallbladder, and bile duct are in-spected and palpated. Although large duodenal ulcers are generally palpable, small lesions may not be so, especially when situated posteromedially. If a large, active duodenal ulcer is present, an inflammatory mass is occasionally encountered; in the absence of bleeding, truncal vagotomy and gastroenterostomy represent a more prudent choice for therapy than gastric resection. The mass may be adherent to the extrahepatic biliary tree or the inferior surface of the liver; when overt bleeding has been the presenting feature, the ulcer will require direct suture, excision, or exclusion. Rarely, ulceration may abut the extrapancreatic common bile duct, requiring meticulous dissection of the duodenum to facilitate separation of the edges of the ulcer from its bed, which is retained in situ contiguous with the bile duct. If previous acute gastrointestinal hemorrhage has occurred, it is important not to overlook the presence of any second ulcer or lesion in the duodenum or stomach.

The right and left gastroepiploic vessels are identified, and small arterial and venous branches extending from the pylorus to the proximal stomach are then ligated and divided between hemostats. This maneuver, which opens wide the lesser sac, permits inspection of the posterior wall of the duodenal bulb with preservation of the main trunks of the right gastroepiploic vessels as the bulb is separated from the head of the pancreas. The duodenum can be mobilized as described by Kocher by division of the peritoneum lateral to its second and third parts. Mobilization of the first part of the duodenum proceeds with division of the branches of the right gastric artery, which arises from the common hepatic. Without gross scarring stump closure is accomplished with no difficulty when 2 cm of proximal duodenum can be freed on duodenal mobilization. This can then be transected with the aid of two Lang Stevenson clamps (Downs, London, England) placed transversally just distal to the pylorus (Fig. 74-6A). Gauze swabs soaked in chlorhexidine hydrochloride (Hibitane blue) are placed behind the duodenum and scalpel duodenal transection is performed between the clamps. The cut ends are swabbed with Hibitane-soaked gauze and a tie is then placed in figure-of-eight fashion to secure an additional small Hibitane-soaked swab to the clamp, which is left in place on the distal portion of the gastric specimen to be resected. This pre-

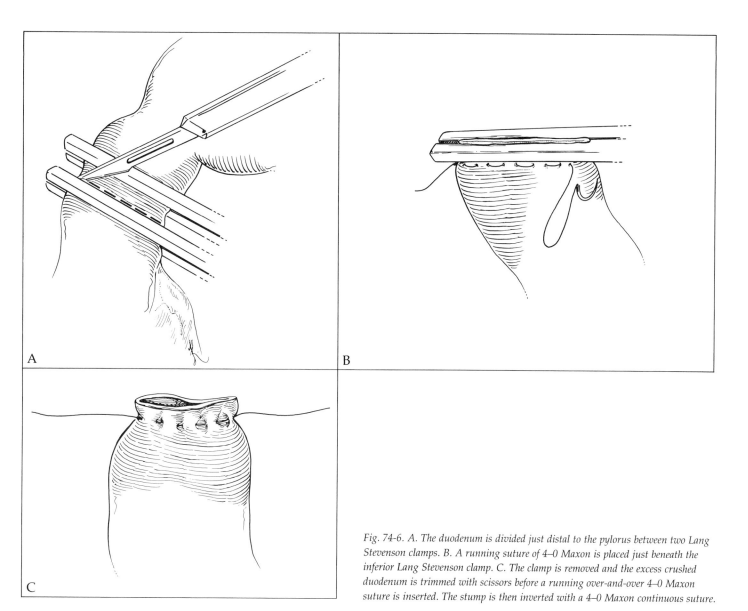

Fig. 74-6. A. The duodenum is divided just distal to the pylorus between two Lang Stevenson clamps. B. A running suture of 4–0 Maxon is placed just beneath the inferior Lang Stevenson clamp. C. The clamp is removed and the excess crushed duodenum is trimmed with scissors before a running over-and-over 4–0 Maxon suture is inserted. The stump is then inverted with a 4–0 Maxon continuous suture.

vents intraperitoneal contamination from the proximal end of the divided duodenum. A 4–0 Maxon suture (Davis and Geck, Manati, PR) is then placed in a continuous fashion beneath the clamp on the duodenal stump (Fig. 74-6B). This suture is run back and forth to close the stump, the clamp is removed, and excess duodenum that has been clamped is trimmed. This first row of sutures is not hemostatic and to ensure that no bleeding will occur from the cut mucosa a second row of sutures is placed in the same plane using the same 4–0 Maxon suture in an over-and-over fashion (Fig. 74-6C). These suture layers are then inverted with the aid of a continuous 4–0 Maxon seromuscular suture placed so as to invert

both corners of the cut edge of duodenum. This layered closure, although it takes a few minutes longer then single-layer or staple closure, has been found to be efficacious, with no leakage observed when it is performed electively for benign disease. Unfortunately, closure is sometimes more problematic without the option of such straightforward suture techniques in healthy tissues. If coincidental gallstones are present in the gallbladder, it is recommended that cholecystotomy and stone removal be performed in preference to cholecystectomy, which is regarded as being more likely to be associated with postoperative digestive sequelae if gastric resection is performed.

Difficult Duodenal Stump Closure

During duodenal mobilization the extrapancreatic common bile duct must be identified and preserved. Inflammation may shorten the duodenum so that the ampulla of Vater is less than 5 cm from the pylorus. If the duodenum is grossly scarred or edematous, it is necessary to assess the feasibility of stump closure before embarking on gastric resection. Occasionally, a penetrating ulcer is encountered that requires scissors dissection to free the edges of the ulcer from the posteromedial duodenal wall, giving rise to a defect that may be several centimeters in size. The ulcer that remains in situ must be plicated adequately to control hemorrhage if it is regarded as the source of previous bleeding. The defect may be very large when ulceration is almost circumferential and the duodenum is divided at the proximal end of the mucosal bridge to facilitate stump closure. When ulceration is so extensive, it is imperative that the ampulla of Vater or any obvious accessory pancreatic duct opening be located by inspection or palpation. Failure to do so can give rise to suture closure of duct(s) with impeded biliary and pancreatic drainage and/or consequent pancreatitis or formation of a pancreatic fistula.

Rarely, if serious doubt exists as to the location of the ampulla it is justifiable to perform a choledochotomy and insert a pediatric infant feeding tube distally into the common bile duct to emerge from the ampulla. This maneuver, described by Longmire, has also been found to be useful in patients with duodenal involvement with antral carcinoma. A small-caliber T tube will subsequently need to be placed for safe duct closure. When a large ulcer has been left in situ, the cut edge of duodenum may be irregular, making it necessary to suture the anterolateral free cut edge to the inferior margin of the ulcer in situ with continuous or interrupted 4–0 Maxon. This excludes the ulcer from the duodenal lumen and a second row of interrupted 4–0 Maxon sutures is placed between the seromuscular layer of the inrolled duodenum and the ulcer base or superior edge depending on its size. When pyloric/duodenal stenosis results in only a pinhole orifice, simple separation of the stomach and duodenum at this site will lessen the difficulties encountered by fibrosis, with the orifice occasionally being more easily identified internally by a small distal gastrotomy.

Closure of the difficult stump may be accomplished by methods described by Nissen, Graham, or Bseth. Nissen and Graham maneuvers involve covering an ulcer left in situ utilizing the anterosuperior duodenal wall, whereas Bseth advocates posteromedial duodenal wall suture for coverage of the ulcer bed. When compared with the Nissen procedure Graham's technique has the disadvantage of requiring a more extensive dissection of the posterior duodenal wall. Nissen effected closure with sutures that incorporated the inferior margin of the ulcer, whereas mobilization

of the duodenum distal to a large ulcer may damage or occlude the accessory pancreatic duct. Graham advocated ulcer exclusion with the duodenum mobilized for 1 to 2 cm distal to the ulcer and subsequent closure with seromuscular suture of the duodenum to the pancreas to cover the ulcer bed. It is not necessary and can be hazardous to attempt to dissect the posterior duodenal wall distal to the inferior border of an ulcer. The secret of successful stump closure is to limit the distal extent of the duodenal dissection. Strauss and others have been proponents of an intramural duodenal dissection with development of a cuff of posterior duodenal wall. A jejunal patch as utilized for repair of traumatic duodenal injuries can also be employed when stump closure appears difficult. Roux en Y duodenojejunostomy can also be considered for the reduction of intraduodenal pressure. An alternative is the Bancroft closure, which suffers the disadvantage of possible retained antral mucosa in the stump and bleeding during separation of the submuscosa from the muscular layer. Following subtotal gastrectomy and end-to-side gastrojejunostomy (Moynihan), Appel has performed duodenojejunostomy with anastomosis of the duodenal stump to the side of efferent loop followed by Braun jejunojejunostomy. It is claimed that this utilizes less duodenal tissue than conventional closure and gives an anastomosis that is tension free, as the duodenum is not mobilized.

Resection of no more than 2 cm of duodenum also obviates excessive devascularization. In circumstances in which one has some reservations regarding the integrity of a proposed or completed closure, other options merit consideration. If the appearance of the transected duodenum and ulceration suggests that the risk of subsequent suture line leakage is probable, then catheter tube duodenostomy is advisable. This may entail the use of a Foley or Malecot catheter in the transected end of the duodenum, secured by means of one or two pursestring sutures and brought out percutaneously in a short straight track. A Malecot catheter is preferred as insufflation of a Foley catheter balloon for retention in situ may cause ampullary or proximal duodenal obstruction if sited distal to the ampulla. End duodenostomy is, however, often accompanied by peritubal leakage of duodenal contents, no matter how secure the nonabsorbable suture purse-

strings appear. Some surgeons hold the view that lateral tube duodenostomy through noninflamed tissue in the second part of the duodenum will allow for earlier healing than end duodenostomy in a scarred stump. For this reason many surgeons opt for a side duodenostomy with latex T-tube drainage via a stab wound in the second part of the duodenum. Most T tubes available today are siliconized and need to remain in situ for 3 to 6 weeks, 10 days being insufficient to enable formation of a satisfactory track. If stump closure can be accomplished, with leakage considered unlikely, then lateral T-tube duodenostomy may suffice (Fig. 74-7). When closure is regarded as unsafe and highly likely to lead to leakage then end tube/catheter is recommended. Personal preference is for end catheter duodenostomy in the most difficult cases.

It is also imperative in the prevention of stump leakage to avoid afferent limb obstruction at the site of subsequent gastrojejunal anastomosis. If duodenal stump closure is difficult, it is necessary to 1) railroad the nasogastric tube well into the afferent limb with or without suturing to the duodenal mucosa with absorbable sutures; 2) meticulously cover the stump with omentum sutured to duodenum or surrounding structures, or both; and 3) insert a drain into the right upper quadrant space for 5 days. Afferent limb intubation in this way stabilizes the loop and is said to prevent kinking of the limb as well as obviating raised intraduodenal pressure, which is detrimental to stump integrity. If stump leakage occurs it is usually evident on the fourth or fifth postoperative day but may occur between the second and seventh days. Any drain placed at operation to deal with stump leakage should this occur must therefore remain in situ for at least 5 days, even if early postoperative drainage is minimal. It is desirable to remove the drain after 5 days, as occasionally small bowel or omentum may become adherent to the drain if it is left for longer, and this may not only make removal difficult even with sedation/analgesia but can result in damage, giving rise to small-bowel fistula or hemorrhage.

Gastric Transection and Reconstruction

Following duodenal stump closure the lesser curvature of the stomach is mobi-

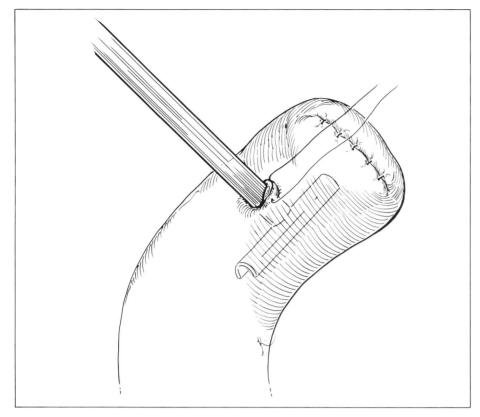

Fig. 74-7. Lateral T-tube duodenostomy. A size 16 T tube is inserted into the already closed duodenal stump through a small opening in the lateral duodenal wall. The horizontal limb of the tube has been trimmed and the roof of this limb has been cut away to facilitate removal.

lized with small anterior and posterior division of branches of the left gastric artery and vein. The dissection is carried superiorly on the lesser curve as the gastrohepatic omentum is divided with electrocoagulation. Branches of the left gastric artery and vein supplying the stomach are divided between hemostats, the dissection proceeding proximally to within 3 cm of the distal esophagus. The stomach is bared on greater and lesser curvatures to such an extent that a two-thirds gastric resection is possible. At least 2.5 cm of bared stomach can be retained on the greater curvature and utilized for anastomosis in the knowledge that intragastric blood supply will be sufficient to maintain viability if short gastric arteries remain intact. Often a natural break in the gastroepiploic arcade will dictate the exact site of gastric transection.

The duodenojejunal flexure is identified and a loop of proximal jejunum is lifted free to lie in juxtaposition to the gastric remnant, being held by two small Babcock clamps at the site proposed for jejunal

anastomosis. It has been emphasized that too long an afferent limb is to be avoided, as this can produce bacterial overgrowth in a blind loop syndrome. Nevertheless, antecolic anastomosis is usually desirable and it is possible to do this without tension on the loop provided a suitable site is chosen to anastomose. It is obviously preferable to make the loop 2 to 5 cm longer than to risk excessive tension. The limb with the screw attachment of a curved Lane twin clamp is applied to the jejunum stretched upward by appropriate placement of two Babcock clamps, the jejunum being grasped across its lumen to within 3 cm of the tip of the instrument. The second limb of the twin clamp is applied to the stomach, which is held caudally by a Babcock clamp attached to part of the bared greater curve that is to be resected. The clamp is applied and closed, taking care not to ensnare the nasogastric tube, which has been passed previously and now withdrawn high in the proximal stomach before application of the clamp, which is again positioned so that the lesser curvature of the

stomach extends to within 3 cm of its tip. The stomach remnant is then lifted anteriorly, permitting the two limbs of the clamps to be apposed behind it utilizing the eye of the inferior clamp, the screw arrangement being tightened to approximate the stomach and jejunum.

A continuous 4–0 Maxon posterior layer seromuscular suture is placed from lesser to greater curvature of the stomach and the suture needle is attached, laid taut to the left side. The jejunum is divided with electrocoagulation for a length that is judged to match the proposed gastric division. This jejunal incision is slightly shorter than the gastric division and can be lengthened if need be during suturing. The stomach to be excised is then clamped inferiorly with a soft bowel clamp 5 cm from the twin clamp attachment. Diathermy is employed to open the gastric wall adjacent to the twin clamp, with Hibitane swabs used to clean the exposed interior of the stomach and jejunum. A continuous 4–0 Maxon suture that includes all coats anastomoses the jejunum and stomach from lesser to greater curvatures. When the greater gastric curvature is reached, the portion of stomach to be excised is lifted anteriorly and division is completed with electrocoagulation in a semicircular fashion to provide a flap; this will enable inner wall gastrojejunal anastomosis without the need to release the twin clamp. The inner layer of the anastomosis is completed and the twin clamp removed from stomach and jejunum. Should there be a small excess of gastric lumen for approximation, this can be directly sutured to itself on the lesser curvature aspect, with subsequent inversion by seromuscular suture application. The anterior outer layer is fashioned by a continuous seromuscular suture employing the previous 4–0 Maxon, which has been laid to the left side. Reinforcement by additional seromuscular sutures between the stomach and jejunum at the vulnerable lateral angles of the stoma has been advocated. The nasogastric tube is manipulated well into the afferent limb. The transverse colon is pulled with gentle traction to the right of the anastomosis, which is inspected, especially posteriorly, to ensure that there is no bleeding from transected extragastric vessels or wall. Patency can be tested by "finger and thumb" opposition between gastric remnant and jejunal loop. The duodenal stump is inspected for leakage or bleeding and then covered with omentum sutured in place to provide a prophylactic patch.

Nonabsorbable mucosal sutures for gastric anastomoses are to be avoided. While absorbable catgut, Vicryl, polyglycolic acid (Dexon) sutures have proved satisfactory, 4–0 Maxon has the ability to slide more easily through tissues, a greater knot pull strength, and a longer absorption time of 180 days. Continuous sutures are favored, as these secure hemostasis. A majority of surgeons continue to use a two-layer continuous anastomosis with a posterior inner layer that incorporates the full thickness of gastric and jejunal walls and an outer seromuscular layer that inverts the inner layer. Recent trends suggest that a one-layer inverting continuous suture that incorporates serosa, muscular, and submucosal coats is gaining popularity despite the risks of gastric suture line hemorrhage.

Stapled Anastomosis

An alternative method of duodenal closure involves placement of a TA30 or TA50 horizontal stapling device positioned across the duodenum just distal to the pylorus (Fig. 74-8). A Lang Stevenson clamp is placed more proximally to avoid leakage on division of the duodenum with a scalpel after the TA stapler has been fired; stay sutures in the duodenum are usually unnecessary. The stomach can be closed with the use of a TA90 transverse stapling device employing 4.5-mm rather than 3.8-mm staples, the former being considered to be more secure and hemostatic. After firing, the stomach can be divided with a scalpel, a soft bowel clamp distally preventing soiling with gastric contents. Following removal of the transverse staplers, on firing the cut ends are inspected for bleeding and integrity; placement of interrupted 4–0 Maxon sutures may be required (Fig. 74-9). The use of electrocoagulation is acceptable for staple lines but is not advisable in the vicinity of a continuous suture line, which may be inadvertently damaged. Many surgeons do not invert transverse staple lines with sutures but continuous suture coverage avoids free leakage should the staple line fail.

The GIA side-to-side stapling device can be used to fashion a gastrojejunostomy after approximation of the posterior stomach

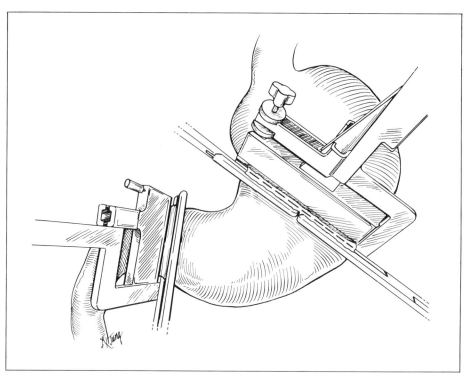

Fig. 74-8. TA30 stapling device is placed on the proximal duodenum. After firing, duodenal division, and mobilization of the stomach, a TA90 stapling device is placed on the proximal stomach.

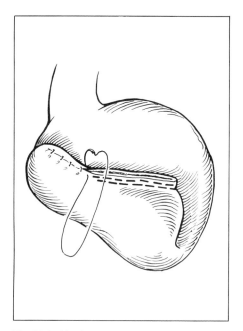

Fig. 74-9. After hemostasis is obtained, the stapled ends of the duodenum and stomach are inverted with continuous 4–0 Maxon sutures.

and jejunum with stay sutures (Fig. 74-10). A small jejunal enterotomy permits placement of one limb of the GIA; the second is introduced via a small, posterior gastric incision appropriately sited to enable a

widely patent anastomosis to be fashioned on firing and located 4 cm proximal to the cut end of the stomach so as to avoid ischemic necrosis of the stomach between the GIA and TA staple lines (Fig. 74-11). The GIA device must provide an anastomosis at least 5 cm in diameter to obviate delayed gastric emptying. The limbs of the GIA device are approximated, and the instrument is fired and withdrawn from the lumen. Active bleeding from the staple line may be difficult to detect through the small stab incisions, which is a distinct disadvantage in gastric surgery, during which continuous spurting hemorrhage may go undetected only to be manifest with persistent heavily blood-stained nasogastric aspirates postoperatively. The conjoined defect at the site of stab incisions is closed with a continuous 4–0 Maxon suture. The GIA can be introduced from the left or the right side, with a left-sided entry often being performed if the remnant is small; right-sided placement is technically more difficult.

A variation in technique incorporates excision of a portion of the TA-stapled greater curvature to provide a gastric opening, which is hand sewn to the jejunal limb in Hofmeister fashion (Fig. 74-12).

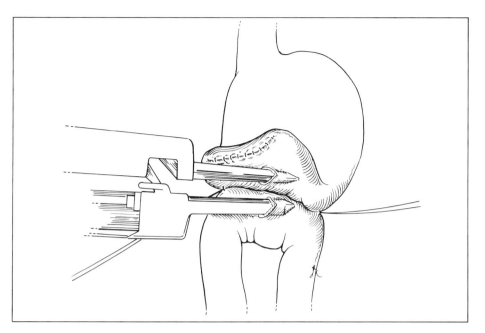

Fig. 74-10. *Small openings in the posterior wall of the stomach and the jejunum enable introduction of the GIA stapler device.*

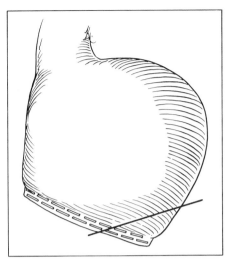

Fig. 74-12. *A wedge of stapled end of the greater curvature is excised to make a gastric opening for a hand-sewn 4–0 Maxon Hofmeister reconstruction.*

Stapling devices are widely employed for duodenal stump closure but are not so favored for gastric resection by most surgeons, with usage being confined to the creation of gastric tubes for esophageal replacement.

Laparoscopic Billroth II Gastrectomy

Laparoscopic exposure of the upper abdomen has been facilitated by the advent of videolaparoscopy, simple retraction techniques of the left lobe of the liver, and patient positioning. Complete expeditious mobilization of the vascular pedicles required the development of the automatic clipping devices and more recently the linear cutter/stapler. This same device has greatly enhanced the surgeon's ability to divide bowel and fashion the anastomosis, essential technical steps performed during gastrectomy. These instruments have only been available since 1991. Along with mechanical devices, suturing techniques have evolved and with current high-quality needle holders standard curved needles can be used. A recently launched suturing device (Endostitch, Auto Suture, Norwalk, CT) has potential to dramatically ease the technical demands on the surgeon during suturing. A variety of procedures to fashion the gastroenterostomy are illustrated to allow surgeons with varying access to

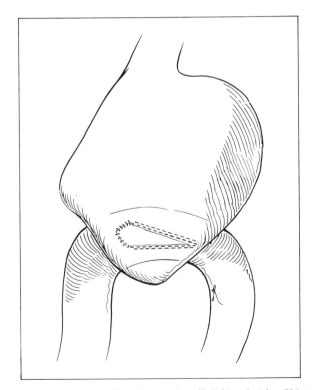

Fig. 74-11. *Billroth II gastrojejunostomy (posterior gastric wall) fashioned with a GIA stapling device.*

expensive technology to choose the most appropriate technique for reconstruction.

Patient Positioning and Port Sites

The patient is positioned supine with varying degrees of head uptilt depending on body habitus, to encourage downward displacement of the transverse colon and omentum. A nasogastric drainage tube decompresses the stomach and antibiotics are routinely administered. The position and sizes of the ports are illustrated in (Fig. 74-13). The epigastric port site, just to the right of the xiphisternum, is used to insert the liver retractor (Wilson Cook, Brisbane, Australia), which is then attached to an external holder ("Iron Intern" or "Omnitract") clamped to the operating table rails. Once positioned and anchored, this system atraumatically elevates the left lobe of the liver for the entire operation, freeing the assistant for other tasks.

Gastric Resection

Dissection begins along the greater curvature of the stomach toward the left, outside the gastroepiploic vascular arcades using sharp scissors dissection of the windows, supplemented with electrocautery. Isolated epiploic vessels are clipped using the 9-mm clip of the automatic clip applier and divided (Fig. 74-14). Attention is then turned to the level of division of the stomach and the posterior aspect is cleared of

any filmy adhesions above the pancreas. A point along the greater curve is chosen for transection of the antrum and sequential applications of the linear cutter are applied until the lesser curvature is reached. The duodenum is next transected in a similar manner (Fig. 74-15). The lesser omentum is now divided using scissors and cautery for small vessels and clips for larger ones. Once this is completed the mobilized antrum is extracted via the 12-mm port site or, if bulky, it can be temporarily placed above the right lobe of liver to await extraction at the end of the procedure. In our view this is best achieved by placement of the specimen in a retrieval bag to minimize bacterial contamination of the abdominal wall during extraction.

Gastric Reconstruction: Stapled/Sutured Anastomoses

The transverse colon is grasped and elevated cephalad with attached greater omentum. The duodenojejunal flexure is located and the jejunum is followed to allow a loop of sufficient length to curve around transverse colon to reach for antecolic anastomosis without kinking. A 2–0 Prolene suture on a curved needle is introduced and passed through the stomach and jejunum, and both ends are removed via the right upper quadrant port site and held with a hemostat. The port at that site is then re-introduced alongside the stay suture and an enterotomy for the

stapling device is created in the jejunum and stomach (Fig. 74-16). Care must be taken to gain access to the thick walled stomach; air insufflation via the nasogastric tube distends and thins out the stomach facilitating this step. For a stapled anastomosis the linear stapler/cutter is introduced and a 60-mm-long anastomosis is created. The residual defect is closed with a single layer of continuous 3–0 PDS, as illustrated in Fig. 74-16C and D. A jamming loop knot enables the commencement of this suture line (Fig. 74-17).

Data for determining an adequate size of stoma are illustrated in Table 74-1. These experimental gastrojejunostomies were created in a piglet model. Those of 40-mm length had a high incidence of stenosis and obstruction at 12 weeks compared with a stoma of 60 mm in length. Of relevance is the thickness of the gastric wall, which produces more scarring than other intestinal anastomoses and subsequent scar contracture during healing, leading to stomal stenosis.

Closure of the residual defect by stapling with the linear cutter is possible. This may, however, very easily cause narrowing of the efferent limb of the jejunum and in our view suturing is safer and more accurate. An aid to simplify technique is available with the Endostitch suturing device; this instrument has only recently become available for clinical practice and shows great promise. With all suture techniques great care must be taken to follow the su-

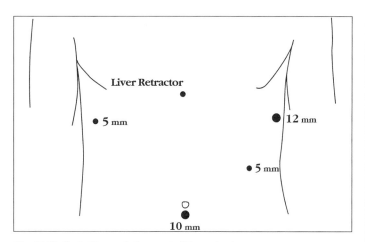

Fig. 74-13. Port siting and placement of liver retractor.

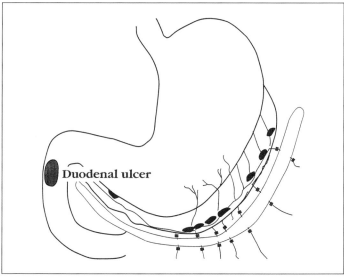

Fig. 74-14. Division of the vascular arcade along the greater curve.

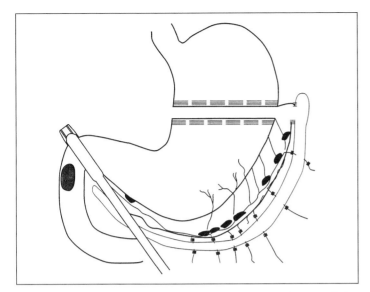

Fig. 74-15. Transection of the antrum and duodenum using the linear stapler/cutter.

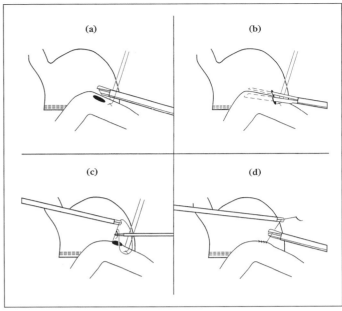

Fig. 74-16. Steps in the gastric anastomosis. (a) Placement of stay suture and creation of enterotomies. (b) Application of the stapler to create 60-mm anastomosis. (c) Suture closure of the residual defect. (d) Completed anastomosis.

ture to ensure that tension is maintained and that the edges of the anastomosis are approximated correctly.

An alternative to the stapled anastomosis is to create an entirely sutured one. This is achieved by placement of the stay suture as illustrated above. The single continuous posterior layer of sutures is then placed as illustrated in (Fig. 74-18). Next, the stomach and jejunum are opened and the anastomosis is completed with the anterior layer of sutures as indicated. Spillage of gastric contents is minimized by aspiration on the nasogastric tube before the stomach is opened. It is important to lock the suture every eight stitches to prevent loosening of the running suture line during peristalsis. The area is lavaged clean with warm Ringer's lactate solution after extraction of the resected antrum if this has not already been performed. The fascia of all ports greater than 5 mm are sutured to prevent port site herniation. A retrocolic anastomosis can be fashioned using the same technique as for antecolic placement. The creation of the window in the transverse mesocolon is sited to the left of the middle colic vessels; the anastomosis is created superiorly and on completion is brought inferiorly below the transverse mesocolon and held in position with a few inter-

rupted 3–0 PDS sutures. A drain is placed to the area of the duodenal stump.

Patients are usually able to tolerate fluids by the third day and solids by the fourth postoperative day. Ambulation is encouraged as soon as possible to minimize the cardiorespiratory complications related to recumbency. Reported series of small numbers of patients demonstrate the feasibility of the technique with the discharge from the hospital between 5 and 12 days after the procedure and return to normal activities in 2 to 3 weeks. Assessment of long-term outcome requires evaluation at further follow-up reviews.

Specific Postoperative Complications

Early postoperative complications include hemorrhage, obstruction, and leakage. Postoperative hemorrhage may be intraperitoneal and the result of splenic injury, which may have been recognized and managed by suture or application of hemostatic agents at operation. Hemorrhage can also occur from small vessels in the omentum or the gastric wall itself. Intraperitoneal hemorrhage is usually manifest within 6 hours after operation and, despite

the temptations of conservative management, often requires relaparotomy for expeditious control. It is important to inspect the bed of the pancreas and celiac axis for any evidence of bleeding before proceeding with restoration of gastrointestinal continuity. In addition, the whole anastomosis must be inspected externally on completion, particularly by elevating and rotating the anastomoses if necessary to identify any bleeding point on the posterior wall consequent to gastric transection. Intraluminal hemorrhage can arise from a suture or staple line and can occur early or a few days later in association with anastomotic dehiscence. A second mucosal lesion overlooked at initial endoscopy and/or laparotomy can also give rise to postoperative hemorrhage. It may be possible to control early suture/staple line or peptic ulcer hemorrhage with injection sclerotherapy but if this is unsuccessful relaparotomy will be necessary. If gentle postoperative endoscopy with minimal insufflation reveals tumor, for example, a small leiomyoma, to be the source of the bleeding, then further surgical intervention is advisable as soon as possible.

Obstruction of the efferent limb of a gastrojejunal anastomosis is unusual but delayed gastric emptying can occur if truncal

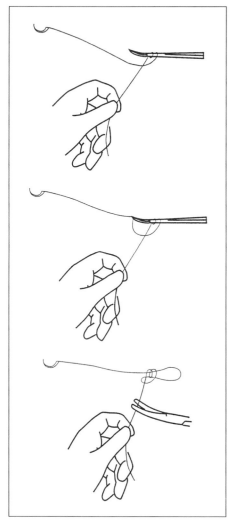

Fig. 74-17. Technique of creating the jamming loop knot before insertion of the suture into the abdomen.

Table 74-1. Stoma Size: Laparoscopic Gastroenterostomy at 12 Weeks in the Piglet Model

Initial Anastomotic Length	Anastomotic Diameter at 12 wk (mean range)
40 mm	4.4 mm (1–10) 2 of 5 stomas obstructed
60 mm	17.5 mm (12-25mm) 0 of 5 stomas obstructed

vagotomy has been previously performed for peptic ulcer disease. This is best managed with conservative measures, with endoscopy serving both to verify that the anastomosis is patent and that no mechanical obstruction is evident in the proximal

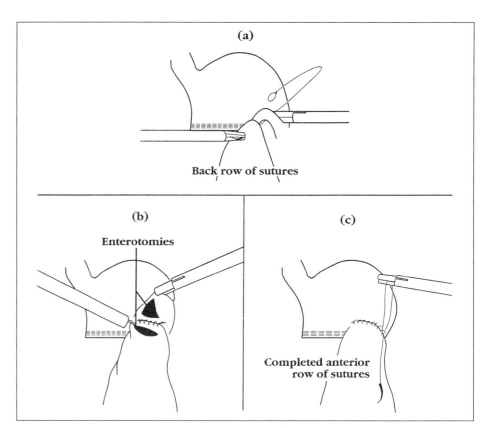

Fig. 74-18. Alternative technique of an entirely sutured anastomosis.

30 cm of the efferent limb. Afferent limb obstruction is suspected if duodenal stump leakage occurs. Not all stump leakage is attributable to afferent limb holdup, and reoperation can often be avoided with successful conservative treatment.

Duodenal Stump Leakage

A gastrojejunal anastomosis is far less likely to be the site of leakage than is the duodenal stump, but if leakage is found at reoperation it can usually be dealt with by omental or jejunal seromuscular patch repair or resection. If upper abdominal pain accompanied by features of tachycardia, fever, or hypotension occurs in the postoperative period, leakage can be confirmed, if it is not overt, with the use of a water-soluble (Gastrografin) study that may identify duodenal stump extravasation. Complete afferent limb obstruction will result in failure to image the duodenum. If afferent limb obstruction is confirmed by the presence of a dilated afferent

limb evident on ultrasound or computed tomography, then reoperation for its correction is essential if the fistula is to heal. In these circumstances the afferent limb can be transected with the GIA stapler close to its junction with the stomach. The gastric staple line is oversewn and the afferent limb reimplanted into the efferent limb in an end-to-side Roux en Y fashion.

Duodenal stump leakage may be associated with 1) inadequate closure of an extensively scarred and edematous duodenum, 2) afferent loop obstruction, or 3) local pancreatitis, this occurring secondary to injury of the main pancreatic duct or substance of the gland, division or ligation of the accessory pancreatic duct, or, less likely, simply excessive handling of the pancreas. The most important cause is inadvertent damage or division of the accessory pancreatic duct, which is vulnerable in a foreshortened scarred duodenum.

Duodenal stump blowout is potentially a major catastrophe with free intraperitonal leakage and peritonism; the reported mortality for stump leakage is 12 to 50 percent. The metabolic effects of external duodenal fistulization can be devastating. End catheter duodenostomy with or without T-tube drainage of the common bile duct or duodenum may salvage the situation. Treatment options for duodenal stump leakage also include reoperation with 1) immediate resuture or covering of the defect with omentum or a seromuscular jejunal patch, 2) resection, 3) additional drainage, or 4) conservative therapy. Management of overt stump leakage includes 1) nasogastric aspiration, 2) stump/right upper quadrant drainage with or without suction, 3) total parenteral nutrition or feeding jejunostomy, 4) H_2 receptor antagonist or proton pump inhibitor, 5) somatostatin infusion, and 6) antibiotic therapy. Strict fluid balance measurements are required with an ongoing evaluation of the volume and nature of the drainage fluid. Blood cultures are necessary in the febrile patient. It is salutary to recall that patients with ongoing leakage who have received antibiotic therapy may often develop systemic infection with Candida. Attention to detail is required with regard to skin protection from pancreatic enzymes and avoidance of excoriation. Culture and sensitivity tests of the fistulous drainage are required at least twice a week. In the presence of ongoing fever despite external drainage, abdominal imaging with ultrasound or preferably computed tomography is indicated. Any localized abscess may require percutaneous drainage under image guidance. Unfortunately, duodenal fistulas are not generally amenable to direct closure but an omental plug can be sutured in place for closure. Once leakage occurs a protracted period of hospitalization is often required before resolution on conservative therapy. Catheter duodenostomy has been recommended if 1) leakage exceeds 200 ml per day when skin excoriation is problematic, 2) drainage is insufficient and bile-stained fluid leaks from the abdominal wound, or 3) features of generalized peritonitis are evident. Subsequent healing can be monitored by contrast studies via the catheter duodenostomy. Extravasation of contrast material will necessitate retention of the catheter for at least 5 days, at which time the study can be repeated. Free passage of contrast into the afferent limb and stomach without extravasation must be observed before clamping of the duodenostomy tube is considered safe. If no features of leakage such as abdominal pain or wound drain-

age arise overnight, the duodenostomy tube can be removed. Bile leakage via the catheter track will usually subside completely within 1 or 2 days; persistent leakage suggests some degree of afferent limb obstruction. When this occurs bile will be conspicuously absent from a nasogastric aspirate and the loop itself will appear dilated on ultrasound or computed tomography. Subphrenic or subhepatic abscess collections are suspected with the onset of pain and fever within 10 days of operation and are usually secondary to suture/staple line leakage or, less commonly, to infected hematoma.

Late sequelae of Billroth II gastrectomy include recurrent duodenal ulceration, chronic reflux gastritis, dumping, gastroesophageal reflux, and remnant cancer. Recurrent ulceration occurs in 5 percent of patients and may be associated with retained gastric antrum with gastrin production in the "duodenal" stump or hypersecretory states such as gastrinoma in the Zollinger-Ellison syndrome, or a mucosal defect. Long-term medical therapy may be advised or, occasionally, if surgical intervention is deemed necessary, a reresection of the stump with excision of the pylorus is performed if retained gastric antrum is confirmed on investigation. Stomal ulceration that fails to heal and merits surgery requires truncal vagotomy for satisfactory control, although the combination of vagotomy and previous resection may give rise to delayed gastric emptying for several weeks. It may well be that thoracoscopic truncal vagotomy alone may yet find a role in the management of stomal ulceration. Reflux gastritis in the remnant is attributable to bile and pancreatic enzyme damage and is perhaps best dealt with by treatment with mucosal cytoprotective agents such as sucralfate. Prostaglandin therapy is an alternative mode of treatment but is often associated with diarrhea and is unsuitable for prolonged usage. Bilious vomiting occurs when some degree of afferent limb obstruction is present and when bile under pressure in a distended intact afferent limb floods into the stomach, overcoming relative gastrojejunal afferent limb holdup. This may be accompanied by marked reflux esophagitis at endoscopy.

Cytoprotective agents may be helpful but if symptoms are troublesome revision gastric surgery with Roux en Y reconstruction

is occasionally recommended. The etiology of postgastrectomy symptoms may be difficult to elucidate and may require endoscopy, 24-hour ambulatory intragastric and esophageal pH monitoring, and perhaps nuclear medicine studies. Early dumping following Billroth II gastrectomy is treated conservatively with small frequent meals and avoidance of liquid intake at mealtimes. Treatment is often unsatisfactory, with drug therapy and antiperistaltic jejunal interposition both proving disappointing; revisional surgery with restoration of gastroduodenal continuity, if technically feasible, is worthy of consideration in the patient with benign disease. Nutritional sequelae relating to iron, B_{12}, and folic acid metabolism require careful follow-up study and monitoring biannually. Supplemental medication and regular B_{12} injections every 3 months are important aspects of care. There is good evidence to suggest that the postgastrectomy patient is at increased risk of gastric cancer, and annual gastroscopy, even in asymptomatic individuals, has been recommended, the risk being greater after a decade.

Summary

A number of technical advances have been introduced to simplify and/or expedite the performance of Billroth II gastrectomy. It is imperative, however, to be aware of the perils of life-threatening surgical complications and to take no risks that are otherwise avoidable. The ideal procedure is one that will provide a successful symptom-free outcome that is lifelong. While various techniques have been described to restore gastrointestinal continuity, there is no strong evidence to suggest that simple Polya reconstruction is inferior for the vast majority of patients. A case for Roux en Y reconstruction may, however, be made in the patient with preexisting troublesome reflux esophagitis. The risk of stomal ulceration is believed to be increased if biliary and pancreatic diversion is performed and many surgeons routinely undertake truncal vagotomy concomitantly. The gastric surgeon must be familiar not only with anatomic choices for restoring continuity but also with the latest developments in minimal access techniques, which are likely to revolutionize surgical management of both benign disease and early gastric cancer.

Suggested Reading

Branicki FJ, Boey J, Fok PJ, et al. Bleeding duodenal ulcer: A prospective evaluation of risk factors for rebleeding and mortality. *Ann Surg* 211:411, 1990.

Branicki FJ, Coleman SY, Lam TCF, et al. Hypotension and endoscopic stigmata of recent haemorrhage in bleeding peptic ulcer: Risk models for rebleeding and mortality. *Gastroenterol Hepatol* 7:184, 1992.

Ellis H. Billroth and the first successful gastrectomy. *Contemp Surg* 15:63, 1979.

Fromm D. Postgastrectomy Syndrome. In GD Zuidema, WP Ritchie Jr (eds), *Shackelford's Surgery of the Alimentary Tract*. Philadelphia: Saunders, 1991.

Goh P, Kum CK. Laparoscopic Billroth II gastrectomy: A review. *Surg Oncol* 2:(Suppl 1):13, 1992.

Lointier P, Leroux S, Ferrier C, Dapoigny M. A technique of laparoscopic gastrectomy and Billroth II gastrojejunostomy *J Laparoendoscopic Surg* 3, 4:353, 1993.

Marshall BJ. *Helicobacter pylori. Am J Gastroenterol*, 89 (Suppl): S116, 1994.

Mulholland MW. Partial Gastrectomy with Gastrojejunal Anastomosis including Roux-en-Y Reconstruction. In GG Jamieson, HT Debas (eds), *Rob & Smith's Operative Surgery. Surgery of the Upper Gastrointestinal Tract* (5th ed). London: Chapman & Hall Medical, 1994. Pp 420–435.

Schreiber HW. Specific Diseases and Methods of Treatment in the Stomach and Upper Duodenum. In K Kremer, W Lierse, W Platzer, et al (eds), *Atlas of Operative Surgery. Oesophagus, Stomach, Duodenum*. Stuttgart, New York: Georg Thieme Verlag, 1989.

Welch C. Gastric Resection for Duodenal Ulcer. In HW Scott, JL Sawyers (eds), *Surgery of the Stomach, Duodenum, and Small Intestine* (2nd ed). Boston: Blackwell, 1992.

EDITOR'S COMMENT

In many parts of the world, gastrectomy ad modum Billroth II remains the operation of choice for both gastric and duodenal ulcer. In my estimation, it continues to serve an important role in our approach to the surgical treatment of ulcer disease, particularly if vagotomy is added when the primary ulcer is in the duodenum. Frank Branicki spent a number of years in Hong Kong with Professor John Wong of the Queen Mary Hospital, University of Hong Kong. The wealth of gastric surgery performed in this famed surgical unit is reflected in this presentation of the Billroth II gastrectomy.

Fortunately, the age-old argument about which is the best surgical treatment of duodenal ulcer, the Billroth I or the Billroth II, no longer continues. With the addition of vagotomy, the recurrent ulcer rate following subtotal gastrectomy is negligible regardless of the type of anastomosis performed.

Because I was trained to perform a Billroth I anastomosis whenever possible, the truism, "if you can close a duodenal stump, you can anastomose to it," was a part of our technique ethic. Yet, of greater importance, whenever an inflamed, phlegmonous duodenal ulcer is found, it would be better to leave the ulcer in place, perform a vagotomy and simple gastrojejunostomy or Jaboulay's gastroduodenostomy, and not insist on performing either type of gastrectomy. Many surgeons would leave the entire antroduodenal complex alone and perform a proximal gastric vagotomy. In other words, a surgeon should not force his or her favorite operation on a patient. The surgeon should be versatile and ready to perform any of a variety of operations, including laparoscopic gastrectomy as presented herein.

L.M.N.

75

Selective Vagotomy, Antrectomy, and Gastroduodenostomy for the Treatment of Duodenal Ulcer

Lloyd M. Nyhus

The surgical treatment of complicated duodenal ulcer has undergone marked change since vagotomy was reintroduced by Dragstedt and Owens in 1943. Subtotal gastrectomy alone had been the mainstay operation for the prior half-century, followed by various surgical procedures, including truncal vagotomy, gastroenterostomy, pyloroplasty, 70 percent subtotal gastrectomy, and antrectomy. My experience with the combined operation of truncal vagotomy, antrectomy, and gastroduodenostomy began in the early 1950s. It became apparent that the method of vagotomy could be improved. Therefore, my associates and I modified our technique of vagotomy to the selective method and changed the name of the procedure to the revised combined operation. Thus, the specific procedure included selective vagotomy, antrectomy (35% distal gastrectomy), and gastroduodenostomy (Billroth I anastomosis). This operation has a good record in terms of ulcer recurrence. The recurrent ulcer rate following this procedure should be no greater than 0.5 percent.

Because of the interest in proximal gastric vagotomy, we have departed from gastrectomy as a routine operative procedure in our clinic. Yet, because of the occasional need to perform a partial gastrectomy or antrectomy, the technical lessons we learned must not be forgotten.

It is for this reason that the classic "revised combined operation of Harkins"* is highlighted in this chapter.

*Modified from H. N. Harkins and L. M. Nyhus. *Surgery of the Stomach and Duodenum*. Boston: Little, Brown, 1962.

Surgical Technique

Failure to appreciate technical details is reflected not only in resultant anatomic disturbances such as postoperative suture line leaks, but also in physiologic effects, for example, recurrent ulcer from incomplete vagotomy.

My experience in performing the revised combined operation (selective vagotomy plus antrectomy plus gastroduodenostomy) has led to the modification of certain steps in the technique.

Surgery is an art and, like all art, it must be developed, not discovered. The technique described is the one that seems to give the best results at the present time. Much of the following surgical technique is applicable to the Billroth II procedure as well as to the Billroth I operation.

General Principles

Sutures

A variety of sutures are used throughout the operation. Whereas fine silk was used predominantly in the past, the new absorbable and nonabsorbable sutures are now being used. Most vessels are simply ligated, but occasionally transfixion sutures are used. An absorbable suture is used for the inner layer of the anastomosis, essentially as a mucosal stitch with inversion. Seromuscular sutures continue to be of 4-0 or 000 black silk. The abdominal wall closure has changed from silk to stainless steel wire sutures to one of several monofilament synthetic sutures.

Open Anastomosis

I prefer the open to the closed type of anastomosis for several reasons. First, there can be no doubt that bleeding from the anastomosis can be entirely prevented by the use of the open technique with the anastomosis under direct visualization at all times. Second, the size of the anastomotic stoma can be assured, and the surgeon can be certain that both the anterior and the posterior walls are not included in one or more sutures. Third, through the open duodenal stump, the ampulla of Vater can be palpated and biliary flow noted; also, the area can be inspected for postbulbar duodenal ulcer and other duodenal abnormalities. I have seen no difficulty arise from soiling of the surgical field with the use of the open technique. The bacterial flora of this portion of the gastrointestinal tract is meager, and adequate protection can be achieved by careful placement of laparotomy pads to protect the remainder of the operative field. An inner mucosal layer of continuous absorbable sutures and an outer seromuscular layer of interrupted silk sutures complete the anastomosis.

Drainage

If it is suspected that the pancreas has been subjected to undue trauma, a Penrose drain or a double-lumen sump-suction catheter can be placed down to the site of suspected trauma and brought out laterally through the abdominal wall by a stab wound (never through the main incision). I sometimes but rarely place a Penrose drain near but not on the anastomosis if some aspect of the coaptation causes concern.

Adequacy of Resection

I adhere inviolably to the dictum that an adequate resection must be done according to the presenting disease before any decision is made to use or not to use any particular type of anastomosis. In fact, this decision is not made until the anastomosis is to be done. If there is any tension whatsoever in attempting to perform a gastroduodenal anastomosis, this method is abandoned and a modification of the Billroth II procedure is used. The anastomosis should not be forced. In general, the resection might be only 35 percent when protected by selective vagotomy.

Protection of Vital Structures

The only way to avoid injury to important structures is to visualize the part of the structure that lies in the field of dissection. The inflammatory reaction and scarring so characteristic of many gastroduodenal lesions can cause distortion of the normal anatomy. This distortion, coupled with the extreme variability in "normal" anatomy, makes dissection in this region extremely hazardous unless good visualization or identification of the vital structures to be preserved is accomplished.

The simple maneuver of intubating the common bile duct in certain instances when the porta hepatis might be involved in ulcer scar or inflammatory reaction is useful. It is important to recognize the possible distortion of normal anatomic configurations of the common bile duct and the pancreatic ducts. Special care should be taken to avoid injury to the common hepatic artery, which sometimes can be retracted near a posterior penetrating duodenal ulcer crater. On the greater curvature side of the pyloric region, the middle colic artery can be so densely adherent to the ulcer scar that it might be easily mistaken for the right gastroepiploic artery.

Caution should be exercised to avoid vigorous palpation or traction in the region of the spleen. The splenic vessels, particularly in older persons, are friable and are quite easily torn. Moderate traction on the greater curvature of the stomach is sufficient to cause tearing of the splenic vessels or of the splenic substance. When such an accident occurs, an attempt should be made to repair the spleen; however, it might be necessary to proceed with splenectomy. Although this incident is not a catastrophic one, it can appreciably increase the morbidity and even mortality.

The tenets of good modern surgery—gentle handling of tissues, avoidance of undue traction, and meticulous identification of adjacent structures to be preserved—are essential to a technically satisfactory operation.

Avoidance of Mass Ligatures

In dividing the blood supply to the portion of the stomach and duodenum to be resected, it is important that small bites of tissue be ligated. Especially in patients with a large quantity of omental fat, there is a tendency, if the vessel ligatures are placed around large quantities of this fat, for the vessels to retract proximal to the ligature and to cause troublesome hematomas or dangerous hemorrhage. Particularly in older people, I have been impressed with the increased quantity of fat that surrounds the left gastric vessels high on the lesser curvature. This situation is observed even in thin elderly patients.

Removal of Ulcer

In association with gastric resection, I regularly remove duodenal ulcers for mechanical rather than physiologic reasons. Only rarely do I leave a duodenal ulcer in situ. However, I do not hesitate to leave the depths of an ulcer crater in the tissue into which it might have penetrated.

Technical Procedure

Only the combined operation of selective vagotomy plus hemigastrectomy (antrectomy) plus gastroduodenal anastomosis will be described.

The sequence of performance of the various steps applies to most operations. However, certain conditions germane to the particular situation can make a somewhat altered sequence more desirable. Step-by-step description of the technique is undertaken merely because it is easier to describe it in this manner. It is the integration of all these steps into a smoothly performed surgical procedure that is productive of technical satisfaction.

The surgical technique (Table 75-1) I prefer at present is described in the following 11 steps.

Incision

An upper midline abdominal incision is used almost exclusively. This incision is begun in the left xiphocostal angle and is extended down the linea alba to the level of the umbilicus or below if necessary. The incision is usually approximately 15 cm long. In patients in whom the distance between the costal arch and the umbilicus is short, I extend the incision inferiorly to one side of the umbilicus. If more room is needed, I excise the xiphoid process. The peritoneum is cut approximately 2 cm to the left and lateral to the skin and fascial incision, giving a "staggered" effect, so that the under part of the fascial closure is protected by intact peritoneum.

Abdominal Exploration

The surgeon must curtail his or her enthusiasm to attack the gastroduodenal disease for which the operation was performed until there is ample opportunity to explore the entire peritoneal cavity. Unless a general exploration is performed as soon as the peritoneal cavity is entered, this important step is apt to be forgotten. In ad-

Table 75-1. Step-by Step Outline of the Combined Procedure for Selective Vagotomy plus Antrectomy plus Gastroduodenal Anastomosis

Step	1.	Incision
Step	2.	Abdominal exploration
Step	3.	Selective vagotomy
Step	4.	Freeing of the greater curvature
Step	5.	Mobilization of the duodenum
Step	6.	Strauss maneuver for division of the duodenum
Step	7.	Division of the gastrohepatic omentum and left gastric vessels
Step	8.	Resection
Step	9.	Closure of the Schoemaker suture line
Step	10.	Anastomosis
Step	11.	Wound closure

dition, it is probably better technique to explore the general peritoneal cavity before the gastrointestinal tract has been entered to avoid the small but ever-present chance of distributing contaminated debris. Two exceptions to the rule of exploring the general abdominal cavity before beginning the gastric procedure are emergency operations for a bleeding gastroduodenal lesion, when control of the hemorrhage should take priority, and operations for obvious perforation of a peptic ulcer.

It is only after adequate inspection of the gastroduodenal disease that the final decision to perform a gastric procedure should be made. This decision should, however, depend on the sum total of information available about the patient and not solely on the findings at the operation. Most often the presence of active ulcer, ulcer scar, or carcinoma of the stomach can be detected by external inspection and palpation. Occasionally, a posterior duodenal or a lesser curvature gastric ulcer can be identified by palpating the crater through the anterior wall of the duodenum or stomach. Often, after rapid withdrawal of the palpating finger, the anterior wall of the duodenum or stomach can be observed to remain depressed into the crater by a suction effect.

Selective Vagotomy

The technique of selective vagotomy is similar to that described by Sawyers in Chap. 76. If an extended highly selective vagotomy is to be performed, without antrectomy, I use the Donahue method (see Chap. 79).

Freeing of the Greater Curvature

The gastrocolic omentum is perforated in an avascular portion by a curved hemostat, thus permitting the lesser peritoneal sac to be entered. Unless care is taken in the execution of this maneuver, the middle colic vessels can be damaged. To minimize the possibility of such an error, it is recommended that the anterior wall of the stomach and the transverse colon be elevated and gently pulled apart to tense the gastrocolic omentum. It is easier to find a good cleavage plane by entering the gastrocolic omentum at the level of the junction of the lower and middle thirds of the greater curvature of the stomach, or even

farther to the left; usually most of the adhesions that tend to obliterate the lesser peritoneal sac are found in the region of the pylorus and lower third of the stomach. At this level, it is easy to identify an avascular area between the main trunk of the gastroepiploic vessels and the colon.

After it is certain that the correct plane has been entered, the defect in the gastrocolic omentum is enlarged superiorly and inferiorly distal to the main gastroepiploic trunk. The avascular portions of the omentum can be divided with scissors without ligation. When vessels have been identified, the omentum is again perforated on the opposite side of the vessel, and ligatures of 4–0 black silk are passed around the vessel. These ligatures are then tied and the vessels are divided between the ligatures. I have found that there is much less chance of losing a vessel and having troublesome bleeding and hematoma formation if the ligatures are tied before the vessels are divided. Often these vessels are so fragile that the slightest tension on a clamp causes tearing. Superiorly, the greater curvature is freed to a point approximately 14 cm proximal to the pylorus or at a point on the greater curvature perpendicular to the lesser curvature incisura. Transection of the stomach between this point and the mid-lesser curvature (proximal to the gastric incisura) ensures an antrectomy (approximately a 35% distal gastrectomy) (Fig. 75-1).

All the freeing of the gastrocolic omentum superior to the point of initial breakthrough is carried out distal to the main gastroepiploic trunk. Inferiorly, the omentum is freed, again distal to the right gastroepiploic trunk, down to a point approximately 5 cm proximal to the pylorus. From this point onward, inferiorly, division of the gastrocolic omentum is carried out between the greater curvature of the stomach and the right gastroepiploic vessel. The main trunk of the right gastroepiploic artery and vein has been transected and ligated previously at approximately 5 cm proximal to the pylorus. From this point onward, special care must be taken to keep the location of the middle colic vessels constantly in mind.

Approximately at the level of the pylorus, the right gastroepiploic artery at its origin is deep to the line of division of the gastrocolic omentum. Unless the right gastroepiploic vessels are intimately adherent in scar tissue in this region, they can and should be preserved to provide an adequate blood supply to the portion of the gastrocolic omentum that is being left behind. However, when the right gastroepiploic vessels are intimately adherent and it is impossible to preserve them, they must be sacrificed. Perhaps attempts to protect this vessel represent unnecessary conservatism, but I believe vessels should be preserved when feasible. At this point, any readily accessible adhesions to the

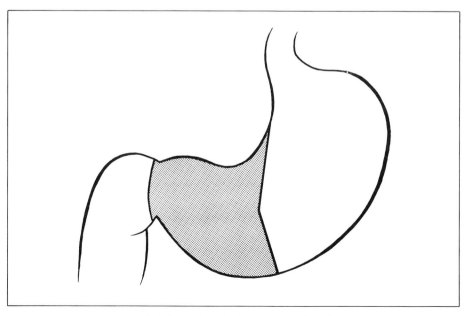

Fig. 75-1. Extent of antrectomy (stippled area). It should represent a 30 to 35 percent gastrectomy.

posterior gastric wall should be divided to allow greater mobility of the stomach.

Mobilization of the Duodenum

One of the most valuable technical contributions to surgery of the stomach and duodenum is the technique of mobilization of the duodenum originally described by Kocher in 1903.

Duodenal mobilization is one of the two phases of the operation best achieved with the surgeon standing on the left side of the operation table. A laparotomy pack is placed on top of the duodenum, the surgeon pulling the other viscera to the left side of the patient and causing the lateral peritoneal reflection of the duodenum to become taut. The peritoneal reflection can then be plainly seen and incised along the lateral margin of the second portion of the duodenum. Then, by gentle blunt dissection, two fingers can be placed superiorly and inferiorly beneath this layer of peritoneum. By tenting the peritoneum with the fingers, the peritoneum can be incised either with scissors or a scalpel, depending on the preference of the surgeon.

The fascia propria (loose areolar tissue) along the lateral and posterior aspects of the second and third portions of the duodenum is divided by sharp dissection. For the most part, this plane is avascular, although occasionally several small bleeding vessels can be encountered.

Mobilization is carried out superiorly and proximally to include the superficial avascular portion of the hepatoduodenal ligament. The duodenum is mobilized distally and inferiorly to the point at which the superior mesenteric vessels cross the third portion of the duodenum. With the duodenum thus mobilized, the second and proximal third portions can be shifted and rotated to the left and superiorly, moving with them the head of the pancreas and the common bile duct. Complete duodenal mobilization should allow visualization of the inferior vena cava. Occasionally the right margin of the aorta can be seen.

The duodenum can usually be mobilized farther than would seem possible. When it appears that the duodenum has been mobilized to its maximal extent, I follow the useful practice of trying again. Usually some additional degree of mobilization can be gained. After complete mobilization of the duodenum, a moist laparotomy pack should be placed beneath the duodenum to elevate it into the more superficial portion of the surgical field.

Mobilization of the duodenum not only facilitates gastroduodenal anastomosis but also serves two other important functions: It minimizes the chance of injury to the common bile duct by allowing better visualization, and it allows the dissection around the proximal duodenum to be performed in a more superficial part of the surgical field.

After its mobilization, the duodenum is freed, first on its greater curvature (caudal) side and then on its lesser curvature (hepatic) side, with division of the right gastric artery and usually of the supraduodenal artery of Wilkie.

Strauss Maneuver for Division of the Duodenum

The proper and safe division of the duodenum is an important and sometimes difficult maneuver, particularly when one is dealing with posterior penetrating duodenal ulcers. I am indebted to the late Alfred A. Strauss of Chicago for the technique of duodenal division that I use for all duodenal ulcers adherent to the pancreas.

This step is best accomplished when standing at the patient's left side. The maneuver consists in elevating the first portion of the duodenum by a finger placed against the posterior wall of the duodenum just to the right of the head of the pancreas. To conserve all duodenal length possible, no resection clamps are placed on the duodenum before division. The anterior wall of the duodenum distal to the ulcer scar is incised first with a scalpel as close to the pylorus as the duodenal lesion allows, and the posterior wall is then incised under direct vision from the internal to the external side and at a level just distal to any possible posterior wall ulcer disease. By incising the posterior wall from the inside out, one can minimize the danger of injuring the subjacent structures. If the posterior wall is adherent to the pancreas because of a posterior penetrating ulcer, the duodenal mucosa proximal to the line of division is shaved off the adherent area, leaving the outer portion of the duodenal wall adherent to the ulcer scar. When a posterior penetrating ulcer is situated immediately distal to the pylorus, it is usually possible to obtain a satisfactorily mobilized end of the duodenum distal to the line of transection, and one that is entirely suitable for end-to-end anastomosis. In brief, the Strauss technique involves a separation of the pylorus from in front and to the left rather than, as is usually done, from behind and to the right.

However, if the posterior penetrating ulcer lies more distally in the duodenum (beyond approximately 2.5 cm), it is usually necessary to leave the posterior wall of the distal duodenal end attached to the posterior penetrating ulcer and to plan a modified closure of the duodenal stump, as will be described. I almost always remove active duodenal ulcers in my resections. However, I occasionally leave active ulcers in situ when they are situated in the more distal parts of the duodenum, and so far I have had no cause to regret doing so.

Under no circumstances must the ulcer crater be excised from the pancreas, since this procedure is dangerous and unnecessary.

In performing the Strauss maneuver, the following anatomic facts concerning the duodenum are worthy of attention. In hundreds of gastric resections, after cutting across the duodenum just distal to the ulcer (that is, approximately 2 cm distal to the pylorus), I have regularly felt for the ampulla of Vater. The index finger of the right hand is used and is inserted with the operator standing on the left side of the table. The distance to the palpated ampulla is then measured; it averages 5.3 cm from the cut end of the duodenum. Thus, the ampulla averages a total of 7.3 cm from the pylorus. Occasionally, the opening of the duct of Santorini or a pancreatic lobule might be mistaken for the ampulla; furthermore, sometimes nothing is palpated, but generally the palpation seems accurate.

Having identified the exact point at which the common bile duct enters the duodenum, the surgeon can proceed with more assurance that he or she will not interfere with this important ostium. After complete division of the duodenum, a sponge is placed in the distal end and another sponge is tied loosely about the proximal end to avoid gross spillage of bile and other contents. As stated before, the final disposition of the duodenal stump is decided *after* an adequate resection has been performed.

With the Strauss maneuver, one can remove the duodenal ulcer in most instances. It has the following advantages: It stops bleeding if present; it removes enough duodenum to give assurance that the antrum is out; it eliminates the indeterminate period an unremoved ulcer takes to heal; and it provides a clean duodenum for anastomosis or closure.

Division of the Hepaticgastro Omentum and Left Gastric Vessels

The hepaticgastro omentum is usually a thin layer of peritoneum with a minimal amount of fat, although the latter is somewhat variable. At a distance of 1.5 to 2.0 cm from the lesser curvature, no sizable blood vessels are encountered until the level of the left gastric vessels, which are in a separate fold placed more posteriorly. A good portion of the dissection of the hepaticgastro omentum can be carried out without ligatures, and usually it is necessary to ligate only two or three rather small vessels before one reaches the left gastric vessels. This part of the dissection is usually easy, but some difficulty can be encountered when there is thickening, scarring, and inflammatory reaction secondary to a gastric ulcer on the lesser curvature. The hepatic branch of the left vagus nerve lies in this curvature just above the level of the left gastric artery. It should not be cut, although cutting this branch makes no difference if a truncal vagotomy is to be done above this level.

The left gastric artery is the largest artery supplying the stomach, and occasionally division of this vessel gives rise to difficulty. It is usually surrounded by a moderate amount of fat, which is increased in elderly people, making it difficult to identify the lesser curvature margin of the stomach. In addition, dissection of this vessel is more hazardous if there is scarring or an inflammatory reaction around it secondary to ulceration on the lesser curvature of the stomach.

A word of caution should be interjected at this point concerning the occasional origin of an aberrant left hepatic artery from the left gastric artery. Sometimes this vessel constitutes the sole blood supply to the left lobe of the liver, and its sacrifice would

almost certainly mean necrosis of the lobe. Therefore, it is worthwhile to examine the configuration of the left gastric artery and its branches carefully and to make certain that the vessel is divided distal to any such possible aberrant hepatic branch. Generally in patients with benign disease, I ligate the left gastric artery, after it has divided, close to the stomach. This method is easier and also avoids unnecessary clamping of the celiac branch of the posterior vagus nerve, although, again, if a truncal vagotomy is to be performed, such clamping makes no difference.

Resection

The lines of resection of the stomach should now be decided. For duodenal ulcer, if selective vagotomy has been performed, 30 to 35 percent distal resection is sufficient (see Fig. 75-1). The extent of resection and exact placing of the line of resection are both important. The antrum is higher along the lesser curvature than along the greater. Thus, it is important to

do a Schoemaker type of tubing of the lesser curvature.

When the site of transection of the stomach has been selected, an Allis clamp is placed on the greater curvature just distal to the selected site. A small Payr clamp is then applied perpendicular to the greater curvature at the selected level and extended across the width of the stomach for a measured distance of 5 cm (Fig. 75-2). The clamp is closed, and a Carmalt clamp is placed just distal to the Payr clamp and parallel to it. The walls of the stomach between the two clamps are incised with a scalpel to a point just distal to the tip of the Payr clamp (Fig. 75-3). The two clamps are separated widely and a von Petz (or other stainless steel clip applicator) sewing clamp is then angled up to the lesser curvature side of the stomach approximately 2 to 3 cm below the esophagogastric junction. A double row of staples is then placed along the line of application of the clamp and the clamp is removed. The anterior and posterior walls of the stomach

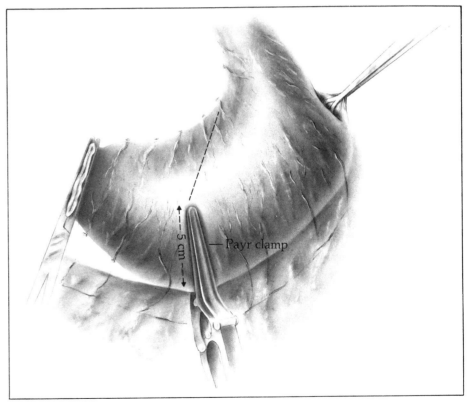

Fig. 75-2. Transection of stomach. For the technique of selective vagotomy, see Chap. 76. A small Payr clamp is placed perpendicular to the greater curvature for a distance of 5 cm across the stomach. To achieve a 30 to 35 percent distal gastric resection (antrectomy), this Payr clamp is placed approximately 14 cm proximal to the pylorus. The broken line shows the proposed line of excision of the lesser curvature.

are then divided between the double row of staples (Fig. 75-4). Just before the division of the upper portion of the lesser curvature of the stomach is completed, a 4–0 silk suture is placed in the form of a Lembert suture just above the most superior clip. Using this suture for traction to prevent the upper portion of the Schoemaker line from springing upward, the remaining distance between the double row of clips is completely incised and the specimen is discarded from the surgical field. Occasionally a few small vessels bleed between the staples. These bleeding points should be clamped and ligated with 4–0 black silk ligatures to achieve complete hemostasis. Otherwise, troublesome hematomas can form and prevent satisfactory closure of the Schoemaker line.

Closure of the Schoemaker Suture Line

The clip closure of the Schoemaker suture line is now closed by interrupted 4–0 black silk Lembert sutures placed close enough to obtain continuous serosa-to-serosa approximation. These reinforcing sutures are placed down to a point 1 cm above the tip end of the Payr clamp. This terminal 1 cm is left unsutured until the anastomosis is completed (Fig. 75-5).

Anastomosis

At this point, the type of anastomosis must be decided. There are few instances in which a gastroduodenal anastomosis cannot be performed, and usually this anastomosis can be of the end-to-end type. In difficult situations, the scope of the Billroth I anastomosis can be greatly extended by use of the von Haberer–Finney end-to-side anastomosis, particularly when the proximal cut end of the duodenum has to be left attached to the distal margin of a posterior penetrating duodenal ulcer.

The anastomosis should not be forced. If the surgeon believes it is technically difficult to use the duodenum in reestablishing gastrointestinal continuity, a gastrojejunal anastomosis should be performed. If the end-to-end type of anastomosis is decided on, the anastomosis is achieved by an outer row of interrupted 4–0 non-inverting black silk sutures. The inner row is closed with a continuous 4–0 absorbable suture that includes only the mucosa and submucosa (Fig. 75-6). During the course of the anastomosis, it might be necessary to

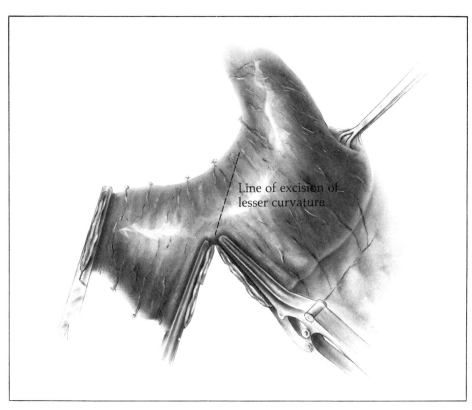

Fig. 75-3. A Carmalt clamp is placed parallel to the Payr clamp. The stomach is divided between the two clamps, and a mechanical stapling device is placed along the proposed line of excision of the lesser curvature.

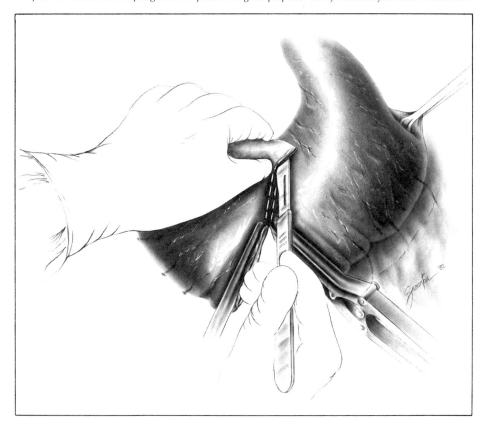

Fig. 75-4. Double row of metallic hemostatic clips. The stomach is divided. Any of a number of modern automatic stapling instruments can be used to close the lesser curvature.

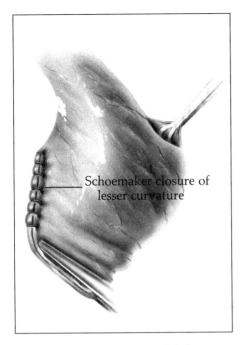

Fig. 75-5. The Schoemaker closure of the lesser curvature with interrupted Lembert sutures of 4–0 black silk.

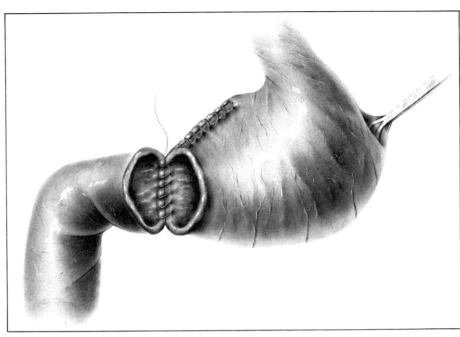

Fig. 75-6. The end-to-end anastomosis. The posterior row of interrupted 4–0 black silk seromuscular sutures has been placed. The inner continuous absorbable hemostatic (baseball stitch) suture is seen.

ligate several bleeding points in the end of the gastric stump.

When the anastomosis is completed, special care is taken to reinforce the critical angle, that is, the point of junction between the Schoemaker suture line and the anastomotic line. The reinforcement consists in the placement of a 000 black silk purse-string suture, taking a bite of the anterior wall of the stomach, the posterior wall of the stomach, and the wall of the duodenum at the critical angle. When this suture is tied down, there is good serosal apposition of all three components: namely, the anterior gastric wall, the posterior gastric wall, and the wall of the duodenum (Fig. 75-7). The completed anastomosis should admit 1½ to 2 fingers.

If the end of the duodenum is unsuitable for end-to-end anastomosis, I prefer to use the terminolateral modification of the Billroth I procedure rather than a Billroth II anastomosis. As stated previously, the main reason for unsuitability of the end of the duodenum for anastomosis is the presence of posterior penetrating ulcer. Under these circumstances, a modified type of duodenal stump closure is achieved, using the method described by Nissen (Fig. 75-8).

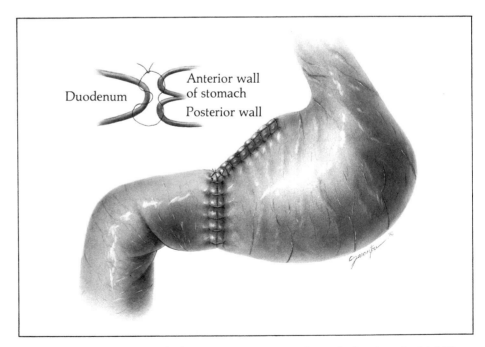

Fig. 75-7. Completed operation—selective vagotomy, antrectomy, and gastroduodenostomy. Inset, infolding of the stomach at the corner of the Schoemaker closure of the lesser curvature and the duodenum at the superior portion of the anastomosis. This suture (usually two bites to the stomach and one or two to the duodenum) protects against an anastomotic leak at this potentially weak part of the closure.

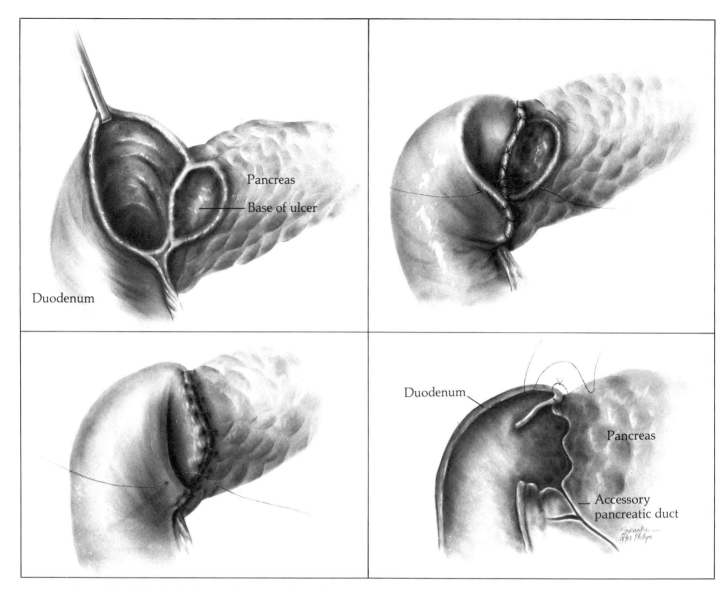

Fig. 75-8. *Closure of the difficult duodenal stump when a terminolateral anastomosis is contemplated (closure after Nissen). A. The distal duodenum is adherent posteriorly to the distal margin of the ulcer bed. B. The anterior duodenal wall is sutured to the distal margin of the ulcer bed and a second row of sutures is begun, suturing the anterior wall to the proximal ulcer margin. C. The second row is completed, and the third and final row is begun, folding the anterior duodenal wall against the capsule of the pancreas proximal to the ulcer. D. Cross-section showing the omission of the first row of sutures when an accessory pancreatic duct opens into the ulcer bed. This omission allows pancreatic juice to drain into the duodenal lumen.*

This method consists of suturing the free anterior wall of the duodenum to the distal margin of the ulcer crater in the pancreas, and then rolling the anterior wall of the duodenum in such a manner that it covers the ulcer crater.

After the closure of the duodenal stump, an end-to-side gastroduodenal anastomosis is performed just distal to the duodenal stump closure. The resultant anastomosis is the same size as, or slightly larger than, the end-to-end anastomosis. When the

end-to-side gastroduodenal anastomosis is used, the ampulla of Vater can be opposite the gastroduodenal stoma.

Wound Closure

I make no attempt to close the peritoneum and have noted no difficulty or complication arising from this omission. It seems that the ligamentum teres of the liver and the falciform ligament quickly adhere and can form a more anatomic peritoneal closure than would be accomplished by su-

ture. The fascia of the linea alba is closed by interrupted nonabsorbable sutures. No subcutaneous sutures are used, and after closure of the fascia of the linea alba, the skin edges are approximated.

Suggested Reading

Donahue PE. Extended Highly Selective Vagotomy. In C Wastell LM Nyhus, PE Donahue (eds.). *Surgery of the Esophagus, Stomach and*

Small Intestine, 5th ed. Boston. Little, Brown, 1995.

Donahue PE, Bombeck CT, Condon RE, Nyhus LM. Proximal gastric vagotomy versus selective vagotomy with antrectomy: Results of a prospective, randomized clinical trial after four to twelve years. *Surgery* 96:585, 1984.

Donahue PE, Nyhus LM. Exposure of the periesophageal space. *Surg Gynecol Obstet* 152:218, 1981.

Donahue PE, Nyhus LM. Surgical excision of gastric ulcers near the gastroesophageal junction. *Surg Gynecol Obstet* 155:85, 1982.

Dragstedt LR, Owens FM Jr. Supradiaphragmatic section of vagus nerves in treatment of duodenal ulcer. *Proc Soc Exp Biol Med* 53:152, 1943.

Harkins HN, Griffith CA, Nyhus LM. The revised combined operation with selective gastric vagotomy. *Am Surg* 33:510, 1967.

Harkins HN, Jesseph JE, Stevenson JK, Nyhus LM. The "combined" operation for peptic ulcer. *Arch Surg* 80:743, 1960.

Kocher T. Mobilisierung des duodenum und gastroduodenostomie. *Zentralbl Chir* 30:33, 1903.

Nissen R. Zur resektion des tiefsitzenden duodenalgeschwurs. *Zentralbl Chir* 60:483, 1933.

Nyhus LM, Donahue PE, Krystosek RJ, et al. Complete vagotomy: The evolution of an effective technique. *Arch Surg* 115:264, 1980.

Waisbren SJ, Modlin IM. The evolution of therapeutic vagotomy. *Surg Gynecol Obstet* 170:261, 1990.

EDITOR'S COMMENT

Doctor Nyhus, whose expertise in the performance of gastrectomy and, especially, vagotomy, is known throughout the world has presented a highly detailed and useful description of the technique of distal gastrectomy. Although gastrectomy is not the most complex operation that we perform in the abdomen, it is one in which the recently trained surgeon has usually had little experience. In our own training program, the average surgical resident's experience with partial gastrectomy of any kind has been involved in fewer than ten procedures. When Dr. Nyhus trained, the average surgical resident performed eight to ten times that number of gastrectomies in the course of a 5-year residency and was far more comfortable with this operation than the current resident or recent graduate.

The incision for this operation is most often a vertical midline from the paraxiphoid area to 2 cm below the umbilicus. I make the incision in a straight line and do not perform a "half keyhole" incision around the umbilicus but sweep the incision approximately 1.5 to 2 cm lateral to the umbilicus, ordinarily on the left side. An excellent alternative incision, if the individual is short and has a wide abdomen, is a long left subcostal incision with a half subcostal extension of the incision on the right, traversing only the rectus muscle on the right but extending the left subcostal component to the anterior axillary line, the entire incision is at least two fingerbreadths below both costal margins. If the esophagogastric junction is difficult to expose for the vagotomy, which is invariably performed for duodenal ulcer disease, a vertical extension from the apex of the "arrowhead" incision superiorly to the paraxiphoid space can be used, which is especially helpful if the liver is somewhat enlarged and it is necessary to retract the left lobe after incision of the falciform ligament.

With endoscopy routinely performed 1 month or less prior to the operation, as is our practice, the presence of the pyloric channel or duodenal ulcer is essentially never in question. With anterior or anterosuperior duodenal ulcers, the operation is simplified and the excision of the ulcer is easily accomplished. The difficult ulcer is the one that has penetrated posteriorly onto the pancreas, and it presents the greatest opportunity for technical mishap if careful attention is not given to the vital structures that are located directly behind the ulcer bed. The author's description of feeling the ulcer crater and actually invaginating the anterior wall into the crater is a very useful maneuver. However, on occasion this sign is not easily demonstrated and stoking the anterior wall of the duodenum with a moist gauze sponge frequently elicits numerous tiny petechial hemorrhages over the anterior surface of the duodenum with stippling of the serosa, referred to as Schoemaker's periduodenitis. This result is usually indicative of an active duodenal ulcer process in the duodenum adjacent to this physical finding. The sign is somewhat less prominent with a posterior duodenal ulcer than with an ulcer of the anterior or superior wall, but with significant inflammation and edema of the duodenum, the sign is likely to be seen regardless of the location of the ulcer.

One area of difference of opinion between Dr. Nyhus and myself is that of the necessity for removing posterior duodenal ulcers that have penetrated deeply. The author states that he "seldom leaves the ulcer in situ," but I have often left it in situ, and if it is greater than 2 cm in diameter, I routinely do so. Even if there is severe acute hemorrhage that requires an emergency operation, I almost invariably attempt to control the bleeding with interrupted permanent sutures in the three branches of the gastroduodenal artery (superior, inferior, and posterior, through the pancreas) and then deal with the ulcer by truncal vagotomy and pyloroplasty. In the less likely event that I resect a patient with a massively bleeding duodenal ulcer (ordinarily this resection would be done only if the patient had been subjected to vagotomy and pyloroplasty in the past, and the treatment had failed so that the bleeding duodenal ulcer was recurrent), I would perform a 60 to 70 percent gastrectomy but would not attempt to remove a large posterior duodenal ulcer. Doing so subjects the pancreas to significant trauma, risks damage to the pancreatic ductal system, and may cause postoperative pancreatitis, which is occasionally fatal. Just as catastrophic, damage to the common bile duct or even the ampulla of Vater has been encountered in referred patients twice in the past year and was a consequence of the surgeon's determination to remove the ulcer.

The management of the ulcer crater often involves sewing the stomach in a Billroth I anastomosis to the distal edge of the ulcer, excluding the ulcer from the gastrointestinal tract, or, under extreme circumstances, sewing the stomach to the proximal edge of the ulcer. Either the proximal or distal edge of a chronic duodenal ulcer is very firm and holds sutures well because of the intense fibrous reaction in the submucosa. Sewing the ulcer to the distal end of the stomach is both easier and safer than attempting to close that duodenal stump. I have never closed a duodenal stump and sewn the stomach to the side of the duodenum just distal to the stump, being persuaded by my long experience observing Dr. Nyhus that the gastroduodenostomy, even if very difficult, is better in terms of its healing than is closure of the friable and seriously diseased duodenal stump.

Although intestinal staplers have almost become the standard for anastomosing most of the gastrointestinal tract, I close the lesser curvature as Dr. Nyhus has described with a GIA stapler but then use a 3–0 absorbable intestinal suture *below* the staple line as a running hemostatic layer. The most common place for postoperative bleeding following gastrectomy is from the lesser curvature closure, and the simple running hemostatic suture below the staple line adds a bit of insurance in preventing that bleeding complication. Following that layer, I fold the staple line under with a series of seromuscular silk Lembert sutures. The purpose of the lesser curvature closure is to convert the remaining stomach to a tube, and so the amount of soft tissue that is enfolded is not important. In the event that we avoid stapling the lesser curvature, most commonly when there is a gastric ulcer in the antrum or at the incisura of the stomach, the same 3–0 absorbable suture is used to undersew a Carmalt clamp applied on the lesser curvature. The clamp is then removed, and a second layer of continuous suture is used to oversew the cut edge, so that there is a double layer that will effectively prevent bleeding from the lesser curvature closure. Obviously, this double closure is then inverted with interrupted permanent sutures, as described previously.

We do not use staplers for anastomosing the stomach to the duodenum, vastly preferring a hand-sewn single- or two-layer anastomosis. If the duodenum is pliable, it is quite easy to use a line of permanent suture material as posterior Lemberts, and then a series of interrupted absorbable sutures as an inner layer on the posterior side. It is just as secure to use full-thickness sutures between the posterior wall of the stomach and the posterior duodenal wall (often the ulcer edge) and then use one or two layers on the anterior aspect. It is quite important to use the U stitch of von Haberer, which Dr. Nyhus has so nicely described in the text. This step closes the Y-shaped corner at the junction of the duodenum and the closure of the lesser curvature of the stomach.

There is currently a rash of enthusiasm for the multiple application of mechanical hemoclips for separating the greater curvature of the stomach from the lienogastric ligament, in which the short gastric vessels are found. Although this method saves a modicum of time, it leaves a large number of clips in the peritoneal cavity, and I have been somewhat disenchanted by the frequency with which laparotomy pads or a surgeon's hand might sweep one or several of these curved hemostatic clips from a short gastric vessel, resulting in delayed bleeding and undue delay. Obviously, such a device also adds to the cost of the operation, whereas hand-tied ligatures have great stability when appropriately applied and produce no complications.

R.J.B.

76

Selective Vagotomy and Pyloroplasty

John L. Sawyers

Selective vagotomy was designed to denervate the stomach without dividing vagal innervation to any other intra-abdominal organs. The technique of selective (gastric) vagotomy was introduced by Jackson and Franksson independently in 1948. Selective vagotomy should not be confused with highly selective vagotomy (parietal cell or proximal gastric vagotomy), which denervates only the acid-secreting parietal cell mass and does not require a drainage procedure. Since selective vagotomy results in division of all parasympathetic nerve branches to the entire stomach, a drainage procedure (pyloroplasty, gastrojejunostomy) or antrectomy is necessary for adequate gastric emptying.

Selective vagotomy is considered to have advantages over truncal (complete abdominal) vagotomy since it obviates the adverse effects of extragastric vagotomy on the biliary tract, pancreas, and intestine. An increased incidence of gallstones and the occurrence of postvagotomy diarrhea are two of the more frequently reported side effects of truncal vagotomy that can be lessened by selective vagotomy.

The increased incidence of diarrhea after truncal vagotomy was a major impetus to the acceptance of selective gastric vagotomy. Burge and Harkins reported an increased incidence rate of diarrhea following truncal vagotomy as high as 68 percent. Diarrhea was markedly reduced after selective gastric vagotomy. The effect of truncal vagotomy on gallbladder disease has been controversial. Disordered gallbladder motility and lithogenic bile have been thought to occur after truncal vagotomy. Studies by Shaffer, however, indicate that truncal vagotomy does not adversely affect gallbladder function and improves cholesterol solubility. Others have found gallbladder dilatation and loss of compliance after truncal vagotomy, which can be secondary to vagally induced alterations in the sphincter of Oddi. Resistance to bile flow through the sphincter of Oddi is increased after truncal vagotomy, whereas gallbladder compliance is reduced. It has been shown that truncal vagotomy induces a delay and decrease in postprandial responses in pancreatic volume and protein outputs, but has no effect on basal and postprandial plasma levels of cholecystokinin.

A prospective randomized clinical study comparing the effects of truncal and selective vagotomy in 143 patients is summarized in Table 76-1. There was no statistically significant difference between the two groups of patients in regard to nutrition, weight gain or loss, anemia, anacidity, and dumping syndrome. Diarrhea occurred more often in patients undergoing truncal vagotomy, but this was not a statistically significant difference. There was an important difference between the two groups of patients in the completeness of gastric vagal denervation as measured by the Hollander test. Postoperative Hollander tests were positive in 19 percent of patients after truncal vagotomy and in only 2 percent of patients after selective vagotomy.

The complementary procedures most frequently used with truncal vagotomy are antrectomy and pyloroplasty. Antrectomy when combined with truncal vagotomy provides protection against recurrent ulcer in 99 percent of patients, whereas pyloroplasty with truncal vagotomy has a reported ulcer recurrence rate ranging from 3 to 22 percent. Most of the patients in whom recurrent ulcers develop have incomplete vagal denervation of the stomach. Pyloroplasty does not afford the additional protection against recurrent ulcer provided by antral resection. On the other hand, truncal vagotomy-antrectomy has a mortality three times higher (1.6 vs. 0.5%) than truncal vagotomy-pyloroplasty. Since selective vagotomy is considerably superior to truncal vagotomy in achieving complete vagal denervation of the stomach, it seemed reasonable to compare the procedures of antrectomy and pyloroplasty with selective vagotomy. A prospective randomized clinical study of patients undergoing selective vagotomy with antrectomy or pyloroplasty resulted in no statistically significant differences between the two groups of patients. Contrary to the results with truncal vagotomy-pyloroplasty, the recurrent ulcer rate remained low (2%). Therefore, selective vagotomy and pyloroplasty is an ideal combination, since the pyloroplasty is technically easier than antrectomy and is usually accompanied by low surgical mortality and morbidity,

Table 76-1. Evaluation of Truncal Versus Selective Vagotomy

	Truncal Vagotomy	Selective Vagotomy
Visick I or II result	93%	96%
Dumping	21%	34%
Small intestine transit time	Normal	Normal
Diarrhea	21%	12%
Gastric anacidity	80%	84%
Positive Hollander test	19%	2%

whereas selective vagotomy, by achieving complete gastric denervation, provides protection against recurrent ulcer.

Enthusiasm for selective gastric vagotomy diminished after proximal gastric vagotomy became widely accepted for the surgical treatment of duodenal ulcer disease. However, the ulcer recurrence rate following proximal gastric vagotomy has been consistently higher in most reported series than that following selective gastric vagotomy with pyloroplasty. For example, the Århus County Vagotomy Trial reported an ulcer recurrence rate for patients with duodenal ulcer treated by proximal gastric vagotomy of 15 percent, compared with 9 percent following selective gastric vagotomy and a drainage procedure. Griffith, in a 12- to 17-year follow-up study of patients undergoing selective vagotomy plus pyloroplasty, reported five ulcerations occurring in 87 patients: one stomal ulcer, two gastric ulcers, and two instances of hemorrhagic gastritis. In his earlier report, Griffith reported only one ulcer recurrence in 103 patients followed for 4 to 9 years after selective vagotomy and pyloroplasty for duodenal ulcer. Three of these gastric ulcers were thought to be secondary to biliary reflux since the insulin test for completeness of vagotomy was negative in these patients. Studies from various groups in Copenhagen report different ulcer recurrence rates following selective vagotomy with pyloroplasty. Madsen and Kronborg reported an ulcer recurrence rate of 14 percent following selective vagotomy and pyloroplasty after 5 to 8 years of a prospective, randomized follow-up study. The ulcer recurrence rate following proximal gastric vagotomy was 26 percent, or almost twice as high. Christiansen reported a 14 percent overall ulcer recurrence rate after selective vagotomy and pyloroplasty, 16 percent after proximal gastric vagotomy, and 10 percent after truncal vagotomy and pyloroplasty in a prospective, randomized study. Later Hoffman and colleagues, of Christiansen's group, in an 11-to 15-year follow-up study, found recurrent ulcer rates of 28.5 percent for truncal vagotomy, 37.4 percent for selective vagotomy, and 39.3 percent for proximal gastric vagotomy. These differences were not statistically significant. The poor long-term results found by Hoffman and colleagues demonstrate a need for many more in-depth studies of this type.

A group from Copenhagen reported in 1994 a 23-year study of patients undergoing parietal cell (selective proximal) vagotomy in 347 patients with a recurrent ulcer rate of 21.9 percent. These investigators concluded that the rate of recurrent ulceration after parietal cell vagotomy is proportional to the duration of follow-up. Almost 80 percent of patients with recurrent ulcer developed their recurrence 10 years or longer after their operation. This increasing incidence of ulcer recurrence with length of follow-up has not been reported after selective vagotomy and pyloroplasty.

Emos and Eriksson from the Karolinska Institute reported in 1992 a 12-year follow-up of a prospective, randomized trial of selective vagotomy with pyloroplasty compared with selective proximal vagotomy with and without pyloroplasty in patients with duodenal, pyloric, and prepyloric ulcers. The ulcer recurrence rate was lower (13%) in patients undergoing selective vagotomy and pyloroplasty. In 143 followed patients, Visick I and II results (excellent or good) were obtained in 75 percent of patients after selective vagotomy with pyloroplasty and in 54 percent after selective proximal vagotomy alone. Seventeen patients from all three groups underwent reoperation. The final clinical results including reoperations were Visick I or II in 85 percent of patients after selective vagotomy with pyloroplasty and selective proximal vagotomy with pyloro-

plasty, but in only 55 percent after selective proximal vagotomy. This significant difference indicated that the addition of pyloroplasty was advantageous. There was no problem with diarrhea in any group. Dumping was more frequent in patients with pyloroplasty, but was stated to be mild and not a serious problem for any patient.

Anatomy

Figure 76-1 demonstrates the vagal nerve supply to the stomach. Two major vagal trunks (anterior and posterior) come through the diaphragm, but there is an esophageal plexus of vagal fibers around the lower esophagus so that fibers are intermingled from the right and left vagus nerves. The anterior vagal trunk gives off the hepatic branch (or branches), which innervates the liver, gallbladder, and pancreas. The anterior vagal trunk then continues along the lesser curvature of the stomach as the anterior gastric nerve of Latarjet. The posterior vagal trunk gives off the celiac branch, which goes to the celiac plexus and provides parasympathetic innervation to the pancreas, duodenum, small intestine, and right half of the colon. The posterior vagal trunk then continues as the posterior gastric nerve of Latarjet, which parallels the anterior gastric nerve but lies in the posterior leaf of the hepatic-gastro ligament.

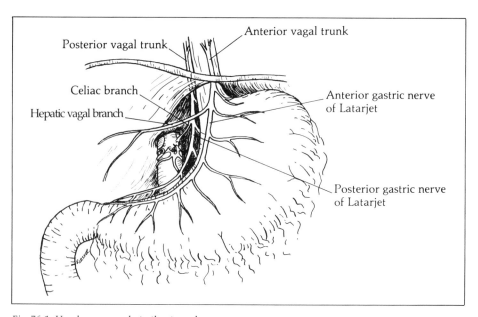

Fig. 76-1. Vagal nerve supply to the stomach.

Selective vagotomy is designed to spare the hepatic and celiac vagal branches but to divide all vagal branches entering the stomach.

Surgical Techniques

Selective Vagotomy

The operation is performed under general anesthesia using an endotracheal tube. A nasogastric tube is then inserted. The peritoneal cavity is opened through an upper midline abdominal incision, beginning to the left of the xiphoid process and extending down to the right of the umbilicus.

After careful abdominal examination, the upper hand retractor is inserted to elevate the xiphoid and rib cage for improved exposure of the upper abdomen. A standard Balfour retractor is also used.

The site of the duodenal ulcer is carefully examined. Any adhesions to the gallbladder or undersurface of the liver are divided. The nasogastric tube is placed along the greater curvature of the stomach and is secured with Babcock clamps to place the stomach on traction and to provide exposure to visualize the hepatic vagal branches and anterior gastric nerve. With traction on the stomach, the anterior vagal trunk can be identified by palpation (it feels like a banjo string) and is encircled with an umbilical tape or vessel loop. The hepatic vagal branch (or branches) is also identified and encircled with a tape (Fig. 76-2).

With gentle traction on the tapes around the hepatic vagal branch and anterior vagal trunk, the origin of the hepatic branch from the anterior trunk is easily visualized. All tissue to the left between these branches and the lesser curvature of the stomach is divided. No attempt is made to identify each gastric vagal nerve branch and divide it individually. Instead, efforts are made to preserve the hepatic vagal branches (Fig. 76-3).

Attention is now directed to finding the posterior vagal trunk. The esophagus can be retracted to the patient's left by a retractor or by encircling it with a Penrose drain and pulling to the left. With traction on the stomach, the posterior vagal trunk is identified and encircled with a tape. The

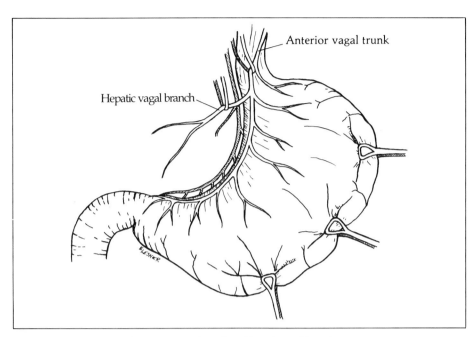

Fig. 76-2. Identification of the anterior vagal trunk and hepatic vagal branches.

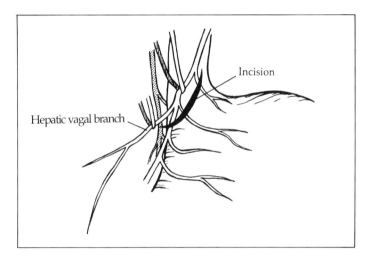

Fig. 76-3. Incision made to preserve the hepatic vagal branches.

celiac branch can then be palpated by the finger. It feels like a taut cord that extends to the celiac plexus. With the posterior trunk and celiac branch identified, all tissue between these nerve trunks and the lesser curvature of the stomach is divided (Fig. 76-4). This step necessitates division of the descending branch of the left gastric artery, which should be carefully ligated. After this maneuver, the lesser curvature of the stomach in the region of the cardia should be completely free.

Because some gastric vagal branches can arise separately from the vagal trunks above the hiatus, dissection around the esophagus should be carried cephalad approximately 5 cm above the esophagogastric junction. Professor Grassi of Rome appropriately named a vagal branch from the posterior trunk to the fundus the "criminal" nerve, since this nerve fiber frequently escapes the surgeon and can result in an incomplete vagotomy with failure to heal the ulcer or in a recurrent ulcer. This

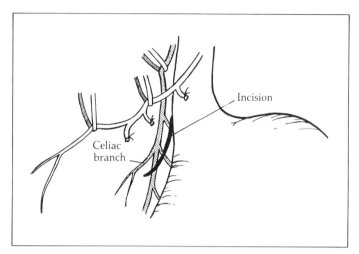

Fig. 76-4. Tissue divided between the posterior vagal trunk and celiac vagal branch.

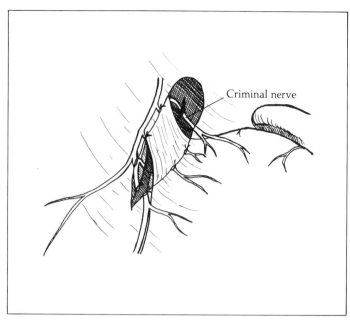

Fig. 76-5. Identification of the criminal nerve.

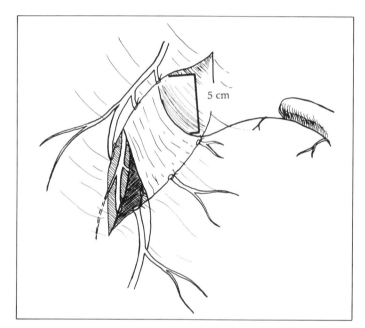

Fig. 76-6. Dissection above the esophagogastric junction.

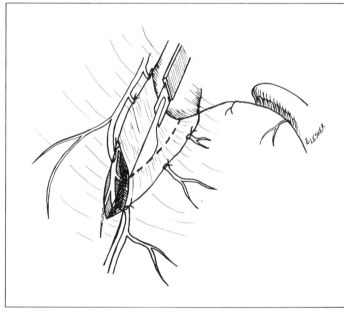

Fig. 76-7. Incision to divide the longitudinal nerve fibrils running distally to the proximal cardia.

vagal fiber is shown in Fig. 76-5. It courses along the left lateral wall of the esophagus to enter the stomach cephalad to the short gastric vessels.

Figure 76-6 shows the dissection above the esophagogastric junction. All tissue around the lower esophagus for a distance of 5 cm above the esophagogastric junction is divided. A superficial incision is then made around the lower end of the esophagus to divide the fine longitudinal nerve fibrils that run distally to the proximal cardia (Fig. 76-7). Some surgeons prefer to omit this step because of concern of incising too deeply into the esophageal wall. An alternative method is to use a fine nerve hook and search carefully for individual vagal fibrils, which can be elevated by the nerve hook and then severed by the scalpel. This maneuver completes the selective vagotomy. If the esophageal hiatus is unusually patulous, one or more nonabsorbable sutures can be placed behind (dorsal to) the esophagus to tighten the hiatus. If the patient has reflux esophagitis in association with a duodenal ulcer, a Nissen fundoplication or Hill median arcuate ligament repair for hiatal hernia can be performed.

After the acceptance of laparoscopic cholecystectomy, surgeons began to use the laparoscopic technique to perform vagotomy as well as pyloroplasty. Most laparoscopic vagotomies have been done for highly selective vagotomy rather than selective vagotomy, but it is possible for an experienced endoscopic surgeon to do the procedure as described above.

Pyloroplasty

Selective vagotomy results in total gastric denervation. When the stomach is vaguely denervated, gastric acidity is controlled, but gastric tone and muscular activity are altered. The stomach loses receptive relaxation with resulting gastric stasis. Pyloroplasty alleviates this side effect of vagotomy and facilitates gastric emptying.

The two most frequently used types of pyloroplasty are the Heineke–Mikulicz pyloroplasty, as modified by Weinberg, and the Finney pyloroplasty. Jaboulay described a gastric drainage procedure (gastroduodenostomy), which is incorrectly called a pyloroplasty since the incision does not extend across the pylorus.

Weinberg Pyloroplasty

Heineke in 1886 and Mikulicz in 1888 independently described a pyloroplasty consisting of a longitudinal incision through the pylorus, which was closed transversely in two layers. Weinberg modified this closure to consist of only one layer of nonabsorbable sutures. This modification resulted in a larger opening with improved gastric drainage.

The Weinberg pyloroplasty is begun by placing two traction stay sutures approximately 1 cm apart on the anterior surface of the pylorus. A longitudinal incision is made between the traction sutures approximately 6 to 7 cm long. The incision extends 3 to 4 cm on the gastric side of the pylorus and approximately 2.5 to 3.0 cm on the duodenal side (Fig. 76-8).

Lateral traction on the divided pylorus with the stay sutures converts the longitudinal incision into a transverse incision. The transverse incision is closed with a single layer of interrupted nonabsorbable sutures, such as 000 silk. The needle enters the serosa of the gastric side approximately 3 to 4 mm from the edge of the incision and passes through the stomach wall in a slanting direction to include the

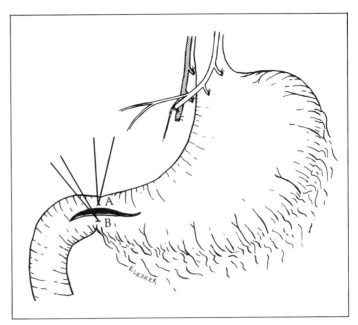

Fig. 76-8. Incision for the Weinberg pyloroplasty and locations of guide sutures (A and B).

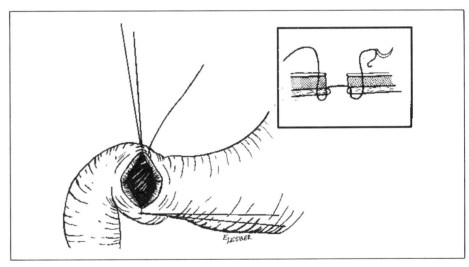

Fig. 76-9. The Gambee suture technique for the Weinberg pyloroplasty.

mucosa near its cut edge. The suture then passes through the duodenal mucosa near the cut edge and is slanted through all layers of the duodenum to emerge approximately 3 or 4 mm from the edge of the wound. Sutures are placed approximately 3 mm apart (Fig. 76-9). All sutures are placed before tying. If placed correctly, mucosa is approximated to mucosa, muscularis to muscularis, and serosa to serosa (Fig. 76-10). The ends of the wound stick out like "dog-ears" and should not be infolded since this can narrow the lumen. Omentum is sutured over the incision to

help prevent leakage from the lumen and to prevent adhesion to the undersurface of the liver.

The Gambee suture can also be used to close the transverse incision. This suture is shown in the inset (see Fig. 76-9) and aids in infolding the mucosa. A few Gambee-type sutures alternating with through-and-through sutures are an effective method of closure.

Experienced endoscopic surgeons have described laparoscopic pyloroplasty using a one-layer Weinberg–type procedure. It is technically possible to perform selective vagotomy and pyloroplasty using the laparoscopic approach, but this approach has been used very infrequently.

Finney Pyloroplasty

The Finney pyloroplasty provides better drainage for a vagotomized J-shaped stomach. The duodenum is mobilized from its retroperitoneal attachments by the Kocher maneuver. A traction suture is placed in the superior margin of the pyloric ring. Upward traction on this suture aids in apposing the anterior wall of the stomach and duodenum, which are sutured together with interrupted 000 silk (Fig. 76-11). A 10-cm inverted U-shaped incision is made into the lumen of the stomach and duodenum transecting the pyloric muscle (Fig. 76-12). The posterior septum between the posterior walls of the stomach and duodenum are sutured with a continuous 0000 chromic catgut suture. This through-and-through suture ensures hemostasis and is begun at the pyloric end of the posterior wall (Fig. 76-13). After the posterior suture is completed, the suture continues anteriorly to close the anterior walls of the stomach and duodenum. The anterior outer layer is completed with a seromuscular layer of 000 silk sutures (Fig. 76-14).

Jaboulay Gastroduodenostomy

Severe scarring or inflammation of the pyloric area can make a Weinberg or Finney pyloroplasty difficult to perform. An alternative gastric drainage procedure is a side-to-side anastomosis between the gastric

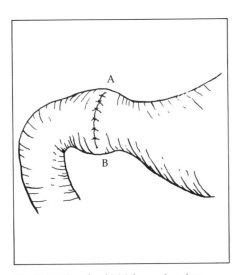

Fig. 76-10. Completed Weinberg pyloroplasty.

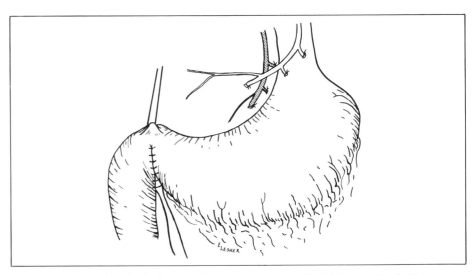

Fig. 76-11. Anastomosis of the duodenum to the greater curvature of the distal antrum for the Finney pyloroplasty.

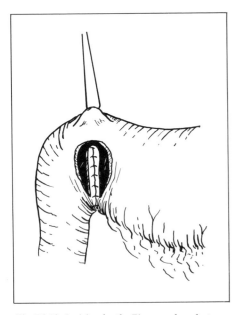

Fig. 76-12. Incision for the Finney pyloroplasty.

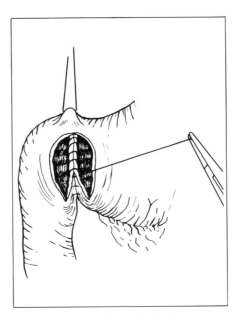

Fig. 76-13. Suture technique for the Finney pyloroplasty.

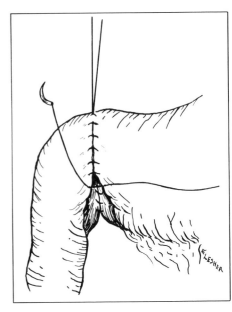

Fig. 76-14. Completed Finney pyloroplasty.

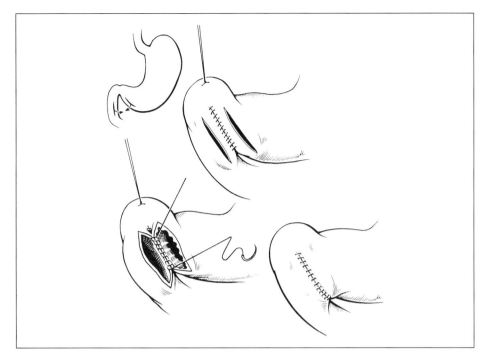

Fig. 76-15. Technique for the Jaboulay gastroduodensotomy.

antrum and the duodenum, as described by Jaboulay in 1892. The Kocher maneuver mobilizes the duodenum. The gastric antrum and duodenum are sutured side to side with nonabsorbable sutures (000 silk). A traction suture in the superior aspect of the pylorus helps to appose the anterior walls of the stomach and duodenum. A 5- to 6-cm incision is made in the antrum and also in the duodenum. An inner layer of continuous 0000 chromic catgut suture completes the second layer of the anastomosis. The outer walls of the anastomosis are secured with interrupted 000 silk sutures (Fig. 76-15).

Since this anastomosis places the ampulla of Vater close to the gastric antrum, bile reflux is frequent. Many surgeons would prefer a gastrojejunostomy placed in a dependent position on the gastric antrum rather than the Jaboulay gastroduodenostomy.

Perforated Duodenal Ulcer

Patients presenting with an acute perforated duodenal ulcer can be managed by selective vagotomy and pyloroplasty if the surgeon wishes to perform a definitive ulcer operation as well as close the perfora-

tion. The site of perforation is debrided and a pyloroplasty is performed. Usually a one-layer Weinberg–type pyloroplasty is easier to do than a Finney pyloroplasty. After thorough irrigation of the abdominal cavity to remove gastric and duodenal contents that might have leaked from the perforated ulcer, selective vagotomy is performed as previously described. The peritoneal cavity is closed without drainage.

Massive Bleeding from Duodenal Ulcer

Patients with persistent, massive hemorrhage from a duodenal ulcer can be managed by selective vagotomy and pyloroplasty. In these patients, the ulcer is usually located on the posterior aspect of the duodenum and can erode into the gastroduodenal artery. A longitudinal incision is made across the pylorus and is enlarged so that nonabsorbable sutures can be placed in the base of the duodenal ulcer to control bleeding. A Weinberg-type pyloroplasty is done followed by selective vagotomy. In elderly or poor-risk patients with massive bleeding, the truncal vagotomy technique might be preferred to the physiologically more ideal but time-consuming selective vagotomy. Truncal

vagotomy can be performed more rapidly than selective vagotomy and is better adapted to the emergency needs of patients with massive bleeding.

Obstruction Caused by Duodenal Ulcer

Patients requiring an operation for persistent pyloroduodenal obstruction can be managed by selective vagotomy and pyloroplasty. These patients usually have a cicatricial stenosis at or just distal to the pylorus. Chronic dilatation and elongation of the stomach often occur. After appropriate preoperative preparation of the patient with nasogastric suction, volume replacement, and electrolyte and nutritional correction, which can take several days, selective vagotomy with pyloroplasty is performed. If the patient has an elongated J-shaped stomach with hypertrophy or edema, or both, of the gastric wall, a Finney-type pyloroplasty is preferred to the Weinberg pyloroplasty, since the Finney pyloroplasty provides better drainage of the stomach in this type of patient.

Suggested Reading

Ami M, Doi R, Inove K, et al. The influence of vagotomy on basal and postprandial pancreatic secretion and plasma levels of gastrointestinal hormones in conscious rats. *Surg Gynecol Obstet* 177:577, 1993.

Christiansen J, Jensen HE, Ejby-Poulsen P, et al. Prospective controlled vagotomy trial for duodenal ulcer: Primary results, sequelae, acid secretion, and recurrence rates two to five years after operation. *Ann Surg* 193:49, 1981.

Emos S, Eriksson B. Twelve-year follow-up of a prospective, randomized trial of selective vagotomy with pyloroplasty and selective proximal vagotomy with and without pyloroplasty for the treatment of duodenal, pyloric and prepyloric ulcers. *Am J Surg* 164:4, 1992.

Franksson C. Selective abdominal vagotomy. *Acta Chir Scand* 96:409, 1948.

Griffith CA. Long-term results of selective vagotomy plus pyloroplasty: 12 to 17 year follow-up. *Am J Surg* 139:608, 1980.

Jackson RG. Anatomic study of the vagus nerves, with a technique of transabdominal selective gastric vagus resection. *Arch Surg* 57:333, 1948.

Laws HL, McKernam JB. Endoscopic management of peptic ulcer disease. *Ann Surg* 217:548, 1993.

Madsen P, Kronborg O. Recurrent ulcer 5 ½ to 8 years after highly selective vagotomy without drainage and selective vagotomy with pyloroplasty. *Scand J Gastroenterol* 15:193, 1980.

Meisner S, Hoffmann J, Jensen HE. Parietal cell vagotomy: A 23-year study. *Ann Surg* 220:164, 1994.

Prietrafitta JJ, Schultz LS, Graber JN, et al. Experimental transperitoneal laparoscopic pyloroplasty. *Surg Lap Endo* 2:104, 1992.

Sawyers JL, Scott HW, Jr, Edwards WH, et al. Comparative studies of the clinical effects of truncal and selective gastric vagotomy. *Am J Surg* 115:165, 1968.

Scott HW Jr, Sawyers JL, Gobble WG Jr, et al. Definitive surgical treatment in duodenal ulcer disease. In *Current Problems in Surgery*. Chicago: Year Book, 1968, (October).

Shaffer EA. The effect of vagotomy on gallbladder function and bile composition in man. *Ann Surg* 195:413, 1982.

Snyders D. Laparoscopic pyloroplasty for duodenal ulcer. *Br J Surg* 80:127, 1993.

Weinberg JA. Pyloroplasty and vagotomy for duodenal ulcer. In *Current Problems in Surgery*. Chicago: Year Book, 1964 (April).

EDITOR'S COMMENT

Selective vagotomy is the catalyst that moved surgeons to turn away from total parasympathetic (and partial sympathetic) denervation of the intraperitoneal organs after truncal or total vagotomy. It was only natural that the next step would be to contract further the scope of the vagal section to include only the fundus and corpus of the stomach.

Although the technique of selective gastric vagotomy was given considerable attention in the United Kingdom, Scandinavia, and the continent of Europe during the 1960s and early 1970s, scant notice was taken of it as a practical technique in the United States. Indeed, in the 1990s the two operations used most frequently in the United States for the treatment of duodenal ulcer are truncal vagotomy plus a drainage procedure or truncal vagotomy plus antrectomy. The number of proximal gastric vagotomies being performed is increasing, but the total still remains at less than 10 percent of all vagotomies performed.

I doubt that selective vagotomy plus a drainage procedure is used by 1 percent of surgeons in the United States. Dr. Sawyers has demonstrated that the procedure does cure the ulcer diathesis with a recurrent ulcer rate of 2 percent. Further, the mortality as reported by Dr. Sawyers should be either nil or no greater than 1 percent. Frankly, selective gastric vagotomy with pyloroplasty has considerable merit as a surgical approach to the treatment of duodenal ulcer. Note the lower recurrent ulcer rate when some type of pyloroduodenal drainage procedure was added to the operative procedure. This finding has also been observed by Holle (*Surg Gynecol Obstet* 167:271, 1988) and by Donahue and colleagues (see Chapter 79).

L.M.N.

77

Proximal Gastric Vagotomy

Keith A. Kelly   BaoLien Nguyen Tu

Proximal gastric vagotomy, also called highly selective vagotomy or parietal cell vagotomy, is now the preferred operation for the elective treatment of chronic duodenal ulcer. This operation interrupts the vagal branches to the acid-producing cells in the fundus and corpus of the stomach, but leaves intact the celiac and hepatic vagal branches and the vagal branches to the antrum and pylorus, the nerves of Latarjet. The reduction in acid secretion is profound and long lasting, and leads to the permanent healing of chronic duodenal ulcers in approximately 90 percent of patients. Additional advantages of this operation are that it is safe and that side effects, such as gastric stasis, bile reflux, and the dumping syndrome and diarrhea that commonly follow truncal vagotomy and "drainage operations" or gastrectomy, seldom occur after proximal gastric vagotomy. Although the technical aspects of proximal gastric vagotomy are more demanding than they are in truncal vagotomy, once mastered and when performed correctly, the advantages of proximal gastric vagotomy outweigh the disadvantages.

In this chapter, we will outline the indications for the operation and present our preoperative, operative, and postoperative management of patients undergoing the operation.

Indications for Operation

Proximal gastric vagotomy is indicated in patients who have chronic duodenal ulcer and who have failed adequate medical treatment for the condition. It is also some-

times the procedure of choice in stable patients with perforated or bleeding duodenal ulcer and in patients who present with gastric outlet obstruction from a stenosing duodenal ulcer. The operation has been used to treat chronic gastric ulcer, but this indication is more controversial.

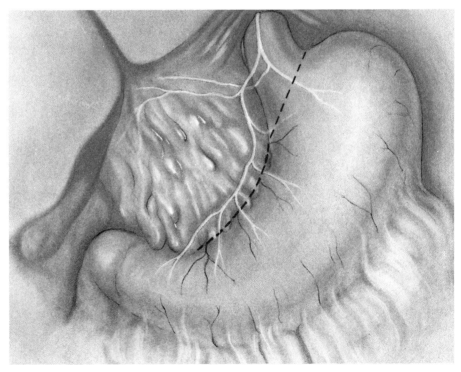

Fig. 77-1. *Anterior view of the stomach with the usual arrangement of the anterior nerve of Latarjet. The dotted line represents the line of the dissection. Note that the last major branch of the nerve of Latarjet is left intact and that the dissection starts 7 cm from the pylorus. Just below the esophagogastric junction, the dissection passes across the front of the stomach, well away from the point of origin of the hepatic branches of the anterior vagi. The line of the dissection passes toward the angle of His on the left-hand side of the esophagogastric junction. (From C Wastell. Proximal Gastric Vagotomy. In LM Nyhus and C Wastell [eds.], Surgery of the Stomach and Duodenum, 4th ed. Boston: Little, Brown, 1986. Reproduced with permission.)*

Preoperative Care

Preoperative antibiotics are usually unnecessary for patients undergoing proximal gastric vagotomy. However, in patients with bleeding or perforated duodenal ulcers and in patients with an obstructing duodenal ulcer when a pyloroplasty is also contemplated, a first-generation cephalosporin should be given before and during the operation to decrease the risk of postoperative intra-abdominal and wound infection. Pneumatic compression boots are applied to prevent deep venous thrombosis in the legs during the operation.

Operation

Positioning, Anesthesia, and Skin Preparation

The patient is placed supine on the operating table. The arms can be tucked along the side of the body or abducted 90 degrees from the body. The operating table is tilted slightly head-up to allow the abdominal viscera to be drawn downward by gravitational forces. General, endotracheal anesthesia with muscle relaxation is used. The patient's lower chest and abdomen are prepped with an antiseptic solution from the nipple line to the pubis. The upper drape should be placed well above the xiphoid.

Incision and Exposure

An upper abdominal midline incision is made from the xiphoid inferiorly, skirting around the umbilicus to the right and ending just below the umbilicus. The peritoneal cavity is entered and the round ligament divided. A "third arm" retractor is inserted to elevate the sternum and anterior costal margin, while a Balfour retractor is used to spread the wound. The liver is retracted anteriorly and to the right with a flat, broad abdominal retractor to expose the stomach, the duodenum, and the esophagogastric junction. Division of the left triangular ligament of the liver is not usually necessary to accomplish good exposure.

Exploration and Ulcer Management

The abdomen is carefully explored to confirm the diagnosis of chronic duodenal ulcer and to rule out other morbid conditions.

Perforated duodenal ulcers should be sutured closed, with the closure reenforced by a Graham patch, if necessary. Bleeding ulcers should be sutured transluminally via an anterior longitudinal duodenotomy

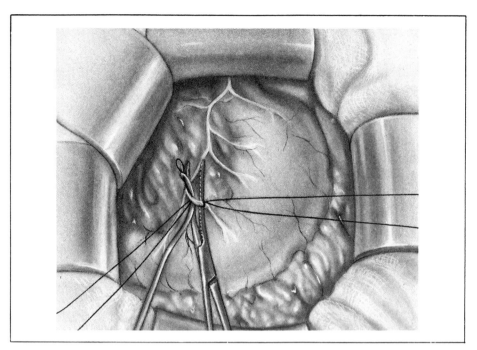

Fig. 77-2. The branches of the vagus nerve entering the lesser curvature of the stomach from the nerve of Latarjet are divided together with the accompanying vessels and ligated. (From C Wastell. Proximal Gastric Vagotomy. In LM Nyhus and C Wastell [eds.], Surgery of the Stomach and Duodenum, *4th ed. Boston: Little, Brown, 1986. Reproduced with permission.)*

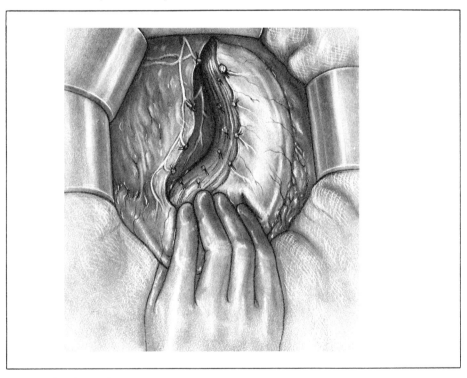

Fig. 77-3. Three layers of vessels enter the lesser curvature—an anterior, a posterior, and a rather irregular intermediate layer. The first part of the anterior dissection has been completed, and the anterior and intermediate vessels have been divided. Note that a nasogastric tube has been passed into the stomach and is being held by the first assistant; it is the most gentle and satisfactory way of drawing the stomach down into the field of vision. (From C Wastell. Proximal Gastric Vagotomy. In LM Nyhus and C Wastell [eds.], Surgery of the Stomach and Duodenum, *4th ed. Boston: Little, Brown, 1986. Reproduced with permission.)*

closed longitudinally. Stenosing ulcers at the pylorus or duodenum should be ruled out by passing a No. 28 French orogastric tube through the pylorus and into the distal second portion of the duodenum. An inflammatory narrowing can usually be easily dilated with the tube or by the index finger passed through a 2-cm anterior antrotomy. A fibrous stenosis should be managed by a Heineke–Mikulicz pyloroplasty, 7 cm in length, centered at the pylorus, or a duodenoplasty. Nonperforated, nonobstructing, nonbleeding ulcers need no operative management.

The orogastric tube used to size the duodenum should next be removed, and a No. 16 French nasogastric tube inserted. The nasogastric tube will facilitate the placement of traction on the stomach later in the operation.

The Vagotomy

The pylorus is identified and a point on the lesser curvature of the stomach 7 cm proximal to the pylorus is marked (Fig. 77-1). This point is where the vagotomy will begin. The vagal branches to the distal 7 cm of the stomach, the antrum, and pylorus are spared.

The first assistant now places the stomach on a stretch by pulling inferiorly on the stomach using the nasogastric tube as a stent. Care must be taken to identify and divide any anterior attachments of the greater omentum to the spleen before this step is performed. Otherwise, the splenic capsule can be torn.

Starting from the previously marked point on the stomach 7 cm proximal to the pylorus and working toward the esophagus, the blood vessels and nerves at the junction of the lesser omentum and the anterior gastric wall are divided and ligated with sutures (Fig. 77-2). It is imperative that these structures be divided close to the wall of the stomach to ensure preservation of the nerves of Latarjet. The nerves of Latarjet course in the lesser omentum approximately 1 cm lateral to the lesser curvature and parallel to it. The nerves of Latarjet and the lesser omentum are retracted to the right, while the stomach is retracted to the left. This dissection continues along the lesser curvature up to the esophagogastric junction.

Once the anterior layer of nerves and blood vessels are divided from the antrum

to the esophagogastric junction, a middle layer of nerves and blood vessels are similarly sought and divided, followed by a posterior layer (Fig. 77-3).

The gastrocolic ligament is next incised, and the lesser sac is entered. The stomach is now retracted upward and to the right to permit visualization of the posterior aspect of the lesser curvature of the stomach. The point 7 cm proximal to the pylorus is again identified on the posterior aspect of the stomach wall. Proximal to this point, any remaining neurovascular bundles entering the gastric corpus and fundus are divided (Fig. 77-3).

Dissection of the Esophagogastric Junction and Esophagus

The first assistant now gently pulls the proximal body of the stomach anteriorly and to the left to provide more exposure to the posterior gastric wall. The esophagogastric junction is freed from its attachments to the diaphragm and retroperitoneum, while retracting the vagal trunks posteriorly and to the right. The dissection is adequate only when the entire junction can be completely lifted anteriorly from its usual position. To avoid injuring the vagal trunks at this point, all dissection around the esophagus should be performed close to the esophageal wall (Fig. 77-4).

The distal 5 cm of esophagus is now freed, moving the anterior and posterior vagal trunks to the right. The distal esophagus is rotated with the fingers of the left hand, while a forceps held in the right hand is used to identify any additional branches coursing from the vagal trunks along the esophagus to the proximal stomach. These branches can be disrupted with the forceps or cut with a scissors or a scalpel. Bleeding can usually be controlled with the cautery.

The first and second short gastric arteries along the greater curvature of the stomach are next divided and any vagal branches from the posterior vagal trunk to the gas-

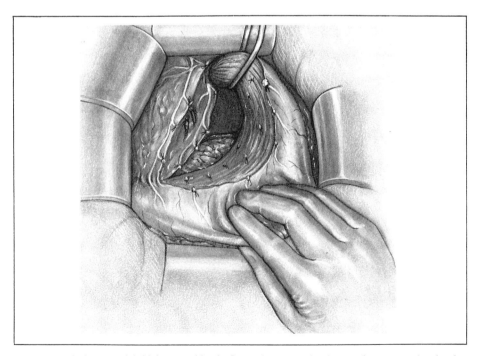

Fig. 77-4. With the stomach held downward by the first assistant grasping it around a nasogastric tube, the remainder of the dissection is performed from the front. When the esophagogastric junction is reached, a soft rubber drain is passed around the esophagus so that it can be held up and to the left. This step makes the division of the last few strands of tissue passing to the right-hand side of the esophagus easier. It is essential to lay bare at least 5 cm of the esophageal muscle and to visualize the posterior vagus as it enters the abdomen between the crura during this part of the dissection. (From C Wastell. Proximal Gastric Vagotomy. In LM Nyhus and C Wastell [eds.], Surgery of the Stomach and Duodenum, 4th ed. Boston: Little, Brown, 1986. Reproduced with permission.)

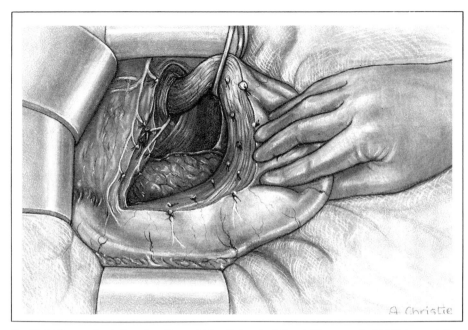

Fig. 77-5. The completed dissection. (From C Wastell. Proximal Gastric Vagotomy. In LM Nyhus and C Wastell [eds.], Surgery of the Stomach and Duodenum, *4th ed. Boston: Little, Brown, 1986. Reproduced with permission.)*

tric fundus and corpus in this region (the nerves of Grassi) are sought and severed. Because recurrent vagal fibers can course along the right gastroepiploic vessels from the antrum to the corpus, these vessels are also divided and ligated at the gastric antrocorporal junction. This step completes the vagotomy (Fig. 77-5).

Completion of the Operation

The lesser curvature of the stomach, the esophagogastric junction, and the distal esophagus should now be carefully inspected for bleeding, and the lesser curvature of the stomach examined for areas of ischemia. Bleeding should be stopped and ischemic areas along the lesser curvature managed by approximating the adjacent anterior and posterior walls of the stomach over the ischemic area with inverting sutures.

The abdomen is irrigated clean with a warm isotonic saline. The abdominal incision is closed without drainage.

Postoperative Care

The nasogastric tube is removed after the patient has recovered from the anesthetic. Postoperative antibiotics are unnecessary.

Oral intake is withheld until postoperative ileus has resolved, which usually occurs by the first or second postoperative day.

Suggested Reading

Amdrup E, Jensen HE. Selective vagotomy of the parietal cell mass preserving innervation of the undrained antrum. *Gastroenterology* 59:522, 1970.

Goligher JA. A technique for highly selective (parietal cell or proximal gastric) vagotomy for duodenal ulcer. *Br J Surg* 61:337, 1974.

Griffith CA, Harkins HN. Partial gastric vagotomy. An experimental study. *Gastroenterology* 32:96, 1957.

Hallenbeck GA, Gleysteen JJ, Aldrete JS, et al. Proximal gastric vagotomy: Effects of two operative techniques on clinical and gastric secretory results. *Ann Surg* 184:435, 1976.

Hom S, Sarr MG, Kelly KA, et al. Postoperative gastric atony after vagotomy for obstructing peptic ulcer. *Am J Surg* 157: 282, 1989.

Johnston D, Wilkinson AR. Highly selective vagotomy without a drainage procedure in the treatment of duodenal ulcer. *Br J Surg* 57:289, 1970.

Johnston D, Lyndon PJ, Smith RB, et al. Highly selective vagotomy without a drainage procedure in the treatment of haemorrhage, perforation and pyloric stenosis due to peptic ulcer. *Br J Surg* 60:790, 1973.

Johnston D, Blackett RL. A new look at selective vagotomies. *Am J Surg* 156:416, 1988.

Miedema BW, Torres PR, Farnell MB, et al. Proximal gastric vagotomy in the emergency treatment of bleeding duodenal ulcer. *Am J Surg* 161: 64, 1991.

Nyhus LM. Proximal gastric vagotomy: Gold or dross. *Arch Surg* 119:1373, 1983.

Shirmer BD. Current status of proximal gastric vagotomy. *Ann Surg* 209:131, 1989.

Soper NJ, Kelly KA, van Heerden JA, et al. Long-term clinical results after proximal gastric vagotomy. *Surg Gynecol Obstet* 169:488, 1989.

Wastell C, Nyhus LM, Donahue PE (eds.). *Surgery of the Esophagus, Stomach, and Small Intestine.* Boston: Little, Brown, 1995.

EDITOR'S COMMENT

Proximal gastric vagotomy (PGV) continues to be the Cinderella operation of surgical gastroenterologists. Conceptually, it should be the answer to our search for an operation with low morbidity and low mortality that removes the stigmata of duodenal ulcer disease from our patients. There is no question that PGV can be performed with totally acceptable short- and long-term morbidity and surgical mortality. An ever-increasing rate of ulcer recurrence was reported in the world literature and was a concern to all of us. When this specter first presented, we were convinced that it was a matter of inadequate or imperfect surgical technique, particularly when subsequent reports from the same authors showed a marked decrease in recurrence following a change in technical approach.

PGV reminds me of another Cinderella operation, namely, simple gastrojejunostomy as first reported by Wolfler in 1881. This procedure also had much lower morbidity and mortality than the subtotal gastrectomies performed then. More important, it cured essentially every patient with duodenal ulcer disease, at least temporarily.

We know that this situation was not the end of the story. Forty-four years later, R. Lewisohn of the Mt. Sinai Hospital in New York City reported a 35 percent incidence rate of gastrojejunal or stomal ulcer (*Surg Gynecol Obstet* 40:70, 1925). It is my contention that 100 patients with simple gastroenterostomy followed for 100 years would have a 100 percent incidence rate of stomal ulcer. We now know that simple gastro-enterostomy is an intrinsically ulcerogenic procedure (Harkins et al. *Arch Surg* 79:981, 1959). I doubt if such a hypothesis will be developed for PGV, that is, that it is an intrinsically ulcerogenic operation.

The doyen of PGV (selective proximal vagotomy), Dr. Fritz Holle of Munich, and his colleagues have studied the patients they operated on from 1969 to 1983 (*Surg Gynecol Obstet* 167:271, 1988). They regularly performed a pyloroplasty at the same operation. Ulcer disease recurred in 6.3 percent of the patients operated on for duodenal ulcer disease and in 8.1 percent of the patients undergoing operations for gastric ulcers. The authors believed the recurrences were the result of technical error, inadequate vagotomy, and incomplete drainage.

The use of pyloroplasty by Holle's group reminds me of the extended proximal vagotomy with drainage practiced in our clinic (see Chap. 79). Our low recurrent ulcer rates after PGV should alert clinics with recurrent ulcer rates greater than 10 percent to consider the main variations in technique proposed by Donahue, namely, regular severance of the gastroepiploic nerve, and more frequent use of pyloroplasty ad modum Holle, Donahue, or Barroso.

L.M.N.

78

Laparoscopic Proximal Gastric Vagotomy and Other Procedures for Peptic Ulcer Disease

Michel Gagner

Several laparoscopic vagotomy techniques have been described in the literature. All reproduce the various approaches used in open surgery. Dubois popularized truncal vagotomies by laparoscopy or thoracoscopy. Although only immediate follow-ups are available, the results of the technique have been good so far. The technique is easy to perform and produces no major complications. Thoracoscopic truncal vagotomy can also be done by single puncture. On the other hand, Katkhouda and Mouiel designed a procedure combining laparoscopic posterior truncal vagotomy with anterior seromyotomy that follows, although not entirely, Taylor's open approach. Anterior seromyotomy is meant to reproduce highly selective anterior vagotomy. Its natural progression is posterior truncal vagotomy with highly selective anterior vagotomy.

Laws has proposed thoracoscopic vagotomy after failed open drainage for recurrent ulcer disease. Perforated duodenal ulcers have even been successfully treated with a laparoscopic closure technique. An endoscopic stapler has been used on the anterior gastric wall along the lesser curvature with associated posterior truncal vagotomy to achieve a quick, highly selective vagotomy. Vagotomy with drainage or pyloroplasty has also been designed and reported. However, it can lead to diarrhea and other complications related to truncal vagotomy. Ultimately, highly selective laparoscopic vagotomy appears to create fewer long-term complications, and, if it fails, there is time to perform truncal vagotomy with a drainage procedure laparoscopically.

Pyloroplasty with a Weinberg- or Heineke–Mikulicz–type stapler has also been recommended. A comparative study of highly selective laparoscopic vagotomy, posterior truncal laparoscopic vagotomy, and highly selective anterior vagotomy was performed by Dudai. Operating time was similar and averaged 120 to 150 minutes. Hospital stay and return to activities were not different. However, there were more complications with the posterior truncal than with the highly selective anterior approach. These complications were mainly diarrhea, transient delayed gastric emptying, and pyloric spasm. This nonrandomized study reported a less complicated course with highly selective complete laparoscopic vagotomy than with posterior truncal laparoscopic vagotomy.

In summary, laparoscopic surgery always returns to the best procedure done conventionally, which really makes sense. Randomized prospective trials should be performed in the future to compare open and laparoscopic methods.

Indications for Laparoscopic Surgical Therapy

Although the annual incidence of duodenal ulcer is in the range of 1 to 3 per 1000, there is a definite trend to less surgical intervention to remedy this disease. Because of the *Helicobacter pylori* hypothesis and treatment, even fewer patients will be candidates for these laparoscopic procedures. More often, surgical therapy is reserved for severe and emergent complications of peptic ulcer disease.

More than 90 percent of patients with duodenal ulcers and 70 percent with gastric ulcers become hosts to gram-negative spiral bacteria. Mucosal invasion triggers an inflammatory response that varies from duodenitis or gastritis to full ulcers. Medical management should always be the first line of treatment with H_2-receptor antagonists or H^+, K-ATPase inhibitors. If *H. pylori* is identified by serodiagnosis or gastric biopsies, treatment to eradicate the bacteria seems reasonable, especially if there is a recurrence after triple therapy involving metronidazole, bismuth, and tetracycline. Cirrhosis, chronic pancreatitis, alcohol abuse, chronic renal failure, and some hematologic abnormalities are associated disorders that increase the frequency of peptic ulcer disease. Upper endoscopy is usually performed to confirm the diagnosis. There might be a need for an upper GI barium series if partial obstruction is seen or malignancy suspected.

Therefore, the indications remain the same as in open surgery, namely failure of medical therapy as mentioned above. The choice of operation should be the least morbid for the patient. To the extent possible, it should be pylorus-preserving surgery with low (zero) mortality and very few side effects. On the other side of the spectrum, partial two-thirds gastrectomy is now rarely indicated. We favor highly selective laparoscopic or proximal gastric vagotomy or if neither is suitable, laparoscopic truncal vagotomy with pyloroplasty. For patients with pyloric stenosis, laparoscopic vagotomy with pyloroplasty is recommended. Alternatively, highly selective laparoscopic vagotomy with pyloroplasty or laparoscopic vagotomy with laparoscopic gastroenterostomy is advisable when there is complete obstruction. If perforation occurs, a laparoscopic omental patch or round ligament patch with simple closure followed by peritoneal lavage is suitable most of the time. If there is sufficient time and the general condition of the patient allows it, a more definite procedure could be performed with minimal peritoneal contamination.

With bleeding ulcers, the aim is to control the bleeding and to save the patient's life. Endoscopic treatment is initiated first, and if unsuccessful then a laparoscopic technique can be tried. However, if the surgeon is not well equipped with a variety of laparoscopic instruments for retraction and suturing, or sufficiently agile with intracorporeal suturing, a quick open technique is preferable. This technique could be pylorotomy with suturing the ulcer, or pyloroplasty and truncal vagotomy if the patient is frail and elderly. Otherwise, a healthy candidate can tolerate highly selective vagotomy after over-sewing the ulcer through a duodenotomy followed by a pyloroplasty.

In general, contraindications to laparoscopic techniques include pregnancy, prior extensive abdominal operations, Zollinger-Ellison syndrome, severe coagulopathies, portal hypertension, and psychiatric instability.

Surgical Technique
Highly Selective Laparoscopic Vagotomy

After proper selection according to strict criteria, patients should be examined preoperatively with barium studies, esophagogastroduodenoscopy, *H. pylori* cultures, stomach biopsy, and serum gastrin assessment. Basal and maximal acid output might be evaluated if patients are on a research protocol.

Once the operative mode is chosen, informed consent should include a discussion of the technique (e. g., trocar position, operating time, and nasogastric tube), possible complications (e. g., diarrhea, delay in gastric emptying, perforation, bleeding, and so forth), the likelihood of conversion to an open method, and ulcer recurrence.

Once anesthetized, the patient should be properly positioned. If the "French" position is used then the patient's legs must be spread apart and not necessarily flexed on stirrups (Fig. 78-1A). A special modified orthopedic table can be used for this purpose because it has the advantage of keeping the patient's legs apart and nonflexed, minimizing the risk of nerve compression or injuries. Both arms are preferably positioned along side the body to allow free movement of both assistants. Right and left monitors are useful on both sides of the patient's head at the level of the surgeon's eyes. A slightly reverse Trendelenburg position of 15 to 30 degrees is helpful to bring the stomach and transverse colon downward with a left tilt for better exposure of the lesser curvature. The standard patient position is also suitable, and the surgeon, instead of being between the legs of the patient, operates from the left side, facing the left lobe of the liver (Fig. 78-1B). The camera operator is on the right, and an assistant is beside the surgeon at the left shoulder level.

A nasogastric tube is inserted by the anesthetist and a Foley catheter positioned for urinary output during the procedure and while the patient stays in the recovery room.

Trocar positioning is shown in Fig. 78-2. Trocars of 10-mm diameter are inserted in

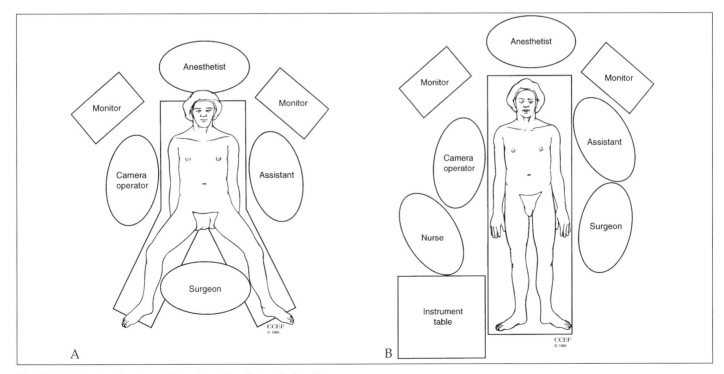

Fig. 78-1. Positioning of patients. A. French position. B. Standard position.

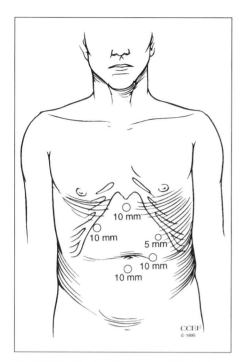

Fig. 78-2. Positioning of trocars: umbilical, left paramedian, right subcostal, epigastric, and left subcostal.

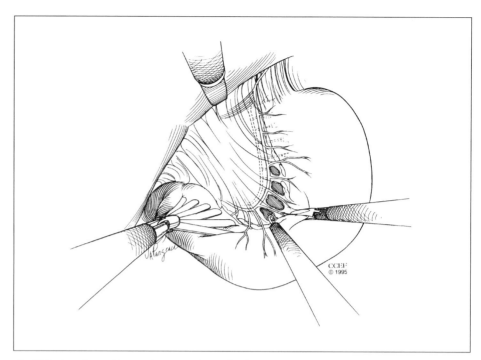

Fig. 78-3. Anterior marking on the antrum (most distal point of dissection).

the umbilicus, left paramedian, right sub-costal, and epigastrium. An additional 5-mm trocar can be inserted in the left sub-costal area. The camera is handled in the umbilicus with the left lobe of the liver re-tractor in the right subcostal port. The sur-geon's operative port for the right hand is the left paramedian with the epigastric port serving the left hand. The 5-mm port is handled by the surgeon's assistant to re-tract the greater curvature of the stomach laterally or inferiorly.

Laparoscopic vagotomy requires almost no special instruments apart from the basic set used for laparoscopic cholecystectomy. Certainly, it is advantageous to use a lap-aroscope of 10 mm with a 30- or 45-degree angle for a view from above and at differ-ent angles. A 10-mm atraumatic liver retractor is important to lift the left lobe of the liver. This retractor could be a simple 10-mm rigid plastic rod or a fan-type re-tractor with large fingers. Any retractor with a sharp end or corner is forbidden since it will lead to liver capsule or dia-phragm damage. A multiple clip applier can decrease operating time but has the disadvantage of being more bulky at the tip, rendering the application of clips less precise. The use of bipolar hooks can speed up highly selective vagotomy on smaller vessels, and ultrasonic instru-

ments can do the same. However, damage from the tip has not been well studied, and there is a possibility of injuring the main vagus trunk or the nerves of Latarjet. An ultrasonic scalpel has been used success-fully on smaller vessels of the greater cur-vature or on short gastric vessels to mo-bilize the gastric fundus.

After proper draping, insufflation is started via an infraumbilical incision with a Veress needle until intra-abdominal pres-sure reaches 15 mm Hg of carbon dioxide. A 10-mm trocar is introduced followed by a 10-mm laparoscope. After proper posi-tioning of the table, the other trocars are inserted under videoscopic vision. The left paramedian 10-mm port is introduced, fol-lowed by the 10-mm trocars in the umbi-licus and right subcostal areas. Finally, the additional 5-mm port is placed in the mid-clavicular left subcostal area, approxi-mately one finger below the costal margin. The liver retractor is given to the camera operator, and the left lobe of the liver is gently retracted upward and toward the right. General inspection of the abdominal cavity is performed to eliminate concomi-tant digestive pathology. The anterior wall of the stomach should be visible and cleared from any adhesions. With a two-handed technique, the surgeon's left hand uses a 5-mm dissector through the epigas-

tric port with a 5-mm curved scissors and cautery in the right hand through the left paramedian trocar. Of course, these trocars are equipped with reducers.

On several occasions, the triangular liga-ment of the liver has been divided to op-timally expose the phrenoesophageal membrane. The scissors and cautery are used for this task. Before anything is done, the nerve anatomy is well identified by magnification with video-endoscopic equipment. The several branches of crow's foot, nerves of Latarjet, and hepatic branch of the anterior vagus can all be readily identified in a nonobese patient. Later, both vagi are identified. Measurements from the pyloric vein of Mayo with a graded palpator (every centimeter) can be taken to mark the most distal point of dis-section with the cautery, that is, 6 cm from the pylorus (Fig. 78-3). This can encompass one branch of crow's foot.

A soft bowel clamp 5 mm in diameter is the best instrument to handle the stomach without creating a serosal tear. It is posi-tioned on the middle of the anterior wall of the stomach through the left subcostal port, and traction is exerted downward and laterally. The assistant must be vigi-lant at all times since the stomach can tear accidentally. Following this maneuver, the surgeon's left hand gently grasps each of the parietal cell branches of the anterior vagus from crow's foot to the distal esophagus. The surgeon's right hand alternates between a Maryland 5-mm dissector to a 10-mm right-angle dissector to a 10-mm clip applier and back to a 5-mm curved scissors (Fig. 78-4). This process is repeated until division of all branches is completed. The same maneuver is repeated for the posterior branches (Fig. 78-5). Dissection is continued by liberating the right side of the esophagus for at least 6 cm from the gastroesophageal junction. The anterior and posterior vagi are identified and left intact. They are retracted medially away from the esophageal wall. Once the right side of the esophagus has been cleared, the anterior wall is next, with the phrenoesophageal membrane being divided with a scissors (Fig. 78-6). The an-

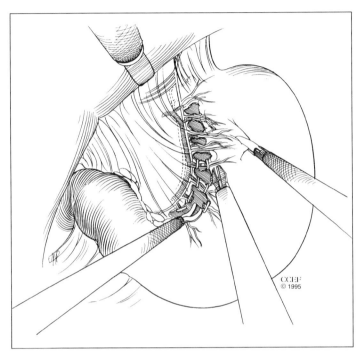

Fig. 78-4. Anterior highly selective vagotomy.

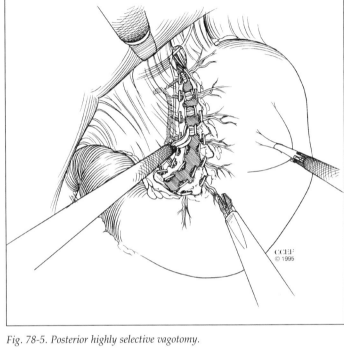

Fig. 78-5. Posterior highly selective vagotomy.

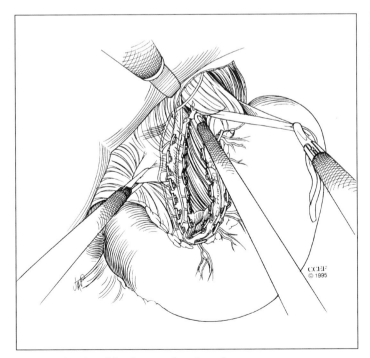

Fig. 78-6. Opening of the phrenoesophageal membrane.

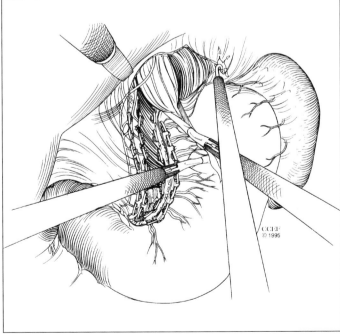

Fig. 78-7. Preservation and identification of the vagal trunks. Distal esophageal mobilization.

78. Laparoscopic Proximal Gastric Vagotomy and Other Procedures for Peptic Ulcer Disease **899**

terior esophagus is then cleared for 6 cm from the gastroesophageal junction.

The surgeon retracts the esophagus laterally with a dissector, and the left hand creates a 1-cm window behind the esophagus over the left crura until it reaches the other side. A 10-cm Penrose drain 1 cm in diameter is introduced via the left paramedian trocar and placed around the distal esophagus. Both ends are clipped anteriorly and the drain used to exert anterior and lateral traction on the distal esophagus to ease posterior dissection from both cruras. With the assistant grasping the Penrose drain from the left subcostal port, the surgeon uses a two-handed technique to complete the esophageal clearance posteriorly. The lesser sac should already have been entered and adhesions from the pancreas and both cruras divided. It is particularly important not to enter the lesser sac medial to both vagi, leaving intact the hepatic and celiac branches. Thus, the peritoneal fold over the left caudate lobe should be intact.

The left side of the esophagus is then completely cleared from the left crus for 6 cm from the gastroesophageal junction (Fig. 78-7). The next step clears the angle of His. The assistant gently grasps the fundus of the stomach close to the angle, and the sur-

geon's left hand holds the Penrose drain. Vessels are often present and must be divided with clips. Short gastric vessels are divided from the fundus. The left diaphragm and the gastrosplenic ligaments are divided with titanium clips or an ultrasonic device. Countertraction with forceps is gently applied by the assistant on the lateral side of this ligament. A right-angle instrument is often used to isolate and perforate the peritoneal folds between each vessel. At least 10 cm of fundus and the greater curvature are cleared in this manner (Fig. 78-8). The patient is often tilted more toward the right in order to place the gastrosplenic ligament under some tension.

After completion of the greater curvature, the Penrose drain is extracted and clips removed (Fig. 78-9). Each site of the operative field is copiously irrigated with saline (heparin, 5000 units per liter) to determine if there is any bleeding. The liver retractor is removed and the inferior capsule of the left liver lobe, the triangular ligament, and left diaphragm are inspected for damage. All cannulas are removed, carbon dioxide evacuated, and all 10-mm fascial defects closed with absorbable 2–0 or 0 sutures with a curved needle. The skin edges are approximated with 4–0 running subcuticular sutures.

Postoperative Care

The nasogastric tube is left in place until the next day, but the Foley catheter is removed in the recovery room. A liquid diet is given and progressively advanced within 3 days. Patients require narcotics either intramuscularly or intravenously via a PCA pump for 24 hours. Oral codeine or a similar type of analgesic is used afterward. Patient discharge is dictated by the judgment of the surgical staff and not according to a precise scheduled day for discharge. In our surgical practice, discharge is usually on the third or fourth postoperative day. During the observation period, patients are examined for signs of gastric perforation, peritonitis, acute gastric distention, delay in gastric emptying, or gastric bleeding. If bleeding occurs, it is usually minor, presenting in the form of melena, and will respond to conservative medical management. A nasogastric tube can be reinserted if there is persistent vomiting or acute gastric atonia. Of course, Gastrografin swallow is recommended and if perforation is suspected, peritonitis warrants emergency laparoscopy or laparotomy. Late complications, such as dysphagia, esophageal stenosis, delay in gastric emptying, or ulcer recurrence, should be investigated thoroughly.

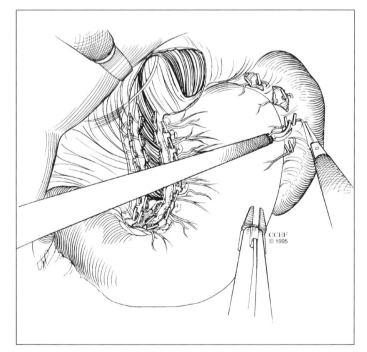

Fig. 78-8. Mobilization of the gastric fundus with ligature of the proximal short gastric vessels.

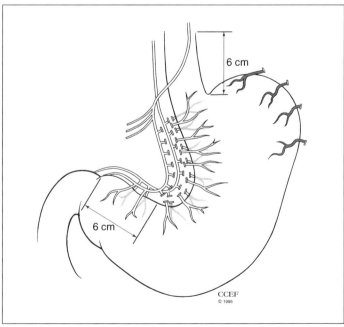

Fig. 78-9. Final aspect of highly selective vagotomy.

More specific to the laparoscopic technique, subcutaneous emphysema can be encountered, but it is usually benign. On a postoperative chest x-ray, this condition can be seen in the mediastinum because of distal esophageal dissection. Occasionally, a patient might have higher endtidal carbon dioxide, and ventilation frequency has to be increased to evacuate and decrease $PaCO_2$. The trocar wounds can cause bleeding and hematomas, usually in the epigastrium or paramedian line. Often, a branch of the epigastric artery is severed, which requires a larger skin opening with direct suturing. Cautery injuries or small bowel lacerations are rare but can occur after this procedure. Most often, a liver laceration from the liver retractor itself can be seen and controlled by laparoscopic monopolar cautery of the liver fracture line.

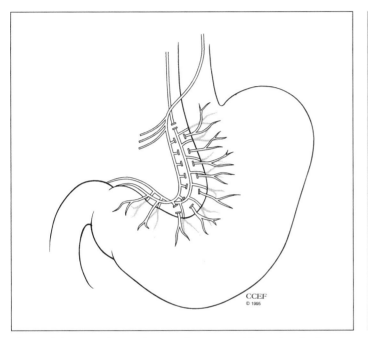

Fig. 78-10. *Laparoscopic posterior truncal vagotomy with anterior selective vagotomy.*

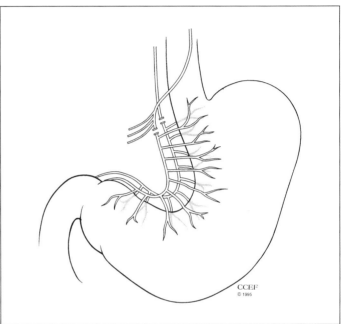

Fig. 78-11. *Bilateral truncal vagotomy with pyloroplasty.*

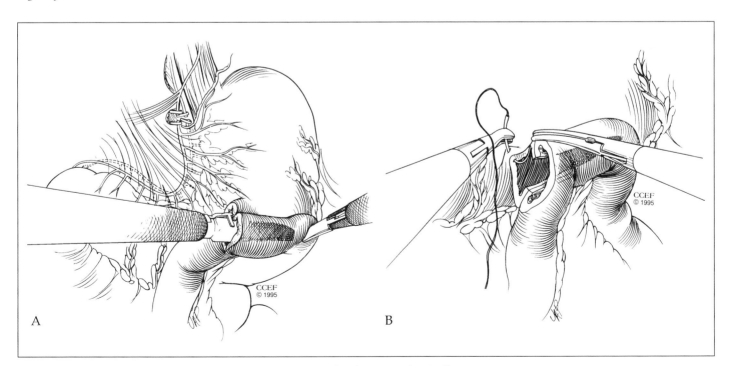

Fig. 78-12. *Laparoscopic gastroenterostomy. A. Creation of enterotomy with endoscopic staplers. B. Closure of enterotomy.*

Other Procedures

Laparoscopic posterior truncal vagotomy with anterior highly selective vagotomy is performed with the same trocar positioning (Fig. 78-10). Highly selective vagotomy is done first, followed by posterior truncal vagotomy by opening the phrenoesophageal membrane with hook cautery or scissors with cautery. The esophagus is then dissected medially from the right crus to expose the posterior vagus. A vagectomy of 1 cm is performed with medium-large titanium clips.

Bilateral truncal vagotomy with pyloroplasty is also performed with the same trocar positioning (Fig. 78-11). Vagotomies are undertaken first with clips, then pyloroplasty is done as with the open procedure. Closure is longitudinal with a running 2–0 silk suture from the superior and inferior borders. If laparoscopic gastroenterostomy is preferred, an endoscopic linear stapler of 30 or 35 cm is fired twice between the antimesenteric side of the proximal jejunum and the greater curvature of the stomach posteriorly (Fig. 78-12A). The enterotomy is then closed with a running 2–0 silk suture after the second cartridge has been fired (Fig. 78-12B). A 12-mm trocar is necessary to insert the stapler so the left paramedian trocar is changed for this purpose.

Suggested Reading

Bailey RW, Flowers JL, Graham SM, et al. Combined laparoscopic cholecystectomy and selective vagotomy. *Surg Laparosc Endosc* 1:45, 1991.

Dubois F. Vagotomies—Laparoscopic or thoracoscopic approach. *Endoscopic Surgery & Applied Technologies* 20:100, 1994.

Dudai M. Laparoscopic modified extended highly selective vagotomy (LMEHSV). Personal communication.

Hannon JK, Snow LL, Weinstein LS. Linear gastrectomy: An endoscopic staple-assisted anterior highly selective vagotomy combined with posterior truncal vagotomy for treatment of peptic ulcer disease. *Surg Laparosc Endosc* 2:254, 1992.

Katkhouda N, Mouiel J. A new technique of surgical treatment in chronic duodenal ulcer without laparotomy with video-endoscopy. *Am J Surg* 161:361, 1991.

Kum CK, Goh P. Laparoscopic vagotomy: A new tool in the management of duodenal ulcer disease. *Br J Surg* 79:977, 1992.

Laws HL, McKernan JB. Endoscopic management of peptic ulcer disease. *Ann Surg* 217:548, 1993.

Laws HL, Naughton MJ, McKernan JB. Thoracoscopic vagectomy for recurrent peptic ulcer disease. *Surg Laparosc Endosc* 2:24, 1992.

McGuire HH, Schubert ML. Laparoscopic treatment of duodenal ulcer: A plea for clinical trials. *Gastroenterology* 101:1744, 1991.

Mouret P, Francois Y, Vignol J, et al. Laparoscopic treatment of perforated peptic ulcer. *Br J Surg* 77:1006, 1990.

Nathanson LK, Easter DW, Cuschieri A. Laparoscopic repair/peritoneal toilet of perforated duodenal ulcer. *Surg Endosc* 4:232, 1990.

Peitrafitta JJ, Shultz LS, Graber JN, et al. Laser laparoscopic vagotomy and pyloromyotomy. *Gastrointest Endosc* 37:338, 1991.

Schurr MO, Buess GL. Wittmoser's technique of thoracoscopic sympathectomy and vagotomy. *Endoscopy Surgery & Applied Technologies* 1:266, 1993.

Snyders D. Laparoscopic pyloroplasty for duodenal ulcer. *Br J Surg* 80:127, 1993.

Taylor TV, MacLeod DAD, Gunn AA, et al. Anterior lesser curves seromyotomy and (posterior truncal vagotomy in the treatment of chronic ulcer disease. *Lancet* ii:846, 1982.

EDITOR'S COMMENT

Laparoscopic vagotomy is one of the newer extensions of minimally invasive operations. The technical approach is well covered in this presentation. Can a complete (total) vagotomy be performed? The devotees of the method believe that because of better visualization, completeness of vagotomy is more likely than with the open approach. Unfortunately, it will be a number of years before we will know the answer. Please remember that the average time interval between performance of simple gastrojejunostomy for the treatment of duodenal ulcer and the development of a recurrent stomal gastrojejunal ulcer was 11 years.

Since our laparoscopic surgeons are in the neophyte stage of this method of treatment of duodenal ulcer, I make a plea for one or more of the investigators to include an arm treatment in each prospective randomized study, namely the extended highly selective vagotomy plus pyloromyotomy of Donahue (see Chap. 79).

For this or any other type of vagotomy used for the treatment of duodenal ulcer, the parasympathic innervation to each parietal cell must be sectioned. This challenge exists for all vagotomists. Parenthetically, the complete severance of the posterior trunk of the vagus nerve to facilitate laparoscopic vagotomy is unfortunate. This maneuver parasympathetically denervates the pancreas, the entire small intestine, and the colon to its mid-transverse part; section of this major vagal trunk destroys the entire concept on which selective vagotomy techniques were promulgated. I am hopeful that a technique can be devised wherein the extragastric branches of the right posterior nerve can be preserved.

L.M.N.

79

Extended Proximal Vagotomy with Drainage

Philip E. Donahue

An ideal operative procedure for obstructing duodenal ulcer must allow adequate gastric emptying, control the primary ulcer diathesis, and be free of late complications. Surgeons disagree, however, about which operation best achieves these ends. Extended proximal vagotomy with drainage (EPV-D) satisfies all requirements for the ideal procedure. The most distinct advantage of EPV-D over vagotomy with resection is that the late complications of gastric resection, which occur in up to 25 percent of patients, are largely avoided. Also, and of extreme importance, the primary ulcer problem is well treated by this approach. In a 20-year period, more than 80 patients have been treated with an average follow-up period of more than 5 years, and none has had a recurrent ulcer.

Proximal gastric vagotomy with drainage (PGV-D) was first used in our clinic in 1968, after the initial experimental description of the procedure in 1957 in Seattle, and the first successful clinical use of this procedure in Munich. Since 1975 the technique of extended proximal vagotomy described herein has evolved as a direct result of research in our laboratory and elsewhere. The scientific basis for extended vagotomy has been placed on firm scientific footing and it can now be considered the gold standard. Proximal gastric vagotomy (PGV) as described in most texts can be considered an earlier version of the definitive operation.

The techniques of drainage used for obstructing ulcers have included all the possible variations, but, of late, the anterior hemipylorectomy has been my favorite approach. I have adopted it as the routine procedure, since it appears to work better than the alternatives. Laboratory evidence

proving the superiority of anterior hemipylorectomy is not yet available, but if patient satisfaction is a valuable criterion, there is no question that this procedure is the optimal form of gastric drainage.

Patient Selection

Drainage procedures are combined with proximal vagotomy when there is objective evidence of gastric outlet obstruction or when there is evidence of pyloric thickening at the time of the primary operation. Most of my patients have had ulcer disease for more than 5 years, and most have had persistent or intermittent vomiting and weight loss. Endoscopic examinations with biopsy of the pyloric mucosa are performed preoperatively in all patients to rule out occult malignant tumors. In the past, the passage of an endoscope past an area of gastric outlet deformity or stenosis was used to rule out the diagnosis of functional pyloric stenosis. Modern endoscopes, however, are small enough (7–9 mm outside diameter) and flexible enough to pass through a partially obstructed pyloric channel, and it is no longer advisable to consider a pylorus that admits an endoscope a functionally normal one. Since anterior pylorectomy does not seem to have the complications associated with traditional pyloroplasty, it is more logical to use this operation liberally whenever the question of pyloric thickening or stenosis is present.

The typical patient has a long history of duodenal ulcer, usually treated for up to 10 years with a combination of medications, including H_2-receptor antagonists after 1976, dietary alterations, and avoid-

ance of noxious stimuli, including cigarette smoking when possible. Patients presenting with obstruction de novo, however, are offered operative treatment without any preliminary medical therapy.

Patients with pyloric obstruction secondary to pancreatic or gastric carcinoma might not have a definite diagnosis of cancer until operative dissection has been performed. The intraoperative diagnosis of unsuspected cancer occurs in approximately 10 percent of patients with outlet obstruction.

Gastric emptying studies with test meals are not yet sensitive enough to be a useful clinical tool. Similarly, the saline loading test and a barium meal cannot clarify the presence or absence of obstruction or pyloric disease in all patients. When an operation is indicated for persistent ulcer disease in a patient with some features of obstruction or with evidence of pyloric scarring, it seems advisable to perform pylorectomy as a definitive means of dealing with a serious potential problem. This statement is especially true in light of the paucity of long-term complications encountered after this operative approach. Further, the established high recurrence rates of pyloric channel ulcer treated by proximal gastric vagotomy alone justify the liberal use of a physiologic drainage procedure.

Surgical Technique
Extended Proximal Vagotomy

Patients who no longer require decompression of the stomach for 4 to 6 days before the operation; instead, they can be operated on at any convenient time. All receive antibiotic prophylaxis (one dose before and two doses after the operation) with cephazolin or cefoxitin.

Extended proximal vagotomy (EPV) consists of the following maneuvers, which denervate the acid-secreting corpus and minimize the chance of late reinnervation. The essential operative steps include:

1. Periesophageal dissection baring 5 to 6 cm of the distal esophagus (Fig. 79-1).
2. Baring of the lesser curve of the stomach from the cardia to the antrum (Fig. 79-2). (followed by re-approximation of the serosa of the lesser curve) (see Fig. 79-6).

3. Division of the gastropancreatic fold from the lesser curve to the first short gastric vessel (Fig. 79-3).
4. Division of the nerves of the greater curvature (right and left gastroepiploic nerves) (Fig. 79-4).
5. Dissection of the heel of the crow's foot, including the "instep" of the crow's foot (Fig. 79-5).

The endoscopic Congo red test (ECRT) was initially found useful at the end of the operation, followed by additional dissection and a second test if evidence of residual innervation was seen. This test is not performed at present because of difficulty obtaining Congo red dye labeled safe for human use.

The dissection along the esophagus is best performed in the periesophageal space, avoiding excessive traction on the esophagus. Attempts to isolate the anterior and posterior nerves are unnecessary and often lead to hematomas, which do not facilitate precise dissection. No attempt is made to visualize vagal trunks, unless previous operations or inflammation lead the surgeon to question whether a nerve trunk might be dangerously close to the gastropancreatic fold. In such situations, it is possible to identify the nerves by the usual methods such as traction on the left gastric artery (a maneuver that stretches the posterior trunk, allowing it to be palpated near the crus of the diaphragm) or traction on the hepatic vagi (a maneuver that stretches

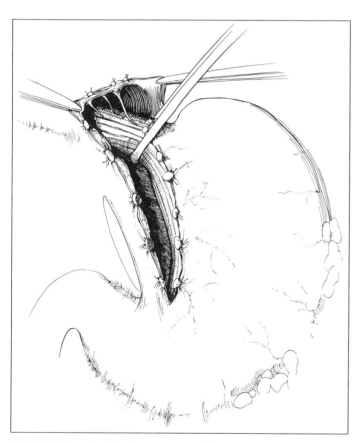

Fig. 79-1. Dissection of the lesser curvature of the stomach as shown results in division of the vagal and sympathetic nerve branches and the blood vessels that supply the proximal lesser curvature of the stomach. Dissection begins proximal to the crow's foot and proceeds toward the esophagus. After the gastric attachments of the phrenoesophageal ligament are incised and elevated (shown elevated by the two forceps), the periesophageal space becomes evident. This potential space is "developed" by blunt dissection along the esophageal wall. It is traversed by neurovascular elements entering from either the right side or closely applied to the posterior and left lateral margin of the esophagus.

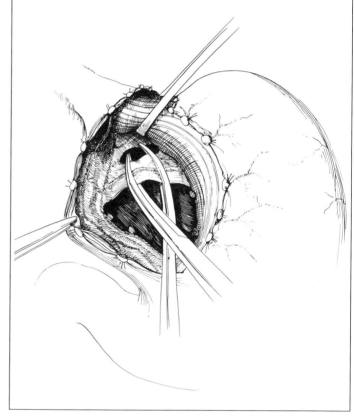

Fig. 79-2. The posterior leaf of the lesser omentum becomes continuous with two structures near the esophagogastric junction: the gastropancreatic fold and the mesoesophagus. After ligation with the clamps, the operator uses blunt dissection with the fingertips to separate areolar connections between these two structures. Figure 79-3 shows the appearance of the gastropancreatic fold after these maneuvers.

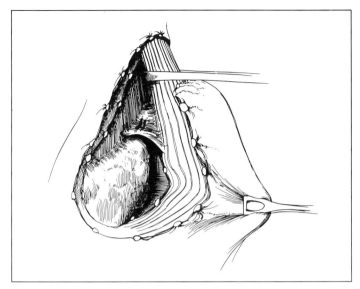

Fig. 79-3. The lesser curvature of the stomach is seen from the patient's right side. Note the gastropancreatic fold, which comprises the peritoneal reflections between the pancreas and the posterior gastric wall. This fold is traversed by the posterior gastric artery and is accompanied by a preganglionic vagus nerve branch supplying the posterior gastric wall. The fold is divided until the spleen is seen. Next, the 5.0 cm of the distal esophagus is bared, completing the proximal dissection.

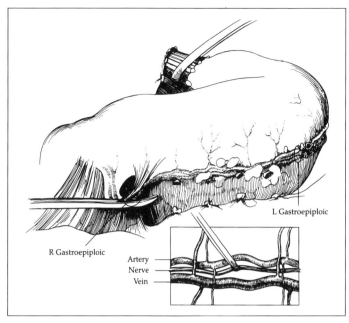

Fig. 79-4. The greater curvature is shown after division of the left gastroepiploic pedicle; the clamp exposes the right gastroepiploic pedicle. It is frequently possible to divide the right gastroepiploic nerve alone, sparing the right gastroepiploic artery and vein. These vessels must be spared if a splenectomy has been performed previously. Inset, the major right gastroepiploic nerve is found between the gastroepiploic artery and vein. To ensure that accessory nerve branches are divided, the omentum between the colon and the greater curvature of the stomach is completely divided.

the anterior vagal nerve branches, allowing them to be palpated on the anterior wall of the esophagus). The posterior trunk must always be identified by palpation before division of the gastropancreatic fold is completed.

After the proximal portion of the dissection is completed, the only attachments of the stomach are the short gastric vessels, esophageal and duodenal connections, the right gastric artery, and the first few branches of the right gastroepiploic artery. The right gastroepiploic arcade continues to supply antral branches, since the gastroepiploic nerve is divided after it gives rise to several branches to the antrum.

Along the distal portion of the lesser curve, some variability in the point of insertion of the crow's foot is frequently noted. The distance between the pylorus and the end point of lesser curve dissection averages 7.0 cm (5.5–7.5 cm) on the anterior wall and 5 cm on the posterior wall of the antrum. At least one large branch and one additional branch of the

anterior and posterior nerves of Latarjet are preserved in each operation. The crow's foot and the instep of the crow's foot are critical areas for precise dissection, as illustrated in Fig. 79-5. The essence of the operative approach illustrated is the anterior rotation of the lesser curve of the stomach, as shown in Fig. 79-5. The instep of the crow's foot (the triangle-shaped mass of tissue between the distal branches of the nerves of Latarjet) is completely dissected, completing the division of nerve branches supplying the corpus of the stomach. In all operations at least two definite branches of the terminal nerve of Latarjet are preserved.

The right gastroepiploic pedicle is usually divided approximately 4 to 6 cm from its emergence at the medial border of the second portion of the duodenum (between the duodenum and the pancreas), after giving off several branches to the antrum. The gastroepiploic nerve can often be divided separately, sparing the gastroepiploic vessels. This approach is mandatory in any person in whom the short gastric

vessels have been previously divided, or if a splenectomy has been performed previously. The left gastroepiploic pedicle is divided beneath the inferior pole of the spleen, with care to avoid trauma to the spleen.

Anterior Hemipylorectomy

Although drainage can be achieved by a variety of techniques, including Jaboulay gastroduodenostomy, Finney pyloroplasty, Heineke–Mikulicz pyloroplasty, duodenoplasty, and gastroenterostomy, I am emphasizing anterior pylorectomy because I believe that it combines the best elements of drainage procedures. Three-fourths of my patients have had stenosis *at* the gastric outlet and have rarely had an isolated duodenal bulb stenosis. Morphometric techniques have shown that the pyloric ring is heavily infiltrated with collagenous tissue and that the precise point of obstruction is at this site. With the precise approach offered by pylorectomy, it is only a rare patient for whom gastroenterostomy is indicated.

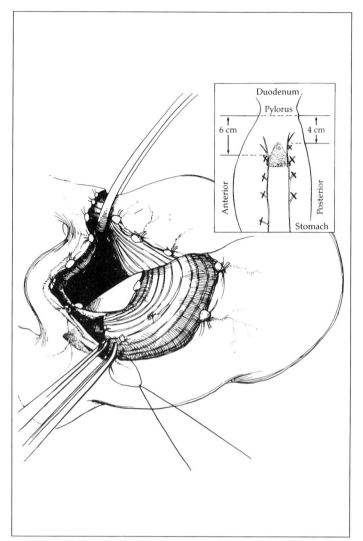

Fig. 79-5. Inset, anterior and posterior relationships. Terminal branches of the anterior nerve enter the antrum approximately 2.0 cm proximal to the terminal branches of the posterior nerve. In this view the stomach has been "turned" clockwise on its longitudinal axis, allowing the surgeon to view the lesser curvature directly. The lesser curvature is displayed as shown, and the insertion of the anterior and posterior nerves of Latarjet is clearly seen. The tissue between the terminal branches of the anterior and posterior nerves of Latarjet (shaded) can now be safely dissected, including any recurrent branches extending toward the corpus. The shaded area between the terminal branches of the crow's foot is termed the "instep" of the crow's foot.

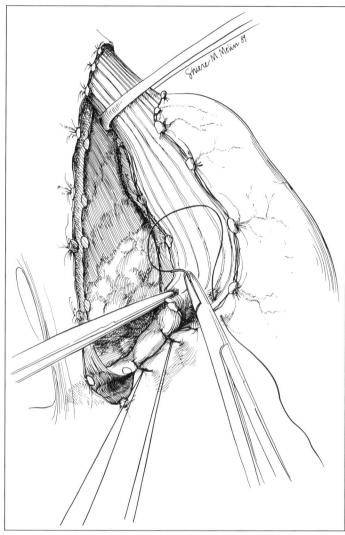

Fig. 79-6. The final maneuver is re-approximation of the serosa of the anterior and posterior gastric walls at the completion of the dissection. The advantages of re-approximating the serosa include prevention of leakage from the lesser curvature if unintentional injury has occurred and, possibly, prevention or retardation of regrowth of vagus nerve fibers.

The hemipylorectomy is planned to include the entire anterior portion of the scarified obstructing lesion. When the pyloric ring itself is the only obstructing element, the block of tissue removed resembles a transversely oriented 1.0 × 2.0 cm rectangle, consisting of the 1.0-cm wide pyloric ring. A needle-tip cautery is used to define the outline of the ring proximal and distal to the pylorus (Fig. 79-7). Excision of the ring is completed by transecting the superior and inferior attachments of the anterior portion of the pyloric ring. When more extensive stenosis is present, the tissue removed is rectangular but is longitudinally oriented. The length of the rectangle conforms to the longitudinal extent of the fibrosis, and the width equals the narrowed pyloric region; the rectangle is usually 3.0 × 1.5 to 2.0 cm in dimension.

In each operation, the first maneuver is to define an area proximal and distal to the stenosis for the first transverse cuts. Then, the ends of these incisions are connected by longitudinal incisions, which remove the entire anterior half of the obstructing area. It is not advantageous or desirable to completely mobilize the pylorus. In patients with severe deformity of the duodenal bulb, a Kocher maneuver allows the

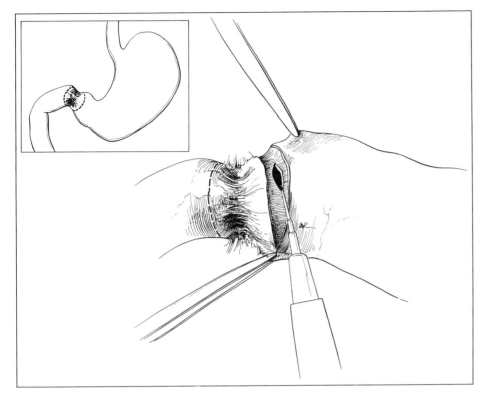

Fig. 79-7. The palpable scar at the gastric outlet is defined by light application of the needle-tip cautery apparatus. It is helpful to plan and define the extent of scar excision before opening the duodenum, since landmarks are easily lost once the lumen is opened. A needle-tipped coagulator is ideal for opening the two layers separately. The seromuscular coat has few blood vessels, whereas the mucosal layer is more richly vascularized. Individual vessels are coagulated as they are encountered.

anastomosis of the proximal and distal margins without tension.

At the conclusion of scar excision, the operative field consists of the posterior mucosal surface of the narrowed gastric outlet, with the open duodenal lumen situated caudally, and the gastric lumen situated cephalad (Fig. 79-8). Simple sutures, which include all layers of the gastric and duodenal wall are used to close the lumen (Fig. 79-9). If there is a discrepancy in size between the gastric and duodenal lumina, a reefing technique is used to conveniently close the defect. Reefing means that a suture is passed through the larger wall of the anastomosis (gastric side) twice, and through the smaller side of the anastomosis (duodenal side) once. Each suture encompasses approximately 5.0 mm of tissue, and each is placed 7 to 8 mm from the edge of the viscus (Figs. 79-10 and 79-11). Each suture is full thickness, and each is driven in perpendicular to the serosal surface, emerging in the submucosa to grasp approximately 2.0 mm of

the mucosal edge. The reefing technique is necessary when a long stenosis is excised: If only pyloric thickening is present, simple sutures achieve a precise anastomosis.

Anastomoses are not drained externally, and all patients have a postoperative nasogastric tube for at least the first 24 hours. In contradistinction to patients with total gastric vagotomy, the gastric drainage during the first 24 hours rarely exceeds 300 ml, and the tube can be removed as soon as active bowel sounds are present.

I have made no mention of manual dilation of the pyloric ring. I believe that the mixed results with this approach do not justify its use and that a more definitive and long-lasting solution to fibrosis of the pyloric ring should be used.

Results

The complications and late morbidity with EPV have been minimal. Rarely, a patient

complains of intermittent dumping, which is not surprising since PGV alone is associated with a small rate of dumping. There have been no deaths and no recurrent ulcers during follow-up periods averaging more than 5 years. No patients had stomal dysfunction.

Discussion

An ideal operative procedure for obstructing duodenal and pyloric channel ulcers must be safe, relatively free of side effects, and effective against the primary disease process. The excellent results that we and others have had make it clear that EPV-D is an approach that deserves wider application. Several points require cautious appraisal before the surgical community will abandon resection in favor of nonresective alternatives such as PGV-D. Foremost among these questions is whether the primary ulcer diathesis is adequately treated. A corollary to this query is whether there is a fundamental difference between the ulcers that cause stenosis of the proximal duodenum and duodenal bulb (DU) and ulcers referred to as pyloric channel ulcers (PCU) or prepyloric ulcers (PPU). There is no clear evidence showing that the pathogenesis of these varieties of ulcer differs. On the other hand, several clinics have achieved excellent results for ulcers causing pyloric stenosis using PGV-D.

What evidence suggests that DU, PCU, and PPU are different diseases? Most of the evidence is inferential, based on the differentially higher recurrence rates for PCU and PPU compared with DU when PGV without drainage was used. These reports are from European centers that have long used PGV, and that have been among the leaders in attempts to study what happens to patients after this operation. For example, the groups from Copenhagen and Lund have reported 16.4 to 33 percent recurrence rates for PPU in contrast to 9.2 to 16 percent recurrence rates for simple DU. In addition, the multicenter trial of PGV, organized in Basle and reported by Müller and colleagues, included 35 PCU, 32 PPU, and 493 DU patients; the ulcer recurrence rates were 35 percent, 33 percent, and 14 percent, respectively. The operations in the Basle series were performed by a technique of PGV reported more than 12 years ago and have relied on a method of vagotomy testing that does not localize the position of undivided nerves.

The technique of EPV that I describe is a modern one based on new scientific evidence. I believe it is now time to distinguish "extended" proximal gastric vagotomy from the other operations, which have not been modified for 20 years and which have been identified with excessive recurrence rates. The success of EPV for obstructing lesions might be related to factors other than the drainage component, since other groups have had success with conventional PGV-D when treating obstructing lesions.

The evidence for the advantage of drainage was first described in Munich, where Holle developed and reported on the first clinical trials of PGV-D. Holle applied this procedure to uncomplicated DU as well as to PCU and PPU (referred to as gastroduodenal ulcers in his text) in a series of more than 2000 patients. The recurrence rate was 1.5 percent in 1202 patients with DU and 1.5 percent in 1454 patients with gastroduodenal ulcers. In the same report, PGV-D was used for 189 of 252 patients with gastric ulcer, who had a recurrence rate of 2.1 percent. These patients had postoperative endoscopic examinations for any type of complaint. Another series was reported from Oslo, where Lunde and colleagues treated 78 patients with pyloric stenosis with only one recurrent ulcer. The same authors found mild early dumping in 5 of 78 patients and an overall satisfaction rate of 93 percent in these patients. The authors compared percentage decreases in postoperative acid secretion in the PGV-D group with decreases in other patients having PGV alone. There was a significantly greater decrease in basal and stimulated secretion 2 months to 5 years after the PGV-D. Similar success with this procedure has been reported from Dublin by Gorey and coworkers, who found that only 1 of 18 patients who had this procedure had a recurrence during a 2-year follow-up period. The major complaint in the patients in Dublin was temporary dysphagia, which occurred in 41 percent of the patients. The absence of serious late sequelae in this group of patients, as in my patients, is another advantage of the nonresectional approach.

On balance, the most attractive feature of PGV-D is the apparent absence of dis-

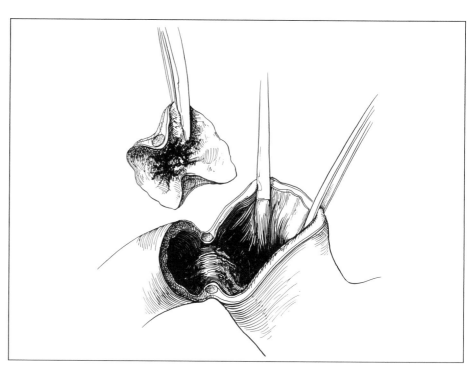

Fig. 79-8. After complete excision of the scarified anterior pyloric ring, the lumens of the stomach and the duodenum are clearly seen. The ends of the severed pyloric muscle are apparent at the superior and inferior portions of the dissection. Before the duodenum and stomach are sewn, digital exploration of the second portion of the duodenum is performed to find occult stenosis.

abling side effects, which occur in a small but predictable number of patients treated by total gastric vagotomy with resection. Parenthetically, a possible reason for the greater efficacy of proximal vagotomy with drainage might be that the intramural nerves that traverse the pylorus are destroyed during pylorectomy or drainage. The findings on this hypothesis have concerned rats, and the hypothesis has yet to be proved in humans.

Whereas many discussions about PGV stress the problem with too high an incidence of recurrent ulcers, the problem with acute and chronic complications after alternative operative procedures such as total gastric vagotomy and resection deserves some mention. A report by Welch and colleagues from Boston describes results in 1068 patients with ulcers, including 113 patients with obstructing duodenal ulcer. There were 45 instances of severe stomal dysfunction among the 531 patients who had vagotomy with resection; there were other acute complications requiring reoperation in 7.4 percent of the group. Although patients who have had a PGV-D are at risk for stoma dysfunction, there

were no such patients in the 133 patients with this procedure treated by Welch and colleagues. Only one patient needed a reoperation for small-intestinal obstruction. Jordan and Thornby compared PGV and selective vagotomy with antrectomy in 200 patients treated prospectively in a randomized trial. Again, excessive recurrence rates were found in patients with PPU and PCU treated with the former. Of interest was that the incidence of serious postoperative complications was much greater in the group that had selective vagotomy with antrectomy. These complications included dumping in 58 patients that was severe enough to account for poor results in 12 patients. Thirteen other patients complained of inability to regain their weight and strength. The same problem did not occur in the group that had PGV. Problems with gastric emptying were serious in five other patients after selective vagotomy with antrectomy compared with one after PGV.

The reports cited give an accurate overview of the type of morbidity that appears to be unavoidable after vagotomy plus resection. Patients with severe nutritional

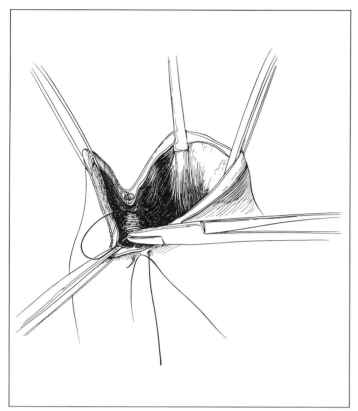

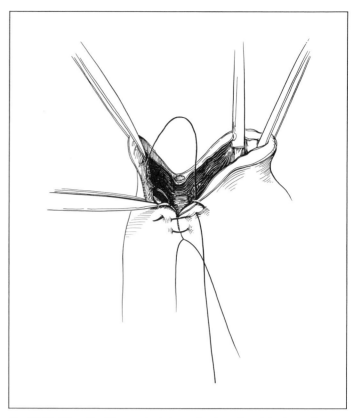

Fig. 79-9. Simple sutures are placed at the corners of the anastomosis without regard to the disparity in size. By focusing on the precise alignment of the corners, any potential for leak is avoided. Sutures include 6.0 mm of the seromuscular layer and are placed perpendicular to the surface of the viscus. Before the needle is inserted, the mucosa is grasped with a forceps, stabilizing the wall for precise suture application.

Fig. 79-10. Disparity of lumen size between the stomach and duodenum is addressed as shown. Two bites of gastric tissue are taken for every one of duodenum, beginning the moment a disparity is noted. In this way, an anastomosis can be made easily with a gastric lumen twice as large as the duodenal lumen.

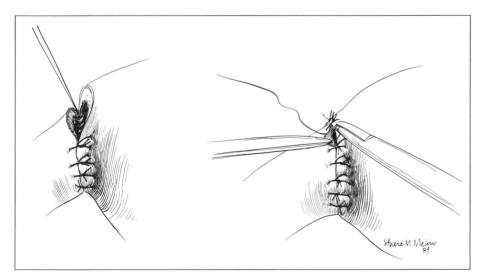

Fig. 79-11. Completion of the anastomosis. The reefing sutures include two applications on the gastric side and one on the duodenal side. Reefing avoids last-minute problems with anastomosis of different-sized openings.

problems and serious postgastrectomy syndromes continue to have serious problems for years if not for their lifetime. In this context, therefore, I conclude that the absence of serious chronic morbidity after PGV-D is as important as the recurrent ulcer rate. For example, even though pyloroplasty destroys an important part of the brake on gastric emptying, the preservation of antral innervation seems to prevent problems associated with poor gastric emptying. Similarly, the absence of bilious vomiting, a common complaint after gastrectomy, suggests that the alkaline reflux syndrome is not a problem when antral innervation is preserved. Another report that deserves consideration is that of Hoffmann and coworkers from Copenhagen, who performed gastric resections on patients who had recurrent ulcers after PGV or total gastric vagotomy plus drainage. Five of 51 patients available for long-term follow-up study needed reoperations for postgastrectomy symptoms within the first 5 years. Twenty-two of these patients had serious or unacceptable postgastrectomy symptoms after the "remedial" operation.

One is forced to question whether the cure of ulcer is worth the risk of postgastrectomy symptoms. The concerns about recurrent ulcer rates after PGV must be addressed, however, since some of the most experienced medical centers have reported alarming recurrence rates. It is curious that one operation should be associated with such a difference in recurrence rates when performed in different medical centers. Furthermore, a number of important areas in the performance of PGV appear to be different in centers performing "complete" PGV from those performing "conventional" PGV. Figures 79-1 to 79-6 illustrate technical details related to the performance of PGV that might explain a difference in the postoperative recurrence rate. My colleagues and I have demonstrated that the nerves of the greater curvature, identified as a concern in achieving a "complete" PGV, are projected from up to 20 percent of the nerve cell bodies of the dorsal motor nucleus of the vagus nerve in the brain stem. At this time, therefore, I believe it is appropriate to adopt the technique of EPV as a means of avoiding the high recurrence rates reported with conventional highly selective vagotomy or PGV. When pyloric stenosis or outlet obstruction is present, anterior hemipylorectomy provides a solution.

Suggested Reading

Donahue PE, Bombeck CT, Condon RE, et al. Proximal gastric vagotomy versus selective vagotomy with antrectomy: Results of a prospective, randomized clinical trial after four to twelve years. *Surgery* 96:585, 1984.

Donahue PE, Yoshida J, Bombeck CT, et al. The endoscopic Congo red test during proximal gastric vagotomy. *Am J Surg* 153:249, 1986.

Donahue PE, Yoshida J, Polley EH, et al. Preganglionic vagal efferent nerves also enter the greater curve. *Gastroenterology* 94:1292, 1988.

Donahue PE, Richter HM, Liu K, et al. Experimental basis and clinical application of extended highly selective vagotomy. *Surg Gynecol & Obstet* 176:39, 1993.

Donahue PE. Invited Commentary—Effects of highly selective vagotomy and additional procedures on gastric emptying in patients with obstructing duodenal ulcer. *World J Surg* 18:137, 1994.

Donahue PE, Yoshida J, Richter HM, et al. Proximal gastric vagotomy with drainage for obstructing duodenal ulcer. *Surgery* 104:757, 1988.

Enskog L, Rydberg B, Adami HO, et al. Clinical results 1-10 years after highly selective vagotomy in 306 patients with prepyloric and duodenal ulcer disease. *Br J Surg* 73:357, 1986.

Gorey TF, Lennon F, Heffernan SJ. Highly selective vagotomy in duodenal ulcer and its complications. *Ann Surg* 200:181, 1984.

Griffith CA, Harkins HN. Proximal gastric vagotomy: An experimental study. *Gastroenterology* 32:96, 1957.

Hoffman J, Hosein Shokouh-Amiri M, Klarskov P, et al. Gastrectomy for recurrent ulcer after vagotomy: Five to nineteen year follow-up. *Surgery* 99:517, 1986.

Holle F. *Spezielle Magenchirurgie*. Berlin: Springer-Verlag, 1968.

Holle F. The why and how of drainage within the nonresective method. In F Holle and GE Holle (eds.), *Vagotomy and Pyloroplasty: Advances 1975–1980*. Berlin: Springer-Verlag, 1980.

Jordan PH Jr, Thornby J. Should it be parietal cell vagotomy or selective vagotomy-antrectomy for treatment of duodenal ulcer. *Ann Surg* 205:572, 1987.

Lunde OC, Liavag I, Roland M. Proximal gastric vagotomy and pyloroplasty for duodenal ulcer with pyloric stenosis: A thirteen-year experience. *World J Surg* 9:165, 1985.

Meisner S, Jorgenson LN, Jensen, HE. The Kaplan and Meier and the Nelson estimate for the probability of ulcer recurrence in 10 and 15 years after parietal gastric vagotomy. *Ann Surg* 207:1, 1988.

Muller C, Liebermann-Meffert D, Allgower M. Pyloric and prepyloric ulcers. *World J Surg* 11:339, 1987.

Welch CE, Rodkey GV, von Ryll Gryska P. A thousand operations for ulcer disease. *Ann Surg* 204:454, 1986.

Yoshida J, Polley EH, Nyhus LM, et al. Pyloroplasty divides vagus nerve fibers to the greater curvature of the stomach. *Ann Surg* 208:708, 1988.

Yoshida J, Polley EH, Nyhus LM, et al. Brain stem topography of vagus nerve to the greater curvature of the stomach. *J Surg Res* 46:60, 1987.

EDITOR'S COMMENT

Extended proximal vagotomy with hemipylorectomy has given very good results in our clinic. This success can be attributed to many factors, including meticulous dissection, recognition of the gastroepiploic nerves as important components of the gastric secretory process, and the performance of an anterior hemipylorectomy in the presence of pyloroantral stenosis.

I continue to be intrigued by the improved results following duodenoplasty associated with proximal gastric vagotomy (Kennedy. *Ann Roy Coll Surg Engl* 58:144, 1976; FL Barroso. In *Mastery of Surgery* (2nd ed.), 1992. Pp 693–694; K Dittrich et al. *J Am Coll Surg* 180:654, 1995). The low ulcer recurrence rate and minimal postgastric operation side effects suggest to me that the pendulum should now swing back to more elective operations being performed to cure the ulcer diathesis. The lifetime control of the patients' painful symptom complex by medical treatment no longer can be justified—with or without *Helicobacter pylori*—with the superb results being reported and including the extended highly selective vagotomy as described by Dr. Donahue.

L.M.N.

80

Pyloroplasty, Vagotomy, and Suture Ligation for Bleeding Duodenal Ulcer

James H. Foster

Indications

With the reduced incidence of peptic ulcer and markedly improved medical management, in recent years there has been a remarkable decrease in the need for emergency operative control.

The title of this chapter implies that an emergency situation exists and that the localization of the point of bleeding has already been made, presumably by endoscopy. It further implies that endoscopic attempts to control hemorrhage have been unsuccessful and that bleeding continues or has recurred. Under these circumstances, an emergency operation should be recommended whenever there is a failure to stabilize the patient's vital signs with rapid volume replacement (exsanguination); when blood loss and transfusion requirement continue in a stabilized patient beyond approximately 2000 ml of blood loss in less than 24 hours; or when considerable hemorrhage recurs in a patient who apparently initially stopped bleeding and who has been on an optimal regimen of medical therapy. An operation should be considered even earlier for elderly and poor-risk patients or for patients who already have a history of enough previous problems with peptic ulcer to justify an elective operation.

There is no place for pitressin infusion or angiographically controlled attempts at arterial occlusion when brisk hemorrhage from a major artery in the first portion of the duodenum has been documented by endoscopy. If the endoscopist can assure the surgeon that there is no diffuse gastric inflammation or erosion and no evidence of portal hypertension, and if the patient's hemostatic mechanisms are intact, the rate and volume of blood loss will determine the urgency of an operation even in patients in whom the endoscopist cannot localize a discrete lesion.

Although emergency antrectomy-vagotomy can be considered for patients whose condition is reasonably stable, and will afford better insurance against recurrent ulceration in the future, it is clear that the operative survival rate in elderly patients and patients for whom the risk of an operation is high will be increased by avoidance of resection. Rebleeding in the immediately postoperative period is not increased after the "lesser" procedure if attention is paid to the details of arterial ligation and if the vagotomy has been adequate.

Choice of Incision

The upper midline incision provides the quickest and driest route into the abdomen and is preferred in the emergency situation. The rare patient with a barrel chest, a nearly horizontal costal margin, and a fairly stable cardiovascular status might warrant a transverse incision, but the additional time required to divide muscle is usually not justified. Proper use of the electrocautery for hemostasis saves additional seconds. A nasogastric tube should be placed to monitor continued bleeding and to aid subsequent dissection around the gastroesophageal junction. When the peritoneal cavity is entered, the round and falciform ligaments should be transected to allow upward retraction of the liver.

Control of Hemorrhage by Suture Ligation

If the bleeding source is known to be a duodenal ulcer, immediate attention should be turned to the pylorus. Two parallel 000 sutures should be placed close together as near to the exact center of the anterior pylorus as possible (Fig. 80-1). These sutures should include a visible pyloric vein. They should be deep enough to include mucosa and should be tied down but not cut. If the ulcer is bulbar and posterior, a Kocher's maneuver does not help exposure and is not needed.

With upward traction and separation of the two stitches, a generous (5–6 cm) longitudinal incision is made in the pylorus, usually 2 cm into the duodenum and 3 or 4 cm into the stomach. I prefer the electrocautery for this procedure because it controls hemorrhage from small vessels, thus aiding visualization; it decreases the requirements for ties, and it can help to seal mucosa to muscularis at the extremities of the incision, thus aiding later repair. Once the lumen is entered, a clamp should elevate the anterior gastric and duodenal mucosa into the cautery, thus protecting the rest of the intestine. It is better to provide adequate exposure with a longer pylorotomy than to tear a fragile duodenum by too vigorous retraction of the edges of a short incision.

If brisk arterial hemorrhage continues, its source is readily found. A few moments of digital compression of a spurting artery

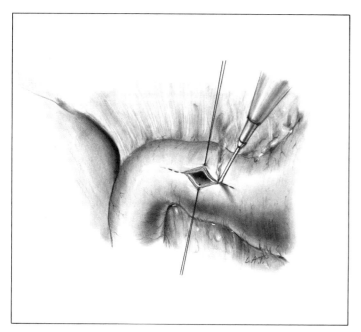

Fig. 80-1. *A longitudinal incision is made into the lumen beginning at the pylorus as it is tented up by the stay sutures, which should include mucosa.*

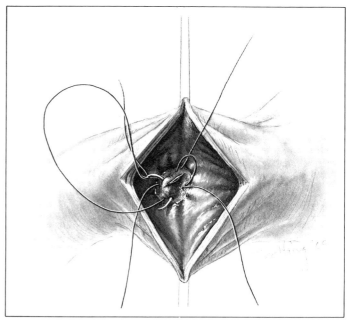

Fig. 80-2. *Transfixion of a bleeding posterior duodenal ulcer through a pyloroplasty incision. The needle should be a full half-circle in shape and sufficiently stout to permit deep penetration into the ulcer bed. Since the bleeding might be coming from a lateral hole in the artery, double ligation is recommended, as shown. (From JH Foster. In JD Hardy [ed.],* Critical Surgical Illness, *1st ed. Philadelphia: Saunders, 1971.)*

can allow the anesthesiologist an opportunity to restore volume in a hypotensive patient before the surgeon proceeds. More often, the bleeding has slowed or stopped before the duodenum is opened. Inspection can be obscured by continued overflow of clotted and unclotted blood from a distended stomach or blood-filled duodenum. Gentle suction using the multiholed, sheathed metal suction tip can be used to empty the stomach or duodenum. Occasionally a small moist gauze can be used to "cork-off" flow from the stomach or distal duodenum. Care should be taken to prevent mucosal injury with these techniques because iatrogenic injury can be difficult to distinguish from acute superficial peptic ulceration in some instances.

The use of ring forceps together with the opposite end of long thumb forceps can aid exposure. A deep chronic ulcer might be hidden under the posterior lip of the pylorus. Occasionally the bleeding ulcer is anterior. It can be transected during pyloroplasty and not be readily visible. Careful palpation usually reveals induration at the site of any chronic inflammation.

If a chronic ulcer is found that is not actively bleeding, any adherent clot should be teased away, and the base should be provoked with a clamp or suction tip to encourage arterial hemorrhage. If arterial hemorrhage does not occur, it may well be that the ulcer under consideration is not the source of the original hemorrhage, and another lesion should be sought elsewhere in the duodenum or in the distal stomach. Once again, palpation of the luminal surface of the lesser curvature of the stomach can be more effective than direct inspection in locating chronic disease.

When an obvious arterial bleeder is found in the base of a chronic duodenal ulcer, it should be controlled with multiple, deeply placed sutures of reasonably heavy material, preferably 00 silk or a synthetic absorbable material (Fig. 80-2). Catgut should not be used. Most arteries require two or three deep needle bites to ensure circumferential control. It is better to risk injury to the common bile duct than to allow recurrent hemorrhage.

Pyloroplasty

After control of the bleeding vessel is achieved and after a finger has been passed distally in the duodenum to rule out any downstream obstruction or a second lesion, the longitudinal pylorotomy is closed transversely in one layer as a Heineke–Mikulicz pyloroplasty. The traction sutures form convenient ends for the suture line. Needle bites include the full thickness of gastric and duodenal walls with only narrow bites in the mucosa. I prefer to use a single-layer closure with interrupted sutures of a synthetic absorbable material placed in a simple manner. More complex suture techniques might provide a more "cosmetic" result but do not improve function or reduce the risk of complications. Technical factors can demand construction of another type of pyloroplasty, but this is unusual for patients with bleeding posterior bulbar ulcers. The Heineke–Mikulicz reconstruction is the easiest and fastest in most emergency situations.

Vagotomy

Rapid, effective truncal vagotomy requires adequate exposure, and surgeons differ on how that exposure can be best obtained. In my experience, the following technique is the most rapid and effective, the safest and simplest. I recommend it for the elective as well as for the emergency situation. Bilateral vagotomy can be accomplished in a few minutes by this method.

First, the operating table should be adjusted to its lowest position for even the tallest surgeon. Short surgeons should get up on a low stand. Second, a Weinberg retractor or similar large, flat-bladed retractor should be placed beneath the left lateral segment of the liver, with the edge of its blade on the diaphragm, centered immediately above where the nasogastric tube can be palpated in the distal esophagus. In thin patients, a wide Deaver or Harrington retractor might suffice, but the retractor must be long enough to reach the diaphragm behind the liver. In any instance, the strongest and surest assistant should be stationed comfortably on the other end of this retractor. The diaphragmatic attachment of the left triangular ligament of the liver is well anterior to the esophageal hiatus, and its lysis is rarely necessary if the retractor is positioned properly. No packs are used in the left upper quadrant.

With gentle caudad traction on the body of the stomach, the surgeon visualizes the *diaphragmatic* peritoneum immediately

above the hiatus (Fig. 80-3), and then makes a 3- to 4-cm transverse incision with scissors or knife. This incision must *not* be made over the fatty areolar tissue that often surrounds the gastroesophageal junction, for several reasons. First, the vagal trunks might have begun to branch at that level and will be difficult to find and define. Second, circumferential dissection of the gastroesophageal junction at this level dislodges a posterior fixation and can allow subsequent reflux; and third, there are small blood vessels here that need not be disturbed. Periesophageal dissection should be done in the mediastinum *above* the diaphragm.

A right-handed surgeon standing on the patient's right side passes his or her right hand into the epigastrium. This hand is not removed again until the vagotomy is completed. The surgeon places his or her right index finger through the peritoneal incision and then slips *beneath* the anterior lip of the esophageal hiatus of the diaphragm *up* into the mediastinum anterior and to the left of the esophagus. The easily palpable nasogastric tube serves to reassure the surgeon about the location of the esophagus. Moving initially to the left of the esophagus, circumferential finger dissection of the esophagus and of all the sur-

rounding tissue anterior to the vertebral body and descending aorta is blindly but easily accomplished *within the mediastinum*. The tip of the index finger then reenters the visible field to the right of the esophagus as it exits the mediastinum under the right crus of the hiatus.

A great deal is accomplished by maintenance of this position of the right hand until the vagotomy is completed. First, the repetitive entrances and exits of hands, instruments, and drains into this area risk injury with every pass. Second, the surgeon's hand is the most sensitive and most flexible instrument to produce the proper amount of downward traction to make the vagi stand out (and is thus much preferable to the drain); and third, the back of the fingers and the right hand hold the spleen tip out of the way to the left and retract the stomach out of the way posteriorly. This positioning eliminates the need for more packs, more retractors, and more hands in the incision—all of which risk injury and get in the surgeon's way.

Now comfortably in place, the right index finger and thumb roll the esophagus and periesophageal tissues at will, and thus discover, define, and deliver the vagal trunks away from the thoracic esophagus,

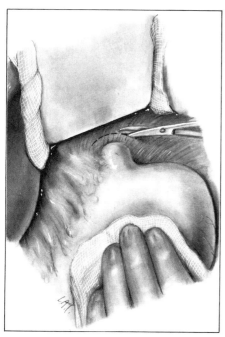

Fig. 80-3. The peritoneal incision is made with a knife or scissors and should be long enough to easily admit the tip of the index finger. Subsequent blunt dissection results in further elongation.

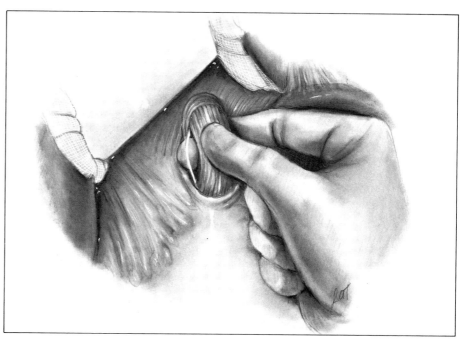

Fig. 80-4. After palpation of the taut right vagus nerve posteriorly, the distal thoracic esophagus, which has been pulled into the abdomen, is rolled to the left by the thumb, thus allowing exposure of the nerve by the tip of the right index finger.

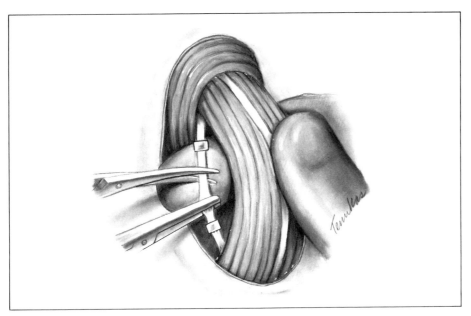

Fig. 80-5. Clip application allows removal of a 2- to 3-cm length of the nerve in most instances. In some instances it is easier to clip and cut one end of the nerve before clipping and cutting the other end. Careful inspection of the removed segment under bright light ensures that neural tissue has been removed.

which has been lifted into the abdomen by anterior pressure of the right index finger.

The right (posterior) vagus is usually found first by palpation alone. If it is not readily apparent, it should be sought in the mediastinum away from the esophagus in the areolar tissue anterior to the vertebral body. The nerve is delivered into sight by the tip of the index finger (Fig. 80-4) and is grasped with the tip of a long clamp held either in the left hand of the surgeon or, preferably, in the dominant hand of a competent first assistant. Once the nerve is grasped, dissection of a length of the nerve with a nerve hook, clipping on either side of the clamp, transection, and then removal of a section of the nerve are all easily accomplished *without using the surgeon's right hand*, which maintains exposure and control (Fig. 80-5). The left vagal trunk lying close to the anterior lateral esophagus might be readily palpable, but also might be easier to see than to feel. Thus a combination of direct vision with a rolling palpation of the esophagus can work best to define this trunk. Occasionally the flattened, folded edge of the esophageal mucosa feels like a vagus nerve, so it is essential to see the nerve clearly before a long clamp is placed on it. Once again, dissection, clipping, and transection are easily accomplished by an assistant (or a left hand). After two discrete

trunks are taken and verified by careful inspection of the removed section under a bright light, scissor transection of any suspicious small fibers should be done as the circumference of the esophagus is rolled and exposed between the right index finger and thumb. Then and only then is the right hand removed. The area is carefully inspected for hemostasis, and the large retractor is removed.

The pyloroplasty is re-inspected to ensure adequate closure and a dry field, and a fold of omentum is placed between the pyloroplasty and the undersurface of the liver. If the patient's condition and the nasogastric aspirate convince both surgeon and anesthesiologist that hemorrhage is controlled, the abdominal incision is closed.

Suggested Reading

Branicki FJ, Coleman SY, Fok PJ, et al. Bleeding peptic ulcer: A prospective evaluation of risk factors for rebleeding and mortality. *World J Surg* 14:262, 1990.

Cochran TA. Bleeding Peptic Ulcer: Surgical Therapy. *Gastroenterol Clin North Am* 22:751, 1993.

Larson G, Schmidt T, Gott J, et al. Upper gastrointestinal bleeding: Predictors of outcome. *Surgery* 100:765, 1986.

EDITOR'S COMMENT

In 1965, my colleagues and I reported a mortality of 34 percent in the surgical treatment of patients with massive upper gastrointestinal hemorrhage from duodenal ulcers or varices (*Am Surg* 31:413, 1965). Naturally, we were impressed with the marked improvement in mortality statistics reported by Foster and Dunphy from the University of Oregon when the surgical approach was changed from gastric resection to vagotomy, pyloroplasty, and suture ligation of the bleeding vessel (*Ann Surg* 161:968, 1965). The incidence rate of recurrent hemorrhage following the suture ligation is approximately 10 percent; however, most of these patients stop bleeding spontaneously. New methods of controlling hemorrhage from esophageal varices, gastric and duodenal ulcers, or stress erosive gastritis, such as sclerotherapy, laser beam, or electrocoagulation, have made it unnecessary to perform emergency operations on many poor-risk patients.

The "T" three-vessel junction in the base of many juxtapyloric posterior penetrating duodenal ulcers was emphasized by Berne and Rosoff (*Ann Surg* 169:141, 1969). They proposed that major rebleeding is most often caused by imprecise application of suture ligatures. This imprecision is caused by failure to recognize that the arterial perforation is frequently located opposite a T juncture of the perforated artery and a major bifurcative branch or an anastomotic artery. Circumferential artery sutures (nonabsorbable) are inserted, and in addition, a U stitch must be placed to ascertain that the "cross" of the T has been ligated.

Most patients stop bleeding spontaneously on hospitalization and standard medical management. There are always a few patients with exsanguination who need an urgent operation after resuscitation. The operative mortality for these patients remains high, approximately 10 percent. How can we determine which patients will rebleed after medical management, necessitating an emergency operation? Patients with increased risk factors who stop bleeding spontaneously or whose bleeding is controlled by therapeutic endoscopy should have an elective operation within 36 hours after admission

(*Surg Gynecol Obstet* 159:113, 1984). We have the operative techniques to prevent rebleeding in an elective setting and to cure the ulcer diathesis at the same time. These goals can be achieved with a very low mortality.

After an in-depth study of patients with massive upper gastrointestinal hemorrhage, I was concerned that surgeons needed guidelines to know when to operate on patients with this difficult problem (*Surgery of the Stomach and Duodenum*, Boston: Little, Brown, 1962). These guidelines from 1962 should be modified as follows:

I. Management should be conservative at the outset.
   A. Adequate and rapid replacement of blood volume is the most important aspect of this phase.
   B. Endoscopy, diagnostic and therapeutic, should be performed early.
II. Operative intervention is indicated when:
   A. There is a need, after initial stabilization, for transfusion of more than 1500 ml of whole blood in any 24-hour period.
   B. Bleeding continues for more than 24 hours from onset (in patients older than 60 years, if bleeding continues for more than 12 hours from onset).
   C. Bleeding in the presence of well-known risk factors, such as a history of shock, advanced age, concomitant disease, or ulcer, has stopped. An elective operation should be performed within 36 hours, following cessation of bleeding.
   D. Bleeding recurs after initial cessation.
   E. There is coincident perforation and hemorrhage.
III. An operation must be seriously considered when:
   A. The patient is older than 60 years.
   B. There is a gastric ulcer.
   C. Hematemesis has occurred during the current episode.
   D. There is a history of chronic ulcer disease or of previous hemorrhage.
   E. Severe pain has preceded the hemorrhage or pain persists during the hemorrhage.

Attention to these guidelines in patients with massive upper gastrointestinal hemorrhage will help to improve the overall results of treatment.

L.M.N.

81

Operation for Acute Perforated Duodenal Ulcer

Robert J. Baker

Surgical treatment of duodenal ulcer complications has diminished drastically in the past two decades, particularly in the past 10 years. The absolute incidence of peptic ulcer, specifically duodenal ulcer and its variant, channel ulcer, is impressive, but the complications of peptic ulcer disease have become extremely rare. Specifically, acute perforation of duodenal ulcers occurs in 5 to 10 percent of all patients with duodenal ulcer disease. The majority are between 40 and 50 years of age, and two-thirds have a history of duodenal ulcer, whereas one-third of patients have no history and no prior treatment. Interestingly, although this phenomenon is most marked in North America, in a number of other countries, including Scandinavia, perforated duodenal ulcer is apparently not significantly changed in incidence, and the number of operations performed for that disease has not been significantly altered. The questions concerning perforated duodenal ulcer have been well outlined by Feliciano and include the following: 1) should the patient be operated on at all; 2) is it sufficient to perform a classic Graham patch, such as will be described, or should a definitive operation to diminish hyperacidity be added; 3) are local conditions satisfactory for a definitive operation, or is the patient in sufficiently satisfactory condition to permit one; 4) if a definitive operation is to be done, which procedure is best under the conditions of an acute perforation; and 5) do the newer agents, specifically omeprazole, provide sufficient protection against recurrent disease so that other operations beyond omental patch closure of the perforated ulcer are unnecessary? A subset of the last question is whether the significance of *Hel-*

icobacter pylori is sufficient to require treatment of that gastric infection in patients with perforated duodenal ulcer. Nonoperative treatment of perforated peptic ulcers has been considered and studied by Donovan, with the conclusion by him and numerous other authors that nonoperative management should be reserved for patients who have a perforation of longer than 24 hours' duration (some authors advocate 48 hours) or for patients whose systemic disease or current state of deterioration militates against operative treatment.

This nonoperative but somewhat radical approach can be used only if a water-soluble contrast study confirms that the ulcer crater is sealed by failure of any contrast medium to leak from the duodenum. Patients with long-standing perforation, shock, or severe concomitant disease of the heart, lung, or kidney represent an unusual group with a very high mortality, approximately 35 to 50 percent. If properly selected patients from that group were treated nonoperatively, the results would probably equal or better the results of standard operative management. Of extreme importance in this method of managing perforated duodenal ulcer is close, accurate reassessment of the patient's general condition and abdominal findings every 2 to 3 hours. If the physical findings of peritonitis have not regressed significantly within the first 12 hours of management, the patient requires an operation to control the acute complication.

It is also important to differentiate perforated gastric ulcer from perforated duodenal ulcer, since gastric ulcers have a

much higher incidence of reperforation, treated with or without an operation, than do duodenal ulcers. Prepyloric and channel ulcers are caused by similar factors and behave like duodenal ulcers, whereas gastric ulcers (perforations more than 2 cm proximal to the pyloric ring) have a higher mortality in part due to the frequency of reperforation for simple closure, which I discourage in favor of resection of the ulcer-bearing portion of the stomach, and in part because the patients with perforated gastric ulcer are much older. The death rate for gastric ulcers was approximately 20 percent as opposed to 6 percent for duodenal ulcers in a large series reported by Kukora. Shock has been suitably emphasized as a major risk factor for mortality after patching or oversewing of perforated duodenal ulcers. The other major risk factor is age; patients 70 years of age or older have three times the mortality of patients younger than 70 years.

As for the second point, there has been a growing trend toward combining closure of the ulcer with interruption of the vagus nerves, primarily by parietal cell vagotomy. However, in patients at poor risk, especially patients who present with sepsis, shock, or generalized peritonitis or who have been treated with large doses of steroids for intercurrent disease, simple closure remains the best choice. Similarly, in elderly patients, patients without symptoms before the perforation, and patients whose treatment is delayed longer than 6 to 12 hours, simple suture with the use of an omental pedicle yields the best results.

Large, chronic, indurated ulcers, especially the ones with a perforation greater than 5 mm in diameter, have a high incidence of reperforation and stenosis and require an adjunctive ulcer operation in addition to or in lieu of the patch closure. In patients with these large ulcers or in patients with simultaneous anterior perforated and posterior penetrating ulcer, truncal vagotomy with pyloroplasty or with antrectomy in acceptable operative candidates can represent the best alternatives. Patients with the following entities require a definitive ulcer operation:

1. Perforated gastric ulcer
2. Combined gastric and duodenal ulcer, one of which has perforated
3. Perforation with preexisting chronic ulcer symptoms
4. Coexistent obstruction and perforation
5. Coexistent hemorrhage and perforation
6. Previous operation for perforated duodenal ulcer

Numerous reports have advocated the use of parietal cell vagotomy and duodenorrhaphy with an omental patch for perforated duodenal ulcer in patients whose general condition and physical findings allow such a maneuver. The caveat here is to rule out duodenal obstruction, which makes this operation unsatisfactory. If selective or truncal vagotomy with pyloroplasty is chosen, the ulcer should be excised in the course of the pyloroplasty if technically feasible; the type of pyloroplasty selected should be one that is simplest to effect adequate drainage without compromising the pyloroplasty suture line. If there is a question about the existence of obstruction, a No. 40 Fr esophageal dilator can be passed by the anesthetist through the mouth, into the stomach, and manipulated by the surgeon past the ulcer site into the duodenum. This maneuver is preferable to performing a gastrotomy to ascertain the size of the pylorus or the duodenal lumen at the site of the perforation.

In the list above, the use of parietal cell vagotomy would be limited to patients who perforated with known, preexisting ulcer disease or in patients who had experienced a previous perforation for perforated duodenal ulcer. Perforated gastric ulcer should be resected, preferably by partial gastrectomy, unless the ulcer is juxtaesophageal, in which case the ulcer should be repaired and a Tanner procedure held in reserve as a secondary choice.

The use of parietal cell vagotomy and patch omental closure of the ulcer has recently been introduced with use of the laparoscope. The technical details of this operation will be discussed elsewhere but are challenging primarily because of the need to mechanically sew the omental patch in place, a skill that not all laparoscopic surgeons have mastered, and because of the desire to extensively irrigate the peritoneal cavity in achieving maximum removal of duodenal content from the various recesses of the abdomen. Probably the real shortcoming of the laparoscopic procedure is the inability to deal with the numerous bursae and recesses of the peritoneal cavity in order to irrigate them optimally. Nevertheless, the reports of the laparoscopic procedure for perforated ulcer to date have shown excellent outcomes, particularly in younger patients with fresh perforations.

Patients in shock, who have severe cardiopulmonary insufficiency or are in renal failure, especially if previous upper abdominal surgery has been performed, are candidates for the simplest possible operation, the Graham patch closure of the duodenal ulcer. Patients over 75 years also need to be viewed with regard to their life expectancy in the context of the need for a definitive ulcer operation. H_2-receptor blockers and omeprazole, the proton pump blocker that works through the ATP-ase enzyme system inhibition, have maximal effect at the parietal cell and block the proton pump. Drugs of this potency forestall further complications of peptic ulcer and very frequently allow peptic ulcers to heal without a definitive procedure, and, in the selected elderly patients alluded to, should be relied on to supplant the more dangerous definitive operative procedure.

Incision

The type of incision is determined to some degree by the body contour and the shape of the abdomen. Patients with a short xiphopubic distance and a wide costal margin can be operated on for perforated duodenal ulcer with a transverse supraumbilical incision extending from 1 inch to the left of the midline to the right beyond the right rectus muscle, cutting that structure. A short incision is undesirable since a most important part of the operation is the ad-

equate visualization, aspiration, and irrigation of the various crevices of the peritoneal cavity. If duodenal content is allowed to remain in the suprahepatic or perisplenic space, or in the pelvis, an abscess is likely to form, and one of the major aims of the operation is defeated.

On the other hand, most patients with a normal habitus and a medium or even somewhat narrow costal margin should be operated on through a vertical midline incision from xiphoid to umbilicus. This incision is more than ample for exposure of the duodenum and, more important, it allows sufficient room to irrigate and evacuate potentially or frankly contaminated material. Several studies have been done comparing the subcostal or transverse incision with the vertical, and the incidence of intra-abdominal infections after the transverse or subcostal approach has been greater than that occurring with the vertical incision. Under either circumstance, an adequately long incision is required to perform the necessary peritoneal cleansing.

Surgical Technique

The perforated duodenal ulcer closure described by Graham has not been improved on in the past 55 years. The perforated ulcer site is visualized; dry laparotomy pads are placed around the site of the perforation to contain any further spill; and three, or occasionally four, 000 silk sutures are placed in the duodenum, passing through the wall of the duodenum from 1.0 to 1.5 cm from the edge of the perforation. These sutures are placed by using a needle with a swaged-on 000 silk suture, first passing the needle through the wall of the duodenum and retrieving the needle through the perforation (Fig. 81-1A and B). The needle is then grasped again in the needle holder and is reintroduced through the perforation to exit from the side of the perforation opposite the point of entry of the suture (Fig. 81-1C). The purpose of this maneuver is to forestall any possibility of catching the posterior duodenal wall with the needle and sewing the posterior duodenal mucosa up to the anterior wall of the duodenum. This risk exists if the needle is passed through both sides of the ulcer at once because there is occasionally poor visibility and some difficulty in doing this maneuver without taking a relatively deep bite. A shallower and safer bite can be

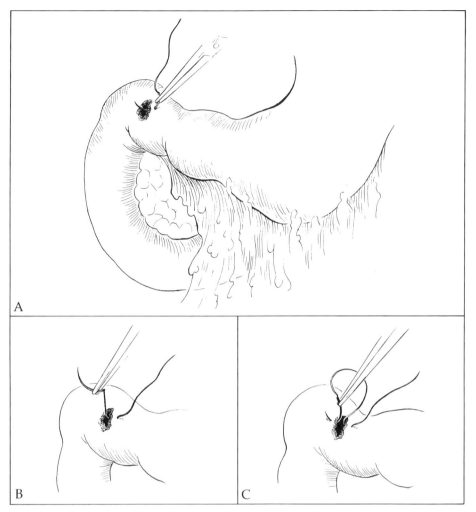

Fig. 81-1. The closure is begun by placing silk sutures through the wall of the duodenum in two steps (A and B), retrieving the needle through the perforation proper between these two steps (C). This technique prevents passing a deeply placed suture into the posterior duodenal wall, causing obstruction.

placed with the needle passed in two stages, especially since a smaller half-circle needle can be used.

The three or four sutures that have been placed should not be tied to approximate the ulcer edges. Rather, the adjacent omentum should be brought up with an intact vascular pedicle (Fig. 81-2). The sutures are then successively tied from the superior to the inferior side of the perforation, so as to tampon the perforation with the living omental pedicle graft (Fig. 81-3). The sutures cannot be tied too tightly because the omentum will be strangulated in those sutures. The initial technique involved an isolated piece of omentum, which had been separated from the main body of the omentum and was used as a free graft; this technique is not as satisfactory as the viable pedicle and is no longer

used. A piece of rectus muscle was also used but has similarly been abandoned.

The disadvantage of sewing the ulcer shut, even if this is technically feasible, is that the omental patch placed over such a closure does not have the surface contact with the anterior duodenal serosa that the initial technique described by Graham permits (Fig. 81-4). If the ulcer edges are soft, they can be coapted, but the tamponade and sealing effect of the viable omental graft is markedly diminished.

After closure of the ulcer, meticulous cleansing of the peritoneal cavity is required, first by passing an appropriate suction tip (Poole or similar fenestrated type) into the retrohepatic, suprahepatic, perisplenic, and retrogastric spaces. The suction tip then is directed distally toward both gutters, adjacent to the ascending and

descending colon, and then into the pelvis. Care should be taken to remove as much of the free peritoneal fluid in the true pelvis as possible. The peritoneal cavity should be irrigated copiously with warm saline solution (5–8 liters is a minimal volume). There is no evidence that has been substantiated by prospective studies that suggests that putting antibiotics of any type into the irrigation fluid is of benefit. Some catastrophic results have been reported with the use of povidone-iodine solutions, even when dilute, as irrigants under these circumstances. One must accept the familiar truism that "dilution is the solution to pollution," attributed to Dr. Simmons, now of Pittsburgh. In general, the mechanical debridement effected by the large volumes of solution used is far more valuable than any other substance introduced into the peritoneal cavity under these circumstances. Obviously, it is necessary to drain any loculated collections of contaminated or purulent fluid, and those areas should be gently debrided if there is a large collection of fibrinous exudate.

Equally questionable is the practice of postoperative peritoneal lavage as a mechanical method of ridding the peritoneal cavity of residual infected material. Peritoneal dialysis catheters were inserted into each flank during the operation, and continuous lavage using approximately 1 liter of peritoneal dialysis fluid per hour was carried out for 24 to 48 hours. This maneuver is not commonly used.

A substantial number of surgeons still believe that it is possible to drain the peritoneal cavity and do not seem to distinguish between draining an abscess cavity, which is frequently desirable, and draining a peritoneal cavity, which is grossly contaminated, as with a patient who has had a perforated duodenal ulcer with wide distribution of duodenal content throughout the peritoneal cavity. Just as we would never drain a perforated appendix unless a definite abscess had been identified or a perforated colon for trauma, drains put into the upper peritoneal cavity in patients appropriately treated for a perforated peptic ulcer are ineffective and probably meddlesome. Draining retroperitoneal structures, such as the pancreas or kidney, is quite another matter; however, in this setting, drains should be avoided under every circumstance, unless one is an advocate of peritoneal dialysis.

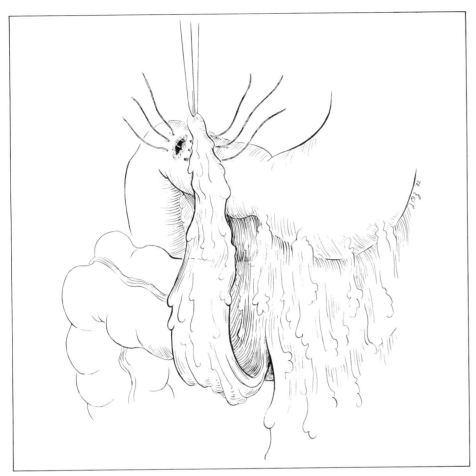

Fig. 81-2. Vascularized greater omentum is used to plug the hole after placement of three silk sutures below the perforation.

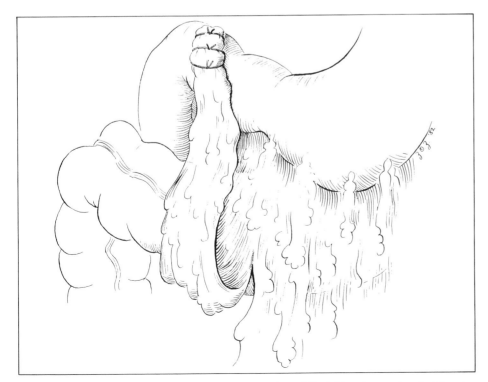

Fig. 81-3. The omentum is held in place by three sutures, each carefully tied loosely enough so that there is no chance of devascularizing the omental patch.

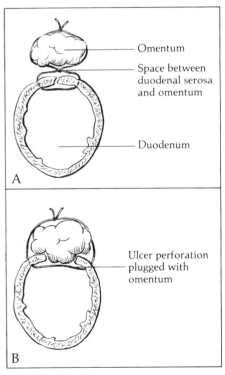

A

Omentum

Space between duodenal serosa and omentum

Duodenum

B

Ulcer perforation plugged with omentum

Fig. 81-4. When the sutures are initially tied to approximate the edges of the ulcer and the omentum is placed above those knots (A), there is a potential space between the duodenal serosa and the omentum. If the procedure is performed as described, the omentum plugs the hole (B) and is closely applied to the serosa, ensuring a watertight closure. In healing, the cicatrix forms on the viable omental bed and mucosa rapidly covers that cicatrix.

Wound Closure and Postoperative Care

It is always desirable to close the incision in one layer, incorporating fascia and peritoneum. A double strand of 3–0 suture material can be used to increase the surface gripped by the suture without increasing the bulk of foreign material left in the wound. The bites should be at least 2 cm from the cut edge of the fascia, and these should be tied in the usual manner. A suitable alternative is single or doubled 00 or 0 polypropylene or polydioxouase, which have become the suture materials of choice. It is important that the skin and subcutaneous tissue not be closed unless the perforation is less than 4 hours old; they should be left open for adequate drainage in most patients. Closure of the skin is occasionally followed by extensive, undermining infection, whereas leaving the wound open allows development of a clean, granulating bed, and delayed primary closure approximately 3 to 5 days after the initial operation is easily accomplished, especially with sterile skin tape strips (Steri-strips). Closing the skin over a subcutaneous drain is to be avoided.

The most common postoperative problems in the first 24 to 48 hours after duodenorrhaphy for perforated duodenal ulcer are inadequate fluid loading and oliguria. Tissue perfusion must be maintained at an optimal level. This perfusion can be monitored with a central venous pressure catheter or, in elderly or debilitated patients, with a pulmonary artery wedge pressure catheter. Thereafter, sepsis becomes the major postoperative problem, and administration of one of the newer broad-spectrum antibiotics (e. g., imipenem) is better and safer than the older triple therapy in this clinical setting. This drug can be continued for 24 to 48 hours after the operation to provide optimal protection. Intravenous hyperalimentation is often required if peritonitis supervenes, and it can be lifesaving.

One of the more recent developments in the consideration of the genesis of the duodenal ulcer, especially perforated duodenal ulcer, is the question of *Helicobacter pylori* infection in patients who have a perforated ulcer. A recent study suggests that the vast majority of patients have a ^{13}C urea breath test and that of patients with the positive urea breath test, over 85 percent had a gastric biopsy done with a positive urease test, both suggesting *H. pylori* infection. Therefore, the suggestion was made to provide triple therapy to eradicate this organism in all patients with perforated peptic ulcer. The recommended treatment is bismuth salts, usually subcarbonate, metronidazole, and tetracycline or amoxicillin, all for 10 days, with omeprazole for 4 weeks. This thesis will certainly require verification by numerous other studies before being universally accepted but is an issue that does need to be addressed.

Suggested Reading

Ball ABS, Thomas PA, Evans SJ. Operative mortality after perforated peptic ulcer. *Br J Surg* 76:521, 1989.

Berne TV, Donovan AJ. Nonoperative treatment of perforated duodenal ulcer. *Arch Surg* 124:830, 1989.

Boey J, Lee NW, Wong J, et al. Perforation in acute duodenal ulcers. *Surg Gynecol Obstet* 155:193, 1983.

Donovan AJ, Vinson TH, Maulsby GO. Selective treatment of duodenal ulcer with perforation. *Ann Surg* 1898:627, 1979.

Feliciano DV. Do perforated ulcers need an acid-decreasing surgical procedure now that omeprazole is available? *Surg Clin North Am* 72:369, 1992.

Graham RR. The surgeon's problem in duodenal ulcer. *Am J Surg* 40:102, 1938.

Horowitz J, Kukora JS, Ritchie, WP Jr. All perforated ulcers are not alike. *Arch Surg* 209:693, 1989.

Jordan PH. Proximal gastric vagotomy without drainage for treatment of perforated duodenal ulcer. *Gastroenterology* 83:179, 1982.

Sebastian M, Chandran VP, Elashaal YI, et al. *Helicobacter pylori* infection in perforated peptic ulcer disease. *Br J Surg* 82:360, 1995.

82

Congenital Pyloric Stenosis and Duodenal Obstruction

Arvin I. Philippart   Diana Farmer

Hypertrophic Pyloric Stenosis

Hypertrophic pyloric stenosis is a common illness with consistent clinical presentation promptly corrected by pyloromyotomy. Although the majority of instances present between 3 and 6 weeks of age, the disease has been documented throughout the spectrum of the first 12 weeks of life, including diagnosis by fetal ultrasound.

The etiology remains unclear. Pathologic studies confirm hypertrophy of muscular fibers rather than hyperplasia. Potential explanations include abnormal autonomic innervation, hypergastrinemia, and work hypertrophy. None of these is convincing. There is a 4:1 male-female ratio and an increased incidence in families in which there are affected members.

Clinical Presentation

The characteristic history is an infant with a progressive increase in frequency, volume, and force of nonbilious emesis associated with weight loss. Symptoms continue despite formula changes. Physical examination should focus on weight, status of hydration, and palpation of the abdomen. Palpation of a pyloric mass in the medial right upper quadrant by an experienced examiner precludes the need for further studies other than electrolytes.

In the absence of a definitively palpable pyloric mass, the currently preferred initial study is an ultrasound. Although operator dependent, accuracy has improved with the establishment of specific criteria. The combination of a pyloric diameter greater than 14 mm, length greater than 16 mm, and muscular thickness greater than 4 mm has been reported to have a 90 percent sensitivity and 100 percent specificity.

If there is a possible history of bile-stained emesis or if the ultrasound is not diagnostic of pyloric stenosis, an upper GI series is appropriate. Findings consistent with the diagnosis of pyloric stenosis include the "shoulders" at the proximal end of the pylorus created by the hypertrophic muscle, a lengthened pyloric channel, and a string sign or double track sign, which results from the compressed pyloric lumen

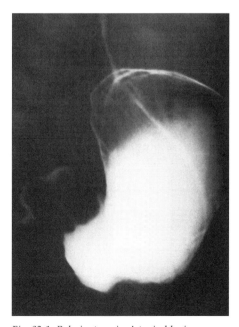

Fig. 82-1. Pyloric stenosis. A typical barium upper GI showing string sign and pyloric shoulders.

(Fig. 82-1). An adequate study requires some barium in the duodenal cap to clearly establish the extent of the pylorus. The additional advantage of an upper GI series is that it allows a diagnosis of malrotation and a presumptive diagnosis of gastroesophageal reflux if characteristic findings of pyloric stenosis are not present.

The pathophysiologic state that results from pyloric stenosis is hypochloremic, hypokalemic alkalosis. The renal response is paradoxic aciduria as a result of selective potassium retention. Any clinically detectable dehydration represents at least a 5 percent decrease in extracellular fluid requiring replacement before operation. Intravenous fluid replacement therapy is initiated with dextrose in normal saline solution, with 5 mEq of potassium chloride per 250 ml added once the child has voided. This solution is used for the first 50 percent of the calculated replacement volume. Dextrose in 0.45 normal saline with potassium is used for the balance of the calculated replacement volume. The operation should be delayed until the serum bicarbonate is less than 30 meq per ml and serum chloride is in the mid 90s. Failure to correct the alkalosis before the operation frequently results in apnea on emergence from anesthesia.

Operative Technique

The preferred incision is a transverse right upper quadrant incision positioned approximately halfway between the xiphoid and the umbilicus and modified to occur at the palpable liver edge. Vertical flaps deep to Scarpa's fascia are raised exposing

921

the anterior rectus sheath and linea alba to allow a subsequent longitudinal incision in the anterior rectus sheath. The rectus muscle is split 2 to 3 mm lateral to the medial rectus margin. Retraction of the rectus muscle laterally is followed by a transverse incision in the posterior rectus sheath and peritoneum. The ligamentum teres is then retracted anteriorly and medially, and the greater curvature of the stomach is delivered into the wound with forceps. This step is performed with rightward traction on the greater curvature until there is adequate stomach to grasp with a moistened sponge, after which leftward traction delivers the pylorus. Failure to easily deliver the pylorus can be the result of an inadequate incision in the abdominal wall or excessive elevation of the abdominal wall by retractors. Before the incision, the pylorus should be stabilized with leftward traction by the assistant and placement of the surgeon's second finger on the duodenal end of the pylorus. The incision is made superficially in the pylorus commencing at the pyloroduodenal junction and carried well onto the wall of the stomach (Fig. 82-2). Muscular disruption results from firm insertion of the blunt end of the scalpel handle to the level of the submu-

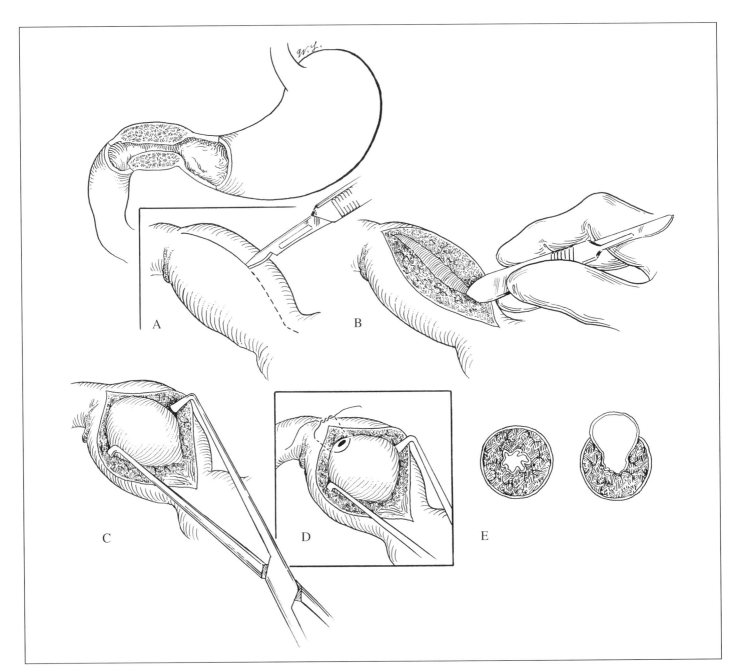

Fig. 82-2. Pyloromyotomy. A. A superficial incision begun on the duodenal end of the hypertrophied pylorus is carried onto the stomach. B. The scalpel handle divides the fibers. C. The pyloric spreader further mobilizes the mucosa. D. A perforation is closed with a horizontal mattress suture. E. Testing for perforation.

cosa in the middle of the pylorus. The scalpel handle is then drawn obliquely to the gastric end of the pylorus until the oblique muscular fibers of the anterior wall of the stomach are exposed. The Benson pyloric spreader is then placed in the pyloromyotomy incision with the blades on the pyloric muscle, not the mucosa, and the cut edges of the muscle are distracted. This additional submucosal dissection plane allows further prolapse of the pyloric mucosa into the defect created. Pyloromyotomy is considered complete when the superior and inferior muscle surfaces sit eccentrically and move independently. With the original incision having been placed in the most avascular portion of the pylorus, attempts at hemostasis of the cut edge are unnecessary. Oozing is a result of venous congestion and stops spontaneously. The divided pylorus is then returned to the abdomen by first placing the duodenal end of the pylorus into the peritoneal cavity.

The only significant complication of pyloromyotomy is mucosal perforation. Perforation should be sought by insertion of 30 to 40 cc of air through a nasogastric tube into the stomach and subsequent manual compression through the pylorus. Bubbles of air recognized at the distal pyloromyotomy are evidence of perforation. If perforation occurs, a single horizontal mattress suture that slides pyloric mucosa distally into the duodenum is preferable to closure of the pyloromyotomy with axial rotation and repeat myotomy.

Postoperatively, the infant is positioned in an infant seat elevated 30 degrees. Feeding is initiated 4 hours after the procedure with rapid progressive increases in volume and consistency of feeds. Postoperative emesis is not infrequent in the first 24 hours.

Duodenal Obstruction

Congenital duodenal obstruction is a sufficiently frequent finding to require a clear understanding by the individual who undertakes surgical correction. The obstruction can be complete (duodenal atresia) or incomplete (duodenal stenosis). These obstructions can be intrinsic to the duodenal wall or the result of extrinsic compression, or a combination of both. In intrinsic obstructions, there is a developmental abnormality of the duodenal wall to include atresia with or without mural continuity and perforated diaphragms referred to as "windsock" deformities. Extrinsic obstructions are the result of compression of an otherwise normal duodenum and include malrotation and preduodenal portal vein or the rare duodenal duplication. Each can be associated with an intrinsic mural abnormality. Annular pancreas is a coincidental anomaly associated with intrinsic duodenal obstruction. Clinical recognition occurs most commonly in the immediate neonatal period, but recognition can be delayed in lesions with lesser degrees of obstruction. Malrotation can present at any age.

Embryology

The widely accepted embryopathologic event leading to intrinsic duodenal obstruction is failure of recanalization. The solid cord stage of duodenal development is followed by vacuolization in the eighth to tenth week. Failure of coalescence of vacuoles results in failure to recanalize and resultant complete or partial obstruction. The temporal relationship to development of the pancreas and pancreaticobiliary ductal system leads to a higher incidence of anomalies in these structures as well. The frequency of an additional more distal duodenal atresia is low (1–3%) in comparison with jejunoileal atresias, in which associated more distal atresias are frequent and often multiple.

Associated anomalies occur frequently in the neonate with congenital duodenal obstruction. Down's syndrome (trisomy 21) and congenital heart disease each have an incidence of 30 to 40 percent in this population. Association with esophageal atresia with tracheoesophageal fistula or imperforate anus, or both, increase the complexity of management and urgency for intervention. Urologic and orthopedic anomalies occur less frequently.

Clinical Presentation

The diagnosis of duodenal atresia can be made on antenatal ultrasound during the third trimester. The finding of a dilated proximal duodenum in a pregnancy complicated by polyhydramnios is highly suggestive. After birth, duodenal atresia presents as emesis within the first 24 hours. In 85 to 90 percent of affected neonates, that emesis is bilious because the obstruc-tion is distal to the ampulla of Vater. The diagnosis can be further delayed in preampullary obstructions because emesis of feedings is nonbilious. In either variation, examination often reveals upper abdominal distention made scaphoid by insertion of a nasogastric tube.

The classic double bubble sign is recognized on plain abdominal x-rays in nondecompressed patients as a consequence of the accumulation of fluid and swallowed air in the enlarged stomach and duodenum proximal to the atresia. If nasogastric tube decompression has occurred before obtaining the films, instillation of 30 to 40 cc of air through the tube before obtaining films will produce the diagnostic findings. Air is a valuable contrast agent in the neonate. Specific attention should be paid to the presence or absence of any air distal to the second portion of the duodenum. Absence of distal air evidences atresia. No further proximally administered contrast agent is necessary or appropriate. If the diagnosis of atresia is certain, the operation can be performed at a convenient time.

If air is seen distal to the obstruction in the second portion of the duodenum, the possibility of complicating events is increased greatly because of the constant specter of malrotation. The duration of the duodenal obstruction can be determined from the plain films and is critical in evaluating the urgency for further roentgenographic evaluation and operation. Long-standing in utero obstruction is associated with marked dilation of the duodenum proximal to the obstruction in the second portion. Small amounts of air distal to a markedly dilated proximal duodenum indicate an intrinsic obstruction rather than a malrotation associated with recent volvulus and mesenteric vascular compromise. If the proximal duodenum is not markedly dilated, either urgent contrast studies or an operation, or both, should be undertaken to avoid delays in malrotation with volvulus.

Preoperative management should include a physical examination for associated anomalies. The dysmorphic features of trisomy 21 are frequently recognizable and a blood sample should be obtained for chromosomal analysis before administration of blood products. Cardiac anomalies should be sought by physical examination, oxygen saturation, chest x-ray, and cardiac ultrasound if readily available. Roentgenographic evidence of a nasogastric tube in the stomach rules out esophageal atresia. Passage of meconium and a patent anus should be documented. Intravenous fluid orders should provide maintenance requirements plus known losses. Broad-spectrum antibiotics are given before the operation.

Operative Technique

The widely accepted approach to each of the anomalies discussed is a generous right upper quadrant transverse incision. The patient is promptly eviscerated for inspection of intestinal viability and mesenteric fixation. Any volvulus is derotated counterclockwise until the mesentery is flat. If intestinal fixation is normal, the small bowel is externally inspected for continuity and patency. The duodenum is then exposed by mobilization of the right colon followed by a Kocher's maneuver with anteromedial rotation of the duodenum to fully expose the nature of the obstruction. This rotation also provides ease in placement of the duodenotomies, which are done laterally and anteriorly to avoid medial extension before identification of pancreaticobiliary ductal anatomy.

Duodenal atresia with mural continuity is now most widely managed by duodenoduodenostomy (Fig. 82-3). This anastomosis has supplanted the previously popular duodenojejunostomy (Fig. 82-4) because it allows earlier postoperative feeding usually obviating the need for total parenteral nutrition (TPN). There are several considerations in the placement of the proximal duodenotomy in Fig. 82-3. The incision is begun laterally for a distance of 3 cm so that no medial duodenum is incised without identification of the duct. The curvlinear nature promotes the rolling of the proximal bulbous duodenum anteriorly and inferiorly onto the distal duodenotomy during the anastomosis. It is important that the proximal duodenotomy be placed sufficiently superior to the proximal level of the obstruction so that the sum of that distance plus the distance between the distal obstruction and distal duodenotomy be greater than not only the length of the intrinsic obstruction but also the extrinsic structures such as an annular pancreas or preduodenal portal vein. In our hands, the use of a minimum 3-cm anastomosis has precluded the need for a lateral tapering duodenoplasty used by some others. Duodenoduodenostomy is also used for duodenal stenotic lesions other than the windsock deformity and for preduodenal portal vein with or without intrinsic obstruction.

Duodenal atresia associated with long gap mural discontinuity is infrequent. Two options exist. If there is associated malrotation and sufficient mesenteric length to the distal duodenum, a duodenoduodenostomy can be performed. If there is normal rotation and fixation, the recommended

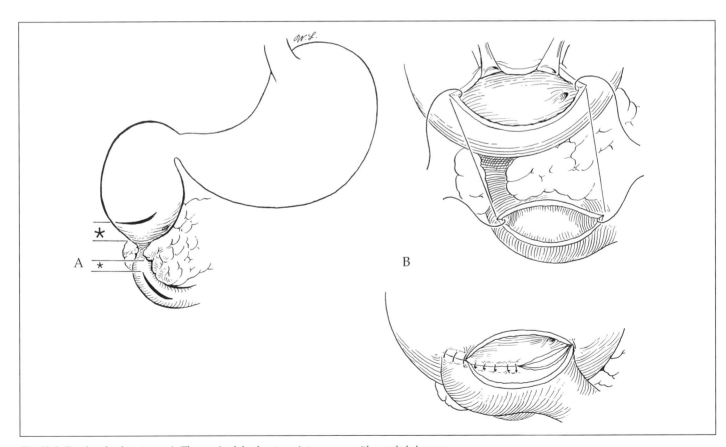

Fig. 82-3. Duodenoduodenostomy. A. The proximal duodenotomy is transverse with a cephalad curve medially. The distance of the proximal duodenotomy to the obstruction (*) is slightly greater than the distance from the obstruction to the distal longitudinal duodenostomy. B. The anastomosis is performed with interrupted full-thickness sutures of 5–0 silk with intraluminal knots.

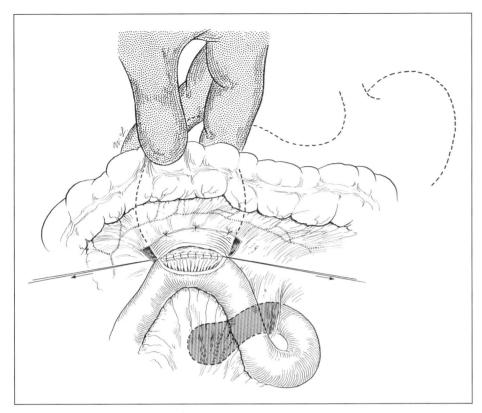

Fig. 82-4. Retrocolic duodenojejunostomy. The proximal duodenotomy is performed as in Fig. 82-2. Incision in the right transverse mesocolon creates a defect, the edges of which are sutured to the duodenum cephalad to the duodenotomy. A proximal loop of jejunum is then incised on the antimesenteric border for a distance of 3 cm. The anastomosis is performed using single layer full-thickness interrupted 5–0 silk suture with knots on the inside.

approach is duodenojejunostomy (Fig. 82-4). This anastomosis has been used for decades with success. Although it is generally accepted that this anastomosis is slower to function, we use neither gastrostomies nor transanastomotic feeding tubes but provide caloric requirements via TPN, if necessary.

Duodenal stenosis resulting from a perforated diaphragm (windsock deformity) is shown in Fig. 82-5. Although there is a broader spectrum of age at presentation, the majority of instances present in the neonatal or early infancy periods. This anomaly can be recognized by duodenal mural continuity, a constriction ring representing the circumferential origin of a conical diaphragm, and a tapered duodenal wall distal to the constriction ring rather than an abrupt transition as seen in Fig. 82-3. If doubt exists, advancement of the nasogastric tube into the duodenum through a patulous pylorus with subsequent downward pressure will exaggerate the constriction ring. Partial excision of this web is important because an ill-advised duodenoduodenostomy can later become partially obstructed by distal progression of the web over time. Although many prefer a transverse proximal duodenotomy for web incision, we prefer a curvilinear vertical duodenotomy on the

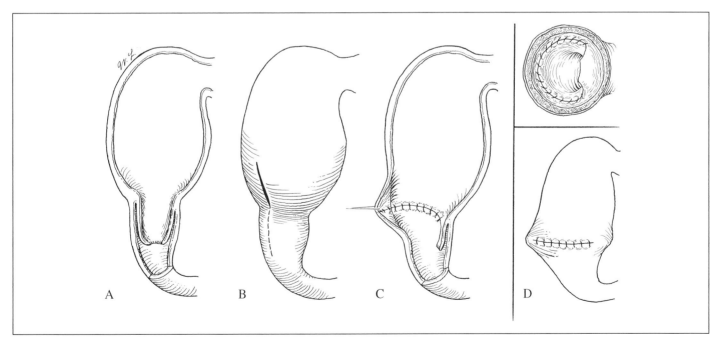

Fig. 82-5. Excision of duodenal windsock. A&B. The anatomic characteristics and external appearance are shown with placement of a curvilinear vertical duodenotomy carried through the constriction ring. C. Excision does not include the medial one-third of the web. D. Completed repair.

anterolateral wall. This duodenotomy is carried through the constriction ring into the duodenum distal to the origin of the web. The web is then excised first posteriorly and then anteriorly. Because of a high association with ductal anomalies, the medial third of the diaphragm is left untouched and hangs distally into the duodenal lumen. The cut edges are oversewn with fine running absorbable suture for hemostasis. The duodenotomy is then closed transversely, further enlarging the lumen at that level.

The same approach is used by others for short transverse imperforate duodenal diaphragms presenting as duodenal atresia unassociated with any extrinsic anomaly. We continue to prefer the duodenoduodenostomy for that lesion to avoid ductal injury.

In all the previously mentioned forms of duodenal atresia or stenosis, surgeons should reassure themselves of proximal and distal patency by passage of a tube or irrigation of saline.

Malrotation

Clinical Presentation

Malrotation is a common anomaly and a common cause of duodenal obstruction. There are two forms of clinical presentation. Malrotation unassociated with midgut volvulus presents as chronic repetitive emesis that is intermittently bile-stained with or without symptoms of colic or abdominal pain. Recognition occurs across the age spectrum from the neonatal period to childhood. Malrotation complicated by mid-gut volvulus is an acute surgical emergency that is a constant element of the differential diagnosis in all children with bilious vomiting. Volvulus with or without antecedent symptoms can occur across the total spectrum from fetal life to adulthood.

Intestinal rotation and fixation occur late in the first trimester of fetal life. There are two consequences of incomplete rotation and fixation. The first is that normal fixation of the small bowel mesentery to the posterior parietes is incomplete. This failure of fixation results in a narrow mesenteric pedicle containing the mesenteric vessels. Torsion or volvulus of that narrow pedicle produces vascular compromise that proceeds to mid-gut infarction without urgent intervention. In that scenario, a diagnosis delayed until there are findings

on physical examination evidencing an intra-abdominal catastrophe is too late.

The second, and frequent, consequence of abnormal rotation and fixation is the development of thickened bands of peritoneum ("Ladd's bands") from the abnormally located cecum to the posterior parietes in the right upper quadrant. The result is extrinsic duodenal compression.

The first step to a correct diagnosis is the constant suspicion that any child with bilious emesis has malrotation with volvulus. There is no consistent diagnostic finding on plain films of the abdomen. The best current diagnostic practice is a limited upper GI series through a nasogastric tube placed through the pylorus for the sole purpose of identifying the presence or absence of the ligament of Treitz. A normal ligament is evidenced by the third and fourth portion of the duodenum crossing the spine with the apex of the duodenojejunal junction occurring at the level of the pylorus. On a lateral view, the duodenojejunal junction should be at or posterior

to the anterior vertebral bodies. Subsequent jejunal loops should be in the left side of the abdomen. Failure of the duodenum to continue to the left side of the spine, failure of the fourth portion to course superiorly, and presence of proximal jejunal loops on the right side of the spine all evidence malrotation. The limited contrast is then aspirated, the nasogastric tube returned to the stomach, and a contrast enema is performed with ileal reflux. In all but the premature, the cecum should be normally located below the iliac crest. The additional value of this roentgenographic approach is that ileal reflux will also detect intussusception, which is part of the differential diagnosis. In any age group, the coexistence of the findings of an acute abdomen on physical examination and malrotation on an upper GI series mandates urgent operation. The contrast enema is not necessary.

Operative Technique

No matter the presentation, the infant or child is approached through a right upper

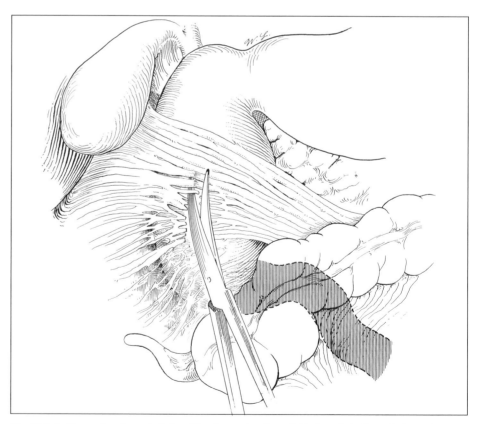

Fig. 82-6. Ladd procedure for malrotation. The abnormal peritoneal attachments to the posterior parietes are first divided by cecal mobilization exposing the anterior wall of the second and third portions of the duodenum. Dissection should occur on the anterior wall of the duodenum to avoid vascular or pancreatic injury.

quadrant transverse incision. A vertical midline incision can be considered for older patients who have evidence of an acute abdomen. The first maneuver is to eviscerate the patient and inspect the mesentery for volvulus. In volvulus, the gut is derotated in counterclockwise fashion until the mesentery is flat. If intestinal ischemia exists, the gut should be packed in warm saline sponges for an adequate period of time to assess the impact of reperfusion. In intestinal necrosis, the choices of resective procedures, stomas, and second look operations should follow sound surgical principles. If after derotation the gut is viable, a Ladd procedure and appendectomy should be performed.

In the patient operated on for malrotation with chronic rather than acute symptoms, the same inspection of the mesentery should be the initial step. One will not infrequently find lesser degrees of mesenteric volvulus that has not resulted in intestinal ischemia. The essence of the procedure for incomplete duodenal obstruction resulting from extrinsic compression is complete division of the abnormal peritoneal bands overlying the duodenum (Fig. 82-6). The abnormally positioned cecum is mobilized by sharp division of its peritoneal attachments superiorly and anteriorly. This mobilization exposes the anterior aspect of the duodenum. All adventitious tissue overlying the anterior duodenum is sharply divided with that dissection occurring on the anterior rather than the medial wall to avoid vascular and pancreatic injury. Complete mobilization of the second portion of the duodenum is commenced laterally and anterior to the inferior vena cava. The third portion of the duodenum can have a variable course, in-

cluding into the route of the mesentery covered by a thin layer of peritoneum. This layer must also be incised. Again, it is important to stay on the anterior wall of the duodenum. At this point, the entire duodenum should be evaluated for possible associated intrinsic obstruction to be dealt with as previously described. In the absence of ischemia, an appendectomy is performed because of the subsequent non-anatomic location of the cecum. The entire mid gut is then laid flat on the abdominal wall to avoid torsion on replacement of the intestine. The second and third portions of the duodenum and proximal jejunum are then carefully positioned along the right gutter into the right lower quadrant, followed by placement of the remainder of the small intestine in the right lower quadrant and pelvis. As a result, the colon will lie on the left side of the abdomen. Final inspection of the base of the mesentery should confirm that it is flat without torsion.

In the absence of intestinal ischemia requiring resection, the GI tract is decompressed with a nasogastric tube postoperatively. In situations in which extensive small intestinal resection is required, a gastrostomy should be placed for postoperative decompression and for the gradual institution of elemental formula once intestinal function returns. Such a feeding regimen can reduce the total time necessary for TPN.

Suggested Reading

Bailey PV, Tracy TF Jr, Connors RH, et al. Congenital duodenal obstruction: A 32-year review. *J Pediatr Surg* 28:92, 1993.

Benson CD. Infantile pyloric stenosis. *Prog Pediatr Surg* 1:63, 1969.

Brown RA, Millar AJW, Linegar A, et al. Fenestrated duodenal membranes: An analysis of symptoms, signs, diagnosis, and treatment. *J Pediatr Surg* 29:429, 1994.

Hight DW, Benson CD, Philippart AI, et al. Management of mucosal perforation during pyloromyotomy for infantile pyloric stenosis. *Surgery* 90:85, 1981.

Keller H, Walderman D, Greiner P. Comparison of preoperative sonography with intraoperative findings in congenital hypertrophic pyloric stenosis. *J Pediatr Surg* 22:950, 1987.

Weber TR, Lewis JE, Mooney D, et al. Duodenal atresia: A comparison of techniques of repair. *J Pediatr Surg* 21:1133, 1986.

EDITOR'S COMMENT

A report from Melbourne, Australia (*J Ped Surg* 30:37, 1995) indicates that 37 infants with infantile hypertrophic pyloric stenosis underwent successful laparoscopic pyloromyotomy. The average age was 6 weeks and average weight was 4.5 kg. Three 4-mm ports were used in each procedure. The average operating time was 29 minutes (range: 7–60 minutes). Feeding was begun an average of 5.2 hours (range: 3–12 hours) postoperatively, and the average time of discharge was 28 hours (range: 16–52 hours) postoperatively. There were no technical failures. One patient had minor surgical emphysema, which resolved spontaneously. It appears that laparoscopic pyloromyotomy can be safe and successful in infants with hypertrophic pyloric stenosis.

L.M.N.

83

Subtotal Gastrectomy for Gastric Cancer

Teruaki Aoki   Sumio Takayama

Preoperative Evaluation and Preparation

Gastric cancer can be diagnosed visually in most patients by means of upper GI series, x-rays, and endoscopy. Figure 83-1 shows the course of diagnosis and clinical evaluation. Definitive diagnosis is made by histologic examination of endoscopic biopsy specimens. In differential diagnosis, the major clinical considerations are lymphoreticular hyperplasia, malignant lymphomas, and submucosal tumors (e. g., leiomyomas, leiomyosarcomas, and so forth).

An accurate diagnosis of the location and site of the primary cancer and the width and depth of the cancerous lesion is important in deciding the extent of the primary resection and in determining the cancer stage. Detailed information about the local area around the lesion can be obtained using the endoscopic contrast dye stain method or endoscopic ultrasonography. With the recent progress made in diagnostic techniques, smaller cancers can be discovered at an earlier stage, and limited surgery such as endoscopic mucosal resection is being widely studied. Therefore, correct diagnosis of the width and depth of the invasion is becoming more important.

The extent of cancerous invasion and metastasis is investigated with CT, ultrasonography, barium enema, and, if required, angiography to detect the presence and extent of liver metastasis, lymph node metastasis, and disseminating peritoneal metastasis (accumulation of ascites), as well

as invasion to contiguous structures. Distant metastatic spread is first evaluated by a careful physical examination and chest x-ray. In instances of advanced cancer, enlargement of the left supraclavicular lymph nodes should be examined carefully. If Virchow metastasis is suspected, biopsy is necessary for histologic diagnosis. A digital examination is also performed to detect the presence of cancer implantation in the cul-de-sac of Douglas. If bone metastasis is suspected, bone scintigraphy is recommended.

The preoperative cancer staging is determined from the localized progression of the primary cancer and the extent of cancerous invasion and metastasis. Our standard method of treatment and operative technique are decided based on the long-term, nationwide clinical data collection in Japan. In most instances, the prognosis can also be predicted according to the preoperative cancer stage.

Patients are instructed in the importance of active respiratory training for postoperative measures against pain and respiratory complications. A catheter for postoperative continuous epidural anesthesia is placed. In the evening of the day before the operation, a laxative is given to cleanse the intestine. A hypnotic is used if required to assure sufficient sleep. On the day of the operation, the patient is placed on nothing per OS (NPO) status and a cleansing enema is given in the early morning. Just before the operation, a nasogastric tube is inserted and the stomach contents are removed. Some patients with advanced lesions in the greater curvature of the stomach require concomitant resection of the transverse colon because of infiltration. In

patients in whom colorectal resection is anticipated, preoperative intestinal preparation is performed.

Indications

Candidates for subtotal gastrectomy are patients who are expected to achieve complete recovery from the disease. Inclusive conditions are the following: 1) no distant metastasis (Virchow metastasis; lung, liver, or bone metastasis); 2) no suspected disseminating peritoneal metastasis or periaortic lymph node metastasis; 3) disseminating peritoneal metastasis seen on laparotomy but limited to P_1 (disseminating peritoneal metastasis around the primary cancer and greater omentum metastasis—hereinafter, grade according to the *General Rules for Gastric Cancer Study*, 12th edition, by Japanese Research Society for Gastric Cancer (Kanehara Publ. Co., Tokyo, 1993); 4) metastasis in a resectable organ in which a surgical cure is considered definitive.

Most surgeons perform the subtotal gastrectomy on the pyloric side together with D_2 lymph node dissection under the following conditions: 1) localized invasion from the center of the stomach to the anal side; and 2) sufficient distance from the tumor margin to the adoral resection line for radical cure (3 cm in the localized type and 5 cm in the invasive type). Total gastrectomy is selected when the invasion extends further on the adoral side. Therefore, in instances of progressive cancer localized on the anal side from the center of the stomach, pyloric subtotal gastrectomy is usually selected. However, the extent of

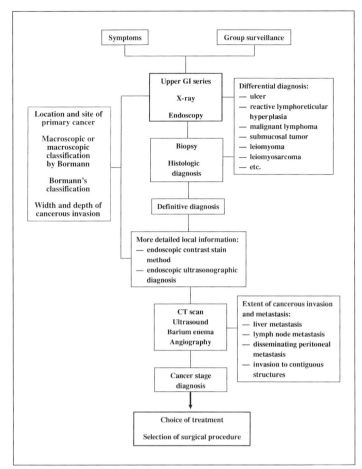

Fig. 83-1. Algorithm for clinical diagnosis of gastric cancer.

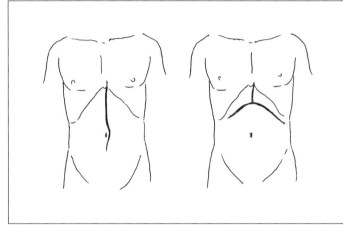

Fig. 83-2. Incisions for subtotal gastrectomy.

the resection can be reduced appropriately in patients with early gastric cancer that is localized, as in the lower part of the stomach.

In instances of progressive cancer, additional lymph node dissection is performed in group 3 or 4 lymph nodes, which show high metastasis rates, such as the lymph nodes behind the common hepatic artery (No. 8p), the retropancreatic lymph nodes (No. 13), the hepatoduodenal mesenteric lymph nodes (No. 12), the mesenteric root lymph nodes (No. 14) on the right side, and the periaortic lymph nodes (No. 16a2, b1) (see Figs. 83-3 and 83-4).

A new approach, preoperative reductive chemotherapy for down-staging of the cancerous lesions, has been advocated recently in patients diagnosed as inoperable because of severe cancerous invasion or in patients who cannot undergo radical operations because of distant metastasis.

Operative Procedures

The principal strategy of radical operations for gastric cancer is adequate resection of the primary cancer and extensive and complete removal of the regional lymphatic system. Therefore, the crux is total lymph node dissection that includes not only the lymph nodes but also the connecting lymphatic ducts, with en bloc resection of the proper range of the arteriolar network extending into the adjacent tissue.

Incision

Laparotomy is usually performed by means of an epigastric median incision from the upper margin of the xiphoid process to 2 to 3 cm below the umbilicus (Fig. 83-2A). In some situations, a combined technique with a transverse incision several centimeters under the xiphoid process is performed depending on the patient's

physique (e. g., thickness of the thorax and degree of obesity) (Fig. 83-2B).

The operative method is decided after examination of the presence and severity of liver metastasis, disseminating peritoneal metastasis and lymph node metastasis, and the possibility of a radical cure. The presence of cancerous lesions in other intra-abdominal organs is investigated at the same time.

Once it is adequately confirmed that a radical surgical cure is possible, the main arteries and veins associated with the primary cancer (bilateral gastric arteries and veins and bilateral gastroepiploic arteries and veins) should be ligated to prevent hematogenous metastasis of the primary cancer during the operative manipulation.

To avoid injury of the spleen during the operation, a towel or sponge pad is inserted at the back side of the spleen to shift the spleen toward the midline.

Extent of Gastrectomy and Lymph Node Dissection

The extent of the gastrectomy and lymph node dissection is shown in Figs. 83-3 and 83-4. The basic operative procedure involves resection with the regional lymphatic system so that the primary cancer is included together with the mesogastrium; it is important to select a free layer of the mesogastrium. This free mesogastrium includes the greater omentum, the frontal layer of the transverse mesocolon, and the anterior surface of the pancreatic capsule, as well as the retroperitoneum, hepatoduodenal mesentery, and lesser omentum, which connect them to the esophageal opening. These structures form the omental bursa. Therefore, the goal is achieved by performing bursectomy together with dissection of the lymphatic system of the celiac arterial system, as well as resection of the enclosed primary cancer en bloc. Generally, a four-fifths gastrectomy on the pyloric side is performed, and the residual gastric circulation is maintained by the left inferior phrenic artery, posterior gastric artery, and short gastric arteries.

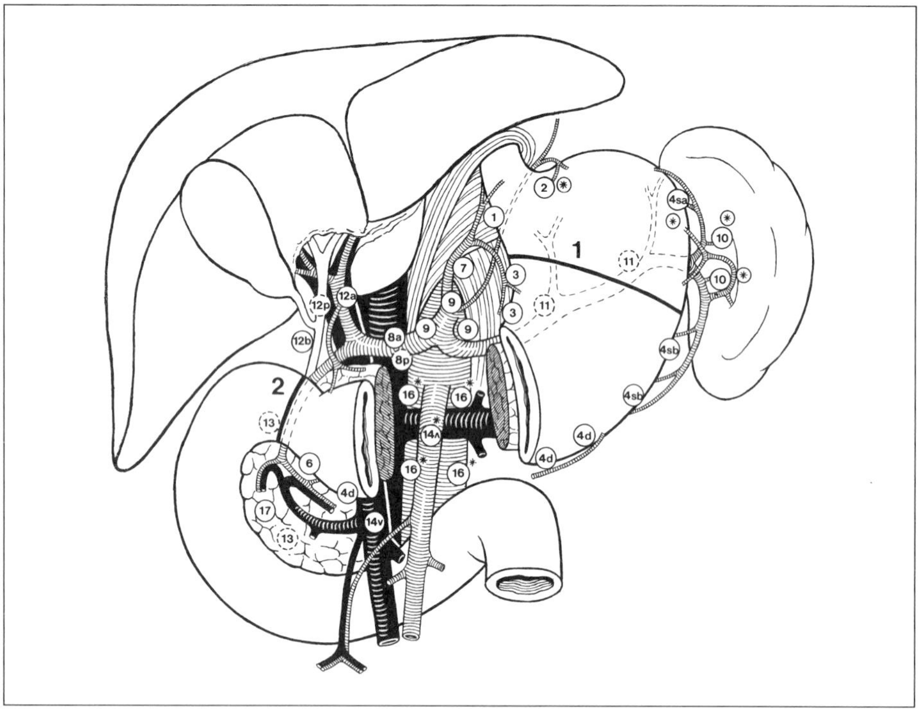

Sequence of Operative Procedures

The operative sequence is shown in Fig. 83-5, as follows: (A) the duodenum is mobilized together with the pancreatic head, and the para-aortic lymph nodes are examined for metastasis; (B) the retropancreatic region and hepatoduodenal region are dissected; (C) the frontal layer of the right transverse mesocolon is freed as far as the sectioned greater omentum, the region around the superior mesenteric artery and vein is dissected, the right gastroepiploic artery and vein are sectioned at the root, and the surrounding tissue is dissected; (D) the frontal layer of the mesocolon is freed from the left side; the root part of the left gastroepiploic artery and vein is identified, sectioned, and dissected; the anterior surface of the pancreatic capsule is freed; and the greater curvature side of the stomach and anterior surface of the pancreas are dissected; (E) the duodenum is sectioned on the anal side just under the pyloric ring; (F) the regions around the common hepatic artery, the upper margin of the portal vein, and the celiac artery are dissected; and the left gastric artery is dissected at the root; (G) the region around the splenic artery is dissected; (H) the lesser curvature side of the stomach is dissected from the junction of the esophagus and the stomach along the stomach wall to the anticipated division line; and (I) the stomach is sectioned with a sufficient distance on the adoral side of the tumor assured. Reconstruction is performed by the Billroth I method.

Mobilization of the Duodenum

The retroperitoneum is sectioned on the side of the descending part of the duode-

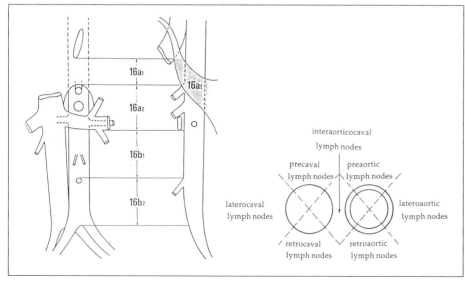

Fig. 83-3. *Margin of gastrectomy and lymph node dissection: (1) gastrectomy line; (2) duodenectomy line; *selective dissection sites; *should not be dissected so as to preserve residual stomach circulation.*

Fig. 83-4. *Abdominal para-aortic lymph nodes.*

num, and the descending part and right side of the horizontal part of the duodenum are turned toward the anterior midline (Fig. 83-6A). The inferior vena cava, left renal vein, and abdominal aorta are adequately separated until they can be observed directly. The upper margin of the retroperitoneal section is left in the same position with the retroperitoneal section on the right side of the abdominal aorta for the later dissection around the celiac artery. Samples are taken of the right para-aortic lymph node No. 16a2, b1 (interaorticocaval, see Fig. 83-4), and a frozen section analysis is performed (Fig. 83-6B). When metastasis is suspected, priority dissection of this region is performed. In instances of progressive cancer of the lower part of the stomach, this route of lymph node metastasis is an important one, and dissection is critically important. When metastasis is confirmed, the radical operation must be abandoned.

Dissection of the Retropancreatic Region and Hepatoduodenal Membrane

With the pancreatic head turned toward the anterior midline, the retropancreatic head lymph nodes (No. 13) are freed and dissected together with the thin capsule in this field of vision. Since the capsule is connected to the hepatoduodenal membrane, the membrane is sectioned along the upper margin of the duodenum. It is then sectioned vertically along the proper hepatic artery to the hepatic portal region, and continued to the section of the lesser omentum at the liver adhesion region (Fig. 83-7A). Once the proper hepatic artery and gastroduodenal artery have been identified, the hepatoduodenal membrane on the right side is first dissected together with the connective tissue toward the left

side (Fig. 83-7B). It is then freed and dissected until the upper margin reaches the level of the cystic duct confluent region so that the common bile duct is exposed. The tissue dissected around the common bile duct and in the retropancreatic head region is subjected to slight traction, and the posterior side of the portal vein is freed and dissected. Isolation of the posterior side of the portal vein is easy, but ligation is carefully performed since there are many small blood vessels flowing in from the lymphatic ducts and the pancreatic parenchyma at the upper margin of the pancreas.

Next, tissue around the proper hepatic artery is freed and dissected on both sides together with the adipose tissue (Fig. 83-7C). The dissection is performed at the upper margin of the duodenal bulb so that the branching part of the right gastric artery and the branching part of the gastro-

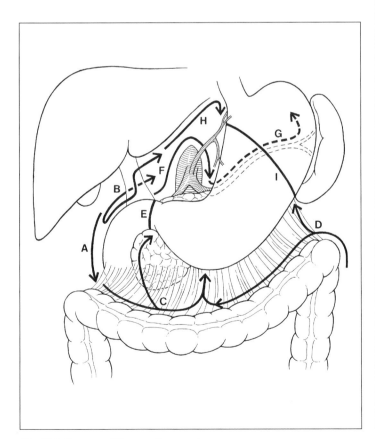

Fig. 83-5. Sequence of the operative procedure.

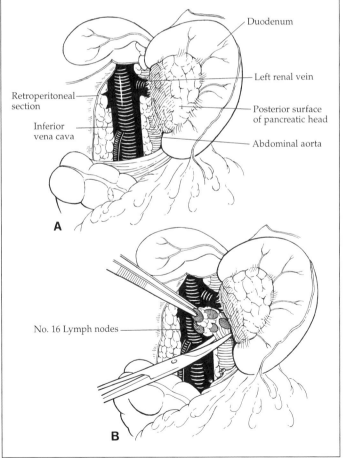

Fig. 83-6. Mobilization of duodenum and sampling of abdominal para-aortic lymph nodes.

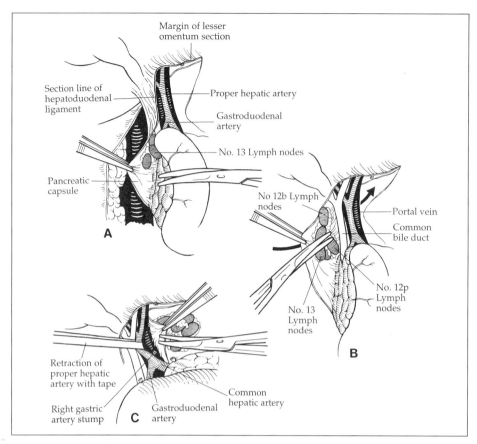

Margin of lesser omentum section

Section line of hepatoduodenal ligament

Proper hepatic artery

Gastroduodenal artery

No. 13 Lymph nodes

Pancreatic capsule

A

No 12b Lymph nodes

Portal vein

Common bile duct

No. 12p Lymph nodes

No. 13 Lymph nodes

B

Retraction of proper hepatic artery with tape

Right gastric artery stump

C

Gastroduodenal artery

Common hepatic artery

Fig. 83-7. Dissection of retropancreatic head region and hepatoduodenal ligament.

duodenal artery from the common hepatic artery are sufficiently exposed. The right gastric artery is sectioned at the root. The proper hepatic artery is then pulled upward using tape, and the anterior surface of the portal vein and posterior surface of the proper hepatic artery are freed and dissected. Since the right gastric vein enters on the anterior surface of the portal vein, it is identified and sectioned at the point of influx. The lymph nodes in the hepatoduodenal membrane and retropancreatic lymph nodes are dissected en bloc with the surrounding connective adipose tissue, which can be pulled out into the omental bursa on the left side of the portal vein.

Dissection on the Greater Curvature Side

The frontal layer of the transverse mesocolon is freed from the posterior layer along the front surface of the descending portion of the duodenum and the hepatic flexure of the colon from the lower direction of the layer of duodenum freed from

the posterior layer. The procedure and identification of the freed layer are relatively easy. When the freed layer is gradually advanced to the distal side, the frontal layer of the mesocolon is freed from the transverse colon without bleeding together with the greater omentum. By extending this freed layer to the left side, the anterior surface of the pancreatic head is exposed. When the greater omentum and frontal layer of the mesocolon are freed, it is easier to identify the freed layer without unnecessary bleeding if the procedure is performed toward the colon rather than starting from the colon side.

As the freed layer is continued to the left, the blood vessels in the mesentery are exposed and the freed layer reaches the lower margin of the pancreas. The right gastroepiploic vein, right gastric and colic venous trunk, and superior mesenteric vein are exposed (Fig. 83-8A). Since this route is an important one in metastasis of cancer of the lower part of the stomach, the region around the superior mesenteric

vein at the lower margin of the pancreas (No. 14v) is dissected, and the right gastroepiploic vein is sectioned at the influx region of the gastrocolic venous trunk. Because the frontal layer of the mesocolon is contiguous to the pancreatic capsule at the lower margin of the pancreas, it is sectioned along the duodenum, the gastroduodenal artery is exposed, and the surrounding tissue is dissected. When the branch of the right gastroepiploic artery has been identified, it is sectioned at the root and dissected as far as the resected stomach together with the surrounding tissue (Fig. 83-8B).

Dissection of the frontal layer of the mesocolon and the pancreatic capsule is continued to the left side. Peeling of the frontal layer of the mesocolon is difficult in the center part, especially on the side of the transverse colon, so it is continued only as long as it remains easy to perform.

Next, the retroperitoneum is sectioned on the side of the descending colon from the splenic flexure of the colon and is freed along the fascial layer of Toldt. This step is continued along the flexure of the colon, which is isolated (Fig. 83-9A). This freed layer is the same as the previously freed layer of the frontal layer of the mesocolon, and it can be easily freed with no bleeding along the lower margin of the pancreas. This step is continued to the right and connects with the layer freed previously from the right. Thereafter, the frontal layer of the mesocolon, which has not been freed, is freed toward the transverse colon so that the whole greater omentum is also easily dissected from the transverse colon. The greater curvature side of the stomach is freed together with the mesentery surrounding the stomach, which forms the omental bursa.

When the freed greater omentum and frontal layer of the mesocolon are pulled upward and the pancreatic capsule is freed toward the pancreatic tail, the left gastroepiploic artery and vein are exposed at the hilum of the spleen. The branches from the splenic artery and vein are identified and sectioned at the root (Fig. 83-9B). The surrounding tissue of the left gastroepiploic vessels is dissected as far as the resected stomach, and the gastric wall along the greater curvature side is freed approximately 5 cm to the anal side from this region for subsequent anastomosis. The pancreatic capsule is freed as far as the upper

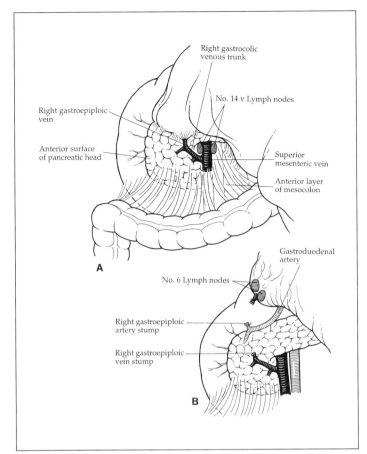

Fig. 83-8. Dissection of greater curvature side.

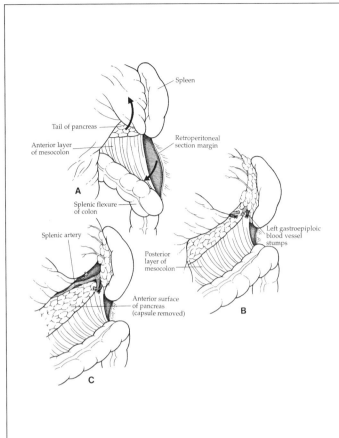

Fig. 83-9. Continued dissection of greater curvature side.

margin of the pancreas until the splenic artery is exposed (Fig. 83-9C).

Sectioning of the Duodenum

To improve the visual field around the common hepatic, celiac, and splenic arteries, and to facilitate dissection of the region, the duodenum is sectioned and the stomach is pulled upward to the left.

The sectioning is usually performed just under the pyloric ring, but when duodenal invasion is suspected, the sectioning is performed at an adequate distance from the tumor. In this situation, reconstruction is performed by the Billroth II method, and the duodenal stump is closed.

Dissection of the Region Around the Common Hepatic Artery

The pancreatic capsule is freed sufficiently as far as the upper margin of the pancreas,

and the tissue between the common hepatic artery and pancreas is sectioned along the upper margin of the pancreas toward the branching part of the splenic artery (Fig. 83-10A). Since there are many small blood vessels from the pancreas, they are carefully ligated because damage to the pancreatic parenchyma might cause future leakage of pancreatic juice. This procedure is easy to perform when gauze is applied to the pancreas and it is pulled gently downward with the other hand. The anterior surface of the common hepatic artery is freed together with the sectioned pancreatic upper margin tissue and is connected with the previously freed layer of the hepatoduodenal membrane (Fig. 83-10B).

The common hepatic artery is taped, traction is applied, and the region between the area around the common hepatic artery and the branching part of the gastroduodenal artery and the portal vein is dissected. The left gastric vein is identified at

the upper margin of the splenic vein on the left side of the portal vein, on the upper margin of the pancreas, or just before influx of the portal vein. Then it is sectioned at the influx region (Fig. 83-10C). The connective tissue at the upper margin of the splenic vein of the portal vein influx region and the left side of the portal vein is freed and dissected, continuing to the freed layer from the posterior part of the pancreatic head in the direction of the posterior surface of the common hepatic artery.

Dissection Around the Celiac Artery

All the tissue that has been dissected so far is pulled up to the left, the retroperitoneum is sectioned on the right side of the aorta, and the retroperitoneum is dissected toward the midline together with the peritoneal adipose tissue so that the diaphragm muscle bundle is exposed. The right celiac artery is then exposed (Fig. 83-11A). The region around the celiac ar-

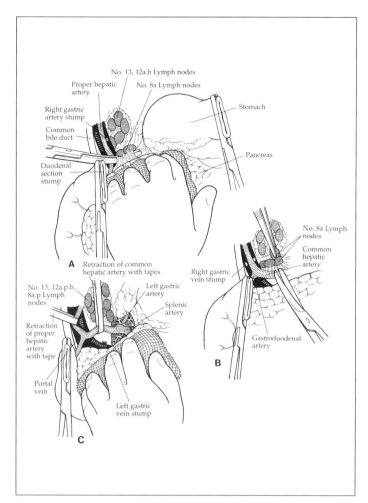

Fig. 83-10. *Dissection around the common hepatic artery.*

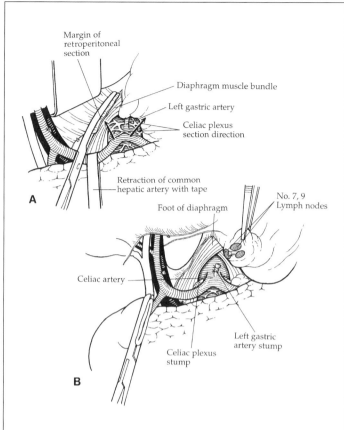

Fig. 83-11. *Dissection around the celiac artery.*

tery together with the superior mesenteric artery is covered with the firm celiac plexus. The dissection around the celiac artery is limited to the anterior surface hemisphere. The branching part of the left gastric artery is exposed and sectioned at the root (Fig. 83-11B).

Dissection Around the Splenic Artery

Dissection of the area around the splenic artery is performed from the branching part of the splenic artery to the splenic hilum in the same manner as dissection of the area around the common hepatic artery. Since the splenic artery shows severe tortuosity and part of it is embedded in the splenic pulp, care is required so as not to damage the pancreatic parenchyma or the blood vessels into the pancreas. The posterior gastric artery is sectioned at the root (Fig. 83-12).

Dissection of the Right Cardiac Region and Lesser Curvature Side of the Stomach

The lesser omentum is sectioned along the liver adhesion region to the junction between the esophagus and stomach. The anterior surface of the abdominal esophagus at this level is freed to avoid damage to the muscle layer and is sectioned in the direction of the angle of His. The anterior surface of esophagus and the anterior wall of the lesser curvature of the stomach are sectioned and dissected along the gastric wall in succession to the anticipated gastric section line (Fig. 83-13A). The posterior surface of the esophagus and posterior wall of the gastric lesser curvature are sectioned and dissected in the same manner. The posterior trunk of the vagus nerve is sectioned at the level of the hiatus and dissected down together with the surround-

ing tissue to the point of the proximal resection line of the stomach (Fig. 83-13B).

Gastrectomy

The line connecting a point approximately 2 cm on the anal side from the esophago-gastric junction on the lesser curvature and a point several centimeters on the anal side from the lowest branch of the short gastric arteries on the greater curvature usually becomes the adoral side gastrectomy line (Fig. 83-14A).

The anastomotic region is preserved. Sectioning and suturing can be performed easily with no bleeding using an automatic suturing device (Fig. 83-14B). After closure of the serosa of the lesser curvature side of the stomach, the anticipated area of anastomosis on the greater curvature side is held by a clamp and is sectioned just beside the clamp (Fig. 83-14C).

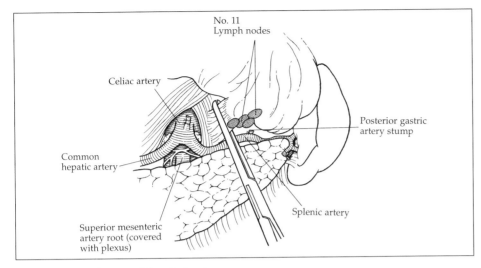

Fig. 83-12. Dissection around the splenic artery.

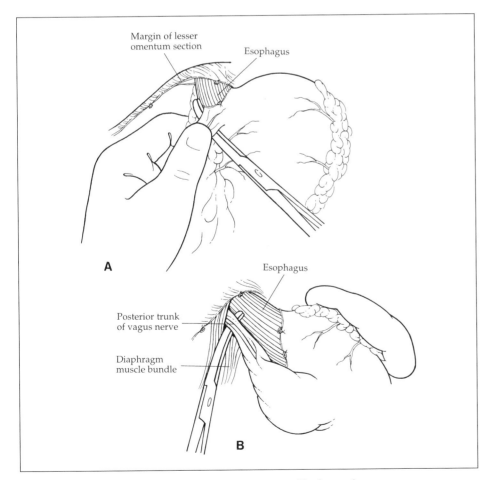

Fig. 83-13. Dissection of right cardiac part and lesser curvature side of stomach.

Reconstruction

Reconstruction is performed by the Billroth I method. The residual stomach is slightly twisted so that the stomach stump suture line is moved toward the posterior wall. Modified layer-to-layer anastomosis as shown in Fig. 83-15 is performed between the residual gastric and duodenal stumps. First, the gastric mucosa and full thickness of the duodenum are sutured around the complete circumference using interrupted sutures. Horizontal mattress suturing is performed to suture the anterior and posterior wall gastric mucosa and the full thickness of the duodenum at the site of the lesser curvature stump suture line (Fig. 83-15A).

Next, the muscle layer of the gastric serosa and the duodenal serosa are sutured around the whole circumference using interrupted sutures. Horizontal mattress suturing is performed to suture the gastric serosal muscle layers of the anterior and posterior walls and the duodenal serosa at the site of the lesser curvature stump suture line (Fig. 83-15B). Figure 83-16 shows the operation completed.

Postoperative Management

The nasogastric tube can usually be removed on day 3 and oral ingestion started on day 4. The drainage fluid must be carefully observed, and the tube can be removed on day 7.

Complications Requiring Caution and the Countermeasures

Continuous epidural anesthesia should prevent postoperative pain, and deep-breathing exercises should be possible. Postoperative continuous epidural anesthesia is performed by: 1) preoperative insertion and anchoring an epidural catheter from T10 to T11 cephalad approximately 5 cm; 2) confirmation of the sufficient scope of analgesia after awakening from the anesthesia; 3) giving a single injection of 5 ml of 0.25% bupivacaine and 0.1 mg of buprenorphine via the epidural catheter before sharp pain appears; 4) after confirmation of the stable vital signs, continuous

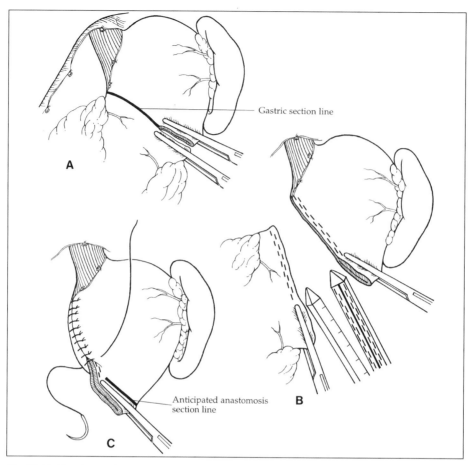

Fig. 83-14. Gastric resection.

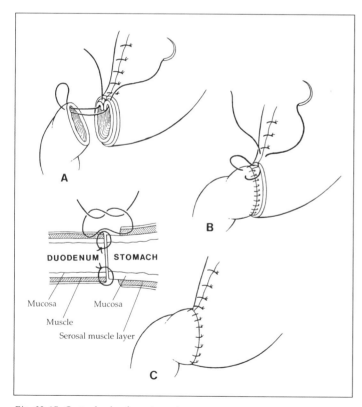

Fig. 83-15. Gastroduodenal anastomosis.

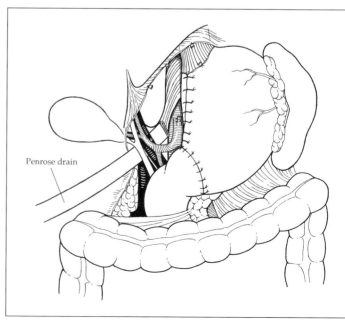

Fig. 83-16. Completed operation with Penrose drain through the hepatoduodenal ligament into the retroperitoneal space.

infusion of 50 ml of 0.25% bupivacaine and 0.2 mg of buprenorphine at a flow rate of 5 ml per hour using an infusion pump, and drip infusion of a low concentration (5 μg/kg) of dopamine to maintain blood pressure. Thereafter, respiratory training (i. e., incentive spirometer, expulsion of sputum, and postural changes) is strongly recommended. Patients can start to walk on the day after surgery. Continuous epidural anesthesia is performed for 3 to 4 days postoperatively, and thereafter only single injections of local anesthesia are given depending on the grade of the pain.

Complications Related to Operative Procedures

Oozing from the freed pancreatic surface and leakage of pancreatic juice associated with lymph node dissection continue in some instances. Oral ingestion is delayed, and antipancreatitis agents and antibiotics are administered for several days. The condition of the drainage is observed, and the timing of oral ingestion and removal of the drain are determined.

Discussion

The operative results for gastric cancer in Japan are excellent. The main reason is extensive and complete resection of the regional lymphatic system en bloc with the primary lesion. However, the postoperative quality of life is often damaged considerably by radical operations. In patients with a lower degree of progression, such as early cancer patients, the type of surgical procedure performed should be determined by the likelihood of effecting a radical cure according to a patient's disease progression, while considering safety and postoperative quality of life. The operative technique introduced here is considered suitable for radical cure of patients with progressive gastric cancer localized in the body or lower part of the stomach with no direct invasion in other organs.

Suggested Reading

Nishi M, Ichikawa H, Nakajima T, et al (eds). *Gastric Cancer*. Tokyo; Springer-Verlag, 1993.

EDITOR'S COMMENT

Doctor Aoki studied with us at the University of Washington in the 1950s. As a student of the famed Minoru Oi (the Rule of Oi: All gastric ulcers are found within 1 cm of a change in the type of gastric mucosa (*Gastroenterology* 36:45, 1959), it is appropriate that he and his colleague Takayama contribute to our monograph on the subject of gastric operations. Because of the respect with which Dr. Aoki is held in the world of surgery, he has served as Secretary General of the Collegium Internationale Chirurgie Digestivae. He now holds the Chair of Surgery at the Jikei Medical School of Tokyo, formerly held by Professor Oi.

We must pay special attention to the details of regional lymph node dissection in the operative treatment of gastric carcinoma. Our coworkers from Japan have shown us the merits of this additional dissection for our patients' long-term well-being.

L.M.N.

84

Total Gastrectomy for Carcinoma

Murray F. Brennan

Complete operative resection remains the only potentially curative modality for gastric adenocarcinoma. The results of resection for early gastric cancer are excellent; however, the majority of patients in the United States present with symptomatic advanced lesions. Operative decisions then focus either on the most effective procedure that offers potential for cure or on how to achieve the maximal palliation with the minimal morbidity.

Four questions must be addressed when considering a patient for gastric resection for adenocarcinoma: 1) Is the patient fit for an operation?; 2) is the operation likely to help?; 3) if operation is to proceed, what is the extent of the gastric resection?; and 4) what is the extent of the nodal dissection? Many patients with advanced gastric adenocarcinoma may not be medically fit for any procedure. More difficult, however, is the patient who can tolerate a procedure and has minimal symptoms, but by preoperative studies (computed tomographic [CT] scan, laparoscopy) has incurable disease (ascites, peritoneal extension, liver metastases). Such patients should be strongly considered for nonoperative treatment. This chapter focuses on the technical issues of resection, when indicated.

Extent of Gastric Resection

The extent of gastric resection for adenocarcinoma of the stomach will be, in the main, predetermined by the site and extent of the primary neoplasm. Total gastrectomy as a routine procedure for gastric ad-

enocarcinoma has not been shown to improve survival, although this has continued to be debated. For those patients in whom adequate (4–6 cm) margins beyond the lesion can be obtained, a more limited gastric resection, such as proximal esophagogastrectomy or distal subtotal gastrectomy, provides the same results for the patient, and diminishes perioperative morbidity. Unfortunately the extent of the margin is rarely the limiting factor in survival. Patients rarely die of local marginal recurrence only, and similarly, patients who are likely to have positive resection margins are usually those with large penetrating (T3) or node-positive lesions. The need for a total gastrectomy, however, to encompass all the disease within the stomach, should never be a factor in precluding proceeding with the operation.

Extent of Lymph Node Dissection

The involvement of lymph nodes will be predicated on the site of the primary lesion within the stomach (Figs. 84-1 to 84-3). Lesions can then be much better defined as to the extent of the dissection (Figs. 84-4 to 84-6). This will be true even in lesions that involve the majority of the stomach. Where the more extensive lesion is identified is the area in which the greater nodal dissection will be required.

The rationale for more extensive nodal dissection continues to be a matter of great debate. Early studies in Western centers suggested a limited advantage to the more extensive operation. This, however, was then neglected as an approach until pop-

ularized by the Japanese with improved morbidity and survival results. The improved survival results seen by the Japanese authors have been suggested to be due in part to the more extended nodal dissection. Whether this is true or whether it is due to more adequate and appropriate staging remains a matter of some controversy. It would seem that biologically, although early forms of the disease are commonly seen in Japan, the nature of the underlying disease process is not different for Asian and Western populations.

Current studies examining the value of the extent of nodal dissection in a randomized fashion are ongoing. Extended node dissection can be performed in experienced hands with only limited morbidity. A recent study from my own institution suggests no increase in morbidity with a more extensive nodal dissection.

Operative Preparation

Total gastrectomy remains a major operation in the hands of all but the experienced gastric surgeon. It is my practice to perform a total gastric resection when 4 to 6 cm of negative margins cannot be obtained from the primary tumor. I believe that an extended R2 dissection (D2) is the nodal dissection of choice.

Diagnosis

Evaluation of the patient with suspected or proven gastric adenocarcinoma is dominated by the use of endoscopic techniques, with or without ultrasound. Endoscopy allows the definition of the extent of the lesion within the stomach along with confir-

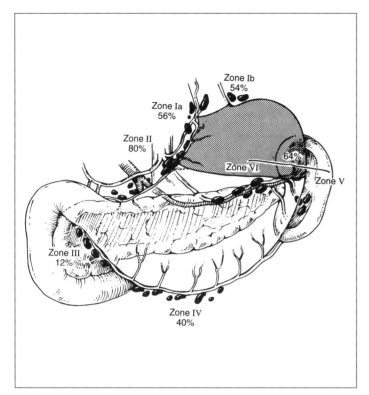

Fig. 84-1. *Proximal gastric cancer, node-bearing areas. (From DA Sutherland. The Lymphatic Spread of Gastric Cancer. In G McNeer, GT Pack [eds], Neoplasms of the Stomach. Philadelphia, Lippincott, 1967. Pp 408–415. Reproduced with permission.)*

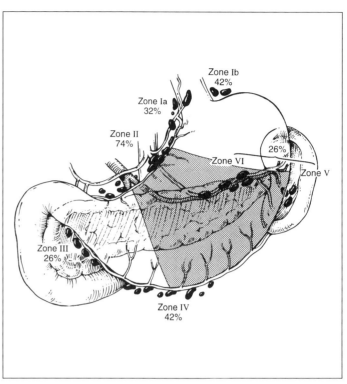

Fig. 84-2. *Midbody cancer, node-bearing areas. (From DA Sutherland. The Lymphatic Spread of Gastric Cancer. In G McNeer, GT Pack [eds], Neoplasms of the Stomach. Philadelphia, Lippincott, 1967. Pp 408–415. Reproduced with permission.)*

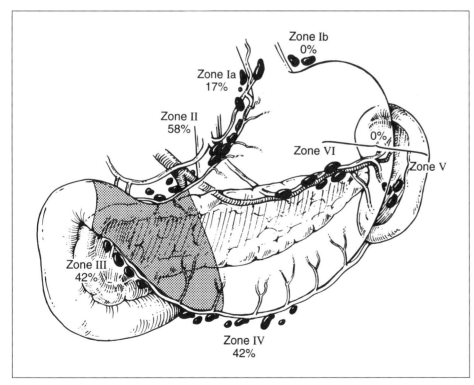

Fig. 84-3. *Distal cancer, node-bearing areas. (From DA Sutherland. The Lymphatic Spread of Gastric Cancer. In G McNeer, GT Pack [eds],* Neoplasms of the Stomach. *Philadelphia, Lippincott, 1967. Pp 408–415. Reproduced with permission.)*

mation of the histopathologic diagnosis. Endoscopic ultrasound allows greater definition of the extent of tumor invasion (T stage) and is the most accurate method for defining T stage. While endoscopic ultrasound provides information on the size of perigastric lymph nodes and can suggest nodal involvement it is not yet definitive. Small amounts of ascites, often unappreciated by other studies, can be seen in the lesser sac with endoscopic ultrasound, and unsuspected small liver metastases in the left lateral segment can also be identified.

Computed tomography remains the only other study of value in defining extent of disease noninvasively. While not as accurate as endoscopic ultrasound for defining T stage, it is more accurate for defining M stage and for detecting ascites and peritoneal or omental deposits. With preoperative staging of this nature, consideration as to curative versus noncurative operation can be embarked on. Investigational studies employ laparoscopy to further determine the possibility of curative resection. Many patients who have disease unresectable for cure can avoid an unnecessary and nonpalliative operation. On occasion, es-

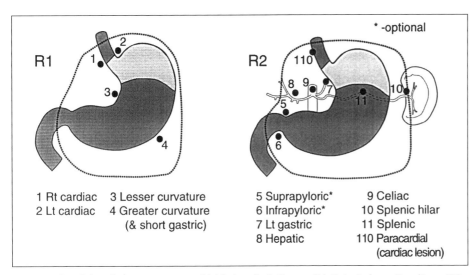

Fig. 84-4. Gastric lymphadenectomy, upper third lesions (including cardia). Extent of resection. (From JW Smith, MH Shiu, L Kelsey, MF Brennan. Morbidity of radical lymphadenectomy in the curative resection of gastric carcinoma. Arch Surg 126:1469, 1991. Reproduced with permission.)

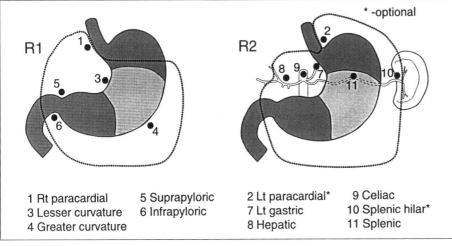

Fig. 84-5. Gastric lymphadenectomy, middle third lesions. Extent of resection. (From JW Smith, MH Shiu, L Kelsey, MF Brennan. Morbidity of radical lymphadenectomy in the curative resection of gastric carcinoma. Arch Surg 126:1469, 1991. Reproduced with permission.)

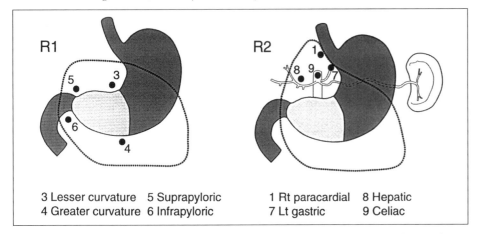

Fig. 84-6. Gastric lymphadenectomy, lower third lesions. Extent of resection. (From JW Smith, MH Shiu, L Kelsey, MF Brennan. Morbidity of radical lymphadenectomy in the curative resection of gastric carcinoma. Arch Surg 126:1469, 1991. Reproduced with permission.)

pecially for distal lesions, despite spread, palliative operations to relieve obstruction are justifiable.

Patients who have undergone endoscopic ultrasound and laparoscopy and have been shown to have advanced T3 lesions apparently confined to the stomach can be considered for investigational regimens of preoperative chemotherapy. This therapy can be delivered safely but with some increase in perioperative morbidity. Given the poor (<20%) long-term (5-year) survival of lesions of T3 or greater, such investigational approaches are justified.

Preoperative Preparation

The patient is evaluated for tolerance of a potential major upper abdominal operation. If the gastroesophageal junction is involved, and there is a likelihood that a thoracic approach will be required, preoperative pulmonary function is determined. Preoperative antibiotics, usually with a cephalosporin, are used at the time of induction, generally for a single dose, dependent on the half-life of the drug employed and the length of the operation, with the intent of diminishing wound infection.

Operative Positioning

The patient is placed supine with consideration given to the possibility of either left or right thoracic approach in proximal gastroesophageal lesions. In both positions the chest is prepared before the patient is allowed to fall back onto a pneumatic mattress, so that reprepping and redraping of the chest can be avoided. A sandbag can be placed beneath the left costal margin to elevate it, and the lower left chest is prepared for an extension directly into the left chest. A split-lumen endotracheal tube is placed in all patients in whom thoracotomy is likely. In the majority of patients undergoing gastrectomy, the lesion will be confined to the stomach and an abdominal approach is adequate.

There is no clear consensus as to whether a long midline incision or a bilateral subcostal incision is preferable. Both provide excellent exposure to the upper abdomen. We tend to use the midline incision when a thoracic extension or second incision is considered, but either approach is adequate. An alternative approach, a left thoracoabdominal incision, is preferred by some for gastroesophageal junction le-

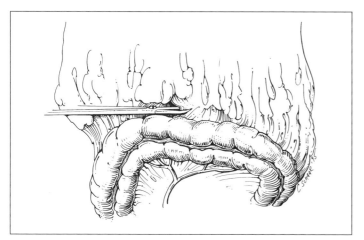

Fig. 84-7. Detachment of the greater omentum from the colon through the avascular plane.

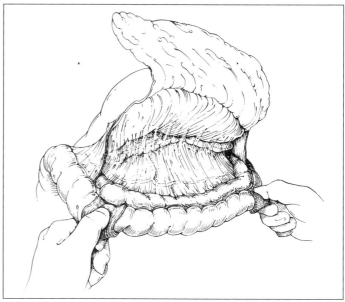

Fig. 84-8. The anterior layer of the mesocolon is sharply dissected from the mesocolonic vessels in an avascular plane.

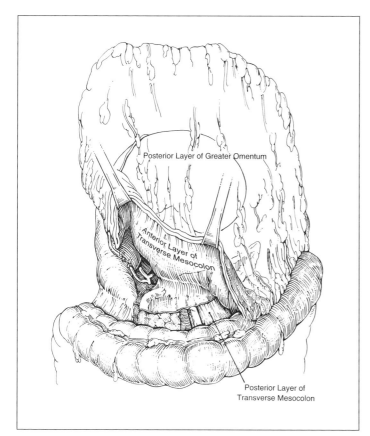

Posterior Layer of Greater Omentum

Anterior Layer of Transverse Mesocolon

Posterior Layer of Transverse Mesocolon

Fig. 84-9. Careful ligation of the gastroepiploic vessels is essential to avoid annoying hemorrhage.

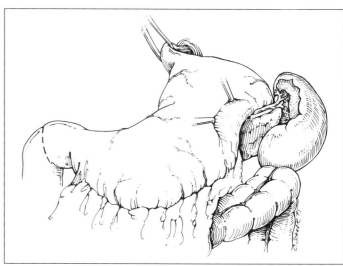

Fig. 84-10. The splenic hilum is carefully dissected, ligating the short gastric vessels.

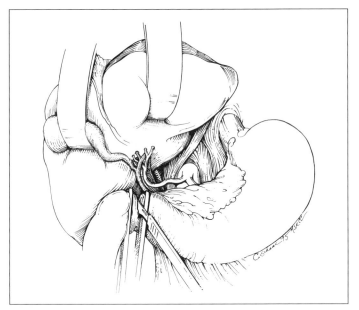

Fig. 84-11. The duodenum is carefully divided between straight clamps or with the GIA stapler.

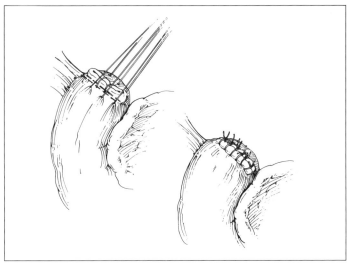

Fig. 84-12. The duodenum is carefully closed with an outer layer of monofilament absorbable interrupted sutures.

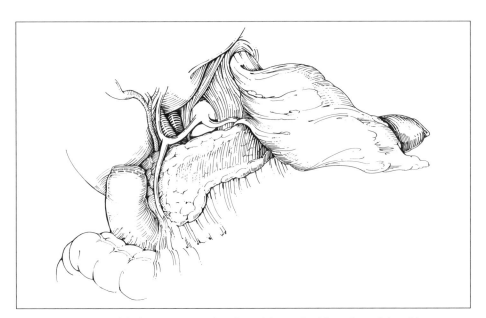

Fig. 84-13. Dissection of the hepatic artery at the celiac axis is completed from above, skeletonizing structures to the left of the left hepatic artery, back to the celiac, and below the common hepatic artery.

sions. Once access to the abdomen is obtained, careful examination for the extent of disease is performed. Important considerations are the presence of peritoneal metastasis or liver involvement. Remote lymph node involvement such as the para-aortic lymph nodes precludes progression to a radical procedure. Lesions involving all of the stomach, but predominantly the proximal stomach with extension to the lymph nodes high in the porta, also pre-

clude the likelihood of any chance for curative resection.

Once formal laparotomy has been employed, fixed retractors are placed. Our first approach in the dissection is section of the greater omentum from the colon (Fig. 84-7). This is performed by using the cautery or the scissors and entering into the anterior leaf of the mesocolon. It can take a small amount of time to obtain the

correct plane and to skeletonize the mesocolonic vessels. Once the correct plane is reached, bleeding should be minimal and the presence of any hemorrhage suggests an incorrect plane. On occasion local invasion or adherence will be present and mesocolonic resection is required. The standard dissection is continued back to the inferior border of the pancreas and the pancreatic capsule is dissected upward (Fig. 84-8). Branches to the right gastroepiploic vessels are divided just at the inferior border of the pancreas, and venous tributaries here should be carefully divided to prevent annoying hemorrhage (Fig. 84-9). The extension is continued out laterally, along with the superior aspect of the pancreas, skeletonizing the splenic artery (Fig. 84-10) and dividing the short gastric vessels close to the spleen. At this point it is often easier to change the approach and begin by dissecting the lesser omentum from the undersurface of the liver, extending back to the right crus and mobilizing the right aspect of the gastroesophageal junction.

At this point division of the duodenum is simple, usually performed with two straight Kocher clamps (Fig. 84-11), taking care to first close the duodenum and then invaginate the closure. We prefer to use running 3–0 absorbable monofilament suture material, but many prefer the use of a stapler (Fig. 84-12). Division of the duo-

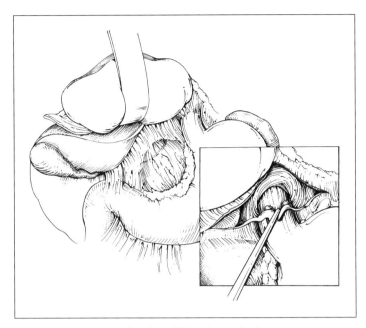

Fig. 84-14. *Mobilization of esophageal hiatus is completed.*

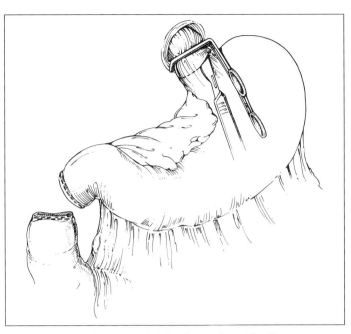

Fig. 84-15. *The esophagus is divided sharply, usually stabilized by a noncrushing vascular clamp.*

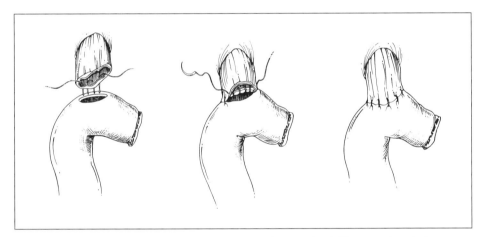

Fig. 84-16. *Standard end-to-side reconstruction, using monofilament absorbable sutures in a single continuous layer.*

denum allows elevation and rotation upward and forward and easy access to the dissection of the node-bearing areas.

Dissection in the porta can begin from above, isolating the bifurcation of the hepatic artery, bringing the node-bearing tissue inferiorly, and dissecting the portal vein, both to the left of the left hepatic artery and in the area between the common hepatic and the superior border of the pancreas (Fig. 84-13). This dissection can be swept back to the celiac axis, picking up

the dissection of the superior border of the pancreas at the junction of the splenic artery with the celiac. The left gastric artery is then divided at its origin.

Dissection from above, along the right crus, allows the aortic junction of the celiac axis to be identified and cleared. The extent of the dissection of the splenic hilum depends on the extent of disease present. We usually preserve the spleen but it can be sacrificed, if necessary. The short gastric vessels are identified and ligated close to the spleen, the colonic attachments to the

spleen having been reflected inferiorly early in the procedure.

The left crus is identified and all tissue is reflected from it. The left adrenal gland should be clearly identified and preserved from harm. At this point, with the entire stomach mobilized, the left gastric artery can be divided at its origin, if this was not done at the time of dissection of the celiac, and the entire stomach is lifted forward. The gastroesophageal junction is mobilized, and we prefer to divide the esophagus, using a soft vascular clamp for stabilization (Figs. 84-14 and 84-15).

Reconstruction

Standard reconstruction is usually by the Roux en Y method, using a loop of jejunum anastomosed from the end of the esophagus to the side of the jejunum. This loop should be at least 40 cm from the subsequent jejunojejunal anastomosis. The length of 40 to 50 cm should minimize esophageal reflux. In preparation of the jejunal loop, we isolate a loop of jejunum with its vascular supply and divide that with the GIA stapler. This then allows the passage through the retrocolic approach to place it in juxtaposition to the esophagus.

Several options exist for anastomosis of the esophagus to the jejunum. I prefer a single layer of running PDS taken with large, full-thickness bites (Fig. 84-16). Of-

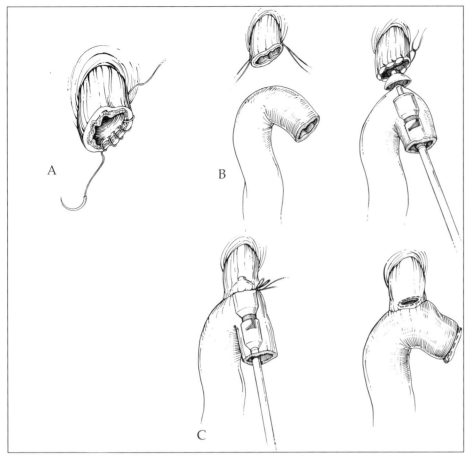

Fig. 84-17. *Reconstruction using the EEA stapler. A. Placement of a full-thickness running suture. B. Placement of the EEA stapler through the divided loop. C. Closure of the end of the loop with a stapler.*

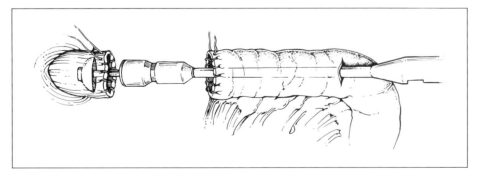

Fig. 84-18. *Alternative reconstruction with the EEA using a separate enterotomy and end-to-end anastomosis.*

ten a stabilizing single suture placed in the posterior aspect of the esophagus, suturing the posterior aspect to the posterior surface of the jejunum, is adequate. Then, beginning in the midline posteriorly, an over-and-over running suture tied anteriorly is more than adequate. An alternative is the use of the end-to-end stapling device, which can be utilized in standard fashion with the entry point either through the end of the jejunum (Fig. 84-17) or through a more distal enterotomy in the jejunal loop (Fig. 84-18).

For the majority of patients with gastric adenocarcinoma, I have not utilized formal pouch creation, as the morbidity and the long-term mortality are usually predicated on the extent of disease rather than on any form of reconstruction (Fig. 84-19).

Postoperative management involves standard maintenance of fluid and electrolyte balance. A nasogastric tube, which may have been passed at the time of the procedure, is removed on the first postoperative day and routine meglumine diatrizoate (Gastrografin) swallow is not performed. While many prefer the use of intra-abdominal drains, I have progressively employed these to a lesser and lesser extent. I now use them only in unusual situations and usually because of concern for the integrity of the pancreas after capsular stripping.

Unless fever or ileus develops, the patient is allowed ice on the second or third day and can be given nutrient by the fifth or sixth day. Any concern clinically for an anastomotic leak can be confirmed by a Gastrografin swallow, which is not routine. If a leak occurs, oral intake is limited until the patient's status is evaluated. Only a clinically significant leak is formally drained.

Results

Radical operations can now be performed for gastric adenocarcinoma. In the 165 patients reported recently, the overall operative mortality was 1.1 percent and no increased morbidity was associated with the extended R2 (D2) dissection. The addition of preoperative and perioperative chemotherapy does appear to increase morbidity and remains an investigational approach. Long-term survival after curative resection remains stage dependent.

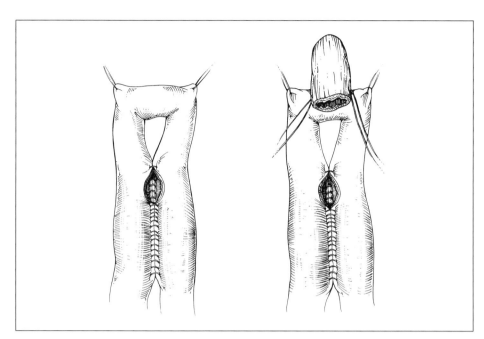

Fig. 84-19. The creation of a pouch is rarely necessary, and not routinely used by me.

Suggested Reading

Botet JF, Lightdale CJ, Zauber AG, et al. Preoperative staging of gastric cancer: Comparison of endoscopic US and dynamic CT. *Radiology* 181:426, 1991.

Brennan MF. Radical surgery for gastric cancer: A review of the Japanese experience (editorial). *Cancer* 64:2063, 1989.

Bunt AMG, Hermans J, Smit VTHBM, et al. Surgical/pathologic-stage migration confounds comparisons of gastric cancer survival rates between Japan and western countries. *J Clin Oncol* 13:19, 1995.

Karpeh M, Brennan MF. Adenocarcinoma of the Stomach. In EM Copeland, RJ Howard, AL Warshaw, et al (eds), *Current Practice of Surgery*. New York: Churchill Livingstone, 1993. Chap XIII, pp 1–24.

Kelsen D, Atiq OT, Saltz L, et al. FAMTX versus etoposide, doxorubicin, and cisplatin: A random assignment trial in gastric cancer. *J Clin Oncol* 10:541, 1992.

Longmire W. Total gastrectomy for carcinoma of the stomach. *Surg Gynecol Obstet* 84:21, 1947.

McNeer G, James A. Resection of stomach and adjacent organs in continuity for advanced cancer. *Cancer* 1:449, 1948.

Noguchi Y, Imada T, Matsumoto A, et al. Radical surgery for gastric cancer: A review of the Japanese experience. *Cancer* 64:2053, 1989.

Reynolds JV, Karpeh MS, Kelsen D, et al. Influence of preoperative and postoperative chemotherapy on perioperative morbidity in patients with gastric adenocarcinoma. Submitted for publication.

Shiu M, Papachristou D, Kosloff C. Selection of operative procedures for adenocarcinoma of the midstomach. *Ann Surg* 192:730, 1980.

Smith JW, Brennan MF. Surgical treatment of gastric cancer. *Surg Clin North Am* 72:381, 1992.

Smith JW, Shiu MH, Kelsey L, Brennan MF. Morbidity of radical lymphadenectomy in the curative resection of gastric carcinoma. *Arch Surg* 126:1469, 1991.

EDITOR'S COMMENT

The pendulum of surgical therapy for carcinoma of the stomach continues to swing toward radical resection, that is, extended total gastrectomy. I held back from this approach after the experience of Appleby (*Cancer* 6:704, 1953) seemed to suggest that the true radical resection did little to improve the overall survival of these patients.

Doctor Brennan gives a fair appraisal of the preoperative and operative approach to this difficult problem. An issue of the *World Journal of Surgery* (19:167, 1995), in its World Progress in Surgery section, presents an up-to-date review of multimodal treatment and prognostic factors in gastrointestinal cancer; these reviews complement the Brennan presentation.

Following total gastrectomy, innumerable techniques are promulgated to improve postoperative nutrition, mainly in the form of pouches formed from small intestine. The poor nutrition is related more often to recurrence of the cancer than to failure to develop an intestinal reservoir. Thus, I am in full agreement that a Roux en Y esophagojejunal reconstruction is satisfactory.

L.M.N.

85

Esophagogastrectomy for Carcinoma of the Abdominal Esophagus and Gastric Cardia

John Wong   Manson Fok

Carcinoma of the abdominal esophagus and gastric cardia causes progressive dysphagia, which, if unrelieved, leads to dehydration, inanition, and death. Because the symptoms are distressing, restoring the ability to swallow as normally as possible is the primary goal of any form of treatment. In patients with resectable tumors, removal of the growth avoids local complications and may result in cure. When resection of the tumor is not possible, a bypass procedure would be an adequate alternative. For patients with very advanced disease or those who cannot tolerate anesthesia, intubation or laser therapy should be contemplated. Patients who are fit enough for esophageal intubation under anesthesia can, as a rule, undergo a bypass operation, which offers better palliation of dysphagia with less risk of gastric reflux.

Carcinoma of the Abdominal Esophagus and Gastric Cardia

The extent of resection depends on the exact location and the size of the tumor, which then determines the level of anastomosis and also the organ to be used for esophagoplasty. If the lesion is situated mainly in the abdominal esophagus, a variable part of the stomach can be preserved for direct anastomosis to the divided esophagus, whether this be in the chest or neck. When the bulk of the tumor is in the cardia, total gastrectomy may be

required, and a loop of colon or jejunum is used for reconstruction. We prefer to use colon rather than jejunum for reconstruction that requires a long length of substitution because the colon has a more reliable vascular arrangement and is easy to prepare; good bowel preparation is essential, however.

Resection and Reconstruction

From experiences learned over the years, we have now limited our practice to the following four operations:

1. Abdominal and right thoracic approach: esophagogastrectomy with intrathoracic esophagogastrostomy or esophagoenterostomy (Fig. 85-1)
2. Abdominal and transhiatal approach: esophagogastrectomy with cervical esophagogastrostomy or esophagoenterostomy (Fig. 85-2)
3. High abdominal approach: esophagogastrectomy with esophagogastrostomy or esophagojejunostomy in the posterior mediastinum (Fig. 85-3)
4. Thoracoscopic approach: thoracoscopic mobilization of the esophagus with cervical esophagogastrostomy or esophagoenterostomy

An upper midline abdominal incision is used in all four procedures and, in addition, the first procedure has a right sixth space thoracic incision; the second procedure has a left supraclavicular incision.

The third procedure is usually reserved for palliative resection in the presence of advanced local disease or distant metastases when cure is not a primary concern. Thoracoscopic mobilization of the esophagus is indicated for patients with tumor confined to the esophageal wall who have increased pulmonary risks for thoracotomy.

The left thoracic approach, alone or in combination with an abdominal or cervi-

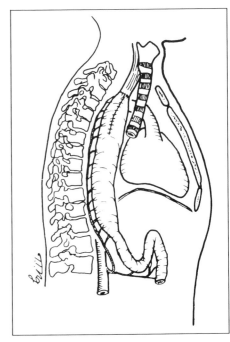

Fig. 85-1. Abdominal and right thoracic approach: intrathoracic esophagogastrostomy after esophagogastrectomy.

946

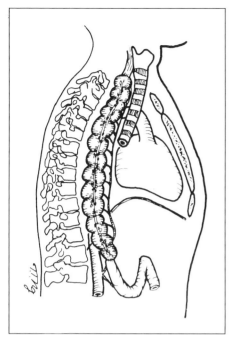

Fig. 85-2. Abdominal and transhiatal approach: orthotopic colonic loop interposition after esophagogastrectomy with cervical esophagocolonostomy.

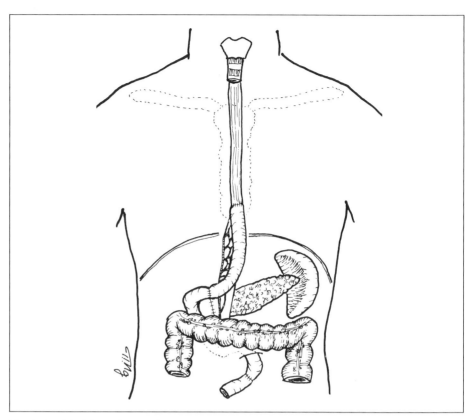

Fig. 85-3. High abdominal approach: jejunal loop interposition in the lower posterior mediastinum after esophagogastrectomy.

cal phase, has fallen out of favor with us because of the limited access to the thoracic esophagus.

Bypass Procedures

For unresectable tumors, a loop of colon or jejunum is used for bypass, the loop being placed in the retrosternal or subcutaneous route. Occasionally, in an otherwise unresectable tumor, sufficient stomach remains uninvolved to allow a tube to be constructed.

The following procedures are used:

1. Retrosternal or subcutaneous colonic or jejunal loop bypass with cervical esophagoenterostomy and abdominal gastroenterostomy (Fig. 85-4)
2. Retrosternal or subcutaneous gastric tube bypass with cervical esophagogastrostomy and abdominal gastrojejunostomy (Fig. 85-5)

Previously described bypass procedures such as abdominal esophagogastrostomy and left intrathoracic esophagogastrostomy are rarely employed.

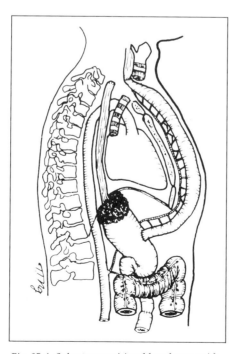

Fig. 85-4. Subcutaneous jejunal loop bypass with cervical esophagojejunostomy for an unresectable tumor of the gastric cardia.

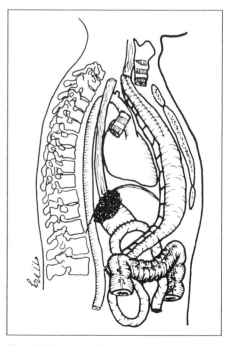

Fig. 85-5. Retrosternal gastric tube bypass with cervical esophagogastrostomy and abdominal gastrojejunostomy.

Resection and Reconstruction

A growth of the abdominal esophagus or cardia is deemed unresectable only when there is local infiltration to the aorta or vertebrae, diffuse peritoneal secondary lesions, bilobar liver metastases, and the presence of ascites. Local invasion that renders resection impossible is uncommon.

Gastric Mobilization

When a growth is large and has involved more than one-third of the stomach, a total gastrectomy is recommended.

Mobilization is begun by freeing the greater omentum from the transverse colon. Because the attachment is devoid of large vessels, separation can be quickly effected by diathermy. The omentum between the spleen and splenic flexure of the colon is divided between clamps and ligated; in obese patients, this process is repeated several times. If uninvolved, the pancreas and spleen are not removed and mobilization of the stomach is achieved by dividing the short gastric vessels.

The gastrohepatic ligament is then detached from the liver and from the portal structures by sharp dissection. Often one set of vessels of considerable size (branch of left gastric artery to left lobe of liver) requires ligation.

The right gastric and gastroepiploic vessels are divided distal to the pylorus. Two pairs of small Payr's clamps are applied to the free first inch of duodenum, and the intestine is transected with a knife. Alternatively, a stapler is used to divide the duodenum. The stomach is turned upward and dissection is begun in the celiac region. The celiac axis is cleared, and the left gastric artery and vein and the posterior vagus nerve are clamped and divided. Continued dissection upward can then be carried along the posterior wall of the abdominal esophagus through the esophageal hiatus along the front of the aorta. Areolar tissues are freed from the aorta and remain attached to the resected specimen.

When the pancreas or the spleen is infiltrated by tumor, or when pancreatic lymph nodes to the left of the celiac axis are involved, splenectomy and pancreatectomy are necessary. The splenic artery is identified to the left of the celiac trunk and clamped and divided.

The spleen is mobilized by freeing the peritoneal attachment between the spleen and the diaphragm. Once this peritoneal adhesion is divided, the spleen and the pancreas are mobilized from the diaphragm, left kidney, and adrenal gland by lifting the spleen and the pancreas to the right, assisted by additional sharp dissection. Care must be taken to avoid damaging the left adrenal gland, since troublesome venous bleeding may ensue. Often, small veins that connect the adrenal gland with the splenic vein can be easily torn, and accurate suturing of these discrete vessels should be done to secure hemostasis.

When the spleen and pancreas are mobilized, the fundus of the stomach is found to be attached to the diaphragm, and freeing of the gastric fundus is accomplished with clamp and ligature. Sometimes brisk bleeding may occur from dividing branches of the inferior phrenic vessels when this peritoneal attachment is cut.

The pancreas is further mobilized by division of the inferior mesenteric veins at the lower border, and the gland is cleared front and back at the region of the neck. The splenic vein is then identified on the posterior surface of the pancreas below the artery; usually it is easy to visualize along its course. This vein is clamped, divided, and ligated. Two Satinsky clamps are applied to the neck of the pancreas, and the pancreas is divided. The distal end is transfixed with a strong, nonabsorbable suture, while the proximal end is closed with continuous 4–0 Maxon (polyglyconate) sutures. The main pancreatic artery near the inferior border often requires a separate suture for hemostasis. Stapling of the pancreatic substances does not achieve satisfactory hemostasis.

Dissection is now directed at the esophageal hiatus. For a tumor of the distal esophagus, a cuff of esophageal hiatus is removed with the tumor. Division of the hiatal musculature is begun on the left side, starting from the freed posterior aspect. Bleeding from the lateral edge is controlled with long hemostats. Division is continued along the front and then to the right side until a cuff of muscle is freed. Bleeding points are controlled by suturing or with electrocautery. Usually when a cuff of muscle from the esophageal hiatus is removed, both pleural cavities are entered. When a transhiatal approach is used, the esophageal hiatus is divided anteriorly as well, the edges being controlled with an artery forceps and then suture ligated.

Right Thoracic Resection

After the abdomen is closed and the patient turned to a right lateral position, a thoracotomy is made through the right sixth intercostal space. Patients who have had previous inflammatory pulmonary disease, especially tuberculosis, may have dense pleural adhesions; these can be time consuming to divide. Bleeding points from the parietal pleura are sutured or coagulated. The right lung is deflated with single-lumen ventilation or alternately can be retracted anteriorly when high-frequency ventilation is used. This enables the exposure of the mediastinum. Since only an apparently normal thoracic esophagus is removed, this part of the operation is straightforward.

The azygos vein is divided and transfixed, and the mediastinal pleura is opened along the whole length of the esophagus if required, both front and back. The esophagus is freed anteriorly from the trachea, both bronchi, pulmonary veins, and pericardium, by sharp dissection. Any fascia, lymph nodes, and connective tissues are removed with the esophagus (Fig. 85-6). Care is taken when mobilizing the proximal end of the esophagus to avoid damage to the left recurrent laryngeal nerve.

By following the front of the azygos vein, the aorta is exposed, and the esophagus is then freed from the front of the aorta by scissors dissection. Just above the diaphragm, the thoracic duct is isolated in front of the aorta and must be ligated; otherwise, chylothorax can develop. A normal thoracic esophagus has only a few small arteries supplying it from the aorta or the bronchial arteries. Only arteries supplying the tumor at the lower esophagus are sufficiently large to require ligation. The proximal end alone of these vessels needs to be ligated since back bleeding from the esophagus is minimal. After the thoracic esophagus is completely freed, the tumor together with the gastric tube or intestinal substitute is pulled up through the hiatus into the right chest. With the substitute sutured to the stomach, the correct orienta-

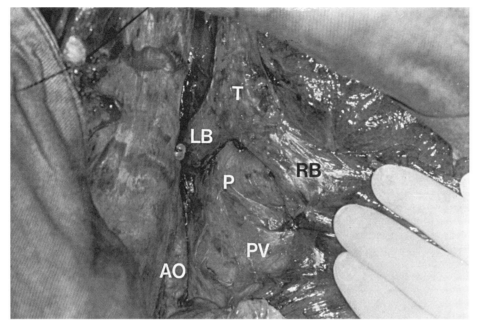

Fig. 85-6. *The mediastinal dissection as seen through a right posterolateral thoracotomy. The esophagus bearing the tumor has been resected, together with the regional lymph nodes, azygos vein, and thoracic duct. The mediastinal structures are bare of all connective tissue attachments. T = trachea; RB = right main bronchus; LB = left main bronchus; P = pericardium; PV = right pulmonary vein; AO = descending thoracic aorta.*

tion of the substitute during its ascent into the chest can be assured.

A Satinsky clamp is then applied across the supra-aortic segment of the esophagus, at least 6 cm from the tumor edge, and the esophagus is divided distal to the clamp. The lower esophagus with the tumor is removed, and the gastric tube or intestinal substitute is placed in the mediastinum ready for anastomosis.

When the tumor is very bulky, the distal esophagus is divided, while in the abdomen the tumor is removed at the abdominal phase. The stomach tube or intestinal substitute is then temporarily anchored to the distal esophageal stump to be pulled up into the chest. After the anastomosis is completed, the chest is closed with drainage.

Transhiatal Resection

Further mobilization of the esophagus from the abdomen can be achieved by inserting long narrow Deaver retractors into the mediastinum, and the soft tissues around the esophagus are clamped and divided under vision up to the level of the inferior pulmonary veins. This dissection is aided considerably by flexible fiberoptic light illumination.

Transhiatal removal of the esophagus is then carried out by inserting the right hand (the surgeon standing on the patient's right side) through the enlarged hiatus into the mediastinum. By using the index and the middle fingers and assisted by the thumb, the connective tissues around the esophagus are stripped off. It is important to keep close to the esophagus to avoid damage to adjacent vessels; otherwise, bleeding can result from tearing of small arterial branches from the aorta. When bleeding is severe, gauze packing is first applied to arrest the hemorrhage and to allow the patient's condition to be stabilized. The incriminating vessel from the distal descending aorta is then clipped and ligated under vision using an extralong hemostat; otherwise, a thoracotomy is required to control vessels located higher up. Venous bleeding can usually be stopped by packing but may occasionally also require a thoracotomy for hemostasis.

It is not easy to bluntly divide the vagal plexus intertwined around the thoracic esophagus, but many of the nerves can be stripped free from the esophagus, pulled down toward the hiatus, and cut under vi-

sion. An important landmark in the hand mobilization of the esophagus is the left main bronchus, which can be recognized by feeling the tips of the characteristic horseshoe cartilaginous rings. At this site and more proximally, great care must be exercised to avoid tearing the thin muscular layer that constitutes the membranous tracheal or bronchial wall posteriorly. A tear in the major respiratory tree is a potentially lethal technical error. Dissection should therefore be close to the esophagus and away from the trachea and bronchus. When both abdominal and cervical mobilization of the thoracic esophagus have been carried out, the site of residual attachment is usually to the pleura on both sides in the upper thoracic cavity, just beyond the reach of the finger from the neck and difficult to free by the hand from the abdomen. Mobilization of this segment is done by the hand from the abdomen but has to be deferred until the cervical dissection is completed and the correct plane is established.

When the hand is in the posterior mediastinum, the anesthetist must be alerted to watch the pulse and blood pressure closely because of the tamponade effect of the hand and forearm on the heart. If hypotension or an arrhythmia occurs, the hand should be withdrawn from the mediastinum to allow the cardiovascular system to stabilize before mobilization of the esophagus is continued.

High Abdominal Resection

This approach is used when a palliative resection is performed for a locally advanced tumor of the cardia or when widespread metastases are present. The distal esophagus is mobilized transhiatally for additional length. A Satinsky clamp is placed at the site of esophageal transection and the esophagus is divided below the clamp. The first Satinsky clamp is replaced by a second one placed more proximally, and moderate traction on this clamp allows the esophagus to descend for easier manipulation. If there is sufficient uninvolved stomach, a tube is constructed for anastomosis; if not, jejunum is used for substitution. When a loop of proximal jejunum is used for reconstruction, it can be placed between the esophagus and the duodenum, or alternatively in a Roux en Y manner. Anastomosis is performed by the hand technique or by using a circular stapler. However, we have not found the use of a stapler to be an easy exercise in this situation. A proximal margin of only 2 to 3 cm may have to be accepted for the anastomosis through the abdomen if it is to be performed safely.

Thoracoscopic Resection

A new alternate approach is now available to remove the thoracic esophagus under vision without the need of a thoracotomy. The risks of a blind dissection of the mediastinum with the transhiatal approach are largely avoided. The technique employs a videoscopic camera and the making of small port holes through which special instruments are passed to mobilize the thoracic esophagus together with the mediastinal lymph nodes. This approach is especially useful for patients with increased pulmonary risks unsuitable for a thoracotomy.

With a double-lumen endobronchial tube inserted for single-lung ventilation, the patient is placed in a left lateral position with the surgeon standing on the right side of the operating table. With the right lung collapsed, five thoracoports are inserted. A 12-mm port is inserted 2 cm behind the posterior axillary line at the fifth intercostal space for the placement of the camera. A 10-mm port is inserted at the anterior axillary line sixth intercostal space for the placement of an endoretractor. The retractor is held by an assistant standing on the left-hand side of the table to retract the lung and mediastinum. Three operator ports are inserted as follows: a 5-mm port at the anterior axillary line fourth intercostal space, a 10-mm port at the tip of the scapular fifth intercostal space, and a 10-mm port at the posterior axillary line eighth intercostal space. No insufflation is necessary for the thoracoscopic mobilization.

The mediastinal pleura is first incised below the level of the azygos vein to expose the esophagus. Using a combination of sharp and blunt dissection, a short segment of esophagus is mobilized. A tape is slung around the esophagus, which enables the esophagus to be lifted outward away from other mediastinal structures that might otherwise be injured during the dissection. These include the azygos vein, pericardium, left and right pulmonary veins, and descending thoracic aorta. When the esophagus is lifted outward, branches of the bronchial arteries and the branches from the aorta that supplies the

esophagus are exposed, and are cauterized or ligated individually under vision.

Mobilization of the esophagus is continued down to the diaphragm reflection. Periesophageal lymph nodes are removed with the tumor. Care is taken when dissecting near the pulmonary veins and the inferior vena cava. Hook cautery is used to lift tissues away from these structures to avoid injuries that can be fatal. The thoracic duct is not identified or ligated.

When the lower thoracic esophagus is completely freed, the next step is the division of the azygos vein. A segment of the vein is freed from its parietal pleura attachment. The vein is ligated with an extracorporal tie using 2–0 Vicryl sutures. Two large clips that self-lock are placed on either side of the suture ties to further secure the vein before its division. Once the azygos vein is divided, the membranous portions of the trachea, bronchus, and carina are exposed. Branches of the bronchial arteries are isolated and ligated. The subbronchial lymph nodes can be dissected with the tumor or can be removed separately.

When the esophagus is lifted away from the aortic arch and the back wall of the trachea, small vessels can be seen and are cauterized. The dissection is continued up to the apex of the thoracic esophagus, and the esophagus is then completely freed. A final inspection of the mediastinum is made to ensure hemostasis. Paratracheal and subbronchial lymph nodes that have not yet been removed are better seen when the mobilized esophagus is retracted away. A size 28 French chest drain is inserted and the lungs are reinflated. The thoracoports are closed in layers.

Mobilization of the Cervical Esophagus

Mobilization of the cervical esophagus is done through a left transverse supraclavicular incision extending from just beyond the sternocleidomastoid muscle to the right of the midline. The left side is chosen because at this level the esophagus is deviated to the left. The skin incision is deepened to the deep fascia, and usually the anterior jugular vein requires ligation and division. The deep fascia along the anterior border of the sternocleidomastoid muscle is divided, and the muscle is retracted laterally with a Czerny retractor.

The ipsilateral strap muscles are divided. Retraction of the divided strap muscles and thyroid gland medially opens up a space between the carotid sheath and the thyroid gland. Usually it is necessary to divide the middle thyroid vein and the inferior thyroid artery. Further medial retraction allows the esophagus to be visualized, and this is picked up by blunt forceps and mobilized by dissecting close to the esophageal wall to avoid damaging the recurrent laryngeal nerves; the left one is always identified.

The index finger of the right hand is inserted into the posterior mediastinum to free the esophagus posteriorly from the vertebral column and to communicate with the free space made by the hand dissection of the esophagus from the abdomen when the transhiatal thoracoscopic approach is used. When it is possible to encircle the esophagus, a tape is passed, and, by traction on the tape, a greater length of esophagus can be freed. Small vessels connected to the esophagus can be ligated or coagulated with diathermy before division.

The upper thoracic esophagus is further mobilized by both finger and scissors dissection. Here also, dissection must be close to the esophagus to avoid recurrent laryngeal nerve damage or tearing the posterior wall of the trachea. By retracting the trachea with fingers and assisted by countertraction on the taped esophagus, dissection under vision can be carried almost to the bifurcation of the trachea. The lateral attachments to the pleura can be separated off by finger as far as possible. The residual attachment to the pleura beyond the finger introduced through the neck has to be stripped from the abdominal approach. This is facilitated by identifying the correct plane established after cervical mobilization. The whole length of the thoracic esophagus is thus freed.

The cervical esophagus is clamped with a Satinsky clamp about 3 to 4 cm from the cricopharyngeus muscle and is divided by a knife above the clamp. This prevents the divided esophagus from retracting behind the sternum. The distal end is then closed to prevent spillage of its contents and a latex drain is attached. The esophagus is then removed with the tumor abdominally, and the drain is left in the mediastinum to serve as a guide for the substitute to be delivered to the neck if this route is used. For the divided cervical esophagus, four to six stay sutures are placed equidistant around its perimeter in preparation for the anastomosis.

Preparation of the Stomach Tube

If the tumor is confined to the distal esophagus or is at the gastroesophageal junction, a stomach tube can be constructed along the greater curvature after adequate resection of the tumor with a distal in situ margin of at least 5 cm. This tube can then be anastomosed to the esophagus in the chest or neck. When the pancreas and spleen are preserved, the stomach is separated from the spleen by dividing the short gastric vessels after the greater omentum has been separated from the splenic flexure. If the pancreas and spleen are also removed, the greater omentum, stomach, spleen, and pancreas are mobilized in the manner described earlier. In addition, the duodenum is freed by Kocher's maneuver.

The gastric tube is prepared by first taking the greater omentum off the greater curvature of the stomach but preserving the gastroepiploic vessels and arcades. Detachment is begun in the pyloric region and continued upward to the short gastric vessels. On the lesser curvature, the right gastric vessels are divided 1 to 2 cm from the pylorus. With a series of intestinal clamps, the greater curvature is divided first at right angles to the gastric border for about 4 cm and then parallel to the greater curvature toward the pylorus onto the lesser curvature, where the right gastric vessels have been divided. The new lesser curvature is then closed with two layers of continuous 4–0 Maxon sutures. To prepare the tube with a stapler, a 90-mm linear stapler is passed across the body of the stomach, from 3 cm proximal to the pylorus on the lesser curve toward the midportion of the greater gastric curvature. Electrocautery is applied to the staple line for hemostasis, and in general, the staple line is not inverted.

When the tumor does not encroach on the stomach, only the cardia is resected and a virtually intact stomach is used for reconstruction (Fig. 85-7). A pyloroplasty is necessary for the vagotomized stomach to avoid gastric outlet obstruction. A Heineke-Mikulicz pyloroplasty is performed using a continuous running absorbable monofilament suture in two

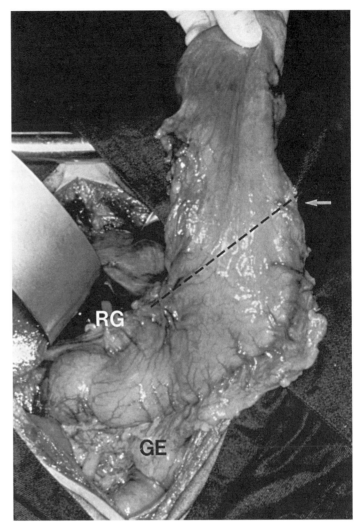

Fig. 85-7. The stomach after mobilization. The source of blood supply is from the right gastroepiploic and the right gastric arcades. If the tumor has extended to involve the proximal stomach, a gastric tube is formed by transection along the dotted line with a 90-mm linear stapler, with the creation of a new lesser curve. The site of the anastomosis will be at the apex of the stomach tube (arrow). GE = right gastroepiploic arcade; RG = right gastric arcade.

layers. The first layer coapts the mucosal and submucosal layers, and the second layer incorporates only the seromuscular layers. This technique allows accurate apposition of individual layers with inversion but minimal infolding.

Preparation of the Colonic Loop

When the stomach is not suitable or available for reconstruction, our next choice is the colon. We have no preference whether this is the ileocolon, right colon, transverse colon, or left colon. The proximal and distal sites of division are often determined by the anastomotic arcade, the feeding ar-

tery, and the draining veins. Whichever part of the colon is used, the same meticulous method of preparation is required. When possible, we would prepare the loop in an isoperistaltic manner.

The steps in the mobilization of either right or left colon are similar. Proper identification of the fusion line between the colon and the peritoneum of the posterior abdominal wall avoids entering the wrong plane and encountering bleeding when the colon is being freed. On the right side, mobilization of the terminal ileum across the iliac vessels and the ureter enables the terminal ileum, cecum, appendix, and ascending colon to be lifted out of the

abdomen. As mobilization proceeds proximally, the duodenum is encountered and
care must be taken not to damage the head
of the pancreas; in this region the main
right colic vessel may be encountered as it
courses over the uncinate process of the
pancreas. Near the liver, it is often necessary to clamp and ligate the more vascular
peritoneal attachment of the hepatic flexure. Adhesions between the gallbladder
and the hepatic flexure also must be released.

Mobilization of the left colon proceeds in
a similar manner as before, and the sigmoid colon is freed from the retroperitoneum toward the midline and can also be
brought out of the abdominal wound.
Proximal extension leads to the splenic
flexure and these peritoneal attachments
also need ligation.

The transverse colon is prepared by detaching the greater omentum from its antimesenteric border. This may be difficult
if the patient has had a previous operation,
but even in an untransgressed abdomen,
natural adhesions may obscure the correct
plane. The omentum is first detached left
of the midline to enter the lesser sac; further separation can then proceed more
readily. Little bleeding should be encountered and only occasionally does a blood
vessel need ligation. It may sometimes be
simpler to leave a small amount of omentum on the colon since a complete removal
would prolong the dissection and can injure the blood supply.

The two areas where separation of the
greater omentum requires additional attention are in the ascending colon, where
the omentum can be attached to any of its
three intra-abdominal surfaces. It is important to free the omentum here to allow
the right colon to be straightened out. On
the left side, detaching the omentum near
the inferior mesenteric vein must be done
with care. When the left colon is chosen for
substitution, this vein must be preserved.
Sometimes the greater omentum is attached very close to this vein, and unintentional ligation eliminates the venous
drainage of the left loop of colon and the
loop has to be discarded.

In preparing the ileocolon, we include the
terminal ileum as part of the loop. The size
of the ileum is similar to that of the cervical
esophagus, which makes it easy to anastomose them end to end (Fig. 85-8). The
size discrepancy for a coloesophageal

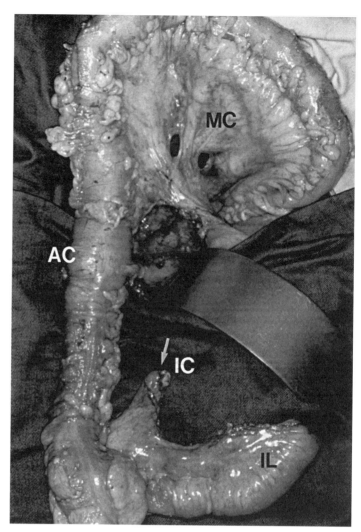

Fig. 85-8. *The ileocolon is prepared for anastomosis to the esophagus. Careful preservation of the marginal
arcade and flush ligation of the ileocolic vessels (arrow) will ensure good vascularization of the colonic loop
based on the middle colic arcades. AC = ascending colon; IL = ileum; IC = ileocolic arcade; MC = middle
colic arcade.*

anastomosis is greater. In the right colonic
mesentery there is usually a large area between the ileocolic and the right colic
branches that is devoid of blood vessels.
We divide the ileocolic vessels near the origin and then follow this down to the ileum about 15 cm from the cecum. If the
ileocolon is used, the middle colic vessels
and, if possible, the right colic vessels also
are preserved. If the right colon is used because the terminal ileum is unsuitable to
be included, the right colic vessels are divided and the middle colic vessels alone
would serve the loop. Additional blood
supply can be obtained by preserving the
marginal arcade supply from the left colic
vessels by carefully separating the colonic

loop left of the middle colic vessels between the bowel wall and its mesenteric
branches for about 8 to 10 cm. The middle
portion of this devascularized loop of
bowel is discarded, and the healthy vascularized end nearest to the middle colic
vessels is used as the distal anastomosis of
the colonic loop (Fig. 85-9). The terminal
ileum, appendix, and cecum are resected
when the length of the right colon alone is
adequate for substitution.

For the left colon, the sustaining arterial
supply is the ascending branch of the left
colic artery, which originates from the inferior mesenteric artery. When this branch
is small and when only the left colon is

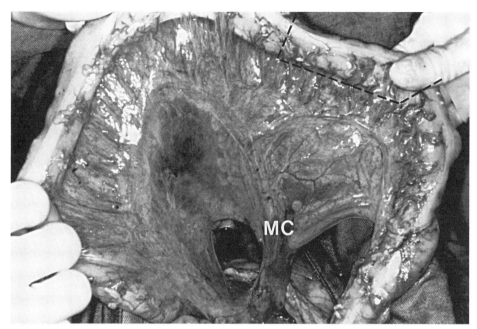

Fig. 85-9. A portion of the transverse colon left of the middle colic arcade is resected (along dotted line) with careful preservation of the marginal arcade. This gives an additional source of blood supply to the right colonic loop via its communication with the blood vessels from the left ascending colonic branches. MC = middle colic arcade.

available, we have used this segment in an antiperistaltic manner with the blood supply based on the middle colic vessels. Usually the ascending branch of the left colic artery is robust and the middle colic vessels can be divided. The venous drainage through the inferior mesenteric vein to the splenic vein has to be safeguarded during the preparation of the left colon, especially when the greater omentum is detached, as mentioned earlier, or during pancreatectomy.

Transection of both ends of a loop of colon is accomplished with staplers, and the ends are thoroughly cleaned with antiseptic swabs. Before transection of the proximal end, a Penrose drain is placed on the surface of the intestine with the long end of the drain on the distal part so that after transection the proximal end of the loop is attached by the drain, which is used to elevate the loop into the neck. After the cervical esophagus and the tunnel have been prepared, the upper end of the loop is brought up and the staple line is resected in preparation for anastomosis.

When the right thoracic approach is used, the loop is sutured to the front of the gastric cardia, in the correct orientation, for placement in the chest. The lower end of the loop is anastomosed to a convenient

part of the upper gastrointestinal tract, whether this be the stomach, duodenal stump, or upper jejunum (if a Polya gastrectomy had been performed previously). If the stomach is intact, the loop is placed in the retrogastric position.

All anastomoses are made using a one-layer, continuous, over-and-over suture technique with a monofilament absorbable material, which is described in detail in Chap. 66.

Preparation of the Jejunal Loop

The duodenojejunal junction is identified, and the proximal jejunum is brought out of the abdomen and placed on a large gauze pack over the abdominal wall so that the mesentery is easily visualized. Two Babcock clamps are placed on the antimesenteric border approximately 10 to 15 cm from the ligament of Treitz to serve as traction and prevent the intestine from retracting back into the abdomen. The vascular pattern of the mesentery is then examined for completeness of arterial and venous arcades. In patients with a thick mesentery, transillumination is a help; in obese patients, the fat in the mesentery has to be removed before the arcades can be observed.

Dissection is begun in the upper jejunum, at a point approximately halfway between the edge of the intestine and the root of the mesentery, proximal to the branching of the main jejunal arteries. The peritoneum is divided and mobilized by gently teasing it off the underlying connective tissue with the convex surface of a pair of Metzenbaum scissors to within 1 to 2 cm of the intestinal edge. Small bleeding points are picked up with fine nontoothed forceps and coagulated. The fat, fascia, lymph nodes, and nerve fibers are then cleared from the arteries and veins. This process is continued for approximately 20 to 25 cm along the mesentery as measured at the point of initial mesenteric dissection. Usually four sets of jejunal arteries and veins have to be divided for a sufficient length of mesentery and intestine to reach the neck. When a shorter length of jejunum is required, such as for intrathoracic anastomosis, meticulous dissection of the mesentery is not required.

The four sets of jejunal vessels are then clamped with bulldog clamps to test the adequacy of the anastomotic arcades. To further ensure that the blood supply is sufficient to support the circulation to the loop, a soft clamp is applied across the intestine at the upper jejunum to abolish any contribution from the proximal arcade. Often the loop of jejunum thus isolated undergoes active peristalsis. After a few minutes, if the color remains pink and the jejunum does not appear congested, and if weak arterial pulsations can be seen in the arcades, the viability of the jejunal loop is assured.

When there is doubt about the vascularity of the loop, as evidenced by flaccidity and congestion of the bowel wall and absence of arterial pulsation, the fourth clamp can be released and the viability reassessed. However, if only three branches are divided, the mesentery may reach the neck only with some tension, which should be avoided. Under these circumstances, mobilization of the entire mesentery by dividing the peritoneum at the root as it crosses over the aorta allows the loop, together with the entire mesentery, to move 4 to 5 cm higher and thus relieve any tension on the anastomosis.

After the adequacy of the blood supply of the jejunal loop has been tested, the bulldog clamps and the soft intestinal clamp are removed. The arterial and venous branches are then cleared of all tissues from the stem to about 1 cm past its bifurcation into the arcades. Because the arteries are more superficial, they are dissected first. After the stem of the jejunal artery is cleaned and separated from the vein, it is clamped 0.5 cm from its bifurcation with mosquito forceps and divided. By gently lifting the artery upward, the back of the artery is mobilized for a similar distance as the front. The divided artery is then ligated with fine silk tie. The vein is treated in a similar manner. Particular care must be exercised to avoid venous damage. Any small bleeding points are coagulated.

By this process, the remaining three jejunal branches are divided and a long length of jejunal loop is thus prepared. The jejunum is then divided proximally and distally with staplers. The leaves of the mesentery are approximated with fine sutures to protect the skeletonized vessels from damage during manipulation.

The freed loop is then placed on the chest wall to determine whether an adequate length has been prepared for cervical anastomosis. Usually, after dividing four jejunal branches, the length is more than sufficient. When the loop is insufficiently long, mobilization of the root of the mesentery may add 4 to 5 cm to the upper reaches of the loop, or an additional jejunal branch will have to be divided. We generally prefer the latter method rather than upward traction of the whole of the mesentery. Before a further branch of the jejunal vessels is divided, the viability of the loop is again tested by temporary occlusion of these vessels. If pulsations can be seen in the arcades of the loop distal to the bulldog clamp, the jejunal loop will be viable after division of that branch.

When a sufficient length of mesentery has been prepared for cervical anastomosis, there is an excess of jejunum in relation to the mesenteric length, with concertina of the intestine. Although moderate excess is harmless, too much redundant jejunum can result in kinking of the loop, which may lead to obstruction. To prevent this complication, a segment of jejunum can be resected, and an end-to-end anastomosis made (Fig. 85-10). Care must be taken to divide the vasa rectae close to the intestinal wall to avoid damaging or angulating the arcade. Midloop resection of redundant jejunum is required only occasionally.

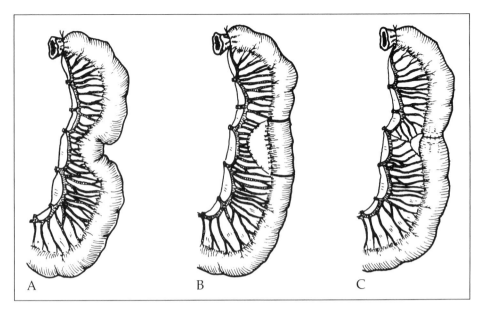

Fig. 85-10. Resection of redundant jejunum in the middle of the loop. A. Excess of jejunum in relation to mesentery. B. Vasa rectae of redundant segment divided close to intestinal wall. C. End-to-end anastomosis resulting in a straight loop.

The loop is then placed in the retrocolic, retrogastric position (when appropriate) before being delivered to the right chest or neck.

Retrosternal and Subcutaneous Tunnels

After resection, the substitute is usually placed in the orthotopic position. For a variety of reasons, it may occasionally be preferable to place it retrosternally or subcutaneously.

To make a retrosternal tunnel, the retroperitoneal space at the back of the xiphoid is entered. A tunnel is opened up behind the sternum initially by blunt dissection using the middle three fingers. Subsequently, a flat malleable retractor is introduced to further open the space behind the upper part of the sternum. Little bleeding occurs if dissection is kept in a plane close to the back of the sternum near the midline.

The upper part of the tunnel is made from the neck. The anterior mediastinum is entered after the sternal heads of the sternohyoid and sternothyroid muscles and the underlying deep fascia are divided with electrocautery. Using the index finger, a space is opened by blunt dissection, again keeping close behind the sternum to avoid injury to various venous structures. A Czerny retractor to lift the manubrium

aids the dissection, and this is continued until the upper tunnel meets with that made from the abdominal dissection. The narrowest part of the tunnel is usually at the thoracic inlet, and a space of three fingers is required to ensure adequate accommodation for the intestinal substitute. Oozing from the tunnel is controlled by gauze packing. There is usually no need to resect the manubrium sterni or the clavicular head to provide sufficient space.

After the tunnel is prepared, the upper end of the intestinal substitute, to which a latex or Penrose drain or a thin malleable retractor has been attached, is placed in the tunnel and the loop is guided into the neck. The loop is preferably pushed up from below rather than pulled up from above. The hand can guide the orientation and the passage of the loop. In the correct position, the mesenteric edge is on the right side.

The subcutaneous route may be selected because growth of metastasis within the thoracic inlet could not compress the loop. Furthermore, if gangrene develops in a loop placed in the subcutaneous tunnel, it would be discovered earlier and be simpler to manage. On the other hand, the subcutaneous route is longer; this is especially important when a stomach tube is used. There is also more angulation of the substitute at the level of the xiphoid, which sometimes causes venous congestion and intestinal obstruction. For this reason, the xiphoid is usually resected. The leakage rate is also higher with the subcutaneous route.

To make the subcutaneous tunnel, the skin at the upper end of the abdominal incision is lifted up, and, with the use of scissors and electrocautery, the subcutaneous plane is opened up. The tunnel is prepared in a similar manner proximally from the cervical incision. The subcutaneous space in the intervening presternal segment is freed by using a pair of long Albee scissors. Bleeding within the tunnel from inaccessible sites may be controlled by gauze packing, but if bleeding persists, the tunnel must be opened and hemostasis secured. If this is required, the bleeding is usually found to be from the upper per-forators of the internal mammary artery, and to gain access to these sites, the cervical incision is extended vertically downward.

The Esophageal Anastomosis (see Chap. 66)

All hand-sewn anastomoses are performed in a standard manner using a single layer of continuous monofilament absorbable sutures, such as 4–0 Maxon (polyglyconate) or 3–0 PDS (polydioxanone) regardless of the level of anastomosis or type of substitute used. The circular stapler (EEA, U.S. Surgical Corp, Norwalk, CT, or ILS, Ethicon, Somerville, NJ) can be used for anastomosis in the chest or abdomen. It is technically difficult to use in the neck because of limited length of bowel and the confined space.

For hand-sewn anastomosis, the esophagus is first prepared in a manner described previously. When a jejunal loop or an ileocolic loop is delivered into the neck, the upper end of the loop (jejunum or ileum) angulates to the right because of a shorter mesentery. This redundant part of the bowel can be straightened by resecting the terminal end for an end-to-end anastomosis, our preferred configuration of establishing continuity. When the stomach is used, a small opening is made on the posterior wall close to the apex, or at the apex itself, for the anastomosis (Fig. 85-11).

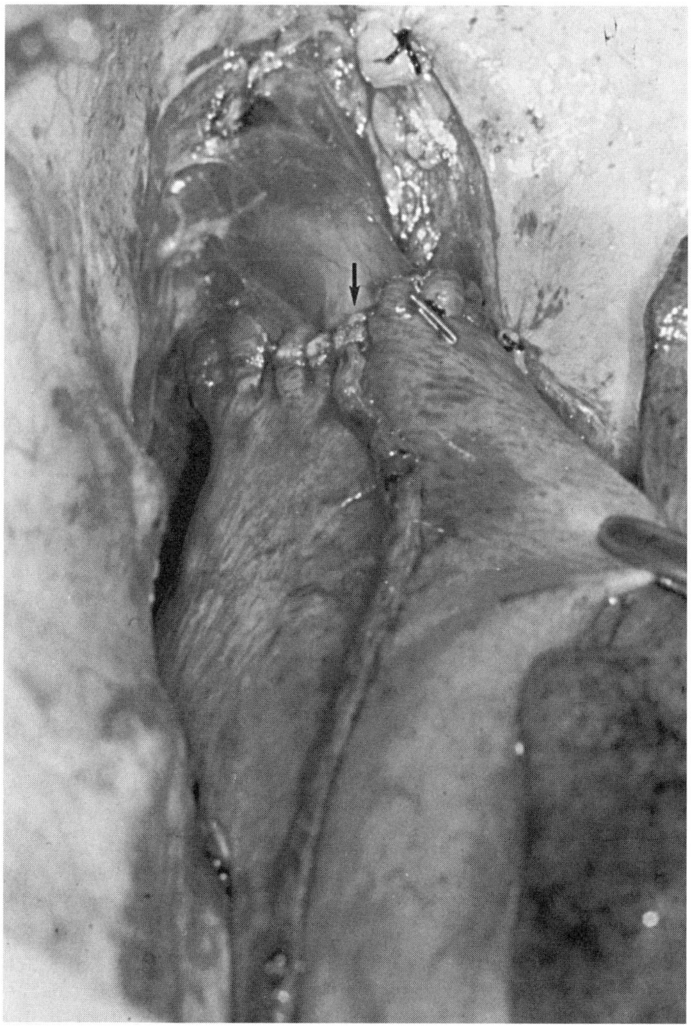

The Abdominal Anastomoses

Anastomoses in the abdomen are necessary only when colon or jejunum is used. The duodenum is usually selected as the site of anastomosis after total gastrectomy. When the colon is used, the distal end of the loop is anastomosed directly to the duodenum. For a jejunal loop, a Roux en Y configuration is an alternative. To select the appropriate site of a jejunal loop for anastomosis to the duodenum, the previously prepared long jejunal loop is placed close to the duodenum, and the site for division is marked by a pair of Babcock forceps. To allow the distal end of the jejunal loop to return to the infracolic compartment, a segment of about 15 to 20 cm of jejunum has to be resected distal to the site of the intended jejunoduodenal anastomosis. The segment for resection is held vertically and the vasa rectae running toward the intestine are clamped and divided close to the intestinal wall to avoid damage to the vascular arcade serving the loop. When an adequate length of the intestine has been removed, the distal end is returned into the infracolic compartment, and the vasa rectae are ligated.

Anastomosis between the colon or jejunum and the stomach or duodenum is by the one-layer method described earlier. Finally, the two ends of the jejunum or the ileum and colon are anastomosed axially and the mesenteric defects are closed (Fig. 85-12).

An inspection for bleeding points is made and hemostasis is secured before closing. The abdomen is closed in layers, but an adequate defect is left in the linea alba

Fig. 85-11. Completed anastomosis lying near the apex of the thoracic cavity. The stomach tube is displaced to show the posterior wall of the anastomosis and the T junction between the line of gastric resection and the esophagus (arrow).

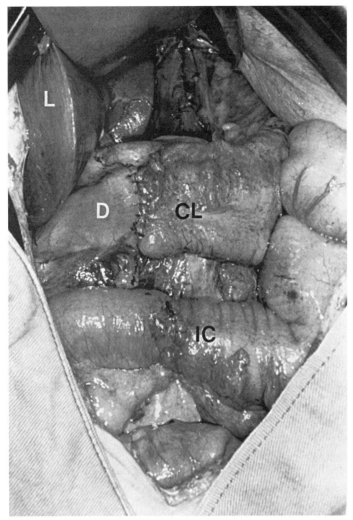

Fig. 85-12. *The completed abdominal anastomoses when a loop of colon is used as substitute. The distal end of the retrosternally placed colonic loop is anastomosed to the duodenum, while the ileocolic anastomosis, which is seen more distally, reconstitutes the continuity of the bowels. L = liver; D = duodenum; CL = retrosternal colonic loop; IC = ileocolic anastomosis.*

when the subcutaneous route is used to allow the substitute and its mesentery to pass without compression.

Bypass Procedures

When the primary tumor is deemed unresectable, a bypass is performed. This may be accomplished by interposition of a loop of colon or jejunum between the cervical esophagus and the gastric antrum, or, when free of tumor, preparation of a stomach tube to anastomose to the cervical esophagus with the remaining proximal stomach defunctioned by a loop of small intestine. In both cases, an end-to-end cer-

vical anastomosis is preferred; the distal end of the divided esophagus is securely closed by continuous suturing or with the use of a linear stapler.

Bypass Using Colon or Jejunum

A loop of colon or jejunum is prepared. When a jejunal loop is used, it is passed in a retrocolic and retrogastric position and then onto the neck along a retrosternal or subcutaneous tunnel. The retrosternal route is preferred. Intrathoracic bypass operations are no longer performed, because patients with very advanced malignant disease tolerate thoracotomy poorly.

After mobilization of the cervical esophagus, an end-to-end esophagoenterostomy is performed. If the cervical esophagus is immobilized by metastatic cervical lymph nodes infiltrating its wall, an end-to-side anastomosis offers the only alternative. The distal end of the intestinal loop is anastomosed to the anterior wall of the stomach or left in a Roux en Y manner. Finally, the mesenteric defects around the vascular pedicle are closed, as is the retrosternal space to prevent herniation of intestine into the chest.

Bypass Using Stomach Tube

The stomach tube is prepared and put aside temporarily. The remaining tumor-bearing proximal stomach is then anastomosed end to side to a loop of jejunum brought up in a retrocolic position. When tumor obstruction is complete, it would be acceptable to close the proximal stomach without draining it.

The stomach tube is passed through the retrosternal or subcutaneous tunnel for anastomosis in the neck. Kocher's maneuver to the third part of the duodenum is desirable to avoid tension at the cervical anastomosis. In the event that the distal cervical esophagus and the remaining proximal stomach are both closed, a mucocele occasionally develops from the blind loop of the intrathoracic esophagus, but even when this occurs, it apparently does not become symptomatic.

Postoperative Management
Respiratory Care

Respiratory failure is the most common postoperative complication and cause of hospital mortality. Selected patients should have prophylactic postoperative ventilatory support and extubation carried out when arterial blood gas results are satisfactory. About 25 percent of our patients are electively ventilated postoperatively. Vigorous physiotherapy is mandatory for all patients. Routine flexible bronchoscopic toilet is carried out in most patients to avoid sputum retention and its consequences. Tracheostomy is performed in about 10 percent of our patients to facilitate bronchial suction; when a cervical anastomosis has been made, a cricothyroidotomy is established instead.

Blood Replacement

Blood transfusion is often not necessary. Very rarely, excessive bleeding resulting in persistent tachycardia or hypotension is an indication for early re-exploration.

Alimentation

Intravenous fluid is given for the first week but oral feeding is commenced by the third or fourth postoperative day. A meglumine diatrizoate (Gastrografin) swallow is performed for documentation only, since anastomotic leakage is now a very rare occurrence and in any event is only relevant when leakage is clinically evident. A solid diet is usually tolerated by the second week postoperatively.

Decompression

Decompression of the substitute is by a nasogastric tube. Distention of the colonic or jejunal loop can compromise its blood supply. The nasogastric tube frequently becomes blocked by intestinal contents and requires flushing regularly.

Anastomotic Leakage

Meticulous attention to technique and the prevention of hypoxia and hypotension in the postoperative period have reduced the incidence of anastomotic leakage following resection from 5 percent overall to 2 percent in the later period. Minor leaks in the cervical anastomosis should be managed conservatively because most heal after local wound treatment. Nasogastric tube feeding may continue even when there is a cervical anastomotic leak, provided that it is small; otherwise, total parenteral nutrition is required.

For intrathoracic anastomotic leakage, adequate drainage must be established together with total parenteral nutrition and antibiotics. When leakage develops in the first 3 or 4 days, exploration is warranted because the leakage may originate from a nonanastomotic site such as the fundus of the stomach or the suture line of the stomach closure. Surgical repair in these situations is mandatory and is usually successful. For anastomotic leaks involving most of the circumference or those associated with gangrene of the substitute, it is necessary to take down the anastomosis, and a cervical esophagostomy and an abdominal gastric or intestinal stoma are established.

Results

Between 1982 and 1994, 1286 patients with carcinoma of the esophagus and cardia were managed at the University of Hong Kong, Queen Mary Hospital. Of these, 962 patients were operated on, while the remaining 324 did not undergo operation because they either declined, were unfit or moribund, or were more suitably treated by nonoperative means, such as by radiotherapy, chemotherapy, prosthetic intubation, or laser because of metastatic disease. Some patients were referred from elsewhere with complications after surgery. Among those who underwent operations at our hospital, there were 788 resections, 139 bypasses, and 35 explorations alone.

Of the 788 patients who underwent resection, 197 had their carcinoma located at the lower third of the esophagus, while another 149 had carcinoma located at the cardia. Of these patients, 185 had squamous cell carcinoma while 143 had adenocarcinomas. The proportion of patients with stage I, II, III, and IV disease was 3.3, 16.4, 64.4, and 15.9 percent, respectively. Resection was considered curative in 42.2 percent while it was palliative in 57.8 percent. Just over half (52%) of all resections for carcinomas of the lower third of the esophagus or cardia were performed by an abdominal and right thoracic approach. A high abdominal approach was used in 25 percent, and the abdominal and transhiatal approach accounted for the remaining 23 percent. Stomach or stomach tube was the most commonly used substitute for reconstruction and was performed in 299 patients (86.4%); there were 28 jejunal (8.1%) and 19 colonic substitutes (5.5%).

Of the 139 patients who had bypasses, 22 had their carcinoma located at the lower esophagus or at the cardia, 14 had squamous cell carcinoma, and 7 had adenocarcinoma. For the bypasses, colon was used in 16 patients and jejunum in 5 patients; only 1 patient was stomach tube appropriate. Altogether, 18 anastomotic leaks occurred in the resection group and 2 in the bypass group. Half of those with anastomotic leakage in the resection group died despite appropriate treatment, while both patients with leakage in the bypass group died from their complications. The 30-day mortality was 4.1 percent in the resection group and 22.7 percent in the by-pass group; the hospital mortality was 11.3 percent in the resection group and 45.5 percent in the bypass group. Many patients remain in the hospital after an operation for socioeconomic reasons rather than for medical reasons. Pulmonary complications and malignant cachexia accounted for most of the deaths.

The median survival time for patients who underwent a curative resection was 22.5 months; for those who had palliative resection, it was 6.6 months. In patients with bypass operations, the median survival time was only 2 months, and no patient lived longer than 8 months. The 30-day mortality and hospital mortality rates were included in all survival results. The 5-year survival rate was 35 percent in patients who had a curative resection and was only 4 percent in patients who had a palliative resection.

Suggested Reading

Akiyama H. Surgery for carcinoma of the esophagus. *Curr Probl Surg* 17:53, 1980.

Ellis FH Jr, Gibb SP, Watkins E Jr. Overview of the current management of carcinoma of the esophagus and cardia. *Can J Surg* 28:493, 1985.

Fok M, Wong J. Oesophageal cancer treatment: Curative modalities. *Eur J Gastroenterol Hepatol* 6:645, 1994.

Fok M, Wong J. Standard oesophagectomy and anastomotic technique. *Ann Chirurg Gynaecol* 84:179, 1995.

Fok M, Cheng SWK, Wong J. Pyloroplasty versus no drainage in gastric replacement of the esophagus. *Am J Surg* 162:447, 1991.

Fok M, Law SYK, Wong J. Operable esophageal carcinoma: Current results from Hong Kong. Progress Symposium on "Squamous Esophageal Carcinoma." *World J Surg* 18:355, 1994.

Fok M, Law SYK, Stipa F, et al. A comparison of transhiatal and transthoracic resection for oesophageal carcinoma. *Endoscopy* 25:660, 1993.

Law SYK, Fok M, Wong J. Risk analysis in resection of squamous cell carcinoma of the esophagus. *World J Surg* 18:339, 1994.

Law SYK, Fok M, Cheng SWK, Wong J. A comparison of outcome after resection for squamous cell carcinomas and adenocarcinomas of the esophagus and cardia. *Surg Gynecol Obstet* 175:107, 1992.

Muller JM, Erasmi H, Stelzner M, et al. Surgical therapy of oesophageal carcinoma. *Br J Surg* 77:845, 1990.

Shao LF, Li ZC, Wang MF. Results of surgical treatment in 6123 cases of carcinoma of esophagus and gastric cardia. *Chin J Surg* 25:449, 1987.

Wang LS, Huang MH, Huang BS, Chien KY. Gastric substitute for resectable carcinoma of the esophagus: An analysis of 368 cases. *Ann Thorac Surg* 53:289, 1992.

Wong J. Management of carcinoma of oesophagus: Art or science? *J R Coll Surg Edinb* 26:138, 1981.

Wong J. Esophageal resection for cancer: The rationale of current practice. *Am J Surg* 153:18, 1987.

EDITOR'S COMMENT

Carcinoma of the distal one-third of the esophagus or proximal stomach, or both, has been and remains a difficult problem with little positive progress in results of therapy. Certainly the operative mortality reported by Drs. Wong and Fok should be emulated. High morbidity and mortality statistics are more common.

Controversy continues as to whether or not to use jejunal pouches in reconstruction following total gastrectomy. Colleagues from Japan (*Ann Surg* 222:27, 1995) have performed a randomized controlled trial comparing the usefulness of three reconstruction procedures:, simple Roux en Y, jejunal pouch and Roux en Y, and jejunal pouch and interposition. This well-controlled study demonstrated that the jejunal pouch with Roux en Y reconstruction was the most useful of the three procedures in improving the postoperative quality of life.

Hölscher and colleagues (*Cancer* 76:178, 1995) have compared the prognosis of patients with T1 squamous cell carcinoma (SCC) of the esophagus with those with T1 adenocarcinoma of the esophagus. I present details of this study to demonstrate how we must continue to search for the finer aspects of this dread cancer. Clinical and histopathologic characteristics, patterns of lymph node metastasis, results of surgery, and long-term prognosis of 47 patients with SCC were compared with those of 30 patients with adenocarcinoma.

The groups with adenocarcinoma and SCC were comparable regarding age, postoperative 90-day mortality (6.6 vs 8.5%), infiltration of submucosa (74.5 vs 80%), and rate of lymph node metastasis (17 vs 16.6%). Cancer limited to the mucosa was not associated with lymph node metastasis in either group, whereas submucosal spread showed lymph node involvement in 21 percent of patients with adenocarcinoma and 26 percent of those with SCC. The 5-year survival rate of patients with complete tumor removal was superior for those with adenocarcinoma (82.5%) compared to those with SCC (59.2%; $P < 0.03$).

Multivariate analysis indicated that the histopathologic type (adenocarcinoma vs SCC) was the only independent prognostic factor. The unfavorable prognosis of patients with T1 SCC was due to a higher recurrence rate and the more frequent development of second primary tumors (21 vs 0%).

Similarly, we now must become au fait with the burgeoning science of molecular biology. Youssef and associates (*Cancer* 76:358, 1995) demonstrated how the monoclonal antibody MIB-1 proliferation index may be a powerful prognostic marker for patients with squamous cell carcinomas of the esophagus.

Particular attention must be paid to the section on the preparation of the jejunal segment. By meticulous attention to the technique described, the jejunum can be regularly brought into the neck for anastomosis to the cervical esophagus. This method of jejunal mobilization has an important use in the treatment of destroyed distal esophagus after alkaline reflux esophagitis. The Merendino jejunal interposition operation (*Ann Surg* 142:486, 1955) after distal esophagectomy for reflux esophagitis suffers at times because neophyte surgeons cannot mobilize a sufficient length of jejunum. If the precepts herein described are followed, technical difficulty should no longer be a concern.

L.M.N.

86

Surgery for Postgastrectomy Syndromes

Stephen B. Vogel

Most patients do quite well following operations on the stomach and proximal small intestine for either benign or malignant disease. In a small percentage, however, debilitating symptoms may develop from alterations in gastrointestinal motility, pathophysiologic conditions, or mechanical problems within the early or late postoperative period. The classic postgastrectomy syndromes have remained relatively unchanged for decades, although recent emphasis now centers on disorders of gastric and upper intestinal motor function. Although the true incidence of these disorders is not increasing, clinicians are becoming more aware of and better able to diagnose them. The advent of gastric and biliary radionuclide scanning has made evaluations more objective. Although elective surgery for peptic ulcer disease has dramatically declined, large numbers of postgastrectomy patients remain from previous decades. Advances in technology have redefined "old syndromes" and led to the diagnosis of new postgastrectomy disorders. Medical treatment, including H$_2$ antagonists, proton pump inhibitors, peptide analogs, and newer prokinetic agents, have had great therapeutic effects on the classic postgastrectomy disorders. The challenge for the surgeon is to identify the patterns of altered motility and pathophysiology, to resist the pressures to "reoperate" when medical therapy will suffice, and finally to choose the appropriate procedure if surgery becomes inevitable.

The overall incidence of postgastrectomy disorders ranges perhaps from 5 to 50 percent but most authors agree that in general 25 percent of patients experience the unpleasant side effects that result from gastric resection and loss of reservoir func-

tion, ablation or bypass of the pylorus, and complete parasympathetic denervation. Since proximal gastric vagotomy (highly selective vagotomy) maintains an intact pylorus and an innervated antrum, the overall incidence of postoperative side effects is less than 5 percent. Following this operation, the classic syndromes of postgastrectomy dumping, alkaline reflux esophagitis/gastritis, early postoperative bilious vomiting, afferent and efferent loop syndrome, and postvagotomy diarrhea are almost completely avoided. During the past decade, the avoidance of postgastrectomy complications was weighed against the higher recurrence rate following highly selective vagotomy. In recent years, however, the dramatic decrease in elective surgery for chronic nonhealing peptic ulcer disease has resulted in fewer operations of this type and eliminated the surgical dilemma.

Patient Evaluation

A careful history is the first essential for establishing the diagnosis of postgastrectomy disorders. Typically, patients will present with one predominant symptom. This may be pain, nausea and vomiting, or cardiovascular vasomotor symptoms. If pain is present, it is important to determine the type of pain, for example, the burning, upper abdominal pain associated with alkaline reflux gastritis. This must be distinguished from the right upper quadrant pain relieved by bilious vomiting in patients with the afferent loop syndrome. Interestingly, patients with very rapid gastric emptying often describe pain immediately after food intake, whereas the pain and distress of chronic gastroparesis usu-

ally occur later in the day after several meals have been ingested.

If nausea and vomiting are present, it is helpful to learn when they occur. Nausea and occasionally vomiting may occur immediately after a meal in the dumping syndrome, whereas these symptoms are usually more prominent later in the course of the meal or even later in the day with chronic gastroparesis. The characteristics of the vomitus may offer clues to the correct diagnosis. Following surgery for peptic ulcer disease, bilious vomiting is not unusual in the early postoperative period, but bilious vomiting, with retained food, may be indicative of an early or late motility disorder. The vomitus of chronic gastroparesis may be diagnostic if the patient describes food that had been ingested a day or more previously. The early symptoms of diaphoresis, dizziness, and syncope often accompany the dumping syndrome. Additionally, diarrhea may be associated with early vasomotor dumping that occurs shortly after the meal, as compared with postvagotomy diarrhea, which occurs throughout the day, unrelated to food intake.

Late in the postoperative period, patients with any postgastrectomy symptom should have a barium upper GI examination and endoscopy. Radiologic examination demonstrates the patency of the gastric outlet and is a "relatively good" test to determine liquid gastric emptying. Endoscopic examination may rule out mechanical or pathophysiologic causes of postgastrectomy disorders, such as strictured anastomosis, intussusception, or marginal ulceration with or without chronic edema. Endoscopic examination can also identify any gross pathologic changes of the gastric mucosa. Punctate gastric ulcerations and limited gastritis surround acute and chronic gastric bezoars. A "beefy" red stomach with or without punctate ulcerations may be seen in patients who suffer from chronic alkaline reflux gastritis. Symptoms in the late postoperative period should prompt a careful search for malignancy. In those patients whose prior gastric surgery was performed 10 or more years before evaluation, endoscopic biopsy of "reddened" areas or obvious gastritis should be performed to rule out dysplastic changes and the potential for early malignancy.

Radionuclide evaluation of gastric emptying and biliary enterogastric reflux is important not only in diagnosing combined disorders but in planning the surgical approach. It is not unusual for patients with dumping symptoms to have associated alkaline reflux gastritis. Similarly, patients with reflux gastritis and bilious vomiting may demonstrate profound gastroparesis documented by radionuclide studies. In this particular case, for example, Roux en Y diversion can be combined with a more extensive gastric resection to eliminate a portion of the chronic atonic stomach. Additionally, and in the face of severe gastroparesis and reflux gastritis, alternative procedures for biliary diversion can be contemplated rather than risking further post–Roux en Y gastroparesis. Quantitative biliary scanning for enterogastric reflux may not only indicate an unsuspected dilated afferent limb in some cases, but may document a prolonged "dwell time" of biliary refluxate in the postgastrectomy stomach even in the absence of bilious vomiting. In evaluating a specific or combined suspected postgastrectomy disorder, objective tests documenting either gastroparesis or alkaline reflux must be considered in planning remedial surgery even if the patient remains relatively asymptomatic for that particular symptom. Further gastric surgery not infrequently leads to a new set of postgastrectomy symptoms and, unfortunately in many patients, further remedial surgery.

The Dumping Syndrome

The dumping syndrome is subdivided into an early and late postgastrectomy complex. The early syndrome is by far the most common and the one most familiar to clinicians. It is also termed "early vasomotor dumping" due to the rapid onset of its symptoms. The late syndrome is extremely rare and is essentially postprandial hypoglycemia occurring approximately 1 to 2 hours following a meal. This is in contrast to the early syndrome, which occurs within minutes after the ingestion of sugars, carbohydrates, or even an ordinary meal.

Early Dumping Syndrome

Some symptoms of early vasomotor dumping occur or can be provoked in up to 25 percent of patients following either vagotomy and pyloroplasty, vagotomy and antrectomy, subtotal gastric resection, or even gastroenterostomy alone. The syndrome usually does not occur after highly selective vagotomy with preservation of antral innervation and an intact pylorus. In most cases, this syndrome will either resolve or respond readily to dietary manipulation as the patients become familiar with provocative foods. Overall, the severe form of this disease occurs in only a small number of patients, probably fewer than 5 percent.

The term *dumping stomach* was coined by Andrews and Mix in 1912 following initial reports of "unfavorable postoperative side effects" in patients who underwent the gastroenterostomy procedure. In 1922, Mix accurately documented that rapid gastric emptying occurred following gastroenterostomy when he performed a barium, upper GI "gastric emptying" study. The symptoms of early vasomotor dumping are classic. Typically, the patient experiences rapid postprandial onset of weakness, dizziness, palpitations, diaphoresis, and an overwhelming desire to lie down. Although nausea, vomiting, and other gastrointestinal symptoms may be present, they are not necessarily a part of the syndrome. Patients occasionally have intense abdominal cramps followed by explosive diarrhea. These symptoms can occur following almost any type of meal but the patients and physicians usually find that a high carbohydrate and sugar intake will precipitate an attack. Abdominal pain is usually absent unless associated alkaline reflux gastritis is present. Even without professional guidance, most patients subtly alter their dietary intake in an attempt to avoid the unpleasant symptoms of rapid gastric emptying. Observations during the past several decades have confirmed that the early dumping syndrome is associated with more than just rapid gastric emptying of hypertonic liquids. Even semisolid and solid foods can produce symptoms. The syndrome is associated with or caused by the release of serotonin, kinins, neurotensin, vasoactive intestinal peptide (VIP), and other gastrointestinal peptides. It is likely that some of the gastrointestinal hormones may play a role in inducing the cardiovascular and plasma volume changes because the severe symptoms of dumping often begin within minutes of eating a meal. Following complete vagotomy and drainage or resection, rapid emptying of liquids can be documented even in those patients who have no early vasomotor symptoms. A careful history, however, will elicit some mild to moderate dumping symptoms in up to 40 percent of patients who have had these procedures even though they are quite satisfied with the results of their operation. Although liquid emptying studies have been the standard in documenting disorders of rapid emptying, we have documented the rapid emptying of radionuclide solid food in patients with the most severe postgastrectomy dumping symptoms.

In patients affected with this syndrome, most symptoms will resolve with time or subtle alteration in dietary intake, or both. For the more severely affected patients, a strict regimen is necessary, including a low-carbohydrate diet and separation of liquids and solids during each meal. If diet alone is ineffective in preventing the dumping syndrome, the addition of gel-forming carbohydrates may modify glucose absorption. Pectin and a similar substance, guar gum, have been reported to alter the dumping effects of a glucose challenge. In our personal experience, pectin has blunted the intense nausea and dizziness in several patients with medically intractable dumping symptoms.

Of recent and perhaps most important interest has been the use of the somatostatin analog octreotide to alter the release of neurotensin, VIP, and enteroglucagon. This analog has proved to be extremely effective in relieving the vasomotor and gastrointestinal symptoms of dumping. It may also have an effect on delaying gastric emptying. Clinically, this substance is administered subcutaneously 15 to 30 minutes before eating in a dose of 50 to 100 μg.

Since the advent of somatostatin treatment, we have only performed surgery for postgastrectomy dumping rarely or when it was associated with alkaline reflux gastritis. Patients with primary dumping symptoms have been adequately treated by this medication in spite of the inconvenience of subcutaneous administration. Alternative delivery systems, including patches, sublingual dosing, nasal spray, or even an oral medication, will vastly improve the treatment of this syndrome.

For those few patients whose conditions do not respond to aggressive medical therapy and dietary manipulation, a variety of surgical procedures have been proposed, but our own experience has documented the efficacy of the Roux en Y procedure in significantly delaying gastric emptying enough to dramatically alter early vasomotor symptoms. Early successful reports of gastroenterostomy takedown were followed by a variety of procedures depending on the original operation, namely, conversion of the Billroth II to Billroth I reconstruction, isoperistaltic and antiperistaltic jejunal interposition, pyloroplasty reversal, and finally Roux en Y diversion. Most of these procedures have resulted in a moderation of the rapid gastric emptying of the dumping syndrome. Criteria for success should be durable, favorable results with minimal secondary postgastrectomy effects. Figure 86-1 outlines some of the surgical procedures used to treat the early vasomotor dumping syndrome.

During the 1970s, we demonstrated that patients with combined alkaline reflux gastritis and postgastrectomy dumping who underwent Roux en Y biliary diversion were pleasantly surprised to note improvement in their dumping symptoms. These observations were followed by experimental and clinical studies that demonstrated that Roux en Y diversion in the presence of complete vagal denervation significantly delays gastric emptying. Since the time of these early observations, we have continued to perform a 50-cm Roux en Y reconstruction for symptomatic, medically resistant dumping.

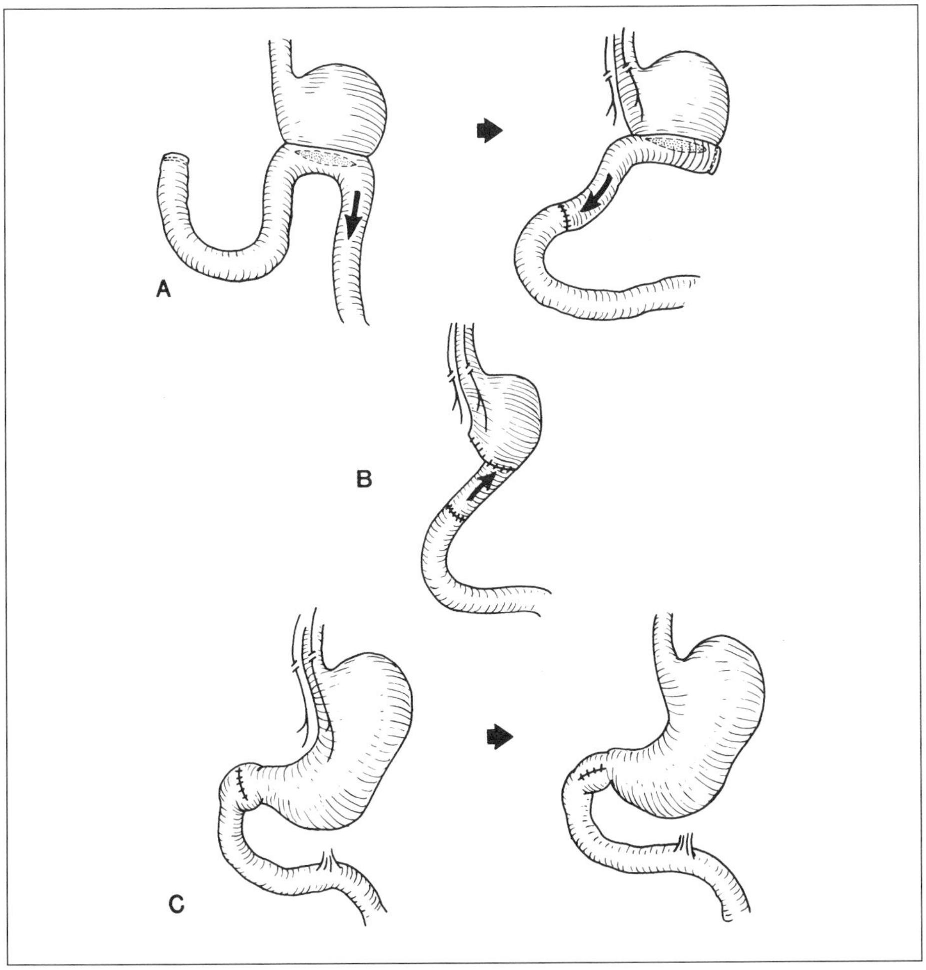

Surgical Strategy

The important history of small-intestinal interposition for the dumping syndrome has been reviewed by Herrington, Sawyers, and Scott. Although conversion to a Henley limb has been a standard for many years, they also reported excellent results using a 10-cm reversed jejunal limb interposed between the stomach and duodenum (Fig. 86-1). Our personal experience with jejunal pouches and interposition between the stomach and duodenum has been less than satisfactory. Many patients seem to develop rather marked gastric retention, alkaline reflux gastritis, or a combination of both disorders requiring further revisional surgery. The operation of pyloroplasty reversal has also been described for early postgastrectomy dumping with moderate success.

Based on early observations (see the section on the Roux syndrome), standard procedure is now revision to a Roux en Y gastroenterostomy with the efferent Roux limb approximately 50 cm in length between the gastroenterostomy and distal Roux enteroenterostomy. The technique depends upon the prior operation. Following a prior vagotomy and pyloroplasty, a distal gastrectomy is performed using the TA90 stapling device. A loop of proximal jejunum is brought up to find the appropriate loop that easily rests against the gastric remnant. In most cases this is performed in an antecolic fashion. There is usually no need to take down arcades of small-intestinal blood supply in performing the Roux. The jejunum is simply transected using the GIA stapling device (Fig. 86-2). The duodenum just distal to the previous pyloroplasty incision is carefully dissected free and stapled closed using a TA50 stapling device. In the presence of marked adhesions or inflammation, or both, care must be taken to avoid injury to the pancreas or distal common bile duct. If necessary, an "on table" cholecystocholangiogram is performed following transection of the duodenum to ensure patency of the distal common duct.

Fig. 86-1. Historical procedures used to treat postgastrectomy dumping. A. Conversion to an isoperistaltic jejunal interposition. B. Antiperistaltic jejunal interposition. C. Pyloroplasty reversal.

Figure 86-3 outlines the procedure when the prior operation was either a Billroth I or Billroth II reconstruction. In the case of a Billroth I operation, the stomach is similarly transected with a TA90 stapling device and the duodenum is closed in the same manner. The Roux limb is usually positioned in an isoperistaltic fashion. If it must be placed in a retrocolic position, the opening in the transverse colon mesentery is tacked closed at the end of the procedure. The distal enteroenterostomy is performed using the GIA stapling device approximately 50 cm distal to the gastroenterostomy. If the prior operation was a Billroth II gastrectomy (Fig. 86-3B), then the afferent limb is transected with the GIA stapling device just proximal to the gastroenterostomy. This portion of the afferent limb is then placed 50 cm distal (or distal small intestine is brought up in close proximity to perform the anastomosis). In the same fashion, the GIA stapling device performs the distal enteroenterostomy.

In spite of documenting an overall high success rate following Roux en Y diversion for postgastrectomy dumping (86%), several patients went from a state of well-documented early vasomotor symptoms and rapid gastric emptying to postoperative gastroparesis that required further revisional surgery and conversion of their Roux en Y gastroenterostomy to subtotal (70%) gastric resection using the same Roux en Y limb. The Roux procedure should be performed in the presence of well-documented symptoms and prior radionuclide studies demonstrating, at the very least, fairly rapid liquid or provocative high-carbohydrate liquid gastric emptying. In general, Roux en Y diversion should not be used as a primary reconstruction in gastric surgery except in the presence of extensive subtotal resection, near-total resection, or total gastrectomy. The procedure is performed primarily in these situations to avoid reflux gastritis and the very debilitating, reflux alkaline esophagitis.

The Late Dumping Syndrome

The late postprandial or hypoglycemic dumping syndrome occurs much less commonly than the early variety. Symptoms appear from 1 to 3 hours after a meal. They are similar to those of early dumping except for the absence of gastrointestinal cramping symptoms. Rapid emptying of soluble carbohydrates into the intestine causes a precipitous rise in postprandial serum glucose, which also reaches higher levels than usual. Hyperosmolar material in the upper intestine causes excessive release of enteroglucagon. This substance

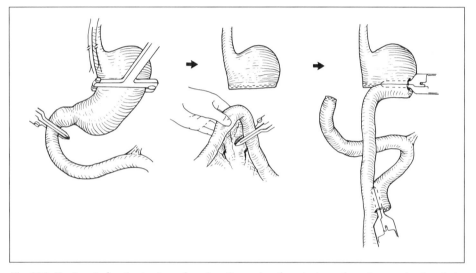

Fig. 86-2. Treatment of postgastrectomy dumping. Conversion of a prior truncal vagotomy and pyloroplasty to a 50-cm Roux en Y gastroenterostomy.

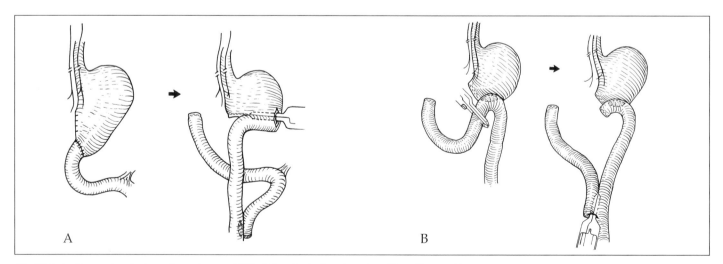

Fig. 86-3. A. Conversion of a truncal vagotomy and Billroth I gastroduodenostomy to a 50-cm Roux en Y gastroenterostomy. B. Roux en Y biliary diversion following a prior Billroth II gastroenterostomy. The afferent limb is transected just proximal to the gastrojejunostomy leaving an intact anastomosis.

sensitizes the beta cells of the pancreatic islet to release excessive amounts of insulin; thus, the postprandial hyperglycemia is overcorrected and is followed by hypoglycemia when high insulin levels persist. Unlike early dumping, symptoms are often relieved rather than aggravated by the ingestion of liquids that contain sugar. Prevention and treatment of the late syndrome is the same as that of the early variety. After several months of a low-carbohydrate diet, the small-bowel mucosa ceases to release excessive enteroglucagon. Patients appear to tolerate larger and larger amounts of carbohydrates in their diet without development of symptoms. Response to medical therapy and dietary manipulation is extremely successful and revisional surgery is almost never necessary.

Postvagotomy Diarrhea

Diarrhea may occur in up to 20 percent of patients following complete vagotomy with gastric drainage or resection. In general, however, only 1 to 2 percent of patients report incapacitating symptoms. Many patients have more frequent bowel movements and may consider this a positive effect after surgery. However, the severe form of this syndrome is characterized by frequent, watery stools, usually unrelated to meals, often occurring at nighttime, and occasionally explosive in character. These few patients often suffer profound weight loss, appear malnourished, and in general are incapacitated by their symptoms. Many undergo extensive medical evaluation for bacterial overgrowth, intestinal parasites, and malabsorption syndromes. The cause of the syndrome is unclear and, although associated with complete vagotomy, it may be related more to the effects of impaired biliary and/or pancreatic function, impaired gallbladder emptying, or perhaps an increase in fecal excretion of bile salts and acids. Conservative medical therapy begins with a dietary change and includes meals with a low fluid content, more frequent smaller feedings, and an increase in dietary fiber to slow intestinal transit. Radionuclide studies may demonstrate a rapid stomach-to-right-colon transit following ingestion of both liquids and solids. When appropriate antibiotics are used to either treat or rule out bacterial overgrowth, antidiarrheal agents and opiates have been em-

ployed to reduce the number of stools and transiently give relief. A dose of 4 g cholestyramine has been used with each meal to bind bile salts and reduce their diarrheagenic effect. Most patients, however, find the chronic oral ingestion of cholestyramine to be unpalatable.

The somatostatin analog octreotide has been used to treat either postgastrectomy diarrhea or combined diarrhea and dumping with overall good results. Certainly, this substance should be administered on a chronic basis before any consideration is given to surgical revision. If patients fail to respond to medical therapy and other associated illnesses are excluded, surgery is indicated.

Surgical Strategy

Sawyers and Herrington originally reported on the successful use of a 10-cm antiperistaltic jejunal segment that was interposed approximately 100 cm distal to the ligament of Treitz for postvagotomy diarrhea. In a recent review, they noted that 14 of 16 patients who underwent this procedure had a successful outcome. We have performed this procedure with "relative success" 12 times during the past 15 years owing to its rarity. The procedure was extremely successful in slowing intestinal transit. The last two patients, however, required removal of this segment for recurrent colicky abdominal pain and intermittent episodes mimicking partial bowel obstruction. Figure 86-4 demonstrates the procedure in a patient with a prior vagotomy and pyloroplasty. At a distance of approximately 100 cm from the ligament of Treitz, a 10-cm section of jejunum is isolated and taken out of continuity. This segment is reversed to place it in an antiperistaltic position. This segment is then sutured both proximally and distally and defects in the mesentery are closed. Although functional end-to-end stapled anastomoses have been performed, we advise performing "hand-sewn" end-to-end sutured anastomoses since experimental observations have documented more profound effects on electrical transmission and motility in the stapled anastomosis compared to the hand sewn.

A procedure reported by Cuschieri in the 1980s consisted of an innovative, reversed ileal onlay graft with the reversed portion encompassing only one-half the diameter of the intestine. In this case, 180 degrees of

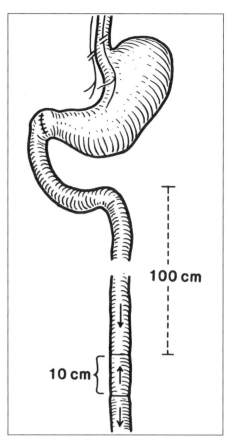

Fig. 86-4. Standard antiperistaltic reversed jejunal segment interposed approximately 100 cm from the ligament of Treitz in treating postvagotomy diarrhea.

the intestine remained isoperistaltic and 180 degrees of diameter remained antiperistaltic. Cuschieri reported excellent results with this innovative procedure but we have had no experience with this form of revisional surgery. It is possible, however, that this form of reconstruction would eliminate some of the recent difficulty reported with a total reversed jejunal interposition.

Postoperative Delayed Gastric Emptying
Acute Gastroparesis

Overall, the incidence of acute postoperative delayed gastric emptying varies between 10 and 30 percent following operations on the stomach that include complete vagal denervation. In special circumstances and even in the absence of vagotomy, acute postoperative gastroparesis can occur in up to 50 percent of patients. The incidence of postoperative delayed gastric emptying has been reported as high as 50 percent following a standard Whipple procedure for pancreatic cancer. Nearly as high an incidence of gastroparesis has also been reported following the pylorus-sparing procedure for pancreatic malignancies. Even palliative gastroenterostomy for unresectable pancreatic cancer often results in marked gastroparesis, with an incidence of 30 to 40 percent being reported in the literature. Complete truncal vagotomy results in some degree of gastric atony to solid food and to a lesser extent to liquids in a large number of patients but it is clinically significant to a lesser extent. Delayed gastric emptying, however, has been reported to occur 2½ times more often in patients with vagotomy and hemigastrectomy than in those without vagotomy; in some series of vagotomy and pyloroplasty, however, the incidence has been reported to be as low as 10 percent. Although controversial, a higher incidence of acute gastroparesis has been reported in the presence of a preoperative diagnosis of acute or chronic duodenal obstruction. The acute form of the disease develops when a patient fails to take or retain adequate oral intake at some arbitrary time during the postoperative period. Adequate oral intake has varied from 5 to 8 days to approximately 2 weeks but most surgeons use 1 week as the cutoff for routine postoperative po intake. Early postoperative vomiting following oral intake or failure of the stomach to adequately empty presents a unique challenge to the surgeon, who is often pressured by the patient, the family, or the referring physician to "do something." In general, the surgeon must reassure all parties involved that this postoperative "inconvenience" or complication usually resolves with time. In general, the causes of this early phenomenon have included stomal edema, kinking, obstruction, acute dense postoperative adhesions, pancreatitis, internal hernia, and overall circumstances usually characterized as acute postoperative ileus.

The treatment of acute delayed gastric emptying is nonsurgical and should include much patience, "tincture of time," appropriate evaluation, and intense medical therapy. After a period of time utilizing nasogastric decompression and correction of any electrolyte abnormalities, a dilute liquid barium study should be performed with the patient in the upright position. If the anastomosis appears patent, then the disorder is considered functional. Functional gastric atony, however, may mimic the radiologic appearance of complete obstruction with pooling of barium in the fundus of a dilated stomach. The radiologist usually reports this as complete gastric outlet obstruction or occasionally a "thin trickle of barium" crossing an "edematous" anastomosis. In these circumstances, endoscopy in a well-sedated patient is mandatory to ascertain whether or not obstruction is present. Fortunately, in most cases the anastomosis is deemed patent. An overall conservative treatment plan includes parenteral hyperalimentation, continued gastric decompression, and pharmacologic therapy. The first major step is removal of the nasogastric (NG) tube. If patients can "tolerate their own secretions," the prognosis is invariably excellent. Our personal experience with pharmacologic therapy is variable and has included the use of the dopamine antagonist metoclopramide, the parasympathetic agent bethanechol, and more recently erythromycin and cisapride. We have recently used the antibiotic erythromycin in an intravenous dose of 1 mg/kg every 6 to 8 hours or, if the patient can be without an NG tube, in a dose of 3 mg/kg po four times a day.

In most patients, acute postoperative gastroparesis will resolve within 3 to 3½ weeks without any specific treatment. In those patients in whom prolonged nasogastric intubation is a problem, we have performed percutaneous gastrostomy to ease the burden of postoperative gastroparesis. In operating on conditions in which the incidence of postoperative delayed gastric emptying is considered high, we have strongly recommended performance of a surgical gastrostomy during the procedure to obviate the necessity of prolonged nasogastric intubation. In cases of pancreatic cancer in which either the Whipple procedure or a palliative gastroenterostomy is performed, surgical gastrostomy greatly increases postoperative patient comfort and is not only readily accepted, but is preferred over the annoying nasogastric tube.

As stated above, the surgeon should resist the temptation to reoperate but if remedial surgery becomes necessary, then a gastrostomy and jejunostomy tube should be inserted at the second operation. If a patent outlet is present, then we would caution against performing an additional gastroenterostomy in the presence of a prior vagotomy and drainage procedure or vagotomy and Billroth I resection. This maneuver seldom results in restoration of gastric emptying except when a further gastric resection is performed and more often results in the additional problem of bilious vomiting in the presence of gastric atony. Occasionally, however, this procedure is the only one available, especially in the presence of dense adhesions and marked inflammation around the gastric outlet found early in the postoperative period. As a general rule, however, and if surgery becomes necessary for acute gastroparesis, further gastric resection to remove a portion of the atonic stomach should result in normal postoperative gastric emptying. Since bilious vomiting is often associated with acute delayed gastric emptying, we would also caution against the use of a Roux en Y procedure in the patient whose primary problem is acute gastric atony. In this circumstance, the Roux en Y reconstruction should only be performed following a more extensive resection and removal of a portion of the atonic stomach. Fortunately, surgical revision is seldom performed for acute postoperative delayed gastric emptying. In the few cases in which remedial surgery is deemed necessary, our procedure of choice is conversion of a prior vagotomy and pyloroplasty or vagotomy and Billroth I reconstruction to a Billroth II hemigastrectomy with a distal (25 cm from the gastroenterostomy) Braun enteroenterostomy. This enteroenterostomy anastomosis decompresses the afferent limb and, at this distance, diverts a considerable amount of bile away from the stomach, thereby decreasing nasogastric or gastrostomy tube output and further bilious vomiting even if the stomach remains atonic. We believe that this maneuver will also prevent future alkaline reflux gastritis.

Chronic Gastroparesis

The chronic form of gastroparesis is characterized by nausea with or without vomiting, abdominal pain, frequent bezoar formation, and postprandial bloating that is more severe in the evening. In the absence of mechanical obstruction, anastomotic stricture, or the edema of chronic marginal ulceration, upper GI barium studies and endoscopy are either normal or demonstrate the presence of chronic bezoars. The treatment of this condition is medical, including frequent endoscopic procedures and breakup of the bezoar, low-residue diet, oral enzyme preparations, and pharmacologic prokinetic agents. Radionuclide gastric emptying studies utilizing either erythromycin or the newer agent cisapride will often document whether the stomach responds to prokinetic stimulation. Most patients, however, are empirically placed on these agents to evaluate their response. For those patients who fail to respond to medical therapy or can no longer tolerate frequent endoscopic procedures, remedial surgery is now becoming more common.

Surgical Strategy

The aim of revisional surgery is to remove a portion of the atonic stomach depending upon the prior gastric operation. In most cases, surgical therapy is not indicated until the patient has been treated with prokinetic agents for many months before revisional surgery. The clinician should be cautious, however, since this field is slowly evolving, and the choice of a revisional reconstruction should be made carefully so as to avoid a second set of postgastrectomy complications.

In patients who have had a prior vagotomy and pyloroplasty, we have performed a hemigastrectomy with a Polya-type Billroth II reconstruction and a distal Braun enteroenterostomy performed approximately 25 cm from the gastroenterostomy (Fig. 86-5). Using quantitative radionuclide biliary scanning, we have documented that this type of reconstruction diverts a major percentage of bile away from the stomach. We have used this technique for many years and recently began documenting its efficacy using quantitative enterogastric reflux scanning. Although not widely used at present, this type of reconstruction at the very least diminishes postoperative nasogastric output; avoids early postoperative bilious vomiting, even in patients with persistent gastric atony; and in all likelihood avoids or dramatically decreases the incidence of chronic alkaline reflux gastritis.

If the patient's prior operation was either an antrectomy or hemigastrectomy, further gastric resection should be performed. The specific type of reconstruction will most definitely depend on the surgeon's "comfort level" and personal experience. The standard approach is conversion of the previous operation to a subtotal gastric resection with Roux en Y reconstruction. We have performed a Billroth II reconstruction with a distal Braun enteroenterostomy following resective procedures

up to 75 percent. With greater resections, there is a tendency to perform a Roux en Y reconstruction to "definitely" divert bile away from the stomach and esophagus. Figure 86-6 demonstrates the two types of reconstruction in the presence of acute or chronic gastroparesis. We have had considerable experience in performing the Billroth II gastroenterostomy with a distal enteroenterostomy in the presence of up to a 75 percent gastric resection. In this case, our "comfort level" is high, as we have demonstrated even in these cases a fairly high percentage of bile being diverted away from the stomach. This is demonstrated in Fig. 86-7 in a patient with a history of significant alkaline reflux gastritis, gastroparesis, and a prior Billroth I antrectomy. The patient underwent conversion of the previous operation to a subtotal Billroth II resection with the distal enteroenterostomy. The radionuclide evaluation demonstrates almost complete diversion of bile away from the stomach. At 90 minutes into the procedure, the area of the remaining gastric pouch is "marked" with a technetium-99 swallow. As the clinician becomes more comfortable with the possibility of biliary diversion without performing the Roux procedure, then this type of reconstruction may be preferable. It is now our standard in the presence of chronic gastroparesis. If, on the other hand, the clinician has no experience with this form of revisional surgery, the stan-

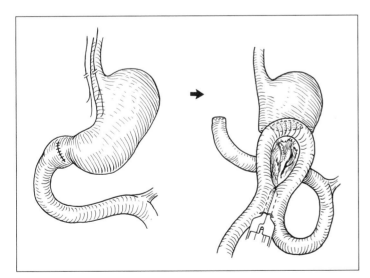

Fig. 86-5. Treatment of chronic gastroparesis. Conversion of a prior truncal vagotomy and pyloroplasty to a hemigastrectomy and Billroth II gastroenterostomy with a distal enteroenterostomy performed at 20 to 25 cm from the gastroenterostomy.

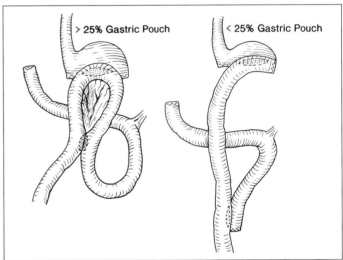

Fig. 86-6. Treatment of chronic medically resistant gastroparesis by conversion to either a subtotal Billroth II gastric resection with distal enteroenterostomy or a near-total Roux en Y gastrojejunostomy.

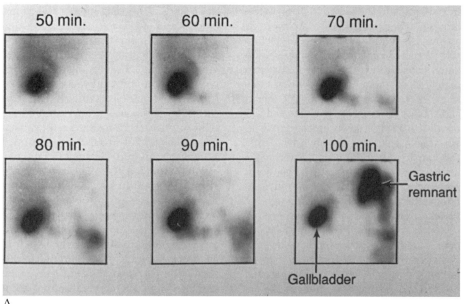
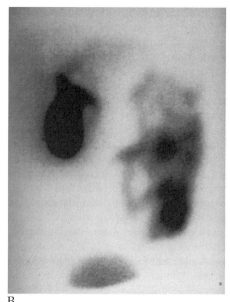

A   B

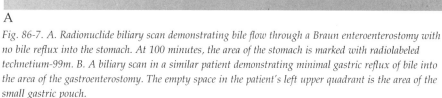

Fig. 86-7. A. Radionuclide biliary scan demonstrating bile flow through a Braun enteroenterostomy with no bile reflux into the stomach. At 100 minutes, the area of the stomach is marked with radiolabeled technetium-99m. B. A biliary scan in a similar patient demonstrating minimal gastric reflux of bile into the area of the gastroenterostomy. The empty space in the patient's left upper quadrant is the area of the small gastric pouch.

dard Roux en Y diversion is not only acceptable but the preferred treatment by many authors in the presence of a subtotal gastric resection. Once again, when a more extensive gastric resection is performed, then the Roux procedure is definitely indicated to absolutely ensure total diversion of bile away from the stomach and esophagus.

Alkaline Reflux Gastritis and the Roux Syndrome

These two conditions are considered together since if it were not for the treatment of one disorder then the second condition would not exist. It has been our belief and experience that the Roux syndrome is a bona fide postgastrectomy complication, but therein lies the clinical paradox since the Roux procedure has been and remains a successful form of biliary diversion when specifically indicated. This entire field as well as alternative procedures to divert bile without altering gastric emptying is undergoing slow but progressive evolu-

tion as continued clinical and experimental observations and procedures are performed.

Alkaline Reflux Gastritis

Postoperative bilious vomiting and abdominal pain are two of the most common postgastrectomy symptoms and have been with us since the early days of gastric surgery, with the first case reports by Billroth in the late 1800s following both the gastroenterostomy and distal gastrectomy procedures. The distinct character of alkaline gastritis as a specific postgastrectomy syndrome was not elucidated until 1965, following the careful observations of Toye and Williams on reproducing the symptoms of postgastrectomy by instillation of alkaline contents into the gastric pouch. Subsequently, this controversial syndrome was popularized in both the British and American literature and diagnosed and treated extensively during the 1970s and early 1980s. It is interesting and perhaps prophetic that early attempts at avoiding bilious vomiting and abdominal pain included Roux en Y biliary diversion

and the Braun enteroenterostomy. Some surgeons even documented a procedure that included suturing of the afferent limb between the stomach and the more distal Braun enteroenterostomy in a further attempt to divert duodenal secretions and keep stomach contents out of the afferent limb. These attempts occurred in the early 1900s but within several decades most were abandoned. The Roux en Y procedure appeared to be associated with a high incidence of marginal ulceration in the era before vagotomy. The enteroenterostomy procedure was also abandoned following the introduction of a "short" Billroth II reconstruction to an area of jejunum just distal to the ligament of Treitz.

The diagnosis of alkaline gastritis has been and, to a certain extent, remains one of exclusion. Patients with this disorder complain of severe burning upper abdominal pain and, not infrequently, bilious vomiting. They usually describe increasing abdominal pain following the ingestion of a meal that is more typical of pain associated with severe gastritis and gastric ulcer than with duodenal ulcer disease. Other etiologies of postgastrectomy symptoms need to be investigated and eliminated as causes of these unfavorable side effects. These include marginal ulceration, afferent loop syndrome, chronic gastroparesis, and anastomotic stricture, among others. Endoscopic examination usually demonstrates marked gastritis with a "beefy red" appearance of the gastric mucosa. Although this syndrome remains controversial, it has always been interesting to surgeons that these endoscopic findings rapidly resolve following Roux en Y diversion of duodenal contents. Similarly, the severe burning upper abdominal pain is noted to completely disappear even in the early postoperative period and even in those patients who subsequently complain of other post–Roux en Y difficulties. Biopsy of the gastric mucosa invariably demonstrates a histologic picture of both acute and chronic inflammation. Although similar to acid reflux esophagitis, histologic inflammation is not necessarily a requirement for diagnosis. Quantitative radionuclide biliary scanning for enterogastric reflux demonstrates an increased percentage of biliary refluxate in the stomach of symptomatic patients compared to asymptomatic Billroth II patients, and additionally real-time scanning demonstrates increased "dwell time" of biliary enterogastric reflux. Radionuclide gastric emptying studies need to be performed since documented abnormalities that may be mimicking some aspects of alkaline gastritis can be treated medically before consideration of revisional surgery.

There is no specific medical treatment for the distinct entity of alkaline reflux gastritis. Most patients have been placed on empiric therapy including H_2 antagonists and more recently prokinetic agents in an attempt to alter the symptom complex and, by treatment, ruling out other associated disorders. Cholestyramine therapy has been used in an attempt to bind bile salts, but with little effect. The most promising therapy has been the use of prokinetic agents to treat chronic gastroparesis when it coexists with alkaline reflux gastritis. This type of treatment may relieve some of the symptoms for a period of time but most patients will continue to complain of upper abdominal burning pain, especially when radionuclide scans demonstrate severe enterogastric reflux. Because of the controversial nature of this syndrome, most patients will have undergone general medical treatment for months and years

before considering revisional surgical therapy.

Roux en Y biliary diversion has been, and in most cases remains, the surgical treatment of choice for medically resistant and well-documented alkaline reflux gastritis. Creation of a 50-cm Roux en Y limb adequately diverts almost all afferent limb secretions away from the stomach, resulting in nearly complete resolution of the burning abdominal pain and intermittent bilious vomiting. This procedure also adequately treats the fairly common associated reflux esophagitis since most patients already have maximal acid suppression with medical therapy, and Roux en Y diversion adequately diverts almost all of the alkaline secretions away from the esophagus in those patients with esophageal reflux.

In the early 1980s, we reviewed the clinical course of 97 patients who underwent Roux en Y diversion for alkaline gastritis during the previous decade and before the advent of radionuclide evaluation of gastric emptying. It is interesting that early results demonstrated complete relief from the pain of alkaline gastritis in almost all patients immediately and in greater than 95 percent of patients at 6 months following the operation. In late follow-up studies, however, 59 percent of patients had excellent (Visick grade I) or good results (Visick grade II), 18 percent were regarded as having only a fair response, and 23 percent were considered complete surgical failures because of severe symptoms of gastric retention. Nearly all of the patients in the groups with fair or poor results readily discriminated between their preoperative burning pain and the more subtle postoperative symptoms of delayed gastric emptying. Of the Visick III patients, almost all were satisfied with the results of Roux en Y diversion. Despite moderate to severe symptoms of delayed gastric emptying in 50 of 97 patients, more than 75 percent believed they had benefited from Roux en Y diversion.

Gastroparesis following the Roux procedure was fairly well documented in the British literature in the 1950s in spite of the fact that the technique was used for "overall" postgastrectomy syndromes before the definitive diagnosis of alkaline gastritis. In our retrospective review, it appeared that a significant percentage of pa-

tients may have had a preexisting chronic gastroparesis, which might, in some cases, have led to unfavorable postoperative results. These suggestions were made by other investigators during the 1970s, but in early 1980, we documented significant delayed gastric emptying using a standard meal as well as radionuclide-labeled food in canine experiments following conversion of a Billroth II gastric resection to Roux en Y biliary diversion. Certainly, in these experiments, no prior motility disorder was present before the primary procedure and all animals were used as their own control. Further clinical studies in postgastrectomy patients demonstrated significant post–Roux en Y gastroparesis in those undergoing Roux en Y diversion with normal preoperative gastric emptying. Although the number of patients affected is controversial, we believe that significant gastroparesis occurs in at least 25 to 30 percent of patients following Roux en Y diversion.

Surgical Strategy

At the present time, Roux en Y diversion is combined with more extensive gastrectomy in those patients with a preexisting motility disorder or radionuclide documentation of significant gastroparesis associated with alkaline reflux gastritis. Based on experience in treating the so-called Roux syndrome, some authors have recommended very extensive gastric resection. At present, however, we convert a prior vagotomy and pyloroplasty or Billroth I antrectomy to approximately a 50 percent gastric resection when performing the Roux en Y procedure for alkaline reflux gastritis only. If the patient had previously documented severe gastroparesis associated with the alkaline gastritis then a further gastric resection is performed up to what is considered subtotal (65–70%). Some authors have recommended near-total resection but we have avoided this extensive a procedure, since in our experience we have noted a small but significant number of patients being converted to marked postgastrectomy dumping with very extensive gastric resection even in the presence of Roux en Y reconstruction.

If the prior operation was a Billroth II gastrectomy and in the absence of any clinical or objective evidence of gastroparesis, the following procedure is performed: If the prior anastomosis is widely patent, the af-

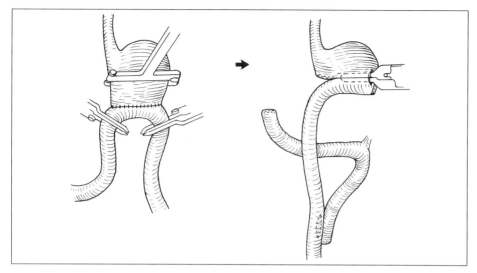

Fig. 86-8. Conversion of a Billroth II gastroenterostomy to a subtotal Roux en Y reconstruction in a patient with combined alkaline reflux gastritis and chronic gastroparesis.

ferent limb is transected using the GIA stapling device just next to the beginning of the gastroenterostomy. The efferent limb is measured to a length of approximately 50 cm and this point is brought up to lie in proximity with the stapled end of the prior afferent limb. A side-to-side anastomosis is performed using the GIA stapling device. This procedure is quick, easy, and an extremely effective form of biliary diversion. The dilemma for the surgeon, however, occurs when a widely patent Billroth II reconstruction is associated with prior clinical and objective evidence of gastroparesis. In the severe form of this disease, we have performed a new anastomosis, resecting the remaining stomach up to the "subtotal" level. The afferent and efferent limbs are transected and a new 50-cm Roux en Y is constructed. Occasionally the gastroenterostomy can be saved with no loss of jejunum. In this case, a simple Roux en Y diversionary procedure is performed. It has always been tempting to maintain the prior Billroth II anastomosis when it is widely patent. Further resection, however, is our attempt to remove some of the atonic stomach and to decrease the incidence of post–Roux en Y gastric retention (Fig. 86-8).

Alternative Procedures to Biliary Diversion

Alternative procedures to Roux en Y gastrojejunostomy have been proposed, such as exclusion, jejunoduodenostomy as reported by Stiegmann and Goff, and the duodenal switch procedure reported by DeMeester and associates. The Tanner 19 modification has anecdotally been reported to be associated with less delayed gastric emptying than occurs after standard Roux en Y gastrojejunostomy although this has not been prospectively evaluated. Gastric emptying into both the afferent and efferent limbs of a Roux en Y in the Tanner 19 procedure might facilitate gastric emptying, although in animal studies we were unable to document any difference between the standard Roux en Y procedure and this form of revisional surgery. A recent procedure reported by Kelly and associates is the "uncut" Roux gastrojejunostomy. This procedure is essentially a Billroth II type of gastrojejunostomy with a distal Braun enteroenterostomy. In this case, however, an incontinuity staple line is placed across the afferent limb, "forcing" afferent limb contents to be diverted through into the efferent limb and away from the stomach. This was one of the types of reconstruction used in the early 1900s with a fair degree of success.

Our experimental and clinical observations have documented that a distal Braun enteroenterostomy adequately diverts most of the bile away from the stomach without a staple line placed on the afferent limb. As previously described in this chapter, this is now our preferred method of reconstruction following primary or revi-

sional gastric resections and for standard Whipple procedures and palliative gastroenterostomies. At the present time, we have a small but significant experience in using this procedure to primarily treat the syndrome of alkaline reflux gastritis either alone or combined with chronic gastroparesis. This procedure has been performed in 12 patients to date. In those with both gastritis and gastroparesis, we have performed a subtotal gastric resection and used the distal Braun enteroenterostomy for biliary diversion. In those without gastroparesis, we perform a hemigastrectomy with the above-described procedure. Early and moderately late results are most gratifying. There is no incidence of recurrent alkaline reflux gastritis, no bilious vomiting in either the early or late postoperative period, and adequate objective documentation of considerable biliary diversion. As described previously, the clinician's "comfort level" will determine whether he or she performs these procedures or the standard Roux.

We suspect that, as experience increases, the distal enteroenterostomy will become a more commonly used procedure in an attempt to avoid some of the unpleasant effects of the Roux syndrome. Since prevention of alkaline reflux gastritis is far more effective than having to treat patients with this disorder, we believe that adequate diversion of bile in the presence of complete vagal denervation in primary gastric operations dramatically decreases the incidence of this syndrome.

The Roux Syndrome

During the 1970s and 1980s, the frequency of diagnosis of alkaline reflux gastritis and treatment by Roux en Y biliary diversion increased dramatically. As described above, the overall results, especially early in the postoperative period, were excellent, but moderate to significant gastroparesis was described late in the postoperative period. In 1975, Davidson and Hurtz suggested that symptoms of alkaline gastritis may be indistinguishable from those of delayed gastric emptying and then suggested that those patients with a preexisting gastric emptying disorder had not benefited from Roux en Y diversion. Other reports have substantiated these suggestions and post–Roux en Y gastroparesis was documented both experimentally and clinically during the 1980s.

We described both an early and late form of this syndrome. The early Roux syndrome is characterized by prolonged hospitalization following Roux en Y diversion and persistent vomiting of either liquids or solids. As described in the section on early postoperative gastroparesis, meglumine diatrizoate (Gastrografin) or barium upper GI evaluation will occasionally suggest complete gastric outlet obstruction. Endoscopic evaluation, however, will demonstrate a widely patent anastomosis. Most patients will respond to "tincture of time," parenteral hyperalimentation, and possibly prokinetic agents. Since 1979, only two patients have undergone revisional surgery for the acute Roux syndrome, converting the Roux en Y procedure with antrectomy to a subtotal gastrectomy with a similar Roux en Y reconstruction. The late Roux syndrome is extremely subtle. This was especially true before the routine use of radionuclide studies. The symptoms are intermittent vomiting, epigastric fullness, and abdominal pain. Most patients have had frequent normal endoscopic procedures and fairly normal upper GI barium evaluations. We and others have demonstrated a massively dilated Roux limb with no evidence of downstream obstruction in some patients who suffer from the late Roux syndrome. Radionuclide evaluation invariably demonstrates significant chronic gastroparesis.

We have had minimal success in treating the chronic syndrome with either metoclopramide or cisapride. Recently, however, we have reported a fair success rate using the prokinetic agent erythromycin. It is interesting that both experimentally and clinically, erythromycin speeds post–Roux en Y gastric emptying when viewed under the gamma camera following the ingestion of a radionuclide-labeled meal. The chronic use of this agent, however, is met with limited success after weeks or months of use.

During the past decade, we and others have demonstrated variable patterns of gastric emptying following Roux en Y diversion. Significant gastric retention is the most common, followed by combined gastric retention in both the stomach and Roux limb, and, finally the most obscure pattern, fairly normal to rapid gastric emptying with prolonged retention of radiolabeled food in the Roux limb. In some patients, it is fairly easy to document a back-and-forth movement of radiolabeled food from the Roux limb to the stomach and back into a dilated Roux limb.

As in most cases of postgastrectomy symptoms, other disorders need to be eliminated. Endoscopic evaluation should include not only the stomach and Roux limb but, if possible, visualization of the downstream enteroenterostomy.

Early on, the etiology of this syndrome was unclear but experimentally it necessitated complete vagal denervation. Certainly, most patients who underwent Roux en Y diversion have had a prior complete vagotomy. We and others initially hypothesized that in the presence of complete vagal denervation, the surgical creation of the Roux limb bypassed the duodenal pacemaker, thereby altering the propagation of myoelectric activity. These initial suggestions have now been well documented clinically and experimentally. It is interesting and part of the overall paradox of this syndrome that although a Roux limb attached to the esophagus following total gastrectomy does not seem to result in significant delay in upper intestinal transit, it is likely that the combination of an atonic gastric pouch and a Roux limb is additive in producing the delayed emptying effect. It has been our experience that this particular postgastrectomy syndrome does not resolve with time in the 25 to 30 percent of patients who suffer from chronic symptoms of gastroparesis.

All patients with the Roux syndrome need to be treated extensively with prokinetic agents before further revisional surgery is considered as described. We have had moderate success using erythromycin but minimal success giving the newer agent cisapride. Before the development of modern agents, we had considerable success using oral bethanechol in a dose of 15 to 20 mg po 30 minutes before each meal. We documented the positive effect of this agent and most patients appear to tolerate this therapy for a period of time. Bezoar formation is fairly common and patients usually undergo frequent endoscopic "breakup" and treatment with low-residue diet and oral enzyme preparations.

Surgical Strategy

The standard operative procedure for treating the Roux syndrome is now removal of a portion of the atonic stomach with Roux en Y reconstruction. We and others have demonstrated the efficacy of further gastric resection in facilitating gastric emptying. Several authors have now recommended near-total removal of the remaining gastric pouch with Roux en Y reconstruction. In view of the fact that the difficulty appears to be in the Roux limb and not necessarily the stomach, we have now "backed off" our original suggestions as to how much stomach should be removed. Based on the old adage that "it is nice to take your stomach to the dinner table," we have avoided converting patients with the Roux syndrome to near-total gastrectomy. If the patient's prior operation was a Roux en Y antrectomy or hemigastrectomy, further gastric resection up to a subtotal is appropriate. Reconstruction is to the same Roux en Y limb if possible. Occasionally, the enteroenterostomy will need to be moved further downstream to maintain the 50-cm distance of the Roux limb. If the prior operation was already a subtotal, then our previous suggestion of removing some of the atonic pouch is still performed. More recently, however, we have performed a different procedure based on previously described observations in an attempt to treat the problem and not risk either further gastric resection or persistent post–Roux en Y gastroparesis. Six patients whose Roux en Y procedure was performed primarily for alkaline reflux gastritis underwent takedown of the Roux en Y gastrojejunostomy and conversion to a Billroth II procedure with a distal Braun enteroenterostomy at approximately 25 to 30 cm. This procedure was performed primarily to treat the Roux syndrome when there was no evidence of gastroparesis before the patient underwent the Roux procedure for alkaline gastritis. The results have been most encouraging, with no symptoms of reflux gastritis and restoration of a fairly normal dietary lifestyle. In several cases and as a part of the technical procedure, 10 to 15 percent of the gastric pouch was removed to facilitate surgical reconstruction. Figure 86-9 demonstrates the standard treatment of the Roux syndrome converting a Roux en Y hemigastrectomy to a subtotal Roux procedure as well as the described conversion to a Billroth II and Braun enteroenterostomy reconstruction. Further time and reports by other investigators will be needed to completely evaluate the efficacy of this procedure in treating patients with the Roux syndrome. The reader should be advised, however, that our prior reports documented that a small but significant

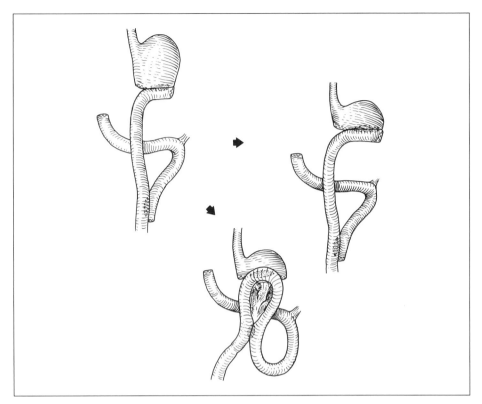

Fig. 86-9. *Two methods of treating the chronic Roux syndrome by either a conversion to a subtotal Roux en Y reconstruction (removing more atonic stomach) or takedown of the Roux and conversion to a Billroth II gastroenterostomy with a distal Braun enteroenterostomy.*

number of patients continue to have symptoms of the Roux syndrome even following extensive gastric resection. When this was documented using radionuclide methods, the patients were converted to a near-total or total gastrectomy. Unfortunately, some of these patients developed severe postgastrectomy dumping syndrome and this in part led to our caution in advising total gastrectomy.

As described, our recent emphasis and clinical observations have been based primarily on the prevention and treatment of alkaline gastritis and use of the same form of treatment in those patients with the debilitating effects of the Roux syndrome.

Afferent and Efferent Loop Syndrome

The afferent loop syndrome does not exist following either vagotomy and pyloroplasty or Billroth I gastric resections. The syndrome is present only following a Billroth II reconstruction and is caused by intermittent obstruction or "kinking" of the afferent limb. Occasionally the syndrome is found to be caused by partial intussusception or even retrojejunal herniation of the loop causing compression of the afferent limb. Early in the 1900s, surgeons found that by performing a "short" afferent limb in the area of the ligament of Treitz, the afferent limb syndrome could be avoided. Interestingly, this surgical approach eliminated the possibility of performing a distal Braun enteroenterostomy.

Patients' symptoms are fairly classic and the syndrome is characterized by intermittent epigastric or right upper quadrant pain relieved by bilious vomiting. The vomiting is quite projectile and often contains only bile with no food. This syndrome must be distinguished from early postoperative gastroparesis, with vomiting of both food and bile but not necessarily severe crampy or colicky pain. In the chronic state, this syndrome must be distinguished from alkaline gastritis. Radionuclide biliary scanning adequately and accurately demonstrates a very dilated afferent limb as opposed to no dilatation in the alkaline reflux gastritis syndrome. Only rarely will a combination of both disorders coexist. The clinician should be aware that the acute postoperative form of this condition may be life threatening and predisposed to duodenal stump dehiscence. Severe pain and bilious vomiting should be immediately evaluated by radionuclide scanning. The chronic form of this syndrome may be associated with rather marked bacterial overgrowth in the chronically obstructed "blind loop." Plain films of the abdomen rarely diagnose a dilated afferent limb but this has been seen on CT examination when this procedure was performed for other reasons. Occasionally, a barium upper GI examination will demonstrate a "trickle" of barium into a dilated afferent limb.

The preferred treatment of this syndrome is always surgical. Several procedures have been recommended but most authors have recommended and continue to recommend conversion of the Billroth II gastroenterostomy to a 50-cm Roux en Y reconstruction. Another common procedure has been to perform a distal enteroenterostomy. This option, however, is limited by the prior operation and reconstruction. In the presence of a "short" afferent limb, this procedure can only be performed following revision of the entire anastomosis. In an attempt to avoid the unpleasant side effects of Roux en Y reconstruction, we have reconstructed several patients by performing a takedown of the prior gastroenterostomy, a Billroth II gastroenterostomy with a distal Braun enteroenterostomy at approximately a 25-cm distance.

The efferent loop syndrome is purely a mechanical problem characterized by relative obstruction at or near the Billroth II reconstruction. As one would expect, partial obstruction of the efferent limb would cause rather profound bilious vomiting, which may be confused with either afferent loop syndrome, alkaline gastritis, or severe postoperative gastroparesis.

The etiology of this syndrome can be kinking or adhesions at the efferent limb or intussusception or internal herniation in the space behind the gastroenterostomy. The diagnosis is difficult but can be aided with the prompt performance of barium upper GI studies and endoscopy. The upper GI examination may fail to demonstrate any emptying into the efferent limb or may document a "thin trickle" into a partially obstructed limb. Upper endoscopy may rule this disorder out if the anastomosis and both limbs appear widely patent. The treatment of this disorder is surgical, often early in the postoperative period. If intussusception, adhesions, or a retroanastomotic hernia is found, the primary anastomosis may be saved following correction of these abnormalities. In most cases, however, a reanastomosis is performed with the placement of a gastrostomy tube to avoid the unpleasant side effects of perhaps further prolonged nasogastric intubation. Our preference is a new Billroth II gastroenterostomy with a distal enteroenterostomy for reasons already described in this chapter.

The chronic form of efferent loop syndrome is extremely rare and infrequently discussed. It may be combined or occasionally confused with chronic anastomotic stricture. Anastomotic strictures, although not considered bona fide postgastrectomy complications, now represent a major form of referral of overall postgastrectomy complications. These appear to occur in a similar proportion to the operations performed for peptic ulcer disease, namely, vagotomy and pyloroplasty, or Billroth I or Billroth II reconstruction. Most patients have subtly altered their diet depending upon the degree of relative obstruction. They seem to tolerate early satiety and occasional vomiting quite well as long as these changes occur slowly. Inter-

estingly, upper endoscopy often fails to diagnose this disorder since the endoscope passes through the anastomosis. It has been our experience, however, that a 1.0- to 1.5-cm opening in the presence of a denervated stomach may be inadequate to allow a normal dietary lifestyle over a period of time. Barium x-ray studies usually delineate the "relative" obstruction of the gastric outlet, especially when the patient's symptoms dictate an appropriate evaluation. Most patients have been treated with prokinetic agents, particularly when radionuclide tests of gastric emptying have documented gastroparesis. The difficulty for the clinician is in distinguishing chronic gastric atony from relative obstruction of the gastric outlet, especially when the anastomoses have strictured to a 1-cm diameter but still appear patent at endoscopy. In recent years, most gastroenterologists have performed frequent balloon dilatations with moderate success. The surgeon's experience is somewhat skewed since referrals are usually those patients in whom either medical or balloon dilatation therapy has failed.

Surgical Strategy

In patients with strictured anastomoses, the surgeon can choose between several strategic approaches. Revision of the previous strictured anastomosis is occasionally successful depending on the prior operation and type of reconstruction. Attempts at performing a "new" pyloro-

plasty or converting a standard pyloroplasty to Finney's procedure are often initially successful. In those patients with a strictured Billroth I anastomosis, reresection and reanastomosis depending on a safe length of proximal duodenum are usually successful. A strictured Billroth II gastroenterostomy can be revised using a unique GIA method if the placement of the prior gastroenterostomy is appropriate (Fig. 86-10). Two puncture wounds are placed in the stomach and one of the gastroenterostomy limbs for placement of the GIA stapling device, and a new anastomosis is performed either distally or proximally depending on prior placement of the anastomosis. In select cases, a "double-length" anastomosis can be performed by replacing the GIA device through the opening and performing a second anastomosis over the first.

The decision to perform a new reconstruction is based on a history of any prior postgastrectomy symptoms. In these cases, however, radionuclide tests for gastric emptying are not helpful since the basic problem is mechanical gastric outlet obstruction. A careful history, however, may document symptoms of gastroparesis in the early postoperative period or years before the stricture was evident. A history of bilious vomiting or burning abdominal pain may necessitate radionuclide scanning to document the presence of a large amount of bile refluxate in the stomach. Most patients with a strictured pyloro-

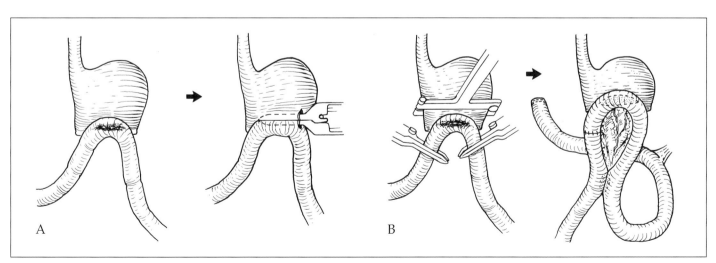

Fig. 86-10. A. Treatment of a strictured Billroth II anastomosis using the GIA stapling device. The GIA instrument is inserted into both the jejunum and the stomach through the strictured area performing a new anastomosis. B. Resection of a strictured Billroth II reconstruction with conversion to a new Billroth II gastroenterostomy with a downstream Braun enteroenterostomy at 20 to 25 cm from the gastroenterostomy.

plasty are usually converted to a Billroth I or Billroth II reconstruction. Our preferred method (as described) is the Billroth II reconstruction with a distal enteroenterostomy in an attempt to avoid future alkaline reflux gastritis. Either revision, however, is appropriate. A small but significant number of patients have been referred with both a prior strictured pyloroplasty (or Billroth I anastomosis) and a second attempt using a gastroenterostomy to bypass the obstructed gastric outlet. Since the tendency of the stomach is to "empty itself" toward the duodenum, symptoms in these patients usually continue. We have made every attempt to convert these patients to a Billroth II reconstruction, stapling off the strictured duodenum and removing the stomach up to the present gastroenterostomy if preoperative endoscopy demonstrated a patent opening. In most of these cases, however, a new anastomosis is performed following distal resection and takedown of the prior reconstruction.

Summary

The diagnosis and treatment of postgastrectomy syndromes have been and continue to be advanced by both experimental and clinical observations as well as technological improvements especially in nuclear imaging. It is interesting, however, that the descriptions and incidence of early and late postoperative food and bilious vomiting, well described in the late 1800s,

remain with us over 100 years later. Although Roux en Y biliary diversion has been and to a certain extent remains the standard surgical approach to postgastrectomy dumping, alkaline reflux gastritis, and, combined with subtotal to near-total resection, the treatment of post–Roux en Y gastroparesis, it is not without its well-described and well-documented difficulties. Emphasis at present, as described in this and other publications, has been and will continue to be development of alternative procedures to divert bile away from the stomach without altering upper gastrointestinal motility and electrical function. Our own emphasis has been toward a more normal gastrointestinal anastomosis combined with the described procedures to divert a significant amount of bile away from the stomach without necessarily transecting the jejunum. Whether this will endure will certainly depend on future studies and evaluation by other institutions and investigators.

Suggested Reading

Eagon JC, Miedema BW, Kelly KA. Postgastrectomy syndromes. *Surg Clin North Am* 445, 1992.

Herrington JL Jr. Remedial Operations for Postgastrectomy and Postvagotomy Syndromes. *In* JL Cameron (ed), *Current Surgical Therapy* (4th ed). St. Louis: Mosby–Year Book, 1992. Pp 86–97.

Hocking MP, Vogel SB, Wicklend E Jr (ed). *Woodward's Postgastrectomy Syndromes* (2nd ed). Philadelphia, Saunders, 1991.

Larson GM. In LM Nyhus (ed), *Problems in General Surgery. Alkaline Reflux Gastritis and Postoperative Gastric Stasis.* Philadelphia, Lippincott, 1993.

McQuarrie DG. Reoperations After Gastric Surgery. *In* DG McQuarrie, EW Humphrey (eds), *Reoperative General Surgery.* St. Louis: Mosby–Year Book, 1992. Pp 242–269.

Ritchie WP Jr, Dempsey DT. Postgastrectomy Syndromes. *In* FG Moody, LC Carey, RS Jones, et al (eds), *Surgical Treatment of Digestive Disease.* Chicago: Year Book, 1990. Pp 236–248.

Ritchie WP Jr, Perez AR. Studies of Gastric Emptying and Motility. *In* HW Scott Jr, JL Sawyers (eds), *Surgery of the Stomach, Duodenum, and Small Intestine.* Chicago: Blackwell, 1987. Pp 319–329.

Sawyers JL, Scott HW Jr. Postgastrectomy Sequelae and Remedial Operations. *In* HW Scott Jr, JL Sawyers (eds), *Surgery of the Stomach, Duodenum, and Small Intestine.* Chicago: Blackwell, 1987. Pp 767–776.

Vogel SB, Hocking MP. Disorders of Altered Gastrointestinal Motility. *In* DG McQuarrie, EW Humphrey (eds), *Reoperative General Surgery.* St. Louis: Mosby–Year Book, 1992. Pp 342–356.

Vogel SB, Hocking MP. Etiology and Treatment of the Roux Syndrome. *In* LM Nyhus (ed), *Problems in General Surgery. Alkaline Reflux Gastritis and Postoperative Gastric Stasis.* Philadelphia, Lippincott, 1993. Pp 308–320.

Vogel SB, Drano WE, Woodward ER. Clinical and radionuclide evaluation of bile diversion by Braun enteroenterostomy: Prevention and treatment of alkaline reflux gastritis. An alternative to Roux-en-Y diversion. *Ann Surg* 219:458, 1994.

87

The Dumping Syndrome and Postvagotomy Diarrhea

Irvin M. Modlin   Gary P. Lawton   Dennis G. Begos

The Dumping Syndrome

The dumping syndrome is a unique and paradoxical entity. Although it is quite common, particularly in its milder forms, it does not often present a major problem. It is frequently spoken of, yet hardly seen; easily recognized, but surprisingly difficult to define. Finally, it is a surgical problem that only rarely requires operation.

Given these contradictions, it is not surprising that reports of the incidence, symptoms, and treatment of the dumping syndrome vary widely, depending on the bias and practice patterns of individual physicians and institutions. The diverse array of symptomatology and disability referred to as the dumping syndrome is a broad spectrum of disease that reflects the vagaries of both the gastrointestinal physiology and hormonal milieu of different patients. In addition, it embraces a variety of individual symptomatic responses (both voluntary and involuntary) engendered by these differences.

Definition

Part of the problem in studying the dumping syndrome is related to the lack of a rigorous definition. Thus, it may be difficult to differentiate predictable alterations in gastric physiology and postcibal sensations consequent on surgery from serious and real disturbances in function associated with disabling symptomatology. Most authors agree that it is a syndrome

characterized by both vasomotor and gastrointestinal components. In general, the condition has been divided into early and late dumping syndromes. Vasomotor and cardiovascular signs and symptoms include flushing, tachycardia, lightheadedness, palpitations, diaphoresis, vertigo, blurry vision, and orthostatic hypotension. Gastrointestinal manifestations may include nausea and vomiting, crampy abdominal pain, diarrhea, bloating, and early satiety. These symptoms are generally initiated during a meal or within the first 5 to 45 minutes after eating, and usually resolve within an hour.

The "late dumping" syndrome predominantly exhibits vasomotor symptoms without significant gastrointestinal disturbance. Symptoms may also include mental confusion and impaired concentration, which occur 2 to 4 hours after a meal and last 10 to 20 minutes. A substantial component of the symptoms of late dumping may involve the consequences of reactive hypoglycemia.

Incidence

In general, the prevalence of this condition is significantly decreasing in concert with the substantial reduction in gastric surgery being undertaken for elective management of duodenal ulceration. The overall incidence of dumping syndrome is unclear, as might be predicted given the difficulty of generating a precise definition of the phenomenon. With rigorous questioning, most patients will report one or more of the symptoms described above after

gastric surgery. The severity and frequency of these symptoms, and the degree to which they incapacitate the patient, are important considerations in establishing a symptom complex consistent with deriving a diagnosis. Thus, reports concerning the frequency of dumping require cautious interpretation, lest institutional or author bias lead to under- or overreporting of symptoms. In the past, the Visick grading system was utilized to provide a clinical scale of objectivity in assessing postgastrectomy symptomatology.

What is clear is that the frequency of occurrence of the dumping syndrome is to a significant level correlated with the degree to which gastric emptying is accelerated. Therefore, more patients will experience dumping symptoms after vagotomy and antrectomy than after highly selective vagotomy, while patients with pyloroplasty may fall somewhere in between. While this is conceptually acceptable, it is not clear what causes one patient to have severe, incapacitating symptoms after a minimally disruptive procedure such as a highly selective vagotomy, while another patient may experience minimal symptomatology after a total gastrectomy. Another poorly understood factor that may variably accentuate or influence symptoms is the extent of the vagotomy. In general terms, it appears that a truncal vagotomy causes more severe symptoms than a less complete vagotomy, but this is not well established or always the case. Alterations in pancreatic, hepatic, and small-bowel neurohumoral responses are predictably accentuated after truncal vagotomy, and this may play a role in amplifying symptomatology.

It is generally accepted that up to 30 to 50 percent of patients will experience symptoms of dumping after truncal vagotomy and pyloroplasty, 20 to 35 percent after selective vagotomy and pyloroplasty, and 5 to 15 percent after more selective vagotomies that do not require a drainage procedure. An equal number of patients in this latter group will experience delay in gastric emptying. Of the patients who suffer symptoms of dumping, the vast majority obtain relief with relatively simple dietary or behavioral alterations such as eating small meals low in carbohydrates and abstaining from liquids during meals. Only 5 percent will have severe symptoms that are refractory to these manipulations and may require more intense dietary or pharmacologic management, or both. About 1 percent fail to benefit from such therapy. These patients develop a fear of food, lose weight, and are unable to lead normal, productive lives because of their malnutrition and associated sequelae. It is this small subgroup of patients who are candidates for surgical management of the dumping syndrome. In some circumstances, a previous history of behavioral or eating-habit disorders may be identifiable. Gastric surgery in such patients appears to amplify an underlying pathophysiologic problem.

A smaller percentage of patients experience the late dumping syndrome. Most studies report an incidence of fewer than 10 percent for this entity. Surgery is not indicated for the treatment of the late dumping syndrome. These patients may benefit from high-glucose snacks 1 to 2 hours after meals.

Pathophysiology

The pathophysiology underlying the signs and symptoms of the early dumping syndrome represents a complex interplay of variables. Mechanical factors include gastric emptying and bowel distention, while dietary factors such as the amount of carbohydrates in a meal and luminal osmolality appear to be of relevance. In addition, enteric and systemic neurohumoral responses modulate the evolution of a complex pattern of visceral and neural sensations that are often poorly accepted by patients. Meals that are hyperosmolar, liquid, and rich in carbohydrates comprise

potent stimuli capable of initiating dumping symptoms.

Gastric function encompasses mechanical digestion of food, as well as maintenance of acceptable osmolality and regulation of emptying (sieving) into the small bowel. In patients with dumping syndrome, these functions are impaired and hyperosmolar chyme is rapidly and prematurely emptied into the proximal small bowel. This event represents a principal component and is a primary inciting factor, leading to a cascade of compensatory physiologic responses that generate the symptomatology classifiable as the dumping syndrome. The hyperosmolar chyme draws extracellular fluid into the bowel lumen, resulting in bowel distention, hemoconcentration, electrolyte abnormalities, and intravascular volume depletion. These factors alone may account for a significant proportion of the early vasomotor and gastrointestinal symptoms.

A wide array of gastrointestinal neurohormonal regulatory peptides are also released. The precise stimulus for this is unclear, and the biologic significance of each hormone is not well understood. Peptides and hormones that have been documented to be elevated in patients experiencing dumping symptoms include neurotensin, glucagon, insulin, pancreatic polypeptide, bradykinin, vasoactive intestinal polypeptide, gastric inhibitory peptide, and serotonin. No single polypeptide has been identified as exhibiting a dominant role in engendering the symptoms of dumping. However, the inhibition of such peptide release by the use of somatostatin may result in significant amelioration of symptomatology.

There are many confounding variables that make this condition a difficult entity to study. It is not known whether these peptides act intraluminally, systemically, or in an autocrine or paracrine fashion. Most studies have measured systemic plasma levels of these agents, which may differ widely from their ambient concentrations in the gut itself. Finally, no appropriate animal model exists to study this phenomenon experimentally.

The late dumping syndrome for the most part comprises an exaggerated insulin response to oral glucose administration. Physiologically, it represents a disturbance in regulation of glucose homeostasis by destabilization of the enteroinsular axis.

Most patients exhibit early postprandial hyperglycemia with delayed hypoglycemia and its attendant symptoms. Response to intravenous insulin is generally normal, as are fasting glucose levels.

Diagnosis

A careful history will identify most individuals with dumping syndrome. In many, however, the symptoms will not be straightforward, or a variety of atypical or confounding symptoms will be present. Various diagnostic studies may be of use in identifying patients whose symptomatology is not overt.

Probably the most useful test is an attempt to reproduce the symptomatology in a clinical environment where the patient can be monitored. Provocative testing with a so-called dumping meal or, more simply, with a hyperosmolar glucose solution is utilized. The dumping meal is, in effect, a high-calorie stress test for the proximal gut. It comprises 700 to 1000 calories, with about 50 percent from carbohydrates and 30 to 40 percent from fat. Alternatively, 250 to 500 ml of a 25% glucose solution can be used. Patients are monitored at 15-minute intervals for at least 2 hours. Vital signs are recorded frequently to detect changes in pulse, respiration, and blood pressure, with special attention to orthostatic changes occurring early after the meal. Serum samples of glucose and potassium as well as the hematocrit should be obtained before the meal and at 10- to 15-minute intervals thereafter. Measuring peptide levels is expensive and labor intensive, and should probably be undertaken only in a research setting. In general, the serum glucose and hematocrit are elevated, while the serum potassium is low in the first 10 to 30 minutes following the meal. Late dumping can be detected by measuring the serum glucose during the symptomatic period.

Another supportive test is the scintigraphic analysis of gastric emptying. Sophisticated nuclear medicine techniques can be utilized to define differential rates of gastric emptying using double-labeled liquid and solid meals. Solids are labeled with technetium-99m colloid, while liquids are labeled with indium-111 diethylenetriamine pentaacetic acid (DTPA). Gamma camera scintigraphic imaging is then performed, using different windows for the two isotopes to simultaneously determine the rates of solid and liquid meal emptying. Patients with dumping syndrome typically exhibit accelerated emptying of both solids and liquids (without discrimination) with a half-emptying time of 10 to 20 minutes. Healthy control subjects exhibit more rapid emptying of liquids as compared to solids, with half-emptying times of 50 minutes for liquids and 2 hours for solids.

Treatment

Management of symptoms of the dumping syndrome fall into three successively more intense regimens: behavior and dietary modification, pharmacologic manipulation, and surgical management.

Behavior/Dietary Management

Many patients who experience dumping symptoms will themselves identify the appropriate basic dietary modifications necessary for relief, and thus never come to medical attention. Eating small meals that are low in carbohydrates and strict abstinence from liquids during meals are the cornerstones of dietary management. Liquids should be hypotonic, calorie free, at room temperature, and taken 30 to 40 minutes before or after solid food. Avoiding salt may also be of some benefit. Other dietary adjuncts include addition of pectin or fiber to food to slow gastric emptying. Lying down after meals may often help alleviate symptoms. Patients with late dumping may benefit from high-glucose snacks taken 1 to 2 hours after large meals, which may effectively blunt the hypoglycemic episodes. Using these relatively simple techniques, the majority of patients with dumping syndrome may either be relieved of symptoms or become symptom free.

Pharmacologic Management

Multiple pharmacologic agents have been evaluated in an attempt to control or modify dumping symptoms. In principle, these agents are intended to either slow gut motility or provide symptomatic relief. For the most part, the utility of such agents has been circumvented by the introduction and availability of the long-acting somatostatin analog, octreotide. Somatostatin is a potent, naturally occurring inhibitor of virtually every known gastrointestinal polypeptide. Studies undertaken in the mid-1980s in patients with the dumping syndrome revealed it to be effective in minimizing symptoms. Somatostatin, however, has a short half-life, requires continuous intravenous infusion, and thus has limited clinical utility. The development of octreotide obviated the problems of bioavailability.

Several blinded and randomized studies of modest size have reported a remarkable benefit of octreotide in 70 to 90 percent of patients with both early and late dumping symptoms. Patients generally require 50 to 100 μg octreotide subcutaneously twice a day, 15 to 60 minutes before meals. The precise dosage may need to be titrated for each patient. Octreotide acts by inhibiting neurohormonal release and consequently downmodulates bowel motility, nutrient absorption, and luminal secretion. Its wide variety of inhibitory effects provide amelioration of symptoms and account for its effectiveness in the management of the dumping syndrome.

Short-term side effects of octreotide may include diarrhea and steatorrhea (possibly due to a degree of malabsorption consequent on inhibition of pancreatic exocrine secretion), nausea, and intermittent abdominal pain. Potential problems with long-term use include gallstone formation in approximately 25 percent of patients secondary to cholestasis. The incidence of cholelithiasis may be accentuated by vagotomy, and cholecystectomy may be necessary if symptoms supervene. Occasionally, hyperglycemia or hypoglycemia due to perturbation of the insulin/glucagon axis is encountered, but it is rarely clinically significant. Pancreatic exocrine enzyme replacement may be necessary in some patients with severe malabsorption.

Surgery

Surgery for early dumping syndrome is indicated after failure of significant and consistent medical therapy in the fully compliant patient. Persistent malnutrition and weight loss are indications of the seriousness of the situation. Before consideration of a patient for surgical revision, a careful and thorough evaluation should be undertaken. This includes exhausting dietary and pharmacologic avenues, and should entail admission to the hospital for a period of supervised adherence to these regimens. Psychosocial evaluation may be necessary in certain patients. Since this is an elective procedure, a full assessment of the patient's perioperative cardiorespiratory risk factors is necessary. Patients who require operative treatment may be malnourished, and preoperative nutritional support (parenterally or enterally) may be necessary.

The operative strategy for treating intractable dumping symptoms embraces two primary principles: 1) restoring the gastric reservoir, or 2) delaying transit of chyme from the stomach into the small bowel, or both. A multitude of procedures have been promulgated over the years. Most have met with only limited success. The procedures that have been proposed can be divided into three main groups.

Reconfiguration of the Anastomosis. Attempts to narrow the gastroduodenal or gastrojejunal anastomosis or the pyloroplasty have met with only marginal success. The inability to precisely define the outlet size and the potential danger of initiating gastric outlet obstruction are significant drawbacks. In addition, the possibility that the revised anastomosis will eventually dilate over time makes this a poor choice of operation. The pylorus represents a complex sieving mechanism capable of monitoring particle size and osmolality in the precise regulation of chyme delivery into the proximal gut. These simplistic attempts at gauging orifice size have predictably been of little benefit.

The conversion of a gastrojejunostomy to a gastroduodenostomy is theoretically attractive since it facilitates modulation of the osmolality of the chyme by the duodenum. However, it ignores the observation that dumping occurs nearly as frequently in patients with Billroth I as with Billroth II reconstructions.

Creation of a Pouch. There are numerous examples of eponymous jejunal pouches that are technically complex and represent a surgical tour de force. While these are often effective in the short term, long-term results have been disappointing due to pouch dilatation and stasis. In addition, they lack coordinated motility-pacemaker activity and do not exhibit the phenomenon of receptive relaxation. Hence stasis, distention, and ulceration supervene.

A double-limb jejunal pouch was described by Poth in which an isoperistaltic jejunal limb (10–12 cm in length) is sutured to the gastric remnant (inlet) and an antiperistaltic jejunal limb (10-12 cm in length) is sutured to the duodenum (outlet). The two limbs are subsequently converted into a pouch (Fig. 87-1). This technique has been used with moderate success (40–50%), but can be complicated by pouch ulcers, stasis, and obstruction.

The Hays pouch (a triple-plicated loop of jejunum) has been employed between the gastric remnant and the duodenum, or in combination with a Roux en Y reconstruction (Fig. 87-2). Such pouches have had some degree of initial success, but the benefit is not durable and the procedures are often complicated by dilatation and stasis.

Interposed Segments. A number of procedures have been described that utilize interposed segments of small or large bowel placed between the stomach and duodenum in order to slow gastric emptying. Initial proposals utilized an isoperistaltic loop of jejunum (20–25 cm) placed

between the gastric remnant and the duodenum (Henley loop). Results have been modest, with most series reporting only 10 to 40 percent success rates. Likewise, antiperistaltic colon interposition has not yielded consistent improvement in dumping symptoms and is associated with ulceration of the interposed segment, vomiting, and bloating.

Recommended Surgical Techniques

The three currently recommended techniques are 1) Roux en Y gastrojejunostomy, 2) antiperistaltic jejunal transfer, and 3) Roux en Y gastrojejunostomy with antiperistaltic jejunal transfer.

Roux en Y Gastrojejunostomy. Roux en Y gastrojejunostomy (Fig. 87-3) was noted to result in delayed gastric emptying in patients who underwent resection for gastric cancer. This procedure has there-

fore been utilized with low failure rates (5–10%) in the treatment of patients with early dumping syndrome. Its effectiveness may reflect the chyme bypassing the pacemaker for the migrating myoelectric complexes in the duodenum and proximal jejunum, thus abrogating excessive motility. This operation must be combined with vagotomy and antrectomy to prevent ulceration of the jejunal Roux limb. An alternative to this added procedure may be long-term modulation of acid secretion by proton pump inhibition. However, the consequences of sustained pharmacotherapy are not yet clearly defined.

Antiperistaltic Jejunal Transfer. Interposition of an antiperistaltic limb of jejunum (8–10 cm) between the gastric remnant and the duodenum has resulted in consistent improvement of the early dumping syndrome (Fig. 87-4). Vagotomy (selective or truncal) must also be per-

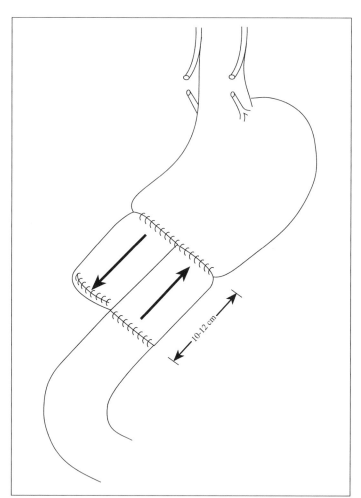

Fig. 87-1. The double-limb jejunal Poth pouch with an isoperistaltic inlet and an antiperistaltic outlet.

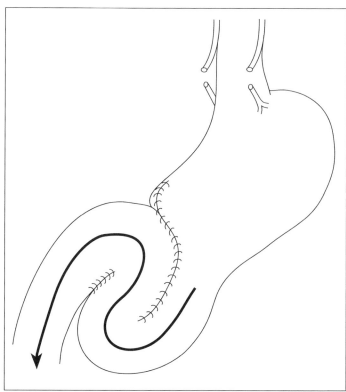

Fig. 87-2. The triple-plication technique utilized to construct the jejunal Hays pouch.

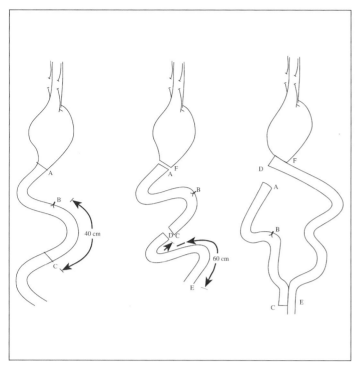

Fig. 87-3. Roux en Y gastrojejunostomy. Left. The jejunum is divided at point C, 40 cm from the ligament of Treitz (B). Middle. A 60-cm Roux limb (D) is created. Right. The transected jejunum (C) is anastomosed at point E, re-establishing continuity of the jejunum. The Roux limb (D) is anastomosed to the gastric remnant (F). The duodenal stump (A) is oversewn.

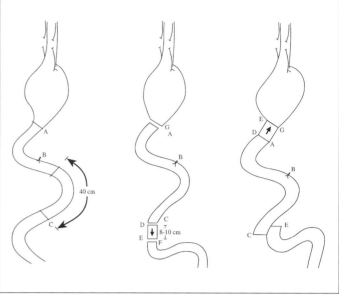

Fig. 87-4. Interposition of an antiperistaltic limb of jejunum (8–10 cm) between the gastric remnant and the duodenum. Left. The jejunal segment is harvested at point C, 40 cm distal to the ligament of Treitz (B). Middle. The duodenal stump (A) is separated from the gastric remnant (G). The proximal end of the jejunal segment (D) is isolated from the proximal jejunal stump (C). The distal end of the jejunal segment (E) is isolated from the distal jejunal stump (F). Right. The isolated jejunal segment is passed through a window in the transverse mesocolon, and rotated counterclockwise 180 degrees on its vascular pedicle. The distal end of the jejunal segment (E) is anastomosed to the gastric remnant (G). The proximal end of the jejunal segment (D) is anastomosed to the duodenum (A). Continuity of the jejunum is then re-established by anastomosing the proximal (C) and distal (F) jejunal stumps.

formed in order to prevent ulceration of the segment of jejunum. Success rates with this procedure range from 70 to 80 percent. Complications include bile reflux, ulceration of the interposed segment, and obstruction at the anastomosis from stricture.

Roux en Y Gastrojejunostomy with Antiperistaltic Jejunal Transfer.
The combination of Roux en Y gastrojejunostomy with an antiperistaltic jejunal transfer between the gastric remnant and the Roux en Y limb (Kennedy operation) has also been shown to be effective (up to 80%) (Fig. 87-5).

Surgical Techniques

Conversion of Billroth I or II Reconstruction to Roux en Y Gastrojejunostomy
For conversion of a previous Billroth I reconstruction after gastric resection to Roux en Y gastrojejunostomy, the anastomosis is taken down and the duodenal stump closed (see Fig. 87-3). Kocher's incision lateral to the duodenum may facilitate mobilization of the anastomosis. Any remaining antrum is resected with the anastomosis. A Dennis clamp is placed proximal to the anastomosis along the greater curvature for a distance of 4 cm. A second clamp is placed distal to the anastomosis across the duodenum. Using the electrocautery, the gastric remnant is divided distal to the first clamp starting from the greater curvature. An additional Dennis clamp is then placed from the tip of the first clamp on the gastric remnant to the lesser curvature. The anastomosis is then resected between the second clamp on the gastric remnant and the clamp on the duodenum using the electrocautery. The lesser curvature portion of the gastric remnant is closed using continuous 3-0 chromic catgut and then an external row of 3-0 Lembert sutures (Hofmeister reconstruction). The Dennis clamp is retained on the greater curvature portion of the gastric remnant for anastomosis to the Roux limb

of jejunum. The duodenal stump is closed with continuous 3-0 chromic catgut followed by interrupted seromuscular 3-0 silk sutures placed from the posterior to anterior walls.

For conversion of a Billroth II reconstruction to a Roux en Y gastrojejunostomy, the anastomosis is resected with the corresponding loop of jejunum. The procedure at the gastric aspect of the anastomosis is the same as described above. Continuity of the proximal jejunum is then restored utilizing a side-to-side technique and an anastomotic stapling device.

After the Billroth I or II anastomosis is taken down, the jejunum is divided using electrocautery 40 cm distal to the ligament of Treitz between a transecting stapler and a Dennis clamp (Fig. 87-6A). Thereafter, the mesentery of the jejunum is divided between clamps using 3-0 silk ties to mobilize the distal segment. The distal segment is closed with interrupted 3-0 silk sutures. Then, the proximal jejunal stump is

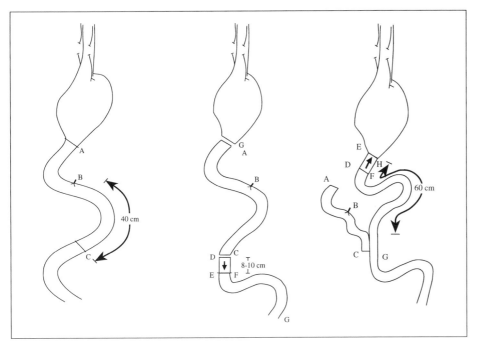

Fig. 87-5. The Roux en Y gastrojejunostomy is combined with the antiperistaltic jejunal transfer (Kennedy operation). Left. The jejunum is transected at point C, 40 cm distal to the ligament of Treitz (B). Middle. The duodenum (A) is separated from the gastric remnant (H). The Roux limb (D) is passed through a window in the transverse mesocolon. An 8- to 10-cm segment of the Roux limb is then isolated by transecting the jejunum at point F. Right. The isolated jejunal segment is then rotated counterclockwise 180 degrees on its vascular pedicle. The distal end of the jejunal segment (E) is anastomosed to the gastric remnant (H). The proximal end of the jejunal segment (D) is anastomosed to the jejunum (F). The duodenal stump (A) is oversewn. Continuity of the jejunum is re-established by anastomosing the proximal jejunal stump (C) to point G.

opposed in a side-to-side fashion along the antimesenteric border of the distal jejunum (60 cm from the distal jejunal stump) (Fig. 87-6B). Two silk stay sutures (3-0) are placed 10 cm apart. The electrocautery is used to enter the two jejunal segments at the proximal stay suture. A stapling device is then introduced through the two enterotomies. After creation of the anastomosis, any bleeding along the suture line can be controlled with 4-0 silk sutures. The enterotomy through which the stapler was removed is closed perpendicular to the long axis of the jejunal anastomosis with interrupted 3-0 silk sutures. The jejunal Roux loop is then approximated to the gastric remnant in a retrocolic fashion using two Allis clamps.

A semiclosed technique is then used to create an end-to-side gastrojejunostomy. The distal jejunal segment at the anastomosis should not be larger than 2 to 3 cm to obviate the formation of a blind loop. The clamps on the gastric remnant and the jejunum are approximated and 3-0 silk stay sutures are placed at the lateral extents of

the proposed anastomosis. A posterior row of interrupted 3-0 silk seromuscular sutures is placed, and then tied. The clamps are removed. Starting from the midpoint of the back wall of the anastomosis, 3-0 chromic catgut is used to create a running closure. The anastomosis is performed in halves, and the catgut tied at the midpoint of the anterior wall. Thereafter, the anterior row of interrupted 3-0 seromuscular sutures is placed and tied. To protect the anastomosis, a 3-0 silk suture is placed between the gastrojejunostomy and the closure of the gastric remnant.

A vagotomy must accompany the Roux en Y reconstruction. This should be undertaken before the resection and anastomosis to decrease the possibility of contaminating the subphrenic spaces.

Antiperistaltic Jejunal Transfer

The interposed jejunal limb should be 8 to 10 cm in length (see Fig. 87-4). Longer segments are prone to ulceration and may cause gastric outlet obstruction, while shorter segments are ineffective in pre-

venting dumping. Patients who have not previously undergone vagotomy and antrectomy should have these performed to decrease acid secretion and prevent ulceration of the jejunal segment. A truncal vagotomy, as some have advocated, is not necessary if the surgeon has experience with selective vagotomy. This may diminish the possibility of initiating further confounding postvagotomy symptoms.

The above-described techniques are used to take down the Billroth I anastomosis. However, the duodenal stump is not closed. In the case of a previous Billroth II anastomosis, the anastomosis is taken down, as described above, and the continuity of the proximal jejunum is restored. The duodenal stump is then mobilized using a lateral Kocher's incision. A Dennis clamp is thereafter placed across the duodenum and the previous stump closure is resected using the electrocautery. Caution should be exercised in identifying the common bile duct and the superior aspect of the pancreas.

The 8- to 10-cm jejunal segment necessary for the interposition is then harvested 40 cm distal to the ligament of Treitz between staplers and Dennis clamps (Fig. 87-7). The segment is maximally mobilized on its vascular pedicle to facilitate tension-free apposition to the gastric remnant. Continuity of the distal jejunum is restored in side-to-side fashion using an anastomotic stapling device. The defect in the mesentery of the reanastomosed jejunum is closed with interrupted 4-0 silk sutures.

An opening is then created in the transverse mesocolon, taking particular care to avoid injury to the vascular arcade. Next, the segment of harvested jejunum is approximated in a retrocolic fashion to the gastric remnant. Once the defect in the transverse mesocolon has been negotiated, the jejunal loop is rotated 180 degrees in a counterclockwise fashion to minimize venous congestion and torsion. The segment is thus placed in an antiperistaltic orientation. An end-to-end two-layer jejunoduodenostomy is then created with 3-0 chromic gut and 3-0 silk suture using the semiclosed anastomotic technique described previously for the creation of the gastrojejunostomy. Thereafter, a gastrojejunostomy is similarly created utilizing the distal component of the interposed segment. Once the anastomoses are complete, the defect in the mesocolon is tacked to the

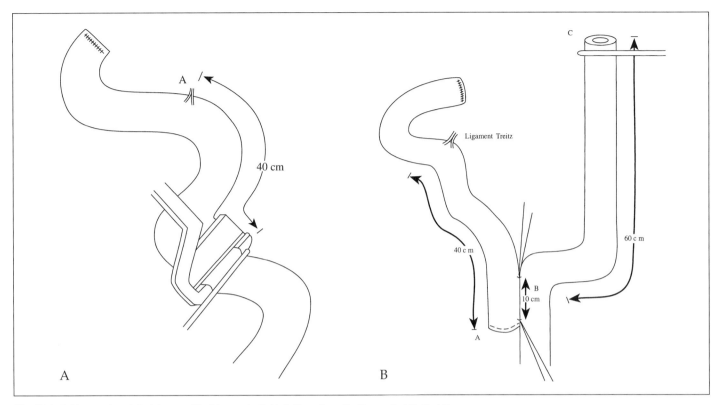

Fig. 87-6. A. Transection of the jejunum. The jejunum is divided 40 cm from the ligament of Treitz (A) between a transecting stapler and a Dennis clamp. B. Re-establishing continuity of the jejunum. The proximal jejunal stump (A) is opposed in side-to-side fashion along the antimesenteric border (B) of the distal jejunum 60 cm from the distal jejunal stump (C). Silk stay sutures are placed 10 cm apart. Continuity is re-established using an anastomotic stapling device.

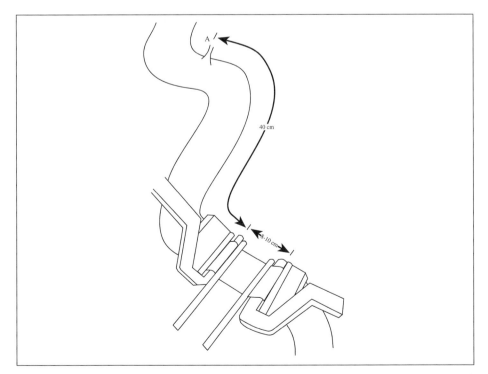

Fig. 87-7. Isolation of the jejunal segment. An 8- to 10-cm jejunal segment for the interposition is harvested 40 cm distal to the ligament of Treitz (A) between staplers and Dennis clamps.

jejunal segment using 4-0 silk suture in order to obviate its displacement and consequent strangulation of the blood supply of the segment. The interposed segment should be carefully observed at the conclusion of the procedure to confirm adequate vascular perfusion and viability.

Combined Antiperistaltic Jejunal Transfer and Roux en Y Gastrojejunostomy (see Fig. 87-5)

First, the previous anastomosis is taken down as described previously. Then, the jejunum is transected 40 cm distal to the ligament of Treitz, as described for the creation of the Roux en Y reconstruction (see Fig. 87-6A). The continuity of the distal jejunum is re-established as previously described (see Fig. 87-6B). Then, the Roux loop is brought through the window in the transverse mesocolon. The proximal 8- to 10-cm segment of the Roux loop is then separated (as above) and rotated 180 degrees in a counterclockwise fashion. Next, the antiperistaltic segment is anastomosed to the gastric remnant, as previously described. An end-to-end jejunal anastomosis is then created using 3-0 chromic catgut and 3-0 silk suture, and the semiclosed technique described previously.

Postvagotomy Diarrhea

Definition

A considerable number of patients will exhibit an alteration in bowel habits following vagotomy. As with the dumping syndrome, the frequency of postvagotomy diarrhea varies depending on the definition of diarrhea. After truncal vagotomy the majority of patients will report occasional loose stools, although only a small minority (<5%) experience incapacitating diarrhea. These individuals may undergo over 20 loose bowel movements per day, and often experience incontinence. There seems to be a markedly lower incidence of diarrhea after selective vagotomy.

Pathophysiology

Numerous mechanisms have been proposed to account for the phenomenon of postvagotomy diarrhea. A number of theories have implicated gastric stasis and a low acid state with consequent bacterial overgrowth and excessive mucosal secretion. The diarrhea does not appear to be related to the type of gastrointestinal reconstruction, but rather to the extent of vagotomy. An alternative possibility is that denervation of the proximal gut interferes with the gastric or duodenal pacemaker, resulting in dysregulation of motility and consequently altered absorption and diarrhea. An increased incidence of postvagotomy diarrhea in patients with cholecystectomy has been suggested as evidence for impaired bile salt absorption in the genesis of this condition.

Diagnosis

Since bowel habits vary widely, diarrhea must be evaluated in the context of the degree of change from the patient's normal pattern. The frequency, volume, and characteristics of the stool, as well as the presence of incontinence, may be useful in the determination of the etiology of the diarrhea. The most common etiology of acute-onset diarrhea is infection, which is often associated with fever, vomiting, malaise, and myalgia. Stool smears and cultures may be useful in the establishment of this diagnosis. Bloody stools, abdominal cramping, tenderness, and fever may indicate ulcerative colitis or Crohn's disease. In addition, diarrhea may accompany the use of a variety of drugs. Conservative treatment is employed first, with further workup including sigmoidoscopy and biopsy initiated in those patients who do not exhibit resolution in one week. A number of features can be used to distinguish postvagotomy diarrhea. These include the explosive onset of up to 20 watery stools per day, the lack of a relationship to meals, occurrence at any time of the day (even during sleep), fecal incontinence, and the absence of associated fever or myalgia. In the evaluation of patients with suspected postvagotomy diarrhea, it is important to consider obscure neuroendocrine tumors of the gut as a possible etiology that may have contributed to symptoms that initiated the original operation. In patients who have refractory symptoms, especially those who had loose stools before vagotomy, [^{111}In-DTPA-D-Phe]-octreotide scintigraphy may detect these otherwise occult tumors.

Treatment

Conservative Management

Management of such patients is initially conservative, since many will improve substantially within 6 to 12 months after the initial procedure. Eliminating agents that are known to promote diarrhea, such as magnesium-containing antacids and caffeine, may also be helpful. Similarly, evaluation of dietary intake utilizing a diary may serve to identify specific foods capable of provoking episodes of diarrhea. Medical therapy may include oral antibiotics such as neomycin or tetracycline. Erythromycin should be avoided because of its enhancement of gastrointestinal motility via activation of motilin receptors. Bulking agents such as cholestyramine or psyllium may help increase intestinal transit time and thus decrease total stool water. Antidiarrheals such as kaolin and opiates play a role in treating symptom exacerbations, but should not be used for long-term therapy. Octreotide does not appear to provide major relief to patients with postvagotomy diarrhea.

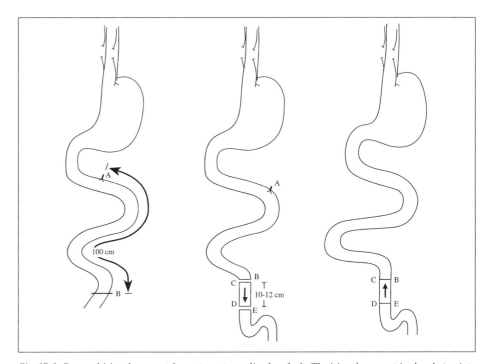

Fig. 87-8. *Reversed jejunal segment for postvagotomy diarrhea.* Left. *The jejunal segment is placed at point B, 100 cm from the ligament of Treitz (A).* Middle. *The proximal end of the 10- to 12-cm segment of jejunum (C) is isolated from the proximal jejunum (B). The distal end of the jejunal segment (D) is isolated from the distal jejunum (E).* Right. *The isolated jejunal segment is then rotated counterclockwise 180 degrees on its vascular pedicle. The distal end of the jejunal segment (D) is anastomosed to the proximal jejunum (B). The proximal end of the jejunal segment (C) is anastomosed to the distal jejunum (E), placing the segment in an antiperistaltic position.*

Surgical Management

Surgical management of postvagotomy diarrhea should be limited to those patients with severely disabling symptoms refractory to medical therapy and in whom all other causes of diarrhea have been eliminated. The primary consideration in the surgical treatment for this syndrome is the reversed jejunal segment. A 10- to 15-cm segment of jejunum 100 cm from the Treitz ligament is utilized. Longer lengths of jejunum may cause excessive stasis or obstructive symptoms. Shorter lengths will not work. The reversed length is placed 100 cm distal to the Treitz ligament. Interposition at shorter or longer distances has been shown to be ineffective. The rationale for this approach is twofold. First, gastrointestinal transit time is increased, thus facilitating increased absorption. Second, the antiperistaltic segment may increase mixing, which may facilitate more complete digestion.

This procedure will not alleviate the symptoms of the dumping syndrome. There are patients who may experience both dumping symptoms and severe postvagotomy diarrhea. In rare situations, it may be appropriate to perform both an antidumping procedure and an antidiarrheal one, provided that the clinical indications are sound. It may be prudent to manage the dumping syndrome before intervening in the postvagotomy problem. More commonly, an initial operation to reverse the dumping syndrome will result in significant amelioration of the diarrheal component of the problem. It is thus inadvisable to perform both procedures simultaneously.

Surgical Technique

The only operation that has been shown to be effective in the reduction of postvagotomy diarrhea is reversal of a 10- to 12-cm jejunal segment 100 cm from the ligament of Treitz (Fig. 87-8). The procedure is similar to that used for the creation of the reversed jejunal segment for the dumping syndrome. A 10- to 12-cm segment of jejunum located 100 cm from the Treitz ligament is harvested between Dennis clamps using electrocautery. The segment is then rotated counterclockwise 180 degrees and anastomosed to the proximal and distal jejunum in end-to-end fashion, utilizing a two-layer closure with 3-0 chromic gut and 3-0 silk suture. Care should be taken to confirm the intestinal viability at the completion of the anastomotic procedures.

Suggested Reading

Carvajal SH, Mulvihill SJ. Postgastrectomy syndromes: Dumping and diarrhea. *Gastroenterol Clin North Am* 23:261, 1994.

Eagon JC, Miedema BW, Kelly KA. Postgastrectomy syndromes. *Surg Clin North Am* 72:445, 1992.

Herrington JL Jr, Edwards WH, Carter JH. Treatment of severe postgastrectomy diarrhea by reversed jejunal segment. *Ann Surg* 168:522, 1973.

Jian R, Lemann M, Flourie B, et al. Clinical relevance of scintigraphic measurement of gastric emptying of a solid-liquid meal in the dumping syndrome. *Hepatogastroenterology* 39:17, 1992.

Kelly KA, Morrison PD. Gastrointestinal Motility Disorders: Pathogenesis, Therapy, and Prevention. In JL Sawyers, LF Williams (eds), *Difficult Problems in General Surgery*. Chicago: Year Book, 1989. Pp 99–116.

Khoshoo V, Reifen RM, Gold BD, et al. Nutritional manipulation in the management of dumping syndrome. *Arch Dis Child* 66:1447, 1991.

Lamers CBHW, Bijlstra AM, Harris AG. Octreotide, a long-acting somatostatin analog, in the management of postoperative dumping syndrome. *Dig Dis Sci* 38:359, 1993.

Lawaetz O, Blackburn AM, Bloom SR, et al. Gut hormone profile and gastric emptying in the dumping syndrome. *Scand J Gastroenterol* 18:73, 1983.

Mackie CR, Jenkins SA, Hartley MN. Treatment of severe postvagotomy/postgastrectomy symptoms with the somatostatin analogue octreotide. *Br J Surg* 78:1338, 1991.

Miedema BW, Kelly KA. The Roux operation for post-gastrectomy syndromes. *Am J Surg* 161:256, 1991.

Miranda R, Steffes B, O'Leary JP, Woodward ER. Surgical treatment of postgastrectomy dumping syndrome. *Am J Surg* 139:40, 1980.

Ramus NI, Williamson RCN. The use of jejunal interposition for intractable symptoms complicating peptic ulcer surgery. *Br J Surg* 69:265, 1982.

Reber HA, Way LW. Surgical treatment of late postgastrectomy syndromes. *Am J Surg* 129:71, 1975.

Sawyers JL. Management of postgastrectomy syndromes. *Am J Surg* 159:8, 1990.

Tytgat GNJ, Offerhaus GJA, Mulder CJJ, van der Berg BT. Consequences of gastric surgery for benign conditions. *Hepatogastroenterology* 35:271, 1988.

88

Gastric Surgery for Morbid Obesity

Harvey J. Sugerman   Eric J. DeMaria

Definition of Morbid Obesity

Obese persons are classified as "morbidly obese" by the arbitrary definition of being more than 100 lb above the ideal body weight (IBW) defined actuarially by the Metropolitan Life Insurance Company 1983 height/weight tables. In order to account for differences in body habitus, patients are classified into small, medium, and large body frame subgroups based on anthropometric assessment. Alternative definitions of morbid obesity include patients who weigh at least 200 percent of their calculated IBW. The most accurate method for the relationship of body weight to frame size is the body mass index (BMI), which is the patient's weight in kilograms divided by the patient's height in meters squared. Obesity is defined as a BMI of more than 30 kg/m^2. A 1991 National Institutes of Health (NIH) Consensus Panel on Gastric Surgery for Severe Obesity concluded that it would be preferable to refer to the problem as clinically severe obesity, rather than using the pejorative term *morbid*, and that the weight for this criterion be a BMI of 35 kg/m^2 or greater with severe obesity comorbidity or 40 kg/m^2 or greater without comorbidity. For an average adult male, a BMI of 40 kg/m^2 is roughly equal to 100 lb over IBW.

Obesity and Disease

Obesity is a significant risk factor that adversely influences the outcome of patients hospitalized for virtually any acute medical illness as well as for those undergoing both elective and emergency surgery, es-pecially for abdominal diseases. Obese patients similarly suffer a significant increased risk of complications and death following relatively minor traumatic injury.

For decades, obese patients have been advised to delay elective surgical intervention until they were able to lose enough weight to decrease perioperative risk. Given the low overall success rate for diet and exercise in producing adequate weight loss in patients with severe obesity, few patients ever "qualified" for an elective treatment, whereas many were converted into an urgent operative intervention for a complication that could have been avoided had elective intervention been deemed safe. An example is the repair of abdominal wall and groin hernias in the obese patient. Since obesity is known to dramatically increase the recurrence risk following elective hernia repair, delay pending satisfactory weight loss may ultimately lead to emergent intervention for incarceration or bowel strangulation.

Severe obesity is associated with a large number of related problems, giving rise to the term *morbid obesity*. Several of these problems are underlying causes for the earlier mortality associated with obesity and include coronary artery disease, hypertension, impaired cardiac function, adult-onset diabetes mellitus, obesity hypoventilation and sleep apnea syndromes, venous stasis and hypercoagulability leading to an increased risk of pulmonary embolism, and necrotizing panniculitis. Morbidly obese patients can also die as a result of difficulties in recognizing the signs and symptoms of peritonitis. They have an increased risk of uterine, breast, and colon cancer. Overall, premature death is much more common in the severely obese individual. There is a 12-fold greater mortality for morbidly obese men as compared to nonobese men in the 25- to 34-year age group.

A number of obesity-related problems may not be associated with death but can lead to significant physical or psychological disability. These include degenerative osteoarthritis, pseudotumor cerebri (idiopathic intracranial hypertension), cholecystitis, skin infections, chronic venous stasis ulcers, stress overflow urinary incontinence, gastroesophageal reflux, sex hormone imbalance with dysmenorrhea, hirsutism, infertility, the nephrotic syndrome, and idiopathic cirrhosis. Many morbidly obese patients suffer from severe psychological and social disability, including a marked prejudice against them regarding employment.

Dietary Treatment

There are a tremendous number and variety of dietary programs for weight reduction, which include hospital-supervised programs, psychiatric behavioral modification programs, commercial organizations, commercial diets, protein-sparing fast programs, and diet pills. Although weight loss programs provide a multimillion dollar industry in the United States, no dietary approach has achieved uniform long-term success for the morbidly obese. Many individuals can lose weight successfully through dietary manipulation, but the incidence of recidivism in the morbidly obese approaches 95 percent. A National Institutes of Health Consensus Conference in 1992 concluded that dietary weight reduction with or without behavioral modification or drug therapy had an unacceptably high incidence of weight regain in the morbidly obese within 2 years after maximal weight loss.

Surgical Treatment
History:
The Jejunoileal Bypass

The first popular surgical procedure for morbid obesity was the jejunoileal bypass. This operation produced an obligatory malabsorptive state through bypass of a major portion of the absorptive surface of the small intestine. The procedure connected a short length of proximal jejunum (8–14 in.) to the distal ileum (4–12 in.) as an end-to-end or end-to-side anastomosis. The end-to-end procedures were associated with a better weight loss but required decompression of the bypassed small intestine into the colon. The jejunoileal bypass was associated with a number of early and late complications. The most serious postoperative complication was cirrhosis, due to either protein-calorie malnutrition and/or to absorption of endotoxin from bacterial overgrowth in the bypassed intestine, a clinical example of bacterial translocation. A rheumatoid-like arthritis also occurred as a result of absorption of bacterial products from the bypassed intestine; antigen-antibody complexes to bacterial antigens were found in the joint fluid of affected individuals. Rapid weight loss, as well as malabsorption of bile salts, increased the risk of cholelithiasis as a result of the decrease in cholesterol solubility. Hypocalcemia was frequent due to chelation of calcium with bile salts and fat, leading to severe osteoporosis. Multiple kidney stones developed as a result of increased oxalate absorption from the colon. Intractable, malodorous diarrhea with associated potassium and magnesium depletion, metabolic acidosis, and severe malnutrition were common, as was vitamin B_{12} deficiency. Bacterial overgrowth in the bypassed intestine also led to vitamin K deficiency, interstitial nephritis with renal failure, pneumatosis intestinalis, and bypass enteritis associated with occult blood in the stools and iron-deficiency anemia. Many of these problems, which are associated with bacterial overgrowth in the bypassed intestine, can be treated with metronidazole.

Some physicians believe that all jejunoileal bypass procedures should be reversed since cirrhosis may develop insidiously in the absence of abnormal liver function tests. Most believe that medical therapy should be tried first. If the medical problems are severe and do not respond to metronidazole, or progressive liver and/or renal dysfunction occurs, the jejunoileal bypass can be reversed. However, if reversed, these patients will invariably regain their lost weight; therefore, conversion to a gastric procedure for obesity should be considered unless the patient is too ill, for example, the patient with severe cirrhosis with portal hypertension. Randomized, prospective studies have shown that the gastric bypass operation is associated with a comparable weight loss and a significantly lower complication rate than jejunoileal bypass. Because of the significant complication rate, the jejunoileal bypass should no longer be performed.

Development of Gastric Bypass and Gastroplasty

In 1966, Mason and Ito reported the results of weight loss using a gastric bypass (GBP) with division of the stomach into a small upper pouch connected to a loop gastroenterostomy. The concept for this procedure was based upon the observation of weight loss that often followed subtotal gastrectomy for duodenal ulcer disease. There was concern that peptic ulcers would develop in the bypassed stomach or duodenum; although these have occurred, the incidence is very low. Serum gastrin levels and acid secretion from the bypassed stomach are low. The technique for GBP was simplified with the use of stapling instruments. The concept of gastroplasty was then proposed as a safer, easier method for restricting food intake. In gastroplasty, the stomach is only stapled, leaving a small opening to permit the normal passage of food into the distal stomach and duodenum.

Surgical Eligibility

Patients are considered eligible for surgery by most insurance companies if they weigh 100 lb or more than the 1983 Metropolitan Life Insurance Company IBW tables. Some payors insist that patients be

both 100 lb over, and 200 percent of, IBW. The 1991 NIH Consensus Conference on Gastric Surgery for Severe Obesity concluded that appropriate surgical candidates are "patients whose BMI exceeds 40 kg/m², [including those with] obesity-induced physical problems that interfere with lifestyle (for example, joint disease that would be treatable but for the obesity, and body-size problems precluding or severely interfering with employment, family function, and ambulation)," or a BMI of 35 kg/m² or more and obesity comorbidity, such as diabetes, hypoventilation, sleep apnea, and so forth.

Gastroplasty
Horizontal Gastroplasty

Gastroplasties have been performed with either horizontal or vertical placement of the staples. Horizontal gastroplasty usually required ligation and division of the short gastric vessels between the stomach and spleen and carried the risk of devascularization of the gastric pouch or splenic injury. Horizontal gastroplasties have been done with a single application of a 90-mm stapling device without suture reinforcement of the stoma between upper and lower gastric pouches or a double application of staples with either a central or lateral polypropylene reinforced stoma. In one study, the failure rates (loss of less than 40% excess weight) for these three horizontal gastroplasty procedures were 71, 46, and 42 percent, respectively. Because of this high failure and complication rate, the horizontal gastroplasty is no longer indicated for the surgical treatment of obesity.

Vertical-Banded Gastroplasty

The vertical-banded gastroplasty (VBG) is a procedure in which a stapled opening is made in the stomach with a stapling device 5 cm from the cardioesophageal junction. One application of a 90-mm "bariatric" stapling device with four parallel rows of staples is made between this opening and the angle of His. Mason insists on measurement of the pouch volume (which should be 15 ml) at this point using an Ewald tube placed by the anesthetist. A strip of polypropylene mesh is wrapped around the stoma on the lesser curvature

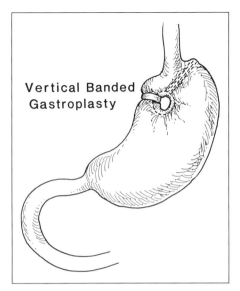

Fig. 88-1. Surgical technique of vertical banded gastroplasty. The vertical gastric staple line is created with a single application of a 90 mm "bariatric" stapling device, which fires four parallel rows of staples. The device is inserted behind the stomach 5 cm below the cardioesophageal junction and directed to the angle of His. The "banding" of the pouch outlet is fashioned by wrapping a 5 cm strip of polypropylene mesh around the pouch outflow tract and suturing it to itself and to the stomach.

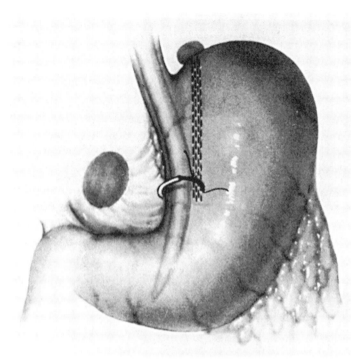

Fig. 88-2. Silastic ring gastroplasty is accomplished by placing a polypropylene or Silastic band around the stomach to calibrate and maintain the outflow tract from the small proximal gastric pouch created by stapling, as in the mesh-banded procedure (see Fig. 88-1). This procedure appears to be the most amenable among the gastric procedures for obesity for adaptation to a laparoscopic approach.

and sutured to itself but not to the stomach, creating a 5-cm circumference outlet of the small upper gastric pouch (Fig. 88-1). Use of a 4.5-cm circumference stomal outlet was not found to produce a better weight loss; in fact, many patients developed maladaptive eating behavior, drinking high-calorie liquids with this small outlet, as meat and chicken would often get caught in the small stoma. The Silastic ring gastroplasty (Fig. 88-2) is a similar procedure that uses a vertical staple line and a stoma reinforced with Silastic tubing.

Gastric Banding

Gastric banding is another form of gastroplasty in which a polypropylene or Silastic band is placed around the stomach just below the gastroesophageal junction. In several series, gastric banding has had markedly variable results in terms of weight loss. Furthermore, the operation can be associated with kinking of the banded "stoma," obstruction, and intractable vomiting. An adjustable, inflatable "band" has been developed and may have more

acceptable results; however, confirmatory data are not yet available. A prospective trial of a laparoscopic adjustable gastric band is currently in progress in the United States, but is a popular procedure in Europe. The current enthusiasm for developing new laparoscopic surgical techniques has led some surgeons to perform this procedure laparoscopically.

Gastric Bypass

Compared with the current standard, the original gastric bypass procedure had a much larger proximal gastric pouch and anastomotic stoma. This was often associated with an inadequate weight loss. The current gastric bypass performed at the Medical College of Virginia is constructed by placing three superimposed 90-mm staple lines in a vertical direction, creating a small gastric pouch (15–30 ml) with a 45-cm Roux en Y limb and the stoma restricted to 1 cm (Fig. 88-3).

The abdomen is entered through a midline incision carried superiorly alongside the xiphoid process and carried inferiorly to just above the umbilicus. The subcutane-

ous fat layer is usually several inches or greater in thickness and can be best divided by equal traction in a lateral direction by the surgeon and assistant across the table using laparotomy pads. Upon entry into the peritoneal cavity a complete exploration is performed to exclude unanticipated pathology before the gastric bypass procedure is begun. Particular attention is paid to the gallbladder given the known high incidence of postoperative gallbladder disease developing in the setting of rapid weight loss induced by gastric bypass. If the gallbladder appears chronically inflamed or if gallstones are palpated, a cholecystectomy should be performed after completion of the bypass procedure. In the absence of visual or palpable gallbladder abnormalities, our group performs an intraoperative ultrasound examination of the gallbladder and cholecystectomy if small stones, sludge, or polyps are identified.

The bypass procedure is initially begun by mobilizing the distal esophagus and encircling it with a one-half–inch soft rubber drain. The gastrohepatic omentum is

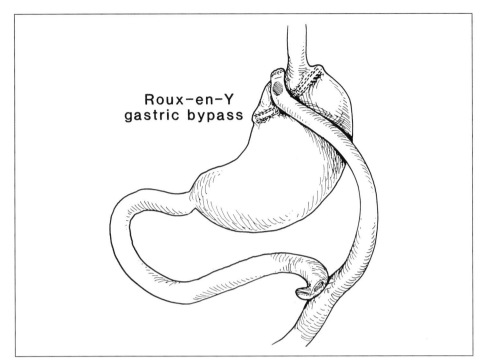

Fig. 88-3. *The current gastric bypass performed at the Medical College of Virginia is constructed by placing three superimposed staple lines in a vertical direction to create a 15- to 30-ml pouch, followed by anastamosis of the pouch to a 45-cm Roux en Y jejunal limb with the stoma restricted to 1 cm. The original proximal gastric bypass procedure for treatment of severe obesity had a much larger proximal gastric pouch and anastomotic stoma.*

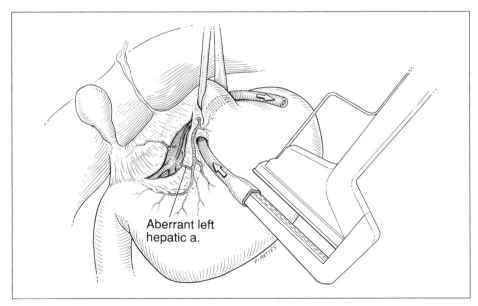

Fig. 88-4. *The blunt tip of a large No. 28 French red rubber tube is passed through the opened gastrohepatic omentum. The tip is guided posteriorly and cranially toward the angle of His along a tract created by blunt dissection with the surgeon's fingers. The open end of the tube is then brought through a dissected opening in the lesser curve mesentery between the first and second branches of the left gastric artery.*

bluntly entered overlying the caudate lobe, taking care to avoid injuring the aberrant left hepatic artery when present. The phrenoesophageal ligament overlying the anterior and lateral distal esophagus is sharply incised to facilitate subsequent blunt mobilization of the distal esophagus. Care must be taken to avoid esophageal injury by carefully identifying the nasogastric tube within the lumen of the esophagus during its mobilization and by bluntly dissecting widely around this important landmark. Laterally, the dissection must be high enough to be at the level of the esophagus. A low dissection laterally can lead to blunt injury to the short gastric vessels, bleeding, and the need for urgent splenectomy (no easy task in the morbidly obese patient) or creation of an inadvertently large pouch by failure to recognize the presence of stomach above the level at which the encircling rubber drain is placed.

After esophageal mobilization, the assistant's left hand is placed through the gastrohepatic omental opening behind the stomach wall on the lesser curvature. The space between the first and second branches of the left gastric artery is then identified as a landmark for creation of the gastric staple line. Using the posterior finger, pressing in an anterior direction to place the tissue under tension, the electrocautery is carefully utilized to divide the mesentery at this level right alongside the stomach wall, and an opening in the mesentery is created that is adequate to admit a large right-angled clamp. Blunt dissection of the avascular tissue on the posterior wall of the stomach is then undertaken between the opening in the gastrohepatic omentum and the lateral angle of His, which is identified by the encircling rubber drain. The blunt tip of a large No. 28 French red rubber tube is then placed in a medial-to-lateral direction behind the stomach along this dissected path to encircle the stomach (Fig. 88-4). The open end of the red rubber tube is subsequently brought through the previously created opening in the mesentery using a large right-angled clamp. The stomach is now ready for stapling and the red rubber catheter serves as a guide for introduction of the device. At this point, all intraluminal tubes and devices (e. g., the nasogastric tube and esophageal stethoscope) must be removed from the esophagus by the anesthetist.

We generally proceed to mobilization of the Roux en Y limb before stapling the stomach to ascertain whether or not the limb can be mobilized adequately to the proximal stomach for anastomosis before we commit to stapling the stomach. In the rare case wherein the mesentery is too foreshortened to reach the proximal stomach without undue tension, we advocate changing the procedure to the vertical-banded gastroplasty rather than creating a gastrojejunal anastomosis under tension with an increased risk of leak. The ligament of Treitz is identified and the jejunum measured to a point 45 cm beyond the ligament where the jejunum is divided with a stapling device. We resect an 8- to 12-cm segment of jejunum at this point in order to create a larger mesenteric defect, which we believe aids in mobilization of the limb to the proximal stomach. The mesenteric dissection is carried posteriorly in the fat with sequential application of clamps until further dissection either appears unnecessary for mobilization or unwise in that mesenteric vascular injury may occur. The jejunojejunostomy is then created with a side-to-side stapling technique 45 cm beyond the initial point of jejunal division for a standard gastric bypass and 150 cm downstream for a long-limb modification procedure, which we use in superobese

patients (BMI ≥ 50 kg/m^2). Care must be taken not to narrow the efferent lumen at the jejunojejunostomy site, particularly when performing the long-limb bypass, in which the distal small-bowel lumen may be quite small in diameter. Closure of the enterotomies for staple device placement can usually be accomplished with a 55-mm horizontal stapler using 3.5-mm staples, but this closure should be hand sewn if undue narrowing may occur with a stapled closure.

The Roux limb is brought through the transverse colon mesentery with blunt dissection and confirmed to be adequate to reach the proximal stomach. The 90-mm stapling device with 4.8-mm staples is guided behind the stomach by inserting its open-mouthed end into the lumen of the previously positioned red rubber catheter. After assuring that the staple line will reach completely across the stomach and that the stomach is not folded on itself, the stomach is stapled three times with superimposed staple applications (Fig. 88-5).

A 1-cm anastomosis is created between the proximal stomach pouch and the Roux limb using an outer layer of interrupted 3-0 silk and an inner layer of continuous 2-0 polyglycolic acid (Dexon) suture (Fig. 88-6). Following completion of the poste-

rior aspect of the anastomosis, a No. 30 French dilator is placed by anesthesia and guided by the surgeon through the anastomosis to define its appropriate dimensions. The dilator is removed after completion of the anastomosis and the tip of an 18 French nasogastric tube is carefully guided through the anastomosis by the surgeon. The Roux limb is occluded with the assistant's left hand and the anesthetist is then instructed to inject successive 10-ml aliquots of a solution of methylene blue dye through the nasogastric tube to assess for possible anastomotic leakage that would require intraoperative repair. A total of 30 ml methylene blue is usually needed to adequately stress the suture line to check for leaks. Following this test, the nasogastric tube tip can be positioned further down in the Roux limb and left to continuous suction overnight. All mesenteric defects are then closed: at the jejunojejunostomy, at the mesocolon, and behind the Roux limb to prevent a Petersen hernia. The abdominal fascia is reapproximated with running No. 2 Dexon, subcutaneous tissues are irrigated with crystalloid solution containing 1% neomycin, and the skin is closed with skin staples. No subcutaneous sutures or drains are used.

Long-Limb Modification

Superobese patients (defined as having a BMI ≥ 50 kg/m^2) have only lost one-half of their excess weight, in contrast to two-thirds of excess in nonsuperobese patients. Extending the Roux limb to 150 cm has increased the percentage of excess weight loss to two-thirds in the superobese patient. The long-limb GBP has not been characterized by an increased difficulty in managing nutritional deficiencies when compared to the standard proximal gastric bypass.

Gastric Transection Versus Stapling

A significant concern for many bariatric surgeons has been a high incidence of staple line disruption causing failed weight loss or weight gain. In a recent series of VBG procedures, a 35 percent incidence of staple line disruption was reported when the TA90B "bariatric stapler" (Autosuture Co, U.S. Surgical Corp, Norwalk, CT) with four parallel rows of 4.8-mm staples was used. Some surgeons advocate transecting the stomach to avoid this risk; others over-

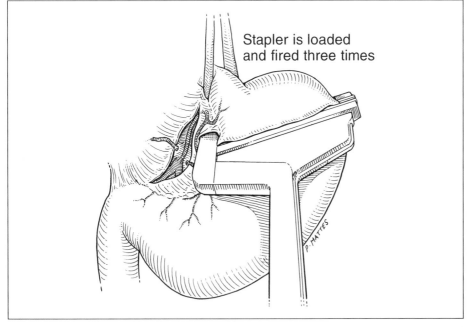

Fig. 88-5. The red rubber tube is used to guide the 90-mm stapling device into position for staple division of the stomach. Three superimposed staple lines form the proximal pouch.

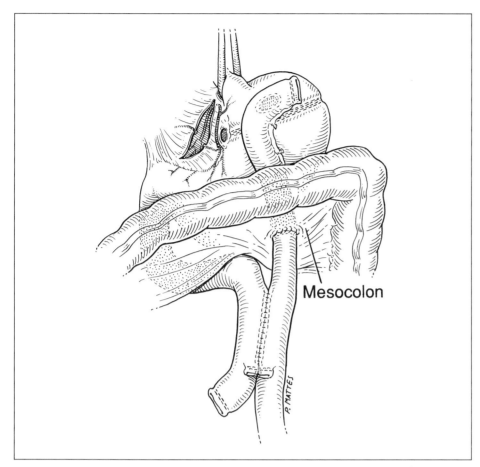

Fig. 88-6. The Roux en Y limb is brought through the transverse mesocolon to reach the proximal stomach. Adequate mesenteric dissection is essential to allow the limb to reach the level of the gastrojejunal anastomosis without tension, which increases the risk of leak. A two-layer hand-sewn anastomosis is constructed over a No. 30 French dilator and is guided gently through the gastrotomy into the enterotomy in the Roux limb after completion of the posterior anastomotic layers. The outer suture line is constructed of interrupted 3–0 silk, with the inner layer of continuous running 2–0 Dexon suture.

sew the staple line. We have decreased the incidence of staple line disruption to less than 2 percent using the technique of three superimposed staple lines, and believe as a result that gastric transection is not necessary and increases the risk of the procedure.

Choice of Operation: Gastroplasty Versus Gastric Bypass

Randomized, prospective trials have documented a significantly better weight loss with gastric bypass than with various types of horizontal gastroplasty procedu-res, in which the poorer results were thought to be secondary to technical causes, such as stomal or pouch enlargement or staple line disruption. The VBG was developed by Mason with the hope that these technical problems would be solved and that the weight loss would be comparable to that seen with gastric bypass without the potential gastric bypass risks of iron, calcium, and vitamin B_{12} deficiencies. In a randomized prospective trial, the GBP was compared with VBG and a significantly better weight loss was again noted with the GBP procedure. On the average, the GBP patients lost two-thirds of their excess weight over 3 years after operation, as compared with about 40 percent for VBG. When patients were di-

vided into eating pathology based upon preoperative dietary interview, it was found that sweets eaters had a markedly decreased weight loss after VBG as compared with GBP. There was no significant difference in weight loss between sweets and non-sweets eaters in the GBP group. The more favorable weight loss results in sweets eaters after GBP appeared to be due to the development of dumping syndrome symptoms with the ingestion of simple carbohydrates, although it is certainly possible that some carbohydrate malabsorption could also be responsible after bypass of the duodenum and upper jejunum. In another study, it was noted that GBP patients had an intolerance of both sweets (including high-calorie beverages) and milk products because of lactose intolerance. Most GBP patients claim that they have lost their craving for sweets. Randomized studies from Sweden and Canada also noted significantly better weight loss with GBP than with VBG. Another randomized study from Australia noted better weight loss with GBP than with vertical gastroplasty; however, this gastroplasty stoma was restricted with two polypropylene sutures rather than mesh or a Silastic band and may not be comparable to either the VBG or Silastic ring gastroplasty. A study from the Mayo Clinic also casts doubts about the effectiveness of the VBG.

Several centers are investigating laparoscopic techniques for performing both VBG and PGB. In the near future, it is likely that laparoscopic VBG techniques will be developed and incorporated into the practice of many bariatric surgeons. Without significant advances in the currently available laparoscopic technology, it is more difficult to imagine that PGB will be done laparoscopically by more than a few surgical pioneers. It remains to be seen whether performing a VBG using less invasive surgical techniques, but with its recognized inferior long-term weight loss, is better than performing an "open" traditional gastric bypass. Furthermore, the low mortality and complication rates for the technically demanding "open" PGB as performed by experienced surgeons will likely be difficult to reproduce with laparoscopic techniques. On the other hand, a laparoscopically placed adjustable Silastic gastric band can be a reasonable alternative to a standard gastric bypass, especially for those who are not superobese.

Postoperative Complications: Abdominal Catastrophe

It may be difficult to recognize an abdominal catastrophe in morbidly obese patients (Table 88-1). They may complain of abdominal pain, and yet on abdominal examination have no evidence of peritoneal irritation (no guarding, tenderness, or rigidity). Symptoms include shoulder pain, pelvic or scrotal pain, back pain, tenesmus, urinary frequency, and, of great importance, marked anxiety. Signs of infection (fever, tachypnea, and tachycardia) may be absent. Patients with peritonitis often have clinical symptoms and signs suggesting a massive pulmonary embolus: severe tachypnea, tachycardia, and sudden hypotension. Such acute pulmonary failure is probably secondary to sepsis-induced adult respiratory distress syndrome (ARDS). Thus, peritonitis must be suspected in any morbidly obese patient with acute respiratory failure. Because a high index of suspicion of peritonitis is required to detect the condition in morbidly obese patients, radiographic contrast studies using water-soluble agents such as meglumine diatrizoate (Gastrografin) may be indicated, even when few clinical signs are present. If a perforated viscus is suspected, an exploratory laparotomy may be necessary despite normal findings on radiographic contrast study.

Table 88-1. Signs and Symptoms of Peritonitis in the Morbidly Obese Patient

Abdominal pain
Absent guarding, tenderness, and rigidity
Shoulder pain
Pelvic pain
Chest pain
Back pain
Tenesmus
Urinary frequency/urgency
Anxiety
Subjective feeling of "impending doom"
Tachypnea
Respiratory failure
Tachycardia
Sudden hypotension

Complications of Vertical-Banded Gastroplasty

Erosion of the mesh into the stomach has been an unusual complication of VBG. Pouch enlargement is much less likely to occur with a vertical staple line in the thicker, more muscular part of the stomach, in contrast to the high incidence in horizontal gastroplasty, and the stomal diameter remains fixed with the mesh band. Should erosion occur, the pouch become enlarged, stomal stenosis develop, or disabling gastrointestinal reflux or recurrent vomiting occur, the patient is probably best converted to a gastric bypass procedure. In patients with a Silastic ring VBG, intractable vomiting of solid foods may develop with no evidence of mechanical obstruction. In our experience, these patients do well with conversion to GBP and the vomiting problem is eliminated.

Complications of Gastric Bypass
Acute Gastric Distention

Following gastric bypass surgery for clinically severe obesity, the distal, bypassed stomach occasionally will develop massive gaseous distention, which can lead to a gastric perforation, dehiscence of the gastric staple line, or disruption of the gastrojejunal anastomosis with leak. The primary symptoms of this complication are the development of hiccups and feeling bloated. Massive gastric dilation can lead to severe left shoulder pain and even shock. The problem is usually secondary to edema at the Roux en Y anastomosis causing afferent limb obstruction, but can be secondary to a mechanical problem. The diagnosis is made with an urgent upright abdominal radiograph that reveals the markedly dilated, air-filled bypassed stomach. Occasionally, the dilated, excluded stomach is filled with fluid and the diagnosis may be more subtle and difficult.

We have treated a few patients with dilation primarily due to gas by percutaneous, transabdominal "skinny"-needle decompression. Subsequent passage of gastric and biliopancreatic juices and gas through the Roux en Y anastomosis may occur after

such decompression, with resolution of the problem. Recurrent dilation or a patient in serious difficulty should lead to an emergent laparotomy with insertion of a gastrostomy tube and evaluation of the jejunojejunostomy. Patients with extensive adhesions from prior abdominal surgery should have a gastrostomy tube inserted at the time of gastric bypass operation to prevent this potentially lethal complication.

Internal Hernia

Following gastric bypass for morbid obesity, patients are at risk for development of an internal hernia with a closed-loop obstruction and bowel strangulation. There are three potential locations for these internal hernias: through the mesenteric defect at the jejunojejunostomy site, through the opening in the transverse mesocolon through which the retrocolic Roux limb is brought, and through the mesenteric defect located behind this Roux limb before it passes through the mesocolon, known as a Petersen hernia. The primary symptom of an internal hernia is periumbilical abdominal pain, which is usually cramping, consistent with visceral colic. Diagnosis may be very difficult. An upper gastrointestinal (UGI) radiographic series is often normal as intermittent spontaneous reduction of the hernia frequently occurs, which may provide a false sense of security that no problem exists. This may be devastating for the patient, should bowel infarction subsequently develop from a closed-loop strangulation obstruction. One should always carefully inspect the plain abdominal radiograph for the abnormal placement or "spreading" of the Roux en Y anastomotic staples. The safest course of action is to subject the patient with recurrent attacks of periumbilical pain to an abdominal surgical exploration.

Complication Rates After GBP

Complications in our series (Table 88-2) included a 1.2 percent incidence of anastomotic leak with peritonitis, 4.4 percent severe wound infection (defined as serious enough to delay hospital discharge), 11.4 percent minor wound infections and seromas (easily treated at home), less than 1 percent incidence of gastric staple line disruption with the use of three superim-

Table 88-2. Complications in 672 Patients Undergoing Proximal Gastric Bypass Surgery to Treat Morbid Obesity

Complication	Percentage of Patients
Operative mortality (2.2% in patients with obesity-related respiratory dysfunction)	0.4
Anastomotic leak with peritonitis	1.2
Severe wound infection (delayed hospital discharge)	4.4
Minor wound infections and seromas (treated at home)	11.4
Gastric staple line disruption (3 superimposed staple rows)	<1
Stomal stenosis	15
Marginal ulcer	13
Incisional hernia	16.9
Cholecystitis	10

posed rows of a 90-mm stapler, 15 percent stomal stenosis, 13 percent marginal ulcer, 16.9 percent incisional hernia, and 10 percent cholecystitis necessitating cholecystectomy. In 32 percent of our GBP patients with a normal intraoperative gallbladder ultrasound, gallstones developed, with sludge occurring in another 10 percent within 6 months of surgery. In a multicenter randomized prospective trial, the frequency of developing gallstones within 6 months of GBP was decreased from 32 to 2 percent with 300 mg ursodioxycholic acid given twice a day. Gallstone formation is very rare beyond 6 months. The operative mortality in our series of 672 gastric bypass procedures was 0.4 percent. Patients with respiratory insufficiency of obesity had a 2.2 percent operative mortality, in contrast to a 0.2 percent mortality in those without pulmonary dysfunction.

The data from both our randomized prospective trial and selective study do not support the contention that VBG is safer than GBP. Although the GBP has an additional anastomosis, complications including leaks and peritonitis occur with both operations. One of the criticisms of GBP is the difficulty in evaluating the distal gastric pouch and duodenum postoperatively. This has been achieved in 75 percent of patients with retrograde passage of an endoscope into the duodenum and stomach, and by others with percutaneous distal distention gastrography. To our knowledge, bleeding from either the distal gastric pouch or a duodenal ulcer has occurred in only 1 of more than 1200 GBP patients. In one patient a gastric perforation developed in his proximal gastric pouch after administration of high-dose nonsteroidal anti-inflammatory medica-

tion. Gastric mucosal metaplasia of the bypassed stomach was noted in 5 percent of patients following retrograde endoscopy, which has raised a concern regarding the risk of carcinoma arising in the bypassed stomach. However, tens of thousands of these procedures have been performed since 1967 and only one case of cancer in the bypassed stomach has been reported to date. We have also had one case that has not yet been published.

Micronutrient Deficiencies After GBP

Both VBG and GBP patients should be advised to take a multivitamin daily for life. When compared with VBG, GBP leads to significantly lower serum hemoglobin and iron concentrations. This is primarily a problem in menstruating women. After GBP all menstruating women should be treated prophylactically with supplemental oral ferrous sulfate, 325 mg per day. As many as six iron tablets per day may be required with heavy menstrual bleeding. On occasion, intramuscular iron (Imferon) injections or, rarely, hysterectomy may become necessary. Vitamin B_{12} deficiency is a greater risk with GBP than with VBG, but can be prevented with supplemental oral vitamin B_{12}, 500 µg per day. A few patients may require, or prefer, monthly B_{12} injections, which they can be taught to self-administer. There is a concern that GBP can lead to other divalent cation deficiencies. We have not found problems with serum levels of magnesium or zinc 5 to 9 years after GBP. However, calcium deficiency may occur, leading to osteoporosis, which may take many years to become manifest and may not be biochemically evident due to normal serum calcium levels;

therefore, we recommend that our patients take oral calcium supplements.

Failed Weight Loss

One of the greatest problems with all gastric procedures for morbid obesity is the risk of failed weight loss or weight regain. Twenty percent of VBG patients have difficulty with solid foods and develop a maladaptive eating behavior with the frequent ingestion of high-calorie liquid carbohydrates. Yale noted that 10 percent of VBG patients failed the procedure for this reason. We have converted 53 VBG patients to GBP. The average loss of excess weight after VBGP was 31 ± 5 percent and reached 67 ± 2 percent at 2 years after conversion to GBP, a value not different from that of our primary GBP group. Thirteen patients became sweets eaters and had lost only 15 ± 5 percent of excess weight beyond 1 year after VBG without any radiographically demonstrated problems with the procedure. One year after conversion to GBP, they lost an average of 78 ± 11 percent of excess weight.

Gastric bypass patients can also suffer from inadequate weight loss. In some patients, stomal dilation will develop over time after the procedure. No correlation between stomal size and weight loss has been demonstrated for GBP. Reoperation to make the pouch or stoma smaller has not been beneficial to the GBP patient who has failed the procedure. In our experience, failure of GBP is most commonly due to either the loss or absence of dumping syndrome symptoms in a small percentage of patients, leading to resumption of high-calorie sweets ingestion or, more often, the frequent ingestion of high-fat junk foods, such as potato or corn chips, microwave popcorn, or peanut-butter crackers. These foods crumble easily and empty quickly from the pouch so that the patient does not feel full. Patients need repeated dietary counseling over years to eat foods low in calories and high in fiber that will stay in the small gastric pouch longer and provide a sensation of early satiety without a large number of calories, for example, raw carrots, broccoli, cauliflower, apples, and oranges. Our philosophy is to make clear to these patients before surgery that the operation is designed to "help you help yourself." Obesity can be easily beaten and they must continue to utilize appropriate food choices and exercise for the rest of their lives. It has been our experience that patients who begin to eat more than 1100 calories per day will begin to gain weight. If they only gain one-half lb per month, this becomes 6 lb per year or 60 lb in 10 years. Bariatric surgical patients need lifelong counseling to optimize the results of their surgery.

Biliopancreatic Diversion

In recent years, investigators from Italy have proposed a combined gastric restrictive and intestinal malabsorptive procedure, known as the biliopancreatic diversion. This procedure does not have a blind intestinal limb and only occasionally produces complications from bacterial overgrowth in the bypassed small bowel (Fig. 88-7). In this operation, a subtotal gastrectomy is performed, leaving a proximal gastric pouch of about 200 ml for superobese (>225% IBW) patients and 400 ml for the others; the distal 250 cm of small intestine is anastomosed with a large 2- to 3-cm stoma to the proximal gastric remnant, and the proximal, bypassed small intestine is reanastomosed to the distal ileum, 50 cm from the ileocecal valve. In this manner, the quantity of food ingested is partially restricted and then passes down the intestine, mostly undigested and unabsorbed until it reaches the bile and pancreatic juices in the terminal 50 cm of ileum (the common absorptive intestinal channel), where digestion and absorption take place. These patients usually have four to six steatorrheic stools per day, which are malodorous and float, reflecting fat malabsorption. In addition to iron-deficiency anemia and vitamin B_{12} deficiency seen with the standard GBP, these patients are at risk for severe protein deficiency and fat-soluble vitamin deficiencies, which lead to osteoporosis secondary to calcium and vitamin D malabsorption, night blindness, and skin eruptions secondary to vitamin A deficiency, as well as a prolonged prothrombin time. This procedure carries a very high incidence of these complications in North American patients. The nutritional complications of this operation may be less severe in Italian patients, whose diet is high in complex carbohydrates (e. g., pasta), as compared to the high fat content of the American diet (e. g., fried foods, potato and corn chips). A number of Italian patients, however, have required rehospitalization for total parenteral nutrition or extension of the "common absorptive channel" from 50 to 150 cm. Although one California group reported favorable results, they also stated that fat-soluble vitamin supplementation was mandatory, osteoporosis and iron deficiency may be severe, and 4.1 percent required reversal for uncorrectable protein-calorie malnutrition.

We have treated a few patients in whom the standard GBP failed by converting them to the partial biliopancreatic procedure with a 50-cm common absorptive ileal channel, which we have called a "distal gastric bypass," since we did not resect the distal stomach. This modification differs from the standard partial biliopancreatic diversion, as the gastric pouch was only 50 ml rather than 200 to 400 ml as originally recommended. Unfortunately, this operation was associated with an unacceptable incidence of severe malnutrition and fat-soluble vitamin deficiencies. More recently, a few superobese patients with significant comorbidity who failed a standard GBP have been converted to a distal gastric bypass with a 150-cm common absorptive intestinal channel, with resumed weight loss. Prophylactic fat-soluble vitamins and pancreatic enzymes have prevented vitamin or protein deficiencies in most of these patients. However, when superobese patients were randomized between a standard GBP and a distal GBP (modified partial biliopancreatic diversion), 25 percent of the distal GBP patients required conversion to a proximal GBP because of severe protein-calorie malnutrition. Those who did not require conversion had a significantly better weight loss at 3 to 5 years after surgery than did the patients randomized to a standard proximal GBP, but they needed more nutritional supplementation in order to avoid fat-soluble vitamin deficiencies or osteoporosis.

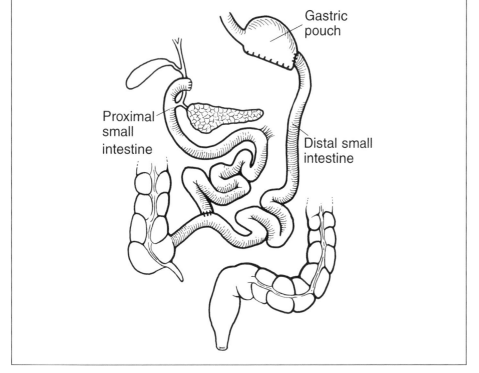

Fig. 88-7. The biliopancreatic diversion procedure combines a subtotal gastrectomy with a small intestinal bypass method. It involves an anastomosis of the distal 250 cm of small bowel to the gastric remnant with anastomosis of the excluded small bowel to the gastrointestinal limb just 50 cm proximal to the ileocecal valve. Thus, a short 50-cm "common absorptive channel" is created to limit the exposure of ingested foodstuffs with the biliary and pancreatic digestive juices.

Suggested Reading

Brolin RE, Robertson LB, Kenler HA, Cody RP. Weight loss and dietary intake after vertical banded gasgtroplasty and Roux-en-Y gastric bypass. *Ann Surg* 220:782, 1994.

Brolin RE, Kenler HA, Gorman JH, Cody RP. Long-limb gastric bypass in the superobese. A prospective randomized study. *Ann Surg* 215:387, 1992.

Foley EF, Benotti PN, Borlase BC, Hollingshead J, Blackburn GL. Impact of gastric restrictive surgery on hypertension in the morbidly obese. *Am J Surg* 163:294, 1992.

MacLean LD, Rhode BM, Forse RA. A gastroplasty that avoids stapling in continuity. *Surgery* 113:380, 1993.

MacLean LD, Rhode BM, Sampalis J, Forse RA. Results of the surgical treatment of obesity. *Am J Surg* 165:155, 1993.

Pories WJ, et al. Who would have thought it? An operation proves to be the most effective therapy for adult-onset diabetes mellitus? *Ann Surg* 222:339, 1995.

Schwartz RW, Strodel WE, Simpson WS, Griffen WO Jr. Gastric bypass revision: Lessons learned from 920 cases. *Surgery* 104:806, 1988.

Scopinaro N, Gianetta E, Friedman D, Adami GF, et al. Surgical revision of biliopancreatic diversion. *Gastroenterol Clin North Am* 16:529, 1987.

Sugerman HJ, Felton WL, Sismanis A, et al. Effects of surgically induced weight loss on pseudotumor cerebri in morbid obesity. *Neurology* 45:1655, 1995.

Sugerman HJ, Fairman RP, Sood RK, et al. Long-term effects of gastric surgery for treating respiratory insufficiency of obesity. *Am J Clin Nutr* 55:597S, 1992.

Sugerman HJ, Kellum JM, Engle KM, et al. Gastric bypass for treating severe obesity. *Am J Clin Nutr* 55:560S, 1992.

Sugerman HJ, Starkey JV, Birkenhauer R. A randomized prospective trial of gastric bypass versus vertical banded gastroplasty for morbid obesity and their effects on sweets versus nonsweets eaters. *Ann Surg* 205:613, 1987.

EDITOR'S COMMENT

Operations for morbid obesity have not been popular in our medical center. This is strange since rotund citizens are not uncommon in Chicago. Thus, it is with a touch of envy that I note the broad experience of 672 patients presented herein by Drs. Sugerman and DeMaria.

We have been concerned with the potential for serious complications following these gastric reservoir manipulations. Indeed, I stated at the outset that the diversion of the gastric acid flow away from the antrum would trigger hypergastrinemia with subsequent marginal or stomal ulceration (*Ann Surg* 170:338, 1969). I note a 13 percent incidence of marginal ulcer in the Sugerman series. In addition, certain of the patients (15%) in whom stomal stenosis developed may have had healing marginal ulcerations as a source of the anastomotic narrowing.

Will there be a move to the use of laparoscopic techniques in performing bariatric surgery? Undoubtedly, there will be a wave of enthusiasm for this "minimally" invasive approach (*Surg Endosc* 8:1354, 1994).

L.M.N.

89

Vascular Compression of the Duodenum

A. Gerson Greenburg   David A. Iannitti

Complete or partial obstruction of the duodenum by the superior mesenteric artery or one of its branches is a clinical entity that has been identified since the mid-nineteenth century. Throughout the years, this syndrome has received various names and a variety of treatment regimens that often reflect the current level of understanding of this disease process. Underlying the disease, in both the acute and chronic form, is the anatomic fact that the superior mesenteric artery arises from the abdominal aorta and crosses the anterior aspect of the third portion of the duodenum. It is here that an obstruction can occur. Diagnosing a patient with vascular compression of the duodenum may be difficult, as the clinical findings are frequently vague and often resemble other forms of high small-bowel obstruction. Fluoroscopic hypotonic duodenography is the important cornerstone of diagnostic imaging. Both nonoperative and operative approaches are used with varying degrees of success. Nutritional support, including nasojejunal feeding, is undertaken as a primary adjunctive management modality. Operative intervention, when indicated, requires division of the suspensory muscle of the duodenum and bypass of the obstruction with a duodenojejunostomy. Accurately diagnosing this syndrome and providing appropriate management of the patient should result in a favorable long-term prognosis.

History

Vascular compression of the duodenum as a disease entity has received a waxing and waning level of interest throughout the years. In 1842, Von Rokitanski proposed that the third portion of the duodenum could be obstructed by compression of the superior mesenteric artery. Later authors proposed other etiologies that included duodenal stasis, dilatation, pseudoobstruction, and compression or traction by the transverse mesocolon. Bloodgood, in 1907, postulated that this syndrome of duodenal obstruction could be surgically treated by duodenojejunostomy, and Stavely first successfully performed this procedure in 1908.

The pathophysiology of vascular obstruction of the duodenum was neither clearly accepted nor understood in the early twentieth century. Procedures including gastroduodenojejunostomy and colonic resections were performed with little success. Wilkie, in 1927, reported a relatively large series of 75 patients, with the greatest success rate associated with duodenojejunostomy. This procedure, once popularized, became the operation of choice for vascular compression as well as other motility disorders of the duodenum.

Over the subsequent decades this disorder continued to receive various levels of attention. Because of overdiagnosis and apparent overuse of duodenojejunostomy, the very existence of vascular compression of the duodenum as an illness once again came into question. In the 1960s, there was a resurgence of interest in this disorder because it was being encountered more frequently in the acute setting. Barner and Sherman, in 1963, provided a comprehensive review from the case reports in the literature to that time. Subsequent additional reports provided further detailed information describing the anatomic, clinical, diagnostic, and pathophysiologic features of vascular compression of the duodenum and their relation to surgical intervention.

The term *vascular compression of the duodenum* is the most appropriate name for this disease process since the middle colic artery or the superior mesenteric artery, or both, may play a role in the etiology of the obstruction. Throughout the century, a variety of names for this syndrome have appeared. Several of these names are listed in Table 89-1.

Anatomy

Precise knowledge of the anatomic relationship among the superior mesenteric artery, middle colic artery, aorta, paraspinal musculature, ligament of Treitz, and third and fourth portions of the duodenum is essential in understanding the etiology of vascular compression of the duodenum and in planning surgical intervention.

The superior mesenteric artery (SMA) originates from the anterior aspect of the abdominal aorta between the celiac axis

Table 89-1. Names Used to Describe Vascular Compression of the Duodenum

Arteriomesenteric duodenal obstruction
Cast syndrome
Cast syndrome incognito
Chronic duodenal ileus
Chronic duodenal pseudoobstruction
Chronic intermittent arteriomesenteric occlusion of the duodenum
Gastromesenteric ileus
Nutcracker syndrome
Superior mesenteric artery (SMA) syndrome
Vascular compression of the duodenum
Wilkie's syndrome

and the renal arteries. It usually arises at the level of the lower aspect of the first lumbar (L1) vertebra; however, this origin can range from T12 to the upper aspect of L3. The SMA leaves the aorta at an acute angle that is much more pronounced in erect humans than in quadrupeds and courses caudally, dorsal to the neck of the pancreas. In sagittal view, the angle between the SMA and aorta contains the left renal vein, the uncinate process of the pancreas, and the third portion of the duodenum (Fig. 89-1). The normal aortomesenteric angle in adults is between 40 and 50 degrees. Also in this area is a retroperitoneal fat pad, surrounding the SMA, that serves to reduce the effect of duodenal compression by these arteries by enlarging the angle. Loss of this fat pad and the resultant change in angle of the SMA over the duodenum is believed to play a role in the etiology of acute vascular compression of the duodenum. This would be especially true of patients experiencing acute rapid weight loss. Branches of the SMA include the middle colic, inferior pancreaticoduodenal, intestinal, right colic, and ileocolic arteries.

The middle colic artery (MCA) arises as a branch of the superior mesenteric artery at the inferior border of the pancreas, cranial to the level of the third portion of the duodenum. It courses caudally and to the right in the transverse mesocolon. The MCA crosses ventral to the duodenum. Compression of the duodenum may occur between the MCA and the right psoas muscle (Fig. 89-2). This relationship may not be appreciated when the transverse colon is reflected cranially.

The duodenum, a structure that received its name from being equal in length to the breadth of 12 fingers (25 cm), is divided into four portions: superior, descending, horizontal, and ascending. The horizontal or third portion of the duodenum is the region most susceptible to vascular compression. It is a retroperitoneal structure, relatively fixed, 5.0 to 7.5 cm in length. The third portion of the duodenum passes from right to left usually with a slight cephalic deviation; it then crosses the vertebral column, generally along the lower border of L3. This vertebral crossing may occur as high as L2 or, more commonly, across L4. It is noted that the lumbar spine reaches its most anterior point at the level of L4. Not only does the third portion of the duodenum cross the vertebral column

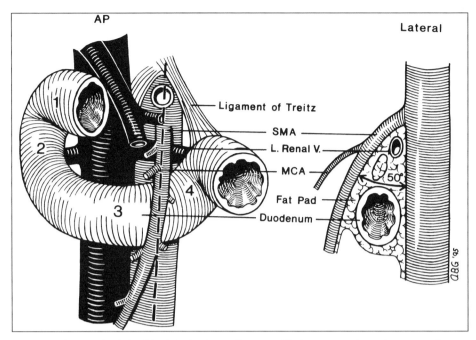

Fig. 89-1. The normal relationship of the duodenum, ligament of Treitz, aorta, and superior mesenteric artery. The SMA crosses the third portion of the duodenum. The lateral view demonstrates the aortomesenteric angle containing the left renal vein, uncinate process of the pancreas, and duodenum. This angle in normal adults is 40 to 50 degrees. AP = anteroposterior; MCA = middle colic artery. Numbers 1 through 4 refer to the first, second, third, and fourth portions of the duodenum, respectively.

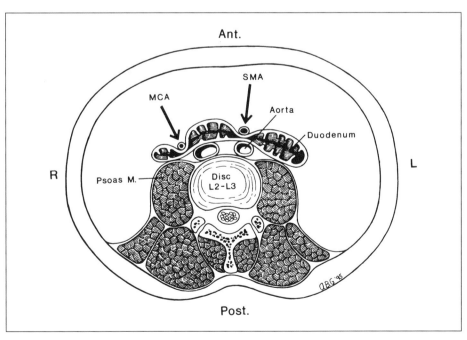

Fig. 89-2. Axial view at the level of the second to third lumbar vertebrae shows the potential points of obstruction of the third portion of the duodenum between the SMA and aorta, or the MCA and right psoas muscle.

in a cephalad direction, it also traverses ventrally, from its relatively dorsal position to the right of the vertebral column. In effect, the junction of the second and third portions of the duodenum is posterior to the plane of the anterior surface of the vertebral column, requiring enteral contents to pass ventrally as well as slightly cephalad before moving caudally. Variations in the aortomesenteric angle when coupled with lesser or greater degrees of lumbar lordosis result in various combinations of open- and closed-angle relationships to the duodenum (Fig. 89-3). When the angle is narrow and lordosis is present, obstruction is more likely to occur.

The ascending or fourth portion of the duodenum is about 2.5 cm in length. It usually rises cephalad to the left of the aorta toward the upper border of L2, where it turns sharply to join the jejunum. The duodenojejunal flexure is held in place by the suspensory muscle of the duodenum, the ligament of Treitz. According to Treitz this structure is composed of smooth-muscle fibers and connective tissue. The ligament originates from the right crus of the diaphragm and passes caudally to insert along the superior aspect of the third and fourth portions of the duodenum and duodenojejunal flexure. There are many possible variations in the attachment of the ligament to the duodenum (Fig. 89-4). A short ligament may pull the third portion of duodenum snugly into the SMA–aortic angle, or may sharply elevate the duodenojejunal flexure without elevating the third portion (Fig. 89-5). These anatomic variations, along with those of the SMA and duodenum, may render some individuals more susceptible to vascular compression of the duodenum.

Clinical Manifestations

Since its clinical presentation is varied, vascular compression of the duodenum is difficult to diagnose. Moreover, there are two manifestations of this syndrome, the more common chronic form and the acute form. Most patients are between the ages of 10 and 40, and 60 percent are female.

Chronic vascular compression symptomatology includes postprandial epigastric discomfort and pain that may be associated with epigastric distention or fullness. Anorexia, early satiety, eructation of foul-smelling gas, nausea, and weight loss are common. Vomiting is usually associated with the relief of these symptoms. Patients often spontaneously assume a knee-chest, left lateral, or prone position to gain postural relief. The symptoms may be intermittent or constant depending on the extent of the obstruction. If protracted vomiting persists, patients may become severely dehydrated and significant fluid and electrolyte imbalances may develop.

Physical examination usually reveals a thin, even cachectic individual often with an asthenic body habitus. Epigastric distention or visible peristalsis may be observed. Right upper quadrant tympany and epigastric tenderness are usually present.

Acute vascular compression occurs in a wide range of clinical scenarios. Acute rapid weight loss is the most consistent predisposing factor. It has been postulated that loss of the retroperitoneal fat pad results in a more acute aortomesenteric angle and duodenal obstruction. This acute weight loss, often in association with significant trauma or burns, supine immobilization, or anorexia nervosa, precipitates acute vascular compression of the duodenum. It has also occurred in adolescents whose growth rate is out of proportion to their weight gain. Placement of a body cast or hip spica cast has been known for decades to induce this syndrome.

The differential diagnosis of this symptom complex includes peptic ulcer disease, biliary disease, duodenitis, and pancreatitis. Obstruction of the distal duodenum is uncommon. Pancreatic cysts or neoplasms, duodenal tumors, para-aortic lymphadenopathy, adhesions, malrotation, and Crohn's disease may present in a similar fashion.

Diagnosis

The diagnosis of vascular compression of the duodenum is made by clinical considerations in conjunction with radiographic studies. Plain abdominal films may demonstrate a dilated stomach and proximal duodenum with air-fluid levels. An acute demarcation of the duodenal dilatation may be visualized.

Although plain films may raise the suspicion of this diagnosis, they are not specific. Contrast studies are needed to confirm the diagnosis. The most sensitive and specific study is hypotonic duodenography performed under fluoroscopic examination. The patient drinks contrast material, or al-

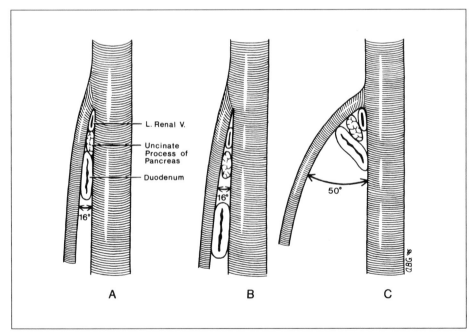

Fig. 89-3. Lateral view of various aortomesenteric angles involved with vascular compression of the duodenum. A. Narrow angle with a high duodenal position. B. Narrow angle with a normal duodenal position. C. Normal angle with a high duodenal position.

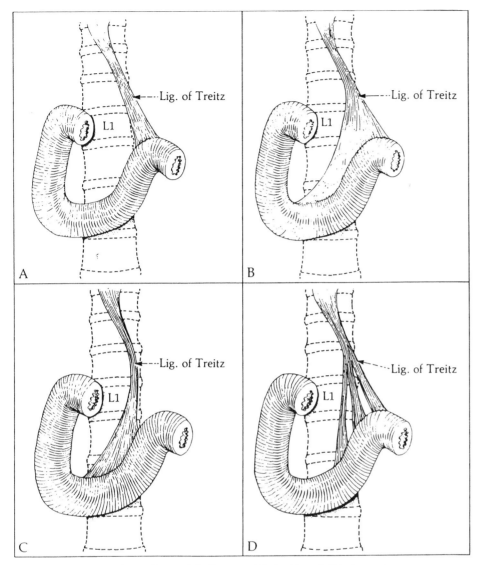

Fig. 89-4. Variations in the attachment of the ligament of Treitz. Example B is the most common configuration. (From JE Skandalakis et al. Vascular compression of the duodenum. Part 2. Contemp Surg *10:33, 1977. With permission.)*

mesenteric artery passing across the duodenum precisely at the point where the GI contrast material is cut off, a finding that clearly confirms the diagnosis.

As technological advances have been made in arteriography, there has been further interest in exploring the role of the aortomesenteric angle. Lateral projection of the aorta during injection of intra-arterial contrast will show the angle of takeoff of the superior mesenteric artery. This angle has been repeatedly studied in cadavers, normal adults, and individuals with vascular compression of the duodenum. The aortomesenteric angle, measured by arteriography in normal individuals, averages 50 degrees with a wide range of 20 to 70 degrees. The angle in cadaveric dissections averages slightly less, at 40 degrees. In affected patients, these studies have clearly documented the average aortomesenteric angle as significantly less, averaging 16 degrees with a range of 12 to 22 degrees.

Mesenteric arteriography does involve certain risks, including allergic contrast reaction, acute renal insufficiency, vessel perforation, bleeding, and embolic events. Although arteriography may reveal a diminished aortomesenteric angle in an individual with suspected vascular duodenal compression, this finding alone would not and should not alter the patient's management. Obstruction of the duodenum to gastrointestinal contrast is essential to establishing the diagnosis. Thus, mesenteric arteriography has a limited role in the diagnosis of vascular compression of the duodenum.

Fluoroscopic hypotonic duodenography is safe, defines the anatomic and physiologic aspects of the obstruction, and should be used as the main diagnostic imaging modality. Mesenteric arteriography with upper GI contrast material should be limited to cases that are difficult to diagnose.

Management

Management of a patient with vascular compression of the duodenum should vary according to the etiology and extent of obstruction. Patients with acute symptomatology can be initially managed conservatively, using a nasogastric tube for gastric and duodenal decompression, and histamine (H₂) antagonists. Thompson

ternatively, it can be infused through a nasogastric tube. The proximal duodenum will be dilated and may have the typical vertical linear cutoff in its third portion. There may be delayed or no passage of contrast material beyond this point (Fig. 89-6). Fluoroscopy is used to observe the characteristic "to-and-fro" peristalsis in the duodenum proximal to the obstruction. Ideally this study is performed while the patient is experiencing acute symptoms to yield a higher diagnostic result. During fluoroscopy the patient can be placed in the knee-chest and left lateral position to facilitate relief of the obstruction. Simultaneous passage of contrast material

past the point of obstruction and sudden relief of symptoms confirm the diagnosis. A conventional barium meal study is not as accurate as hypotonic duodenography and is associated with a higher false-negative rate.

Aortic and selective superior mesenteric arteriography is another diagnostic imaging study used to evaluate patients with suspected duodenal vascular compression. This study can be performed with or without upper gastrointestinal contrast material. If intraluminal and arterial contrast is used, the anteroposterior (AP) projection will demonstrate the superior

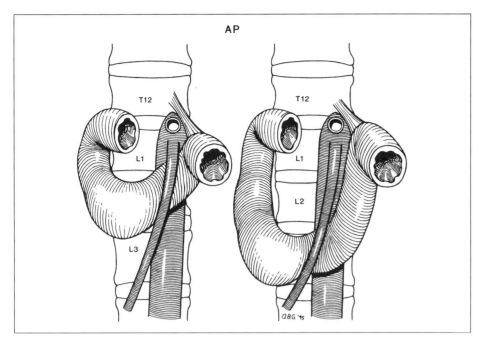

AP

Fig. 89-5. *Examples of a short ligament of Treitz resulting in a highly positioned duodenum held snugly in the aortomesenteric angle, and a normally positioned duodenum with a sharply elevated duodenojejunal flexure.*

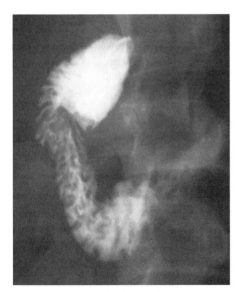

Fig. 89-6. *Hypotonic duodenography demonstrating a cutoff of contrast material in the third portion of the duodenum where it is crossed by the SMA in a patient with vascular compression of the duodenum.*

and Stanley have documented an increased incidence of peptic ulcer disease associated with vascular compression of the duodenum; thus, prophylaxis against ulceration appears warranted. These patients can also become severely dehy-

drated with significant electrolyte disturbances. Aggressive intravenous hydration and electrolyte replacement should be carried out promptly before further diagnostic or therapeutic interventions are performed.

Removal of aggravating factors is essential. If a body or hip spica cast is the predisposing factor, it must be completely removed. To do this may require initiation of alternative orthopedic management such as internal fixation. Removal of a window or section of the cast is considered inadequate. Usually alleviation of the obstruction is observed with body cast removal.

Most patients with vascular compression of the duodenum have some element of acute or chronic malnutrition. In the acute form, most cases are preceded by significant weight loss. Reckler reported an average 25 percent weight loss of initial body mass in burn patients in whom this syndrome developed. Nutritional intervention and restoration of body weight may help re-establish the retroperitoneal fat pad and aortomesenteric angle. Nasojejunal feedings are used for this purpose. A small-caliber, soft, flexible feeding tube can be introduced past the point of obstruction by a variety of techniques. Fluoroscopic or

endoscopic guidance is most commonly used to achieve this goal. Isotonic enteral feedings are then instituted for nutritional support. Parenteral hyperalimentation is rarely indicated for this purpose.

Patients with the chronic form of duodenal compression are less likely to respond to conservative measures. Individuals with milder symptomatology should be instructed to assume the knee-chest and left lateral or prone positions in the postprandial period. When patients do not improve or worsen with conservative measures, continue to demonstrate severe symptomatology, or have progressed to an advanced state of weight loss and malnutrition, conservative measures are likely to fail and surgical intervention is recommended.

Surgical Technique

The surgical treatment for patients with vascular compression of the duodenum consists of two principles: 1) divide the suspensory muscle of the duodenum and 2) bypass the point of obstruction by duodenojejunostomy. Preoperatively, it is essential to prepare the patient by replacement and correction of any fluid and electrolyte imbalances that may be present.

The abdomen is entered through a midline vertical incision or a right transverse abdominal incision. The transverse incision is preferred as it is better tolerated and has a lower risk of incisional hernia development. This incision extends from the midline, two fingerbreadths above the umbilicus, to the midpoint between the costal margin and the anterosuperior iliac spine in the right anterior axillary line. The transverse incision provides adequate access to both the duodenum and transverse mesocolon.

Following exploration of the abdomen, the diagnosis of vascular compression of the duodenum is confirmed. The gastrocolic omentum and transverse colon are elevated through the incision and retracted inferiorly and to the left. This exposes the distal stomach, pylorus, and proximal duodenum. The duodenum may appear dilated at this level. However, the use of a nasogastric tube and traction of the transverse mesocolon may leave the proximal duodenum decompressed. The nasogastric tube can then be used to instill 150 to 300 ml air. If the diameter of the second portion of the duodenum increases by 3 to 4 cm after insufflation, the diagnosis is confirmed.

The next step is to divide the suspensory muscle of the duodenum, effectively lowering the distal third and fourth portions of the duodenum from the aortomesenteric angle. The omentum and transverse colon are retracted superiorly exposing the posterior surface of the transverse mesocolon. The duodenojejunal flexure is identified as the jejunum exits at the base of the transverse mesocolon to the left of the spine. The proximal jejunum is gently retracted caudally as the peritoneum along its left side is incised (Fig. 89-7A). The sus-

pensory muscle (ligament of Treitz) can be divided along the anterior cranial aspect of the third and fourth portions of the duodenum (Fig. 89-7B). Adequate mobilization should allow passage of two fingers between the duodenum and the origin of the superior mesenteric artery (Fig. 89-7C). Dissection of this area can be complicated by significant bleeding, as the inferior mesenteric vein and superior mesenteric, middle colic, and inferior pancreaticoduodenal arteries are close and susceptible to injury.

Mobilization of the duodenojejunal flexure may at times be limited as there are multiple anatomic configurations and attachments of the suspensory muscle to the duodenum. The attachments may also be vascular. Multiple small branches from the

inferior pancreaticoduodenal artery may also limit the mobilization of the duodenum. These technical and anatomic difficulties may contribute to or directly lead to the mixed and generally poor outcomes when this procedure is used alone to alleviate the obstruction. An enteral bypass is required to assure relief of the obstruction.

Side-to-side duodenojejunostomy is the preferred bypass procedure. The omentum and transverse colon are retracted superiorly and to the left. The distal second and proximal third portions of the duodenum may appear distended, underlying the peritoneum caudal to the base of the transverse mesocolon. This peritoneum is incised transversely for approximately 10 cm

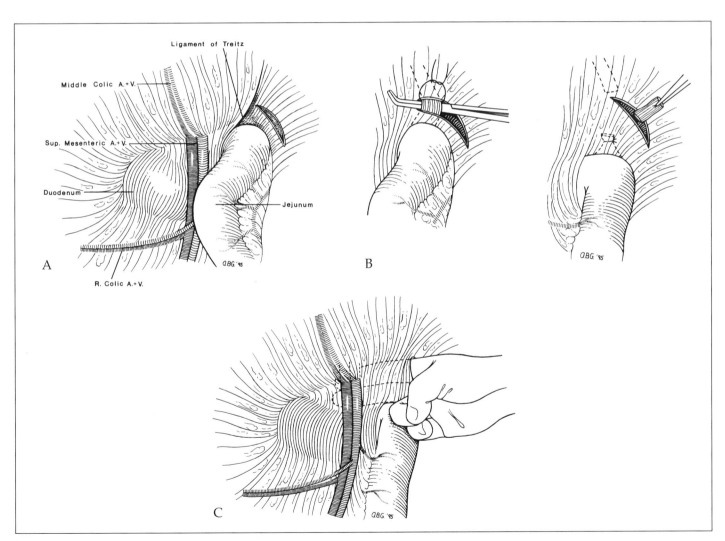

Fig. 89-7. A. Division of the ligament of Treitz begins by incising the peritoneum along the left side of the duodenojejunal flexure. B. Division and ligation of the ligament of Treitz to mobilize the duodenojejunal flexure out of the aortomesenteric angle. C. Following mobilization of the duodenojejunal flexure, two fingers should be able to pass between the duodenum and the origin of the SMA.

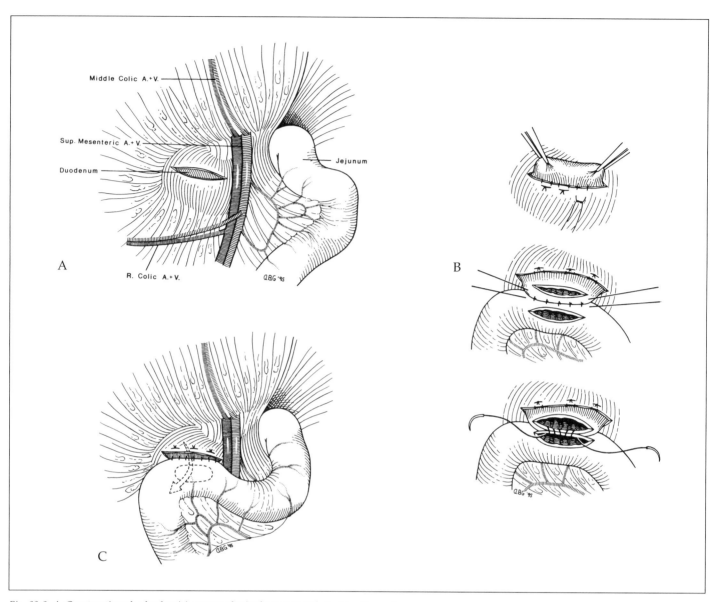

Fig. 89-8. A. Construction of a duodenojejunostomy begins by transversely incising the peritoneum overlying the junction of the second and third portions of the duodenum. B. Continued construction of the duodenojejunostomy is carried out by mobilizing the second and third portions of the duodenum. The peritoneal edges are sutured to the duodenum. A posterior row of seromuscular 3-0 silk sutures is placed between the duodenum and jejunum. Running absorbable sutures are used to create the inner layer. The side-to-side anastomosis is completed with an anterior row of reinforcing 3-0 silk seromuscular sutures. C. The completed duodenojejunostomy.

(Fig. 89-8A). This is an avascular space; however, care should be taken to avoid injury to the middle colic vessels. The duodenum is mobilized by incising its lateral and posterior attachments. The duodenum is retracted caudally through the peritoneal incision. At this point, the peritoneum is sutured circumferentially to the seromuscular layer of the duodenum with simple interrupted 3-0 silk sutures to prevent herniation. The proximal 10 to 15 cm of jejunum is brought to the right to lie in a side-to-side fashion and a hand-sewn, two-layer anastomosis is performed (Fig. 89-8B). A posterior row of 3-0 silk, simple, interrupted seromuscular sutures is placed between the duodenum and jejunum. Longitudinal full-thickness incisions are made along the antimesenteric borders of the duodenum and jejunum. These should be incised sufficiently to ultimately create a 5-cm anastomosis. The inner layer of suture is a running 3-0 absorbable suture. Two suture lines are begun posteriorly, and run circumferentially to be secured on the anterior surface. This closure is reinforced with an anterior layer of 3-0 silk interrupted seromuscular (Lembert) sutures (Fig. 89-8C).

An alternative option is a Roux en Y duodenojejunostomy from the junction of the second and third portions of the duode-

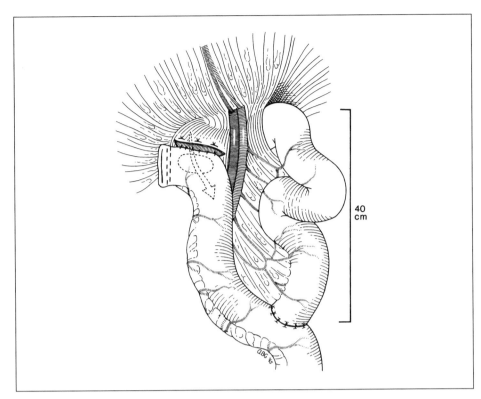

Fig. 89-9. A Roux en Y duodenojejunostomy.

num (Fig. 89-9), or the low second portion of the duodenum. The only real disadvantage of this approach is the use of two suture lines with an increased risk of dehiscence.

Patients undergoing duodenojejunostomy for vascular compression of the duodenum can be expected to have a favorable outcome. This procedure can be performed with minimal perioperative morbidity and mortality. Division of the suspensory muscle of the duodenum alone has been advocated by Akin and associates. Review of the world literature reveals an 83 percent success rate, while 17 percent of these patients had fair to poor results. Patients subsequently underwent duodenojejunostomy with an excellent outcome. When division of the ligament of Treitz is performed in conjunction with a duodenojejunostomy, according to a 30-year review, a 98.5 percent success rate will result. Patients usually have immediate relief of symptoms and enjoy rapid weight gain in the following weeks and months.

Suggested Reading

Akin JT, Gray SW, Skandalakis JE. Vascular compression of the duodenum: Presentation of ten cases and review of the literature. *Surgery* 79: 515, 1976.

Akin JT, Milsap JH, Gray SW, et al. Vascular compression of the duodenum. Part 3. *Contemp Surg* 10: 52, 1977.

Anderson JR, Earnshaw PM, Fraser GM. Extrinsic compression of the third part of the duodenum. *Clin Radiol* 33: 75, 1982.

Barner HB, Sherman CD. Vascular compression of the duodenum. *Int Abstracts Surg* 117: 103, 1963.

Duvie SO. Anterior transposition of the third part of the duodenum in the management of chronic duodenal compression by the superior mesenteric artery. *Int Surg* 73: 140, 1988.

Gray SW, Akin JT, Milsap JH, et al. Vascular compression of the duodenum. *Contemp Surg* 9: 37, 1976.

Gray SW, Skandalakis LJ, Rowe JS, et al. Vascular compression of the duodenum. In LM Nyhus, R Baker (eds), *Mastery of Surgery* (2nd ed). Boston: Little, Brown, 1992.

Gustafsson L, Falk A, Lukes PJ, et al. Diagnosis and treatment of superior mesenteric artery syndrome. *Br J Surg* 71:499, 1984.

Jones AS, Carter R, Smith LL, et al. Arteriomesenteric duodenal compression. *Am J Surg* 100: 262, 1960.

Mansberger AR, Hearn JB, Byers RM, et al. Vascular compression of the duodenum. *Am J Surg* 115: 89, 1968.

Reckler JM, Bruck HM, Munster, AM. Superior mesenteric artery syndrome as a consequence of burn injury. *J Trauma* 12: 979, 1972.

Skandalakis JE, Akin JT, Milsap JH, et al. Vascular compression of the duodenum. Part 2. *Contemp Surg* 10: 33, 1977.

Thompson NW, Stanley JC. Vascular compression of the duodenum and peptic ulcer disease. *Arch Surg* 108: 674, 1974.

Ylinen P, Kinnunen J, Hockerstedt K. Superior mesenteric artery syndrome. A follow up of 16 operated patients. *J Clin Gastroenterol* 11: 386, 1989.

III

The Liver and Biliary Tract

90

Surgical Anatomy of the Liver and Bile Ducts

Henri Bismuth   Denis Castaing   Joseph S. Raccuia

Modern surgery of the liver is dependent on the concepts initiated by Couinaud (1957) and developed by Ton That Tung and Bismuth. Surgical anatomy of the liver based on precise knowledge of its natural divisions and complete understanding of these basic components is an essential requisite for any surgeon who is performing an operation on the liver. These concepts can be described in two aspects: one concerns the morphologic anatomy and the other the functional anatomy. Improvements in imaging technology with ultrasound, computed tomography (CT), and magnetic resonance imaging (MRI) have provided two- and three-dimensional interpretations of the liver anatomy preoperatively and have added a third, more recent scope capable of accurately portraying the "real" or actual liver anatomy of individual patients with all their particular variations. This full picture enables the surgeon to consider an individual patient's anatomy, an element that can often have a major effect on the extent and type of procedure to be performed.

Morphologic Anatomy

Classic morphologic anatomy examines the external appearance of the liver and ligamentous attachments, such as when seen topographically at laparotomy. The liver, an intrathoracic organ that lies behind the ribs and costal cartilages, is separated by the diaphragm, pleura, and lung. Only a small epigastric portion lies behind the anterior abdominal wall. The anterior concave surface forms a fissure, or hilus, for the passage of the major vessels and bile ducts. The posterior surface is primarily retroperitoneal and lies in contact with the inferior vena cava, enclosed by

leaves of the coronary and triangular ligaments. The four peritoneal folds, including the falciform ligament, suspend the liver from the anterior abdominal wall and diaphragm. The round ligament, a fibrous cord formed from the obliteration of the umbilical vein, arises at the level of the end of the left portal vein branch.

The anterior surface of the liver, as seen at laparotomy, seems to divide the liver into two parts, or classic lobes, with the falciform ligament. The right is considerably larger than the left (Fig. 90-1). Inferiorly, this apparent division corresponds with the round ligament and umbilical fissure forming the posterior part of the right lobe, which appears to be divided posteriorly by the transverse fissure of the hilus. The right lobe has a convex superior surface, which lies under the diaphragm. The anterior margin is divided by the anterior portion of the gallbladder fossa. The quadrate lobe lies at the inferior surface of the right lobe, anterior to the hilus, to the right of the umbilical fissure, and to the left of the gallbladder fossa. The left lobe, the smaller portion of the liver, lies to the left of the falciform and round ligaments, and to the left of the hilus. The caudate (Spigel) lobe, the fourth lobe of the liver, is posterior to the transverse fissure of the hilus, which is delineated by the ligament of Arantius to the left. That ligament is formed from the insertion of the lesser omentum on the left. This lobe surrounds the inferior vena cava and is not apparent when viewing the liver from the anterior surface. Hence, the liver is composed of two main lobes, the right and the left; and two accessory lobes, the quadrate and the caudate, which are all divided by fissures. The "lobar" description corresponds to the Stedman's medical dictionary terminology

of a "true" lobe, which is defined as a "part of parenchyma limited by fissures or grooves."

Functional Anatomy

The other, more recent concept, concerning the functional anatomy of the liver was first initiated by Cantlie in 1898 and was enhanced with the efforts of McIndoe and Counseller in 1929, Ton That Tung in 1939, Hjörstjö in 1931, Couinaud in 1957, and Goldsmith and Woodburne in 1957. Although seemingly complex, the concept of Couinaud is the most exact and complete description of liver anatomy and has distinct and useful application for the functional aspects of liver operations, which has been verified by extensive clinical application over the years. This functional anatomy accurately describes the segmentation of the liver in a manner that is very similar to the lobar anatomy of the lungs. Segmental liver anatomy, based on the distribution of the glissonian pedicles and the hepatic veins, has been the foundation of modern hepatic surgery. The portal pedicle or "triad," for example, is enclosed by an expansion of Glisson's capsule and contains the portal vein, hepatic artery, and bile ducts. The portal vein, within this investment, divides into right and left branches just to the right of the hilus. The left branch is longer, remains extrahepatic for a distance, and curves forward at the left border of the hilus along the umbilical scissurae before penetrating the hepatic parenchyma at the level of the recessus of Rex (an area inside the liver delineated by the left portal scissura). Conversely, the shorter right branch penetrates directly into the hepatic parenchyma immediately after the bifurcation. According to this con-

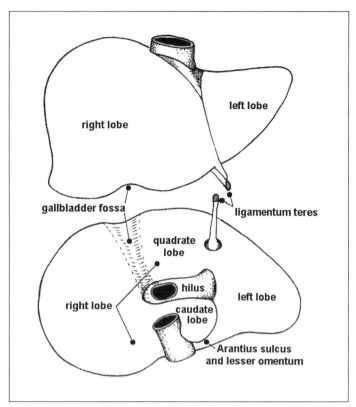

Fig. 90-1. *The classic morphologic liver with division into right and left lobes, as seen topographically. These true lobes are bound toward the inferior aspect by the transverse fissure posteriorly. The portion of the right lobe anterior to this point is the quadrate lobe, limited on the left by the umbilical fissure (ligamentum teres) and on the right by the gallbladder fossa. Posterior to the right lobe is the fourth lobe, the caudate (Spigel) lobe, separated by the lesser omentum in the sulcus of Arantius.*

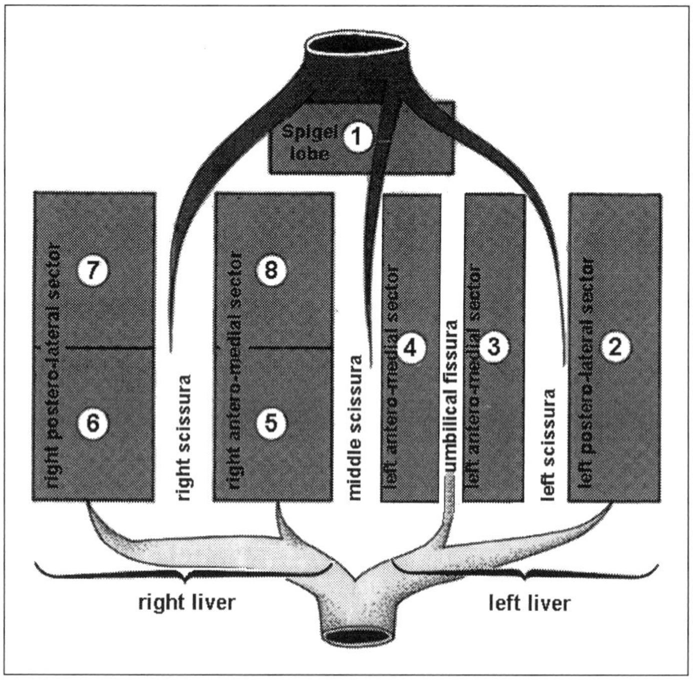

Fig. 90-2. *The functional anatomy in this schematic represents the division by the three hepatic veins that lie within the liver scissurae like fingers of the hands. Each receives a portal pedicle.*

cept, the liver appears to be separated into two livers, or right and left hemilivers, by the main portal scissura, which is also called Cantlie's line. We prefer the terms *right* and *left* livers, rather than lobes, which we consider erroneous since there are no identifiable surface markers to distinguish these sections as true lobes. Furthermore, our nomenclature does not cause confusion with the lobes of the classic morphologic liver anatomy previously described.

The three main hepatic veins divide the liver into four sectors, each of which receives an alternating glissonian (portal) pedicle, somewhat similar to the fingers of the hand (Fig. 90-2). The four sectors, individualized by the three hepatic veins, are called portal sectors and are independent portions of parenchyma supplied autonomously by glissonian pedicles. Similarly, the scissurae containing the hepatic veins are called portal scissurae, whereas the

scissurae containing the portal pedicles are called hepatic scissurae. For example, the umbilical fissure corresponds to the plane of the hepatic scissura where the left hepatic vein lies, while the main portal scissura begins at the middle of the gallbladder bed anteriorly to the left of the vena cava posteriorly. This scissura follows an angle of 75 degrees with the horizontal plane opened toward the left side, thus delineating the right and left livers. Each contains independent portal, arterial, and biliary structures. The middle hepatic vein is within the plane of the main portal scissura. The left and right livers divide further into two separate portions by two other portal scissurae, with the right and left hepatic veins, respectively, within their planes.

The parenchymal zones in between these scissurae consist of four subdivisions called segments in the Anglo-Saxon nomenclature. However, according to Coui-

naud's nomenclature, used here, they are called sectors (one sector equals two segments of Couinaud). In Couinaud's description, the right portal scissura divides the right liver into two sectors consisting of anteromedial and posterolateral components, as clearly seen when the liver is autopsied and placed on a flat table known as the "bench position" (Fig. 90-3A). Along the right portal scissura lies the right hepatic vein, which inclines approximately 40 degrees to the right. When the liver is in its usual place, within the abdominal cavity, the posterolateral sector is behind the anteromedial sector, almost in a frontal plane. When the liver is in the normal in situ position (Fig. 90-3B) at laparotomy and when referring to all morphologic examinations such as ultrasound, CT, angiography, and MRI, we prefer to call these portions of the liver the right *anterior* and *posterior* sectors, according to their actual orientation within the abdominal cavity. The exact location of the right

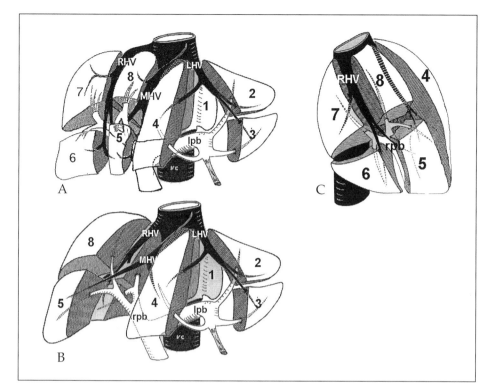

Fig. 90-3. A. Couinaud's original drawings depicted the liver in the "bench" or autopsy position. Misinterpretation of the actual plane of the anterormedial and posterolateral sectors along with the orientation of the portal structures has persisted. B. The actual orientation of the functional anatomy of the liver with the anterior and posterior right sectors almost in a frontal plane. Similarly, the portal structures to segments 5 and 8 are anterior and those structures supplying segments 6 and 7 are posterior. C. The right and left livers are divided by the right portal scissura in an oblique plane extending from the anterior surface of the liver, to the right of the gallbladder fossa, to the confluence between the vena cava and the right hepatic vein posteriorly. The left liver comprises the anterior portion of the liver to the left of the right portal scissura and the left lobe. Note that the posterior sector (segments 6 and 7) is considerably more posterior than the IVC. RHV = right hepatic vein; MHV = middle hepatic vein; LHV = left hepatic vein; lpb = left portal branch; rpb = right portal branch; = inferior vena cava.

portal scissura is not well defined because there is no external landmark. According to Couinaud, it extends from the anterior surface of the liver at the anterior border, to midway from the right angle of the liver and the right side of the gallbladder fossa, to the confluence between the inferior vena cava and the right hepatic vein posteriorly (Fig. 90-3C). In contrast, the description of Ton That Tung places this scissura in a line following parallel to the right lateral edge of the liver, three finger breadths from the lateral liver margin.

The left portal scissura (Fig. 90-4) divides the liver into two sectors, which were called anteromedial and posterolateral in Couinaud's first description. However, when the liver is in the in situ position, with a slightly different orientation than when in the bench position, we prefer to use the terms left *anterior* and *posterior* sectors.

In this circumstance, it is important that this left portal scissura is not mistaken for the umbilical fissure. The left portal scissura lies within the left liver, posterior to the ligamentum teres, and the presence of the left hepatic vein distinguishes this scissura from the umbilical fissure, which contains the left portal pedicle. Thus, the anterior sector of the classic morphologic left lobe is composed of the portion of the right lobe that is to the left of the main portal scissura and the anterior part of the left lobe.

It must be emphasized that Couinaud's description, although accurate, was made with autopsy specimens and all the drawings were made in the bench position. However, when the liver is examined in situ, at laparotomy, the right and left an-

terior and posterior sectors are truly almost completely one behind the other. When one examines these sectors in the autopsy specimen on a flat table, the orientation is changed to almost completely medial and lateral. Therefore, many have misinterpreted the orientation of structures within the parenchyma when image studies have been described. In another misconception, the vena cava is on the same plane as the most posterior portion of the right posterior sector (segments 6 and 7*), when, in fact, this portion of the liver parenchyma is significantly more posterior than the vena cava by virtue of its intra-abdominal position (Fig. 90-5).

The Organization of the Right Liver

The right portal pedicle divides into anterior and posterior portions. The anterior branch arises immediately from the upper right pedicle running in a frontal plane before it divides into ascending and descending branches for segment 5 (inferior) and segment 8 (superior) (Fig. 90-6). The posterior branch curves toward the superior convexity of the liver and divides into ascending and descending branches for segment 6 (inferior) and segment 7 (superior). The two right sectors are divided by the right scissura, within which lies the right hepatic vein. These two sectors are divided into two segments. However, there are no scissurae between segments 5 and 8 or between segments 6 and 7.

The Organization of the Left Liver

The segmental portal branch that supplies the posterior portion of the left lobe delineating segment 2 arises from the left portal pedicle, at the left end of the hilus. After curving for a short distance, this branch terminates 1 to 2 cm from the anterior edge of the liver, the recessus of Rex, where the round ligament is joined anteriorly. Here, at the intrahepatic portion of the left portal pedicle is where structures to segments 2, 3, and 4 originate before branching into their respective segments. This point is a clinically important ultrasound landmark. From the left side, a branch arises for the anterior portion of the left lobe, referred to as segment 3. Another branch arises from

*To facilitate distinction, we prefer to use the Arabic numbers instead of the previously used Roman numerals when describing the liver segments.

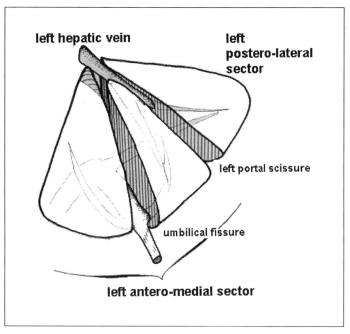

Fig. 90-4. The left liver is divided into the left anterior sector (segments 3 and 4) and the left posterior sector (segment 2 only). It is important to distinguish the left portal scissura from the umbilical fissure. Note the arrangement of the segment in relation to the portal and hepatic venous vasculature.

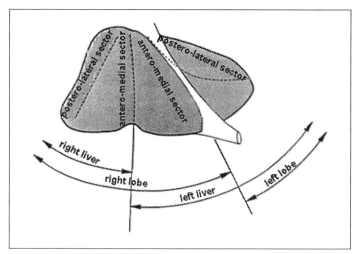

Fig. 90-5. The orientation of the right posterior sector is actually more posterior than the vena cava when viewed in the abdominal cavity.

the left side for the portion of the liver situated to the right of the umbilical fissure, referred to as segment 4, which corresponds to the quadrate lobe of the classic morphologic anatomy. The portion to the left half of the gallbladder bed is known as segment 4a (inferior), and the tissue above the left portal pedicle and caudate (Spigel) lobe is known as segment 4b (superior). Thus, the anterior left sector is composed of segments 3 and 4, while the posterior sector is formed from only segment 2 (the only exception to the nomenclature when each sector is divided into two segments), which constitutes the whole posterior sector of the left lobe.

The Organization of Segment 1 (Caudate Lobe)

Functionally, segment 1 must be considered an autonomous segment because the vasculature is independent of the glissonian division and the three hepatic veins. Segment 1 is supplied by two or three branches from the portal vein that exit from the bifurcation of the portal pedicle or directly from the left branch, or both, and less often from the right branch. Similarly, hepatic veins to segment 1 are independent of the three main hepatic veins and drain directly into the inferior vena

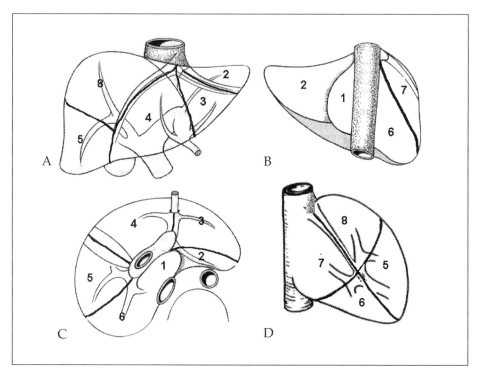

Fig. 90-6. The actual in situ position of the liver as viewed in A) anterior, B) posterior, C) inferior, and D) lateral orientations. The segments are viewed in relation to their respective portal and hepatic venous vasculature.

cava. The anatomy of this "third" liver is revealed in certain pathologic conditions such as Budd–Chiari disease, in which the hepatic blood outflow is ensured through direct connections to the inferior vena cava because of obstruction of the three main hepatic veins, resulting in significant caudate lobe hypertrophy. Furthermore, this particular arrangement makes resection of lesions involving segment 1 a considerably more advanced and technically demanding intervention.

The Arterial Blood Supply

The hepatic artery supplies the liver with arterial blood through branches that run in close approximation to the portal branch and bile duct within the investment (portal triad) of the hepatic pedicle. Then these branches follow with the expansion of Glisson's capsule entering into the hepatic parenchyma. Embryologically, there are three hepatic arteries: a left artery, which arises from the left gastric artery, a middle from the celiac axis, and a right from the superior mesenteric artery. Usually, the left and the right disappear, leaving the embryologic middle branch from the celiac axis, which is the classic proper hepatic artery in the adult. This artery divides, usually at the level of the left side of the hilum, into a left branch and a right branch (which is longer) supplying the respective hemilivers. Multiple combinations of these embryologic arteries have been described in the adult; usually however, only one of the left or the right artery persists. Therefore, the origin of the hepatic artery is subject to considerable variation outside of the liver (Fig. 90-7).

The Hepatic Veins

The hepatic veins arise from the central lobar veins within the hepatocytes, which drain into the larger segmental and sectorial branches before forming the main hepatic vein branches. These veins are solitary vessels without accompanying elements and are in direct contact with the hepatic parenchyma. The *right hepatic vein*, in general, is formed from three veins that are divided into superior, middle, and inferior branches from the right liver. The inferior branch of the right hepatic vein, which is present in 20 percent of patients, drains two or three segments of the right liver directly into the vena cava. The middle branch of the right hepatic vein runs in a transverse direction and enters the vena cava slightly above the superior branch. The superior branch of the right hepatic vein, although short (1–2 cm), is the largest of the branches. In many instances, one or two veins arise from the posterior surface of the liver (segments 7 and 8) and join the main trunk close to the vena cava, where they sometimes can enter the vena cava separately. The right hepatic vein trunk joins at the right margin of the vena cava at a point separate from and slightly above the trunk formed by the middle and left hepatic veins. The *middle hepatic vein* is formed from two veins arising from segments 4 and 5, where the confluence of these vessels lies within the main portal scissura in a frontal plane passing through the hilus. Superior to this confluence is a consistently present branch from the posterior portion of segment 8, and less consistent is a branch from the posterior portion of segment 4. The middle hepatic vein joins the left hepatic vein to form a common trunk just before draining into the inferior vena cava in approximately 90 percent of instances. However, sometimes the two vessels enter separately. The formation of the *left hepatic vein* is somewhat more variable with many different configurations. One arrangement consists of a short trunk made from the combined tributaries of intersegmental branches of segments 4, 3, and 2; and in another scenario, there is a long trunk with two or three veins draining segment 2. Whatever the organization, the position of the left hepatic vein is extremely posterior in the left lobe, and dissection of the left hepatic ligament at this level must be performed with caution to avoid injury to this vessel. Of surgical significance is the small caliber of the left hepatic vein trunk, and the diversity and variability of the branches entangled with portal branches making the scissura between the left anterior and posterior sectors unrecognizable, therefore,

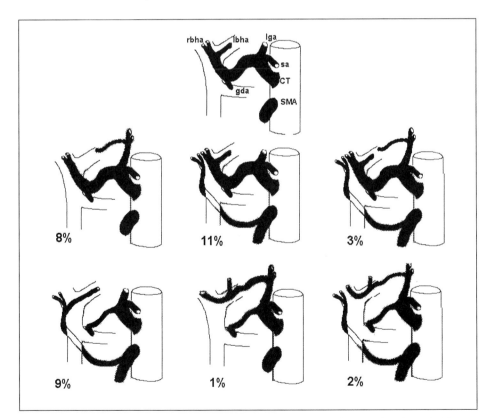

Fig. 90-7. The anatomic variations of the right and left hepatic arteries in relation to the celiac axis. The most common arrangement arises from the celiac axis and branches to form the gastroduodenal artery (inferiorly) and the main hepatic artery branch (superiorly). CT = celiac trunk; SMA = superior mesenteric artery; sa = splenic artery; rbha = right branch of middle hepatic artery; lbha = left branch of middle hepatic artery; gda = gastroduodenal artery; lga = left gastric artery. Percentages indicate the instances of anatomic variation.

rendering it impossible to perform an isolated segment 2 resection. In regard to all the hepatic veins, anastomoses are common, often numerous, and can occur randomly at the level of the main vessels or the smaller tributary branches of the same vein, or both.

Bile Ducts

Intercellular passages join to form interlobar bile ducts, which drain directly into the same glissonian pedicles containing the afferent vessels. In the right hemiliver, the ducts of segments 6 and 7 form the posterior right duct, and the ducts of segments 5 and 8 form the anterior right duct, which combine at a confluence to form the main branch of the right bile duct, which is approximately 1 cm in length (Fig. 90-8). The right posterior duct reaches the hilum by passing superiorly (epiportal) to the right anterior portal vein, a line sometimes visible on x-ray examination. However, this epiportal position is inconsistent, and in approximately 20 percent of instances the right posterior duct passes inferiorly (hypoportal) to the anterior portal vein. The left duct is formed from the ducts of segments 2 and 3 to the left of the intrahepatic portion (recessus of Rex) of the left portal branch within the umbilical fissure, and it also receives a branch from segment 4 to the right of the left portal branch. This duct is longer than the right with an average length of approximately 2.5 cm. However, the size can vary from 1 to 5 cm, a factor that is dependent on the size of the quadrate lobe. The biliary confluence is formed outside of the hepatic parenchyma in the hilum, which then forms the common (proper) hepatic duct. This classic junction occurs in approximately 56 percent of instances. However, other anatomic variations are known to occur (Fig. 90-9). Segment 1 is drained by two or three ducts, which enter both the right and left hepatic ducts close to the confluence.

The Extrahepatic Bile Ducts

The extrahepatic bile ducts are composed of the segments originating from the right and left hepatic ducts, which join to form the biliary confluence and the main biliary channel, which drains into the duodenum. The accessory biliary apparatus comprises the gallbladder and cystic duct.

The Biliary Confluence

The confluence of the right and left hepatic ducts occurs at the right of the hilus of the liver, along and anterior to the origin of the right branch of the portal vein, where the duct is actually displaced superiorly and medially to the left of the main portal vein branch. Exposure of the biliary confluence begins with dissection and lateral traction of the gallbladder bed plus outward and upward traction of the round ligament (ligamentum teres). Thus, the contents of the hepatic duct confluence unfold like an accordion. This maneuver is an essential one, especially in the reoperated on patient. Good exposure, primarily of the left hepatic duct, which is mostly extrahepatic, can be obtained by incising the hilar plate at the junction with the liver capsule. The dissection plane is extrafascial and exists between the plate and the parenchyma of segment 4 (quadrate lobe). The extrahepatic segment of the right duct is very short and runs vertically and almost immediately enters the hepatic parenchyma. The left duct has a much longer extrahepatic course along the left portal branch, horizontally. The biliary ducts are enclosed within the connective tissue (Glisson's capsule) of the hilar plate. Occasionally, small vessels or biliary radicals can enter or leave along this margin. Once the hilar plate is opened, the contents of the portal pedicle are displaced inferiorly and segment 4 can be lifted to gain further exposure. Normally, the confluence actually exists in only 57 to 72 percent of instances. The anatomic variations that exist are numerous (Fig. 90-9), and one involves a right sectorial duct that joins the main bile duct directly in 25 percent (in 16% the right posterior duct and in 9% the right anterior) of instances. This variation is known as an "étagée" or shelved confluence. A triple confluence of the right posterior duct, the right anterior duct, and the left hepatic duct, without a right hepatic duct occurs in 12 percent of instances, whereas in 4 percent a right sectorial duct can join the left hepatic duct (the right posterior duct in 3% and the right anterior duct in 1%). Other variations (3%) include an absence of the hepatic duct confluence or a right sectional duct (2%) can join the neck of the gallbladder or the cystic duct or a right sectional duct can join the main bile duct. There are several variations. However, since they exist within the glissonian sheaths, maintaining this plane

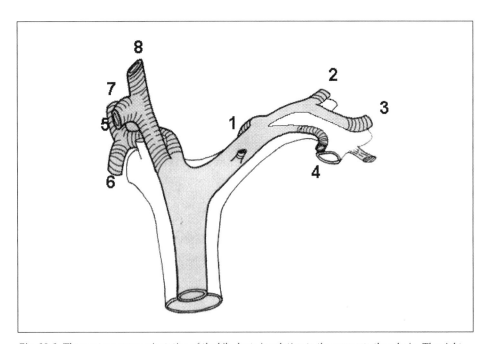

Fig. 90-8. The most common orientation of the bile ducts in relation to the segments they drain. The right anterior sector is drained by segments 5 and 8, the right posterior by segments 6 and 7, the left anterior by segments 3 and 4, the left posterior by segment 2 only, and small branches mostly from the left hepatic duct drain segment 1. However, some branches from the confluence and right duct are also common. Percentages indicate the incidences of anatomic variation.

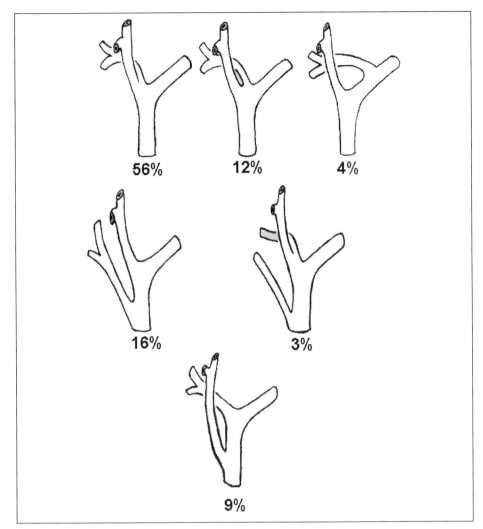

Fig. 90-9. *The most common arrangements of the bile ducts in relation to the right and left hemilivers. Note that the most common arrangement consists of a single main right branch, which divides into right anterior and posterior sectorial branches. The left main branch is usually a single trunk before entering the main hepatic duct. (Percentages indicate the incidence of anatomic variation.)*

during dissection can avoid surgical misadventure before a variant structure is properly identified. Once the plane is properly dissected, the sheath can be opened from the superior surface, and the left duct can be easily exposed. The exposure of the right pedicle is more limited but can be increased by incising the posterior extremity of the cystic plate at the junction of the biliary plate. However, this step is performed only after cholecystectomy.

The Main Bile Duct and the Sphincter of Oddi

The common (proper) hepatic duct is situated just distal to the biliary confluence and joins of the cystic duct to form the common bile duct or "choledochus." The site of the insertion of the cystic duct is variable and most commonly occurs between the biliary convergence and the retroduodenal region. This variability must be carefully considered during gallbladder operations, and cystic duct ligation should be as close as possible to where it exits from the gallbladder. The mean diameter of this duct is approximately 6 mm, but it enlarges with age. The common bile duct courses downward and anterior to the portal vein joining its left margin in the middle part of the hepatic pedicle. The hepatic artery, which runs upward, is usually to the left. The right branch of the hepatic artery crosses the common hepatic duct posteriorly, although sometimes it can exit anterior to the superior part of the hepatic pedicle. The cystic artery, arising from the right branch of the hepatic artery crosses the common hepatic duct posteriorly or anteriorly. The common hepatic duct constitutes the left border of the triangle of Calot. The other parameters were originally described as the cystic duct below and the cystic artery above; however, today it is universally accepted to be the inferior surface of the right lobe of the liver as the upper border and the cystic duct as the lower margin. The union between the cystic duct and the common hepatic duct can be located at various levels and forms the choledochus. At its lower extrahepatic portion, the common bile duct crosses posterior to the pyloric vessels and the pancreaticoduodenal arteries, then traverses the posterior part of the head of the pancreas running in a groove of the pancreatic parenchyma. This "retropancreatic" portion of the common bile duct approaches the second portion of the duodenum obliquely and is accompanied by the terminal part of the duct of Wirsung for approximately 2 cm where it is separated from it by the transampullary septum before it enters the duodenum after traversing the sphincter of Oddi. There is a small common duct: the ampulla of Vater. The ampullary papillae of Vater protrude into the duodenal lumen at the papilla of Vater and are marked by a longitudinal fold of duodenal mucosa. The usual position of the papilla of Vater (major papilla) is in the second portion of the duodenum, approximately 8 cm from the pylorus. The duct of Wirsung forms a confluence with the bile duct in 85 percent of instances and enters the duodenum independently in 10 to 13 percent of patients, whereas in only 2 percent it is replaced by the duct of Santorini.

Gallbladder and Cystic Duct

The gallbladder is a reservoir located on the surface of the inferior face of the right lobe within the gallbladder fossa and separated from the hepatic parenchyma by the cystic plate, which is composed of connective tissue intimately associated with Glisson's capsule. This area is a prolongation of the hilar plate. Sometimes the gallbladder is deeply embedded into the liver, but occasionally it can be almost completely detached and surrounded by its own peritoneum. The gallbladder consists of a fundus, a body, and an infundibulum, with the tip of the fundus usually, but not always, reaching the free edge of the liver where it is closely attached to the cystic plate.

The cystic duct lengthens the infundibulum of the gallbladder and joins the common hepatic duct to form the choledochus. The lumen is usually 1 to 3 mm in diameter. Its length is variable, depending on the type of insertion with the common hepatic duct. The insertion can be angular (75%), parallel (20%), or spiral (5%), and usually exists at the supraduodenal part of the common hepatic duct in 80 percent of patients. However, it can extend downward to the retroduodenal or even retropancreatic area. Occasionally, the cystic duct joins the right hepatic duct or a right hepatic sectorial duct, particularly in étagée or shelved confluence. The mucosa of the cystic duct is arranged in spiral folds known as the valves of Heister, and its wall is surrounded by a sphincteric structure called the sphincter of Lutkens.

Bile Duct Blood Supply

The blood supply of the supraduodenal duct arises from the retroduodenal artery, the right branch of the hepatic artery, the cystic artery, the gastroduodenal artery, and the retroportal artery. An average of eight small arteries, each measuring approximately 0.3 mm in diameter, supply the supraduodenal duct. The most important of these vessels runs along the lateral borders of the duct. The majority (60%) course upward from the major inferior vessels, while only a few (38%) course downward. They originate from the right branch of the hepatic artery and other vessels, and only 2 percent arise directly from the main trunk of the middle hepatic artery. The hilar ducts receive a copious supply of arterial blood from surrounding vessels (left and right branches of the middle hepatic artery), forming a rich plexus on the surface of the ducts in continuity with the vessels around the supraduodenal duct. The source of the blood supply of the retropancreatic common bile duct is the retroduodenal artery, which provides multiple small vessels running around the duct into mural planes. The arrangement of the blood supply to the extrahepatic bile ducts has important surgical significance and recommendations in achieving proper

exposure of the main bile duct and performance of cholecystectomy have been made: The main bile duct should never be stripped for exposure. It should be opened longitudinally through an area devoid of vessels leaving the fascial envelope intact (when resutured all vessels should be avoided), and the cystic artery should always be ligated close to the gallbladder. Furthermore, since the cystic artery and the right branch of the proper hepatic artery are smaller and less likely to sustain adequate lengths of bile duct, the surgical implication would dictate that when it is necessary to cut the main bile duct (e. g., with a pancreaticoduodenectomy) it is best to do so closer to the hilum.

The veins draining the bile ducts usually exit in parallel to the corresponding described arteries along the borders of the common bile duct. Veins draining the gallbladder terminate into the right portal branch and into the hepatic parenchyma in the branch of the right portal vein or the middle suprahepatic vein. In patients with portal hypertension, these veins can be particularly large and the source of unwanted hemorrhage. In portal thrombosis, the large collateral venous channels in the portal pedicle are hypertrophied veins of this system.

Lymphatic Drainage

The lymphatic drainage of the extrahepatic biliary tract distributes into two principal pathways. One exists superiorly with nodes along the cystic duct, hepatic artery, medial aspect of the portal vein, and celiac axis; and another inferiorly with nodes along the cystic duct, anterolateral aspect of the portal vein, posterior pancreas, between the aorta and vena cava, and the left para-aortic area under the left renal vein. In gallbladder carcinoma, metastasis to the parenchyma of the liver by lymphatic spread alone occurs in up to 16 percent of patients. Tumors of the gallbladder and bile ducts can be extensive and, therefore, difficult to treat for cure.

In summary, the functional anatomy divides the liver into two hemilivers by the main hepatic scissura within which the middle hepatic vein runs. In many countries, segmental anatomy has become very popular among surgeons. The definition of these segments according to Couinaud's nomenclature is different from concepts described by Healey and Schroy and Gold-

smith and Woodburne in that the Anglo-Saxon literature refers to Couinaud's sector as a "segment" and his segments become "sub-segments." Finally, Couinaud initially described anatomy in the "bench" or "table" position, and the anatomy must be conceptualized in the in situ position for proper interpretation of imaging studies and operative anatomy. These last two misconceptions are implicated as the main causes for the discrepancies in the interpretation and use of the Couinaud segmental anatomy by many Anglo-Saxon surgeons.

The Real Anatomy

The arterial and portal blood supply to the liver is terminal and the scissurae are interposed only by hepatic sinusoids. Therefore, if a vascular pedicle has been interrupted, the hepatic parenchyma at the scissural limits is devascularized. This devascularization causes a distinct and quite remarkable change in the color of the parenchyma because there are no anastomotic collaterals to maintain the blood supply to that particular segment. Portal segmentation is absolutely independent of the gross liver surface anatomy as in the classic morphologic description. Conversely, the functional anatomy honors the segmental parenchymal vascularization, and subsequent transection of a portal scissura respects the vessels and bile ducts within that segment. Since the main portal scissurae remain constant, without anatomic markings to locate other scissurae, the knowledge of the real anatomy as opposed to the theoretical anatomy is the fundamental basis for all modern hepatic surgery.

Recent progress with imaging techniques, particularly intraoperative ultrasound, has allowed surgeons to know the precise or real anatomy of the individuals they operate on, including variations that could alter the operative technique. Recognition of the vascular distribution within the liver is the first major step before initiating liver resection. The three hepatic veins and the portal scissurae can be accurately located and their positions marked with small incisions on Glisson's capsule. Intraoperative ultrasound is even more useful for locating the main portal branches inside the liver and thus facilitates true segmental resection, for example, when isolated segmental resection is contemplated. Similarly, the knowledge that there is an inferior branch to the right hepatic vein might significantly change the operative approach in certain situations. Frequent and repeat intraoperative ultrasound evaluation of the margin of resection in relation to both the lesion and hepatic vasculature has contributed to refinements in the techniques of hepatobiliary surgery. In addition, more precise definition of the individual segments to be resected can be performed with ultrasound-guided dye injection into the appropriate segmental portal branch or by balloon catheter occlusion. These particular techniques make indispensable comprehension of the real anatomy possible.

Anatomic Surgery of the Liver

Classification of the Hepatectomies According to the Anatomy

Liver resections can be separated into two groups with the first termed *typical hepatectomies* ("réglées"), which are defined as resection of a portion of hepatic parenchyma following one or several anatomic scissurae. These resections can be referred to as hepatectomies (left or right), sectorectomies, and segmentectomies, according to the Couinaud classification, depending on which segment or groups of segments are resected. The second group is called *atypical hepatectomies* and consists of resection of a portion of parenchyma not limited by anatomic scissurae. This resection should be differentiated from wedge resections, which are considered *minor* hepatectomies.

The most common types of *typical* hepatectomies can be separated into two groups. First, there is the right hepatectomy consisting of four segments (segments 5, 6, 7, and 8) and the left hepatectomy consisting of three segments (segments 2, 3, and 4). Both are determined by the line of transection of the main portal scissurae, which functionally separate the right and left livers as described by Couinaud. Second, there is the right lobectomy consisting of five segments (segments 4, 5, 6, 7, and 8) and the left lobectomy consisting of two segments (segments 2 and 3), which are both determined by the line of

transection of the umbilical fissure, first described by Lortat–Jacob. The Anglo-Saxon literature frequently uses the terms right or left lobectomy to define what is, in fact, a right or left hepatectomy according to the Couinaud classification. In our opinion, it is preferable not to use the term lobectomy when referring to a resection of a portion of the liver that does not correspond to the anatomic definition of a lobe as previously described. In order to maintain the terminology of the functional anatomy and avoid confusion, we have recently proposed to completely avoid the term right lobectomy for any type of *right* liver resection and use the term right hepatectomy extended to segment 4 (segments 4, 5, 6, 7, and 8 or right and quadrate lobe), which is equivalent to the right lobectomy or trisegmentectomy of Starzl and colleagues. A right hepatectomy extended to segments 4 and 1 (segments 1, 4, 5, 6, 7, and 8 or the right, quadrate and caudate lobes) is not distinguished in the Anglo-Saxon literature. This combination is frequently overlooked when larger series of liver resections are reviewed, as any hepatic resection to include segment 1 is a considerably more technically involved procedure and a considerable technical task even in the hands of a trained hepatobiliary surgeon. In regard to the left liver, when describing resection of the classic left lobe, it seems difficult to avoid mention of the left lobectomy since the term left lateral segmentectomy is anatomically inaccurate because the true left posterolateral segment (the only sector of Couinaud composed of one single segment) consists only of segment 2.

The typical hepatectomies can be divided into four groups according to the number of resected segments. The first group is the *extended* hepatectomies (superextended and extended), the second group includes the *major* hepatectomies, the third is the *limited* hepatectomies, and the fourth is the *segmental* hepatectomies.

Superextended hepatectomies correspond to resection of *six or more* segments on the right, which is the right hepatectomy (segments 5, 6, 7, and 8) extended to include segments 1 and 4 (Fig. 90-10). Similarly, they correspond to at least *five or more* segments on the left, for example, a combination that includes the left hepatectomy (segments 2, 3, and 4) extended to segment 1 and segment 5 or 8. *Extended hepatectomies* correspond to resection of *five* seg-

ments on the right such as the right hepatectomy (segments 5, 6, 7, and 8) extended to segment 4 or 1 and at least *four* segments on the left such as the left hepatectomy (segments 2, 3, and 4) extended to segment 1 or 5 or 8. *Major hepatectomies* consist of *four* segments (Fig. 90-11) on the right such as right hepatectomy (segments 5, 6, 7, and 8) and *three* left or central segments such as left hepatectomy (segments 2, 3, and 4) and central hepatectomy (segments 4, 5, and 6). *Limited hepatectomies* include resection of *two* segments (Fig. 90-12) such as with left lobectomy (segments 2 and 3) or bisegmentectomy (segments 4 and 5 or 6 and 7 or 5 and 8). *Segmentectomies* are resection of one single Couinaud segment and *subsegmentectomy* refers to the partial anatomic resection of a portion of a segment such as anterior (subsegment 4b) or inferior (subsegment 4a) quadrate subsegmentectomy. This last classification should not be mistaken for *atypical* hepatectomy, which is not determined by anatomic scissurae and describes removal of a lesion with a margin of normal parenchyma. Furthermore, the term *minor* hepatectomy should be used to describe a *wedge resection* and not be confused with an *enucleation* or a *biopsy specimen*, which are not considered hepatectomies according to our classification. The other liver resection combinations are theoretically numerous and any combination of individual or associated segmentectomies can be described. Although there are many different methods to describe hepatectomies in the literature, which often makes comparisons between series very difficult, application of the numeric segments as described by Couinaud according to our classification permits universal application regardless of the terminology used (Fig. 90-13).

Classification According to Surgical Technique

Several technical conceptions of typical hepatectomies can be described (see Fig. 90-14) which utilize knowledge of the liver's functional and real anatomy.

Hepatectomy with Preliminary Vascular Ligation

This technique was first described by Lortat–Jacob and colleagues and consists of ligating and dividing the portal pedicle and hepatic vein before the parenchymal transection. The right portal pedicle (vein and artery) is ligated en bloc and sectioned

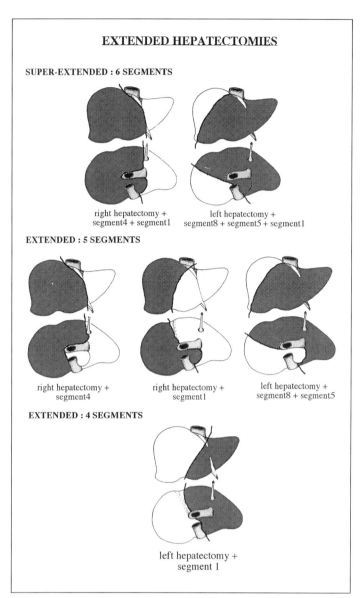

EXTENDED HEPATECTOMIES

SUPER-EXTENDED : 6 SEGMENTS

right hepatectomy +
segment4 + segment1

left hepatectomy +
segment8 + segment5 + segment1

EXTENDED : 5 SEGMENTS

right hepatectomy +
segment4

right hepatectomy +
segment1

left hepatectomy +
segment8 + segment5

EXTENDED : 4 SEGMENTS

left hepatectomy +
segment 1

Fig. 90-10. Superextended hepatectomies include resection of at least six segments on the right and at least five on the left. Extended hepatectomies include five on the right and four on the left.

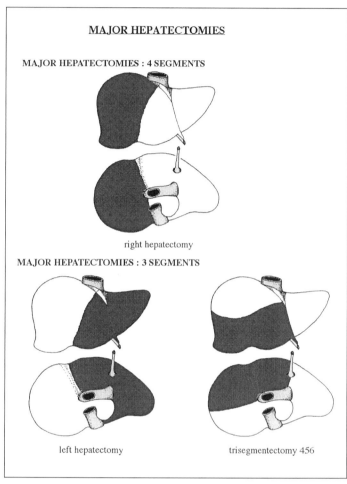

MAJOR HEPATECTOMIES

MAJOR HEPATECTOMIES : 4 SEGMENTS

right hepatectomy

MAJOR HEPATECTOMIES : 3 SEGMENTS

left hepatectomy

trisegmentectomy 456

Fig. 90-11. Major hepatectomies include resection of four segments on the right and three segments on the left. Note that the term trisegmentectomy *refers to three Couinaud segments.*

at the hilus, then continues with ligation and section of the right hepatic vein before the parenchymal transection. This technique of primary devascularization permits demarcation of the border between the two livers and facilitates resection to decrease intraoperative bleeding from the portal and arterial branches. Unfortunately, the dissection of the hepatic vein can be dangerous and can lead to disastrous consequences with a major risk of inadvertently tearing or penetrating this large vein or the vena cava itself, a complication that can be difficult to control and

can cause an air embolism. Subsequently, for this reason, Lortat–Jacob suggested that dissection of the right hepatic vein be preceded with control of the inferior vena cava above and below the liver. This technique of primary vascular control of the liver affords two distinct advantages by permitting the exact border between the right and left liver to be visualized by parenchymal devascularization, and the complete vascular control results in decreased operative bleeding. However, the disadvantages of this technique include the risk of causing injury to the hepatic

vein, inability to easily control the middle and inferior branches of the right hepatic vein, and the danger of devitalizing a portion of the remaining liver by erroneous ligation of an element in the porta hepatis (such as the biliary confluence), a hazard that is increased by the frequency of anatomic variations.

Hepatectomy by Primary Parenchymal Transection

The principle of this technique, described by Ton That Tung, begins initially with an

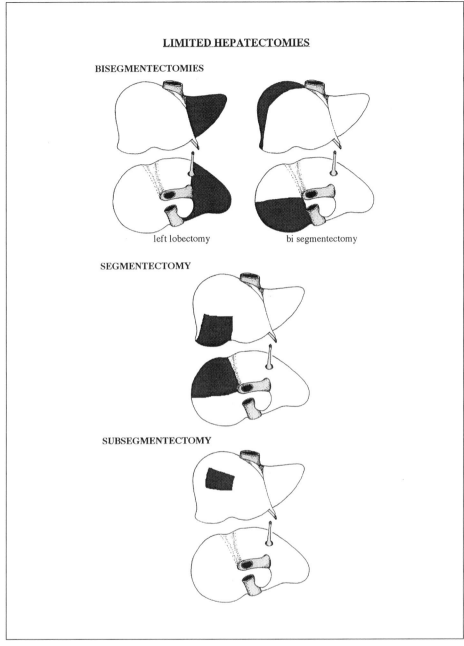

LIMITED HEPATECTOMIES

BISEGMENTECTOMIES

left lobectomy   bi segmentectomy

SEGMENTECTOMY

SUBSEGMENTECTOMY

Fig. 90-12. Limited hepatectomies include resection of two segments such as a left lobectomy (segments 2 and 3) and bisegmentectomy (such as segments 6 and 7 or 5 and 8) (central bisegmentectomy).

able intraoperative bleeding because of the lack of primary vascular control, which mandates expeditious completion of the procedure. Secondary intermittent clamping of the porta hepatis might be necessary to control bleeding.

Hepatectomy by Selective Clamping

This procedure, which the authors use, has been previously described and is characterized by a combination of the previous two techniques, while seeking to avoid their disadvantages. The principle of this technique begins with the hilar dissection in order to obtain isolated control of the arterial and portal elements of the right pedicle (for a right hepatectomy), and these structures are clamped without initial ligation. The right side of the retrohepatic vena cava (including the inferior vena caval ligament) is freed without attempting to dissect the vena cava and the right hepatic vein. Once this step is completed and the appropriate portions of the liver are mobilized, the parenchyma is opened along the plane of the main portal scissurae, as in the Ton That Tung technique, and the portal elements are located and divided through a superior approach from within the parenchyma. Ligation of the vessels is performed distal to the clamped portal pedicle, and the hepatic vein is ligated from inside the liver at the completion of the parenchymal transection. This technique combines the advantages of the Lortat–Jacob technique with control of the vessels before liver resection but without transection, and the benefit of the technique of Ton That Tung, which individually divides and ligates the vessels from within the hepatic parenchyma, a feature that permits surgical modification for potential anatomic variations. We refer to this technique as hepatectomy by *selective* (right or left) *clamping.*

Hepatectomy Under Total Vascular Occlusion

Resection of large central tumors close to the vena cava or the hepatic veins might be facilitated by the use of total vascular occlusion. This procedure, initially described by Heaney and Jacobson, is achieved by simultaneous clamping of the hepatic pedicle and vena cava above and below the liver after full mobilization of

incision into the parenchyma along the line of the scissura, the hilar elements are approached and ligated from within the liver during the parenchymal transection, and the procedure is completed with section of the hepatic vein as previously described but from inside the liver. The advantages to this technique are twofold: first, it excises the liver parenchyma *à la*

demande according to the nature and location of the lesion; and second, the ligation of the vessels is not hampered by anatomic abnormalities since the vessels are approached from above the hilus within the liver—only the vessels in direct relationship to the resected portion of the liver are ligated. The disadvantages to this technique include the possibility of consider-

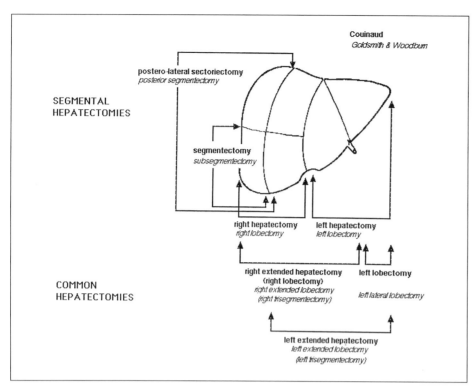

SEGMENTAL
HEPATECTOMIES

Couinaud
Goldsmith & Woodburn

postero-lateral sectoriectomy
posterior segmentectomy

segmentectomy
subsegmentectomy

right hepatectomy
right lobectomy

left hepatectomy
left lobectomy

COMMON
HEPATECTOMIES

right extended hepatectomy
(right lobectomy)
right extended lobectomy
(right trisegmentectomy)

left lobectomy
left lateral lobectomy

left extended hepatectomy
left extended lobectomy
(left trisegmentectomy)

Fig. 90-13. The various hepatectomies as described by the two most commonly used descriptions in the literature: Couinaud (bold) and Goldsmith and Woodburne (italic). Note that the sectors of Couinaud are composed of two segments.

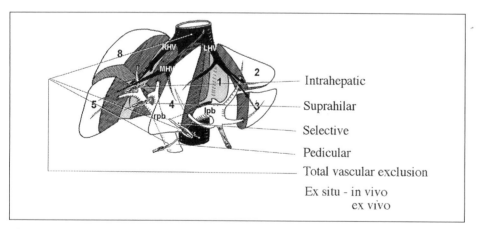

Intrahepatic
Suprahilar
Selective
Pedicular
Total vascular exclusion
Ex situ - in vivo
ex vivo

Fig. 90-14. Various modalities of obtaining vascular control during the parenchymal dissection. Pedicle clamping or the Pringle maneuver, selective clamping of either the right or left portal pedicle, suprahilar clamping for sectorial devascularization, and intrahepatic clamping are all methods that can be applied. The total vascular exclusion is obtained after dissection and clamping the IVC above and below the liver, combined with main portal pedicle clamping. All these clamping procedures offer control without ligation. RHV = right hepatic vein; MHV = middle hepatic vein; LHV = left hepatic vein; rpb = right portal branch; lpb = left portal branch; IVC = inferior vena cava. Each number represents the corresponding segment.

the liver plus ligation and division of the right adrenal vein (Fig. 90-14). The liver parenchyma can tolerate 60 to 90 minutes of devascularization in normothermic conditions. However, with this technique, the anatomic margins are not visible, a considerable disadvantage when an extended hepatectomy is being performed since only the main scissurae are easily located. In addition, any injury to the hepatic veins and retrohepatic vena cava can often go unnoticed until liver reperfusion is initiated.

Hepatectomy with Intermittent Pedicle Clamping

Pringle was the first to describe en bloc portal pedicle clamping to control hepatic bleeding during liver trauma. This technique interrupts all the inflow to the liver parenchyma while leaving the hepatic vein outflow intact. This technique can be very useful with all types of hepatectomies; however, the anatomic markings are not evident. In the normal noncirrhotic liver, intervals of intermittent clamping for 15 minutes are well tolerated. However, in the cirrhotic liver, alternate clamping for up to 10 minutes before reperfusion can be performed with no upper limits to the amount of time the pedicle can be clamped. This technique can be very useful in the cirrhotic patient when the parenchyma tends to bleed profusely. Application of gentle pressure on the liver will control the bleeding during the reperfusion intervals. During these reperfusion periods, we recommend frequent and repeat intraoperative ultrasound assessment with attention to the line of transection relative to the hepatic vasculature, thus continuously applying the real liver anatomy in a dynamic fashion.

Hepatectomy by Suprahilar Clamping

This technique offers the possibility to obtain super-selective (suprahilar) clamping by dissecting the hilar plate and exposing the sectorial branches of the portal pedicle (Fig. 90-14). The easiest branch to control is the anterior right sectorial portal branch. At this branch, sectorial devascularization can be accomplished with resultant demarcation on the liver surface, a maneuver that can greatly facilitate right anterior or posterior bisegmentectomies.

Hepatectomy by Intrahepatic Portal Control

Occlusion of the portal vein branch to the segment (Fig. 90-14) to be resected can be achieved by transhepatic balloon catheter placement under ultrasound control combined with selective hepatic artery clamping. Segmental or subsegmental devascularization is attained with clear demarcation on the liver surface of the corresponding parenchymal distribution. This technique is particularly useful for anatomic segmentectomy or subsegmentectomy. A similar technique involves the ultrasound control to locate the segmental portal branch, and with a needle methylene blue dye is injected into a small tributary near the lesion. This technique elegantly demarcates, with a conspicuous blue color, the functional parenchymal segment or subsegment branch, thus mapping out the area of resection before transection.

In parenchymal transection, the quality of the liver can vary greatly depending on the underlying diseases, such as steatosis and cirrhosis. However, neoadjuvant chemotherapy also affects the parenchyma, and the quality of parenchyma and capacity for bleeding varies from patient to patient even when the parenchyma is normal. These differences require the surgeon to be able to adapt different techniques of vascular control as dictated by a particular situation. The parenchymal transection techniques include crushing techniques using finger-fracture (digitoclasy) or a Kelly clamp (Kellyclasy). In our experience, ultrasound dissection is very useful and allows meticulous dissection of small vessels and bile ducts and permits elective ligation. It must be emphasized that this technique removes a portion of the liver parenchyma within the plane of dissection, a factor that must be considered when tumor margins are evaluated. This situation becomes especially relevant for large tumors when the margin on the final pathology specimen might not accurately reflect the true margin known to have been obtained during the actual resection.

In conclusion, intimate knowledge of the morphologic, functional, and real anatomy is a prerequisite for anatomic liver resection. A surgeon must be able to determine which type of resection is warranted, and depending on the amount of tissue to be resected, appropriate choice of vascular control and parenchymal transection must be adapted. There are many different types of liver resections, depending on the amount of tissue to be resected and the surgical technique selected. In this regard, we believe that operative ultrasound has a fundamental role in the effective application of the Couinaud segmental anatomy, the basic functional unit of all anatomic descriptions. Information obtained with intraoperative ultrasound can supplement preoperative investigations by adding the element of anatomic reality to the individual patient and aid in refining the techniques of a successful anatomic resection.

Suggested Reading

Appleby CH. Indwelling common duct tubes. *J Int Coll Surg* 31:631, 1959.

Bismuth H. Surgical anatomy and anatomical surgery of the liver. *World J Surg* 6:3, 1982.

Bismuth H, Houssin D, Castaing D. Major and minor segmentectomies "reglées" in liver surgery. *World J Surg* 6:10, 1982.

Bismuth H, Castaing D, Garden OJ. Major hepatic resection with total vascular exclusion. *Ann Surg* 210:13, 1989.

Castaing D, Emond J, Kunstlinger F, et al. Utility of operative ultrasound in surgery of liver tumors. *Ann Surg* 204:600, 1986.

Castaing D, Garden J, Bismuth H. Segmental liver resection using ultrasound-guided selective portal venous occlusion. *Ann Surg* 210:20, 1989.

Couinaud C. Le Foie-Études Anatomiques et Chirurgicales. Paris: Masson, 1957.

Goldsmith NA, Woodburne RT. Surgical anatomy pertaining to liver resection. *Surg Gynecol Obstet* 195:310, 1957.

Healey JE, Schroy P. The anatomy of the bile ducts within the human liver: An analysis of the prevailing patterns of branching and their major variations. *Arch Surg* 66:599, 1953.

Heaney JP, Jacobson A. Simplified control of upper abdominal hemorrhage from the vena cava. *Surgery* 78:138, 1975.

Hodgson W, Delguergio L. Preliminary experience in liver surgery using ultrasonic scalpel. *Surgery* 95:230, 1984.

Hörstjö CH. The topography of the intrahepatic duct system. *Acta Anat* 11:599, 1931.

Huguet C, Nordlinger B, Galopin JJ, et al. Normothermic hepatic vascular exclusion for extensive hepatectomy. *Surg Gynecol Obstet* 147:389, 1978.

Lin YT. Results of 107 hepatic lobectomies with a preliminary report on the use of a clamp to reduce blood loss. *Ann Surg* 177:413, 1973.

Lortat-Jacob JL, Robert HG, Henry C. Un cas d'hépatectomie droite reglée. *Mem Academie Chirurgie* 78:244, 1952.

Makuuchi M, Hasegawa H, Yamasaki S, et al. The inferior right hepatic vein: Ultrasonic demonstration. *Radiology* 148:213, 1983.

McIndoe AH, Counseller VX. A report on the bilaterality of the liver. *Arch Surg* 15:589, 1927.

Moosman DA. The surgical significance of six anomalies of the biliary duct system. *Surg Gynecol Obstet* 131:665, 1970.

Northover JMA, Terblanche J. A new look at the arterial blood supply of the bile duct in man and its surgical implications. *Br J Surg* 66:379, 1979.

Padbury R, Azoulay D. *Anatomy: Surgery of the Biliary Tract*. Edinburgh: Churchill-Livingstone, 1993.

Phillip J, Koch H, Classen M. Variations and anomalies of the papilla of Vater, the pancreas and the biliary duct system. *Endoscopy* 6:70, 1974.

Pringle JH. Note on the arrest of hepatic hemorrhage due to trauma. *Ann Surg* 48:541, 1908.

Rocko JM, Swan KG, Di Gioia JM. Calot's triangle revisited. *Surg Gynecol Obstet* 153:410, 1981.

Starzl TE, Bell RH, Beart RW, et al. Hepatic trisegmentectomy and the other liver resection. *Surg Gynecol Obstet* 14:429, 1975.

Tung TT. Chirurgie d'exerese du Foie. Paris: Masson, 1962.

Tung TT. La Vascularisation Veinuese du Foie et ses Applications aux Résections Hépatique. Hanoi: These, 1939.

Tung TT, Dong Quang N. L'hépatectomie par ligature vasculaire transparenchymateuse. *Presse Med* 73:3015, 1965.

Wood D. Eponyms in biliary tract surgery. *Am J Surg* 138:746, 1979.

91

Diagnostic Considerations in Liver Disease

Byers W. Shaw, Jr.   Rakesh Sindhi   Thomas G. Heffron

Optimizing the care of patients with liver disease involves establishing the most accurate diagnosis possible. As in many areas of medicine, surgeons tread cautiously on a fine line between a shotgun approach to diagnostic evaluations and overly prejudicial presumptions regarding the probable diagnosis. A happy medium provides optimum care in a situation complicated by the fact that many patients have already undergone a partial work-up of their chief complaint before they see the surgeon. In such instances, the focus of the diagnostic evaluation has already been narrowed, and the journey the surgeon travels with the patient has already been steered in a certain direction. The journey must begin with a careful history, physical examination, and review of all available records. Surgeons should narrow their diagnostic hunches substantially before they order that first additional test.

Biliary Tract Disease

The patient with biliary tract disease most often presents with pain or jaundice, or both. Other presenting complaints can include fever, weight loss, pruritus, a palpable mass in the right upper quadrant, or a change in stool color or consistency. Figure 91-1 illustrates some of the early diagnostic considerations in evaluating patients who are referred to the surgeon for evaluation of possible biliary tract disease.

Cholecystitis and Cholelithiasis

Biliary colic characteristically follows a fatty meal, is crampy in nature, is located in the right upper quadrant, and can ra-

diate into the right shoulder or subscapular region. It can persist for several minutes to several hours, but rarely longer unless acute cholecystitis or, more ominously, cholangitis develops. The student of surgery is well versed in the identification of the classic risk factors for cholelithiasis, commonly referred to as the four-F's: fat, female, fertile, and forty.

One wonders whether the cost-conscious surgeon with a patient who satisfies all the risk factor demographics and has the typical history should proceed with any additional evaluation beyond what is necessary to prepare for surgery, particularly since the laparoscopic approach has so dramatically eased the difficulty of recovery for most patients. Often, however, neither the history nor the risk factors are all classic, and additional tests might be warranted.

Most of us obtain a routine liver function panel to determine whether the patient has evidence of hepatitis masquerading as acute biliary colic or cholecystitis. Although any of these illnesses can elevate the serum transaminase levels slightly, dramatic elevations, on the order of 10 to 20 times normal or more, should raise the surgeon's suspicions of a different diagnosis or an additional diagnosis beyond cholelithiasis. The additional diagnosis of acute cholecystitis is entertained if fever is present. If the patient also has an elevated serum bilirubin level or is jaundiced, acute cholangitis should be suspected. In the face of biliary obstruction, ascending cholangitis can develop, requiring urgent intervention.

Virtually every patient who undergoes an operation for cholelithiasis or acute cho-

lecystitis has had an abdominal ultrasound. In most patients, routine abdominal ultrasound carries a high degree of sensitivity and specificity in diagnosing either cholelithiasis or acute cholecystitis. The success of ultrasound is dampened by obesity, large amounts of air (usually intraluminal), or situations that block adequate access to the optimum scanning site, such as large wounds or dressings. Under optimal conditions, stones as small as 3 mm can be identified with modern ultrasound. Ultrasound can also identify dilatation of the intrahepatic biliary tract, a finding that should alter one's approach, as we will note later.

If cholelithiasis or evidence of cholecystitis (thickened gallbladder, pericholecystic fluid, or, in more severe cases, gas in the gallbladder wall) is identified by routine ultrasound, if the bile ducts do not appear to be dilated, and if no other lesions are found, no further diagnostic tests are necessary before undertaking the surgical procedure. However, if biliary tract dilatation is noted and is associated with jaundice, with or without the onset of fever, the surgeon might want to evaluate the presence of biliary tract obstruction as discussed below.

The advent of laparoscopic cholecystectomy in combination with advanced techniques for endoscopic evaluation and treatment of biliary tract lesions has dramatically altered the routine diagnostic approach to biliary tract obstruction. Specifically, if the obstruction can be relieved before cholecystectomy, routine laparoscopic cholecystectomy in a stable, nonseptic patient can usually be accomplished.

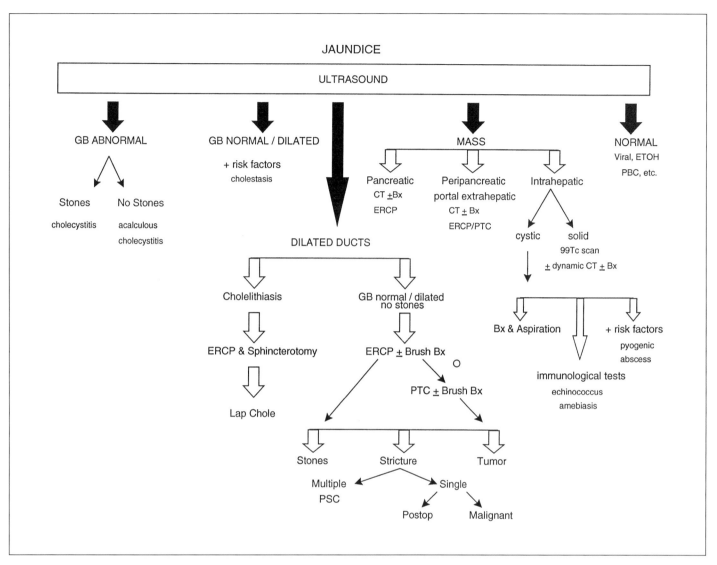

Fig. 91-1. Algorithmic approach to evaluation of biliary tract disease. GB = gallbladder; CT = computed tomography; ERCP = endoscopic retrograde pancreaticocholangiograph; PSC = primary sclerosing cholangitis; ETOH = ethanol; PBC = primary biliary cirrhosis; Bx = biopsy; PTC = percutaneous transhepatic cholangiography.

Surgeons should be cautious when a patient presents with fever, right upper quadrant pain, and an ultrasound that does not show stones. The level of concern should be further raised if the patient has AIDS or is a victim of major trauma or burns, particularly if there is an antecedent history of hemodynamic instability, prolonged mechanical ventilation, total parenteral nutrition, or recent episodes of sepsis. If, on examination, the patient is exquisitely tender below the right costal margin, a diagnosis of acalculous cholecystitis should be entertained, particularly if there is a palpable mass.

The ultrasound can be helpful in this situation if it shows gallbladder wall edema or pericholecystic fluid. However, remember that the patient with congestive heart failure, or ascites and hypoalbuminemia from liver disease or nephrotic syndrome, might have a swollen gallbladder in the absence of acute infection. CT scans offer little additional information. Cholescintigraphy can be helpful, but in our experience, many patients in the intensive care unit have abnormal examinations merely on the basis of bile stasis, viscid bile, and poor gallbladder contractility. A normal scan, however, is inconsistent with acalculous cholecystitis.

Acalculous cholecystitis probably accounts for fewer than 5 to 10 percent of instances of cholecystitis in adults but up to 30 percent of instances in children. Although most cases of cholecystitis in children are related to stone disease and occur more commonly in patients with hemolytic disorders (e. g., sickle cell disease), congenital cystic duct stenosis, acute streptococcal infections, and even (as we saw during the summer of 1995) tick-borne relapsing fever (*Borrelia recurrentis*) can be causative.

One should have a sense of urgency in making a diagnosis of acalculous cholecystitis and proceed to emergency treatment, primarily because the mortality in patients who are already quite ill is very high, almost twice the rate associated with acute calculous cholecystitis. The incidence of gangrene of the gallbladder and perforation is also much higher in this disease. In the unstable patient, percutaneous cholecystostomy under ultrasound or CT guidance can be lifesaving.

Choledocholithiasis and Biliary Strictures

If routine ultrasound reveals dilatation of the intrahepatic bile ducts, one should evaluate the presence and possible causes of biliary tract obstruction. In the face of typical biliary colic with or without an acute cholecystitis, the most likely diagnosis is choledocholithiasis. Dilatation of the intra- and extrahepatic biliary tree suggests a distal location of an obstructing stone. In this instance, provided the services of an experienced endoscopist are available, endoscopic retrograde cholangiography will reveal the location of the obstruction and suggest its treatment, including sphincterotomy with endoscopic stone extraction. Except in instances in which stones are extremely large, endoscopic extraction should be successful in most patients. Transhepatic cholangiography might reveal the presence of the stone, but because removal of the stone from this approach requires pushing it out from above, rather than pulling it from below, this test is usually not the best for evaluating the patient who might need intervention. If the stone can be removed and the obstruction relieved before laparoscopic cholecystectomy, classic common bile exploration can be avoided.

Returning to Fig. 91-1, we need to consider the rest of the differential diagnosis in a patient who presents with jaundice. Once again, we review the available records to narrow the list of possibilities.

Does the patient have a history of significant alcohol abuse, a prior history of pancreatitis, or any other risk factors for pancreatitis such as hypercholesterolemia, medications (glucocorticoids, oral contraceptives, thiazide diuretics, azathioprine and acetaminophen)? Subacute or chronic pancreatitis, with or without pancreatic pseudocyst, can present with jaundice, which is less painful than one would expect with full-blown acute pancreatitis.

Again, a search in the records for the liver function panel might provide important clues, including confirmation that one is dealing with obstructive jaundice, rather than jaundice associated with one of the various causes of hepatitis (e. g., viruses, drugs, or other toxins).

Assuming that the history, physical examination, and initial screening laboratory tests continue to support a diagnosis of biliary tract obstruction, we once again move toward our standard use of abdominal ultrasound to identify biliary tract dilatation. One could again argue that in a more cost-conscious atmosphere, one might actually be able to omit the ultrasound and proceed directly to endoscopic cholangiography, since there can be fairly overwhelming evidence that the patient has obstructive biliary tract disease. However, ultrasound might give some indication of the location of the obstruction as well the likelihood of success with either transhepatic or endoscopic cholangiography.

Dilated intrahepatic ducts with a normal extrahepatic duct might lead one to consider an initial transhepatic approach to cholangiography, particularly if endoscopic expertise is not readily available. However, in most larger hospitals, good endoscopic cholangiographic services are available and would be our first choice, almost regardless of what the ultrasound showed. The ultrasound can be helpful in rare instances in identifying a mass lesion, either within the liver or the pancreas, associated with obstructive jaundice. In this situation, the decision to perform either ultrasound or CT scan imaging of the liver before cholangiography is best guided by the surgeon's notion of the most likely diagnosis after obtaining the history and performing the physical examination.

For example, the 58-year-old man with painless jaundice, palpable mass, and marked weight loss probably has pancreatic carcinoma. In this circumstance, an ultrasound might reveal a mass in the head of the pancreas that would make an endoscopic approach to the bile duct difficult, if not impossible, leading one to perform percutaneous cholangiography first, particularly when there is intrahepatic ductal dilatation present. In contrast, the 55-year-old man with a long-standing history of ulcerative colitis, with or without a known diagnosis of primary sclerosing cholangitis, most likely requires cholangi-

ography and would not be likely to have a mass lesion on routine ultrasound that would alter the initial diagnostic approach.

Because of the need to use both oral and intravenous contrast in performing CT scan evaluation of the liver, we do not view it as the best initial screening tool for biliary tract lesions. Instead, we reserve CT scanning for the definitive evaluation of mass lesions initially seen on ultrasound or in the performance of a metastatic work-up for either primary or secondary hepatic malignancies. We believe that CT scanning is notoriously inaccurate in evaluating lesions in the hilum of the liver and in the distal common bile duct.

An initial endoscopic approach to the evaluation of biliary tract lesions should include the possibility of therapeutic intervention at the same setting. As mentioned, stone extraction, with or without sphincterotomy, can provide immediate relief of obstructive jaundice and cholangitis. Similarly, temporary stenting of obstructive distal bile duct lesions associated with primary sclerosing cholangitis, or even malignancy, can provide immediate relief of the symptoms of obstructive jaundice.

Of equal value, the endoscopist should be able to perform both biopsy and brush cytology of any suspicious lesions within the bile ducts on initial evaluation, including lesions up to and above the right and left hepatic ducts. One should remember, however, that cytologic specimens must be obtained before the placement of indwelling stents because of the frequent association of cytologic atypia in patients who have had a stent in place for more than a few days. The best chance of obtaining a proper diagnosis of a suspected biliary tract malignancy is during the initial encounter with the lesion, before endoscopic or percutaneous placement of stents. The exceptions to this rule are patients with obvious acute cholangitis, especially patients with hemodynamic instability associated with overt sepsis, in whom the first goal is to relieve biliary obstruction.

Of further concern, exploratory surgery is not justified until an effort has been made to make a diagnosis by nonoperative means. The presence of enlarged lymph nodes in the area should prompt CT-guided percutaneous biopsy of these nodes as well. Obtaining a specific tissue diagnosis and a metastatic work-up before undertaking any surgery will avoid surprises at the time of laparotomy and make it more likely that definitive treatment can be accomplished in a single operation. Another concern of importance is that in our experience, cholangiocarcinoma is associated with a high risk of intraperitoneal spread from operative biopsy or from exploration of the bile duct when intraluminal tumor is present.

Patients with jaundice and serum liver function studies suggesting an obstructive cause, but in whom initial screening ultrasound does not show stones or dilated ducts, might have other causes of severe intrahepatic cholestasis. For instance, a woman in her early-to-late fifties with the insidious onset of itching, fatigue, and painless jaundice and with liver function studies that reveal low-grade elevations of serum transaminases alone and marked elevations of the γ glutamyl transpeptidase (gGTP) might have primary biliary cirrhosis. In this situation, before ordering more invasive tests, the surgeon should consider obtaining serum antimitochondrial antibody titers, antinuclear antibodies, and anti-smooth-muscle antibodies. If these serologic tests are positive, the surgeon should suggest liver biopsy to confirm the diagnosis. One might be even more suspicious of this diagnosis if, on examination, the patient has noticeable hepatosplenomegaly.

Surgeons at a secondary or tertiary care center might have a jaundiced patient who has undergone recent cholecystectomy referred to them. In this instance, diagnostic considerations narrow considerably. An ultrasound is an important initial screening tool to rule out the presence of a biloma or an abscess and to look for ductal dilatation as well. If a fluid collection is seen that raises suspicions about a biloma and if there is ductal dilatation, an initial percutaneous approach might allow one to both drain the biloma and obtain transhepatic control of the injured bile duct. This point is particularly relevant since the injury is most likely near the confluence of the right and left hepatic ducts or in the right hepatic duct itself.

Many iatrogenic bile duct injuries require direct surgical intervention. Once again, initial control with a transhepatic tube can make surgical reconstruction that much easier. Furthermore, in complete obstruction of the bile duct, a transhepatic approach provides initial drainage while preparing the patient for surgery. This step might be very important in the patient who presents with a septic course and obstructive jaundice. Thus, in most instances, the diagnostic evaluation of a patient with iatrogenic bile duct injury is better facilitated by a transhepatic, as opposed to an endoscopic, approach to initial cholangiography (Fig. 91-2).

Although it is not a focus of this chapter, congenital biliary tract anomalies must also be considered in a patient whose initial evaluation does not suggest more common diagnostic possibilities. The presentation of intermittent episodes of jaundice in an adolescent might make one consider a choledochal cyst. Although rare, Alagille's syndrome (arterohepatic dysplasia) might not cause jaundice until late childhood or even young adulthood. This au-

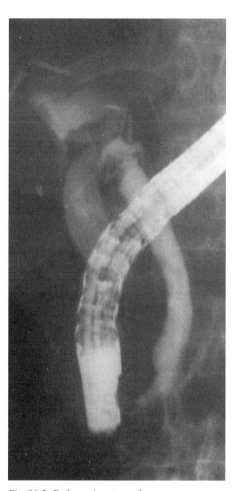

Fig. 91-2. Endoscopic retrograde pancreaticocholangiograph (ERCP) showing extravasation from transected (extrahepatic) CBD after laparoscopic cholecystectomy. The intrahepatic bile ducts are not visualized.

tosomal dominant syndrome with variable expression and penetrance is identified by a paucity of intrahepatic bile ducts associated with characteristic facies, hepatosplenomegaly, eye and bone disorders and, occasionally, mental retardation.

In summary, the surgeon should be able to narrow the diagnostic considerations dramatically after an initial review of the referred patient's records. Although the standard approach to evaluation of biliary tract disease can and has been well-defined by standard algorithms, some of the expensive or invasive diagnostic steps can be omitted when the initial clinical evidence is overwhelmingly in favor of a specific diagnosis. In this regard, the risk of omitting an important diagnostic test is proportional to the surgeon's diagnostic skills of examination and history-taking.

Mass Lesions

A surgeon is often called to see a patient who has a mass lesion of the liver after the lesion has been identified by ultrasound. Many times, ultrasound was obtained as part of the investigation of the cause of abdominal pain.

The surgeon's first step is to determine whether the lesion requires removal. The pertinent questions, in order, are: 1) what is the specific tissue diagnosis of the mass lesion?; 2) does this specific type of lesion require routine resection, regardless of whether any symptoms are attributed to it?; 3) if routine resection is not required, does this patient have symptoms related to the presence of this liver mass that are severe enough to warrant resection?

Most of the time, the initial studies with which the patient comes to the surgeon give significant clues about the most probable diagnosis. The ultrasound can show, with a high degree of accuracy, whether the lesion is cystic or solid. If the lesion is cystic and small, it might represent a simple cyst that is unlikely to require further treatment. However, a large cystic lesion requires further definition. In areas in which such infections are endemic, amebic abscesses and echinococcal cysts are appropriate to consider. Polycystic liver disease, Caroli's disease, pyogenic abscess, cystadenoma, and cystadenocarcinoma are also in the differential diagnosis.

Amebic abscesses, found primarily in the tropics and subtropics, such as Africa, Southeast Asia, Mexico, Venezuela, and Colombia, are generally approximately 5 cm in diameter and are usually located in the right lobe, superoanteriorly, often just below the diaphragm. On CT scan (considered more sensitive than ultrasound for small abscesses), they show an irregular, enhanced rim around a center with lower attenuation than the surrounding liver. The diagnosis can be confirmed by a positive result on indirect amebic hemagglutination tests.

An infestation of the tapeworm *Echinococcus granulosus*, echinococcal cysts are endemic in sheep-raising areas such as South Australia, New Zealand, Africa, South America, southern Europe, and the Middle and Far East. They are usually found in the right lobe of the liver, either anteroinferiorly or posteroinferiorly. Indirect hemagglutination, ELISA, and complement fixation testing provide a diagnosis in approximately 85 percent of instances, with the occurrence of some false negatives and false positives. Initially, these cysts fragment, creating a multiloculated appearance. When old and inactive, they can develop calcification.

Pyogenic abscesses are more likely to be present in patients with a history of previous biliary surgery or in intravenous drug abusers. There is an important association with ascending cholangitis, cholecystitis, obstructive neoplasm, or penetrating injury. Abscesses are more likely to be multiple. Blood cultures are positive in approximately 50 percent of instances, so, when possible, culture of the abscess itself is helpful. Computed tomography can assist both the diagnosis and treatment with percutaneous drainage.

Several syndromes are associated with multiple cysts. For example, multiple intrahepatic cysts with evidence of infection and stones are suggestive of Caroli's disease (congenital hepatic biliary dilatation), a diagnosis that can be confirmed by percutaneous transheptic cholangiogram (PTC) or, as is our usual preference, by endoscopic retrograde pancreatocholangiography (ERCP). Generally, the common bile duct appears normal, but the intrahepatic ducts have bulbous dilatations with normal ducts between.

In autosomal dominant polycystic disease, the liver is diffusely involved with cysts that generally range in size from 1 to 10 cm. Women outnumber men slightly in asymptomatic instances and account for 80 percent of symptomatic instances, which are far more likely to be associated with larger cysts. Single congenital cysts also occur and have been found as large as 15 cm. Fifty percent are associated with smaller adjacent cysts.

Malignant transformation of cysts is rare in association with nonparasitic cysts or polycystic liver disease, occurring more often when the epithelium is exposed to bile. When they do occur, cystic liver tumors are much more likely to be metastatic than primary, occurring commonly with primary tumors of the ovaries, stomach, or hepatobiliary system. The imaging characteristics of malignant cystic tumors resemble the characteristics of benign cysts. Three-fourths occur in women over the age of 40 and are associated with a slight increase in serum transaminase levels. Ultrasound can show septations, mural nodules, or calcification, all of which occur rarely in simple cysts.

When the lesion in question appears to be solid on ultrasound, the first diagnostic consideration is whether the lesion is benign or malignant. Again, examination of the patient's history might be particularly useful. For example, in a patient with known cirrhosis associated with chronic type B or type C hepatitis or alcohol abuse, primary hepatocellular carcinoma becomes a consideration. In any adult with a solid liver lesion, an elevated serum level of alpha-fetoprotein should also create a high degree of suspicion for hepatoma. A history of intra-abdominal malignancy, breast or lung cancer, or malignant skin cancers, particularly melanoma, raises the possibility that the solid lesion in the liver is metastatic.

However, the surgeon should remember that these lesions generally do not present as an incidental solid hepatic mass discovered on routine ultrasound. Instead, they are more likely found as part of routine follow-up examinations for the primary cancer.

Hemangioma is the most common benign neoplasm of the liver. Sometimes, distinguishing these lesions from other solid liver tumors can be challenging. Conventional CT scan can detect lesions as small as 1 to 2 cm but is not very reliable in confirming the diagnosis of hemangioma. A

more appropriate course is to ask the radiologist to perform dynamic CT scanning with delayed images at 30 minutes. Detection and diagnosis of small lesions can require multiple slices at many levels using very rapid scanners. Technetium 99–labeled radionuclide studies have the highest accuracy for lesions greater than 2.0 cm and should be considered the method of choice for noninvasive diagnosis of a large hemangioma. Pooling of radioactive tracer on delayed ^{99m}Tc injections is pathognomonic.

Magnetic resonance imaging (MRI) can be used for lesions too small for detection with radionuclide scanning and for lesions adjacent to the heart or blood vessels. Without requiring contrast, MRI can characterize multiple hemangiomas at multiple levels with greater than 85 percent accuracy in differentiating these lesions from multiple metastases. The T2-weighted images can be used to enhance resolution, creating the classic "light bulb" appearance of a hemangioma (Fig. 91-3). Magnetic resonance angiograms using superparamagnetic iron oxide can allow lesion detection and characterization to the 2 to 4 mm level, thus eventually replacing contrast-dependent vascular imaging in the evaluation of solid liver masses.

Aside from hepatoma and hemangioma, the other diagnostic considerations for a single solid mass in the liver include adenoma, focal nodular hyperplasia, hematoma, focal fatty degeneration, regenerating nodule (in a patient with cirrhosis), and a host of other, less common possibilities. Adenomas and focal nodular hyperplasia occur in premenopausal women more frequently than in men. Adenomas appear to be associated with history of prior use of birth control pills.

If directed use of ultrasound and CT scanning has not yielded a diagnosis with satisfactory certainty, the surgeon has three options: 1) obtain a tissue diagnosis, preferably with CT-guided needle biopsies; 2) explore the patient with a mind toward resection; and 3) follow the lesion for 2 to 3 months to determine whether it is growing.

In reality, the surgeon should have a reasonable hunch about the identity of the lesion at this stage. If there is overwhelming evidence that this is an hemangioma, one proceeds with surgery only if the patient is symptomatic. These lesions do not carry

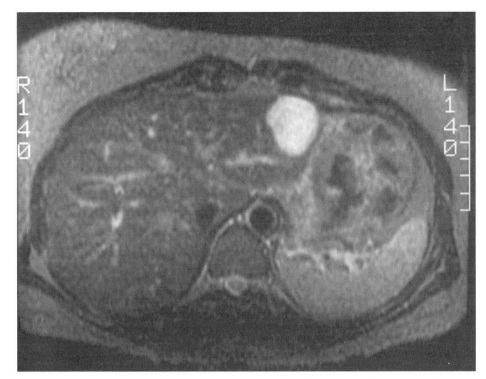

Fig. 91-3. T2-weighted image shows the classic MRI appearance of a hemangioma. The lesion is well defined with very high signal intensity.

malignant potential and rarely cause bleeding.

Since an adenoma carries a risk of eventual hemorrhage and focal nodular hyperplasia does not, we normally proceed with fine-needle biopsy of the lesion and base subsequent therapy on the results. If, even after this study, the diagnosis remains in doubt, we normally proceed with liver resection.

If the remaining distinction is between benign and malignant tumor, then waiting for the lesion to grow might not be wise. Again, CT-guided needle biopsy is warranted to relieve patient anxiety and to proceed to definitive treatment.

In evaluation of multiple lesions in the liver, tissue diagnosis is even more important. If the lesions appear to be metastatic adenocarcinoma, then one's greatest concern should be the extent of the metastatic disease. In this situation, observation of the patient for 2 to 3 months to determine whether new lesions develop in the liver is usually warranted.

Before beginning any resectional therapy for primary or secondary hepatic malignancy, a complete metastatic work-up, including CT scan of the head and chest and bone scan, is warranted. If all these tests are normal, if there is no evidence of continued tumor spread beyond the limits of safe resection, and if no lymph nodes appear to be enlarged enough to warrant percutaneous biopsy, we proceed with exploratory laparoscopy. Perihilar and celiac lymph nodes are examined as well as the diaphragmatic and peritoneal surfaces. Any suspicious lesions are biopsied for immediate frozen section examination. Direct placement of a specialized ultrasound probe on the liver through a laparoscopic portal can result in detection of metastatic lesions in the portion of the liver not known to be affected. One can also gain valuable information regarding the proximity of the known tumor to vascular and biliary structures within the liver. If microscopic examination does not reveal any evidence of metastatic spread and confirms that the tumor remains resectable, then we proceed with open laparotomy and resection.

Bleeding Varices

When we evaluate a patient with bleeding varices, we focus on the issues of their etiology, perhaps already identified by the referring physician, and the severity and pattern of bleeding. Once the etiology is established, our attention turns to such questions as: 1) Is the patient a candidate for something other than standard medical treatments of sclerotherapy or endoscopic ligation? or 2) has such treatment already failed and therefore the patient needs surgical treatment?

Portal hypertension usually follows obstruction to the portal blood flow anywhere along its course and is generally thought of as falling into one of three categories: 1) presinusoidal (changes in the portal vein or its branches within the liver); 2) sinusoidal; and 3) postsinusoidal (obstruction of venous blood flow at or beyond the terminal hepatic venule). Portal hypertension can result from a mixture of these types of lesions (Fig. 91-4).

The origins of presinusoidal portal hypertension include noncirrhotic causes such as portal vein thrombosis associated with hypercoagulable state, infection, pregnancy, tumors, or cirrhosis. Other causes of presinusoidal portal hypertension include schistosomiasis, nodular regenerative hyperplasia, and granulomatous liver disease such as sarcoidosis. Presinusoidal portal hypertension might not be associated with severe liver disease and might not result in other manifestations of portal hypertension, such as ascites or hepatic encephalopathy, until late in its course.

Sinusoidal portal hypertension, resulting from compression or obliteration of hepatic sinusoids, is most often associated with alcoholic cirrhosis or drug-induced liver disease. It is characterized by replacement of the hepatic lobular architecture with regenerating nodules and the replacement of sinusoids by portal-hepatic venous shunts (Fig. 91-4).

Postsinusoidal portal hypertension, a consequence of resistance to outflow from the sinusoids, can follow compression or occlusion of the terminal hepatic veins from a variety of causes, including cirrhosis, alcoholic hepatitis, veno-occlusive disease and thrombosis of the hepatic veins (Budd–Chiari syndrome). It can also result from nonhepatic causes such as constrictive pericarditis and congestive heart failure.

When patients present with esophageal or gastric varices, cirrhosis is the most probable diagnosis. Variceal bleeding tends to be of large volume, and other signs of liver

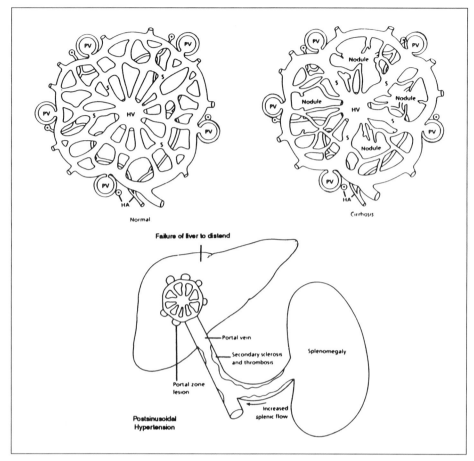

Fig. 91-4. Cirrhosis of the liver. The formation of portal venous (PV), hepatic venous (HV) anastomoses or internal Eck fistulas at the site of preexisting sinusoids (S). Note that the regeneration nodules are supplied by the hepatic artery (HA). Factors concerned in so-called idiopathic primary portal hypertension (bottom). (From S Sherlock, and J Dooley. Diseases of the Liver and Biliary System. *Oxford: Blackwell, 1993. Reproduced with permission.)*

disease can be present, such as splenomegaly, ascites, prominent abdominal wall venous collaterals, and a venous hum above the umbilicus.

Esophageal and gastric varices can be well demonstrated by a barium swallow and upper gastrointestinal (UGI) series, in which esophageal varices appear as curvilinear, serpiginous filling defects in a barium-filled esophagus. The UGI is more sensitive than ultrasound or CT scan for esophageal varices, but less so for gastric lesions. Definitive diagnosis is made by esophagogastroduodenoscopy (EGD).

In the absence of active bleeding, EGD can assess the size of varices and changes suggestive of potential bleeding, such as red wales and lines, adherent clots, thinning varix walls, and erosive mucosal changes. Large varices are more often associated with bleeding than are small ones.

Ultrasound assesses the flow characteristics in the portal, hepatic arterial, and vena caval circulations and determines portal and splenic vein patency. Doppler ultrasound can reveal spontaneous reversal of flow in the portal, splenic, and superior mesenteric veins. This finding correlates with the severity of portal hypertension. Doppler studies are also useful for assessing the patency and flow characteristics of previous portosystemic shunts. Duplex Doppler allows assessment of hepatic vein flow in the evaluation of possible veno-occlusive disorders and is a routine method for evaluating the patency of hepatic arterial and portal vein anastomoses after liver transplantation.

Although some authorities claim that CT scanning allows better definition of the portal vein anatomy and patency than does ultrasound, we seldom find Doppler

ultrasound lacking. However, CT angiogram can be used in some circumstances to supplement ultrasound such as in the case of presinusoidal portal hypertension, which might be caused by splenic vein thrombosis.

In most patients with bleeding esophageal varices, the demonstration of portal hypertension and underlying liver disease is straightforward. However, occasionally the type and cause of portal hypertension are unclear. Further characterization can then require direct measurement of hepatic venous and wedged hepatic venous pressures. Normal wedged hepatic vein pressures, reflecting portal vein pressures, are 7 to 12 mm Hg with a gradient between the wedge and unwedged readings of 4 mm Hg. Gradients in excess of 12 mm Hg in the alcoholic cirrhotic are said to be associated with a very high risk of variceal bleeding.

Of course, the wedged pressures do not reflect portal vein pressures in the face of presinusoidal portal hypertension. Direct splenoportography with pressure measurements has been advocated in the past, but we have no experience with this technique. However, if Budd–Chiari syndrome or veno-occlusive disease of the liver is suspected, both hepatic venograms plus direct hepatic vein and vena caval pressure measurements will help define the anatomy and the location of important gradients.

In preparation for shunt surgery, the surgeon is well advised to obtain angiographic delineation of splanchnic and systemic venous anatomy, at least if a distal splenorenal shunt is proposed. If ultrasound suggests that flow in the main portal vein is antegrade into the liver (hepatopetal), then the venous phase of a superior mesenteric arteriogram might define portal venous anatomy adequately. Splenic and renal vein anatomy can similarly be determined by watching for the venous phase after simultaneous celiac and aortic injections or an aortic flush. If portal vein or mesenteric vein flows are reversed on Doppler ultrasound, direct hepatic or splenic portography might be required to visualize portal or splenic vein anatomy (Figs. 91-5 and 91-6). MRI angiography has the potential to replace conventional angiography for some of these procedures.

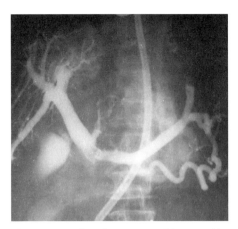

Fig. 91-5. Transhepatic portogram. A 71-year-old cirrhotic male undergoing transhepatic embolization of varices. A catheter has been introduced into the portal system through the right lobe. Two coronary veins have been embolized.

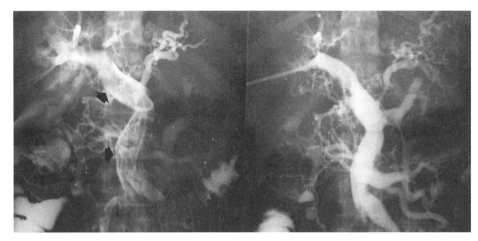

Fig. 91-6. Transhepatic portogram and aspiration of thrombus. A 31-year-old female spontaneously developed a clot in her superior mesenteric and portal veins. A catheter has been introduced into the portal system through the right lobe. The initial contrast study (left) shows extensive clot (arrows). After clot aspiration through the catheter, patency of major veins was restored (right).

Hepatic venography is essential to establish the diagnosis of Budd–Chiari syndrome, characterized by the inability to advance a hepatic venous catheter more than a few centimeters into the liver. In Budd–Chiari syndrome, venography can reveal absent or narrowed hepatic veins, or a patent inferior vena cava with retrohepatic narrowing caused by compression by an enlarged caudate lobe. Surgeons should remain alert for the possibility of this syndrome in a patient with a myeloproliferative disorder who also has an enlarged liver with venous outflow obstruction. In this circumstance, determination of liver size, portal vein anatomy, and vena caval flow, best achieved through ultrasound, is crucial.

Assessing the Adequacy of Liver Function

The surgeon with a patient with portal hypertension requiring surgical intervention must be able to make a reasonably accurate assessment of the degree of liver dysfunction before recommending the best surgical course. The essential question is often whether to offer a shunt or refer the patient for liver transplantation. Although some authorities have advocated any number of tests of hepatic function (e. g., aminopyrine breath test, galactose elimination capacity, indocyanine green clearance, amino acid profiles, caffeine clearance, lidocaine clearance) as a means of assessing liver function, we have never found them to be of much added value when the patient's clinical history, physical examination, and routine laboratory evaluation are reviewed.

We base our preoperative assessment of patients requiring surgical intervention for bleeding varices on an estimation of their clinical course over the ensuing 2 to 5 years. A patient who is already beginning to experience quality of life issues (e. g., severe fatigue, pruritus, muscle wasting, malnutrition, or moderate ascites) and who has a progressive liver disease, can be a candidate for transplantation rather than shunt, even though bleeding varices are the only life-threatening complication to date. Obviously, a patient who has other manifestations of advanced disease (encephalopathy—either clinical or subclinical as shown by careful psychomotor testing—moderate to severe ascites, jaundice, hypoalbuminemia, and coagulopathy) and who has no contraindications, is a candidate for transplantation rather than a type of surgical shunt. Transjugular intrahepatic portosystemic shunt has become a popular means of supporting a patient with bleeding varices requiring surgical intervention during the wait for a suitable donor organ.

Evaluation of the Living Related Donor

In July 1992, living related transplantation was incorporated into our pediatric liver transplantation program as a response to the shortage of donors for small children. It involves a left lateral hepatectomy, usually from a parent, to yield a graft for his or her child with end stage liver disease. Over a 35-month period, 28 percent (25/90) of pediatric transplants at the University of Nebraska Medical Center had been from living related donors (LRD). Living related donation has been used most frequently for the very small pediatric recipient, median age 8 years and median weight 8 kg, for whom the shortage of donors is most problematic. We will briefly discuss the diagnostic considerations used in evaluating potential living donors for liver transplantation.

Donors should be 18 to 55 years of age, be ABO compatible with the recipient, and have no medical or surgical illnesses that would increase operative risk. A hepatologist conducts an extensive history and physical examination of the donor. Normal results of hematologic and serum chemistry studies as well as exclusion of transmissible viral illness is required. A complete psychosocial assessment evaluates the psychological fitness of the donor, the donor's ability to fully understand the risks and benefits of the LRD hepatectomy procedure, and the social support systems of the donor's family.

The second part of the donor evaluation consists of assessing the suitability of the proposed hepatic graft for LRD hepatectomy (Fig. 91-7). Volumetric CT scanning determines liver volume of the segment to

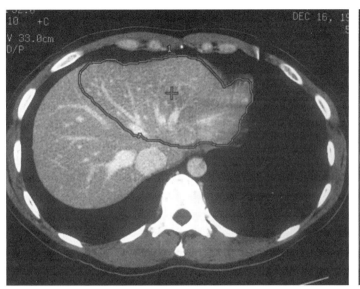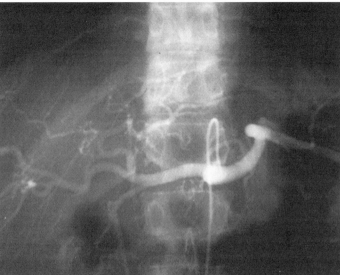

Fig. 91-7. Computed tomographic volumetry and angiography illustrating arterial supply and parenchymal volume (white line) of a left lobe graft (normal anatomy).

be resected and excludes abnormal parenchyma or space-occupying lesions within the liver (Fig. 91-8). Continuous 10-mm–thick axial slices are obtained through the liver following intravenous contrast administration. The segments to be resected are electronically outlined on the CT console, and the measured area of the liver slice is multiplied by its known thickness. Individual volumes are then added to determine the total volume. Computed tomographic volumetry has proved to be both accurate and reproducible. At the time of the operation, the actual volumes of the resected segments are quantified by the weight of the liver and by measurement of its volume of displacement before implantation into the recipient.

Accurate estimation of volume preoperatively is vital for donor and recipient safety. A donor graft of inadequate parenchymal volume relative to the recipient leads to postoperative liver failure culminating in retransplantation or recipient death. A graft that is too large can lead to portal vein or hepatic artery thrombosis or respiratory compromise in the recipient secondary to abdominal compression. The actual lower limit of liver graft parenchyma necessary for survival is unknown and can vary with the condition of the recipient at the time of surgery. For example, a patient in acute fulminant hepatic failure

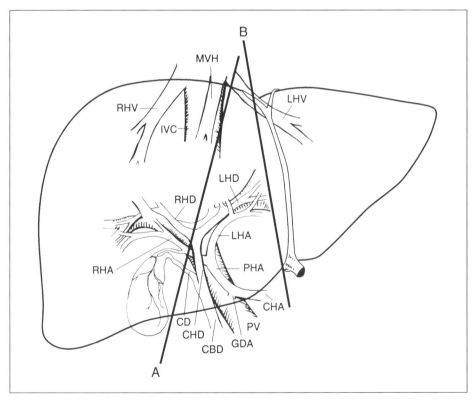

Fig. 91-8. Parenchymal division lines for hepatic resection. Line B represents left lateral hepatectomy; line A, full left hepatectomy. MHV = middle hepatic vein; RHV = right hepatic vein; IVC = inferior vena cava; LHV = left hepatic vein; LHD = left hepatic duct; RHD = right hepatic duct; RHA = right hepatic artery; LHA = left hepatic artery; CD = cystic duct; PHA = proper hepatic artery; CHD = common hepatic duct; CBD = common bile duct; GDA = gastroduodenal artery; PV = portal vein; CHA = common hepatic artery.

might not tolerate a marginal amount of tissue as well as a more stable patient undergoing less urgent transplantation would. It is also important to consider that postoperatively acute rejection can rapidly decrease available hepatic functional reserve. For patients undergoing elective procedures, 1 percent of the recipient's weight is believed to be a safe lower limit.

The maximal donor-to-recipient ratio has been reported to be 15:1. As such, a 5-kg child could theoretically accept a left lateral segment graft from a donor up to a weight of 75 kg. However, in our experience, left lateral segment parenchymal volume correlates very poorly with donor weight. For example, we successfully transplanted a graft into a 3.9-kg child with biliary atresia using an 82-kg father as the donor (greater than 20 times the weight of the recipient). The left lateral segment of the donor was estimated at 186 grams, but the actual weight was 240 grams. Abdominal closure with mesh graft was used to avoid graft compression postoperatively.

Angiography is used as a road map to minimize dissection and decrease the risk of hepatic artery thrombosis (Fig. 91-8). We attempt to avoid using donor segments with multiple arteries to the left lateral segment or with hepatic arteries smaller than 2 mm in diameter. We have used this approach in the first 25 patients and have lost only one graft (4%) from hepatic artery thrombosis. There has been no long-term morbidity or mortality among living related liver donors at the University of Nebraska Medical Center.

Conclusion

The ease, sensitivity, and specificity of diagnostic modalities for evaluating liver disease will probably improve dramatically in the next decade. At the same time, the expense associated with these new and wonderful tests will likely skyrocket. Because they will be less invasive and therefore better tolerated by patients, expense might be the only factor limiting widespread use of shotgun techniques in diagnosis. However, the availability of such "harmless" modalities does nothing to detract from the value of a directed and thoughtful approach to tailoring the workup to the individual patient. The surgeon who can narrow the diagnostic possibilities to a likely few by the time the history and examination are completed will be more valuable when we finally discover the price of diagnostic excess.

Acknowledgment: The authors would like to acknowledge Elizabeth H. Tape, M.D. for her valuable editorial assistance.

Suggested Reading

Babineau TJ, Lewis, WD, Jenkins, RL, et al. Role of staging laparoscopy in the treatment of hepatic malignancy. *Am J Surg* 67:151, 1994.

Child CG, Turcotte JG. Surgery and Portal Hypertension. In CG Child (ed.), *The Liver and Portal Hypertension*. Philadelphia: Saunders, 1964.

Ferrucci JT. Liver tumor imaging. *Radiol Clin North Am* 32:39, 1994.

Forse RA, Babineau TJ, Bleday R, et al. Laparoscopy/thoracoscopy for staging: Staging endoscopy in surgical oncology. *Semin Surg Oncol* 9:51, 1993.

Gazelle GS, Lee MJ, Mueller PR. Cholangiographic segmental anatomy of the liver. *Radiographics* 14:1005, 1994.

Gitnick G (ed.). *Diseases of the Liver and Biliary Tract*. St. Louis: 1992. Mosby,

Heffron TG, Langnas AN, Fox IJ, et al. Preoperative evaluation of the living related donor in pediatric liver transplantation. *Transplant Proc* 27:1180, 1995.

Infante-Rivard C, Esnaola S, Villeneuve JP. Clinical and statistical validity of conventional prognostic factors in predicting short-term survival among cirrhotics. *Hepatology* 7:660, 1987.

Jakimowicz, JJ. Review: Intraoperative ultrasonography during minimal access surgery. *J R Coll Surg Edinb* 38:231, 1993.

Johansen K, Paun M. Duplex ultrasonography of the portal vein. *Surg Clin North Am* 70: 181, 1990.

Kawasaki S, Makuuchi M, Ishizone S, et al. Liver regeneration in recipients and donors after transplantation. *Lancet* 339:580, 1992.

Pugh RNH, Murray-Lyon JL, et al. Transection of the oesophagus for bleeding oesophageal varices. *Br J Surg* 60:646, 1973.

Schiff L, Schiff ER (eds.). *Diseases of the Liver*, 7th ed. Philadelphia: Lippincott, 1993.

Sherlock S, Dooley J. *Diseases of the Liver and Biliary System*, 9th ed. London: Blackwell, 1993.

Shortell CK, Schwartz SI. Hepatic adenoma and focal nodular hyperplasia. *Surg Gynecol Obstet* 173:426, 1991.

Ward BA, Miller DL, Frank JA, et al. Prospective evalutaion of hepatic imaging studies in the detection of colorectal metastases: Correlation with surgical findings. *Surgery* 105:180, 1989.

Hilson AJW, Fleming JS. Radionuclide Investigations of the Liver. In McIntyre, JP Benhamou, J Bircher, et al (eds.), *Oxford Textbook of Clinical Hepatology*. New York:Oxford University Press, 1991.

EDITOR'S COMMENT

Doctor Shaw and coworkers argue elegantly for the surgeon playing a major role in the diagnostic and judgmental acumen of patients with liver disease. Far from relying on third-generation tests, such as galactose elimination tests or antipyrine clearing tests, Dr. Shaw's group emphasizes no-nonsense patient observation, patient course, and simple liver chemistries. It also emphasizes the need for surgeons to develop judgmental skills with respect to liver disease. Although there are some newer modalities such as MRI with iron oxide and, more recently mentioned in the literature, superparamagnetic iron oxide (Saini et al., *Am J Roentgenol* 164:1147, 1995), most of the tests advocated by Dr. Shaw and coworkers involve more simple and straightforward judgments. This approach, in the old days, used to be known as good surgical judgment.

In describing the minimally invasive surgical approach through laparoscopic ultrasound, Dr. Shaw and his group also make an inadvertent argument for surgical expertise in diagnostic and therapeutic manipulation of the lower end of the common duct, that is, ERCP. At a time when surgeons are doing increasingly more to the biliary tree in a minimally invasive manner, it makes little sense not to have the ability to assess the lower end of the common duct through ERCP. We hope that in the future, more surgeons will become expert at this important diagnostic modality so that they know not only the technique but also the shortcomings of these procedures.

The alcoholic with cirrhosis has long been the subject of an attempt to determine which patients are at risk for bleeding esophageal varices. In a previous study of prophylactic portacaval shunts, Conn and his colleagues noted that despite the very high operative mortality, the alcoholic patient with tight ascites was at risk for bleeding esophageal varices, and perhaps a side-to-side decompression was appropriate. In this manuscript, the figure of 12 mm of differential between the portal vein and the zero point in the vena cava is offered. This group is probably the same group of patients. Temporary techniques that one might yet again attempt include a side-to-side type of decompression. Although my own favorite might be a central splenorenal shunt, others might favor an interposition shunt using a 10-mm graft. Since many of these patients are likely to need transplantation if and when the disease becomes progressive, and they have abstained from alcohol, it is best to stay out of the porta.

J.E.F.

92

Drainage of Hepatic, Subphrenic, and Subhepatic Abscesses

Jonathan L. Meakins   Andrew Seely

Hepatic Abscesses

Hepatic abscesses are an uncommon yet potentially lethal clinical entity; if prompt diagnosis and treatment are not begun, the condition is uniformly fatal. Liver abscesses represent 6 to 7 per 100,000 adult admissions to hospitals in the United States. Pyogenic hepatic abscesses reflect the major contribution to the incidence of liver abscesses (over 80%); the remainder are amebic in origin. The treatment, diagnosis, and prognosis of liver abscesses have evolved remarkably over the past 6 decades. Diagnosis improved first with the advent of technetium liver scans and then with the use of ultrasound and CT. In addition, radiologic imaging has altered therapeutic strategy with the possibility of percutaneous drainage. The concept of minimally invasive drainage has been and continues to be of paramount importance in the treatment of hepatic abscesses. With the advances in diagnostic imaging and drainage procedures, prognosis has dramatically improved. The diagnosis, distinction between pyogenic and amebic abscesses, pathogenesis, treatment, and prognosis of both abscesses will be examined.

Diagnosis

The diagnosis of hepatic abscesses based on history and physical examination is exceedingly difficult given the multiplicity and variability of complaints, as well as the common association with other intra-abdominal processes. Fever, chills, and abdominal pain are the most common symptoms; fever, hepatomegaly, and right upper quadrant tenderness are the most common signs. Table 92-1 displays the different signs and symptoms associated with hepatic abscesses. It is of note that no particular sign or symptom is correlated to number, microbiology of abscesses, or outcome.

Patients with liver abscesses usually present with abnormalities on routine hematologic and liver function tests. Elevated white blood cell count, anemia of chronic disease, and high alkaline phosphatase are commonly found. Table 92-2 displays the incidence of abnormal laboratory studies in 73 patients with liver abscesses. In addition, transaminase levels can be slightly elevated, depending on the amount of hepatic parenchyma involved. Mischinger has recently shown that a high WBC count, hyperbilirubinemia, anemia, and a high APACHE II score are significant predictors of increased morbidity and mortality.

Ultrasound and computed tomography (CT) scans are the imaging modalities of choice in the diagnosis of hepatic abscesses. Hepatic scans with radioisotopes, although exceedingly useful in the past, are now obsolete. The sensitivity of ultrasound is 85 to 90 percent, whereas the sensitivity of CT is approximately 95 percent. Although sensitivity is excellent, specificity is not; thus aspiration of the abscess is necessary for confirmation of the diagnosis and the microbiology.

Table 92-1. Signs and Symptoms Associated with Hepatic Abscess

Sign/Symptom	No.	%
Initial Complaint		
Fever/chills	31	38
Abdominal pain	29	36
Anorexia/malaise	9	12
Symptoms		
Fever/chills	55	75
Anorexia/malaise	42	58
Abdominal pain	40	55
Nausea/vomiting	20	27
Weight loss	21	29
Night sweats	7	10
Diarrhea	6	8
Signs		
Fever (T > 38)	45	61
Hepatomegaly	28	38
RUQ tenderness	26	36
Weight loss	23	31
Right basilar rales	18	25
Jaundice	17	23
Diffuse abdominal tenderness	11	15
Ascites	3	4

RUQ = right upper quadrant.
Adapted from GD Branum, GS Tyson, MA Branum, et al. Hepatic abscess: Changes in etiology, diagnosis and management. *Ann Surg* 212:655, 1990.

Table 92-2. Laboratory Data from 73 Patients with Liver Abscesses

Laboratory Value	No.	%
Hematocrit < 40 mg %	49	67
WBC > 10,000/mm	50	68
Bands > 10%	29	40
Alkaline phosphatase > 110 IU	57	78
SGOT > 35 IU/dL	42	57
Bilirubin > 1.5 mg/dL	26	36

WBC = white blood cell count; SGOT = serum glutamic oxaloacetic transaminase.
Adapted from GD Branum, GS Tyson, MA Branum, et al. Hepatic abscess: Changes in etiology, diagnosis and management. *Ann Surg* 212:655, 1990.

Amebic Versus Pyogenic Hepatic Abscesses

Despite considerable attempts to distinguish the two entities, there are no reliable clinical features that are specific for amebic versus pyogenic hepatic abscesses. Younger age, recent travel to endemic areas, diarrhea, and marked abdominal pain raise the clinical suspicion of amebic abscess; however, serology is necessary to confirm the diagnosis. Indirect hemagglutination is the most sensitive and specific laboratory test available but requires 24 to 48 hours for processing. Although aspiration is unnecessary if there is a high suspicion of amebic abscess, if it is performed, the aspirate is classically reddish brown, "anchovy-paste"–like material with a negative gram stain. Prompt resolution of symptoms after the onset of metronidazole supports the diagnosis of amebic abscess.

Amebic Liver Abscess

Pathogenesis

The protozoa *Entameba histolytica* is distributed worldwide; however, it is most commonly found in tropical climates and in societies with poor sanitation. Cysts containing the parasite are transmitted via the fecal-oral route. Trophozoites are released in the intestinal tract after ingestion of cysts and then reside primarily in the large intestine. Amebic abscesses in the liver form when the amebic trophozoites invade through the colonic mucosa and spread via venules or lymphatics from the colon to the liver. *Entameba histolytica* can live within the lumen of the colon and might or might not be invasive. The liver is the most common extraintestinal site of amebic invasion.

Treatment

The treatment of amebic liver abscess is primarily noninterventional. Metronidazole remains the drug of choice; it is highly effective, inexpensive, and has the advantage of being effective for intestinal as well as extraintestinal amebiasis. The dose regimen is 750 mg tid for 10 days. Chloroquine can be added if defervescence does not occur in 72 hours or if a patient is acutely ill.

Percutaneous aspiration of amebic abscesses is unnecessary unless: 1) there is suspicion of bacterial suprainfection; 2) a pyogenic liver abscess is suspected; or 3)

the abscess is left-sided (segments 2 and 3) and large such that the risk of rupture into the pericaridium is significant. Normally, the amebic liver abscess will respond to amebicides promptly (48–72 hours) without the need for aspiration or surgical drainage. Most authorities agree that laparotomy is indicated for ruptured amebic abscesses into the pericardium; however, recent series propose a nonoperative approach and simply follow the clinical response to amebicides. Rupture into the pleura or pericardium can be treated with amebicides and pleuricentesis or pericardiocentesis as necessary. If laparotomy is performed, a midline incision should be used.

Prognosis

The prognosis for uncomplicated amebic liver abscesses is excellent. Possible complications with an increased morbidity and mortality include rupture into the pleura, peritoneum, and pericardium, and secondary bacterial infection. Rupture into the pericardium is the most significant complication and is associated with a mortality of at least 30 percent. If all instances are included, the mortality is approximately 4 percent, as Pitt found with a review of data collected between 1950 and 1980 from over 3000 instances.

Pyogenic Abscesses

Pathogenesis

The exact pathogenesis of a pyogenic liver abscess is unclear; however, several mechanisms of infection have been discussed. There are five possible etiologic mechanisms (Fig. 92-1):

1. Transportation of virulent organisms through the portal system from the GI tract
2. Trauma
3. Spread of infection from the biliary tract
4. Bloodborne infection via the hepatic artery
5. Extension from contiguous disease process

Gastrointestinal causes, including appendicitis, were by far the most common etiologic factor in Ochsner and DeBakey's series of 1938 and were presumed to be secondary to septic emboli and portal thrombophlebitis. Recent series indicate that the biliary tree is most often the etiologic factor involved in pyogenic liver abscesses (approximately 35%). Direct extension from active cholecystitis, a biliary stasis secondary to benign or malignant obstruction with infection, and previous biliary enteric bypass are most commonly found to be the underlying factors in-

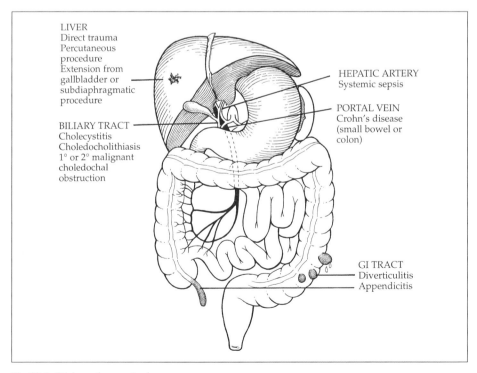

Fig. 92-1. Etiology of pyogenic abscess

volved. GI disease such as diverticulitis, inflammatory bowel disease, adenocarcinoma of the colon, and appendicitis are also associated with hepatic abscesses, although much less commonly. Of particular importance for patients with pyogenic hepatic abscesses is the increasing number of patients with malignancies or immunosuppressed states, or both. Recent studies demonstrate an increased association between malignant disease and liver abscesses as well as increased mortality in patients with malignancies. Notwithstanding tremendous advances in diagnostic imaging, cryptogenic hepatic abscesses (no source identified) still represent a significant percentage (up to 30%) of liver abscesses.

Bacteria and Choice of Antibiotics

The organisms most commonly cultured from pyogenic hepatic abscesses are gram-negative aerobic rods (most commonly *Klebsiella* and *E. coli*), gram-negative anaerobes (*Bacteroides fragilis*) and gram-positive aerobes (enterococcus, micro-aerophilic streptococcus). The majority of abscesses are polymicrobial containing anaerobes and thus require broad-spectrum antibiotics. A good choice of antibiotics involves the use of a penicillin, an aminoglycoside, and metronidazole. Clindamycin can be used to replace the penicillin if the patient is allergic to penicillin. Imipenem can also be used as the sole agent in the treatment of pyogenic liver abscesses.

Treatment

The principles of management of pyogenic liver abscess must be cartesian; there are generally two problems that must be resolved. First the abscess must be managed, most often with a drainage procedure, accompanied by antimicrobial therapy. Second, the initiating process must be identified and managed to ensure that there will be no recurrence or persistence of infection. Therefore, the guiding principles for surgical management of infection prevail: diagnosis, drug(s), and drainage.

The Abscess. There has been great evolution in the treatment of pyogenic liver abscesses since 1938 when Ochner and DeBakey demonstrated the reduction in mortality associated with operative drainage for all liver abscesses. A completely extraperitoneal approach was later described to minimize intra-abdominal contamina-

tion in the preantibiotic era. However, with the use of perioperative parenteral antibiotics, it has been shown that a transperitoneal approach can be safely used, although extraperitorial drainage is preferred. Since MacFadzean first published a series of pyogenic liver abscesses treated with needle aspiration and antibiotics alone in 1953, there has been a shift toward nonoperative management of liver abscesses.

A series by Berger and Osborne in 1982 demonstrated treatment of 62 patients with hepatic abscesses with antibiotics and needle aspiration, and a mortality of 4 percent. It is important to emphasize that percutaneous aspiration and drainage are simply extensions of standard surgical principles. As Gerzof has pointed out, the routes of percutaneous drainage are similar to minimally invasive surgical routes of drainage. The principles involved are to minimize spillage of abscess contents and decrease hematogenous spread with the least insult to the patient as possible.

Once the diagnosis of a single or multiple liver abscesses is made, broad-spectrum parenteral antibiotics should be started. Routine hematologic blood work, liver function tests, indirect hemagglutination to rule out an amebic abscess, and blood cultures before onset of antibiotics should be performed.

There are four treatment modalities for pyogenic liver abscesses. They are indicated in different clinical scenarios; however, in general, they represent a sequential approach to the treatment of pyogenic hepatic abscesses.

1. parenteral broad-spectrum antibiotics alone
2. needle aspiration and antibiotic therapy
3. percutaneous catheter drainage and antibiotics
4. laparotomy with intraoperative drainage and antibiotics

A trial of antibiotics alone should be reserved for patients with multiple small abscesses, low risk of abscess rupture, and lack of toxemia (i. e., no hemodynamic instability, patient does not feel acutely ill, and so forth). Once committed to the antibiotic regimen, clinical response is gauged by defervescence, fall in leukocytosis, and resolution of symptoms and should be reassessed frequently. Imaging

with ultrasound or CT can be used to assess resolution of abscess(es). No improvement after a reasonable course (10–14 days) indicates failure of treatment. Oral antibiotics should be continued for at least 4 weeks after discontinuing parenteral antibiotics. Worsening fever, leukocytosis, and symptoms at any time also indicate failure of treatment and immediately qualify the patient for a more aggressive treatment regimen involving a drainage procedure.

The first-line treatment for most patients with a pyogenic liver abscess should be needle aspiration and antibiotic therapy. Aspiration involves as complete as possible evacuation of the abscess cavity, and no catheter is left within the cavity. The patient's symptoms will normally improve immediately following aspiration. The aspirated fluid should be sent for aerobic and anaerobic cultures. Clinical response is again measured by fall in fever, leukocytosis, and symptomatic improvement. It might be necessary to repeat aspiration when follow-up imaging is performed. Worsening clinical features or failure to improve after a reasonable time (10–14 days) qualifies the patient for percutaneous catheter drainage. The number of patients who fail needle aspiration and antibiotic therapy will be approximately 15 to 20 percent.

Percutaneous catheter drainage with ultrasound or CT guidance is indicated for patients who fail aspiration and for whom percutaneous drainage is not contraindicated. Contraindications include coagulopathy and the lack of a safe or appropriate access route. It is of note that the septae visualized within the abscess cavity on CT or ultrasound are not a contraindication to catheter drainage, because they rarely represent separate localized abscesses. Using a modified Seldinger technique, the catheter is placed into the abscess cavity and left to straight drainage in a position as dependent as possible to facilitate drainage. This technique is discussed in detail by Clark and Towhin. The catheter is flushed one to three times daily with 25 cc of sterile saline solution depending on the viscosity of the aspirate. The patient is again monitored for clinical improvement and cessation of drainage from the abscess (the catheter is slowly removed as the cavity shrinks). Sinograms must be performed if drainage persists or if an enteric or biliary fistula is suspected; otherwise they are not routinely required. Approximately 10 to 15 percent of patients fail percutaneous drainage and require intraoperative drainage.

Operative drainage of pyogenic hepatic abscesses is indicated for the following patients: 1) patients who require laparotomy for any other associated intra-abdominal process; 2) patients who fail percutaneous catheter drainage; and 3) patients with contraindications to percutaneous drainage. Patients who rupture liver abscesses into the peritoneum also require laparotomy. A midline or subcostal incision is performed, although the occasional patient will benefit from a posterolateral eleventh rib approach. Intraoperative ultrasound can be useful to help determine the ideal site for abscess drainage and can be used to identify the portal structures and hepatic veins. Needle aspiration is used to precisely localize the abscess. The hepatotomy is then performed with electrocautery in order to open the abscess cavity. Drains (preferably closed suction) should be placed into abscess cavity(ies) and exited via a separate abdominal stab wound. Thorough irrigation of the peritoneal cavity is performed before closure. If there is diffuse contamination from abscess perforation in the peritoneum, closure should not be attempted. Once drainage is sufficiently low (<30 cc/8 hours) and the drainage does not contain bile, the drains can be removed over 2 to 3 days.

The Underlying Disease. As previously mentioned, the most common underlying cause is biliary pathology usually related to a benign or malignant obstruction. Generally, malignant obstruction does not produce cholangitis or abscesses because the obstruction has developed in the presence of sterile bile. However, modern techniques (e. g., ERCP and percutaneous cholangiogram) have led to increased manipulation, use of contrast material, and needle aspiration of the biliary tree, all of which contribute to the possibility of subsequent cholangitis. A percutaneous catheter guarantees contamination and infection, if drainage is compromised.

The relief of biliary obstruction or correction of stenosis is imperative. This step usually requires common duct exploration, clearing of stones if feasible and T-tube drainage. The use of choledochoscopy, extensive exploration and manipu-

lation, or bypass depends on the patient's clinical status. In our enthusiasm to correct all defects, we should not lose sight of the objective: drainage and relief of obstruction. Further operative therapy can be required after recovery from the acute process. These procedures can include biliary-enteric bypass or its redo, resection of the liver for ductal obstruction, or sphincterotomy.

Abscess via direct extension is usually secondary to acute cholecystitis. Cholecystectomy is required with appropriate drainage and operative cholangiography to ensure that the common duct is not obstructed. If portal vein dissemination is the problem, although less common, the focus (usually appendicitis or diverticulitis) must be managed; resection is best if possible. Hepatic artery bacteremia requires the identification of the focus (e. g., TPN line, endocarditis, or tuberculosis). Hepatic trauma that leads to abscess can require evacuation of the hematoma or debridement of necrotic hepatic parenchyma, or both. Failure to resolve the underlying process leads to persistence or recurrence of the infection.

Prognosis

The prognosis of patients with hepatic abscess has improved dramatically with concurrent advances in diagnostic and treatment modalities. Sepsis and multiple organ system failure are now the most common cause of death in patients with liver abscesses. Although there are reports of lower rates, mortality for hepatic abscesses is approximately 20 percent.

Subphrenic and Subhepatic Abscesses

Diagnosis

As is true for liver abscesses, the presentation of intraperitoneal abscesses surrounding the liver is variable and nonspecific. The majority of patients present with fever and chills, as well as right or left upper quadrant pain. Other less common symptoms include weight loss, nausea, and vomiting. Physical signs include right or left upper quadrant tenderness, local drainage of pus, or a palpable mass. Laboratory tests are not helpful except to demonstrate an elevated leukocyte count.

Ultrasound and CT remain the imaging procedures of choice in the diagnosis of in-

traperitoneal abscesses. In addition to diagnostic value, ultrasound and CT can be used to guide percutaneous drainage, which will be discussed subsequently. It is nevertheless important to recall some of the useful indirect diagnostic aids in finding subphrenic collections. Abdominal series can be helpful, displaying an air fluid level or gas within the abscess, a mass effect, or an ileus. However, the abdominal series is normal in approximately 25 percent of patients. It is particularly important to note that the chest roentgenogram is abnormal more often than the abdominal study. Subphrenic abscesses clearly present as a thoracoabdominal process and should be treated as such. A majority of patients (85%) have an abnormal chest roentgenogram, most commonly a pleural effusion, and possibly an elevated hemidiaphragm and atelectasis.

Etiology

The majority of patients with suprahepatic or infrahepatic intraperitoneal abscesses present following an operation. In a series of 196 cases by Serrano and colleagues, only 20 percent of patients presented without history of an operation. Hepatic, gastric, biliary, and colonic surgery constitute the majority of operations leading to the development of a suprahepatic or infrahepatic abscess. Technical errors, such as anastamotic disruptions, lead to perihepatic abscesses. Appendicitis was responsible for a great number of abscesses in the past but is no longer a significant etiologic factor in modern series. The prevalence depends on the reporting center, however, post-traumatic abscesses unfortunately are increasing in importance in North American urban centers. Right-sided abscesses are most commonly associated with hepatic and biliary surgery, whereas left-sided are associated with gastric and pancreatic surgery, as well as splenectomy.

Microbiology

The microbiology of intraperitoneal extrahepatic abscesses is very similar to intrahepatic abscesses. The organism(s) of the abscess generally reflects the operation of which the abscess is a complication. The most common organisms identified are streptococci, bacteroides, *E. coli*, and *Klebsiella*, and less commonly, staphylococci, *Proteus*, and *Pseudomonas*. Broad-spectrum antibiotics are exceedingly important, as with liver abscesses. The discussion of antimicrobial therapy for liver abscesses can be applied to intraperitoneal abscesses surrounding the liver.

Anatomy

There are five intraperitoneal spaces surrounding the liver: two on the right and three on the left. The classification is a slight modification of Boyd's, and is presented and discussed in more detail by Harley. To avoid confusion, abscesses or spaces lying superior to the liver and immediately inferior to the diaphragm will be referred to as suprahepatic, and abscesses or spaces lying inferior to the liver will be termed infrahepatic. Although the term subphrenic is normally used synonymously with suprahepatic, the term is misleading and will not be used in this discussion. On the right, there are the right suprahepatic and the right infrahepatic spaces. They are separated by the coronary and right triangular ligaments. The left is divided into a suprahepatic space, and posterior and anterior infrahepatic spaces. The left suprahepatic space is separated from the right by the falciform ligament, and from the left posterior inferior space (the lesser sac) by the left triangular ligament. The anterior and posterior left infrahepatic spaces are separated by the stomach and the lesser omentum. The suprahepatic and infrahepatic spaces communicate. However, fluid collects in one or perhaps two and subsequently leads to an abscess. The most common site is the right subhepatic space, which is responsible for approximately 30 to 40 percent of all intraperitoneal abscesses surrounding the liver.

Treatment

As is true for liver abscesses, the treatment of suprahepatic and infrahepatic abscesses has changed dramatically over recent decades. In the past, extraserous operative drainage was the only sensible option in the preantibiotic era; however, operative intervention is now clearly the exception, not the rule in the treatment of intraperitoneal abscesses surrounding the liver. Percutaneous drainage is performed in the same manner as it is for hepatic abscesses. Note that aspiration alone (i. e., no catheter left within the abscess) is not indicated for suprahepatic and subhepatic abscesses.

Percutaneous catheter drainage has become the standard of treatment for almost all suprahepatic or infrahepatic abscesses. This technique has repeatedly been shown to be effective in treating abdominal abscesses of all types. Gerzof, Robbins, and colleagues have shown decreased rates of complications, decreased rates of inadequate drainage, and shorter duration of drainage with percutaneous versus open drainage.

Although less common, operative drainage of suprahepatic and infrahepatic abscesses might be required in selected instances. The indications for operative drainage include the following:

1. Contraindication to catheter drainage (i. e., no safe route or coagulopathy)
2. Multiple abscesses
3. Active intra-abdominal pathology requiring laparotomy
4. Failure of catheter drainage

Failure of catheter drainage is evidenced by worsening of fever, leukocytosis, right upper quadrant pain, and other symptoms at any time, or lack of resolution of signs and symptoms after a reasonable time (10–14 days). As is the case with liver abscesses, septae visualized within the abscess cavity on CT or ultrasound are not a contraindication to catheter drainage. If there are contributing factors in the subphrenic abscess—foreign body, necrotic tissue, hematoma, fistula with obstruction, and so forth—the initiating or perpetuating process must be properly managed.

Operative Treatment

Historically, the extraserous approach was exceedingly important to minimize intraperitoneal and intrapleural contamination. After the onset of antibiotic therapy, it became evident that a transperitoneal approach could be performed safely. Given that the transperitoneal approach allows for drainage of multiple abscesses if present, as well as examination of the entire peritoneal cavity, this approach has become more popular, accounting for 65 percent of the approaches in the series by Serrano and colleagues.

The extraserous approach is still indicated for a single abscess readily accessible to anterior or posterior drainage and when there is no indication for laparotomy. The anterior approach allows the surgeon to

reach the suprahepatic spaces on both sides, the right infrahepatic space, and the left anterior infrahepatic space. Although very popular in the past, the posterior approach should not be used except for right posterior infrahepatic abscesses. It has been shown that this approach is not adequate for right suprahepatic abscesses because of the presence of the bare area of the liver, which lies in the way. However, the benefit to the posterior approach is that it allows for dependent drainage in the bedridden patient. Extraserous approaches have become relatively rare because they have been replaced by percutaneous drainage.

Transperitoneal Approach. A midline incision is used to enter the peritoneal cavity. The abscess cavities are punctured and suctioned, minimizing bacterial contamination. Gram stain and cultures are sent to the lab. Cultures are important. Resistant flora from the original abscess are usually associated with recurrence. Thorough irrigation of the cavity is performed, as well as irrigation of the peritoneal cavity. Exploration of the peritoneal cavity to find the source of the abscess can be performed at this stage.

Anterior Extraserous Approach. An oblique incision is made one finger breadth beneath the costal margin from the lateral edge of the rectus abdominis muscle and extended laterally (Fig. 92-2). The incision is deepened through the three muscular layers of the abdominal wall until the properitoneal fat is reached. Care is taken not to enter the peritoneum. Using blunt dissection with the fingertips, the peritoneum is gently peeled from the underside of the diaphragm. The incision should be wide enough to admit three fingers and a sponge stick. Dissection is continued until the abscess is reached, and opening of the cavity is accomplished with the finger. After cultures and gram stain of the contents are taken, the abscess cavity is emptied completely and all loculations removed. Thorough irrigation of the cavity is then performed.

Posterior Extraserous Approach. The incision is made 2 cm from the midline over the bed of the eleventh or twelfth rib and extended laterally past the tip of the rib (Fig. 92-3). The latissimus dorsi and serratus posterior muscles must be di-

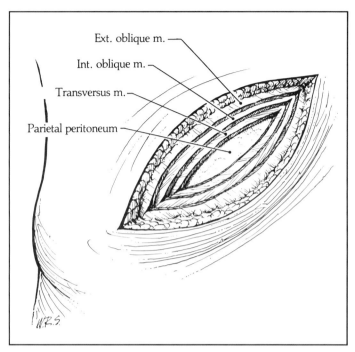

Fig. 92-2. *Drainage of anterior liver abscesses. Division of the abdominal musculature is shown. The parietal peritoneum is not opened. This approach is useful for left or right subdiaphragmatic abscesses.*

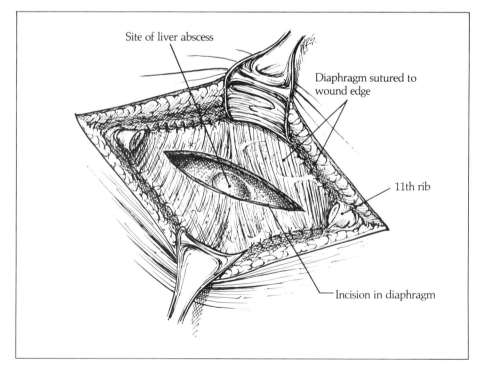

Fig. 92-3. *Drainage of posterior liver abscesses. The rib has been resected. The diaphragm is then sutured to the parietal pleura surrounding the incision and incised. The liver abscess can be seen as a slight prominence in the liver parenchyma.*

vided to gain access to the periosteum of the twelfth rib. The periosteum is divided in the middle of the rib and then stripped from the underlying bone. The rib can then be removed. The bed of the periosteum is subsequently incised longitudinally at the level of the spinous process of L1. Care is taken not to open the pleura during the removal of the rib or dissection of the periosteum. If entered, it can be excluded from the drainage tract by a running suture. The attachments of the diaphragm must be divided under the periosteum. The subcostal and iliohypogastric nerves must be preserved. The perinephric fat will lie under the incision, and blunt exploration with the fingers between the renal and diaphragmatic fasciae will allow access to the right posterior infrahepatic space.

Drainage and Closure. Regardless of the surgical approach, a closed suction drainage system should be used (Fig. 92-4). The number of drains used depends on the size and number of the cavity(ies) and the nature of contents following drainage. "Less is more" remains a fundamental principle of drain management. Closure is completed using interrupted monofilament nonabsorbable sutures in layers. Skin closure with intermittent sutures and packing or leaving the subcutaneous tissue packed open is appropriate.

Postoperative Care

The patient must be kept on parenteral broad-spectrum antibiotics until the gram stain and subsequent culture results allow for more specific antibiotic coverage. The parenteral antibiotics should be maintained until the patient is no longer febrile (48 hours) and the white blood cell count is normal. Oral therapy can be started, if desired. Generally, further antibiotic therapy is not required if the white blood count is normal and the patient is afebrile.

The catheter within the abscess cavity should be monitored for quantity and quality of drainage fluid. Irrigation with 25 cc of sterile normal saline (NS) can be performed one to three times a day depending on the viscosity of the contents. The catheters can be removed if the drainage fluid is no longer purulent and the quantity is no longer significant (< 30 cc/8 hours). If drainage persists after 7 to 10 days, or if the patient fails to defervesce, a sinogram with repeat CT should be performed in or-

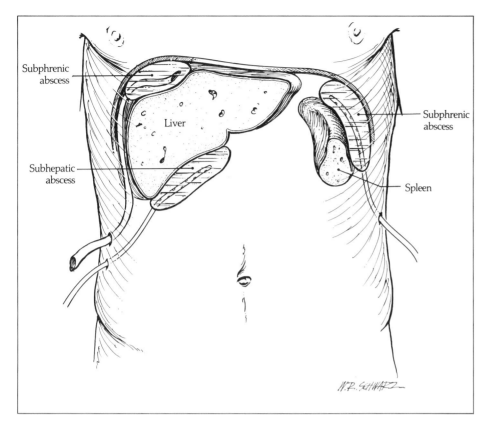

Fig. 92-4. *Transperitoneal drainage of subphrenic and subhepatic abscesses. Schematic position of drains is shown. Closed drainage should be used.*

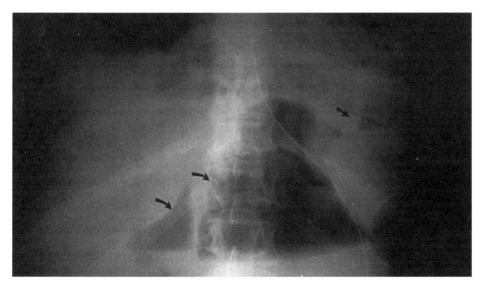

Fig. 92-5. *The upright film of an abdominal series showing most of the signs of subphrenic abscesses. The chest is abnormal with consolidation and a small amount of fluid. There is free air in the abdomen with multiple shadows under the right and left (straight arrow) diaphragm, in the subhepatic space (lower curved arrow) and separate from it, and in the stomach there is a large collection of free air (upper curved arrow). Clearly, laparotomy is required.*

der to recognize an inadequately drained abscess or to diagnose a separate undrained collection.

Conclusion

Although percutaneous drainage has had a salutary effect on the management of patients with subphrenic abscesses, there are pitfalls in relying solely on roentgenographic intervention. The following situation illustrates several points. A patient 5 days after low anterior resection had developed fever, leukocytosis, and worsening upper abdominal pain. Figure 92-5 shows the upright film of an abdominal series. Note the air fluid levels under the diaphragm as well as elevated diaphragms and pleural effusions. Computed tomography confirmed the presence of a large intra-abdominal abscess. It is notable that the CT was not required to make the diagnosis given the findings on abdominal series. The patient was managed with percutaneous drainage and antibiotics. However, the symptoms did not resolve, and the patient progressed into renal failure. Laparotomy was then performed, which revealed a disrupted anastomosis.

This situation illustrates several important points. First, early diagnosis of both the abscess and the cause, early drainage, and prompt use of drugs (antibiotics) are of paramount importance. Second, hepatic, suprahepatic, or infrahepatic abscesses present as a thoracoabdominal process, with abnormal findings on chest roentgenogram. Third, the management of hepatic, suprahepatic, or infrahepatic abscesses must always take into account the management of the cause of the abscess. Although consultation with an interventional radiologist is essential, management of hepatic, suprahepatic, or infrahepatic abscesses is surgical, and responsibility cannot be abdicated. Finally, "never let the sun set on intra-abdominal abscess," is an old adage that is still valid. Maintenance of these surgical principles allows for the successful management of most suprahepatic, hepatic, and infrahepatic abscesses.

Suggested Reading

Andersson R, Forsberg L, Hederstrom E, et al. Percutaneous management of pyogenic hepatic abscesses. *HPB Surg* 2: 185, 1990.

Berger LA, Osborn DR. Treatment of pyogenic liver abscesses by percutaneous needle aspiration. *Lancet* 1:132, 1982.

Bertel CK, Van Heerden JA, Sheedy PF. Treatment of pyogenic abscesses, surgical vs. percutaneous drainage. *Arch Surg* 121:554, 1986.

Boyd DP. The subphrenic spaces and the emperor's new clothes. *New Engl J Med*, 275:911, 1966.

Branum GD, Tyson GS, Branum MA, et al. Hepatic abscess: Changes in etiology, dignosis and management. *Ann Surg* 212:655, 1990.

Clark RA, Towhin R. Abscess' drainage with CT and U/S guidance (Review) *Radiol Clin North Am* 21:445, 1983.

Dietrick RB. Experience with liver abscess. *Am J Surg* 147:288, 1984.

Donavan AJ, Yellin AE, Ralls PW. Hepatic abscesses. *World J Surg* 15:162, 1991.

Gerzof SG, Robbins AH, Johnson WC, et al. Intrahepatic pyogenic abscesses: treatment by percutaneous drainage. *Am J Surg* 149:487, 1985.

Gerzof SG, Robbins AH, Johnson WC, et al. Percutaneous catheter drainage of abdominal abscesses: A five-year experience. *N Engl J Med* 305:653, 1981.

Levision MA. Percutaneous vs. open operative drainage of intraabdominal abscesses. *Inf Dis Clin North Am* 6:525, 1992.

McFadzean AJS, Chang KPS, Wong CC. Solitary pyogenic abscess of the liver treated by closed aspiration and antibiotics: a report of 14 consecutive cases of recovery. *Br J Surg*, 41: 141, 1953.

Mischinger HJ, Hauser H, Rabl H, et al. Pyogenic liver abscesses: Studies of therapy and analysis of risk factors. *World J Surg* 18:852, 1994.

Mueller PR, Simoone JF, Burn RJ, et al. Percutaneous drainage of subphrenic abscesses: a review of 62 patients. *Am J Roentgenol.* 147:1237, 1986.

Ochsner A, Debakey M, Murray S. Pyogenic abscess of the liver. *Am J Surg* 40:292, 1938.

Pitt HA. Surgical management of hepatic abscesses. *World J Surg* 14:498, 1990.

Serrano A, Dahl EP, Rubin RM, et al. Eclectic drainage of subhpepatic abscesses. *Arch Surg* 119:942, 1984.

Shimada H, Ohta S, Maehara M, et al. Diagnostic and therapeutic strategies of pyogenic liver abscesses. *Int Surg* 78:40, 1993.

Stain SC, Yellin AE, Donovan AJ, et al. Pyogenic liver abscesses: Modern treatment. *Arch Surg* 126:991, 1991.

EDITOR'S COMMENT

Doctors Meakins and Seely have presented a well-reasoned and orderly approach to the diagnosis and therapy of hepatic, subphrenic, and subhepatic abscesses. They emphasize the difference between hepatic pyogenic abscesses, in which single aspiration can be sufficient, and subphrenic and subhepatic abscesses, in which closed catheter drainage is the standard. This point is still a matter of some controversy within the radiology literature. Georgio and coworkers (*Radiology* 195:122, 1995) presented 115 patients treated over 13 years with ultrasound-guided percutaneous needle aspiration. In what they say was long-term follow-up, 98 percent of the patients were successfully treated with a single aspiration. Unfortunately, there is no evidence in the paper of follow-up 1 or 2 years later, which would probably be necessary to declare this technique a successful one. In contrast, Hashimoto and colleagues (*Am Surgeon* 61:407, 1995) argued, on the basis of the review of their patients, that CT-guided catheter drainage with operative drainage should be reserved for patients who failed to respond to percutaneous drainage or for patients in whom an operation is indicated for other purposes (e. g., treatment of the primary disease, such as malignancy). However, they did conclude that aspiration without catheter drainage, while possibly efficacious, needed long-term follow-up and could not be advocated at that point. I tend to agree, although undoubtedly some patients will respond favorably.

I'd like to make a few comments on the subject matter of the chapter. Irrigation for catheter drainage is appropriate. There is some evidence that irrigation with antibiotic solution can be superior to irrigation with saline and should be used.

The diagnosis of subphrenic abscesses is of course much simpler now with the capability of CT scans. Nonetheless, one can take advantage of physical examination by percussing the diaphragm and its movement on simple physical examination. If one suspects a subphrenic abscess, it is highly unlikely that the diaphragm will move a great deal on physical examination, and one can confirm this supposition by auscultation.

The extraperitoneal approach to drainage of subphrenic abscesses was always complicated for me. However, as Drs. Meakins and Seely point out, if one resects the eleventh rib, makes a short incision, and peels the peritoneum away from the diaphragm, when one reaches the abscess there will be sufficient inflammation that the entire area will be edematous and one can palpate the fluctuant nature of the abscess, at which point it can be drained by the finger. It is still a useful technical exercise, fortunately not necessary very often, because of the success of percutaneous catheter drainage.

J.E.F.

93

Treatment of Echinococcal Cysts

Farrokh Saidi

Hydatid disease, or echinococcosis, is a parasitic condition of worldwide distribution, recognized since ancient times. The organism involved, *Echinococcus granulosus*, belongs to the order of cestodes or flatworms of the family *Taenia*. The biologic characteristics of the parasite greatly favor its survival in nature, and in a pastoral setting the parasite continuously repeats its life cycle between the domestic dog and sheep. Humans happen to be an accidental or incidental intermediate host, and from the parasite's viewpoint a dead end. The disease can be brought under control by such simple public health measures as not feeding entrails of slaughtered sheep to stray or shepherd dogs. In industrialized countries, hydatid cysts are much rarer now than they were in the past. In endemic areas of the world where proper zoonotic conditions prevail, however, echinococcosis remains a major economic problem.

Hydatid cysts can occur in any organ system of the body. As a chronic and well-localized affliction, they are unaffected by age, sex, or other intercurrent disorders. While the cystic parasite enlarges slowly in quest of living space, the infected patient suffers no serious constitutional reactions. Nevertheless, the disease continues as a serious combat between the host and parasite, and in the end one or the other must die.

The clinical signs and symptoms can be affected by the setting in which the disease occurs. In endemic areas of the world, primarily the Near and Middle East, Greece, North Africa, and South America, almost everyone is familiar with the "cystic condition." Physicians recognize it promptly,

and surgeons generally know how to deal with it. By contrast, in hospitals of the industrialized Western world, the disease is usually a surprise finding and is overtreated more often than not.

Echinococcosis need not be either mysterious or difficult to manage. The parasitology is easy to grasp and the pathology is straightforward. An understanding of both is fundamental to a proper surgical approach. This chapter presents the basics, allowing the surgeon to deal logically, simply, and effectively with any hydatid cyst of any organ of the body.

Parasitology

The adult worm of the parasite is a little less than 1 cm long and attaches itself to the intestinal mucosa of its definitive host, the dog and related carnivores. Each adult worm is a true hermaphrodite, the next to last of four separate segments bearing both the male and female reproductive organs. The last segment is the uterus, gravid with approximately 1000 eggs. Each time a heavily infested but otherwise healthy dog defecates, countless highly infective ova of the parasite are set free in the surrounding environment. These microscopic eggs, approximately 30 μ in size, are ingested by grazing sheep, goats, and cattle. In the intestinal tract of these intermediate hosts, the eggs hatch, penetrate the host's intestinal wall to reach the liver by the portal system, and from there are distributed in the bloodstream to the lungs and thereafter other organs.

Once it has reached its definitive organ of the intermediate host's body and has over-

come local defensive reactions, the parasite's egg becomes transformed into the larval stage, called the protoscolex, or scolex for short. A scolex can multiply asexually ad infinitum in the intermediate host but is always confined within a well-circumscribed sphere, the hydatid cyst. The natural life cycle of the parasite is completed when a hydatid cyst with its viable scoleces is devoured by the dog, in whose intestines the scoleces are transformed once again into adult worms.

The definitive and the intermediate hosts cannot exchange their places in the parasite's life cycle. Humans are only an accidental intermediate host, harboring one or more of the larval hydatid cysts. The usual mode of acquiring the infection is through ingestion of contaminated vegetables. No amount of washing with any known detergent can reliably eradicate the parasite's sturdy eggs from contaminated material. The best protection against the disease in endemic areas is to completely avoid eating vegetables and fruit harvested at ground level.

Pathology

The highly infective eggs of the parasite, once ingested, lose their protective shell in the upper GI tract and penetrate the small-intestinal mucosa to be carried in the portal blood to the liver. Most are filtered out in the liver sinusoids, but quite a few reach the lungs. Some pass this second filtering sytem as well. Eventually, no more than 5 to 10 percent of ingested eggs reach peripheral organs by the arterial bloodstream. No organ of the body is immune

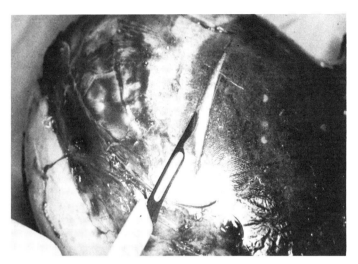 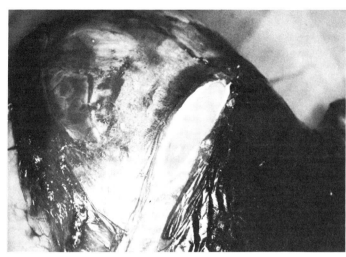

Fig. 93-1. A spleen, enlarged because of hydatid cyst, has been surgically removed. Its surface has been incised down to the whitish adventitial pericystic layer.

Fig. 93-2. The pericystic layer of the same specimen as in Fig. 93-1 has been further opened down to the glistening laminated membrane of a single intact hydatid cyst.

to invasion, but the local reaction is the same in all soft tissues.

The pathology of echinococcal disease is simply the expression of an obligatory multiplication of the larval scoleces, reflected in a slow but steady physical enlargement of the whole cystic colony, which means that any viable hydatid cyst situated in any organ of the body is bound to grow in size. For the parasite, this mechanism is necessary for adaptive survival. For the human host, however, it implies the forced surrender of organ space. Enlargement of the cyst is very gradual, so the patient's symptoms are rarely acute. Since the host and parasite are organically separated by the cyst's chitinous outer shell, there are no attending systemic reactions.

The first cellular response of host tissue, if the newly arrived egg is not killed outright, is to wall it off by an encasing fibrous tissue in an adventitial reaction. The parasite in turn begins to form around itself a spherical enclosure of inert chitinous material with central vacuolization, and the first phase of a viable hydatid cyst is established. Over succeeding weeks and months—but more likely years—there develops a typical and characteristic cystic structure, which is the same in all soft-tissue host organs.

Two distinct anatomic layers are encountered in dissecting down on a hydatid cyst. The first is the pericyst (ectocyst) ad-

ventitial layer of host origin (Fig. 93-1). This area is a relatively thin zone of compressed and nonepithelialized fibrous tissue and is never anatomically separable from the surrounding normal parenchyma of the host organ. It provides some measure of mechanical support for the hydatid cyst. However, its far more important function is exchange of nutrients and waste material between host and parasite through its multitude of capillaries and vascular spaces. This exchange is contingent on the nonepithelialized inner surface of the pericystic layer being in complete contact at all times with the next layer encountered by the surgeon, the outer covering of the parasite itself, the so-called laminated membrane (Fig. 93-2). This pure white, opaque, glistening, quite elastic, but very fragile membrane cannot be mistaken for anything else. It is never thicker than 1 or 2 mm, regardless of the size of the cyst itself, because further thickening would interfere with osmotic transfer of substances across it. Its chitinous nature makes it impervious to many substances as well as bacteria. When fully intact, the laminated membrane assumes a near-perfect spherical shape easily recognized as a typical hydatid cyst.

At no time is there any organic connection between the host and parasite, which means that a hydatid cyst always separates from, or can be readily lifted out from within, a surgically exposed pericystic cavity (Fig. 93-3). Filling an intact hydatid cyst and stretching it maximally is the crystal-

clear hydatid fluid (Fig. 93-4). Lining the inside of the laminated membrane, but rarely recognized as a distinct anatomic layer, is the germinative membrane. This extremely thin and transparent layer, as the name implies, is the template on which scoleces are born, nurtured, and released into the fluid interior of the cyst. Broken-off portions of the germinative membrane are capable of becoming closed off into small spheres floating in the cyst's interior and in time form daughter cysts, which are replicas of the mother cyst. Such daughter cysts do not have a pericyst of their own and are presumably nourished through the medium of the hydatid fluid itself.

The hard skeletal tissue of bones does not allow the formation of grossly discernible cysts. Instead, the trabecular architecture of affected bone is slowly destroyed by the insinuating and advancing small cyst-like lesions.

Progressive accumulation of hydatid fluid is clearly a biologic response to the ever-increasing population of scoleces, and the fluid pressure within a cyst can be as high as 100 cm of water. It is the single most reliable indicator of overall viablity of the cyst. Actively growing cysts feel tense, whereas recently ruptured, degenerating, or dead cysts feel soft to a palpating finger. It is also the high intracystic fluid pressure that, on rupture of a cyst at operation, leads to explosive discharge of hydatid fluid and scoleces, with resulting contamination of the surrounding surgical field.

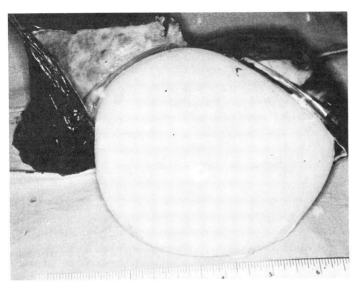

Fig. 93-3. The whole pericystic cavity of the same specimen as in Figs. 93-1 and 93-2 has been laid open, allowing extrusion of an unruptured, intact hydatid cyst.

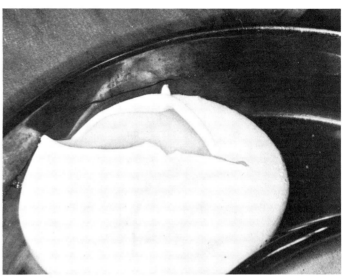

Fig. 93-4. Puncture of the same cyst as in the previous figures has resulted in a long tear of the laminated membrane, allowing the scolex-rich, crystal-clear hydatid fluid to flow out. The veil-thin germinative membrane lining the everted edges of the torn laminated membrane can be seen only if it is specifically sought.

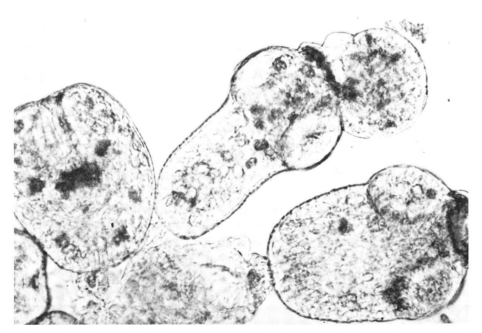

Fig. 93-5. A group of viable scoleces in different stages of inversion and eversion of their heads. Each scolex is covered by a birefringent hyaline cuticle ($\times$ 250).

The scoleces are responsible for all the clinical manifestations of echincoccal disease, including recurrence after local spillage. A larval scolex is a complex organism, approximately 150 µ long (Fig. 93-5). It has a number of unusual characteristics: It is sturdy and mobile, inverting and everting its head actively. It has respiratory functions but does not ingest particulate matter. It thrives in its laminated membrane housing, leisurely floating and multiplying in the fluid medium. Once set free from within the hydatid cyst, it can implant on any exposed tissue surface of the body, serosal surfaces preferred, and re-create a new hydatid cyst or cysts. However, it cannot settle and regrow on epithelial surfaces.

Scoleces are too small to be seen readily by the naked eye unless they form an aggregate called a brood capsule or settle to the bottom of the interior of the cyst, forming what is called hydatid sand. It is always safer to assume that any amount of hydatid fluid, no matter how clear, contains many viable and potentially infective scoleces.

All clinical signs and symptoms of hydatid disease are based on the single-minded craving of the parasite, that is, the sum total of its viable scoleces, for living space and the local havoc it creates in the process. Peaceful coexistence between the host and parasite is eventually upset by the parasite's outgrowing available host organ space, violating the host's structural integrity.

Hydatid fluid is antigenic. This antigenicity is rarely of any great clinical significance. Previously sensitized patients can have high levels of immunoglobulin E (IgE) in their sera, and sudden massive reexposure to the antigen(s), as can happen with internal (intrapericystic) or external (outside the involved organ) rupture of a large cyst, can precipitate an anaphylactic reaction. The antigenicity of hydatid fluid is the basis for a number of diagnostic serologic tests, some of high sensitivity and specificity. However, these tests, whether positive or negative, cannot determine what should or should not be done surgically for a patient suspected of having echinococcal disease.

One final pathologic aspect of the parasite greatly affects its surgical management: Occasionally, the adventitial pericystic layer becomes at first more fibrotic, then more dense, next calcareous, and finally calcific. This stage signifies the beginning of the parasite's end: The host is no longer able to support the parasite nutritionally through the now hardened and avascular pericystic layer. However, until this structural change of the pericystic layer becomes circumspherically complete, there is no assurance that all of the myriad scoleces are dead. The underlying cause of such a spontaneous, although slowly progressive abortion, is unknown. In any case, such dying cysts usually do not grow in size when followed over months and years, and are generally of no further threat to their host.

This short review of the parasitology and pathology of echinococcal disease permits a clearer discussion of the clinical manifestations and surgical treatment of all hydatid cysts, focusing on these organs most commonly affected.

Hydatid Cysts of the Liver

Presentation

Since the liver is the first filter in the way of ingested eggs, approximately 75 percent of all hydatid cysts are found in this organ. There seems to be no limit to the number of cysts a liver can accommodate. However, note that these cysts do not destroy but slowly displace normal liver substance over succeeding months and years. At any time, however, any one particular hydatid cyst can, independent of the rest, undergo any of the complications discussed in the following sections.

Internal Rupture

Approximately one-half of all liver cysts, on incising their pericystic layer, are found to have the expected intact laminated membrane. This membrane is the so-called univesicular cyst and is the usual conception of a liver hydatid as diagrammatically

depicted in Fig. 93-6. Just as often, however, no laminated membrane is encountered when the pericystic layer is opened. Instead, there are literally hundreds and thousands of small- and medium-sized daughter cysts floating in a pool of turbid, yellowish fluid and gelatin-like amorphous material. This cyst is a so-called multivesicular cyst, as shown in Fig. 93-7. (This term is not to be confused with "multilocular cyst" of an altogether different type of echinococcal disease.) There are no telltale marks on the surface of the liver to distinguish an intact univesicular cyst from a previously ruptured multivesicular one, since the pericystic layer looks the same from the outside in both situations.

What has happened is that at some indeterminate time in the past the laminated membrane of the univesicular cyst ruptured within its own pericystic cavity, and liberated scoleces have had time to grow into many daughter cysts occupying the original space available. The torn laminated membrane was not absorbed but became part of the debris filling the pericystic cavity. The important fact is that growth and expansion of the parasite as a whole continued unabated, the daughter cysts exerting, in the aggregate, the same pressure on surrounding host tissues as the original single univesicular cyst.

Rupture of the laminated membrane can be caused by trauma to the liver. However, it is more likely that relentless expansion of the cyst causes pressure necrosis of the wall of a nearby major bile duct. The resulting leakage of bile into the potential space between the pericyst and laminated membrane separates the two and eventually brings about rupture of the latter. The yellowish tinge of the fluid medium of a multivesicular hydatid cyst attests to the previous, and no doubt continuing, entry of bile into the pericystic cavity. Any multivesicular hydatid cyst, by virtue of the growth potential of its many intact daughter cysts, is capable of damaging its host in exactly the same way as an intact univesicular cyst.

Two special features of a multivesicular cyst deserve to be mentioned: First, with rupture of the laminated membrane the spilled hydatid fluid is absorbed into the circulation, establishing a sensitivity to the hydatid antigen, if such did not exist before. Second, the fluid medium of a multivesicular cyst has, for all practical pur-

poses, the gross appearance of thin pus. This characteristic might prompt the surgeon to think that secondary bacterial infection has set in. Unless a Gram stain on this purulent material shows actual bacteria or many white blood cells, or both, one can safely assume that the particular multivesicular cyst is bacterially as sterile as a univesicular cyst with an intact laminated membrane.

Intraperitoneal Rupture

Following the line of least resistance, hydatid cysts of the liver grow centrifugally toward the surface of the organ. The most superficial portion of the covering fibrous pericystic layer becomes thinned out and blanches to the point of being mistaken for the pericystic layer. Eventually, the stretched pericystic layer tears apart. Intraperitoneal rupture is inevitable for a cyst reaching the anterior or inferior surface of the liver, regardless of whether it is uni- or multivesicular. The stage is set for the condition known as abdominal echinococcosis—liberated scoleces from a univesicular cyst develop into a variable number of hydatid cysts anywhere within the abdominal cavity. Freed daughter cysts of a multivesicular cyst continue their leisurely growth, creating new pericystic spaces for themselves within the folds of the intestine and omentum. The emptied pericystic cavity of the liver is resorbed into a fibrous scar, often leaving no obvious trace on the liver surface.

Intrathoracic Rupture

A hydatid cyst in the superior and posterior portions of the right or left lobe of the liver is more apt to grow cephalad. Relentless pressure on the diaphragm lifts it upward in a dome-shaped manner into the chest cavity. The muscular diaphragm is stretched and eventually eroded through by the advancing liver cyst. This process is usually clinically silent or at most attended by ill-defined chest or shoulder pain. Free intrapleural rupture of the invading liver hydatid cyst is unlikely, since the drawn-out process of diaphragmatic penetration leads to a local inflammatory pleural reaction, leaving the lung as the point of least resistance against the invading cyst.

Intrabiliary Rupture

As already described, erosion into small bile ducts results in the conversion of a univesicular into a multivesicular cyst. Pressure necrosis of larger bile ducts can

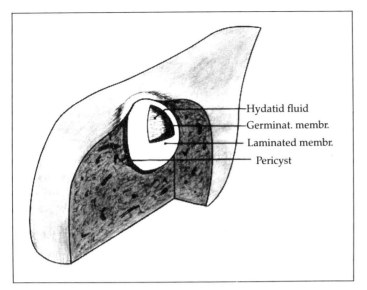

Fig. 93-6. A perspective view of a single univesicular hydatid cyst surfacing at the top of the right lobe of the liver. At its most superficial part the pericystic layer has been thinned out to a blanched circular area on the liver surface. The laminated membrane has been schematically cut open to depict the germinative layer and the hydatid fluid inside the cyst.

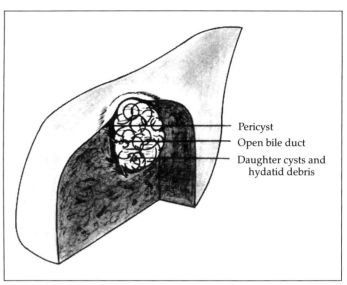

Fig. 93-7. Perspective view of a multivesicular hydatid cyst of the liver. The laminated membrane is no longer present as such and the whole pericystic cavity is filled with innumerable daughter cysts and hydatid debris. The latter consists of ruptured daughter cysts, degenerating fragments of the original laminated membrane, and bilious material. Invariably, one or more small bile ducts open into the multivesicular pericystic cavity.

create an opening large enough to allow the escape of some of the smaller daughter cysts and fragments of laminated membrane into the biliary tract. This process does not lead to spontaneous cure of the cyst; the bile duct aperture created is rarely large enough to allow a full evacuation of cyst contents. Instead, the situation changes from a relentlessly enlarging cyst to an unresolving and often secondarily infected pericystic cavity. Additionally, intermittent jaundice can dominate the clinical picture as parasitic debris escapes the pericystic space into the common duct system.

Secondary Bacterial Infection
This complication is theoretically possible but is uncommon. Its true incidence is unknown since in many reported instances the diagnosis is made on the basis of the gross appearance of a multivesicular cyst and not on the basis of a Gram stain or bacterial culture. It should be reiterated that bacterial and echinococcal infections are not mutually exclusive, each following their own natural dictates.

Spontaneous Abortion
Last, and from the host's point of view a very fortunate turn of events, is spontaneous abortion of the parasite. How,

when, and why it occurs is unknown. The breakdown is in the pericystic layer, which thereafter stops being fully functional. This process is undoubtedly very protracted, the final phase of which is total calcification of the pericyst.

Diagnosis

History and Physical Examination
The diagnosis of any of the six possible complications, or for that matter the diagnosis of an uncomplicated univesicular hydatid cyst, rests heavily on a strong clinical suspicion. The history of having resided or traveled in an endemic area is always a strong diagnostic lead. The diagnosis of hydatid disease of the liver with all its protean manifestations can become an intriguing and sometimes delightful clinical exercise. Intrabiliary rupture, for example, can be puzzling because internal decompression of the cyst itself is clinically silent. The cause of expectoration of bilious material requires some clinical acumen to unravel. The history and physical examination, conducted in the traditional and thorough manner, remain the foundation of clinical diagnosis of hydatid disease of the liver. What is remarkable but often not apparent at first, is that the patient is gen-

erally healthy despite the extent of the lesion, namely the multiplicity of cysts, and the severity of the complications. This, of course, is because of the absence of any generalized systemic ill effects of the echinococcal infection.

Because of its leisurely rate of growth, a hydatid cyst of the liver does not stretch the liver capsule acutely enough to cause severe right upper quadrant pain. More commonly, the patient volunteers a vague and poorly localized ache or fullness in the general area of the liver. Not uncommonly, an asymptomatic mass is palpated accidentally in the right upper quadrant if a large cyst happens to be located in the inferior portion of the liver. Small or deeply situated hydatid cysts are completely asymptomatic. The history of sudden urticaria following a fall, with or without a mild and transient abdominal pain, suggests the possibility of internal rupture of the univesicular hydatid cyst.

Routine Laboratory Tests
These tests do not confirm or rule out the clinical diagnosis of liver echinococcosis. Eosinophilia, for example, is a nonspecific laboratory finding that is found particularly in endemic areas where other parasitic infestations coexist.

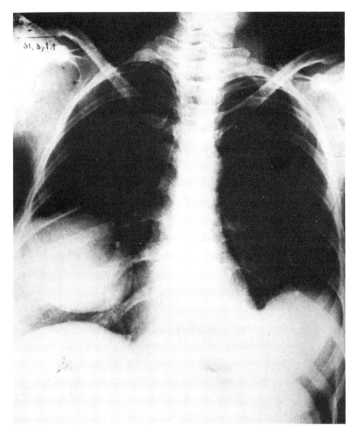

Fig. 93-8. A posteroanterior chest roentgenogram of a young woman shows bilateral, intact hydatid cysts in the lower lung fields. This finding would strongly favor a diagnosis of hydatid cyst of the liver as the cause of the elevated right hemidiaphragm. (In this patient, the right lung cyst and the liver cyst could both be managed surgically through a right posterolateral incision.)

Roentgenographic Examination

The *plain roentgenogram* of the abdomen is not revealing, since the radiodensity of noncalcified cysts is the same as the radiodensity of the rest of the liver substance. However, a chest roentgenogram, posteroanterior and lateral, is essential for two reasons: First, the unexpected finding of an asymptomatic hydatid cyst of the lung confirms the diagnosis (Fig. 93-8). More important is the finding of an elevated hemidiaphragm. The degree of diaphragmatic elevation and its configuration relate to the size, location, and number of hydatid cysts situated in the superior aspect of the underlying liver. Unexplained calcification of any roentgenographic pattern in the liver area should also suggest the presence of an aborted hydatid cyst. This finding might be no more than a calcified streak, or a very telling round calcification (Fig. 93-9).

Computed tomography (CT) scanning has opened new dimensions in the diagnosis of hydatid disease of the liver. However, the radiologist and the surgeon must have some familiarity with the tomographic appearance of liver hydatids to even consider that they might be present. A round area of homogeneous density always raises such possibility. In the instance of a multivesicular hydatid cyst, the central homogeneous density can appear broken up by curved thin-lined partitions, denoting the walls of the larger daughter cysts. The pericystic layer is rarely visible as such. A special value of CT scanning is the discovery of calcific areas of the pericystic layer, often changing the overall configuration of the lesion from a completely circular to an oval or irregular one (Fig. 93-10).

Sonography is a simple and noninvasive diagnostic technique for liver hydatid cysts.

It can readily make a distinction between uni- and multivesicular cysts (Fig. 93-11). However, it does have one disadvantage: It cannot accurately localize the position of the cyst within the liver substance or pinpoint its most superficial area for proper surgical exposure.

Scintigraphy is a reliable way of detecting any space-occupying lesion within the liver substance that is greater than 4 cm in diameter. This size limitation does not detract from its value since deep lying cysts of this size do not usually require surgical intervention. Scintigraphy performed in the anterior, lateral, and posterior view is more helpful than sonography in localizing the cysts, a necessary step in surgical management.

Angiography is too invasive to be used routinely. However, in nonendemic areas, it often is used anyway as a supplementary diagnostic test. It does provide spectacular and quite useful diagnostic images by showing large areas devoid of any circulation. In the late venous phase, the pericystic layer appears as a distinctive halo around a central avascular area (Fig. 93-12).

Surgical Treatment

Surgical intervention remains the principal form of definitive treatment of hydatid cysts of the liver. However, in two distinct situations hydatid cysts of the liver need not necessarily be approached surgically when they are first encountered.

1. Hydatid cysts of the liver should not be operated on when they are relatively small, that is, less than approximately 4 cm in diameter, or when they are situated deep within the liver substance, that is, more than approximately 4 cm beneath the liver capsule. The reason is that the surgeon must cut through a thick layer of normal liver tissue to reach the cyst, only to lose the intact cyst, which readily bursts on contact and is no longer palpable within its thin-walled pericystic cavity. It would be better to wait months or years until the cyst has surfaced and can be readily evacuated through its most superficially presenting part on the liver capsule. The slow course of the cyst's development can be followed by sonographic examinations at 6-month intervals.

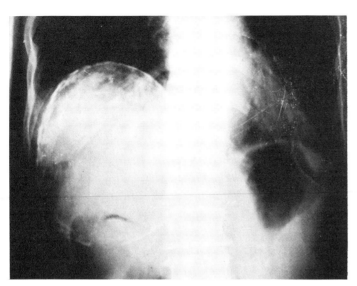

Fig. 93-9. A very large but remarkably asymptomatic calcified hydatid cyst of the liver.

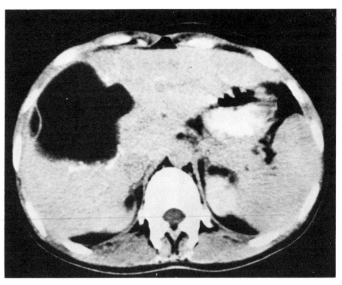

Fig. 93-10. An irregular outline of a cystic lesion seen on CT suggests degeneration of the hydatid cyst. Indeed, the lower margin shows calcification of the pericyst. More laterally, the outline of a single daughter cyst is clearly visible.

2. Because most calcified hydatid cysts of the liver have stopped growing and do not pose any danger for the host, most of them can be treated expectantly. Another valid reason for not attacking them is that their stiff-walled calcareous or calcified pericystic cavity cannot collapse and become obliterated after its contents are fully evacuated. If a secondary bacterial infection surpervenes, the stage is set for a never-healing abscess cavity.

All other hydatid cysts of the liver, regardless of whether they are simple and univesicular, or multivesicular and complicated, can be managed according to a clear operative plan, following certain basic rules. It might be prudent to administer 100 mg of hydrocortisone just before the operation to prevent intraoperative anaphylactic reaction secondary to spillage and absorption of hydatid antigens in a previously sensitized patient.

Approach
All hydatid cysts of the liver should be visualized mentally as being situated either above or below a horizontal plane that passes through the body at the level of the xiphoid, as depicted in Fig. 93-13. Cysts lying above this imaginary plane are best approached through the chest, and cysts ly-

ing below through the abdomen. The reason for this is twofold: Entry into the pericystic cavity is least traumatic if it is through its most superficially presenting part, since the least amount of normal liver substance is traversed. More important, unless the whole interior of a multivesicular pericystic cavity is laid wide open to inspection, fragments of the laminated membrane or daughter cysts, or other hydatid debris, can be overlooked. This situation will most certainly lead to local persistence of the disease, local recurrence, an infected foreign-body cavity, or all three.

Cysts localized to the superior aspect of the liver should always be approached through the chest. The thoracic incision can be a standard posterolateral one, usually in the eighth or ninth interspace. The diaphragm is opened peripherally in a semicircular manner away from the well-marked central area involved by the underlying hydatid cyst.

Cysts that can be palpated on the abdomen beneath the costal margin or cysts that have been localized to a position below the imaginary plane are approached through a midline or paramedian incision. A subcostal incision precludes proper exploration of the abdominal cavity and management of intraperitoneal cysts, which might also be present.

A thoracoabdominal incision, or the conversion of a thoracic or abdominal incision into a thoracoabdominal one, should rarely be necessary if the principal location of the cyst has been determined beforehand on the basis of a physical examination and a plain roentgenogram of the chest. There can be two cysts, one surfacing beneath the diaphragm and the other pushing out onto the inferior aspects of the liver. If both cannot be reached readily and safely through one incision, it would be easier on the patient to manage one of the two cysts properly through the chosen incision, and attack the other at a second sitting through the more appropriate incision. Patients with hydatid disease can tolerate any number of operations because of their basically normal liver status. It would be poor surgical judgment to leave behind hydatid material with resulting secondary infection simply because an ill-chosen surgical approach did not allow full evacaution of all parasitic material.

Decompression
The most superficial part of a liver cyst is readily seen or felt as a firm area quite distinct from the surrounding liver parenchyma. This area is now fully exposed and walled off from the rest of the operative field by appropriately placed gauze pads. The edges of the chest or abdominal inci-

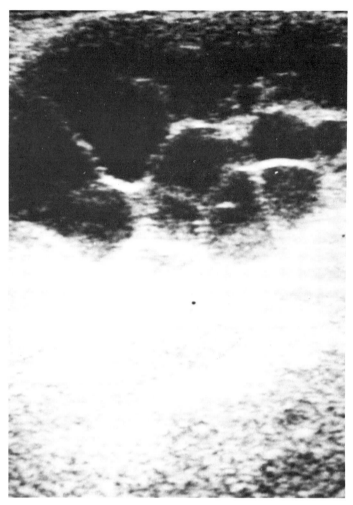

Fig. 93-11. Sonogram of a large, multivesicular hydatid cyst of the liver showing a multitude of daughter cysts within a large multivesicular pericystic cavity. The exact location of the cyst within the liver is difficult to ascertain by sonography.

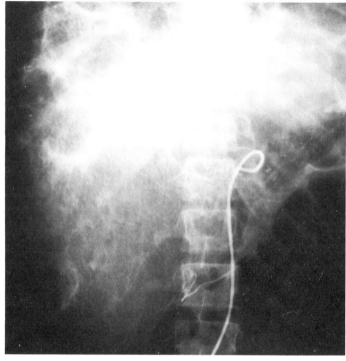

Fig. 93-12. Late venous phase of selective hepatic artery angiography showing halos around separate hydatid cysts of the liver as the vascular spaces of the pericyst are filled with contrast medium. (From F Saidi, Surgery of Hydatid Disease. London: Saunders, 1976. Reproduced with permission.)

sions must also be covered to protect against possible spillage of scolex-bearing hydatid fluid. The first step in the evacuation of the cyst is to lower its high internal fluid pressure. Decompression can be done in one of three ways.

1. A large-bore angiocatheter needle can be inserted and the hydatid fluid aspirated with a syringe. The diagnosis of a univesicular hydatid cyst is made on aspiration of crystal-clear hydatid fluid. This technique fails if the cyst is multivesicular, because only one or two of its daughter cysts are punctured.
2. The cyst can be punctured with a suction trocar. This method works well for univesicular cysts and is of some value for multivesicular ones when a number of daughter cysts can be punctured in succession.
3. One of a number of decompression devices can be used. These instruments consist of a cone, the lower end of which is placed on the superficial part of the cyst and kept fastened there either by a rapid freezing mechanism incorporated into the circular open end of the cone, or by a simple suction attachment of the cone end to the liver surface. An even simpler instrument consists of two concentric cylinders with separate suction arrangements (Fig. 93-14). The outer open-ended cylinder fastens itself to the liver surface by simple suction. The inner open-ended cylinder suctions off cyst contents after the pericyst is broken into with a long-handled knife inserted at the top from within the inner cylinder.

Regardless of the decompression device used, as soon as some decompression has taken place, the adjacent pericystic wall is grasped with Kocher clamps and strongly lifted upward, thereby preventing any escape of parasitic elements into the surrounding surgical field.

Evacuation

The opening into the pericystic cavity can now be enlarged for proper access to its interior. This step is readily performed by excising the thinned-out excess rim of the pericystic layer. Evacuation of cystic contents can be a straightforward maneuver of pulling out the punctured and collapsed laminated membrane of a univesicular

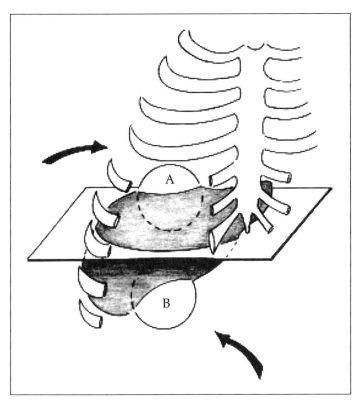

Fig. 93-13. *Two large hydatid cysts of the liver, cyst A advancing upward into the chest, cyst B surfacing on the inferior portion of the liver. Regardless of its size and contents, cyst A lies above an imaginary plane at the level of the xiphoid and should be approached through a thoracotomy incision. Cyst B lies below such a plane and is best approached through the abdomen.*

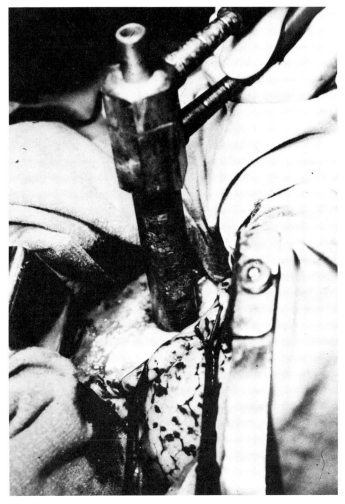

Fig. 93-14. *A simple device for preliminary decompression of hydatid cysts. It is approximately 14 cm long and consists of two concentric cylinders with separate suction outlets. The outer cylinder attaches by suction to the surface of the host organ over the most superficially presenting part of the pericyst. A long-handled knife inserted from above into the inner cylinder punctures the cyst, allowing its fluid to be aspirated through a separate suction line. This device can be manipulated more easily than a cone device to reach the cyst lying more laterally in the liver. (Courtesy Mr J Ali Mohammadi-Parsa, Medical Student, Beheshti University of Medical Sciences.)*

cyst, or it might be a tedious process of bailing out a seemingly endless collection of jelly-like material and a host of small and large solitary daughter cysts from within the huge and bottomless pericystic cavity of a large multivesicular cyst (Fig. 93-15). In either situation, nothing of parasitic nature must remain behind.

What might defeat the clearing-out process is if one or more small fragments of laminated membrane or tiny daughter cysts get lost in the folds and crevices of the collapsed walls of the pericystic cavity. These fragments or cysts can be swept out of their hiding places by using a dry gauze sponge to wipe the surface of the pericystic cavity.

At the end of the procedure, obvious bile duct openings are closed with fine chromic catgut sutures, although there is no guarantee that they will remain closed.

Killing the Scoleces

Because a univesicular cyst is first ruptured and then removed from the pericystic cavity, it is always possible that many scoleces can escape and become implanted somewhere on the surface of the emptied pericystic cavity. Leaving these scoleces in their homeground invites regrowth of new cysts. The best way of killing these unseen scoleces, whose presence can only be surmised, is to fill the entire emptied pericystic cavity with an effective scolecidal solution. I have found a freshly prepared solution of 0.5% silver nitrate to be an inexpensive, readily available, and nontoxic effective scolecidal agent. Use of formalin solution is to be decried since a number of instances of a sclerosing-cholangitis type of bile duct damage have been observed, the formalin solution having apparently entered the biliary system. Hypertonic sa-

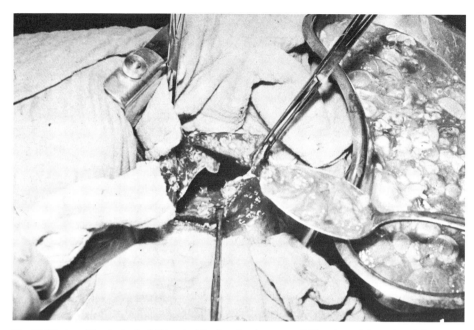

Fig. 93-15. A multivesicular hydatid cyst of the liver has been opened. The edges of the pericystic layer are held up with clamps, while spoonfuls of its contents are evacuated into a nearby receptacle.

line has its advocates. However, it can only be effective against scoleces if the concentration of salt is well above 15 percent, which has quite a desiccating effect on most normal tissues. Iodine solutions in any form and alcohol have no scolecidal properties because scoleces are not unicellular organisms. The scolecidal effectiveness of any agent must first be verified in the laboratory by intraperitoneal murine inoculation techniques. As a last maneuver, the cavity is filled with sterile saline to neutralize the effects of any residual scolecidal agent used.

In the past, it was customary to puncture the cyst ritualistically with a needle attached to a three-way stopcock, aspirate a syringeful of hydatid fluid, and then instill formalin solution in the hope of sterilizing the scoleces before entry into the cyst. This gesture is futile since not enough formalin can be injected to reach all the scoleces floating inside a large univesicular cyst. The univesicular cyst would be broken up by the needle puncture anyway, releasing its scolex-rich fluid outside the laminated membrane. For a multivesicular cyst, it is a patently ineffective maneuver.

A last look into the evacuated pericystic cavity will ensure complete clearance of all parasitic material. Finally, it is worthwhile to palpate with fingertips the walls of the pericystic cavity, feeling for additional hy-

datid cysts lying just outside. These cysts can often be easily managed from within the pericystic cavity of the one already evacuated.

Managing the Residual Pericystic Cavity

Next to the manner of evacuating the pericystic cavity, managing it afterward is a matter of some controversy among surgeons. Postoperative morbidity and sometimes even mortality hinge on how the evacuated liver pericystic cavity is handled. A number of techniques are available depending on the size of the cavity, its location, and personal preference of the surgeon. Usually, the simplest method based on the pathology observed at the operation works best. The options available are as follows:

1. The opening into the pericystic cavity through which its contents were evacuated can be sutured watertight and without any drainage whatsoever. The cavity can be filled with sterile saline or left empty. This approach works well for small- and medium-sized cysts. It is suitable for univesicular cysts because no major bile duct openings are present. In fact, closure of the pericystic opening without any drainage often works quite well even for large multivesicular cysts. Fluid left behind or accumulating later

on will drain off through existing small- and medium-sized bile duct openings. As a whole, this method of managing all pericystic cavities that are not bacterially infected is very appealing in that the patient can be discharged without bothersome long-term drainage. There is, however, a small and unpredictable risk of having fluid reaccumulate in the closed pericystic cavity, which might become secondarily infected. This complication would necessitate a second procedure for drainage, usually under general anesthesia, although simple needle drainage with sonographic guidance can be tried.

2. A second method of managing the emptied pericystic cavity is to leave it wide open to the peritoneal cavity. The rim of the cavity opening is overrun with catgut sutures but otherwise left open. This method is safe if the pericystic cavity is shallow or not large enough to allow small intestinal loops to fall into the cavity and create intestinal obstruction. A more important prerequisite is that the evacuated pericystic cavity be a univesicular one. Leaving the pericystic cavity of a multivesicular hydatid cyst open would be inviting free leakage of bile into the peritoneal cavity. This unfortunate course of events has happened even with modest sized univesicular hydatid cysts that did not show large bile duct openings at operation.

3. Many expert surgeons from Turkey and Greece with experience in echinococcocal disease prefer omentoplasty. In this method, a viable flap of omentum is brought to rest within the pericystic cavity on the assumption that the omentum is of material help in sealing off small biliary fistulas. I have not had much experience with this technique, but it would seem that here the omentum simply preempts a space that might be filled by small intestinal loops.

4. A compromise solution would be to suture close the pericystic opening with a Foley catheter inserted for prolonged drainage. This procedure is the safest method of managing the pericystic cavity. It has the great drawback, however, of committing the patient to a variable period of tube drainage, which might not be uncomfortable but is still inconvenient.

In short, good judgment is necessary in deciding how to technically manage a fully evacuated pericystic cavity. The size of the cavity, its location, contents, and pliability or rigidity of its pericystic walls must all be taken into consideration. Two other methods are mentioned, one of which is to be condemned outright: Marsupialization, that is, suturing of the edges of the opening of the pericystic cavity to the skin, is absolutely unsafe. It invariably results in a large, open, infected, bile-draining, and excoriating skin wound, which cannot be closed afterward in any readily conceivable manner. Capitonnage, the approximation of the opposite pericystic walls with a series of catgut sutures, can fail if the pericystic edges are stiff.

I have no fixed method of managing a completely evacuated pericystic cavity, but in general I prefer the following technique: For very large cavities, that is, the ones measuring 15 cm or more in diameter, especially if multivesicular and particularly if a Gram stain of the contents is reported to show bacteria, a large-sized Foley catheter is inserted into the pericystic cavity after closure of its initial opening. The catheter is brought out somewhere on the abdomen where it can be conveniently handled by the patient for a period of weeks. At biweekly or monthly intervals, as seems appropriate, sinograms are taken and the catheter is pulled out when the cavity has shrunk to a small tract. Prolonged drainage, regardless of the size of the cyst, is mandatory if the walls of the cavity appear stiff. I leave smaller pericystic cavities of univesicular hydatid cysts open if they are located on the dome of the liver. I alway close smaller pericystic cavities of multivesicular cysts to avoid free peritoneal bile leakage.

Liver resection of any magnitude, either to avoid inadvertent spillage of cyst contents or to circumvent altogether the problem of managing the residual pericystic cavity, creates more problems than it solves. It is too radical an approach for a basically benign condition.

A special problem arises in intrabiliary rupture of hydatid cysts of the liver. Both the biliary obstruction and the multivesicular cavity discharging into the biliary system must be managed in one sitting. The approach is, of necessity, always an abdominal one. The common duct is first explored in a standard manner. The finding of dark colored plaques or other amorphous material in the common duct not resembling stones is taken as strong evidence of a previous intrabiliary rupture of a hydatid cyst lying somewhere within the liver substance. The offending cyst can be small or large, palpable and visible, or it might have been detected preoperatively by appropriate roentgenographic studies. When more than one hydatid cyst is present, it can be difficult to know which one is discharging its contents into the biliary system. The simplest method of locating the responsible cyst during the operation is to perform retrograde operative cholangiography.

The guilty pericystic cavity itself is next managed according to the plan previously outlined. Sphincterotomy has been advocated as a final measure, based on the theory that if overlooked parasitic material enters the biliary system afterward, it can escape into the duodenum. This step is unncecessary if the basic principle of always evacuating completely all pericystic cavities has been followed. Irrigating the common duct and the emptied pericyst with saline helps in flushing out all gross hydatid debris. The use of scolecidal agents, especially formalin, can be very damaging to the biliary tract and is completely irrelevant, since scoleces do not implant on mucosally lined surfaces.

When hydatid cysts of the liver have penetrated the diaphragm to enter the chest cavity, the lungs must first be handled in an appropriate manner through a thoracotomy. The liver cyst itself can be managed through an incision in the diaphragm. This step often requires no more than enlarging the small diaphragmatic hole or vent through which the liver cyst had initially penetrated the diaphragm. Such liver cysts are always multivesicular and usually not very large because they have already decompressed themselves across the diaphragm. The pleural space does not present any particular problems but should be drained in the standard manner.

It bears reemphasis that calcified hydatid cysts should not be surgically attacked if at all possible. If such cysts have been entered into unintentionally, their pultaceous contents are evacuated and primary closure without drainage is effected in the hope of not having to deal with secondary bacterial infection afterward. Sometimes there might be no alternative but to bluntly scrape off the hardened pericystic layer, stanching ensuing bleeding from raw liver surface as best as possible.

There is a temptation, in this era of minimal access surgery, to somehow attempt evacuating liver hydatids percutaneously. No particular technical problems are involved in entering into and sucking out the cyst without opening the abdomen. However, the proper treatment of liver hydatids entails more than emptying the cyst. Walling off the surgical field, avoiding spillage, searching for and removing all parasitic elements, and sterilizing and suitably managing the residual pericystic cavity are manipulations more safely accomplished under direct vision with full exposure.

Hydatid Cysts of the Lung
Presentation

Structurally and in terms of an obligatory enlargement, a hydatid cyst of the lung is in every way similar to one of a liver, the only significant difference being that lung hydatids can enlarge much more rapidly. This difference is readily explained by the lesser resistance offered by lung tissue as compared with the relatively nonyielding liver substance. Approximately 15 to 20 percent of all hydatids seen in endemic areas are located anywhere in the lung. These cysts can be assumed to be descendants of the initially ingested hydatid eggs, which have passed through the liver sinusoidal filtering system but could not negotiate the pulmonary capillary circulation.

Once established in the lung parenchyma, a viable hydatid cyst keeps growing in size until it impinges on nearby structures. Blood vessels are pliant and are pushed aside. Bronchi, on the other hand, are nonyielding and suffer pressure necrosis of their walls. All pulmonary hydatid cysts larger than approximately 2 to 4 cm can be assumed to have already caused such bronchial side openings. Under ordinary circumstances, these small bronchial ports are mechanically plugged up by the impinging laminated membrane. At some point in the course of the parasite's enlargement, air escapes into the potential space between the parasite and host, leading to rupture of the laminated membrane. From that point on, the clinically silent host-parasite relationship is terminated.

Internal rupture of lung cysts is invariably symptomatic, but rarely does it lead to the formation of a multivesicular lung cyst. For one thing, the actual rupture of the intact lung cyst brings about a sudden coughing spell, often with expectoration of the salty-tasting hydatid fluid. Most of the liberated scoleces are also expelled at the same time. Remaining scoleces have almost no chance to grow into mature daughter cysts, since they are readily discharged through the patent bronchial openings, which brought about rupture of the cyst in the first place. The pericystic cavity persists, however, because the torn laminated membrane is too large to escape through the bronchial openings. On rupture, a lung cyst essentially becomes an indolent lung abscess and stops enlarging. However, the persistent bronchial communications allow enough drainage to prevent the development of a truly septic abscess cavity. The patient is never ill and never well.

For purposes of diagnosis and treatment, hydatid cysts of the lung can be grouped into three distinct categories: 1) intact cysts, 2) ruptured cysts, and 3) intrapleural extrusion.

Diagnosis

History and Physical Examination

The finding of an *intact hydatid cyst* on a chest roentgenogram often comes as a surprise, because many of these patients have no specific clinical signs or symptoms. Not infrequently, however, the patient has mild hemoptysis, which is usually small in amount, streaked, and bright red. Why there should be any bleeding in the case of an intact hydatid cyst is not quite clear. It is not related to the size or location of the cyst. Whether this finding indicates impending rupture of the intact cyst cannot be known, since such bleeding usually leads to discovery of the cyst and its surgical removal. Vague chest pains and some shortness of breath can be present at times, but these symptoms are rarely so prominent as to have the patient seek medical attention.

In the case of *ruptured hydatid cysts*, one would expect a whole range of signs and symptoms depending on the pathology that has evolved after rupture. This is indeed the case. The initial episode attending rupture of the cyst might have long been forgotten, and the patient's presenting problem is usually a persistent cough or intermittent hemoptysis, or both. It is rare, although not unheard of, for a patient to actually expectorate the grapeskin-like pieces of laminated membrane and come in with the diagnostic evidence in hand.

Intrapleural extrusion of a lung hydatid cyst is uncommon, even in endemic areas. However, it is easy to predict that the clinical signs and symptoms will be those of sudden pneumothorax, followed by pleural effusion with appropriate respiratory signs and symptoms. Over time, the acute episode changes into that of a chronic empyema. The patient will not recover fully, however, until the parasite is removed and the pleural space managed appropriately.

Roentgenographic Examination

The roentgenographic picture of an *intact hydatid* cyst rarely presents any diagnostic problems in endemic areas. In nonendemic areas, the list of differential diagnoses for a spherical, sharply demarcated, and homogeneous lesion must include pericardial cyst (if the lesion is near the heart border), dermoid cyst, hamartoma, fibroma or lipoma, bronchogenic cyst, and possibly even small-cell carcinoma of the lung. Bronchogenic cysts are rarely dense, and hamartoma is uncommonly of a near-perfect spherical configuration. In children, metastatic sarcomas always remain a distinct possibility.

Fortunately, none of the aforementioned conditions obviates operative intervention. For this reason, it is useless to pursue a complicated and expensive diagnostic track, which might be educational for the surgeon but hardly is profitable for the patient. Neither CT nor radionuclide scans, nor plain tomography nor bronchography will pinpoint the diagnosis if the clinician has not taken the trouble to obtain a proper history.

The roentgenographic diagnosis of a *ruptured hydatid cyst* can be easy, difficult, or impossible, depending on whether the presentation is that of an abscess, a quiescent lesion, or of a progressive and cicatrizing process. The clinical history is helpful, and the presence of hydatid cysts in the liver even more so.

The roentgenographic picture can be pathognomonic if the radiologist is familiar with the unique appearance of a thin-walled abscess cavity showing the so-called water lily sign with the collapsed cyst rising somewhat above the flat fluid level. Even rarer and more transient, but just as picturesque, is the roentgenographic appearance of two concentric empty or fluid-filled thin-walled balloons, variously called double-domed arch or pericystic pneuma (Fig. 93-16). In this instance, the entry of bronchial air, which first led to rupture of the cyst, has also caused partial insufflation of the collapsed cyst.

The lung parenchyma surrounding the ruptured cyst cavity remains remarkably thin because the pericystic layer is an effective barrier against extension of bacterial reaction into surrounding lung tissue. Another helpful roentgenographic sign is the constantly changing appearance of the lesion, especially the more solid-looking ones. The pericyst becomes inflamed with accumulation of purulent secretions, only to be relieved again by their escape into the bronchial system. Resulting roentgenographic changes take place much more rapidly than one would expect with an ordinary inflammatory lesion or even a malignant tumor.

Tomography might or might not reveal the collapsed and fragmented laminated membrane within the center of the nondescript lesion; its roentgenographic density is too similar to that of the host tissue. Bronchography usually shows no more than an irregular nonhealing cavity, the real nature of which remains a mystery until it is surgically exposed.

With *intrapleural extrusion* of a lung cyst, the peripherally located and now emptied pericystic cavity might be visible roentgenographically depending on how long ago the extrusion occurred. The pneumothorax is usually well established by the time the patient is seen, and there is invariably some pleural effusion. The intact but usually ruptured hydatid cyst might or might not be apparent roentgenographically because it can be partially hidden by the effusion (Fig. 93-17).

Bronchoscopy

It can seem heretical to suggest that bronchoscopy should not be done at any time for *intact hydatid cysts* of the lung; this is, however, the most likely way of rupturing such cysts. It would be most fortuitous but

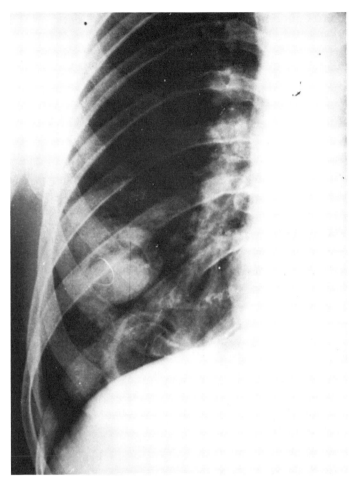

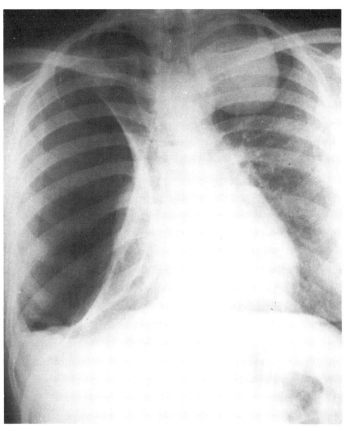

Fig. 93-16. Two ruptured small hydatid cysts of the lung. The lower one shows clearly the ballooned-out laminated membrane within the air-filled pericystic cavity, giving the appearance of a double-domed arch.

Fig. 93-17. A right-sided pneumothorax has developed after an intrapleural rupture of a pulmonary hydatid cyst. The collapsed laminated membrane is barely visible at the costophrenic angle. A separate intact hydatid cyst is located at the apex of the left lung.

unrealistic to expect to see the surface of the whitish laminated membrane through one of the minute side openings of a small- or even medium-sized bronchus. On the other hand, insertion of the tip of a bronchoscope into a lobar or segmental bronchus can provide just the needed trauma to bring about sudden rupture of an intact cyst. If the intact cyst is a very large one, the great quantity of escaping hydatid fluid can flood the bronchial tree faster than can be aspirated by available means of suctioning. A calamity can ensue, which can well be avoided by thinking beforehand about the possibility of a hydatid cyst and by having reviewed mentally its structural configuration.

For *ruptured hydatid cysts*, especially long-standing ones, diagnostic bronchoscopy is unavoidable. There is a chance, occasionally, of actually seeing and retrieving a part of the fragmented laminated membrane and thereby making the diagnosis.

Surgical Treatment

The operative management of either *intact* or *ruptured* hydatid cysts of the lung is generally the same, and the basic approach to both can be discussed together. A clear-cut diagnosis might not have been made preoperatively in either situation. However, the patient's general condition and the often unexplained roentgenographic picture, if not the surgeon's curiosity, eventually prompt operative intervention.

Certain preoperative steps are superfluous: The risk of bronchoscopy in instances of *intact lung cysts* has already been mentioned. The next to consider is chest physiotherapy. Chest percussion can be helpful in clearing secretions, but there is always the danger of precipitating rupture of an *intact cyst*. For long-standing ruptured cysts, no amount of physiotherapy will bring about evacuation of parasitic material. As for liver hydatids, the possibility always exists of an anaphylactic reaction during the operation as a result of rupture of a large intact cyst with rapid absorption of hydatid fluid in a previously sensitized patient. The most likely manifestation would be bronchospasm. This complication can be avoided by preoperative medication with approximately 100 mg of intravenously administered fast-acting corticosteroids.

I have never felt the need for one-lung anesthesia. Recall that liberated scoleces do not get a foothold on bronchial mucous membranes. Therefore, there is no need for separate control of the two-stem bronchi in the hope of averting any possible contamination of the bronchial tree during an operation. Expanding the lung at will during the operation greatly facilitates not only entry into the cyst but also identification of all bronchial openings into the pericystic cavity.

Exposure

The standard posterolateral incision provides the best access to hydatid cysts anywhere in the lung. There might be overlying vascular pleural adhesions, especially in the instance of previously ruptured cysts. When there are no pleural adhesions, the characteristically round and whitish or grayish surface discoloration, representing the most superficial portion of the pericystic layer, leaves no doubt as to the diagnosis. Less superficial cysts might have no special surface markings and the surgeon can only feel a firm tumefaction. With experience, the surgeon can distinguish the fluid sensation of an intact cyst from the soft feel of a ruptured one. Long-standing and chronically inflamed cysts impart a feeling of hardness no different from that of a lung tumor.

The first effort must be directed toward freeing up the whole lung by taking down all pleural adhesions without much manipulation of the involved lobe or a premature entry into the pericystic cavity. Once the lung has been fully freed up, nearby pleural surfaces as well as the thoracotomy wound edges must be carefully walled off with appropriately placed gauze pads. The surgeon is now ready to attack the lesion itself, often without being absolutely certain of the diagnosis.

Entry and Evacuation

The surgical approach advocated in this situation is evacuation of the parasite with conservation of lung tissue, the implication being that no intact hydatid cyst of the lung, no matter how large, requires any type of resectional therapy. With reasonable care, spillage of hydatid fluid and contamination of the surgical field with viable scoleces can be avoided. Resection is justified only in the uncommon situation of a ruptured cyst having caused progressive fibrous destruction of a significant portion of the lung.

Entry into an intact cyst should be preceded by decompression of its internal fluid pressure. This step is performed exactly as has been described for liver hydatid cysts. The pericystic cavity is next laid wide open (Fig. 93-18). The punctured and partially collapsed laminated membrane is now extracted, and any hydatid fluid still within the pericystic cavity is sucked away.

The idea, still encountered in some texts, of carefully cutting lung tissue until the laminated membrane is exposed and then gently enucleating the intact cyst and having it fall into a water-filled basin—a maneuver assisted by having the anesthetist fully inflate the lungs—is appealing. It rarely succeeds, however, and it is usually disastrous in terms of unexpected rupture of the partially exposed or partly delivered laminated membrane.

Preliminary decompression hardly matters in instances of previously ruptured hydatid cysts. Therefore, the first step is to cut directly into the pericystic cavity at the point on the surface of the lung that seems closest to the lesion. Once the center of the lesion is reached, the distinctive white piece of laminated membrane comes into view, establishing the diagnosis. The whole of the cavity, which might not be very large, is laid open. There are rarely any daughter cysts to worry about, and once the parasite has been extracted, the first phase of the operation is over.

Managing the Residual Cavity

Management of the residual cavity consists of closure of the bronchial openings and obliteration of the emptied pericystic cavity. It would at first seem quite feasible to take a number of deep suture bites into the pericystic wall and obliterate the pericystic cavity in layers, closing the bronchial openings at the same time. This technique, called capitonnage, cannot be counted on to work all the time. Some of the smaller bronchial openings are not readily visible and have to be carefully sought. Since all these openings are of such a size as to have cartilage in their walls, their closure must be effected in the proper manner, that is, careful and atraumatic approximation of their edges. Closure of bronchial openings and obliteration of the pericystic cavity must remain two separately executed operative steps.

Holding the edges of the pericystic opening wide apart for proper inspection, one can find a number of small- and sometimes even medium-sized bronchial openings. The anesthetist can help in this search by increasing the intrabronchial air pressure. In instances of long-standing ruptured cysts, the bronchial apertures sometimes appear grossly inflamed and set within a

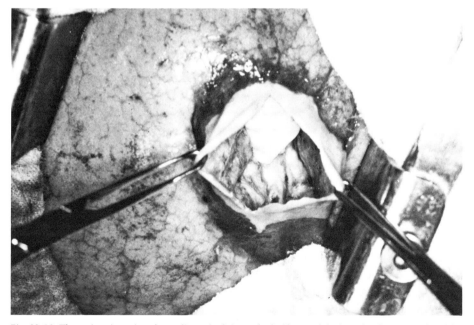

Fig. 93-18. The pericystic cavity of a medium-sized, intact hydatid cyst of the lung has been opened widely after a preliminary decompression, which has also caused rupture of the cyst. The edges of the pericystic layer are held apart with Allis clamps. The collapsed laminated membrane rests in the upper part of the pericystic cavity. At the bottom of the pericystic cavity can be seen one medium-sized bronchial opening. There are undoubtedly other smaller bronchial openings in the folds of the pericystic cavity.

field of granulation tissue. It seems against all good surgical principles to suture such bronchial openings and expect them to remain closed. However, gentle and not-too-tight closure with fine nonabsorbable suture material is effective regardless of the gross appearance of such a bronchial opening.

Bronchial openings larger than 4 to 5 mm in diameter, usually seen in ruptured cysts of long standing, cannot be closed from within the pericystic cavity. There is commonly gross destruction of lung tissue as well. In this circumstance, resectional therapy does have a place. The size of the cystic lesion itself is not the crucial factor.

It should be clear that resectional therapy for lung cysts is never necessary for intact hydatid cysts regardless of their size. It should not be undertaken to avoid spillage of cystic contents. Resection becomes necessary only when primary closure of bronchial openings cannot be safely achieved and the surrounding lung tissue is irreversibly damaged.

Killing of Scoleces

Only after all bronchial openings have been closed can one attempt to kill the scoleces that might have been lost within the fine interstices of the pericystic surface lining. A scolecidal agent such as 0.5% silver nitrate solution, which I prefer because of its effectiveness and lack of toxicity, is poured into the pericystic cavity. This solution stays within the pericystic cavity once all bronchial escape holes have been sutured shut. The cavity is further washed out with normal saline solution. For each washing, the anesthetist increases the airway pressure to reveal additional small bronchial openings, which might have been overlooked. For hydatid cysts that have ruptured for a period longer than just a few days, the use of any scolecidal agent is of doubtful value, because spilled scoleces are either well established or have already been expectorated.

Closure

The edges of the pericystic cavity opening are now trimmed and oversewn with running fine catgut suture material. This step stops bleeding and leakage of alveolar air from the edges of the cavity, ensuring at the same time that the cleaned-out pericystic cavity will remain widely open into the pleural space. A chest tube leading to an underwater seal is inserted and the

chest closed. Prompt and full expansion of the lung is the best guarantee of a smooth postoperative course. There is no need to apply continuous controlled suction to the chest tube. In fact, it is preferable to allow lung expansion by the patient's own effort, assisted by vigorous chest physiotherapy. Any major air leak that persists postoperatively beyond 2 or 3 days might be a sign that a bronchial opening has been overlooked. This finding calls for re-exploration and closure.

Intrapleural Extrusion

The surgical treatment of intrapleural extrusion, which is rare, is management of the contaminated pleural space and the pericystic cavity at the same time. A great deal depends on how soon after extrusion of the cyst the pleural space is surgically exposed. This event would depend on the severity of the attending signs and symptoms as well as the correct diagnosis having been made. Patients with intrapleural extrusion of hydatid cysts are prone toward secondary pleural hydatid cysts months or years after their initial operation. Such cysts are remnants of scoleces implanted on the pleural surfaces at the time of the initial rupture of the cyst. Therefore, these patients should have follow-up chest roentgenograms at 6-month intervals for approximately 3 years.

Intrabronchial Embolization

A potentially disastrous intraoperative complication, usually encountered with long-standing intrathoracic rupture of liver hydatid cysts, is intrabronchial embolization of daughter cysts or fragments of laminated membrane to the opposite lung. When this occurs, the anesthetist is suddenly unable to expand the opposite lung since the solid parasitic fragments cannot be extracted even with suctioning. The use of a double-lumen endotracheal tube or blocking the bronchus on the operative side does not necessarily avert the problem. In fact, solid fragments of the parasite can escape unnoticed into the nonfunctioning bronchial tree of the operative side, only to enter the opposite lung after extubation. The best way to deal with such a serious complication is to be alert to the possibility when dealing with pericystic cavities containing many small daughter cysts and fragments of laminated membrane, usually following chronic intrathoracic rupture of liver cysts. Too much pressure on the involved lung

should be avoided. Prior control of the stem bronchus before actual entry into the pericystic layer is also helpful. The latter step permits rapid bronchotomy for evacuation of parasitic debris, should it become necessary.

Intra-Abdominal Hydatid Cysts

The Setting

Next to the liver and the lung, the abdominal cavity is the most common site of hydatid cysts. Theoretically, there can be no such thing as a primary peritoneal cyst since the peritoneum does not have a distinct arterial circulation of its own. All hydatid cysts within the free abdominal cavity are, indeed, secondary to intraperitoneally ruptured liver hydatids. Their number can vary from one or more large- or medium-sized cysts anywhere in the abdominal cavity to literally hundreds or thousands of small cysts disseminated among the viscera (Fig. 93-19). There might be no evidence of the initial liver cyst whose intra-abdominal rupture at some time in the past had seeded the abdominal cavity. Each individual intra-abdominal cyst, regardless of size or location, is encased within a very vascular fibrous tissue pericystic layer contributed by the serosal surfaces of adjacent viscera.

The management of intra-abdominal cysts rests on a clear understanding of the pathology involved. As elsewhere in the body, hydatid cysts in the abdomen are bound to grow in size, sooner or later creating pressure symptoms along with local or general abdominal enlargement. Remarkably enough, the parasite is not known to cause pressure necrosis of the nearby intestinal wall or directly enter the intestinal lumen. Hydatid cysts of the spleen are not rare at all. They are always primary cysts but for treatment purposes can be considered along with intra-abdominal hydatids. Intraperitoneal rupture of splenic cysts is possible, but most of the time such cysts remain within the confines of the spleen, reaching sometimes enormous dimensions, or they might calcify and stop growing.

The diagnosis of intra-abdominal or splenic cysts is made, again, mainly on the basis of the history and other circumstantial evidence. The physical examination

Nonsurgical Treatment of Hydatid Disease

Until approximately 15 years ago, there was no alternative to surgical treatment of echinococcal disease. Even radiation therapy and immunotherapy had been tried without any benefit. Most patients afflicted with echinococcal disease, especially in endemic areas of the world, are generally young and healthy, and can be operated on with an acceptably low morbidity and mortality. However, there are exceptions, and some patients would be better off without surgery if a truly effective drug regimen were available. Hydatid cysts of certain organs such as the bones and especially the vertebral column are inherently difficult to treat, bordering on incurability. For these situations, especially if the patient is otherwise debilitated, medical treatment would be preferable to any surgical intervention. The difficulty has always been the inability to transport large molecular substances across the impervious laminated membrane.

Effective medical treatment seems now available with mebendazole, a well-known but poorly absorbed benzimidazole antihelminthic. Perhaps no more than 5 percent of the oral dose of this drug is absorbed from the intestinal tract, but strangely enough, what does reach the laminated membrane seems to go across it and effectively interfere with the glucose metabolism of the germinative layer. For reasons not known, however, not all viable cysts are adversely affected by mebendazole. My experience is that no more than one-half of patients respond to long-term mebendazole treatment. A more recent drug of the same generic family, albendazole, is more readily absorbed from the intestine. It is understandably difficult and impractical, especially in nonendemic areas of the world, to conduct controlled clinical trials to establish the true value of such drug therapy.

These drugs are reasonably well tolerated, except for occasional leukopenia or erythropenia, or both, and a reversible change in liver function tests. The real problem, however, lies in not being able to predict which patients will respond and which will not. In practice, whenever operative intervention seems contraindicated, me-

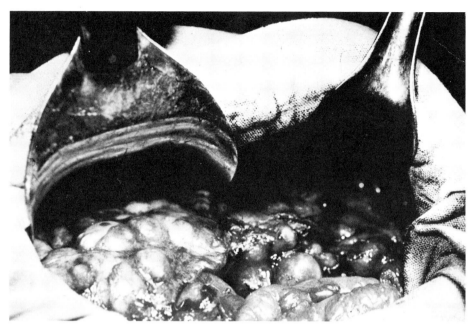

Fig. 93-19. The peritoneal cavity of a patient with diffuse abdominal echinococcosis has been opened, showing innumerable small- and medium-sized intra-abdominal hydatid cysts matted together and interspersed among the viscera.

can only corroborate the clinical suspicion, and sonography and CT should readily support the clinical diagnosis.

Surgical Treatment

Once the abdomen has been opened and the diagnosis verified, it becomes tempting to deliver each cyst in an intact manner by dissecting all around its pericystic layer. This procedure is practicable for a few pedunculated cysts. More often, many large and small cysts are matted together or are located deep in the recesses of the abdominal cavity, their pericystic layer being part of the nearby intestinal wall. The risk of local spillage of hydatid fluid does rise in proportion to the number of cysts removed. However, it is less dangerous than trying to dissect out the cysts intact, thereby unintentionally entering the intestinal lumen. Furthermore, dissecting outside the pericystic layer of such cysts can become a very bloody procedure. More and more cysts are encountered as dissection proceeds, the removal of each becoming a challenge to remove the rest as well. The total blood loss can be considerable. It is best to be conservative and remove as many intra-abdominal cysts in one operation as seems safe and reasonable, leaving the rest for another session.

Single large cysts that are not pedunculated are best treated as if they were lung or liver cysts: The area around the cyst is isolated, and then decompression is carried out in the prescribed manner. The pericyst is next opened, the collapsed laminated membrane extracted, and the lining of the pericystic cavity sterilized with a scolecidal solution. When there are many small cysts all matted together, the surgeon might have no choice but to remove a number of them as a single specimen. All possible precautions against uncontrolled spillage should be taken routinely. (Silver nitrate solution, 0.5%, is very hypotonic and should, therefore, not be poured too liberally into the abdominal cavity as a general washing-out maneuver.)

In instances of splenic cysts, it only needs to be emphasized that there is no need to remove the whole spleen. Splenectomy does obviate all risks of rupture and spillage of cystic contents. However, if a splenic hydatid is managed as outlined for liver and lung cysts, there should be little or no risk of local recurrence, and the spleen can be saved. After the excess pericystic layer is trimmed at the edges of the opening, the pericystic cavity can be left wide open to the peritoneal cavity.

Table 93-1. Essential Points in the Surgical Management of all Hydatid Cysts

Rules	Reasons
1. Only the parasite needs to be removed, there being no need to remove all or part of the affected organ	1. The host organ parenchyma is displaced but not damaged
2. The most superficial part of the cyst should be approached, exposed, and used for decompression and evacuation	2. This reduces surgical trauma to the host organ and allows complete evacuation of all parasitic elements
3. The operative site should first be isolated from the surrounding operative field	3. Uncontrolled release of high intracystic pressure can lead to contamination of nearby areas
4. The first step should always be decompression of the internal pressure of the cyst	4. See reason 3
5. Intact removal of a large univesicular hydatid cyst from within the pericystic cavity should rarely be attempted	5. The intact laminated membrane is fragile and is easily ruptured during its delivery
6. There is no need to remove the pericystic layer	6. The pericystic layer is host tissue and not separable from the rest of the host organ
7. An opened pericystic cavity must be well inspected and thoroughly emptied of all parasitic material	7. Residual parasitic material, whether fragments of laminated membrane or daughter cysts, remains unabsorbable foreign matter
8. A fully evacuated pericystic cavity must be washed out with an appropriate scolecidal agent	8. During extraction of the cyst, viable scoleces can be released and implanted within the pericystic cavity
9. A calcified hydatid cyst, or one beginning to calcify, does not necessarily have to be removed surgically	9. Such cysts are dead or dying; they do not grow and are usually no longer of any danger to the host
10. There is no need for special precautions against contamination of personnel in the operating room	10. Transfer of larval infection from person to person does not take place through intact skin or mucous membranes

bendazole in a dosage of 50 mg/kg body weight on an empirical basis (albendazole, 10 mg/kg body weight) can be prescribed and its effectiveness reevaluated clinically in 3 to 6 months. Reductions both in the size of intact cysts and in the pain of bone involvement are reliable criteria of drug effectiveness. Serum levels of the drug can be measured to make certain that minimally effective amounts are present in the circulation. It should not be forgotten, however, that the laminated membrane is not dissolved by antihelminthics and remains behind as a foreign body.

Summary

The essential points in the surgical management of all hydatid cysts of soft-tissue organs can be summarized as certain simple and basic rules. For each rule there is practical reason (Table 93-1).

Suggested Reading

Deve F. Experiments proving that ingestion of echinococcus by way of digestive tract does not cause secondary echinococcosis. *Compt Rendu de la Societe Biologie*. 114:669, 1933.

Dew H. *Hydatid Disease: Its Pathology, Diagnosis and Treatment*. Sydney: Australasian Medical Publishing Co., 1928.

Doty JE, Tompkins RK. Management of cystic disease of the liver. *Surg Clin North Am* 69:285, 1989.

Golematis B, Delikaris P. Treatment of Echinococcal Cyst. In LM Nyhus and RJ Baker (eds.), *Mastery of Surgery*. (1st ed). Boston: Little, Brown, 1983.

Morris DL, Dykes PW, Marriner S, et al. Albendazole—objective evidence of response in human hydatid disease. *JAMA* 253: 2053, 1985.

Mottaghian H, Saidi F. Postoperative recurrence of hydatid disease. *Br J Surg* 65:237, 1978.

Romero-Torres R, Campbell JR. An interpretive review of surgical treatment of hydatid disease. *Surg Gynecol Obstet* 121:852, 1965.

Saidi F. *Surgery of Hydatid Disease*. Philadelphia: Saunders, 1976.

Saidi F, Rezvan-Nobahar M. Intraoperative bronchial aspiration of ruptured pulmonary hydatid cysts. *Ann Thorac Surg* 50:631, 1990.

Stamatakis J. Hepatic Hydatid Disease. In CD Johnson and I Taylor (eds.), *Recent Advances in Surgery—17*. London: Churchill-Livingstone, 1994.

Thompson RCA (ed.). *The Biology of Echinococcus and Hydatid Disease*. London: Allen & Unwin, 1986.

EDITOR'S COMMENT

As travel becomes more widespread, physicians in developed countries will need to have the same degree of suspicion and expertise as in countries such as Iran, Turkey, and Greece, in which this disease is endemic.

Doctor Saidi's chapter emphasizes several points concerning this disease. First, that it is generally benign. Dr. Saidi as well as other authorities in the field emphasize that radical procedures such as hepatic resection are almost never necessary. Second, that surgery is the primary mode of treatment in any patient who can withstand the surgical procedure. Similar conclusions were reached by Golematis and Peveretos (*Mount Sinai J Med* 62:71, 1995).

These patients are generally not ill unless there is bacterial superinfection, in which case one has a set-up for a chronic, low-intensity infection, which is usually treated with external drainage. All authorities emphasize that albendazole is the appropriate antibiotic of choice.

In most series, resection and subtotal resection are possible in less than one-half of patients. The remainder are treated with aspiration, cyst obliteration, and external drainage. The scolecidal activity of 0.5% silver nitrate seems to be recognized by most. Hypertonic saline, which has been a standard, apparently is not efficacious unless it reaches a 15% solution.

The principal problem, especially in developed countries, remains the diagnosis of this disease, particularly when individuals do not have a high index of suspicion. Even in Saudi Arabia, von Sinner and associates (*Acta Radiologica* 36:168, 1995) pointed out that the diagnostic value of fine-needle aspiration biopsy was limited, especially when there was a low index of suspicion. In only 7 of 31 patients were the specimens obtained of value in the ability to make the diagnosis of hydatid disease. An occasional patient had an anaphylactic reaction. Thus, fine-needle aspiration biopsy at this point in time does not appear to have a great role in the diagnosis of this disease. Similarly, although one might be tempted to pursue a minimally invasive approach, the dangers of uncontrolled spillage of scoleces would seem to be an important and absolute contraindication to this approach.

J.E.F.

Major Hepatic Resection
for Primary and Metastatic Tumor

Leslie H. Blumgart   Yuman Fong

Hepatic resection for the treatment of tumors involving the liver can be necessary for the removal of primary benign or malignant tumors of the liver or biliary tract or for secondary neoplasms. Hepatic resection for the removal of gallbladder carcinoma and cholangiocarcinoma at the confluence of the bile ducts is a special subject and will not be dealt with in this chapter.

General Principles

Partial hepatectomy for the removal of *benign tumors* of the liver should, in general, be performed only for symptomatic patients, in the presence of doubt as to the diagnosis, or for tumors with known malignant potential. Removal of liver tissue should be minimal. The use of techniques for enucleation of such tumors is often appropriate in the management of hemangioma, adenoma, or fibronodular hyperplasia but is not described in this chapter.

On the other hand, partial hepatectomy as treatment for *malignant tumors* of the liver must be guided by the principle of complete tumor removal with a margin of parenchymal transection clear of the tumor. Current evidence suggests that this margin should ideally be no less than 1 cm. Frequently, practical considerations, particularly in the removal of large tumors, dictate that the clearance is less than this optimal margin. Since long-term survival has been recorded even with close margins, inability to obtain wide clearance should not restrain the surgeon.

The main problems in achieving adequate clearance margins in *wedge resections* for tumors apparently situated peripherally in the liver should not be underestimated. In the latter situation, adequate clearance is often compromised in the depth of the wedge. Indeed, it has been demonstrated that wedge resections carry an unacceptable local recurrence rate and that anatomically based resection yields better results. Another factor that can compromise resection is the presence of a very hard tumor, which is often the case with metastatic colorectal carcinoma, residing in a soft and easily fractured liver. Extreme care should be taken that, at the point of closest parenchymal transection, the liver does not tear open and split along the tumor-liver interface at the time of transection.

The *main hazards* of hepatic resection are biliary leakage and bleeding. In particular, bleeding from the hepatic veins and inferior vena cava during parenchymal transection is a major problem. This hazard is especially likely to occur during major resection for high and posteriorly placed tumors where there is little clearance between the tumor margin and the passage of the hepatic veins into the vena cava or when tumors are closely adherent to or adjacent to the inferior vena cava.

In this chapter, the description of techniques in the performance of hepatic resection concentrates on the removal of minimal liver tissue with the achievement of adequate margins of resection in malignant disease and on the simultaneous prevention of hemorrhage, particularly from the hepatic veins or inferior vena cava. The

performance of formal resection guided by the anatomic configuration of the liver is important.

Anatomy and Classification

Precise knowledge of the surgical anatomy of the liver, its blood vessels, and biliary channels is essential for the performance of safe liver resection.

Lobes

The ligamentum teres enters the umbilical fissure of the liver where it joins the termination of the left portal vein. The liver is divided by the umbilical fissure and by the prolongation of the ligamentum teres as the falciform ligament into two lobes, a right and a left (Fig. 94-1). At the inferior surface of the right lobe, the transverse hilar fissure constitutes the posterior limit of this lobe. The portion of the right lobe anterior to the fissure is called the quadrate lobe and is limited on the left by the umbilical fissure and falciform ligament and on the right by the gallbladder fossa. Posterior to the hilar transverse fissure is a fourth lobe, the caudate lobe. All these lobar areas are demarcated by visible and well-defined fissures in the liver surface.

Sectors and Segments

The gross division of the liver into lobes, which can be observed on inspection, hides within the liver substance a much more complex segmental organization. The description of Couinaud (1957) is the

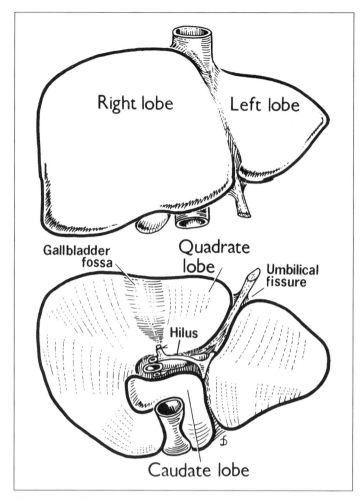

Fig. 94-1. Morphologic aspect of the liver. Note that the liver is divided into right and left lobes as seen from the anterior aspect. From the inferior aspect, the right lobe is bounded posteriorly by the transverse fissure, the portion of the right lobe lying anterior to this being the quadrate lobe limited on the left by the umbilical fissure and on the right by the gallbladder fossa. Posterior to the hilar fissure is the caudate lobe. (From H Bismuth, D Castaing, and F Emond. Intraoperative Ultrasound and Liver Surgery. In LH Blumgart [ed.], Surgery of the Liver and Biliary Tract, 2nd ed. London: Churchill-Livingstone, 1994. Reproduced with permission.)

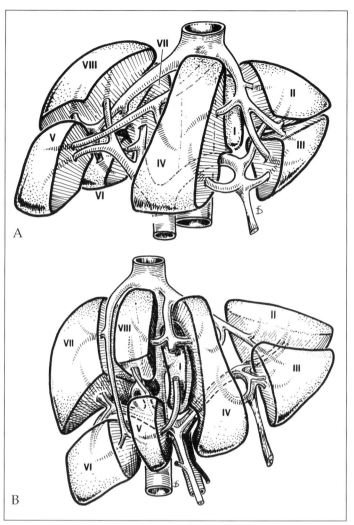

Fig. 94-2. The functional division of the liver into sectors and segments according to Couinaud's nomenclature. A. As seen in the patient. B. In the ex-vivo position. There are three main hepatic veins lying within the liver scissurae and dividing the liver into four sectors, each receiving a portal pedicle. The portal pedicles subdivide and pass to the individual segments. (Note that in the nomenclature of Goldsmith and Woodburne [1957] the sectors are referred to as segments (see text and also Figures 94-3A and 94-4). The hepatic veins and portal pedicles interdigitate as the fingers of two hands. (From H Bismuth, D Castaing, and F Emond. Intraoperative Ultrasound and Liver Surgery. In LH Blumgart [ed.], Surgery of the Liver and Biliary Tract, 2nd ed. London: Churchill-Livingstone, 1994. Reproduced with permission.)

most useful and is now widely accepted. The portal triads composed of the hepatic artery, portal vein, and biliary ducts enter the liver at the hilus contained in a sheath of fibrous tissue as the portal pedicles (vide infra) and blood are drained to the vena cava via the hepatic veins. Distribution of the main portal pedicles and the location of the major hepatic veins allow description of the sectors and segments of the liver. The three main hepatic veins di-

vide the liver into four sectors*, each of which receives a portal pedicle. The four sectors demarcated by the hepatic veins are called the portal sectors, and these portions of parenchyma are supplied by independent portal pedicles. The divisions

*It should be noted that in the nomenclature described by Goldsmith and Woodburne (1957), the major subdivisions of the liver are usually called segments, whereas according to the nomenclature of Couinaud they are called sectors.

separating the sectors are called portal scissurae and contain the hepatic veins. The segmental structure of the liver (which makes up the sectors) is based on the distribution of the portal pedicles (Fig. 94-2).

The anatomic division between the right and left liver is not at the falciform ligament but follows a line projecting through a plane (the principal plane or Cantlie's line) running from the medial margin of

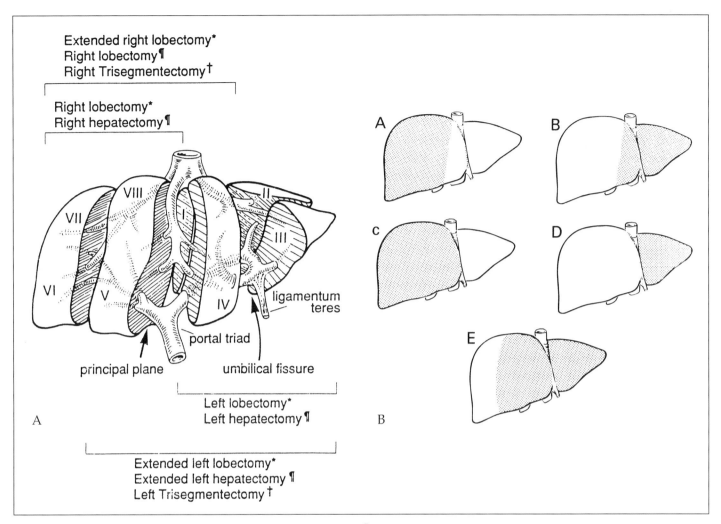

Extended right lobectomy*
Right lobectomy¶
Right Trisegmentectomy†

Right lobectomy*
Right hepatectomy¶

VIII

VII

I

II

III

VI

V

IV

ligamentum
teres

portal triad

principal plane

umbilical fissure

A

B

Left lobectomy*
Left hepatectomy¶

Extended left lobectomy*
Extended left hepatectomy¶
Left Trisegmentectomy†

A

B

C

D

E

Fig. 94-3. A. The various major hepatectomies with the nomenclature of Couinaud,¶ Goldsmith and Woodburne,* and Starzl† indicated. Left lobectomy (Couinaud) (left lateral segmentectomy) is not shown here but is indicated in part B. B. The major hepatic resections are indicated: A, right hepatectomy; B, left hepatectomy; C, right lobectomy; D, left lobectomy; E, extended left hepatectomy (Couinaud 1957). (From LH Blumgart. Liver Resection—Liver and Biliary Tumours. In LH Blumgart [ed.], Surgery of the Liver and Biliary Tract, 2nd ed. London: Churchill-Livingstone, 1994. Reproduced with permission.)

the gallbladder bed to the left side of the vena cava posterosuperiorly. This line marks the main scissura of the liver and contains the middle hepatic vein. Each of these major right and left portions of the liver is further divided into sectors and segments. The *segments* (Fig. 94-2) are numbered one through eight for convenience of description. Thus, segment I is used to describe the caudate lobe. Segments II and III constitute the left lobe of the liver, and because the left hepatic vein courses between these two segments forming the left scissura, it demarcates segment II as the only unisegmental sector of the liver. Segments III and IV (or the quadrate lobe), separated by the umbilical fissure,

together constitute the medial sector of the left liver, being themselves demarcated by the main scissura containing the middle hepatic vein from the right liver. The right liver is composed of an anterior sector comprising segments V and VIII separated from a posterior sector, comprising segments VI and VII, by the right hepatic vein lying within the right scissura. The symmetry of this organization is well illustrated in Figs. 94-2 through 94-4.

Pedicles

The portal veins and hepatic artery divide into major right and left branches outside the liver substance below the hilus. The

branches of the hepatic artery and portal vein together with the accompanying bile ducts form triads, and as they pass into the liver tissue take a prolongation of Glisson's capsule with them so that within the liver these structures are contained in a well-formed fibrous sheath forming the portal pedicles, which are of surgical importance. Beneath the liver in the hilus, no such dense sheath exists, but here after dividing the peritoneum, the major branches of the portal vein and hepatic artery and, indeed, tributaries of the bile ducts can be individually dissected. On the right, the short course of the extrahepatic structures beyond their bifurcation and the variable anatomy of the biliary tree make them vul-

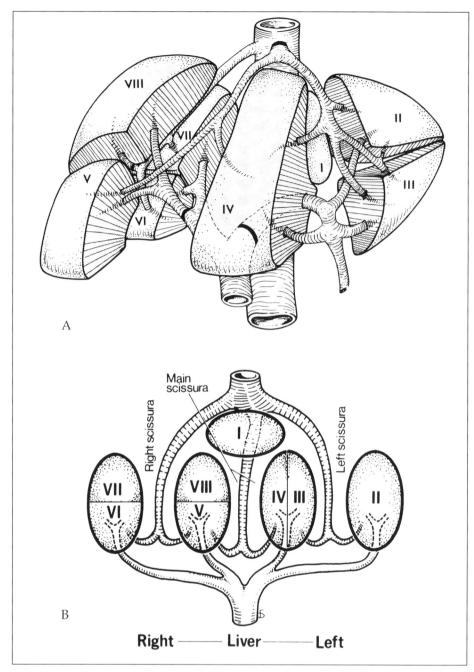

Fig. 94-4. A. Exploded view to show the sectors and segments of the liver. Extended left hepatectomy involves removal of segments II, III, IV, V, and VIII, and sometimes of segment I. The segments in dark shading to be removed are illustrated. The solid lines on the right anterior sectoral pedicle and the left portal triad illustrate the devascularization necessary. The solid lines on the middle and left hepatic veins illustrate the point of hepatic venous transection. Note that the right posterior sectoral triad is preserved supplying segments V and VIII, as is the right hepatic vein. B. A diagram of the liver's structure. (From LH Blumgart. Liver Resection—Liver and Biliary Tumours. In LH Blumgart [ed.], Surgery of the Liver and Biliary Tract, 2nd ed. London: Churchill-Livingstone, 1994. Reproduced with permission.)

nerable and more easily damaged during dissection. By contrast, the left branch of the portal vein and left hepatic duct pursue a longer, more horizontal extrahepatic course beneath the quadrate lobe (Figs. 94-2 and 94-3) and are more easily dissected. The ligamentum teres runs sharply into the umbilical fissure of the liver, and within the fissure the left branch of the portal vein curves caudally and in its passage through the fissure gives branches not only to the left lobe (segments II and III) but together with branches of the left artery gives rise to "feedback vessels" to segment IV (quadrate lobe) of the left liver (Figs. 94-2 and 94-3).

Hepatic Veins

The liver lies astride the inferior vena cava immediately below the diaphragm, and the hepatic veins run a short extrahepatic course before emptying into the vena cava. The hepatic veins are not invested with a fibrous sheath as are the pedicles. The right hepatic vein emerges from the right scissura and enters the vena cava separately, but the left hepatic vein, which runs in the left scissura between segments II and III, is frequently joined by the middle hepatic vein, which importantly occupies the principal scissura as already described (Fig. 94-2). The left hepatic vein can enter the vena cava independently. Smaller veins drain from the posterior surface of the liver into the inferior vena cava and particularly from the caudate lobe, which is closely applied to the left of the vena cava. Occasionally, a large inferior right hepatic vein is present and can be of importance in some major resections (vide infra).

In essence, major hepatic resection is carried out by isolating the vessels supplying the area to be removed (Fig. 94-5). This isolation can be done by dissection of the relevant portal pedicle at the hilus and outside the liver substance. Alternatively, the major branches can be controlled within the liver by division of the liver tissue so as to allow isolation of the intrahepatic pedicles. In practice, most surgeons use a combination of techniques in hepatic resection. Initial isolation of the vessels at the hilus and outside the liver substance followed by ligation and division of these structures and subsequent parenchymal transection is the most commonly performed approach and

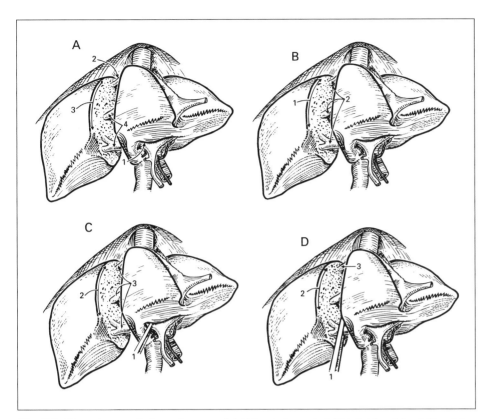

Fig. 94-5. Alternative steps in the performance of right hepatectomy. A. Initial division of the right portal triad (1) and of the right hepatic vein (2) and then subsequent transection of the liver substances (3) with intrahepatic isolation of vessels (4). B. Initial parenchymal dissection (1) with intrahepatic control of the vessels (2). C. Initial dissection of the portal triad and clamp (1) followed by parenchymal transection (2) with intrahepatic control of the vessels (3). D. Intrahepatic control of the portal pedicles (1) followed by parenchymal transection (2) with subsequent intrahepatic control of the hepatic veins (3). Most experienced surgeons use a combination of these techniques as dictated by the particular case. (From LH Blumgart. Liver Resection—Liver and Biliary Tumours. In LH Blumgart [ed.], Surgery of the Liver and Biliary Tract, *2nd ed. London: Churchill-Livingstone, 1994. Reproduced with permission.)*

is important for large tumors encroaching on the hilus, but extrahepatic dissection can be followed by temporary clamp occlusion of the relevant vessels until major structures are isolated within the liver structure and secured.

Major hepatic veins can be secured within the liver substance during the process of parenchymal transection but retrohepatic dissection and control of the major veins outside the liver substance are our preference and are essential if tumor clearance is to be obtained for large tumors lying high within the liver and close to the vena cava.

Classification

For practical purposes, there are five types of major resection (Fig. 94-3). The nomen-clature of these major resections is based on the anatomic description of Couinaud but the alternative terminology described by Goldsmith and Woodburne is also used and shown in Fig. 94-3A. It should be noted that the terms right trisegmentectomy and left trisegmentectomy coined by Starzl are, in fact, inappropriate and the operations described conform more closely to descriptions of trisectorectomy.

Preoperative Investigation

Preoperative investigation is directed first at anatomic definition of the liver lesion and second at determining, as far as possible, the presence or absence of extrahe-patic disease. The *extent of tumor involvement of the liver* is important since it can influence the decision to operate and the operative approach.

Computed tomographic (CT) scans give valuable preliminary information. Peripherally placed lesions never involve the hilar structures or vena cava and CT scanning, by demonstrating such lesions, indicates freedom from involvement and can obviate the necessity for other studies. More centrally situated lesions can involve major vessels close to the hilus, and CT scanning with dynamic portography can be most helpful in creating an image of the extent of vascular compromise caused by the tumor. Most metastatic lesions tend to respect intersegmental planes and push structures away rather than directly invade them. Even when very large lesions shown on CT scan seem to involve the hilar structures or inferior vena cava, they often do not and such appearances should not preclude consideration for resection. Involvement of the diaphragm can also be suggested by CT scanning, but similarly, should not deter the surgeon since such apparent diaphragmatic involvement in metastatic colorectal cancer is almost always the result of adhesion at the site of previous infarction of the tumor.

Magnetic resonance imaging (MRI) can also be valuable in the demonstration of the mass or the presence of additional lesions not shown at CT. In particular, MRI angiographic images recently have been shown to be of value in the demonstration of major hepatic vessels and their relationship to tumor masses. Nevertheless, and despite this demonstration, ultrasonography, particularly duplex ultrasonography, is readily performed, much cheaper, and can yield the same information.

Ultrasonography provides information regarding the size of the tumor and extent of liver involvement. It is of special value in the preoperative assessment of multiple tumors and particularly in the demonstration of small additional tumors. Duplex ultrasonography by demonstrating vascular structures including the hepatic veins and the vena cava obviates the need for angiography in some instances.

Hepatic angiography and inferior vena cavography are no longer essential in all situations and indeed should not be used for the preoperative assessment of peripherally placed tumors. For large tumors or lesions close to the midline, hepatic angiography with late-phase portography and for inferior vena cavography can be useful, although modern advances in duplex ultrasonography and MRI imaging make the necessity for these studies increasingly less frequent.

In our practice, the indication for hepatic angiography is usually the preoperative demonstration of *extrahepatic arterial anatomy* in patients in whom the insertion of a hepatic infusion pump for postoperative adjunctive chemotherapy is contemplated.

Assessment of resectability of solitary large tumors has in recent years become a question of judgment for the individual surgeon as to the ability to remove lesions involving hilar structures or the major hepatic veins. Large tumors expand, compress, and displace surrounding vessels and only occasionally is there direct vascular invasion. The size of a tumor alone is not a contraindication to resection. Indeed, techniques are now available to resect and repair the portal vein and inferior vena cava even when major vessels are involved. If there are multiple or bilateral tumors, their disposition and number can indicate clear irresectability, but frequently final decisions must be delayed until the operation.

In summary, with increasing experience, we have come to rely on CT images and ultrasonography as the major preoperative investigative modalities of value in allowing preoperative assessment of resectability and of the likely difficulties to be encountered during an operation.

Extrahepatic disease is sought by a series of studies including colonoscopy, CT images of the abdomen, chest x-ray, and more recently, CT images of the chest. Bone scans are not essential except in an investigative setting.

It should, of course, be emphasized that the presence of lymph nodes on CT scanning does not imply nodal involvement by a tumor and such studies are notoriously unreliable. Thus, the presence of demonstrable nodes on CT scanning should not deter the surgeon from an operation. However, evidence or suggestive evidence of pulmonary involvement, particularly on CT scanning, must be taken seriously; we

proceed to video thoracoscopy or guided-needle aspiration of lung lesions for definition of intrapulmonary pathology.

Assessment of associated parenchymal disease of the liver is important, particularly for patients with primary hepatocellular cancer. Indeed, cirrhosis should be considered in every patient presenting with primary hepatocellular carcinoma, and all such patients should be tested for the presence or absence of hepatitis antigenemia and carefully assessed using the well-known Child's Pugh criteria to determine liver functional status. Although we do not advocate biopsy of all lesions of the liver, and we do not proceed to such biopsy in patients in whom resection is contemplated, it can be reasonable to biopsy the liver tissue outwith the tumor in order to assess the presence or absence of cirrhosis. Accompanying complications of the cirrhotic liver, in particular evidence of portal hypertension, must be carefully sought. Computed tomographic scans should be examined for evidence of splenomegaly, collateral circulation, and ascites. Esophageal varices can be detected at endoscopy.

The potential for primary liver tumors to directly invade the portal vein or the biliary system should also be considered before surgery. Such changes are often visible on high-quality CT scans provided the index of suspicion is high. Confirmatory studies in the form of duplex ultrasonography, late phase portography, or endoscopic retrograde cholangiography (ERCP) are occasionally necessary.

In the assessment of patients with metastatic disease from neuroendocrine tumors, angiography is important since it might demonstrate multiple small lesions not shown by other methods. In addition, angiography offers consideration of transarterial embolization in the management of such tumors.

Selection for Operation

In general, all patients who are fit to undergo an operation and who present with potentially resectable liver tumors are candidates to be considered for hepatic resection.

Preoperative Preparation

Preoperative preparation involves the correction of anemia and of coagulopathy and appropriate single-dose antibiotic prophylaxis. All patients with a history of cardiorespiratory disease and all patients over the age of 65 are submitted to full cardiorespiratory investigation.

We encourage all patients, particularly patients with metastatic colorectal cancer to the liver, to donate two units of blood before their operation, in case a transfusion is needed.

Anesthetic Considerations

Anesthetic techniques should take into account the possibility of major intraoperative hemorrhage. Suitable monitoring and facilities for rapid transfusion should be set up, and the possibility of a thoracoabdominal incision should be allowed.

Hemorrhage during hepatic resection usually arises from the major hepatic veins or vena cava, and we have pursued a policy of deliberate retrohepatic dissection of the minor and major hepatic veins before commencing parenchymal transection. This procedure is carried out using a controlled central venous pressure, which is not permitted to rise above 5 mm Hg. To obviate air embolism, the dissection is performed with the patient approximately 15 degrees in the Trendelenburg position. Control of the central venous pressure is maintained at the desired level using a combination of anesthesia and early intraoperative fluid restriction. The minimum accepted intraoperative urine output is 25 ml per hour.

We now limit intraoperative blood transfusion, the indications being a decrease in the hematocrit to 24 percent in patients without antecedent cardiac disease or a decrease to 29 percent in patients with cardiac disease. Other indications include a total volume blood loss estimated at 20 percent or more or hemodynamic instability, or both. For vascular isolation of the liver, the anesthetic requirements are different and require the maintenance of cardiac output during cross-clamping of the vena cava. We have seldom performed vascular isolation of the liver even during the removal of very large tumors close to or involving large veins or the inferior vena cava. In a recent series of more than 250 patients, we considered the technique on only two occasions, in one of which the operation was abandoned because of extrahepatic disease. To date, no patient has been deemed irresectable because of vascular involvement alone.

A prolonged operation with wide abdominal exposure can result in hypothermia, and the body temperature should be carefully monitored and maintained. Blood and other infusion fluids should be warmed.

Operative Procedures

Position of the Patient

The patient should be supine with the right arm extended at a right angle to the body. ECG leads should be kept clear of the right chest wall and the presternal area. Preparation and draping should allow for the exposure of the lower chest and entire upper abdomen to below the umbilicus. For some large right-sided tumors a thoracoabdominal incision or median sternotomy might be necessary, and in this instance the draping should expose the right chest and the entire presternal area as far as the suprasternal notch. A crossbar or similar device should be fitted to the table, which holds self-retaining retractors used to elevate the costal margin.

The Incision

For most hepatic resections, a bilateral subcostal incision extended in a vertical manner to the xiphisternum is adequate (Fig. 94-6). As already discussed for large tumors of the right lobe, a thoracoabdominal incision might be necessary. However, in a recent series of 100 patients of whom 52 were submitted to extended hepatic resection, a thoracoabdominal incision was used on only three occasions.

Abdominal Exploration and Intraoperative Ultrasound

The falciform ligament is divided (Fig. 94-7), and the liver is bimanually palpated. The lesser omentum is incised and a finger is introduced into the lesser sac to allow palpation of the caudate lobe.

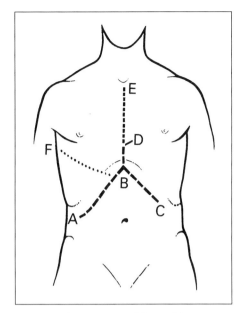

Fig. 94-6. The incisions used for partial hepatectomy. A, B, C, D, "rooftop" incision with vertical extension; F, right thoracic extension; D, E, median sternotomy. (From LH Blumgart. Liver Resection—Liver and Biliary Tumours. In LH Blumgart [ed.], Surgery of the Liver and Biliary Tract, 2nd ed. London: Churchill-Livingstone, 1994. Reproduced with permission.)

Intraoperative ultrasound (Fig. 94-8). is systematically carried out to identify all possible lesions and their relationship to major vascular structures. Several studies attest to the ability of intraoperative ultrasound to identify small lesions that might have been missed at preoperative study and by palpation of the liver. We do not find that intraoperative ultrasound is of particular value in guiding parenchymal transection in the normal liver or in obtaining adequate clearance, but we have found it to be useful in the delineation of additional disease not demonstrated by preoperative investigations. In the cirrhotic liver, intraoperative ultrasound is of value in guiding parenchymal transection to allow minimal removal of tissue, particularly for resection of small tumors.

The hilar lymph nodes are palpated and any suspicious nodes are removed for frozen section study. The lower abdomen is palpated for evidence of recurrent tumor. Very frequently, full abdominal exploration is difficult to perform in a thorough manner particularly if there are dense adhesions in the infracolic compartment of

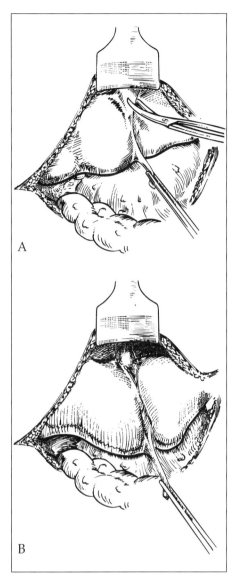

Fig. 94-7. A. The ligamentum teres is secured, and division of the falciform ligament is commenced. B. The falciform ligament is divided backwards to expose the suprahepatic inferior vena cava and hepatic veins. (From LH Blumgart. Liver Resection—Liver and Biliary Tumours. In LH Blumgart [ed.], Surgery of the Liver and Biliary Tract, 2nd ed. London: Churchill-Livingstone, 1994. Reproduced with permission.)

the abdomen as a result of previous colonic resection.

Once the surgeon decides to proceed, the liver is fully mobilized by detaching all ligamentous attachments and, in particular, the suprahepatic area. The subdiaphragmatic inferior vena cava and the hepatic veins above the liver are dissected (Fig.

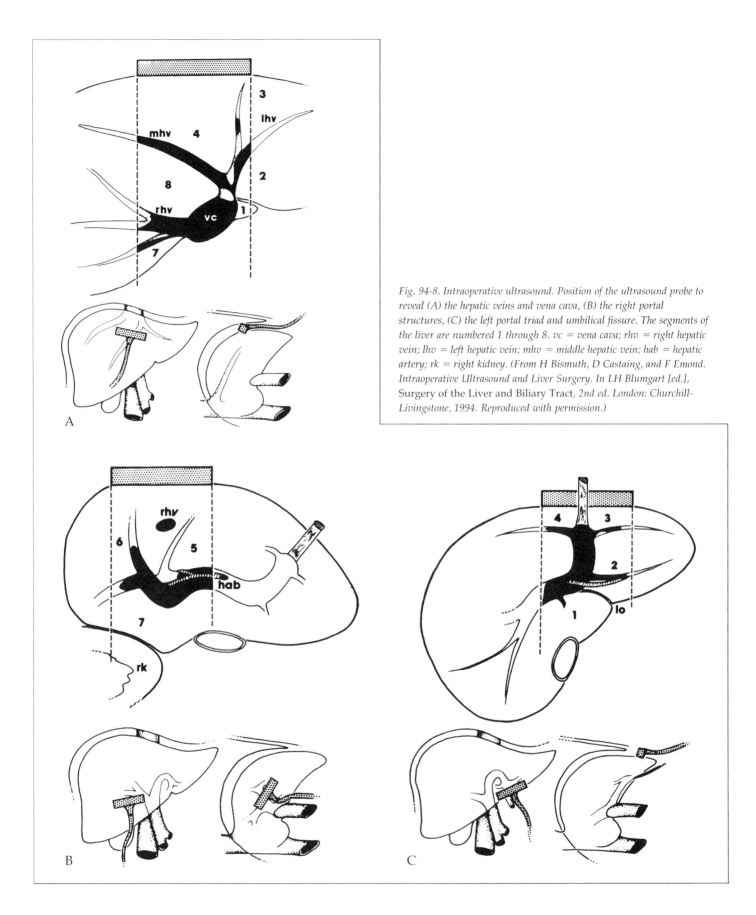

Fig. 94-8. Intraoperative ultrasound. Position of the ultrasound probe to reveal (A) the hepatic veins and vena cava, (B) the right portal structures, (C) the left portal triad and umbilical fissure. The segments of the liver are numbered 1 through 8. vc = vena cava; rhv = right hepatic vein; lhv = left hepatic vein; mhv = middle hepatic vein; hab = hepatic artery; rk = right kidney. (From H Bismuth, D Castaing, and F Emond. Intraoperative Ultrasound and Liver Surgery. In LH Blumgart [ed.], Surgery of the Liver and Biliary Tract, 2nd ed. London: Churchill-Livingstone, 1994. Reproduced with permission.)

94-7). Once mobilized further, palpation of the liver is performed to detect any small lesions that might have been obscured initially. This step is particularly important since the posterior parts of the liver are initially blind to palpation, and small lesions in this area can be missed at intraoperative ultrasound. If during dissection, the tumor is found attached to the diaphragm, it is usually only over a limited distance and the affected area of diaphragm is either separated or a segment of the diaphragm excised and subsequently repaired.

Techniques of Major Hepatectomy

The precise steps in the performance of the various major hepatectomies are described in this section. We have developed new techniques for cryo-assisted hepatic resection.

Parenchymal transection is performed using a Kelly clamp to crush the tissue and isolate vessels for control, but more elaborate techniques using the ultrasonic dissector or a jet dissector are preferred by some surgeons.

Drainage of the subdiaphragmatic space after resection has long been considered mandatory, but some surgeons have suggested that this measure is not necessary. We have performed a prospective study of this problem in 120 patients and now recommend no drainage after major hepatic resection except when a thoracoabdominal incision is used or when the operation has involved biliary reconstruction, for example, after hepatic resection for hilar cholangiocarcinoma.

Right Hepatectomy

The hilar structures are controlled by lowering the hilar plate (Figs. 94-9A, B and 94-10) and extrahepatic dissection of the porta hepatis (see Fig. 94-9A–F). An important alternative to the extrahepatic dissection of the vascular and biliary structures of the hilus of the liver has recently been proposed. This method relies on intrahepatic definition and control of the portal triads to the area to be removed and on the fact that the structures of the portal triad (portal vein, hepatic artery, and bile duct) take Glisson's capsule with them

into the liver so that within the parenchyma they are contained in a well-formed sheath as portal pedicles (Fig. 94-11).

If this technique is used, there are several important guiding principles. First, the hepatic pedicle outside the liver is encircled with a vessel loop to facilitate occlusion during liver resection (the Pringle maneuver). No attempt is made to dissect these structures individually. If present, the gallbladder is dissected away from the liver and can be later removed, but it can be used to provide downward traction on the right hepatic pedicle and help orientate the surgeon in the region of the porta hepatis.

It is important to dissect the lowermost hepatic veins behind the liver (vide infra) before performing the maneuver since they are a potential source of hemorrhage in the area of incision of the caudate hepatotomy, which forms part of the procedure. Incisions are now made in the liver capsule (Fig. 94-12) in two areas. The first is made in the caudate process immediately parallel to and to the right of the inferior vena cava. The full thickness of the caudate process is divided using diathermy, crushing, and ligation. The second incision is made almost vertically in the medial part of the gallbladder bed and is continued from the gallbladder bed above the hilum of the liver and just above the hilar plate. These incisions must be fairly substantial and reasonably deep. The only bleeding encountered might come from terminal branches of the middle hepatic vein close to the gallbladder fossa. Using either finger dissection or the passage of a large curved clamp, a tape is placed around the right main sheath (Fig. 94-13). This sheath is invariably close to the confluence, and it is necessary to dissect the sheath a little further to the right before declamping the main pedicle and clamping the right sheath. After clamping, the right liver is devascularized and the color change in the line of the principal plane indicates that the clamp is correctly placed. We find it convenient at this stage to pass a vascular stapler around the whole sheath and to staple the sheath closed until later into the dissection.

Any bleeding from the hepatotomy wound is usually minor and ceases spontaneously. The passage of Surgicel into the wound usually causes cessation of any oozing during subsequent dissection.

Our experience using this technique includes approximately 70 instances of right hepatectomy or right lobectomy. It has been a valuable and rapid approach and has the great advantage that there is almost no chance to damage the biliary structures. They can be damaged during extrahepatic dissection.

We have *never used* the pedicle ligation technique when tumor extends close to the hilus on the right side since it is impossible to simultaneously adhere to the principle of securing an adequate clearance margin. Furthermore, mobilization of the gallbladder can expose the underlying tumor.

Control of Hepatic Veins

For right-sided hepatic resections, the hepatic veins are divided commencing at the inferior border of the liver and then progressing upward to expose the right hepatic vein (Fig. 94-14). The right hepatic vein is usually easily exposed if all lower veins are initially freed and the vena cava dropped away from the posterior surface of the liver. This method is particularly important for tumors close to the vena cava. There is usually no direct invasion of the vena cava even if the tumor appears to involve the vena cava or displace it at preoperative imaging studies. The right hepatic vein is then isolated, cross-clamped, divided, and oversewn (Fig. 94-15). The middle hepatic vein is usually not controlled extrahepatically for right-sided resections, and if necessary, it is easily secured during parenchymal transection.

If difficulty is encountered in gaining control of the hepatic veins and vena cava (which might be the case in very large tumors lying high in the right lobe within segments VII and VIII), there should be no hesitation in extending the incision to the right chest or vertically by median sternotomy. This possibility will usually have been considered on the basis of preoperative investigation. It is dangerous to persist through an abdominal incision in an attempt to mobilize a rigid right lobe of liver containing a large tumor since the right hepatic vein can tear posteriorly. Once the chest is opened, the vena cava can be more easily approached. If a median sternotomy is used, the pericardium can be opened and control of the inferior vena cava gained within the pericardial sac. This step is usually unnecessary, and in most in-

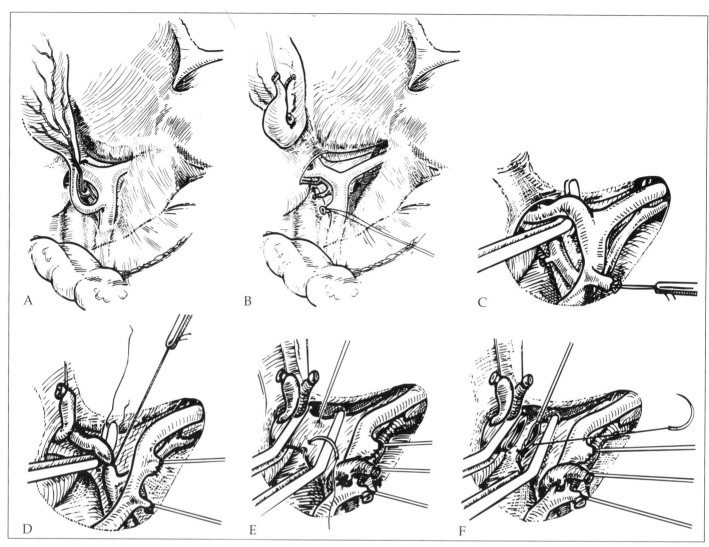

Fig. 94-9. *A. The hilar plate is lowered to expose the left hepatic duct and the confluence of the bile ducts (see Fig. 94-10), and dissection of the right hepatic duct is commenced. B. The peritoneum overlying the common bile duct on the free edge of the lesser omentum and extending up into Calot's triangle is incised and the common bile duct, common hepatic duct, and Calot's triangle are exposed. The cystic duct and cystic artery are secured and divided. A tie is left on the cystic duct for later retraction. C. The right hepatic duct is dissected. Note that the confluence of the hepatic ducts and the origin of the left hepatic duct are clearly demonstrated. D.* The right hepatic duct has been transfixed with absorbable suture material, divided, and ligated or oversewn. Alternatively, it can be simply divided under direct vision and then oversewn. In any event, the suture is held and retracted toward the left. Traction on the sutures attached to the cystic duct and the right hepatic duct stump allows retraction of the common hepatic duct and common bile duct to the left and assists display of the vessels beneath. The right hepatic artery is dissected, ligated, and divided usually to the right (as shown) but sometimes to the left of the common hepatic duct. E. The right portal vein is dissected, and forceps are gently passed beneath it. Special care is taken not to damage the first branch of the right portal vein, which comes off early and posteroinferiorly. This branch is initially sought and either ligated and divided or avoided. Straight-bladed vascular clamps are then applied to the right portal vein. Note the retaining sutures used to secure the vein before division. F. The vein is divided and its proximal stump oversewn using a vascular suture. The distal stump is transfixed and ligated. Note again that light traction on the cystic duct, right hepatic duct stump, and the right hepatic artery assists display. (From LH Blumgart. Liver Resection—Liver and Biliary Tumours. In LH Blumgart [ed.],* Surgery of the Liver and Biliary Tract, *2nd ed. London: Churchill-Livingstone, 1994. Reproduced with permission.)*

*It might be safer and easier to control the right hepatic artery and the right branch of the portal vein and leave the right hepatic duct to be secured within the liver substance during parenchymal transection.

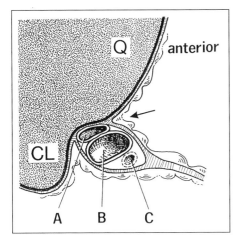

Fig. 94-10. Lowering of the hilar plate. Glisson's capsule is incised at the base of the quadrate lobe (segment IV), and the structures of the left portal triad are lowered from beneath the overhanging quadrate lobe, thus exposing the left hepatic duct. Q = quadrate lobe; CL = caudate lobe; A = left hepatic duct; B = left portal vein; C = left hepatic artery (usually only near the base of the umbilical fissure); and arrow = point of peritoneal incision. (From LH Blumgart and HU Baer. Hilar and Intrahepatic Biliary-enteric Anastomosis. In LH Blumgart [ed.], Surgery of the Liver and Biliary Tract, 2nd ed. London: Churchill-Livingstone, 1994. Reproduced with permission.)

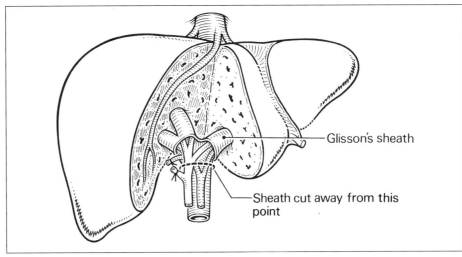

Fig. 94-11. The anatomy of the left and right portal pedicles at the hilus. Note that Glisson's capsule is prolonged into the liver surrounding the portal triads to form portal pedicles within the liver. (From LH Blumgart. Liver Resection—Liver and Biliary Tumours. In LH Blumgart [ed.], Surgery of the Liver and Biliary Tract, 2nd ed. London: Churchill-Livingstone, 1994. Reproduced with permission.)

stances the inferior vena cava and right hepatic vein can be dissected through an abdominal incision alone. The liver tissue is now divided in the principal plane and the right liver is excised.

Right Hepatic Lobectomy (Right Trisegmentectomy)

The initial steps of this operation are the same as for right hepatectomy, but the operation involves further and continued mobilization to devascularize the quadrate lobe (segment IV) of the liver. The first essential steps are to lower the hilar plate (Figs. 94-9 and 94-10) and to locate and display the umbilical fissure of the liver. In many instances, the lower part of the umbilical fissure is concealed by a bridge of liver tissue fusing segments II and III to segment IV. This tissue is easily divided by passing a curved director beneath it and dividing it with diathermy. The ligamentum teres can now be visualized running into the fissure. We identify any visible recurrent vessels from the umbilical fissure

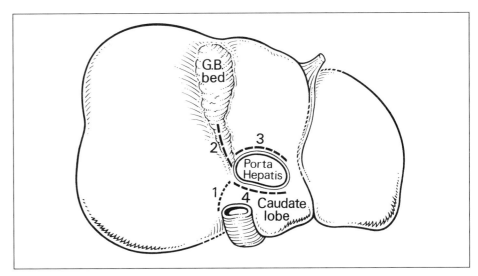

Fig. 94-12. Lines of incision to allow isolation of the portal pedicles. For an operation on the right liver, the pedicles can be approached by one of two methods. The first is to make an incision in the caudate process parallel to and 5 mm to the right of the inferior vena cava (1). The full thickness of the caudate process is divided. The second incision is made more anteriorly in the central part of the gallbladder bed near the hilum (2). A second method is more frequently used, consisting of an anterior incision in front of the hilum (3) and extending up into the gallbladder bed (2). For operations on the left side, a similar approach can be used, although the left main sheath can usually be dissected at the base of the caudate lobe near the umbilical fissure without the need for a posterior approach (see Fig. 94-16). (From LH Blumgart. Liver Resection— Liver and Biliary Tumours. In LH Blumgart [ed.], Surgery of the Liver and Biliary Tract, 2nd ed. London: Churchill-Livingstone, 1994. Reproduced with permission.)

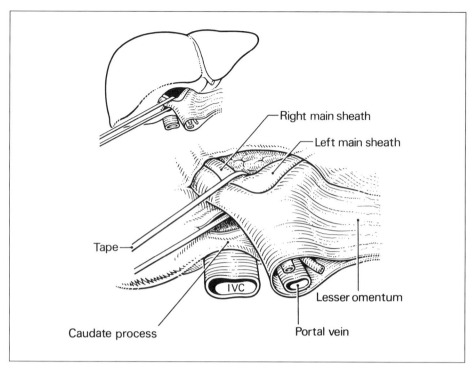

Fig. 94-13. A large curved clamp has been used to place a tape around the right main sheath (pedicle). The right pedicle can now be clamped or controlled with a vascular stapler. IVC = inferior vena cava. (From LH Blumgart. Liver Resection—Liver and Biliary Tumours. In LH Blumgart [ed.], Surgery of the Liver and Biliary Tract, *2nd ed. London: Churchill-Livingstone, 1994. Reproduced with permission.)*

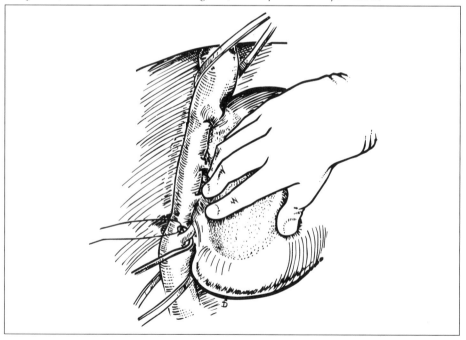

Fig. 94-14. Short hepatic veins issuing from the caudate lobe and the right liver are individually secured using aneurysm needles to pass fine sutures around the vessels, which are then tied and cut. Smaller veins can be controlled with clips. This procedure is carried upward beneath the liver until the right lobe is mobilized and the vena cava displayed up to the right hepatic vein. This step is necessary for subsequent safe dissection of the right hepatic vein. It is usually unnecessary to fully dissect and encircle the vena cava with vessel loops as shown. (From LH Blumgart. Liver Resection—Liver and Biliary Tumours. In LH Blumgart [ed.], Surgery of the Liver and Biliary Tract, *2nd ed. London: Churchill-Livingstone, 1994. Reproduced with permission.)*

to segment IV and underrun them with a 3–0 Prolene suture (Fig. 94-16).

The liver tissue is now divided just to the right of the falciform ligament progressing backward toward the point of transection of the right hepatic vein to the vena cava (Fig. 94-17). The middle hepatic vein is encountered in the upper part of this dissection and is easily controlled. We usually do so by passing a 3–0 Prolene suture around the vein and securing it by direct suture ligation.

Left Hepatectomy

Left hepatectomy involves a similar dissection to the method described for right hepatectomy. Our preference is to perform this dissection at the base of the umbilical fissure (Fig. 94-16). First, the left hepatic artery is divided. If the caudate lobe is to be removed, then the point of ligation of the portal vein is proximal to the takeoff of the caudate venous branches of the left portal vein. The left branch of the portal vein is easily identified at the base of the umbilical fissure, and if the caudate lobe is to be preserved, the left portal vein is divided just distal to its caudate branch. The left hepatic duct is identified beneath the quadrate lobe after lowering of the hilar plate and is similarly secured. Alternatively, the pedicle ligation technique can be used following hepatotomy above the left portal structures at the base of segment IV and after incision posterior to the hilus (see Fig. 94-12).

In all instances of left hepatic resection, it is our practice to gain control of the left and middle hepatic veins by mobilizing the left lobe of the liver. The gastrohepatic ligament is divided and dissection at the upper end of the ligamentum venosum, just at the upper border of the caudate process, usually identifies a passage beneath the left and middle hepatic veins and anterior to the inferior vena cava (Fig. 94-18). The left and middle hepatic veins can then be easily clamped, divided, and sutured. The liver tissue is divided in the principal plane, and the left liver is removed.

Left Lobectomy (Left Lateral Segmentectomy)

If present, the bridge of tissue between segment IV and the left liver is divided as

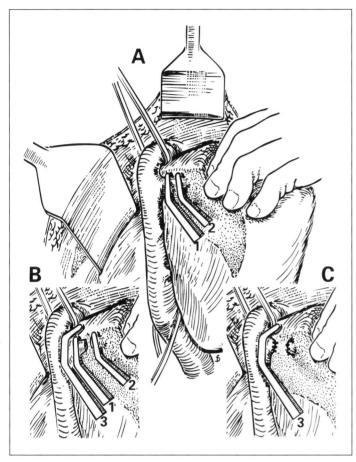

Fig. 94-15. A. Approach to the right hepatic vein. Note that the inferior vena cava is encircled with tapes, although this is usually not necessary. The right liver has been extensively mobilized and the inferior vena cava exposed up to the right hepatic vein. The right hepatic vein is dissected and a vascular clamp applied on the caval side. There is usually space for the application of a second clamp on the hepatic side, although it is not essential since, if the vein is divided after the portal triad at the hilus, bleeding from the exposed venous orifice can be readily controlled with a suture after division of the vein. If possible, another clamp should be applied on the caval side before division of the vein, but there might not be a space for it. In this event, a second clamp is applied immediately after the vein is divided. B. The initial clamp has been removed. The right hepatic vein has been divided and its stump closed with an over-and-over 3–0 vascular suture (C). (From LH Blumgart. Liver Resection—Liver and Biliary Tumours. In LH Blumgart [ed.], Surgery of the Liver and Biliary Tract, 2nd ed. London: Churchill-Livingstone, 1994. Reproduced with permission.)

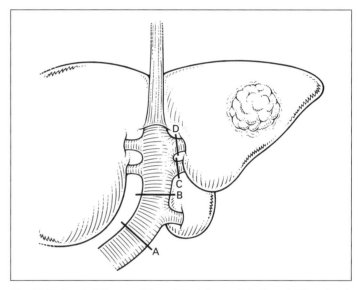

Fig. 94-16. Detailed diagram of the umbilical fissure of the liver. A. The point of division of the left portal triad to devascularize the left liver and the caudate lobe (segment I). B. The point of division to preserve the blood supply to the caudate lobe. C. The point of division of the pedicle to segment II. D. The point of division of the pedicle to segment III. Note that the pedicles to segments IV-A and IV-B issue from the right side of the left portal triad within the umbilical fissure and can be controlled there during extended right hepatic lobectomy. Alternatively, they can be controlled within the liver tissue just to the right of the falciform ligament (Fig. 94-17).

already described. The left lobe is mobilized.

Dissection is performed within the umbilical fissure to the left of the main triad. The pedicle to segments II and III can usually be dissected and controlled (Fig. 94-16). This approach is important in allowing tumor clearance for lesions close to the um-

bilical fissure. Alternatively, the liver can be split anteroposteriorly just to the left of the ligamentum teres and falciform ligament, and as this split is done, the vessels are encountered and divided serially. As the liver is opened posteriorly, the left hepatic vein is identified and controlled and the left lobe removed.

Extended Left Hepatectomy (Left Trisegmentectomy)

In some instances, large tumors occupying the left half of the liver cross the principal scissura into the anterior sector of the right liver (segments V and VIII). In such situ-

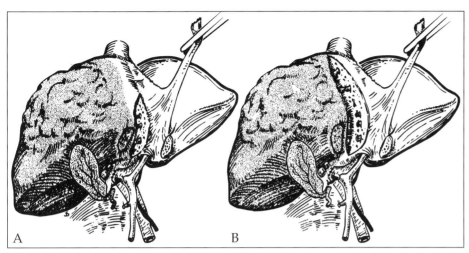

Fig. 94-17. A. Feedback vessels from the left portal triad are secured just a little to the right of the falciform ligament. This dissection can also be done to the right within the umbilical fissure (Fig. 94-16), but the procedure indicated here is also performed. This procedure deprives segment IV of its blood supply. B. Division of the liver substance is developed backwards toward the vena cava just to the right of the falciform ligament. (From LH Blumgart. Liver Resection—Liver and Biliary Tumours. In LH Blumgart [ed.], Surgery of the Liver and Biliary Tract, 2nd ed. London: Churchill-Livingstone, 1994. Reproduced with permission.)

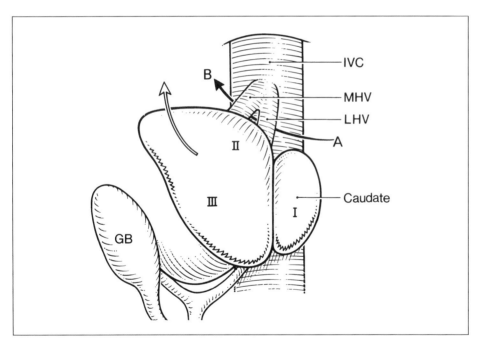

Fig. 94-18. The approach to dissection of the left and middle hepatic veins. The left lobe of the liver (segments II and III) is completely mobilized from the diaphragm and turned to the right (open arrow) and the gastrohepatic ligament is divided. The line of the ligamentum venosum is exposed. It can be necessary to mobilize the upper part of the caudate lobe from the vena cava, and this maneuver is often of assistance in exposing the window between the vena cava and the left hepatic vein, which lies at the upper limit of the caudate lobe. By dissection in this window, it is possible to dissect free the left and middle hepatic veins, as illustrated, and to pass a director between these structures and the inferior vena cava (A–B). Clamps can then be applied and the left and middle hepatic veins divided. This approach to the left and middle hepatic veins is relevant for left hepatectomy and extended left hepatectomy. IVC = inferior vena cava; MHV = middle hepatic vein; LHV = left hepatic vein; and GB = gallbladder.

ations, left hepatectomy can be carried out with an extension of the procedure to remove segments V and VIII in continuity with the remainder of the left liver with or without excision of the caudate lobe (see Fig. 94-4). The procedure is extensive, and the indications for its performance are either large solitary tumors extending from left to right or left-sided tumors with additional lesions that lie within the right anterior sector of the liver. Difficulty in defining a plane of parenchymal transection on the right side and in controlling hemorrhage and biliary complications have been recognized as the major hazards. Experience with this operation remains modest, but as reported by Blumgart and colleagues, recent experience has addressed the main problems and, in particular, outlined techniques for defining the plane of parenchymal transection and for controlling blood loss.

Preoperative evaluation is especially important before undertaking the procedure. Roentgenographic investigations are directed to display the gross morphologic anatomy of the tumor and related vessels and biliary structures. In a previous report by Blumgart, liver tumors have been classified into pushing, hanging, and invading types. This simple classification has particular value in assessment for extended left hepatectomy. The pushing variety of tumor, even when the lesion is seen to be extremely large on initial CT scan, tends *not to* invade surrounding structures but to displace the portal pedicles and hepatic veins. This expansion compresses a layer of atrophic liver tissue in advance of the tumor that lies between the lesion and the vascular structures. This compression is of importance during later parenchymal transection. Appreciation of the pushing nature of the lesion means that even very large and apparently irresectable tumors can be removed. We advocate angiography before extended left hepatectomy for large tumors, which frequently encroach on the portal triad at the hilum of the liver and lie adjacent to or compress the inferior vena cava. Doppler ultrasonography or MRI can be of considerable value in demonstrating the patency of major vessels before an operation.

In our experience, *preoperative studies can dictate one of two different approaches to the procedure*. When the tumor is very large and is compressing and displacing vessels as previously described, the line of parenchymal transection is *primarily dictated by the tumor itself* and is essentially performed within the peripheral fibrous atrophic zone surrounding the lesion. For such large tumors, extrahepatic dissection and preparation of the hilar structures are usually necessary. However, a less extensive tumor that does not impinge on the right posterior sectoral triad allows transection within normal parenchyma and permits greater tumor clearance. In such situations, the control of the anterior and posterior right sectoral portal pedicles described in the following discussion facilitates dissection.

After division of the falciform ligament back to the vena cava, intraoperative ultrasonography is performed to confirm the anatomic configuration of the tumor and major hepatic veins. In particular, an attempt is made to identify a large inferior right hepatic vein, the presence of which augments draining of segment VII and can even allow the right main hepatic vein to be sacrificed during the operation. The liver must be fully mobilized by division of the left triangular ligament, but also there should be complete division and mobilization of the ligament on the right. This maneuver not only allows palpation of segment VII for the presence of additional tumor but also is essential later in the procedure for the identification and dissection of the correct plane of parenchymal dissection.

Initial dissection is the same as for left hepatectomy. The liver is turned to the right side and the portal triad approached from the left. The point of ligation of vessels to the left liver is dictated by tumor involvement of the caudate lobe (segment I) (Fig. 94-19). If segment I requires resection the left hepatic artery, the bile duct and portal vein must be ligated close to the hilum to interrupt the blood supply to segment I as well as to the left liver. However, when segment I is to be preserved, the structures of the left portal triad are secured in the base of the umbilical fissure to leave the blood supply to segment I intact (Figs. 94-16 and 94-19).

After vascular control at the hilum has been achieved, the left hepatic vein and the left subdiaphragmatic inferior vena cava are dissected. It is usually possible to control the left and middle hepatic veins in their extrahepatic portion (Fig. 94-18). *Every effort should be made to do so since it renders the final stages of the parenchymal transection easier, and there is much less intraoperative bleeding* than if these veins were exposed at a late stage during parenchymal transection.

In the past, there has been some difficulty in defining the line of incision of the liver capsule, which lies well to the right of the principal scissura. The plane of transection is horizontal, lateral to the gallbladder fossa, and parallel and just anterior to the right scissura. It is important to define this plane, which passes anterior to the right hepatic venous trunk and allows division of the anterior sectoral part of the right portal triad while preserving and avoiding damage to the posterior triad. Although there are no reliable surface markings, a plane extending from the anterior border of the right hepatic vein above and extended horizontally to emerge well to the right of the gallbladder fossa designates the correct position within the parenchyma. This line can be accurately defined by clamping the portal pedicle to the anterior right sector of the liver. This step is

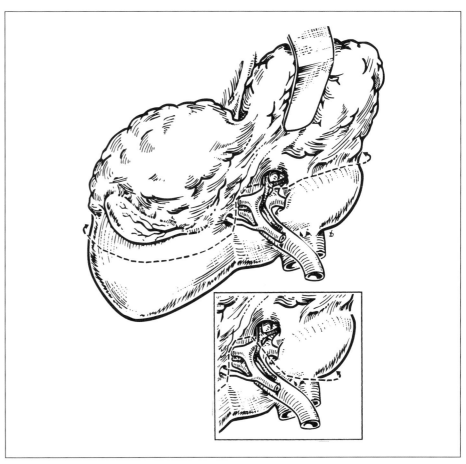

Fig. 94-19. The initial approach during extended left hepatectomy allowing dissection of the portal triad or structures from the left posterolateral aspect. The line of future transection is indicated. If the caudate lobe is to be preserved, the left portal vein is ligated beyond its caudate branch. If the caudate is to be removed as well, then the portal vein can be ligated more proximally (inset) (see also Figs. 94-4 and 94-16). Note that the line of transection runs along the obliterated ligamentum venosum, then across the base of the quadrate lobe and hilus, and curves to the right extending into the right scissura lateral to the gallbladder fossa. The dissection as illustrated in the main diagram would preserve the caudate lobe, but in the inset the caudate lobe is also removed. (From LH Blumgart. Liver Resection—Liver and Biliary Tumours. In LH Blumgart [ed.], Surgery of the Liver and Biliary Tract, 2nd ed. London: Churchill-Livingstone, 1994. Reproduced with permission.)

possible in patients in whom the tumor does not extend so near to the right main pedicle that it makes access impossible without compromising tumor clearance. If the right anterior sectoral pedicle is clamped and the right posterior sectoral pedicle left intact, a line of demarcation extending along the right scissura rapidly develops.

The parenchymal phase is now performed from below upward (Fig. 94-20). Hemorrhage is controlled by using an intermittent Pringle maneuver. *The techniques for control of central venous pressure referred to previously are especially important in this operation.* For very large tumors, the parenchymal transection is carried out in the narrow zone of compressed liver tissue as already described. The parenchymal transection proceeds upward and medially. If

not previously secured, the middle hepatic vein is encountered and controlled within the line of transection, as is the left hepatic vein. If removal of the caudate lobe is envisaged as part of the total resection, the caudate draining veins must be controlled by retrohepatic dissection before parenchymal transection.

Segmental Resection

Hepatic segmentectomy involves removal of one or more of the eight segments of the liver. The more commonly used segmental resections involve removal of segments I, IV, or bisegmental resection of segments IV and V and of IV, V, and VI. Resection of segments VI and VII (right posterior sectorectomy) is now commonly used for small posteriorly located tumors in the right liver.

Segment IV resection is of value in the management of metastatic lesions occupying the quadrate lobe. Resection of segment I can be necessary when this segment is involved by tumor either on its own or in continuity with right or left hepatectomy, right lobectomy, or extended left hepatectomy.

Segmentectomy I (Caudate Lobe Resection)

Resection of the caudate lobe (segment I) presents particular problems since it is closely applied to the retrohepatic inferior vena cava and approach to the draining caudate veins can be difficult and hazardous, whether the lobe is to be resected alone or as part of a major hepatic resection. The approach to the hepatic veins of the caudate lobe can be anterolaterally from the left or more readily using a technique that allows an approach from the right side. With this method, the right and left lobes of the liver are mobilized from the diaphragmatic attachment. The right lobe of the liver is turned medially, and the hepatic veins are dissected proceeding from below upward to free the entire posterior liver from the retrohepatic vena cava as high as the insertion of the three main hepatic veins. The dissection is pursued over the anterior surface of the vena cava to its left side where access to the draining veins of the caudate lobe of the liver is obtained allowing division of all such veins under direct vision. After completion of this maneuver, the liver remains attached only by the major hepatic veins and the portal triad. The portal vein and hepatic artery are dissected at the hilus in order to ligate branches supplying the caudate lobe of the liver. These branches are found close to the base of the umbilical fissure of the liver and just before the main portal triad on the left enters the fissure (Fig. 94-16). Vascular inflow occlusion is now performed, and the lobe is removed and separated from its attachment to the right liver. In this manner, the caudate lobe or a lesion within it can be removed leaving the remaining hepatic tissue intact. If difficulty is encountered in removing a large tumor in the caudate lobe, the liver can be opened along the principal plane to provide access for caudate lobectomy without loss of functional hepatic parenchyma. This approach requires preliminary dissection of the retrohepatic veins as already described. Temporary occlusion of the left

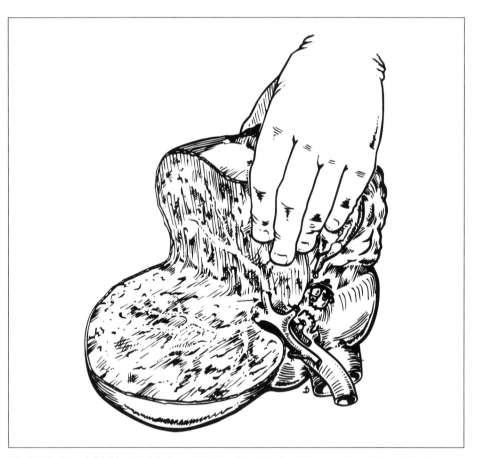

Fig. 94-20. Extended left hepatic lobectomy. The liver tissue is entered for parenchymal transection just anterior to the lower limit of the right scissura. This plan of dissection is then followed, the surgeon working toward the base of the gallbladder fossa and the point of entry of the right hepatic duct into the liver substance. The anterior sectoral vessel of supply and the bile ducts are identified in the liver substance (arrow) and can be ligated. (From LH Blumgart. Liver Resection—Liver and Biliary Tumours. In LH Blumgart [ed.], Surgery of the Liver and Biliary Tract, *2nd ed. London: Churchill-Livingstone, 1994. Reproduced with permission.)*

and middle hepatic veins can help control venous bleeding.

An anterolateral approach to segment I can also be carried out by exposing the caudate lobe through the gastrohepatic ligament and then after division of the hepatic arterial and portal venous branches, ligating the caudate hepatic veins commencing at the inferior and lateral margin of the caudate lobe and progressing superomedially. This approach is more difficult since the caudate lobe hugs the vena cava anteriorly and on the left and visualization for dissection is impaired. In any event, final dissection from the left across the lesser sac of the peritoneum is necessary, and segment I is removed. In many instances, alternating dissection from the right and left retrohepatic areas is necessary. We have removed segment I alone or in combination with major hepatic resection in 26 instances, and all were carried out with minimal loss of blood and without mortality.

Segment IV (Quadrate Resection)

The blood supply of segment IV arises in the umbilical fissure from the left portal vein and left hepatic artery. The venous drainage is via branches of the middle hepatic vein on the medial side and an umbilical hepatic vein that courses beneath the falciform ligament to drain into the left or middle hepatic vein. Segment IV is divided into two portions, segment IV-A posterosuperiorly and segment IV-B anteroinferiorly. All of segment IV can be removed, or segment IV-A or segment IV-B can be removed separately. If segment IV-A is removed together with the right liver, the middle hepatic vein can be sacrificed and venous drainage to segment IV-B preserved through the umbilical vein as described by Scheele.

The operation comprises essentially four maneuvers. It is important to lower the hilar plate (Figs. 94-9A, B and 94-10). Second, the liver parenchyma is divided to the right of the ligamentum teres with control of the feedback vessels as they are for lobectomy. Third, division of liver tissue is made in the principal plane. It is possible to preserve the middle hepatic vein by pushing it laterally, or it can be sacrificed without affecting venous drainage from the remaining liver. Finally, transection of

the liver substance is made between these two previous parenchymal incisions.

The initial step is the division of the bridge of parenchyma that joins segments III and IV at the base of the umbilical fissure (Fig. 94-16). The hilar plate is then lowered. The peritoneum is opened along the right border of the ligamentum teres, and several arterial and portal branches passing from the umbilical portion of the left portal vein and the accompanying arteries and ducts feeding back to segment IV are divided. The parenchymal dissection is then deepened backwards extending toward the vena cava. For removal of segment IV-B, the parenchymal dissection need not extend as far back as the cava, but for complete removal it must be extended fully. A similar parenchymal incision is then made along the main scissura of the liver commencing anteriorly at the gallbladder fossa and progressing backwards in the principal plane. During this stage of the operation, the middle hepatic vein must be dealt with as previously described. After these two initial incisions, a transverse incision is made above joining the two previously made parenchymal splits. This incision is deepened, and branches of the middle hepatic vein are divided as encountered. For complete removal of segment IV, it is usually necessary to ligate the middle hepatic vein and to divide the parenchyma separating segments IV and I.

Bisegmentectomy VI and VII (Right Posterior Sectorectomy)

In some patients with metastatic deposits in segments VI and VII only, it is possible to perform a limited resection posterior to the right hepatic vein, thus avoiding dangerous attempts at wedge resection in this area and the necessity for complete right hepatic lobectomy.

In this operation, we mobilize the right lobe of the liver completely from the diaphragm and divide all minor veins draining the liver posteriorly to the vena cava on the right to allow access to the right hepatic vein. This step enables clamping of this vein during removal of the posterior sector and ready repair if it is damaged.

After this retrohepatic preparation, the portal pedicle on the right is exposed as already described, and the right anterior and posterior sectoral portal triads are

identified. Clamping of the posterior portal triad reveals a line of demarcation running just in the line of the right hepatic vein, the maneuver being similar to the one described for extended left hepatectomy. The right posterior sectoral triad can then be controlled at the hilus, and the right posterior sector can be removed during temporary cross-clamping of the right hepatic vein.

Special Problems and Techniques
Hepatic Veins and Inferior Vena Cava

For tumors, particularly very large tumors, compromising the vena cava or the hepatic veins, special techniques might be appropriate.

Before proceeding to describe these techniques, it is important to emphasize that even severe distortion of the vena cava by large tumors seldom indicates direct invasion by carcinoma, and in most instances, the cava can be separated without violating the tumor. The techniques for controlling the vena cava and hepatic veins described previously are sufficient in most instances. In 100 consecutive major hepatic resections performed at Memorial Sloan–Kettering Cancer Center, 52 of which were extended hepatectomies and many of which involved tumors compromising the vena cava, we had no recourse to complex measures of vascular control on any occasion.

However, complete vascular *isolation* of the liver with clamping of the hepatic arterial and portal inflow and of the inferior vena cava above and below the liver (Fig. 94-21) can be performed. This technique is based on the fact that the liver will tolerate total normothermic ischemia for 30 to 60 minutes. The liver can also be isolated by control of the inferior vena cava, portal vein, and hepatic artery, and the liver can be *perfused* with cold solutions during this period. Such techniques are not associated with an improvement in resectability rate. More recently, liver isolation with a venovenous bypass (vide infra) and complete or partial explantation of the liver have been used by some surgeons in the performance of complex hepatic resections involving the major vessels. These approaches have come primarily from and

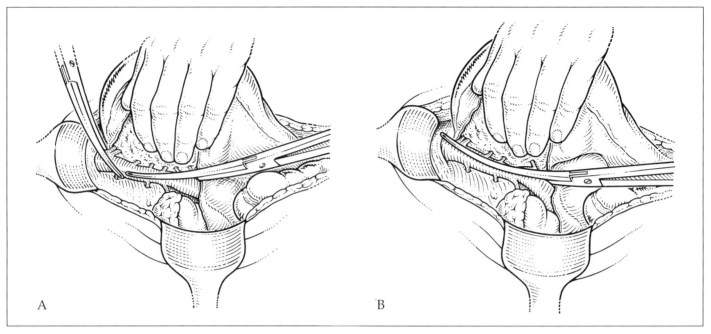

Fig. 94-21. Position of the vascular clamps using (A) two clamps and (B) one long clamp to allow control of the retrohepatic inferior vena cava during vascular exclusion of the liver. (From LH Blumgart. Liver Resection—Liver and Biliary Tumours. In LH Blumgart [ed.], Surgery of the Liver and Biliary Tract, *2nd ed. London: Churchill-Livingstone, 1994. Reproduced with permission.)*

been developed within hepatic transplantation units.

It must be emphasized that despite the fact that temporary occlusion of the inferior vena cava is usually reasonably well tolerated, it does cause a decrease in venous return. This decrease together with cross-clamping of the hepatic arterial and portal venous inflow results in a situation not very different from the anhepatic phase of liver transplantation. There is a marked reduction in cardiac output and an increase in systemic vascular resistance. Although arterial blood pressure is reasonably well maintained, cardiac output is reduced, and this reduction occurring with an increase in peripheral resistance and a decrease in central venous volume is not tolerated by many patients and can result in the development of cardiac failure with marked hypotension, cardiac arrhythmia, and cardiac arrest. In addition, when the circulation is released, stagnant blood rich in potassium suddenly returns to the systemic circulation and aggravates the situation. For these reasons, a number of attempts have been made to monitor hemodynamic and biochemical parameters during major liver resection using a variety of vascular exclusion techniques.

It must be recognized that hepatic vascular isolation can be associated with a high incidence of morbidity. Recent studies of patients for whom hepatic vascular exclusion was used in the resection of liver or extrahepatic tumors invading the vena cava report vascular isolation being abandoned in up to 19 percent because of poor hemodynamic tolerance. Hospital mortality is reported at 6 percent, 30-day mortality at 8 percent, and complications at 60 percent. Reoperation is necessary in 23 percent, and the average hospital stay is 24 days. These results were obtained by investigators with extensive experience in these isolation techniques.

The value of *venovenous bypass* in clinical liver transplantation using a pump that does not require systemic heparinization has been demonstrated. The system has been used in the approach for extracorporeal resection.

While recognizing that there is an occasional place for vascular isolation and venous bypass methods, we believe that they are very rarely required. We have resected portions of the vena cava without any form of isolation, and involvement of the retrohepatic vena cava at a level below the

major hepatic veins can be treated by simple excision of the affected segment without replacement, if there is already an established collateral circulation. Indeed, resection of the retrohepatic inferior vena cava has been combined with right hepatic lobectomy for liver tumor in the absence of an established collateral circulation without subsequent venous reconstruction.

Cryo-assisted Resection

The cryoprobe can be used as a physical aid in hepatic resection. After placing the probe within the tumor and freezing the tumor, the cryoprobe can be used as a "handle" for resecting the liver tumor. The rationale for using this technique includes improved tumor clearance for wedge resections and the performance of minor resection contralateral to major lobe resection. Colorectal metastases to the liver tend to be hard tumors. Therefore, when manipulating these tumors, there is a tendency for the specimens to fracture along the interface of the hard tumor and soft liver. This fracturing accounts, in part, for the high incidence of positive margins (up to 40%) when wedge resections of these le-

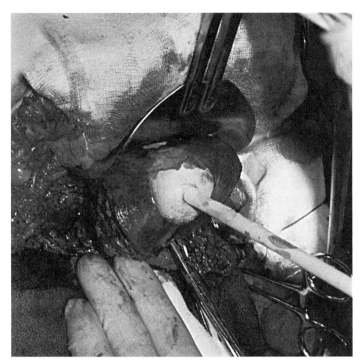

Fig. 94-22. Cryo-assisted resection of a metastatic tumor of the liver. The cryoprobe is placed into the tumor under ultrasound guidance and the tissue frozen until a 1- to 1.5-cm rim of ice is formed around the tumor. Resection is then performed with the handle of the probe used for traction.

sions are attempted. With cryo-assisted resections, the specimen can be frozen to 1 or 2 cm beyond the tumor, and this freeze margin can be confirmed by ultrasound. Resection of this iceball (Fig. 94-22) then increases the chance for a negative margin. Even if the specimen is fractured along the ice-liver interface, the margin is well beyond the tumor.

Blood Loss and Transfusion

An inherent risk in hepatic surgery is the need for homologous blood transfusion because of significant intraoperative blood loss. The risks of homologous blood transfusions are well known and include transmission of disease, alloimmunization, transfusion reactions, and an increased risk of postoperative infectious complications. It has been suggested that blood transfusion has an adverse effect on disease-free and overall survival for patients undergoing hepatic resection for colorectal metastases. These are compelling reasons for the hepatic surgeon to minimize operative blood loss and to use au-

totransfusion to prevent the use of homologous transfusion. With this in mind, *our current surgical attitude to hepatic resection is to limit blood loss and to have all patients donate 2 units of autologous blood, if possible, before the surgical procedure.* In December 1991, we instituted a program to assess the results of such an approach. Hepatic resection and anesthesia were carried out by the techniques outlined previously.

Of 100 patients submitted to hepatic resection over a 14-month period, four were discharged from the Post-Anesthesia Care Unit (PACU) within 8 hours after their operation, 94 spent one night in the PACU and were then transferred to the floor, and two were transferred from the PACU to the ICU for an additional night of observation. Only two patients were subsequently transferred from the floor to the ICU, and both remained in the ICU until death, 10 and 14 days following admission to the ICU. The median length of hospital stay was 13 days. The in-hospital mortality was 3 percent.

Blood loss was proportional to the amount of liver tissue resected. Segmental resections included one bisegmentectomy,

three left lateral segmentectomies, and eight segmental resections, which accounted for a median blood loss of 450 ml. Patients who underwent six atypical resections (major resections), eight enucleations, and five wedge resections had a median blood loss of 700 ml. Lobectomy, extended right resection, and extended left resection accounted for a median blood loss of 1000 ml, 1100 ml, and 1500 ml, respectively. Median blood loss for the entire series was 1000 ml.

In major resections, 41 of 69 (59%) patients were transfused, compared with only 12 of 31 (39%) minor resections ($P = 0.009$). The overall transfusion rate was 59 percent. Two patients required more than 10 units of blood, and 44 percent were transfused only 1 to 2 units. Patients were more likely to be transfused if they had undergone a major resection (46 of 69) (67%) than if they had a minor resection (13 of 31) (42%) ($P = 0.04$). The use of homologous blood transfusion was reduced during this study to an overall rate of 38 percent.

The uniform approach to our patients made them a homogeneous group for evaluation. The distribution of patients was heavily weighted toward major resections, 52 percent of instances being extended hepatic resections. The median length of hospital stay was 13 days. Further evidence of the effectiveness of the technique is reflected by the fact that only four of 100 patients required transfer to the ICU during hospitalization. In this time of cost consciousness, the techniques have to be cost effective and allow acceptable morbidity and mortality during the hospital stay and minimization of ICU care.

Hemodilutional techniques have not reduced the operative blood loss during hepatic resection but have been proven to decrease the need for perioperative transfusion. Major drawbacks of this method are the time and resources required to withdraw, store, and retransfuse blood, and in our studies, 75 percent of our patients would have gone through the process of hemodilution for no reason.

Suggested Reading

Baer HU, Dennison AR, Mouton W, et al. Enucleation of giant hemangiomas of the liver Amer. *Ann Surg* 216:673, 1992.

Baer HU, Gertsch PH, Matthews JB, et al. Resectability of large focal liver lesions. *Amer J Surg* 141:18, 1987.

Bismuth H, Castaing D, Emond F. Intraoperative ultrasound and liver surgery. In LH Blumgart (ed.), *Surgery of the Liver and Biliary Tract*, 2nd ed. London: Churchill-Livingstone, 1994.

Bismuth H, Houssin D, Castaing D. Major and minor segmentectomies ''reglees'' in liver surgery. *World J Surg* 6:10, 1982.

Blumgart LH. Liver Resection—Liver and Biliary Tumours. In LH Blumgart (ed.), *Surgery of the Liver and Biliary Tract*, 2nd ed. London: Churchill-Livingstone, 1994.

Blumgart LH, Baer HU, Czerniak A, et al. Extended left hepatectomy: Technical aspects of an evolving procedure. *Br J Surg* 80:903, 1993.

Couinaud C. Bases anatomiques des hepatectomies gauche et droite reglees. Techniques qui en decoulent. *J Chirurgie* 70:933, 1954.

Couinaud C. *Etudes Anatomiques et Chirurgicales*. Paris: Masson, 1957.

Cunningham JD, Fong Y, Shriver C, et al. One hundred consecutive hepatic resections: Blood loss, transfusion and operative technique. *Arch Surg* 129:1050, 1994.

Goldsmith NA, Woodburne RT. The surgical anatomy pertaining to liver resection. *Surg Gynecol Obstet* 105:310, 1957.

Hepp J, Couinaud C. *L'abord et L'utilisation du Canal Hepatique Gauche dans les Reparations de la Voie Biliare Principale*. Paris: Presse Medicale, 1956.

Huguet C, Addario-Chieco P, Gavelli A, et al. Technique of hepatic vascular exclusion for extensive liver resection. *Am J Surg* 163:602, 1992.

Huguet C, Gavelli A, Addario-Chieco P, et al. Liver ischemia for hepatic resection: Where is the limit? *Surgery* 111:251, 1992.

Jamieson GG, Corbel L, Campion JP, et al. Major liver resection without blood transfusion: Is it a realistic objective? *Surgery* 112:32, 1992.

Launois B, Jamieson GG. The importance of Glisson's capsule and its sheaths in the intrahepatic approach to resection of the liver. *Surg Gynecol Obstet* 174:7, 1992.

Morris DL, Horton MDA, Dilley AV, et al. Treatment of hepatic metastases by cryotherapy and regional cytotoxic perfusion. *Gut* 34:1156, 1993.

Pichlmayr R, Broelsch CH, Wonigeit K, et al. Experience with liver transplantation in Hannover. *Hepatology* 4:56, 1984.

Polk W, Fong Y, Karpeh M, et al. A technique for the use of cryosurgery to assist hepatic resection. *J Amer Coll Surg* 2:171, 1995.

Ravikumar TS, Kane R, Cady B, et al. A 5-year study of cryosurgery in the treatment of liver tumors. *Arch Surg* 126:1520, 1991.

Ravikumar TS, Steele G Jr, Kane R, et al. Experimental and clinical observations on hepatic cryosurgery for colorectal metastases. *Can. Res.* 51:6323, 1991.

Scheele J, Stangl R. Segment orientated anatomical liver resections. In LH Blumgart (ed.) *Surgery of the Liver and Biliary tract* 2nd ed. London: Churchill-Livingstone, 1994.

Starzl TE, Bell RH, Beart RW, et al. Hepatic trisegmentectomy and other liver resections. *Surg Gynecol Obstet* 141:429, 1975.

Starzl TE, Koep LJ, Weil R III, et al. Right trisegmentectomy for hepatic neoplasms. *Surg Gynecol Obstet* 150:208, 1980.

Starzl TE, Iwatsuki S, Shaw BW, et al. Left hepatic trisegmentectomy. *Surg Gynecol Obstet* 155:21, 1982.

EDITOR'S COMMENT

Doctor Blumgart and his coworkers at Memorial Sloan-Kettering Hospital have extended the technique of hepatic resection and combined it with a variety of reconstructions of both the vascular system and the biliary tree. This tradition is different from that of most American hepatic resections, many of which have developed in liver transplantation units. Nonetheless, the inclusion of this chapter has enabled us to evaluate adventurous techniques in performing a series of resections for hepatic neoplasms.

A number of techniques are emphasized. Particularly important, in my view, are the lowering of the hilar plate, enabling adequate dissection of both the right and left vascular structures as an initial maneuver. I enthusiastically agree with Drs. Blumgart and Fong about rotating the liver to the patient's left before performing hepatic resections and left hepatectomies. This maneuver minimizes blood loss. Dissection of the hepatic veins in the extrahepatic plane is well worth the time one spends in preventing hemorrhage during transection of the parenchyma.

Doctor Blumgart and I disagree with respect to sternal splitting, only in the matter of emphasis. Doctor Blumgart, with his vast experience, appears to persist longer in an effort not to split the sternum and gain access to the inferior vena cava from above. In a bulky, stiff right lobe, splitting the steinum early can save a good deal of time and enable the resection to proceed safely. It does not in itself result in much morbidity.

I am undecided as to whether the inclusion of Glisson's capsule in the extension along the major vascular pedicles represents an advance in technique. It presumably saves time. Whether it gives one a feeling of assurance during the resection is unclear to me. Emre and colleagues (*Ann Surg* 217:15, 1993) have described 16 instances of liver resection under total vascular isolation. As Drs. Blumgart and Fong state, techniques of total vascular isolation, venovenous bypass, and bench surgery on livers in which difficult dissections are managed on the back bench and the liver is reinserted into the patient seem to have arisen in transplantation units that are more comfortable with the technique. Greater comfort would appear to be present in surgeons who use these techniques on a weekly basis.

Zulim and colleagues (*Arch Surg* 128:206, 1993) questioned the rate of pulmonary metastases following intraoperative autotransfusion in hepatic resection for malignancy. The working hypothesis was to question whether humoral emboli would result more frequently in patients in whom hepatic tumors were resected. Presumably, tumor cells would be shed in the blood, particularly if the margins were clear. In their paper, no evidence was elicited for increased implantation of tumor cells following autotransfusion and hepatic resection.

J.E.F.

95

Treatment of Major Hepatic Trauma

Donald D. Trunkey

Before World War II, major injuries to the liver were only occasionally resected and hepatorrhaphy was somewhat primitive. Abdominal packs were often used to control hemorrhage and almost all injuries were drained. Based on World War II experience, Madding and Kennedy recommended liver resection as a primary treatment for major hepatic injuries. Over the next few years, large trauma centers reported extensive experience with hepatic resections, with mortalities that averaged approximately 50 percent. Debridement and hepatorrhaphy had more acceptable survivability; however, complication rates were high. As a consequence of the high mortality associated with resection, packing of liver injuries was re-introduced in the 1980s.

More recently two significant events have changed the approach to major hepatic trauma. As a consequence of some pioneering work in the anatomy of the liver there has been a surge of operative techniques for elective hepatic resection. An understanding of the segmental anatomy has allowed segmental resection and innovative procedures to be developed for handling tumors and obstruction of the porta hepatis. The second factor influencing liver surgery has been liver transplant operation. This has furthered our understanding of the anatomy and has particularly influenced surgeons in their ability to perform hepatic isolation procedures.

Anatomy

Repair and resection for treatment of hepatic trauma demand a working knowledge of the anatomy of the liver. The seg-
mental approach to liver anatomy that is presented here is valuable for the surgeon for prediction of the locations of vascular structures within the liver substance. While small segmental resections are feasible in elective surgery, liver resection for trauma is almost exclusively restricted to nonanatomic debridement of nonviable liver tissue, left lateral segmentectomy, and formal right or left hepatic lobectomy.

The liver has three major surfaces: superior, inferior, and posterior. Both the superior and posterior surfaces rest against the diaphragm; however, the inferior surface is more complex, containing the gallbladder, hepatic ducts, hepatic arteries, and portal veins (Fig. 95-1). The liver is attached to surrounding structures by ligaments, the reflexion of parietal peritoneum (Fig. 95-2). The coronary ligament is formed along the superior surface of the right lobe and secures the liver to the diaphragm posteriorly and superiorly. The two leaves of the coronary ligament join at the extreme left to form the triangular ligament. The falciform ligament and ligamentum teres (obliterated umbilical vein) provide anterior attachment of the midportion of the liver to the anterior abdominal wall.

Morphologically the liver is described as two main (right and left) and two accessory (quadrate and caudate) lobes. The right and left lobes are divided by the ma-

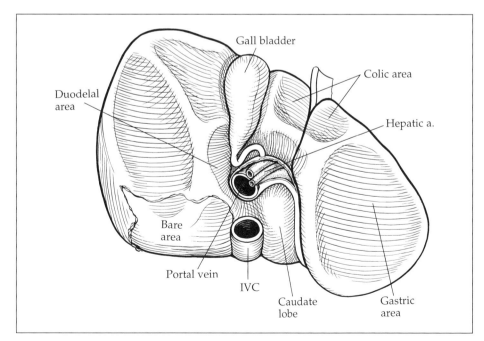

Fig. 95-1. Anatomy of the inferior surface of the liver.

jor fissure with the right being larger. The quadrate lobe is that portion of the right lobe lying anterior to the transverse hilar fissure, medial to the gallbladder fossa, and lateral to the umbilical fissure. The caudate lobe lies posterior to the transverse liver fissure.

Surgical treatment of traumatic injuries relies on a functional anatomic description of the liver. Segmental and anatomic resection has been well documented by Bismuth using an anatomic description from Canad. Hepatic segmentation based on the distribution of the portal pedicle and location of hepatic veins defines the functional anatomy (Figs. 95-3 and 95-4). The three main hepatic veins (right, left, and middle) divide the liver into four sections: right posterior lateral, right anterior medial, left anterior, and posterior. Each of these sectors receives a portal pedicle. Sectors of the right liver are further divided into two segments each: the anterior medial sector, segment IV anteriorly and segment VIII posteriorly; and the posterior lateral sector, segment VI anteriorly and segment VII posteriorly. The left anterior sector is divided by the umbilical fissure into segment IV, the anterior portion of the quadrate lobe, and segment III, the anterior portion of the left lobe of the liver. The posterior sector is comprised of only one segment (II) and lies in the posterior portion of the left lobe. The caudate lobe is considered independently as segment I.

The hepatic artery supplies 25 percent of the blood flow to the liver and 50 percent of the oxygen. In 55 percent of cases, the hepatic artery supply is exclusively from the celiac trunk (Fig. 95-5). The common hepatic artery is the contribution of the celiac trunk after the left gastric and splenic arterial branches. The common hepatic artery traverses along the upper border of the head of the pancreas, then turns to ascend in the lesser omentum. It lies to the left of the common bile duct and anterior to the portal vein. The gastroduodenal artery arises from the distal horizontal position of the common hepatic artery. The right gastric artery arises from the proper hepatic (40% of cases) or left hepatic artery (40% of cases).

The hepatic artery bifurcates in the porta hepatis to give rise to the right and left hepatic arteries. The right hepatic artery courses to the right behind the common bile duct. The anterior and posterior seg-

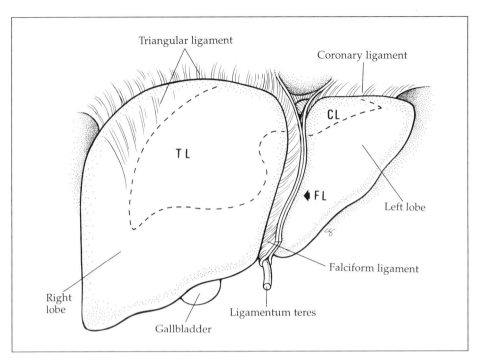

Fig. 95-2. Superficial anatomy of the liver showing the ligaments. TL = triangular ligament; CL = coronary ligament; FL = falciform ligament.

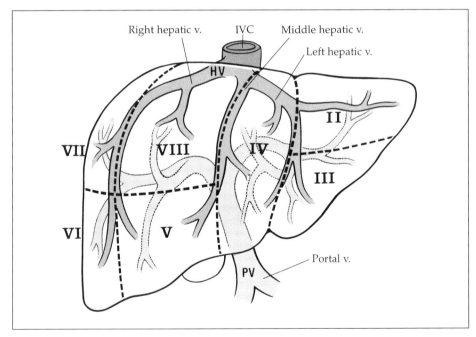

Fig. 95-3. Anterior view of segmental anatomy. HV = hepatic vein; PV = portal vein; IVC = inferior vena cava.

mental arteries of the right lobe take separate origin from the right hepatic artery. The anterior segmental branch courses along the gallbladder fossa in close proximity to the cystic duct. The left hepatic artery runs upward obliquely to the left and divides into its two terminal branches, the medial and lateral segmental arteries. The medial segmental artery descends into the quadrate lobe (segment IV). The lateral segmental artery travels obliquely toward the upper, outer aspect of the lateral seg-

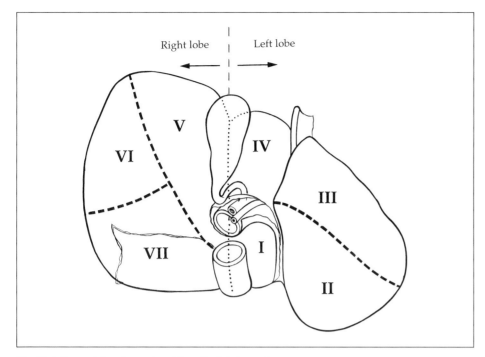

Fig. 95-4. Segmental anatomy viewed from the inferior surface.

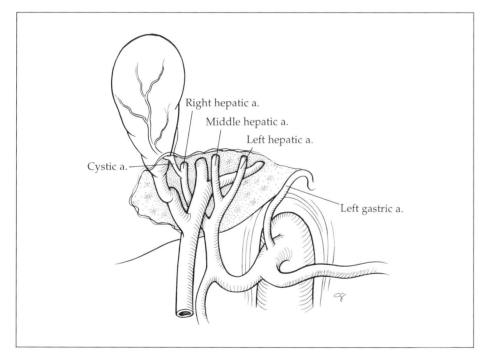

Fig. 95-5. Most common hepatic artery configuration.

ment, where it divides into the superior and inferior branches. The blood supply to the caudate lobe (segment I) is variable. In approximately 35 percent of cases, the entire blood supply of the caudate lobe comes from the right hepatic artery, and in 12 percent entirely from the left hepatic artery. In the majority, however, the blood supply is from both. Aberrant hepatic arteries occur frequently in 40 to 50 percent of cases. The most frequent anomaly is the left hepatic artery arising from the gastric artery (25–30%) (Fig. 95-6A). This includes a 10 percent incidence of a totally replaced left hepatic artery and a 15 percent incidence of an accessory left hepatic artery. The right hepatic artery originates from the superior mesenteric artery in 17 percent of cases: 10 percent total replacement and 7 percent accessory (Fig. 95-6B). The middle hepatic artery arises from the left or right hepatic artery with equal frequency. The cystic artery usually is a branch of the right hepatic artery. It reaches the gallbladder behind the common hepatic duct after traversing the cyst-hepatic triangle to the right of the common hepatic duct. In 85 to 90 percent of cases, there is a single cystic artery.

The portal vein carries 75 percent of the blood flow to the liver and 50 percent of the oxygen. The portal vein is formed by the confluence of the superior mesenteric vein and the splenic vein behind the neck of the pancreas. Approaching the liver within the porta hepatis, the portal vein lies anterior to the inferior vena cava and to the left of the common bile duct and the hepatic artery. The portal vein is 7 to 10 cm in length and bifurcates into the left and right portal veins. The portal lobar veins lie posterior to the hepatic veins and bile ducts. The right portal vein is short and divides into anterior and posterior segmental vessels. Each of these segmental vessels further divides into inferior and superior subsegmental branches. The right portal vein sends a branch to the right side of the caudate lobe (segment I).

The left portal vein is longer than the right and courses to the left in the hilar plate from the bifurcation. It then turns inferiorly in the liver at the umbilical fossa. The superior and inferior subsegmental veins of the lateral segment (segments II and III) arise from the left side of the umbilical portion of the left portal vein. The medial segmental veins rise from the right side of the umbilical portion of the left portal vein. This is of importance when performing a left lateral segmentectomy (segments II and III) as the umbilical portion of the left portal vein should be left intact.

Venous drainage of the liver is quite simple. The hepatic veins lie in the planes dividing the segments of the liver. There are three major veins: right, middle, and left. The right hepatic vein is the largest and drains the anterior and posterior portions of the right lobe of the liver (segments VI, VII, and VIII). The middle and left hepatic veins frequently enter the inferior vena

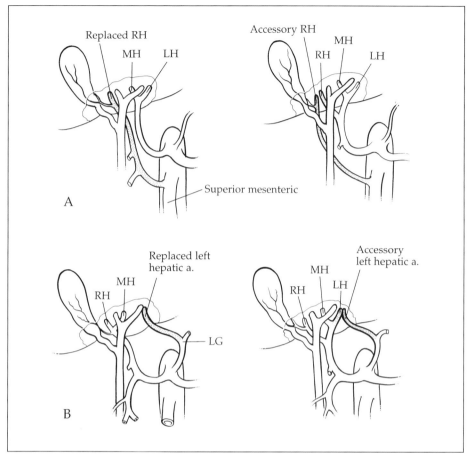

Fig. 95-6. A. *Various anomalies of the hepatic artery circulation.* Left. *Replaced right hepatic (RH) artery off superior mesenteric artery.* Right. *Accessory right hepatic artery. MH = middle hepatic; LH = left hepatic. B. Anomalies of the left hepatic artery.* Left. *Replaced left hepatic (LF) artery. LG = left gastric.* Right. *Accessory left hepatic artery.*

odenum and superior edge of the pancreas. The gastroduodenal artery lies to the left and the posterosuperior pancreatic duodenal artery lies anterior to the bile duct. The pancreatic portion of the common bile duct passes from the upper margin of the head of the pancreas obliquely to the right posterior portion of the pancreas to its entrance into the duodenum. The intramural portion of the common bile duct travels an oblique path approximately 1.5 cm long through the duodenal wall. It joins with the main pancreatic duct inferiorly.

Pathophysiology

In general the amount of damage caused by penetrating missiles to the liver is determined by the kinetic energy. This kinetic energy is a reflection of the mass of the missile, the differential of the velocity of the missile as it enters the tissue, and the velocity of the missile as it exits the tissue. In the past decade trauma centers have seen an increasing number of medium velocity injuries. Typically, these are caused by large-caliber semiautomatic and automatic weapons. More extensive injuries are seen following a shotgun blast and occasional assault rifle injuries.

Blunt trauma typically results from direct compressive forces or shear forces. The elastic tissues within arterial blood vessels make them less susceptible to tearing than any other structure within the liver. Venous and biliary ductal tissue is moderately resistant to shear forces; the liver parenchyma is the least resistant of all. Thus, fractures within the liver parenchyma tend to occur along segmental fissures or directly into the parenchyma. This causes shearing of lateral branches of the major hepatic vein and portal veins. With severe deceleration injury the origins of the hepatic veins may be ripped from the cava causing devastating hemorrhage. Similarly, the small branches from the caudate lobe entering directly into the cava are at high risk for shear and thus a linear tear appears on the anterior caval surface. Direct compressive forces usually cause tearing between segmental fissures in an anteroposterior sagittal orientation. Horizontal fracture lines into the parenchyma give the characteristic burst pattern to such liver injuries. These usually underlie the ribs and costal cartilage. Fracture lines that

cava as a single trunk. The middle hepatic vein drains the superior aspect of the anterior segment of the right lobe (segment V). The left hepatic vein drains the superior aspect of the medial and lateral segments of the left lobe (segments II, III, and IV). The caudate lobe (segment I) usually drains directly into the inferior vena cava via multiple small branches.

The biliary drainage of the liver follows a segmental and lobar pattern and shares a common pathway with the blood supply (portal triad). The right hepatic duct is formed by the joining of the anterior and posterior segmental ducts of the porta hepatis. In 30 percent of cases, one of the two ducts, usually the posterior, crosses the segmental fissure to drain in the left hepatic duct.

The left hepatic duct is formed by the confluence of the medial and lateral segmental ducts. This is in the left segmental fissure in 50 percent of cases and to the right of the fissure in 42 percent. In the caudate lobe (segment I) drainage is variable and may flow into either the left or right duct. The common hepatic duct is formed by the confluence of the right and left hepatic ducts in the transverse fissure of the liver. Its distal end is defined by the junction of the cystic duct and may range from 1.0 to 7.5 cm in length. The normal diameter is 4 mm. The common bile duct is a continuation of the common hepatic duct, distal to the cystic duct. It ranges in length from 2 to 7 cm. It has a very consistent course and is divided into four portions: supraduodenal, retroduodenal, pancreatic, and intramural. The supraduodenal lies between layers of the hepatic duodenal ligament, anterior to the foramen of Winslow. The retroduodenal portion is between the superior margin of the first portion of the du-are parallel have been dubbed "bear-claw"–type injuries. Occasionally, there will be a single fracture line across the horizontal plane of the liver usually between the anterior and posterior segments. Since this involves both lobes of the liver it can cause significant hemorrhage if there is direct extension or continuity with the peritoneal cavity.

Knowing the mechanism of injury articulated by the paramedics allows the surgeon to anticipate certain patterns of injury. Compressive forces caused by the steering wheel or the shoulder belt of a three-point restraint system can result in extensive bear-claw–type injuries to the liver and even transections of the liver (Fig. 95-7). Another example is the so-called T-bone auto crash, which is a crash of two vehicles in a perpendicular fashion. Extensive injury can occur to the liver, usually when the T-bone is into the passenger side. This causes extensive right lateral rib fractures and compression of the right lobe of the liver. An extreme form of this lateral compressive injury is a transverse fracture through both lobes of the liver (Fig. 95-8). Shear injuries are usually associated with deceleration from falls (greater than two floors) or unrestrained occupants in high-speed motor vehicle accidents. The abrupt deceleration tends to tear the "relatively" heavy liver from its attachments, such as hepatic veins, veins from the caudate lobe, and lacerations into parenchyma at the ligamentum teres. These are often associated with exsanguinating hemorrhage.

Diagnosis

The liver is at high risk for injury from penetrating wounds since it is the largest parenchymatous organ and its anatomic location is at the junctions of the upper one-third and middle one-third of the torso. Major hepatic trauma is usually associated with medium-and high-velocity wounds. Occasionally, major vessel injury (usually hepatic vein) can be caused by stab wounds, and the author has seen several, with large knives such as bayonets or bowie-type weapons. If a patient with penetrating wound to the torso, particularly the midportion, is in hemodynamically unstable condition, he or she requires no diagnostic studies except a chest x-ray, which may help the surgeon in deciding which torso cavity to open first. If one of the hemithoraces is full of blood, as determined by chest x-ray, it may be prudent to open that cavity first. The pitfall is that a hole in the diaphragm with injury to either the left or right lobe of the liver can be the source of exsanguination. This makes the point that the trauma patient should never be in any other position than the supine one. The surgeon must be prepared to deal with exsanguination on both sides of the diaphragm. Rarely, a patient with major hepatic trauma can present in hemodynamically stable condition from penetrating wounds. If there is a high index of suspicion of penetration into the abdominal cavity or peritoneal signs are present, exploratory celiotomy is indicated. If in doubt, the surgeon can use diagnostic peritoneal lavage or ultrasound as a diagnostic adjunct to confirm that intraperitoneal blood is present. It must be emphasized that in the hemodynamically unstable patient with penetrating wounds to the torso, there is no diagnostic challenge. The patient requires immediate surgery.

From a diagnostic standpoint, major hepatic injury from blunt trauma can be more vexing than trauma from penetrating wounds, particularly in the young healthy adult who can compensate for significant blood loss. Physical examination, even in an alert patient, is accurate in only one-half of cases and carries a 56 percent false-positive rate and a 34 to 46 percent false-negative rate. The introduction of diagnostic peritoneal lavage in 1965 dramatically improved the surgeon's ability to diagnose intra-abdominal injury. It is rapidly performed and highly sensitive. More recently, CT scan has been shown to be an even more valuable diagnostic tool since it allows the surgeon to make judgments as to whether or not the patient requires operative intervention. This is true for even very extensive liver lacerations. If these lacerations are contained and there

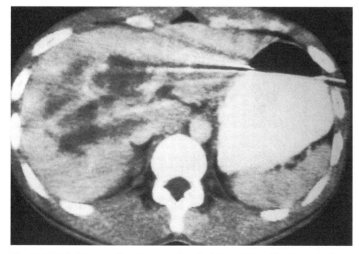

Fig. 95-7. This 25-year-old patient was involved in a "T-bone" motor vehicle accident. He has extensive transverse lacerations across both lobes of the liver. The patient was managed nonoperatively.

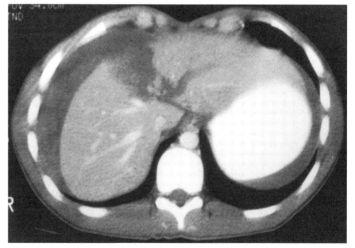

Fig. 95-8. This 19-year-old patient was wearing three-point restraints when involved in a high-speed motor vehicle accident. The chest portion of the restraint has caused almost complete transection of the liver in its anatomic plane. Left hepatic lobectomy was performed.

Table 95-1. Grading of Liver Injuries

	Grade	Injury Description
I.	Hematoma	Subcapsular, nonexpanding, <10% surface area
	Laceration	Capsular tear, nonbleeding, <1 cm deep parenchymal disruption
II.	Hematoma	Subcapsular, nonexpanding, hematoma 10–50%; intraparenchymal, nonexpanding, <2 cm in diameter
	Laceration	<3 cm parenchymal depth, <10 cm in length
III.	Hematoma	Subcapsular, >50% of surface area or expanding; ruptured subcapsular hematoma with active bleeding; intraparenchymal hematoma >2 cm
	Laceration	>3 cm parenchymal depth
IV.	Hematoma	Ruptured central hematoma
	Laceration	Parenchymal destruction involving 25–75% of hepatic lobe
V.	Laceration	Parenchymal destruction >75% of hepatic lobe
	Vascular	Juxtahepatic venous injuries (retrohepatic cava/major hepatic veins)
VI.	Vascular	Hepatic avulsion

From EE Moore, SR Shackford, HL Pachter, et al. Organ injury scaling: Spleen, liver, and kidney. *J Trauma* 29:1664, 1989. © by Williams & Wilkins, 1989. With permission.

is minimal blood into the peritoneal cavity, it may be more prudent to treat the patient nonoperatively.

Ultrasound has also been advocated as a diagnostic adjunct. It has an 85 to 90 percent sensitivity in picking up intraperitoneal blood but it does not meet the high-resolution standards of CT. Because of its relative simplicity and low cost it has been advocated as a useful technique.

The American Association for the Surgery of Trauma has recently developed a grading of organ injuries including the liver. This classification is depicted in Table 95-1. Recent studies have confirmed the utility of this classification and it has a good correlation with operative management.

Initial Operative Approach

The trauma patient who requires celiotomy should be prepared and draped from the midneck to the midthighs anteriorly and from tabletop to tabletop laterally. In a patient in unstable condition, the preparation and draping optimally should be done before the induction of anesthesia since the administration of a muscle relaxant can lead to a significant drop in blood pressure. The surgeon should be prepared to open the abdomen as soon as possible after the induction of anesthesia.

A generous midline incision is made from the xiphoid to below the umbilicus (Fig. 95-9). Once the abdomen is open and it has been determined that there is a large amount of blood within the peritoneal cavity, this incision should be carried down to the suprapubic area. My initial approach is to immediately evacuate as much clot as possible and then to pack all quadrants of the abdomen. This will usually temporarily control hemorrhage and allow the anesthesiologist to replace needed volume. The surgeon should make some critical decisions at this juncture. Every effort to keep the patient warm must be done. This includes turning the thermostat in the operating room up to 85°F. There should be an adequate blood-warming device and the humidifier on the ventilator should be turned up to 105°F. It should also be determined at this time whether more access lines to the circulation are needed. If the hospital has a massive transfusion protocol it should be initiated.

The surgeon should then remove the packs from the lower abdominal quadrant, checking for associated injuries, particularly those that can cause fecal contamination. If no fecal soilage is present, the surgeon can then use autotransfusion devices. The packs in the left upper quadrant are removed and if there is associated injury to the spleen, it should be promptly removed in order to reduce associated hemorrhage while the liver injury is being

addressed. Finally, the packs in the right upper quadrant are removed (Fig. 95-10). At this juncture I usually do a diagnostic maneuver by gently retracting the dome of the liver rostrally. If a gush of blood emanates from the central area this is a presumptive diagnosis of hepatic vein injury. Packs are replaced and the surgeon must decide what isolation technique will be used. If there are obvious parenchymatous deep lacerations into the liver substance and blood is coming from the depths, another diagnostic maneuver is to apply a vascular clamp across the porta hepatis. If this controls the hemorrhage it eliminates the hepatic veins as a source of the major bleeding and one should presume that it is either hepatic arterial or portal venous bleeding. This may lead to further dissection within the distal porta hepatis to isolate the left and right portal vein and the left and right hepatic artery in order to selectively control them and to determine which one is the source of bleeding.

Although it has been advocated that a left anterior thoracotomy be done and the descending thoracic aorta clamped, this has not been useful in my experience and in fact can be harmful. The single exception is the patient with penetrating gunshot wound to the midline in whom an associated abdominal aortic injury within the lesser sac is suspected. Clamping the descending thoracic aorta to control liver bleeding does not work and simply aggravates the metabolic acidosis and reperfusion injury that ensue when the clamp is removed.

Operative Management

After temporary control of hemorrhage has been achieved by packs or compression, the first priority is to mobilize the liver. This includes sharply dividing the falciform ligament, taking down both leaves of the coronary ligament, and dividing the triangular ligament on the left lobe. If not already performed, the lesser sac should be entered by dividing the avascular area or the gastrohepatic ligament (Fig. 95-11). With these ligamentous attachments divided, the surgeon can mobilize the individual lobes in order to compress and get access to the injuries.

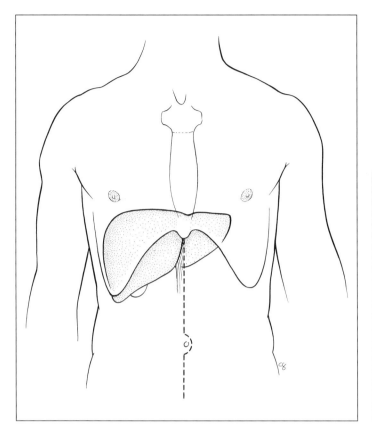

Fig. 95-9. An extensive midline incision is preferred for all major hepatic injuries with an option of extending the incision up the sternum.

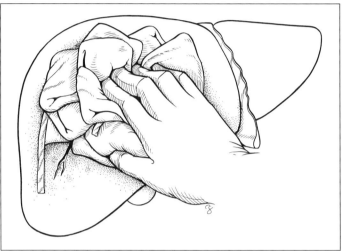

Fig. 95-10. Hemostasis of liver fracture. Direct pressure with packs is usually sufficient to control the majority of liver parenchymal bleeding.

The most common major hepatic injuries that surgeons will be called on to treat are deep lacerations into the parenchyma, usually involving the right hepatic lobe or segment IV (quadrate lobe) proximate to the falciform ligament (Fig. 95-12). Controlling the bleeding is best achieved by the assistant who stands on the left side of the patient. He or she can extend the left hand underneath the right lobe and can compress the dome or the uninjured part with the right hand. This allows the surgeon to deepen the laceration, using a finger fracture technique and clamping the bleeding vessels and bile ducts; this is followed by suture ligation with 3–0 or 4–0 silk. Although clips have been recommended, the author prefers suture ligation since these sutures are less likely to fall off with ventilatory movement of the liver. Deep liver sutures or mattress sutures are rarely indicated for control of hemorrhage, as they can lead to hematobilia, hepatic necrosis, abscess, and hematoma formation within the liver parenchyma. Once hemorrhage has been controlled with suture li-

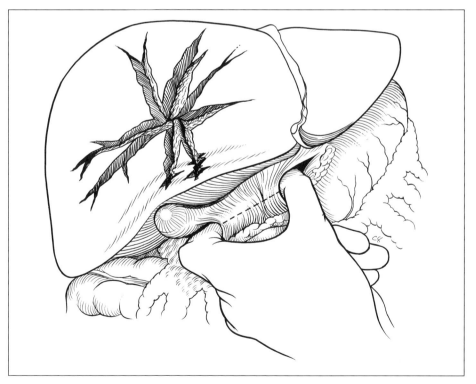

Fig. 95-11. Access to the porta hepatis is achieved by inserting the index finger into the foramen of Winslow and the thumb through the avascular portion of the gastrohepatic ligament.

gation of the individual vessels the margins are checked for viability. The use of a viable pedicle of omentum is a useful technique to help with hemostasis and to close the dead space. The omentum also aids wound healing and reduces sepsis. If compression by the assistant is inadequate to control bleeding from the laceration, a vascular clamp can be placed across the porta hepatis (Pringle's maneuver) (Fig. 95-13). Once hemostasis is achieved this clamp should be removed as soon as possible. Although the Pringle maneuver has been used for up to one hour in elective hepatic surgery, the safe limit in the hypovolemic trauma patient has not been established. In general, I prefer to limit warm ischemia to 15 minutes but would accept up to 30 minutes.

Resectional debridement is the next most common procedure performed in major hepatic injuries. Resection is not determined by segmental anatomy but by the extent of injury and liver viability. Most often these injuries are caused by shotgun blasts or large lacerations from blunt trauma that have lateral extensions. The general principles are straightforward. All nonviable liver tissue is resected using a finger fracture technique or the back of the scalpel handle. When resistance is encountered with either technique this usually indicates the elastic tissue of vessels or biliary ducts. These are doubly clamped, divided, and suture ligated. Nonpulsatile oozing from the parenchyma can be controlled with the electrocautery unit or the argon beam coagulator. Fibrin glue, thrombin-soaked Gelfoam, and infrared diathermy are all techniques that have been described to control oozing. I prefer the electrocautery unit since it is invariably available.

If there is any question about the viability of the margins of the tissue after resectional debridement, a second-look operation should be scheduled in 24 to 36 hours. In my opinion, removal of necrotic tissue is mandatory and reduces the incidence of systemic inflammatory response syndrome (SIRS).

In a very few cases (less than 1%), bleeding will continue to vex the surgeon during hepatorrhaphy or resectional debridement. In these instances, it is worthwhile to dissect out the right and left hepatic arteries and portal vein in the porta hepatis.

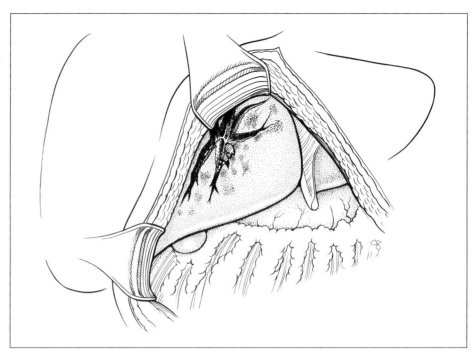

Fig. 95-12. Approach to liver fracture. A typical stellate laceration of the right lobe of the liver extending into segment IV is shown. The falciform and triangular ligaments must be incised to mobilize the liver into the midline, in order to control and treat the hemorrhage.

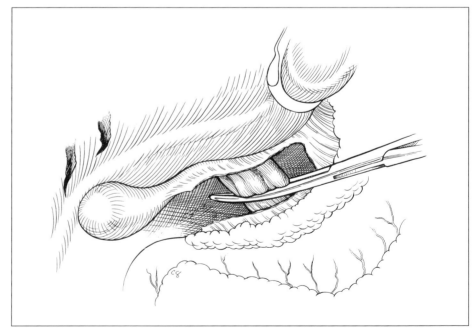

Fig. 95-13. Pringle's maneuver.

If application of a vascular clamp to one of these four vessels stops the hemorrhage, it is worthwhile to consider ligating one vessel and one vessel only. Ligating both the portal vein and hepatic artery to one lobe will ensure nonviability. Ligation of the common hepatic artery has been described with maintenance of liver function since there is adequate collateral through the gastroduodenal artery. Ligation of the proper hepatic artery is contraindicated.

Hepatic lobectomy is indicated in 2 to 4 percent of all patients with liver trauma; however, in major liver trauma it is indicated in approximately 20 percent of cases. Usually the extent of injury has made it obvious to the surgeon that a formal lobectomy will be necessary to control the hemorrhage. I start the lobectomy by incising the liver capsule with a scalpel or the electrocautery unit in the anatomic plane (Fig. 95-14). The blood loss is minimized by compression of the liver between the assistant's hands. As described above the liver parenchyma is divided by the finger fracture technique or the blunt end of a scalpel handle. As vessels and bile ducts are encountered they are individually ligated with 3–0 or 4–0 silk. For a left lateral segmentectomy (segments II and III), resection is carried down to the left of the falciform ligament (Fig. 95-15). Care must be taken not to divide vessels that may be supplying segment IV. Care must also be exercised when one reaches the proximal part of the left hepatic vein to make sure that the middle hepatic vein is not divided. The left hepatic vein stump is oversewn with 4–0 vascular silk suture. The arterial supply to segments II and III is ligated to the left of the falciform ligament with 2–0 silk and the branch of the portal vein to segment II is also ligated with 2–0 silk.

The line of resection for a left lobectomy should be carried out to the left of the gallbladder fossa (Fig. 95-16). It is important to identify the middle hepatic vein during resection since it drains the superior segment of the right lobe and commonly drains into the left hepatic vein. The left hepatic vein should be ligated and divided distal to the junction with the middle hepatic vein. The left portal vein should not be ligated until it is well exposed within the hilum because it might give off a branch to the anterior segment of the right lobe. Care should also be taken when dividing the left hepatic duct because a seg-

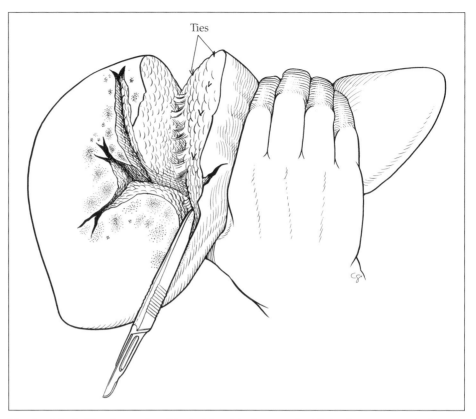

Fig. 95-14. Scalpel-handle resection. After incision of the liver capsule with the electrocautery unit, finger fracture technique or the scalpel handle can be used to dissect through the parenchyma to expose the hepatic vessels and biliary radicals, which are individually suture ligated with 2–0 or 4–0 silk.

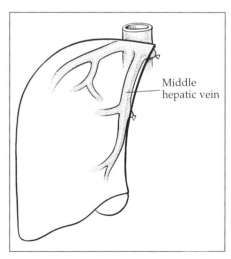

Fig. 95-16. Left hepatic lobectomy.

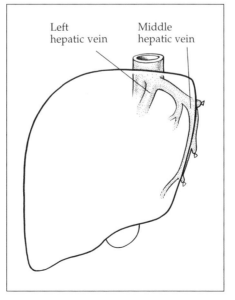

Fig. 95-15. Left lateral segmentectomy (II, III).

mental hepatic duct from the right frequently crosses the segmental fissure to drain into the left hepatic duct. The left hepatic artery supplies only the left side and can be readily ligated.

In performing a right hepatic lobectomy, the line of resection should be carried to the right of the gallbladder fossa (Fig. 95-17). The middle hepatic vein should be divided early and proximately to avoid injury to the left hepatic vein. The dissection should then be carried cephalad and posteriorly toward the vena cava to the right of the middle hepatic vein. The right hepatic artery and portal vein can be dissected early in the dissection and ligated to decrease blood loss. Care should be taken to avoid damage to the occasional branch of the right hepatic artery that may supply the medial segment of the left lobe. Following either right or left hepatic lobectomy, there is a large raw surface over which I prefer to place omentum that is sutured to the capsule at the cut margins.

A useful adjunct in a small number of patients who require lobectomy, resectional debridement, or hepatorrhaphy is vascular isolation. At least three methods are currently in use: Heaney's maneuver, atriocaval shunting, and venovenous bypass. Of these three techniques I prefer Heaney's maneuver and would only rarely use venovenous bypass (Fig. 95-18). Atriocaval shunting has been abandoned by most surgeons.

Heaney's maneuver is performed by clamping both the suprahepatic and infrahepatic inferior vena cava while simultaneously applying Pringle's maneuver. During Heaney's maneuver, it is crucial

that central pressures are monitored and that fluid replacement is adequate when the inferior vena cava is clamped.

The second most common method of hepatic vascular isolation is venovenous bypass using a centrifugal pump that was initially described by Starzl. The modification of this technique is to simply cannulate the femoral vein in the groin and the axillary vein in the upper arm (Fig. 95-19). Heparin-coated tubing connects the two cannulas. The centrifugal pump is used to assist flow. Complete hepatic vascular in-flow can then be accomplished by clamping the suprahepatic vena cava at the diaphragm, suprarenal vena cava, and porta hepatis. It is not necessary to place a portal vein catheter as originally described by Starzl.

As was mentioned earlier, packing was popular before World War II but the results were poor. More recently it has been recognized that packing of liver injuries cannot only buy time to mobilize resources but can be definitive treatment in certain injuries. Such injuries usually are crush injuries to the liver that involve both lobes. It is particularly useful in those injuries in which the bleeding is primarily venous. In the author's experience it is not successful

when ongoing surgical bleeding from arteries is present. Packing is probably the only way of salvaging a patient who is coagulopathic or hypothermic, or both, during operation. The intent here is to pack temporarily, resuscitate and rewarm the patient in the intensive care unit, and return to the operating room as soon as possible. When packing is being used as definitive treatment with a transverse fracture through both lobes, it will often require repacking at 12 to 24 hours following the initial packing and even repacking a third time 24 hours later.

The technique does not involve simply stuffing laparotomy sponges around the liver. Some surgeons have advocated placement of plastic between the gauze and the liver, but in my experience plain gauze is equally effective. The goal is to pack the perihepatic area so that closure of the injury is accomplished (Fig. 95-20). The rib cage provides a rigid strut so that circumferential compression of the liver is accomplished. The intent is to place the packs so that the diaphragm is not unduly elevated and the inferior vena cava is not compromised. The latter can be assessed by having the anesthesiologist give the central venous pressure values and blood

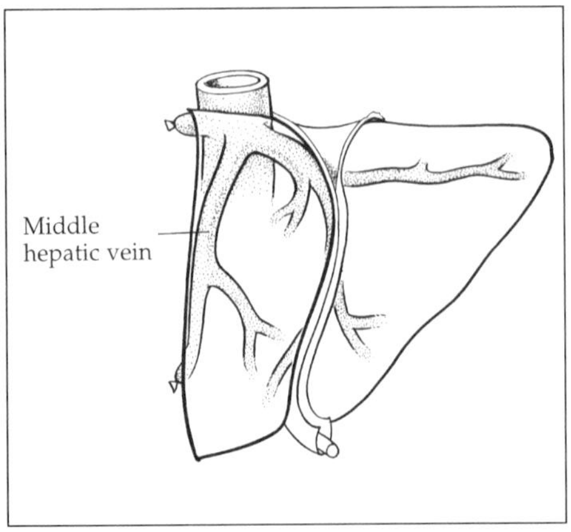

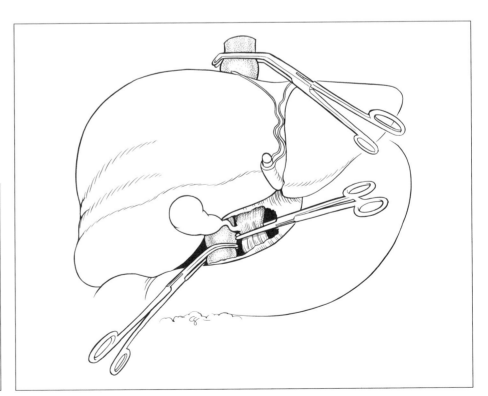

Fig. 95-17. Right hepatic lobectomy.

Middle hepatic vein

Fig. 95-18. Heaney's maneuver for vascular isolation of the liver.

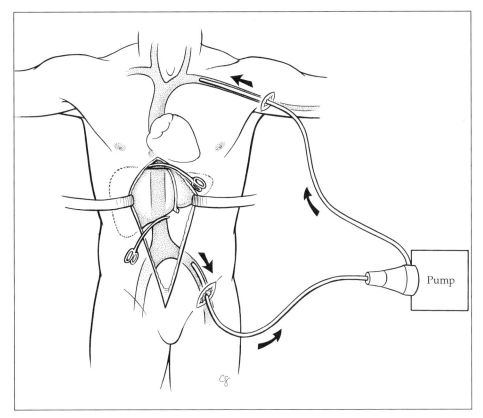

Fig. 95-19. Venovenous bypass. Note the placement of the suprahepatic inferior vena cava clamp and the intrahepatic suprarenal venous clamp.

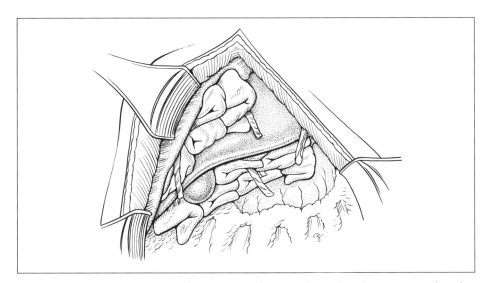

Fig. 95-20. Circumferential packs of the liver. Care must be exercised not to impede venous return from the inferior vena cava or to push the diaphragm cephalad, which will compromise ventilation.

pressure during the packing. If either of these values falls, compromise of the inferior vena cava is usually indicated. Once the circumferential packs are placed, packs are gently placed against the base of the liver and closure of the abdomen is accomplished. During the time that the patient is being resuscitated in the intensive care unit, preparation for the next operation is carried out. This would include anticipa-

tion of using venovenous bypass to facilitate hepatic vascular isolation and to mobilize the massive transfusion protocol. It is also possible after packing to transport the patient to a different center that has more resources.

Drainage of the liver is controversial following repair of injury. In general, I prefer to drain only for biliary leak; thus, the most severe injuries are the ones that will require drainage. I prefer closed drainage systems and drain not only in proximity to the injury but also posterior in order to provide dependent drainage of fluid collections.

A final therapeutic modality that has to be considered in the context of modern surgery is hepatic transplantation. There have been several successful reported cases after major hepatic trauma. The indication for hepatic transplantation secondary to trauma is a severe nonreconstructible injury to the porta hepatis or bilobar nonreconstructible injuries. Other intra-abdominal injuries and head injuries are relative contraindications. The availability of an appropriate donor is unpredictable and every effort should be made to consult a liver transplant center as soon as possible so that the anhepatic period is minimized.

Repair of Injuries to the Porta Hepatis

Most of the injuries to the porta hepatis are from penetrating causes. Control of hemorrhage is the first priority. I prefer to perform an extended Kocher's maneuver, taking down the entire right colon and mobilizing it toward the midline along with the duodenum. This exposes the portal vein and a significant portion of the inferior vena cava and infrarenal aorta, which may also be injured. In a few instances it may be necessary to divide the neck of the pancreas in order to visualize the proximal portion of the portal vein at the junction of the splenic vein and the superior mesenteric vein. Although successful ligation of the portal vein has been reported, I would make an extra effort to repair it or to do an interposition graft using harvested internal jugular vein from one side of the patient's neck. If the spleen has been injured, it may also be possible to use a portion of the splenic vein as an interposition graft. Injuries to the hepatic artery are problematic. As was noted previously ligation of the proper hepatic artery is not recommended. Every effort should be made to repair this or replace it with an interposition saphenous vein graft. I prefer to repair most with lateral sutures of 5–0 or 6–0 Prolene.

Injuries to the extrahepatic biliary tree are also usually associated with penetrating trauma; however, blunt trauma can cause stretch or avulsion injuries. When the injury is to the common duct, repair must be meticulous. The normal common duct is approximately 4 mm in diameter. Lateral repair is possible provided that there is no segmental loss. If segmental loss is present, and involves the proximal common bile duct, biliary drainage can be accomplished using a Roux en Y procedure to either the common hepatic duct or the gallbladder. This Roux en Y can be difficult to perform with a normal-sized common bile duct, and to make this anastomosis technically easier I use a modification of the vascular Carrel patch (Fig. 95-21). A one-centimeter length of cystic duct is preserved after cholecystectomy and the side wall is opened into the common bile duct remnant. This patch of bile duct is then used to anastomose in an end-to-side fashion to the Roux limb. In the unstable pa-

tient temporary biliary drainage can be accomplished by placing catheters into the right and left hepatic ducts or the common duct, which are then brought out of the abdomen laterally. Delayed reconstruction of the biliary systems can be accomplished after the patient recovers from other injuries.

Postoperative Management and Complications

Massive blood loss, transfusion, tissue trauma, shock, hypothermia, and liver dysfunction contribute to coagulopathy, both intraoperatively and postoperatively. Treatment of the coagulopathy requires rewarming of the patient as well as replenishment of clotting factors using transfusion of either fresh whole blood or fresh frozen plasma in conjunction with cryoprecipitate and platelets. Hematocrit, platelet count, and prothrombin time should be measured frequently as a guide to therapy for coagulopathy. If the coagulopathy has been corrected and the patient continues to hemorrhage, re-exploration is indicated. For complex liver injuries

(classes IV and V), I would advocate second-look reoperation at 24 to 48 hours.

Postoperative pulmonary failure is frequent after major trauma. Tissue trauma, large-volume fluid resuscitation, and associated injuries (e.g., rib fracture) contribute to pulmonary failure. The patient should be managed with endotracheal intubation and positive-pressure ventilation until hemodynamically stable. The patient should be extubated as soon as possible, but with the knowledge that reintubation may be necessary.

Jaundice occurs frequently after liver trauma. This may be a sign of severe hepatic dysfunction but usually is related to resorption of hematomas, breakdown of transfused red cells, and mild hepatic dysfunction from central lobular necrosis secondary to shock. Hepatic function returns to normal promptly, although elevated bilirubin levels in the serum may persist for weeks.

Bile leaks and fistulas can usually be detected when the perihepatic area has been drained. Unless these leaks are from a major bile duct, they generally close spontaneously.

Hematobilia is an uncommon complication, occurring in fewer than 1 percent of complex injuries. The typical presentation is days to weeks after the injury and can be manifest by melena, upper gastrointestinal bleeding, hypotension, or biliary colic. The diagnosis is confirmed by visualizing blood coming from the ampulla during upper gastrointestinal endoscopy. Treatment is preferentially by percutaneous transvascular selective embolization of the involved artery.

Sepsis after hepatic trauma occurs in 7 to 12 percent of patients and is related to intra-abdominal abscess, pneumonia, acalculous cholecystitis, and ischemic bowel. Risk factors associated with intra-abdominal abscess postoperatively include associated splenectomy, liver packing to control hemorrhage, class IV or V injury, large transfusion requirement, and colon injury. Subphrenic and subhepatic abscesses are usually marked by fever 4 to 7 days after operation. Pleural effusion may be noted on chest radiography. Diagnosis can be made by ultrasound or CT scan. Treatment includes percutaneous or surgical drainage and intravenous antibiotics. Prophylactic antibiotics are not rec-

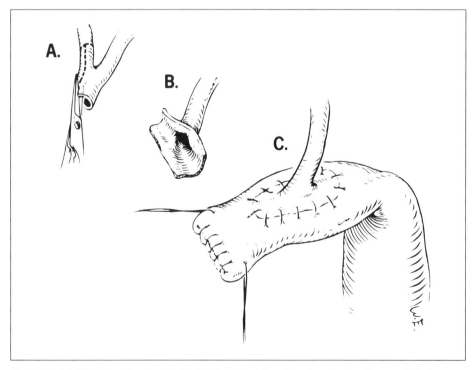

Fig. 95-21. Modification of the Carrel patch for choledochojejunostomy in patients with normal-sized common ducts.

ommended postoperatively unless an associated bowel injury is present.

Suggested Reading

Bismuth H. Surgical anatomy and anatomical surgery of the liver. *World J Surg* 6:3, 1982.

Burch JM, Feliciano DV, Mattox KL. The atriocaval shunt: Facts and fiction. *Ann Surg* 207:555, 1988.

Cogbill TH, Moore EE, Jurkovich GJ, et al. Severe hepatic trauma: A multicenter experience with 1,335 liver injuries. *J Trauma* 28:1433, 1988.

Fabian TC, Stone HH. Arrest of severe liver hemorrhage by an omental pact. *South Med J* 73:1487, 1980.

Heaney J, Scanton W, Halbert D, et al. An improved technique for vascular isolation of the liver: Experimental study and case reports. *Ann Surg* 163:237, 1966.

Kudsk KA, Sheldon FG, Lim RC. Atrial caval shunting after trauma. *J Trauma* 22:81, 1982.

Mavroudis C, Trunkey DD. Choledochoplasty for choledochojejunostomy: Variations on a theme by Carrel. *Am J Surg* 142:305, 1987.

Moore EE. Critical decisions in the management of hepatic trauma. *Am J Surg* 148:712, 1984.

Ochsner MG, Jaffin JH, Golocovsky M, Jones RC. Major hepatic trauma. *Surg Clin North Am* 73:337, 1993.

Pringle JH. Notes on the arrest of hepatic hemorrhage due to trauma. *Ann Surg* 48:541, 1908.

Shaw BW, Martin DJ, Marquez JM, et al. Venous bypass in clinical liver transplantation. *Ann Surg* 200:524, 1984.

EDITOR'S COMMENT

As evacuation techniques, including air evacuation, and more practiced communication between the EMT teams and trauma surgeons have become common, more patients with severe hepatic injuries are reaching the accident floors and the operating room. Injuries that previously would have been fatal have now at least a reasonable chance of being salvaged. However, a systematic approach is critical.

Because of this, a number of organizations, such as the American Association for the Surgery of Trauma, have proposed classification of hepatic injuries both for comparison of purposes and results, but also for approaches.

The careful reader of this volume will note that there are no fewer than three different expositions of hepatic anatomy, which could be attributed to poor editing. While the space occupied by these different versions of hepatic anatomy by Drs. Blumgart, Bismuth, and Trunkey may be considered by some to be slightly wasteful, each of these authorities in his specific areas of liver expertise offers a somewhat different approach to the usual classical anatomy. Doctor Trunkey's orientation, for example, is that of a nonstructured injury based on acceleration or deceleration, shearing forces, or compression injury. Thus, one's interest in hepatic anatomy is tempered by that aspect of the approach.

There are a number of gems in this chapter, including the reminder that prepping of the patient should be extremely wide and should be carried out before the induction of anesthesia so that if the administration of muscle relaxant results in loss of blood pressure, one can intervene promptly. The necessity for maintaining normothermia and the inability to achieve hemostasis in hypothermia with the attendant coagulopathy have been realized by all surgeons who deal extensively with trauma. It is far better to pack, go to the ICU, warm the patient, and correct the coagulopathy than it is to persist in the face of failing coagulation factors.

The major problem of massive liver injury remains the retrohepatic caval injury. Doctor Trunkey is correct that when the pack is removed and dark blood wells up from the depths of the wound, one is likely dealing with a retrohepatic caval injury. At that point, the critical decision the trauma surgeon must make is to prepare right then and there for the repair of the retrohepatic caval injury, by instituting a shunt, either a femoral-atrial or caval-atrial exclusion (the "Schrock shunt"). While Dr. Trunkey has abandoned the caval-atrial shunt, our own trauma group seems to have had reasonable success with it, probably by not persisting in trying to identify the injury, but by immediately splitting the sternum, cannulating the right atrium, and isolating the liver with total hepatic isolation, before one is down 10 or 12 units and before the patient is cold and coagulopathic. I do not argue with the approach, merely that the decision must be made quickly.

Chen and colleagues (*J Trauma* 38:886, 1995) failed to achieve salvage in combined right and left hepatic injuries despite the use of various shunts. All four patients with combined right and left hepatic vein injuries died despite one receiving total hepatectomy and a liver transplant and the liberal use of cavalatrial shunts in the right hepatic vein injuries. As they themselves point out, the optimal approach to right and mixed hepatic venous injuries has not been found in this series. Most trauma surgeons would agree. The only chance the patient has is for early recognition and rapid movement to up the level of repair without hesitation in the decision-making process.

Croce and coworkers (*Ann Surg* 221:744, 1995) argue cogently for the use of nonoperative observation management of hemodynamically stable patients with blunt hepatic injury regardless of the level of severity. There were fewer abdominal complications and fewer transfusions (1.9 vs 4.0 units, $P < 0.02$) in the nonoperative-treated group when compared to a matched cohort of operated patients. Computed tomographic scan or admission characteristics did not make it possible to predict failures. Obviously, intensive care unit monitoring is required.

Liver trauma is a devastating injury that still carries a very high mortality. The evolution of the treatment of these patients over the past 5 to 10 years continues and has already resulted in higher salvage rates.

J.E.F.

96

Cholecystostomy, Cholecystectomy, and Intraoperative Evaluation of the Biliary Tree

E. Christopher Ellison   Larry C. Carey

Operations on the biliary tree are among the most common abdominal procedures performed in the United States, with approximately 650,000 cholecystectomies done each year.

Eighty-five to 90 percent of cholecystectomies are performed by the laparoscopic approach. However, the surgeon must be facile with open biliary surgery for several reasons. First, the conversion rate to open cholecystectomy remains approximately 2 to 5 percent in most series. This is more common in the elderly and in those who have acute cholecystitis. In these situations cholecystectomy will be more difficult and therefore experience and proper care are necessary to avoid technical errors that could lead to devastating complications. Secondly, there are specific instances when open surgery should be considered a wiser choice.

Indications for Open Biliary Surgery

Table 96-1 highlights the conditions that, in our experience, should be treated by open cholecystectomy or, in some instances, cholecystostomy. The general categorization of these indications is made on the basis of certain preoperative conditions and then certain intraoperative findings during laparoscopic cholecystectomy.

The first consideration is the patient in whom there is a prohibitive risk for general anesthesia. In these patients, who have serious symptomatic biliary tract disease, and perhaps acute cholecystitis, cho-

lecystostomy should be considered. This procedure can be performed safely under local anesthesia with appropriate intraoperative monitoring. The second condition is the situation of ascending cholangitis and/or the presence of common bile duct stones without cholangitis. In many instances these conditions can initially be handled by endoscopic papillotomy and clearance of the bile duct. In some cases this is unsuccessful or perhaps the technology is unavailable and then open cholecystectomy and common bile duct exploration and appropriate decompression are mandatory. Presently, some surgeons are doing laparoscopic common bile duct exploration but we think in general that the techniques and appropriate instrumentation are still in the developmental phase, and they are not currently performed by a large number of general surgeons. In these situations if the surgeon is uncertain about the endoscopist's availability or ability it is best to proceed with open surgery.

A clear contraindication to laparoscopic cholecystectomy is the presence of cirrhosis that is complicated by clinically apparent portal hypertension. These are patients who have had previous bleeding from esophageal varices or have marked esophageal and gastric varicosities on endoscopy. These patients may have a variety of other associated problems such as ascites or hepatorenal syndrome. The reasons to avoid laparoscopic cholecystectomy in this group of patients are twofold: 1) Bleeding, when encountered, will be difficult if not impossible to control by current laparoscopic technology, and 2) the firm, shrunken, cirrhotic liver is difficult to mo-

bilize and therefore exposure of the porta hepatis will be less than satisfactory, as cephalad retraction of the liver is frequently not possible. If varices are encountered during the operative procedure in their usual location overlying the portal hepatis then conversion to the open operation should follow.

The final preoperative indication for open cholecystectomy is cholecystitis or severe biliary colic occurring in late pregnancy. This is largely a matter related to the size of the uterus. We would prefer to perform laparoscopic cholecystectomy when the uterus is not above the umbilicus in order to have a larger area to work in and to avoid possible injury to the uterus as well. In addition, during late pregnancy premature labor can be induced in the third trimester. If an elective cholecystectomy is indicated during pregnancy it is best to

Table 96-1. Indications for Open Biliary Surgery

PREOPERATIVE
Contraindication to general anesthesia
Inability to obtain endoscopic papillotomy in
    Cholangitis
    Common bile duct stones
Cirrhosis complicated by portal hypertension
Late pregnancy
Suspected gallbladder cancer

INTRAOPERATIVE
Inability to identify anatomy
Multiple omental adhesions secondary to
    previous surgery
Biliary ductal abnormality on cholangiogram
Intraoperative metabolic acidosis

perform it during the second trimester or early third trimester in order to avoid the complication of premature labor. Later than this open cholecystectomy is best.

In specific instances conversion to an open operation is indicated after laparoscopic cholecystectomy has commenced. The first of these is the inability to identify appropriate anatomy. This can occur as a result of severe inflammation in the porta hepatis or adhesions in the area either from previous surgery or from multiple attacks of cholecystitis or acute cholecystitis. In addition, exposure may be made difficult by an enlarged fatty liver, again precluding cephalad retraction and making exposure of the porta hepatis less than optimal. The second reason for opening a patient would be biliary ductal abnormalities that are seen on cholangiography that could lead to hepatic duct injury. Such anomalies would be absence of a cystic duct, or the presence of a right hepatic duct entering into the gallbladder directly from the liver surface. In addition, the presence of a choledochocyst on cholangiography would warrant open surgical treatment. Furthermore, if the patient had previous upper abdominal surgery and if after insertion of the laparoscope one observes multiple omental adhesions overlying the liver secondary to this previous operation, one would best consider open conversion. Our experience in these particular cases has been the development of bleeding from taking down these omental adhesions by sharp dissection with hot scissors or by electrocautery. Use of the ultrasonic dissector may facilitate this but we have not had extensive experience with its utilization.

Finally, the development of intraoperative metabolic acidosis as a consequence of the carbon dioxide pneumoperitoneum is an indication for open conversion. This usually manifests as an elevated end-tidal carbon dioxide that cannot be corrected by hyperventilation. This must be confirmed by measurement of arterial blood gases.

A final comment perhaps should be made about the use of laparoscopic cholecystectomy in acute cholecystitis. In general, most surgeons would favor inserting the laparoscope to get a preliminary look at the gallbladder to determine if safe laparoscopic cholecystectomy can be done. Studies have demonstrated that there is no predictor as to the success of laparoscopic cholecystectomy in these patients other than the duration of the patient's symptoms. Patients who have symptoms for longer than 3 to 4 days before presentation and surgical treatment have a statistically significantly higher open conversion rate than do those who have a shorter duration of symptomatology. Even ultrasound-measured wall thickness, the presence of abnormal liver tests, or the presence of previous pancreatitis is not a good indicator of successful laparoscopic cholecystectomy in this setting. We have been concerned with the application of laparoscopic cholecystectomy in acute cholecystitis in the geriatric population. It has been our impression that most of the patients who are older than 65 will need to be converted to open operations. Laparoscopic cholecystectomy in this setting was found not to differ from open cholecystectomy in terms of hospital costs, duration of hospitalization, or morbidity from the operative procedure. In addition, it is our belief that the operating time of failed laparoscopic attempts, which is significantly higher than that of open cholecystectomy, would outweigh any theoretical advantage of the laparoscopic procedure.

Cholecystostomy

Cholecystostomy has been considered a procedure to be performed when cholecystectomy is deemed unsafe. The reason for selecting cholecystostomy may be related to the severity of systemic illness; recent myocardial infarction is a classic example. A local condition precluding safe cholecystectomy is another circumstance that may dictate cholecystostomy. As surgical training has improved and become more widely available, cholecystostomy is done with ever-diminishing frequency.

The presence of threatening systemic illness generally leads to cholecystostomy under local anesthesia. It is quite helpful to know the size and locations of the gallbladder when planning the incision. Ultrasonography is helpful and also provides information concerning dilatation of the extrahepatic bile ducts, which when present suggests common-duct obstruction.

Once the decision is made to proceed with cholecystostomy under local anesthesia, a transverse muscle-splitting incision is preferred. As was previously stated, ultrasonography is invaluable in helping select the optimum incision site.

The anesthetic chosen may be $\frac{1}{4}$ or $\frac{1}{2}$ % lidocaine since infiltration rather than nerve block will be used. Infiltration of the skin with a 27-gauge needle minimizes patient discomfort. Abdominal operations under local anesthesia are possible but depend on the skill and experience of the surgeon.

A skilled anesthetist should be in attendance. Large-bore intravenous lines should be in place and monitoring used as the situation dictates.

The patient should be well sedated and well oxygenated. Hypoxia leads to restlessness and must be avoided. Noise in the operating room must be kept to an absolute minimum. There is no need to ask the patient about pain, the presence of which will be clear. Ideally, in addition to being well sedated and well oxygenated, the patient should be carefully monitored and undisturbed. Instruments should be passed with a minimum of oral communication. All movements should be slow and deliberate. Ample local anesthetic should be infiltrated and special attention given to the peritoneum. If the incision site has been well chosen, when the peritoneum is opened the gallbladder will be seen immediately and will be tense and distended. The technique of cholecystostomy is shown in (Fig. 96-1).

A pursestring suture should be placed in the fundus of the gallbladder. Suture gauge should be at least 00 to avoid cutting through the edematous tissue. Silk is preferred, but polyglycolic acid monofilament is quite good. Moist surgical pads are placed to isolate the area of the pursestring suture. A trocar is introduced into the gallbladder through the pursestring suture. It is essential to make certain that the trocar is very sharp. If it is not, an incision should be made in the gallbladder and the contents aspirated with a standard suction tip. Cultures of the bile should be obtained. An effort should be made to remove all stones, but this may be very difficult. Once the stones are removed, a catheter should be placed through the pursestring and the pursestring tied snugly. The catheter may be a Foley with a 5-cc balloon or a Pezzer catheter; size 16 to 20 French is usually adequate. Ideally, a contrast study should be done before the operation is over to demonstrate patency of the cystic and common

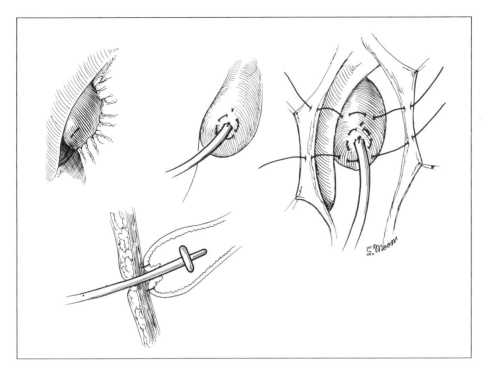

Fig. 96-1. The technique of cholecystostomy. A pursestring suture of 00 silk is used to secure the tube in the gallbladder. The gallbladder is sutured to the peritoneum and posterior rectus fascia to prevent leakage of bile into the peritoneal cavity if the catheter becomes dislodged.

ducts. If the patient's systemic illness is sufficiently serious to preclude a cholecystectomy, it is unlikely that stones of the cystic or common duct can be managed at the time of cholecystectomy. After placement of a tube in the gallbladder, the gallbladder is sutured to the peritoneum and the incision is closed.

In instances in which local factors preclude a safe cholecystectomy, general anesthesia is usually used. An effort has been made to remove the gallbladder, and the surgeon has concluded that pursuit of the definitive procedure is unsafe. This decision is generally evidence of maturity and experience rather than the contrary. The technical procedure is usually not different from that of the planned operation under local anesthesia.

It is not unexpected that cholecystostomy is associated with higher mortality and morbidity than cholecystectomy. Inevitably, it is planned in patients who are at high surgical risk or chosen when local conditions are quite bad. A mortality of 9.2 percent and a morbidity of greater than 20 percent are common.

A matter of some continuing controversy is what to do with the gallbladder once the

patient has recovered. If patency of the biliary tract can be demonstrated, the cholecystostomy tube can be removed, usually after 6 to 12 weeks. If residual stones are present, several options are available. Common-duct stones can be removed by endoscopic papillotomy. Stones in the gallbladder can be removed percutaneously with urologic instruments.

A variety of compounds have been used in attempts to dissolve stones. Without discussing the advantages and disadvantages of the various compounds, it is clear that methyl tert-butyl ether is the best material currently available.

Once the biliary tree has been cleared of stones, it is probably best to remove the gallbladder. In very old patients or those in whom associated illness precludes a safe elective operation, cholecystectomy can be deferred indefinitely.

Cholecystectomy

There are two prevailing reasons why the technical aspects of cholecystectomy deserve attention. The first is that the operation is very common. The second is that technical errors in cholecystectomy are of-

ten devastating. The possibility of technical error is enhanced by a remarkable inconsistency in the anatomy of the biliary tree and the vascular structures of the porta hepatis.

In the century since the first cholecystectomy, the indications for the operation are still not completely settled. The presence of gallstones in the gallbladder is most often the condition that leads to cholecystectomy. Ultrasonography has largely replaced oral cholecystography as the principal diagnostic measure for gallstones. Ultrasonography has the advantage of being safe, fast, painless, and highly accurate.

Most surgeons and nonsurgeons agree that patients with symptomatic gallstones should have an elective cholecystectomy. The controversy arises concerning how to manage patients who have gallstones without symptoms. The evidence is contradictory. Some studies show a risk of the development of complications of the stones, supporting cholecystectomy. Other studies show no significant risk, thus supporting continued observation. In general asymptomatic patients should not have cholecystectomy unless one of the following conditions is present: 1) insulin-dependent diabetes, 2) concurrent elective abdominal surgery, and 3) porcelain gallbladder (cancer risk estimated at 20%).

An occasional patient has classic symptoms of biliary colic and both an ultrasonic examination and oral cholecystogram are normal. A biliary drainage procedure may be helpful in demonstrating microstones or cholesterol crystals. Cholecystokinin hepatobiliary (CCK-HIDA) scintigraphy can be used to sort out patients with biliary tract symptoms who may have acalculous disease and benefit from cholecystectomy. Correlation with surgical and histologic findings and clinical follow-up suggest that a gallbladder ejection fraction of less than or equal to 35 percent is a reliable and accurate indicator of acalculous gallbladder disease. In 80 percent or more of these patients, cholecystectomy will achieve symptomatic relief. Endoscopic cholangiography with filling of the gallbladder may show stones which are otherwise unapparent. When the patient's symptoms are typical of biliary colic and when all attempts at demonstrating stones fail to produce a diagnosis, a cholecystectomy is indicated. When patients are selected carefully, removal of a normal gallbladder rarely occurs.

Technique

Incision

The more frequently used incisions for cholecystectomy are subcostal, transverse, and midline. There is no rational defense for the use of a paramedian incision. A transverse incision provides the best cosmetic result and is especially useful in younger patients for whom cosmetic appearance is a consideration. A very narrow angle at the xiphoid process, usually in tall esthenic patients, may make a subcostal incision preferable. In recent years we have used fewer subcostal and more transverse incisions, finding the exposure adequate.

Vertical midline incisions are useful when speed is an important factor, when there has been a previous upper midline incision, or when an additional operation, such as a splenectomy or fundoplication, is contemplated. It is also the preferred approach in patients taking anticoagulants or those who have bleeding disorders.

When converting from laparoscopic to open cholecystectomy, a large subcostal or midline incision is used. It is not necessary to "connect the dots" created by the laparoscopic incision (Fig. 96-2).

The incision should be of sufficient size to provide adequate exposure and to admit the examining hand. Some have argued that manual exploration of the abdomen at the time of cholecystectomy is not useful and may cause unnecessary adhesions. That argument seems hollow, and failure to take advantage of the opportunity to discover unexpected pathology by manual exploration is not sensible, especially since the evidence that harm done by such exploration is purely speculative.

Dissection

Once the abdomen has been explored, the gallbladder is exposed and a few filmy adhesions to adjacent structures may require division. Moist gauze pads are used to control exposure. One is used to block the right paracolic gutter, one is used to hold the stomach to the left, and one is used to allow traction in a caudal direction, placing the porta hepatis on tension. A Kelly clamp is placed on the gallbladder near the ampulla, with the assistant providing exposure and traction inferiorly and toward the left (Fig. 96-3). The Kelly clamp on the gallbladder is used to create traction inferiorly and to the right, placing the peritoneum overlying the cystic duct and cystic artery on tension. This peritoneum is carefully incised with curved scissors. With blunt dissection and a right-angled clamp, the cystic artery is identified and traced onto the gallbladder far enough to be certain that it is not the right hepatic artery.

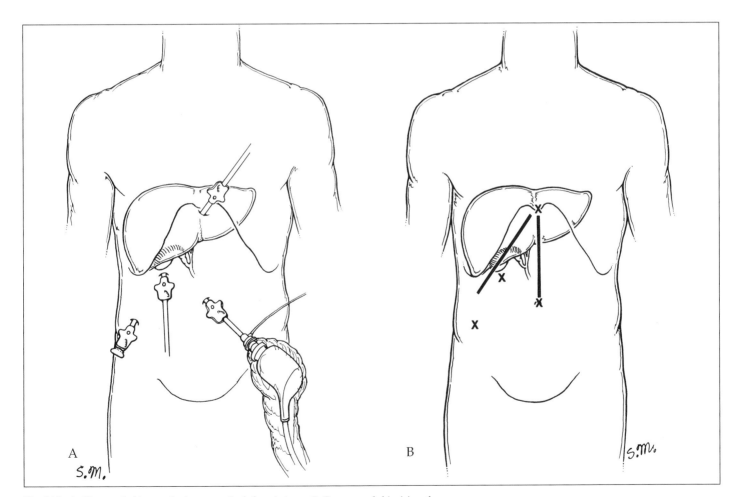

Fig. 96-2. A. Placement of trocars for laparoscopic cholecystectomy. B. Recommended incisions for conversion of laparoscopic to open cholecystectomy.

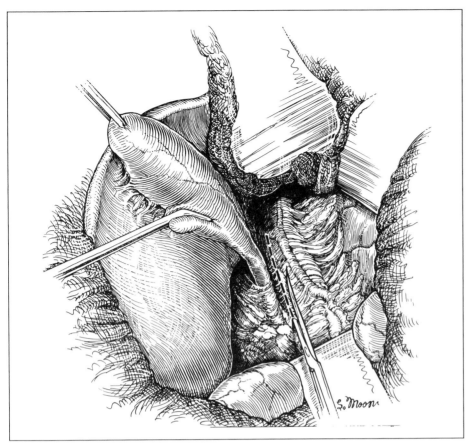

Fig. 96-3. *A right-angled clamp is placed on the gallbladder near the ampulla with traction inferiorly and to the left, and the peritoneum over the cystic duct and cystic artery is divided.*

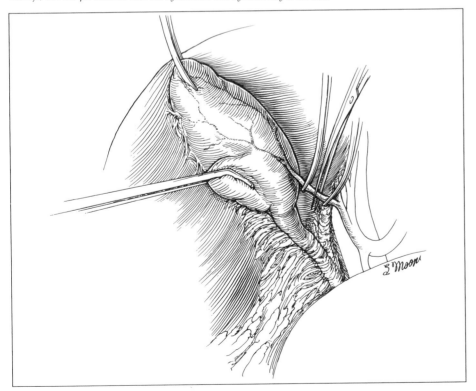

Fig. 96-4. *The cystic artery is dissected and clamped for ligature.*

In patients with arteriosclerotic vascular disease, the right hepatic artery may elongate and be easily mistaken for the cystic artery. After the cystic artery is clearly identified, a tie is passed around it and it is ligated; 00 or 000 silk is suitable (Fig. 96-4). A hemoclip is placed on the cystic artery well up on the gallbladder, and the vessel is divided.

The dissection is resumed with a right-angled clamp. The cystic duct is identified and encircled with a ligature, which is tied snugly enough to produce occlusion with a single half-hitch knot (Fig. 96-5). The course of the cystic duct may be variable. Several common variations are shown in Fig. 96-6.

An incision is made with a scissors in the peritoneum between the gallbladder and the liver. It has been tradition to score this peritoneum with a scalpel before dissecting the gallbladder from the liver. This unnecessary step, however, has been abandoned. The entire dissection of the gallbladder from the liver is now done with a scissors, and small vessels are managed by electrocautery as they are encountered. As the dissection continues toward the hepatic hilus, great care and excellent exposure are essential. As the dissection approaches the common hepatic duct, the scissors are replaced by a right-angled clamp, and blunt dissection is used to clearly identify the junction of the cystic and common ducts. This is the most dangerous part of the dissection. The course of the cystic duct parallels that of the common hepatic duct, which varies in length from 1 to 3 cm. When the dissection is complete, the cystic duct is seen to enter the common duct at a right angle. This dissection is facilitated by removing the previously placed Kelly clamp from the ampulla of the gallbladder and moving it to the fundus, allowing for an improved line of traction.

Once the junction of the cystic and common ducts is identified with traction on the gallbladder, the scissors is used to make a small incision in the cystic duct about 2 cm from the common duct. Though this maneuver can be done with a scalpel, the scissors produces a small flap on the cystic duct that facilitates cannulation.

Intraoperative Evaluation

A blunt probe is introduced into the cystic duct and passed into the common duct.

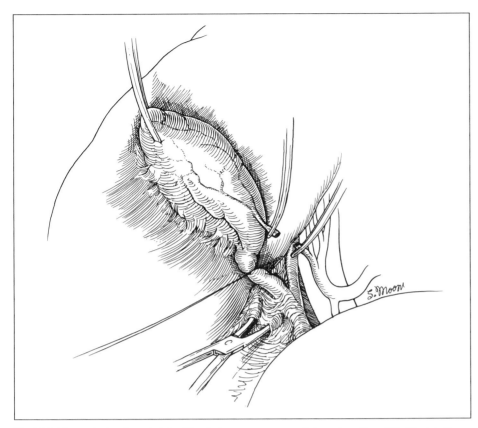

Fig. 96-5. The cystic duct is encircled with a tie to prevent passage of stones from the gallbladder into the common bile duct during dissection of the gallbladder.

Note is taken of the direction that allows easy passage of the probe. With a commercially made, metal-tipped catheter, the cystic duct is cannulated and the cannula is held in place with a large hemoclip (Fig. 96-7). As the cannulation is performed, saline solution is injected continuously to avoid air bubbles. Two 20-ml syringes connected to the cannula with a three-way stopcock greatly lessen the problem of air bubbles. One syringe contains saline solution, and the other contrast medium diluted 1 : 1 with saline solution. Dilute contrast medium is best, as undiluted contrast material obscures small (< 2 mm) stones. The entry site is examined for extravasation and if none is evident, the cholangiogram proceeds. At this point the gallbladder is removed and all packs are taken from the abdomen. A sterile towel is placed over the wound. Operative fluoroscopy has many advantages over still roentgenograms: One is able to examine the ductal system as it fills. One can control the flow of dye and watch the dynamics of ductal emptying. The time required to perform cholangiography is greatly reduced, the quality of the examination is improved, and the need for repeated roentgenograms is eliminated. For these reasons, we now use a C-arm device to do all operative cholangiograms by fluoroscopy.

If the necessary equipment is not available, still roentgenograms are used. A preliminary roentgenogram should be taken to establish the roentgenographic technique to be used. A single roentgenogram is

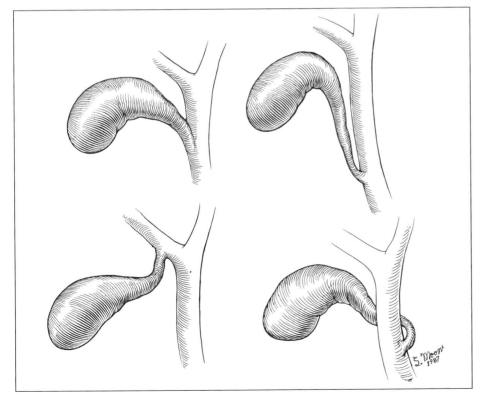

Fig. 96-6. Frequently observed variations in the course of the cystic duct. One must always assume variations in the anatomy of the cystic duct.

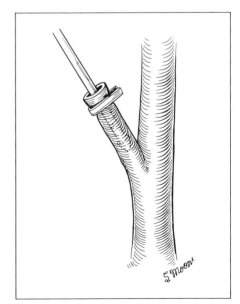

Fig. 96-7. Cholangiocath in the cystic duct.

taken after injection of 8 ml contrast material. If that roentgenogram is adequate, the examination is complete. If not, the necessary technical adjustments are made before a second roentgenogram is done. Our previous routine of taking two roentgenograms before seeing one developed has been abandoned.

Although we have altered our indications for operative cholangiography, we still use the test frequently. A patient with a single large nonfaceted stone, a small cystic duct, a normal common duct, and no clinical or chemical evidence of common-duct disease does not need an operative cholangiogram. However, in most instances and when any doubt about common-duct stones is present, operative cholangiography is performed. In addition, cholangiography will help to identify biliary ductal anatomy and detect unrecognized injuries to the bile duct.

If there is no evidence of stones, and dye enters the duodenum, the hemoclip holding the cannula is removed and the cystic duct is ligated. Excessive tension on the cystic duct may produce tenting of the common bile duct, resulting in injury when the cystic duct is ligated. If in every patient the common hepatic duct and common bile duct were clearly seen before the cystic duct were divided, common-duct injury would be eliminated.

In an occasional patient there is no obvious abnormality but no dye is seen to enter the duodenum. If there is no common-duct dilatation and the distal common duct is smoothly tapered, no abnormality is present. Administration of cholecystokinin (CCK-OP, 20 mg/kg) or inhalation of amyl nitrate usually results in opening of the sphincter of Oddi, with flow of contrast material into the duodenum. Glucagon, 1 mg intravenously, also relaxes the sphincter of Oddi. Intraoperative ultrasound can be used to detect common-duct stones. The technology has not become popular, probably because of the well-established use of and comfort with cholangiography.

Exploration of the Common Duct

When the common duct is dilated, when a stone is palpable, or when there is evidence of a stone on cholangiogram, common-duct exploration is indicated. The duct is exposed just distal to the entrance of the cystic duct. This site is chosen because of the possibility that choledochoduodenostomy may be required. A choledochotomy in the proximal portion of the duct may make a subsequent anastomosis to the duodenum difficult and produces an unnecessarily long segment of bile duct distal to the anastomosis.

Stay sutures of 4–0 silk are placed in the anterior surface of the common bile duct about 3 mm apart. With a No. 11 blade, the sharp edge toward the anterior abdominal wall, a longitudinal opening about 1.5 cm long is made in the bile duct. Bleeding is rarely a problem. A moderately stiff, tapered urologic catheter of 12 or 14 French is introduced distally in the bile duct and into the duodenum. Before introduction, the peritoneum lateral to the duodenum is incised and the duodenum is mobilized by manual dissection. Adequate mobilization exposes the left renal vein as it crosses the aorta.

With the duodenum adequately accessible, the catheter is advanced into the duodenum, where it can be seen to tent the duodenal wall opposite the papilla of Vater. Using a 50-ml syringe with an adapter, normal saline solution is injected as the catheter is withdrawn back into the duct. If the catheter is properly placed, no saline solution refluxes from the duct, and the duodenum distends with the initial injection. As the catheter is withdrawn into the duct, saline solution leaks from the choledochotomy. Stones are often dislodged and flushed out with this maneuver.

The catheter is then removed and a choledochoscope is used to examine the ductal system. Both flexible and rigid scopes are available; both have advantages and disadvantages. Having worked with both, we find the rigid scope to have superior optics and a slightly larger operating channel. For stones in the secondary hepatic radicals, the flexible scope is superior.

Stone Removal

Occasionally, a stone is so firmly lodged in the distal duct that it cannot be easily removed. A series of devices have been devised by Glassman, and these may relieve difficult common-duct obstruction.

With a tightly impacted stone, one can move to the left side of the operating table and, with the duodenum well mobilized, palpate the stone with the left hand. Using a right-angled stone forceps introduced into the duct and held in the right hand, the left hand holding the head of the pancreas, the surgeon can feel the stone in the distal duct, place the stone in the open forceps, and remove it. Very rarely a stone cannot be removed and a sphincterotomy must be performed.

Sphincterotomy

One does a sphincterotomy by palpating in the groove between the pancreas and the duodenum to locate the papilla of Vater. A longitudinal duodenotomy about 5 cm long is made opposite the papilla. With a probe in the papilla, two stay sutures of 4–0 silk are placed 2 mm apart on the cephalad portion of the papilla. The accuracy of the placement of these sutures is essential to avoid injury to the pancreatic duct. A fine-pointed scissors or No. 11 blade is used to cut between the sutures. As the sphincter is cut, the impacted stone can be seen and removed from below or pushed back into the duct and removed from above. A formal sphincteroplasty is usually not required. The duodenotomy is closed longitudinally, never transversely, with a single layer of interrupted 000 silk Lembert sutures. If a sphincterotomy has been done, the choledochotomy can be closed with interrupted 4–0 sutures of absorbable or nonabsorbable material. Sutures must not be placed through the ductal mucosa.

T-Tube Insertion

If a sphincterotomy has not been done, a T tube should be inserted through the choledochotomy. The size of the tube is not critical, but if there is any concern that stones have been left, a Wahlen-Moss T tube is used. The stems of these tubes are larger than the Ts, allowing ease of stone removal percutaneously should it be necessary. The stem of the tube is brought out in as straight a path as possible. The choledochotomy is closed about the T tube with interrupted Lembert sutures, care being taken to avoid penetrating the ductal mucosa. A closed suction drain is placed in the area of the choledochotomy and brought out through a separate stab wound.

A T-tube cholangiogram is obtained before closure and again on the seventh or eighth postoperative day. If there are stones in the duct, the tube is left in place for 5 to 6 weeks and then removed by a radiologist in order to extract retained stones percutaneously.

Postoperative Care

In routine cholecystectomy, no drain and no nasogastric tube are used. The patient resumes eating on the first postoperative day and is usually discharged in 3 to 5 days.

Complications may necessitate transient nasogastric intubation for a few days. Drains of the closed suction type are used when the common duct has been opened. These drains are removed when drainage falls to a minimum volume (less than 100 ml/24 hr).

Suggested Reading

Allen MJ, Borody TJ, Bugliosi TF, et al. Rapid dissolution of gallstones by methyl tert-butyl ether. *N Engl J Med* 312:217, 1985.

Flowers JA, Bailey RW, Zucker KA. Laparoscopic management of acute cholecystitis. *Am J Surg* 161:388, 1991.

Gilliland TM, Traverso LW. Modern standards for comparison of cholecystectomy with alternative treatments for symptomatic cholelithiasis with emphasis on long-term relief of symptoms. *Surg Gynecol Obstet* 170:39, 1990.

Glenn F. Cholecystectomy in the high risk patient with biliary tract disease. *Ann Surg* 185:185, 1977.

Henry ML, Carey LC, Complications of cholecystectomy. *Surg Clin North Am* 63:1191, 1983.

Middleton GW, Williams JH, Is gallbladder ejection fraction a reliable predictor of acalculous gallbladder disease? *Nucl Med Comm* 13:894, 1992.

Peters JH, Ellison EC, Innes JT, et al. Safety and efficacy of laparoscopic cholecystectomy—a prospective analysis of 100 initial patients. *Ann Surg* 213:3, 1991.

Sackman M, DeLuis M, Sauerbach T, et al. Shockwave lithotripsy of gallbladder stones. *N Engl J Med* 318:393, 1988.

EDITOR'S COMMENT

Doctors Ellison and Carey have given us an excellent chapter on open cholecystectomy, cholecystostomy, and exploration of the common duct, which, although less often performed than in the past, nonetheless are a necessary part of the surgeon's armamentarium.

A number of comments are appropriate.

First, for indications, there is the usual problem patient who has all the symptoms of cholelithiasis, but does not have stones. The use of very sophisticated labeling techniques with emptying studies is perfectly reasonable. If, however, these studies prove to be normal, it is my view that the most likely diagnosis is biliary dyskinesia. In these patients, cholecystectomy is often not followed by any relief of symptoms. One hesitates to advocate primary sphincteroplasty in these patients, but often these are individuals who end up with a biliary and pancreatic sphincteroplasty.

I am very pleased to see Drs. Ellison and Carey advocate the transverse incision, which is also much more comfortable for the patient and much more cosmetically acceptable. Increasingly, I perform transverse incisions for many procedures for which others use midline incisions, such as Whipple procedures, right colectomies, pyloroplasties, and various operations on the stomach, including those performed on the occasional bariatric patient. If one is using a transverse incision for cholecystostomy in a patient who is a poor candidate for elective cholecystectomy, I would suggest that the local anesthetic contain not only lidocaine but also 0.5% bupivacaine (Marcaine). This will give long-standing local anesthetic relief of up to 8 hours, and the patient may not require very many narcotics in the postoperative period. The initial pain that accompanies the injection of local anesthetic can be completely obviated by the use of sufficient bicarbonate to neutralize the acidity of the lidocaine

and Marcaine mixture. Blocking two or three of the intercostal nerves with this long-acting mixture may help completely obviate the need for postoperative narcotics.

Finally, after cholecystostomy, if no stones remain and the patient is asymptomatic, in my view cholecystectomy is not indicated and I believe that this view is supported by the literature.

I have a few differences with the authors in technique in the traditional open cholecystectomy. After the cystic artery is dissected free, I prefer to ligate it in continuity, placing two ties of 2–0 or 3–0 silk proximally and one where it joins the gallbladder before dividing it. This is much less likely than the clamp technique to result in inadvertent avulsion of the cystic artery from the hepatic artery with the resulting bleeding, which is most commonly responsible in open cholecystectomy for damage to the common duct. In open cholangiography, which I perform routinely, I prefer two injections: the first with 3 ml of a 50% diluted dye, and the second with 7 to 8 ml if the fluoroscopic equipment is not available and still radiographs must be obtained. Fluoroscopic equipment with selected "hard copy" is a great advance in cholangiography and will provide much greater information. In exploring the common duct, the insertion of the scoop gently may enable one to retrieve a stone that is lodged in the distal common duct that one cannot get with the stone searcher.

Finally, if a sphincterotomy is required to dislodge an impacted stone, it is much easier, in my view, to make a transverse incision over the papilla, which is almost always at the junction between the second and third portions of the duodenum and which usually can be palpated, especially when an impacted stone is present. In my review of a series of cases concerning gastroduodenal fistulas, longitudinal duodenotomy in the performance of sphincteroplasty figures very prominently.

J.E.F.

97

Nonoperative Treatment of Residual Biliary Tract Stones

Thomas R. Gadacz

In 5 to 15 percent of cases following exploration of the common bile duct, a retained common-duct stone will be found on T-tube cholangiography. This is somewhat distressing for the surgeon; however, several options are available. These include

1. Observation
2. Endoscopic retrograde cholangiography (ERC) and endoscopic papillotomy (EP)
3. Extraction through the T-tube tract
4. Dissolution
5. Reoperation

Observation

In patients with small stones (1–2 mm in diameter), the stones will generally pass through the common bile duct and the sphincter of Oddi into the duodenum. This usually occurs within a 6- to 8-week period. If the stones are still present after this time, they should be extracted or dissolved. This approach is supported from the experience of extracorporeal shock wave lithotripsy. Patients with small stones proximal to the T tube may require removal of the tube before these stones are passed. Various kinds of drugs have been given to promote passage of the stones. Bile salts not only promote a choleresis, which may flush the stones out of the duct, but also serve as a cholesterol solvent to dissolve small cholesterol stones. Various drugs have been given to relax the sphincter of Oddi; however, there are no scientific data to attest to their efficacy.

Endoscopic Retrograde Cholangiography and Endoscopic Papillotomy

Endoscopic retrograde cholangiography (ERC) and endoscopic papillotomy (EP) consist of passing a side-viewing endoscope orally into the duodenum. The ampulla is identified and cannulated. Cholangiography is performed to confirm cannulation of the bile duct and to document the size and position of the stones. A sphincterotome (wire in a sheath) is passed into the common bile duct and is tented up with the wire placing tension on the ampullary area. An electric current (cautery) is passed through the wire, which incises and coagulates the area. Generally, a 1.0- to 1.5-cm cut is made into the ampulla. This is generally sufficient to enlarge the ampullar area and allow the passage of intermediate-sized stones. Patients with a small (3–8 mm) common bile duct and multiple intermediate-sized stones (3–10 mm in diameter) are good candidates for ERC and EP. Interrupting the sphincter of Oddi can result in passage of these stones into the duodenum. The advantage of this approach is that it can be performed relatively soon after cholecystectomy when the stones are discovered on T-tube cholangiography. The disadvantage is the interruption of the sphincter and the potential long-term effects of direct reflux in the biliary tract.

In special situations, such as in very elderly or high-risk patients, a *biliary stent* can be placed into the duodenum and common duct around the stones. The stent allows bile to pass around the stone preventing obstruction and cholangitis. Generally, this is reserved for very unusual circumstances such as in a patient with especially significant risk factors or when a papillotomy cannot be performed because of technical problems or the presence of a duodenal diverticulum.

Extraction

A very effective method of removing common-duct stones is extraction of the stones using the T-tube tract for access into the common bile duct (Fig. 97-1). The T tube should be at least No. 14 French in size and exit the lateral abdominal wall. Smaller T-tube tracts can be dilated. To perform percutaneous extraction, the T-tube tract must be allowed to mature for 6 to 8 weeks. This permits a fibrous tract to be formed between the skin and the choledochotomy. At 6 to 8 weeks, the T-tube cholangiogram is repeated and if stones are seen, the T tube is removed over a guidewire. The guidewire is used to pass a ureteral stone basket or Dormia stone basket (Fig. 97-2) into the common bile duct. The basket is closed and remains in its sheath until the basket is passed beyond the stones. Once the basket is past the stones, one opens it by extruding it from its sheath. It is pulled back with a gentle

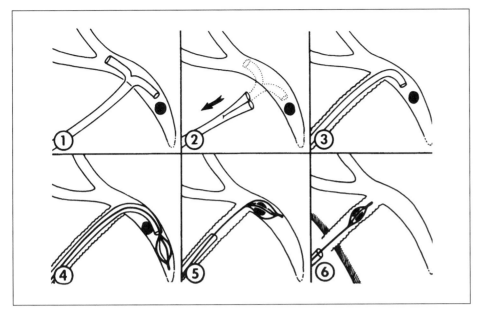

Fig. 97-1. Technical steps for retained common-duct stone extraction. 1) After the T-tube tract matures for 5 to 6 weeks, a cholangiogram confirms the presence of a stone in the common bile duct. 2) The T tube is removed. 3) Using the mature tract, the Burhenne catheter (or a ureteral stone basket) is passed into the common bile duct. 4) Once the tip of the catheter is advanced beyond the stone, the basket is inserted through the catheter and opened. 5) The basket engages the stone and the catheter is withdrawn. 6) The stone is extracted through the drain tract. (From RN Berk, AR Clemett. Radiology of the Gallbladder and the Bile Ducts. Philadelphia: Saunders, 1977. With permission.)

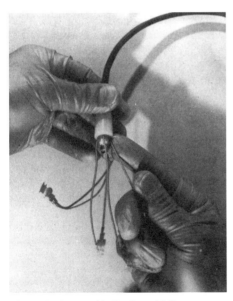

Fig. 97-2. The steerable (Burhenne) biliary catheter. The four wires are attached to a control plate and allow multidirectional steering. (From RN Berk, AR Clemett. Radiology of the Gallbladder and the Bile Ducts. Philadelphia: Saunders, 1977. With permission.)

twisting motion, which will trap the stones in the basket. The basket is closed and it and the stones are extracted. This procedure may be required multiple times to remove all of the stones. It is usually performed by an interventional radiologist using fluoroscopy. The advantages of this approach are a rapid extraction of sometimes very large stones and the avoidance of a papillotomy. The disadvantage of this approach is the 6- to 8-week period of waiting until the T-tube tract matures. Stone extraction can also be performed under direct visualization using a choledochoscope. The T-tube tract must be mature and the tract large enough to accommodate the scope. The bile duct is irrigated with saline through one of the ports to distend the duct and visualize the stones. A basket is passed through a port and, using the technique described above, stones are trapped in the basket, and the scope, basket, and stones are removed.

Special approaches to very large common-duct stones include fragmenting the stone with such modalities as electrohydraulic lithotripsy. The voltages used to perform electrohydraulic lithotripsy have been outlined in one of our studies, which is cited

in the references. This technique is generally safe as long as the tip of the probe does not make excessive contact with the wall of the common bile duct. Generally, the stones are fragmented into multiple pieces and can then be extracted by a basket or, if the fragments are small enough, they can pass into the duodenum. Other modalities for fragmentation have been used such as the laser, especially the tunable dye laser. Extracorporeal shock wave lithotripsy has also been used to fragment large stones, which can then be extracted with a basket or allowed to pass spontaneously.

Dissolution

When stones are discovered on a T-tube cholangiogram, an attempt can be made to dissolve them, especially if no distal obstruction is present. The solutions used to dissolve stones include bile salts and monooctanoin. Monooctanoin is a medium-chain diglyceride that dissolves cholesterol stones in 3 to 7 days. Only cholesterol stones are amenable to dissolution. Some of the stones should be kept following cholecystectomy and analyzed for cholesterol or incubated in monooctanoin at 37°C. If the cholesterol content of the stones is greater than 60 percent, they will dissolve. If the stones incubated in monooctanoin dissolve in the test tube within 3 to 5 days, a high cholesterol content is indicated. The details for the clinical use of monooctanoin are described in one of our papers, which is referenced (Fig. 97-3). A solution buffered to pH 7.4 of monooctanoin is infused into the common bile duct through the T tube at a rate of 3 to 10 ml per hour. This rate will vary from patient to patient and depends upon tolerance. It is recommended that a 30-cm in-line manometer be used to monitor the pressure. If excessive pressure develops in the common bile duct the infusion will overflow the manometer. The 30-cm manometer serves as a safety precaution to avoid infusing monooctanoin or any solution under pressure, thereby causing cholangitis.

Bile salts such as sodium cholate have been infused into the bile duct to dissolve cholesterol stones; however, dissolution may require a week or two.

Solutions such as methyl tert-butyl ether (MTBE) have been used to dissolve gallstones in the gallbladder. Generally, it is

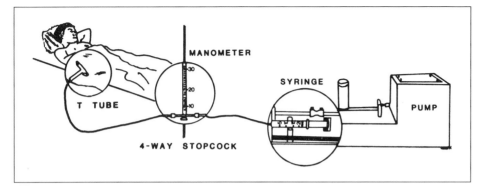

Fig. 97-3. Safe infusion technique for topical administration of monooctanoin or other gallstone-dissolving agents. Note that the system has a manometer to monitor and prevent excessive intrabiliary pressures. (From HA Pitt, DW McFadden, TR Gadacz. Agents for gallstone dissolution. Am J Surg 153:233, 1987. With permission.)

not recommended that MTBE be instilled into the common bile duct since it is such a good lipid solvent that it can produce very significant duodenitis. If it gets into the liver, cholangitis and respiratory failure can occur.

Other solutions such as heparin and ethylenediaminetetraacetic acid (EDTA) have been reported to be effective, but these findings have not been confirmed and the author has not had any success with these agents.

The advantage of using an agent such as monooctanoin to dissolve retained common-duct stones is its simplicity and low cost. Infusion can begin as soon as the stones are discovered as long as there is no leak from the choledochotomy site. It is very economical to treat patients with monooctanoin, especially if they are reliable and can monitor their biliary pressure as an outpatient. The disadvantages include the length of time of infusion (3–7 days) and the precautions that need to be taken to avoid cholangitis.

Re-Exploration

Occasionally, a few patients will have many stones in the bile duct. Generally, the bile duct is enlarged to 2 cm or greater in size. Some of the patients may have ampullar stenosis; however, the majority have a motility dysfunction of the bile duct. These individuals may return with recurrent common bile duct stones even though the stones are successfully removed by nonoperative methods. It is recommended in this group of patients that a choledochoduodenostomy or Roux en Y choledochojejunostomy be performed. A Roux en Y choledochojejunostomy is usually preferred since this procedure has the advantage of successfully decompressing the bile duct and preventing intestinal reflux into the biliary system. In general, the functional results from the Roux en Y and choledochoduodenostomy have been excellent and the stricture rate following either reconstruction is relatively low.

Suggested Reading

Baker AR, Neoptolemos JP, Leese T, et al. Long-term follow-up of patients with side to side choledochoduodenostomy and transduodenal sphincteroplasty. *Ann R Coll Surg Engl* 68:253, 1987.

Callans LS, Gadacz TR. Fragmentation of human gallstones using ultrasound and electrohydraulic lithotripsy: Experimental and clinical experience. *Surgery* 107:121, 1990.

Nishioka NS, Levins PC, Murray SC, et al. Fragmentation of biliary calculi with tunable dye lasers. *Gastroenterology* 93:250, 1987.

Orii K, Ozaki A, Takase Y, et al. Lithotomy of intrahepatic and choledochal stones with YAG laser. *Surg Gynecol Obstet* 156:485, 1983.

Panis Y, Fagniez P, Brisset D, et al. Long term results of choledochoduodenostomy vs. choledochojejunostomy of choledocholithiasis. *SGO* 177:33, 1993.

Pitt HA, McFadden DW, Gadacz TR. Agents for gallstone dissolution. *Am J Surg* 153:233, 1987.

Sauerbruch T, Stern M. Fragmentation of bile duct stones by extracorporeal shock waves after failure of routine endoscopic measures. *Gastroenterology* 94:A401, 1988.

Stain SC, Cohen H, Tsuishoysha M, et al. Choledocholithiasis: Endoscopic sphincterotomy or common bile duct exploration. *Ann Surg* 213:627, 1991.

Way LW, Admirand WH, Dunphy JE. Management of choledocholithiasis. *Ann Surg* 176:347, 1972.

EDITOR'S COMMENT

Doctor Gadacz has clearly outlined the various options for use in patients with retained common-duct stones. He is correct in that it appears that the pendulum has swung away from allowing the T-tube site to mature for 6 to 8 weeks and using the Dormia basket in the tract, to endoscopic papillotomy or extracorporeal piezolithotripsy, or both. Previous experience, when we used Bakes dilators and disrupted the sphincter at the lower end of the common duct during common-duct explorations, revealed that there was a finite incidence of stenosis, perhaps about 2 to 3 percent, following the forcible use of Bakes dilators. It appears that endoscopic papillotomy, at least initially, has a similar incidence of perhaps 2 percent in the early results. I am concerned about this because a papillotomy is not a sphincteroplasty. While Dr. Gadacz speaks of a 1.0- to 1.5-cm papillotomy, in my experience it is rarely that large. Consequently, stenosis and scarring may result from the normal healing.

The repeated use of stents has not, in my experience, been very satisfactory. I have even seen one patient, whom I operated on for cholangitis in the presence of repeated stents, who had a radiolucent 3-cm stone in which there was a doughnut opening through which the stent had been exchanged. One wonders how often this occurs.

Sheen-Chen and coworkers (*Arch Surg* 130:430, 1995) compared intraoperative choledochoscopic electrohydraulic lithotripsy in difficult-to-retrieve impacted common-duct stones to sphincteroplasty. The two groups were not historically concurrent, but relatively recent. Length of stay was diminished by approximately 4 days and complications were fewer in the electrohydraulic lithotripsy group.

Most studies in the literature show that sphincteroplasty and Roux en Y choledochojejunostomy have identical outcomes. However, I have recently seen a number of cases of Roux en Y choledochojejunostomies in which the common duct was anastomosed side to end to the Roux en Y, with the result that a sump syndrome developed. Sphincteroplasty and the revision of the Roux en Y succeeded in alleviating the sump syndrome. Thus, while the initial results may be identical, long-term follow-up may reveal an advantage for sphincteroplasty.

J.E.F.

98

Laparoscopic Cholecystectomy, Intraoperative Cholangiography, and Common Bile Duct Exploration

John G. Hunter   Ted Trus

Laparoscopic Cholecystectomy and Intraoperative Cholangiography

History

In 1882, Carl Langenbuch performed the first open cholecystectomy for gallstone disease. In 1987, 105 years later, Philipe Mouret performed the first laparoscopic cholecystectomy in Lyon, France. Working independently, two groups of American surgeons performed laparoscopic cholecystectomy in early 1988. In 1990, 10 percent of cholecystectomies were being performed laparoscopically in the United States, and by 1992, this percentage had risen to 90 percent. Never before has a surgical revolution occurred so fast. Laparoscopic cholecystectomy was a significant advance, removing many of the objections that patients had to open cholecystectomy. Prospective randomized trials were late and largely irrelevant because advantages were clear: Pain was less, recovery was faster. This cataclysmic change took its toll. Training of surgeons to perform the procedure was frequently inadequate, and early complications gave birth to the phrase "learning curve." It is the intention of this chapter to review the lessons of the last 5 years and to detail current techniques for laparoscopic cholecystectomy, intraoperative cholangiography, and common bile duct exploration.

Indications and Contraindications

With rare exception the sole indication for laparoscopic cholecystectomy (LC) is symptomatic cholelithiasis. Classic symptoms present in the majority of patients include stabbing (colicky) pain in the right upper quadrant radiating to the back and to the shoulder. While it is often taught that this pain occurs after the patient eats a fatty meal, the pain pattern is not always so predictable. Frequently, the pain will come on in the middle of the night, usually between the hours of 12:00 and 3:00 AM. After awakening the patient from sleep, the pain will generally last from a few minutes to a few hours. Usually the pain will pass within 30 minutes to an hour and the patient will return to sleep. Frequently, the pain is associated with nausea and vomiting but is rarely accompanied by jaundice, fevers, or chills, unless acute cholecystitis or cholangitis is present. When the pain is most severe and unrelenting, an emergency room visit is prompted. Myocardial infarction is often suspected, but "ruled out" with an ECG and, in those emergency rooms so equipped, "cardiac enzymes." If a sonogram demonstrates cholelithiasis in this setting, elective laparoscopic cholecystectomy is indicated. Occasionally, the presentation will be less characteristic of biliary colic. The patient may only complain of a nagging dull pain in the right side, epigastrium, or back without the severity of colic. In this setting,

the association of gallstones and right upper quadrant pain that cannot be attributed to another cause merits consideration of laparoscopic cholecystectomy.

Complicated gallstone disease is usually handled laparoscopically in the same manner as it was handled during the era of open cholecystectomy. Acute cholecystitis (fever, leukocytosis, and right upper quadrant tenderness and gallstones) demands more immediate attention than biliary colic. Laparoscopic cholecystectomy in patients with acute cholecystitis may be significantly more difficult and associated with conversion rates of 10 to 50 percent (depending on surgeon experience), but is nonetheless worth pursuing in patients without severe concomitant risk factors.

Biliary pancreatitis (mild) is approached by allowing the amylase level to return to the normal level before performing laparoscopic cholecystectomy, during the initial hospitalization. In this setting many surgeons will choose to perform a preoperative endoscopic retrograde cholangiogram (ERC) and endoscopic sphincterotomy (ES) (if a stone is detected on ERC) before laparoscopic cholecystectomy. Bile duct stones will be found in only 10 to 15 percent of these patients, subjecting the remaining 85 percent to an unnecessary procedure and the risk of recurrent pancreatitis. It is our practice to perform an intraoperative cholangiogram at the time of laparoscopic cholecystectomy and to remove bile duct stones through the cystic duct or through a choledochotomy. For a surgeon inexperienced in laparoscopic bile duct exploration, conversion to open cholecystectomy or postoperative ES are both reasonable options when a stone is discovered intraoperatively.

Cholangitis (jaundice, shaking chills, right upper quadrant pain and tenderness) should be treated with preoperative ES and stone extraction unless the cholangitis is easily controlled with intravenous antibiotic therapy (it often is). ERC and ES should be successful at removing all common bile duct stones in more than 90 percent of patients with cholangitis. Laparoscopic bile duct exploration and stone extraction in this setting may be difficult because the stone is often impacted and the bile duct is inflamed and friable. If the cholangitis is easily cleared with antibiotics, and the patient's symptoms resolve, it may be appropriate to perform elective LC, operative cholangiography, and transcystic bile duct exploration if a stone is detected. Alternatively, LC can be performed shortly after the common bile duct has been cleared through ERC and ES. The appropriate management of common bile duct stones in the era of laparoscopic cholecystectomy is fertile soil for good clinical studies.

The absolute contraindications to laparoscopic cholecystectomy are few. Certainly, a patient who is unable to tolerate general anesthesia, a patient with gallbladder cancer (suspected or confirmed), and a patient with a "frozen upper abdomen" because of previous surgery or peritonitis are all individuals who should not undergo laparoscopic cholecystectomy. In addition, relative contraindications include any previous right upper quadrant surgery, portal hypertension, coagulopathy, cholecystoenteric fistula, advanced acute cholecystitis, and pregnancy. While successful management of gallstone disease has been achieved in all of these patient groups, these procedures should be left for the surgeon who makes laparoscopy the majority of his or her practice and is technically gifted in these areas.

Preoperative Evaluation of a Patient with Gallstone Disease

In addition to a careful history and physical examination, preoperative testing for 90 percent of patients with gallstone dis-

ease is minimal. An ultrasound of the right upper quadrant will usually confirm the diagnosis, and the hepatic biochemical profile (alkaline phosphatase, SGOT, bilirubin, lactic acid dehydrogenase [LDH]) will usually determine the likelihood that common bile duct stones are present. Striking abnormalities in the hepatic profile, or an ultrasonographically dilated common bile duct, may warrant a preoperative ERC or abdominal CT scan, or both, to search for the cause (e.g., neoplasm or stricture) of bile duct obstruction.

The diagnosis of acute cholecystitis, when the diagnosis is in doubt, can be made with a nuclear hepatobillary scan. Nonfilling of the gallbladder in one hour, especially after administration of intravenous morphine (which contracts the sphincter of Oddi) is a highly accurate predictor of acute cholecystitis. When the ultrasound demonstrates nonuniform thickening of the gallbladder wall or pancreatic head, a CT scan should be performed to assess the likelihood of the presence of gallbladder cancer. Intravenous cholangiography,

rarely performed in the US, is popular in Europe for detecting common bile duct stones preoperatively in patients with abnormal liver function studies.

Patient Preparation, Equipment, and Anesthesia

The first step in successful laparoscopic cholecystectomy is the recruitment of a good operating team. This will include a well-trained laparoscopic surgeon, a first assistant with equivalent skills, and a camera operator familiar with the anatomy and technique of laparoscopic cholecystectomy. With a well-choreographed operation, the first assistant can also be the camera operator. The elimination of a dedicated "camera operator" can only be achieved if the surgeon uses a two-handed operating technique. Ideally, the patient is placed on a fluoroscopic table with the table turned around backward for easy C-arm access to the midabdomen. Two monitors are placed at the 10:00 and 2:00 position with respect to the patient's head (Fig. 98-1). Generally the surgeon stands to

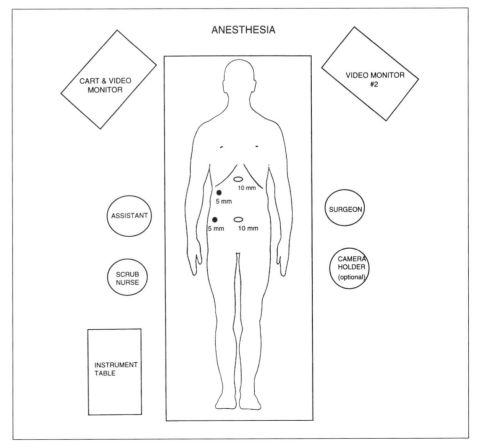

Fig. 98-1. Room setup for laparoscopic cholecystectomy.

the patient's left and the first assistant to the patient's right. If a dedicated camera operator is used that person will stand at the surgeon's left.

Anesthetic techniques for laparoscopy are quite different than those used for open surgery. Generally, nitrous oxide is avoided to minimize the likelihood of bowel distention. Since insensible fluid losses through the closed abdomen are minimal, intravenous fluids should be run more frugally than during open surgery. In addition, the pneumoperitoneum is a strong stimulus to antidiuretic hormone (ADH) release, decreasing intraoperative urine output. If the anesthesiologist responds to oliguria with fluid boluses in the absence of fluid losses, pulmonary edema may result. Lastly, the anesthesiologist must be acutely attuned to ventilatory function, as the carbon dioxide pneumoperitoneum will occasionally lead to hypercarbia and acidosis if close attention is not paid to the carbon dioxide concentration of expired gas (end-tidal PCO_2). In addition, we ask our anesthesiologists to minimize the use of narcotics and to request that a powerful antiemetic be given to lessen postoperative nausea. Once the patient is anesthetized and intubated, a Foley catheter, sequential compression boots, and an orogastric tube are generally placed. Decompression of the stomach and bladder minimizes the opportunity for their injury during establishment of abdominal access.

The equipment for laparoscopic cholecystectomy is quite simple. The only rigid requirements are that a high-quality videolaparoscope with a 300-W light source be coupled to two high-resolution monitors. A high-flow carbon dioxide insufflator, four trocars (two 10-mm trocars, two 5-mm trocars), and approximately 10 specialized laparoscopic hand instruments are required. The necessary hand instruments include a monopolar electrode (L hook) with suction and irrigation capacity, a fine-tipped dissector, two gallbladder graspers, a large gallbladder extractor, a pair of scissors, and a medium to large hemoclip applier. If a cholangiogram is to be performed, instrumentation should include a small "microscissors," a specialized cholangiogram clamp, and a No. 4 or 5 French tapered catheter. Techniques of

cholangiography are discussed in a later section.

Pneumoperitoneum

Laparoscopic cholecystectomy is generally performed with a carbon dioxide pneumoperitoneum at 15 mm Hg pressure. There is no evidence that lower pressures confer a significant safety advantage, but there is much interest in the use of alternative gases (e.g., N_2O, helium, argon) for patients in whom excessive amounts of carbon dioxide may be detrimental. Generally, the pneumoperitoneum is obtained by sliding a specialized needle (Veress needle) through the umbilicus, testing its position by allowing saline to run through the needle from a plungerless syringe, and then attaching the needle to tubing from the carbon dioxide insufflator. Initially the flow rate of carbon dioxide is kept below two liters per minute to assure that proper placement has occurred before a large volume of gas is insufflated. Confirmation of intra-abdominal position of the needle can be obtained by observing for uniform abdominal distention, tympany, and the ability to vary the intra-abdominal pressure by raising and lowering the abdominal wall. Initial pressures greater than 10 mm Hg nearly always reflect preperitoneal placement of the needle. Once the surgeon is comfortable that the needle is in the abdomen, the flow rate can be increased until an intra-abdominal pressure of 15 mm Hg is achieved.

The alternate method for establishing the pneumoperitoneum is to use an open laparoscopy technique, whereby the abdominal cavity is directly entered with a scalpel, electrocautery, and scissors. The initial trocar is placed directly in the abdomen and its position is secured with two stay sutures. The abdomen can then be rapidly insufflated with carbon dioxide. Either pneumoperitoneum technique is acceptable, but there appear to be fewer major vessel injuries when a novice or occasional laparoscopic surgeon uses an open access technique.

Trocar Placement

Once the pneumoperitoneum has been established the primary trocar is placed through the umbilicus. This will be a 10-mm trocar. Trocars are placed with a screwing, not a plunging, motion. It is generally a good idea to apply a second hand

to the barrel of the trocar to prevent the inadvertent plunge that leads to intestinal or vascular injury. The assistant should provide countertraction on the abdominal wall during placement of the first trocar. If the patient is morbidly obese, a primary trocar position above the umbilicus allows better access to the right upper quadrant. If previous abdominal surgery has been performed through a vertical midline incision, an alternate site for primary puncture is chosen. In this situation we insufflate through a site adjacent to the umbilicus, then place the primary trocar, a 5-mm trocar, in the right upper quadrant and pass a 5-mm telescope. The 10-mm umbilical trocar is then placed under direct vision, avoiding the adhesions from previous operation. Many surgeons prefer to use the open laparoscopy technique when previous abdominal surgery precludes primary puncture through the umbilicus. Again, there are no prospective data establishing one method as safer than the other. If bowel is adherent to the undersurface of a previous midline incision, open laparoscopy risks intestinal injury during the abdominal access maneuvers.

Once the umbilical trocar is established, a 10-mm telescope is passed through the primary trocar. An angled (30 degree) telescope allows a better view of the common bile duct, the posterior wall of the gallbladder, and Calot's triangle than does a straight (0 degree) telescope. Next, a 10-mm trocar is placed in the epigastrium, usually starting from the midline and angling toward the gallbladder. This trocar should enter at the level of the inferior liver edge. If this trocar is too low, the surgeon will be working parallel with his or her operating telescope. If this trocar is placed too high, segment IV of the liver will impede the surgeon's ability to get to the gallbladder fossa. The third trocar is a 5-mm trocar, which is generally placed immediately over the fundus of the gallbladder. If the fundus rides high, under the costal margin, this trocar is placed very close to the costal margin, usually near the anterior axillary line. The fourth trocar is located in a variable position, generally in the anterior to midaxillary line, several centimeters below the fundus of the gallbladder. If this port is placed too low, it will be impossible to lift the gallbladder up sufficiently to expose the porta hepatis (Fig. 98-2).

Dissection Technique

Exposure of the Porta Hepatis

Exposure of the porta hepatis requires maximal elevation of the gallbladder fundus and liver edge. This is usually achieved by placement of a ratcheted, aggressive clamp on the fundus of the gallbladder from the lateralmost trocar, and cephalad displacement is initiated until the infundibula of the gallbladder, the duodenum, and the porta hepatis are well exposed (Fig. 98-2.) If exposure of the porta is inadequate, the patient can be placed in a more severe reverse Trendelenburg position, the fundic grasper can be moved further down the gallbladder to better elevate the liver, or a fifth trocar can be introduced from the patient's left side to push down on the duodenum. This last technique is rarely necessary.

Stripping the Peritoneum

Using a two-handed technique the surgeon grasps the gallbladder infundibulum with an instrument in his or her left hand and retracts it laterally. With a fine dissector, the peritoneum is torn at the interface between the gallbladder and periportal fat. The peritoneum is teased toward the common duct until the cystic duct, cystic artery, or lymph node of Calot is identifiable. Complete stripping of the posterior cystic duct is facilitated if the surgeon pushes the infundibulum medially to strip the peritoneum off the posterior aspect of the gallbladder and cystic duct. This to-and-fro retraction of the infundibulum assures circumferential visualization and dissection of the gallbladder infundibulum (Fig. 98-3.)

Pedunculation of the Gallbladder

Stripping of the peritoneum over the gallbladder should reveal the presumed insertion of the cystic duct into the gallbladder. Continued dissection at this interface, first with a fine dissector and then with a monopolar L hook between the cystic artery and cystic duct, will provide the anatomic definition of important cystic duct anatomy. Complete dissection in this region will allow the gallbladder to appear like a polyp on a stalk (the cystic duct). The cystic artery and lymphatics crossing Calot's triangle may impede this pedunculation effort and may be divided near the

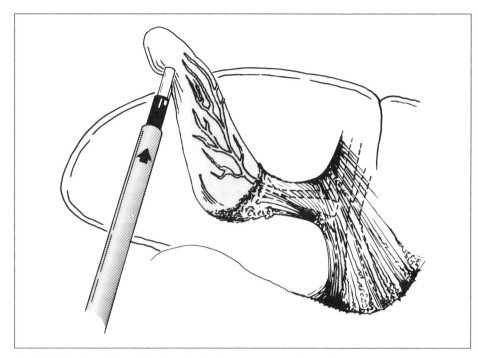

Fig. 98-2. Elevation of the gallbladder infundibulum and exposure of porta hepatis.

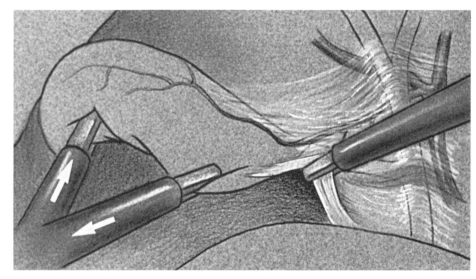

Fig. 98-3. The cystic duct is visualized by retracting the gallbladder infundibulum laterally, and then stripping the peritoneum off the gallbladder.

gallbladder if necessary. It is unnecessary to continue the dissection any farther down the cystic duct than is needed to get two clips on the structure. The common bile duct is usually seen with the angled scope, and it is almost never necessary to dissect the cystic duct down to its junction with the common bile duct. To do so is to risk injury to this structure (Fig. 98-4.)

Control of the Cystic Duct and Cystic Artery

Generally, the cystic duct is narrow enough that an 8-mm (medium large) hemoclip can be passed around it and slid up to the infundibulum of the gallbladder, where it is closed. If cholangiography is to be performed (see below), it is done now. If a cholangiogram is not to be performed, two clips are placed on the cystic duct immediately below its junction with the gallbladder, and the cystic duct is divided. A long cystic duct remnant is not a concern as long as no stones are retained in this duct. Two hemoclips are placed on the cystic artery as it crosses onto the gallbladder, and the cystic artery is divided (Fig. 98-5.)

Resection of the Gallbladder

If adequate pedunculation has been performed before cystic duct division, the gallbladder should already be dissected off the liver a quarter of the way to the fundus. Gallbladder resection is facilitated by strong use of the retracting (left) hand to pull the gallbladder away from the liver. As the gallbladder is pulled away from the liver the monopolar electrode is used to coagulate the small bridging veins and areolar tissue connecting the gallbladder to the liver. If hemorrhage occurs during this dissection, it usually means the surgeon is not in the right tissue plane, most frequently in the hepatic parenchyma. Holes in the gallbladder occur in nearly 30 percent of all dissections at this stage, and can usually be controlled with a pretied chromic ligature (EndoLoop, Ethicon Endosurgery, Cincinnati, OH). When the fundus of the gallbladder is reached, the majority of the gallbladder is flipped over onto the anterior surface of the liver, and hemostasis of the liver bed is checked (Fig. 98-6.) The remaining peritoneum connecting the gallbladder and liver is then divided with electrosurgery to disconnect the gallbladder from the liver.

Removal of the Gallbladder

At this point, the telescope is moved to the epigastric trocar, the gallbladder is grasped with a 10-mm grasper introduced through the umbilicus, and the gallbladder and trocar are removed. If the gallbladder does not come out easily the bile is generally removed from the gallbladder with a small suction device passed into the gallbladder, below the level of the fascia. When large stones are present, it may be necessary to dilate the fascial opening with a Kelly clamp or to enlarge the fascial incision with a pair of curved Mayo scissors to facilitate gallbladder removal (Fig. 98-7). The umbilical fascia is then closed with an interrupted or figure-of-eight suture and the abdomen is reinflated. With the telescope through the epigastric trocar, the right upper quadrant is thoroughly irrigated and all fluid is removed from the

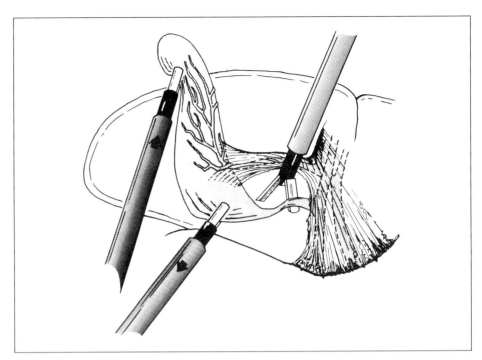

Fig. 98-4. Pedunculation of the gallbladder.

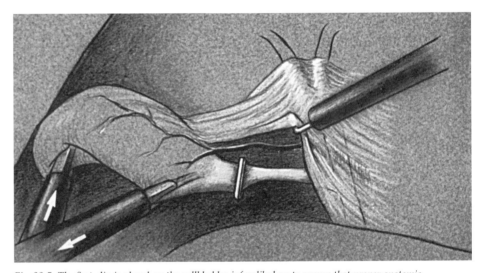

Fig. 98-5. The first clip is placed on the gallbladder infundibulum to ensure that proper anatomic identification has occurred.

subphrenic space. Then the remaining trocars are all removed under direct vision, the skin is closed with a subcuticular suture, and Steri-Strips are placed.

Additional Operative Maneuvers

Intraoperative Cholangiography.
Whether intraoperative cholangiography should be performed routinely or selectively is still a matter of great debate. When a surgical resident is present, we

perform cholangiography routinely to ensure that all residents are familiar with this technique. Outside of this setting, a policy of *liberal* selective cholangiography is probably appropriate.

Two methods are available for performance of cholangiography. In the first method, a specialized cholangiogram clamp (Olsen Clamp, Karl Storz, Inc, Tuttlingen, Germany) is passed through the subcostal trocar, and a saline-flushed, 60-

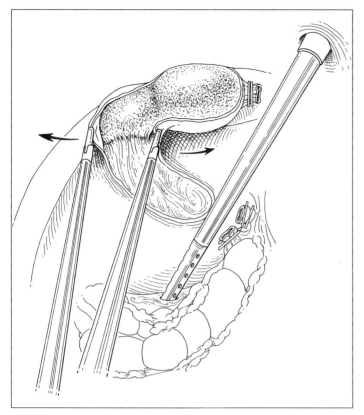

Fig. 98-6. Excellent exposure of the gallbladder bed and remaining peritoneum is gained by "flipping" the gallbladder over the liver edge and stretching apart the last bit of peritoneum with two graspers.

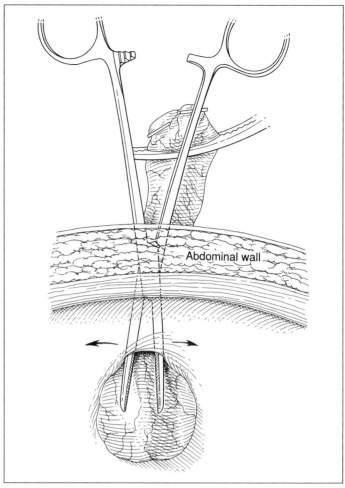

Fig. 98-7. Removal of the gallbladder with a large stone burden.

cm, tapered No. 5 French catheter is advanced directly into the cystic duct. Surgeons find this technique difficult if they have not placed the middle trocar immediately beneath the ribs and close to the anterior axillary line. Introduction of the catheter will occasionally require a hydrophilic guidewire to get through the valves of Heister. Once the catheter is in the cystic duct, the jaws of the Olsen clamp are closed around the cystic duct.

The second method for performing cholangiography, a percutaneous cystic duct access technique, appears equally efficacious. With this method a separate small puncture is made in the abdominal wall, over the cystic duct, with a two-inch, 14-gauge IV catheter. A No. 5 French cholangiocatheter is then slid directly through the intravenous catheter into the cystic duct by the surgeon with a grasper in his or her right hand. Once the catheter is in

the cystic duct, it is held in place with a hemoclip.

Before cholangiography is performed, all instruments are removed and the trocars are positioned so as not to obscure the cholangiogram. A small lead screen with a sterile table cover over it is then rolled up to the right side of the patient, and the surgeon stands behind this screen. The C-arm is introduced from the patient's left and positioned over the right upper abdomen. A slow injection of 60% meglumine diatrizoate (Renografin) under fluoroscopic control will assure an initial dilute injection to look for small stones in the common bile duct. After complete imaging of the distal bile duct, sphincter of Oddi, and duodenum has been attained, a second injection, usually under pressure, will delineate the proximal biliary radicals. The surgeon must identify the two major ductal systems in the right lobe of the liver, as low

inserting ducts from hepatic segments VII and VIII have frequently been injured during laparoscopic cholecystectomy. Selected images are saved from the C-arm and high-quality prints are made from a laser printer or high-quality dot matrix printer. If bile duct stones are seen on the cholangiogram, they can be addressed with transcystic extraction techniques (see below).

Hydrops of the Gallbladder. If the gallbladder is so tense that it cannot be grasped, it is decompressed through a cholecystotomy made with electrosurgery. This hole is controlled with an EndoLoop, after decompression of the gallbladder. An aggressive clawed grasper is then used to elevate the gallbladder.

The Wide-Mouthed Cystic Duct. One of the more difficult challenges in laparoscopic cholecystectomy is the short, wide cystic duct. Clips will usually not reach across this duct, and even if they do, may risk narrowing the common bile duct (Fig. 98-8A). Under these circumstances, there are four acceptable techniques for closing the cystic duct. If the duct is long and wide, it can be transected and a pretied ligature (EndoLoop) can be applied to the cystic duct stump. Alternatively, two ties can be passed around the cystic duct, in continuity, and secured with extracorporeal knotting techniques. Occasionally, there is concern that this technique might narrow the common bile duct. Under these circumstances the cystic duct is transected with an endoscopic stapling device, or is simply divided and oversewn with an intracorporeal suturing technique (Fig. 98-8B and C). All of these methods have been applied successfully. A critical factor in avoiding bile duct injury in these circumstances is understanding the anatomy. While a cholangiogram may be difficult to obtain in these circumstances, it is just these situations that demand the accurate anatomic detail provided by cholangiography.

Conversion to Open Cholecystectomy

The decision to convert to open cholecystectomy should be made before a complication occurs. The two most frequent indications for conversion currently are dense upper abdominal adhesions or a necrotic gallbladder wall that precludes grasping and elevation with a grasper. If exposure and retraction are accomplished, yet the dissection in the region of the gall-bladder neck is tedious and bloody, consideration should be given to conversion. As a general rule, if we have not identified the junction of gallbladder and cystic duct within 30 minutes of the start of the operation, we will convert to open cholecystectomy. Otherwise this tedious dissection can "go on all day" and still require conversion for bleeding or complication. A conversion rate of less than 5 percent can be expected in the hands of a well-trained laparoscopic surgeon.

Postoperative Care

Following laparoscopic cholecystectomy, postoperative care is simple. We usually start these patients on a clear liquid diet as soon as they awaken. If there is no nausea or vomiting, we proceed immediately to a regular diet. No postoperative blood tests are required. The patient can usually be discharged several hours after operation. For successful performance of outpatient cholecystectomy, patients must be aware of potential postoperative complications, including bile leak, bleeding, pancreatitis, intestinal perforation, and ileus. Family members must be able to recognize these complications immediately, before life-threatening consequences occur. At least half of all patients have an indication for overnight hospitalization.

Complications and Management

Serious complications of laparoscopic cholecystectomy occur in fewer than 2 percent of all cases. Intestinal injury may occur during establishment of abdominal access, adhesiolysis, or dissection of the gallbladder away from the duodenum. If an accidental enterotomy is made during access with open laparoscopy (Hasson technique), this hole can usually be repaired through the fascial incision and the operation continued. If an accidental intestinal puncture is made by the Veress needle, no treatment is generally necessary. An accidental electrosurgical injury to the colon or duodenum should be treated by conversion to laparotomy, and careful two-layer suture repair of the enterotomy.

Large-vessel vascular injury usually occurs at the time of initial abdominal access and is a result of inadequate anterior abdominal wall distraction or excessive thrusting of the trocar by the surgeon. These may be lethal complications. An unexplained retroperitoneal hematoma or hypotension should be immediately treated by conversion to laparotomy.

In the infancy of laparoscopic cholecystectomy, common bile duct injury occurred more frequently during laparoscopic cholecystectomy than during open cholecystectomy. The reason for this injury was usually a confusion in anatomy. Inadequate videooptics and improper dissection techniques rendered the common bile duct more susceptible to injury. This should be a completely avoidable complication if the surgeon follows the dissection techniques that we have mentioned previously. If a lateral injury to the common bile duct occurs, repair over a T tube is acceptable. Complete division or excessive devascularization of a very small bile duct should be treated by drainage and immediate transfer to a large institution that special-

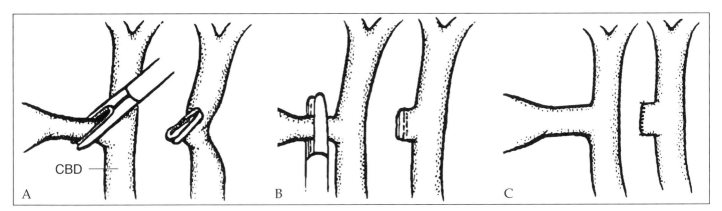

Fig. 98-8. Techniques for managing the short, wide cystic duct. When clips are too short or risk common bile duct (CBD) narrowing (A), the cystic duct is controlled with an endoscopic stapler (B) or sutured closed (C).

izes in care of these injuries. Primary repair by surgeons inexperienced in these techniques usually leads to further complications or operations, or both.

Excessive bleeding in the region of the porta hepatis should not be treated laparoscopically. Attempts at clipping or cauterizing large-volume bleeding will usually lead to more large-volume bleeding or hepatic artery ligation. If a bleeding site the size of the cystic artery or smaller can be identified by irrigation, and the location of hepatic artery and common bile duct is well known, bleeding may be controlled with electrocautery or clips. Bleeding in the gallbladder bed can usually be controlled by fulguration of the bleeding site. If a larger intrahepatic sinus has been entered, hemostatic agents (e.g., microfibrillar collagen) can be placed laparoscopically in the liver bed and pressure can be held with a clamp.

Stone spillage during gallbladder dissection should be avoided by closing gallbladder holes when they occur. If a few small stones are spilled from an uninfected gallbladder no further attention is needed. Attempts to remove large stones with collecting bags are appropriate. The only circumstance in which conversion to an open procedure should be considered is when stones are spilled in the presence of infected bile. Under these circumstances occult abscesses have been reported to occur in many locations around the abdomen, presenting between 12 days and 12 months after operation.

Laparoscopic Common Bile Duct Exploration

In 1890, Ludwig Courvossier was the first to perform a choledochotomy and remove a common bile duct stone. One hundred years later, laparoscopic cholecystectomy was in its infancy. The intraoperative detection of common bile duct (CBD) stones

with cholangiography led many surgeons to develop techniques for removing these stones at the time of laparoscopic cholecystectomy. Initially these techniques were borrowed from retrograde biliary endoscopy (ERCP) and involved the use of baskets passed into the CBD under fluoroscopic guidance. A technique from endourology that has been very valuable is the use of small-caliber flexible endoscopes to retrieve stones. Other borrowed techniques from retrograde biliary endoscopy include the use of balloon dilators, and intraoperative sphincterotomy. Choledochotomy, borrowed from traditional open surgery, is rarely necessary and can delay hospital discharge by the necessity of T-tube drainage. An algorithm for addressing common bile duct stones starts with the operative cholangiogram (Fig. 98-9). The variables that determine the best approach to each common bile duct stone are the size of the stone, the number of stones, the size of the cystic duct, whether the stone is impacted or freely floating,

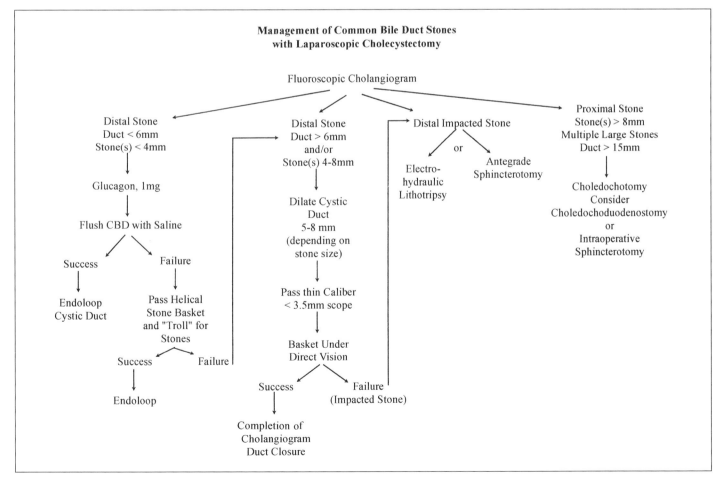

Fig. 98-9. Management of common bile duct (CBD) stones with laparoscopic cholecystectomy.

and whether the stone is in the common hepatic or common bile duct.

Normal Common Bile Duct (<6 mm), Small Stone (<4 mm)

Stones less than 2 mm in diameter will *usually* pass on their own. The best treatment strategies for these small stones are either to merely observe, or to dilate the sphincter of Oddi with glucagon and flush the bile duct vigorously with normal saline. We prefer to clear the CBD before leaving the operating room, as even these small stones may cause excruciating colic or pancreatitis when they pass through the papilla. If the stone does not pass with flushing (e.g., stones > 2–4 mm), these stones can usually be basketed with a six-wire helical stone basket (with filiform tip), which is either passed alongside the cholangiocatheter or passed through a No. 6 French introducer that has replaced the cholangiocatheter after CBD stone detection (Fig. 98-10.) All catheter exchanges are performed over a hydrophilic guidewire. The basket is opened in the ampulla of Vater and is trolled backward entrapping the small stone. One must be careful not to open the basket in the duodenum or else papillary elements will be ensnared and the basket will become entrapped.

Dilated Common Bile Duct (>6 mm), Medium Stone (4–8 mm)

This is the most common situation, and rarely amenable to flushing techniques or fluoroscopic basketing. The usual problem with fluoroscopic basketing is that the wires are too close to allow entrapment of these larger stones. Under these circumstances a direct-vision basketing approach is preferred. We use a slim-caliber flexible choledochoscope (Karl Storz, Inc, Tuttlingen, Germany) and a second video cart, including light source, video monitor, video camera, and VHS recorder. In the majority of circumstances, it is necessary to dilate the cystic duct to a minimum size of 5 mm to introduce the choledochoscope. If the bile duct stone is substantially larger than 5 mm, we will dilate the cystic duct up to 8 mm using a balloon dilator. The choledochoscope is passed through the valves of Heister into the common bile duct. Frequently we will make a second cystic ductotomy close to the common bile duct to bypass most of the valves of Heister. Once the common bile duct is achieved, the choledochoscope will almost always drop into the distal duct, where the majority of bile duct stones are located. A No. 2.4 French flat wire Segura basket is then advanced through the operating channel of the choledochoscope with saline running at low pressure around the basket. The basket is opened, the stone is entrapped, and the apparatus is pulled out. If multiple stones are present the procedure is repeated. This will generally work for stones up to 8 mm in diameter.

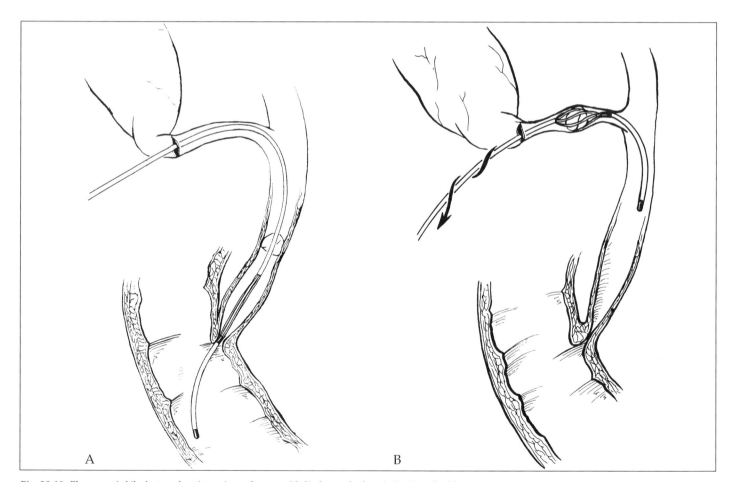

Fig. 98-10. Fluoroscopic bile duct exploration using a C-arm and helical stone basket. A. Positioned with closed basket in distal CBD. B. Removing entrapped stone with clockwise rotation.

Stones Greater than One Centimeter

Very large stones and those above the cystic duct entrance will not be amenable to any of these previous techniques. In order to adequately remove these stones, a choledochotomy must be made, the stone must be fragmented, or a sphincterotomy must be made. If the surgeon is extremely skilled in laparoscopic techniques, a curved microscissors can be used to make a small anterior choledochotomy, 1 to 2 cm in length. Again, a choledochoscope (generally a standard choledochoscope) is advanced through the choledochotomy, and the stones are entrapped with a Segura basket and pulled out the choledochotomy. Irrigation and Fogarty catheters can also be used. If the bile duct is larger than 2 cm in diameter, or if there are more than five stones, the patient will be at high risk for recurrent primary bile duct stones. Under these circumstances the surgeon should consider more permanent biliary drainage with a choledochoduodenostomy or endoscopic sphincterotomy.

The Impacted Stone

When stones are impacted in the ampulla of Vater, they cannot be removed with any of the techniques mentioned previously, as it is impossible to get a basket beyond these stones and even an inflated Fogarty balloon will rarely dislodge them. Under these circumstances there are three acceptable options.

Option 1 is to do nothing further; a drain, either a straight tube or T tube, is placed through the cystic duct into the common bile duct and then the operation is completed. The drain is secured in the cystic duct stump with a pretied loop (Endo-Loop). At a later date a guidewire is passed through the drain into the duodenum and a retrograde sphincterotomy is performed over the guidewire. Alternatively, using this technique some surgeons prefer to perform an endoscopic retrograde sphincterotomy on the operating table. This requires exquisite communication and a large degree of expertise on the part of the biliary endoscopist.

Option 2 is a similar technique that is easier for the biliary endoscopist, anterograde sphincterotomy. A guidewire is passed beyond the stone into the duodenum and a wire-guided endoscopic sphincterotome is

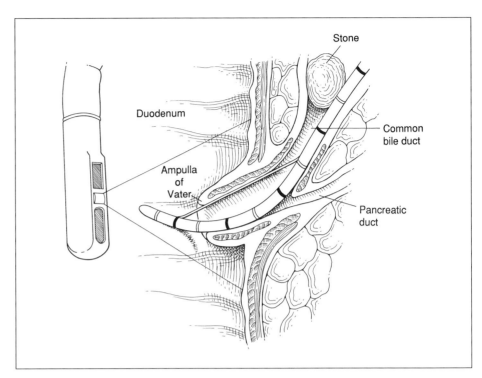

Fig. 98-11. *Anterograde sphincterotomy performed with the guidance of a side-viewing duodenoscope.*

passed over the guidewire across the sphincter of Oddi. In order to make sure that the sphincterotome is well oriented, a duodenoscope is passed through the mouth into the duodenum. After sphincterotomy, the bile duct stone is pushed into the duodenum with a choledochoscope or an inflated balloon extractor (Fig. 98-11.)

Option 3 is electrohydraulic lithotripsy. Through the choledochoscope, a very fine lithotripsy probe, No. 1.8 to 2.8 French, is passed through the operating channel. Under direct vision the bile duct stone is fragmented into pieces. The fragments are extracted with baskets or pushed into the duodenum. This technique seems to work best with the smaller impacted stones as large stones make large fragments that are difficult to remove through the cystic duct and similarly difficult to push through the ampulla of Vater without a sphincterotomy.

Common Bile Duct Closure

If the common bile duct has been explored through the cystic duct, and if the completion cholangiogram demonstrates duodenal filling, the cystic duct can usually be closed with a single EndoLoop. Drainage

of Morrison's pouch is unnecessary under this circumstance. Patients are usually discharged the next day as if only a laparoscopic cholecystectomy had been performed. If spasm, edema, or obstruction of the sphincter of Oddi is present, a straight latex drain is passed into the CBD and secured in place with an EndoLoop. If a choledochotomy was necessary, a small (No. 12–14 French) T tube is passed through a 10-mm trocar and placed in the common bile duct. The common bile duct can be closed with two or three interrupted absorbable (4–0 Vicryl) sutures. Under these circumstances a Jackson Pratt drain is usually also placed and brought out through one of the lateral trocar holes. The disadvantage of this technique is that more extended hospitalization is usually required.

Complications

It appears from several large series that the complications of laparoscopic bile duct exploration run in the range of 5 to 7 percent, similar to that of endoscopic sphincterotomy. The complications of this procedure include cholangitis, pancreatitis, bile leak, entrapped baskets, and retained stones. While rare mechanical damage to the CBD may be incurred with instrumentation, the advantage of laparoscopic CBD exploration is that it can be performed at the same time as laparoscopic cholecystectomy, rendering a second procedure on another day unnecessary. As well, failure to "clear the duct" can be immediately remedied by converting to an open procedure, or leaving guidewire access to the CBD for future endoscopic sphincterotomy.

Summary

Laparoscopic cholecystectomy has largely replaced open cholecystectomy for the treatment of symptomatic cholelithiasis. The advantages of rapid recovery are clear. With careful, meticulous technique, the complications of this procedure should be fewer than with open cholecystectomy. Appropriate treatment of the common bile duct stone is the next frontier. At this time, the best management will depend on local expertise, but it behooves the next generation of surgeons to achieve the expertise with transcystic bile duct exploration, which will allow the surgeon to remain the primary physician caring for diseases of the biliary tract.

Suggested Reading

Deziel DJ, Millikan KW, Economou SG, et al. Complications of laparoscopic cholecystectomy: A national survey of 4292 hospitals and an analysis of 77604 cases. *Am J Surg* 165:9, 1993.

Dubois F, Icard P, Berthelot G, Levard H. Coelioscopic cholecystectomy. *Ann Surg* 211:60, 1990.

Hunter JG. Avoidance of bile duct injury during laparoscopic cholecystectomy. *Am J Surg* 162:71, 1991.

Hunter JG. Laparoscopic transcystic common bile duct exploration. *Am J Surg* 163:53, 1992.

Legorreta AP, Silber JH, Costantino GN, et al. Increased cholecystectomy rate after the introduction of laparoscopic cholecystectomy. *JAMA* 270:1429, 1993.

National Institutes of Health Consensus Development Conference Statement on Gallstones and Laparoscopic Cholecystectomy. *Am J Surg* 165:390, 1993.

Nenner RP, Imperato PJ, Alcorn CM. Serious complications of laparoscopic cholecystectomy in New York State. *NY State J Med* 92:179, 1992.

Petelin JB. Laparoscopic approach to common duct pathology. *Am J Surg* 165:487, 1993.

Peters JH, Ellison EC, Innes JT, et al. Safety and efficacy of laparoscopic cholecystectomy: A prospective analysis of 100 initial patients. *Ann Surg* 213:3, 1991.

Soper NJ, Brunt LM, Kerbl K. Laparoscopic general surgery. *N Engl J Med* 330:409, 1994.

Southern Surgeons Club. A prospective analysis of 1518 laparoscopic cholecystectomies. *N Engl J Med* 324:1073, 1991.

Steiner CA, Bass EB, Talamini MA, et al. Surgical Rates and Operative Mortality for Open and Laparoscopic Cholecystectomy in Maryland. *N Engl J Med* 330:403, 1994.

EDITOR'S COMMENT

Doctors Hunter and Trus are recognized experts in the area of laparoscopy in general and laparoscopic cholecystectomy in particular. Their chapter is most welcome from the standpoint of someone who is experienced and a pioneer in the field.

Doctors Hunter and Trus are correct in that laparoscopic cholecystectomy has taken the market by storm, and that its success is patient driven. There is little question that patient recovery is quicker with this technique. However, the cost-effectiveness has been more difficult to establish. Also, despite the fact that patient recovery is quicker, it has been difficult to establish that the degree of trauma is less, and that laparoscopic cholecystectomy is, for example, accompanied by a less negative nitrogen balance than is open cholecystectomy. In contrast to colectomy, in which a laparoscopic-assisted colectomy has been shown to result in more positive nitrogen balance because of earlier return to oral intake (Sinagore et al, *Ann Surg* 221:171, 1995), similar studies in laparoscopic cholecystectomy have failed to reveal such an advantage. Despite this, the surgeon who ignores obtaining expertise in laparoscopic cholecystectomy does so at his or her peril.

The technique described by Drs. Hunter and Trus should be contrasted with the technique portrayed in Drs. Fingerhut and Millat's chapter (Chap. 17) for comparison.

Doctors Hunter and Trus raise a number of cogent issues: first, the need for preoperative endoscopic retrograde cholangiopancreatography (ERCP). As they point out, this is very much dependent on the operator's ability to carry out laparoscopic manipulation of the common bile duct, in which case ERCP is unnecessary.

Second, the learning curve is, of course, well known. What continues to be disturbing is that while the incidence of common-duct injury after laparoscopic cholecystectomy decreases, it still remains fairly high in some hands. The technique described here by Drs. Hunter and Trus will help minimize that, but one wonders whether injury to the common duct, the mortality of which is approximately 25 percent over 5 years, is part and parcel of this technique.

Third, the comment concerning fluid losses being minimal is well taken. Although the physiology of pneumoperitoneum has not been well worked out, the comments concerning acidosis and the need to be more frugal as far as fluid replacement is concerned are also well taken and directed at the anesthesiologist.

Fourth, one hesitates to abandon lessons learned the hard way from the earlier days of open cholecystectomy. The arguments concerning whether or not cholangiography should be routine are very reminiscent of the arguments of the 1960s. Suffice it to say that in patients in whom routine cholangiography is not carried out, an incidence of retained common-duct stones of between 3 and 9 percent can be expected. This, in my view, is excessive. It is also important for individuals to become expert at cholangiography so that it does not take a great deal of time.

Likewise, I am not ready to accept without at least some challenge the statement that a long cystic duct stump is of no consequence. I would be the first to admit that I do not know what a long cystic duct stump does, and whether it may serve as a nidus for stones; I suspect that it does, but I cannot prove it. On the other hand, the evils that may befall someone who takes the cystic duct too short far outweigh the necessity for having a minimal cystic duct stump. In view of the drastic consequences of narrowing the duct or injuring the hepatic duct, it is probably best to allow cystic duct stumps to be longer than they would have been in open cholecystectomy.

Finally, Drs. Hunter and Trus raise a very important issue concerning the division of labor that currently exists between gastroenterologists or biliary endoscopists (as they are called) and surgeons. It would seem to me that it is most effective to have a single individual experienced in all manipulations of the common duct, whether open, laparoscopic, or endoscopic. The challenge for surgeons to become expert in all aspects of clearing the duct of common-duct stones (at the time of surgery!) is an essential one. This will, I believe, inevitably require that surgeons who become expert common-duct stone extractors via laparoscopic techniques will also be required to become expert in endoscopic techniques. Surgical training programs should be modified, in my view, to train the next generation and leaders of the current generation in these techniques.

J.E.F.

99

Repair of Acute Hepatic Duct Injury and Hepatic Duct Stricture

John W. Braasch

Damage to or strictures of the biliary tract are unfortunate complications of operations in the right upper quadrant of the abdomen. In particular, injury during cholecystectomy is the cause in about 95 percent of patients. The incidence of this type of problem occurring during cholecystectomy, as far as can be estimated, is about 0.05 percent. Most complications are preventable by a few simple precautionary measures, such as adequate visualization of the common hepatic and common bile ducts before clamping or ligation of the cystic duct. When visualization of these structures is obscured, cholecystostomy is a valid temporizing and safety maneuver. In a few patients, the common hepatic or common bile duct can be damaged by erosion from calculi or external blunt or penetrating trauma, but these situations are unusual. The frequency of acute ductal injury, about 0.5 percent, dramatically increased with the pandemic of laparoscopic surgery. Injury rates during the learning curve period range from 2 to 7 percent and remain at approximately 0.3 to 1.0 percent even after learning is complete.

The injuries following laparoscopic cholecystectomy tend to be more extensive. Most injuries involve complete resection of the common hepatic duct, necessitating repairs in the hilum.

Reconstruction of the Biliary Tract

Several basic considerations are fundamental to biliary tract reconstruction. The acuteness and the extent of the injury have great bearing on the type of procedure that should be performed. Acute injury to the hilar biliary tract can be repaired without too much of a problem, but an injury in this location can be difficult to expose and repair when a chronic stricture is present because of scarring and an overhanging obstructed liver.

In most instances of segmental or lobar obstruction of the bile duct, no disability results when one lobe of the liver drains normally into the gastrointestinal tract. However, when infection is present in the obstructed lobe or segment, cholangitis and jaundice can occur. Therefore, all segments and lobes of the liver must be drained adequately by the operative anastomosis. Surgeons of experience can usually prove satisfactory drainage from both lobes of the liver by probing the ductal system. In some patients, however, it may be necessary to prove this by operative cholangiography. Imaging of proximal ducts may be afforded by injecting contrast material through a small Foley catheter, which can occlude the lumen and permit contrast filling of the duct in question.

Injection corrosion studies of the arterial supply of the bile duct have indicated that a submucosal plexus is fed by twigs from two longitudinal arteries, one on either side, which in turn are supplied by branches of the hepatic artery proximally and the gastroduodenal artery distally (Fig. 99-1). In preparation for any anastomosis, devascularization of the ductal system must be avoided. Ischemic necrosis of

the suture line can result in stricture, and, therefore, no more than just enough length of duct must be freed up to accommodate a single row of interrupted sutures for anastomosis, that is, no more than 1 or 2 mm.

In some anastomoses, the use of stents is important to aid in the symmetrical placement of sutures for the repair. Their long-term use is helpful for maintaining access to the biliary tract for contrast imaging studies of the anastomosis and biliary tree, percutaneous manipulation of the anastomosis, or extraction of calculi. Also, long-term stenting of up to 6 months may help to prevent stricture formation, although disagreement exists on this point, and it has never been studied satisfactorily. In any case, the ideal stent is a large-sized T tube, the vertical limb of which is brought out above the anastomosis. For high anastomoses at the bifurcation of the common hepatic duct, a percutaneous transhepatic tube through the left lobe of the liver or a T tube, the vertical limb of which is brought out through the left hepatic duct, is a satisfactory stent. The material from which the stent is constructed is probably not of great importance, but latex rubber seems to be as satisfactory as Silastic. Percutaneous stents can be changed after a tract is formed by withdrawing the tube and soon thereafter passing another tube down the tract. Replacement of a T tube requires the use of a flexible wire technique.

The repair is best accomplished with interrupted sutures placed in one layer

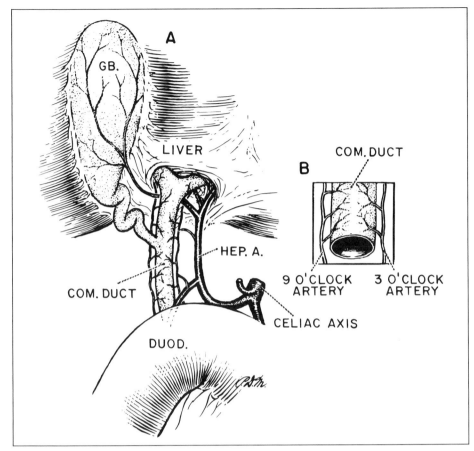

Fig. 99-1. A. Arterial blood supply to bile ducts from hepatic and gastroduodenal arteries to longitudinal extraductal arteries to submucosal plexus. B. Close-up of longitudinal arteries and plexus. (From JS Bolton, JW Braasch, RL Rossi. Management of benign biliary stricture. Surg Clin North Am *60:323, 1980. Reproduced with permission.)*

through all layers, making sure that the scar has been dissected from the proximal duct. These sutures may be fine chromic catgut sutures or a fine, either permanent or absorbable, monofilament type of suture. Two-layer anastomoses are not useful because the inner layer often sloughs, and the addition of a second layer does not decrease the rate of leakage, which should be minimal with the appropriate placement of sutures.

The recipient of the proximal bile duct can be distal duct, duodenum, or jejunum. The jejunum may be in the form of a Roux en Y loop or a simple loop with a side-to-side anastomosis at its base. It makes little difference whether duodenum or jejunum is used and in what configuration, except that if the anastomosis is made to the duodenum, it is available for inspection through the endoscope and possible manipulation should it become narrowed. A Roux en Y loop of jejunum is more complicated than a simple loop and requires dissection into the mesentery. Whether any reflux occurs though the loop into the biliary tree is not clinically important, provided that drainage of bile is unimpeded, to prevent cholangitis. End-to-end anastomoses are useful mainly at the time of acute injury to the biliary tract if the ductal system is of fairly large diameter with a wall of reasonable thickness for suturing.

Acute Hepatic Duct Injury

Damage to the biliary tract during cholecystectomy usually goes unrecognized. However, in the 10 percent of patients in whom it is recognized, repair is possible at the time of the original operation. Understandably, this problem has not been documented in large numbers of patients. Therefore, treatment of patients with acute biliary tract damage observed for an appropriate length of time is based on limited documented experience.

When the common hepatic or common bile duct has been ligated, simple deligation and placement of a T tube, one limb of which goes through the area of the damage, suffices. The T tube should be kept in place for approximately 6 months. When a clamp has been applied across the common hepatic or common bile duct and the width of the clamp area is more than 1 mm, excision of this area of the duct, a Kocher's maneuver, and end-to-end anastomosis seem appropriate. When the duct is thin or small, a loop of jejunum should be brought up for anastomosis to the proximal segment. This anastomosis should be stented with a T tube for 6 months. When a long portion of the common bile duct has been excised, the proximal segment is anastomosed to either the jejunum or duodenum.

In small numbers of patients, the literature indicates that an approximately 50 percent satisfactory result is possible after the repair of an acute hepatic duct injury.

Hepatic Duct Stricture

Hepatic duct stricture is characterized by the onset of jaundice within a day or two of cholecystectomy or many days after cholecystectomy. An alternative presentation can be an immediate external bile fistula permitting leakage of appreciable amounts of bile. An external fistula might close with the subsequent development of jaundice in a few days. With this sequence of events, almost all patients have a biliary stricture. Imaging studies of this stricture can be obtained by retrograde endoscopic cholangiography or by percutaneous transhepatic cholangiography (Fig. 99-2). The latter examination is probably more valuable than the former because it defines the length of proximal duct available for an anastomosis. It also enables passage of ring or similar catheters, which may help in the identification of the duct in a difficult situation, as well as in providing postoperative stenting or drainage, or both. It also shows whether the bifurcation of the common hepatic duct has been destroyed,

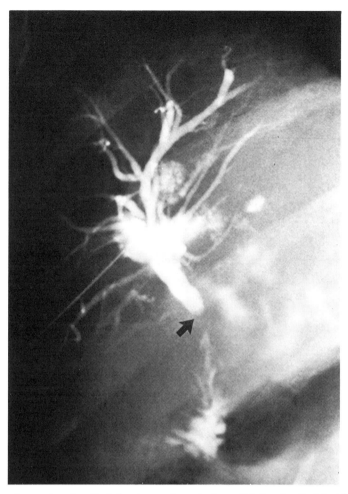

Fig. 99-2. Percutaneous transhepatic cholangiogram demonstrating satisfactory length of duct for anastomosis. Stricture at arrow. (From JW Braasch. Postoperative Strictures of the Bile Duct. In SI Schwartz [ed], Maingot's Abdominal Operations [8th ed]. Norwalk, CT: Appleton & Lange, 1985. P 1956. Reproduced with permission.)

a situation that presents special problems for the operator.

Preparation of the Patient

Infection is the most common and most lethal complication of repair of biliary tract strictures. The organisms involved are gram negative, such as *Escherichia coli* and *Pseudomonas*. Antibiotics are given before, during, and after the operation, and these agents must be effective against these organisms. Treatment should be continued for several days after the operation.

Often, patients with strictures have no compromise of the clotting mechanism. However, with long-term jaundice and with established biliary cirrhosis, liver dysfunction can be evidenced as clotting dysfunction. Preoperative treatment with

vitamin K serves to replete the missing components of the clotting mechanism.

With long neglect, biliary cirrhosis and portal hypertension can be complications. In the presence of severe grades of portal hypertension, bleeding during the operative repair can be so severe as to impair the quality of the anastomosis or even prevent the accomplishment of the anastomosis. In these patients, sometimes a first-stage portal shunt is necessary to permit the performance of the anastomosis as a second procedure.

Preoperative biliary tract drainage has been advocated to improve liver function and to lower morbidity and mortality. To date, however, evidence is not adequate to recommend drainage. It may take 2 or 3 weeks for drainage to lower the bilirubi-

nemia appreciably, and certain major complications from tube placement must be recognized. Possibly, with serum bilirubin levels of 25 to 40 mg per deciliter, this technique may have some merit.

The entire question of preoperative drainage and whether it was efficacious enjoyed a great deal of popularity in the early to mid 1980s. Two initial reports from two different organizations at approximately the same time suggested that preoperative drainage improved the outcome. Subsequent randomized trials, however, failed to confirm an improved outcome. The only trial in which improved outcome might have been suggested was in a situation where preoperative drainage was associated with nutritional repletion.

One of the problems with this whole area is that most of the data concerning preoperative drainage come from malignant disease, either tumors at the hilar bifurcation or tumors of the pancreas or ampullary region. Thus, the presence of malignancy usually adds a metabolic, anorectic, and, to a considerable extent, cachectic component. Therefore, whatever results are obtained in preoperative drainage in malignancy cannot be automatically transposed to the benign circumstance. If there is a group who will benefit from preoperative drainage, it is the group with a very high bilirubin, between 25 and 40 mg per deciliter. In this group, one occasionally sees postoperative central lobular necrosis, sepsis, and hepatic failure, with death approximately 1 or 2 months after operation. Preoperative drainage may evert this unfortunate outcome. At the very least, if the liver is damaged to the point where preoperative drainage will not reduce the bilirubin, then long-term stenting should probably be used instead of operation since mortality from the operative procedure is likely to result.

Perhaps a larger question is that of percutaneous transhepatic or endoscopic dilatation as it compares to operative repair. Certainly, in poor-risk patients, in patients who refuse surgery, and in patients with diffuse cholangiocarcinoma, for example, there is a place in the armamentarium for percutaneous transhepatic or endoscopic dilatation and stenting. The major question is the comparability of stenting versus operative repair. There is little question that a number of technologic improvements have been made in both the equipment (Guelrud, Mendoza, Gelrud, *Gastrointest Endosc* 41:246, 1995) and in techniques (Perry et al, *Radiology* 195:163, 1995) by which access to strictures can be gained in nonconventional fashion. Of particular interest is the percutaneous access by puncture of the antecolic jejunal loop, which, in skilled hands, can be done frequently. Thus far, such access is dependent on the antecolic position of the Roux en Y loop. Many surgeons prefer a retrocolic loop, as it gives more direct drainage when one is performing a Roux en Y.

Percutaneous access to strictures and stenting may be useful when the patient is septic with cholangitis. Dilatation and stenting may allow the cholangitis to subside so that the patient can recover for a definitive repair.

To sum up, percutaneous and endoscopic dilatation and stenting tend to be temporizing measures and do not give the same long-term beneficial results as does operative repair. However, the two techniques should not be used as competitive but rather as complementary, employed conjointly to obtain a long-term beneficial outcome. Unfortunately, there are no or few adequate studies of dilatation of strictures available.

Technique of Reconstruction for Stricture

The incision of choice for most repairs is a high right rectus muscle-splitting incision that permits access to the ligament of Treitz and establishment of a jejunal loop for anastomosis, if this is chosen by the surgeon. After the incision has been made and after the usual adhesions of the omentum and the hepatic flexure to the peritoneum or the right lobe of the liver are released, the duodenum must be rolled off from its position anterior to the distal common duct and the injured duct by sharp dissection. Kocher's maneuver is performed, which permits adequate palpation and the opening of the foramen of Winslow. The hepatic artery is identified, and pressure control of arterial bleeding is made possible during dissection of the difficult strictured area.

The proximal duct must be located for anastomosis, which can be easy or difficult. Usually, the proximal duct is found in a palpable scar, or it might be enveloped by an enlarged liver. The presence of clips, sutures, or a bulging proximal duct (Fig. 99-3) calls attention to this scar. Palpation of the hepatic artery guides the surgeon to the probable location of the common hepatic duct about 1 cm lateral to the artery and at the hilus of the liver. Direct dissection into the scar frequently is rewarded by a gush of bile. The proximal duct and its branches may be identified by suitable probing or, when necessary, by operative cholangiography. Previous placement of transhepatic catheters may also aid in identifying the hepatic end of the duct, although the catheter should be placed only 24 to 48 hours before the operation. Catheters left in place for longer may elicit a fibrotic reaction. The scar should be trimmed back so that normal biliary mucosa is available for construction of the anastomosis. The blood supply to the proximal end of the duct must be preserved by limiting the proximal dissection to no more than 1 or 2 mm. For the anastomosis, a jejunal loop almost always can be brought anterior to the colon and easily reaches the hilus of the liver. In obese patients, this loop must be brought through the transverse mesocolon, and in some patients, only a Roux en Y jejunal loop brought through the transverse mesocolon reaches the hilus of the liver for construction of the anastomosis. This problem is avoided when the duodenum is chosen for the recipient of the proximal duct. However, when the duodenum is used and a second procedure is necessary, disconnection of this hepatoduodenostomy can leave a defect in the side wall of the second portion of the duodenum that is difficult to repair.

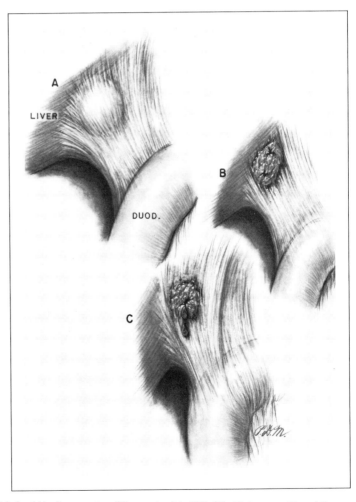

Fig. 99-3. A bulge (A), clips or suture (B), or a droplet of bile (C) aids in recognition of the proximal duct in scar tissue. (From JW Braasch. Current considerations in the repair of bile duct strictures. Surg Clin North Am 53:427, 1973. Reproduced with permission.)

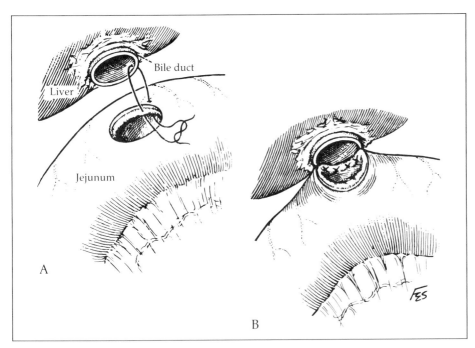

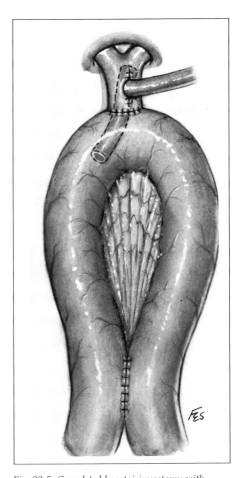

Fig. 99-4. Posterior anastomotic suture has been placed (A), and row has been tied (B) for hepatojejunostomy. (From JW Braasch. Postoperative Strictures of the Bile Duct. In SI Schwartz [ed], Maingot's Abdominal Operations [8th ed]. Norwalk, CT: Appleton & Lange, 1985. P 1965. Reproduced with permission.)

Fig. 99-5. Completed hepatojejunostomy with T-tube stent. (From RL Rossi, M Gordon, JW Braasch. Intubation techniques in biliary tract surgery. Surg Clin North Am 60:300, 1980. Reproduced with permission.)

In most patients, the choice of procedure is hepatojejunostomy. The proximal duct is freed appropriately, the jejunum is brought in apposition to the duct, and a short jejunotomy incision is made about half the length of the diameter of the proximal common duct. The posterior row of interrupted sutures is placed, the jejunum is railroaded down these sutures to the proximal duct, and the sutures are tied (Fig. 99-4). A T tube is placed with a vertical limb emerging from the common hepatic duct about 1 cm proximal to the anastomosis. The proximal duct is snugged around the vertical limb of the T tube, and the anterior row of sutures is placed to complete the anastomosis (Fig. 99-5). The anastomosis is checked for leakage, and additional sutures are placed when necessary. When a simple loop of jejunum has been used, an enteroenteroanastomosis is made at the base of the loop. This anastomosis aids in reducing the amount of leakage (if any) from the hepatojejunostomy.

When the hepatic bifurcation has been destroyed, the right and left hepatic ducts can be approximated side to side to make a new septum that can be crushed with a narrow hemostat, producing a new com-

mon hepatic duct (Fig. 99-6). In this way, just a single anastomosis is necessary. When the two proximal hepatic ducts are too far apart, it is necessary to perform two hepatojejunostomies. In this instance, it is usually difficult to stent these anastomoses with a proximal T tube, and transhepatic tubes are suitable. Use of transhepatic tubes is avoided in patients with biliary cirrhosis because spontaneous cessation of arterial bleeding from the passage of the tube sometimes does not occur. The transhepatic tube is easily placed through the left hepatic ductal system because the tube emerges from the superior surface of the left lobe and can be brought out through the abdominal wall with a straight course. The posterior part of the liver and the major hepatic veins must be avoided. Transhepatic tubes are placed by plunging an instrument retrogradely through the liver to grasp the transhepatic tube and draw it back down through the biliary tract. The tissue around the site of emergence of the transhepatic tube from the surface of the liver must be sutured to decrease fistulous drainage at this point, and a drain is placed in the subphrenic area (Fig. 99-7).

Sometimes the stricture in the bile duct is minimal with regard to narrowing and

length, and a Heineke-Mikulicz type of plastic procedure is useful (Fig. 99-8). It is seldom, however, that such an enviable situation is found. This procedure should also be stented by a T tube, the vertical limb of which is brought out elsewhere through the biliary system.

Operative dilation of strictures is useful only for right hepatic duct strictures that cannot be treated easily by excision and anastomosis at this high level. Dilated strictures should be stented for at least 6 months. The Smith mucosal graft technique has been advised for high strictures in which direct suturing is not possible. However, almost all strictures are reparable by direct suturing. The mucosal graft technique is illustrated in Fig. 99-9.

The worldwide experience in stricture repair is presented in Table 99-1. With a 3-

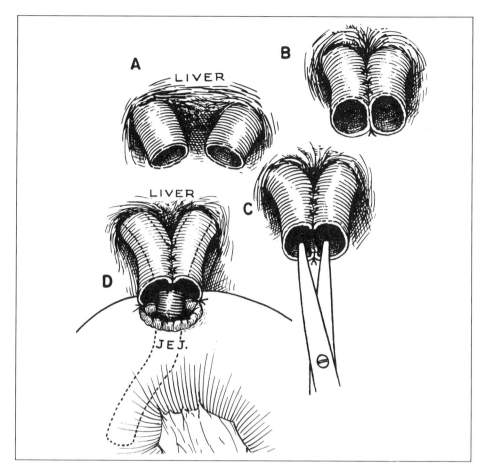

Fig. 99-6. Construction of hepatic duct bifurcation to permit only one anastomosis. A. The two hepatic ducts. B. Joined position. C. Cut septum. D. One anastomosis. (From RB Cattell, JW Braasch. Repair of benign strictures of the bile duct involving both or single hepatic ducts. Surg Gynecol Obstet 110:57, 1960. By permission of Surgery, Gynecology & Obstetrics.)

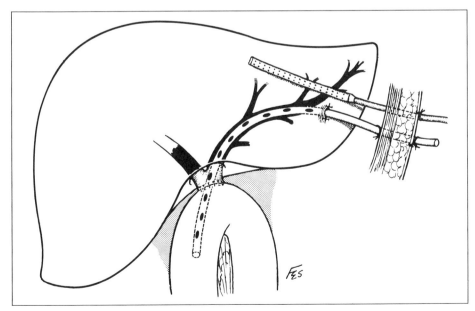

Fig. 99-7. High hepatojejunostomy with transhepatic tube in place. (From RL Rossi, M Gordon, JW Braasch. Intubation techniques in biliary tract surgery. Surg Clin North Am 60:304, 1980. Reproduced with permission.)

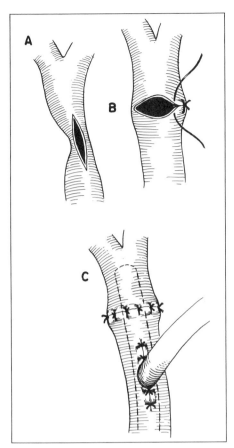

Fig. 99-8. Heineke-Mikulicz plastic repair of stricture. A. Longitudinal incision. B. Transverse closure. C. Completed and stented anastomoses. (From DT Moorhead, KW Warren. Changing patterns of surgery of the gallbladder, bile ducts, and liver. Surg Clin North Am 56:657, 1976. Reproduced with permission.)

to 13-year follow-up period, the satisfactory result reported from several centers is approximately 80 to 85 percent. The mortality should be about 2 percent and will be less when liver disease has not developed.

A great deal of interest has been shown in percutaneous dilation of benign biliary strictures, but until recently no sizable series of patients followed for 3 to 5 years had been reported in the literature. Preliminary studies performed so far show that percutaneous dilation is useful only in patients who have a short segmental stricture, usually after a biliary-enteric anastomosis. Percutaneous dilation should not be used as a primary repair in patients with a long tortuous stricture. Repeated dilations are necessary, with stents left in place between dilations.

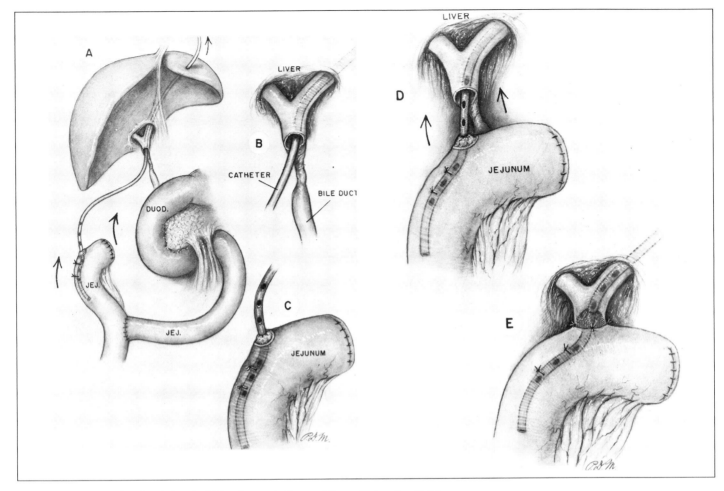

Fig. 99-9. *Smith mucosal graft technique for high strictures. A. Roux en Y loop with transhepatic tube. B. Close-up of proximal dissection. C. Close-up of jejunal mucosa and tube. D. Jejunum being pulled up to proximal duct. E. Completed anastomosis. (From JW Braasch. Liver, Gallbladder, Biliary Tract, Pancreas, and Spleen. In OH Beahrs [ed], Therapy Update Service: General Surgery. Media, PA: Harwal Medical Publications, 1978. Pp 6–10. Reproduced with permission.)*

Table 99-1. Results of Operative Treatment for Benign Biliary Strictures

Author	Year	No. of Operations	Mortality (%)	No. of Biliary-Enteric Anastomoses	Recurrent Anastomotic Strictures (%)	Mean Follow-Up (mo)
Bismuth et al	1978	125	0	123	0.8	66
Braasch et al	1981	49	2	39	13	36*
Kalman et al	1982	103	2	63	13	27
Pitt et al	1982	172	2	160	21	36
Pellegrini et al	1984	66	4	55	27	102
Blumgart et al	1984	63	3	61	10	40
Genest et al	1986	129	4	72	19	60
Pain et al	1988	163	—	163	28	133
Csendes et al	1992	99	9	99	20	85
Matthews et al	1993	24	4	24	29	12
Jedrezjczyk et al	1994	81	4	81	12	66
Kozicki et al	1994	101	1	101	27	154

*Minimum follow-up time.

Suggested Reading

Andrén-Sandberg A, Johansson S, Bengmark S. Accidental lesions of the common bile duct at cholecystectomy. II. Results of treatment. *Ann Surg* 201:452, 1985.

Bade PG, Thomason SR, Hirschberg A, Robbs JV. Surgical options in traumatic injury to the extrahepatic biliary tract. *Br J Surg* 76: 256, 1989.

Bismuth H, Franco D, Corlette MB, Hepp J. Long term results of Roux-en-Y hepaticojejunostomy. *Surg Gynecol Obstet* 146:161, 1978.

Braasch JW, Bolton JS, Rossi RL. A technique of biliary reconstruction with complete follow-up in 44 consecutive cases. *Ann Surg* 194:635, 1981.

Genest JF, Nanos E, Grundfest-Broniatowski S, et al. Benign biliary strictures: An analytic review (1970 to 1984). *Surgery* 99:409, 1986.

Kalman PG, Taylor BR, Langer B. Iatrogenic bile-duct strictures. *Can J Surg* 25:321, 1982.

Mueller PR, vanSonnenberg E, Ferrucci JT Jr, et al. Biliary stricture dilatation: Multicenter review of clinical management in 73 patients. *Radiology* 160:17, 1986.

Pellegrini CA, Thomas MJ, Way LW. Recurrent biliary stricture: Patterns of recurrence and outcome of surgical therapy. *Am J Surg* 147:175, 1984.

Pitt HA, Miyamoto T, Parapatis PA, et al. Factors influencing outcome in patients with postoperative biliary strictures. *Am J Surg* 144:14, 1982.

Smith R. Obstructions of the bile duct. *Br J Surg* 66:69, 1979.

EDITOR'S COMMENT

The Lahey Clinic has a long and fine tradition for repairing operative and other strictures of the common bile duct. The emphasis has always been on careful mucosa-to-mucosa anastomosis as being the technique most likely to give superior results. Doctor Braasch's admonition concerning the blood supply to the common hepatic duct as coming from the two lateral arteries is well taken, and data from the transplantation literature with respect to operative strictures and devascularized common duct bear this out.

The anastomosis is carried out with a single layer. There seems to be no advantage to a double layer unless the common hepatic duct is very large, in which case a two-layer anastomosis, with the outer layer being a nonabsorbable type of suture and the inner layer being an absorbable type of suture such as fine chromic, may have some place. If one is using a single-layer technique, experience and reports from the older literature suggest that a nonabsorbable suture is better. I personally prefer Prolene or a fine, relatively long-term absorbable suture such as PDS. The knot should be placed outside, as silk sutures with knots inside very frequently have given rise to concretions.

The controversy of stenting versus nonstenting continues. I personally much prefer the use of transhepatic tubes to use as stents. This obviates the problem of making an additional hole in what is often a very short duct, or in the bowel, and threading the stent through retrograde. In this fashion, the U tubes or Silastic stents can be changed frequently if necessary, preserving the diameter of the anastomosis. To my knowledge, there has been no satisfactory study that has answered the question of whether long-term stenting adds anything in the way of patency, although my impression is that stenting is useful.

Although there has been tremendous growth in the technology involved in percutaneous transhepatic drainage, such as the use of a "mother-baby" drainage catheter (Tsai et al, *Eur J Radiol* 18:6, 1994), the long-term results of balloon dilatation continue to be unsatisfactory. Jan and coworkers (*Int Surg* 79:103, 1994) reported a 45 percent restenosis rate with pain and cholangitis with long-term follow-up of 5 to 7½ years. This compares poorly with what is thought to be a 75 to 85 percent satisfactory long-term result in patients repaired operatively.

Stenting is not completely complication free either. Costa and associates reported an intestinal perforation following endoscopic biliary stenting (*Br J Radiol* 67:1270, 1994). In my experience, one may see some rather interesting results of stenting. In one particular patient who had repeated episodes of cholangitis despite repeated changes of stents through a choledochoduodenostomy, at laparotomy a 3-cm stone was found at the anastomosis that had not been visualized by x-ray. The stents had been passed through the doughnut hole in the stone, which clearly was ineffective in obtaining bile drainage. Thus, despite advantages in technology, operative repair can be aided by a variety of new innovations, but remains the cornerstone of repairing common-duct injuries.

J.E.F.

100

Current Application of Lateral Choledochoduodenostomy and Transduodenal Sphincteroplasty

E. Christopher Ellison   W. Scott Melvin   Stephen G. Moon

Transduodenal sphincteroplasty and lateral choledochoduodenostomy are complementary procedures used for dealing with distal common bile duct obstruction either due to stones, stricture, or, in some cases, motor dysfunction of the sphincter of Oddi. Surgical drainage procedures have in many instances been replaced by endoscopic papillotomy or sphincterotomy. However, there remain situations where surgical therapy is needed. Each of the procedures has specific indications, contraindications, advantages, and disadvantages. This chapter considers each operation and discusses applications so that the surgeon can make a rational choice concerning which technique is appropriate to a given clinical circumstance. Before proceeding with discussion of the surgical techniques, the anatomy and physiology of the distal common bile duct and pancreatic duct are addressed.

Anatomy of the Distal Common Bile Duct and Pancreatic Duct

The common bile duct and main pancreatic duct run in parallel as they enter the duodenum (Fig. 100-1). It is important to recognize the anatomic relationship between the common bile duct and the insertion of the main pancreatic duct in order to avoid damage to the latter structure during sphincteroplasty. As the common bile duct courses through the muscle layers of the duodenum its caliber tapers markedly, producing the characteristic narrowing seen during cholangiography. This tapering is the result of a complex sphincteric mechanism surrounding the distal common bile duct. The main pancreatic duct opens into the bile duct at a variable distance from the major duodenal papilla. A common channel is present in approximately 85 percent of cases. In these situations, dissections have demonstrated that the pancreatic duct is usually located on the medial aspect of the common duct, entering 2 to 3 mm proximal to the papilla of Vater. In about 6 percent of patients, the ducts open close to one another but separately on the papilla of Vater. The pancreatic and bile ducts open into the duodenum at separate points in 9 percent of cases.

Control of the flow of bile and pancreatic juice is regulated by a complex sphincteric mechanism that consists of four sphincters of smooth muscle surrounding the intramural portion of the common bile duct,

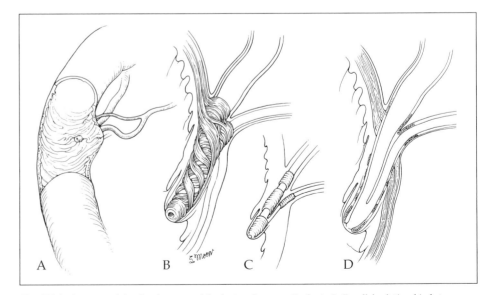

Fig. 100-1. Anatomy of the distal common bile duct and pancreatic duct. A. Parallel relationship between bile duct and pancreatic duct as they enter the duodenum. B. The sphincteric mechanism. C. The four components of the sphincteric mechanism. D. Cross-sectional view of the sphincter of Oddi.

main pancreatic duct, and ampulla (Fig. 100-1B, C, and D). This collection of musculature was first noted by Oddi in 1888 and was expanded upon by Boyden's anatomic descriptions in 1936. This complex is functionally separate from the duodenal musculature. The bile duct sphincter itself consists of three interconnected sphincters: 1) the superior sphincter surrounding the bile duct for 0.5 cm just proximal to its passage through the duodenal wall, 2) a submucosal portion surrounding the intramural duct, and 3) the inferior portion, or the sphincter of the hepatopancreatic ampulla located within the ampulla itself. A pancreatic sphincter is described surrounding the intramural portion of the pancreatic duct as well. Depending on the angle at which the biliary and pancreatic ducts pass through the duodenal wall, the total sphincteric complex may be as short as 6 mm or as long as 30 mm.

Physiology of the Sphincter of Oddi

Physiologic studies have demonstrated that the sphincter of Oddi generates a resistance of approximately 5 mm Hg at the opening of the bile duct and pancreatic duct. The basal pressure measured manometrically is usually 5 to 15 mm Hg greater than the common bile duct pressure and 15 to 30 mm Hg greater than the duodenal pressure. Superimposed on this tonal pressure are prominent phasic contractions (100–150 mm Hg), which occur at a frequency of two to six per minute and are propagated in an anterograde direction (from bile duct to duodenum). Bile flows mainly between these phasic contractions through a relaxed musculature. However, the contractions do propel a small bolus of fluid allowing clearance of the ductal opening, but the major portion of bile flow occurs by passive means.

The frequency of contractions of the sphincter of Oddi varies between the fed or fasted state. During fasting, contractions of the sphincter increase just before phase III duodenal activity. After feeding, the amplitude of contractions decreases and the tone is reduced. This facilitates passive bile flow. Neuronal and hormonal mechanisms are involved with the fine tuning of sphincteric contractions yet many of the precise details of this interplay have not been fully elucidated.

Pathophysiology

Successful miniaturization of manometry catheters so that they can be used through side-viewing endoscopes has permitted measurement of sphincter of Oddi pressures. This has not only enhanced our understanding of normal physiology, but has allowed accurate manometric definition of disorders of the sphincter complex. These triple-lumen catheters are either made of polyethylene or Teflon with an outer diameter of 1.5 to 1.7 mm. Side holes are oriented so that the lumens record across a length of 5 mm. The catheters are placed with a side-viewing scope before other instrumentation of the papilla. A patient undergoing endoscopic sphincter of Oddi manometry is prepared somewhat differently than for standard endoscopic retrograde cholangiopancreatography (ERCP). After topical anesthesia of the oropharynx, mild sedation is achieved with either intravenous diazepam or midazolam. It is important to avoid anticholinergics, such as atropine, or opiate analgesics, such as morphine, as they reproducibly alter sphincter of Oddi pressures. (Figure 100-2A shows a normal motility of the sphincter.

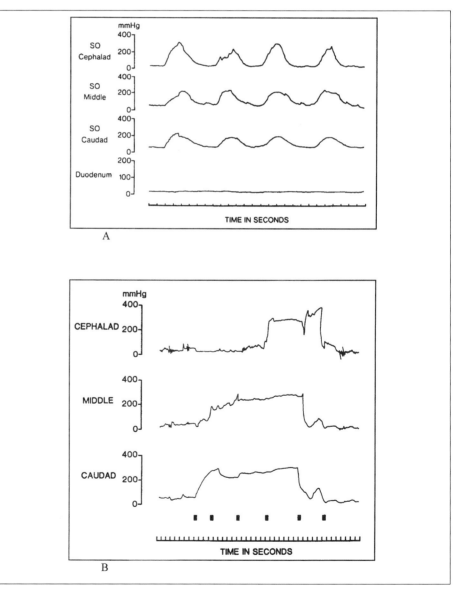

Fig. 100-2. Manometric recording of the sphincter of Oddi (SO). A. Normal manometry with phasic contractions superimposed on low basal pressure. B. Manometry in sphincter of Oddi stenosis characterized by high basal pressure.

Four manometric abnormalities have been categorized. The first abnormality is increased basal pressure in the sphincter of Oddi (basal pressure >40 mm Hg). This abnormality has been further subdivided into two entities: 1) papillary stenosis, which occurs if the increased basal pressure does not relax after the administration of smooth-muscle relaxants such as nitrates, and 2) dyskinesia, when the basal pressure does respond to smooth-muscle relaxants. The second condition is termed "tachyoddia" and is evidenced manometrically by an increased number of phasic contractions (>38/min). The third abnormality is an increased number of retrograde waves (from duodenum to bile duct) with a corresponding decrease in the number of anterograde waves. The fourth abnormality is a paradoxical response to cholecystokinin (CCK)-octapeptide. Ordinarily, CCK-octapeptide, when given intravenously, should cause a decrease in sphincter of Oddi basal pressure and phasic wave pressures. The paradoxical response occurs when CCK causes an increase in basal and phasic wave pressures.

These classifications of motility disorders correlate with a spectrum of clinical syndromes. It is postulated that disordered motility causes poor emptying of the biliary tree, ductal dilatation, and pain. Most patients have had cholecystectomy and the symptoms are nearly identical to those produced by cholelithiasis and dyskinesia of the gallbladder. Abdominal pain can be constant or intermittent, and may not be temporally associated with dietary intake. Elevation of liver function tests is often seen in these disorders but the abnormalities may be mild, and in some patients transient, correlating with their episodes of pain.

Lateral Choledocho- duodenostomy

Lateral choledochoduodenostomy can be done as a primary procedure at the time of cholecystectomy or for recurrent common bile duct stones occurring remotely following cholecystectomy that cannot be treated by endoscopic papillotomy. In the past the frequency of the necessity of this drainage procedure has been about 1 percent of all biliary operations, 38 percent of patients having a primary operation, and 62 percent having a secondary procedure. It is

more often necessary in the elderly; the mean age of patients reported in the literature is 61 years.

The surgeon should consider performing a lateral choledochoduodenostomy in patients with a dilated common bile duct secondary to distal obstruction from a benign process. A large duct, measuring greater than 2 cm, is an indication of prolonged obstruction or loss of tone leading to biliary stasis. Biliary stasis results in a potential for primary stones within the duct and, therefore, size alone is a relative indication for this operative procedure. The presence of primary common bile duct stones, numerous common bile duct stones (>15), or intrahepatic duct stones, especially in any patient who has undergone a previous choledochotomy, usually requires choledochoduodenostomy. Distal obstruction from strictures secondary to a primary benign process such as chronic pancreatitis is also treated appropriately with choledochoduodenostomy. Lateral choledochoduodenostomy is contraindicated in patients with a common bile duct less than 15 mm or a stone impacted in the ampulla.

A minimum stoma size of 2.5 cm should be achieved in all cases. If a large stoma is created, the results are usually satisfactory and late stenosis or cholangitis is rare. If the stoma is small, stenosis or the "sump" syndrome may occur. The "sump" syndrome is the collection of vegetable debris in the distal segment of the bile duct below the anastomosis (Fig. 100-3). This can eventually produce obstruction with cholangitis, jaundice, or even pancreatitis. Overall, the reported incidence of this complication is less than 1 percent. The advantages of lateral choledochoduodenostomy over sphincteroplasty to drain the biliary system are speed, the ease of performance, and decreased incidence of perioperative morbidity. It is particularly applicable in the poor-risk patient or in the patient with a long stricture who cannot undergo a sphincteroplasty. The main disadvantage of a lateral choledochoduodenostomy is the potential development of the "sump" syndrome. Additionally, there is decreased visualization of the papilla to exclude malignancy although this can be done with choledochoscopy or direct visualization through the duodenotomy.

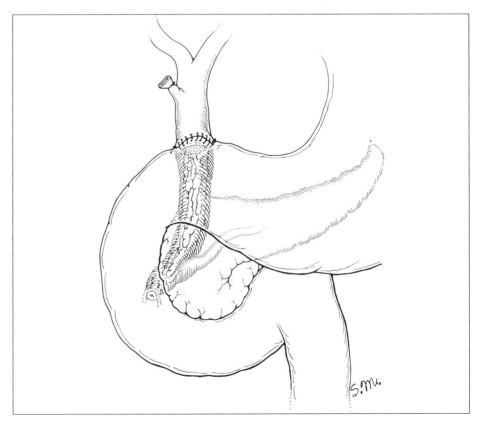

Fig. 100-3. Example of "the sump syndrome" with debris filling the distal bile duct.

Technique

After the gallbladder is removed, the common bile duct is exposed by incising the overlying peritoneum. The common bile duct is opened in a longitudinal fashion in the supraduodenal location. An extended Kocher's maneuver is routinely performed to enhance exploration of the common bile duct and performance of the choledochoduodenostomy (Fig. 100-4). If findings are compatible with the indications for choledochoduodenostomy, the incision in the common bile duct is extended to 2.0 to 2.5 cm in the longitudinal axis (Fig. 100-5). This incision usually will extend up to the common hepatic duct. After having completed the common-duct exploration and obtained proper mobilization and exposure, a longitudinal incision is made in the postbulbar duodenum (Fig. 100-5). It is wise to make this incision somewhat smaller than the expected stomal caliber because the elasticity of duodenal incision can result in excessive stretching and technical difficulty. Stay sutures are placed at the corners of the planned choledochoduodenal anastomosis. These sutures pass from the end of the duodenal incision to the midpoint of the choledochal incision (Fig. 100-6). The duodenal incision is bi-

sected with a suture placed at the lower aspect of the choledochotomy in the midpoint of the adjacent duodenum (Fig. 100-6). The posterior row of sutures is then placed with a 4–0 absorbable material, preferably polyglycolic acid, so that knots are placed on the internal aspect of the anastomosis. The anterior row of sutures is then placed, without tying (Fig. 100-7). Traction is used to hold the sutures until all are placed; this prevents inadvertent closure of the posterior wall. Then they are tied, beginning at the medial side of the anastomosis (Fig. 100-8). It is unnecessary to use a double-layer closure since a second layer would only cause narrowing of the anastomotic orifice. We routinely place a closed suction-type drain posterior to the choledochoduodenostomy.

Transduodenal Sphincteroplasty

The usual indications for surgical decompression of the bile duct are anatomic causes of obstruction. It is important, however, to be aware of the various treatments employed for sphincter of Oddi dysfunc-

tion. The classification proposed by Geenen and Hogan, which separates patients with unexplained biliary pain into subgroups based on the number of clinical laboratory and radiologic parameters, is used to guide diagnosis and therapy (Table 100-1). Type I patients usually have ampullary stenosis. Routine need for sphincter of Oddi manometry is not necessary in this group. If an endoscopic papillotomy cannot be performed then surgical sphincteroplasty is necessary. Types II and III patients often need motility studies to further clarify the pathophysiology. Sphincter of Oddi basal pressure is greater than 40 mm Hg in 16 to 68 percent of type II patients and 0 to 55 percent of type III patients, with tachyoddia being present in about 1 percent of each group (see Fig. 100-2B). The wide variety of findings among the reports reflect variations of patient selection.

The initial treatment of type II and III sphincter of Oddi dysfunction is the oral administration of smooth-muscle relaxants, such as dicyclomine hydrochloride, cycline trinitrate-sorbide nitrate, and nifedipine. However, the most effective definitive therapy is either endoscopic papillotomy or surgical sphincteroplasty. It should be emphasized that those patients in whom recurrent pancreatitis has developed as a result of sphincter of Oddi dysfunction need both division of the choledochal and pancreatic duct components of the sphincter of Oddi. This should be performed by transduodenal sphincteroplasty and septectomy. Most of the patients, however, do not have pancreatitis and can be treated with endoscopic papillotomy.

Type II patients with elevated basal sphincter pressure have a good response to papillotomy in 80 to 90 percent of reported cases, compared to 50 to 60 percent in those without a hypertensive sphincter. In a few studies no correlation was seen between the clinical response to papillotomy and sphincter of Oddi motility abnormalities. Type III patients have about a 50 percent response rate when they have manometric evidence of dysfunction.

The indications that will commonly be encountered for performing a transduodenal sphincteroplasty are stones impacted in the ampulla of Vater, papillary stenosis, and recurrent pancreatitis with multiple common bile duct stones. In general, surgical sphincteroplasty can be applied for

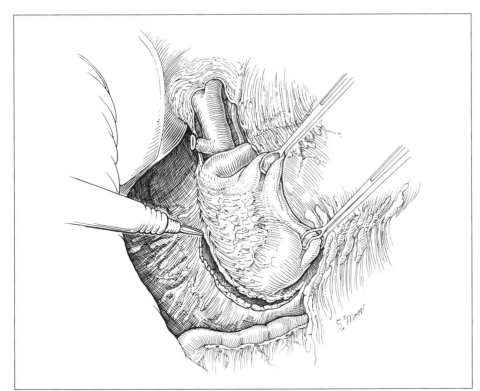

Fig. 100-4. A wide Kocher's maneuver is necessary for common-duct exploration, choledochoduodenostomy, and sphincteroplasty.

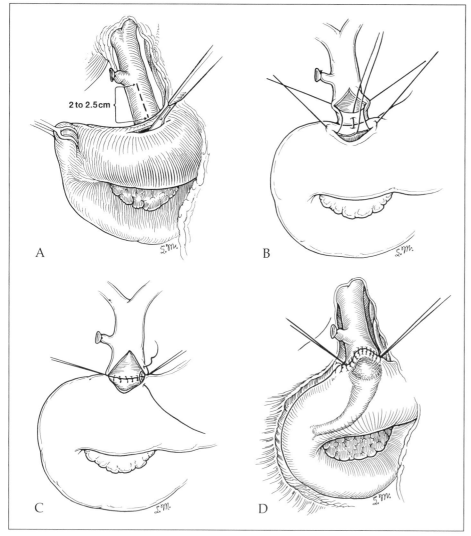

Fig. 100-5. A. Proper incision of bile duct for creation of choledochoduodenostomy. B. Initial sutures for choledochoduodenostomy. C. Posterior row of choledochoduodenostomy is completed. Anterior row is placed, but not tied, until all sutures are completed. D. Completed choledochoduodenostomy.

ported in 20 percent of patients, compared to 11 percent for choledochoduodenostomy.

Technique

Precise terminology should be used in describing the various operations on the sphincter of Oddi. A sphincterotomy is essentially a cut made into the sphincter with no suturing of bile duct mucosa to the duodenal mucosa. A sphincteroplasty is the incision of the common portion of the sphincter of Oddi with suturing of the mucosa of the common bile duct to the duodenum. The patient with recurrent pancreatitis may need to undergo further a septectomy and septoplasty of the septum between the pancreatic duct and common bile duct. These variations are illustrated in Fig. 100-6.

The patient is operated on in the supine position. Use of the radiolucent table will facilitate fluoroscopic cholangiography or pancreatography if needed. The incision can be either midline or subcostal although we prefer a subcostal incision. After removal of the gallbladder, an extended Kocher's maneuver is performed. The assistant retracts the second portion of the duodenum medially and inferiorly. The peritoneum is incised along the lateral edge of the duodenum. Blunt dissection is used to develop a plane posterior to the head of the pancreas with countertraction provided by the assistant. This is an avascular space between the posterior pancreatic head, the perinephric fat, and the inferior vena cava. It is important to sufficiently mobilize the third portion of the duodenum to allow surgical access to the papilla and for closure of the duodenotomy without tension.

The papilla is normally located at the junction of the lower third and upper two-thirds of the second portion of the duodenum. Identification of its precise location is assisted by passing a balloon-tipped No. 4 or 6 French biliary Fogarty catheter through the cystic duct stump into the common duct and into the duodenum. By inflating the balloon with a small amount of saline the surgeon can palpate the exact location of the sphincter mechanism. This allows for accurate placement of the duodenotomy and will diminish the length of this incision that is required. We perform a longitudinal duodenotomy, which will

Table 100-1. Geenen-Hogan Classification of Patients with Unexplained Right Upper Quadrant Pain

	Type I	Type II	Type III
Twofold elevation of liver enzymes (×2)	+	±	−
Delayed biliary drainage (>45 min)	+	±	−
Common duct > 12 mm	+	±	−

+ = presence of designated abnormality; − = absence of designated abnormality; ± = may be present or absent.

treatment of sphincter of Oddi dysfunction; however, it is usually recommended that this be treated by endoscopic papillotomy unless specific contraindications to its performance exist or previous endoscopic treatment has failed. Transduodenal sphincteroplasty is contraindicated in patients with a common bile duct with a diameter greater than 2 cm, a long distal common bile duct stricture, a perivaterium duodenal diverticulum, or severe inflammatory changes involving the duodenal wall or the head of the pancreas. This procedure is more often performed in younger patients than is choledochoduodenostomy. Major morbidity has been re-permit extension of the incision either in the cephalad or caudad direction, if necessary. In addition, when retractors are introduced or stay sutures are placed on the cut edge of the duodenum, any inadvertent increase in the size of the incision would be in a longitudinal dimension rather than medially into the pancreas. Once the duodenotomy is made, the balloon-tipped Fogarty will be seen coming out of the papilla (Fig. 100-7). If the balloon-tipped Fogarty cannot be placed, the papilla can be identified either by palpation or by manual inspection of the duodenal mucosa. The minor papillary orifice of the accessory pancreatic duct is located cephalad approximately 2 cm.

When the sphincter of Oddi is identified, traction sutures are placed into the duodenal wall adjacent to, but not into, the ampullary complex to elevate and expose the ampulla. Care must be taken to avoid injury to the duct of Wirsung, which will enter on the medial aspect of the ampulla. We prefer to perform all of the subsequent steps with loupe magnification. The goal is to completely incise the intraduodenal portion of the distal bile duct and approximate the mucosa to the duodenal mucosa. The ampulla should be viewed longitudinally with the cephalad end at the top—12 o'clock—and caudad end at 6 o'clock. At approximately 11 o'clock a needle-tipped electrocautery is used to make an initial incision in the sphincter over the Fogarty catheter (Fig. 100-10B). Absorbable sutures, 5–0 or 4–0, are then placed on each side of this incision and held with fine hemostats and not tied. The incision is continued for about 5 mm with placement of sutures approximately every 1.5 mm, being held with slight traction to open the bile duct (Fig. 100-8A). At this point the balloon on the biliary Fogarty is deflated and the catheter pulled back proximally, and a grooved director is passed into the sphincteric opening. The incision in the sphincter is then continued for the length of the intramural common bile duct, which may vary from as short as 6 mm to as long as 3 cm. The incision is stopped proximally, at the point that the common bile duct leaves the wall of the duodenum. Sutures are continued up to the apex stitch. The apex stitch is very important as this closes the opening on the most outside wall of the duodenum where the bile duct becomes extramural. Failure to accurately

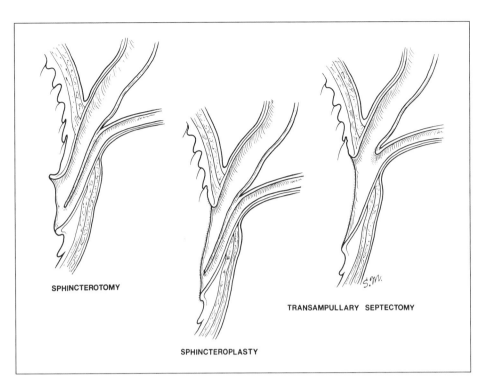

Fig. 100-6. Various operations on the sphincter of Oddi.

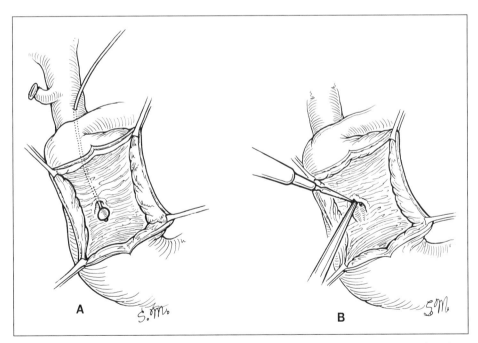

Fig. 100-7. A. Identification of the ampulla of Vater with a biliary Fogarty catheter either passed through the cystic duct or the common duct. B. The initial incision is in the ampulla at 11 o'clock.

place this stitch can result in leakage of the sphincteroplasty. The grooved director is removed and the opening of the pancreatic duct is identified between 4 and 6 o'clock on the medial aspect of the opening; only after the duct is visualized are the medial sutures placed above the pancreatic ductal opening, so as not to occlude it. The pancreatic duct orifice usually appears as a slitlike aperture. It frequently is necessary

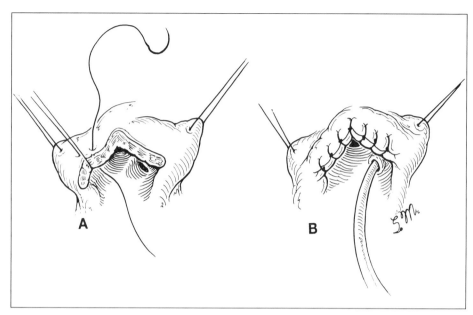

Fig. 100-8. A. Initial sutures for the sphincteroplasty are placed 1.5 mm apart. B. Precise localization of the pancreatic duct.

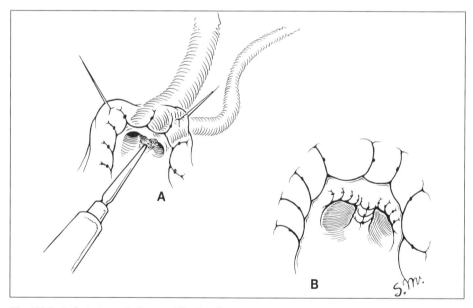

Fig. 100-9. A. Septectomy. B. Sutures following the septectomy.

to cannulate the pancreatic duct opening with a lacrimal duct probe for precise localization (Fig. 100-8B). If the pancreatic duct cannot be identified, it may be necessary to give secretin (75 units per kilogram intravenously) in order to induce pancreatic secretion so that the orifice can be found. Precise localization is mandatory, as inadvertent closure of the main pancreatic duct orifice will result in serious postoperative pancreatitis. If the pancreatic duct cannot be precisely identified,

medial sutures are avoided between 3 and 6 o'clock.

If the patient has had recurrent pancreatitis and stricturing of the orifice of the pancreatic duct or sphincter dysfunction is thought to exist, a septectomy is performed (Fig. 100-9). Although usually not necessary pancreatography can be done to exclude other pancreatic duct abnormalities, if not accomplished preoperatively. This is performed by backloading a 22-

gauge angiocatheter onto a lacrimal duct probe. After the tip of the probe is inserted in the duct the angiocatheter can easily be placed into the duct using the stiffer probe as a guide. Pancreatography is then performed, preferably under fluoroscopic guidance, by a gentle infusion of contrast, introduced by gravity with an elevation of the syringe to no more than 25 cm. The ductal septectomy is done by inserting the lacrimal duct probe into the pancreatic duct and making an incision over this, removing the septum between the common bile duct and the pancreatic duct. Sutures are placed between the cut edge and the duodenal mucosa. Some surgeons do not use sutures unless bleeding is present. We prefer to complete a septoplasty with sutures. Care must be taken not to expand the incision in the septum into the pancreas in order to avoid focal postoperative pancreatitis. If this does occur, the defect can be repaired by reapproximating the edges of the duct and the duodenum.

Once the sphincteroplasty is completed, the common bile duct can be explored in a retrograde fashion if it has not already been explored. Choledochoscopy can also be done through the sphincteroplasty. Placement of a T tube is not usually necessary even if a supraduodenal choledochotomy has been made, although it may be advantageous if a stone was impacted in the ampulla, resulting in edema and swelling.

Duodenal closure is accomplished in a longitudinal fashion with a single layer of 3–0 silk Lembert sutures in normal cases (Fig. 100-10). Transverse closure is not necessary and in our experience it has been associated with more complications, particularly anastomotic leak, and possible duodenal stenosis, as transverse closure may require a two-layer anastomotic technique.

Early complications of sphincteroplasty include acute pancreatitis (0.6%), bleeding of the incised papilla (0.3%), and leakage of the duodenal suture line (0.6%). However, other major morbidity is reported in about 20 percent of patients. Late sequelae include routine asymptomatic pneumobilia. Importantly, air in the biliary tree indicates a patent sphincteroplasty. Duodenal biliary reflux may occur but usually does not cause symptoms or problems. Recurrent papillary stenosis may occur, but

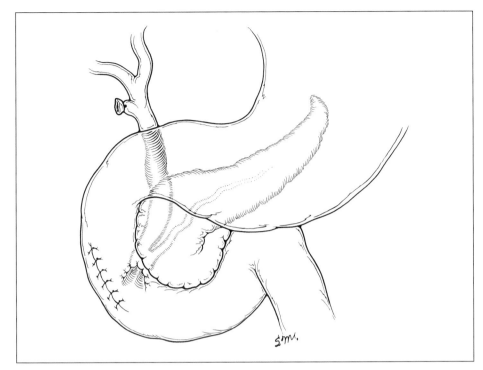

Fig. 100-10. Completed sphincteroplasty with longitudinal closure of the duodenum.

is rare; if it is suspected, the patient should initially have an upper gastrointestinal barium study to look for barium reflux into the biliary system. If none is detected, stenosis of the sphincteroplasty is suggested and ERCP is warranted.

Historically the application of sphincteroplasty became more common after original observations of sphincterotomy done surgically showed poor results. The introduction of endoscopic papillotomy has allowed a larger study of simple sphincterotomy. The overall stenosis rate in these cases is approximately 2 percent. Surgical sphincterotomy is not the same as endoscopic sphincterotomy. The length of endoscopic sphincterotomy is shorter, and theoretically there is more edema that could result in early stenosis or occlusion, accounting for the historically less satisfactory results. Therefore, when indicated, surgical sphincteroplasty is still preferred over surgical sphincterotomy, and may be appropriate in some patients rather than endoscopic sphincterotomy.

Postoperative Care

The patient normally has a nasogastric tube in place for approximately 3 days. It is removed on the third or fourth postop-erative day depending on the output. A diet is then initiated, first with liquids, with advancement to solid food as tolerated. The drain is checked for amylase content 24 hours after initiation of oral intake. It is removed if the amylase is normal. For patients who have had a sphincteroplasty, we check the amylase on the first and third postoperative days. If pancreatitis occurs, postoperative care is altered accordingly and bowel rest is prolonged. The normal hospital stay is approximately 6 days although in the elderly with intercurrent conditions length of stay may be as long as 7 to 10 days.

Summary

The availability of endoscopic retrograde cholangiopancreatography and hence endoscopic papillotomy has limited the necessity for lateral choledochoduodenostomy or transduodenal sphincteroplasty; however, specific instances occur when the surgeon needs to perform these operations. The operations should be considered complementary. The lateral choledochoduodenostomy is preferred for larger bile ducts, greater than 2 cm, or if there is a perivaterium duodenal diverticulum of considerable size that would make perfor-

mance of the transduodenal sphincteroplasty difficult. The exact choice of the above operations depends on specific clinical situations.

Suggested Reading

Anderson TM, Pitt HA, Longmire WP. Experience with sphincteroplasty and sphincterotomy in pancreaticobiliary surgery. *Ann Surg* 201:299, 1985.

Baker AR, Neoptolemos JP, Carr-Locker DL, Fossard OD. Sump syndrome following choledochoduodenostomy and its endoscopic treatment. *Br J Surg* 72:433, 1985.

Cubillos L, Fiallo R, Rodriguez F. Is choledochoduodenostomy in the treatment of stones in the common bile duct an obsolete technique? *World J Surg* 484, 1985.

Geenen JE, Hogan WJ, Dodds WJ, et al. The efficacy of endoscopic sphincterotomy after cholecystectomy in patients with sphincter of Oddi dysfunction. *N Engl J Med* 320:82, 1989.

Moody FG, Becker JM, Potts JR. Transduodenal sphincteroplasty and transampullary septectomy for post cholecystectomy pain. *Ann Surg* 197:627, 1983.

Stuart M, Hoerr SO. Late results of side to side choledochoduodenostomy and of transduodenal sphincteroplasty for benign disorders. *Am J Surg* 123:67, 1972.

Steinberg WM. Sphincter of Oddi dysfunction: A clinical controversy. *Gastroenterology* 95:1409, 1988.

EDITOR'S COMMENT

As Dr. Ellison and his co-authors so nicely point out, the sphincteroplasty is not interchangeable with sphincterotomy, and they make the additional well-indicated point that septoplasty is not a necessary part of sphincteroplasty. The additional information offered since the publication of the last edition of this volume on the different types of sphincter of Oddi dysfunction is most welcome, as the authors have begun to make sense of the clinical syndrome of pain indistinguishable from that of cholelithiasis, but with no stones in the gallbladder. Many of the patients have had their gallbladders out regardless of the fact that no pathology is demonstrated in the gallbladder. It is persistence of the pain that is then referred to as the postcholecystectomy syndrome, interchangeable with sphincter of Oddi dysfunction, biliary dyskinesia, and the other wastebaskets. It would take some courage to carry out sphincteroplasty as an initial procedure; if one does this, one must be certain of the diagnosis based on endoscopic and manometric characteristics, and a cholecystectomy is indicated as well.

Endoscopic sphincterotomy and stenting have been offered as alternatives to biliary and pancreatic sphincteroplasty. The two are not interchangeable. While Maxton and coworkers (*Gut* 36:446, 1995) have reported a fairly large series of patients with retained common-duct stones following endoscopic sphincterotomy, a No. 7 French double-pigtail stent was inserted. Common bile duct stone extraction was achieved endoscopically in 50 of 79 patients after a mean of 4.3 months. The main complication was persistent cholangitis in 13 patients.

Our own experience with stents has not been that happy. I do remember the patient with a huge common-duct stone not visible on x-ray who had a stent replaced through a hole in the middle of the stone. She was operated on when her cholangitis became uncontrollable. The stone measured 2.5 cm. When Bakes dilators were used in common-duct exploration initially, surgeons learned the hard way that trauma to the sphincter would result in late scarring, and the use of dilators to cal-ibrate the duct was abandoned. Although the stenosis rate thus far following sphincterotomy has been reported in the range of 2 percent, it is likely that in time this will go much higher. Unfortunately, the follow-up period is rather brief, as most "lesser invasive procedures" tend to be.

With respect to the indications, although Table 100-1 suggests that there are transient abnormalities in the liver function tests, our own experience (*Am J Surg* 157:38, 1989) indicates that the elevations are very transient, if at all, and may be limited to a slight elevation in alkaline phosphatase. Patients with pancreatitis, unless it is accompanied by common-duct stones, do not benefit from this procedure. Similar findings were presented in the original re-evaluation of sphincteroplasty by S. Austen Jones (*Surgery* 71:565, 1972).

The technique described by Dr. Ellison and colleagues is a fairly standard method with which I differ only slightly. I make a transverse incision that can be extended across the midline if necessary, but which rarely is. The sphincter can be palpated without opening the common duct. It is, of course, helpful to have something through the sphincter, but it generally is at the junction of the second and third portions of the duodenum. I find a transverse duodenotomy more convenient, and place stay sutures and tie at the anterior and posterior portions of the duodenotomy to prevent additional tearing. Doctor Ellison and coworkers are correct in saying that, if a longitudinal duodenotomy is carried out, it is inappropriate to close it transversely. I always perform a pancreatic septoplasty, since I believe that the postoperative swelling may result in an increased incidence of postoperative pancreatitis if it is not carried out. I also utilize a gastrostomy and a feeding jejunostomy, since if patients do develop postoperative pancreatitis, their postoperative course may be prolonged and nutrition may become a problem.

Lateral choledochoduodenostomy has been shown to give results equivalent to sphincteroplasty.

Ramirez and coworkers (*Br J Surg* 81:121, 1994) have presented the latest in a series of reviews, indicating that 71 percent of patients who underwent choledochoduodenostomy and 75 percent of patients with transduodenal sphincterotomy (not sphincteroplasty) were asymptomatic, and the remainder suffered from dyspepsia, colicky pain, or episodes of cholangitis. In my own practice in patients who have a long stenosis for stricture of the bile duct because of chronic pancreatitis, the loop that is used for the Peustow procedure is then positioned past the choledochus so that a choledochojejunostomy can be done as the second (lower) anastomosis.

J.E.F.

101

Treatment of Sclerosing Cholangitis

R. Scott Jones

Primary sclerosing cholangitis is a rare chronic disease characterized by patchy progressive inflammatory sclerosis of the intrahepatic or extrahepatic biliary ducts. Dilbay first described this disease in 1924 and by 1958 the details of only 13 patients had been published. With increased recognition of the disease, follow-up studies suggest a poor long-term prognosis.

Incidence and Associated Conditions

Sclerosing cholangitis develops two to three times more commonly in men than in women and those who develop the disease usually do so in their 20s or 30s. However, it has developed in patients aged 2 to 82 years. Sclerosing cholangitis develops in between 5 and 15 people per 100,000. In the 1980s, the disease appeared more commonly, probably because of the general application of endoscopic retrograde cholangiopancreatography (ERCP), increased physician awareness of the disease, and the realization that liver transplantation improves patient survival.

Chronic inflammatory bowel disease, especially chronic ulcerative colitis, is the most common disease associated with sclerosing cholangitis. Between 35 and 72 percent of patients with sclerosing cholangitis will also have inflammatory bowel disease, and a small portion of these will have Crohn's disease. About 1 to 4 percent of patients with chronic inflammatory bowel disease will develop sclerosing cholangitis before or after the onset of inflammatory bowel disease. Colectomy

does not alter the progression of sclerosing cholangitis.

Other associated conditions include retroperitoneal fibrosis, sarcoidosis, celiac sprue, mediastinal fibrosis, retractile mesenteritis, Peyronie's disease, pancreatitis, submandibular gland fibrosis, Riedel's thyroiditis, pseudotumor of the orbit, bile duct cancer, Weber-Christian disease, histiocytosis X, rheumatoid arthritis, systemic lupus erythematosus, hemolytic anemia, and various immunodeficiency states. The associated immunodeficiency states are hyperimmunoglobulin deficiency, chronic granulomatous disease of childhood, and angioimmunoblastic lymphadenopathy. Patients with AIDS have developed bile duct abnormalities resembling primary sclerosing cholangitis.

The relationship between sclerosing cholangitis and bile duct carcinoma deserves special mention. Bile duct carcinoma develops in as many as 10 percent of patients with sclerosing cholangitis. The development of cancer is particularly difficult to recognize because the clinical symptoms and the radiographic findings of sclerosing cholangitis mask the developing cancer. Most patients in whom bile duct carcinoma develops have a long history of bile duct disease and many have associated inflammatory bowel disease. A worsening of jaundice or the development of thrombophlebitis in patients with sclerosing cholangitis should raise the suspicion of bile duct carcinoma. Those patients should undergo evaluation by cholangiography and bile duct brushings when cancer is suspected. A rising Ca 19-9 concentration in the serum in a patient with sclerosing cholangitis can detect cancer in the bile ducts.

Pathophysiology

The cause of sclerosing cholangitis remains unknown. Chronic low-grade bacterial or viral infections of the biliary ducts were once thought to produce the disease. While bacterial infection of the biliary ductal system occurs in primary sclerosing cholangitis, the infection probably results from rather than produces the disease. Although bacterial infection of the biliary system and inflammation or infection of the colon frequently accompany primary sclerosing cholangitis an etiologic role for bacterial infection has not been established. Hepatitis virus does not cause primary sclerosing cholangitis.

Familial concordance and documentation of circulating immune complexes support an autoimmune mechanism of pathogenesis. Patients with primary sclerosing cholangitis exhibit marked reduction in the clearance of immune complexes, whereas the clearance of immune complexes remains unchanged in people with other forms of liver disease and in normal control subjects.

Patients with chronic ulcerative colitis and primary sclerosing cholangitis demonstrate the HLA-B8 antigen in 60 to 80 percent of cases. This and the observation that ulcerative colitis patients with spondylitis have the HLA-B27 antigen suggest that genetic factors play a role in the susceptibility of patients with ulcerative colitis to sclerosing cholangitis. Several studies have reported a familial occurrence of primary sclerosing cholangitis and ulcerative colitis. The HLA-DRw52a antigen was found in all of 29 patients with sclerosing

1127

cholangitis, compared to a control population frequency of 35 percent. Patients with primary sclerosing cholangitis have an increased frequency of HLA-B8 antigen and a decreased frequency of HLA-B12 antigen. Also bile duct epithelium shows no class II antigen expression and high concentrations of HLA-DR. There may be a disease susceptibility gene associated with the B locus of the major histocompatibility complex.

Primary sclerosing cholangitis may mimic bile duct cancer, gallstones, primary biliary cirrhosis, or cryptogenic cirrhosis. One must differentiate between primary sclerosing cholangitis and the sclerosing cholangitis secondary to biliary obstruction and recurrent biliary infections. In addition, metastatic cancer can infrequently mimic primary sclerosing cholangitis.

Fibrous thickening of the intrahepatic and extrahepatic bile ducts with the formation of multiple strictures and "beading" of the biliary ducts characterize primary sclerosing cholangitis. The disease probably originates in the intrahepatic ducts with progression to involvement of the extrahepatic ducts in over 90 percent of cases. Approximately 10 percent of the patients exhibit a single dominant stricture. Primary sclerosing cholangitis preferentially involves the confluence of the right and left lobar ducts.

Upon biopsy the intrahepatic and extrahepatic bile ducts of patients with primary sclerosing cholangitis exhibit no pathognomonic features. Concentric layering of connective tissue with a mixed inflammatory infiltrate occurs. The histology of liver biopsies in primary sclerosing cholangitis exhibits nonspecific changes, such as periductal concentric fibrosis of the small intralobular ducts, cholangiolar or small ductal proliferation, cholestasis, and degeneration of bile duct epithelium with inflammatory infiltration. Piecemeal necrosis and Kupffer cell hyperplasia also may occur. Copper accumulation in the liver invariably accompanies primary sclerosing cholangitis.

The four stages of progressive pathologic change in liver biopsies in patients with primary sclerosing cholangitis include *stage 1*: enlargement of periportal triads with connective tissue and edema fluid; *stage 2*: the spread of connective tissue into the periportal parenchyma; *stage 3*: the formation of fibrous septi; and finally, *stage 4*:

the formation of cirrhosis. Obliteration of intralobular bile ducts by solid cords of fibrous tissue occurs early in the disease and is the most characteristic finding of primary sclerosing cholangitis on liver biopsy. Unfortunately, this occurs in only 10 percent of biopsies with the disease.

Clinical Features

The symptoms of primary sclerosing cholangitis include malaise, jaundice, abdominal pain, anorexia, weight loss, fever, pruritus, nausea, vomiting, and cholangitis. Most patients have physical findings, such as hepatomegaly, jaundice, splenomegaly, and signs of liver failure.

There are three general clinical syndromes of primary sclerosing cholangitis. The most common manifests recurrent episodes of acute cholangitis. The recurrences may occur sporadically and episodically over many years. Late in the course of the disease, persistent cholestatic jaundice develops. Signs of secondary biliary cirrhosis

may develop later. The fluctuating course of primary sclerosing cholangitis with relapses and remissions makes evaluation of treatment difficult. The second important syndrome is portovenous hypertension, which occurs in about 14 percent of cases. Patients present with bleeding esophageal varices or hepatosplenomegaly and have minimal signs of cholestasis. Thirdly, about 7 percent of patients with primary sclerosing cholangitis will be asymptomatic. Their disease will be detected by investigation of a persistently elevated serum alkaline phosphatase occurring in a patient with ulcerative colitis.

Forty-five patients with asymptomatic sclerosing cholangitis underwent serial evaluations to study the progress of their disease. During a median follow-up period of 75.2 months, 34 patients had evidence of disease progression and 14 developed liver failure that resulted in death or referral for liver transplantation. Sclerosing cholangitis is a progressive disease with significant morbidity and mortality even when detected before symptoms occur.

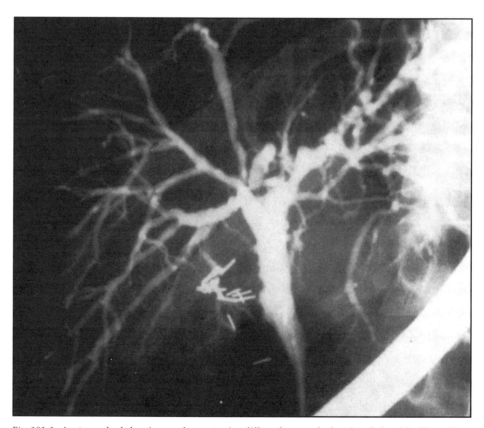

Fig. 101-1. A retrograde cholangiogram demonstrating diffuse changes of sclerosing cholangitis. (From PB Cotton, N Nickl. Endoscopic and radiologic approaches to therapy in primary sclerosing cholangitis. Semin Liver Dis 11:40, 1991. Reproduced with permission.)

The laboratory tests in patients with primary sclerosing cholangitis characteristically exhibit a cholestatic pattern with a markedly elevated serum alkaline phosphatase. Hyperbilirubinemia is very common but the serum bilirubin concentration fluctuates during the course of the disease. Many patients may have normal serum bilirubin concentrations at times during their illness. The serum transaminase concentration will be mildly or slightly elevated. About 50 percent of patients with primary sclerosing cholangitis will have elevations in serum immunoglobulin M (IgM) concentrations, but alterations in serum IgA and IgG concentrations occur less commonly. The serum antimitochondrial antibody is invariably absent in primary sclerosing cholangitis. Bile cultures, when available, generally reveal contamination with *Klebsiella*, coliforms, and *Bacteroides*. Some patients may have fungal organisms, particularly *Candida*.

Cholangiography, preferably ERCP, is essential in evaluating patients suspected of having primary sclerosing cholangitis (Fig. 101-1). When evaluating cholangiograms, one should serially and systematically inspect the intrahepatic ducts, the proximal extrahepatic ducts, and the distal extrahepatic ducts. Diffuse multifocal strictures involving both intrahepatic ducts and extrahepatic ducts comprise the most common findings. Nearly all patients have intrahepatic disease. The short strictures alternate with normal-appearing segments of bile duct to give a beaded appearance. The short strictures and normal segments produce outpouchings like diverticula, which, in the extrahepatic ducts, characterize sclerosing cholangitis. Longer confluent strictures occur later in the disease. Mural irregularities occur commonly. Usually the extrahepatic and intrahepatic ducts are involved, but in a small number of cases, the disease may be confined either to the intrahepatic or the extrahepatic ducts.

The diagnosis of primary sclerosing cholangitis is based on clinical suspicion confirmed by cholangiographic demonstration of the typical pattern of bile duct scarring. The clinical and histologic patterns of this disease overlap considerably with those of primary biliary cirrhosis, although the latter disease typically affects middle-aged women with keratoconjunctivitis sicca, hyperpigmentation, and high titers of antimitochondral antibodies.

Cholangiography allows differentiation between these two diseases, as primary biliary cirrhosis never involves extrahepatic ducts.

A suggestive history coupled with a typical cholangiogram affords reasonable certainty for the diagnosis, particularly when liver biopsy offers confirmatory evidence. The diagnosis of sclerosing cholangiocarcinoma may be extremely difficult to exclude. Extrahepatic or hilar cholangiocarcinoma produces general or diffuse intrahepatic bile duct dilatation while sclerosing cholangitis does not.

Management

There is no effective medical treatment for primary sclerosing cholangitis, and patients who suffer from this disease most often experience liver failure and develop cirrhosis and portal hypertension, eventually dying of these conditions. The mean duration from diagnosis to death lasts from 4 to 7 years with wide individual variations. Some patients with mild forms of the disease may experience minimal disability and live a relatively normal life for as long as 15 years. Some patients have been treated with corticosteroids, but no firm evidence supports this therapy. Likewise, azathioprine and bile acid binding

agents lack effectiveness. A careful clinical trial of penicillamine therapy showed no benefit. Because of penicillamine's toxicity it should be avoided. The oral administration of ursodiol shows promise as a treatment for sclerosing cholangitis. Several studies provide evidence that ursodiol reduces serum bilirubin, decreases clinical jaundice, decreases serum transaminase levels, improves symptoms, and in some cases improves the cholangiographic appearance of the disease. A prospective randomized trial using ursodiol to treat sclerosing cholangitis showed marked improvement in liver tests in the treated groups but symptoms were not relieved. Whether ursodiol prolongs life in sclerosing cholangitis is not known.

Many years ago surgical treatment consisted of T-tube drainage of the common bile duct to palliate the jaundice produced by lower ductal strictures. More recently biliary enteric anastomoses can palliate those patients with a predominant single stricture or disease localized to the lower tract, and about three-fourths of these patients achieve satisfactory symptomatic improvement.

Cameron and associates advocate bilateral hepaticojejunostomy with transhepatic stenting to bypass the strictured lobar duct confluence. The patients chosen for this therapy had persistently elevated serum

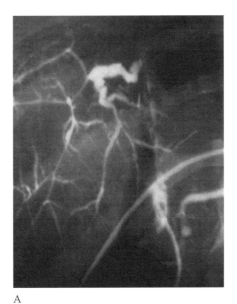 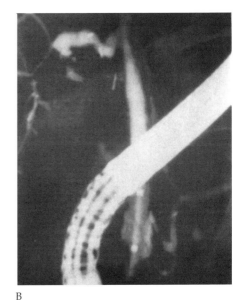

A   B

Fig. 101-2. A. A very severe stricture of the bile duct in a patient with sclerosing cholangitis. B. Dramatic improvement in the bile duct appearance after balloon dilatation. (From PB Cotton, N Nickl. Endoscopic and radiologic approaches to therapy in primary sclerosing cholangitis. Semin Liver Dis 11:40, 1991. Reproduced with permission.)

bilirubin and no evidence of cirrhosis on biopsy. Thirty-one patients underwent excision of the extrahepatic bile ducts, Roux en Y hepaticojejunostomy, and long-term transhepatic stenting for persistent jaundice or recurrent cholangitis. The 1-, 3-, and 5-year survival rates of patients with cirrhosis were 20, 20, and 20 percent. The 1-, 3-, and 5-year survival rates for patients with hepatic fibrosis were 92, 87, and 71 percent, respectively. Two of the long-term survivors subsequently underwent liver transplantation. Symptomatic palliation has been accomplished in the majority of these patients; however, longer follow-up will be necessary to demonstrate any alteration in the natural history of the disease.

Percutaneous or endoscopic dilatation of predominant strictures may play a role in the palliation of primary sclerosing cholangitis (Figs. 101-2 to 101-4). Successful nonoperative dilatation of dominant strictures in patients with sclerosing cholangitis has been reported from several centers. This treatment reduced the episodes of bacterial cholangitis, serum bilirubin, and pruritus. Thirteen of fourteen patients with sclerosing cholangitis experienced improvement following percutaneous balloon dilatation of dominant strictures and insertion of transhepatic stents. The use of balloon dilatation, endoscopic stenting, and ursodiol administration has been reported to improve the condition of patients with sclerosing cholangitis.

Liver transplantation is the only effective treatment for end-stage liver disease. Since its introduction, improved surgical technique, venovenous bypass, improved organ harvesting techniques, improved organ preservation, and improved patient selection have provided a treatment that improves the natural history of sclerosing cholangitis. Two hundred sixteen adult patients with advanced primary sclerosing cholangitis underwent liver replacement and survived. These patients were compared to a group of 392 conservatively treated patients observed at five centers in England and North America. The workers at the Mayo Clinic analyzed these nonoperatively treated patients to estimate survival probabilities without liver transplantation. Within 6 months of follow-up, the Kaplan-Meier survival probability after liver transplantation (0.89) was already higher than predicted by the Mayo model (0.83). At 5 years the Kaplan-Meier actual

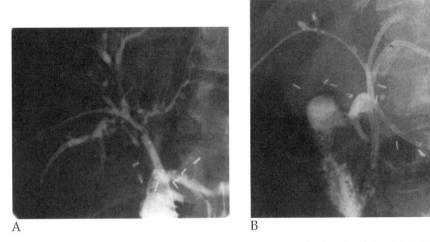

Fig. 101-3. A. Percutaneous access to hilar stricturing in a patient with sclerosing cholangitis. B. Combined percutaneous and endoscopic stenting in the same patient. (From PB Cotton, N Nickl. Endoscopic and radiologic approaches to therapy in primary sclerosing cholangitis. Semin Liver Dis 11:40, 1991. Reproduced with permission.)

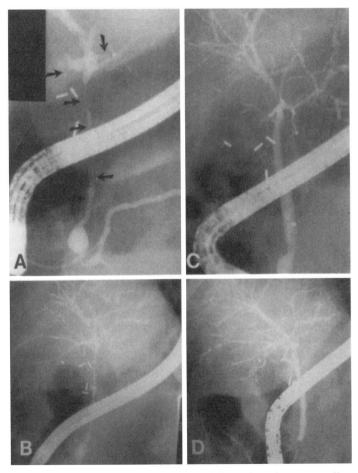

Fig. 101-4. A. ERCP of a patient with sclerosing cholangitis before endoscopic treatment. Six stricture sites noted. B. ERCP 1 year after endoscopic treatment. C. ERCP 2 years following endoscopic treatment. D. ERCP 3 years following treatment. The patient remained symptom free. (From GK Johnson, JE Geenen, RP Venu, et al: Endoscopic treatment of biliary tract strictures in sclerosing cholangitis: A larger series and recommendations for treatment. Gastrointest Endosc 37:38, 1991. Reproduced with permission.)

survival with transplantation was 0.73 compared with 0.28. Liver transplantation is effective therapy for sclerosing cholangitis. Disease gravity and unsuspected bile duct carcinoma adversely affected the outcome of transplantation.

Because sclerosing cholangitis is a progressive lethal disease for which there is no proven effective medical therapy, patients should be considered for transplantation early enough to minimize both the development of bile duct cancer and the operative risks that accompany prolonged liver failure. Although operative management of the biliary obstruction of sclerosing cholangitis provides palliation for the jaundice, such procedures increase the technical complexity of liver transplantation. Patients with persistent cholestasis due to sclerosing cholangitis should be considered for transplantation.

A recent study of 22 patients who received liver grafts for the treatment of sclerosing cholangitis included serial liver biopsies following transplantation. Seven patients had biopsies that showed features of biliary obstruction, 6 demonstrated fibrous cholangitis, and 3 showed classic fibro-obliterative lesions. These findings suggest that sclerosing cholangitis may recur in the liver allograft.

Liver transplantation has provided an effective definitive therapy for patients with primary sclerosing cholangitis. Because this disease can be mild and characterized by variable natural history of exacerbations and remissions, it remains difficult to decide properly when to recommend transplantation for the patient. Most patients who require surgical treatment for sclerosing cholangitis should undergo liver transplantation.

Operative Treatment

As was discussed previously selected patients have been treated surgically by excision of the extrahepatic bile ducts, intraoperative dilatation of intrahepatic strictures, insertion of bilateral transhepatic stents, and hepaticojejunostomy. The indications for this procedure in sclerosing cholangitis include unrelenting jaundice with serum bilirubin concentrations over 5 mg %, cholangitis, and the absence of cirrhosis.

The procedure begins with a right subcostal incision, which permits identification of the liver edge and dissection of the subhepatic space for exposure of the porta hepatis and the gastroduodenal ligament. Removal of the gallbladder enhances exposure of the bile ducts (Fig. 101-5). The

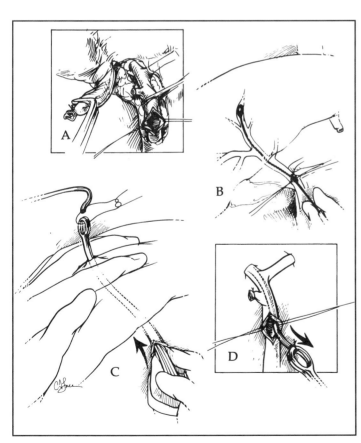

Fig. 101-5. Exposure of the extrahepatic bile ducts, dilatation of strictures, and intraoperative insertion of a transhepatic biliary stent. (From RS Jones. Atlas of Liver and Biliary Surgery. *Chicago: Year Book, 1990. Reproduced with permission.)*

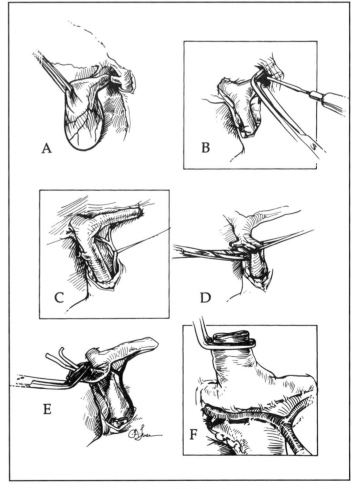

Fig. 101-6. Excision of the extrahepatic bile ducts. (From RS Jones. Atlas of Liver and Biliary Surgery. *Chicago: Year Book, 1990. Reproduced with permission.)*

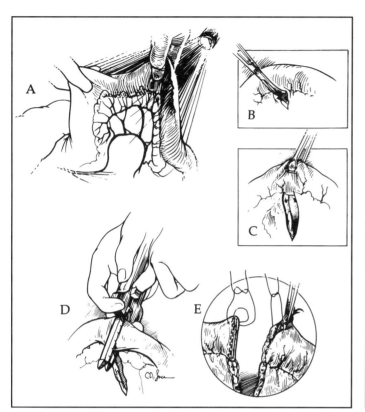

Fig. 101-7. Preparation of a jejunal loop for construction of a Roux en Y hepaticojejunostomy. (From RS Jones. Atlas of Liver and Biliary Surgery. Chicago: Year Book, 1990. Reproduced with permission.)

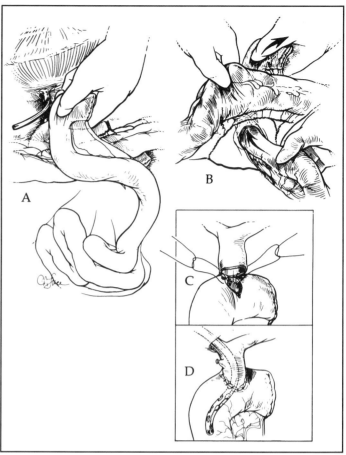

Fig. 101-8. Positioning a Roux en Y limb in the subhepatic space for biliary enteric anastomosis. (From RS Jones. Atlas of Liver and Biliary Surgery. Chicago: Year Book, 1990. Reproduced with permission.)

extrahepatic bile duct anatomy should be evaluated carefully. In this situation many patients will have a percutaneous transhepatic tube, which helps to identify the common bile duct.

Today we infrequently place transhepatic stents in the operating room because in most instances they are inserted preoperatively in the radiology suite. Several techniques allow intraoperative placement of transhepatic stents. When treating sclerosing cholangitis the ducts are probed with Bakes dilators to delineate the anatomy and dilate strictures. Choledochoscopy may be difficult or impractical in severe sclerosing cholangitis. After the strictures are dilated, the liver is palpated carefully. Then the dilated duct is explored for stenting with a Bakes dilator to assess the configuration of the duct and to plan the trajectory of the tube. One should choose a stone forceps with the proper curve and

pass it into the chosen hepatic duct and along the route previously selected. After passing the forceps into the duct until it will go no further with gentle pressure, the instrument is passed with one hand and the surface of the liver palpated with the other hand. With bimanual guidance and palpation, the tip of the stone forceps is forced through the hepatic parenchyma and through Glisson's capsule. The stent tube is affixed to the forceps and the forceps and stent are withdrawn gently so that the stent passes through the liver into the hepatic duct and out through the extrahepatic duct (Fig. 101-6). The common bile duct is encircled and retracted anteriorly to find the plane dorsal to the duct.

After the extrahepatic bile ducts are dissected to the point where they enter the liver, the suprapancreatic bile duct is transected and the distal end is oversewn with

interrupted sutures. One should choose a site on the right and left lobar ducts, transect them, and remove the specimen from the field (Fig. 101-7). The ligament of Treitz is identified and a suitable loop of proximal jejunum is selected for the construction of a Roux en Y segment. The overhead light is directed away from the operative field to transilluminate the mesentery, preferably using the assistant's headlight. One or two of the straight mesenteric vessels are divided and ligated adjacent to the bowel. The mesentery is scored at right angles to the bowel and transected, and the mesenteric vessels are doubly ligated. This allows sufficient length of jejunum to reach the subhepatic space easily without tension. The prepared bowel is transected with a GIA stapler and the stapled closure reinforced with a row of Lembert sutures (Fig. 101-8). One should assess the mobility of the Roux en Y limb by temporarily approximating the proximal end to the bile

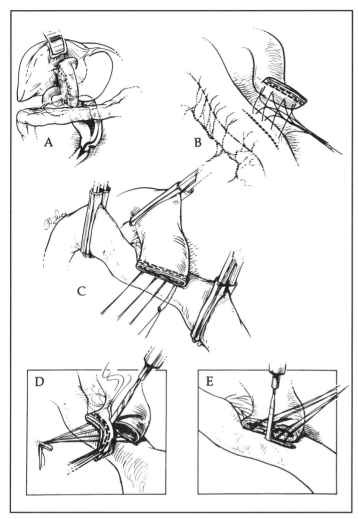

Fig. 101-9. Restoring intestinal continuity to complete the construction of a Roux en Y hepaticojejunostomy. (From RS Jones. Atlas of Liver and Biliary Surgery. *Chicago: Year Book, 1990. Reproduced with permission.)*

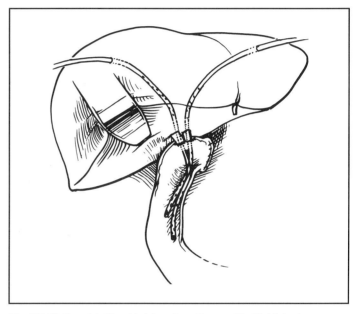

Fig. 101-10. Completed hepaticojejunostomy Roux en Y with bilateral transhepatic stents. (From RS Jones. Atlas of Liver and Biliary Surgery. *Chicago: Year Book, 1990. Reproduced with permission.)*

duct stumps in the subhepatic space. Then the transverse colon is held superiorly and anteriorly to locate the middle colic vessels. One should find an avascular clear space in the mesocolon, make a small incision there, and advance the Roux en Y limb through the mesocolon so that it lies easily without torsion or tension in the subhepatic space. Using interrupted sutures a single-layer anastomosis is constructed between the ends of the prepared bile ducts and the antimesenteric side of the proximal part of the Roux en Y limb. The transhepatic stents should be positioned properly across the anastomosis so that the tip lies in the Roux en Y limb (Fig. 101-9). Then 40 cm is measured along the mesenteric border of the Roux en Y limb and that point is marked with a suture as

the point for restoration of gastrointestinal continuity. The relationships between the proximal jejunal loop and the Roux en Y limb and their mesenteries are checked so that an anastomosis will lie comfortably with no kinks or tension. This enteroenterostomy can be done either with the GIA stapler or with a hand-sewn anastomosis. Figure 101-10 depicts the initial steps of a two-layered anastomosis using interrupted sutures (Fig. 101-10). This illustration shows the completed operation for sclerosing cholangitis. It includes bilateral transhepatic stents through bilateral hepaticojejunostomies Roux-en-Y. The tip of a closed suction drain is left beneath the biliary anastomosis and the drain tube exits through a small stab wound beneath the incision.

Suggested Reading

Abu-Elmagd KM, Malinchoc M, Dickson ER, et al. Efficacy of hepatic transplantation in patients with primary sclerosing cholangitis. *Surg Gynecol Obstet* 177:335, 1993.

Cameron JL, Pitt HA, Zinner MJ, et al. Resection of hepatic duct bifurcation and transhepatic stenting for sclerosing cholangitis. *Ann Surg* 207:614, 1988.

Dickson ER, Murtaugh PA, Wiesner RH, et al. Primary sclerosing cholangitis: Refinement and validation of survival models. *Gastroenterology* 103: 1893, 1992.

Harrison RF, Davies MH, Neuberger JM, et al. Fibrous and obliterative cholangitis in liver allografts: Evidence of recurrent primary sclerosing cholangitis? *Hepatology* 20:356, 1994.

Johnson GK, Geenen JE, Venu RP, et al. Endoscopic treatment of biliary tract strictures in sclerosing cholangitis: A larger series and recommendations for treatment. *Gastroenterol Endosc* 37:38, 1991.

Martin FM, Rossi RL, Nugent FW, et al. Surgical aspects of sclerosing cholangitis. *Ann Surg* 212:551, 1990.

Prochazka EJ, Terasaki PI, Park MS, et al. Association of primary sclerosing cholangitis with HLA-DRw52a *N Engl J Med* 322:1842, 1990.

Rosen CB, Nagorney DM, Wiesner RH, et al. Cholangiocarcinoma complicating primary sclerosing cholangitis. *Ann Surg* 213:21, 1991.

Springer DJ, Gaing AA, Siegel JH. Radiologic regression of primary sclerosing cholangitis following combination therapy with an endoprosthesis and ursodeoxycholic acid. *Am J Gastroenterol* 88:1957, 1993.

Stiehl A, Walker S, Stiehl L, et al. Effect of ursodeoxycholic acid on liver and bile duct disease in primary sclerosing cholangitis. A 3-year pilot study with a placebo-controlled study period. *J Hepatol* 20:57, 1994.

EDITOR'S COMMENT

As Dr. Jones points out, sclerosing cholangitis is probably an autoimmune disease that complicates inflammatory bowel disease, among others. The presentation of the disease may not involve inflammatory bowel disease. Indeed, I have personally seen patients who have presented with cirrhosis and ascites without any previous evidence of clinical inflammatory bowel disease, only to be diagnosed with very mild ulcerative colitis that has been misdiagnosed in the past. Doctor Jones is correct in that colectomy does not alter the progression of sclerosing cholangitis once it is established. There remains some controversy, however, that if one performs a colectomy on a patient who has not manifested sclerosing cholangitis, the latter may not develop. The literature is not clear on this because, as Dr. Jones points out, the classic findings on liver biopsy of sclerosing cholangitis are only present in 10 percent of the patients in early disease. On routine liver biopsies in patients with ulcerative colitis on whom I have done pullthrough procedures, infiltration of lymphocytes and macrophages always occurs. It is difficult to know how to interpret these findings.

The difficulty in patients with sclerosing cholangitis is the incidence of carcinoma. This is particularly difficult to diagnose because cholangiography does not readily differentiate between the two conditions. Because of this, various investigators have attempted to find prognostic features that may point to one or the other. While serum antigen 19-9 may result in the diagnosis of a cholangiocarcinoma that was not clinically apparent, this is probably true in the late phases of the disease. Indeed, Schrumpf and colleagues (*J Hepatol* 21:1061, 1994) followed a group of 77 consecutive patients with sclerosing cholangitis. The bilirubin level was found to be an independent risk factor for both mortality and the necessity for transplantation and the appearance of cholangiocarcinoma. Thus, one uses the bilirubin as a marker for the necessity for transplantation when one may in fact be transplanting a patient with a cholangiocarcinoma.

The relative roles of biliary surgery and transplantation are not yet elucidated. We have had a number of patients on whom we have performed restorative proctocolectomy and anal pouch/anal anastomosis procedures who have had subsequent liver transplantation. Farges and coworkers (*Surgery* 117:146, 1995) compared the actuarial symptom-free survival of patients treated by nontransplantation biliary surgery with those undergoing transplantation. While cumulative actuarial incidence of cancer 5 and 10 years after the onset of primary sclerosing cholangitis was 13 and 31 percent, respectively, symptom-free survival in patients treated by nontransplantation biliary surgery was 35 percent at 10 years. Actuarial patient survival 5 years after transplantation was 89 percent, much greater than the 31 percent expected from prognostic models. The results suggest to the authors that liver transplantation improves the prognosis of patients with primary sclerosing cholangitis. Liver transplantation should be undertaken early after onset of symptoms since it is difficult to identify patients who will benefit from nontransplantation therapeutic interventions or those in whom a cancer will develop.

Clearly, our job in these patients is to identify those in whom nontransplantation biliary surgical intervention will prolong life. Doctor Jones, in his fine chapter, has summarized some hints as to how this might happen.

J.E.F.

102

Treatment of High Malignant Biliary Tract Obstruction

Keith D. Lillemoe

Malignant obstruction of the biliary tree can occur at any point along its length from the intrahepatic bile ducts to the ampulla of Vater. Relief of biliary obstruction, to prevent progressive liver failure or biliary sepsis, is an essential aspect of any treatment plan. The specific management of each patient, however, is dictated primarily by the location of the obstruction. High malignant biliary tract obstruction at or proximal to the hepatic duct bifurcation can be one of the most difficult challenges facing a general surgeon. These tumors are difficult to diagnose, are frequently quite advanced at the time of presentation, and are technically difficult to treat either for palliation or cure. A number of options exist for the management of high malignant biliary obstruction. The technique of resection and reconstruction of proximal biliary cancers using Silastic transhepatic biliary stents, however, offers several technical advantages at the time of the operation, provides short-term biliary decompression in the postoperative period, and maintains long-term access to the biliary tree for postoperative adjuvant radiation therapy and to prevent or treat late obstruction caused by progressive or recurrent tumor.

Etiology and Pathology

Carcinoma of the hepatic duct bifurcation was first described by Altemeier and colleagues in 1957, and subsequently, a series of 13 patients with this diagnosis was reported on by Klatskin in 1965. Since then, cholangiocarcinomas at this location have been known as Klatskin tumors. Approx-

imately 15,000 new cases of liver and biliary tract carcinoma are diagnosed annually in the United States, with roughly 10 percent of these carcinomas being Klatskin tumors. Although these tumors are often considered to be slow-growing malignancies, death caused by progressive hepatic failure occurs quickly unless adequate biliary decompression is achieved.

Although cholangiocarcinoma is the most common tumor resulting in obstruction of the proximal biliary tree, other malignancies must also be considered. Primary hepatocellular carcinoma located in the hilum of the liver, extension of gallbladder cancer to involve the biliary tree, lymphoma or metastatic cancer to the periportal lymph nodes, and cystadenomas or cystadenocarcinomas of the liver can also cause proximal biliary obstruction. In addition to malignant causes, at least two benign processes must also be included in the differential diagnosis of proximal biliary obstruction. First and most important, primary sclerosing cholangitis can frequently present with an isolated dominant stricture at the hepatic duct bifurcation. Distinguishing primary sclerosing cholangitis based on clinical and roentgenographic criteria can be very difficult. Furthermore, the development of cholangiocarcinoma in patients with sclerosing cholangitis has been well documented. Finally, benign strictures involving the proximal biliary tree can present with a clinical and roentgenographic picture similar to that of primary biliary malignancies. The use of tissue cytology or direct cholangioscopic biopsies via transhepatic or endoscopic techniques can be helpful in distin-

guishing the benign from malignant conditions.

Diagnosis and Staging

Most patients with proximal biliary cancer are between the ages of 50 and 70 years, with a slight male predominance. Progressive jaundice is the presenting complaint in over 90 percent of patients. Pruritus, weight loss, and abdominal pain are seen less frequently. Cholangitis is uncommon unless prior biliary tract manipulation has occurred. Rarely, either the right or left hepatic ducts might obstruct before progressive involvement at the bifurcation leads to jaundice. Such patients can experience mild abdominal discomfort, unilobular liver enlargement, and elevation of serum alkaline phosphatase or γ-glutamyltransferase.

The evaluation of any jaundiced patient should begin with either an abdominal ultrasound or computed tomography (CT) scan. The findings on either study that are suggestive of a proximal cholangiocarcinoma include a dilated intrahepatic biliary tree, a normal or collapsed gallbladder and extrahepatic biliary tree, and a normal pancreas. The primary tumor mass is rarely visualized. Early experience suggests that magnetic resonance imaging (MRI) can be somewhat more sensitive in detecting these tumors.

After biliary ductal dilatation has been demonstrated by imaging studies, it is imperative that cholangiography be performed for proximal biliary tumors. Cholangiography should not only define the location but also visualize the uppermost extent of the tumor to determine the limits of resectability. Percutaneous transhepatic cholangiography (PTC) is favored over endoscopic retrograde cholangiography because it better defines the proximal extent of the tumor involvement and allows placement of percutaneous transhepatic catheters (Fig. 102-1). In most patients with proximal biliary cancers, both the right and left hepatic ducts must be intubated to establish adequate biliary drainage.

Preoperatively placed biliary catheters serve a number of roles in the management of proximal malignant biliary tract obstruction. As discussed earlier, transhepatic catheters allow access for obtaining a preoperative tissue diagnosis using either scrape biopsy or brushings or direct cholangioscopic biopsy. These catheters also serve a valuable role at the time of the operation. They are also used primarily to assist in the identification and dissection of the hepatic duct bifurcation and the individual right and left hepatic ducts. In addition, the biliary catheters greatly facilitate the placement of large bore Silastic stents used for reconstruction. Finally, although prolonged biliary decompression to improve jaundice is not indicated routinely, patients with significant malnutrition, biliary sepsis, or medical problems

such as renal failure, can benefit from biliary drainage to allow an opportunity for recovery before a planned surgical procedure.

In patients who are candidates for surgical resection, preoperative staging should be completed. Findings on CT scan such as extrahepatic disease or bilobar liver metastasis preclude curative resection. Extensive bilobar proximal extension into the hepatic parenchyma on cholangiography also indicates unresectability. Finally, involvement of the major hepatic portal vessels (hepatic artery and portal vein) with tumor encasement or occlusion preclude resection. Currently, hepatic arteriography with venous phase studies are the gold standard for determining major vessel involvement. Magnetic resonance imaging or spiral CT scan with bolus contrast holds promise as noninvasive tools in assessing tumor extent and invasion of major portal vascular structures.

A recent retrospective review from the Johns Hopkins Hospital has compared the results of cholangiography and angiography over an 8-year period in patients with pathologically proven hilar cholangiocarcinomas. Overall, 28 of the 65 patients (43%) were resected for cure. Cholangiographic involvement of four or more ductal systems or extensive right intrahepatic ductal encasement was observed in 12 patients, and none of these patients was resectable. Cholangiography predicted the clinical management in 62 percent of the patients. Angiographic findings of arterial or venous encasement was observed in 38 percent of patients, and only one of these patients, with a left portal vein encasement, was resected for cure. Angiography predicted the clinical management in 80 percent of the patients. When combined, cholangiography and angiography predicted the clinical management in 86 percent of patients, emphasizing that these studies should be performed routinely in the preoperative staging of perihilar cholangiocarcinomas.

Operative Management

At completion of preoperative staging, approximately two-thirds of patients with proximal cholangiocarcinomas will be considered operable. Resectability is fur-

ther assessed during the operation by careful exploration for peritoneal implants, hepatic metastases, and regional lymph node involvement. Finally, careful assessment of the extent of tumor along the bile duct must be completed. The operative approach for bifurcation tumors should include hilar resection with reconstruction as a bilateral hepaticojejunostomy using transhepatic Silastic stents. Typically, the abdomen is entered by a right subcostal or midline vertical incision. After thorough exploration, dissection of the hepatic duct bifurcation can be facilitated by two maneuvers. First, early mobilization of the gallbladder helps to expose the extrahepatic biliary tree and the hepatic duct bifurcation, which can be palpated using the preoperatively placed transhepatic catheters. Second, early division of the distal extrahepatic biliary tree below the tumor aids in the technical aspects of the proximal hepatic bile duct dissection. The distal extrahepatic biliary tree is sutured closed, and the proximal bile duct is reflected cephalad, freeing the biliary tree from the portal vein and hepatic artery under direct vision (Fig. 102-2A). Once the hepatic duct bifurcation is visualized, the surgeon palpates the transhepatic catheters and the hepatic ducts above the tumor to determine if a tumor-free segment is present. If so, the right and left hepatic ducts are then divided (Fig. 102-2B), leaving the transhepatic catheters exiting through each of the lobar hepatic ducts (Fig. 102-2C). If gross tumor extends along either the right or left hepatic duct into the hepatic parenchyma, appropriate hepatic lobectomy can be considered.

Following resection of the tumor at the hepatic duct bifurcation, the previously placed transhepatic catheters are used to pull progressively larger coudé catheters and eventually Silastic transhepatic biliary stents into each of the lobar hepatic ducts (Fig. 102-3). The Silastic transhepatic stents are in proper position when all of their side holes reside in the intrahepatic biliary tree and in the upper portion of a 50-cm retrocolic Roux en Y jejunal limb that is used for the biliary enteric anastomosis. Normally, two separate end-to-side hepaticojejunostomies are performed over the Silastic stents. Interrupted 4–0 or 5–0 polypropylene or synthetic absorbable sutures are used for the hepaticojejunal anastomoses. The free ends of the stents exit

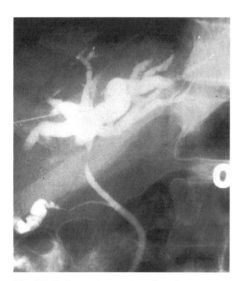

Fig. 102-1. A percutaneous transhepatic cholangiogram in a patient with hilar cholangiocarcinoma (From CJ Yeo, HA Pitt, and JL Cameron. Cholangiocarcinoma. Surg Clin North Am 70:1429, 1990. Reproduced with permission.)

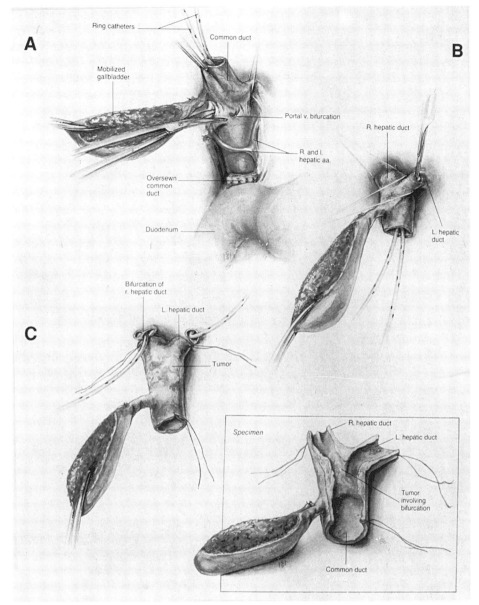

Fig. 102-2. A. During exploration and resection of a hilar carcinoma, early gallbladder mobilization and transection of the distal common bile duct are recommended. These steps allow cephalad reflection of the common bile duct, using the preoperatively placed transhepatic (Ring) catheters for traction, and facilitate hilar dissection of the common hepatic duct and tumor off the portal vein. B. The right and left hepatic ducts are then identified by palpation of the Ring catheters and divided above the tumor. C. The specimen is resected and all margins are identified and submitted to pathologic examination Insert, resected specimen. (From JL Cameron. Resection of a Proximal Cholangiocarcinoma with Reconstruction Utilizing Silastic Transhepatic Biliary Stents and Bilateral Hepaticojejunostomies. In JL Cameron [ed.], Atlas of Surgery, Vol. I Toronto: Decker, 1990. Reproduced with permission.)

through the upper aspect of the liver capsule and are then brought out through separate stab wounds in the abdominal wall. Closed suction drains are placed in the area of the anastomosis and over the dome of the liver at the exit sites of the Silastic stents. The latter drains are useful to drain

bile that might leak around the catheter exit site.

The use of Silastic transhepatic stents in the surgical management of proximal biliary cancers offers many advantages. Silastic (polymeric silicone) stents are usu-

ally 70 cm long, with side holes extending over 40 percent of the length of the catheter. Various diameters are available (Fig. 102-4). Silastic stents allow healing of the biliary enteric anastomosis with a minimum of foreign body reaction. Since the stents exit through the liver and not through the biliary tree, the diameter can be large, thus ensuring a large anastomosis. The thickness of the wall of the stent prevents compression by tumor, and, therefore, maintains patency of the biliary tree even with extensive local tumor growth.

In instances in which hilar cholangiocarcinoma extends either along the left or right hepatic duct into the hepatic parenchyma, appropriate hepatic lobectomy can be considered in addition to hilar resection (Fig. 102-5). The major indication for hepatic lobectomy can be suspected at the time of preoperative cholangiography with proximal tumor involvement extending into the hepatic parenchyma in either the right or left hepatic duct. The hepatic resection is preformed using standard techniques. After resection of the hepatic duct bifurcation, biliary enteric continuity is restored using a hepaticojejunostomy performed over a Silastic transhepatic stent.

Other Surgical Options

Recently, a more aggressive approach to hepatic resection has been advocated by groups in Europe and Japan. Through the use of anatomic and pathologic studies these groups have recognized that tumor involvement at or above the bifurcation is almost always accompanied by extension into the biliary ducts draining the caudate lobe (segment I). Therefore, these groups advocate resection of segment I for all tumors involving the hepatic bifurcation. Furthermore, these authors advocate caudate lobe resection and formal hepatic lobectomy for any tumor extension above the bifurcation because of concerns for secondary ductal involvement on the involved side. Although this approach has been associated with reports of favorable survival, this technique has not been used frequently in the United States.

A final, more controversial resectional option for patients with hilar cholangiocarcinoma is that of total hepatectomy and

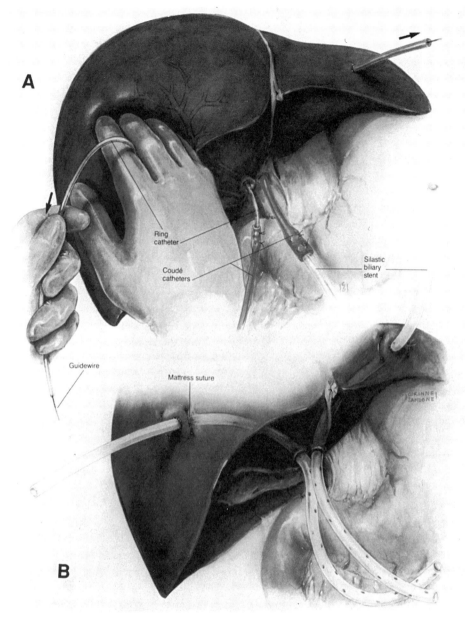

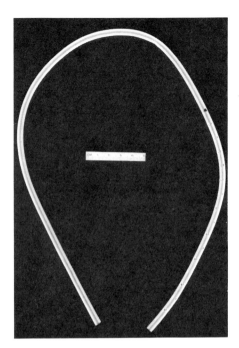

Fig. 102-4. The Silastic transhepatic stent is 70 cm long with side holes extending over 40 percent of the length of the catheter. Various diameters are available. The stent pictured here is 8 mm in outside diameter, which is the size most commonly used. The junction of the side holes, the initial stent, and the intact stent is marked by a radiopaque marker. This marker is used by radiologists to ensure proper position during stent manipulation under fluoroscopy.

Fig. 102-3. A. After resection of the tumor at the hepatic duct bifurcation, the preoperatively placed percutaneous catheters are used to place the Silastic transhepatic stents. A 14Fr coudé catheter is first sutured to the 8Fr Ring catheter, and this catheter is withdrawn through the top of the liver, leaving the coudé catheter in the transhepatic tract. This step dilates the transhepatic tract and corrects the size discrepancy between the 18Fr preoperative catheter and the 16Fr–18Fr Silastic transhepatic stent. The Silastic transhepatic stent is sutured to the widened flange of the coudé catheter and then pulled out the top of the liver. B. The Silastic stents are positioned so that the portion of the stent with the side holes lies entirely within the hepatic parenchyma and extends outside the porta hepatis to be placed through the anastomosis. (From JL Cameron. Resection of a Proximal Cholangiocarcinoma with Reconstruction Utilizing Silastic Transhepatic Biliary Stents and Bilateral Hepaticojejunostomies. In JL Cameron [ed.], Atlas of Surgery, Vol 1. Toronto: Decker, 1990. Reproduced with permission.)

liver transplantation. Although, initially the presence of a bile duct cancer was considered a contraindication for liver transplantation, some centers consider it an option in selected patients. The indication for this approach is bilateral extension of the tumor into the hepatic parenchyma or involvement of the main trunk of the hepatic artery or portal vein. Most protocols also include aggressive preoperative chemo- and radiation therapy. The results of liver transplantation for perihilar cholangiocarcinoma have been disappointing, however, with early and widespread recurrence precluding tumor-free survival in most patients. Survival rates of less than 10 percent have been reported among all patients who undergo liver transplantation for cholangiocarcinoma. Therefore, liver transplantation should be considered primarily as an option only as part of an investigative protocol.

Palliative Therapy

Palliative therapy in patients with proximal biliary cancers can be accomplished either nonoperatively or by biliary enteric bypass. If preoperative staging suggests unresectable disease or if the patient is not a suitable surgical candidate, a nonoperative approach is indicated. Although endoscopically placed biliary catheters are preferred for mid- and distal bile duct ma-

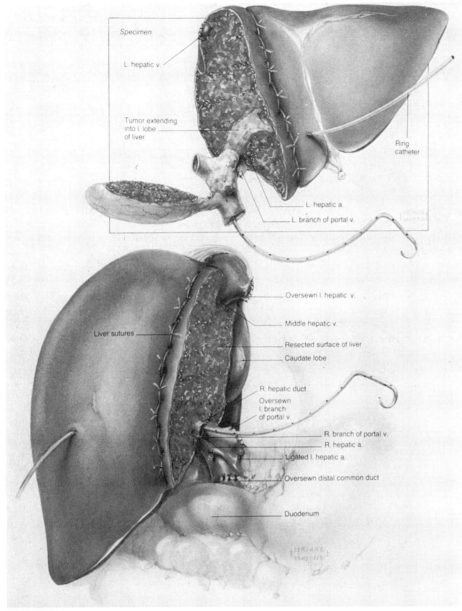

Fig. 102-5. When a hilar cholangiocarcinoma extends along either the left or right hepatic duct into the hepatic parenchyma, the appropriate hepatic lobectomy can be considered to obtain an adequate margin on the tumor. Hepatic lobectomy is performed in a standard manner. When the division of the parenchyma has been completed, the specimen is removed from the operative field. The entire extrahepatic biliary tree including the bifurcation has been resected, along with the left lobe of the liver (insert). The tumor involves the bifurcation and clearly extends into the left hepatic parenchyma. Hemostasis is completed on the raw area remaining on the right lobe of the liver and figure-of-eight sutures of 3–0 synthetic absorbable material. Because the stay sutures are compressing hepatic parenchyma, very little hemostasis is generally required. (From JL Cameron. Resection of a Proximal Cholangiocarcinoma with Reconstruction Utilizing Silastic Transhepatic Biliary Stents and Bilateral Hepaticojejunostomies. In JL Cameron [ed.], Atlas of Surgery, Vol 1. Toronto: Decker, 1990. Reproduced with permission.)

be easily externalized to treat biliary sepsis, which frequently accompanies the advanced stages of this disease. Expandable metallic endoprostheses have recently become popular in the management of unresectable biliary malignant tumors, since such stents are entirely internal and have prolonged patency (often exceeding life expectancy).

In patients who do undergo abdominal exploration for attempted surgical resection but are found to have unresectable tumors, there are two options. In patients with widespread intraperitoneal tumor, minimal operative manipulation should be performed. Transhepatic catheters placed preoperatively are left in position for palliation of biliary obstruction. A cholecystectomy should be performed to prevent the development of acute cholecystitis from cystic duct obstruction from tumor or related to the in-dwelling catheter. Postoperatively, the transhepatic catheter can be exchanged fluoroscopically for a larger diameter soft Silastic catheter or a metallic endoprosthesis.

In patients with locally advanced, unresectable tumor at the porta hepatis, a biliary enteric bypass can be performed. A cholecystectomy is performed and the bile duct distal to the tumor is divided. The malignant stricture can be dilated using progressively larger coudé catheters, and eventually a Silastic transhepatic stent is positioned into the right and left ductal systems. A choledochojejunostomy to a Roux-en-Y jejunal limb is completed. The advantages to this approach over simply leaving the percutaneous stents include: 1) removal of the gallbladder, 2) placement of larger stents, and 3) positioning the stents into a Roux-en-Y jejunal limb. Although it is difficult to document, larger stents that drain into a defunctionalized limb of jejunum should reduce the incidence of cholangitis.

Postoperative Care

The Silastic transhepatic stents are left to dependent bile bag drainage for 5 days after the operation. At that time, cholangiography is performed through the stent. If there are no leaks at the site of the anastomosis or at the exit site of the stent at the top of the liver, the stent can be internalized, and thus allow biliary drainage to return to the GI tract. If, at the initial post-

lignant obstruction, proximal cholangiocarcinomas at the bifurcation usually require intubation of both the right and left ducts to avoid complications of recurrent cholangitis or liver abscess, or both. Therefore, percutaneous transhepatic catheters provide the best long-term palliation for inoperable hilar cholangiocarcinomas. These catheters are readily exchangeable in the event of catheter sludging and can

operative cholangiography, a bile leak is demonstrated, dependent external drainage should be maintained until cholangiography subsequently demonstrates complete healing. Whenever biliary anastomotic integrity can be confirmed on cholangiography, and there has been 24 hours of internal drainage without demonstration of bile leakage via the closed suction drains, the drains can be removed. After internalization of the stents, the patient should be instructed in irrigating the stent two to three times a day with 10 to 20 cc of a sterile saline solution.

In patients with proximal biliary carcinomas, the stents are generally left in place permanently. After hospital discharge, the stents should be changed periodically with fluoroscopic guidance to prevent side hole occlusion with resultant cholangitis. The stents are generally changed fluoroscopically over a guidewire on an outpatient basis. The role of long-term antibiotics for suppression of infection has not been proven. However, in many patients with a persistent or recurrent tumor, episodes of cholangitis can be frequent, and therefore, periodic courses of antibiotics can be useful in avoiding hospitalization.

Adjuvant Therapy

The use of chemotherapy alone, using 5-fluorouracil, and other drugs has not been known to improve survival in patients with resected or unresected proximal biliary cancers. Radiation therapy has been evaluated by many investigators using a variety of methods including external beam radiotherapy, intraoperative radiotherapy, internal radiotherapy, and radioimmunotherapy. External beam therapy is most frequently delivered through multiple fields with a total dose of 50 to 60 Gy. Internal radiotherapy is normally delivered by percutaneous or endoscopically placed biliary stents, using [192]iridium, or [60]cobalt as the radiation source. Radiotherapy has been thought to be useful in this disease because of the high incidence of microscopic tumor found at the resection margins and the tendency of the tumor to invade through the ductal wall into the surrounding portal structures. Prospective trials designed to evaluate the role of radiation as an adjuvant are currently underway. A troublesome complication of

duodenal obstruction from severe postradiation peptic ulceration has been noted in a number of series.

Results

Survival for patients with proximal cholangiocarcinoma is highly dependent on whether they are treated by palliative stenting or tumor resection. At the Johns Hopkins Hospital between 1973 and 1989, 96 patients with such tumors were operated on with curative intent. At the time of laparotomy, disseminated tumor was identified in 15 percent of patients, 30 percent had locally unresectable tumor, and the remaining 55 percent were initially believed to be resectable. At the end of the resection, 14 of these 53 patients had gross tumor remaining, and 39 of the 53 patients were believed to have undergone curative resection. Eight of these 39 patients had a hepatic lobectomy added to their bifurcation resection. Postoperative mortality was 4 percent. All deaths resulted from biliary sepsis. Postoperative radiation therapy with a total dose of 50 to 60 Gy was delivered to 63 patients (66%). In addition, internal radiotherapy using ^{192}Ir was delivered via Silastic transhepatic stents to the area of the hepaticojejunostomy with a total boosting dose of 20 Gy. The 1-, 2-, 5-, and 10-year actuarial survivals for all 96 patients were 49 percent, 20 percent, 15 percent, and 2 percent, respectively. Considering only these 53 patients treated by resection, the 39 patients who were completely resected had an increased survival rate compared with the 14 patients who underwent only a partial resection (Fig. 102-6). The partially resected patients had a course similar to that of the patients undergoing palliative stenting alone.

During this time period, 65 patients with unresectable proximal biliary carcinomas from the Johns Hopkins Hospital were treated for biliary obstruction. Twenty-one patients were managed completely nonoperatively, and 44 underwent a laparotomy. The mean survival in the nonoperative group was 5 months and in the operative group 8 months. There was

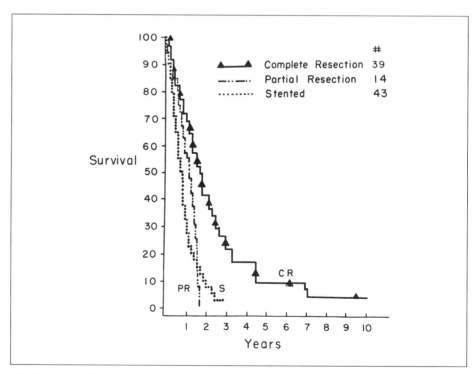

Fig. 102-6. Actuarial survival curves for patients undergoing partial and complete tumor resection. Patients undergoing partial resection followed a clinical course closer to patients who were merely stented than to patients undergoing complete resection. (From JL Cameron, HA Pitt, MJ Zinner, et al. Management of proximal cholangiocarcinomas by surgical resection and radiotherapy. Am J Surg 159:91, 1990. Reproduced with permission.)

a significant difference in survival at 6 months when comparing the nonoperative group (30%) with the operative group (64%). The incidence of cholangitis following initial treatment was 50 percent in each of the two groups. There were no differences between the two groups in the number of readmissions to the hospital, however, there were fewer unscheduled emergency stent changes in the operative group than in the nonoperated group. These results tend to favor an operative approach to patients with unresectable hilar carcinoma. However, these differences might reflect bias and patient selection in this retrospective analysis.

The role of postoperative radiation therapy for perihilar cholangiocarcinoma was recently evaluated in a prospective, nonrandomized study of patients managed at the Johns Hopkins Hospital between 1988 and 1993. Fifty patients with localized disease were considered eligible for postoperative radiation therapy. Thirty-one of these patients (62%) had complete or partial tumor resection, whereas 19 patients (38%) had undergone palliative surgical procedures. Surgical resection improved the length of survival compared with patients undergoing surgical palliation (24.2 ± 2.5 vs. 11.3 ± 1.0 mo, p < 0.05). Furthermore, survival quality as determined by standard quality of life measurements was improved in patients undergoing resection. Radiation therapy, however, did not improve survival in patients undergoing resection or palliation. The mean survival in resected patients receiving postoperative radiation therapy was 23.9 ± 4.4 months vs. 24.5 ± 3.3 months in patients not receiving radiation therapy. In patients receiving palliative therapy, postoperative radiation therapy also had no effect on mean survival (9.8 ± 1.4 vs. 12.7 ± 1.3 mo). There was no difference in quality of life or late toxicity in either the resected or the palliated patients receiving radiation therapy. This prospective study suggests that postoperative radiation therapy has no effect on either length or quality of survival. Therefore, to improve outcome, newer agents or strategies to deliver adjuvant therapy are needed.

Suggested Reading

Bengmark S, Ekberg H, Evander A, et al. Major liver resection for hilar cholangiocarcinoma. *Ann Surg* 207:120, 1988.

Bismuth H, Nakache R, Diamond T. Management strategies in resection for hilar cholangiocarcinoma. *Ann Surg* 215:31, 1992.

Cameron JL. Resection of a proximal cholangiocarcinoma with reconstruction using Silastic transhepatic biliary stents and bilateral hepaticojejunostomies. In JL Cameron (ed.), *Atlas of Surgery*, Vol 1. Toronto: Decker, 1990.

Cameron JL, Broe P, Zuidema GD. Proximal bile duct tumors: Surgical management with Silastic transhepatic biliary stents. *Ann Surg* 196:412, 1982.

Cameron JL, Gayler BW, Zuidema GD. The use of Silastic transhepatic stents in benign and malignant biliary strictures. *Ann Surg* 188:552, 1978.

Cameron JL, Pitt HA, Zinner MJ, et al. Management of proximal cholangiocarcinoma by surgical resection and radiotherapy. *Am J Surg* 159:9198, 1990.

Crist DW, Kadir S, Cameron JL. Proximal biliary tract reconstruction: The value of preoperatively placed percutaneous biliary catheters. *Surg Gynecol Obstet* 165:421, 1987.

Iwatsuki S, Gordon RD, Shaw BW, et al. Role of liver transplantation in cancer therapy. *Ann Surg* 202:401, 1985.

Klatskin G. Adenocarcinoma of the hepatic duct at its bifurcation within the porta hepatis. An unusual tumor with distinctive clinical and pathologic features. *Am J Med* 38:241, 1965.

Nagorney DM, Donohue JH, Farnell MB, et al. Outcomes after curative resections of cholangiocarcinoma. *Arch Surg* 128:871, 1993.

Nimura Y, Hayakawa N, Kamiya J, et al. Hepatic segmentectomy with caudate lobe resection for bile duct carcinoma of the hepatic hilus. *World J Surg* 14:535, 1990.

Norback IH, Coleman JA, Venbrux A, et al. Palliative treatment of biliary obstruction in unresectable hilar cholangiocarcinoma. *Surgery* 115:597, 1994.

Pitt HA, Nakeeb A, Abrams RA, et al. Perihilar cholangiocarcinoma: Postoperative radiotherapy does not improve survival. *Ann Surg* 221:788, 1995.

Yeo CJ, Pitt HA, Cameron JC. Cholangiocarcinoma. *Surg Clin North Am* 70:1429, 1990.

EDITOR'S COMMENT

Doctor Lillemoe is correct in that my predecessor, Dr. Altemeier, should receive credit for the description of what is now known as Klatskin tumor. However, there were three authors and not a single author, and so the tumor is referred to as the Klatskin tumor, but the priority is correct.

Once the tumor is identified, various steps in management continue to be controversial. Preoperative decompression has been argued for well over 15 years. I am aware of no study, or perhaps one, in which decompression was combined with preoperative preparation and nutritional support in which any difference in outcome was seen. Most studies fail to reveal any difference in outcome. The exception to this rule, as Dr. Lillemoe has pointed out, is where there are significant medical problems such as renal failure secondary to obstructive jaundice, which might remit when the jaundice is relieved, as well as a patient with long-standing obstruction, perhaps, as I have occasionally seen it, unfortunately attributed to hepatitis. Operating on a patient with prolonged biliary obstruction without drainage can result in late hepatic failure and lack of recovery even when good drainage is instituted. I believe that preoperative drainage is useful in these patients. If the bilirubin level comes down, the patient will begin to eat, feel better, and be a better operative candidate. Since these tumors are slow-growing and since, in my view, almost all of these operations are palliative because cholangiocarcinoma tends to be a multifocal disease, there is little to be lost by allowing the patient to get into shape. In the patient in whom obstruction is relieved and the bilirubin level does not go down significantly, there is seemingly (and rarely) an irreversible case of hepatic failure secondary to obstruction; these patients will die if operated on. Thus, preoperative biliary decompression might select patients who will not do well following surgery.

In all areas of liver surgery, there appears to be a dichotomy between surgeons who believe that one should know as much as possible about a patient with a liver tumor before operating, and surgeons whose attitude seems more like a "macho" approach, which is, "I don't need an angiogram to tell me what to do at the time of surgery." While I admire the technical expertise of individuals who do not prefer angiography, I believe it is a surgeon's obligation to know as much as possible about the local situation with the patient before an operation. The operative procedure will be shortened because the decision-making process will have been aided by preoperative angiography and a valid estimation of the anatomic situation. Ego should not get in the way of doing the best possible thing for the patient.

Finally, the combination of hepatic lobectomy in association with resection of the bifurcation is a technical tour de force. Lobectomy is relatively safe now and has a hospital mortality of 1 to 4 percent, depending on the patient population. However, it is my impression that patients who undergo lobectomy for cholangiocarcinoma rarely survive without recurrence. However, the median life expectancy for resection has increased from approximately 9 months to 24 to 25 months, not an insubstantial increase.

J.E.F.

103

Cholecystojejunostomy and Choledochojejunostomy

Herbert R. Freund   Yacov Berlatzky

Cholecystojejunostomy

In recent years, some promising data have been published concerning curative surgery of carcinoma of the pancreas. The operative mortality of pancreatoduodenectomy, reported recently, ranges below 3 to 5 percent and morbidity dropped to 25 to 30 percent. Even in nonmajor referral centers, operative mortality (7–10%) and morbidity (30–45%) are significantly reduced. Five-year survival rates are approaching 12 to 24 percent for patients undergoing curative resection compared with a 6-month survival average for patients undergoing bypass surgery or stent endoscopic retrograde cholangiopancreatography [ERCP] or percutaneous transhepatic cholangiography [PTC] procedures. However, in various large reports, only 5 to 22 percent of patients have resectable pancreatic tumors, the remaining requiring some sort of palliation for relief of jaundice, actual or pending duodenal obstruction, or pain.

Decompression of the biliary tract obstructed by malignant periampullar lesions is indicated for the relief of obstructive jaundice and its ensuing severe and often intolerable pruritus. Three viable options are available today for the palliation of obstructive jaundice caused by periampullary malignant lesions in patients whose disease was determined to be unresectable:

1. Percutaneous transhepatic external or internal permanent catheter drainage of the biliary system.

2. Endoscopic papillotomy with insertion of an internal biliary-duodenal stent-catheter.
3. Operative biliary-enteric bypass by either cholecysto-or choledochojejunostomy with or without a gastroenteric bypass.

Without getting into the yet unresolved dispute whether roentgenographic or endoscopic stents are superior to a biliary-enteric surgical bypass, we believe that a surgical biliary-enteric bypass has a viable role in the palliation of patients with periampullary carcinomas, particularly in younger, more fit patients who are likely to survive a reasonable length of time. These patients are also the ones in whom an additional gastrojejunostomy is advocated for actual or pending mechanical duodenal obstruction. Because comparable postoperative morbidity and mortality have been reported following "double bypass" or biliary diversion only, we routinely perform a "double bypass," namely, a cholecysto-, choledocho-, or hepaticojejunostomy and a gastrojejunostomy.

The use of the gallbladder for internal biliary drainage is quick, simple, effective and safe, and is the biliary conduit of choice when the cystic duct is patent and enters the common duct well away from the tumor mass. The gallbladder should not be used if it is previously diseased (chronic cholecystitis or cholecystolithiasis, or both), or when the cystic duct is narrow or enters the common duct close to the tumor. In such situations, the common hepatic duct is the preferred conduit for bypass, and the gallbladder is to be re-

moved. When creating a cholecystojejunostomy, a loop of jejunum is the preferred enteric component of the bypass, whereas with a hepaticojejunostomy, the Roux en Y technique is applied.

Cholecystojejunostomy with a simple loop bypass is almost exclusively used in patients who were operated on for cure and found to have locally advanced disease, possibly liver metastases or peritoneal implants. The first loop of jejunum that easily and comfortably reaches the subhepatic space is passed in an antecolic manner without tension and approximated to the gallbladder with a posterior row of seromuscular interrupted silk (4–0 or 3–0) sutures (Fig. 103-1A, B). On the jejunum, the sutures are placed parallel and adjacent to the edge of the mesenterium. Using electrocautery, an incision as long as possible, is made in the body of the gallbladder, the bile evacuated and sent for culture. A similar, but a bit shorter incision is made on the antimesenteric part of the approximated jejunum (Fig. 103-1B). Beginning in the middle and suturing toward the corners, the full thickness of the gallbladder and of the jejunum are anastomosed with 3–0 or 4–0 monofilament absorbable interrupted sutures. This creates the posterior wall of the anastomosis with all sutures tied on the inside (Fig. 103-1C). Turning both corners, sutures are placed from both sides of the anterior wall with ties on the inside (Fig. 103-1C). The last sutures on the anterior wall (simple or gumby sutures) are all placed before tying them with their knots on the outside (Fig. 103-1D). We rarely approximate the anterior serosal layer, although, if the gallbladder is big

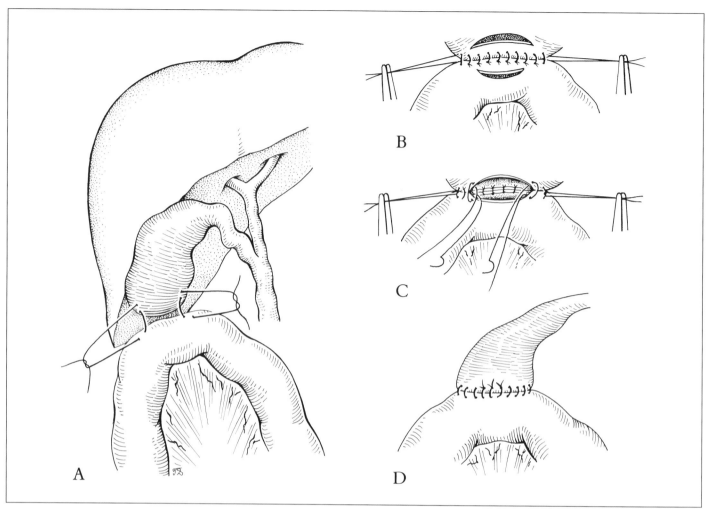

Fig. 103-1. Side-to-side cholecystojejunostomy. A. The first loop of jejunum is approximated to the gallbladder with a posterior row of interrupted silk sutures, which is seen completed in B. B. Following completion of the posterior layer, both jejunum and gallbladder are incised and opened to the maximal length possible to create a good size anastomosis. C. A full thickness posterior wall anastomosis between jejunum and gallbladder is constructed with the sutures tied on the inside and continued in a similar manner on the anterior part of the anastomosis. D. The last sutures of the anterior wall are all tied on the outside to complete the cholecystojejunostomy.

enough and redundant, it could be done. In our experience, leakage from a cholecystojejunostomy is extremely rare, but we still leave a closed suction drainage for 3 to 4 days. It is our practice to always add a small, sutured, or stapled (GIA) gastrojejunostomy distal to the cholecystojejunostomy.

Recent advances in laparoscopic surgery make it possible to safely perform the double bypass procedure laparoscopically. The procedure requires advanced laparoscopy skills and suturing capabilities. It takes longer to accomplish than the traditional "open technique," but results in reduced

operative injury and possibly in a shorter and easier postoperative course and more rapid convalescence.

Choledochojejunostomy

The main indications for a choledochojejunostomy are benign biliary strictures and malignant obstruction of the biliary system caused by pancreatic or duct wall tumors. Rare indications for choledochojejunostomy are direct trauma to the biliary system and select instances of sclerosing cholangitis in which areas of dilatation occur. Because biliary tract strictures are essentially iatrogenic in 97 percent of instances and each unsuccessful repair poses increased morbidity and mortality, reconstruction should restore long-lasting primary functional and anatomic integrity.

Preoperative Evaluation

The diagnosis should be established, and the anatomy of the biliary duct system and the nature and location of the obstruction should be characterized by percutaneous transhepatic cholangiography, endoscopic retrograde cholangiography, or both. At

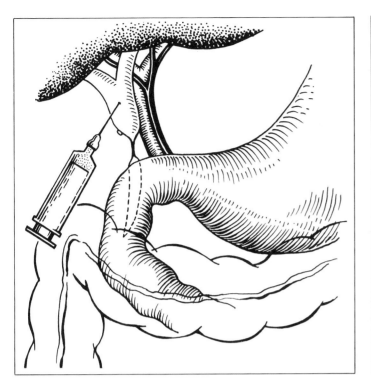

Fig. 103-2. *The location of the hepatic artery to the left of the common duct and exploratory aspirations with a fine needle are of great assistance in locating the common duct.*

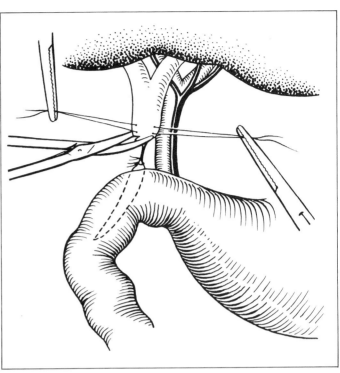

Fig. 103-3. *The distal part of the duct is doubly ligated, and the proximal part is trimmed to achieve maximal diameter, good blood supply, and viable duct tissue.*

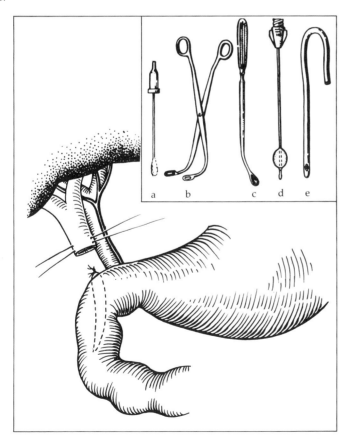

Fig. 103-4. *After opening the common duct, a bile specimen is sent for culture (a); the duct is cleaned out by forceps (b), scoops (c), or Fogarty catheter (d), and is irrigated (e).*

the same time, jaundiced patients can undergo drainage by either a percutaneous catheter or an endoprosthesis. The presence of such catheters, although reported to carry an increased operative morbidity, is a tremendous help for the surgeon exploring a previously damaged or transected ductal system, particularly if this attempt to repair is not the first.

If no stent is placed during surgery, the transhepatic catheter might eventually be left in place during an operation and removed only after the safety and patency of the anastomosis are proved by injection of contrast material 1 to 2 weeks following repair.

Preoperative Preparation

Most patients who require a choledochojejunostomy have experienced cholangitis and jaundice, and should therefore receive antibiotics, parenteral vitamin K, and fresh frozen plasma perioperatively. Nutritional support should be offered when and where indicated. We have found that most patients with a diseased biliary system have infected bile, the most common pathogens being *Escherichia coli*, *Klebsiella*, and streptococci. However, because many of these patients have had previous biliary tract operations and interventions, infections with hospital-acquired or resistant bacteria should be considered in the choice of antibiotics. Our preference is the combination of gentamicin and ampicillin, amikacin and ampicillin, or a third-generation cephalosporin. Because the colon can be densely adherent to the gallbladder bed and liver, requiring meticulous separation, bowel preparation is advised.

Surgical Procedure

The biliary tract can be approached through a right subcostal or a right paramedian incision. However, the best possible exposure is offered by the bilateral subcostal, better known as the "Buckethandle," incision. Figure 103-2 indicates the anatomic situation following release of adhesions, dissection of the area of the hepatoduodenal ligament, and kocherization of the duodenum. It is important at this stage to perform meticulous dissection of the area between the undersurface of the right lobe of the liver and the duodenum. Sometimes, aspiration with a 25-gauge needle attached to a syringe can be helpful in locating the dilated common duct. Recently favorable results have been reported with intraoperative sonographic detection of dilated common ducts, ductal stones, and pancreatic tumors. In dissecting out the common bile duct, the hepatic artery lying to its left is an important anatomic landmark (see Fig. 103-2). However, one should be aware of the fact that this "textbook" arrangement of the common hepatic artery originating from the celiac trunk, firing off the left and right hepatic arteries is found in only 55 percent of instances. In 45 percent of patients, variations in the hepatic arterial supply exist. Of particular importance in this respect is the right hepatic artery arising from the superior mesenteric artery, which usually passes to the liver along the right side of the portal vein and the common bile and common hepatic ducts. Also frequent are anatomic variations in the extrahepatic biliary tree, most of them related to the confluence of the right and left hepatic ducts and of the cystic duct with the common hepatic duct.

Once the common duct has been identified, two traction sutures (4–0 silk) are placed through the dilated common-duct wall just above the stricture. The common duct is ligated below the stricture with two 00 silk ligatures and is divided below the traction sutures (Fig. 103-3). The proximal end of the common duct is trimmed to achieve maximal diameter, good blood supply, and viable duct tissue for anastomosis. Because the common hepatic and

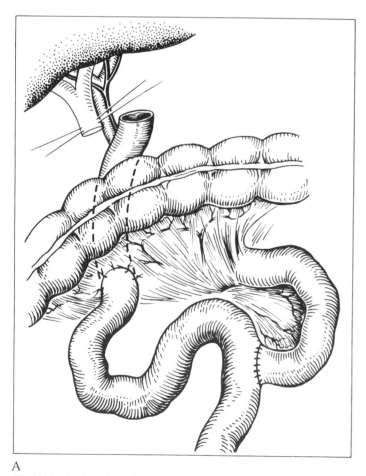

A

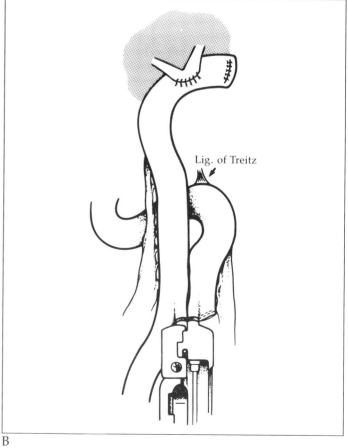

B

Fig. 103-5. A. The end-to-side anastomosis of the Roux-en-Y is constructed, and the ascending limb of jejunum measuring approximately 45 cm is brought through the mesocolon toward the severed common duct. B. The construction of a Roux-en-Y enteroenterostomy using the GIA stapler and the completed end-to-side hepaticojejunostomy.

upper common bile ducts depend on two axial arteries located along the lateral and medial borders of the ducts, undue mobilization and dissection should be avoided to ensure good blood supply to the anastomotic site.

Once the biliary system is opened, a bile specimen is sent for culture and sensitivity testing (Fig. 103-4, inset a). Next, stones and debris are evacuated using Randall forceps (b), scoops (c), or a biliary Fogarty balloon catheter (d). After removal of stones, the duct system is irrigated with copious amounts of saline solution through a No. 8 or 10 French soft rubber catheter (e).

The first jejunal loop adjacent to the ligament of Treitz that comfortably reaches the subhepatic space is used to create a Roux-en-Y conduit. It is divided, using the GIA stapler, and the distal part of it is brought through a window in the transverse mesocolon toward the severed common duct. The proximal afferent loop is sutured in a one- or two-layer end-to-side manner to the ascending limb of defunctionalized jejunum (Fig. 103-5A), or is stapled with a GIA stapling instrument (Fig. 103-5B). The ascending limb is anchored to the mesocolon with few 000 silk sutures to avoid internal hernias. Care should be taken to use a limb of intestine 45 to 75 cm long between the biliary-enteric and the Roux-en-Y anastomosis to avoid reflux of gastrointestinal content and resulting cholangitis (Fig. 103-5A, B).

When dealing with benign biliary tract strictures, two kinds of anastomoses are commonly used. A greatly dilated biliary system is amenable to an end-to-end choledochojejunal anastomosis. This anastomosis is performed with one layer of interrupted 00 or 000 synthetic absorbable sutures (mono- or polyfilament), which offer favorable tissue drag, elasticity, and gradual loss of tensile strength. First to be placed are the two corners (Fig. 103-6A, a and b) and center (Fig. 103-6A, c) sutures of the posterior anastomotic wall. Each such interrupted suture is tied and used as a holding suture. The rest of the posterior wall is completed with sutures placed every 3 mm, care being taken to include the full thickness of both jejunum and common duct. The knots of the posterior wall are all tied inside toward the lumen (Fig. 103-6B).

The anterior wall of the end-to-end anastomosis is constructed in a similar manner. Starting on each corner, sutures are placed in an inside-outside–outside-inside manner so as to position the knots inside the lumen, gradually working from both sides toward the center (Fig. 103-6C). The last sutures in the center of the anterior wall are placed to be tied on the outside. These sutures are all placed before being tied to achieve secure closure and to avoid damage to the posterior wall (Fig. 103-6D). When doing an end-to-end anastomosis, we find it unnecessary to stent the stoma by a T-tube or any other kind of prosthesis.

More commonly performed is the end-to-side mucosa-to-mucosa choledochojejunostomy or hepatojejunostomy, which facilitates adjusting the size of the anastomosis to the diameter of the bile duct (Fig. 103-7). It is our conviction that all mucosa biliary-enteric anastomoses should be performed under magnification. The proximal end of the jejunal limb, which was stapled by the GIA stapler, is secured with a second layer of 000 silk su-

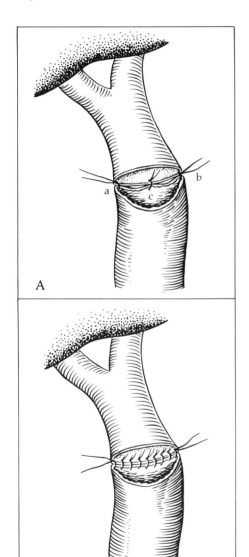

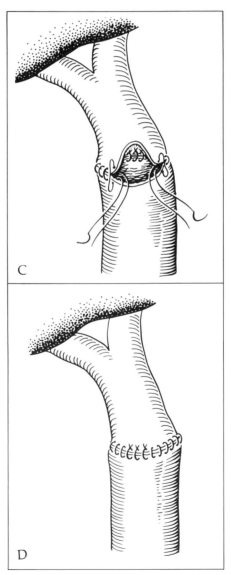

Fig. 103-6. Construction of an end-to-end biliary-enteric anastomosis in a very dilated biliary system. A. Placing of the first anchoring sutures. B. The knots of the posterior wall are all placed inside toward the lumen, 2 to 3 mm apart. C. Note the inside-outside-outside-inside sutures when advancing toward the anterior wall. D. The last sutures in the center of the anterior wall are knotted on the outside.

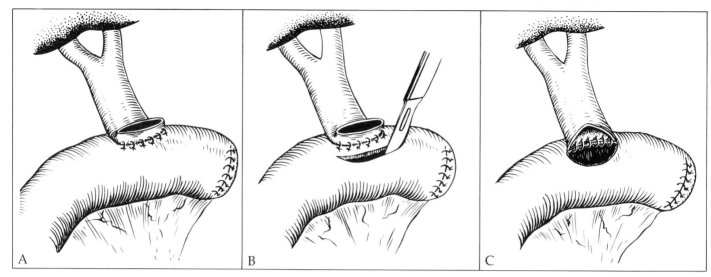

Fig. 103-7. *Construction of an end-to-side choledochojejunostomy. The proximal end of jejunum is closed. A. Seromuscular layer of posterior wall, for approximation and anchoring. B. Construction of a longitudinal opening on the antimesenteric part of intestine. C. Inner layer of the posterior wall using full thickness of duct and intestine with mucosa-to-mucosa approximation.*

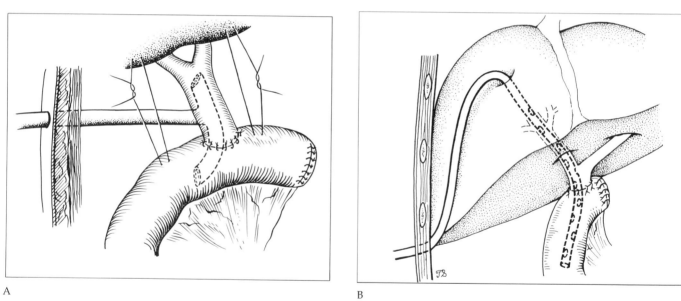

Fig. 103-8. *A. If required, a loosely fitting T-tube can be inserted through anterior wall of bile duct and passed through the biliary-enteric anastomosis into the intestine. The vertical portion of the T-tube is passed through a separate incision in the abdominal wall. The jejunal limb is anchored by two sutures to the undersurface of the liver or to surrounding structures. B. Another option to stent a biliary-enteric anastomosis is to pass a long silicone tube with several holes cut along it through the liver into the biliary ductal system and past the anastomosis into the intestine.*

tures (Fig. 103-7). Approximately 5 cm proximal to this closure, on the antimesenteric aspect of the intestine, a one-layer biliary-enteric anastomosis is constructed. The seromuscular layer of the bile duct and the jejunum serosa might be approximated by a few or 4–0 silk sutures (Fig. 103-7A). Using electrocoagulation, the jejunum is opened longitudinally to accommodate the width of the bile duct (Fig. 103-7B). The inner layer of the posterior wall is placed next, using interrupted 3–0 or 4–0 synthetic absorbable (preferably monofilament) sutures (Fig. 103-7C). Starting in the middle of the posterior wall, sutures are placed on alternate sides until reaching the anterior wall with just 2 or 3 sutures yet unplaced in the center of the anterior wall. The last few sutures are tied only after all of them have been placed with their knots on the outside. Meticulous mucosa-to-mucosa approximation without tension is of prime importance for a safe and long-lasting patent anastomosis.

This anastomosis is rarely stented, particularly in a small caliber duct, in difficult repairs or with thin-walled bile ducts, to prevent postoperative stricturing of the

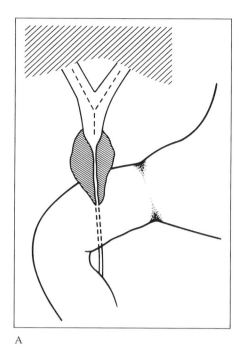

A

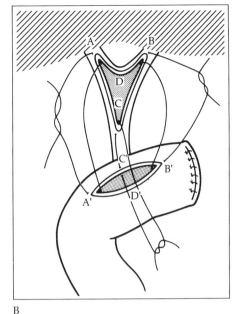

B

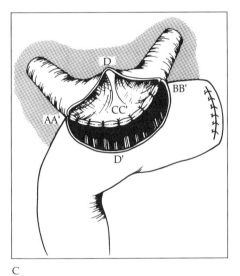

C

Fig. 103-9. A. The Y-shaped incision is made above the point of obstruction with two arms extending into the right and left hepatic ducts and the third arm extending into the common hepatic or if feasible even the common bile ducts. B. A longitudinal incision is performed in the defunctionalized loop of jejunum. The Y-shaped incision opens up into a three-angled opening. The posterior layer of the hepatocholedochojejunostomy is constructed by first attaching points A to A', B to B', and C to C'. C. The posterior layer of the hepatocholedochojejunostomy is completed. The anterior layer will be fashioned by attaching D to D' and then suturing of the rest of the distance between AA' and BB'.

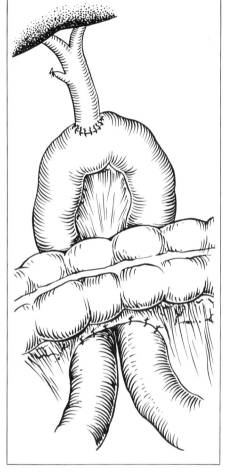

Fig. 103-10. End-to-side choledochojejunostomy using a loop of proximal small intestine.

anastomosis. If needed, our preference is a T-tube with its short arm in the bile duct and the long one in the lumen of the intestine (Fig. 103-8A). The loosely fitting T-tube should be brought out through a stab wound in the anterior wall of the bile duct, if possible. Bringing out the T-tube limb through a small incision in the jejunal loop is less desirable because it can be dislodged by intestinal peristalsis. The external limb of the T-tube should never be passed through the anastomotic line. The long vertical portion of the T-tube is brought out through a separate stab wound in the abdominal wall (Fig. 103-8A) and should have some intra-abdominal re-

dundancy to prevent traction on the tube if the patient becomes distended. Another option to stent the biliary-enteric anastomosis is to pass a long silicone tube with many holes cut along it via the liver into the biliary system and through the anastomosis (Fig. 103-8B). After placement of the T-tube or the long silicone tube, the anterior half of the anastomosis is completed in a similar manner with interrupted 3–0 or 4–0 sutures. Again, care should be taken to meticulously approximate mucosa to mucosa. At the completion of the anastomosis, the jejunal limb should be anchored to surrounding structures, mainly the hepatoduodenal ligament and capsule of the

liver at the hilus, to avoid unnecessary tension on the biliary-enteric anastomosis (Fig. 103-8A).

If the biliary ductal system is narrow, we advocate the use of the side-to-side Y-type biliary-enteric bypass (hepatocholedochojejunostomy). A Y-shaped opening is made with two arms extending into the right and left hepatic ducts and the third arm extending longitudinally into the common hepatic and common bile ducts. All limbs of the Y-shaped incision should be as long as possible (Fig. 103-9A). A 2- to 3-cm longitudinal incision is performed in the jejunal loop brought up to the hilus

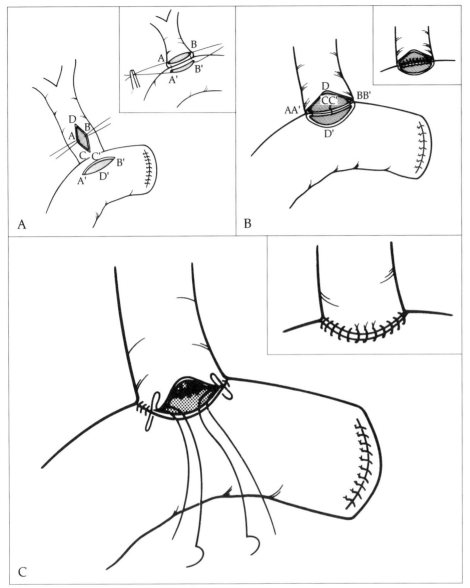

Fig. 103-11. Side-to-side choledochojejunostomy. A. The longitudinal incisions in the common duct and adjacently placed loop of excluded jejunum are converted by placing two anchor sutures into transverse incisions (inset). The diameter of the anastomosis should be made as large as possible, depending on the size of available common duct. B. The posterior wall of the choledochojejunostomy is initiated by placing the corner (AA' and BB') and center (CC') sutures. The posterior wall is a one- or two-layer anastomosis of interrupted synthetic absorbable sutures 2 to 3 mm apart (inset). C. The anterior wall is sewn by interrupted inside-outside–outside-inside sutures. The last sutures in the center of the anterior wall are placed and knotted on the outside (inset).

of the liver, care being taken not to open too much mucosa (Fig. 103-9B). A one-layer biliary-enteric anastomosis is constructed with 4–0 or 5–0 monofilament synthetic absorbable sutures. The posterior layer is created by first attaching points A to A', B to B', and C to C' (Fig. 103-9B), and the rest of the posterior wall is completed with sutures placed approx-

imately every 2 mm (Fig. 103-9C). The anterior layer is created by attaching D to D' and suturing the rest of the distance between AA' and BB'. The completed anastomosis should be anchored with a few sutures to the hilus and capsule of the liver.

By patching the jejunum into the widest area of a narrow biliary ductal system,

namely, at the confluence of the right, left, and common hepatic ducts, a wide-open and effective biliary-enteric anastomosis is achieved.

When dealing with malignant obstructions of the biliary system, for which a bypass procedure seems advisable, we tend to use a simpler and less time-consuming biliary-enteric anastomosis. Either the dilated common duct proximal to the site of obstruction is divided and anastomosed in an end-to-side manner to the first loop of jejunum (Fig. 103-10), or an even simpler side-to-side choledochojejunostomy can be fashioned (Fig. 103-11). Both procedures can be performed as a one- or two-layer anastomosis, depending on the diameter and wall thickness of the common duct (Figs. 103-10 and 103-11). These two techniques of choledochojejunostomy offer better decompression and drainage of the biliary tract than does a cholecystojejunostomy and are thus preferable if the general condition of the patient and the local findings during the operation make it feasible. As a rule, we do not stent this anastomosis. In most of these patients we advocate the addition of a gastrointestinal bypass to avoid subsequent gastric outlet obstruction.

Postoperative Care

A closed system soft drain is placed in the foramen of Winslow and brought out through the abdominal wall, to be removed approximately 5 to 7 days after the operation. If there is leakage of bile, the drain is left in place as long as necessary. Almost all such biliary fistulas close within 2 to 3 weeks. We use nasogastric suction and intravenous therapy for 3 to 5 days, depending on the general condition of the patient and the resumption of peristalsis and bowel movement. Antibiotic treatment is continued for 3 to 5 days and is adjusted in accordance with the cultures obtained during the operation.

EDITOR'S COMMENT

Doctors Freund and Berlatzky have provided a series of techniques for dealing with a most difficult area, the right upper quadrant. As patients get older and as evaluative procedures improve, it is inevitable that more and more bypass procedures will be performed to the common duct. Although some surgeons have advocated endoscopic stenting, my experience with endoscopic stenting in patients with carcinoma, either as preparation or as definitive therapy, is such that a good part of the time the stent slips and the jaundice does not abate. A cholecystojejunostomy is rather quick and easy, and, if the patient is not in good condition and if the life expectancy is short, when combined with a gastric bypass should remediate the patient's condition quite easily and efficaciously.

For the more complicated procedures, I prefer a transverse incision if the patient is of the proper habitus. If the costal angle is narrow, one will probably have to use a vertical incision. The advantages of a transverse incision are comfort and cosmesis. In addition, transverse incisions rarely disrupt unless they become infected, and the hernia incidence is quite a bit lower than it is for the other incisions described.

There are a few technical points in my own practice that are somewhat different than those of Drs. Freund and Berlatzky. Although stapling is useful for the end of the Roux-en-Y, most stapling devices are not hemostatic. An occasional bleed from the end of the staple has made it my practice to oversew the staple line with an underrunning continuous suture of 4–0 absorbable suture followed by a second row of Lemberts to turn in the staple line. A few nonabsorbable sutures complete this effort; it does not take long, and the nonabsorbable sutures provide a handle. The stapled anastomosis at the lower end of the Roux-en-Y is usually quite awkward and lends itself to intestinal obstruction, as pointed out elsewhere in my comments in this volume. It is far better to do a sutured anastomosis in an antimesenteric manner, because the Roux-en-Y will lie better.

In Fig. 103-6, the last sutures in segment D are tied externally. It is certainly possible to use a Connell suture as the last suture and reinforce it with a small serosal suture. The technique described by Drs. Freund and Berlatzky is certainly adequate, but it is not my practice.

There is the controversy concerning stenting or not stenting of biliary reconstructions, which unfortunately are becoming more rather than less common as the learning curves of laparoscopic cholecystectomy continue. The sine qua non of an excellent repair is a good mucosa-to-mucosa anastomosis with an adequate blood supply, as Drs. Freund and Berlatzky have pointed out. It does appear from reading the older literature that if one stents, prolonged stenting is appropriate. The question is where to stent. My own view is that despite the argument, which I accept, that a T-tube that is placed in the intestine can be dislodged, it is possible to place a T-tube in the intestine, thus not compromising the choledochus (which may be required in the future), by taking a nonabsorbable suture and placing it through the T-tube and through the wall of the common duct. A silk suture will keep the T-tube in place for 6 to 9 months, which is what is recommended, and the duct will be stented. After that period of time, the suture generally is extruded and one can remove the T-tube.

Finally, one should not overlook the appropriateness of tube enterostomy in patients with complicated upper abdominal procedures. Many of these patients have lost weight and require nutritional support. The 4- to 7-day period of poor intake does not help the effort of these already depleted patients. A No. 12 to 14 catheter placed 20 cm from the ligament of Treitz or below the last anastomosis will help avert further weight loss.

J.E.F.

104

Operative Treatment for Choledochal Cyst

Lester W. Martin   Moritz M. Ziegler

Choledochal cysts (CDCs) are rare, with an estimated occurrence rate of 1 per 150,000 population. They can occur at any age but are most common in infants, with one-half of all patients being under 10 years of age. They occur more frequently in Asians, particularly Japanese, in whom there is no sexual predilection. In the Western hemisphere, 85 percent of patients are female.

Choledochal cysts are generally referred to as "congenital" with numerous theories proposed regarding their etiology. It is the current belief that CDCs develop secondary to an anomalous insertion of the pancreatic duct into the common bile duct proximal to the sphincter of Oddi (Fig. 104-1), instead of the normal arrangement whereby both ducts pass through the sphincter. With this anomalous insertion of the pancreatic duct proximal to the sphincter of Oddi, contraction of the sphincter forces digestive enzymes from the pancreas to reflux up into the common bile duct. These digestive enzymes then cause irritation, inflammation, and partial digestion of the wall of the bile duct, resulting in a localized weakness with subsequent dilatation of the weakened area. Some authorities believe that an extreme variant of this same mechanism might explain the entity of "idiopathic perforation of the common bile duct in the neonate." The other end of the spectrum could be the CDC that does not develop until the patient is 30 or more years of age.

Pathology

Choledochal cysts can be separated into five distinct types. Type I, which is the most common, is a localized uniform, fu-

siform dilatation of the common bile duct (Fig. 104-2). The common hepatic duct proximal to the cystic duct is only minimally dilated, and intrahepatic ducts are normal in size. Distally, the dilatation of

the duct tapers rapidly down to a normal diameter before entering the duodenum. The wall of the dilated area is greatly thickened and the mucosa severely inflamed or even completely destroyed and

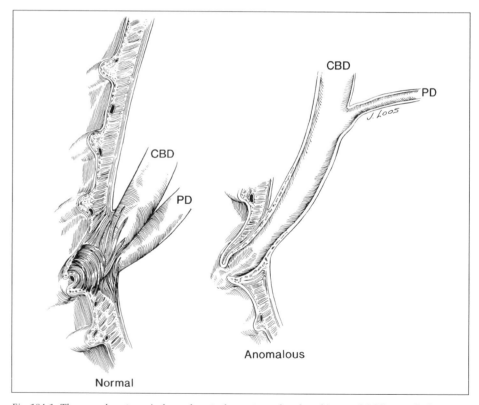

Fig. 104-1. The normal anatomy is drawn here to demonstrate that the sphincter of Oddi controls the emptying of both the common bile duct and the pancreatic duct. Both enter the duodenum together but empty independently. The anomalous entrance of the pancreatic duct into the common bile duct, proximal to the sphincter of Oddi, permits pancreatic enzymes to enter the lumen of the bile duct. Therefore, contraction of the sphincter of Oddi can cause reflux of pancreatic enzymes further proximally in the biliary ducts. The delicate bile duct mucosa, unlike that of the duodenum, contains no Brunner's glands or other means of protection from the digestive action of the pancreatic enzymes. This enzymatic digestive process leads to localized weakness of the bile duct wall and expansion to form the choledochal cyst. CBD = common bile duct. PD = pancreatic duct.

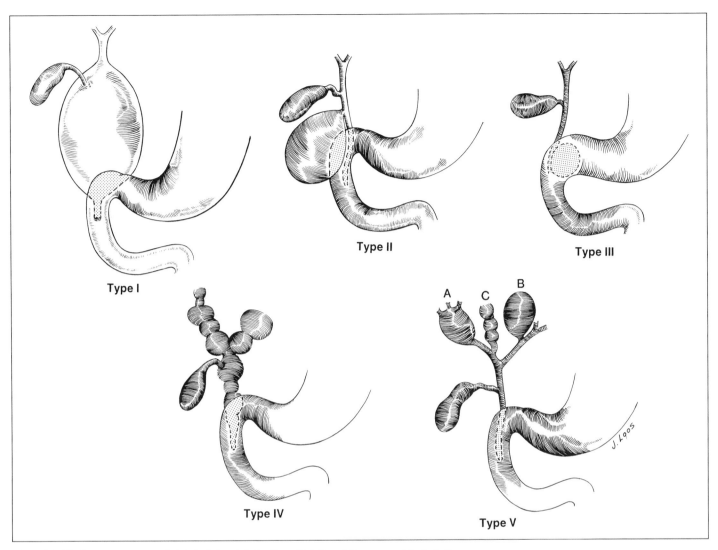

Fig. 104-2. The five common types of choledochal cyst. I. Fusiform dilatation of the common bile duct. II. Localized, almost polypoid configuration. III. Choledochocele—the weakness of the duct wall involves only the intramural portion, and the cyst protrudes into the duodenal lumen. IV. Multiple small fusiform dilatations separated by strictures—Caroli's disease. V. Intrahepatic choledochal cyst—can be of either type I, II, or IV.

replaced by granulation tissue. The gall-bladder and cystic duct can appear normal with no dilatation. The degree of cystic dilatation of the common bile duct can sometimes be extreme, and clinically the resultant abdominal distention has masqueraded as ascites, which in at least one reported instance after failure of more conservative, noninvasive measures, was erroneously treated by repeated percutaneous abdominal paracentesis. The diagnosis of CDC was not suspected before postmortem examination. The liver is usually normal except in far advanced stages of the condition.

Type II consists of a diverticulum of the wall of the bile duct (Fig. 104-2). Presumably, this type results from a localized weakness of the side of the duct wall. In this rare variety of CDC, isolated instances have been reported of a cyst attached by a pedicle to the common duct with the duct otherwise appearing normal.

Type III is a choledochocele, which consists of a dilatation of the distal end of the common duct with the dilatation protruding into the lumen of the duodenum similar in appearance and pathology to that of a ureterocele (Fig. 104-2). The dilated cho-ledochocele often contains gallstones, partially obstructs the duodenum, and often is difficult to differentiate from an intra-mural duodenal duplication. The exact pathologic physiology remains uncertain, although it would appear that any portion of the bile duct wall could become digested and weakened, even the intramural duodenal portion, which could cause the choledochocele.

Type IV, or Caroli's disease, is characterized by multiple cystic dilatations of the bile ducts, often with strictures between the cysts (Fig. 104-2). The etiology of this

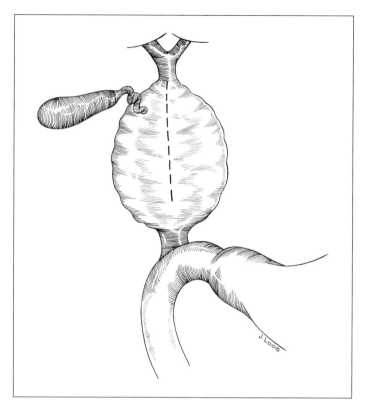

Fig. 104-3. *After obtaining a cholangiogram and a bile sample for culture and amylase determination, we prefer a longitudinal incision to provide decompression and facilitate excision of the cyst.*

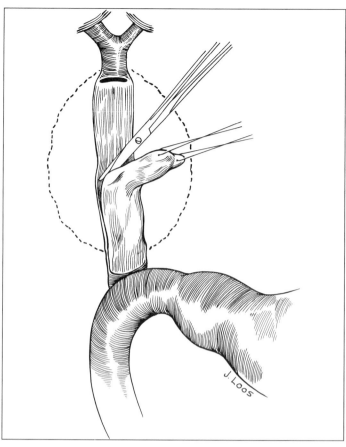

Fig. 104-4. *If the cyst is adherent to the portal vessels, the mucosa can be stripped away leaving the fibromuscular portion of the posterior cyst wall adherent to the portal vein and hepatic artery.*

extremely rare variety has not been clarified, but it is probably the same as that of types I and II.

The type V variety is entirely intrahepatic in location (Fig. 104-2) and can be fusiform, pedunculated, or of the Caroli variety with multiple cysts and strictures. The pathology, however, can be located entirely within the liver with no dilatation of the extrahepatic ducts. In fact, it would be possible for the intrahepatic variety to include examples of fusiform enlargement, tangential or pedunculated cysts, and Caroli's disease all within the same patient, although to our knowledge this situation has not been reported.

A sixth variety would be the CDC that involves the cystic duct only. We are aware of only two reported instances of CDCs involving the cystic duct only. Because of its rarity, this variety is generally not included in the usual classification. Nevertheless, its occurrence lends further credence to the

theory that when digestive enzymes from the pancreas reflux into the biliary ducts, no portion of the duct wall is immune to the digestive process.

Diagnosis

Patients with CDC typically present with the classic triad of:

1. Jaundice (often recurrent and sometimes associated with fever).
2. Abdominal pain that is generally recurrent and crampy.
3. Palpable right upper quadrant abdominal mass. The mass can also be intermittently palpable.

The CDC is sometimes associated with intermittent common duct obstruction. In fact, one of our patients was referred by a family physician because the jaundiced 8-year-old child presented to him with a

third attack of "hepatitis." He suspected an intermittent obstruction because of the associated crampy abdominal pain.

Laboratory studies are often indeterminate and of little help since the biliary obstruction is both incomplete and intermittent. Ultrasound studies are generally sufficient to confirm the diagnosis and delineate the anatomic type of choledochal malformation. Other studies including radionuclide excretions studies (DISIDA), computed tomography (CT), endoscopic retrograde cholangiopancreatography (ERCP), and percutaneous transhepatic cholangiography (PTC) can provide additional helpful anatomic detail but are not always necessary. Both oral and intravenous cholangiography have been largely replaced by contrast-enchanced CT, which can sometimes be helpful, but unless the clinician believes that additional information can be gained that would alter the treatment, it cannot be justified.

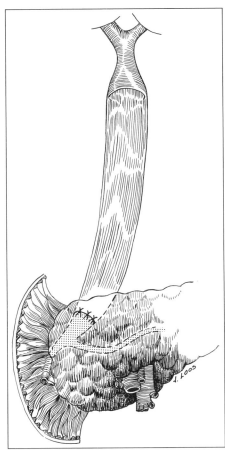

Fig. 104-5. Cyst mucosa must be removed distally beyond the point of dilatation and near to the entrance of the pancreatic duct because of the malignant potential of any residual damaged mucosa.

Associated splenomegaly can indicate portal hypertension that developed secondary to inflammation and obstruction of the portal vein caused by spread of the inflammatory process from the closely approximated inflamed CDC. Since it is possible that the associated esophageal varices could be injured by a nasogastric tube and cause bleeding, a gastrostomy should be considered as an alternate means of postoperative gastrointestinal decompression. In one of our patients several years ago, the CDC was first discovered during a shunt operation that was being performed because of recurrent bleeding from esophageal varices. Portal hypertension is reported to occur in 12 percent of patients with CDC.

Prenatal diagnosis of CDC is occurring with greater frequency associated with the expanding use of ultrasound examinations during pregnancy. The luxury of this early diagnosis provides the surgeon the opportunity to balance the degree of biliary obstruction against the overall condition of the infant in choosing the optimum time for an operation.

Treatment

Our preferred treatment for types I, II, and IV CDC is total excision of the cyst with Roux-en-Y drainage of the proximal bile ducts. There is some difference of opinion regarding type II CDC. Some authorities advise excision of the diverticular cyst only and reconstruction of the duct wall. They believe that the increased morbidity of the Roux-en-Y procedure is greater, particularly in the infant, than the risk of subsequent duct dilatation.

We prefer a transverse incision well above the umbilicus transecting both rectus abdominus muscles and extending laterally through the oblique muscles on the right side. Following operative identification of the cyst, we routinely obtain an operative cholangiogram through the gallbladder or through the cyst wall after partial decompression. A bile sample is submitted for culture and for analysis for amylase. The cholangiogram provides additional anatomic detail and roentgenographic confirmation of the anomalous high insertion of the pancreatic duct into the common duct and, therefore, helps prevent damage to the pancreatic duct during cyst excision. A generous vertical incision into the cyst accomplishes decompression and facilitates dissection of the cyst from any inflammatory adherence to the underlying hepatic artery and portal vein (Fig. 104-3). In the event of significant such adherence, it is preferable to leave the attached posterior fibromuscular wall of the cyst in place and just remove the inner layer of the cyst wall, leaving the outer layer of the posterior wall, which is adherent to the hepatic artery and portal vein (Fig. 104-4). It is important to remove all the cyst lining because of its well-known malignant potential. The gallbladder and cystic duct are removed along with the cyst. Even though the gallbladder appears normal and could be preserved, there is a reported high instance of subsequent stasis and gallstone formation when it is not removed. Dissection of the cyst mucosa is continued distally behind the pancreas to a point where it narrows down to approximately 1 cm in diameter (Fig. 104-5). Care must be taken at this point to avoid injury to the pancreatic duct, although it is generally not visualized. The distal mucosal lining of the cyst can be simply ligated, or it can be closed with inverting nonabsorbable Lembert sutures or an inverting pursestring suture. The use of nonabsorbable sutures is mandatory since absorbable sutures could be digested within only a few hours by the refluxing pancreatic enzymes. It is important that the common hepatic duct above the CDC be transected in an area well above the dilated portion and in an area where the mucosa appears normal. The surgeon must resist temptation to leave a small segment of the cyst under the mistaken belief that doing so will provide a larger lumen for the anastomosis to the intestine. This fallacious reasoning can result in late anastomotic stricture, which is the most common long-term postoperative complication of this operation. The inflamed and damaged or more often completely destroyed mucosa of this small button of residual cyst will subsequently scar down, causing the lumen to become completely obliterated. Therefore, it is necessary that the duct be transected proximal to the inflamed dilated thickened area. The anastomotic lumen can be enlarged by spatulation if desired. An attractive alternate method designed to enlarge the anastomotic lumen consists of transection of the common hepatic duct where the right and left hepatic ducts join. The lumen is then further enlarged by spatulating both sides (Fig. 104-6). This enlarged lumen will provide a better fit for an end-to-end anastomosis to the jejunal segment, which some surgeons prefer, and the greater diameter will minimize the likelihood of subsequent stricture. However, the anastomosis at this level can require extension of the laparotomy incision in order to provide adequate exposure.

We prefer to construct an isoperistaltic retrocolic Roux-en-Y limb, which in infants is approximately 15 to 20 cm in length and in older children approximately 30 to 40 cm. The entire Roux limb is passed through the surgically created defect in the transverse mesocolon, and the edges of the mesenteric defect are then sutured to the small intestinal wall at the level of the enteroenterostomy. The space behind the proximal jejunal segment is then obliterated by suturing to the posterior peritoneum to minimize the risk of subsequent

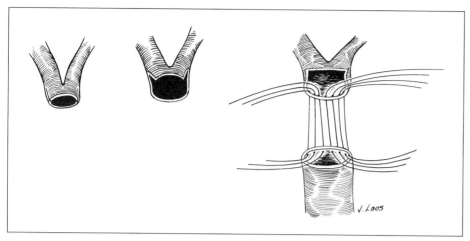

Fig. 104-6. *To enlarge the anastomotic lumen and minimize the incidence of stricture formation, some surgeons prefer to transect the hepatic duct at its bifurcation, then enlarge it further by spatulation. The diameter of the lumen can then be similar to that of the jejunum, therefore, permitting a safe end-to-end anastomosis.*

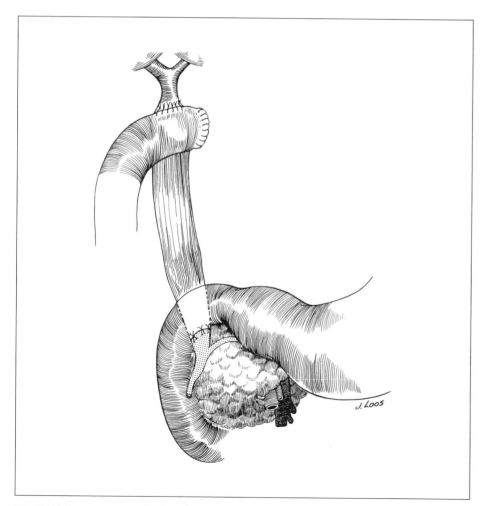

Fig. 104-7. *Some surgeons prefer the end-to-side anastomosis, particularly for adult patients. Of far greater importance, however, is the necessity for a tension-free, accurate mucosa-to-mucosa anastomosis.*

herniation and volvulus. The anastomosis of the bile duct to the jejunal segment is accomplished as either end-to-end or end-to-side, depending on any size discrepancy of the two structures. For the adult patient, we often prefer the end-to-side method following closure of the proximal end (Fig. 104-7). It is important to anchor the Roux loop to the periductal tissues with three or four sutures, and then assess the position and configuration of the loop. A meticulous one layer mucosa-to-mucosa anastomosis is then accomplished with simple interrupted sutures. Three or four additional anchoring sutures are placed anteriorly to relieve any tension from the mucosal suture line. We routinely use absorbable sutures for the mucosal anastomosis and nonabsorbable for the anchoring seromuscular sutures.

In small infants or in patients with associated esophageal varices, we generally perform a gastrostomy for postoperative gastrointestinal decompression. Otherwise, a nasogastric tube is generally adequate.

Several alternative treatment methods are of interest. Of historic interest, from 1920 to 1930, the use of cholecystogastrostomy or cholecystoenterostomy to provide biliary tract decompression resulted in frequent unsatisfactory results with continued symptoms and in many patients, the need for additional surgery. A simple anastomosis of the cyst to the duodenum was popular in the 1940s and 1950s but has largely been abandoned because of the high incidence of postoperative ascending cholangitis and subsequent liver damage. Simple Roux-en-Y drainage of the cyst, leaving the cyst in place, produced results superior to cyst duodenostomy, but still one-third of the patients developed stricture requiring surgical revision. In addition, there was a significant risk of carcinoma developing in the retained cyst in later years.

Other procedures have been developed with the goal to further minimize the chances for reflux of intestinal contents into the biliary ducts. Satisfactory short-term results have been achieved by simply interposing an isolated segment of small intestine between the hepatic duct and the duodenum after excision of the CDC. Other surgeons have created a permanent intussusception within this small intestine conduit to further minimize reflux. Such direct bile drainage into the duodenum can enhance the pancreaticoduodenal physiology of motility, digestion and absorption; it connects the biliary tree into a site, the duodenum, with a reduced bacteriologic flora; and it places the biliary anastomosis at a site amenable to endoscopic examination through the gastrointestinal tract. The long-term follow-up of the intussuscepted valves suggest that they are usually effective in preventing retrograde gastrointestinal regurgitation into the biliary tree. Another method is to use a segment of terminal ileum and right colon whereby the ileocecal valve serves to prevent or minimize reflux. The appendix was first recommended approximately 20 years ago as a replacement for the common duct. The appendix, with its active peristalsis and with its small diameter, which is very similar to that of the common bile duct, would appear to be a satisfactory conduit from the hepatic duct to the duodenum. There have been sporadic reports of satisfactory short-term results. However, further experience and a longer follow-up will be required before these procedures can be generally recommended.

For the type II CDC, simple excision of the pedunculated cyst has been recommended, and satisfactory results with short-term follow-up have been reported. If the current common channel theory of etiology is accepted, however, one would expect simple excision to be followed by a high instance of recurrence of the cyst. For this reason, we recommend simple excision of the cyst and Roux-en-Y drainage of the proximal bile duct, the same as for the type I malformation.

For type III CDC, or the choledochocele, authorities differ on their recommendations. Satisfactory short-term results have been reported in at least one patient by simple endoscopic "sphincterotomy," or "meatotomy" to enlarge the opening and relieve any obstruction decompressing the cyst. In one of our patients, age 32 years, the cyst wall was an estimated 0.4 cm in thickness, and a muscular wall divided the spherical cyst into two halves. The pancreatic duct entered one-half. The common duct entered the other half, and it contained numerous gallstones. Since neither the common duct nor the pancreatic duct were found to be dilated, we excised the septum and evacuated the stones and constructed a wide "sphincteroplasty" mar-

supializing the cyst to the duodenum from a transduodenal approach. The patient was symptom-free 16 years later. Our recommended treatment for a choledochocele for infants and for small children is a generous transduodenal sphincteroplasty to provide decompression and drainage. For the older child and for the adult, endoscopic sphincterotomy might provide satisfactory results. However, because of the rarity of choledochocele, its questionable etiology, and confusion with duodenal duplications, if this approach is elected, at least yearly follow-up by examination and by ultrasound for a number of years will be an essential part of the therapeutic regimen. In the event of recurrence of the choledochocele, open surgical transduodenal sphincteroplasty would be recommended. The malignant potential of the choledochocele has not been documented but continues to be a matter of concern. For the more complicated variety of choledochocele or in the event of subsequent ascending cholangitis or other complications of the more "simple" treatment, the Roux-en-Y procedure would be recommended.

Type IV (Caroli's disease) because of its rarity has been subjected to insufficient study to fully understand its etiology and pathophysiology. It is believed that it is simply another form of CDC and should be treated accordingly with excision and Roux-en-Y drainage plus dilatation of any remaining strictures above the anastomosis. Our experience with one patient, a 2-year-old child treated by this method, resulted in an asymptomatic patient 24 years later.

Type V, the intrahepatic CDC can be of either the type I, type II, or type IV variety, the only difference being that it is located entirely within the liver. Because of the rarity of this type, experience has been limited. Our two patients were both treated with simple Roux-en-Y drainage and are free of symptoms after 4 years and 20 years. We are aware of one report of a type II pedunculated intrahepatic cyst that was treated by complete excision but with a short follow-up. It is probable that patients with intrahepatic CDC possess the same common channel anomaly and simply represent a variant of the same entity, although we have been unable to find reports documenting this belief. If analysis of the bile demonstrated the presence of amylase, a Roux-en-Y choledochoenterostomy would be the logical consideration.

Unfortunately, this data is usually not available to the surgeon at the time of the operation.

Our recommendation, therefore, on the basis of our own experience combined with available reported experience is a simple Roux-en-Y drainage for any intrahepatic choledochal cyst. It is important that a bile sample be submitted for amylase determination, and in the event of a positive report, we would recommend follow-up examination with physical examination and ultrasound study at yearly intervals for 10 years and then every 5 years thereafter.

Postoperative Care and Follow-up

Postoperative gastrointestinal decompression is essential until active peristalsis has returned. For infants, we prefer use of a gastrostomy tube. For older children and adults, a nasogastric tube is usually adequate unless contraindicated because of associated esophageal varices.

We routinely use perioperative antibiotic prophylaxis followed by suppressive treatment with broad-spectrum antibiotics for 1 month postoperatively in order to minimize the incidence of ascending biliary tract infection. At the present time, we prefer sulfamethoxazole/trimethoprim for this purpose.

A mild degree of biliary cirrhosis is sometimes encountered in older patients, but it is usually not progressive once satisfactory biliary drainage has been established.

The need for long-term follow-up is emphasized for all patients with CDC because of possible late complications of an anastomotic stricture as well as malignancy in any retained cyst mucosa. Follow-up is particularly important for the rare types III, IV, and V because of limited experience with these varieties.

The most frequent long-term complication is anastomotic stricture, which is closely related to the operative technique. This complication can be virtually eliminated by using the technique of hepaticoplasty (Fig. 104-6), with a wide anastomotic lumen of 10- to 30-mm diameter for the hepaticojejunostomy to the Roux-en-Y limb.

In a long-term follow-up of 28 patients who had undergone cyst excision with

Roux-en-Y hepaticoenterostomy, Chijiiwa found three patients, 3, 5, and 12 years following their operations who had developed intrahepatic gallstones. In all three, the bile was infected, and in one there was residual dilatation of intrahepatic ducts that had been dilated before the operation. A fourth patient developed clinical cholangitis 5 years following the operation. The symptoms cleared promptly in response to antibiotic therapy. None of the four patients had anastomotic stricture.

Yoshikawa reported a patient who developed carcinoma arising in the intrapancreatic terminal choledochus 12 years following primary excision of a giant choledochal cyst. This report underscores the importance of removal of the mucosa of the distal end of the cyst to include all the dilated portion.

Long-term follow-up is of particular importance if the operation left the patient with an intact common bile duct and the potential for continued reflux of pancreatic enzymes, which could cause a recurrence of the CDC. For these patients, it is our current policy to examine the liver and bile ducts by ultrasound at least every 5 years.

Suggested Reading

Alonzo-Lej F, Rever WB, Pessagno DJ. Congenital choledochal cyst, with report of two, and an analysis of 94 cases. *Surg Gynecol Obstet* 108:1, 1959.

Babbitt DP. Congenital choledochal cyst: New etiologic concept based on anomalous relationship of common bile duct and pancreatic bulb. *Ann Radiol* 12:231, 1969.

Bancroft JD, Bucuvalas JD, Rickman FC, et al. Antenatal diagnosis of choledochal cyst. *J Pediatr Gastroenterol Nutr* 18:142, 1994.

Chijiiwa K, Tanaka M. Late complications after excisional operation in patients with choledochal cyst. *J Am Coll Surg* 179:139, 1994.

Flanigan DP. Biliary cysts. *Ann Surg* 182:635, 1975.

Gross RE. The Surgery of Infancy and Childhood. In *Choledochal Cysts*. Philadelphia: Saunders, 1953.

Hays DM, Goodman GN, Snyder WH, et al. Congenital cystic dilatation of the common bile duct. *Arch Surg* 98:457, 1969.

Kasai M, Asakura Y, Taira Y. Surgical treatment of choledochal cyst. *Ann Surg* 172:844, 1970.

Kim SH. Choledochal cyst: Survey by the Surgical Section of the American Academy of Pediatrics. *J Pediatr Surg* 16:402, 1981.

Ladd WE, Gross RE. Idiopathic Dilatation of the Common Bile Duct. In *Abdominal Surgery of Infancy and Childhood*. 1947.

Lilly JR. The surgical treatment of choledochal cyst. *Surg Gynecol Obstet* 149:36, 1979.

Lujan-Mompean JA, Torralba-Martinez JA, Parilla-Paricio P, et al. Quantification of duodenogastric reflux in patients with choledochoduodenostomy. *J Am Coll Surg* 179:193, 1994.

Martin LW, Rowe GA. Portal hypertension secondary to choledochal cyst. *Ann Surg* 190:638, 1979.

O'Neill JA. Choledochal cyst. *Pediatric Surgery* (4th ed.). KJ Welch, JG Randolph, MM Ravitch, et al (eds.) In Chicago: Year Book, 1986.

O'Neill JR, Clatworthy HW. Management of choledochal cysts: A fourteen year follow-up. *Ann Surg* 37:230, 1971.

Shamberger RC, Lund DP, Lillehei CW, et al. Interposed jejunal segment with nipple valve to prevent reflux in biliary reconstruction. *J Am Coll Surg* 180:10, 1995.

Todani T, Watanabe Y, Fujii T, et al. Anomalous arrangement of the pancreaticobiliary ductal system in patients with a choledochal cyst. *Am J Surg* 147:672, 1984.

Todani T, Watanabe Y, Toki A, et al. Carcinoma related to choledochal cysts with internal drainage operation. *Surg Gynecol Obstet* 164:61, 1987.

Zinninger MM, Cash JR. Congenital cystic dilatation of the common bile duct. *Arch Surg* 24:77, 1932.

EDITOR'S COMMENT

Choledochal cysts remain an interesting and intriguing congenital anomaly. Now classified, there seems to be general agreement that excision of the inflamed mucosa of the choledochal cyst is essential to prevent carcinoma in the late postoperative period. Doctors Martin and Ziegler stress the necessity for leaving excellent biliary duct epithelium in order to do the anastomosis to the Roux-en-Y limb or the interposed loop. This important point has been learned the hard way by various biliary surgeons over the years. Regardless of whether one stents or does not stent, the sine qua non of trouble-free anastomoses is good biliary epithelium and a clean mucosa-to-mucosa anastomosis.

Recently, there have been arguments for the interposed jejunal segment with a nipple valve reconstruction in order to prevent reflux in biliary reconstruction. In a recent paper, Shamberger and associates (*J Am Coll Surg* 180:10, 1995) reported on 12 cases in which a Roux-en-Y hepaticojejunoduodenostomy was performed with an interposed nipple valve. The claim for this operation, as originated by Raffensberger and colleagues in 1981, is that it creates a more "physiologic" reconstruction and has a lower incidence of cholangitis. If one examines the incidence of cholangitis in Shamberger's series (3 out of 12), the series quoted by Drs. Martin and Ziegler, and also the recent report by Chijiiwa and Tanaka (*J Am Coll Surg* 179:139, 1994), one sees there were only four cases of cholangitis, generally associated with strictures. Thus, the incidence of cholangitis was no greater than it was in the nipple valve reconstruction and, although not statistically significant, possibly a little less. The claim, therefore, that cholangitis occurred less often in the group receiving nipple valve reconstruction is unproven. Of greater concern might be the width of the anastomosis, which it appears is best handled by a spatulated hepaticojejunostomy, since in the series by Chijiiwa and Tanaka, all instances of cholangitis were associated with stricture formation.

Complications of hepaticojejunoduodenostomy include both bile reflux gastritis, as reported by Okada and colleagues (*Surg Gynecol Obstet* 174:313, 1992), and gastric and duodenal ulceration. The latter probably relates to the length of the Roux-en-Y bypass. The longer the bypass, the higher the gastric acid secretion, a phenomenon first reported by Mann and Williamson in the early 1920s and the ulcer of which bears their names.

The use of the appendix as an interposed segment between the top and the bottom segments of the bile duct remains an intriguing possibility. A few authors have reported the use of the appendix and its blood supply, primarily in association with the right colon. The appendix has also been recently used as a substitute for the ureter. It has vigorous peristalsis and a good blood supply, and is approximately the diameter of the common bile duct. Its use as a substitute should be further explored.

J.E.F.

105

Surgical Treatment of Jaundice in Newborn Infants

Joseph P. Vacanti   Kaoru Sano

Jaundice in newborn infants can be caused by many diseases such as infectious hepatitis, metabolic diseases caused by liver enzyme deficiency, idiopathic intrahepatic diseases (neonatal hepatitis), or extrahepatic diseases (biliary atresia). Surgical treatment is indicated in the diseases that are caused by mechanical impairment of bile flow. The differentiation between functional and mechanical impairment of bile flow is sometimes difficult. Exploratory laparotomy including intraoperative cholangiogram and liver biopsy might be necessary to evaluate the cause of disease. It is of great importance to make the correct diagnosis early and start the appropriate treatment as soon as possible. It is especially crucial to differentiate between biliary atresia and other diseases, because the timing of an operation for biliary atresia greatly influences the prognosis of this disease.

Extrahepatic Biliary Atresia

Biliary atresia is the most common cause of jaundice in newborn infants that needs surgical treatment. In 1891, this disease was described by Thomson as a "progressive inflammatory lesion of the bile duct." In 1916, the possibility of surgical treatment for biliary atresia was first discussed by Holmes. Despite widespread efforts, the etiology of biliary atresia has not been elucidated. This fundamental lack of understanding has hindered the development of a safe and efficacious treatment. A correctable type of biliary atresia, which

had a bile cyst at the liver hilus, was reported by Ladd in 1928 as the first successful surgical treatment for biliary atresia. Unfortunately, this type constitutes less than 10 percent of instances of biliary atresia. In 1959, Kasai reported his successful operation for this disease—a hepatic portoenterostomy (Kasai's operation). This surgical treatment has gradually been accepted worldwide. With its acceptance, the number of survivors has increased remarkably. Portoenterostomy should be undertaken by 3 months of age, before the liver changes become irreversible. If it is performed by this age, approximately 80 percent of patients will have their jaundice corrected. Despite the success of Kasai's operation, many patients develop progressive cirrhosis, which leads to failure of treatment. The survival ratio 5 years after Kasai's operation (without liver transplantation) is 30 to 60 percent. Twenty percent of the patients can survive more than 10 years without jaundice after Kasai's operation, but most of them have portal hypertension or abnormal liver function, and only 10 percent have normal liver function. Most patients with biliary atresia might need organ replacement for liver dysfunction, recurrent gastrointestinal bleeding, or hypersplenism.

Since the 1980s, liver transplantation has made great progress. Because of the acceptable morbidity and mortality of liver transplantation in small children, liver transplantation has been proposed as the initial surgical treatment for biliary atresia. However, Kasai's operation clearly delays the need for transplantation and gives the benefits of growth and development in

many patients. In addition, donor organ scarcity limits the role of transplantation in this population. We believe that combining Kasai's operation with liver transplantation as needed is an effective therapy for children with biliary atresia.

Pathology

Macroscopically, biliary atresia presents with obliteration of either the common bile duct or the common hepatic duct, or both. The location and degree of obliteration, however, can be quite variable. Usually, an anatomic classification is used to express the type of disease (Fig. 105-1). Types A and B were previously referred to as "correctable cases," because the patients have a cyst at the liver hilus that can be used for bile drainage. Types C and D represent a complete obliteration of the extrahepatic biliary tree. In type E, the gallbladder and common bile duct are patent.

Microscopically, biliary atresia is characterized by a dynamic process of progressive inflammatory destruction of the extrahepatic bile ducts. The process begins with periductal inflammation with necrosis and sloughing of epithelial cells. Eventually, the biliary tracts are replaced with fibrous scar and an obliterated lumen. In most instances, at the time of the operation microbiliary tracts are appreciated in the fibrous scar tissue of the liver hilus.

Etiology

The precise etiology of this disease is still unknown. Biliary atresia was considered a congenital malformation of the biliary sys-

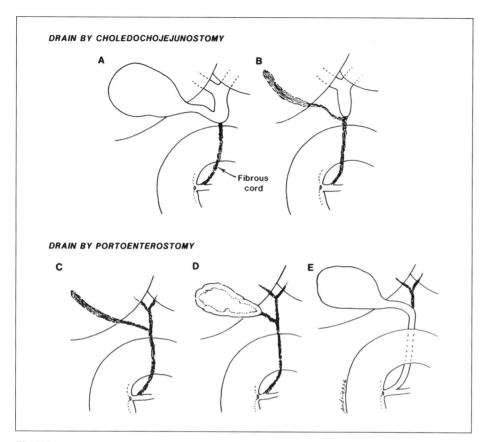

DRAIN BY CHOLEDOCHOJEJUNOSTOMY

A

B

Fibrous cord

DRAIN BY PORTOENTEROSTOMY

C

D

E

Fig. 105-1. Most common types of biliary atresia and method for drainage. (From WH Hendren and JP Vacanti. Pediatric Liver Surgery. In WV McDermott Jr. [ed.], Surgery of the Liver. *Boston: Blackwell, 1989. Reproduced with permission.)*

tem. But, in some instances, patients have no jaundice at birth and only later develop jaundice. Obliteration can occur in either a caudal or cranial component of the hepatic diverticulum, or occasionally, even both components can be impaired. In some instances, biliary atresia accompanies malformations of other organs that develop during the differentiation of the hepatic diverticulum. This phenomenon suggests perturbation of embryologic events occurring at 4 to 6 weeks of embryonic life. Retrovirus type 3 infection has been suggested as a possible etiologic agent in the cause of biliary atresia, but this explanation remains controversial.

Diagnosis

When presented with an icteric infant, it is imperative to make a diagnosis as soon as possible. Radioisotope imaging with 99m technetium iminodiacetic acid (IDA) agents is useful for rapid screening for flow into the intestine. Ultrasonography is useful and might show a small, shrunken, and noncontractile gallbladder and enhanced hepatic parenchymal echoes in patients with biliary atresia. Choledochal cyst can be differentiated from biliary atresia using ultrasonography.

Preoperative Management

Coagulation abnormalities, hypoproteinemia, and anemia should be corrected before the operation. Vitamin K is administered for coagulation abnormalities, and unabsorbable antibiotics such as kanamycin are administered orally to prepare the intestine before laparotomy. Skillful pediatric anesthetic management (safe depth of anesthesia, careful control of blood volume, normalization of acid-base status, oxygen saturation, and temperature regulation) is critical.

Operation

In types C, D, and E biliary atresia, there are no patent bile ducts at the liver hilus

macroscopically. In these instances, hepatic portoenterostomy (Kasai's operation) is required. In types A and B patients, who have a cyst at the hilus, bile flow can be maintained via the cyst. If the jejunal conduit is anastomosed to the cyst wall, bile stasis and anastomotic stricture often occur postoperatively because there is no epithelial lining in the cyst wall. The cyst should be removed as close as possible to the liver. In most types A and B biliary atresia, portoenterostomy is required. Only in patients with a patent hepatic duct can a hepatojejunostomy be performed.

In portoenterostomy, microbiliary tracts should be exposed by cutting the liver surface at the hilus. If the liver surface is dissected into parenchyma too deeply, microbiliary tracts cannot be identified. If dissection is not sufficient, the bile flow might not be initiated. The jejunum is not anastomosed directly to the biliary mucosa. The anastomosis will be covered by epithelium after healing by secondary intention. Cholangitis is the major cause of an inflammatory reaction around the anastomosis and leads to obliteration of the microbiliary tracts because of the formation of granulation tissue. Several variations on this surgical technique offer theoretical means of preventing this complication (Fig. 105-2). These include conduit exteriorization, nipple valve creation, and determination of an optimal length of conduit. Therefore, Kasai's operation requires surgical skill and experience to achieve good results. Loupe magnification can greatly aid in the dissection and reconstruction. Before portoenterostomy, an intraoperative cholangiogram should be performed in order to differentiate this disease from other causes of jaundice and to determine the type of biliary atresia.

Intraoperative Cholangiogram

The patient is placed in the supine position and widely draped to expose the entire abdomen. A small right subcostal skin incision is made. The subcutaneous tissue and muscle layers are cut with the electrocautery after the skin is incised with a scalpel. Once the gallbladder is identified, a tube is inserted into the fundus of the gallbladder and secured with a 5–0 Prolene purse-string suture (Fig. 105-3). If the gallbladder is atretic and invisible, a cholangiogram is unnecessary (Fig. 105-4). Intraoperative cholangiography is undertaken with appropriately diluted contrast medium in or-

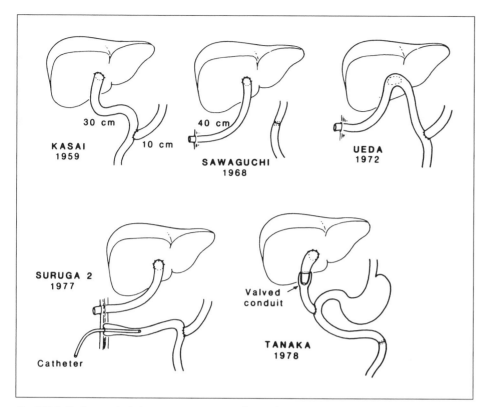

Fig. 105-2. Various methods for portoenterostomy to drain bile and avert ascending cholangitis. (From WH Hendren and JP Vacanti. Pediatric Liver Surgery. In WV McDermott Jr. [eds.], Surgery of the Liver. Boston: Blackwell, 1989. Reproduced with permission.)

der to detect the biliary tree. If both the extrahepatic and intrahepatic biliary trees are normal, a liver biopsy is performed, and the abdomen is closed. If the biliary tree is abnormal, a cholangiogram is obtained while gently compressing the common bile duct in order to evaluate the patency of the common hepatic and intrahepatic bile ducts. If the biliary tree cannot be visualized with this maneuver, we proceed to the reconstructive Kasai procedure.

Hepatic Portoenterostomy (Kasai's Operation)

The skin incision is extended laterally and medially to the left subcostal margin. The round and falciform ligaments are divided. In order to rotate the liver anteriorly for optimal exposure of the liver hilus, the left and right triangular ligaments are also divided (Fig. 105-5). It should be noted that rotation of the liver can cause compression of the vena cava leading to hypotension. After the tube is removed from the fundus, the gallbladder is dissected from the liver bed with the electrocautery. The cystic duct leads to a fibrous cord along the hepaticoduodenal ligament. This

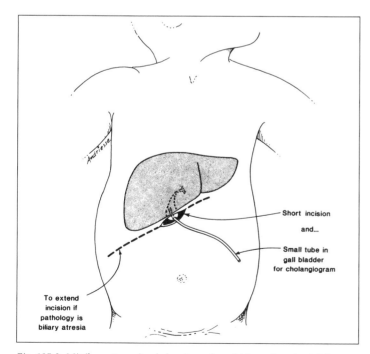

Fig. 105-3. Minilaparotomy for cholangiography, which can be extended for biliary exploration. (From WH Hendren and JP Vacanti. Pediatric Liver Surgery. In WV McDermott Jr. [eds.], Surgery of the Liver. Boston: Blackwell, 1989. Reproduced with permission.)

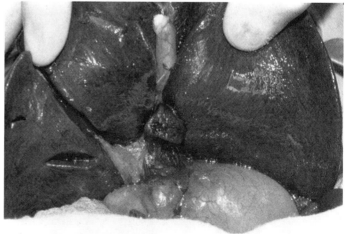

Fig. 105-4. Operative photograph of biliary atresia. The gallbladder is atretic and invisible. In this instance, a cholangiogram is unnecessary. A Kasai procedure is indicated.

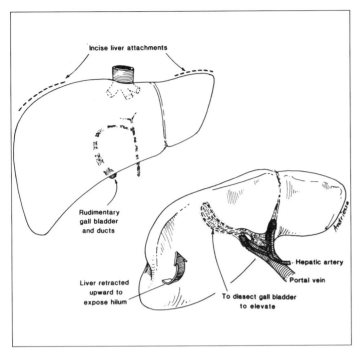

Fig. 105-5. Portoenterostomy operation. Liver attachments are incised, and the liver is retracted to expose the hilum. (From WH Hendren and JP Vacanti. Pediatric Liver Surgery. In WV McDermott Jr. [eds.], Surgery of the Liver. Boston: Blackwell, 1989. Reproduced with permission.)

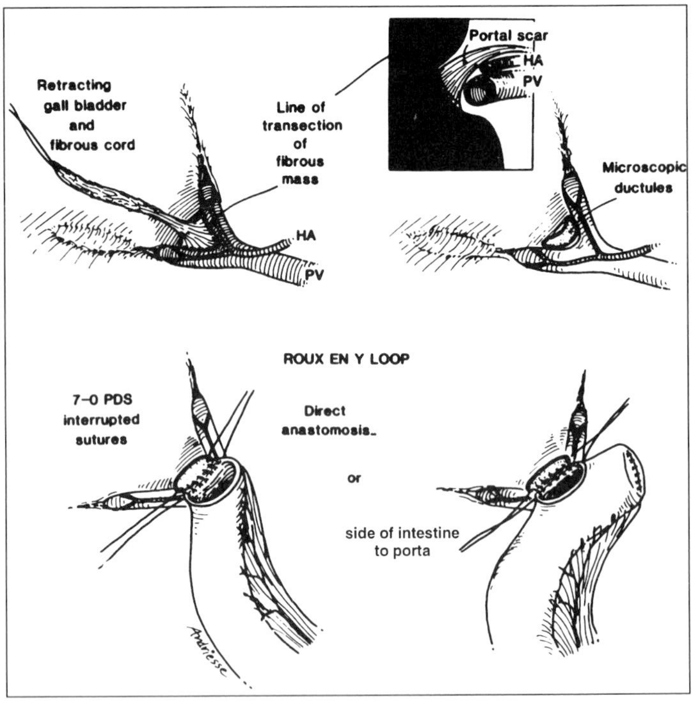

Fig. 105-6. Portoenterostomy operation. Dissecting into the hilum to expose microscopic ductules and drainage by a Roux-en-Y loop. (From WH Hendren and JP Vacanti. Pediatric Liver Surgery. In WV McDermott Jr. [eds.], Surgery of the Liver. Boston: Blackwell, 1989. Reproduced with permission.)

fibrous tissue is composed of the biliary radicles and leads to the liver hilus where the microbiliary tracts might be open.

While retracting the gallbladder, the fibrous cord is dissected from the portal vein and the hepatic artery toward the duodenum. At the superior surface of duodenum, the distal portion of this fibrous tissue is suture ligated with 5–0 Prolene.

This dissection is undertaken toward the liver hilus. At the liver hilus, the hepatic artery and portal vein should be dissected carefully from this fibrous tissue so as not to damage them. The broad fibrous scar tissue is appreciated at the liver surface at the bifurcation of the portal vein (Fig. 105-6). If both vessels are retracted downward, we usually find one branch of the hepatic artery and a few branches of the portal vein entering into this scar tissue. These branches should be ligated and divided. The portal vein should be dissected to the back wall. The broad fibrous scar tissue is sharply dissected with a scalpel. There should be numerous microbiliary tracts. The dissection should be performed 1 to 2 mm in thickness and be very wide at the entrance of the right and left hepatic arteries (Fig. 105-7). After this procedure, bile flow is often appreciated. Before removing

this scar tissue, some stay sutures with 5–0 Prolene are placed on the posterior edge of the dissection. These stitches are helpful for the posterior wall anastomosis. A frozen section of this resected scar tissue is immediately checked by a pathologist to determine if the microbiliary ducts are present and their approximate dimensions.

To make a jejunal conduit, a Roux-en-Y is made from the jejunum with a stapler at approximately 10 cm distal to the ligament of Treitz. This limb is brought up in a retrocolic manner through the transverse mesocolon. The end of the limb is sutured with 5–0 Vicryl interrupted Lembert sutures to overlap the staples. Approximately 3 cm distal to the end of the limb, a 3-cm longitudinal incision is made along the antimesenteric border.

Interrupted sutures with 6–0 PDS are placed between the cut edge of the hilus and the whole layer of jejunum (Fig. 105-8). When sewing the posterior wall, it is helpful to retract the stay sutures that were previously placed at the posterior edge of the cut surface. The length of the Roux-en-Y limb should be longer than 30 to 35 cm to help prevent cholangitis. Jejunojejunostomy is performed with a single layer of

5–0 Vicryl suture. Backflow of intestinal contents into the conduit can cause elevation of internal pressure and bacterial contamination in the conduit. A 1 to 1.5 cm intussuscepted nipple valve can be made in the middle of the conduit to prevent reflux (Fig. 105-9). Many types of exteriorization of conduit have been developed. We do not recommend exteriorization because this procedure does not improve the results of portoenterostomy and makes liver transplantation difficult because of varices around the stoma. Liver biopsy is performed to evaluate the extent of liver damage.

A closed-suction drainage catheter is left in Morison's pouch and is brought out through a separate stab incision. The abdominal wall is closed in layers.

Postoperative Management

Postoperative management concentrates on monitoring and preventing cholangitis. Stool color and body temperature are good barometers. Liver function is frequently monitored with biochemical tests. Broad-spectrum antibiotics are prophylactically given because cholangitis usually occurs secondary to bacteria in the intestinal conduit. Good bile flow might wash out the

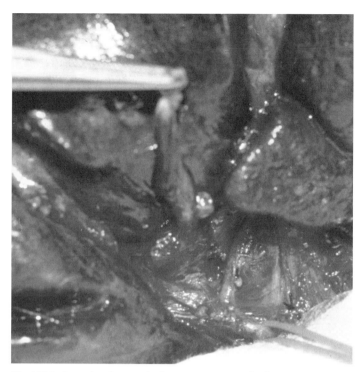

Fig. 105-7. Operative photograph of portoenterostomy. The fibrous tissue is retracted upward, and the broad scar tissue is sharply dissected widely at the liver hilus. A vessel tape is placed around the proper hepatic artery.

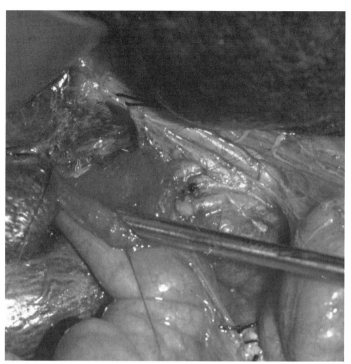

Fig. 105-8. Operative photograph of portoenterostomy. The jejunum is anastomosed to the cut edge of the hilus.

bacteria around the anastomosis, and so choleretics (phenobarbital) are administered. Steroids can also be used in an attempt to decrease scarring at the hilar anastomosis.

Complications

Cholangitis

Cholangitis is the major risk factor associated with failure of Kasai's operation. Even in patients with good bile flow, cholangitis can lead to cessation of bile flow by causing scar formation of the microbiliary ducts at the liver hilus. Fever, acholic stool, and elevation of serum bilirubin level are signs of cholangitis. If cholangitis develops, additional antibiotic administration should be started immediately. In recurrent jaundice caused by recurrent cholangitis, a second Kasai's operation (conduit revision, hilar debridement) can be considered. In instances in which bile is not demonstrated at the time of the first portoenterostomy, a second operation should not be attempted because bile flow after the second operation is unlikely. In addition, repeated operations can endanger the success of future transplantation procedures.

Portal Hypertension

At the time of Kasai's operation, some degree of hepatic fibrosis is usually found. Hepatic fibrosis is one of the major causes of portal hypertension. Portal hypertension often persists for several years after a successful Kasai's operation. Postoperative cholangitis also leads to portal hypertension. The manifestations of portal hypertension include splenomegaly, hypersplenism, esophageal varices with potential bleeding, and subcutaneous varices.

Other Complications

Fat-soluble vitamin deficiency is commonly found both before and after Kasai's operation because of lack of bile in the enteric tract. Administration of these vitamins is required.

Liver Transplantation

In 20 percent of patients undergoing portoenterostomy, bile drainage is not obtained. Organ replacement should be planned. Recurrent cholangitis and persistent jaundice lead to chronic liver failure. Recurrent gastrointestinal bleeding caused by portal hypertension or hypersplenism is also an indication for liver transplantation. In small children, cadaveric split liver or living related partial liver transplantation is useful, in addition to cadaveric whole organ transplantation.

Prognosis

In infants with biliary atresia who do not undergo either Kasai's operation or liver transplantation, survival of less than 2 years is expected. Kasai's operation can greatly lengthen survival. However, treatment only with Kasai's operation shows a 10-year survival of 10 to 20 percent. By combining Kasai's operation with liver transplantation, 10-year survival might reach 89 percent (Fig. 105-10).

Congenital Dilatation of the Bile Ducts

In newborn infants with choledochal cyst, the clinical manifestations are similar to those of biliary atresia: obstructive jaundice, acholic stool, and hepatomegaly. The classic triad of pain, mass, and jaundice is rarely seen in infants. This disease is categorized into five classes (Fig. 105-11):

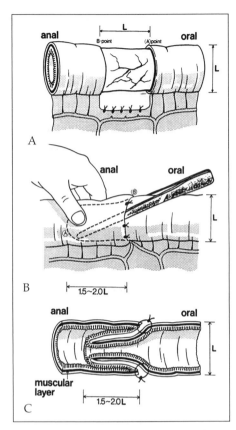

Fig. 105-9. Construction of an intussuscepted muscular valve. A. Removal of the seromuscular layer. B. Intussusception and valvular fixation. C. Cross-section of the valve. (From K Tanaka, I Shirahase, H Utsunomiya, et al. A valved hepatic portoduodenal intestinal conduit for biliary atresia. Ann Surg 213: 1991. Reproduced with permission.)

Type I. Segmental or diffuse fusiform dilatation of the extrahepatic bile duct

Type II. Diverticulum of the extrahepatic bile duct

Type III. Choledochocele

Type IV. Multiple cysts of the intrahepatic or extrahepatic duct, or both

Type V. Single or multiple intrahepatic cysts (Caroli's disease)

This classification is based on cholangiographic findings. Over 90 percent of these patients have the type I variety.

Pathologically, choledochal cysts have a thick wall that lacks a mucosal layer and consists of dense connective tissue, except in the case of a choledochocele. The etiology is still unknown. Obstructive factors at the distal portion, and weakness or ab-

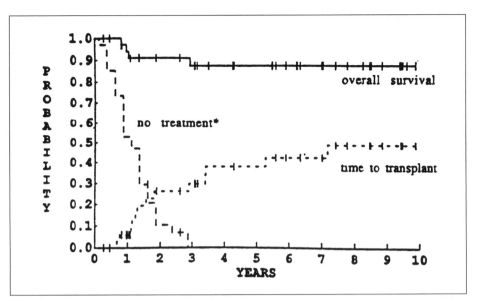

Fig. 105-10. Actuarial survival (Kaplan–Meier method) of children with biliary atresia treated at Children's Hospital, Boston, from 1981 to 1991, compared with survival of patients without surgical treatment.* Addition of liver transplantation into therapy is also shown. (*Adapted from DM Hays and WH Snyder. Life-span in untreated biliary atresia. Surgery 54:373, 1963.) (From JP Vacanti, AM Leichtner, RC Shamberger, et al. The Surgical Management of Biliary Atresia at Children's Hospital, Boston. In R Ohi [ed.], Biliary Atresia. Proceedings of the 5th International Sendai Symposium on Biliary Atresia. Tokyo: ICOM Associates, Inc., 1991. Reproduced with permission.)

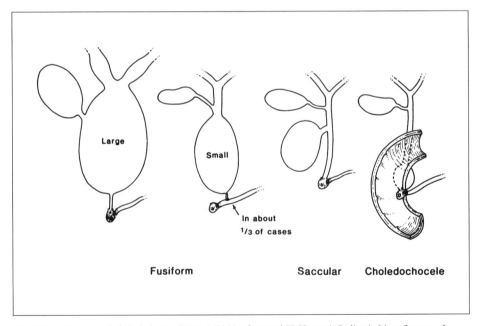

Fig. 105-11. Types of choledochal cyst. (From WH Hendren and JP Vacanti. Pediatric Liver Surgery. In WV McDermott Jr. [ed.], Surgery of the Liver. Boston: Blackwell, 1989. Reproduced with permission.)

normality of the bile duct at the pathologic site have been considered as possible causative factors of cyst formation. Reflux of pancreatic juice into the common bile duct because of an anomaly of choledochal-

pancreatico-ductal junction can act as an etiologic agent by dissolving the bile duct wall. This disease is found in the Orient (especially in Japan) much more frequently than in the West, suggesting that

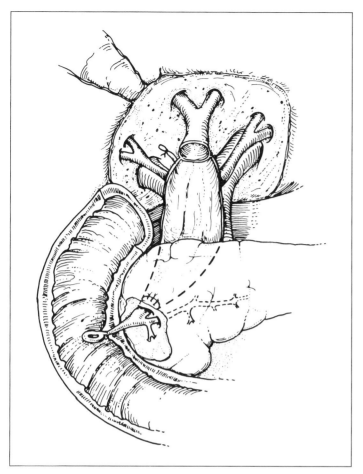

Fig. 105-12. Internal excision of a cyst. (From KW Aschcraft. Atlas of Pediatric Surgery. *Philadelphia: Saunders, 1994. Reproduced with permission.)*

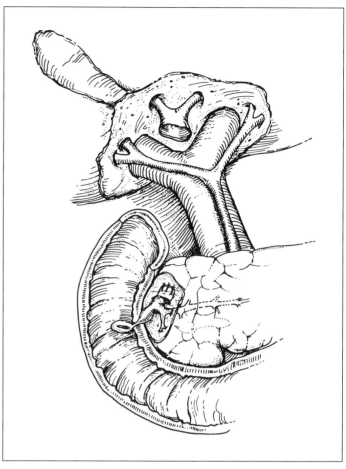

Fig. 105-13. External excision of a cyst. (From KW Aschcraft. Atlas of Pediatric Surgery. *Philadelphia: Saunders, 1994. Reproduced with permission.)*

a viral infection might be the cause. The differential diagnosis between choledochal cyst and biliary atresia can be made using both a 99m technetium IDA scan and ultrasonography.

Treatment

Formerly, cyst enterostomy was performed for this disease. But the anastomosis between jejunum and diseased cyst was found to cause complications such as anastomotic stricture, biliary stasis, and carcinoma. Therefore, except when it is technically unfeasible, cyst excision should be undertaken at the original operation.

The patient is placed in the supine position. A right subcostal skin incision is made. An intraoperative cholangiogram should be undertaken to confirm the entrance of the pancreatic duct and the existence of intrahepatic cystic disease.

A tube is inserted into the fundus of the gallbladder and fixed with a 5–0 Prolene pursestring suture. An intraoperative cholangiogram is performed with appropriately diluted contrast medium. After cholangiography, the tube is removed, and the gallbladder is dissected from the liver bed. The dissection of the cystic duct leads to the choledochal cyst. While retracting the cystic duct or gallbladder, the dissection between the cyst (common bile duct), portal vein, and hepatic artery must be performed with care. If the inflammation around the cyst is not severe, the dissection between the cyst and vessels can be performed bluntly at the level of the external layer of cyst. However, if the inflammation is severe, it is unnecessary to dissect the external layer. In this situation, it is satisfactory to perform the dissection leaving the outer layer at the cyst wall in place (Fig. 105-12), thereby protecting the vascular structures. After finishing the blunt dissection posterolaterally, the com-

mon bile duct is transected. While picking up the edge of the distal common bile duct, dissection around the bile duct is undertaken inferiorly. While dissecting the intrapancreatic bile duct, bleeding from pancreas tissue occurs easily. Careful hemostasis should be achieved with the electrocautery. The bile duct is divided proximal to the site of the pancreatic duct. Care should be taken not to damage the pancreatic duct. To prevent postoperative leakage of pancreatic secretion, the stump of the bile duct should be suture ligated with 5–0 Prolene. The dissection toward the liver hilus is advanced, while picking up and retracting the end of the proximal bile duct. The dissection should be performed up to the level where the hepatic duct is normal. At this level, the hepatic duct is transected (Fig. 105-13). If the cyst extends into the liver, the bile duct should be transected as near as possible to the normal intrahepatic duct with extension of the incision into the primary ducts to remove

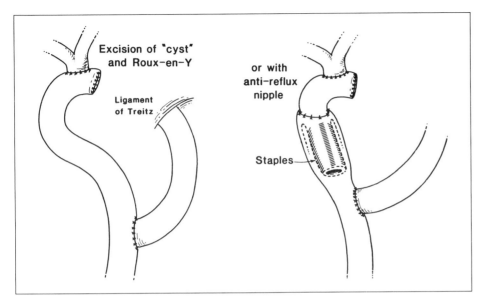

Fig. 105-14. Roux-en-Y drainage of biliary tract after excision of a choledochal cyst. (From WH Hendren and JP Vacanti. Pediatric Liver Surgery. In WV McDermott Jr. [ed.], Surgery of the Liver. Boston: Blackwell, 1989. Reproduced with permission.)

the dilated bile duct as much as possible. At approximately 10 cm distal to the ligament of Treitz, the jejunum is divided as the end of a Roux-en-Y limb with a stapler. This limb is brought up in a retrocolic manner through the transverse mesocolon. The staples are oversewn using 5–0 Vicryl interrupted Lembert sutures. At 2 to 3 cm distal to the end of the limb, a hole slightly smaller than the hepatic duct is made at the antimesenteric side. An interrupted anastomosis with 5–0 Vicryl sutures between the hepatic duct and full thickness of jejunum is performed. The length of the limb should be at least 30 cm. Additional procedures such as a nipple valve creation can be considered, but bile flow is usually sufficient to prevent cholangitis. Jejunojejunostomy is performed with a single layer 5–0 Vicryl anastomosis (Fig. 105-14).

A closed-suction drainage catheter is left in Morison's pouch and is brought out through a separate stab incision. The abdominal wall is closed in a two-layer manner. The skin is closed with staples.

Complications

Cholangitis, obstructive jaundice, and carcinoma are possible complications. If the diseased bile duct is not resected and is anastomosed to the intestine, anastomotic stricture and cholangitis frequently occur. In the remaining cyst wall, there is an increased risk of carcinoma. Complications are unusual if the operative resection and reconstruction are performed properly.

Other Diseases
Paucity of Interlobular Bile Duct (Biliary Hypoplasia)

The diseases that are characterized with an absence or marked reduction in the number of interlobular bile ducts in the portal triads, are referred to as biliary hypoplasia. These diseases have manifestations similar to those of biliary atresia, including jaundice and acholic stool, and it can be difficult to make the diagnosis without laparotomy. Alagille syndrome is the most common syndrome with intrahepatic bile duct paucity and has typical symptoms such as facial characteristics, ocular abnormalities, and vertebral arch defects. An intraoperative cholangiogram and liver biopsy are necessary to make this diagnosis. Prognosis is variable. Liver transplantation is curative in these patients.

Inspissated Bile Syndrome

Inspissated bile syndrome results from massive neonatal hemolysis caused by Rh and ABO blood group incompatibility between the patient and mother. Elevation of conjugated bilirubin in bile will cause bile sludge or calculi formation, which can cause bile duct obstruction. Intraoperative irrigation of the bile duct is sufficient to resolve this situation in most instances, but it can occasionally be necessary to remove the calculi from the biliary system manually. Blood exchange or phototherapy can obviate the need for operative treatment if they are performed early enough in the disease process.

Idiopathic Perforation of the Extrahepatic Bile Ducts

The cause of bile duct perforation in neonates is unknown. Perforation is primarily found at the union of the common bile duct and cystic duct. This phenomenon suggests that a developmental weakness at this site might be present. Patients with this disease have sterile bile ascites and can form pseudocysts around the perforation site. Drainage around the area of the perforation is usually all that is required because the perforation site heals spontaneously several weeks after the operation. A cholecystostomy catheter is recommended to evaluate healing of the bile duct perforation postoperatively by cholangiography.

Suggested Reading

Adelman S. Prognosis of uncorrected biliary atresia: an update. J Pediatr Surg 13:389, 1978.

Hendren WH, Vacanti JP. Pediatric liver surgery. In WV McDermott, Jr. (ed), Surgery of the Liver. Boston: Blackwell Scientific, 1989.

Hoffman MA. Current Controversies in Biliary Atresia. Austin: R. G. Landes Company, 1992.

Kalayoglu M, D'Alessandro AM, Knechtle SJ, et al. Long-term results of liver transplantation for biliary atresia. Surgery 114:711, 1993.

Kasai M, Kimura S, Asakura S, et al. Surgical treatment of biliary atresia. J Pediatr Surg 3:665, 1968.

Meister RK, Esquivel CO, Cox KL, et al. The influence of portoenterostomy with stoma on morbidity in pediatric patients with biliary atresia undergoing orthotopic liver transplantation. J Pediatr Surg 28:387, 1993.

Miyano T, Fujimoto T, Ohya T, et al. Current concept of the treatment of biliary atresia. World J Surg 17:332, 1993.

Ryckman F, Fisher R, Pedersen S, et al. Improved survival in biliary atresia patients in the present era of liver transplantation. *J Pediatr Surg* 28:382, 1993.

Suruga K, Tsunoda S, Deguchi E, et al. The future role of hepatic portoenterostomy as treatment of biliary atresia. *J Pediatr Surg* 27:707, 1992.

Tan CEL, Driver M, Howard ER, et al. Extrahepatic biliary atresia: A first-trimester event? Clues from light microscopy and immunohistochemistry. *J Pediatr Surg* 29:808, 1994.

Tanaka K, Shirahase I, Utsunomiya H, et al. A valved hepatic portoduodenal intestinal conduit for biliary atresia. *Ann Surg* 213:230, 1991.

Tanaka K, Uemoto S, Tokunaga Y, et al. Surgical techniques and innovations in living related liver transplantation. *Ann Surg* 217:82, 1993.

Toyosaka A, Okamoto E, Okasora T, et al. Outcome of 21 patients with biliary atresia living more than 10 years. *J Pediatr Surg* 28:1498, 1993.

Vacanti JP, Shamberger RC, Eraklis A, et al. The therapy of biliary atresia combining the Kasai portoenterostomy with liver transplantation: A single center experience. *J Pediatr Surg* 25:149, 1990.

Vacanti JP, Leichtner AM, Shamberger RC, et al. The surgical management of biliary atresia at Children's Hospital, Boston. In R Ohi (ed.), *Biliary Atresia*. Proceedings of the 5th International Sendai Symposium on Biliary Atresia. Tokyo, 1991. (ICOM Associates Inc.)

EDITOR'S COMMENT

Doctors Vacanti and Sano have given us an excellent review of the surgical treatment of jaundice in newborn infants, ranging from biliary atresia to choledochal cyst (also well covered in this volume by Dr. Grosfeld, Chap. 155), and some other miscellaneous conditions leading to neonatal jaundice.

The diagnosis may be difficult, even with current techniques. Ben-Haim and co-workers from the Department of Radiology at the University of Iowa College of Medicine (*Clin Nucl Med* 20:153, 1995), reported on a series of 36 infants with hyperbilirubinemia with and without phenobarbital inducement. Technetium-99m mebrofenin was used as the agent of biliary excretion. Twenty-four hours was used as the cut-off point for detection of Technetium in the bowel. Of the 28 patients without biliary atresia, 26 had bowel activity within 24 hours. Unfortunately, two patients had no bowel activity and subsequently were shown to have cystic fibrosis and neonatal hepatitis. Thus, in those patients in whom it is most difficult to make the diagnosis, there continue to be difficulties in assessing biliary excretion of dye.

The therapy of jaundice in newborn infants, particularly that of surgical disease, must be looked at as a continuum of procedures, including portoenterostomy, Kasai's procedure, and liver transplantation. The long-term results of Kasai's procedure are still somewhat controversial, with many authorities believing it has a real place in the management of these patients, at least as a temporizing measure and perhaps in a few patients to a permanent outcome. The differences in permanent outcome appear to be somewhat different between Japan and the United States. Ohi and colleagues of Tohuku University, Sendai, Japan *J Ped Surg* 25:442, 1990) appear to believe that Kasai's procedure offers a long-term solution to the problem. They reviewed 48 patients after a follow up of 10 to 33 years after the procedure and found that 37 of 48 patients were leading "normal" lives. Some had jaundice and portal hypertension, however, and undoubtedly were in need of liver transplan-

tation. The results in the United States are not as good, with up to 50 percent requiring liver transplantation in childhood. However, the Kasai procedure does provide a valuable temporizing procedure so patients can grow and mature. Synthetic failure, growth failure, and bleeding and sepsis relating to hepatic compromise should lead one, however, to the relatively quick conclusion that the patient is heading toward transplantation. Figure 105-10 is particularly revealing. For those patients without treatment, the survival curve is dreadful. The overall survival of close to 90 percent of patients who were treated with the Kasai procedure and subsequently underwent transplant when necessary, is rather dramatic.

As to the technique, as Dr. Blumgart points out in Chap. 94 on hepatic resection, the principle of lowering the hepatic plate is graphically illustrated in Fig. 94-6, 94-7, and 94-8. The Roux length is something to which one needs to pay careful attention. Doctors Vacanti and Sano advocate a Roux length of 30 to 35 cm, at the very least. They are less insistent on the long length following portoenterostomy following surgery for choledochal cyst, because in the latter there is good bile flow. Following the Kasai procedure, it is particularly important to have a sufficient length of the Roux loop that will grow to 60 cm, which seems to be the magic number in adults at the present time to prevent the reflux of intestinal contents. Yet, the longer the Roux length that one uses, one gets into the problem of the type of Mann-Williamson ulcer preparation. The longer the segment of the small bowel from which bile is diverted, the more frequent the incidence of ulceration. Thus, one must plan a balance between the two.

J.E.F.

106

Liver Transplantation

Douglas W. Hanto

Indications for Liver Transplantation and Selection Criteria

In general, liver transplantation is indicated in children and adults suffering from irreversible liver injury after alternative medical and surgical treatments have been exhausted and the patients are approaching the terminal phase of their illness. More specifically, liver transplantation is indicated when:

1. The patient has end-stage liver disease with a life expectancy of 12 months or less and currently has no medical or surgical alternatives to a liver transplant.
2. The expected mortality of the patient's liver disease is greater than the expected mortality of liver transplantation.
3. The patient has a high likelihood for a successful outcome with an improved quality of life.
4. The patient and the family are capable of understanding the indications, potential benefits, risks, and potential complications of liver transplantation.
5. The patient is believed to be compliant and able to adhere to the follow-up medical regimen, including taking medications indefinitely.
6. The patient with alcoholic cirrhosis, currently the most common indication for liver transplantation, or a history of substance abuse meets the criteria established by the Ohio Solid Organ Transplant Consortium (OSOTC).

These OSOTC criteria were designed to reduce the risk of recidivism and to optimize the fair and equitable use of a scarce resource. There are six screening guidelines

for liver patients with histories of chemical dependency:

1. Patients are to be abstinent for 3 to 6 months and actively participating in a chemical dependency recovery program if abstinent for less than 2 years at the time of referral.
2. Patients must consent to unannounced, random urine or blood tests.
3. The patient and family must agree that, if the patient begins drinking or using drugs again, the patient or family, or both, will provide this information to the transplant team, who will report it to the chemical dependency program.
4. The patient should have a history (past and current) of stable personal relationships.
5. The patient should have a stable work history.
6. Both the patient and family must acknowledge that alcohol or substance abuse is or has been a problem.

All patients undergo a detailed psychiatric evaluation to assess whether they meet these screening guidelines. There is some flexibility for patients with severe encephalopathy or who are critically ill and have not already entered a recovery program as described above and are, therefore, unable to form a treatment alliance with the transplant team. All patients being considered for liver transplantation in Ohio, regardless of the specific indication, must be approved by a local institutional multidisciplinary committee and by the OSOTC Liver Selection Committee before listing with the United Network for Organ Sharing (UNOS). The Liver Selection Committee is composed of surgeons, physicians,

ethicists, and lay representatives from the public.

Specific disease indications for liver transplantation include extrahepatic biliary atresia or hypoplasia, chronic active hepatitis (A, B, C, or acute autoimmune), primary biliary cirrhosis, inborn errors of metabolism (α_1-antitrypsin deficiency, Crigler–Najjar disease, Type I, Byler's disease, glycogen storage disease [0 and IV], Wilson's disease, hemochromatosis, tyrosinemia, and so forth); sclerosing cholangitis, hepatic vein thrombosis (Budd–Chiari syndrome), secondary biliary cirrhosis (Caroli's disease, choledochal cyst, trauma, postnecrotic cirrhosis, and congenital biliary cirrhosis), congenital hepatic fibrosis, cystic fibrosis, and acute fulminant hepatic failure (acetaminophen overdose, hepatitis, ischemia, and so forth). Relative indications for liver transplantation include hepatocellular carcinoma, cholangiocarcinoma, slow-growing metastatic leiomyosarcoma, neuroendocrine tumors including carcinoids, and hemangioendotheliomas. Contraindications to liver transplantation include hepatitis B in association with stage III or IV hepatocellular carcinoma, HBV-DNA positive and HBeAg positive hepatitis B, HIV infection, active alcohol or drug abuse, active infection outside the hepatobiliary system, active ulcer disease, unstable psychotic disease (preliver failure), uncontrolled malignancy, and other imminent life-limiting illness. In most instances, although the disease is important in the decision-making process, the actual indications for liver transplantation relate to the complications of end-stage liver disease. For example, the most common complication of liver failure leading to liver transplantation is intractable ascites, often in association with episodes of spontaneous bacterial peritonitis. Other common complications include bleeding esophageal or gastric varices in patients with poor hepatic reserve who are not candidates for surgical shunt procedures and have failed medical management, hepatic encephalopathy, reduced hepatic synthetic function (coagulopathy and hypoalbuminemia), malnutrition, fatigue, hepatorenal syndrome, and recurrent cholangitis in patients with sclerosing cholangitis. With the increasing shortage of cadaver donor livers and the longer waiting periods that result, patients are being listed earlier in the course of their disease. It is usually in the patient's best interest to err on the side of transplanting too early, rather than too late, because of the greater morbidity and mortality in patients with far advanced liver disease who have multiple simultaneous complications.

Preoperative Evaluation and Management

Potential liver transplant recipients can undergo initial evaluation as an outpatient or as an inpatient depending on the disease and its severity. A complete history is obtained along with previous laboratory studies, x-rays, biopsies, endoscopy studies, and so forth so that unnecessary repetition of previously performed studies is avoided. As part of the patient's initial evaluation the following studies are obtained: routine CBC, platelet count, renal profile, hepatic profile, prothrombin time (PT), partial thromboplastin time (PTT), hepatitis serology (A, B, and C), viral serology (HSV, CMV EBV, HIV, and VZV), infectious serology (RPR, toxoplasmosis, rubella), AFP, CA 19-9 (in patients with suspected cholangiocarcinoma or sclerosing cholangitis) chest x-ray, ECG, MRI of the abdomen (for vessel patency, liver volume, and to rule out hepatic tumors), upper GI endoscopy, dental evaluation, pap smear, mammogram (in females over the age of 40 years), and prostate specific antigen (PSA) (in males over the age of 40 years). Other studies that are obtained less frequently, depending on the patient's history and disease, include pulmonary function tests, colonoscopy (in patients over

the age of 40 years), echocardiogram, dipyridamole stress thallium study, cardiac catheterization with coronary angiography, and psychiatric evaluation (for all patients with a history of substance abuse, alcohol abuse, or psychiatric illness). Patients whose MRI reveals suspected portal vein thrombosis undergo visceral angiography to assess patency of the portal, splenic, and mesenteric veins. Appropriate consultations from physicians in cardiology, pulmonary disease, neurology, and infectious diseases are obtained as needed.

Once a patient is listed for liver transplantation, it might be several months before the transplant is performed. During this period, close patient follow-up and careful management of complications of the liver disease is mandatory to maintain the patient in optimal medical condition for transplantation. Intractable ascites is usually managed with intermittent large volume paracentesis, spontaneous bacterial peritonitis with intravenous antibiotics followed by oral antibiotics for long-term prophylaxis, esophageal or gastric varices with sclerotherapy or transjugular intrahepatic portal systemic shunts (TIPS), hepatic encephalopathy with lactulose and protein restriction, malnutrition with oral nutritional supplements or feeding tube placement, and hepatorenal syndrome with dialysis if required. In patients with cardiac or pulmonary disease, periodic re-evaluation is mandatory, and the patency of the portal vein should be assessed at intervals.

Patients admitted to the hospital with acute fulminant hepatic failure or decompensation of chronic liver disease require urgent inpatient evaluation and listing for liver transplantation, if indicated. The principles of management of patients with acute fulminant hepatic failure are similar to the principles for patients with primary nonfunction after transplantation and include 1) protection against and treatment of critical cerebral edema; 2) maintenance of other organ system function (cardiovascular, respiratory, renal, and so forth); 3) protection against complications of coagulopathy; 4) prevention of sepsis; and 5) prevention of hypoglycemia. Patients in stage III or IV coma are intubated when there is concern regarding respiratory insufficiency or a risk of aspiration. All patients undergo placement of a Swan–Ganz catheter, arterial line, and Foley catheter for appropriate fluid management. An at-

tempt is made to partially correct the patient's coagulopathy so that the PT is less than or equal to 15 seconds. If stable, patients undergo a CT scan of the head before placement of an intracranial pressure monitor. An EEG is also performed. An epidural or subdural intracranial pressure monitoring device is placed in order to monitor the intracranial pressure (ICP) and the cerebral perfusion pressure (CPP). Cerebral edema is managed by the use of hyperventilation, intravenous mannitol, and fluid restriction. An attempt is made to maintain the serum osmolality at approximately 325 mosm/dl. The patient's coagulopathy is closely monitored and treated as needed with fresh frozen plasma, cryoprecipitate, and platelets. If the patient requires large amounts of blood products, diuretics are administered as necessary to avoid cerebral edema. Patients are treated with prophylactic antibiotics to prevent sepsis. They are also started on lactulose via a nasogastric tube. Patients undergo very close neurologic monitoring and are aggressively treated for any evidence of increase in ICP or decrease in CPP (less than 60 mm Hg). A full transplant evaluation is completed as quickly as possible, and patients are activated on the UNOS waiting list if they are acceptable candidates.

Intraoperative Management

Patients are admitted to the hospital emergently for liver transplantation when a donor liver becomes available. They are then taken to the operating room where they undergo induction of general anesthesia, often with a full stomach. Therefore, a rapid sequence induction with cricoid pressure is used for intubation. General anesthesia is maintained with an inhalation agent, a neuromuscular blocking agent, and intravenous narcotics. Monitoring and infusion lines are placed, including two radial arterial lines (one for continuous measurement of arterial pressure and one for intermittent blood drawing), a right internal jugular vein Swan–Ganz catheter for hemodynamic monitoring, a 9Fr trauma catheter for use with the rapid infuser placed in an internal jugular or a subclavian vein, and two 14-gauge peripheral intravenous lines. As is standard for any general anesthetic, continuous ECG, pulse oximetry, capnography, and core temperature monitoring are performed. A Foley catheter and nasogastric tube are placed, and a forced air warmer is attached to the lower extremities to help maintain the body temperature. Intraoperatively, close monitoring of arterial blood pressure, central venous and pulmonary artery pressures, cardiac output, systemic vascular resistance, stroke volume, and urine output is critical during the recipient hepatectomy when the blood loss can be significant. Laboratory studies are measured at least hourly, including hemoglobin, hematocrit, platelet count, electrolytes, ionized calcium, PT, PTT, factor and fibrinogen levels, fibrin degradation products, and arterial blood gases.

There are several major events that occur during liver transplantation that require attention. During the recipient hepatectomy, it is critical to carefully replace ongoing blood loss and to maintain normal fluid, electrolyte, and coagulation homeostasis. The goal is to maintain all values as normal as possible throughout the operative procedure, particularly the coagulation studies. The hemoglobin should be maintained at over 10 g per dl, the platelet count at over 100,000 mm^3, the fibrinogen level at over 150 mg per dl, and the prothrombin time at less than 15 seconds by replacing the intraoperative losses with the appropriate units of packed red cells, platelets, cryoprecipitate, and fresh frozen plasma. After initiation of venovenous bypass and just before removing the liver, additional replacement of intravascular volume is usually required because of a decrease in venous return that occurs when portal and vena caval blood return to the heart is interrupted. Increasing the venovenous bypass flow rate after the liver is removed is usually helpful. During the anhepatic phase, while hemostasis is achieved in the retroperitoneum and the liver is sewn in place, careful attention to hemodynamic changes, electrolyte abnormalities (hypocalcemia and hyperkalemia), and coagulation abnormalities (decreased fibrinogen, increased PT, and ↑ fibrin degradation products [FDP]) is important, and appropriate measures to correct any deviations from normal are taken. Before unclamping the liver, additional calcium, sodium bicarbonate, and fluid or blood products are administered. After the liver is unclamped, there can be a brief period of hyperkalemia, hypocalcemia, metabolic acidosis, depressed cardiac output and hypotension, pulmonary hypertension and right ventricular dysfunction, and fibrinolysis that require careful correction. Once the patient is stabilized and all bleeding is controlled, overcorrection of minor abnormalities in the PT and PTT or platelet count should be avoided to minimize the risk of subsequent hepatic artery or portal vein thrombosis.

Surgical Technique
Cadaver Donor Hepatectomy

The donor is placed in the supine position on the operating table with the arms extended. A midline incision is made from the suprasternal notch to the symphysis pubis. A sternal retractor is placed, which improves the exposure in the upper abdomen, along with a wide abdominal re-

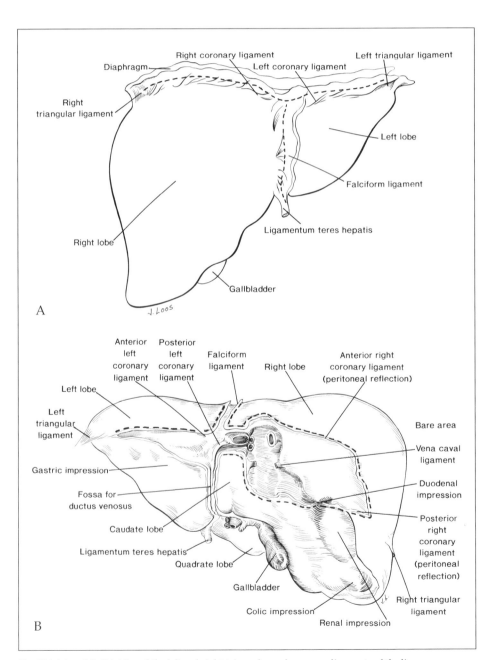

Fig. 106-1A and B. Division of the left and right triangular and coronary ligaments of the liver.

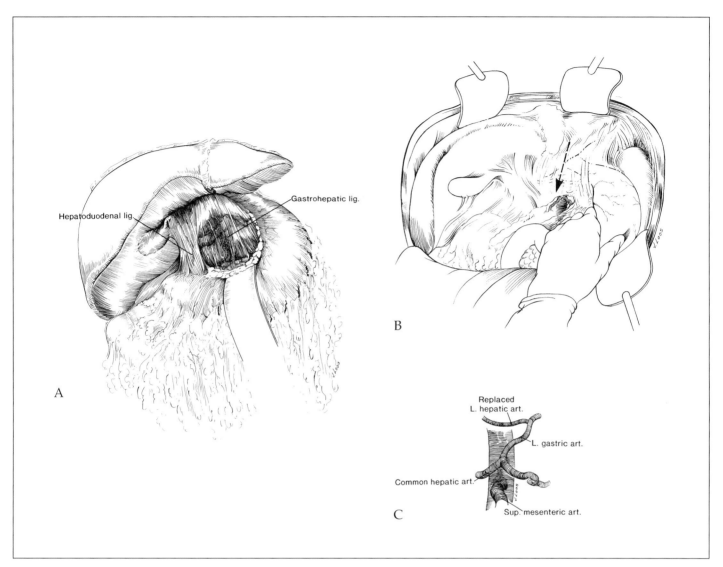

Fig. 106-2. A. The gastrohepatic and hepatoduodenal ligaments. B. Division of the gastrohepatic ligament exposing the lesser sac and the medial aspect of the inferior vena cava and caudate lobe. C. Anatomy of the replaced left hepatic artery originating from the left gastric artery.

tractor with sharp penetrating blades. In obese patients, a transverse abdominal incision at the level of the umbilicus can facilitate exposure. The liver and the remainder of the abdominal cavity should be thoroughly examined visually and manually to exclude any unsuspected infections, malignancies, or other disease processes that would preclude organ retrieval. The falciform ligament should be divided superiorly to the level of the suprahepatic vena cava. The left and right lobes of the liver are mobilized by dividing the left and right triangular and coronary ligaments (Fig. 106-1A and B). These maneuvers allow the liver to be freely retracted during

the portal dissection and reduce the risk of capsular tears or subcapsular hematomas caused when attachments to the liver capsule are torn by excessive retraction.

The dissection begins in the gastrohepatic ligament. The liver is retracted cephalad and to the right while the stomach is retracted downward and to the left, placing the gastrohepatic and hepatoduodenal ligaments on tension (Fig. 106-2A) The almost transparent gastrohepatic ligament is incised from the superior border of the porta hepatis to the diaphragm, thereby exposing the lesser sac and the medial aspect of the inferior vena cava and caudate

lobe (Fig. 106-2B). A replaced left hepatic artery arising from the left gastric artery occurs in approximately 17 percent of donors, usually passes through the superior portion of the gastrohepatic ligament to the liver, and must be carefully preserved (Fig. 106-2A, C). At this point, it is usually preferable to isolate the supraceliac aorta, to identify the origins of the celiac axis and superior mesenteric artery, and to separate the left gastric artery and replaced left hepatic artery from the lesser curvature of the stomach if present. The tissue and blood vessels, including branches of the left gastric artery, should be divided along the lesser curvature of the stomach to the

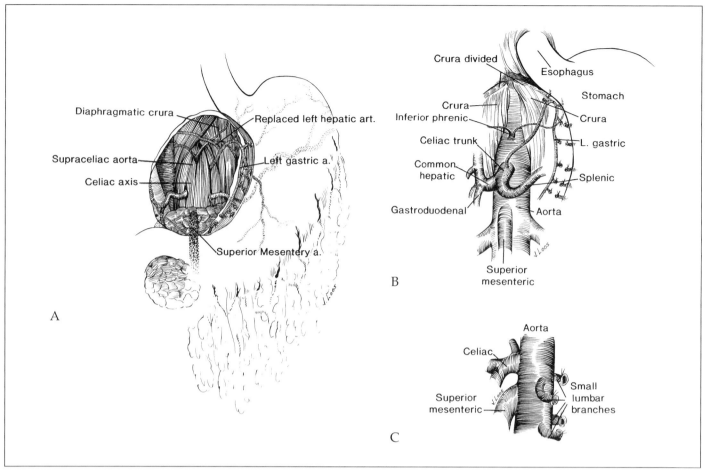

Fig. 106-3. A. Diaphragmatic crura overlying the supraceliac aorta. B. Division of the diaphragmatic crura exposing the aorta. C. Mobilization of the left side of the aorta.

level of the gastroesophageal junction superiorly and to the incissura inferiorly. This step preserves the left gastric artery and exposes the diaphragmatic crura overlying the supraceliac aorta (Fig. 106-3A). The crura are divided, exposing the aorta (Fig. 106-3B). The left side of the aorta should be mobilized first to avoid inadvertent injury to the celiac axis or superior mesenteric artery that comes off the aorta anteriorly and continues to the right (Fig. 106-3C). Small lumbar arteries can be ligated and divided. The origins of the celiac axis and superior mesenteric artery should be isolated by division of the overlying tissue of the celiac plexus. The aorta should be mobilized so that clamps can be placed above the celiac axis, which allows perfusion of the liver and kidneys without perfusing the heart, and between the celiac axis and superior mesenteric artery (or below the superior mesenteric artery if a replaced right hepatic artery is present),

which allows continued perfusion of the kidneys while the liver is being removed (see below).

The dissection then continues in the hepatoduodenal ligament. The tissue of the hepatoduodenal ligament is incised close to the duodenum. The common bile duct is identified inferiorly, and the proper hepatic artery is identified at the superior aspect of the porta hepatis (Fig. 106-4A). The proper hepatic artery is dissected free circumferentially of the surrounding lymph nodes with particular care being taken to avoid excessive stretching of the artery, which can disrupt the intima and lead to an arterial dissection. The artery is followed proximally along the superior border of the pancreas, and the gastroduodenal and right gastric arteries are ligated at a distance from the hepatic artery to avoid compromising its lumen or disrupting the intima (Fig. 106-4B). The splenic artery is

identified and preserved if the pancreas is being retrieved and ligated and divided if it is not. The hepatic artery is then freed to the level of the celiac axis.

The tissue between the hepatic artery and common bile duct overlying the portal vein is incised, and the anterior surface of the portal vein exposed. The portal vein is mobilized circumferentially by clearing the surrounding adventitial and lymphatic tissue and separating the portal vein from the common bile duct, while preserving the periductal tissue containing its blood supply, ligating the left gastric (coronary) vein along its superior aspect, and ligating the pancreaticoduodenal vein branch that is usually on the anterior or inferior aspect of the portal vein. The portal vein is isolated to the junction of the splenic vein and superior mesenteric vein (Fig. 106-5). If the pancreas is not being retrieved, the neck of the pancreas can be divided to expose the

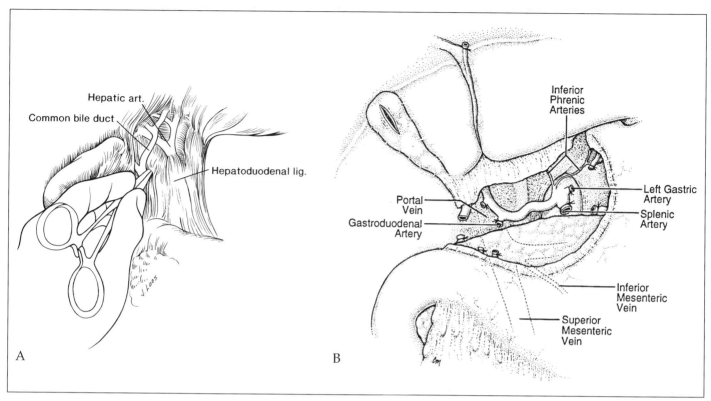

Fig. 106-4. A. Isolation of the hepatic artery at the superior aspect of the porta hepatis. B. Dissection of the hepatic artery along the superior border of the pancreas to the celiac access. (From S Emre, ME Schwartz, CM Miller Jr. The Donor Operation. In RW Busuttil and GB Klintmalm [eds.] Transplantation of the Liver. Philadelphia: Saunders, 1996. P. 396. Reproduced with permission.)

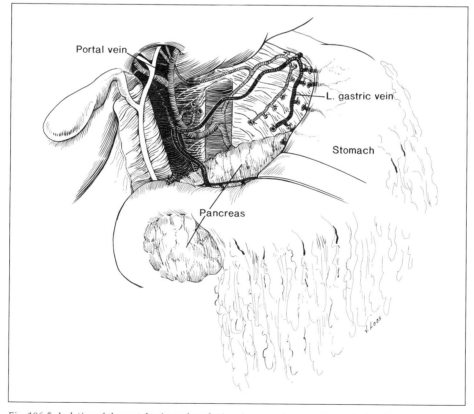

Fig. 106-5. Isolation of the portal vein at the splenic vein—superior mesenteric vein junction.

junction of the splenic and superior mesenteric veins (Fig. 106-6A). The splenic vein is ligated, and a portal perfusion cannula is secured in the splenic vein with a ligature (Fig. 106-6B). A slow infusion of room temperature lactated Ringer's solution is begun. If the pancreas is being retrieved, the portal perfusion cannula is placed in the inferior mesenteric vein. The common bile duct can now be ligated distally adjacent to the pancreas and divided. An incision is made in the fundus of the gallbladder and the biliary tree irrigated with saline. This step prevents necrosis of the biliary tract mucosa caused by bile remaining in contact with the mucosa during cold storage. If a replaced right hepatic artery arising from the superior mesenteric artery is present, it will be found posterior to the common bile duct and portal vein and must be preserved and kept in continuity with the superior mesenteric artery. The infrahepatic vena cava is mobilized above the level of the renal veins. If easily visualized, the right adrenal vein can be ligated and divided at this time. Any remaining ligamentous attachments to the right lobe of the liver are then divided.

The root of the small intestine mesentery, cecum, right colon, and hepatic flexure are then mobilized and reflected medially and superiorly by incising the lateral peritoneal reflection, thereby exposing the retroperitoneum, inferior vena cava, and distal aorta. The anterior surface of the aorta is exposed to the level of the left renal vein with division of the inferior mesenteric artery and identification of the superior mesenteric artery. The inferior mesenteric vein near the ligament of Treitz is identified and cannulated for portal vein flushing if the pancreas is being procured or divided if it is not. The inferior vena cava is also mobilized anteriorly to the level of the infrahepatic cava previously mobilized. During this portion of the operation, particular care must be taken to avoid compromising portal flow by retracting and twisting the small intestine and its mesentery.

The patient is then systemically heparinized (10,000 units iv), and the distal aorta is ligated with an umbilical tape. The aorta is compressed against the vertebral column by the assistant, an aortotomy is made, and a perfusion catheter inserted into the aorta and secured with an umbilical tape. The distal inferior vena cava is then ligated with a heavy ligature, occluded proximally, and a drainage catheter is inserted into the vena cava and secured with an umbilical tape. This step should be the last one before clamping the aorta and perfusing because the decrease in venous return can lead to a drop in blood pressure.

If the donor is in stable condition, cold lactated Ringer's is infused into the portal cannula while preparing for clamping of the aorta. The cardiac surgeons begin the infusion of cardioplegia solution and removal of the heart. The supraceliac aorta is cross-clamped at this point, and infusion of cold University of Wisconsin (UW) solution through the aortic and portal cannulae is begun. The inferior vena cava drainage catheter is unclamped and placed to gravity drainage. If the pancreas is not being retrieved and a replaced right hepatic artery is not present, the superior mesenteric artery can be ligated to prevent perfusion of the intestines and minimize UW wastage. The superior mesenteric vein is ligated and divided if the portal cannula is present in the splenic vein. Surface cooling of the liver, pancreas, and kidneys is achieved by placing cold slush solution in the abdomen. Usually, 2 liters of UW are infused into the aorta (500–1000 cc in children) and 500 to 750 ml into the portal vein (100–250 cc in children) over approximately 10 minutes (Fig. 106-7). The liver edges should be carefully observed for signs of overperfusion manifest by a liver tense to palpation with rounding of the liver edges. The liver can then be removed. An aortic clamp is placed between the celiac axis and the superior mesenteric artery, or distal to the superior mesenteric artery if a replaced right hepatic artery is present. In both situations, care must be taken to clamp proximal to the take off of the renal arteries. Infusion of UW solution and cooling of the kidneys can be continued while the liver is being removed.

The liver is excised by dividing the aorta proximal to the celiac axis and distal to either the celiac axis or superior mesenteric artery, depending on whether a replaced right hepatic artery is present. The splenic and superior mesenteric veins have already been divided if the pancreas is not being retrieved. If the pancreas is being removed, then the portal vein is divided to provide an adequate length of vein for the liver and for the pancreas. The inferior vena cava is divided proximal to the renal veins. The suprahepatic vena cava will have been divided above the diaphragm by the cardiac surgeon. The diaphragm is divided around the suprahepatic vena cava and the liver taken to the back table and placed in cold UW solution. An additional 250 to 500 cc of UW are infused into the hepatic artery and 500 to 750 cc into the portal vein. The effluent from the hepatic veins should be clear. The liver is then packaged in UW solution for transport.

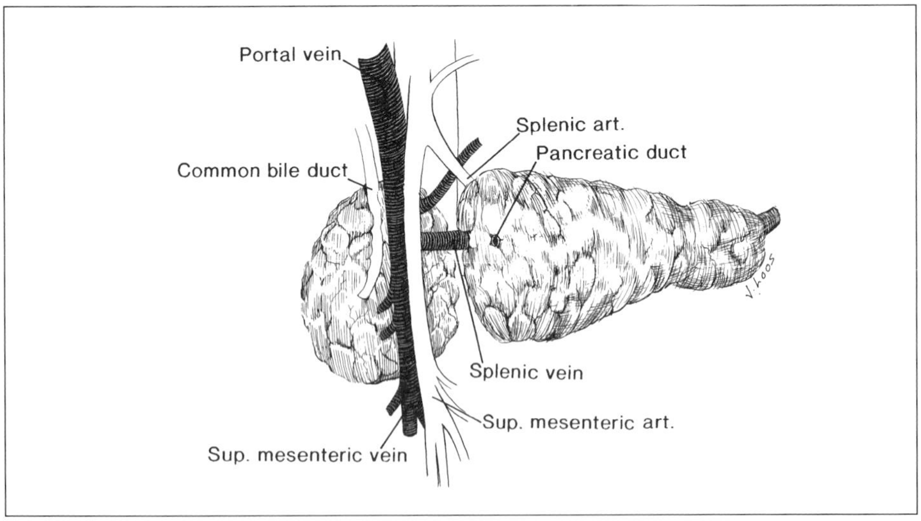

Portal vein
Common bile duct
Splenic art.
Pancreatic duct
Splenic vein
Sup. mesenteric art.
Sup. mesenteric vein

Fig. 106-6. Division of the neck of the pancreas when the pancreas is not being retrieved.

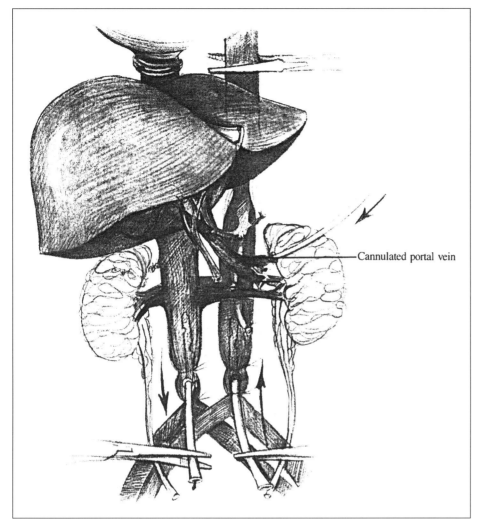

Fig. 106-7. *Perfusion of the intraabdominal organs at the time of cadaver donor retrieval. (From NL Archer. Multiple organ donation from a cadaver. In RL Simmons, et al. [eds.],* Manual of Vascular Access Organ Donation and Transplantation. *New York: Springer, 1984. P. 135. Reproduced with permission.)*

Before transplantation into the recipient, the cadaver liver must be prepared on the back table. This preparation is usually performed by a second surgeon during the recipient hepatectomy. The diaphragm left on the liver is dissected free, and the suprahepatic vena cava isolated. The three phrenic veins entering the suprahepatic vena cava must be identified and suture ligated to prevent bleeding after unclamping. The infrahepatic vena cava is cleaned of its attachments, the right adrenal vein ligated, and any other small branches that were divided during retrieval ligated. The portal vein and hepatic artery are isolated and the gallbladder removed after ligation of the cystic artery and duct. UW solution is infused into the hepatic artery, portal vein, and vena cava to check for leaks.

Recipient Hepatectomy

A bilateral subcostal skin incision is made approximately 4 to 6 cm from the costal margin. The incision should be made lower in patients with massive ascites or the incision will rest over the lower ribs when the abdomen is decompressed and closed. The incision is carried from the lateral border of the left rectus muscle to a point beyond the right rectus muscle approximating the anterior axillary line. In many patients, exposure of the suprahepatic vena cava is facilitated by a midline extension of the incision to the xiphoid process and in some instances resection of the xiphoid, although this resection results in a significant incidence of wound complications (infection, dehiscence, and inci-

sional hernia) in this region. The falciform ligament is clamped, divided, and ligated. The falciform ligament is divided with electrocautery cephalad until the anterior surface of the suprahepatic vena cava is identified. A Thompson self-retaining retractor is then placed. The left lobe of the liver is mobilized by dividing the left triangular and coronary ligaments. The gastrohepatic ligament is incised, which defines the upper border of the porta hepatis. If a replaced left hepatic artery is present in the gastrohepatic ligament, it is ligated and divided because it is almost always too small to use for the hepatic artery anastomosis.

The hilar dissection begins by incising the peritoneum overlying the cystic duct-common bile duct junction. The cystic duct and cystic artery are identified, ligated, and divided. Three retractors are then placed to retract the liver cephalad; the hepatic flexure caudad; and the stomach, duodenum, and transverse colon to the left and caudad. This retraction places the porta hepatis on tension and allows easier dissection of the portal structures. The left and right hepatic arteries are located along the superior border of the hilum and divided close to the liver to provide adequate length for a branch-patch anastomosis to the donor hepatic artery. It is critical to avoid excessive traction on the hepatic artery to avoid disruption of the intima and subsequent arterial dissection, which can preclude the use of the recipient artery for anastomosis. Vessel loops should not be used. In addition, careful identification and ligation of small branches are necessary to avoid the need for direct suture ligation on the hepatic artery of small branches torn from the vessel, which can compromise the arterial lumen. The hepatic arteries are then dissected free proximally to the bifurcation and a length of the common hepatic artery cleared that is sufficient to allow a clamp to be placed later. In some instances, neither the right and left hepatic arteries nor the common hepatic artery is suitable for anastomosis and further dissection to or beyond the take off of the gastroduodenal artery might be necessary.

The tissue posterior to the hepatic artery is then divided, exposing the anterior aspect of the portal vein. The portal vein is most easily mobilized first anteriorly and distally to its bifurcation into the left and right branches and proximally to the head of the pancreas. There is usually a pancreatico-duodenal vein branch of the portal vein anteriorly or inferiorly that should be identified and divided. The lymph node tissue along the superior border of the portal vein is divided. The lymph node tissue inferolateral and posterior to the common duct is divided, and the posterior aspect of the portal vein is identified. An opening anterior to the portal vein and posterior to the common duct is then made leaving much of the surrounding tissue adjacent to the bile duct intact to avoid devascularization of the bile duct. Dissection to close to the common bile duct can also lead to bleeding from large venous collaterals that can be difficult to control and might require suture ligation and compromise of the bile duct lumen. Occasionally, the common bile duct cannot be used because of the large size of the venous collaterals. The common bile duct is ligated adjacent to the liver and divided. A bulldog vascular clamp is placed on the distal duct to control oozing from the cut surface, or small veins are suture ligated with 5–0 monofilament absorbable sutures.

The tissue overlying the anterior surface of the infrahepatic vena cava is then divided. In some instances, exposure of the vena cava can be easier after dividing the portal vein and placing the patient on venovenous bypass. Initiation of venovenous bypass can also reduce blood loss at this stage by reducing portal pressure and decreasing blood loss from retroperitoneal collaterals that might be injured during mobilization of the infrahepatic vena cava and the right lobe of the liver. Mobilization of the right lobe of the liver by dividing the right coronary and triangular ligaments, exposing the bare area of the retroperitoneum, is then performed. Significant bleeding can occur from the retroperitoneum between the superior aspect of Gerota's fascia and the adrenal gland and the diaphragm if the dissection proceeds too deeply. The infrahepatic vena cava is then isolated above the renal veins and looped with an umbilical tape. It is important not to mobilize the vena cava more caudad because oozing that is difficult to control can occur in the adventitial tissue posterior to the vena cava. The tissue along the right side of the vena cava is then divided cephalad to the level of the suprahepatic vena cava. The right adrenal vein is doubly ligated and divided, along with any other lumbar branches. It is im-

portant to identify the right adrenal gland and to avoid injury to it because hemorrhage that is difficult to control can result. The tissue along the left side of the vena cava is also divided so that the entire vena cava is separated from the retroperitoneum. The liver is then ready for removal. In patients with severe portal hypertension or when exposure of the vena cava is difficult, isolation of the entire length of the vena cava is not necessary and in fact should be avoided to prevent hemorrhage from the retroperitoneum. The infrahepatic and suprahepatic vena cavae can simply be isolated enough to allow clamping and the back wall of the vena cava left in place when the liver is excised. Alternatively, the hepatic veins entering the liver posteriorly from the anterior surface of the inferior vena cava can be divided and the liver dissected off the vena cava. Using this technique, the inferior vena cava can be left in situ, which eliminates the need for venovenous bypass to maintain venous return from the lower extremities.

In order to remove the liver once the patient is on venovenous bypass (see the following discussion), the infrahepatic vena cava is horizontally clamped with a straight or angled vascular clamp to preserve its orientation for subsequent anastomosis. If the patient remains in a hemodynamically stable condition, the suprahepatic vena is clamped with a German vascular clamp. The liver parenchyma is incised caudad to the German clamp to be certain that the suprahepatic cava is not cut short. Next, the infrahepatic vena cava is divided and the liver removed. If the retrohepatic vena cava has not been isolated, the vena cava is incised anteriorly leaving the posterior wall of the vena cava intact. Suture ligation of backbleeding lumbar veins and the right adrenal vein is then accomplished. Hemostasis in the retroperitoneum is then achieved using the argon beam and silk suture ligatures (other materials including chromic, Vicryl, Prolene, neurolon, and so forth are melted by the argon beam). The suprahepatic and infrahepatic vena cavae are trimmed and prepared for anastomosis.

Venovenous Bypass

The primary advantage of venovenous bypass is the maintenance of venous return and splanchnic venous drainage during the anhepatic phase with improved he-

modynamic stability and a reduction in mesenteric edema. Other benefits include improved renal perfusion as a consequence of lowered renal venous hypertension and the provision of additional time to obtain hemostasis in the retroperitoneum for placement of vascular grafts when necessary and for performance of the vascular anastomoses. The implementation of venovenous bypass has contributed to a decline in early morbidity and mortality after liver transplant, although it is not routinely used by all liver transplant surgeons. Venovenous bypass has typically been performed by the placement of heparin-bonded cannulae into the axillary and femoral veins using cut-downs. Complications of femoral and axillary cut-downs include wound infections, hematomas, and lymphoceles. Recently, the percutaneous placement of both cannulae have been described with maintenance of flow rates and a reduction in the incidence of lymphoceles (Fig. 106-8).

Open Bypass Technique
Heparin-bonded Gott shunts #7 (Sherwood Medical, St. Louis, MO) are placed into the left saphenous and axillary veins, using a cut-down. Occasionally, a smaller aortic cannula is used for venous return in patients with small axillary veins. The portal vein is cannulated with a No. 9 Gott shunt. The portal and femoral vein lines are coupled with a Y-connector (Gish Biomedical, Santa Anna, CA) and then connected to the return line via a Bio-medicus pump (Medtronic Bio-Medicus, Inc., Eden Prairie, MN). More recently, a heparin-coated pediatric heat exchanger (Bentley, Irvine, CA) is included in the circuit. At the completion of the bypass, the greater saphenous vein is doubly ligated. The axillary vein is repaired with 7–0 Prolene if it is of sufficient caliber, or ligated if it cannot be repaired. The wounds are meticulously closed with at least three layers of running absorbable suture.

Percutaneous Bypass Technique
Either 17F or 14F catheters are placed in the left femoral and subclavian veins via a double Seldinger technique as follows. Using a 16F introducer kit (Denver Shunt, Evergreen, CO) for the 17F cannula and a 13F introducer kit (Bard Introducer kit, Salt Lake City, UT) for the 14F cannula, a needle stick of the left femoral vein is performed and the J-wire is passed, followed by the dilator or introducer with a tear-

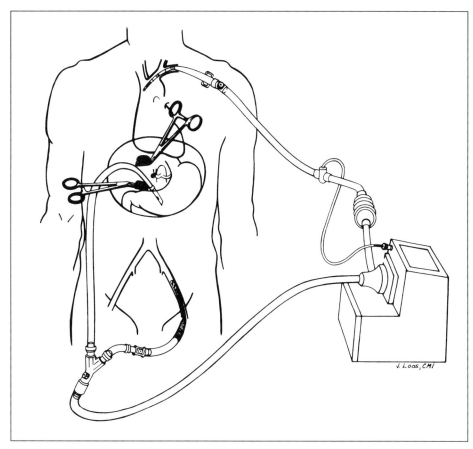

Fig. 106-8. Technique of percutaneous venovenous bypass.

away sheath. After the dilator is removed, a 17F or a 14F cannula (DLP, Inc., Grand Rapids, MI) with an inner introducer is passed over the J-wire into the tear-away sheath. The sheath is removed as the cannula and introducer are advanced. The inner introducer and J-wire are removed, and the cannula is clamped and irrigated with heparinized saline. The femoral cannula is attached to the bypass pump tubing via a Y-type connector (Gish Biomedical, Santa Ana, CA). A left subclavian triple lumen catheter is placed percutaneously before the transplant when the patient can be properly positioned. This catheter is subsequently removed over a guidewire for placement of the bypass cannula, using the same technique described for the femoral cannula. The subclavian cannula is attached directly to the pump tubing. Air is removed from the system.

A modification of this procedure was made after the superior vena cava was perforated in one patient by the stiff inner introducer of the cannula with subsequent development of a right hemothorax. Now,

a 3-mm (0.038 in., 150 cm) Teflon coated J-wire (Cordis Co., Miami, FL) is passed through the inner introducer and through the dilator within the vein. The cannula or introducer is then advanced over this larger, longer J-wire into the tear-away sheath to prevent the stiff inner introducer from puncturing the superior vena cava. This J-wire has also been used to facilitate placement of the femoral cannula. Currently, we are using a 15F femoral cannula (DLP, Inc., Grand Rapids, MI) with wire reinforcement to prevent kinking or collapsing of the tubing.

Cadaver Donor Liver Transplantation

The donor liver and cold UW solution are transferred to a basin and brought to the operating table. The suprahepatic vena caval anastomosis is performed first. The donor vena cava should be trimmed to avoid redundancy. Leaving the donor suprahepatic vena cava too long can theoretically lead to twisting of the suprahepatic cava

and obstruction of the vena cava or hepatic veins, especially when the donor liver is much smaller than the recipient liver or when a segmental graft is being used. Everting corner sutures from the donor to recipient vena cava are placed using 3–0 Prolene with the liver still in the basin (Fig. 106-9). Ice cold laparotomy packs are placed in the abdomen, the liver is removed from the basin, and the suture on the patient's left side is tied, while the ends of the suture on the right are left untied and clamped with rubber shod clamps to maintain better exposure of the back wall. The back wall is sewn using an everting running stitch that is tied at the corner. A size discrepancy between the donor and recipient vena cava can be compensated for by using horizontal everting mattress sutures on the larger vessel. The anterior wall is then sewn and tied.

The donor infrahepatic vena cava is trimmed to an appropriate length to avoid redundancy that can lead to kinking and obstruction. An end-to-end anastomosis to the recipient suprarenal inferior vena cava is performed. Everting corner sutures of 5–0 Prolene are placed with the two vessels properly oriented (Fig. 106-10). The corner sutures are tied and the back wall sewn using an everting running stitch. At the same time, an infusion of 1 liter of cold lactated Ringer's solution is begun through the portal vein cannula. This infusion clears the liver of UW solution, which is high in potassium and contains heparin. It also flushes air from the liver and reduces the risk of air emboli. The anterior wall is sewn as the infusion is completed.

The portal vein venovenous bypass cannula is clamped and removed from the recipient portal vein, which is clamped. The donor and recipient portal veins are trimmed to avoid redundancy that can lead to kinking. Everting corner sutures of 6–0 Prolene are placed. The back wall is sewn using an everting running stitch. The anterior wall is sewn without exerting excessive tension on the suture line that can pursestring the anastomosis. The suture is tied loosely at the corner (a "growth stitch") (Fig. 106-11).

In instances in which the portal vein is thrombosed, a long donor iliac vein graft can be sewn end-to-side to the superior mesenteric vein, which is isolated in the mesentery of the transverse colon. The superior mesenteric vein is thin, easily torn,

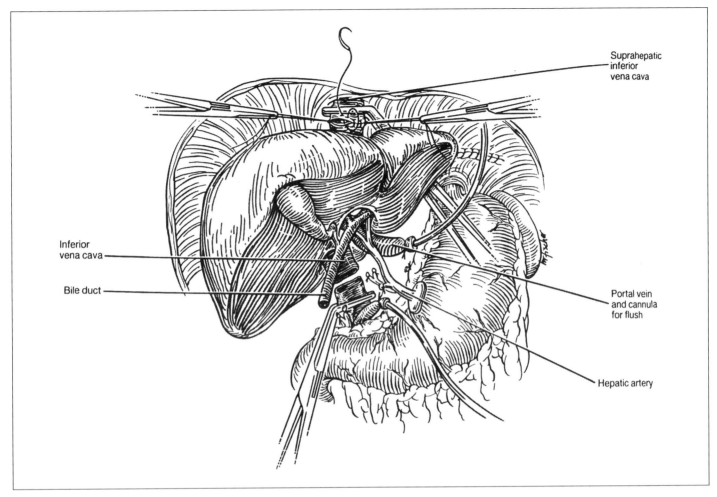

Fig. 106-9. *Suprahepatic vena caval anastomosis during implantation of the donor liver. (From JM Henderson and LF Rikkers. Atlas of Liver Surgery. In RH Bell Jr, LF Rikkers, MW Mulholland [eds.], Digestive Tract Surgery: A Text and Atlas. Philadelphia: Lippincott-Raven, 1996. P. 300. Reproduced with permission.)*

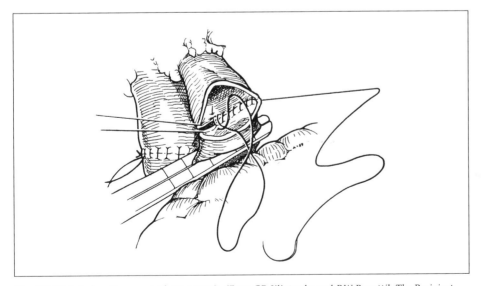

Fig. 106-10. *Intrahepatic vena caval anastomosis. (From GB Klintmalm and RW Busuttil. The Recipient Hepatectomy and Grafting. In RW Busuttil and GB Klintmalm [eds.], Transplantation of the Liver. Philadelphia: Saunders, 1996. P. 413. Reproduced with permission.)*

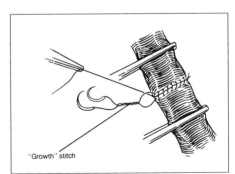

Fig. 106-11. *Portal vein anastomosis with a growth stitch. (From JM Henderson and LF Rikkers. Atlas of Liver Surgery. In RH Bell Jr, LF Rikkers, MW Mulholland [eds.], Digestive Tract Surgery: A Text and Atlas. Philadelphia: Lippincott-Raven, 1996. P. 801. Reproduced with permission.)*

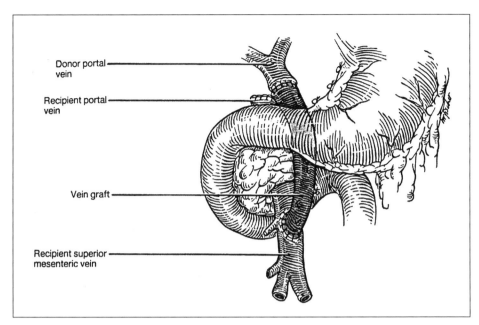

Fig. 106-12. Donor iliac vein graft from the recipient's superior mesenteric vein to the donor portal vein. (From JM Henderson and LF Rikkers. Atlas of Liver Surgery. In RH Bell Jr, LF Rikkers, MW Mulholland [eds.], Digestive Tract Surgery: A Text and Atlas. Philadelphia: Lippincott-Raven, 1996. P. 801. Reproduced with permission.)

and must be handled carefully. Small branches should be ligated and divided to provide an adequate length of vein for the anastomosis. A Statinsky clamp is placed, a venotomy is made, and the donor iliac vein is sewn as an end-to-side anastomosis to the superior mesenteric vein using 5–0 Prolene. Two sutures are placed in the corners of the free end of the donor vein to maintain its orientation as it is tunnelled retrocolic, posterior to the antrum, and anterior to the pancreas for anastomosis to the portal vein (Fig. 106-12). The Statinsky clamp is removed from the superior mesenteric vein, and the donor vein graft is clamped in the porta hepatis. The orientation of the vein should be rechecked to be certain there are no twists in the tunnel.

There are several techniques for performing the arterial anastomosis, depending on the size of the vessels and the arterial anatomy. The arterial anastomosis can be performed as an end-to-end anastomosis between the recipient proper hepatic artery and the donor common hepatic artery using interrupted or running 6–0 Prolene. Our preferred technique is to longitudinally open the recipient right and left hepatic artery branches using a Potts scissors

to create a "branch patch." An end-to-end anastomosis of the branch patch to the donor celiac axis with a Carrel patch is completed using running 6–0 Prolene (Fig. 106-13). This technique has the lowest risk of subsequent hepatic artery stenosis or thrombosis. Alternatively, the donor common hepatic artery or Carrel patch can be sewn end-to-side to the junction of the common hepatic artery and the gastroduodenal artery (Fig. 106-14). When there is a replaced right hepatic artery from the superior mesenteric artery, a cuff of superior mesenteric artery can be sewn end-to-end to the stump of the splenic artery using interrupted 6–0 Prolene, or if the replaced right hepatic artery has been divided, it is sewn directly to the splenic artery stump. Alternatively, if a cuff of aorta with the orifices of the celiac axis and superior mesenteric artery is preserved, the aortic patch can be folded and the edges sewn together and the distal superior mesenteric artery used for anastomosis to the recipient hepatic artery (Fig. 106-15). If there is inadequate inflow via the recipient hepatic artery or celiac axis, a donor iliac arterial graft can be placed to the supraceliac or infrarenal aorta as an end-to-side anastomosis using 5–0 Prolene. In the latter sit-

uation, the arterial graft is usually tunnelled anterior to the pancreas posterior to the antrum.

After completion of the vascular anastomoses, the clamps are removed sequentially. First, the portal vein clamp is removed and the liver perfused. Once the liver is filled, the suprahepatic vena cava clamp is removed. Next, the hepatic artery clamp is removed. The inferior vena cava clamp is removed only when the patient's condition is stabilized after removal of the first three clamps. Hemostasis is obtained, and the patient is taken off venovenous bypass.

The bile duct is usually reconstructed as an end-to-end choledochocholedochostomy using interrupted 5–0 monofilament absorbable sutures (Fig. 106-16). Two sutures between the donor and recipient bile ducts are initially placed, one in the center of the posterior duct and one opposite it anteriorly. The posterior suture is tied, and interrupted sutures are then placed superiorly and then inferiorly, leaving the anterior half of the anastomosis open. An 8Fr T-tube is brought out through a separate choledochotomy in the recipient common bile duct with one limb crossing the anastomosis. The choledochotomy is repaired around the T-tube with interrupted 5–0 monofilament absorbable sutures. The anterior row of sutures is then completed. The T-tube is injected with saline to identify and allow repair of any leaks. An intraoperative cholangiogram is obtained. The bile duct anastomosis is then covered with saline and air injected into the T-tube to further identify any leaks.

If the recipient bile duct is not usable secondary to disease (e.g., sclerosing cholangitis or large periductal varices) or a marked size discrepancy with the donor duct, an end-to-side Roux-en-Y choledochojejunostomy should be performed (Fig. 106-16). A 60-cm Roux-en-Y loop is created. The jejunum is divided using a GIA stapler and the end oversewn with 4–0 interrupted silk sutures. Intestinal continuity is reestablished with a two-layer end-to-side jejunojejunostomy 60 cm from the end of the Roux-en-Y loop. The inner layer is completed using a running 3–0 monofilament absorbable suture with a Connell stitch anteriorly. The outer layer is completed using 4–0 silk interrupted stitches. The Roux-en-Y loop is brought retrocolic. An end-to-side choledochojejunostomy is

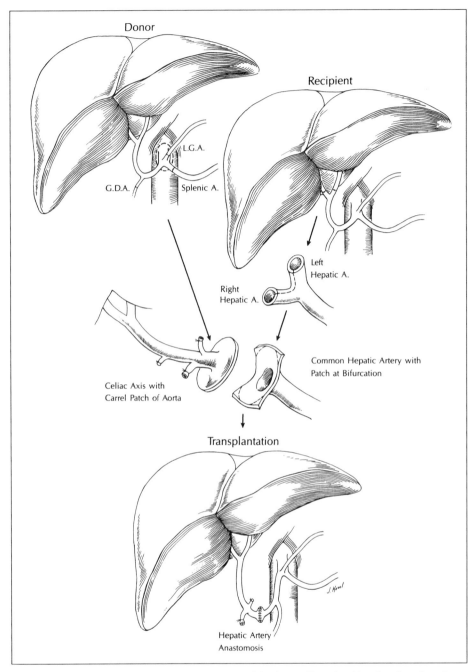

Fig. 106-13. "Branch patch" technique for anastomosis of the donor celiac axis with a Carrel patch to the longitudinally opened recipient right and left hepatic artery branches. (From M Kalayoglu and FO Belzer. A new technique for arterialization of the hepatic duct. Surg Gynecol Obstet 164:564, 1987. Reproduced with permission.)

and left untied. A posterior row of stitches is then placed inside-out on the intestine and outside-in on the common bile duct with the knots tied on the inside for simplicity. The knots can also be tied on the outside by placing the sutures outside-in on both the bile duct and intestine using double-armed sutures, but it is unnecessary. The anterior row of sutures is then placed outside-in on the intestine and inside-out on the bile duct with the knots tied on the outside. The anastomosis is checked as already described, and an intraoperative cholangiogram obtained.

After hemostasis has been obtained, all anastomoses are examined again. The abdomen is irrigated with antibiotic-containing saline solution. Two Jackson–Pratt drains are placed: One subphrenically and posterolateral to the right lobe of the liver with the end adjacent to the suprahepatic vena cava, and one subhepatically posterior to the porta hepatis and anterior to the infrahepatic vena cava. The drains and T-tube or biliary stent are brought out through separate stab incisions in the abdominal wall and secured to the skin with 3–0 nylon horizontal mattress sutures. The abdominal incision is closed with running No. 1 Novafil for the posterior layers and interrupted No. 1 Novafil for the anterior fascia and linea alba. The subcutaneous tissue is reapproximated with 3–0 absorbable sutures, and the skin is closed with staples.

Infection Prophylaxis

A variety of infectious complications can occur following liver transplantation. Many can be prevented or their severity reduced by appropriate prophylaxis. When liver transplant candidates are listed for transplantation, they are placed on Mycelex troches three times per day to reduce fungal colonization in the gastrointestinal tract. After liver transplantation our anti-infective prophylactic regimen includes 1) ampicillin or sulbactam 3.0 g preoperatively and 1.5 g intravenously every 6 hours for 5 days postoperatively, 2) ganciclovir 5 mg per kg intravenously twice a day for 14 days, followed by acyclovir 800 mg orally four times a day for 3 months, 3) fluconazole 400 mg orally every day for 3 months, and 4) Bactrim DS one tablet orally twice a day for 2 weeks, followed by one tablet orally every day indefinitely.

performed in a single layer using interrupted 5–0 Maxon sutures over a 5Fr feeding tube as a biliary stent. Two enterotomies are made near the end of the Roux-en-Y loop, and a 5Fr feeding tube is passed and secured to the intestine with a 5–0 Maxon pursestring suture. Interrupted 4–0 silk sutures are placed to create a tunnel for the feeding tube to prevent any leakage of intestinal contents. Two corner sutures of 5–0 Maxon are placed between the common bile duct and the intestine

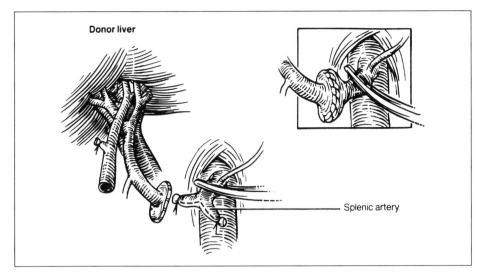

Fig. 106-14. Anastomosis of the donor celiac axis with a Carrel patch to the junction of the recipient's common hepatic artery and gastroduodenal artery. (From JM Henderson and LF Rikkers. Atlas of Liver Surgery. In RH Bell Jr, LF Rikkers, MW Mulholland [eds.], Digestive Tract Surgery: A Text and Atlas. Philadelphia: Lippincott-Raven, 1996. P. 803. Reproduced with permission.)

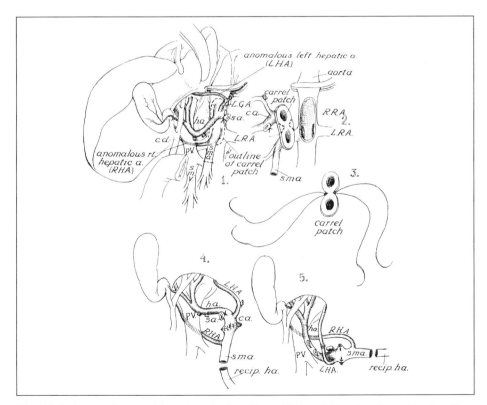

Fig. 106-15. 1. Anomalous arterial supply to the donor liver with the right hepatic artery arising from the superior mesenteric artery. LGA = left gastric artery; sa = splenic artery; LRA = left renal artery; sma = superior mesenteric artery; smv = superior mesenteric vein; PV = portal vein; ha = hepatic artery; cd = common duct; LHA = left hepatic artery; RHA = right hepatic artery. 2. Removal of an aortic Carrel patch with the celiac axis and superior mesenteric artery orifices. RRA = right renal artery. 3. Folding of the aortic patch. 4. The superior mesenteric artery distal to the right hepatic artery is used for anastomosis to the recipient hepatic artery. 5. The newly constructed arterial supply can be rotated to approximate the orientation of the recipient vessel. (From RD Gordon, et al. A simplified technique for revascularization of homographs of the liver with a variant right hepatic artery from the superior mesenteric artery. Surg Gynecol Obstet 160:474, 1985. Reproduced with permission.)

Immunosuppressive Protocol and Results

Our current induction immunosuppressive protocol uses quadruple therapy, including the intraoperative administration of azathioprine (4 mg/kg iv), methylprednisolone (1 g iv), and OKT3 (5 mg iv), an anti-CD3 monoclonal antibody. In order to minimize the cytokine-release syndrome caused by OKT3, patients receive acetaminophen (650 mg/NG [nasogastric]), indomethacin (50 mg/NG), and diphenhydramine (50 mg iv) in addition to the Solu-Medrol 30 minutes before OKT3 administration. Postoperatively, patients receive azathioprine (1 mg/kg), prednisone (1.0 mg/kg tapering to 0.3 mg/kg by 1 month post-transplant), and OKT3 (5 mg/day for 7 days). On postoperative day 5, Neoral (8–10 mg/kg/day in two divided doses po) is started and the dose adjusted to maintain a cyclosporine level of 350 to 450 ng per ml for the first month post-transplant. The cyclosporine levels should be in the therapeutic range for 2 days before discontinuing the OKT3. Patients with acute renal failure or hepatorenal syndrome preoperatively are maintained on OKT3 until renal function improves (Cr < 3.0), or for a maximum of 14 days, before starting Neoral. Daily CD3 counts and weekly antimurine antibody titers are obtained while patients are on OKT3. If the absolute CD3 count increases significantly (usually > 50), the OKT3 dose is doubled to 10 mg per day and an antimurine antibody titer is repeated. If the antimurine antibody titer is greater than 1:100, OKT3 is discontinued to prevent the development of xenotypic antimouse antibodies. Patient survival using this protocol is 87 percent, 84 percent, and 82 percent at 1, 2, and 3 years, respectively. Graft survival is 79 percent, 74 percent, and 74 percent, respectively. The incidence of rejection has been decreased from 65 to 75 percent using triple therapy (azathioprine, prednisone, and cyclosporine) to 36 percent using this quadruple therapy protocol without a concomitant increase in infectious complications. The incidence of second and third rejection episodes is 15 percent and 11 percent, respectively. Approximately 81 percent of rejection episodes respond to antirejection therapy with prednisone only (2.0 mg/kg/day tapering to 0.3 mg/kg/day by 1 month), and 19 percent require OKT3 treatment.

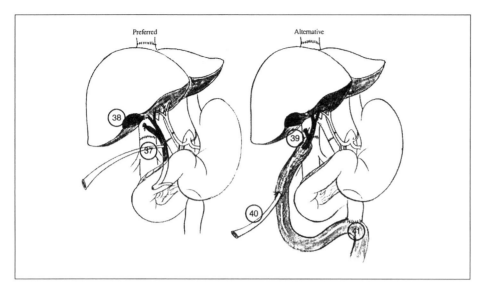

Fig. 106-16. End-to-end choledochocholedocostomy over a T-tube or Roux en Y hepaticojejunostomy. (From NL Archer. Multiple Organ Donation from a Cadaver. In RL Simmons, et al. [eds.], Manual of Vascular Access Organ Donation and Transplantation. New York: Springer, 1984. P. 275. Reproduced with permission.)

Suggested Reading

Broelsch CE. *Atlas of Liver Surgery.* New York: Churchill-Livingstone, 1993.

Gordon RD, Shaw BW Jr, Iwatsuki S, et al. A simplified technique for revascularization of homografts of the liver with a variant right hepatic artery from the superior mesenteric artery. *Surg Gynecol Obstet* 160:474, 1985.

Kalayoglu M, Belzer FO. A new technique for arterialization of the hepatic graft. *Surg Gynecol Obstet* 1664:564, 1987.

Johnson SR, Marterre WF, Alonso MH, et al. A percutaneous technique for venovenous bypass in orthotopic cadaver liver transplantation (OLTx) and comparison with the standard open technique. (Submitted.)

Simmons RL, Finch ME, Ascher NL, Najarian JS. *Manual of Vascular Access, Organ Donation, and Transplantation.* New York: Springer, 1984.

Starzl TE, Shapiro R, Simmons RL. *Atlas of Organ Transplantation.* New York: Gower, 1992.

Stewart MT, Millikan WJ Jr, Henderson JM, et al. Proximal abdominal graft for arterialization during hepatic transplantation. *Surg Gynecol Obstet* 169: 261, 1989.

Tzakis A, Todo S, Starzl TE. Orthotopic liver transplantation with preservation of the inferior vena cava. *Ann Surg* 210: 649, 1989.

Tzakis A, Todo S, Stieber A, Starz TE. Venous jump grafts for liver transplantation in patients with portal vein thrombosis. *Transplantation* 48:530, 1989.

EDITOR'S COMMENT

In a relatively long transition from the initial days of liver transplantation, liver transplantation has become accepted and widely performed with the expectation that survival rates of upwards to 80 percent, as Dr. Hanto documents, can be expected after 1, 2, and 3 years. As such, the controversies of liver transplantation no longer concern the procedure but rather a few technical components such as the bile duct, perhaps the hepatic artery, but more important in the nature of the recipient population. Until such a time as xenografts or hepatocytes, grown on a matrix and either implanted in the liver or in a structure become available, there will always be a shortage of donors. The greatest controversy concerning hepatic transplantation involves patients with substance abuse, as evidenced by the controversy concerning Mickey Mantle, who in addition to his substance abuse, manifested a malignancy. The outcome, rather occurrence or persistence of malignancy within 2 months of the transplant, suggests once again that malignancy may not be the most favorable of diagnoses for which to transplant patients. Likewise, societal pressures may continue to mitigate against transplantation for patients with substance abuse, particularly when a prolonged period of abstinence and family support is not present.

My own experience in patients with liver disease undergoing splenorenal or portacaval shunt suggests that the use of psychiatric services, even when carefully structured, are not ideal for the prevention of recidivism. Indeed, many studies show that there is little added value to psychiatric therapy in patients with alcoholism, provided they do not wish to make the break with substance abuse themselves. In my experience, Alcoholics Anonymous is the only group that has shown consistent ability to maintain abstinence from alcohol.

Some technical matters are of interest. The artery of Hyrtl is present in a remarkably large number of cases and is rarely referred to in the other general surgical literature. One must be careful in doing a high gastrectomy not to devascularize the left lobe of the liver. I agree with Dr. Hanto that the artery's small size usually precludes its use during an anastomosis.

The everting mattress suture, such as described, is a valuable suture to bear in mind not only in liver transplantation, but in surgery for portal hypertension, particularly in relatively small-size splenorenal shunts. Doctor Linton was a champion of this approach, and his text for splenorenal shunts is particularly useful (*Atlas of Vascular Surgery.* Philadelphia: Saunders, 1973). Closure of the fascia following portal hypertension surgery and/or (I assume) liver transplant surgery, in which ascites may occur, leads me to use an entirely different type of closure on the fascia. I use a closure with a running nonabsorbable suture such as Prolene and then place interrupted nonabsorbable sutures between the running nonabsorbable suture. I do not believe that an interrupted closure has much advantage for prevention of ascitic leakage.

Another concern is fulminant hepatitis, which has recently become an indication for liver transplant surgery, particularly in the younger patient. Here urgency is essential, since cerebral edema and breakdown of the blood-brain barrier may result in irreversible damage to the central nervous system, even if a successful liver transplantation occurs. In addition, Bismuth and coworkers (*Ann Surg* 222:109, 1995) found that survival was 83 percent in patients with grade 1 and 2 comas, versus 56 percent in patients with grade 3 comas. Patients with high-risk grafts had a lower survival (51%) versus low-risk grafts (81%), which did not have incompatible, split, or steatotic livers. However, in a patient who was deteriorating rapidly from fulminant hepatitis, non-ideal livers must often be used. In Bismuth's series of 139 patients, 22 died before transplantation, 1 recovered, and 116 underwent transplantation with a 1-year survival rate of 68 percent. Use of high-risk livers permitted transplantation in 83 percent of patients. As stated previously, a higher mortality accompanied the use of these high-risk livers.

Finally, in all surgery of patients with portal hypertension and/or liver disease, it is essential to suture-ligate the lymphatics of the retroperitoneum, particularly in the area around the cisterna chyli. The lymphatics do not clot and a significant amount of morbidity, if not some mortality, is present following failure to ligate these lymphatics in the form of a lymphatic leak or tense ascites, which requires a whole series of management maneuvers. It is far better to prevent lymphatic leaks by suture ligation of these lymphatics in the retroperitoneum.

J.E.F.

Index

Index

Amebic abscess of liver, 1020, 1028
Amino acids
  branched-chain
    in multiple organ dysfunction syndrome,
        162, 164
    as nutritional supplements, 19
    in parenteral nutrition, 65
  dietary
    in acute renal failure, 131
    assessment of requirements, 59
ε-Aminocaproic acid
  in fibrinolysis, 119
  in hemangiomas, 392
  in post-Leveen shunt coagulopathy, 1320,
      1326, 1328
Aminoglycosides, toxicity of, 139
Ampulla of Vater, 1194–1195
Amputations of lower extremity, 2114–2123
  above-knee, 2120–2122
    disarticulation of knee joint in, 2120–2121
    Gritti-Stokes, 2120
    short, 2122
    supracondylar, 2121–2122
  below-knee, 2118–2120
  causes of, 2113–2115
  Chopart, 2116
  determination of surgical level in, 2115–2116
  hip disarticulation, 2122
  Lisfranc, 2116
  surgical technique, 2116–2122
  Syme, 2116–2117
  transmetatarsal, 2116
Amrinone for cardiovascular support, 94–95
Amylase levels in pancreatic injuries, 1256
Anal conditions. See Anus
Anderson-Hynes dismembered pyeloplasty,
      1629–1630
Anemia
  in hemorrhoids, 1568
  splenectomy in, 1269–1270, 1274
Anesthesia
  in carotid body tumor removal, 402
  continuous epidural, postoperative, 935, 937
  in hepatectomy, 1058–1059
  in laparoscopic cholecystectomy, 1100
  local
    in chest tube insertion, 606
    in facial soft-tissue injuries, 458
    maximum dosage in, 459
    in thoracentesis, 603
  in radical neck dissection, 375
  in Shouldice inguinal herniorrhaphy, 1827,
      1829
Aneurysm
  abdominal aortic, 1951–1956
    ruptured, 1981–1989
  autotransfusion technique for
      endoaneurysmorrhaphy, 2004, 2006
  carotid, 2008–2013
  femoral, 1957–1961
  hepatic artery, 1997–2000
  iliac artery, 1986, 2001–2007
  popliteal, 1958, 1961–1962
  renal artery, 1990–1993
  splenic artery, 1993–1997
  thoracoabdominal, 1965–1980
Angina pectoris, partial ileal bypass affecting,
      1364
Angiofibroma of nasopharynx, juvenile, 364
Angiography
  after partial ileal bypass, 1364
  cerebral, in carotid body tumors, 399–400
  in echinococcal cysts of liver, 1040

in hilar cholangiocarcinomas, 1136, 1141
in liver tumors, 1057–1058
magnetic resonance, of portal system, 1291
in pancreatic disease, 1204, 1235–1236
in penetrating neck trauma, 465
preoperative, in trauma to thoracic great
    vessels, 1939–1940
transhepatic portograms in, 1022
in vascular compression of duodenum, 995
Angioplasty, balloon, in subclavian artery
    occlusion, 1916
Anorectal disorders, 1560–1580
  abscess, 1561–1563
    clinical features, 1561
    conservative treatment, 1563
    diagnosis, 1562
    etiology, 1562
    intersphincteric, 1563
    ischiorectal, 1563
    perianal, 1563, 1579
    submucous, 1564
    supralevator, 1563
    surgical drainage of, 1563, 1579–1580
  Crohn's disease, 1392–1398
    perianal, 1578–1579
  fissure in ano, 1560–1561
  fistulas, 1564–1567
    causes of, 1564
    clinical features, 1564
    diagnosis, 1564–1565
    fistulectomy in, 1567
    fistulotomy in, 1565–1566
    Goodsall's rule in, 1565
    mucosal advancement flap in, 1567
  hemorrhoids, 1567–1572
  hidradenitis suppurativa, 1575–1576
  in immunosuppressed patients, 180
  pilonidal sinus, 1573–1575
  rectovaginal fistula, 1576–1577
  warts, 1573
Anorectal manometry in Hirschsprung's
    disease, 1596
Antenatal diagnosis. See Prenatal diagnosis
Anterior commissure procedure in glottic
    cancer, 419
Anthropometry, 54
Antibiotic prophylaxis, 40–44, 134–142
  in bowel preparation, 43
  in bowel surgery, 142–143
  in cardiothoracic surgery, 141
  in cesarean delivery, 1738
  in choledochal cysts, 1157
  in clean surgery, 140–141
  complications of, 139–140
  in diverticulitis, 1466
  dosage in, 138
  in enterocutaneous fistulas, 1379
  in esophageal and gastric surgery, 142
  in head and neck surgery, 141–142
  in liver transplantation, 1180
  misconceptions in, 144
  in obstetric and gynecologic surgery,
      143–144
  recommendations for, 145
  resistance to, 139–140
  selection of patients for, 140–144
  in small bowel obstruction, 1344
  timing of, 137–138
  topical administration of, 138–139
  in toxic megacolon, 1438
  in transplant recipients, 173
  in vascular surgery, 141
  in ventral abdominal hernia repair, 1878

Antibiotic therapy, antitumor, toxicity of, 177
Anticoagulation
  in deep venous thrombosis, 2125–2126
  preoperative management of, 40
  in prophylaxis of thromboembolism, 35
  in pulmonary embolism, 2130
Antimetabolic agents, toxicity of, 177
Antireflux surgery
  biomechanics of, 729–731
  choice of procedure in, 731
  Hill repair in, modified, 758–762
  indications for, 727–729, 743–744, 764
  in infants and children, 708–715
  laparoscopic, 265–269, 273, 763–770
  migration of wrap in, 756
  Nissen-Rossetti fundoplication in, 743–757
  in paraesophageal hernias, 701–702, 707
  perforation of esophagus in, 750, 756
  retractors used in, 756
  transthoracic, 727–742
    Belsey partial fundoplication in, 731–736
    Collis gastroplasty in, 736–737
    indications for, 731
    Nissen fundoplication in, 737–741
  vagotomy in, 752–753, 758–759
Antithrombin III replacement therapy, 122
α₁-Antitrypsin replacement therapy, 122
Antrectomy with selective vagotomy and
      gastroduodenostomy for duodenal
      ulcer, 873–882
Anus. See also Anorectal disorders
  coloanal anastomosis
    in Delorme operation for rectal prolapse,
        1551
    in perineal rectosigmoidectomy for rectal
        prolapse, 1552–1553
    in total proctectomy, 1533, 1538
  colon J-pouch reconstruction, 1533, 1538
  dilatation, 1561
    in hemorrhoids, 1569
    in perianal Crohn's disease, 1579
  ectopic, rerouting of, 1585
  encirclement procedure in rectal prolapse,
      1549
  ileal pouch-anal anastomosis, 1447–1455
    with total proctocolectomy in ulcerative
        colitis, 1482–1488
  sphincter in fecal continence, 1581–1582
  sphincterotomy for fissure in ano, 1561
  transanal-abdominal-transanal
      proctosigmoidectomy, 1524–1531
Aorta
  abdominal aneurysms, 1951–1956
    diagnosis of, 1951–1952
    endovascular grafting technique in, 1955
    inflammatory, 1956
    mycotic, 1956
    postoperative care, 1955
    preoperative preparation in, 1952
    proximal control of aorta in, 1952–1953
    repair of aneurysm in, 1953–1955
    ruptured, 1981–1989
      exposure and control in, 1982–1984
      iliac arteries in, 1986
      operative complications, 1986–1987
      postoperative care, 1987
      preoperative preparation in, 1981–1982
      repair of, 1984–1986
      results of repair, 1987–1988
    surgical technique in, 1852–1955
  ascending aortobifemoral graft, 2035–2038
  in cadaver donor hepatectomy, 1172
  descending thoracic, trauma of, 1942–1944

Ischemia
    cerebral, assessment of, 1901
    in continent ileostomy, 1372
    and reperfusion injury, 159
    visceral, chronic, 2045–2053
Ischiorectal abscess, drainage of, 1563
Islet cell tumors, pancreatic, 544–548
Isoproterenol for cardiovascular support, 94

J pouch
    colon, in anal reconstruction, 1533, 1538,
        1539, 1540
    ileal, anal anastomosis to, 1449–1450, 1455,
        1486–1487, 1489
Jaboulay gastroduodenostomy, 888–889
Jammerecke in Billroth I operation, 852
Janeway gastrostomy, 840
Jaundice
    after hepatic trauma, 1084
    in choledochal cysts, 1154
    in high malignant biliary tract obstruction,
        1135
    neonatal, 1159–1167
        in biliary hypoplasia, 1164
        in congenital dilatation of bile ducts,
            1163–1166
        in extrahepatic biliary atresia, 1159–1163
        in idiopathic perforation of bile ducts, 1164
        in inspissated bile syndrome, 1164
Jejunoileal bypass in obesity, 983
    complications from, 1365
Jejunostomy, 1350–1352
    catheter, 1350
    for enteral nutrition, surgical technique in,
        74–77
    feeding tube, 1350, 1357
        in pancreatic trauma, 1255, 1257
        in pancreaticoduodenectomy, 1243–1244,
            1249, 1255
    needle catheter, 1351, 1357
        in colonic resection for diverticulitis,
            1467–1468, 1480
    proximal, with distal mucous fistula, 1345
Jejunum
    cholecystojejunostomy, 1143–1144
    choledochojejunostomy, 1144–1150
        in pancreaticoduodenectomy, 1243
    cystojejunostomy in pancreatic pseudocysts,
        1229
    duodenojejunostomy, retrocolic, 925
    esophagojejunal anastomosis in total
        gastrectomy, 943–944
    gastrojejunostomy
        in Billroth II operation, 858–872
        in Crohn's disease, 1385
        in pancreaticoduodenectomy, 1243
    hepaticojejunostomy
        in biliary tract strictures, 1114
        in choledochal cysts, 1155, 1158
        in high malignant biliary tract obstruction,
            1136–1137
        in sclerosing cholangitis, 1129–1130,
            1131–1133
    interposition procedures
        in alkaline reflux gastritis, 857
        in dumping syndrome, 961, 976–977,
            978–979
        in esophageal reconstruction, 802–812
        in open gastrostomy, 841
        reversed segment for postvagotomy
            diarrhea, 963, 981
        with Roux en Y gastroenterostomy,
            979–980

lateral pancreaticojejunostomy for chronic
    pancreatitis, 1205–1214
loop preparation in esophagogastrectomy,
    947, 953–954, 956, 958
pancreaticojejunostomy, 1248
    with distal pancreatectomy, 1219–1220
    in pancreaticoduodenectomy, 1243
    in portoenterostomy, 1162
    pouch construction in dumping syndrome,
        975–976
    reservoir as gastric substitute, 208–211
Jugular lymph nodes, 356–357
Jugular vein
    anterior, 353
    external, 295, 296, 353
    internal, 294, 296, 353
        catheterization, 83
        in LeVeen shunt, 1323
    ligation in radical neck dissection, 378,
        382
Juxtavisceral lymph node chain, 357

Karapandzic flap in lip reconstruction, 330
Kasabach-Merritt syndrome, 391
    treatment of, 392
Kasai operation in biliary atresia, 1159,
    1161–1162
Kehr incision for splenic repair, 1277
Ketoacidosis, diabetic, 45–46
Kidneys
    acute failure, 125–132
        atrial natriuretic peptide in, 130
        calcium antagonists in, 130
        cellular damage in, 126
        cytoprotective agents in, 130–131
        diagnosis of, 128–129
        dialysis in, 132
        diuretic phase of, 128
        diuretics in, 129–130
        electrolyte levels in, 131–132
        functional recovery in, 128
        incidence of, 125
        initial phase of, 127
        intrinsic, 127
        in multiple organ dysfunction syndrome,
            164–166
        nutrition and metabolism in, 130
        oliguric phase of, 127–128
        polyuria in, 128
        postrenal, 127
        prerenal, 126–127
        radiologic studies in, 129
        renal blood flow in, 126
        risk factors for, 125–126
        treatment of, 129–132
        vasodilators in, 130
    acute tubular necrosis, 127
    anatomy of, 1613–1615, 1617
    Anderson-Hynes dismembered pyeloplasty,
        1629–1630
    calculi
        after partial ileal bypass, 1363
        in hyperparathyroidism, 508, 516
        open operative procedures in, 1622–1628
    chronic failure, secondary
        hyperparathyroidism in, 517
    Culp-DeWeerd pelvic flap pyeloplasty, 1631
    Davis intubated ureterotomy, 1631–1633
    fascia of, 1613–1614
    Foley YV-plasty, 1630–1631
    function studies with monitoring of urinary
        output and electrolytes, 92
    hepatorenal syndrome, 1320

insufficiency from calculous disease, 1621,
    1628
lymphatic drainage of, 1615
nephrolithotomy, 1625
    anatrophic, 1625–1628
nephrotoxic agents, 127
preoperative management in uremia, 36
pyelolithotomy, 1624–1625
    extended, 1625
relationships with other structures, 1613
in renal artery aneurysms, 1990
renal cell carcinoma, 1635–1645
    aortic disease with, 1645
    causes of, 1635
    classification of, 1635
    diagnosis, 1635–1636
    locally extensive, 1637
    metastatic, 1637–1638
    partial nephrectomy in, 1637, 1641
    pathology, 1635
    radical nephrectomy in, 1638–1644
    staging of, 1636–1637
    surgical anatomy in, 1638
    treatment of, 1638–1644
    vena caval tumor thrombus in, 1637
        surgical management of, 1641–1644
revascularization of, 2053–2059
structure of, 1614
in thoracoabdominal aneurysmectomy, 1969
trauma of, 1699–1700
    vascular injuries, 1699
ureteropelvic junction surgery, 1629–1634
vascular supply of, 1614–1615
Wilms tumor, 1685–1697
Klatskin tumor, 1135, 1141
Klippel-Trenaunay syndrome, 393
Knee disarticulation amputation, 2120–2121
Kocher incision, 188–189, 196
    in portacaval shunt procedure, 1295
Kocher maneuver
    in Billroth I gastrectomy, 849
    in Billroth II gastrectomy, 862
    in duodenal obstruction management, 924
    in lateral choledochoduodenostomy, 11211
    in pancreatic cystoduodenostomy, 1228
    in pancreatic trauma evaluation, 1251, 1256
    in pancreaticoduodenectomy, 1237, 1293
    in portacaval shunt procedures, 1295, 1300,
        1301, 1307
    in reoperative surgery, problems with, 1248
    in selective vagotomy, 876
Kock ileostomy, 1366–1376
    with proctocolectomy in ulcerative colitis,
        1482
Kock pouch for bladder replacement,
    1723–1725
Kupffer cells, interaction with hepatocytes, 10
Kwashiorkor, 51, 56
    marasmic, 51, 56

Labial arteries, 325, 326
Labial veins, 325
Lacrimal duct, trauma of, 460
Lactation, breast in, 553, 561
Lactiferous ducts, 561
Ladd's procedure
    in Bochdalek hernia, 676
    in malrotation, 926
Lahey neck incision, 350
Laparatomy, second-look, in ovarian cancer,
    1770–1771
Laparoscopic surgery, 255–269, 272–273
    in adrenalectomy, 541–542

Metabolism—Continued
 resting metabolic expenditure, 55, 58, 70
 stress assessment, 55
Metalloproteinase, tissue inhibitor of, 396
Metanephrines, urinary, in
  pheochromocytoma, 535–536
Methotrexate toxicity, 177
Metronidazole
 in diverticulitis, 1464
 in perianal Crohn's disease, 1394
Midazolam in mechanical ventilation, 110
Miles operation, 1507–1516
 colon mobilization in, 1509
 colostomy preparation in, 1511
 division of lateral ligaments in, 1510–1511
 incision in, 1508–1509
 mesorectum in, 1510–1511, 1515
 pelvic floor reconstruction in, 1511
 perineal phase of, 1511–1515
 position of patient in, 1508
  in perineal phase, 1511
 preoperative preparation in, 1508
 rectum mobilization in
  anterior, 1509–1510
  posterior, 1509
 two-team approach in, 1508, 1515
 in women, 1509–1510, 1515
Milrinone for cardiovascular support, 95
Mitomycin-C toxicity, 177
Molybdenum, recommended daily allowance,
  52
Monitoring
 after thromboembolectomy, 1896
 cardiovascular, 82–92
 cerebral
  in carotid body tumor removal, 402–403
  in carotid endarterectomy, 1906
 in enteral nutrition, 71
 in mechanical ventilation, 111
 in parenteral nutrition, 64
Monoclonal antibody therapy
 in multiple organ dysfunction syndrome,
  166
 OKT3 in liver transplantations, 1181
Monooctanoin to dissolve biliary stones,
  1095–1096
Morgagni foramen, 655, 661
 herniation through, 652, 654, 679–680
  surgical repair of, 680
Morphine in mechanical ventilation, 110
Mouth. See Oral cavity
Mucosal advancement flap
 in anorectal fistula, 1567
 in perianal Crohn's disease, 1579
 in rectovaginal fistula, 1577
Mucosal graft of Smith in biliary tract stricture
  repair, 1114
Mucosal sleeve resection in rectal prolapse,
  1549–1551, 1554
Mucosectomy, rectal, 1537
Multiple endocrine neoplasia
 gastrinoma in, 544–545
 hyperparathyroidism in, 509, 516, 523
 insulinoma in, 546
 thyroid carcinoma in, 497
Multiple organ dysfunction syndrome, 153–169
 characteristics of, 153–154
 endotoxin in, 160
 epidemiology of, 155
 hepatic dysfunction in, 166
 immunotherapy in, 166
 and inflammatory response to injury, 3–6,
  157–161

ischemia-reperfusion injury in, 159
management of, 161–167
metabolic and nutritional support in,
  161–162
neutrophil-endothelial cell interactions in,
  159–160
nitric oxide in, 160
oxygen kinetics in, 155–157, 161
pathogenesis of, 155
prevention of, 160–161
primary, 152
pulmonary dysfunction in, 155, 162–164
renal dysfunction in, 164–166
role of gut in, 160
secondary, 153, 154
Murphy's sign, posterior, 1204
Muscle flaps in chest wall reconstruction,
  621–622, 624, 625, 626
Muscle protein metabolism in trauma and
  infection, 8–9
 regulation of, 14–15
Musculophrenic artery, 664
Musculophrenic veins, 664
Myasthenia gravis, 527–528
 thymectomy in, 529–539
Myectomy, anorectal, in outlet obstruction,
  1593
Myenteric nervous system in Hirschrpung's
  disease, 1594
Mylohyoid muscle, 297, 310
Mylohyoid nerve, 298, 299
Myocutaneous flaps
 gluteus maximus, in sacral ulcers, 275
 transverse rectus abdominis, in breast
  reconstruction, 275–280
Myo-osseous graft in mandibular
  reconstruction, 341

Narcotics in mechanical ventilation, 110
Nasoenteric tubes, 71
Nasofrontal duct injuries, 461
Nasogastric tubes, 71
Nasopharynx, juvenile angiofibroma of, 364
Nasotracheal intubation, 104
Neck
 abscesses of, imaging of, 363
 in actinomycosis, 368
 anatomic landmarks, 349
  and zones used in trauma patients, 813
 branchial cleft anomalies, 385–388, 389
  imaging of cyst, 363
 congenital anomalies of, 366, 383–389
 cystic hygromas of, 369
 cysts of, 368
 dermoid cysts, 367
 diagnostic approach to masses in, 359–372
  fine-needle aspiration biopsy in, 360–361
  imaging in, 361–365
  open biopsy in, 361
  physical examination in, 359–360
 esophagus in, 464
  vasculature in, 464–465
 fascia of, 351
 fascial spaces in, 351–352
 in Hodgkin's disease, 371, 373
 infections
  acute, 367
  chronic, 367–368
 lipomas of, 368–369
  imaging of, 363
 lymphatics of, 354–358
  classified by levels, 358

and location of tumors, 361, 371
 in tuberculosis, 367–368
lymphomas of, 371
management in lip cancer, 327
metastases to, 371
modified dissection in thyroid malignancies,
  496, 502–506
muscles of, 350–351
nerves of, 353–354
paragangliomas of, 369
parotid gland tumors, 370
penetrating trauma, 463–472
 in asymptomatic patients, 463
 carotid exposure and repair in, 466–467
 classification by zones, 563
 diagnosis of, 464–465
 esophageal exposure and repair in, 470–471
 incisions for exposure in, 465
 indications for exploration in, 465
 larynx in, 464
 selective management of, 465, 472
 surgical techniques in, 465–471
 venous repair in, 470
 vertebral artery exposure and repair in,
  467–470
radical dissection, 373–384
 adjunctive radiation therapy, 382
 advice to patients, 374–375
 anesthesia in, 375
 chylous fistulas from, 381
 closure of, 380
 complications of, 381
 flap development in, 376–377
 hemostasis in, 376
 incisions in, 375–376
 indications for, 373–374
 jugular vein ligation in, 378, 382
 modified, 374
 in parotid tumors, 303–308
 positioning of patient in, 375
 posterior triangle dissection in, 377–378
 postoperative care in, 380–381
 seromas from, 381
 spinal accessory nerve in, 375, 382
 sternocleidomastoid muscle in, 378–379,
  382
skin of, 349–350
submandibular gland enlargement, 370
thyroglossal duct cysts, 366–367, 383–385,
  389
thyroid gland enlargement, 369–370
thyroid surgery, 488–506
tumors, 368–372
 benign, 368–370
 imaging of, 364
 invasion of carotid artery, 372
 malignant, 370–371
vasculature of, 352–353
Necrosis
 of abdominal wounds, after pancreatic
  anastomosis leak, 287
 of hepatic left lobe, hepatogastric artery in,
  835
 omental, after gastric resection, 829–830
 renal tubular, acute, 127
 of stomach
  in lesser curve, after proximal vagotomy,
   835
  in remnants, 935
 of valve in continent ileostomy, 1372
Necrotizing pancreatitis
 debridement in, 1204
 operative care of, 1221–1223